Clinical Nuclear Medicine

Hojjat Ahmadzadehfar
Hans-Jürgen Biersack
Leonard M. Freeman
Lionel S. Zuckier
Editors

Clinical Nuclear Medicine

Second Edition

Springer

Editors
Hojjat Ahmadzadehfar
Department of Nuclear Medicine
Klinikum Westfalen -
Knappschaftskrankenhaus
Academic teaching hospital of the Ruhr
University
Dortmund, Nordrhein-Westfalen
Germany

Leonard M. Freeman
Division of Nuclear Medicine
Department of Radiology
Montefiore Medical Center
Bronx, NY
USA

Albert Einstein College of Medicine
Bronx, NY
USA

Hans-Jürgen Biersack
Department of Nuclear Medicine
Beta Klinik Bonn
Bonn, Germany

Lionel S. Zuckier
The Ottawa Hospital
Division of Nuclear Medicine
Department of Radiology
Bronx, NY
USA

Albert Einstein College of Medicine
Bronx, NY
USA

1st Ed published 2007 Springer-Verlag Berlin Heidelberg
ISBN 978-3-030-39455-4 ISBN 978-3-030-39457-8 (eBook)
https://doi.org/10.1007/978-3-030-39457-8

This Springer imprint is published by the registered company Springer Nature Switzerland AG
The registered company address is: Gewerbestrasse 11, 6330 Cham, Switzerland

Preface

After several years of concerted effort, we are pleased to present the second edition of *Clinical Nuclear Medicine*. In the years following the publication of the first edition, groundbreaking developments have taken place in the field of nuclear medicine. Among those developments are the increasing use of hybrid imaging as well as the revolutionary progress that has been made in radiochemistry and radiopharmacy. Imaging of prostate cancer using PSMA ligands was a game changer in terms of the available diagnostic approaches to prostate cancer. The treatment of neuroendocrine tumors using peptide receptor radionuclide therapy with [^{177}Lu]Lu-DOTA-TATE is now an approved therapy under marketing authorization. The treatment of prostate cancer using PSMA ligands will become an approved therapy in the near future as well, joining ^{223}Ra-dichloride, used to treat bony prostate metastases.

Compared to the first edition of *Clinical Nuclear Medicine*, we have added several new chapters to this edition, while some of the original chapters have been completely rewritten. Chapter Two, "Radiopharmaceutical Sciences," could be described as a textbook within a textbook. Radiochemistry/Radiopharmacy is one of the most important fields of our specialty, and therefore, we invited a group of experienced experts to help update this chapter. We would like to express our thanks and respect to all the authors and contributing colleagues of this chapter, and especially to Prof. Dr. Klaus Kopka for his fantastic work in harmonizing this topic for the current *Clinical Nuclear Medicine*. He assembled this group of expert scientists who contributed to their distinct subtopics for this chapter. Radionuclide therapy in general, and theranostics in particular, will become an increasingly important field of our specialty over the next 20 years. Hence, the therapy section has been completely updated in this edition. With respect to the topics of nuclear hematology, and the application of nuclear medicine diagnostic techniques to various miscellaneous applications, readers are referred to the excellent and comprehensive chapters which appeared in the first edition of the textbook.

We wish to thank all the contributors to this book for their efforts. It has been a privilege to work with them. We are aware that this book, similar to other textbooks, will require continuous updating. Therefore, we invite all readers to email their comments and suggestions to the authors at nuclearmedicine@gmail.com, under subject "CNM." We will use your comments and suggestions when preparing the third edition of *Clinical Nuclear Medicine*.

Dortmund, Germany	Hojjat Ahmadzadehfar
Bonn, Germany	Hans-Jürgen Biersack
Bronx, NY, USA	Leonard M. Freeman
Bronx, NY, USA	Lionel S. Zuckier

Contents

Part III Nuclear Medicine Therapy

Part I

Basics

Physics, Instrumentation, and Radiation Safety and Regulations

1

Pat Zanzonico

1.1 Introduction

Nuclear Medicine imaging utilizes unsealed sources of radioactivity administered in the form of radiopharmaceuticals; the ionizing radiations which accompany the decay of the administered radioactivity can be detected, measured, and localized with specially designed instrumentation. This chapter begins with atomic and nuclear structure, radioactivity and radioactive decay, and interactions of radiation with matter. This is followed by a discussion of techniques for detection and measurement of radiation, the design and operating principle of detection and imaging instruments, instrument quality control, and radiation protection.

1.2 Basic Physics

1.2.1 Atomic and Nuclear Structure

Matter is, of course, comprised of atoms, which represent the smallest indivisible sub-unit of an element which retain the characteristic physical and chemical properties of that element. Atoms are comprised of a nucleus surrounded by orbital electrons, with the atomic structure maintained by electrostatic forces of attraction between the positively charged nucleus and the negatively charged electrons. Nuclei are comprised of positively charged protons and electrically neutral neutrons, which are collectively referred to as nucleons. Orbital electrons are negatively charged; in an electrically neutral, or uncharged, atom, the number of negative orbital electrons equals the number of positive nuclear protons, the charge on these respective particles being equal in magnitude. The properties of these fundamental building blocks of matter – electrons, protons, and neutrons – are summarized in Table 1.1. In addition, positively charged electrons (referred to as "positrons") can be produced during certain modes of radioactive decay (described below).

Nuclei are structurally characterized by three parameters: atomic number (Z), representing the number of protons; neutron number (N), representing the number of neutrons; and the mass number (A), representing the number of nucleons (i.e., neutrons and protons) and equal to $Z + N$. The atomic number, Z, thus indicates the positive charge of the nucleus and the chemical identity of the element. For example, an atomic number of "6" defines the atom as carbon. The most abundant naturally occurring isotope of carbon, carbon-12, has a mass number $A = 12$ and is composed of six protons ($Z = 6$) and six neutrons ($N = 6$); it is fully represented by its chemical

P. Zanzonico (✉)
Memorial Sloan Kettering Cancer Center,
New York, NY, USA
e-mail: zanzonip@mskcc.org

H. Ahmadzadehfar et al. (eds.), *Clinical Nuclear Medicine*,
https://doi.org/10.1007/978-3-030-39457-8_1

Table 1.1 Properties of the fundamental particles of matter

Particle	Symbol[a]	Mass		Rest mass energy, E_o[b]		Charge	
		Universal mass unit, u[c]	Gram, g	keV[d]	MeV[d]	Elementary charge	Coulomb, C
Electron	e						
Negatron	e^-	5.486×10^{-4}	9.110×10^{-28}	511	0.511	−1	-1.602×10^{-19}
Positron	e^+	5.486×10^{-4}	9.110×10^{-28}	511	0.511	+1	$+1.602 \times 10^{-19}$
Proton	p/p^+	1.007	1.673×10^{-24}	938,000	938	+1	$+1.602 \times 10^{-19}$
Neutron	n/n^o	1.009	1.675×10^{-24}	939,000	939	0	0

[a]In representing particles, the charge is often not explicitly indicated. In the case of electrons, the symbol e (without the charge indicated) is generally interpreted as identifying a negatron (e^-)

[b]From Einstein's special theory of relativity, the rest mass energy E_o of a particle of mass m is given by the equation, $E_o = mc^2$, where c is the speed of light in vacuum, 3×10^8 m/s

[c]In atomic and nuclear physics, energies are commonly expressed as universal mass units (u), 1/12 of the mass of a carbon-12 atom, 1.66054×10^{-27} kg

[d]In atomic and nuclear physics, energies are commonly expressed as multiples of an electron volt (eV), the kinetic energy of an electron after passing through a potential difference of 1 volt (V). An MeV, or megaelectron volt, equals one million eV, and a keV, or kiloelectron volt, equals 1000 eV

symbol and mass number, that is, as ^{12}C. Based on the foregoing structural parameters, different nuclear "families" have been defined: "isotopes" (e.g., $^{10}_{5}B^{5}$ and $^{11}_{6}B^{5}$) are nuclei having the same atomic number, *Z*, and thus are nuclei of the same element; "isobars" (e.g., $^{11}_{5}C^{6}$ and $^{11}_{6}B^{5}$) have the same mass number, *A*; and "isotones" (e.g., $^{11}_{5}C^{6}$ and $^{10}_{5}B^{5}$) have the same neutron number, *N*. A useful graphical representation of the atomic nuclei, the so-called chart of the nuclides, is shown in Fig. 1.1, plotting the neutron number, *N*, versus the atomic number, *Z*. For relatively small nuclei ($Z < 20$), the nuclei are clustered around the line of identity (i.e., the line $N = Z$); for larger nuclei, they cluster about a steeper line (i.e., the line $N = 1.5\ Z$).

In the parlance of modern physics, atoms and nuclei are "quantum" systems: the values specifying the positions and energies of particles comprising atoms and nuclei are discrete. Thus, orbital electrons are found only in orbits, or shells, at discrete distances from the nucleus, as shown diagrammatically in the Bohr (or "planetary") model of the atom (Fig. 1.2). Nucleons (i.e., protons and neutrons) are likewise arranged in discrete energy levels, or shells, within the nucleus. The electron's binding energy decreases, and its potential energy increases, with increasing distance from the nucleus. Atoms are on the order of 10^{-10} m in diameter and nuclei only one-thousandth of that, 10^{-13} m, in diameter. Nuclear volumes are therefore only ~1 billionth of atomic volumes. The atom and therefore matter in general is thus almost entirely empty space! Nucleon masses, on the other hand, are more than 1000 times the mass of electrons (Table 1.1), and therefore virtually all (>99%) of the "mass" of the atom and of matter generally is found in the nucleus.

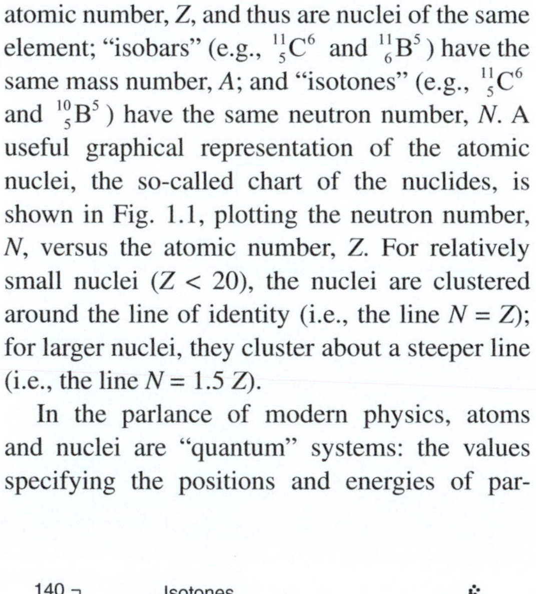

Fig. 1.1 The chart of the nuclides, a scattergram of neutron number, *N*, versus atomic number, *Z*, for all nuclides. Note that isotopes, isobars, and isotones lie along vertical, diagonal, and horizontal lines, respectively. Note further that structurally stable and therefore nonradioactive nuclei lie along the so-called line of stability, which runs through the center of this scattergram. The line of stability is biphasic, corresponding to the line of identity, $N = Z$, for small nuclei ($Z \leq$ ~20) and to a steeper line, $N = 1.5\ Z$, for larger nuclei (~$20 \leq Z \leq$ ~80), and ends at $Z \approx 80$

In so-called "ground-state" atoms, orbital electrons occupy the shells (i.e., energy levels) closest to the nucleus, that is, the lowest-energy levels. Likewise, in ground-state nuclei, nucleons occupy the lowest-energy shells. Orbital electrons and nucleons may transition to higher-energy shells, creating vacancies among the inner shells and producing non-ground-state, or "excited," atoms and nuclei, respectively. In such instances, electrons or nucleons will spontaneously move inward to fill these vacant, lower-energy shells. In the process, energy is released from the atom in the form of electromagnetic radiation (Table 1.2). This photon energy is equal to the difference between the initial and final potential energies of the electron or nucleon (Fig. 1.3a). In an atom, electron transitions from one shell to a lower-energy shell result in the emission of characteristic photons; if such a transition involves the inner shells of atoms in higher-*Z* elements, the photons will have relatively high energy and may correspond to X-rays. The energy of the emitted photons is generally expressed in units of electron volts, or eV; an eV is the increase in kinetic energy as an electron (or other unit-charge particle) is accelerated through a potential of 1 V. Likewise, in a nucleus, nucleon transitions result in the emission of characteristic nuclear

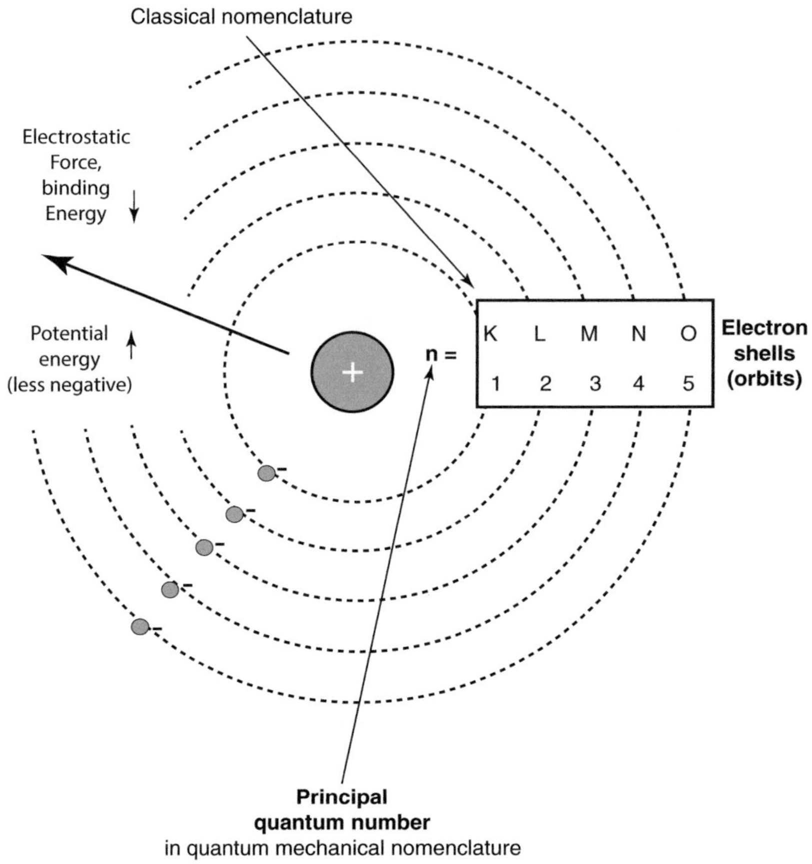

Fig. 1.2 In the Bohr (or planetary) model, the atom is depicted as a miniature solar system, with a positively charged nucleus at the center and negatively charged orbital electrons at discrete (or quantized) radial distances away. Each electron's radial distance from the nucleus and therefore its shell (or orbit) and its potential energy are indicated by its principal quantum n (beginning with the value 1 for the innermost, or lowest (most-negative)-potential energy, shell and ascending in numerical order for further, higher-potential energy shells). An alternative designation of the respective electron shells begins with the letter K for the innermost shell, ascending in alphabetical order for the further shells. Although not shown, each shell is comprised of more closely spaced subshells and ultimately orbitals (designated, in order of increasing potential energy as s, p, d, and f). There may be up to two electrons—one with spin "up" and the other with spin "down" (corresponding to spin quantum numbers +1/2 and −1/2, respectively)—per orbital. A shell with principal quantum number n may contain up to n^2 orbitals and therefore up to $2n^2$ electrons

Table 1.2 The electromagnetic (EM) spectrum

	Energy, E			Frequency, ν		Wavelength, λ	
	eV	keV	MeV	Hz[a]	MHz[a]	m	nm
Radio, TV	10^{-8}	10^{-11}	10^{-14}	10^{6}	1	10^{2}	10^{11}
Microwave	10^{-4}	10^{-7}	10^{-10}	10^{10}	10^{4}	10^{-2}	10^{7}
Infrared	0.1	10^{-4}	10^{-7}	10^{13}	10^{7}	10^{-5}	10^{4}
Visible	1	10^{-3}	10^{-6}	10^{14}	10^{8}	10^{-6}	10^{3}
Ultraviolet	10	10^{-2}	10^{-5}	10^{15}	10^{9}	10^{-7}	10^{2}
X- and γ-rays	10^{3}	1	10^{-2}	10^{18}	10^{12}	10^{-10}	10^{-1}

[a]Frequencies are typically expressed in units of Hertz (Hz), equal to 1 cycle/s (or 1 s^{-1}). The unit of MHz, or megahertz, equals one million Hz and is commonly used to express frequencies of EM radiations

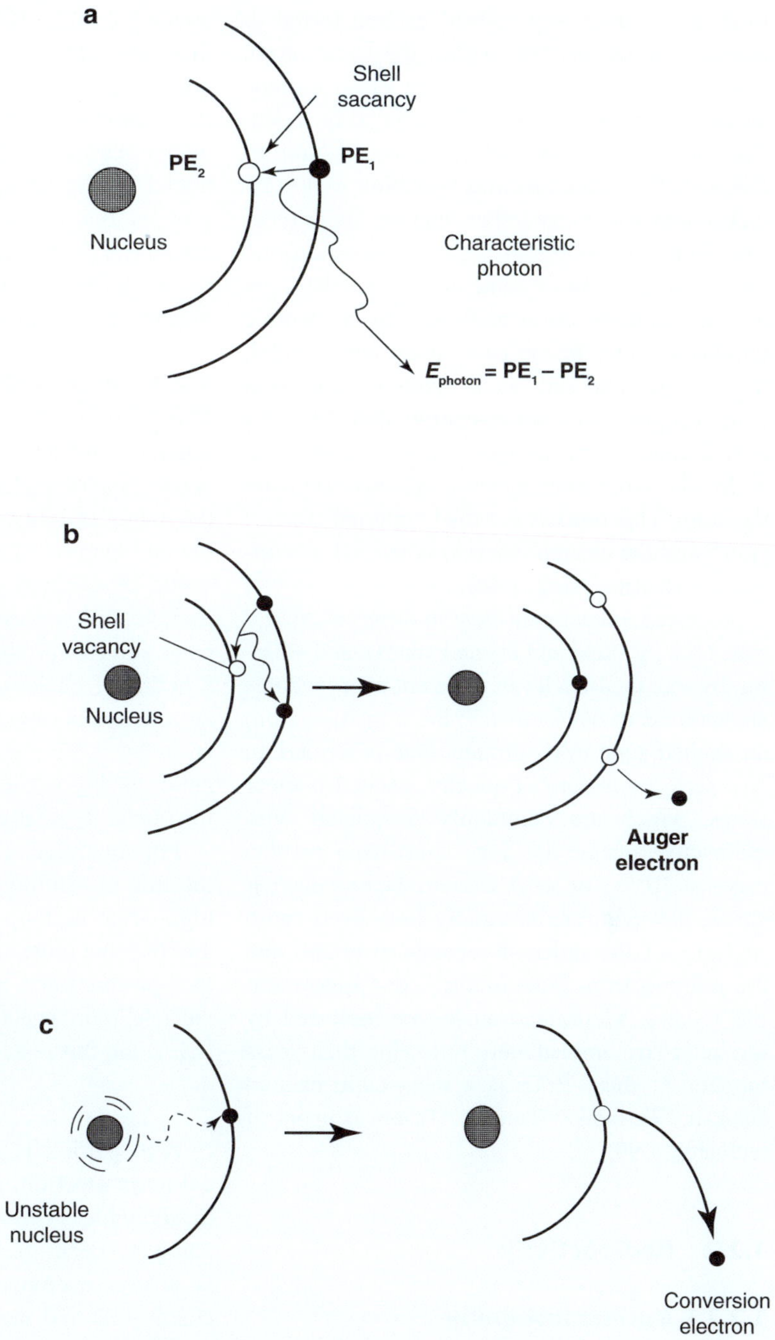

Fig. 1.3 (**a**) Emission of characteristic atomic radiation (i.e., photon) resulting from a shell-to-shell transition of orbital electrons. The photon energy, E_{photon}, equals the difference in potential energies of the electron in its initial and final energy levels, PE_1 and PE_2. Analogous processes, shell-to-shell nucleon transitions, occur in atomic nuclei and result in the emission of characteristic nuclear radiations (i.e., γ-rays). (**b**) Auger electron emission. (**c**) Internal conversion, with emission of a conversion electron (Adapted from [1])

photons, or gamma (γ) rays. These photons have energies on the order of kiloelectron volts or keV (1 keV = 10^3 eV) to megaelectron volts or MeV (1 MeV = 10^6 eV); the energies of X-rays are typically only in the range of keV. The defining difference between X- and γ-rays is related to where they originate—X-rays from outside the nucleus and γ-rays from within the nucleus.

Excited atoms and nuclei do not always result in the emission, respectively, of X- and γ-rays. In the case of excited atoms, the energy released as an orbital electron transitions from an outer to an inner shell may instead be transferred to another orbital electron within the same atom, ejecting the latter electron. The electron thus ejected is termed an "Auger electron" (Fig. 1.3b). The "fluorescent yield (ω_K)" is the probability that a shell-to-shell electron transition will yield a characteristic X-ray rather than an Auger electron. This ratio increases with increasing atomic number and reaches a value of ~1 (i.e., all X-ray and no Auger-electron emission) by an atomic number of ~50. In the case of unstable nuclei, the energy released as a nucleon transition from a higher- to a lower-energy shell likewise may instead be transferred to an orbital electron within the same atom, ejecting that electron from the atom. This process is called "internal conversion," and the ejected electron is termed a "conversion electron" (Fig. 1.3c).

As noted, nuclei may exist in different energy states (i.e., ground and excited states), and structurally identical nuclei in different energy states are referred to as "isomers"; the transition from an excited state to its ground state is termed an "isomeric transition." Typically, excited nuclear states, which are commonly associated with radioactive decay, are very short-lived (of the order of 10^{-12} s or less). Certain excited nuclear states, however, are unusually long-lived (with lifetimes of the order of seconds to hours) and are referred to as "metastable" (or "almost-stable") states. Metastable nuclei are indicated by the letter "m" immediately following their mass number *A*; thus, ^{99m}Tc is a metastable excited state of ^{99}Tc, and ^{99m}Tc and ^{99}Tc are isomers of technetium-99.

1.2.2 Radioactivity

1.2.2.1 Nuclear Instability

Radioactivity is a property of atomic nuclei and may be defined as the spontaneous transformation of a structurally unstable nucleus to a structurally more stable nucleus, with the emission of energy in the form of ionizing radiation. Two features largely determine the structural stability of a nucleus, the size (i.e., atomic number, *Z*) and the neutron-to-proton (*N*-to-*Z*) ratio. All large nuclei (i.e., $Z \geq$ ~80) are structurally unstable and therefore radioactive. For nuclei with an atomic number $Z \leq$ ~80, structural stability depends on the neutron-to-proton (*N*-to-*Z*) ratio. For small nuclei (i.e., $Z \leq$ ~20), stability is achieved for nuclei having an equal number of neutrons and protons, that is, an *N*-to-*Z* ratio of 1. For larger nuclei (i.e., ~20 $\leq Z \leq$ ~80), stability is achieved for nuclei having three neutrons for every two protons or an *N*-to-*Z* ratio of 1.5.

1.2.2.2 Modes of Radioactive Decay

The position of a nuclide on the chart of the nuclides indicates its mode(s) of radioactive decay. Nuclei of elements with $Z \geq$ ~80 lie *above* the line of stability, and all such nuclei are unstable and therefore radioactive; they become more stable by generating and emitting an alpha (α) particle. An α-particle, consisting of two neutrons and two protons, is structurally identical to a helium-4 nucleus, ${}_2^4He^2$, and α-decay reduces atomic number by 2 and the mass number of the atom by 4. Emitted α-particles are monoenergetic, having a kinetic energy that is specific to the nuclei (typically of the order of 5 MeV).

For small nuclei ($Z \leq$ ~80) lying to the *left* of the line of stability, the *N*-to-*Z* ratio is unstably high—that is, they have an excess of neutrons-and become more stable by converting a neutron to a proton and a negative electron (or beta (β) particle, more specifically, a beta minus (β^-) particle), and this results in beta decay:

$$ {}_N^A X^Z \rightarrow {}_{N-1}^{A} Y^{Z+1} + {}_0^0\beta^{-1} + \overline{\nu} \quad (1.1)$$

A β^--particle is, of course, structurally identical to an electron, e^-, and β^- decay reduces the unstably high *N*-to-*Z* ratio to a lower, more stable value, $N - 1/Z + 1$. The emission of a β^--particle is always accompanied by the emission of a charge-less and mass-less particle known as an antineutrino, $\overline{\nu}$.

For small nuclei ($Z \leq$ ~80) lying on the opposite side—to the *right*—of the line of stability, the *N*-to-*Z* ratio is unstably low, that is, they have a deficiency of neutrons and become more stable by converting a proton to a neutron and generating a positive electron (i.e., a beta plus (β+) particle or positron); this results in positron decay:

$$ {}_{N}^{A}Y^{Z} \rightarrow {}_{N+1}^{A}Y^{Z-1} + {}_{0}^{0}\beta^{+1} + \nu \quad (1.2) $$

A β^+-particle is also referred to as a positron and has the same mass as a negative electron. For those nuclei with an unstable, low *N*-to-*Z* ratio, there is an alternative mode of decay called electron capture (EC), in which an intranuclear proton literally captures (i.e., combines with) an orbital electron and is thereby converted to a neutron:

$$ {}_{N}^{A}X^{Z} + {}_{0}^{0}e^{-1} \rightarrow {}_{N+1}^{A}Y^{Z-1} + \nu \quad (1.3) $$

Importantly, β^+ decay is only possible if the "transition energy, *Q*," the difference between the total mass plus nuclear binding energies between the two nuclei, exceeds an energy threshold of 1.022 MeV (= 1022 keV). If the transition energy of the decay is less than 1.022 MeV, then *only* electron capture can occur. If, however, $Q > 1.022$ MeV, then both β^+ decay and electron capture can occur. Both β^+ decay and electron capture increase an unstably low *N*-to-*Z* ratio to a more stable value, $N + 1/Z - 1$, and are accompanied by the emission of a charge-less and mass-less neutrino, ν.

In beta (either β^- or β^+) decay and electron capture, the mass number, *A*, does not change. Therefore, beta decay and electron capture are known as "isobaric transitions," since the parent and daughter nuclei are isobars of each other. In beta (β^- or β^+) decay of a particular radionuclide, the electrons or positrons are emitted over a range of kinetic energies from 0 to a radionuclide-specific maximum energy known as the "end-point energy, $(E_\beta)_{max}$." A useful rule of thumb is that, for a particular radionuclide, the average β-ray energy, $\bar{E}_\beta$, is approximately 1/3 of the end-point energy.

As noted, radioactive decay generally yields daughter nuclei in excited states, with dissipation of excess energy either by the emission of γ-rays or by internal conversion and emission of the resulting conversion electrons. The electron shell vacancies which result from internal conversion (or from electron capture), in turn, lead to electrons entering these inner shells and the emission of characteristic X-rays and Auger electrons. Thus, radioactive decay typically results in a complex cascade of events, beginning with the transformation of one nuclide to another and culminating in the emission of γ-rays, X-rays, and/or electrons.

1.2.2.3 Mathematics of Radioactive Decay

The physical quantity "activity, *A*," specifies the amount of radioactivity and is the number of radioactive disintegrations (or decays) which occur per unit time. Activity is commonly expressed in disintegrations per second (dps) or disintegrations per minute (dpm):

The conventional unit of activity is the "curie (Ci)," corresponding to 3.7×10^{10} dps. (This somewhat odd value is the number of dps in 1 g of radium.) Relative to the amounts of radioactivity used clinically in Nuclear Medicine, 1 Ci is a very large activity. Accordingly, submultiples of the curie are often used: 1 mCi (millicurie), 3.7×10^7 dps, is one one-thousandth of 1 Ci, and 1 μCi (microcurie), 3.7×10^4 dps, is one one-millionth of 1 Ci. The System International (SI) unit of activity is the "becquerel (Bq)," which corresponds to 1 dps. In contrast to 1 Ci, 1 Bq is a very small activity, and so multiples of the becquerel are often used clinically: 1 kilobecquerel (kBq), 1×10^3 dps, is 1000 Bq, and 1 megabecquerel (MBq), 1 10^6 dps, is 1 million Bq. Note that 1 μCi = 37 kBq and 1 mCi = 37 MBq.

The mathematics of radioactive decay are well characterized and allow calculation of activities as a function of time. Radioactive nuclei decay in an exponential manner as a function of time, that is, for a given radionuclide, the *fraction* of the number of such nuclei decaying per unit time is constant. The physical decay constant, λ, is the fraction of radioactive nuclei decaying per unit time (e.g., 0.1 s^{-1} or 10% decaying per second). The practical form of the exponential law of radioactivity is written as:

$$ N(t) = N(0)e^{-\lambda t} \quad (1.4) $$

$$ A(t) = A(0)e^{-\lambda t} \quad (1.5) $$

where

$N(t)$ = the number of radioactive nuclei remaining at the time t.
$N(0)$ = the number of radioactive nuclei at time 0.
$A(t)$ = the activity remaining at time t.
$A(0)$ = the activity at time 0.

Note that $A(t) = \lambda\ N(t)$. The quantity $e^{-\lambda t}$ is the so-called decay factor, the fraction of activity remaining at time t. The appearance of the exponential law of radioactive decay (Eq. 1.4) on various types of graphs is presented in Fig. 1.4. Note, in particular, that such an exponential function appears as straight line when plotted on a semilog graph (Fig. 1.4c).

In addition to the physical decay constant, λ, there are other quantities which express the rate of decay of a given radionuclide: the half-life, $T_{1/2}$, which is the time interval for the activity (or the number of radioactive atoms) to decrease by 50% and the mean life, τ, which is the average time

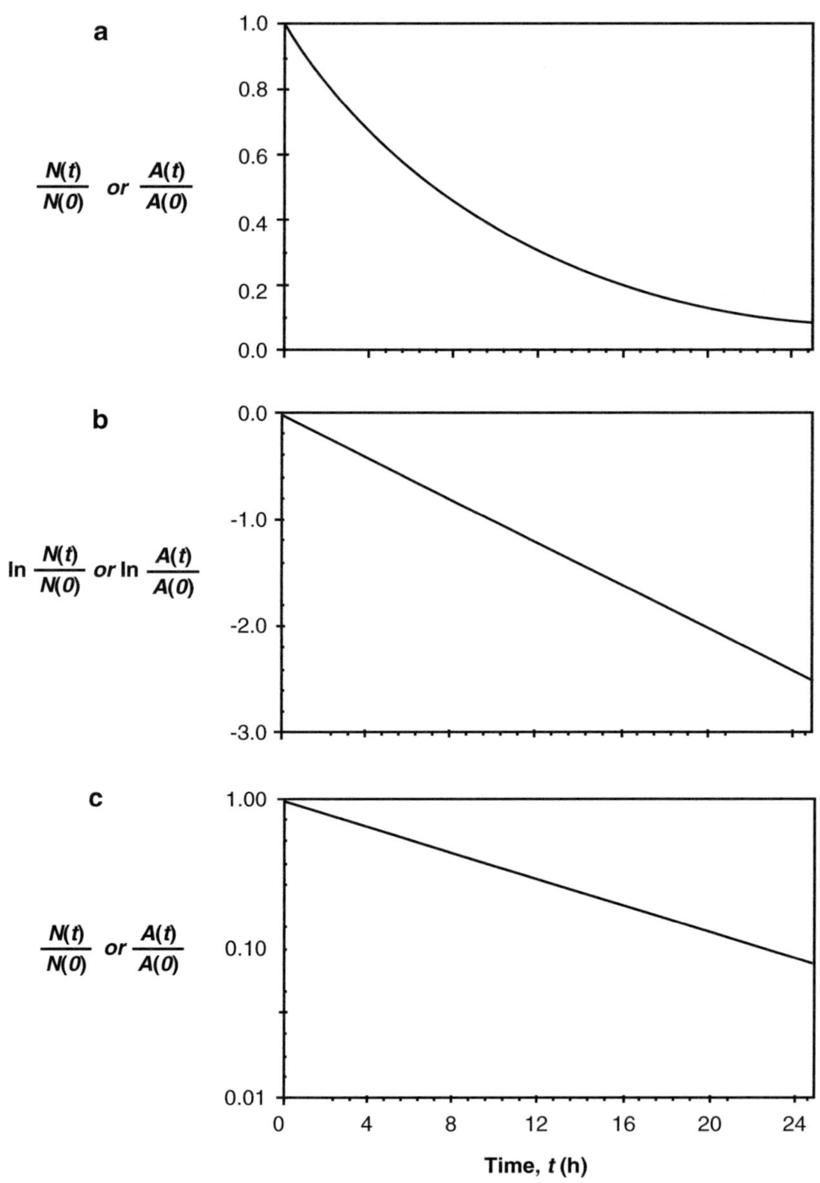

Fig. 1.4 Graphs of the exponential law of radioactive decay (Eqs. 1.4 and 1.5): the fraction of the number of radioactive nuclei [$N(t)/N(0)$] or of activity [$A(t)/A(0)$] versus time (in h), t, for a decay constant $\lambda = 0.1\ h^{-1}$. (**a**) Plotted on a linear-linear graph. (**b**) Plot of the log transform of the exponential law of radioactive decay, that is, the natural logarithm of $N(t)/N(0)$ or of $A(t)/A(0)$ plotted on a linear-linear graph. It appears as a straight line with a slope of λ and a y-intercept of 0. (**c**) When $N(t)/N(0)$ or $A(t)/A(0)$ is plotted on a semilogarithmic ("semilog") graph, it again appears as a straight line

interval over which the radioactive nuclei decay. The decay constant, λ, half-life, $T_{1/2}$, and mean life, τ, are mathematically related as follows:

$$\lambda = 0.693 / T_{1/2} \tag{1.6}$$

$$T_{1/2} = 0.693 / \lambda \tag{1.7}$$

and

$$\tau = 1.44 T_{1/2} \tag{1.8}$$

The factor 0.693 equals the natural logarithm of 2, ln(2).

Combining Eqs. (1.5) and (1.6) yields the following form of the decay equation:

$$A(t) = A(0)e^{-0.693t/(T_{1/2})} \tag{1.9}$$

Radionuclides often decay not to a stable (i.e., nonradioactive) nuclide but rather to another radionuclide. The resulting radionuclide, of course, will itself undergo radioactive decay. Such sequences of parent (p), daughter (d), granddaughter (g), and other radionuclides are known as radioactive "families" and are the basis of radionuclide generators. The most important radionuclide generator is, of course, the molybdenum-99/technetium-99m (^{99}Mo/^{99m}Tc) generator. The daughter activity is continuously replenished by the decaying parent. The parent ^{99}Mo half-life (66 h) is much longer than that of the ^{99m}Tc daughter (6 h), and generators are generally used for 1–2 weeks; thereafter, the ^{99}Mo has itself decayed to the point where the amounts of ^{99m}Tc the generator produces are prohibitively low for most clinical applications. Other important radionuclide generator systems in Nuclear Medicine include the strontium-82 (25 days)/rubidium-82 (1.3 min) (^{82}Sr/^{82}Rb) generator and the germanium-68 (271 days)/gallium-68 (1.3 h) (^{68}Ge/^{68}Ga) generator.

1.2.3 Interactions of Radiation with Matter

1.2.3.1 Elastic and Inelastic Interactions

Radiation interacts with matter by either elastic or inelastic interactions. In an elastic interaction, the incident radiation is scattered in a different direction but does not lose energy. In contrast, in an inelastic interaction, energy is lost. X- and γ- rays, α- and β-particles, and Auger and conversion electrons are sufficiently energetic to ionize atoms of a stopping medium, ejecting an electron and producing an ion pair (i.e., a free negative electron and a positive ion), and are thus referred to as ionizing radiations.

1.2.3.2 Photon (X- and γ-Ray) Interactions

X- and γ-rays undergo inelastic interactions by one of several mechanisms: the photoelectric effect, Compton scatter, pair production, and photodisintegration. Pair production, in which an X- or γ-ray interacts with an atomic nucleus and produces a positron-electron pair, has an energy threshold of 1.022 MeV (to account for the combined rest mass energies of the positron and electron created). Photodisintegration, in which an X- or γ-ray interacts with and fragments the nucleus, has an even higher energy threshold of at least several MeV. Pair production and photodisintegration are therefore not energetically possible for the range of relatively low-energy X- and γ-rays encountered in Nuclear Medicine and will not be considered further. In the photoelectric effect (Fig. 1.5a), the X- or γ-ray energy is completely transferred to an orbital electron in an atom of the stopping medium, some of the energy ejecting the electron from the atom and the balance providing kinetic energy to the ejected electron. In Compton scatter (Fig. 1.5b), only a portion of the incident photon's energy is transferred to an orbital electron, which is likewise ejected from the atom. The scattered photon's energy is therefore less than that of the incident photon, and it travels in a different direction. The *relative* probability of the photoelectric effect increases as the incident photon energy, E_γ, decreases and the effective atomic number, Z_{eff}, of the stopping medium increases (i.e., approximately in proportion to E^3/Z^3). Conversely, the *relative* probability of Compton scatter increases as E_γ increases and Z_{eff} decreases. For X- and γ-ray energies typically encountered in Nuclear Medicine, the predominant mode of interaction in soft tissue (low Z) is Compton scatter.

The mathematics of X- and γ-ray attenuation follows an exponential relationship (similar in mathematical form to that for radioactive decay).

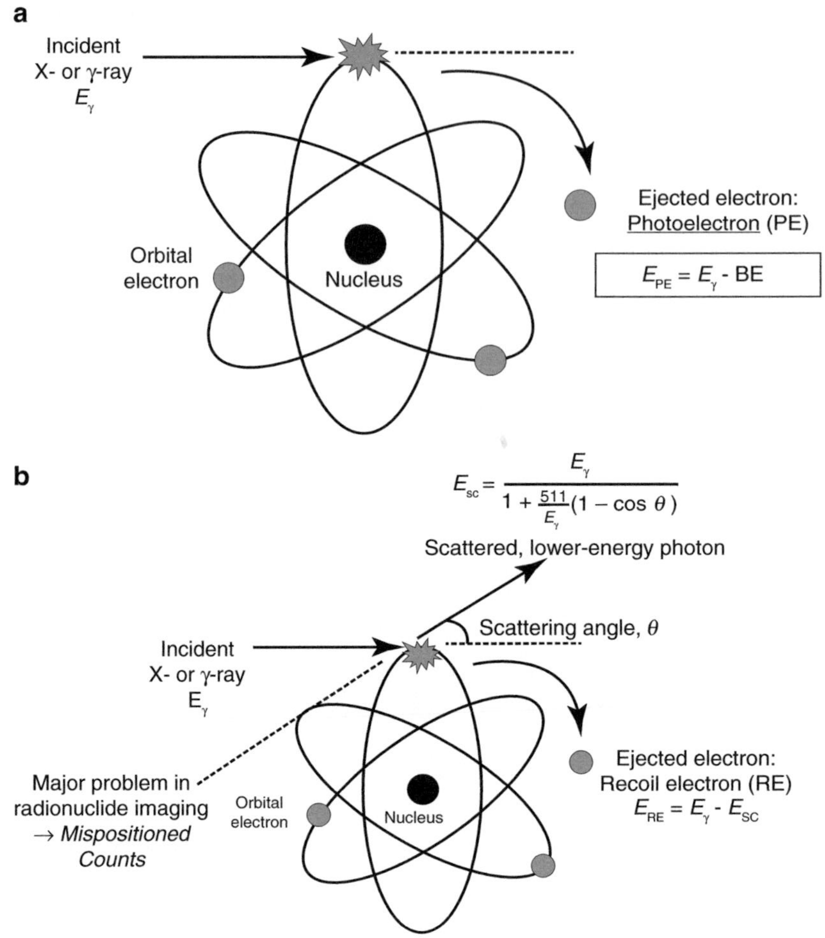

Fig. 1.5 Interactions of X- and γ-rays in matter in the energy range encountered in Nuclear Medicine. (**a**) In the photoelectric effect, the energy, E_{PE}, of the ejected electron, termed the photoelectron (PE), is E_γ − BE where E_γ is the energy of the incident photon and BE was the binding energy of that electron in the atom. Note that the incident photon disappears completely. (**b**) In Compton scatter, the photon does not disappear but is scattered with a lower energy (in keV), E_{SC}; E_{SC} is a function of the energy (in keV) of the incident photon, E_γ, and the scattering angle, θ, as indicated by the equation shown. The energy of the recoil electron (RE), E_{RE}, is therefore E_γ − E_{SC}. Compton scatter generally involves outer-shell orbital electrons with binding energies, BEs, negligibly small compared to typical values of E_γ and E_{SC}; the binding energy, BE, is therefore ignored in calculating the energy of the recoil electron (Adapted from [4])

For an attenuating medium of thickness x, this relationship is:

$$I(x) = I(0)e^{-\mu x} \tag{1.10}$$

where

μ = the linear attenuation coefficient
= the fraction of photons attenuated per unit thickness of stopping material (e.g., in cm^{-1})
$I(x)$ = the photon intensity transmitted through a thickness x of stopping material.
$I(0)$ = the incident photon intensity.

The linear attenuation coefficient, μ, is a property of both the photon energy and the stopping material: μ increases (i.e., photons become less penetrating) as photon energy decreases and as the mass density and atomic number of the stopping medium increase.

In addition to the linear attenuation coefficient, μ, other quantities expressing the attenuation of X- and γ-rays are the half-value layer, HVL (or half-value thickness, HVT), which is the thickness required to reduce the photon intensity by one-half, and the mean free path, MFP, the thickness a photon travels, on average, before interacting. The linear attenuation coefficient, μ, half-value layer, HVL, and mean free path, MFP, are mathematically related as follows:

$$\mu = 0.693 / \mathrm{HVL} \quad (1.11)$$

$$\mathrm{HVL} = 0.693 / \mu \quad (1.12)$$

$$\mathrm{MFP} = 1.44\,\mathrm{HVL} \quad (1.13)$$

and

Combining Eqs. (1.10) and (1.11) yields the following form of the attenuation equation:

$$I(x) = I(0)\mathrm{e}^{-0.693x/\mathrm{HVL}} \quad (1.14)$$

Note that when the absorber thickness, x, is equal the HVL, the equation correctly predicts that 50% of the incoming radiation is stopped by the absorber. Another term commonly used when dealing with greater thicknesses of attenuating material is the tenth-value layer (TVL) or (tenth-value thickness, HVT), referring to a thickness which permits only 10% of the incident radiation to penetrate a medium. The TVL is related to the HVL by TVL = 3.32 HVL.

1.2.3.3 Particulate-Radiation Interactions

Particulate radiations (i.e., β-rays, Auger and conversion electrons) interact with matter by one of the two mechanisms: collisional interactions and radiative interactions. Collisional interactions are somewhat analogous to Compton scatter: an incident β-ray or electron "collides" with and transfers sufficient energy to an orbital electron to eject it from the atom and, in the process, is scattered with a lower energy. In radiative interactions, on the other hand, the β-ray or electron penetrates the electron "cloud" surrounding the nucleus and thus reaches and interacts with the atomic nucleus. However, because of the large mass disparity (of the order of a thousand-fold) between electrons and nucleons, the energy lost by the incident β-ray or electron in this interaction appears as X-rays, or *bremsstrahlung* (or "brake radiation"), rather than as kinetic energy of the nucleus. The emitted *bremsstrahlung* exhibits a broad energy spectrum, with X-ray energies ranging from zero to a maximum value equal to the kinetic energy of the incident particle. For the range of β-ray and electron energies (up to approximately several hundred keV) typically encountered in Nuclear Medicine, the predominant type of interaction in soft tissue (which has a relatively low Z_{eff}) is overwhelmingly collisional interactions, with less than 1% of the interactions attributable to radiative interactions.

There is a large disparity in penetrabilities between photon and particulate radiations. X- and γ-rays typically encountered in Nuclear Medicine have energies on the order of several hundred keV, and thus a significant proportion of such radiations can penetrate soft-tissue thicknesses of the order of 10 cm or more. As a result, X- and γ-ray-emitting radionuclides in vivo can be detected and imaged externally. In contrast, α- and β-particles and electrons are non-penetrating radiations; electrons typically encountered in Nuclear Medicine have ranges in soft tissue on the order of only 1 mm or less and α-particles even shorter ranges, of the order of 100 μm or less. Thus, α- and β-particles- and electron-emitting radionuclides in vivo cannot be detected and imaged noninvasively. On the other, since all their energy and radiation dose are deposited locally, α- and β-particle- and electron-emitting radionuclides are well-suited for radionuclide therapy.

1.3 Radiation Detection and Measurement

1.3.1 Statistical Considerations

Radioactive decay is a random process, and therefore statistical fluctuations will occur in the measured counts or count rates. Such random fluctuations complicate the accurate detection, measurement, and imaging of radioactivity. If a detector were used to repeatedly measure the counts or count rates from a given activity, slightly different values would be obtained from measurement to measurement. If an average of N counts is obtained, the standard deviation, σ, of the number of counts is

$$\sigma = \sqrt{N} \tag{1.15}$$

and the percent standard deviation (or "noise"), $\%\sigma$, is

$$\%\sigma = \frac{100\%}{\sqrt{N}} \tag{1.16}$$

As an example, if a sample count were 100, the $\%\sigma = 10\%$. For a normal bell-shaped distribution, this can be interpreted this as follows: if we counted a radioactive sample many times, 2/3 of the measured counts would be within 10% of the true value. If, on the other hand, we counted for a longer time and measured 1000 counts, the $\%\sigma = 3.3\%$; 2/3 of the time, the measured counts would then be within 3.3% of the true value. Measuring for a longer time and obtaining more counts thus produces less random variation in the measurement, and any one measured value would be closer to the "true" value. This principle applies to the counting of radioactive samples or to planar radionuclide imaging (i.e., to the counts per unit picture element (or pixel) in a planar image). In other words, the statistical quality of higher-count images is better than that of lower-count images.

1.3.2 Radiation Detector Performance

Radiation detectors may be quantitatively characterized by many different performance parameters. Among the most important of these, however, are sensitivity (or efficiency), energy resolution, and, for devices which localize (image) as well as count radiation, spatial resolution and uniformity.

Sensitivity (or efficiency) is the detected count rate per unit activity. Because the count rate detected from a given activity is highly dependent on the source-detector geometry and intervening absorbing media, characterization of sensitivity can be ambiguous. There are two components of sensitivity: geometric sensitivity and intrinsic sensitivity. Geometric sensitivity is the fraction of emitted radiations which intersect, or strike, the detector, that is, the fraction of the total solid angle subtended by the detector. It is therefore directly proportional to the radiation-sensitive detector area and, for a point source, inversely proportional to the square of the source-detector distance. Intrinsic sensitivity is the fraction of radiations intersecting the detector which is stopped within the detector. Intrinsic sensitivity is directly related to the detector thickness, effective atomic number, and mass density and decreases with increasing photon energy, since higher-energy photons are more penetrating and are more likely to pass through a detector without interacting.

Characteristic X-rays and γ-rays are emitted from radioactively decaying atoms with well-defined discrete energies. Due to photon scatter from intervening material (i.e., a patient) and even in the absence of scatter, output electrical pulses from absorption of these radiations will appear corresponding to a range of energies. This reflects the finite *energy resolution* of detection systems. Many radiation detectors employ some sort of energy-selective counting: an energy range, or window, is selected such that radiations are counted only if their detected energies lie within that range. Commonly (at least for scintillation detectors such as gamma cameras (see below)), a so-called 20% photopeak energy window, $E_\gamma \pm 10\%$ (e.g., 126–154 keV for the 140-keV γ-ray of ^{99m}Tc), is employed, where E_γ is the photopeak energy of the radiation. For such energy-selective counting, overall sensitivity appears to increase as the photopeak energy window is widened. However, this results in acceptance of more scattered as well as primary (i.e., unscattered) radiations. Energy resolution quantifies the ability of a detector to separate, or discriminate, radiations of different energies. As illustrated in Fig. 1.6a, energy resolution is generally specified as the full width at half-

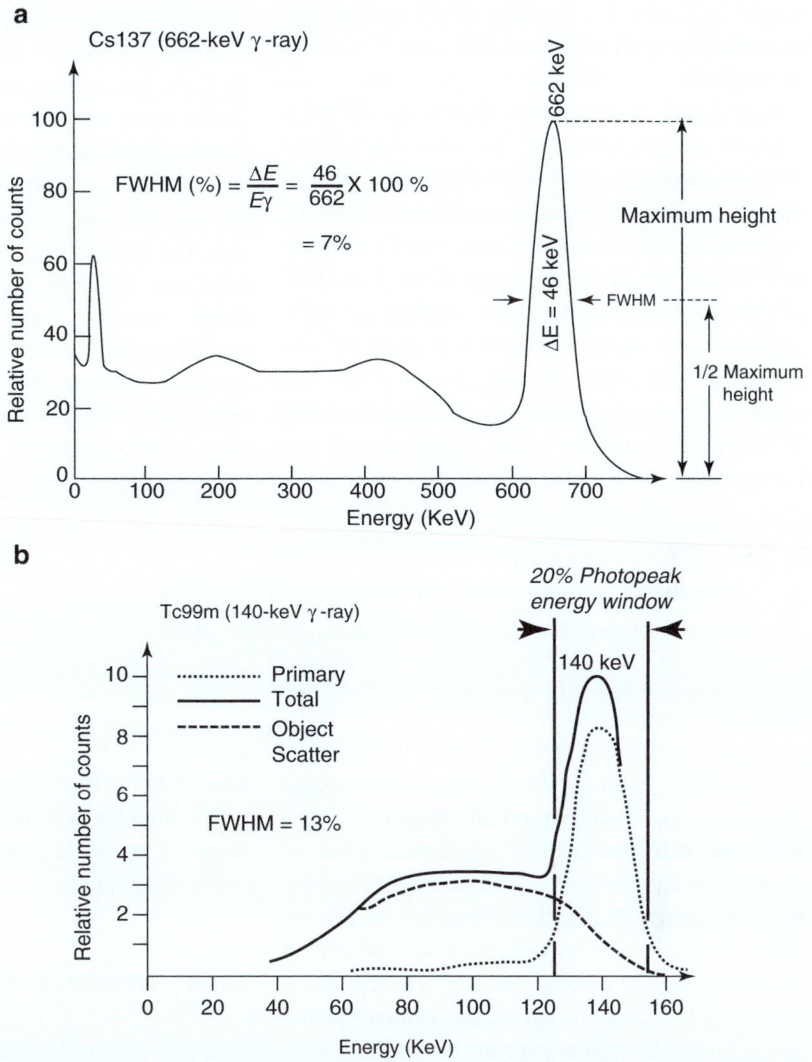

Fig. 1.6 (**a**) Energy spectrum for the 662-keV γ-rays emitted by Cs137, illustrating the definition of the measure of energy resolution "full width at half maximum (FWHM)" of the photopeak energy, E_γ. (**b**) Energy spectrum for the 140-keV γ-rays emitted by Tc-99m, illustrating the contributions of primary (unscattered) and scattered radiation counts. In (**a**) and (**b**), the energy spectra were obtained with a thallium-doped sodium iodide (NaI(Tl)) scintillation detector (see text) (Adapted from [1])

maximum height (FWHM = ΔE) expressed as a percentage of the photopeak energy (E_γ) of the bell-shaped photopeak, FWHM (%) = $\frac{\Delta E}{E_\gamma}100\%$. The importance of energy resolution lies in scatter rejection, particularly for imaging detectors. Radiation loses energy when scattered, and the lower-energy scattered – and therefore mispositioned—radiations may therefore be discriminated from the primary radiations. However, the finite energy resolution of radiation detectors (i.e., the width of the photopeak in the energy spectrum) means that there will be overlap of scattered and primary radiations, as illustrated in Fig. 1.6b. For systems with superior energy resolution (i.e., the FWHM (%) decreases and the photopeak becomes narrower), the separation of primary and scattered radiations is such that more scattered radiation is excluded while still accepting more counts corresponding to primary radiation.

For detectors such as gamma cameras where radiation is localized (imaged) as well as detected and counted, *spatial resolution* is a critical performance parameter. It reflects the ability of the detector to accurately determine the location of a source or, similarly, the ability to visually separate two closely spaced point sources. This is usually measured by imaging a line or point source and examining the dispersion of the source as it appears in an image. The detector's spatial resolution can then be expressed as the full width at half-maximum height (FWHM) of this line or point spread function (LSF or PSF, respectively). Spatial resolution generally worsens with increasing source-to-detector distance. There is a trade-off between sensitivity and resolution, as they are inversely related: sensitivity is reduced as spatial resolution improves, and spatial resolution is degraded as sensitivity increases.

Uniformity is likewise a critical parameter of gamma cameras and other imaging devices. In principle, a uniform source of radioactivity (such as large disk with cobalt-57 (^{57}Co) uniformly embedded in plastic) should yield a uniform image (i.e., an image in which the counts per unit picture element (or pixel) is constant over the entire image). In practice, this is never achieved—even if one discounts the effects of count statistics (noise)—because of inevitable point-to-point variations in sensitivity of an imaging detector. For gamma cameras, uniformity (actually, the deviation from uniformity) may be expressed by a quantity known as the "integral uniformity (IU)":

$$\mathrm{IU} = \frac{\text{Maximum counts per pixel} - \text{Minimum counts per pixel}}{\text{Maximum counts per pixel} + \text{Minimum counts per pixel}} \times 100\% \quad (1.17)$$

To reliably estimate the IU, a very-high-count image (e.g., a 15-million-count image) of a uniform source minimizes the quantitative effect of count statistics (noise). Acceptable uniformity is 5% or better, although uniformities of 3% are generally achievable nowadays. A second related parameter widely used to characterize uniformity (specifically, gamma camera uniformity) is the so-called differential uniformity (DU), the maximum value of the expression on the right side of Eq. (1.17) determined among all 1 × 5-pixel regions of interest over the entire field of view.

1.3.3 Basic Design and Operating Principles of Radiation Detectors

Radiation detectors are generally characterized as either scintillation or ionization detectors (Fig. 1.7). In scintillation detectors, visible light is produced as radiation interacts with atoms of a crystal and converted to an electronic signal, or pulse, and amplified by the photomultiplier tube (PMT). In ionization detectors, free electrons, directly produced as radiation ionizes a stopping material, are collected to produce an electronic signal.

1.3.4 Ionization Detectors

Detector materials in the most common ionization detectors are gaseous, and such detectors are therefore often known as "gas-filled detectors." The two most important gas-filled ionization detectors for Nuclear Medicine are dose calibrators and Geiger counters. The principal difference among such detectors is the magnitude of the voltage between the anode and cathode, as indicated in Fig. 1.8 and in Table 1.3. In the 300- to 600-V range, the so-called "ionization chamber" region, all of the electrons produced directly by ionization of the detector material by an incident radiation are collected at the anode and produce a fixed detector signal per radiation. In the 300- to 600-V range, the overall signal thus corresponds to the number of primary elec-

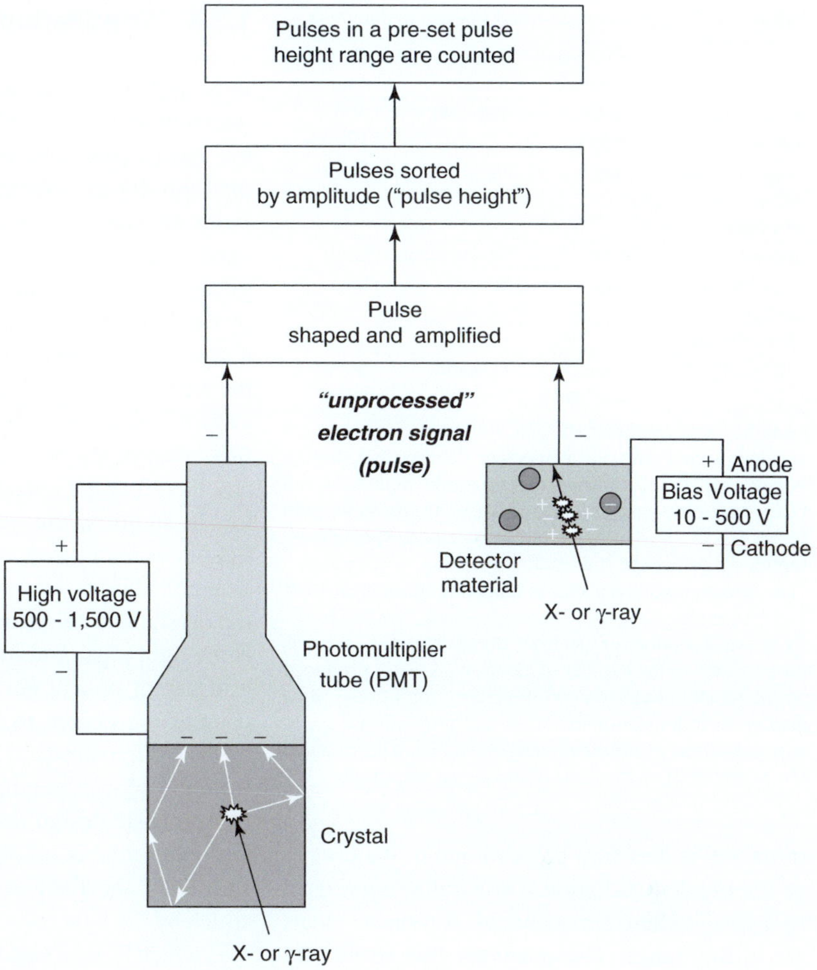

Fig. 1.7 The basic design and operating principle of (**a**) scintillation and (**b**) ionization detectors

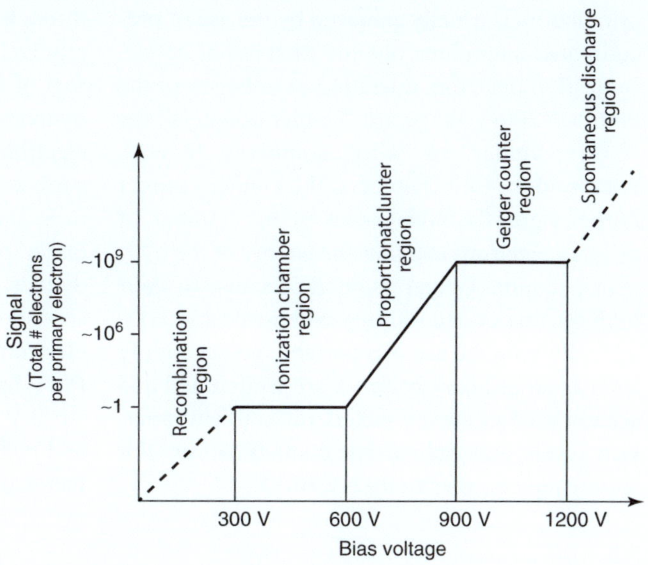

Fig. 1.8 The signal (expressed as the amplification factor, that is, the total number of electrons per primary electron produced in the detector material) as a function of the bias voltage for gas-filled ionization detectors. The principal difference among such detectors is the magnitude of the bias voltage between the anode and cathode. The amplification factors and the voltages shown are approximate

Table 1.3 Properties of gas-filled ionization detectors

	Ionization detector	Proportional counter	Geiger counter
Bias-voltage operating range	300–600 V	600–900 V	900, 1200 V
Response stable with respect to voltage?[a]	Yes	No	Yes
Sensitivity[b]	Low	Intermediate	High
Capable of energy discrimination?	Yes	Yes	No
Applications	Dose calibrator	Research	Survey meter

[a]Stability with respect to the bias voltage corresponds to a constant signal over the respective detector's operating voltage range. In contrast to ionization detectors and Geiger counters, proportional counters are unstable with respect to the bias voltage and thus require specialized, highly stable voltage sources for constancy of response
[b]The sensitivity of a detector is related to its amplification factor (see Fig. 1.7)
[c]If the total number of electrons comprising the signal is proportional to the number of electrons directly produced by the incident radiation and therefore proportional to its energy, as in ionization detectors and proportional counters, radiations of different energies can be discriminated (i.e., separated) on the basis of the signal amplitude

trons and is therefore proportional to the energy of the incident radiation. Dose calibrators, used to assay radiopharmaceutical activities, operate in this range. The relatively low sensitivity of such devices is not a major disadvantage, as radiopharmaceutical activities are typically rather large (i.e., in the mCi range). Isotope discrimination is usually achieved by the use of pre-calibrated amplifiers, one for each radionuclide. Ionization detectors operating at voltages in the 900- to 1200-V range are "Geiger counters" (or "Geiger-Muller" or "GM" counters). In contrast to ionization chambers, the Geiger counter output signal is independent of the number of primary electrons and thus the energy of the incident radiation. Geiger counters, because of their high sensitivity and stability with respect to voltage (allowing the use of a portable power supply such as an ordinary battery), are well-suited and widely used as survey meters for ambient radiation levels and radioactive contamination. For survey meters, sensitivity is critical.

1.3.5 Scintillation Detectors

In scintillation detectors (Fig. 1.9a), radiation interacts with and deposits energy in a scintillator, most commonly, a crystalline solid such as thallium-doped sodium iodide (NaI(Tl)). The radiation energy thus deposited is converted to visible light. Because the light is emitted isotropically (i.e., in all directions), the inner surface of the light-tight crystal housing is coated with a reflective material so that light emitted toward the sides and front of the crystal is reflected back toward a photomultiplier tube (PMT) (Fig. 1.9b); this maximizes the amount of light collected and therefore the overall sensitivity of the detector. In addition, this insures that the amount of light detected is proportional to the energy of the detected photon. Interposed between the back of the crystal and the entrance window of the PMT is the light pipe, nowadays simply a thin layer of transparent optical gel. The light pipe optically couples the crystal to the PMT and thus maximizes the transmission (>90%) of the light signal from the crystal into the PMT.

The basic design and operation of the photomultiplier tube is as follows. Coated on the inner surface of the PMT is the photocathode. When struck by the light from the crystal, the photocathode, which is at ground (i.e., 0 V), emits electrons. Immediately beyond the photocathode is the focusing grid, maintained at a relatively low positive voltage of the order of 10 V. Electrons pass through the focusing grid and are attracted by a relatively large positive voltage, ~300 V, on the first of a series of small metallic elements called dynodes. The resulting high-speed impact of each electron results in the ejection from the dynode surface of an average of three electrons. The electrons thus ejected are then attracted by the even larger positive voltage, ~400 V, on the second dynode. The impact of these electrons into the second dynode surface ejects an additional three electrons for each incident electron. Typically, a PMT has 10–12 such dynodes (or stages), each ~100 V more positive than the preceding dynode and resulting in an overall electron amplification factor of 3^{10}–3^{12} for the entire PMT. At the last

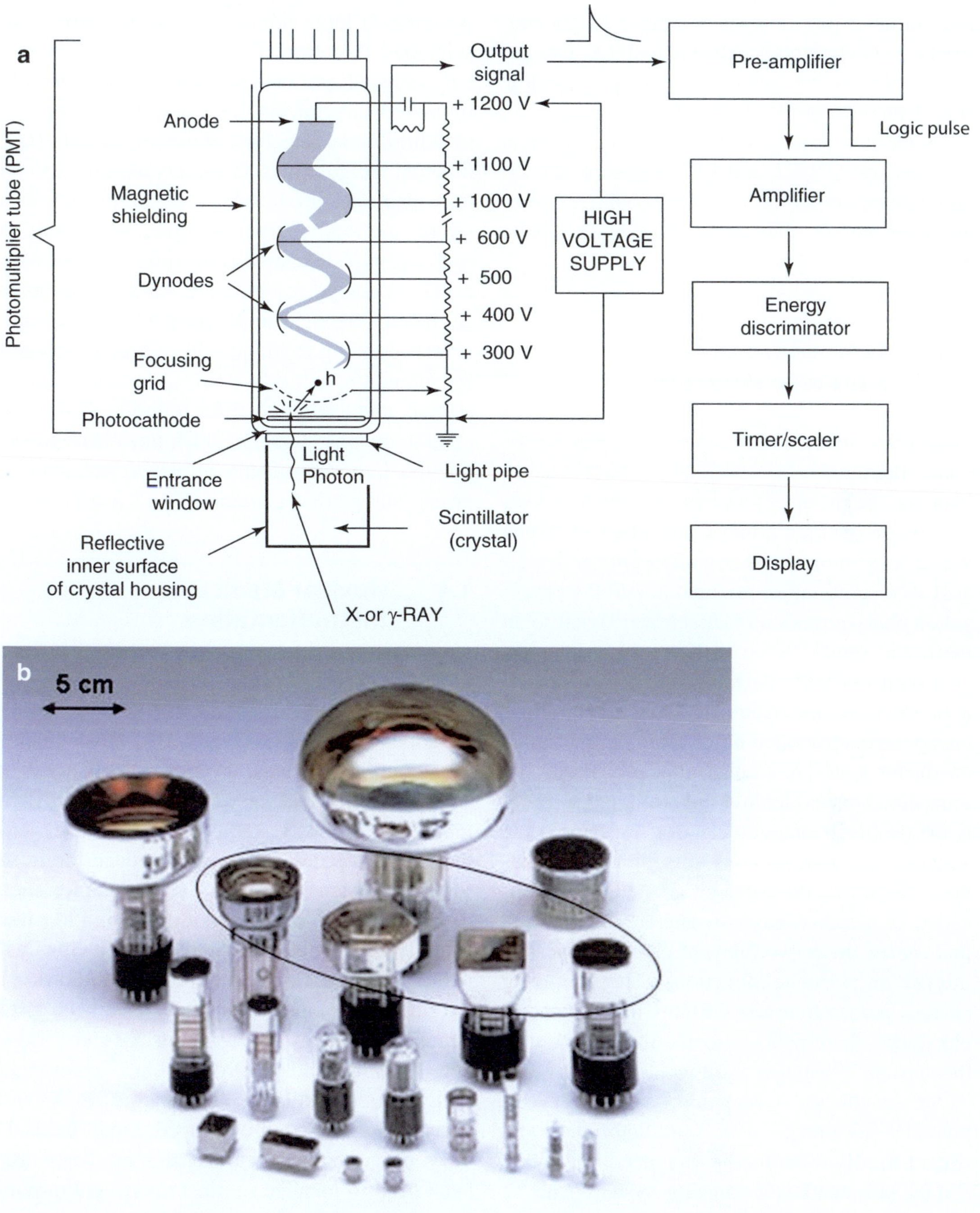

Fig. 1.9 (**a**) The basic design and operating principle of PMTs and scintillation detectors (Adapted from [1]). (**b**) Photographs of PMTs. The PMTs circled are typical of those used in gamma cameras

anode, an output signal is generated. The irregularly shaped PMT output signal is then shaped by a preamplifier and further amplified into a logic pulse that can be electronically manipulated. The resulting electronic pulses, whose amplitudes (or "heights") are proportional to the number of electrons produced at the PMT photocathode, are therefore also proportional to the energy of the incident radiation. These pulses can then be sorted according to their respective heights by an energy discriminator (also known as a pulse-height analyzer), and those pulses with a height (i.e., energy) within the preset photopeak energy window (Fig. 1.6b) are counted by the timer/scaler.

In addition to their widespread use in gamma cameras and SPECT and PET scanners, scintillation detectors are used in well counters, intraoperative probes, and organ ("thyroid") uptake probes.

1.3.6 Semiconductor-Based Ionization Detectors

Semiconductor radiation detectors represent the main alternative to scintillator detector-based systems. Such detectors are so-called direct-conversion devices, a major advantage of which is that they minimize the random effects associated with scintillation production and the propagation and conversion of the optical signal to an electronic signal. When an X- or γ-ray interacts in a semiconductor detector, one or more energetic electrons are created and subsequently lose energy through ionization of atoms in the semiconductor material, among other processes. The ionization creates electron-hole (e-h) pairs; a hole is the positively charged electron vacancy in the valence band that remains after an electron has been raised into the conduction band. The application of a bias voltage creates an electric field that causes these two types of charge carriers to migrate in opposite directions. These moving charges induce transient currents in the detector electrodes, thereby allowing the measurement of the detector's response to an incident X- or γ-ray.

Semiconductor detectors offer several potential advantages over scintillator detectors (Eq. 1.8). By eliminating the need for bulky PMTs, semiconductor imaging systems can be made much more compact than PMT-based systems. More importantly, the direct conversion of energy deposited by X- or γ-rays into electron-hole pairs eliminates the light-to-electrical signal transduction step and the associated loss of signal. Further, since the energy required to create an electron-hole pair in most semiconductors is small (typically 3–5 eV), each incident photon generates a large number of charge carriers. In principle, therefore, Poisson noise is considerably reduced and energy resolution considerably improved in semiconductor detectors compared to scintillation detectors. However, defects (i.e., inherent irregularities in the crystal lattice) can trap electrons produced by radiation and thus reduce the total charge collected. As a result of such incomplete charge collection, the otherwise excellent energy resolution of semiconductors is degraded. Practical and reasonably economical crystal-growing techniques have been developed for cadmium telluride (CdTe), mercuric iodide (HgI_2), and cadmium zinc telluride (CdZnTe) (also known as "CZT"), which have been incorporated into commercial intraoperative gamma probes and gamma cameras (Eqs. 1.8 and 1.9).

1.4 Nuclear Medicine Instrumentation

1.4.1 Intraoperative Probes

Intraoperative probes (Fig. 1.10), small, hand-held counting devices, are now widely used in the management of cancer, most commonly, to more expeditiously identify and localize sentinel lymph nodes and thereby reduce the need for more extensive surgery. In principle, such devices can also be used to identify and localize visually occult disease at surgery following systemic administration of a tumor-avid radiotracer. (Although intraoperative probes have been used almost exclusively for counting X- and γ-rays, beta (electron and positron) probes constructed with plastic scintillators "transparent" to X- and γ-rays have also been developed. Small field-of-view intraoperative gamma cameras have also been used to localize sentinel nodes and tumors intraoperatively.) Intraoperative gamma probes are available with either scintillation or semiconductor (ionization) detectors. Scintillation detector-based probes have the advantages of relatively low cost and high sensitivity (mainly because of their greater thickness, ~10 mm, versus only ~1 mm in ionization detectors), especially for medium- to high-energy photons.

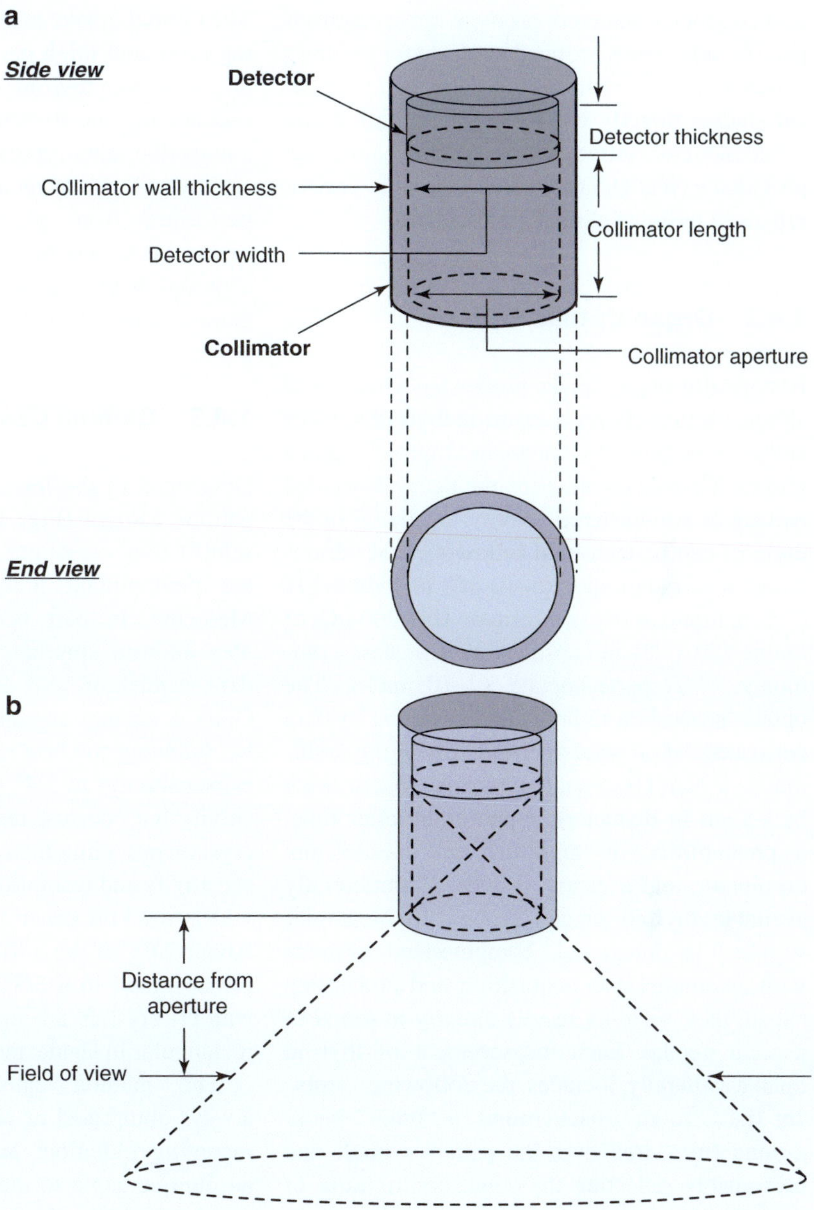

Fig. 1.10 (**a**) Basic design of a gamma probe. The collimator may be thought of as an extension of the detector shielding in the forward direction, that is, beyond the detector face in the desired counting direction. A collimator may be characterized by its aperture (generally, but not necessarily, equal to the width of the detector), its length, and its wall thickness. (**b**) The probe's field of view, that is, the area of tissue from which unscattered X- or γ-rays may reach the detector, increases with increasing distance from the collimator aperture. The volume of tissue from which unscattered X- or γ-rays may reach the detector is thus a three-dimensional cone diverging outward from the collimator (the dotted line) (Adapted from [7])

Disadvantages include bulkiness and relatively poor energy resolution and scatter rejection relative to semiconductor-based probes. In some scintillation-detector intraoperative probes, the light signal from the crystal is guided to a remote PMT through a flexible fiber-optic cable, allowing the probe assembly to be made relatively light and compact and more like a surgical instrument but with some loss of light in the long cabling. On the other hand, semiconductor-based probes are compact and have excellent energy resolution and scatter rejection. To minimize degradation of energy resolution, semiconductor detectors are made relatively thin (only ~1 mm) but at the cost of lower intrinsic sensitivity. The main disadvantage of semiconductor detectors remains their limited thickness and resulting lower sensitivity, especially for medium- to high-energy X- and γ-rays. Nonetheless, while scintillation detectors can be made thicker and therefore more sensitive, semiconductor detectors produce more electrons per X- and γ-ray stopped and therefore have superior energy resolution. To date, the few clinical studies directly comparing scintillation and semiconductor intraoperative probes have not provided a clear choice between the two types of probes in terms of clinical performance.

1.4.2 Organ Uptake Probes

Historically, organ uptake probes have been used almost exclusively for measuring thyroid uptakes and are thus generally known as "thyroid" uptake probes. Thyroid uptake (i.e., the decay-corrected percent of administered activity localizing in the thyroid) can be measured following oral administration of radioiodide (5–10 μCi of iodine-131 (^{131}I) in liquid or capsule form or 100–200 μCi of iodine-123 (^{123}I) in capsule form) or, less commonly, ^{99m}Tc-pertechnetate (2–10 mCi). The uptake probe is a radionuclide counting system consisting of a wide-aperture, diverging collimator, a NaI(Tl) crystal (typically ~5 cm thick by ~5 cm in diameter), a photomultiplier tube, a preamplifier, an amplifier, an energy discriminator, and a gantry (stand). Commercially available thyroid uptake probes are generally supplied as integrated, computerized systems with automated data acquisition and processing capabilities, yielding results directly in terms of percent uptake. Each measurement of thyroid uptake generally includes the following: ambient (i.e., "room") background, a "thigh" background (measured over the patient's thigh and presumably reflecting the count contribution of extra-thyroidal neck activity), thyroid (i.e., neck) activity, and a standard (which may be counted in a Lucite neck phantom simulating the thyroid/neck anatomy) activity. By including measurement of a standard activity with each uptake determination, corrections for radioactive decay and day-to-day variation in system sensitivity are automatic. (Alternatively, one may measure the administered activity itself in a phantom immediately prior to patient administration and then correct for radioactive decay when comparing with subsequent thyroid uptake measurements.) The thyroid uptake is then calculated by subtracting room and thigh background counts from the phantom and thyroid counts, respectively, and normalizing the thyroid counts to the phantom counts (the latter representing 100% uptake).

Thyroid uptake measurements are now often performed from planar scintigraphic images of the neck and of a standard (i.e., phantom) acquired with a gamma camera fitted with a parallel-hole collimator.

1.4.3 Gamma Cameras

Developed in the late 1950s by Hal Anger, the gamma camera (Fig. 1.11), also known as the scintillation or Anger camera, has long been the predominant imaging device in Nuclear Medicine, in part because its large detector area allowed simultaneous and therefore rapid data acquisition over a large area of the body. Gamma camera crystals vary in thickness from ¼″ (yielding the best spatial resolution but lowest sensitivity) to 3/4″ (yielding the highest sensitivity but coarsest resolution), with 3/8″-thick crystals providing the optimum balance between sensitivity and resolution and remaining the most widely used for general gamma camera imaging. About 95% of the 140-keV photons from ^{99m}Tc are absorbed in a 3/8″ crystal. Gamma camera NaI(Tl) crystals are nowadays most commonly rectangular in shape and ~50 × 60 cm in area.

The gamma camera collimator, almost always comprised of lead, "directionalizes" the incoming radiation: any radiation traveling at an oblique angle to the axes of the holes (apertures) will strike the lead walls (septa) between the holes and not reach the crystal, thereby allowing only radiation traveling perpendicular to the crystal surface to pass through the apertures and contribute counts to the resulting image. Of course, a certain fraction of photons striking the septa will nonetheless pass through them and reach the crystal (about 5%); this phenomenon, which degrades image quality, is known as septal penetration. The large majority of collimators are parallel-hole collimators, in which the apertures and septa are parallel to one another. In addition,

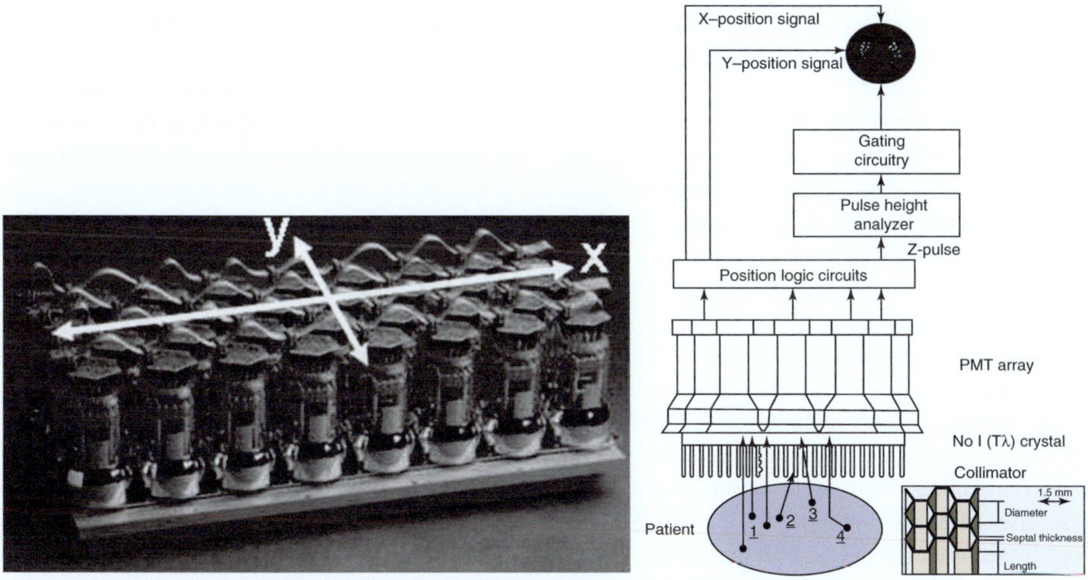

Fig. 1.11 Basic design of a gamma camera, consisting of a multi-hole collimator, a thin large-area NaI(Tl) crystal, a two-dimensional array of PMTs and associated electronics (high-voltage power supply, preamplifier, and amplifier), position logic circuitry, energy discriminator, and image display. Note that there are actually two position logic circuits—for the determination separately of the *x*- and *y*-positions of the scintillation within the crystal. Note further that the output signal from each PMT is actually split into three parts, one (the *z* pulse) for the determination of the energy of the incident radiation as well as one each for the determination of its *x*- and *y*-positions. The left inset shows a photograph of the two-dimensional PMT array backing the crystal in a typical rectangular field-of-view gamma camera. The right inset shows a drawing of a portion of a parallel-hole collimator, identifying the dimensions—aperture diameter, septal thickness, and septal length—of such a collimator. The "desirable" events (arrows labeled "1") are unscattered (i.e., photopeak) photons traveling in a direction parallel or nearly parallel to the axes of the apertures and thus yielding correctly positioned counts in the gamma camera image. "Undesirable" events include scattered as well as unscattered photons traveling in a direction oblique to the axes of the apertures (2) and thus eliminated by attenuation by one or more collimator septa; septal penetration (3), that is, unscattered photons traveling in a direction oblique to the axes of the apertures yet passing through the septa and yielding mispositioned counts; scatter (4), that is, photons undergoing Compton scatter within the patient and either eliminated by energy discrimination or not eliminated and yielding mispositioned counts (Fig. 1.6b) (Adapted from [1])

single-aperture pinhole collimators, most commonly used for thyroid imaging because of their pronounced magnifying effect, are available as well. Pinhole collimators, however, suffer from geometric distortion, that is, image magnification varies with both distance and lateral distance from the center of field.

Gamma camera collimators are "rated" with respect to photon energy and resolution/sensitivity. Low-energy, or "technetium," collimators, referred to as "low-energy all-purpose" (LEAP) collimators or "low-energy high-resolution" (LEHR) collimators, are designed to image radionuclides emitting X- and γ-rays less than 200 keV in energy, including, most notably, ^{99m}Tc (photopeak energy: 140 keV) as well as thallium-201 (^{201}Tl) (68–80 keV), ^{123}I (159 keV), and ^{57}Co (124 keV). Medium-energy, or "gallium," collimators are designed for radionuclides emitting X- and γ-rays 200–300 keV in energy, including gallium-67 (^{67}Ga) (93, 185, and 300 keV) as well as indium-111 (^{111}In) (172 and 247 keV). High-energy, or "iodine," collimators are designed to image radionuclides emitting X- and γ-rays greater than 300 keV in energy, including iodine-131 (^{131}I) (364 keV). Some departments no longer have a high-energy collimator and use a medium-energy collimator for imaging ^{131}I, accepting the increased septal penetration but achieving higher sensitivity. In progressing from low- to medium- to high-energy collimation, the collimators are made longer and the septa thicker in order to interpose more lead between the patient and the crystal and to thereby maintain septal penetration (i.e., the percent of counts in an image attributable to photons penetrating the septa) at or below an acceptably low level, typically set at 5%. This, in turn, reduces the overall fraction of emitted X- and γ-rays reaching the crystal. To compensate, at least in part, for the resulting lower sensitivity, the apertures are typically made wider progressing from low- to medium- to high-energy collimators. This, however, degrades spatial resolution. Overall, therefore, gamma camera images are progressively poorer in quality for radionuclides emitting low- versus medium- versus high-energy X- and γ-rays because of a combination of increased septal penetration with increasing photon energy, lower sensitivity because of the longer collimation, and coarser resolution because of the wider apertures. For each energy rating, collimators may also be rated as "general-purpose" (or "all-purpose"), "high-resolution," or "high-sensitivity." High-resolution collimators have narrower apertures (and therefore lower sensitivity), and high-sensitivity collimators have wider apertures (and therefore coarser resolution), respectively, than general-purpose collimators. Finally, in instances where a radionuclide emits a number of photons in significant amounts, it is the highest-energy photon which dictates the collimator to be used. For example, a medium-energy collimator must still be used to image ^{67}Ga (93, 185, and 300 keV) even if only the two lower-energy (i.e., the 93- and 185-keV) photons are used for imaging. (For some older systems, only two, rather than three, photon energies can be imaged simultaneously.)

Once the incident radiation passes through the collimator aperture, it strikes and may produce a scintillation within the crystal. The resulting light signal is distributed among the PMTs in a two-dimensional array backing the crystal, the intensity varying inversely with the distance between the scintillation and the respective PMT: the further the PMT is from the scintillation, the less light it receives and the smaller its output pulse. This inverse relationship is the basis of the Anger position logic circuitry for determining the precise position of a scintillation within the crystal. In the older gamma cameras, the *x*- and *y*-coordinates were calculated by analog circuitry, that is, using matrices of resistors and capacitors. In newer models, this is done by digitizing the output signal from each PMT with an analog-to-digital converter (ADC) and using digital electronics.

1.4.4 Tomographic Scanners

1.4.4.1 Introduction

A "tomogram" is literally a picture of a slice. Tomography may be characterized as either transmission or emission tomography depending on the origin of the radiation. In transmission tomography (i.e., computed tomography (CT)), X-rays are transmitted through the patient; in emission tomography, X- or γ-rays are emitted from within the patient. Emission tomography can be further characterized on the basis of the nature of the emitted radiation. Single photons, such as gamma rays associated with isomeric transition and X-rays associated with electron capture or internal conversion, form the basis of single-photon emission computed tomography (SPECT). The two 511-keV annihilation photons simultaneously emitted following positron-electron annihilation and associated with positron emission form the basis of positron emission tomography (PET).

The basic paradigm includes acquisition of images from multiple angles around a patient (multiple projections), correction of the acquired data for nonuniformity, and mathematical reconstruction of thin (several-millimeter-thick) transverse tissue-section images. In both SPECT and PET, the reconstructed transverse-section images are essentially contiguous, with no inter-section gaps, and therefore the reconstructed three-dimensional array of volume elements, or voxels, may be rearranged at any angle relative to the longitudinal axis of the patient and thus yield coronal, sagittal, or oblique images. The principal advantage of tomography thus lies in its improved image contrast: by eliminating the count contribution from activities in tissues above and below the section of interest, the target (e.g., tumor)-to-background count ratio may dramatically improve.

1.4.4.2 SPECT Data Acquisition

SPECT, like PET, is now a mature but continually improving technology. Although there are many possible combinations of detector number, geometry, and motion that can acquire the necessary projection data, rotating gamma camera-based SPECT systems occasionally use one or three detectors but most commonly use two detectors. The raw data are acquired as a series of discrete planar images at multiple angles about the longitudinal axis of the patient (Fig. 1.12). The number of counts recorded in each projection-image pixel represents the ray sum, or line integral, of the sampling line perpendicular to and extending from the detector through the patient. The following are typical SPECT acquisition parameters: 20–30 min for data acquisition; ~60 to ~120 projection images (corresponding to angular increment between successive projection images of 6–3°, respectively); and a 360° rotation. An angular increment in excess of 6° between successive projection images will result in prohibitive under-sampling artifacts in the reconstructed images.

Because of the length of time required for a single SPECT study (20–30 min), dynamic SPECT and whole-body SPECT remain largely impractical. It should be emphasized that SPECT images can in principle be quantitative in absolute terms, with voxel values representing the local activity concentration. However, in contrast to PET, this is often not the case in routine practice because of the confounding effects of scatter and attenuation. Accurate correction for these effects is advancing but remains more challenging in SPECT than in PET.

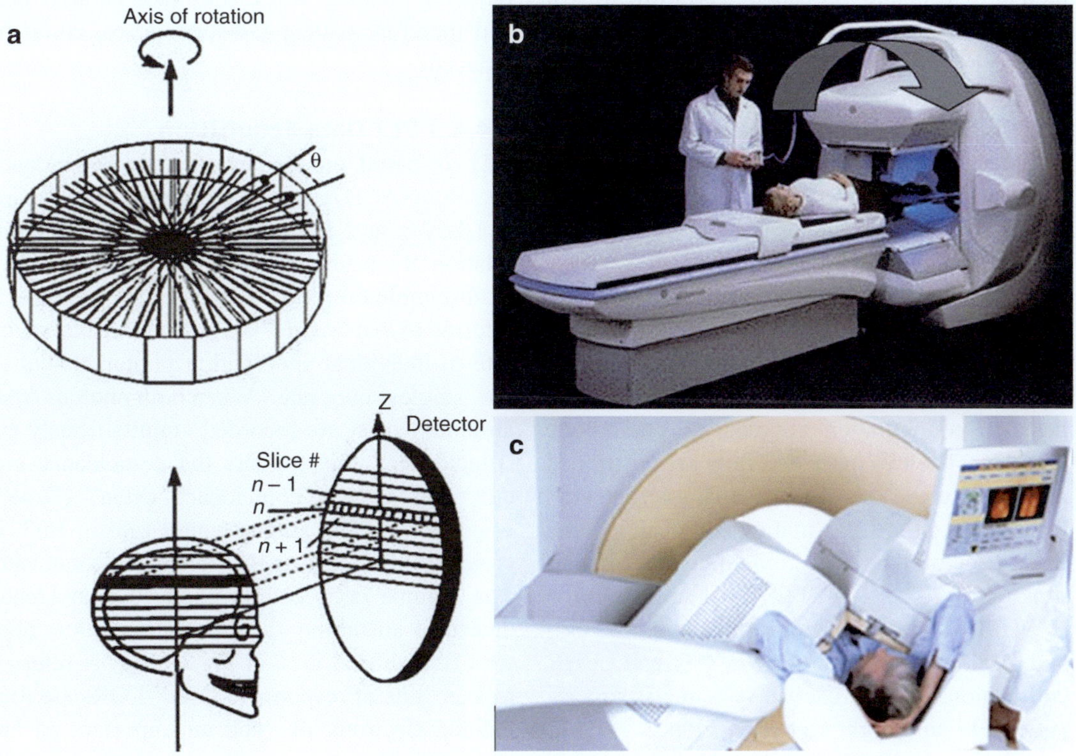

Fig. 1.12 (**a**) The basic data acquisition paradigm in rotating gamma camera SPECT. Photographs of modern dual-detector gamma cameras, with (**b**) the two detectors in opposed positions, as routinely used for a 360° rotation and general (non-cardiac) SPECT, and (**c**) the two detectors perpendicular to each other, as routinely used for a 180° rotation and cardiac SPECT (from approximately right anterior oblique to left posterior oblique). The obvious advantage of such two-detector systems is that two projection images can be acquired simultaneously and the acquisition time therefore halved (Reprinted with permission from [5])

Among the most noteworthy refinements in SPECT technology in recent years have been the application of solid-state ionization detector (i.e., semiconductor)-based gamma cameras, the introduction of novel, application-specific detector and collimator configurations (particularly in nuclear cardiology), and (as noted) improved quantitative accuracy. Cardiac imaging typically involves acquisition of projection data over only a 180° orbit (instead of the 360° orbit used for general SPECT imaging) – from right anterior oblique to left posterior oblique—because of the left, anterior position of the heart within the thorax (Fig. 1.12c). By positioning the two detectors at a right angle to one another, both detectors can simultaneously acquire usable data over the 180° orbit. Dedicated cardiac SPECT scanners with two scintillation detectors *fixed* at a right angle to one another (Eqs. 1.7 and 1.8) are commercially available. So-called "cardio-focal" (or "astigmatic") collimators are comprised of converging collimation at the field of view (FOV) to provide magnification in both the axial and transaxial directions and diverging collimation at the periphery of the FOV to provide coverage of the entire body and thereby avoid truncation artifacts commonly seen with fanbeam collimators when imaging the torso.

One dedicated cardiac scanner employs one, two, or three pixilated CsI(Tl) scintillation detectors and images of patients in an upright seated position. It uses fanbeam collimators in the three-detector configuration coupled to photodiode detectors. The two outer detectors are positioned at a 67.5° angle relative to the central detector. Data are acquired by rotating the chair (rather than detectors) by 67.5°, yielding an acquisition arc of 202.5°. Its SPECT spatial resolution (FWHM) is 11.0 mm (radius of rotation: 20 cm) and sensitivity 160 cpm/μCi for ^{99m}Tc and LEHR collimation. Another cardiac system also images patients in an upright seated position. It is comprised of three curved stationery NaI(Tl) crystals backed by three rows of 20 PMTs, with a thin curved lead collimator having six vertical slots for horizontal collimation and rotating slowly back and forth every 10 s. Its spatial resolution varies from 3.6 mm at an 82-mm source-to-detector distance to 7.8 mm at a 337-mm source-to-detector distance. Several vendors have introduced CZT-based cardiac SPECT systems. In these systems the detector gantry does not rotate or otherwise move. Their high sensitivity is not related to the intrinsic sensitivity of the CZT detectors but rather the high-sensitivity geometric arrangement and collimation of the detectors.

The foregoing dedicated cardiac scanners provide better spatial resolution and higher sensitivity than conventional gamma cameras. These systems provide up to a sevenfold increase in sensitivity and twofold improvement in reconstructed image resolution compared with those of conventional dual-head systems. Cardiac imaging times with these scanners thus range from 2 to 3 min for systems with solid-state detectors to 4 min on scintillation-detector systems with cardio-focal collimation. As an alternative to reducing imaging times, administered activities, and therefore patient radiation doses, could be reduced.

1.4.4.3 PET Data Acquisition

PET is based on the annihilation coincidence detection (ACD) of the two colinear (180° apart) 511-keV γ-rays resulting from the mutual annihilation of a positron and an electron (Fig. 1.13). Each annihilation photon recorded by a detector is referred to as a "single" event, and the total count rate of individual annihilation photons is called the "singles count rate." When both photons from an annihilation are recorded simultaneously (in coincidence), this triggers the coincidence circuit, and a "true coincidence event" ("true") is generated. The singles count rate in PET is typically much higher than the trues count rate. The volume between the opposed coincidence detectors absorbing the two annihilation photons (the shaded area in Fig. 1.13a) is referred to as a "line of response (LOR)." LORs are thus defined electronically, and an important advantage of ACD is that a collimator is not required. As a result, the sensitivity of PET is 2–3 orders of magnitude higher than that of gamma camera imaging. As shown in Fig. 1.13b, modern PET scanners employ a series of rings of discrete, small-area detectors (i.e., scored block detec-

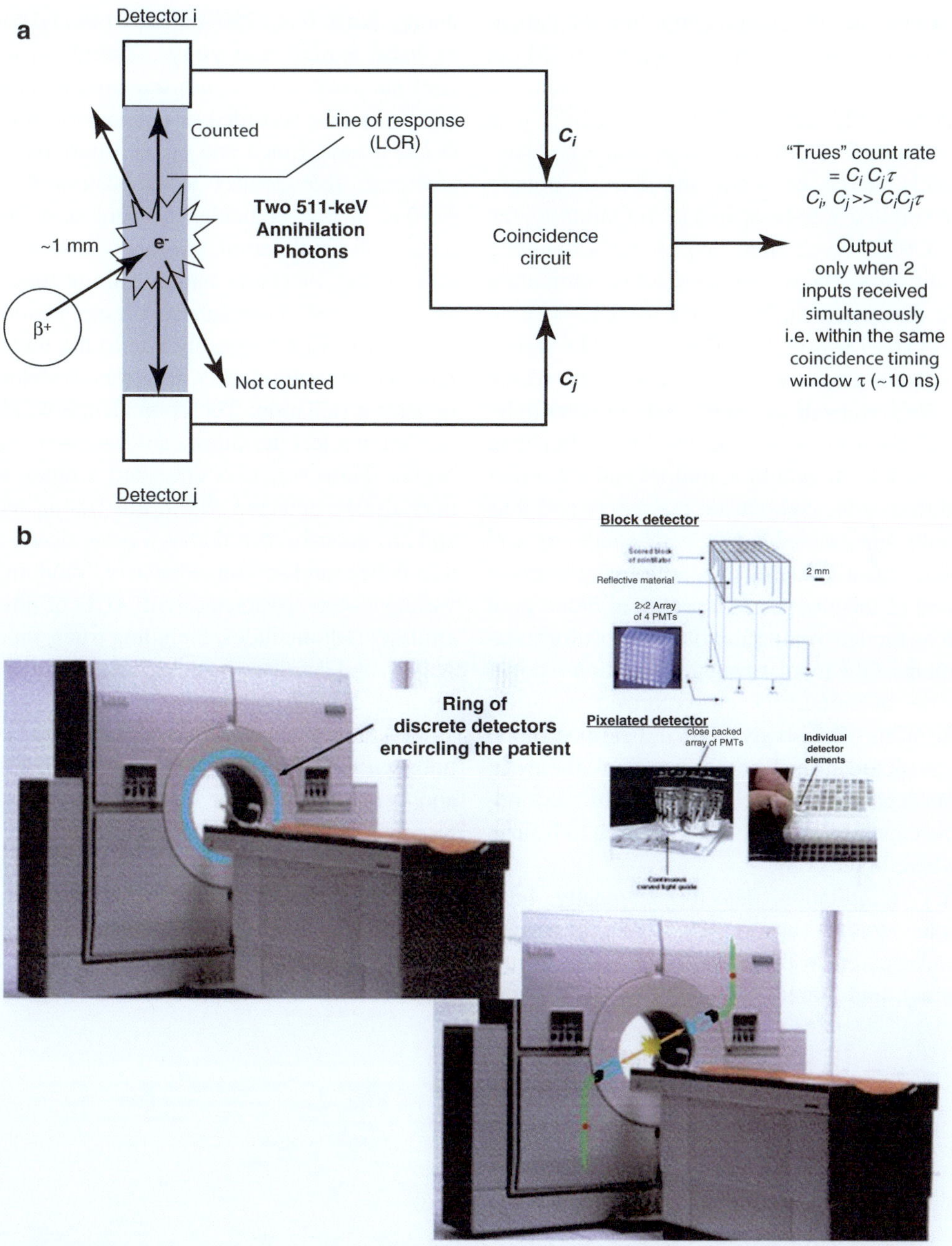

Fig. 1.13 (**a**) Annihilation coincidence detection (ACD) of the two opposed 511-keV γ-rays resulting from positron decay and positron-negatron annihilation. Note that the true coincidence (or "trues") count rate, given by the product of the singles count rates, C_i and C_j, and the coincidence timing window, τ, is much less than C_i and C_j—the coincidence timing window, τ, is short (<10 ns) to minimize the number of random coincidence events (Fig. 1.15), and most of the annihilation photons therefore do not produce coincidence events. (**b**) A photograph of a modern PET, illustrating one of a number of rings of discrete detectors encircling the patient (left-hand panel) and ACD of an annihilation photon by a pair of these detectors. In the insert are shown a block detector (top) and pixelated detectors (bottom) currently used in PET scanners. The block detector consists of a cubic piece of scintillator scored to variable depths into a two-dimensional array of detector elements, typically backed by a 2 × 2 array of position-sensitive PMTs. Pixelated detectors consist of individual scintillator detector elements backed by a continuous light guide and a close-packed array of PMTs. For both the block and pixelated detectors, the individual detector elements are typically ~2 × 2 mm in area (Adapted from [6])

tors or pixelated detectors) encircling the patient and typically spanning a distance of 10–20 cm in the patient's longitudinal direction. Thus, a whole-body PET scan will typically require data acquisition at 6–7 discrete bed positions and subsequently merge, or "knit," the discrete images into a single whole-body image. Importantly, the EXPLORER consortium, led by the University of California, Davis, has completed fabrication of the first true total-body PET system, with an axial FOV of nearly 2 m (Fig. 1.14). The resulting 40-fold improvement in sensitivity would allow PET scans of the entire body to potentially be performed in as little as 15–30 s rather than in 10–20 min. In addition, tumors and other diseased tissues located outside the thorax and thus generally not amenable to kinetic modeling and absolute quantitation of metabolic parameters—because of the absence of a proximal blood pool (such as the left ventricular blood pool) for measurement of the input, or supply, function—could now be quantitatively characterized noninvasively. With whole-body PET, the cardiac blood pool is included in dynamic imaging studies of tumors regardless of their location, thus extending the capabilities of kinetic modeling to lesions anywhere in the body.

PET scintillation detectors typically have a rather coarse (up to 30%) energy resolution (compared to 8–9% for traditional gamma cameras), and therefore photons within a broad energy range (e.g., 250–650 keV) can be counted as valid annihilation γ-rays. Therefore, significant numbers of Compton-scattered annihilation γ-rays may be recorded as mispositioned coincidence events. Since one or both may have been scattered, this creates a mispositioned event. Further, a true coincidence event is defined as a pair of annihilation photons counted by the coincidence detectors within a finite time interval called the "coincidence timing window τ," typically 6–12 ns—mainly due to the finite time required for scintillation detectors to detect and register a radiation. The coincidence window is needed to reject the significant fraction of singles events. However, two unrelated singles events may also be detected within this timing window and erroneously recorded as a coincidence event, a so-called random coincidence or "random." The various events associated with ACD of positron-emitting radionuclides, including trues, randoms, scatter, and spurious coincidences or singles, are illustrated in Fig. 1.15.

PET ring scanners originally employed lead or tungsten walls, or the septa, positioned between and extending radially inward from the detector elements (Fig. 1.16a). Removing the septa altogether and including coincidence events from all of the LORs among all the detectors significantly increases PET detector sensitivity (Fig. 1.16d)—a system with ~10,000 detector elements has approximately 100 million

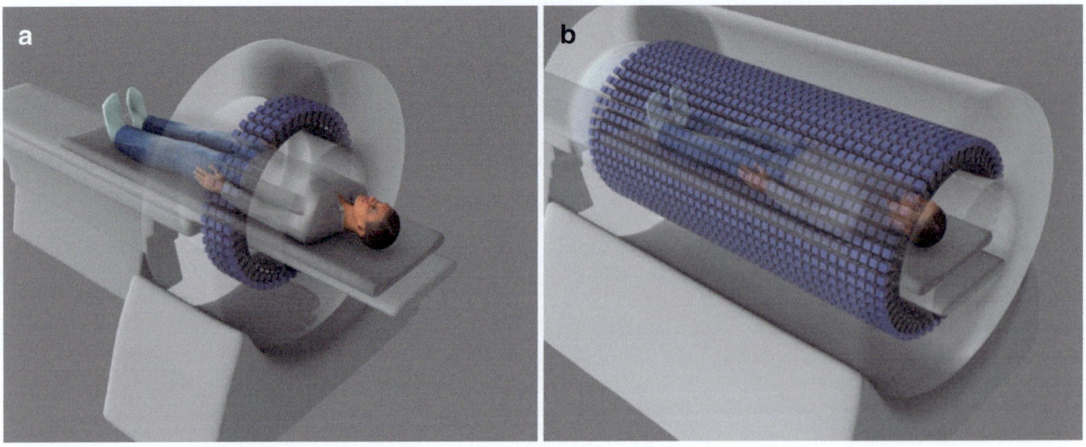

Fig. 1.14 (**a**) Conventional (i.e., limited-FOV) versus (**b**) whole-body PET (Reprinted with permission from [8])

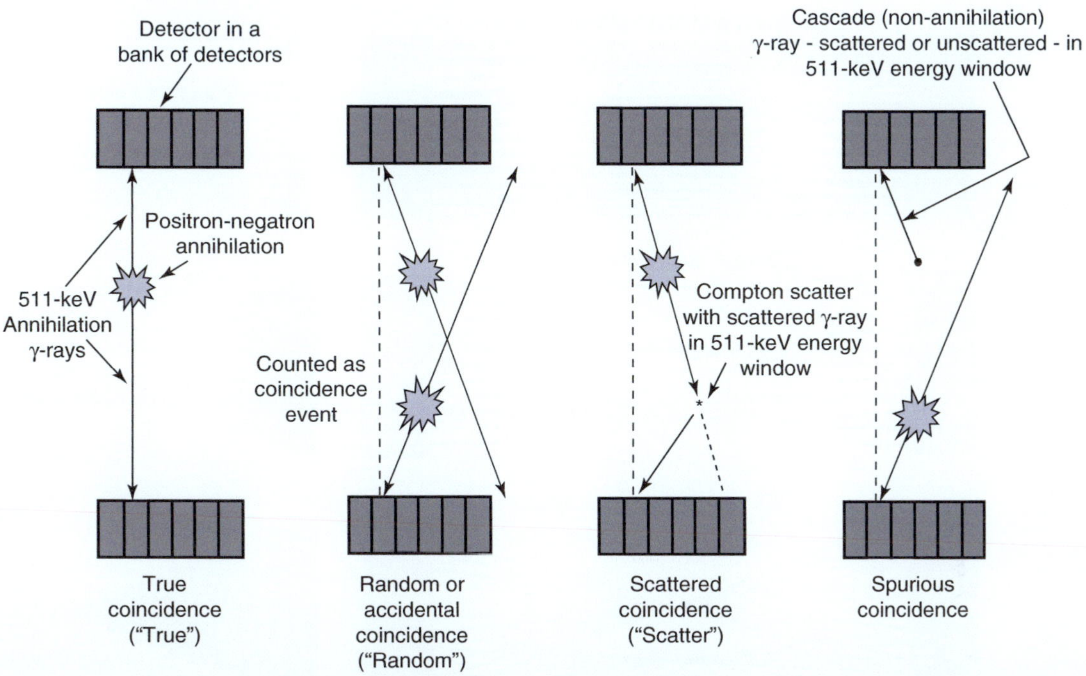

Fig. 1.15 The various events associated with ACD of positron-emitting radionuclides, illustrated for two opposed banks of coincidence detectors and assuming only one opposed pair of detectors is in coincidence. A true coincidence ("true") is counted only when each of the two 511-keV annihilation γ-rays for a single positron-negatron annihilation is not scattered and is detected within the timing window τ of the two coincidence detectors. A random or accidental coincidence ("random") is an inappropriately detected and positioned coincidence (the dashed line) which arises from two separate annihilations, with one γ-ray from each of the two annihilations detected within the timing window τ of the coincidence-detector pair. A scattered coincidence ("scatter") is a mispositioned coincidence (the dashed line) resulting from a single annihilation, with one of the γ-rays undergoing a small-angle Compton scatter but retaining sufficient energy to fall within the 511-keV energy window. A spurious coincidence is an inappropriately detected and positioned coincidence (the dashed line) which arises from an annihilation and a cascade γ-ray, scattered or unscattered but having sufficient energy to fall within the 511-keV energy window. Spurious coincidences occur only for radionuclides which emit both positrons and high-energy prompt cascade γ-rays, that is, γ-rays with energies (either scattered or unscattered) lying within the 511-keV energy window (Adapted from [6])

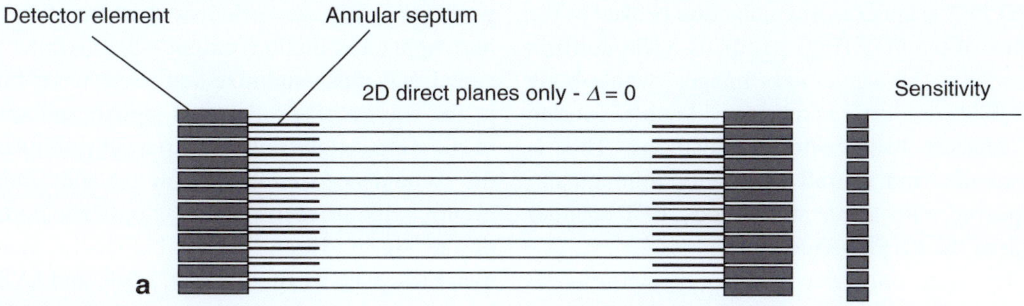

Fig. 1.16 Two-dimensional (2D) and three-dimensional (3D) PET data acquisition schemes (axial cross-sectional views of a multi-ring scanner) and the corresponding axial sensitivity profiles. (**a–c**) 2D data acquisition with a ring difference Δ of 0 (direct planes only), 1, and 3, respectively. (**d**) 3D (septa-less) data acquisition. The sensitivity profiles show the nonuniformity of response as a function of position along the axial FOV (Adapted from [1])

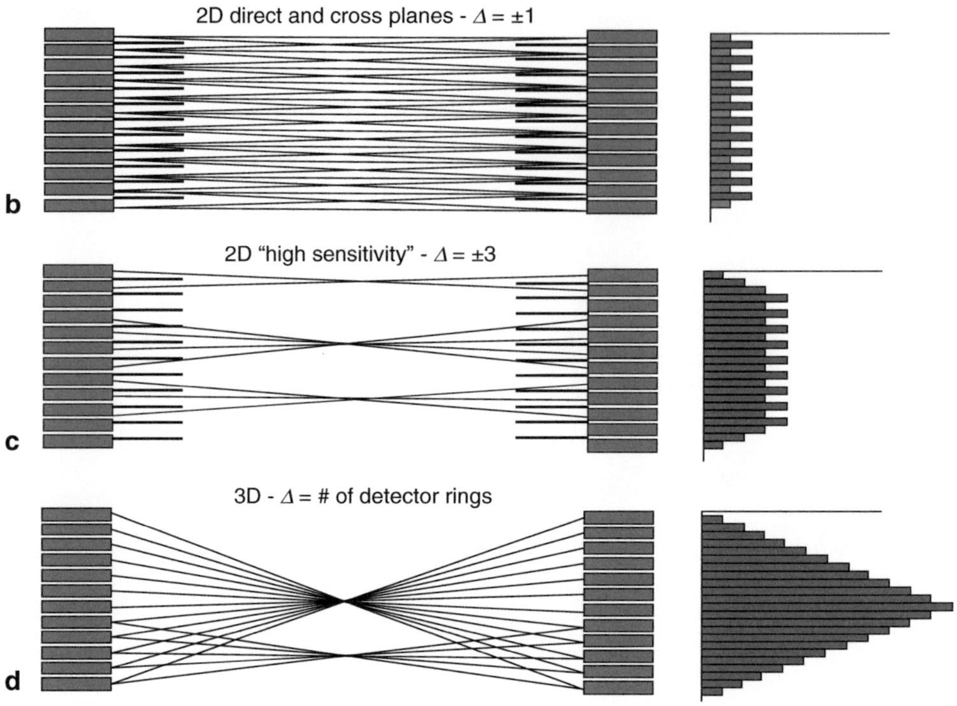

Fig. 1.16 (continued)

LORs. This is known as three-dimensional (3D) PET, and commercially available PET scanners are now exclusively 3D devices. Sensitivity is increased approximately fivefold in 3D relative to 2D PET but with a considerable increase in the randoms and scatter count rates. Axial sensitivity is also affected by removing the inter-ring septa: in contrast to the relatively uniform axial sensitivity for 2D PET, the axial sensitivity profile for a 3D PET scanner is triangular and peaked at the center of the FOV (Fig. 1.16d). To yield uniform sensitivity for whole-body images, whole-body 3D PET studies require considerable overlap of adjacent bed-position acquisitions. This is overcome, and overall sensitivity dramatically improved with a true whole-body PET scanner such as the EXPLORER.

To date, only five detector materials—all inorganic scintillators—have been widely used in PET scanners: bismuth germanate (BGO, $Bi_4Ge_3O_{12}$), cerium-doped gadolinium oxyorthosilicate (GSO(Ce) or GSO, Gd_2SiO_5:Ce), cerium-doped lutetium oxyorthosilicate (LSO(Ce) or LSO, Lu_2SiO_5:Ce), and cerium-doped lutetium-yttrium oxyorthosilicate (LYSO(Ce) or LYSO, Lu_2YSiO_5:Ce) as well as thallium-doped sodium iodide (NaI(Tl)). Although used in some of the very first PET scanners, NaI(Tl) is really sub-optimal for PET and has not been used in PET devices for many years. The most important practical features of scintillation detectors include high mass density (ρ) and effective atomic number (Z_{eff})—to maximize the photon stopping power (i.e., intrinsic efficiency) of the detector; high light (scintillation) output—to maximize the signal and thus minimize statistical uncertainty in the energy of the detected signal; and speed of the output light pulse—to permit minimizing the coincidence timing window (τ) and random events, without sacrificing a significant portion of the signal. Higher-ρ and higher-Z_{eff} atomic materials, such as BGO, GSO, LSO, and LYSO, have emerged as the detectors of choice for PET because of their greater stopping power for 511-keV annihilation γ-rays. GSO, LSO, and LYSO have faster light output—nearly tenfold faster—than BGO, with LSO having a much greater light output, approximately threefold greater than either BGO or GSO. GSO has somewhat better energy resolution, and scatter rejection capability, than BGO, LSO, or LYSO. A notable disadvantage of LSO and LYSO is the presence of a naturally occurring long-lived radioisotope of lutetium, lutetium-177. Lutetium-177 (^{177}Lu) has an isotopic abundance of 2.6% and a half-life of ~4 × 10^{10} years and emits two prompt γ-rays (88% abundance) of 201 and 306 keV in energy; the summed energy of 507 keV falls well within the 511-keV energy windows commonly used in PET scanners. The presence of ^{177}Lu results in a measured background count rate of 240 cps/cm^3 of LSO and singles and trues count rates of 100,000 and 10,000 cps, respectively, in clinical LSO PET scanners. This has a negligible effect on typical PET scans, however.

1.4.4.4 Data Processing and Tomographic Image Reconstruction

Normalization/Nonuniformity Correction

Even optimally performing SPECT or PET scanners exhibit some nonuniformity of response. Among the thousands of pixels in a SPECT projection image and the thousands of detector elements (and therefore LORs) in a PET scanner, slight variations in detector thickness, light emission properties, electronics performance, etc. result in slightly different measured count rates for the same activity. In principle, such nonuniform response can be corrected by acquiring data from a uniform flux of X- or γ-rays and normalizing to the *mean* count rate from all the pixels in SPECT or LORs in PET. This "normalization" table, or "uniformity map," corrects for the nonuniform count rate among the individual pixels or LORs to thereby yield a pixel-by-pixel or LOR-by-LOR uniformity correction. For planar gamma camera imaging as well as SPECT, such a correction table may be acquired using either a uniform flood source placed on the detector or a point source placed sufficiently far (typically ~2 m) from the uncollimated detector to approximate a uniform photon flux (see below). For PET, it may be acquired using a positron-emitting rod source (e.g., germanium-68) spanning the entire axial FOV and rotating it around the periphery of the FOV, exposing the detector pairs to a uniform photon flux per revolution. Alternatively, a uniform cylinder of a positron-emitting radionuclide can be scanned, with the data thus acquired corrected for attenuation. For both planar imaging and SPECT and PET, acquisition of the data required for uniformity correction is somewhat problematic in practice because of statistical considerations: tens of millions (SPECT) to hundreds of millions (PET) of counts must be acquired to avoid possible "noise"-related artifacts in the uniformity correction table.

Dead Time Correction

Scintillation detectors have a finite dead time and associated count losses. The dead time is the length of time required for a counting system to record an event, during which additional events cannot be recorded. As a result, the measured count rate is lower than the actual count rate. Such count losses are significant, however, only at "high" count rates and are generally minimal at clinical administered activities. Nonetheless, a real-time correction for dead time count losses is routinely applied in PET (though not in SPECT) to the measured count rates, most commonly by scaling up the measured count rate based on an empirically derived mathematical relationship between measured and trues count rates.

Center-of-Rotation Misalignment Correction (SPECT)

In rotating gamma camera SPECT, the location of the projection of the center of rotation (COR) on the projection-image matrix must be constant. If the mechanical and electronic CORs are aligned, the pixel location of the projection of the COR onto the projection-image matrix will be the same for all projection images, and, for all such images, the counts in each pixel will then be projected across the appropriate row of pixels in the tomographic image matrix. If, however, the mechanical and electronic CORs are not aligned, the pixel location of the COR will vary among the projection images, and the counts in each projection-image pixel will be projected across different locations in the tomographic image matrix, and blurred images will result (Fig. 1.17a). In today's SPECT systems, COR misalignment may

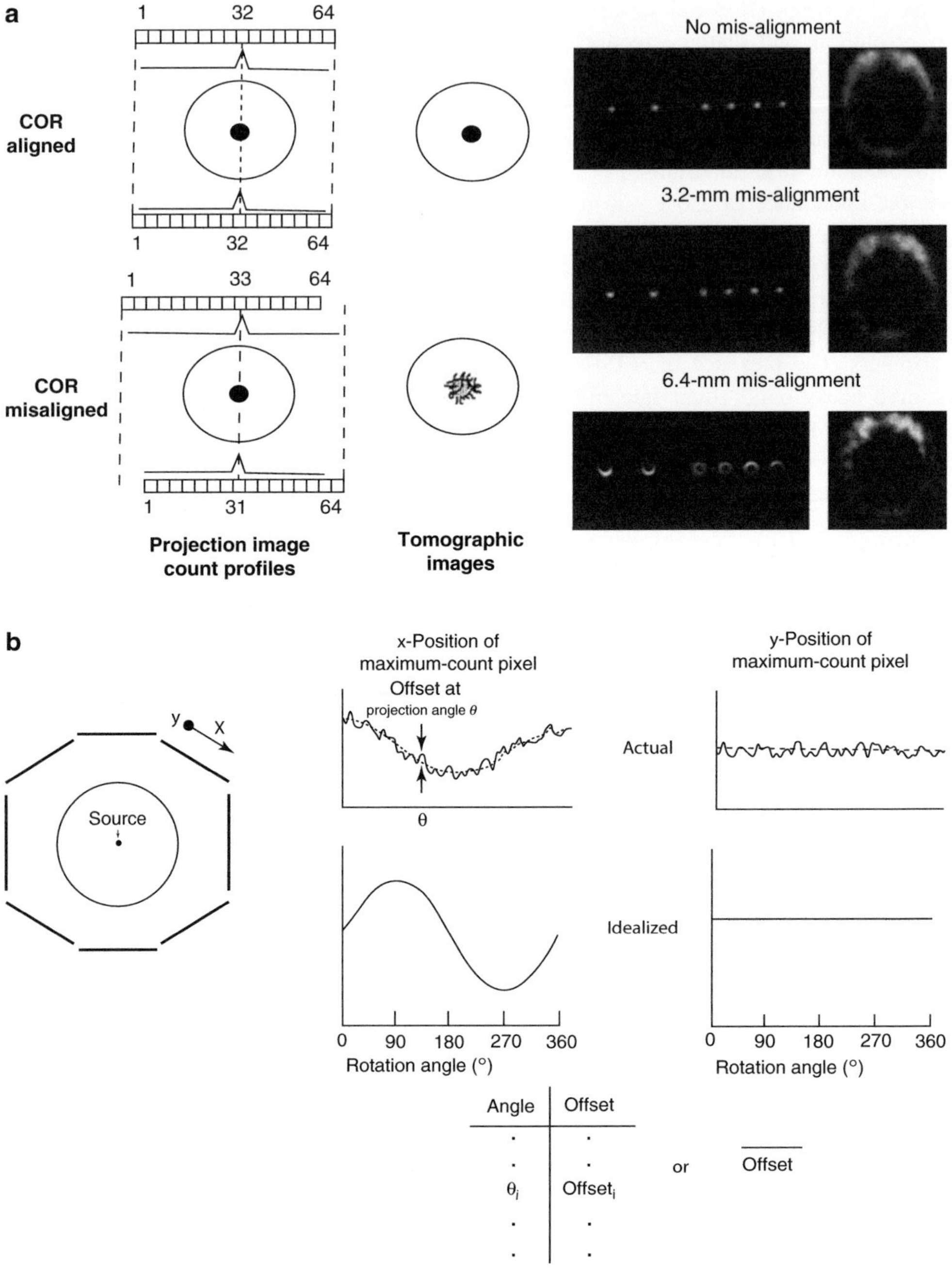

Fig. 1.17 (**a**) Center-of-rotation (COR) misalignment and resulting image-blurring artifacts in rotating gamma camera SPECT. The degree of blurring is related to the magnitude of the spatial misalignment of the mechanical and electronic CORs. A misalignment as small as 3.2 mm (or ½ a pixel for a 64 × 64 image matrix) can produce perceptible blurring in SPECT images, with the blurring substantially worse for a misalignment of 6.4 mm (1 pixel). (**b**) COR misalignment can be measured and corrected based on acquiring a 360° circular SPECT study of a ^{99m}Tc point source and constructing graphs of the *x*- and *y*-positions (perpendicular and parallel to the axis of rotation, respectively) of the position of the maximum-count pixel in each projection image versus angular position. The *x*- and *y*-position-versus-angle graphs should be a sinusoidal curve and a straight line, respectively. The angle-by-angle deviation between the *x*-position on the best-fit sine curve and the *x*-position of the actual maximum-count pixel thus yields a correction table indicating the offset by which each projection image must be shifted at each angular position to align the CORs. Alternatively, the average of the offsets may be used at each angular position (Adapted from [5])

be easily measured and corrections created and automatically applied using the system's software (Fig. 1.17b).

Randoms Correction (PET)

In PET, randoms increase the detected coincidence count rate by introducing mispositioned events and thus reduce image contrast and distort the relationship between image intensity and activity concentration. The standard approach to randoms correction, the "delayed-window" method, is based on the fact that the random coincidence γ-rays are temporally uncorrelated (i.e., not simultaneously emitted). Briefly, once singles in the coincidence timing window (typically 6–12 ns) are detected, the number of singles in a timing window equal in duration to, but much later (>50 ns later) than, the coincidence timing window is determined. The number of events in the delayed timing window provides an estimate of the number of randoms in the coincidence timing window. Real-time subtraction of the delayed-window counts from the coincidence-window counts for each LOR thus corrects for randoms.

Scatter Correction

Scatter results in mispositioned counts in reconstructed images, reducing contrast and distorting the relationship between image intensity and activity concentration. In PET in general, scatter correction is rather straightforward. Once the randoms correction has been applied, the peripheral "tails" in the projection-image count profiles, presumably due exclusively to scatter, are fit to a mathematical function and then subtracted (deconvolved) from the measured profile to yield scatter-corrected profiles for tomographic image reconstruction. Other scatter corrections for 3D PET include dual energy window-based approaches; convolution/deconvolution-based approaches (analogous to the correction in 2D PET); direct estimation of scatter distribution (by Monte Carlo simulation of the imaging system); and iterative reconstruction-based scatter compensation approaches (also employing Monte Carlo simulation). The Monte Carlo simulation and subtraction of scatter have been implemented in commercial PET scanners.

The most widely used approach to scatter correction in SPECT is the "triple-energy-window" method in which two "scatter" energy windows (equal in width (in keV)) are created which bracket and are immediately adjacent to the photopeak energy window. Three separate images, two scatter images and a photopeak image, are simultaneously acquired. The scatter image is then multiplied by fractional weighting factors, to estimate the pixel-by-pixel scatter counts appearing in the photopeak image, and the weighted scatter image is then subtracted from the photopeak image.

Attenuation Correction

Attenuation correction is generally the largest correction in tomographic imaging. In contrast to SPECT, one of the most attractive features of PET is the relative ease of applying accurate and precise corrections for attenuation, based on the fact that attenuation depends only on the total thickness of the attenuation medium. For a positron-emitting source and a volume of thickness L, the attenuation factor is $e^{-\mu L}$ and the attenuation correction factor $e^{\mu L}$ regardless of the position of the source. Accordingly, the attenuation correction factor (ACF) can be derived as follows:

$$\mathrm{ACF}_{\mathrm{ij}} = e^{\mu L}{}_{\mathrm{ij}} \tag{1.18}$$

$$= \frac{\left[(C)\mathrm{Blank}\right]_{\mathrm{ij}}}{\left[(C)\mathrm{Trans}\right]_{\mathrm{ij}}} \tag{1.19}$$

where ACF_{ij} is the attenuation correction factor between coincident detectors i and j, L_{ij} the thickness of the volume between coincident detectors i and j, and $[(C)_{\mathrm{Blank}}]_{\mathrm{ij}}$ and $[(C)_{\mathrm{Trans}}]_{\mathrm{ij}}$ the external-source counts between detectors i and j in the blank and transmission scans, respectively. In practice, a blank scan is acquired only once a day. In PET-CT scanners attenuation correction is, of course, performed using CT. A CT image is basically a two-dimensional map of attenuation coefficients at the CT X-ray energy (~80 keV). For attenuation correction of the PET emission data, however, these must be appropriately scaled to the 511-keV energy of the annihilation γ-rays. The mass-attenuation coefficients (μ_m) for CT X-rays (~80 keV) and for 511-keV annihilation γ-rays are 0.182 and 0.096 cm²/g, 0.209 and 0.093 cm²/g, and 0.167 and 0.087 cm²/g in the soft tissue, bone, and lung, respectively. The corresponding μ_m ratios are therefore 1.90, 2.26, and 1.92, respectively. Thus, ACFs derived from CT images cannot be scaled to those for 511-keV annihilation γ-rays simply using a single, or global, factor.

Like scatter corrections, attenuation corrections in SPECT are not yet as well developed as those in PET. With the growing deployment of SPECT-CT scanners, however, CT-based attenuation correction in SPECT is becoming more commonplace.

Image Reconstruction

In SPECT and PET, the raw data are essentially same (though acquired with very different detector geometries): one-dimensional projections (sets of parallel line integrals or ray sums) of the radiations emitted from the patient. In order to convert these data into a usable form, they must be mathematically transformed and reconstructed into a set of transverse images. These may then be reformatted into coronal, sagittal, and even oblique images. (Raw PET data must undergo several reformatting steps in order to create the one-dimensional projection data for image reconstruction.)

Historically, one of the most widely used algorithms for the reconstruction of tomographic images was filtered back projection (FBP). The basic procedure is as follows. Each projection is Fourier transformed into spatial-frequency space. The projection is mathematically filtered to amplify certain spatial frequencies and to dampen or eliminate other spatial frequencies. The filtered projection is inverse Fourier transformed from frequency back to real space. The filtered projection data in real space are then distributed (or back-projected) over the reconstructed image matrix. To eliminate spatial frequencies beyond the maximum frequency imageable by the scanner (i.e., the Nyquist frequency, ν_N) and thereby eliminate certain artifacts as well as excessive statistical uncertainty (noise or mottle), filters (known as Hanning, Butterworth, etc.) with cutoff frequencies, ν_c, set equal to ν_N or some fraction thereof are used. Although the resulting reconstructed images have somewhat degraded spatial resolution, they are far less "noisy" (mottled). The filter and the value of the cutoff frequency may be selected by the user. Care should be exercised in doing so, however, as these parameters affect the appearance and quantitative accuracy of the reconstructed images. Scanner manufacturers generally provide recommended values for the filters and filter parameters for different types of studies; in SPECT, for example, the recommended filter and cutoff frequency will depend on the radionuclide and the region of the body imaged.

Iterative reconstruction algorithms have almost entirely replaced FBP in SPECT and, in particular, in PET. Iterative algorithms attempt to progressively refine estimates of the activity distribution (rather than directly calculate the distribution) by maximizing or minimizing some "target function." The solution is said to "converge" when the difference of the target function between successive estimates (iterations) of the activity distribution is less than some prespecified value. Importantly, iterative reconstruction algorithms allow for the incorporation of realistic modeling of the data acquisition process (including effects of attenuation and scatter), the modeling of statistical noise, and the inclusion of pertinent a priori information (e.g., only nonnegative count values). Widely used iterative reconstruction algorithms include the maximum-likelihood expectation maximization (MLEM) and the ordered-subset expectation maximization (OSEM) algorithms. The OSEM algorithm, which is actually a modified version of the MLEM algorithm, converges more rapidly than MLEM and is now the most widely used iterative reconstruction method in PET as well as SPECT.

Quantitation

Once the PET emission data have been corrected for dead time, randoms, system response (by normalization), scatter, and attenuation, the count rate per voxel in the reconstructed tomographic images is proportional to the local activity concentration and is finally converted to activity concentration using a measured system calibration factor, (MBq/cm^3)/(cps/voxel). As noted, SPECT images can be made quantitative in an analogous manner. In practice, however, the pertinent corrections (especially scatter and attenuation corrections) are currently not as routine in SPECT as in PET. To make the images quantitative, then, the count rate per voxel (cps), $\dot{C}_{ijk}$, in voxel ijk should be divided by the measured system calibration factor, CF (MBq/cm^3)/(cps/voxel), to yield the activity concentration:

$$[A]_{\text{ijk}} = \frac{\dot{C}_{\text{ijk}}}{CF} \quad (1.20)$$

where $[A]_{\text{ijk}}$ is the activity concentration (MBq/cm^3) in voxel ijk. The calibration factor (CF) can be derived by scanning a calibrated standard, that is, a water-filled or water (tissue)-equivalent volume source with all linear dimensions at least twice that of the system spatial resolution (FWHM) and with a uniform, well-defined activity concentration at the time of the scan. The requirement for water equivalence is to ensure that effects such as scatter and attenuation are comparable in both the patient and the standard. And the requirement for linear dimensions at least twice that of the system spatial resolution is to ensure that the effect of partial-volume averaging and associated underestimation of local count rates are negligible. Clinical expression of activity concentration is in terms of the decay-corrected fraction or percent of the administered activity per cubic centimeter (cc) or, more commonly, in terms of the standard uptake value (SUV):

$$\text{SUV} \equiv \frac{\text{MBq / cm}^3 \text{ of tissue}}{\text{MBq injected / g body mass}} \quad (1.21)$$

1.4.4.5 Time-of-Flight (TOF) PET

Time-of-flight (TOF) PET is based on the measurement of the difference between the detection times of the two photons arising from the positron-negatron annihilation. Currently, this allows spatial localization of the annihilation event along the LOR with a spatial resolution of ~100 mm assuming a coincidence time resolution (τ) of ~1 ns. Though a considerably coarser resolution than that of the conventional PET scanner (~5 mm), this approximate localization reduces the random coincidence rate and improves the signal-to-noise ratio (SNR), especially for large objects. For the original TOF scanners developed in the 1980s, the SNR gain was offset by the low stopping power of the scintillation crystals (barium fluoride (BaF_2) and cesium fluoride (CsF)) used at the time, and TOF PET was largely abandoned. Today, however, faster electronics and crystals such as LSO and LYSO have made TOF PET feasible, and TOF scanners are commercially available.

1.4.5 Gamma Camera Performance and Quality Control

Quality control (QC), a critical component of analytical procedures and instrumentation in general and medical devices in particular, is an established set of ongoing measurements and analyses designed to ensure that the performance of a procedure or instrument is within a pre-defined acceptable range. An extensive series of parameters have been developed over the years to characterize gamma camera, SPECT scanner, and PET scanner performance, and detailed data acquisition and analysis protocols have been promulgated by the National Electrical Manufacturers Association (NEMA), the American Association of Physicists in Medicine (AAPM), and others for this purpose. In practice, however, less extensive and less rigorous procedures are used for day-to-day QC.

To understand gamma camera performance and routine QC, several pertinent terms—intrinsic versus extrinsic (or system) performance and the useful versus the central field of view—must be understood. Intrinsic performance refers to gamma camera performance without a collimator in place, while extrinsic (or system) performance refers to that of the entire gamma system, including collimation. The useful field of view (UFOV) of a gamma camera is essentially the entire detector (i.e., crystal) area, while the central field of view (CFOV) corresponds to the inner, or central, three-quarters of the crystal area. The periphery of the gamma camera detector suffers from artifacts (e.g., edge packing) and poorer image quality in general, in part because light reflected from the mirror-like inner surface of the detector housing makes it appear that a disproportionate amount of light is emanating from this peripheral area. Accordingly, the periphery of the crystal is masked (or shielded), often by lead built into the edges of the collimator housing. Thus, the CFOV is the portion of the detector actually used in clinical imaging.

The performance parameters most commonly evaluated as part of a routine gamma camera QC program include uniformity, spatial resolution, and energy resolution. (See above.) Uniformity (the so-called "daily flood") should be evaluated each day either intrinsically or extrinsically (Fig. 1.18). Either ^{99m}Tc (intrinsic) or ^{57}Co (extrinsic) is used on a daily basis. Periodically (e.g., monthly), however, intrinsic uniformity for other radionuclides used clinically (e.g., ^{67}Ga, ^{111}In, and ^{131}I) should also be evaluated. Integral uniformities (Eq. 1.17), or IUs, up to 5% are acceptable, although nowadays IUs of 3% or better are routinely achievable. If the uniformity for any radionuclide is out of tolerance (i.e., >5%), that radionuclide's uniformity (or sensitivity) correction table should be updated. The necessary data may be acquired using the same setup as for the daily uniformity test, except that a much larger number of counts (60–100 million) must be acquired. In today's gamma cameras, uniformity correction tables may be easily updated and the corrections created, processed, stored, and automatically applied using the system's integrated software. In addition to an outdated uniformity correction table, there are other causes of gamma camera nonuniformity (Fig. 1.19): mistuning (detuning), uncoupling of a PMT; a cracked crystal; or corruption or switching off one or more

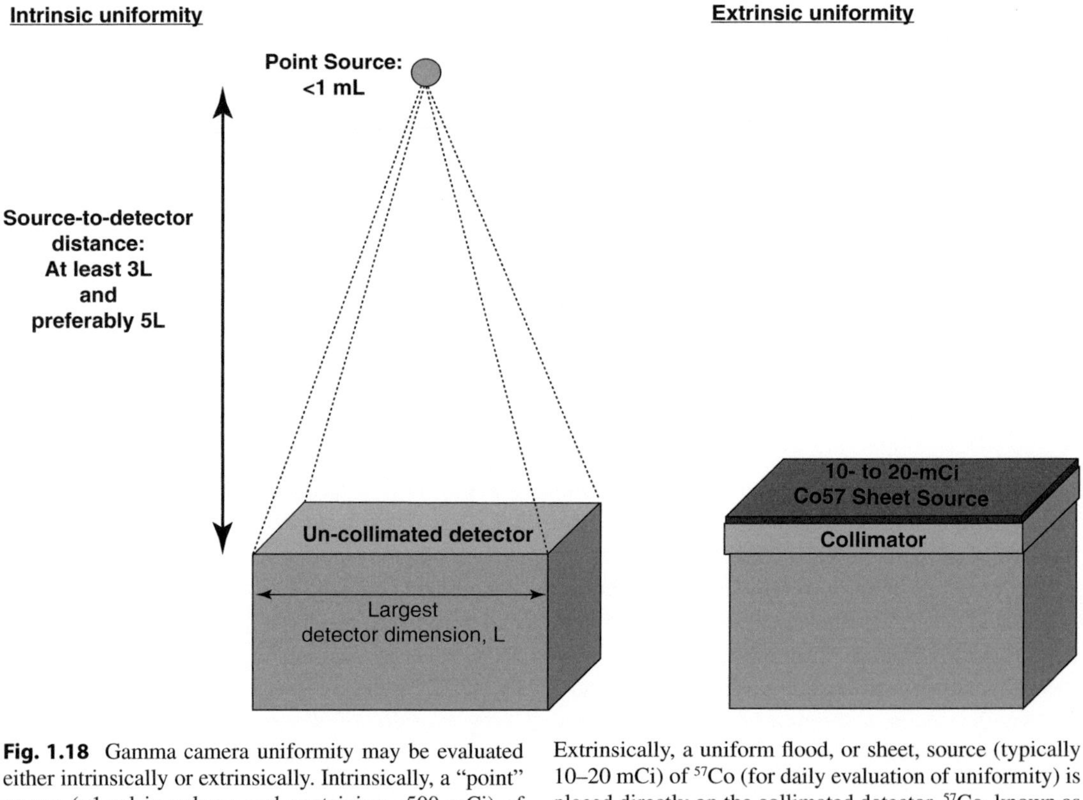

Fig. 1.18 Gamma camera uniformity may be evaluated either intrinsically or extrinsically. Intrinsically, a "point" source (<1 ml in volume and containing ~500 mCi) of ^{99m}Tc (at least for daily evaluation of uniformity) is placed at least three and preferably five crystal dimensions from and centered over the uncollimated detector to approximate a uniform photon flux. If necessary, the activity should be adjusted to yield a measured count rate no greater than 25,000 cps (to avoid dead time counting losses and count rate-related image degradation). Extrinsically, a uniform flood, or sheet, source (typically 10–20 mCi) of ^{57}Co (for daily evaluation of uniformity) is placed directly on the collimated detector. ^{57}Co, known as "mock Tc99m," has a half-life of 270 days and emits a 122-keV γ-ray and is thus a convenient, long-lived alternative to ^{99m}Tc. Such ^{57}Co sheet sources are available commercially. A total of 10–15 million counts should be acquired and uniformity evaluated quantitatively (e.g., in terms of the integral and differential uniformities) (Adapted from [2])

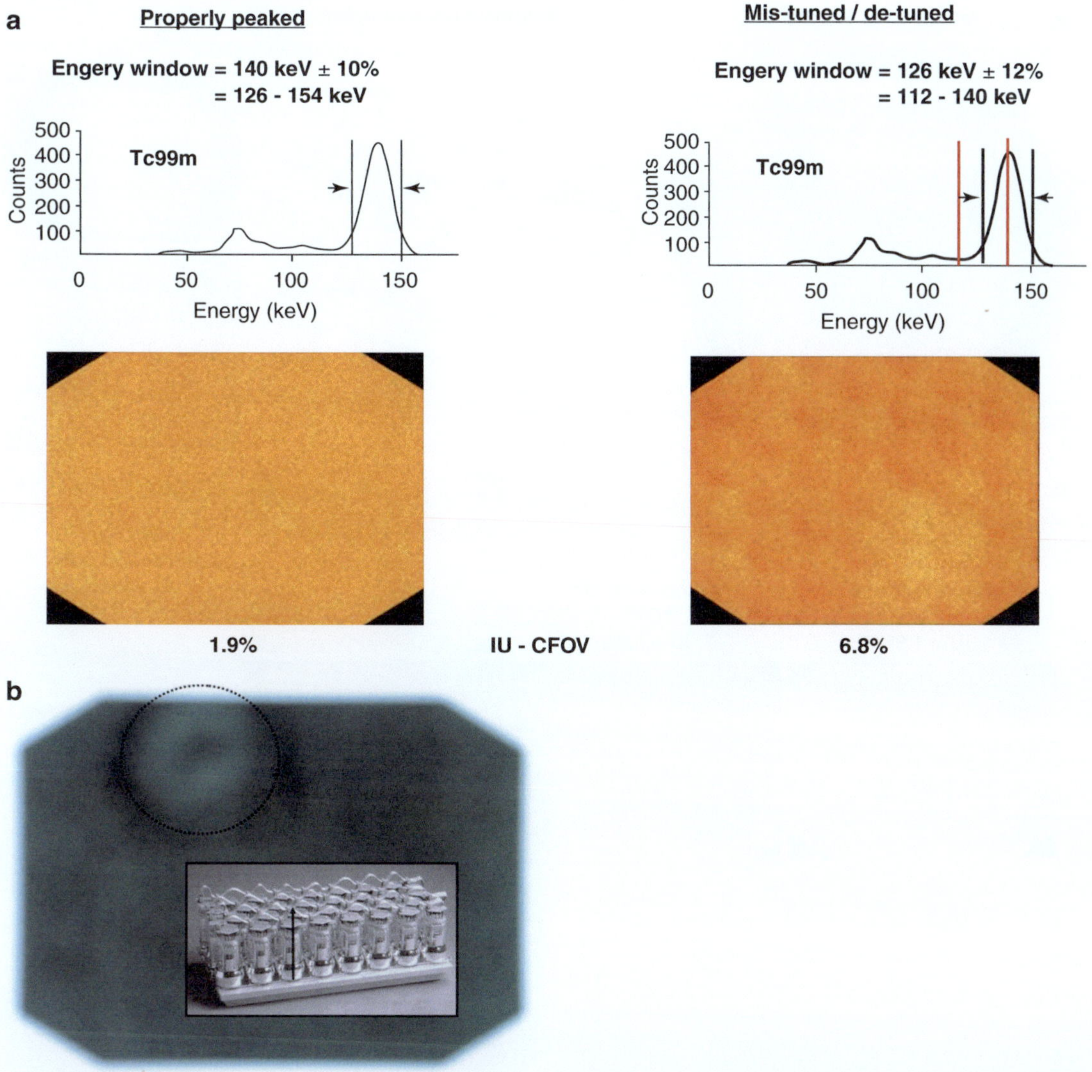

Fig. 1.19 Sources of gamma camera nonuniformity. (**a**) Mistuning (or detuning), meaning that the radionuclide's photopeak does not coincide with the camera's photopeak energy window, perhaps because the photopeak energy window (as shown) and/or the PMTs' high voltages are not set correctly. (**b**) Uncoupling of a PMT from the crystal, resulting in loss of all or part of the light signal in the resulting air gap between the PMT entrance window and the crystal. (**b**) Cracked crystal, either due to mechanical trauma (an impact) or a temperature incursion (i.e., a temperature increase *or* decrease at a rate faster than ~5 °C per hour causing the crystal to expand or contract, respectively, to the point of cracking). Note that it is the *rate* of the temperature change which is critical. The photographs on the right shows the cracked crystal which produced the "temperature-excursion" image. Even though the cracks are grossly imperceptible, the artifacts produced are very dramatic. (**d**) Corrupted, deleted, or switched-off software correction tables. Even perfectly functioning gamma cameras have some nonuniformity due to point-to-point variations in the energy spectra; greater sensitivity at and lower sensitivity between the PMTs; and residual nonuniformity due to ill-defined factors such as variations in crystal thickness. The associated nonuniformities are measured and used to create energy, linearity, and uniformity (or sensitivity) correction tables, respectively. Note that the linearity correction table has the biggest impact on uniformity: if corrupted, deleted, or switched off, the PMT pattern becomes grossly apparent, and the IU approached 20%. Fortunately, in contrast to the uniformity correction table and, to a lesser extent, the energy correction table, the linearity correction table rarely needs to be updated once a gamma camera is installed; if it becomes necessary, it is almost always done by field service personnel, not the end user (Adapted from [2])

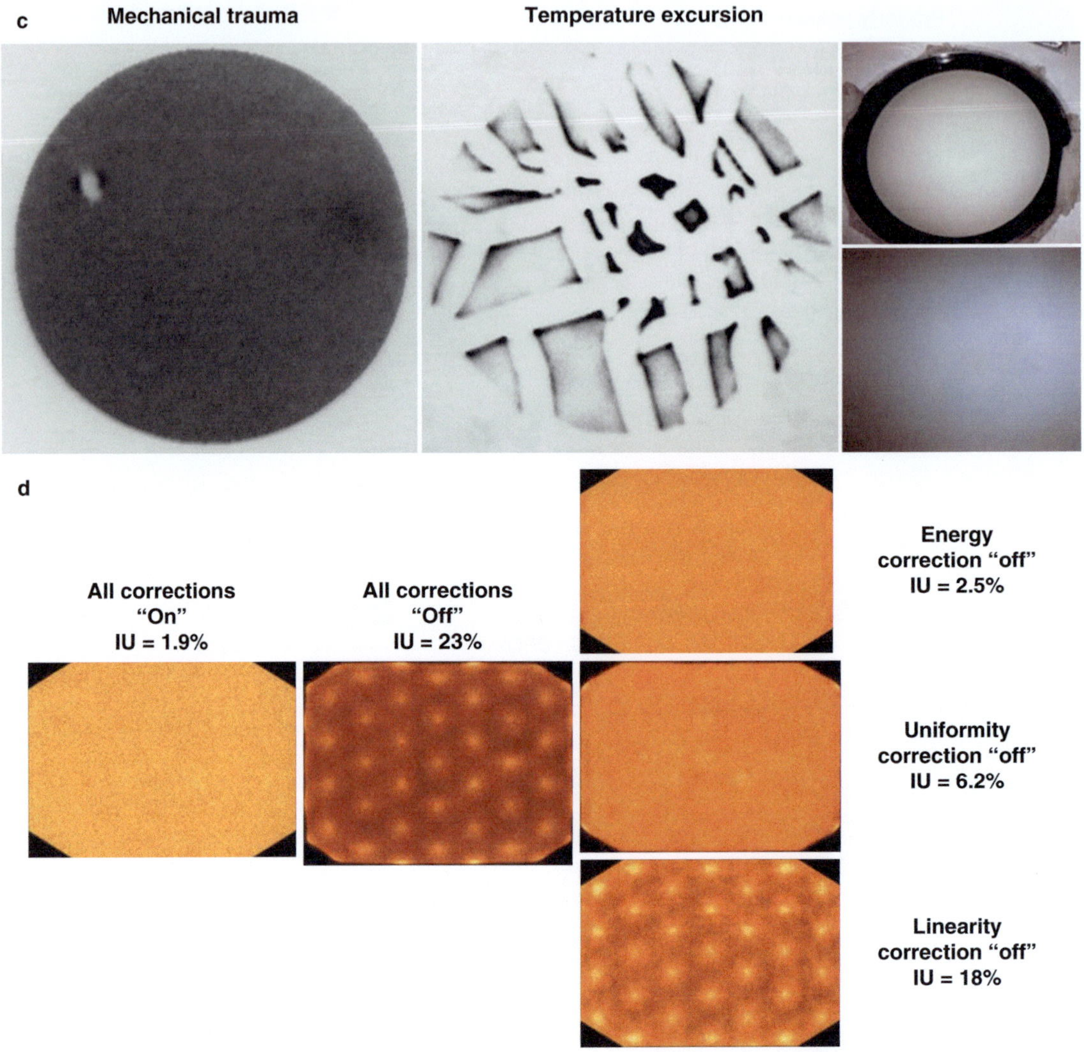

Fig. 1.19 (continued)

of the camera's correction tables (i.e., its energy, uniformity, and/or linearity correction tables).

Spatial resolution, in practice, is generally assessed using some sort of resolution phantom (or mask), the four-quadrant bar phantom perhaps being the one most widely used (Fig. 1.20). This should be done at least weekly. Gamma camera energy resolution per se is not generally evaluated on a routine basis. However, the energy spectrum for each radionuclide used clinically should be checked at least once a day to verify that the photopeak(s) is (are) centered in the photopeak energy window(s) currently set (Fig. 1.6b). Ideally, the energy spectrum should be checked for each patient.

In addition to the foregoing QC procedures for gamma camera imaging generally, rotating gamma camera SPECT requires QC as well. Among the components of a routine SPECT QC program are periodic assessment of COR alignment (Fig. 1.17), tomographic uniformity, and, for lack of a better term, overall system performance. As described above and in Fig. 1.17, proper alignment of the mechanical and electronic CORs is critical in rotating gamma camera SPECT and should be checked and, if neces-

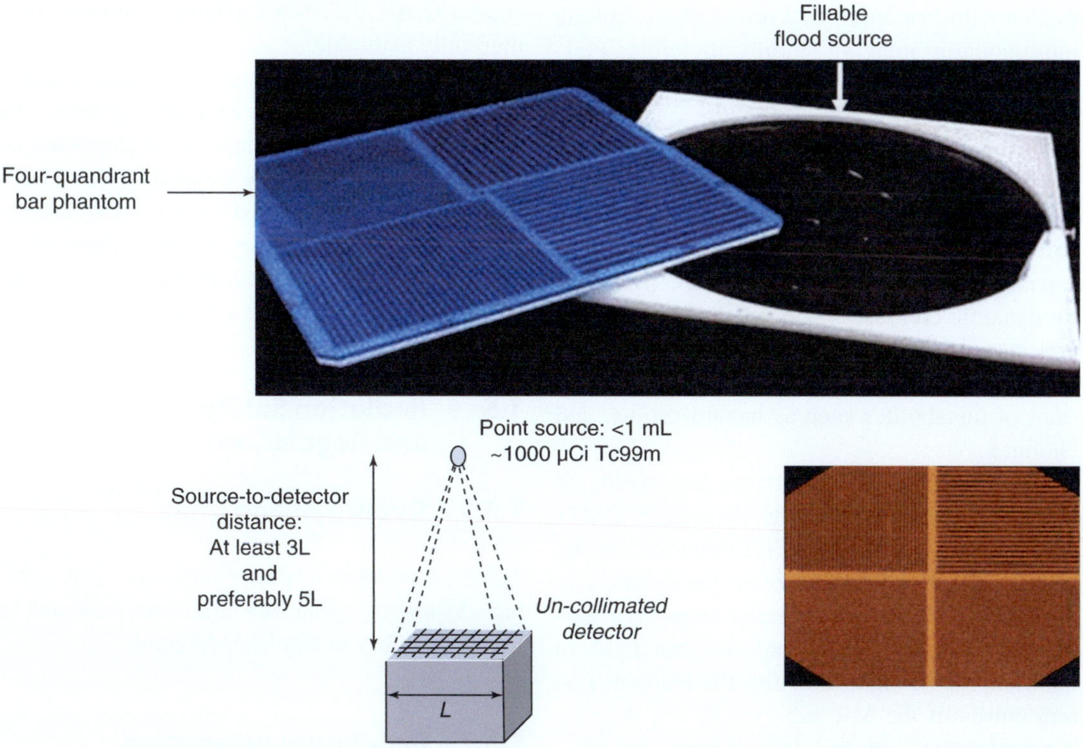

Fig. 1.20 In practice, intrinsic gamma camera resolution is often evaluated using a four-quadrant bar phantom, consisting of radiopaque lead bars and intervening radiolucent plastic strips 2, 2.5, 3, and 4 mm in width. A "point" source (<1 ml in volume and containing ~1000 μCi) of ^{99m}Tc is placed at least three and preferably five crystal dimensions from and centered over the uncollimated detector, with the phantom placed directly over the detector. A 5- to 10-million-count "transmission" image is then acquired and visually inspected. The lead bars in at least the two coarsest quadrants (i.e., with the 3- and 4-mm-wide bars) should be visually resolvable (A fillable sheet source, which may be filled with different radionuclides and used to evaluate extrinsic uniformity (see Fig. 1.19), is also shown in the photograph) (Adapted from [2])

sary, the COR misalignment correction updated at least weekly. Tomographic uniformity may be evaluated by imaging a uniform cylinder source (at least 20 cm in diameter) and visually inspecting the resulting images for the absence of rings, or "bull's-eye," attributable to system nonuniformity. Overall system performance may be evaluated using any number of commercially available fillable phantoms containing nonradioactive ("cold") inserts of different sizes and by visually inspecting the resulting images to determine the size of the smallest insert that is visible. Typically, such a phantom will include a uniform portion that can be used to simultaneously evaluate tomographic uniformity. PET tomographic uniformity and overall system performance may also be evaluated using such phantoms.

1.4.6 Multimodality Devices

The major manufacturers of Nuclear Medicine instrumentation now market multimodality scanners, combining high-performance state-of-the-art PET and CT scanners and, more recently, SPECT and CT scanners in a single device. These instruments provide near-perfect registration of images of in vivo function (PET or SPECT) and anatomy (CT). PET scanners are now marketed exclusively as multimodality devices, that is, PET-CT devices.

Compared to CT, MRI provides not only better contrast among soft tissues but also functional imaging capabilities. The combination of PET-MRI may thus provide advantages which go well beyond simply combining functional information with structural MRI information. Among multimodality imaging studies, therefore, PET-MRI may ultimately provide the greatest yield of information by combining the quantitative molecular imaging capabilities of PET (including the large number and variety of radiotracers) with the excellent anatomic resolution, marked soft-tissue contrast, and functional imaging capabilities provided by MRI (e.g., perfusion by dynamic contrast-enhanced (DCE) imaging) and magnetic resonance spectroscopic imaging (MRSI) (e.g., quantitation of regional concentrations of metabolites such as lactate, citrate, and choline).

The effects of the high magnetic fields of the MR sub-system exclude the use of PMTs employed in conventional PET detectors, as the path of the electrons between the dynodes in the evacuated PMT is deflected from their normal trajectory by the external magnetic field. In addition, the RF fields and also the gradient system pulses of the MR sub-system can degrade the performance of and even damage the PET electronics. One approach to overcoming this limitation is the use of long optical fibers (up to several meters in length) to couple the detector crystal to a PMT positioned outside the MR sub-system's fringe field (i.e., at magnetic fields of no greater than 10 mT). In this way, only the X- and γ-ray detection elements lie within the magnetic field, and the scintillations are directed out of the field by the fibers. Despite the challenges presented by such systems, including the large number of optical fibers required (one per detector element) and partial loss of the light signal over the length of the fibers, several prototypes of such PET-MRI scanners (with field strengths up to 3T) have been fabricated. An alternative, and ultimately more practical approach, to PET-MRI is elimination of the PMTs altogether by using solid-state scintillation detectors such as APDs or SiPMs. APDs and SiPMs are relatively insensitive to magnetic fields and thus can be coupled directly to the scintillation detector blocks via conventional (i.e., short) light guides. It is still important, however, to provide RF shielding of the PET sub-system components within the magnetic field, for example, using copper mesh. PET-MRI scanners are now commercially available.

MR images do not directly provide attenuation information, and in PET-MR systems, the attenuation correction maps must therefore be estimated indirectly. Software methods have been proposed and implemented for MR-based attenuation correction, based on image segmentation or co-registration of templates with pre-assigned tissue-specific attenuation coefficients.

1.5 Radiation Safety and Regulations[1]

1.5.1 Quantities and Units

Table 1.4 presents a tabular summary of the various dosimetric quantities and units relevant to radiation safety in Nuclear Medicine.

1.5.2 Regulatory Jurisdiction and Licensure

The use of radioactivity, particularly in medicine, is highly regulated, and extensive institutional as well as regulatory policies and procedures have been promulgated to ensure its safe and compliant use. In the United States, the use of radioactivity is primarily regulated by a federal agency, the Nuclear Regulatory Commission (NRC), pursuant to Title 10, Part 35 of the Code of Federal Regulations (10CFR35). As stated in 10CFR35, "This part contains the requirements and provisions for the medical use of byproduct material and for issuance of specific licenses authorizing the medical use of this material. These requirements and provisions provide for the radiation safety of workers, the general public, patients, and human research subjects." However, in well over half of the states—so-called Agreement States—the NRC has agreed to delegate its regulatory authority to the state; in Agreement States,

[1]The dose limits and other regulatory values cited in this section are those currently in effect in the United States. These are subject to change and may be different in other jurisdictions.

Table 1.4 Quantities and units in radiation dosimetry

Quantity	Symbol	Definition	Conventional unit (abbreviation)	System International (SI) unit (abbreviation)	Units conversions
Exposure	X	Electric charge produced per unit mass of air by X- or gamma rays	Roentgen(R)	Coulomb per kilogram (C/kg)	$1\ R = 2.58 \times 10^{-4}$ C/kg 1 C/kg $= 3.94 \times 10^{3}$ R
Absorbed dose	D	Energy deposited per unit mass	rad	Gray (Gy)	1 rad = 1×10^{2} erg/g 1 Gy = 1 J/kg 1×10^{2} rad = 1 Gy 1 cGy = 1 rad
Kerma	K	Kinetic energy released per unit mass	rad	Gray (Gy)	1 rad = 1×10^{2} erg/g 1 Gy = 1 J/kg 1×10^{2} rad = 1 Gy 1 cGy = 1 rad
Dose equivalent[a]	H	$w_R \cdot D$	rem	Sievert(Sv)	1×10^{2} rem = 1 Sv 1 cSv = 1 rem
Effective dose[b]/effective dose equivalent[c]	H_E	$\sum_{\text{Tissue,T}} W_T \cdot H_T$	rem	Sievert(Sv)	1×10^{2} rem = 1 Sv 1 cSv = 1 rem

[a]The radiation weighting factor, w_R, reflects differences among radiations (R) in their ionization density and therefore their biological effectiveness, with more densely ionizing radiations such as alpha particles having a greater probability of producing biological damage and/or producing more severe biological damage than less densely ionization radiations such as X- and gamma rays. The currently assigned values of w_R are as follows: 1 for X- and gamma rays and for beta particles and other electrons, 2 for protons, ≥5 for neutrons (depending on their energy), and 20 for alpha particles

[b]The tissue weighting factor, w_T, reflects differences among human tissues (T) in their sensitivity to stochastic radiation damage (i.e., cancer induction and germ cell mutagenesis and resulting heritable genetic damage). The currently assigned values of w_T range from 0.01 for brain and other "radioresistant" tissues to 0.12 for lung and other "radiosensitive" tissues. Note that $\sum_{\text{Tissue,T}} w_T = 1$. In principle, the effective dose provides a single-value metric of overall stochastic risk for any given irradiation

[c]The effective dose equivalent is a quantity similar in concept to the effective dose. It is an older quantity than the effective dose but is still found in regulations (e.g., to express the maximum permissible dose for occupationally exposed individuals) issued by the Nuclear Regulatory Commission (NRC). In addition to subtle technical differences, the effective dose equivalent differs from the effective dose in that fewer tissues are included in the summation and the tissue weighting factors have somewhat different values

therefore, the use of radioactivity is directly regulated by a state agency rather than the NRC. In addition, the Food and Drug Administration (FDA), the US Department of Transportation (US DOT), and other federal agencies maintain regulatory authority over certain aspects of the medical use of radioactivity. In any medical or other facility in which radioactive materials are used, the radiation safety officer (RSO), in conjunction with a Radiation Committee and individual authorized users (AUs), is charged with ensuring that all such materials are used in a manner which is safe and compliant with all applicable regulations. Among the regulatory activities of the NRC and their Agreement-State counterparts are the licensing of physicians to possess radioactive materials for medical use and stipulation of the training-and-experience requirements for such licensure.

1.5.3 Sources of Radiation Exposure and Dose Limits

Everyone is constantly and universally exposed to background radiation – from cosmic radiation from outer space, naturally occurring radionuclides in our environment and our own bodies, and other sources (Fig. 1.21). In the United States, the total exposure (actually, effective dose) averages

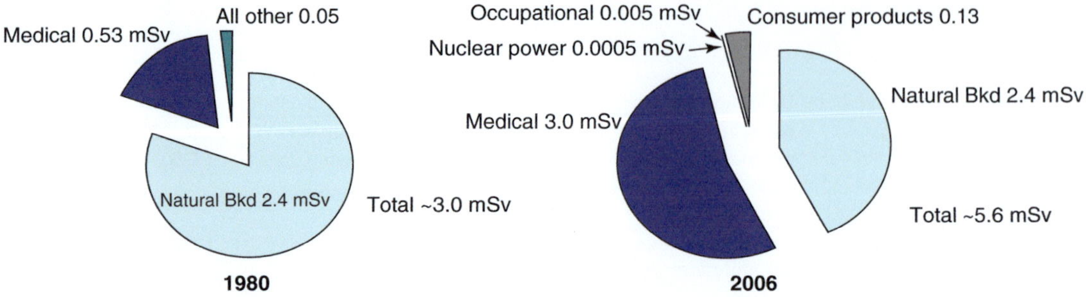

Fig. 1.21 Average annual per capita radiation exposure of the US population in 1980 and in 2006 (Reprinted with permission from [3])

5.6 mSv, or 560 mrem, per year (ca. 2006). This represents a dramatic increase over the prior estimate of 3.0 mSv, or 300 mrem, per year (ca. 1980). Specifically, as a result of the introduction and widespread use of spiral CT combined with the growth of nuclear cardiology and fluorine-18 fluorodeoxyglucose (^{18}F-FDG) PET, the average per capita medical dose increased from 0.53 mSv (53 mrem) to 3.0 mSv (300 mrem). The large majority of natural background radiation results from inhalation of naturally occurring radon gas and decay in situ to its alpha particle-emitting daughters.

Diagnostic medical exposures (in terms of effective dose) range from less than 10 mrem for a chest X-ray at the low end to nearly 1000 mrem for a chest CT at the high end, with Nuclear Medicine exposures (e.g., that from a Tc99m bone scan) generally in the middle of this range. Miscellaneous nonmedical exposures range from 6 mrem for a transatlantic commercial airline flight to 400 mrem per year from natural background radiation in Denver, CO. The foregoing dose estimates provide some perspective on radiation exposures.

10CFR35 stipulates radiation protection standards for occupationally exposed individuals (such as Nuclear Medicine technologists and physicians) as well as for non-occupationally exposed individuals. These standards are based on the assumption—the no-threshold hypothesis—that any radiation dose above natural background may create some additional risk of damage, hereditary defects, potential life-span shortening, and, in particular, cancer. Thus, radiation safety programs are designed to maintain radiation doses to workers and the public not just below the regulatory limit but as low as reasonably achievable (ALARA). The annual maximum permissible doses (MPDs) for radiation workers are currently as follows: effective dose equivalent, 50 mSv = 5 rem; dose equivalent to any one tissue or organ except the eye, 500 mSv = 50 rem; and dose equivalent to eye, 150 mSv = 15 rem. The respective MPDs to non-occupationally exposed individuals are one-tenth of the corresponding MPD for occupationally exposed individuals, including an effective-dose-equivalent limit of 5 mSv, or 0.5 rem, per year. Regulations also stipulate an annual MPD of 1 mSv, or 0.1 rem, for the general public. Unlike the MPD for non-occupationally exposed individuals, which is a dose limit for specific individuals (such as a secretary in a radiology department), the general-public MPD serves instead as a design goal. For example, the shielding and other design features for a CT installation adjoining a public corridor are dictated by the annual 1-mSv (0.1 rem) general-public MPD; this dose limit does not actually apply to any identifiable individual, however. Finally, for a declared pregnant worker (i.e., an occupationally exposed individual who has informed her employer of her pregnancy), the MPD over the total duration of her pregnancy is the same as that of a non-occupationally exposed individual, 5 mSv (0.5 rem).

1.5.4 Personnel Dosimetry

For occupationally exposed individuals, personnel monitors provide estimates of external exposure. Personnel monitors typically achieve an accuracy of ±30% and a precision of ±10% over an exposure range of 10 mR (the lowest detectable exposure) to 2000 R with constancy (i.e., constant signal per unit exposure) over a wide X- and γ-ray energy range. For many years, commercially supplied and processed "film badges" consisted of plastic holders containing a small piece of X-ray film in a light-tight seal. The optical density, or opacity ("blackening"), of film is directly related to its exposure. Thermoluminescent dosimeters (TLDs) and optically stimulated luminance (OSL) dosimeters have replaced film in personnel monitors. TLDs are essentially storage phosphors in which electrons are raised to excited energy states by the incident radiation, a fraction of which remains trapped in these excited states. When the dosimeters are subsequently heated, these trapped electrons are released and return to their ground state, with the emission of light. The amount of light emitted is related to the number of trapped electrons and, in turn, to the radiation doses delivered to the TLD. Optically stimulated luminance (OSL) dosimeters, composed of crystalline aluminum oxide activated with carbon (AL_2O_3:C), are now used as an alternative to TLDs. OSL dosimeters work in a similar manner to TLDs except that laser light rather than heat frees the trapped electrons. While film-based dosimeters provide a permanent dose record, the fact that TLDs and OSL dosimeters are reusable offers significant cost savings, and most personnel dosimeters now use TLDs or OSL dosimeters.

Personnel dosimeters typically have a metallically filtered area (to provide an estimate of the "deep" dose) and an unfiltered area (to estimate the shallow, or "skin," dose). Both film and TLDs as well as OSLs are "integrating" detectors and thus yield the total dose up to the time the film is developed or the TLD or OSL is read. Personnel dosimeters are generally changed monthly. Most radiation workers wear a single dosimeter, typically on the trunk of the body. Certain cohorts of workers such as radiopharmacists may wear additional dosimeters (e.g., ring and eye glass dosimeters).

1.5.5 Receipt, Transport, Storage, and Inventory of Radioactive Materials

Radioactive packages should be examined and opened on disposable pads wearing disposable gloves. Packages should be inspected immediately upon receipt for any sign of damage such as breakage, moisture, or discoloration of the outer packing. As soon as possible after receipt, packages should be monitored for external radiation levels using a survey monitor and possible surface contamination determined by wipe testing (see below). If the measured exposure rate is not consistent with the package label or if it appears that the package is damaged, the radiation safety officer (RSO) shall be contacted immediately. Once a package is opened, the inner container should be inspected for any breakage or leakage and wipe tested for contamination. The inner container label and the packing slip should be cross-checked to verify the vendor, the identity and physical and chemical forms of the radionuclide, the activity present, and date and time of calibration. Any deviations should be reported to the shipper and resolved. The packing material and empty package should also be monitored for radioactive contamination using a survey meter before disposal. If radioactively contaminated, these materials should be treated as radioactive waste. If free of contamination, the radiation/radioactivity labels should be removed or obliterated before appropriate disposal as nonradioactive waste.

Radioactive packages cannot be transported in the same manner as nonradioactive packages and must be shipped by UD DOT-authorized "dangerous-goods" carriers. A completed "dangerous-goods" manifest, listing the names and addresses of the shipper and the consignee, the radionuclide and its activity and chemical and physical forms, a 24-hour emergency contact telephone number, and the transport index (see below), must accompany the shipment. In addition, US DOT-authorized "radioactive shipment" labels must be completed and affixed to at least two surfaces of the radioactive package (Fig. 1.22).

All vials or other vessels that contain radioactive materials should be labeled appropriately

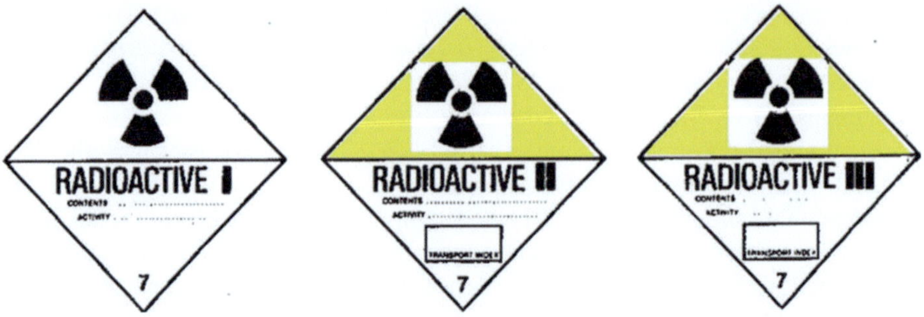

Color	**White**	**Yellow**	**Yellow**
Exposure rate (mR/h)			
On Surface	**< 0.5**	**0.5–50**	**50–200**
At 1 m	**0**	**< 1**	**1–10**
Type of shipment	Diagnostic unit doses	Therapy unit doses	Generators

Fig. 1.22 US DOT labels required for shipment of radioactive packages. The particular label required is dictated by the package's "transport index (TI)," defined as its exposure rate in mR/hr. measured at a distance of 1 m from the package surface: TI = 0 (i.e., a measured exposure rate at 1 m equal to the background exposure rate) "White I"; TI < 1 "Yellow II"; TI = 1–10 "Yellow III"

with "Caution Radioactive Material" warnings and provide the identity of the radionuclide, physical and chemical forms of the radionuclide, activity, and date and time of calibration. Such items should be stored in shielded (lead) containers and the containers stored in shielded cabinets or drawers or behind lead shielding. For certain radiopharmaceuticals that must be stored at low temperatures, a refrigerator may be lined with lead or located in an appropriately shielded area. Radioactive materials should be stored in secure, controlled areas, such as a radiopharmacy, posted with "Caution Radioactive Material" warning signs. If personnel inside these areas could receive a dose rate of 0.05 mSv/h (5 mrem/h) or more, the door should be posted with a "Caution Radiation Area" sign. Items such as food, beverages, and medications shall not be stored in the same area as radioactive materials. A running inventory of radioactive materials must be maintained. This inventory should include the identity of the radionuclide, physical and chemical forms of the radionuclide, activity, date and time of calibration and of receipt, activities dispensed and the dates and times of dispensing and the patient or other purpose for which it was dispensed, and the activity, date and time, and method of disposal.

1.5.6 Radiation Surveys

Radiation surveys should be performed using a survey meter (such as a Geiger counter) calibrated in absolute exposure rate or absorbed dose rate units (mR/h or mrad/h, respectively). Because of the limited penetration of β-rays and other particulate radiations, the ability of each type of survey meter to detect these radiations should be clearly understood. The use of beta shields or caps may allow for measurements in fields of mixed radiations. Survey meters should include a "battery check" function. Some models may include a low-activity "check source" to provide a check on operation of the instrument immediately prior to use. These devices shall be calibrated at least annually, and records of the calibrations shall be maintained.

Removable radioactive contamination can be deposited on the skin or enter the body and irradiate an individual internally. Therefore, assay of removable radioactive contamination on all potentially contaminated surfaces and on sealed radioactive sources must be performed at regular intervals and whenever contamination is suspected. Nonremovable radioactive contamination, that is, fixed contamination, contributes only to external exposure, and its contribution is reflected in the radiation surveys. Assay of removable radioactive contamination is typically performed using a "wipe test." In such a test, a representative area of approximately 100 cm^2 of a potentially contaminated surface is wiped with a dry piece of paper, and the wipe is counted in a counting system. The resulting gross count rates are converted to net count rates by subtracting a background, or blank, count rate and the net count rates converted to activity using the counting system's measured calibration factors.

In controlled, or restricted, areas, surveys should be performed daily and wipe tests weekly. In other (uncontrolled or unrestricted) areas, surveys should be performed weekly and wipe tests monthly.

1.5.7 Waste Disposal

Nuclear Medicine generates low-level radioactive waste, mostly in the form of dry waste (such as empty vials, syringes, intravenous tubing, disposable gloves, absorbent pads, paper toweling, gauze, contaminated disposable eating utensils, and partially decayed sources). Regulations concerning disposal of radioactive or radioactively contaminated waste are stringent: no waste which is detectably radioactive (i.e., yields a count rate significantly greater than the background count rate when assayed with a high-sensitivity survey meter) may be disposed of as nonradioactive waste. Depending on a facility's volume of radioactive waste and its capacity for waste storage, disposal may be accomplished by one or more of the following methods: return to vendor, decay-in-storage, transfer to a radioactive waste facility (commercial disposal), and, for liquid waste, dilution and dispersal.

Radioactively contaminated dry waste that will decay to background levels within a reasonably short period of time (i.e., up to several months) should be stored for decay. Such storage locations should be in a low-occupancy, secure, and posted area of the facility and adequately shielded as required. Prior to disposal or recycling of decayed radioactive waste, such materials should be monitored with a suitable survey meter to verify that radioactivity is undetectable, and all "radioactive-material" labeling should be removed or obliterated prior to disposal or recycling. Radioactive or radioactively contaminated waste should be segregated by physical half-life to facilitate final disposal. Many hospitals have installed high-sensitivity counting systems to monitor *all* waste exiting the facility and, if necessary, divert at that point radioactively contaminated waste for decay-in-storage. Low-level, noninfectious liquid radioactive waste as well as excreta (including excreta collected in urine bags and bedpans) from Nuclear Medicine patients generally may be disposed of by dilution or dispersal, that is, disposal down a waste drain or toilet. The facility's RSO must assure that liquid radioactive waste discharged into the sewer does not exceed regulatory limits. Radioactivity and radioactively contaminated waste too long-lived to be practically held for decay-in-storage (such as carbon-14 (half-life: 5730 years) and tritium (12.3 years)) must be disposed of commercially (for eventual encasement, transport to, and long-term burial at one of only several low-level radioactive waste sites nationwide). Commercial disposal is extremely expensive but, fortunately, is rarely required in Nuclear Medicine.

1.5.8 Emergency (i.e., Spill) Procedures

When working with radiopharmaceuticals and other unsealed sources of radioactivity, the possibility of spills exists. The emergency procedures for dealing with spills of radioactive materials differ depending upon whether the spill is a minor or a major spill and are detailed in Table 1.5.

Table 1.5 Emergency procedure for radioactive spills

• Notify all personnel in room that a spill has occurred and instruct all uninvolved individuals to exit the area
• Restrict entry to room
• Don 2 pairs of disposable waterproof gloves (so that the outer, contaminated gloves can be removed and replaced while avoiding hand contamination)
• Upright the container from which the spill occurred
• Cover the spill with absorbent sheets having a water-impermeable plastic coating facing the spill
For a "minor" spill, proceed to the next steps
For a "major" spill or if in doubt as to the severity of a spill or how to proceed, contact the institutional Radiation Safety Office for further remediation
Spills of technetium-99 m, indium-111, and thallium-201 activities in excess of 100, 10, and 100 mCi, respectively, are considered major; spills of lesser activities of these respective radioisotopes are considered minor
• Decontaminate the area, discarding cleanup materials in a plastic bag for disposal as radioactive waste
– Wipe the spilled liquid toward center of the spill area with dry paper toweling, then with moist paper toweling, and then with dry paper toweling, taking care not to flood the area and spreading the spill
• Survey the spill area, clothes, and hands and feet
– With a survey meter for gamma and X-ray-emitting radioisotopes
– By wipe testing for a pure beta particle-emitting radioisotope
– Contaminated shoes and clothing should be removed, placed in plastic bags, appropriately labeled, and held for decay-in-storage
• As a rule of thumb, continue decontamination until the results of the post-contamination surveys are no greater than twice the background count rate. If this level of decontamination cannot be achieved, the contaminated area may need to be shielded with lead and labeled as "contaminated" until the remaining radioactivity is eliminated by physical decay
• Report the spill and remedial actions taken to the institutional Radiation Safety Office

1.5.9 Release Criteria for Radionuclide Therapy

Historically, the NRC and Agreement States required radionuclide therapy patients to remain hospitalized until the retained activity in the patient was less than 1110 MBq (30 mCi) or the dose rate at 1 m from the patient was less than 0.05 mSv/h (5 mrem/h). However, the NRC amended its regulations concerning radionuclide therapy patients through the issuance of new rules that appeared in the *Federal Register* on January 29, 1997. The new NRC regulations, revised 10CFR 35.75 effective May 1997, allow for the release from medical confinement of patients if the expected total effective dose equivalent to individuals exposed to the patient is not likely to exceed 5 mSv (500 mrem). Guidance on determining when patients may be released based on the new criteria, when written instructions on post-release radiation precautions must be provided, and when records related to the release of the patient must be maintained is provided in NRC Regulatory Guide 8.39. A licensee may release from his control any patient administered (diagnostic or therapeutic) radiopharmaceuticals or therapeutically implanted with sealed radioactive sources if the TEDE to any individual from exposure to the patient after release is not likely to exceed 5 mSv (500 mrem). Compliance with this dose limit may be demonstrated using either (a) a default table in Regulatory Guide 8.39 for activity (e.g., <33 mCi of iodine-131 retained by the patient) or dose rate (e.g., <7 mrem/h at 1 m from an iodine-131-containing patient) or (b) patient-specific kinetic data using effective halftimes or residence times and dose rate measurements and a patient-specific projected dose calculation. The use of method (b) will generally result in patients being released with substantially higher activities—up to several hundred mCi—than would method (a). Importantly, in basing release on patient-specific information (method (b)), the NRC regulations allow for representative kinetic data such as effective halftimes or residence times for a particular population of patients (e.g., hyperthyroid patients) to be applied to an individual patient in that population, thus obviating the need in certain cases for measurement of kinetic data on an individual patient basis. The revised NRC regulations require that the licensee provide written instructions to the released patient regarding radiation precautions. Post-release radiation safety instructions to the patient should address maintenance of distance from other persons; separate sleeping arrangements; minimization of time in public places including public transportation facilities such as buses, trains, and planes; and measures to reduce environmental contamination. In the case of nursing mothers, recommendations on discontinuation of breastfeeding should be included as well. Information on the duration of post-release radiation precautions must also be provided. The revised NRC regulations impose, under some circumstances, certain record-keeping requirements. If patient release is based on method (a), records are not required. However, if release is based on method (b), a record of the basis for release including patient-specific factors and dose-calculation equations must be prepared and maintained for 3 years from the date of release.

1.5.10 Record-Keeping

Written and/or computerized records, maintained for periods established by regulatory agencies and/or the facility, are required. The required records and other documentation include the radioactive materials receipt, inventory, distribution, and disposal, including radiopharmaceutical prescriptions; radiation survey data, including measurements of ambient radiation levels and surface radioactive contamination, and annotated facility diagrams indicating the sites of such measurements; monitoring records for all occupationally exposed personnel, including any bioassay data; written policies and procedures for the clinical and the radiation safety program; description of the radiation safety training program; the Radiation Safety Committee membership and minutes; and reports of any unusual, radiologically significant occurrences.

1.5.11 "Sensitive" Patient Populations

The administration of radioactive materials, even in diagnostic amounts, to certain "sensitive" populations—pregnant women, nursing mothers, and prospective parents—remains a matter of concern in Nuclear Medicine.

1.5.11.1 Pregnant Women

Increasingly accurate anatomic models of the fetus and pregnant woman have been developed, including models of the pregnant female at the beginning of pregnancy (representing the embryo as a small unit density sphere located at the uterus) and at the end of the first and third trimesters. Radiopharmaceutical kinetic data in utero and therefore fetal dose estimates are quite limited, however. Published fetal absorbed dose estimates are generally of the order of or less than 0.1 cGy (0.1 rad) per 37 mBq (1 mCi) administered to the mother. A particularly worrisome issue, however, is radioiodine administration to pregnant women. The fetal thyroid begins concentrating iodine at the 12th–15th week of gestation. At 16–24 weeks, ^{131}I-iodide delivers a very large absorbed dose of 1500–6000 cGy/37 MBq (rad/mCi) to the fetal thyroid and an absorbed dose of 3–5 cGy/37 MBq (rad/mCi) to the fetal total body, depending on maternal thyroid uptake. For a hyperthyroid therapy administration of 185 MBq (5 mCi), 7500–30,000 cGy (rad) would therefore be delivered to the fetal thyroid and 15–25 rad to the fetal total body. Not surprisingly, with radiogenic destruction of the fetal thyroid and thyroid hormone deficiency in utero, fetal hypothyroidism and congenital cretinism have been shown to result following radioiodine therapy of hyperthyroidism or thyroid cancer in pregnant women. It is therefore critical to avoid radioiodine administration to the pregnant patient, even in diagnostic amounts.

1.5.11.2 Nursing Mothers

Diagnostic radiopharmaceuticals administered to lactating women can achieve rather high concentrations in breast milk and potentially deliver significant radiation doses to nursing infants.

For example, the cumulative breast milk activity ranged from 0.03% to 27% of ^{131}I-iodide administered to six women for thyroid uptake studies. Using a variety of dosimetric criteria (e.g., an effective dose equivalent to the nursing infant of 0.1 cSv (0.1 rem)), a number of authors have recommended different interruption periods prior to resuming breast-feeding following administration of radiopharmaceuticals. While there is no absolute consensus, the following are representative of the published recommendations: 24 h following any administration of ^{99m}Tc or ^{18}F, 2–4 weeks following administration of ^{67}Ga-gallium citrate, and permanently for the current nursing infant following any administration of ^{131}I-iodide.

1.5.11.3 Prospective parents

No evidence of significant germ cell damage (indicated by an increased risk of birth defects among subsequently conceived offspring) has been observed among A-bomb survivors (average gonadal absorbed dose: >30 cGy) and exposed human cohorts, and no such damage is expected, therefore, among diagnostic Nuclear Medicine patients. Nonetheless, demonstrable gonadal damage, specifically, *transiently* impaired fertility, may occasionally occur among thyroid cancer patients treated with much larger amounts (>100 mCi) of I131 followed by full recovery of fertility. While it is difficult to rationally formulate guidelines on the basis of the limited human data available, it is perhaps prudent that patients forego starting a family for at least several months following such high-dose radioiodine therapy.

1.5.12 Concluding Remarks

In diagnostic Nuclear Medicine, the activities used and the associated radiation doses are generally so low that there appears to be no practical possibility of any short- or long-term demonstrable harm to patients, staff, and other individuals. However, because of the large relative increase in the risk of childhood cancer following even low-level exposures in utero, radiation (including Nuclear Medicine) procedures in pregnant women must be based on an informed and documented decision regarding medical necessity. This, and *not* the possibility of inducing fetal death or congenital abnormalities, is why females of childbearing age are routinely queried about the possibility of being pregnant prior to undergoing a radiological or Nuclear Medicine procedure.

References

1. Cherry SR, Sorenson JA, Phelps ME. Physics in nuclear medicine. 3rd ed. Philadelphia, PA: Saunders; 2003.
2. Zanzonico P. Routine quality control of clinical nuclear medicine instrumentation: a brief review. J Nucl Med. 2008;49:1114–31.
3. Mettler FA Jr, Bhargavan M, Faulkner K, Gilley DB, Gray JE, Ibbott GS, Lipoti JA, Mahesh M, McCrohan JL, Stabin MG, Thomadsen BR, Yoshizumi TT. Radiologic and nuclear medicine studies in the United States and worldwide: frequency, radiation dose, and comparison with other radiation sources – 1950–2007. Radiology. 253:520–31.
4. Zanzonico PB. Radionuclide imaging. In: Cherry SR, Badawi RD, Jingi Q, editors. Essentials of in vivo biomedical imaging. Boca Raton, FL: CRC Press; 2015.
5. Zanzonico P. Instrumentation for single-photon emission imaging. In: Strauss HW, Mariani G, Volteranni G, Larson SM, editors. Nuclear oncology: from pathophysiology to clinical applications. 2nd ed. New York, NY: Springer; 2017.
6. Zanzonico P. Instrumentation for positron emission imaging. In: Strauss HW, Mariani G, Volteranni G, Larson SM, editors. Nuclear oncology: from pathophysiology to clinical applications. 2nd ed. New York, NY: Springer; 2017.
7. Zanzonico P. Instrumentation for intraoperative detection. In: Strauss HW, Mariani G, Volteranni G, Larson SM, editors. Nuclear oncology: from pathophysiology to clinical applications. 2nd ed. New York, NY: Springer; 2017.
8. Cherry SR, Jones T, Karp JS, Qi J, Moses WW, Badawi RD. Total-body PET: maximizing sensitivity to create new opportunities for clinical research and patient care. J Nucl Med. 2018;59:3–12.

2 Radiopharmaceutical Sciences

Johannes Ermert, Martina Benešová, Verena Hugenberg, Viplav Gupta, Ingo Spahn, Hans-Jürgen Pietzsch, Christos Liolios, and Klaus Kopka

2.1 Introduction

Radiopharmaceutical sciences summarizes all scientific aspects comprising chemistry, physics, and biology/pharmacology that deal with incorporating a suitable radionuclide into a pharmaceutical or other biologically active molecule or molecular entity. The resulting radiopharmaceuticals are used in nuclear medicine applications both for diagnosis [meaning noninvasive scintigraphic imaging] and for internal radiotherapy [1]. Internal radiotherapy is nowadays called radioligand therapy (RLT) or endoradiotherapy and altogether, i.e., noninvasive scintigraphic imaging and therapy, is summarized under the term radiothera(g)nostics.

For each of these applications, special types of radionuclides are demanded depending on their decay properties. For diagnostic purposes, the radiation dose to the patient should be as low as possibly achievable, and the radiation can leave the body almost unhindered, which is fulfilled by short-lived gamma emitters or with the annihilation rays of positron (beta$^+$) emitters. The radiation of these

J. Ermert · I. Spahn
Institut für Neurowissenschaften und Medizin, INM-5: Nuklearchemie, Forschungszentrum Jülich GmbH, Jülich, Germany

M. Benešová
Junior Research Group Molecular Biology of Systemic Radiotherapy, German Cancer Research Center (DKFZ), Heidelberg, Germany

V. Hugenberg
Heart and Diabetes Center North Rhine Westphalia, Institute for Radiology, Nuclear Medicine and Molecular Imaging, University Hospital, Ruhr University Bochum, Bad Oeynhausen, Germany

V. Gupta · C. Liolios
Radiopharmaceutical Chemistry, German Cancer Research Center (DKFZ), Heidelberg, Germany

H.-J. Pietzsch
Institute of Radiopharmaceutical Cancer Research, Helmholtz-Zentrum Dresden-Rossendorf (HZDR) e.V., Dresden, Germany

K. Kopka (✉)
Institute of Radiopharmaceutical Cancer Research, Helmholtz-Zentrum Dresden-Rossendorf (HZDR) e.V., Dresden, Germany

Radiopharmaceutical Chemistry, German Cancer Research Center (DKFZ), Heidelberg, Germany
e-mail: k.kopka@hzdr.de

H. Ahmadzadehfar et al. (eds.), *Clinical Nuclear Medicine*,
https://doi.org/10.1007/978-3-030-39457-8_2

kinds of radionuclides can be efficiently detected from outside of the body finding application in single-photon emission computed tomography (SPECT) and the latter in positron emission tomography (PET). Caused radiation dose is not significant thereby justifying the administration of corresponding radiopharmaceuticals within the radiotracer/radioindicator principle at the microdosing level [2] (cf. Sects. 2.3 and 2.4).

On the other hand, in RLT the ionizing radiation of corpuscular radiation emitters like alpha-, beta^{-}-, or Auger electron emitters are used to achieve the desired therapeutic effect in malignant or inflammatory tissues. Therefore, a localized, well-defined radiation dose needs to be deposited in the desired tissue region [2] (cf. Sect. 2.5).

Primordial and cosmogenic radionuclides are typically not applied for diagnostic and therapeutic applications due to their not suitable decay characteristics. Radionuclides for medical applications are produced artificially by fission, neutron activation, or (commonly cyclotron-based) particle "bombardment" of corresponding target material. Some of these radionuclides are easily made accessible to nuclear medicine clinics by so-called generator systems. For that purpose, the production of radionuclides requires an exact knowledge of the relevant nuclear data in order to maximize the yield of the desired product and to minimize the impurity level (cf. Sect. 2.2).

The relatively short physical half-life of the radionuclides requires fast and efficient radiolabeling strategies. As a rule-of-thumb, a total radiosynthesis time of approximately three radionuclide half-lives should not be exceeded [3]. Even if high radiation exposure is given, radiolabeling procedures are performed in lead-shielded "hot cells" on fully automated computer-controlled radiosynthesizers [4].

Quality criteria have to be fulfilled even before human applications. This includes the radionuclide purity, the radiochemical and chemical purity, and absence of microbiological impurities of the radiopharmaceutical. Due to its relatively long testing time, long-lived radionuclide impurities or even the sterility of the composed injection solutions, in which normally the radiotracer is formulated predominantly for intravenous injection, can only be determined after human application. It is therefore absolutely necessary to validate the whole radiosynthesis process to exclude these impurities. Depending on the specific international and national regulations affecting radiopharmaceutical production, numerous and complex criteria have to be fulfilled in any case under conditions of good manufacturing practice (GMP) [5].

A further criterion for the quality of a radiopharmaceutical is the amount of radioactivity per gram (termed as specific activity; Bq/g) or the amount radioactivity per mol (termed as molar activity; Bq/mol) [6], which depends on the amount of a respective carrier. The carrier type can be divided in a:

- Non-isotopic carrier, that has very similar chemical properties compared to the produced radionuclide or the radiolabeled compound
- Isotopic carrier, which differs only in isotopic composition of the corresponding molecule [7]

Depending on the amount of carrier intended, radiosyntheses can be classified into three types that are termed as:

- Carrier-free (c.f.)
- No-carrier-added (n.c.a.)
- Carrier-added (c.a.)

In order to avoid pharmacodynamic effects as well as toxic and immunological reactions, even PET radiopharmaceuticals are preferably administered in the no-carrier-added state with tracer substance amounts in the subnanomolar range [8, 9].

The major challenges in the development of a new radiopharmaceuticals include:

(a) The identification of an adequate ligand that specifically binds to the biological target of interest
(b) The chemical modification of the ligand to enable radiolabeling while preserving the binding affinity to the biological target

(c) The synthesis of an appropriate radiolabeling precursor
(d) A successful radiolabeling strategy yielding the radiopharmaceutical in high activity amounts and high molar activities
(e) Preclinical evaluation of the potential radiopharmaceutical by in vitro assays and in vivo (small) animal imaging
(f) The translation of validated animal studies into first in-human studies and in best case into first prospective clinical trials [10–12]

2.2 Clinically Relevant Radionuclides

2.2.1 Introduction

Since the discovery of the first nuclear reaction by Ernest Rutherford in 1919 [13], and the epoch-making discovery of artificial radioactivity by Irène Curie and Frédéric Joliot [14], a vast expansion in the field of nuclear chemistry and radiochemistry has taken place. To date the research and development activities in this field are mostly related to medical applications.

The production of radionuclides is complementarily done using nuclear reactors and accelerators which also provide the basis for radionuclide generator systems with ^{99}Mo and ^{68}Ge. The neutron-induced production at nuclear reactors generally leads to the formation of neutron excess radionuclides which mostly decay via β^- or α-particle emission making them especially suitable for radiotherapy. The accelerator-produced radionuclides, on the other hand, are mainly neutron deficient and decay via electron capture (EC) or β^+ emission. The bulk of those radionuclides are applied for diagnostic purposes, namely PET and SPECT (cf. Sects. 2.3–2.5).

The production routes and methods for radionuclides commonly used in diagnosis and internal radiotherapy or radioligand therapy (RLT) (also called endoradiotherapy) are generally well established [2]. The medical radionuclide production technology is well developed and is pursued at commercial centers and research institutes. Nonetheless, constant research work is ongoing to improve existing production methodologies as well as to develop compounds based on rarely available radionuclides for new medical applications like multimodal imaging or dual-tracer PET applications. To date about 250 [15] operational research reactors and about 1200 cyclotrons exist in the world [16]. However, the recently decreasing number of nuclear reactors suitable for radionuclide production induces alternative strategies for the production of β^- emitters using cyclotrons and modern high-intensity γ-ray sources [17]. In recent years, proton-induced spallation reactions have also been utilized for the production of some nonstandard potential medical radionuclides like ^{44}Ti for alternative radionuclide generator systems [2].

This field of work has to comply with certain economic and technical constraints, e.g., type of production facility, yield of nuclear reaction, and enrichment of the target material. It calls upon interdisciplinary studies comprising nuclear data measurement, high-current targetry, chemical processing, recovery of the enriched target material, automation of the entire production processes, measurements against hazardous radiation exposures and quality control of the produced radionuclide.

Over the years, intensive efforts have been made in investigation of various medically relevant radionuclides and their respective production routes. This chapter focuses mainly on the essential aspects of radionuclide production and will introduce the important medical radionuclides. Furthermore, an outlook on future prospects on medically relevant radionuclides is discussed.

2.2.2 Properties of Radionuclides for Medical Application

Even though endoradiotherapy and noninvasive scintigraphic imaging are complementary approaches within nuclear medicine, the demands on the radionuclides involved are rather different. The radiation of therapeutic radionuclides is meant to deposit sufficient energy within the targeted area to destroy malignant tissue. This can be achieved by soft γ-ray and β^- emitters as well as by α-particle emitting radionuclides. Early success of ^{131}I in combination with ^{123}I for the treatment of the diseased thyroid motivated researchers to focus more on investigations of therapeutic radionuclides that could be well utilized for treatment. The field of radionuclide therapy can be divided into the two subfields, namely brachytherapy which utilizes mostly β^- emitter in the form of sealed sources and endo- (or internal) radiotherapy, in which the energy dose is delivered by radiolabeling small drugs, peptides, or antibodies.

The major criteria to select a radionuclide for medical applications are its physical characteristics, nuclear decay properties, feasible radiochemistry, molar/specific activity, emitted γ-ray energies, and biochemical kinetics in the body. The respective physical half-lives of the therapeutic radionuclides are normally in the range between a few hours and several days. The biological half-life plays a vital role in medical application and hence has to be determined for each individual system. The effective range of the emitted particles from the applied parent radionuclides needs to be suitable and, in case of endoradiotherapy, needs to possess a sufficient linear energy transfer (LET) value. The assessment and determination of radiation dose is hereby of utmost importance to balance the therapeutic effect, caused by the irradiation of malignant tissue, against harmful effects on adjacent normal tissues.

Regarding diagnostic applications, i.e., planar scintigraphy, SPECT, or PET, the resulting radiation exposure to the patient needs to be as low as possibly achievable. The utilized radionuclides should ideally be pure and decay with high-intensity positrons or single γ-ray emission with physical half-lives in the range of a few minutes to several hours. Especially for PET and SPECT diagnosis, any highly branched decay schemes should be avoided to assure optimum image quality.

The selection of radiotracers, especially radiometals like technetium or lanthanides for medical application, calls for developing complexes which are not only thermodynamically stable but also sufficiently kinetically stable or inert in vivo, as in vivo dissociation of the complexes would contribute to a high radiation dose of healthy organs and tissues without any therapeutic effect.

2.2.3 Nuclear Data

The basis for all applications of radionuclides is comprehensive knowledge of the relevant nuclear reactions and their corresponding nuclear data. This knowledge is important not only for an efficient production of radionuclides but also to guarantee the generation of chemically pure end-products with well-defined decay properties to ensure maximum benefit and in parallel minimum hazards for the patient due to radioactive and nonradioactive impurities. To achieve these goals, the excitation functions of the most promising radionuclides for this purpose have to be measured. This is achieved by determining the nuclear reaction cross sections, which are usually specified in milli-barn (mb)[1]1, a non-SI unit. The determination of the cross-sectional data against the energy of the interacting particle then makes it possible to identify the optimal energy range for radionuclide production.

2.2.4 Reactor-Based Radionuclide Production

Concerning the production of certain SPECT radionuclides like ^{99m}Tc and the majority of therapeutic radionuclides, which are mostly neutron-deficient β^-- and α-particle emitters, dedicated nuclear reactors remain the most important production sites (Fig. 2.1). Due to the large irradiation geometries and the deeply penetrating nature of the neutron beam, large amounts of radioactivity can be generated. The most commonly used (n,γ)-reaction generally shows high cross sections and allows a highly efficient production of radionuclides in very high yields. However, this pro-

[1]Nuclear reaction cross section: 1 barn (*b*) = 10^{-28} m^2.

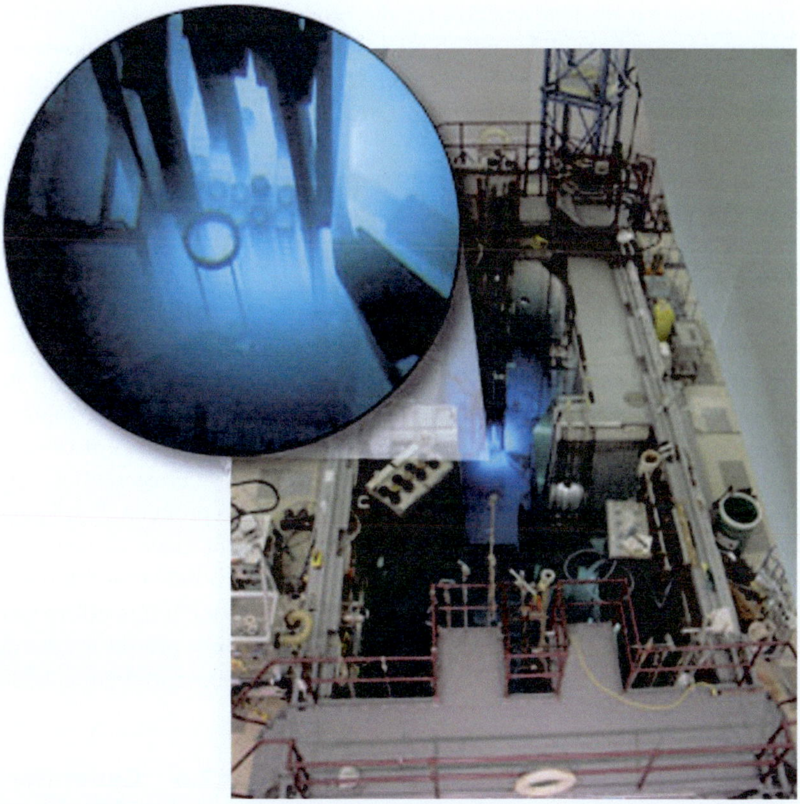

Fig. 2.1 Top view of a research reactor with reactor pool (zoomed) (Source: McMaster University)

duction route comes with the disadvantage of a limited specific activity, as the produced radionuclides are (radio)isotopes of the (normally stable) target element. This problem can only be solved if indirect production routes are available. A good example of such a case is the production of ^{131}I, which is produced via β^- decay of both metastable and ground state of ^{131}Te formed via neutron irradiation of ^{130}Te in a nuclear reactor (see Sect. 2.2.11.19 on ^{131}I below).

Nuclear reactors are supporting the radionuclide production since 60 years. Until 2016 there were around 770 research reactors that have been commissioned out of which roughly 60% have been shut down and/or decommissioned [15]. The declining number of nuclear reactors is due to the high fabrication costs and an increasing demand on safety and safeguard to match the state of the current art. Hence, reactor-based radionuclide production poses an increasing limitation and therefore prompting researchers to investigate alternative methods to produce radionuclides. Thus, the reactor-based radionuclide production will be more and more restricted to the remaining facilities, resulting in an increasing centralization. Currently some research effort is put in the investigation of new methods for the production of radionuclides derived by neutron irradiation including accelerator-based neutron and high-intensity X-ray sources (see below).

2.2.5 Accelerator-Based Radionuclide Production

The use of charged particle accelerators is essential for the production of diagnostic, especially PET, radionuclides. The ongoing propagation of neutron-deficient radionuclides for medical imaging is accompanied by an increasing number of accelerators, especially cyclotron facilities. This increase is based on the one hand on the necessity of a decentralized radionuclide distribution network due to the shorter physical half-lives of the diagnostic radionuclides and on the other hand on the fact that the (p,n)-process is the most important nuclear reaction for the production of those radionuclides which allows the service ability of compact cyclotrons with less than 18 MeV which are operable at comparatively low costs and manpower.

Due to the charged nature of the projectiles and the point-shaped irradiation of the target material, the production conditions are very different to those at a nuclear reactor. During the irradiation of the target material, a lot of heat is generated due to the high beam current and necessary particle energy. This heat accumulation inside the target body has to be dealt with by running effective cooling systems during irradiations for the large-scale production of radionuclides. As the kinetic energy of the projectiles is absorbed by the constant interaction with target atoms on its path, the reaction cross section of a respective nuclear reaction is constantly changing, too. Thus, the thickness of the irradiated target materials should be as thin as feasible to cope with the selective energy window which is needed for the production of the desired certain radionuclide. The limitation on the resulting production yield is a disadvantage compared with the reactor-based radionuclide production. However, the introduction of one or more protons into a target nucleus mostly lead to the formation of a non-isotopic reaction product, which can be radiochemically separated. Thus, the use of an accelerator allows the production of radionuclides with highest specific activity and even in no-carrier-added (n.c.a.) form.

Accelerators exist in different energy ranges depending on the scientific program of the respective research facility or medical institution. For medical radionuclide production, especially, cyclotrons are used. Currently, the smallest cyclotrons dedicated to clinical radionuclide production purposes possess the maximum proton energy (E_p) of 7.5 MeV (e.g., BG-75™, ABT Molecular Imaging Inc., and GENtrace™ PT 600, GE Healthcare) (see Fig. 2.2a, b). On the other hand, the largest cyclotron for radionuclide production ranges up to 520 MeV at TRIUMF, Canada (Fig. 2.2c).

Apart from other nuclear physics research projects at TRIUMF, one of the beam lines from this 520 MeV cyclotron is installed for the production of radiometals needing high energies for, e.g., production of ^{82}Rb as a parent generator radionuclide for ^{82}Sr.

The majority of medically relevant accelerator radionuclides are produced via proton-induced nuclear reactions using small (up to 18 MeV) (Fig. 2.2d) and intermediate energy cyclotrons (up to 30 MeV) (Fig. 2.2e).

Nevertheless, the options of deuteron- and alpha particle-induced reactions should not be forgotten. Some of these radionuclides, e.g., ^{15}O and ^{43}Sc, have arguably better yields via deuteron routes since it offers comparatively higher reaction cross sections. Also, the most feasible route to produce ^{211}At is via alpha particle irradiations, but since deuterons and alpha particles are not available on the majority of medical cyclotrons, continuous efforts are made in the direction of only proton irradiations to produce most of the relevant radionuclides.

2.2.6 Generator-Based Production of Radionuclides

The first radionuclide generator for life science application was developed in 1920 for the generation of ^{222}Rn as daughter radionuclide of ^{226}Ra [18]. Later in 1957, the breakthrough of this concept was achieved with the development of the ^{99}Mo/^{99m}Tc generator at Brookhaven National Laboratory by Stang et al. [19].

Generator systems (Fig. 2.3) are of special interest predominantly for the diagnostic application of radionuclides. The basic principle of a medical generator system is the state of a transient[2] or secular[3] radioactive equilibrium between a sufficiently long-lived (T_1) parent radionuclide and suitably short-lived (T_2) daughter radionuclide. A more detailed essay on the states of radioactive equilibrium, i.e., transient and secular, is given by Hendee et al. [21]. A generator

[2]Transient equilibrium: Physical half-life of parent radionuclide T_1 is longer than daughter T_2 ($T_1 > T_2$).

[3]Secular equilibrium: Physical half-life of parent radionuclide T_1 is much longer than daughter T_2 ($T_1 \gg T_2$).

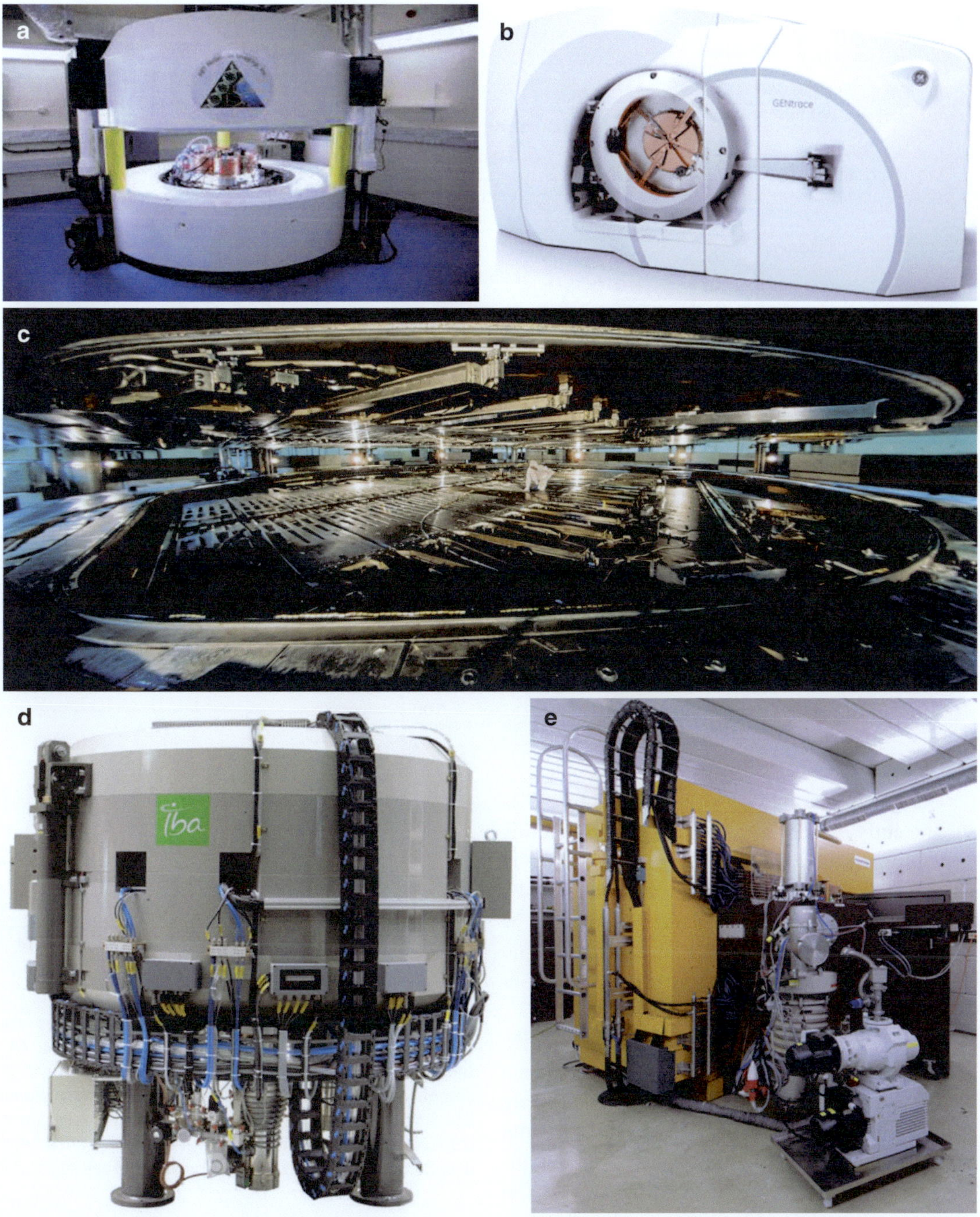

Fig. 2.2 (**a**) BG-75 7.5 MeV. (Source: ABT). (**b**) GENtrace PT 600 7.8 MeV. (Source: GE Healthcare). (**c**) Insight of the tank of TRIUMF 520 MeV cyclotron (Source: TRIUMF). (**d**) IBA CYCLONE™, 18 MeV (Source: IBA). (**e**) Scanditronix™ MC32NI, 32 MeV (Source: DKFZ)

system with a state of secular equilibrium, in which the physical half-life of the parent radionuclide is much longer than that of the daughter radionuclide ($T_1 \gg T_2$), can be operated over a long period of time. However, it is limited by the fact that the radioactivity of the daughter radionuclide cannot exceed the parent radionuclide activity. The maximum activity of the

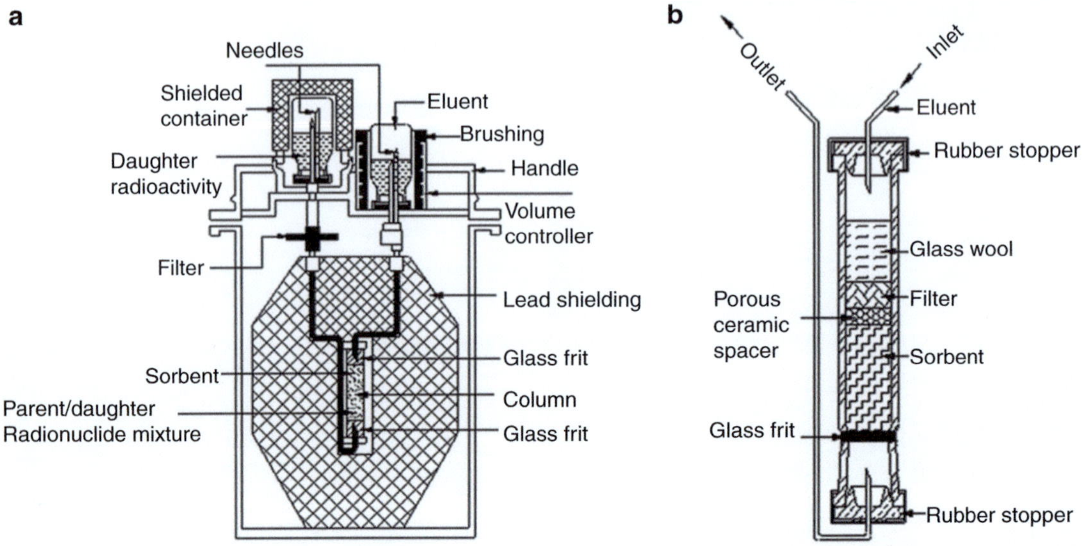

Fig. 2.3 Schematic diagram of a typical radionuclide generator system. (**a**) A column chromatography generator housed in a lead shielded container to provide short-lived radionuclides for industrial radiotracer investigation. (**b**) A chromatography column of a typical radionuclide generator (Source: Dash and Chakravarthy 2014 [20])

daughter radionuclide occurs at the time t, according to the equation:

$$t = \frac{1}{\lambda_1 - \lambda_2} \bullet \ln\left(\frac{\lambda_2}{\lambda_1}\right) \quad (2.1)$$

One such example of secular equilibrium is the recently widely used medical radionuclide generator system ^{68}Ge ($T_{1/2}$ = 270.8 days)/^{68}Ga ($T_{1/2}$ = 68.3 min) in which the ratio of the half-lives of the parent to daughter radionuclide is (270.8 × 24 × 60) min/68.3 min = 5709. The kinetics of secular equilibrium is illustrated in Fig. 2.4.

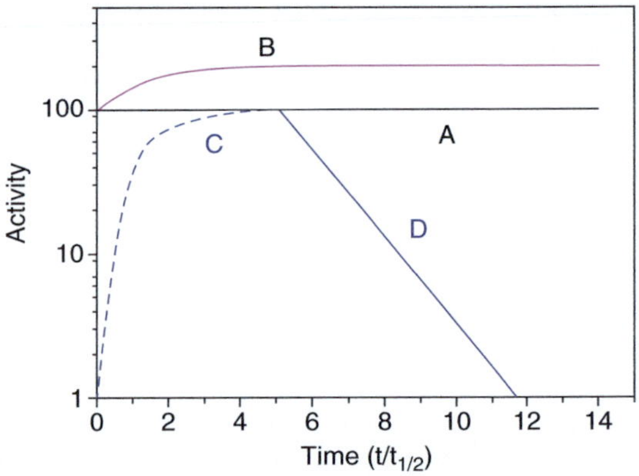

Fig. 2.4 Secular radionuclide generator kinetics for radionuclide generator kinetics the system ^{68}Ge/^{68}Ga. (**A**) Independent activity of the parent nuclide; (**B**) growth of cumulative parent and daughter activity in a pure parent fraction; (**C**) growth of daughter activity in a pure parent fraction; (**D**) independent decay of the separated pure daughter fraction at maximum of generated activity

In the case of a transient radioactive equilibrium, at which the parent radionuclide still has a longer half-life than the daughter but its decay cannot be neglected within a respective time interval ($T_1 > T_2$), the radioactivity of the daughter radionuclide maybe greater than that of the parent radionuclide. The ratio of the absolute activities of the two radionuclides is described by the equation:

$$\frac{A_1}{A_2} = \frac{\lambda_2 - \lambda_1}{\lambda_2} = 1 - \frac{\lambda_1}{\lambda_2} \quad (2.2)$$

Whereas:

A_1, A_2: radioactivity of the daughter and mother radionuclides

λ_1 and λ_2: decay constants of daughter and parent radionuclides

The most prominent radionuclide generator system ^{99}Mo ($T_{½}$ = 65.945 h)/^{99m}Tc ($T_{½}$ = 6.006 h)

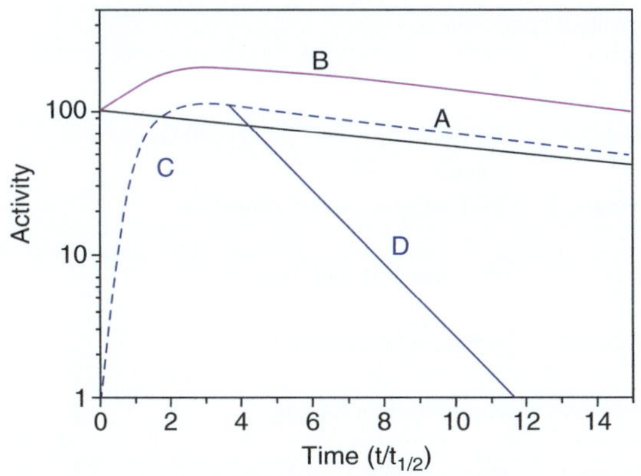

Fig. 2.5 Transient for the system ^{99}Mo/^{99m}Tc. (**A**) Independent activity of the parent nuclide; (**B**) growth of cumulative parent and daughter activity in a pure parent fraction; (**C**) growth of daughter activity in a pure parent fraction; (**D**) independent decay of the separated pure daughter fraction at maximum of generated activity

comes under the transient equilibrium category. Here, the ratio of the physical half-lives of the parent to daughter is 11, and its corresponding kinetics is shown in Fig. 2.5. The difference between the two equilibrium kinetics can easily be compared in the above examples given in Figs. 2.4 and 2.5 [22]. The elution process of the generated radioactivity is described in more detail in Sect. 2.3.1.1.

Although the lifetime of the latter class of generator system is limited, it can be operated more frequently due to the shorter recharge time of the diagnostic daughter. This is making it more favorable for clinical use, where the elution process can be repeated periodically, allowing multiple applications over a certain period of time.

The radioactive decay of the mother radionuclide leads to the formation of the diagnostic radionuclide (see Eq. 2.2), e.g., ^{99m}Tc, in no-carrier-added form, which then can be purely eluted due to its different chemical behavior. The chemical and technical concept of the separation method has to be highly optimized to warrant high yield of the daughter radionuclide in minimum volumes and highest radionuclidic and radiochemical purity.

The parent radionuclide is produced either by means of a cyclotron or a nuclear reactor. The radiochemical separation, isolation, and subsequent preparation of the generator are done at a few specialized facilities, such as Brookhaven National Center, USA. Ideally the daughter radionuclide can be simply eluted as radiotracer solution ready for injection into a patient.

The technical and legal demands on a radionuclide generator are comparably small, and it can be shipped to most clinics worldwide without need of any advanced local radiochemical infrastructure. Thus, a radionuclide generator system is, if available, a rather cheap and convenient alternative compared to other in-house production facilities.

Today, a few generator systems have been clinically approved, and rather a large number of potential generator pairs are under investigation. Table 2.1 below gives an overview of existing and potential generator systems for medical application.

A novel concept for the medical applications of generator radionuclides is the development of in vivo generators. Such generator systems involve labeling of a suitable carrier or tracer, e.g., radiolabeled antibodies, metal complexes, peptides, etc., with intermediate physical half-life parent radionuclides, which decay to much shorter-lived daughter radionuclides after accumulation in the targeted tissue. This approach allows the medical application of radionuclides which would otherwise be too short-lived for clinical use. A possible example of an in vivo generator for therapeutic use is the decay of ^{212}Pb ($T_{½}$ = 10.64 h) to ^{212}Bi ($T_{½}$ = 60.55 min). By chelating the parent ^{212}Pb radionuclide, the effective radiation dose delivered to the targeted tumor can be significantly increased [23], because the effective half-life of the ^{212}Bi decay product is then dependent on the half-life of the parent radionuclide according to Eq. 2.2. However, the application of the in vivo concept is accompanied by some disadvantages, i.e., the biochemical and biological behavior of both the parent and the daughter radionuclide has to be considered, the administered radiometal-bearing compound and composition has to meet higher demands on its radiometal chelating agent moiety, and not only

Table 2.1 Established and potential generator systems for medical applications

Generator system	Parent	Daughter	Equilibrium	Application
$^{82}Sr/^{82}Rb$	^{82}Sr $T_{1/2} = 25.6$ days	^{82}Rb $T_{1/2} = 1.27$ min	Secular[a]	PET imaging, esp. myocardial perfusion imaging (MPI)
$^{62}Zn/^{62}Cu$	^{62}Zn $T_{1/2} = 9.26$ h	^{62}Cu $T_{1/2} = 9.74$ min	Transient[b]	PET imaging and diagnostics
$^{68}Ge/^{68}Ga$	^{68}Ge $T_{1/2} = 270.8$ days	^{68}Ga $T_{1/2} = 68.3$ min	Secular[a]	PET imaging and diagnostics
$^{228}Th/^{212}Pb$	^{228}Th $T_{1/2} = 1.91$ years	^{212}Pb $T_{1/2} = 10.64$ h	Secular[a]	Radioimmunotherapy
$^{212}Pb/^{212}Bi$	^{212}Pb $T_{1/2} = 10.64$ h	^{212}Bi $T_{1/2} = 1.01$ h	Transient[b]	Radioimmunotherapy
$^{90}Sr/^{90}Y$	^{90}Sr $T_{1/2} = 28.6$ years	^{90}Y $T_{1/2} = 64.1$ h	Secular[a]	Therapy: e.g. liver cancer therapy
$^{188}W/^{188}Re$	^{188}W $T_{1/2} = 69$ days	^{188}Re $T_{1/2} = 16.9$ h	Transient[b]	Therapy, imaging, biodistribution and absorbed radiation dose studies
$^{99}Mo/^{99m}Tc$	^{99}Mo $T_{1/2} = 65.9$ h	^{99m}Tc $T_{1/2} = 6.0$ h	Transient[b]	Various body organs like liver, kidney, thyroid as well as neuroendocrine tumors imaging
$^{44}Ti/^{44}Sc$	^{44}Ti $T_{1/2} = 60.3$ years	^{44}Sc $T_{1/2} = 3.93$ h	Secular[a]	Primary and metastatic neuroendocrine tumors imaging, bone studies
$^{166}Dy/^{166}Ho$	^{166}Dy $T_{1/2} = 3.4$ days	^{166}Ho $T_{1/2} = 1.12$ days	Transient[b]	Therapy: e.g. radiation radiosynovectomy, myeloablative therapy of multiple myeloma
$^{225}Ac/^{213}Bi$	^{166}Ac $T_{1/2} = 10$ days	^{213}Bi $T_{1/2} = 45.6$ min	Transient[b]	Therapy: e.g. treatment of myelogenous leukemia

[a]Secular equilibrium according to Eq. 2.1
[b]Transient equilibrium according to Eq. 2.2

the parent radionuclide has to be stable under in vivo conditions but also the respective decay products, which is additionally complicated by the decay process itself.

2.2.7 High-Intensity γ-Ray Sources for Photonuclear Radionuclide Production

This novel concept of radionuclide production only became possible, because very brilliant γ-ray sources have been developed, where the γ-rays are produced by Compton backscattering of laser light from brilliant high-energy electron bunches [17]. Such a facility will typically consists of a high-performance electron accelerator from which intense laser beams are Compton backscattered. A 50 MeV electron beam from an accelerator falling on a heavy metal target delivers photons with an energy spectrum extending from about 0.1 to 50 MeV [24]. Nuclear model calculations on medium mass nuclei show that the threshold of a (γ,n)-reaction lies at approximately 8 MeV and the maximum of the excitation function at about 15 MeV with a maximum cross section around 150 mb [25]. In comparison the threshold of a (γ,p)-reaction in the same mass region lies at about 10 MeV with an estimated maximum cross section of about 10 mb between 20 and 30 MeV [25].

Such facilities may allow the production of radionuclides with high specific activity by new photonuclear reactions. Foremost, the use of photonuclear reactions can be a promising alternative for the reactor-based production of radionuclides. Besides the possibility of performing photofission reactions, some special applications have been considered. It is discussed in particular for the production of ^{99}Mo via the (γ,n)-reaction on ^{100}Mo. Other promising photonuclear reactions discussed for medical application could be $^{68}Zn(\gamma,p)^{67}Cu$ and $^{124}Xe(\gamma,n)^{123}Xe \rightarrow {}^{123}I$ [2]. In addition metastable isomers are advantageously produced via (γ,γ′)-reactions, e.g., $^{195}Pt(\gamma,\gamma')^{195m}Pt$ in higher specific activity [17].

Currently, there is a strong deficit in photonuclear cross sections, and for irradiation, a further narrowing of the γ-ray bandwidth would be needed in order to exploit nuclear-level resonances. Also the low-reaction cross sections make the large-scale production of radionuclides inefficient at presence. However, given time to further develop the accelerator technology to provide higher beam currents, this novel approach can be a powerful complement for radionuclide production.

2.2.8 Spallation Neutron Sources for Radionuclide Production

In the wake of the development work on accelerator-driven spallation neutron sources suggested as alternative technology to nuclear fission reactors, studies have been done on radionuclide production using spallation neutrons.

The irradiation of a heavy mass target with protons of energies above 150 MeV leads to a spallation neutron spectrum, which has a strong component covering the energy region of 0.5–10 MeV. Due to this energy range, it would be possible to induce several threshold reactions, in particular the (n,p)-reaction, which in some cases show up to three times higher cross sections than those with fission neutrons [26, 27]. The production potential of several medically interesting radionuclides using spallation neutrons neutrons like ^{47}Sc was recently discussed by DeLorme et al. [28].

In a high-intensity spallation neutron source, about 1000 MeV protons at a beam current of about 1 mA fall onto a Pb/U target, whereby the neutron fluxes generated are comparable to those in a medium to high flux reactor [29].

However, before future radionuclide production can be efficiently done at a spallation neutron source, extensive amount of nuclear data will be needed to characterize and standardize the neutron spectra prior to measurement and validation of the production-related integral data.

2.2.9 Medical Applications of Radionuclides

The scope of radionuclide applications in nuclear medicine is well defined. Since years, radioactivity generated by radionuclides find continuous increase in application in the two complementary major fields of nuclear medicine, i.e., diagnosis (noninvasive imaging) and therapy (endoradiotherapy). Each application, however, requires specific radionuclides depending on its physical, chemical, and biological characteristics. In this context, the following chapter discusses well-established and rarely available radionuclides together with their respective production methods for their use in nuclear medicine. Recent advancement in cancer research is made with the introduction of the theranostic approach which is a combination of diagnostics and endoradiotherapy realized with on and the same class of radiopharmaceuticals (cf. Sect. 2.5). The theranostic approach from the perspective of feasible radionuclides is discussed in detail as follows in Sect. 2.2.10 together with an outlook on possible future trends in the application of radionuclides in medicine.

2.2.10 Outlook on Future Radionuclides of Clinical Relevance

The use of radioactive agents for medical applications has been constantly growing during the past decades, and there is no indication that this trend is going to change in the near future.

Upcoming questions on biological processes and on unmet clinical needs are currently inducing new developments of radiochemistry methodologies and of new suitable radionuclide probes. In this respect the technological evolution moving away from nuclear reactor-based production toward on-site solutions and new accelerator-driven production facilities demands for new target designs and production routes for medical radionuclides in general.

A promising example for a novel approach to radionuclide production is the use of proton-induced spallation reactions on a tantalum target to produce the medically interesting radioisotopes ^{149}Tb ($T_{½}$ = 4.12 h), ^{152}Tb ($T_{½}$ = 17.5 h), ^{155}Tb ($T_{½}$ = 5.32 days), and ^{161}Tb ($T_{½}$ = 6.89 days), which can find application in therapy and diagnosis [30, 31].

The ongoing progress in targeted cancer therapy (belonging to precision medicine) is directly connected to the availability of diagnostic probes which are able to guide these efforts. Furthermore, the merge of diagnosis and endoradiotherapy under the concept of theranostics demands of matching radionuclide pairs or dual-use radionuclides. Combining a β^- (or Auger electron) and β^+ emitting pair of radionuclides, it is possible to measure the uptake kinetics by PET imaging, thereby allowing an accurate dosimetric calculation related to therapy. The principle was firstly applied in the case of endoradiotherapy with ^{90}Y in combination with the positron emitter ^{86}Y [32, 33]. Today, there several corresponding pairs, e.g., $^{47}Sc/^{44}Sc$; $^{67}Cu/^{64}Cu$; $^{67}Ga/^{66}Ga$ or ^{68}Ga, and $^{131}I/^{124}I$, are discussed. This concept of theranostics could also be extended by radiolabeling of therapeutic agents used in chemotherapy. In order to reach the stage of clinical application, considerable radiochemical efforts and work related to nuclear data are demanded.

In recent years, medical multimodal imaging methods like SPECT/CT, PET/CT, and PET/MRI gain more and more importance and fuel the development of new radiotracers. Multimodal imaging is defined as the combination of two or more diagnostic imaging methods to simultaneously measure complementary information. The combination of these radiological imaging methods allows benefiting of the individual assets, namely the high resolution of computed tomography (CT) and magnetic resonance imaging (MRI) and the extraordinary sensitivity of PET and SPECT. For example, PET/CT hybrid systems deliver higher morphological contrast in a shorter measurement time by use of the CT for the attenuation and scatter correction necessary for quantitation with PET making additional transmission source measurements redundant. After its introduction in 1998 [34] and its commercial availability in 2001, the number of deployed hybrid systems rose significantly [35]. A similar approach was taken to combine PET and MRI systems, pairing the high soft tissue contrast of MRI with the quantitative assessment of biochemical functions by PET. A first prototype for humans was developed in 2007 [36], and a first clinical PET/MRI system (*Biograph mMR*, Siemens) has been available since 2011 [37].

A new class of contrast agents utilizing the full potential of this multimodal imaging is presently emerging and is called *responsive* or *smart* contrast agents [38]. Promising examples of bimodal imaging probes are the radionuclides ^{52g}Mn and ^{147}Gd.

2.2.11 Radionuclides for Diagnosis and Therapy

The most important "standard" short-lived positron emitters for routine positron emission tomography (PET) investigations are ^{18}F, ^{11}C, ^{13}N, and ^{15}O. Their production routes and respective applications are well established and have been described comprehensively in the literature [39–42]. In the following sections, a selection of radionuclides is highlighted, and their current status is summarized. The special focus of this brief overview is on available radionuclides of emerging clinical demand or of potential clinical interest. Their production methods are correspondingly described in detail. Additional radionuclides of interest might be not covered in this overview. However, comprehensive reviews on radionuclides can be found also elsewhere [2, 41, 43, 44].

2.2.11.1 The "Standard" PET Radionuclides ^{11}C, ^{13}N, ^{15}O, and ^{18}F

The radionuclides ^{11}C ($T_{½}$ = 20.38 min), ^{13}N ($T_{½}$ = 9.96 min), ^{15}O ($T_{½}$ = 2.03 min), and ^{18}F ($T_{½}$ = 109.728 min) can successfully be introduced into biochemically active organic compounds and in case of ^{11}C and ^{15}O often allow even authentic radiolabeling. Their respective production with small "medical" cyclotrons (<18 MeV proton beams) using gas or water targets is well established [2, 41]. In Table 2.2 a short overview of the production of the "standard" PET radionuclides is given.

For production of ^{11}C and ^{15}O, generally pressurized gas targets are used, from which the product activity is led to reaction vessels where the

Table 2.2 Production of standard PET radionuclides

Radionuclides	Nuclear reaction	Energy range [MeV]	Batch yield [GBq]
^{11}C	$^{14}N(p,\alpha)$	13 → 3	100
^{13}N	$^{16}O(p,\alpha)$	16 → 7	30
^{15}O	$^{14}N(d,n)$ $^{15}N(p,n)$	8 → 0 10 → 0	100 50
^{18}F	$^{18}O(p,n)$ $^{20}Ne(d,\alpha)$	16 → 3 14 → 0	100 30

conversion to the radiolabeling precursor takes place. The chemical form of the radioactive compound leaving the target depends upon the additive, e.g., given to the N_2 gas target and in the case of ^{11}C also on the radiation dose effective in the target [41].

Carbon-11 is mostly obtained and applied as $[^{11}C]CO_2$. Only for some applications, ^{11}C is converted to $[^{11}C]$methane [45]. Although the production and clinical use of ^{11}C is well established, the preservative problem of ensuring high molar/specific activity has to be taken care of and precautions regarding gas composition, construction material, and chemicals are needed [46, 47].

The very short-lived PET radionuclide ^{15}O is generally produced in-target as $[^{15}O]O_2$ and either can be directly used for metabolic oxygen consumption measurements or can be chemically processed to form $[^{15}O]CO$, $[^{15}O]CO_2$, and especially $[^{15}O]H_2O$ [48] which finds clinical applications in lung perfusion studies and regional cerebral blood flow measurement [49]. The most efficient production of ^{15}O demands a cyclotron-derived deuteron beam (Table 2.2). Since deuterons are not available in many medical cyclotrons, successful efforts have been made [48, 49] to produce ^{15}O in sufficient yields using low-energy proton accelerators ($E_p < 15$ MeV) following the $^{15}N(p, n)^{15}O$ nuclear reaction. However, this route requires highly enriched ^{15}N for irradiation to avoid radioactive by-products. Thus, this route is more expensive compared to the production via deuterons, and the recovery system for the enriched ^{15}N [49] has to be set up.

The nitrogen isotope ^{13}N is mostly used as ammonia or nitrate. The latter, however, is only used as radiotracer in research on plant physiology [50]. The radionuclides ^{13}N and ^{18}F are commonly produced using water targets, of which several types have been developed in the past [41, 51].

The dominant role of radiofluorinated PET tracers will not diminish. For all radiosyntheses, either aqueous $[^{18}F]$fluoride or gaseous $[^{18}F]F_2$ is used as starting material. Both chemical forms are generally produced with a cyclotron via the $^{18}O(p,n)^{18}F$ nuclear reaction [41].

The nucleophilic $[^{18}F]$fluoride ion is available in no-carrier-added (n.c.a.) form which allows the synthesis of radiotracers with high molar/specific activity. The electrophilic $[^{18}F]F_2$, on the other hand, is available only in carrier-added (c.a.) form which leads to radiotracers with low molar/specific activity [39].

The production of electrophilic ^{18}F is usually carried out using a gas target. However, the formation of $[^{18}F]F_2$ and the subsequent removal of the activity from the target demand addition of some F_2 carrier. The carrier is either added directly to the target gas, when the $^{20}Ne(d,\alpha)^{18}F$ reaction is used, or it is introduced in a second step, in case an ^{18}O target is used for production [41]. Studies showed that the production via the $^{18}O(p,n)$ reaction leads to higher yields and better molar/specific activity of $[^{18}F]F_2$ [52–54]. However, the achievable molar activity of about 600 GBq per mmol is still about a factor of 50 lower than needed for some CNS receptor radiopharmaceuticals. In 1997 Bergman and Solin therefore introduced a conversion method of $[^{18}F]$fluoride into $[^{18}F]$fluorine gas using an electrical discharge chamber [55].

2.2.11.2 ^{44g}Sc ($T_{½}$ = 3.97 h)

The potential PET radionuclide ^{44g}Sc is currently gaining increasing interest. Its physical half-life and average positron energy of 632.0 keV marks it as suitable for medical imaging. A drawback, however, is the appearance of the strong 1157 keV γ-ray emission. The possibility of fast and efficient complexation of $[^{44}Sc]Sc^{3+}$ using different medically interesting chelators like DOTA (1,4,7,10-tetraazacyclododecane-1,4,7,10-tetraacetic acid) and AAZTA (1,4-bis (carboxymethyl)-6-[bis(carboxymethyl)]amino-6-methylperhydro-1,4-diazepine) was demonstrated, and the potential of the radionuclide for PET imaging was shown [56–59].

The radionuclide can be obtained either via cyclotron irradiation of an isotopically enriched Ca target or as the daughter radionuclide of a $^{44}Ti/^{44}Sc$ generator system. However, the experimental cross-sectional data are not that comprehensive for neither the $^{44}Ca(p,n)^{44}Sc$ reaction nor the $^{45}Sc(p,2n)^{44}Ti$ reaction. A disadvantage of the direct production is the co-production of ^{44m}Sc ($T_{½}$ = 58.61 h) in small amounts <10%. In contrast the generator-produced ^{44}Sc has very high radionuclidic purity. However, the physical half-life of 59.1 years of the mother radionuclide ^{44}Ti demands a very high starting radioactivity and high amount of beam time for production. Recent work therefore is focusing on the investigation of cyclotron-produced ^{43}Sc for PET. Carzaniga et al. [60] reported on measurements on the $^{46}Ti(p,\alpha)^{43}Sc$ and $^{43,44}Ca(p,xn)^{43}Sc$ reactions with maximum cross-sectional values of about 40 and 250 mb, respectively, at proton energies below 18 MeV. A more detailed discussion on the production of ^{44g}Sc is given by Synowiecki et al. [61].

2.2.11.3 ^{52}Mn ($T_{½}$ = 5.591 Days)

Manganese has gained more attention in the last two decades due to its increasing use in MEMRI (manganese-enhanced magnetic resonance imaging) [62]. In the past radioisotopes of manganese were mainly used in the form of $MnCl_2$ for imaging studies. However, in combination with the propagation of multimodal imaging technologies, the development of radiomanganese-labeled PET tracers may lead to new high-potential radiopharmaceuticals.

The main production route of ^{52g}Mn is the irradiation of elemental chromium or compounds thereof with charged particles leading to ^{51}Mn, ^{52g}Mn, and ^{54}Mn. Although its decay is connected to the emission of several γ-rays (1434.09 keV, 935.54 keV, etc.) and the positron emission probability is only 29.4%, the radioisotope ^{52g}Mn is highly suitable for PET. This is especially due to its low average positron energy of only 241.59 keV, which allows a PET image resolution close to that of ^{18}F. Furthermore, ^{52g}Mn can be produced via the (p,n)-reaction with a medium-energy cyclotron ($E_p \leq 18$ MeV). The physical half-life of about 5.6 days is a downside, limiting repetition experiments in conjunction with the biological half-life of the respective compound but allowing observation of slower biochemical processes. Even so, ^{52g}Mn seems to be the most suitable manganese radioisotope for PET, and a first study was already conducted by Topping et al. [63] showing its applicability in PET. Integral yields of 4.5 MBq/μA h (16 MeV) and 21.0 MBq/μA h (22 MeV) have been reported by Abe et al. [64] and Dmitriev et al. [65]. The existing experimental cross section is, however, rather inconsistent and poorly investigated above 10 MeV.

Another downside in the application of ^{52g}Mn is the need of excessive radiochemical work to separate the irradiated chromium bulk for subsequent radiosynthesis of the aimed-at radiotracer.

2.2.11.4 ^{64}Cu ($T_{½}$ = 12.7 h)

Copper forms stable coordination complexes, and together with its suitable physical half-life, ^{64}Cu is very useful for studying slow functional processes. In the form of $[^{64}Cu]CuCl_2$, ^{64}Cu is commercially available for radiolabeling of pharmaceutical compounds under the trade name Cuprymina™. The radionuclide ^{64}Cu emits low-energy positrons with an average energy of 278 keV and has no disturbing γ-rays. Due to its low β^+ energy, the resolution of reconstructed PET images after ^{64}Cu administration is comparable to that of ^{18}F-derived images. Due to the rather small positron branching (17.8%), either much higher radioactivity has to be injected or longer counting time is needed to achieve an imaging quality comparable to that of ^{18}F-labeled radiopharmaceuticals. In addition, the remaining 82.2% decay branching (β^-, EC) induces a non-negligible radiation dose to the patient. However, these decay characteristic makes it suitable for its use in diagnostic PET investigations. Moreover, besides ^{64}Cu, the copper radioisotopes ^{61}Cu ($T_{½}$ = 3.339 h, β^+) and ^{62}Cu ($T_{½}$ = 9.67 min, β^+) are considered for diagnostic applications as well. In combination with neutron-rich ^{67}Cu, copper radioisotopes offer high potential for the theranostic approach.

Table 2.3 Comparison of production routes of ^{64}Cu[a]

Nuclear process	Optimum energy range (MeV)	Thick target yield (MBq/μA)[b]
^{64}Ni(p,n)^{64}Cu	12 → 8	304
^{64}Ni(d,2n)^{64}Cu	17 → 11	430
^{68}Zn(p,αn)^{64}Cu	30 → 21	116
^{66}Zn(p,2pn)^{64}Cu	52 → 37	316
^{64}Zn(d,2p)^{64}Cu	20 → 10	27.1
^{66}Zn(d,α)^{64}Cu	13 → 5	13.8
^{nat}Zn(d,x)^{64}Cu	25 → 10	57.0

[a]Aslam and Qaim [66]
[b]Calculated for 1 h of irradiation time

Table 2.4 Overview of the relevant nuclear reactions for the production of ^{66}Ga

Nuclear reaction	Energy range (MeV)	Max. cross section (mb)	Reference
^{66}Zn(p,n)	29.0 → 4.5	644	Szelecsényi et al. [70]
^{67}Zn(p,2n)	29.0 → 14.0	477	Szelecsényi et al. [70]
^{68}Zn(p,3n)	100 → 20	120–250	cf. EXFOR [71]
^{nat}Cu(α,xn)	48.0 → 13.0	306	Takács et al. [72]

Several routes have been investigated for the production of no-carrier-added ^{64}Cu. Initially, ^{64}Cu was produced via the ^{64}Zn(n,p)^{64}Cu reaction in a nuclear reactor. However, the yield and purity of the product obtained via this route do not meet the present demands for medical applications.

Thereafter, production routes of ^{64}Cu using proton- and deuteron-induced reactions were investigated with up to 80 MeV beams. In Table 2.3 a comparison of the most promising methods is given based on a critical review of the published nuclear reaction cross-sectional data [67]. Of all the investigated processes, the (p,n)-reaction on enriched ^{64}Ni, initially reported by Szelecsényi et al. [68], was found to be the best regarding both yield and specific activity. Batch yields of about 40 GBq ^{64}Cu can be achieved, and the enriched target material ^{64}Ni can almost quantitatively be recovered. An advantage of this production route is that it can be utilized at a small-sized cyclotron. Small amounts of ^{64}Cu have also been produced using the nuclear processes ^{64}Zn(d,2p)^{64}Cu and ^{68}Zn(p,αn)^{64}Cu. The radiochemical separation of ^{64}Cu and its by-products, e.g., activation products from the irradiated ^{64}Ni target (^{55}Co, ^{57}Co, ^{57}Ni, ^{61}Co), was achieved by using anion and cation exchange chromatography [69].

2.2.11.5 ^{66}Ga ($T_{½}$ = 9.49 h)

Next to ^{99m}Tc, the radioisotopes of Ga are currently the second most important radiometals used for clinical diagnostics. Although the nuclear properties of ^{66}Ga, i.e., the low positron branching of 51% and the affiliated 2751 keV γ-ray, do not recommend that radionuclide for PET imaging, its longer physical half-life allows the investigation of slower metabolic processes.

Several production routes for ^{66}Ga have been studied and evaluated. The most relevant nuclear reactions are given in Table 2.4. These nuclear processes have been well studied and evaluated [70, 72]. Nevertheless, the ^{68}Zn(p,3n)^{66}Ga reaction shows some discrepancies between the different obtained data sets. The maximum cross sections show that the (p,n) and (p,2n) as well as the (α,xn) reactions are suitable production routes for ^{66}Ga. However, the data also show that the use of enriched target material is mandatory to avoid the formation of the longer-lived ^{67}Ga.

2.2.11.6 ^{67}Ga ($T_{½}$ = 3.2617 Days)

In spite of its rather long physical half-life, ^{67}Ga is an important SPECT radionuclide. It decays exclusively via electron capture to the stable ^{67}Zn, and its predominant γ-rays, i.e., 93.310 keV (38.81%) and 184.576 keV (21.41%), are close to the efficiency maxima of conventional SPECT cameras. The most important ^{67}Ga agent is [^{67}Ga]Ga-citrate, but over the years, many other gallium-based radiopharmaceuticals have been developed [42]. Besides its clinical application, the formation of ^{67}Ga via the ^{nat}Cu(α,x) process is an important monitor reaction for the determination of beam currents and projectile energies of α-particle-induced nuclear reactions [72].

A number of nuclear reactions have been studied for the production of ^{67}Ga, and an overview of the most relevant is given in Table 2.5.

Table 2.5 Overview of the relevant nuclear reactions for the production of ^{67}Ga

Nuclear reaction	Energy range (MeV)	Max. cross section (mb)	Reference
$^{67}Zn(p,n)$	25.5 → 2.5	615	IAEA [43]
$^{68}Zn(p,2n)$	45.0 → 12.0	725	IAEA [43]
$^{nat}Zn(d,xn)$	48.3 → 5.7	106	Tárkányi et al. [73]
$^{nat}Zn(d,xn)$	23.2 → 2.6	116	Khandaker et al. [74]
$^{nat}Cu(\alpha,x)$	48 → 13	300	Takács et al. [72]
$^{65}Cu(\alpha,2n)$	75 → 7	500–900	cf. EXFOR [71]
$^{nat}Zn(\alpha,x)$	96.5 → 8.8	200–290	Cf. EXFOR [71]

2.2.11.7 ^{68}Ga ($T_{½}$ = 68.3 min)

The use of ^{68}Ga in PET imaging can be considered as advancement of the well-established ^{67}Ga applications. ^{68}Ga shares the chemical properties of its lighter radioisotope but comes with two major advantages concerning application and production: The β^+ emission of 0.836 MeV (avg.) with the intensity of 87.72% allows for quantitative PET studies. Furthermore, its shorter physical half-life results in a short scanning time, and combined with very low γ-ray emission of less than 3.5%, this leads to a reduced radiation exposure of the patient, in spite of the rather high energy of the emitted photons of 1077.34 keV. The high potential of ^{68}Ga PET is especially recognized, namely in oncology as well as in infection and cardiology research.

The production of ^{68}Ga can be achieved not only via direct processes with an accelerator analog to that of ^{67}Ga, but it can also be provided by corresponding $^{68}Ge/^{68}Ga$ generator systems. With regard to the type and the usually low energy of medical accelerators available for on-site production, basically two nuclear reactions are used to efficiently produce ^{68}Ga, namely the $^{65}Cu(\alpha,n)^{68}Ga$ reaction ($E_{threshold}$ = 6.18 MeV) and the $^{68}Zn(p,n)^{68}Ga$ reaction ($E_{threshold}$ = 3.76 MeV). Among those the proton bombardment of enriched ^{68}Zn results in the highest yields and the lowest amount of longer-living impurities.

However, the possibility of producing ^{68}Ga via a radionuclide generator is still the most attractive for clinical use due to the considerably easier handling. With the availability and reliability of commercial generator systems, the worldwide interest toward ^{68}Ga strongly has increased the last decade [75].

As reviewed by Isabel and Prata in 2012, there exist two main strategies to design $^{68}Ge/^{68}Ga$ generators giving ^{68}Ga in corresponding eluates in high purity, namely the use of:

- Organic matrices bearing phenolic groups
- Inorganic oxide matrices, such as Al_2O_3, SnO_2, Sb_2O_5, ZrO_2, and TiO_2

This allows the elution of $[^{68}Ga]Ga^{3+}$ by using HCl, citrate solution, or EDTA as eluent [76–78].

There are some common concerns toward all generator systems, which have to be dealt with. First of all this is the potential breakthrough of ^{68}Ge but also large eluate volumes and the presence of metallic impurities like Zn^{2+}, Ti^{4+}, and Fe^{3+} that may disturb the radiolabeling with $[^{68}Ga]Ga^{3+}$ by competing for the same chelator. Different strategies have been developed to overcome these drawbacks [75], and Zhernosekov et al. published a post-processing method on a cation exchanger in hydrochloric acid/acetone media to concentrate and purify generator-derived ^{68}Ga eluates [79].

A limiting factor for the extension of this generator technology, however, is the production of the long-lived electron-capture radionuclide ^{68}Ge ($T_{½}$ = 270.93 days). The most efficient way for its generation is the (p,2n) reaction on ^{69}Ga with intermediate energy proton beams of 30–35 MeV, which has been evaluated by Takács et al. [80]. It requires a long irradiation time at a large accelerator facility. The long physical half-life of ^{68}Ge, on the other hand, allows for worldwide shipping of radionuclide generators without significant loss.

2.2.11.8 ^{72}As ($T_{½}$ = 26.0 h)

Arsenic is an element of relevance in environmental and toxicological sciences. For tracer studies in those two areas, the radionuclides ^{76}As

($T_{½}$ = 26.4 h) and ^{74}As ($T_{½}$ = 17.77 days) have been suggested [81]. In addition, the radioisotopes of arsenic are promising for applications in the fields of (radio)pharmacology, diagnostics, and cancer treatment [82, 83].

^{72}As is an interesting radionuclide for PET, as it is an intense β^+ emitter with three significant maximum β^+-particle energies at 2.499 MeV (64.2%), 3.334 MeV (16.3%), and 1.870 MeV (5.82%). Given the role of arsenic compounds in tumor treatment, such PET measurements can be very valuable for therapy control. Different methods of production and separation of ^{72}As have been reported. ^{72}As is generally obtained via the ^{72}Se/^{72}As generator system [84]. An overview of the direct production methods of ^{72}As via proton-, deuteron-, and α-particle-induced reactions is given in Table 2.6. However, the direct production route demands for the use of enriched target material to avoid the formation of longer-lived radionuclides. Furthermore, validation and extension of those data seems necessary for more precise calculation of production yields.

Concerning the proton-induced formation of ^{72}As experimental batch yields have been reported, which amounted up to 90.3 MBq/μA h (1 h irradiation time) in the energy range 44 → 28.5 MeV and 79.2 MBq/μA h (1 h irradiation time) at 25.5 → 0 MeV [90].

2.2.11.9 ^{73}Se ($T_{½}$ = 7.1 h)

Selenium is an essential element and is also an analog of sulfur which itself does not provide a suitable positron-emitting radionuclide. The positron endpoint energy of ^{73}Se (β^+ = 65.4%, EC = 34.6%) amounts to 1.3 MeV. Although a few γ-rays are also emitted, the decay parameters suggest its suitability for PET studies. However, due to the difficulty in production and radiochemistry of ^{73}Se, its medical application has been very limited so far.

Several production routes have been investigated for ^{73}Se using proton-, deuteron-, ^{4}He- and ^{3}He-induced reactions. A brief overview is given in Table 2.7. A critical analysis of the available cross-sectional data has been published by Qaim et al. [95].

The highest-reaction cross sections are connected to the (α,n) process. However, due to the very short range of α-particles, the resulting thick target yields are rather low. With regard to the possible batch yields and the levels of associated longer-lived impurities, i.e., ^{75}Se ($T_{½}$ = 120.0 days) and ^{72}Se ($T_{½}$ = 8.5 days), it was concluded that the ^{75}As(p,3n)^{73}Se reaction over the energy range of E_p = 40 → 30 MeV is most suitable for its production. The yield of ^{73}Se amounts to 1400 MBq/μA h, and the levels of ^{75}Se and ^{72}Se impurities are 0.05% and 0.11% of the amount of ^{73}Se, respectively. This method also has the advantage that the arsenic target material is monoisotopic. For the irradiations using protons, two target materials have been utilized, namely As_2O_3 and Cu_3As alloy, of which the latter is more suitable for high-current

Table 2.6 Direct production of ^{72}As

Production route	Energy range (MeV)	Max. cross section (mb)	Latest references
^{nat}Ge(p,xn)^{72}As	50 → 8	ca. 250	Horiguchi et al. [85], Spahn et al. [86])
^{nat}Ge(d,xn)^{72}As	49.9 → 9.3	ca. 190	Takács et al. [87]
^{nat}Ga(α,xn)^{72}As	31.5 → 7.5	ca. 750	Didik et al. [88]
^{nat}Ge(α,x)^{72}As	50.7 → 12.9	ca. 130	Takács et al. [89]

Table 2.7 Production of ^{73}Se via different routes

Nuclear reaction	Energy range [MeV]	Yield [GBq/μA]	Reference
^{75}As(p,3n)^{73}Se	40 → 30	1.41[a]	Mushtaq et al. [91]
^{nat}Br(p,x)^{73}Se	62 → 42	0.087[a]	Faßbender et al. [92]
^{75}As(d,4n)^{73}Se	56 → 26	1.18[a]	Mushtaq et al. [91]
^{72}Ge(^{3}He,2n)^{73}Se	36 → 13	0.004[b]	Mushtaq and Qaim [93]
^{70}Ge(α,n)^{73}Se	28 → 10	0.003[b]	Blessing et al. [94]

[a]Calculated for 1 h of irradiation time
[b]Using natural Ge (20.57%)

irradiations above 3 μA/h. For the isolation of the pure positron emitter, several radiochemical separation methods have been introduced using dry distillation, ion exchange, and liquid extraction procedures [96].

The use of the $^{75}As(p,3n)^{73}Se$ reaction for the production of ^{73}Se is very advantageous, and batch yields of up to 5 GBq were reported [91, 97]. However, the optimum production of ^{73}Se demands proton energy of about 40 MeV. Thus, an intermediate energy accelerator is needed which is not commonly available.

2.2.11.10 ^{76}Br ($T_{½}$ = 16.2 h)

The neutron-deficient nonmetal radiohalogen ^{76}Br, with a physical half-life of 16.2 h and a β^+-branching of 58.2% (β^+_{max} = 3.4 MeV; stable daughter ^{76}Se) [98], lends itself as potential "non-standard" PET radionuclide for imaging of slow(er) metabolic processes (cf. 2.2.11.4 ^{64}Cu) and of slow clearance from nonspecific binding sites [99], as well as for drug development purposes. Also, ^{76}Br has, over the years, found versatile applications like radiolabeling of antibodies for tumor imaging or radiolabeling of receptor ligands for brain studies [100]. Radiobromine is of interest for radiolabeling of tracer molecules, because there are isotopes available which are suitable for both molecular imaging approaches and endoradiotherapy, like ^{76}Br and ^{77}Br, respectively [96]. The rather high endpoint energy of the emitted positrons and several high-energy γ-rays (E_γ > 500 keV) lead to some limitations, concerning spatial resolution and image quality [98, 99], but may be reduced by appropriate specific corrections in the image reconstruction.

Several routes for the production of ^{76}Br had been investigated until 1986 [101]. They included direct formation of the radionuclide as well as formation via the precursor ^{76}Kr, respectively, obtained through irradiations with protons, deuterons, ^{3}He and ^{4}He particles, which yielded maximum quantities of about 0.5 GBq ^{76}Br [102]. Use of the reaction $^{78}Kr(d,\alpha)^{76}Br$ [103] led only to limited quantities of about 10 MBq of ^{76}Br. More attention has been paid to the production of ^{76}Br via the $^{76}Se(p,n)^{76}Br$ reaction [104]. Recently, further developmental work was realized on the processing of NiSe-alloy as improved target material for high-current irradiations [105].

2.2.11.11 ^{82m}Rb ($T_{½}$ = 6.472 h) and ^{82}Sr ($T_{½}$ = 25.35 Days)

Although ^{82m}Rb is not a pure β^+ emitter with a maximum of 19.7% emission intensity of its main positrons at 353 keV, the radionuclide has been routinely used for blood flow measurements, especially myocardial perfusion imaging [106]. This is mainly due to the fact that rubidium shows a biochemical activity very similar to that of potassium. Its suitable physical half-life and its efficient chemistry lead to the establishment of [^{82m}Rb]RbCl as imaging agent. The ground-state ^{82}Rb has a physical half-life of 1.2575 min and decays via EC and positron emission to the stable ^{82}Kr. Compared to corresponding ^{99m}Tc-radiopharmaceuticals, it shows better diagnostic accuracy and the advantage to quantify the myocardial blood flow [107]. The radionuclide ^{82m}Rb is exclusively produced by the decay of ^{82}Sr. A generator system $^{82}Sr/^{82}mRb$ (CardioGen-82®) was approved in the USA in 1989.

The parent radionuclide ^{82}Sr is generally produced via the ^{nat}Mo(p,spall) or the $^{85}Rb(p,4n)$ reaction [108, 109]. The spallation process demands a high-energy accelerator and is used only at a few places in the world (e.g., Los Alamos, TRIUMF, Dubna). The yield data are well known, but a drawback of the method is the occurrence of long-lived isotopic impurities, e.g., ^{90}Sr ($T_{½}$ = 28.6 a), ^{89}Sr ($T_{½}$ = 50.5 days), and ^{85}Sr ($T_{½}$ = 64.9 days). In particular ^{85}Sr is formed in large amounts. This impurity decays via EC (100%) and emits 514 keV γ-rays energy (96.4%). This demands not only extra shielding of the generator but also creates some difficulty in the quality control of the separated ^{82m}Rb, in case some breakthrough of radiostrontium has occurred.

The $^{nat}Rb(p,xn)^{82}Sr$ reaction for the production of ^{82}Sr is now more commonly employed. A cyclotron with incident proton energies of ca. 70 MeV is adequate and can produce about 14.8 MBq/μA (for 1 h irradiation) [80]. The corresponding cross-sectional data have been evaluated and show a maximum reaction cross section of 98.2 mb [80] . The by-product ^{83}Sr ($T_{½}$ = 32.4 h) is formed in large amounts, but decays out within a week. The level of the ^{85}Sr impurity can be controlled through the use of enriched target material and adapting the beam energy range (E_p = 70 → 50 MeV). However, the high cost of the enriched material, the effort involved in the recovery of the target material after irradiation, and the chemical processing impel several laboratories to rather use the $^{nat}Rb(p,xn)^{82}Sr$ process. The purified ^{82}Sr is then distributed worldwide to prepare generators.

2.2.11.12 ^{86}Y ($T_{½}$ = 14.7 h)

The radionuclide ^{86}Y is the most important imaging radionuclide for radiation dosimetry that was used in combination with ^{90}Y-labeled therapeutics [33]. This matched-pair combination was one of the first applications of the theranostic concept (after radioiodine). Currently the demand for this radionuclide is continuing, and its large-scale production is established at several centers.

^{86}Y ($\beta^+ \approx 33\%$) decays with six possible end-point positron energies up to 3153 keV and is connected to the emission of more than 12 γ-rays. These decay characteristics do not qualify ^{86}Y as a most suitable PET radionuclide but when developed and administered together with ^{90}Y, it allows an exact estimation of the dose from the ^{90}Y-labeled compound in terms of mGy per MBq. The historical development has been described in the literature [33].

Several nuclear reactions have been investigated for the formation of ^{86}Y. A critical evaluation of data for some of the important reactions was performed by Zaneb et al. [110]. The most feasible method recommended for the production of ^{86}Y is via the $^{86}Sr(p,n)^{86}Y$ reaction [111] on a highly enriched target material in the energy range E_p = 14 → 7 MeV. The cross-sectional data show considerable spread, but the production methodology is established using enriched [^{86}Sr] $SrCO_3$ (96–97% enrichment) as target material. Extensive efforts devoted to chemical separation of radioyttrium have been made involving coprecipitation and ion-exchange chromatography, electrolysis, single-column chromatography, multiple-column chromatography, solvent extraction, and precipitation of the target element [33]. The best result so far obtained a maximum batch yield of about 3.5 GBq [112, 113]. In recent years, the production of ^{86}Y via the $^{86}Sr(p,n)$ reaction at small hospital-based cyclotrons has been investigated utilizing liquid targets for irradiating a solution of the target nuclide [114]. The yield of ^{86}Y achieved using a liquid target is generally low, but it may be enough for local use.

2.2.11.13 ^{89}Zr ($T_{½}$ = 78.41 h)

At first glance ^{89}Zr (β^+(avg.) 395.5 keV) appears unsuitable for PET application due to its rather low positron intensity of 22.74% and the emission of the rather high-energetic γ-ray of 909.15 keV (0.04%). Nevertheless interest in this radionuclide has increased over the last couple of years as it exhibits a rather longer physical half-life compared to other clinically relevant positron emitters, making it ideally suited for imaging studies with slowly accumulating bioactive molecules, allowing for imaging of biological processes at late time points after radiotracer application. Furthermore, Zr(IV) (oxidation state +4) has a high affinity for its corresponding chelating agents such as deferoxamine (DFO) [115] (cf. Sect. 2.5.4.2) and remains stable in its coordination cavity in vivo [116, 117]. ^{89}Zr has therefore been one of the most popular PET radionuclides for radiolabeling of monoclonal antibodies (mAbs), which have typical circulation times of 1–3 weeks [116]. Up to date the number of ^{89}Zr-based immuno-PET probes in the clinics has grown to about 22 ^{89}Zr-mAbs which are currently undergoing or have completed clinical trials [118]. The production technology for medical use of ^{89}Zr is well established and can be achieved by means of small medical cyclotrons [119].

Typically, ^{89}Zr is created by proton bombardment of natural ^{89}Y. The isotopic abundance of the natural target is 100%, making the production affordable and alleviating the need for complicated target recycling procedures. Besides commercial yttrium foils, several groups use sputtered targets with gold or copper backings to improve heat dissipation during irradiation. Additionally, powder targets of both yttrium metal and Y_2O_3

have been suggested [119]. Omara et al. [120] measured the cross sections for the production of ^{88}Zr, ^{88}Y, and ^{89}Zr from proton irradiation of metal yttrium. They concluded that the optimum energy for proton bombardment is 14 MeV resulting in a batch yield of 58 MBq/μA h. Above the threshold incident energy of 13.1 MeV, proton irradiation also produces the isotopic impurity ^{88}Zr, which needs to be avoided.

The most established radiochemical separation procedure of ^{89}Zr from yttrium is the weak cation exchange method using a hydroxamic acid resin developed by Meijs et al. [117]. The product is finally eluted with oxalic acid.

2.2.11.14 ^{90}Y ($T_{½}$ = 64.00 h) and ^{90}Sr ($T_{½}$ = 28.79 Years)

The radionuclide ^{90}Y decays almost exclusively via β^- emission with the maximum particle energy of 2.28 MeV that allows a high dose deposition when used for endoradiotherapy. The medical application of ^{90}Y has been discussed in detail by Wright et al. [121]; the physical half-life of ^{90}Y makes it amenable for a variety of targeted endoradiotherapy applications like ^{90}Y-labeled colloid, tumor-targeting antibodies, and resin/glass microspheres for treatment of hepatic malignancies and metastases [121].

Due to the lack of any significant γ-ray emission of ^{90}Y, until recently activity quantification was performed using the Bremsstrahlung spectrum of ^{90}Y captured with single-photon emission computed tomography (SPECT) [122]. However, the SPECT-based method suffers from inaccuracies in quantification due to its low spatial resolution, photon scatter, and collimator septal penetration [123].

The production of ^{90}Y is done using ^{90}Sr/^{90}Y generators of which various forms have been available for a number of years. However, due to the safety issues connected to the use of ^{90}Y and ^{90}Sr, those generators are typically installed at specialized processing units, at which the no-carrier-added products are prepared by batch solvent extraction methods and then distributed. A detailed discussion on the making of the ^{90}Sr/^{90}Y generator was published by the IAEA [124]. The parent radionuclide ^{90}Sr is a pure β^- emitter (E_{max} = 546.0 keV (100%), no γ-ray) and is a product of nuclear fission. For thermal neutron fission as in typical nuclear power plants, the fission product yield from ^{235}U is 5.7% and from ^{233}U 6.6%. It decays via the emission of β^--particles of 195.8 keV (average) and does not emit any γ-rays.

2.2.11.15 ^{94m}Tc ($T_{½}$ = 52.0 min)

The positron emitter ^{94m}Tc attracted interest as potential PET radionuclide in the wake of the ^{99m}Tc shortage during the late 2000s initiated by the unexpected shutdown of the most important production site, the National Research Universal (NRU) nuclear reactor in Canada. Although its average positron energy of 1094.2 keV (67.6%) and the simultaneous emission of several γ-rays are not ideal for positron emission tomography, it could be a suitable alternative for ^{99m}Tc due to the fact that it does not demand for development of new radiopharmaceutical labeling methods

For the production of ^{94m}Tc, several routes have been investigated including proton-, deuteron-, ^{3}He- and α-particle-induced reactions on natural and enriched Mo as well as on ^{93}Nb. With regard to a possible clinical use, the (p,n) reaction on enriched ^{94}Mo targets appears to be the most promising, because it provides the highest yields at a rather low incident energy below 15 MeV. However, only few research groups worked on this topic, and the nuclear data measurements on that reaction are inconsistent [125–128].

2.2.11.16 ^{99m}Tc ($T_{½}$ = 6.0072 min)

This highly established SPECT radionuclide continues to be the most widely used radioisotope in nuclear medical imaging today [129]. A variety of ^{99m}Tc complexes have been established and described in more detail in the literature [42]), and the global consumption of this radionuclide was estimated to exceed 40 million scans per year in 2009 [130].

Up to date ^{99m}Tc is typically obtained from the in situ decay of ^{99}Mo on a ^{99}Mo/^{99m}Tc generator, which contains high specific activity ^{99}Mo embedded onto a small alumina column [22] allowing daily extraction of [^{99m}Tc]TcO_4^-

(cf. Sect. 2.3) The parent radionuclide is currently produced in nuclear reactors by the fission ^{235}U and the subsequent recovery of ^{99}Mo. The apprehension of shortage in the supply of this most important SPECT radionuclide [131, 132], due to possible shutdown of nuclear research reactors, has led to considerable scientific effort to develop alternative production methods for the parent radionuclide ^{99}Mo as well as the desired product ^{99m}Tc.

For the production of ^{99}Mo, several alternative routes are being considered [2]. One option would be the use of high-intensity γ-ray sources, enabling the photon-induced reactions $^{nat}U(\gamma,f)^{99}Mo$ and $^{100}Mo(\gamma,n)^{99}Mo$. However, further development of the production technology will be needed. A second alternative to the reactor-based production would be the utilization of fast or spallation neutrons, aiming either for the $^{100}Mo(n,2n)^{99}Mo$ reaction or the $^{nat}U(n,f)^{99}Mo$ and $^{232}Th(n,f)^{99}Mo$ reactions, respectively. These routes, however, demand intense fast or spallation neutron sources. Furthermore, the ^{99}Mo parent radionuclide can be produced by the charged-particle-induced reactions $^{100}Mo(p,pn)^{99}Mo$ and $^{100}Mo(d,p2n)^{99}Mo$. Reaction cross-sectional data on these processes were done [2]. Regarding all the above options, it should be pointed out that the production of ^{99}Mo from a ^{100}Mo target always leads to low specific activities.

In contrast to the production of ^{99}Mo discussed above, presently the direct production of ^{99m}Tc at a cyclotron has come into focus. The production reaction $^{100}Mo(p,2n)^{99m}Tc$ was first suggested by Beaver and Hupf in 1971 [133]. Over the last few years, a large number of measurements have been reported [2], and a critical evaluation of all data has been carried out [134]. From the evaluated excitation function of this reaction, the possible production yield of ^{99m}Tc over the suitable energy range of $E_p = 22 \rightarrow 10$ MeV was calculated as 700 MBq/μA h. Inspired by this promising results, the Canadian federal government initiated programs that have led to the development of large-scale production methods using small medical cyclotrons with proton energies of about 16.5 MeV [135, 136]. Figures 2.6 and 2.7 show a medical cyclotron and a Cu-Mo target disc for the large-scale production of ^{99m}Tc.

Despite the promising nature of the $^{100}Mo(p,2n)^{99m}Tc$ reaction, the formation of a higher level of radioactive and nonradioactive metallic impurities needs to be considered [2]. In particular the level of ^{99g}Tc and ^{98}Tc may exceed the critical value allowed by the present-day pharmacopeia rules, especially if incident proton energies above 20 MeV are used.

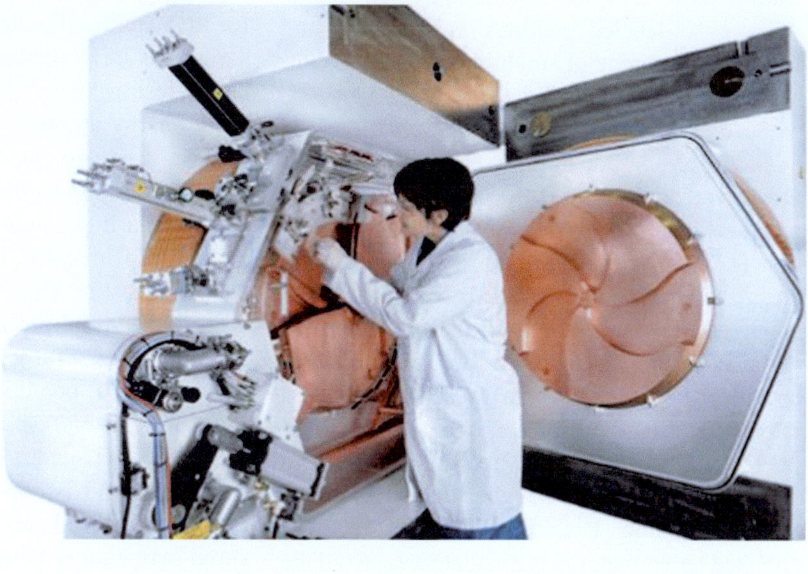

Fig. 2.6 GE PETtrace 800 cyclotron [136]

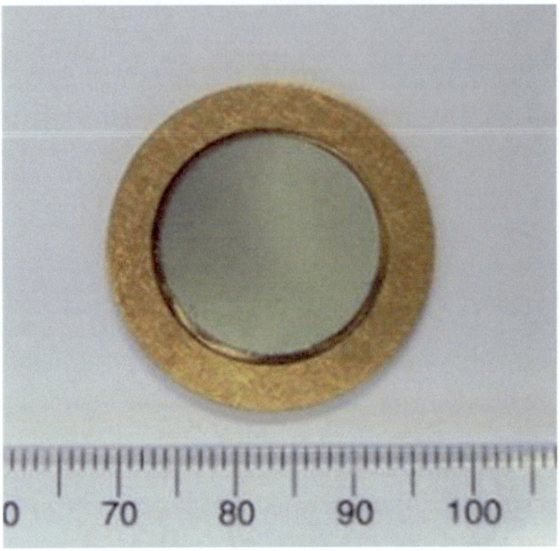

Fig. 2.7 Pressed-sintered and brazed Cu-Mo target disc for irradiation [136]

2.2.11.17 ^{111g}In ($T_{½}$ = 2.8047 Days)

Decaying solely via electron capture in combination with two γ-rays of 245.35 keV (94.1%) and 171.28 keV (90.6%), ^{111g}In is an important SPECT radionuclide. With its rather longer physical half-life, it is especially useful for radiolabeling of biomolecules with relatively slow in vivo kinetics and thus is often applied for radiolabeling of antibodies and peptides. The most prominent radiopharmaceutical up to date is OctreoScan® (cf. Sects. 2.3 and 2.5) used in somatostatin receptor scintigraphy. In recent years, ^{111g}In-labeled peptides were investigated for SPECT imaging of amyloid beta plaques connected to Alzheimer's disease [137].

Several production routes have been discussed including proton-, deuteron-, ^{3}He- and α-particle-induced reactions. The 1^{11}Cd(p,n) and ^{112}Cd(p,2n) reactions were finally recommended for production [138]. The (p,n) reaction has a maximum cross section of about 740 mb with protons of about 12 MeV, thus allowing the production of ^{111g}In in sufficient amounts at small medical cyclotrons. The ^{112}Cd(p,2n) reaction shows a maximum cross section of about 986 mb at 20 MeV. Utilizing the (p,2n) reaction leads to yields about three times higher compared to the yield using the 1^{11}Cd(p,n) reaction. Use of enriched target material is mandatory to avoid the formation of the longer-lived isotopic impurity ^{114m}In ($T_{½}$ = 49.51 days).

2.2.11.18 ^{123}I ($T_{½}$ = 13.2235 h) and ^{124}I ($T_{½}$ = 4.18 Days)

The physical and chemical properties of iodine make the radioisotopes ^{123}I and ^{124}I very attractive for radiolabeling of pharmaceutical compounds. The radioisotope ^{123}I decays exclusively via electron capture, having its most intensive γ-ray at 158.97 keV (83.3%), what makes it an ideal SPECT nuclide. At present the preferred route for ^{123}I production is bombardment of highly enriched ^{124}Xe gas with medium energy protons of 30–35 MeV incident energy. The triggered ^{124}Xe(p,2n)^{123}Cs reaction allows taking advantage of the subsequent decay chain ^{123}Cs → ^{123}Xe → ^{123}I. After irradiation the gas target is allowed to cool for several hours ensuring optimal in-growth of ^{123}I from its precursors. The produced radioiodine can then be rinsed from the target vessel with aqueous solution as described in detail by Coenen et al. [139]. The cross-sectional maximum of the reaction involved occurs around 25 MeV [140]. The direct production of ^{123}I via α-particle-induced reactions on antimony has been investigated more recently by Hassan et al. showing that its production is possible but the resulting radionuclide yields are low [141].

The radionuclide **^{124}I** (β^+ = 22.0%) is not ideal for PET studies, but detailed PET phantom measurements have shown that it is able to provide better results than ^{86}Y-PET [142]. The β^+ endpoint energy amounts to 2.13 MeV, and several γ-rays are also associated with its decay. Nevertheless, up-to-date γ-ray scattering corrections make it possible to use ^{124}I even in small animal PET imaging. The radionuclide is widely used in targeting tumor cells as well as in thyroid dosimetry. Initial production of ^{124}I involves the reaction route ^{124}Te(d,2n)^{124}I. Later on, cross sections of other potential nuclear reactions, i.e., ^{124}Te(p,n)^{124}I, ^{125}Te(p,2n)^{124}I, ^{126}Te(p,3n)^{124}I, as well as of ^{3}He- and α-particle-induced reactions on natural and isotopically enriched antimony, i.e., ^{nat}Sb(α,xn)^{124}I and ^{123}Sb(α,3n)^{124}I, were measured over energy ranges of up to 100 MeV. The alternative production route via the α-particle-induced reaction on ^{121}Sb, $^{121}Sb(\alpha,n)^{124}I$ also results in a high-purity product. However, due to the low batch yield, this method did not find much practical application [143]. It was concluded that the $^{124}Te(p,n)^{124}I$ reaction using highly enriched target material in the proton energy range of 12 → 8 MeV is the most suitable for the production of ^{124}I [144]. The mean nuclear reaction cross section in this energy range is not very high, but experimental studies and theoretical calculations showed that the product obtained is of the highest radionuclidic purity. Especially the longer-lived radioimpurity ^{125}I ($T_{½}$ = 60.0 days), which is mainly produced via the (p,γ) reaction, is lower than 0.1%. Today, after clinical upscaling batch yields of a few GBq are obtained via the $^{124}Te(p,n)^{124}I$ process. The produced ^{124}I can be radiochemically separated from the enriched [^{124}Te]TeO_2 target material using a dry distillation process. The product obtained is in (basic) iodide form which is very suitable for subsequent radiosynthesis procedures. The enriched target material can be recovered nearly quantitatively for reuse.

2.2.11.19 ^{125}I ($T_{½}$ = 59.407 Days) and ^{131}I ($T_{½}$ = 8.0252 Days)

Radioactive ^{131}I is the first radionuclide ever used clinically (1940s) for the treatment of thyroid cancer, and its success had served as a platform of motivation for further investigations on new therapeutic radionuclides in nuclear medicine. Na[^{131}I]I is the most commonly used for the treatment of thyroid-related diseases like hyperthyroidism due to toxic diffuse goiter (Graves' disease) but is also applied for different kinds of thyroid cancer [145]. As meta-[^{131}I]iodobenzylguanidine ([^{131}I]MIBG), it is used for imaging and treating pheochromocytoma and neuroblastoma [146].

^{131}I is produced either by neutron irradiation of [^{235}U]UAl_3 via the (n, fission) process or by neutron irradiation of ^{130}Te via the (n,γ) reaction in nuclear reactors. However, due to the need of sophisticated equipment and waste handling facilities, the former method has been abandoned, and now the bulk production is carried

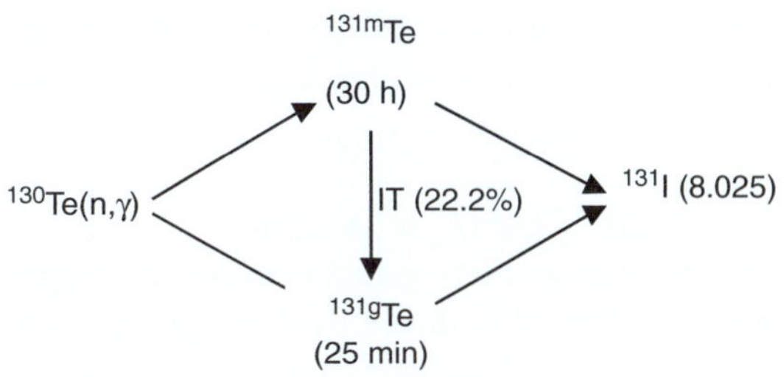

Fig. 2.8 Production scheme of ^{131}I

out by the latter route. Today, the production of ^{131}I is well established, and numerous radioiodinated compounds are available [139]. The target material for irradiation can be either Te in metallic form if the wet distillation method is employed or TeO_2 if the dry distillation method is applied [147]. By the neutron irradiation of ^{130}Te, both metastable and ground state of ^{131}Te are formed which further decay by β^--particle emission into ^{131}I (Fig. 2.8).

^{131}I decays with β^- emission with a maximum β^- energy of 610 keV (89%) and γ-ray emission with principle gamma energy of 364 keV (81%). The latter emission can contribute to unwanted whole-body radiation burden, and hence it is very important to adapt dosimetric approaches to precisely determine the amount of ^{131}I dose to be injected into a patient at various stages of the treatment.

The radioactive iodine-isotope ^{125}**I**, on the other hand, also finds clinical application in brachytherapy [148]. In recent years, computed tomography (CT)-guided ^{125}I seed implantation has received much attention in the field of medical science. It is a minimally invasive technique that ensures protracted cell killing over a period of several months through targeted delivery of high-dose radiation [149].

The decay of ^{125}I via pure electron capture (100%) leads to the intensive emission of soft X-rays as well as Auger and conversion electrons, and whereas the electrons cannot leave the implanted seeds, the emitted X-rays allow for the use of this radionuclide for therapy. Although proton- and α-particle-induced reactions have been investigated for direct production, the indirect reactor-based production via the $(n,\gamma)^{125}Xe(EC) \rightarrow {}^{125}I$ process is by far the most effective method, leading to good yields and highest specific activity.

2.2.11.20 ^{147}Gd ($T_{½}$ = 38.06 h)

The development of a gadolinium-based imaging agent for SPECT is driven by the ongoing development of hybrid scanners (bimodal imaging systems). In spite of its toxicity, there are a few clinically approved contrast agents for MRI, i.e., Gd-1,4,7,10-tetraazacyclododecane-1,4,7,10-tetraacetic acid (Gd-DOTA) [DOTArem®, Guerbet, France] and Gd-diethylenetriaminepentaacetic acid (Gd-DTPA) [Magnevist®, Bayer Healthcare, Germany]. Although both complexes possess very high thermodynamic stability constants (>1020) and a high degree of kinetic inertness, complications in using these contrast agents are possible, like the rare disease of necrosis systemic fibrosis (NSF) in patients with kidney insufficiency [150]. The radiosynthesis of an authentic SPECT or PET tracer would be a valuable amend to this technology.

The only radioisotope of Gd with a physical half-life suitable for in vivo studies is ^{147}Gd. The emitted high-intensity γ-rays of this radioisotope have higher (rather suboptimal) energies which are still useful for SPECT. Unfortunately, only few studies describe the examination of the production and separation of ^{147}Gd until now. This owes to the intermediate particle energies or uncommon projectile types needed for the production. The necessary radiochemistry for the isolation of ^{147}Gd is, as in the case of most lanthanides, rather complex, but Denzler et al. [151] and Nayak et al. [152] published the successful separation procedures of no-carrier-added radiogadolinium. In Table 2.8 an overview of the possible production routes of ^{147}Gd is given.

Table 2.8 Possible nuclear reactions for the production of ^{147}Gd

Reaction channel	Threshold (MeV)	Reference
$^{151}Eu(p,5n)^{147}Gd$	32.6	West et al. [153]
$^{151}Eu(d,6n)^{147}Gd$	35.0	Takács et al. [154]
$^{153}Eu(p,7n)^{147}Gd$	47.5	Takács et al. [153]
$^{153}Eu(d,8n)^{147}Gd$	50.1	Takács et al. [154]

2.2.11.21 ^{153}Sm ($T_{½}$ = 46.284 h)

This soft β^--emitter (100%) finds popular application in internal radiotherapy/endoradiotherapy, especially in the palliative treatment of bone metastases it substitutes meanwhile ^{90}Y and ^{32}P. It is mainly used in form of EDTMP (ethylenediamino-tetrakis-methylenediphosphonic acid), also known as samarium (^{153}Sm) lexidronam or by its trade name Quadramet®.

The radionuclide is commonly produced in a nuclear reactor via the $^{152}Sm(n,\gamma)^{153}Sm$ reaction. Because of the relatively high-reaction cross section of 473 mb (30 keV spectrum temperature) [155], the radionuclide yield is high, but the specific activity is limited due to the isotopic target material. Due to the demand for this radionuclide, coordinated research was realized to optimize its production [156]. More recently alternative production routes, i.e., the reactions $^{153}Eu(n,p)^{153}Sm$ and $^{150}Nd(\alpha,n)^{153}Sm$, were investigated, to assess their potential for the production of high molar/specific activity ^{153}Sm [157]. However, the resulting production yields using these nuclear reactions are too low for efficient medical application.

2.2.11.22 ^{177}Lu ($T_{½}$ = 6.647 Days)

^{177}Lu is a widely used radionuclide for targeted endoradiotherapy in nuclear medicine (cf. Sect. 2.5). It emits several β^- particles with maximum energies of 498.3 keV (79.4%), 385.4 keV (9.0%), and 177.0 keV (11.61%) and low-abundance, low-energy γ-rays (113 keV (6.6%) and 208 keV (11%)) which make it also suitable for in vivo imaging and quantification of radiotracers.

^{177}Lu is produced in nuclear reactors either directly by neutron irradiation of natural Lu or enriched ^{176}Lu or indirectly by first neutron irradiation of natural or enriched Yb leading to the formation of ^{177}Yb followed by its decays into ^{177}Lu: $^{176}Yb(n,\gamma)^{177}Yb \rightarrow {}^{177}Lu$. The latter indirect production route has a disadvantage over the direct production route due the lower neutron reaction cross section (2.5 barns) as compared to the direct route via the $^{176}Lu(n,\gamma)^{177}Lu$ reaction (ca. 2100 barns) [158]. Due to this very high cross section, ^{177}Lu can be produced at research reactors in bulk quantities with very high specific activities, which can be shipped globally. However, unlike the indirect production route starting from ^{176}Yb, this high yielding route also produces small amounts (<1%) of the long-lived isomeric contaminant ^{177m}Lu ($T_{½}$ = 160.44 days). Hermanne et al. [159] and Manenti et al. [160] have also reported the possibility of deuteron-induced production of ^{177}Lu with a cyclotron; however, this method is not suitable for large-scale production due to the poor nuclear reaction cross section.

Owing to the multiple preclinical studies and clinical trials in the last few decades, ^{177}Lu has been proved as one of the most successful candidates for treatment of various cancer types. Several publications have already established the important role of ^{177}Lu and its application in nuclear medicine [161]. Recently, Kratochwil et al. have shown the successful application of ^{177}Lu for therapy of prostate cancer metastases [162]. It is highly expected that in the near future, ^{177}Lu will be a competing radionuclide similar to already clinically established ^{131}I (cf. Sect. 2.5.4.1, VISION trial).

2.2.11.23 ^{186}Re ($T_{½}$ = 3.7183 Days) and ^{188}Re ($T_{½}$ = 17.0040 h)

The radionuclide ^{186}**Re** shows two different decay paths: one via emission of soft β^--particles (92.53%) to the stable daughter ^{186}W and the other via electron capture to the primordial nuclide ^{186}Os. Those decay characteristics identify it as a potential agent for internal radiotherapy/endoradiotherapy, which was discussed for palliative treatment of bone metastases in the late 1980s. ^{186}Re was used as HEDP ([^{186}Re]Re-1,1-hydroxyethylidene-diphosphonate) in phase-III clinical trials in 2002 [163]. Due to its physical half-life, ^{188}Re also lends itself for the radiolabeling of antibodies.

The intensities of the weak γ-rays emitted during the decay were remeasured by Miyahara et al. [164], and there is optimism that the uptake of this therapeutic radionuclide could be quantified through SPECT imaging using these γ-ray emission [165]. The chemistry of Re is similar to that of Tc; however, the tendency of rhenium complexes toward reoxidation leading to the presence of high radiochemical impurities in the final product makes the development of rhenium radiopharmaceuticals more challenging [166].

^{186}Re is one of the radionuclides that can be prepared in nuclear reactors with reasonably high specific activities via the (n,γ) reaction by using enriched target material [167]. The production of ^{186}Re in no-carrier-added form has hitherto been investigated using two accelerator-driven methods, namely $^{186}W(p,n)^{186}Re$ and $^{186}W(d,2n)^{186}Re$. A critical analysis of data [168] showed that, for obtaining a high-purity product, an enriched ^{186}W target is absolutely necessary. The calculated yield of ^{186}Re from the evaluated excitation function of the $^{186}W(p,n)^{186}Re$ reaction amounts to 4.4 MBq/μA h (E_p = 18 → 8 MeV) and from the $^{186}W(d,2n)^{186}Re$ reaction to 15.8 MBq/μA h (E_d = 18 → 8 MeV). A clinical upscale production using a cyclotron has hitherto not been reported [96].

Like its isotope the radionuclide ^{188}Re is highly suitable for radiotherapeutic applications as well. In analogy to ^{186}Re, different radiotracers, like [^{188}Re]Re-HEDP, have been synthesized and clinically evaluated. ^{188}Re is a pure β^- emitter, and although its main beta energies of 2118 keV and 1962 keV are significantly higher than those of its sister isotope, ^{188}Re comes with the advantage of being a potential generator nuclide.

For the production of ^{188}Re, the $^{188}W/^{188}Re$ generator was described already in 1966 by Lewis and Eldridge [169]. Present systems of this generator are mainly based on the separation chemistry similar to that of the $^{99}Mo/^{99m}Tc$ generator and include the adsorption of tungstic acid at an alumina-based matrix [170]. The production of the parent radionuclide ^{188}W might be a limiting factor, as it is achieved by double neutron capture of enriched ^{186}W via the route $^{186}W(n,\gamma)^{187}W(n,\gamma)^{188}W$. This process calls for the availability of a high-flux reactor and even then produces only a modest specific activity of about 180 GBq/g [170].

2.2.11.24 ^{193m}Pt ($T_{½}$ = 4.3 Days) and ^{195m}Pt ($T_{½}$ = 4.010 Days)

Platinum complexes, e.g., cisplatin, have been used in chemotherapy as potent antitumor agents since late 1970s. Therefore, the pure X-ray and Auger electron emitters ^{193m}Pt and ^{195m}Pt have great potential in Auger electron therapy. For example, each decay of ^{193m}Pt leads to more than 30 secondary electrons with kinetic energies ranging between 10 and 130 keV [2]. A major impediment for its widespread use, however, is its nonavailability with high specific activity.

Regarding ^{193m}Pt, the product yield using the ^{192}Pt(n,γ)^{193m}Pt reaction is very satisfactory; however, the specific activity is low even while using enriched target material. The production via the ^{192}Os(α,3n)^{193m}Pt reaction on a highly enriched target appears to be very promising [171] to solve this problem. Due to the favorable population of the high-spin (13/2+) ^{193m}Pt, the cross section of the reaction is high showing a maximum of about 1500 mb at 36 MeV. Over the energy range E_{α} = 40 → 30 MeV, the yield of ^{193m}Pt amounts to 10 MBq/μA h. Regarding the production data, there is considerable need of new measurements as well as of evaluation of the existing data [2, 172]

Similar to its lighter isotope, the radioisomer ^{195m}Pt can be produced only with low specific activity via ^{194}Pt(n,γ)^{195m}Pt reaction [172]. Takács et al. showed that the production using a 35 MeV α-particle beam on an iridium target, i.e., via the ^{nat}Ir(a,x)^{195m}Pt reaction, provides a pure product with high specific activity; however, the cross sections proved to be low [173]. Alternatively ^{195m}Pt could be produced via the double neutron capture following the route ^{193}Ir(n,γ)^{194}Ir(n,γ)^{195m}Ir → ^{195m}Pt. However, this route needs additional experimental investigation before it can be thoroughly evaluated.

2.2.11.25 ^{211}At ($T_{½}$ = 7.214 h)

Among the α-emitting radionuclides which are connected with targeted endoradiotherapy, ^{211}At probably is the most versatile based on its physical half-life, decay scheme, and chemistry [174, 175]. ^{211}At decays via electron capture (58.20%) and α-particle emission (41.80%) with very little γ-ray emission (<1%). Being a halogen, it can often be incorporated into biomolecules of interest by adapting radioiodination chemistry. A wide spectrum of compounds from the simple [^{211}At]astatide ion to small organic molecules, peptides, and large proteins radiolabeled with ^{211}At have been investigated [176]. However, the use of ^{211}At is constrained on the one hand by its rather short physical half-life excluding slow metabolic processes to be targeted and on the other hand by its limited availability.

^{211}At can be produced in reasonable yield from natural bismuth targets via the ^{209}Bi(α,2n)^{211}At nuclear reaction [177]. The excitation function of this reaction has been well determined over the past seven decades indicating a maximum cross section of about 950 mb at 31 MeV α-particle energy. Hermanne et al. investigated the optimum incident particle energy for maximizing the ^{211}At yield while minimizing production of ^{210}At and ^{210}Po [178]. They concluded that the α-particle energy should be limited to 29 MeV to avoid the formation of contaminants and producing about 32 MBq/μA h ^{211}At. Although the number of capable cyclotrons is currently increasing, the need of a medium energy α-particle beam up to 30 MeV for its production poses an impediment.

2.2.11.26 ^{225}Ac (9.9203 Days)

^{225}Ac is a pure α-particle emitter (100%) and decays into several daughter radionuclides, of which the α-particle emitter ^{213}Bi ($T_{½}$ = 45.59 min; E_{α} = 5875 keV) is the most important. Both radionuclides are very promising candidates for targeted alpha therapy (TAT). ^{225}Ac has found a relevant place in targeted alpha-immunotherapy [179] and prostate-specific membrane antigen (PSMA)-TAT for the treatment of metastatic castration-resistant prostate cancer (mCRPC) with [^{225}Ac]Ac-PSMA-617 [180]. Figure 2.9 shows the decay chain of ^{225}Ac.

Notwithstanding, the rather low amount of radioactivity which is needed because of the potency of α-particle emitters for endoradiotherapy, the production of ^{225}Ac faces some challenges.

Currently, all available ^{225}Ac for preclinical and clinical trials is produced from "milking"

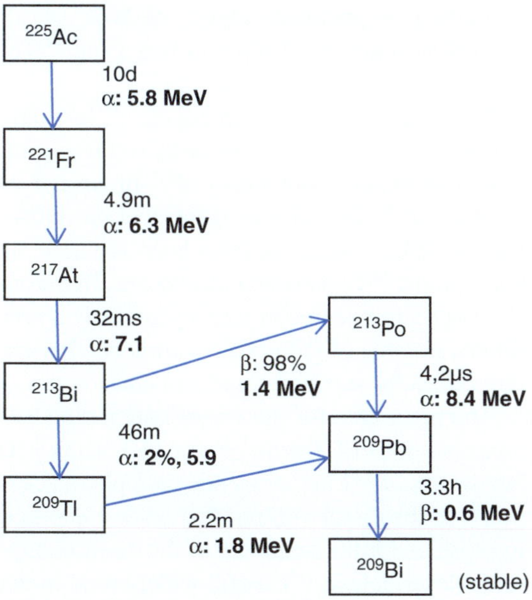

Fig. 2.9 Radioactive decay chain of ^{225}Ac

^{229}Th ($T_{1/2}$ = 7340 a) which is isolated either from nuclear waste or as the decay product of ^{233}U. The latter is obtained from the (n,γ)-reaction on ^{232}Th and the follow-up of two subsequent β^--decays. In the 1960s ^{233}U was produced mainly in the USA up to one ton, and since then ca. 4 × 1011 Bq of ^{229}Th were built up from it. However, today the irradiation of ^{232}Th with neutrons in order to produce ^{233}U almost stopped [181].

Presently, extensive effort is being devoted to the production of ^{225}Ac. On the one hand, its separation from nuclear waste has been optimized [182] and, on the other, two accelerator-driven nuclear routes, namely ^{226}Ra(p,2n)^{225}Ac and ^{232}Th(p,spall)^{225}Ac, have been investigated: Apostolidis et al. [183] reported a successful approach of producing about 480 MBq of ^{225}Ac by irradiation of radioactive ^{226}Ra (ca. 30 mg) with 16.5 MeV protons with a medical cyclotron. The calculated yield via the spallation process amounts to about 4 MBq/µA h (E_p = 140 → 60 MeV) [184].

Another approach was shown in 2007 by Melville et al. [185] for the production of ^{225}Ac in MBq quantity by photon-induced transmutation of ^{226}Ra via ^{226}Ra(γ,n)^{225}Ra with an 18 MV electron linear accelerator. This reaction produces ^{225}Ra, which subsequently decays to ^{225}Ac through beta decays. These modern alternative production routes require further experimental research work, but the continuous effort in this field ensures a bulk production of ^{225}Ac independent of ^{229}Th in coming years.

2.2.11.27 ^{223}Ra ($T_{½}$ = 11.43 Days) and ^{224}Ra ($T_{½}$ = 3.6319 Days)

The radionuclide ^{223}Ra is a pure (100%) α-particle emitter. Its importance has grown in recent years, and it is approved under the tradename XOFIGO® for use in the form of [^{223}Ra]RaCl$_2$ injection solution. It is used for the treatment of blood cancer and especially for the treatment of mCRPC with bone metastases. In contrast to the use of ^{223}Ra in chloride form, the delivery of ^{223}Ra to cancer cells in radioimmunotherapy for treating soft tissue malignancies requires a suitable bifunctional chelating agent. Ionizable calixarene crown ether ionophores were found to exhibit high selectivity for radium over lighter alkaline earth metal ions [186]. Moreover, ^{223}Ra is used as a generator for the production of ^{211}Pb [187]. The radium isotope ^{224}Ra has been used for clinical applications as well, especially for palliative treatment [188]. The use of this radionuclide is less common due to its limited availability. The enhanced use of radium for therapeutic application is hampered by the difficulty of synthesizing in vivo stable bifunctional chelating agents for this element [188].

^{223}Ra can be obtained $_{\beta}$via the chain ^{226}Ra(n,γ)^{227}Ra (42.2 min) $\xrightarrow{\beta-}$ ^{227}Ac (21.8 a) $\xrightarrow{\beta-}$ ^{223}Ra or via the decay of ^{235}U. However, the ^{227}Ac activity is available only in limited quantity. In view of the increasing significance of this radionuclide, a potentially interesting production route involving the irradiation of ^{232}Th with intermediate energy protons was recently investigated [184]. Another production source of ^{223}Ra involves ^{227}Ac and ^{227}Th isolation from ^{231}Pa ($T_{1/2}$ = 32,760 years). A miniaturized production scale of the ^{223}Ra generator has been established utilizing traces of ^{227}Ac (kBq scale) produced as a by-product from cyclotron production of ^{225}Ac. This method provides a supply of ^{223}Ra in amounts sufficient for preclinical studies [189].

Due to the scarcity of ^{227}Ac, a highly efficient radiochemical separation method for obtaining high-purity ^{223}Ra from ^{227}Ac and recovering the parent radionuclide was developed utilizing ion exchange resins [190, 191]. A novel approach for the application of ^{223}Ra is the production using an in vivo generator system based on the administration of complexed ^{227}Th [192].

The radioisotope ^{224}Ra can either be produced using the proton-induced reaction on thorium, i.e., the ^{232}Th(p,x)^{224}Ra reaction, or via the ^{223}Ra(n,γ)^{224}Ra process at a nuclear reactor.

2.3 Clinically Relevant SPECT Tracers

The radionuclides most often used for SPECT applications, ^{99m}Tc, ^{111}In, and ^{123}I, are summarized in Table 2.9.

The key advantages of ^{99m}Tc, such as its physical decay characteristics, on-demand availability by commercially available radionuclide ^{99}Mo/^{99m}Tc-generators, kit preparations of the radiopharmaceuticals, and lower cost, overshadow the possible use of ^{111}In- or ^{123}I-labeled radiotracers. Furthermore, the rich coordination chemistry of technetium allows incorporation of this transition radiometal into a wide variety of ligands stabilizing the radionuclide at different oxidation states such as +5, +3, and +1. Thus, many ^{99m}Tc-radiopharmaceuticals have been developed, and some have gained significant clinical relevance and market success. Even though nuclear medicine diagnostic scans by means of PET/CT and PET/MRI have gained increasing importance, about 70–80% of all diagnostic scans are still performed using ^{99m}Tc-labeled radiopharmaceuticals [193].

Table 2.9 Radionuclides most frequently used for SPECT and their decay modes

Nuclide	$T_{1/2}$	Decay mode (% abundance)	Photon emission (keV) (% abundance)
^{99m}Tc	6.0 h	IT (100)	141 (87%)
^{111}In	2.83 days	EC (100)	247 (94%); 173 (91%)
^{123}I	13.1 h	EC (100)	159 (83%); 528 (1.4%)

In contrast, fully approved ^{111}In- and ^{123}I-labeled SPECT radiopharmaceuticals are rare. The imaging properties of ^{111}In are not as good as for ^{99m}Tc and thus agents that prove useful for SPECT imaging have been replaced by appropriate ^{99m}Tc-labeled radiotracers. Therefore it is not a surprise that in recent years only a very limited number of ^{111}In-labeled compounds were introduced for use in nuclear medicine.

The main area for the use of radioiodine isotopes is not SPECT with ^{123}I (or PET using ^{124}I) but the use of ^{131}I in therapeutic radiopharmaceuticals, starting with sodium [^{131}I]iodide composed in capsules for the treatment of the diseased thyroid. Nevertheless, ^{123}I is still widely used in the development of new tracers. Because of the necessity of crossing the blood-brain barrier (BBB), the majority of CNS ligands are radiolabeled with the halogen ^{123}I, in order to avoid major alterations of the unlabeled lead structures which would occur after introduction of chelating moieties which are used to bind radiometals such as ^{99m}Tc and ^{111}In.

As follows basic aspects of the radiopharmaceutical chemistry of ^{99m}Tc, ^{111}In, and ^{123}I will be described and illustrated by selected examples of clinically relevant radiotracers.

2.3.1 Technetium-99m (^{99m}Tc)

2.3.1.1 ^{99}Mo/^{99m}Tc-Generator

^{99m}Tc decays with a physical half-life of 6.0 h by isomeric transition to ^{99g}Tc, thereby emitting a single photon with an energy of 141 keV. This energy almost ideally meets the sensitivity maximum of modern SPECT camera systems. Another advantage is the low radiation burden to patients due its short physical half-life. Furthermore, the decay within hours also facilitates the handling of radioactive waste. However, the main reason for the special role of technetium in nuclear medicine is probably the cost-effectiveness and the on-demand availability of the radiometal through the ^{99}Mo/^{99m}Tc generator system (cf. Sect. 2.2.6). The cross section of a typical ^{99}Mo/^{99m}Tc generator is given in Fig. 2.10. The eluant (physiological saline, 0.9% NaCl in water) is driven by vacuum-driven elution of the saline solution through a small chromatography column, which is loaded with [^{99}Mo]molybdate by an evacuated eluation (normally 10 mL) vial. Typically, the [^{99}Mo]molybdate is bound strongly to the aluminum oxide matrix used as the solid phase. The radioactive daughter nuclide ^{99m}Tc is eluted in the chemical form of sodium [^{99m}Tc]pertechnetate (Na[^{99m}Tc]TcO_4), which is weakly bound on Al_2O_3 so that it is easily eluted with saline. After elution, the ^{99m}Tc activity will regrow (transient equilibrium) to close to its maximum value within ca. 24 h (Fig. 2.11). After 5 days the nominal ^{99}Mo activity ($T_{1/2}$ = 66 h) will be around one-fifth of the initial activity, and usually ^{99}Mo/^{99m}Tc generators will be replaced on a weekly schedule.

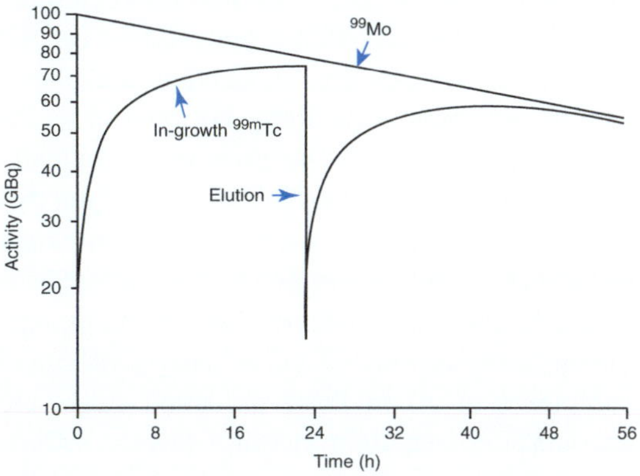

Fig. 2.11 Elution profile of a ^{99}Mo/^{99m}Tc generator

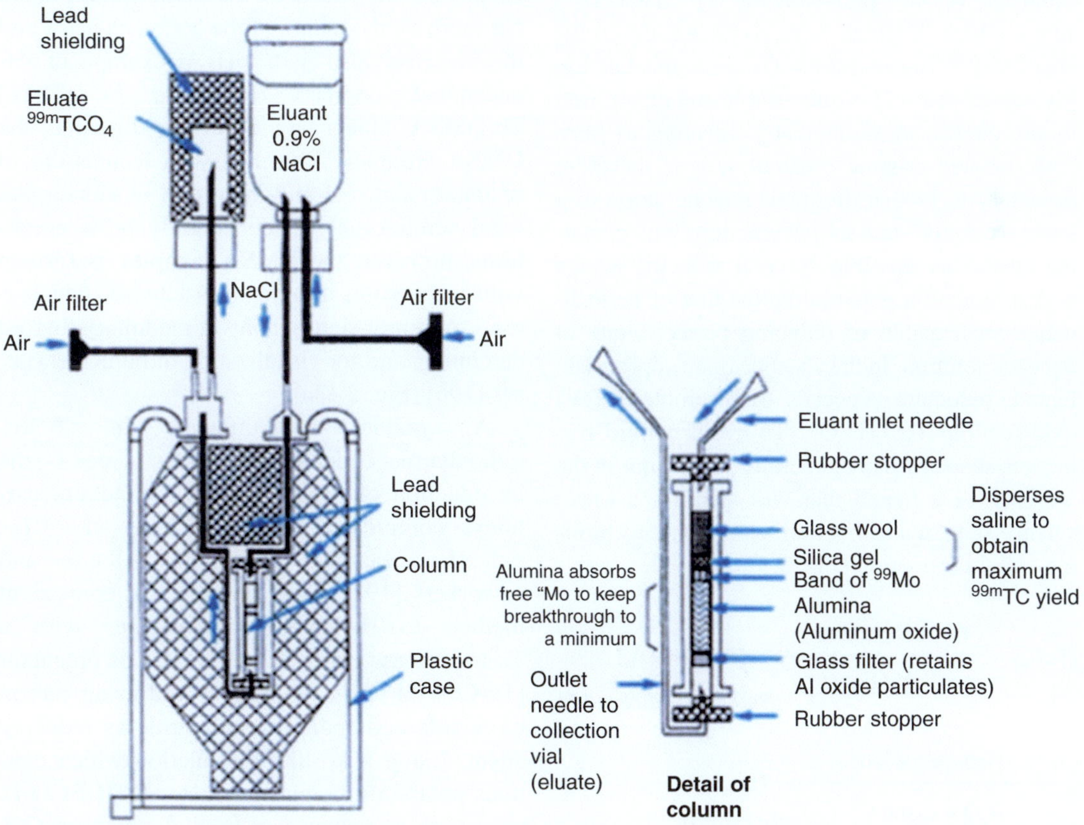

Fig. 2.10 Cross section of a typical ^{99}Mo/^{99m}Tc generator

2.3.1.2 Basic Aspects of ^{99m}Tc-Radiopharmaceutical Chemistry

The transitional metal technetium (element 43) is located in the seventh subgroup of the periodic system of elements and is located between manganese and rhenium of the same subgroup. All technetium isotopes are radioactive, and therefore this element is naturally not present in the earth's crust. It has to be prepared technically (this fact led to the name "technetium"), and this fact of course delayed the chemical development of technetium until the respective technology was available. As with manganese and rhenium, oxidation states between +7 and −1 are possible, and complexes at all of these oxidation states are known. However, their stability greatly differs, and therefore in radiopharmaceuticals the oxidation states +5, +3, and +1 are dominant [194].

The basis for all ^{99m}Tc-labeled radiopharmaceuticals is the pertechnetate ([^{99m}Tc]TcO_4^-) anion, which is eluted from commercially available ^{99}Mo/^{99m}Tc generators. The pertechnetate ion [oxidation state +7] is quite stable and rather inert to any coordination chemistry. In order to form ^{99m}Tc-labeled organic molecules, it is therefore necessary to reduce the pertechnetate anion to a lower oxidation state so that reactions with chelating agents are possible. Several reducing agents with a reduction potential below that of pertechnetate are capable of reducing pertechnetate in aqueous solution. In the absence of an appropriate ligand, reduction proceeds to insoluble Tc(IV) oxide/colloid $TcO_2(H_2O)_x$. To avoid colloid formation, reductions are generally carried out in the presence of a ligand that will stabilize a lower valence state of a technetium complex, thus limiting colloid formation (Fig. 2.12).

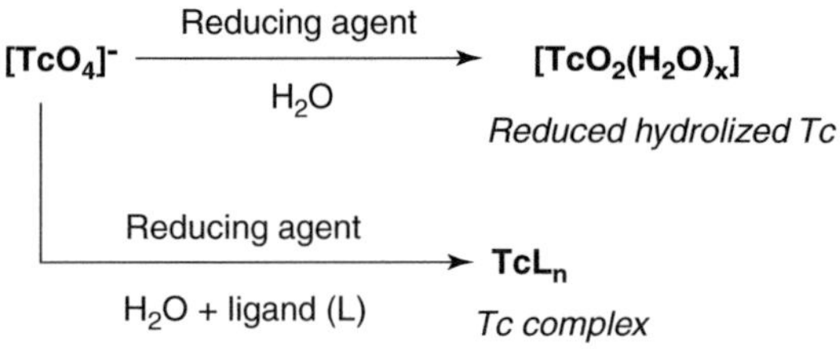

Fig. 2.12 General principle of reduction and complex formation starting from pertechnetate

A variety of reducing agents have been used for pertechnetate reduction such as ferric chloride, ascorbic acid, or sodium dithionite. However, stannous(II) ions are commonly used in all commercial kit preparations as they are nontoxic, water soluble, and stable when lyophilized.

Chelating agents possess several heteroatoms geometrically arranged in such a way that 5- or 6-membered rings are formed after binding to the ^{99m}Tc core [194, 195]. Optimal heteroatoms for binding of technetium are:

- Nitrogen (in amines, amides, imines, oximes, and aromatic rings)
- Sulfur (in thiols and thioethers)
- Phosphorus (in phosphines)
- Oxygen (in carboxylates, phenols, alcohols, enols, and phosphonates)

The oxidation state in the final complex is usually not dependent on the used reducing agent but more on the nature of the bound chelator and in some cases also on the pH. An example of pH-dependent complex formation is [^{99m}Tc]Tc-DMSA. Under slightly acidic condition, the DMSA complex is formed with technetium in oxidation state +3 and then used in kidney and renal scintigraphy. Under slightly basic conditions, however, the DMSA complex is formed with technetium in oxidation state +5, which is used for tumor scintigraphy of medullary thyroid carcinoma and for visualization of bone metastases [196] (Fig. 2.13a).

A major breakthrough in ^{99m}Tc-radiopharmaceutical chemistry was the introduction of organometallic technetium carbonyl complexes as a new kind of ^{99m}Tc-radiopharmaceutical design by Alberto and coworkers [197]. They developed a convenient method to radiolabel biomolecules with a Tc-tricarbonyl core [$^{99m}Tc(CO)_3$]$^+$. The precursor $[Tc(CO)_3(H_2O)_3]^+$ can be prepared using carbon monoxide and sodium borohydride as reducing agent. Using a kit-like formulation which contains potassium boranocarbonate ($K_2[H_3BCO_2]$), used both as reducing agent and source of CO, the precursor formation proceeds even more easily, reproducibly, and safely [198].

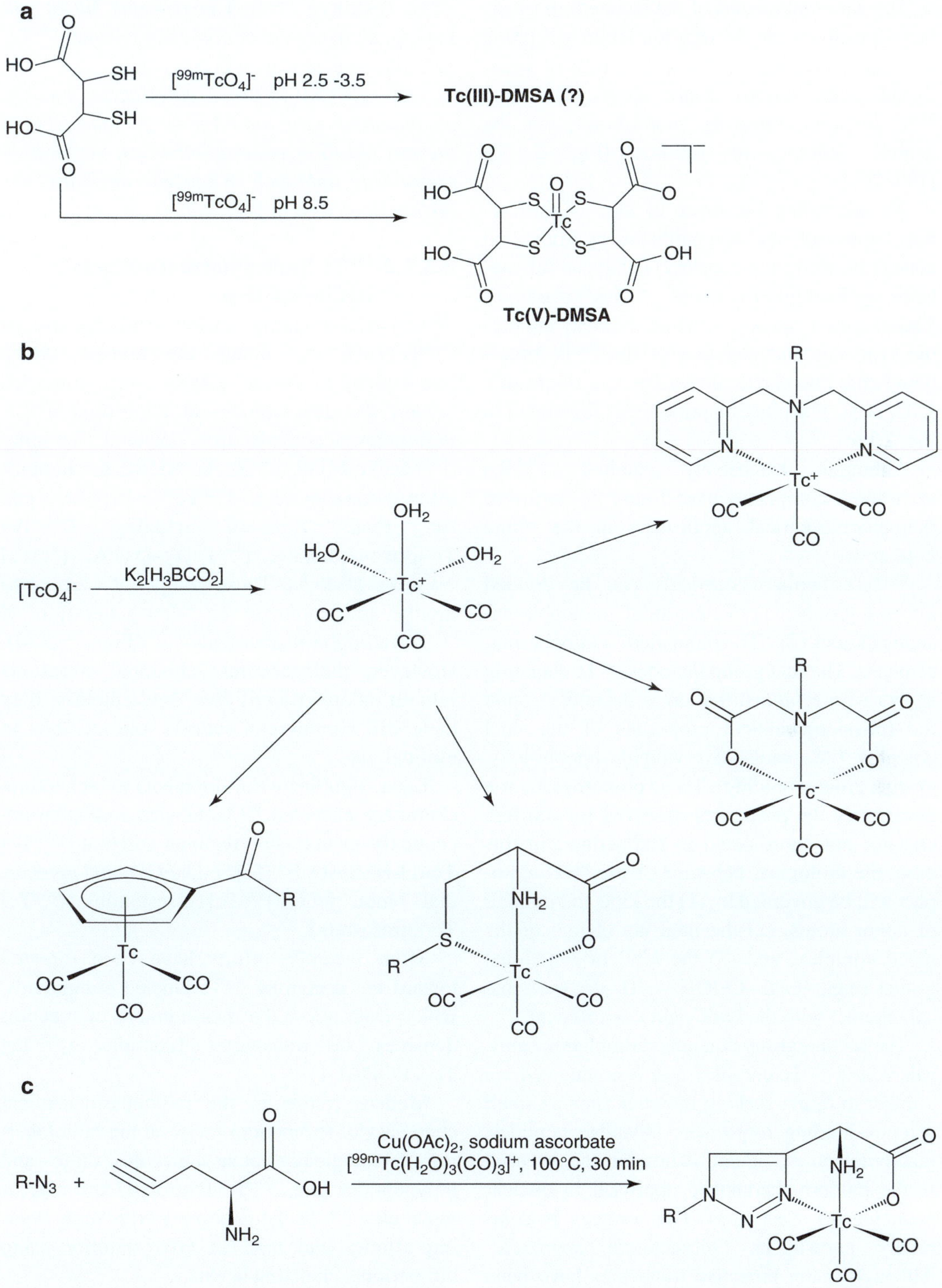

Fig. 2.13 (**a**) The pH value determines valence of reduced Tc and nature of formed complex in the case of ^{99m}Tc-DMSA (the structure of Tc-DMSA with technetium in oxidation state +3 is still unknown). (**b**) Selection of prototypic ^{99m}Tc tricarbonyl complexes starting from $[Tc(CO)_3(H_2O)_3]^+$. (**c**) "Click-to-chelate" approach: synthesis and insertion of the ^{99m}Tc tricarbonyl core into carrier molecules in a single step (R = e.g., small molecules, oligopeptides)

The water molecules of the technetium tricarbonyl precursor are substitution labile and prone to chelator exchange with a wide variety of donor ligands with varying donor atoms. The final ^{99m}Tc-tricarbonyl-bearing biomolecule can be neutral, anionic, or cationic (Fig. 2.13b) [199–201].

An interesting follow-up of the ^{99m}Tc tricarbonyl approach has been published by Mindt and coworkers using the copper(I)-catalyzed alkyne-azide cycloaddition (CuAAC, "click" reaction). The so-called "click-to-chelate" strategy enables the synthesis and insertion of the ^{99m}Tc tricarbonyl core into carrier molecules in a single step [202, 203]. The reaction principle is illustrated in Fig. 2.13c.

Although extensively studied, ^{99m}Tc-tricarbonyl complexes have found no approved radiopharmaceutical application in the clinic until now.

^{99m}Tc-radiopharmaceuticals can be divided into two groups: (1) "Tc-essential" radiopharmaceuticals and (2) "Tc-conjugated" radiopharmaceuticals. The first group includes ^{99m}Tc chelating agents whose biodistribution is dependent upon the (physico)chemical properties of the final complex (i.e., molecular weight, lipophilicity, charge, protein binding). These properties are not necessarily the properties observed for the free chelator not coordinated to technetium. In this case, the biological behavior of the ^{99m}Tc complex will be governed by (1) the kind and number of donor atoms, (2) the final net charge of the metal complex, and (3) the kind of functional groups (e.g., –OH, –COOH, $–NH_2$, –F, etc.) that can interact with the biological environment.

The second group contains radiopharmaceuticals whose ^{99m}Tc complex unit is conjugated via a linker to target-seeking moieties such as small receptor-binding molecules, bioactive peptides, macromolecules, or antibodies, nowadays used in the modern theranostic approach in nuclear medicine (cf. Sect. 2.5). This strategy is commonly known as "bifunctional approach." Although many bioactive molecules have been successfully conjugated with ^{99m}Tc, only a very small number of compounds could be translated into the clinic until now (e.g., ^{99m}Tc-TRODAT-1, ^{99m}Tc-Tektrotyd, ^{99m}Tc-Tilmanocept). In the following, an overview of clinically relevant ^{99m}Tc-radiopharmaceuticals will be given.

The relevant SPECT radiotracers used in combination with radiotracers for radioligand therapy (RLT) or endoradiotherapy, the modern theranostic approach in nuclear medicine, are further described in Sect. 2.5.

2.3.1.3 ^{99m}Tc-Radiopharmaceuticals in Clinical Use

^{99m}Tc-based imaging started with the use of $[^{99m}Tc]TcO_4^-$ to image the thyroid [204]. Subsequently, major efforts were directed toward the development of additional ^{99m}Tc-radiopharmaceuticals for skeletal imaging ([^{99m}Tc]Tc-MDP, [^{99m}Tc]Tc-HDP), for hepatobiliary imaging (e.g., [^{99m}Tc]Tc-EHIDA), and for renal function imaging ([^{99m}Tc]Tc-glucoheptonate, [^{99m}Tc]Tc-DTPA, [^{99m}Tc]Tc-meso-DMSA). These compounds are commonly apostrophized as "first-generation of ^{99m}Tc-radiopharmaceuticals" (Fig. 2.14). However, their absolute chemical structures remain unknown until now. Nevertheless, they have still commercial success and are thus in clinical use.

Later, significant developments in technetium chemistry provided ^{99m}Tc-labeled radiopharmaceuticals for assessing regional cerebral ([^{99m}Tc]Tc-d,l-HMPAO, [^{99m}Tc]Tc-l,l-ECD) and myocardial blood flow ([^{99m}Tc]Tc-sestamibi, [^{99m}Tc]Tc-tetrofosmin).

More recently, efforts have been directed toward the design of ^{99m}Tc-labeled compounds, which even allow the measurement of receptor densities or transporter functions ([^{99m}Tc]Tc-TRODAT-1).

Modern trends in the radiopharmaceutical chemistry of technetium focus on the radiolabeling of biologically active molecules, oligo- and polypeptides (e.g., ^{99m}Tc-Tektrotyd) and macromolecules (^{99m}Tc-Tilmanocept) with high binding affinity and high in vivo stability using bifunctional chelating agents.

Corresponding receptor-targeted ^{99m}Tc-radiotracers which can be used with radiotracers for radioligand therapy (RLT) (called

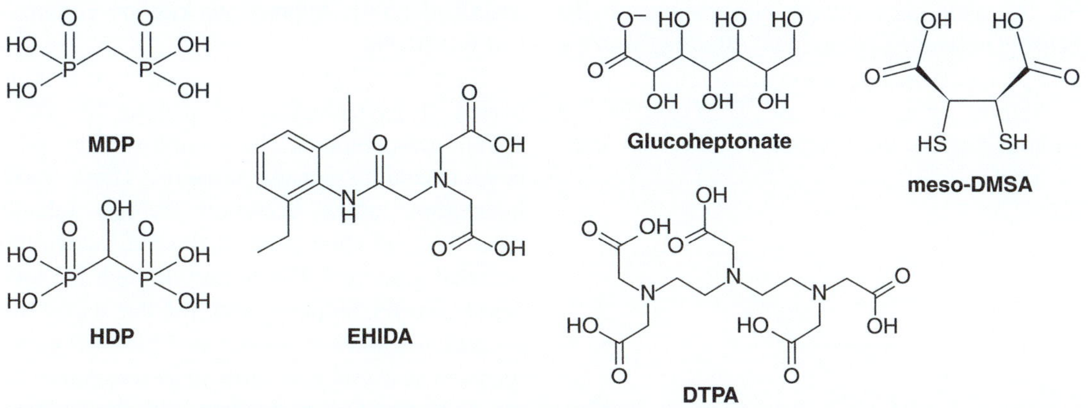

Fig. 2.14 Ligands forming ^{99m}Tc-radiopharmaceuticals for skeletal imaging ([^{99m}Tc]Tc-MDP, [^{99m}Tc]Tc-HDP), for hepatobiliary imaging ([^{99m}Tc]Tc-EHIDA), and for renal function imaging ([^{99m}Tc]Tc-glucoheptonate, [^{99m}Tc]Tc-DTPA, [^{99m}Tc]Tc-meso-DMSA)

endoradiotherapy) are further described in detail in Sect. 2.5 in which the modern theranostic approach in nuclear medicine is discussed.

2.3.1.4 Inorganic ^{99m}Tc- Compounds

Sodium [^{99m}Tc]pertechnetate

The first inorganic technetium compound used in nuclear medicine is the negatively charged technetium oxo complex sodium pertechnetate. Because of the similar size of iodide and pertechnetate ions, it can be used as a surrogate for iodide in the diagnosis of thyroid disorders. Pertechnetate addresses the Na^+/I^--symporter and therefore is actively transported into the thyroid [205]. Of course it does not participate at the thyroid hormone metabolism like iodide. However, the determination of the local iodide uptake (substituted by pertechnetate) is sufficient enough for almost all diagnostic indications. In addition, the radiation exposure on the patient is much lower than that obtained with sodium [^{123}I] iodide.

[^{99m}Tc]Tc_2S_7 ([^{99m}Tc]Technetium-Sulfur Colloid)

The physiological mechanism behind static liver scintigraphy using [^{99m}Tc]Tc-sulfur colloid is the rapid clearance by the reticuloendothelial system/monocyte-macrophage system. Uptake of the radioactive colloid by organs of the reticuloendothelial system is dependent on both their relative blood flow rates and the functional capacity of the phagocytic cells [206]. The preparation of the sulfur colloid is usually achieved by thiosulfate in acidic media as a source of sulfide ions which also serve as reductant.

^{99m}Tc on Carbon as Aerosol ([^{99m}Tc]Technegas)

The conversion of sodium [^{99m}Tc]pertechnetate at 2500 °C in the presence of crucible graphite leads to ^{99m}Tc on carbon as an aerosol. The particles have nm size. The aerosol is used for inhalation to perform lung ventilation studies. Therefore a special *Technegas generator* system is required for the aerosol formation [207].

2.3.1.5 ^{99m}Tc-Complexes

Imaging of Renal Excretion

[^{99m}Tc]Tc=O-mercaptoacetyltriglycine ([^{99m}Tc]Tc-MAG3) was developed as radiotracer to examine the renal tubular function (Fig. 2.15). The complexing agent MAG3 is used either as its S-benzyl-protected derivative or as deprotected thiolate. If the ligand is present in protected form, complex formation proceeds upon heating at

95 °C with concomitant elimination of the benzoyl protecting group [208]. Starting from the S-unprotected mercaptoacetyltriglycine, a more convenient preparation of [^{99m}Tc]Tc-MAG3 without heating the reaction mixture has been described [209]. Appropriate kits are commercially available.

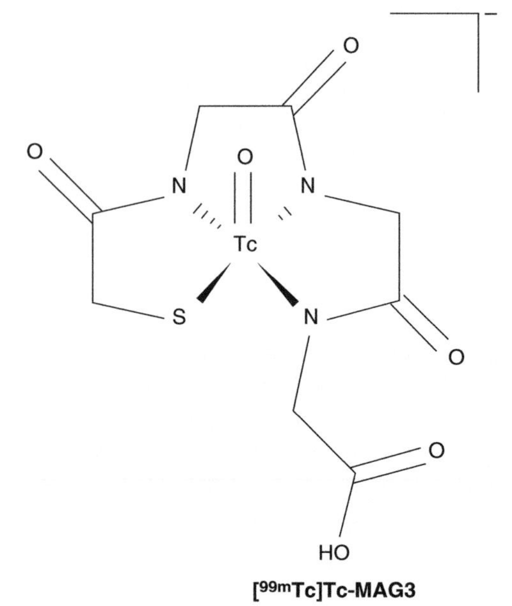

Fig. 2.15 Structure of the renal function and imaging agent [^{99m}Tc]Tc=O-mercaptoacetyltriglycine ([^{99m}Tc]Tc-MAG3)

The carboxyl group of the complex is deprotonated at physiological pH making the compound monoanionic. The complex binds to a large extend to plasma proteins. These weak interactions allow excretion through tubular secretion, and about 50% of the radioactivity is excreted after each blood pass through the kidneys. Like for hippuric acid, for this excretion, the presence of a non-coordinated carboxyl group seems to be essential in order to be recognized by the corresponding transporters in the kidneys [210–212].

Imaging of Myocardial Blood Flow

The finding that unipositive cations such as K^+, Rb^+, and Tl^+ accumulate in the myocardium suggested monocationic technetium complexes to be promising candidates for myocardial uptake. As a result of systematic investigations, [^{99m}Tc]Tc-sestamibi and [^{99m}Tc]Tc-tetrofosmin have been approved as commercial radiopharmaceuticals for myocardial perfusion imaging (Fig. 2.16). These monocationic ^{99m}Tc complexes contain ether-like bonds (C-O-R) and are excreted through the hepatobiliary system due to their high lipophilicity [213–216].

[^{99m}Tc]Tc-sestamibi can conveniently be synthesized in a "kit-like" preparation from [^{99m}Tc]

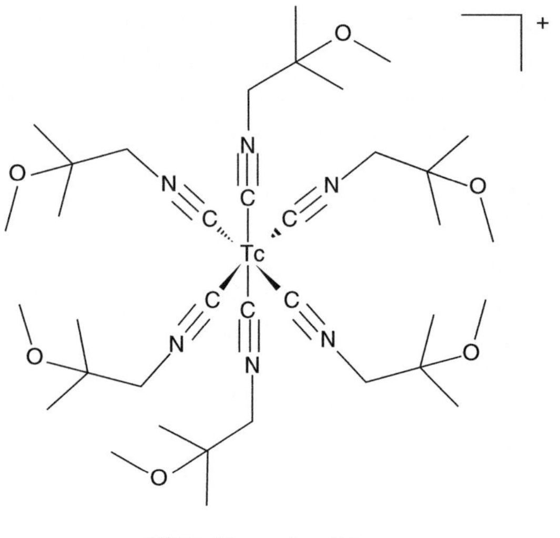

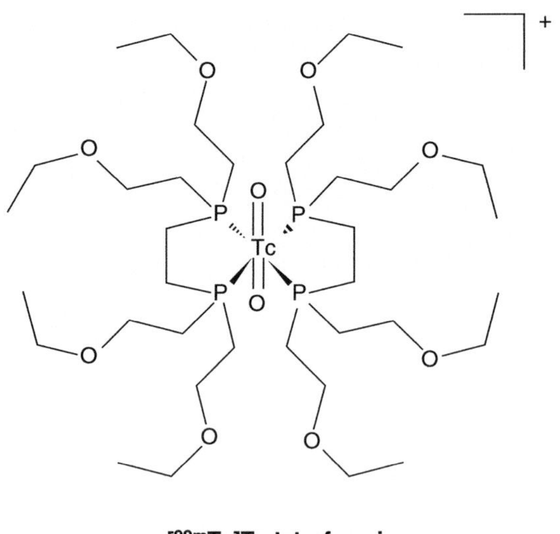

Fig. 2.16 [^{99m}Tc]Tc-sestamibi and [^{99m}Tc]Tc-tetrofosmin for myocardial perfusion imaging and blood flow quantification

TcO_4^- in saline with $SnCl_2$ as the reducing agent. The isocyano ligand is supplied in the form of its cationic copper(I) complex $[Cu(mibi)_4]^+$. The presence of the methoxy groups on the periphery of the cationic complex provides optimal lipophilicity and allows for enzymatic in vivo cleavage of the ethers to the respective alcohols which may increase the clearance rates from blood and liver [217, 218].

$[^{99m}Tc]$Tc-tetrofosmin is the first and so far only example of a technetium(V) trans dioxo entity bearing technetium complex $[[^{99m}Tc]Tc(O)_2]^+$ which shows substantial myocardial uptake and retention in combination with fast nontarget washout. The eight ethoxyethyl groups of the ligands apparently contribute to efficient clearance of background activity from nontarget tissues. There is no evidence for in vivo reduction of ^{99m}Tc(V) to lower oxidation states [219, 220].

Imaging of Cerebral Blood Flow

Aiming at the development of ^{99m}Tc agents capable of penetrating the intact blood-brain barrier (BBB), during the 1980s and 1990s, neutral and lipophilic technetium complexes were synthesized and evaluated as brain perfusion imaging agents. This effort resulted in the development of two radiopharmaceuticals, $[^{99m}Tc]$Tc-d,l-HMPAO [221] and $[^{99m}Tc]$Tc-l,l-ECD [222–224] (Fig. 2.17). Both complexes penetrate the intact BBB and are accumulated into the brain through complex rearrangement of ^{99m}Tc-d,l-HMPAO or saponification of ^{99m}Tc-l,l-ECD, respectively.

It is hypothesized that the retention of $[^{99m}Tc]$Tc-d,l-HMPAO is related to its chemical instability. After the penetration of BBB $[^{99m}Tc]$Tc-d,l-HMPAO undergoes a rearrangement to a more hydrophilic species rendering it unable to rediffuse through the BBB so that it is trapped in the brain. The redox status of the tissue and the concentration of glutathione have been identified as critical parameters for this conversion [225, 226].

It is interesting to note that the HMPAO chelator has chiral centers and only its d,l-form leads to a technetium complex that is suitable for clinical brain imaging. Complexes with the meso-form of the ligand show a different biological distribution behavior. In particular, they are more resistant against conversion into the hydrophilic species, and, therefore, their redistribution is much faster.

Retention of $[^{99m}Tc]$Tc-l,l-ECD is attributed to the enzymatic hydrolysis of the ester groups and the formation of a hydrophilic metabolite, which cannot diffuse back across the BBB and thus is trapped in the brain allowing for SPECT brain perfusion imaging. The distribution of $[^{99m}Tc]$Tc-d,l-HMPAO and $[^{99m}Tc]$Tc-l,l-ECD into the brain is well correlated with regional cerebral blood flow (rCBF), and their use is based on monitoring the changes of rCBF in various neurological disorders like dementia, Alzheimer's disease, epilepsy, stroke, and Parkinson's disease.

Receptor-Specific Targeting for Measurement of the Dopamine Transporter (DAT) Density and Function

$[^{99m}Tc]$Tc-TRODAT-1 (Fig. 2.18), a cocaine derivative combined with a $[^{99m}Tc]$Tc(V)-oxo-

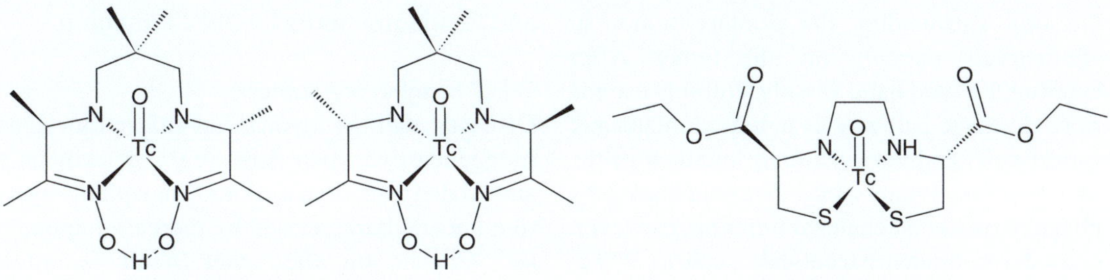

[99mTc]Tc-d,l-HMPAO **[99mTc]Tc-l,l-ECD**

Fig. 2.17 $[^{99m}Tc]$Tc-d,l-HMPAO and ^{99m}Tc-l,l-ECD for imaging regional brain perfusion

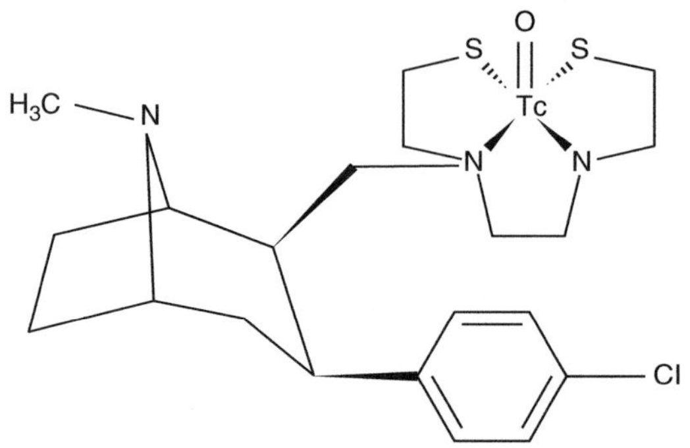

^{99m}Tc-TRODAT-1

Fig. 2.18 ^{99m}Tc-TRODAT-1 for SPECT measurement of the dopamine transporters

diaminodithiol moiety, was developed by Kung and coworkers [227–229]. Its usefulness for the diagnosis of Parkinson's disease was established in clinical studies which have proven the binding affinity [^{99m}Tc]Tc-TRODAT-1 for the dopamine transporter [230, 231]. Interestingly, this ^{99m}Tc-labeled compound is the first and so far only technetium complex penetrating the BBB and thus applicable for receptor studies in the CNS.

^{99m}Tc-Radiopharmaceuticals for Sentinel Lymph Node (SNL) Localization

Detection of the sentinel lymph node (SNL), the first node to receive lymphatic flow as well as metastatic cells from the primary tumor site is currently employed for planning the therapeutic treatment of cancers such as breast cancer and skin melanoma. Commonly, ^{99m}Tc-labeled colloids in combination with blue dyes are used to detect the sentinel lymph node. The labeled colloids are injected beneath the skin surrounding the primary tumor or alternatively directly into the tumor. After entering the lymphatic vessels, colloids use the same drainage pathway as potential metastatic cancer cells and are eventually retained in the first draining lymph node (sentinel node) by phagocytosis or mechanical trapping. However, colloidal radiopharmaceuticals such as ^{99m}Tc-sulfur colloid, ^{99m}Tc-antimony trisulfide, and ^{99m}Tc-labeled albumin microcolloids have disadvantages, like slow elimination rates from the injection site and migration to secondary nodes [232]. Thus, noncolloidal particles have been developed as alternatives such as ^{99m}Tc-labeled human serum albumin and ^{99m}Tc-labeled dextran.

A fluorescence-labeled ^{99m}Tc-HSA derivative (indocyanine green ICG-^{99m}Tc-NanoColl) was used to improve the surgical accuracy of laparoscopic lymph node (LN) dissection by integration of molecular imaging and intraoperative image guidance [233]. The authors could demonstrate that multimodal ICG-^{99m}Tc-nanocolloid, in combination with a laparoscopic fluorescence laparoscope, can be used to facilitate and optimize dissection of SLNs during robot-assisted laparoscopic prostatectomy.

2.3.1.6 Receptor-Targeted ^{99m}Tc-Radiopharmaceuticals Based on Bifunctional Chelators

^{99m}Tc-Tilmanocept

A tailor-made ^{99m}Tc-radiopharmaceutical for SLN diagnosis based on dextran has been approved by the FDA in 2013 (^{99m}Tc-tilmanocept) [234–237]. It is a macromolecule (18 kDa, 7 nm size) composed of a dextran backbone and multiple subunits of DTPA and mannose (Fig. 2.19). ^{99m}Tc-tilmanocept belongs to the class of receptor-binding radiopharmaceuticals. The mannose residues serve as ligands for receptors expressed on myeloid cells for recognition and binding. ^{99m}Tc-labeling of the macromolecule is performed via diethylenetriaminepentaacetic acid (DTPA).

^{99m}Tc-Labeled Peptides and Peptidomimetics for SPECT Imaging

SPECT Imaging of Apoptosis

Diseases such as myocardial infarction, neurodegenerative disorders (e.g., Parkinson's and Alzheimer's disease) and transplant rejection are all characterized by increased apoptosis. Cancer on the other hand is often characterized by minimal apoptosis and by the capacity to evade programmed cell death [238, 239]. This is known as one of the hall-

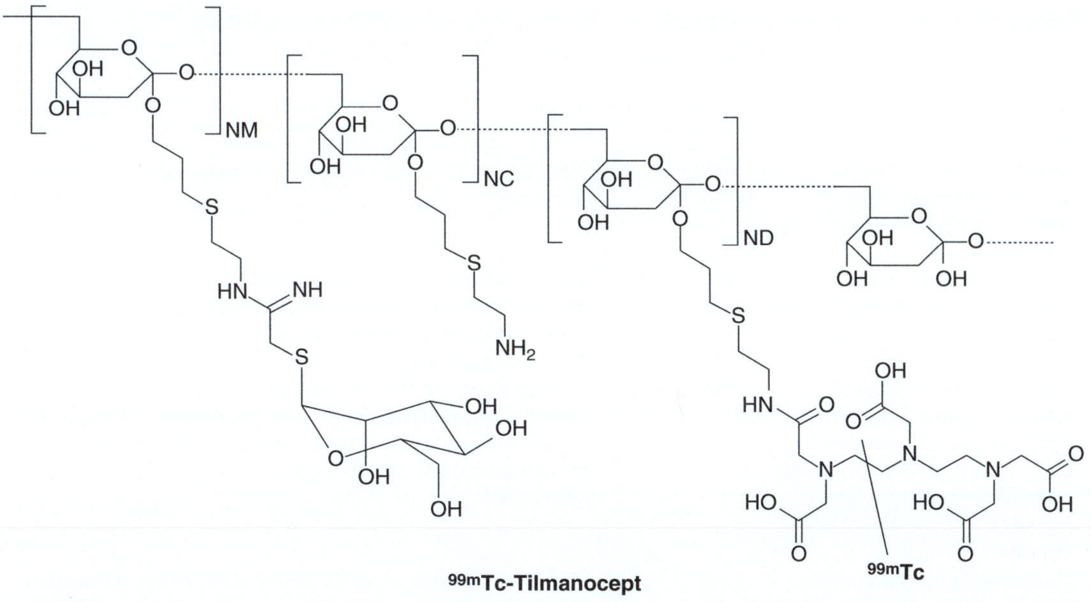

Fig. 2.19 Schematic representation of ^{99m}Tc-tilmanocept for lymphatic mapping and sentinel lymph node (SNL) localization. The unlabeled DTPA-mannosyl-dextran has a molecular weight of 35,800 g/mol and a molecular diameter of 7.1 nm. The final amino (NC), mannose (NM), and DTPA (ND) densities were 23, 55, and 8 mol per dextran [237]

marks of cancer and associated with cancer development [239]. Several radiopharmaceuticals including ^{99m}Tc-annexin V, [^{18}F]ML-10, [^{18}F]CP18, and [^{18}F]ICMT-11 (cf. Sect. 2.4.6.8) have been developed and are currently or were under clinical investigations in phase-I/phase-II or phase-II/phase-III clinical trials for imaging apoptosis [240]. A vast majority of the work on apoptosis-targeted radiotracers has focused on annexin V and its derivatives, which have been radiolabeled with a wide variety of radionuclides including radioiodine (e.g., ^{123}I, ^{124}I, ^{125}I, ^{18}F, ^{99m}Tc, ^{111}In, ^{11}C, ^{64}Cu). Annexin V (= annexin A5) is a member of the calcium- and phospholipid-binding superfamily of annexin proteins and displays selective, nanomolar binding affinity (K_d ~ 0.5–7 nM) toward phosphatidylserine (PS) residues, which are exposed on the cell surface of apoptotic (still living) cells [240–242].

Among these tracers, especially with the ^{99m}Tc-annexin V radiopharmaceuticals, more than 17 clinical trials have been conducted investigating apoptotic tumor responses in patients before and after the first course of chemotherapy and/or radiotherapy [242]. [^{99m}Tc]Tc-4,5-bis-(thioacetamido)pentanoyl-annexin V (also named [^{99m}Tc]Tc-BTAP-annexin V or ^{99m}Tc-apomate) was the firstly described ^{99m}Tc-Annexin V radiopharmaceutical which was evaluated in humans [243], while later [^{99m}Tc]Tc-hydrazinonicotinamide-annexin V ([^{99m}Tc]Tc-HYNIC-annexin V or ^{99m}Tc-annexin A5, Theseus Imaging Corporation, Boston, USA) and [^{99m}Tc]Tc-(N-1-imino-mercaptobutyl)-annexin V ([^{99m}Tc]Tc-i-annexin V, Mallinckrodt, Petten, The Netherlands) were also developed, each with improved radiolabeling yields [240]. Recently, ^{99m}Tc-rh-annexin A5–128 (Advanced Accelerator Applications, Canada), a mutant form of annexin A5 has been designed for phase-I/phase-II clinical trials. This tracer has twice as high sensitivity for detection of apoptosis than that of [^{99m}Tc]Tc-HYNIC-rh-annexin A5 so that increased tumor-to-background ratios are expected [242]. A summary of the clinical studies with ^{99m}Tc-Annexin V analogs is included in Fehler! Verweisquelle konnte nicht gefunden werden (Table 2.10).

Table 2.10 Clinical trials/clinical studies (phases I–III) with ^{99m}Tc-annexin V analogs in humans

Aim of the study	Tumor type (number of patients)	Results	References
^{99m}Tc-labeled recombinant human (rh) annexin V for imaging apoptosis immediately after completion of the first course of chemotherapy	NSCLC (7), SCLC (3), BC (2), L (3)	Tumor response and survival time were significantly correlated with the ^{99m}Tc-annexin V uptake	Belhocine et al. [244]
[^{99m}Tc]Tc-HYNIC-annexin A5 baseline imaging before platinum chemotherapy and 24 h after the first dose	NSCLC (46)	Early posttreatment change in [^{99m}Tc]Tc-HYNIC-annexin A5 uptake is associated with an improved response rate to platinum-based chemotherapy	Steinmetz [245]
Identifying the relationship between baseline quantitative [^{99m}Tc]Tc-HYNIC-annexin A5 tumor uptake and the number of apoptotic cells derived from histologic analysis after surgical resection	HNC (18)	Quantitative [^{99m}Tc]Tc-HYNIC-annexin A5 tumor uptake correlated well with the number of apoptotic cells if only tumor samples with no or minimal amounts of necrosis were considered	Van de Wiele et al. [246]
Estimation of the intra-, inter-, and day-to-day reproducibility of quantitative [^{99m}Tc]Tc-HYNIC-annexin A5 tumor uptake values	HNC (13)	The mean differences for the intra-, inter-, and day-to-day measurements were −3.4%, 2.4%, and −6%, respectively	Vermeersch et al. [247]
[^{99m}Tc]Tc-HYNIC-annexin A5 visualization of primary HNC lesions and lymph nodes before surgical resection and lymph node dissection	HNC (18)	[^{99m}Tc]Tc-HYNIC-annexin A5 allowed for the visualization of all primary HNC tumors identified by CT scan but failed to identify most of the sites of lymph node involvement	Vermeersch et al. [248]
Evaluation of [^{99m}Tc]Tc-HYNIC-Annexin A5 imaging for monitoring radiation-induced apoptotic cell death	FL (11)	In ten patients, posttreatment cytology matched [^{99m}Tc]Tc-HYNIC-annexin A5 uptake ASOT. Baseline uptake was weak or absent	Haas et al. [249]
Predicting outcome of various treatments by [^{99m}Tc]Tc-HYNIC-annexin A5 imaging	ML (26), NSCLC (5), HNC (2), Le (1), H&NSCC (1)	Complete or partial TRR was associated with a marked increase of [^{99m}Tc]Tc-HYNIC-annexin A5 accumulation early during treatment compared to baseline values. In case of SD or PD, pretreatment scans demonstrated predominantly low [^{99m}Tc]Tc-HYNIC-annexin A5 tumor uptake and no significant increase early after treatment	Kartachova et al. [250]
Predicting outcome of chemotherapy by [^{99m}Tc]Tc-HYNIC-annexin A5 imaging	M (3), Bl (1), BC (5), HNC (2), Other (6)	[^{99m}Tc]Tc-HYNIC-annexin A5 imaging allowed for separation of responders and nonresponders to treatment in 16/17 patients	Rottey et al. [251]
Predicting outcome of (radio) chemotherapy by baseline uptake of [^{99m}Tc]Tc-HYNIC-annexin V	HNC (8), BC (6), M (2), Other (7)	Significantly higher pretreatment tracer uptake was found in therapy responders (CR, PR) compared to nonresponders (PD, SD)	Rottey et al. [252]
Predicting outcome of platinum-based chemotherapy by [^{99m}Tc]Tc-HYNIC-annexin A5 imaging	NSCLC (14)	Patients with notably increased [^{99m}Tc]Tc-HYNIC-annexin A5 uptake showed CR or PR. SD or PD showed less prominently increased or decreased tracer uptake	Kartachova et al. [253]
Identifying the reliability of visual analysis of [^{99m}Tc]Tc-HYNIC-annexin A5 tumor uptake compared to quantitative tracer uptake evaluation	NSCLC (4), HNC (3), FL (26)	Both visual ($r = 0.97$, $P < 0.0001$) and quantitative ($r = 0.99$, $P < 0.0001$) analysis of [^{99m}Tc]Tc-HYNIC-annexin A5 tumor uptake significantly correlated with TRR	Kartachova et al. [254]

Table 2.10 (continued)

Aim of the study	Tumor type (number of patients)	Results	References
Predicting outcome of cisplatin-based chemoradiation by [^{99m}Tc]Tc-HYNIC-annexin A5 imaging	HNC (13)	[^{99m}Tc]Tc-HYNIC-annexin A5 imaging showed a radiation-dose-dependent uptake in parotid glands. No correlation could be established between baseline- or treatment-induced tracer uptake and TRR, DFS, or OS	Hoebers et al. [255]
Identifying prognostic value of baseline [^{99m}Tc]Tc-HYNIC-annexin A5 imaging	HNC (29)	[^{99m}Tc]Tc-HYNIC-annexin A5 pretreatment uptake was inversely correlated with DFS and OS	Loose et al. [256]
Determining the influence of chemotherapy on the biodistribution of [^{99m}Tc]Tc-HYNIC-annexin A5 in healthy tissues	HNC (4), BC (2), Other (5)	No significant differences in [^{99m}Tc]Tc-HYNIC-annexin A5 uptake in healthy tissues were found between patients who received chemotherapy and who did not	Rottey et al. [257]
Imaging tumor cells undergoing apoptosis in breast cancer patients with [^{99m}Tc]Tc-EC-annexin V	BC (10)	[^{99m}Tc]Tc-EC-annexin V could localize and image primary invasive BC with a median signal ratio which was double compared with normal tissue (internal control). 9/10 cases showed detectable [^{99m}Tc]Tc-EC-annexin V uptake in tumor. Higher values of T/N ratios are associated with patient after treatment	Kurihara et al. [258]

ASOT after start of therapy, *BC* breast cancer, *Bl* bladder cancer, *CR* complete response, *DFS* disease-free survival, *FL* follicular lymphoma, *HNC* head and neck cancer, *H&NSCC* head and neck squamous cell carcinoma, *HL* Hodgkin's lymphoma, *L* lymphoma, *Le* leukemia, *M* melanoma, *ML* malignant lymphoma, *NSCLC* non-small cell lung cancer, *NHL* non-Hodgkin's lymphoma, *OS* overall survival, *PD* progressive disease, *PR* partial response, *SCLC* small cell lung cancer, *SD* stable disease, *TRR* tumor response rate

The results of the clinical trials/clinical studies conducted so far indicate that ^{99m}Tc-annexin V scintigraphy might be a valuable predictive test for therapy response during radio- and/or chemotherapy. In addition, ^{9m}Tc-annexin V scintigraphy could be an alternative to insufficient [^{18}F]FDG PET to specifically image apoptosis induced by chemotherapy or radiotherapy, helping distinguishing imaging patterns of reactive inflammation versus residual tumor lesions [240, 242, 259].

Apoptosis plays a dominant role in typical pathologic processes of cardiovascular diseases (myocardial infarction, heart failure, and atherosclerosis), thus several clinical trials with ^{99m}Tc-annexin V imaging in patients with cardiovascular diseases have been conducted [240]. According to the results of these studies, ^{99m}Tc-annexin V imaging has proven valuable for patients with myocardial infarction, acute stroke, Alzheimer dementia, and non-Alzheimer dementia [240]. Despite these encouraging results, the wide clinical use of ^{99m}Tc-annexin V imaging remains a challenge, due to the following limitations: (i) the limited specificity of ^{99m}Tc-annexin V for apoptotic cells (it cannot discriminate apoptosis and necrosis in certain cases) and (ii) limited sensitivity of SPECT imaging [240].

Imaging (Neo)angiogenesis with SPECT

Angiogenesis, the formation of new blood vessels from preexisting blood vessels, is a fundamental process occurring during tumor progression. Among the factors regulating angiogenesis are integrins [239, 260]. Integrins are a family of heterodimeric transmembrane glycoproteins involved in a wide range of cell-extracellular matrix and cell–cell interactions. Overexpression of integrins on endothelial cells modulate cell migration and survival during angiogenesis, whereas overexpression of integrins on cancer cells potentiate metastasis by facilitating invasion and movement across the blood vessels [261].

Imaging the $a_v\beta_3$ Integrin with RGD Peptide Analogs

The tripeptide sequence of arginine-glycine-aspartic acid (RGD) can specifically bind to the integrin $\alpha_v\beta_3$ receptor. A variety of radiolabeled RGD-based peptides have been developed for noninvasive imaging of integrin $\alpha_v\beta_3$ expression with SPECT or PET [241, 262–264]. Among all the RGD radiotracers studied, several RGD analogs have been radiolabeled with SPECT radionuclides and have been investigated in clinical trials/clinical studies (Table 2.11) [264, 265].

One of these RGD analogs is ^{99m}Tc-NC100692 (also known as maraciclatide, GE Healthcare), a synthetic cyclic peptide (Fig. 2.20) with high binding affinity for specific integrins, such as $\alpha_v\beta_3$. Several phase-I clinical trials have been completed so far mainly focusing on breast cancer (BC) detection (Table 2.11). In these studies ^{99m}Tc-maraciclatide, has shown 81–86% efficacy for BC lesions, with mild non-serious AEs [267, 268]. In another study with NSCL and BC patients, ^{99m}Tc-NC100692 scintigraphy was considered safe and well tolerated. While detection of lung and brain metastases was feasible, detection of liver and bone lesions was poor [266]. In another study ^{99m}Tc-maraciclatide was compared with [^{99m}Tc]Tc-sestamibi showing that lesion uptake was comparable (efficacy 86% and 90%, respectively), in both malignant and benign BC lesions, while there was good correlation between lesion extent and uptake measured from both radiopharmaceuticals. ^{99m}Tc-maraciclatide offered a marginal (but not significant) improvement in sensitivity over [^{99m}Tc]Tc-sestamibi [265].

Recently, several RGD multimeric peptides have been studied. The new types of RGD peptides showed much higher in vitro integrin $\alpha_v\beta_3$-binding affinity than the single RGD tripeptide sequence, and importantly, they exhibited a significantly increase in tumor uptake than their monomeric counter parts [264, 275–279]. Among these a dimeric peptide with PEG linkers [^{99m}Tc]Tc-HYNIC-PEG$_4$-E[PEG$_4$-c(RGDfk)]$_2$ ([^{99m}Tc]Tc-HYNIC-3P-RGD$_2$) has moved forward in clinical studies (Fig. 2.20) [264, 269, 273, 280]. Several clinical studies are currently running in China with this cyclic RGD dimer in different cancer types (esophageal, lung, breast) and rheumatoid arthritis (Table 2.11). In 2012 the results of the first multicenter study investigating the efficacy of [^{99m}Tc]Tc-HYNIC-3P-RGD$_2$ for the evaluation of patients with lung cancer were published. Seventy patients (51 men, 19 women; 63 ± 9 years old) with a suspected lung lesion and for whom a definite pathologic diagnosis was finally obtained (malignant, $n = 58$; benign, $n = 12$) were recruited from six centers. Whole-body planar scanning and chest SPECT were performed at 1 and 4 h, respectively, after intravenous injection of 11.1 MBq/kg (0.3 mCi/kg) of [^{99m}Tc]Tc-HYNIC-3P-RGD$_2$. The radiotracer [^{99m}Tc]Tc-HYNIC-3P-RGD$_2$ showed low background in the lungs and mediastinum; most lung malignancies were prominent on the 1 h images (T/B ratio, 1.65 ± 0.47 for the planar imaging and 2.78 ± 1.52 for SPECT). The T/B ratios were significantly lower in the benign lesions. The sensitivity was 88% for semiquantitative analysis and can reach 93–97% in visual analysis when considering the volume effect, necrosis, and metastasis. However, the specificity was only 58–67%. Most lymph node and bone metastases could be also detected [269].

Later in another multicenter study (four centers), [^{99m}Tc]Tc-HYNIC-3P-RGD$_2$ was evaluated for imaging of bone metastasis in patients with lung cancer in comparison with conventional [^{99m}Tc]Tc-MDP bone scans. A total of 44 patients (29 male, 59 ± 10 years old) with suspected lung cancer were recruited. Patients underwent whole-body scan and chest tomography successively at both 1 h and 4 h after intravenous injection of 11.1 MBq/kg [^{99m}Tc]Tc-HYNIC-3P-RGD$_2$. [^{99m}Tc]Tc-MDP whole-body bone scan was routinely performed within 1 week for comparison. Eighty-nine bone lesions in 18 patients were diagnosed as metastases, and 23 bone lesions in

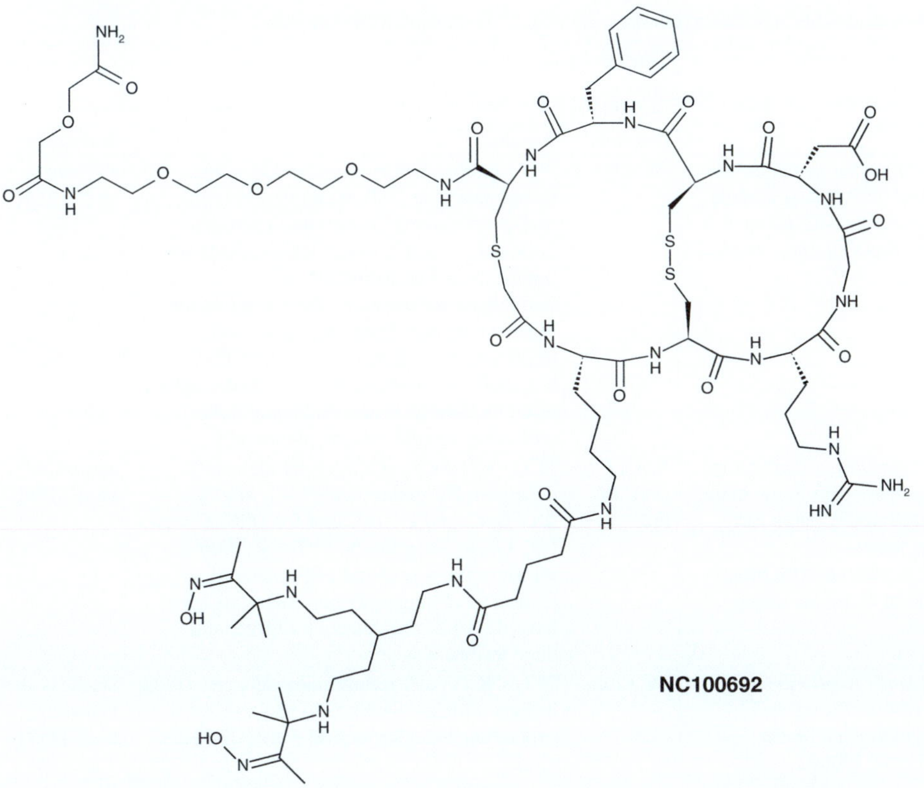

NC100692

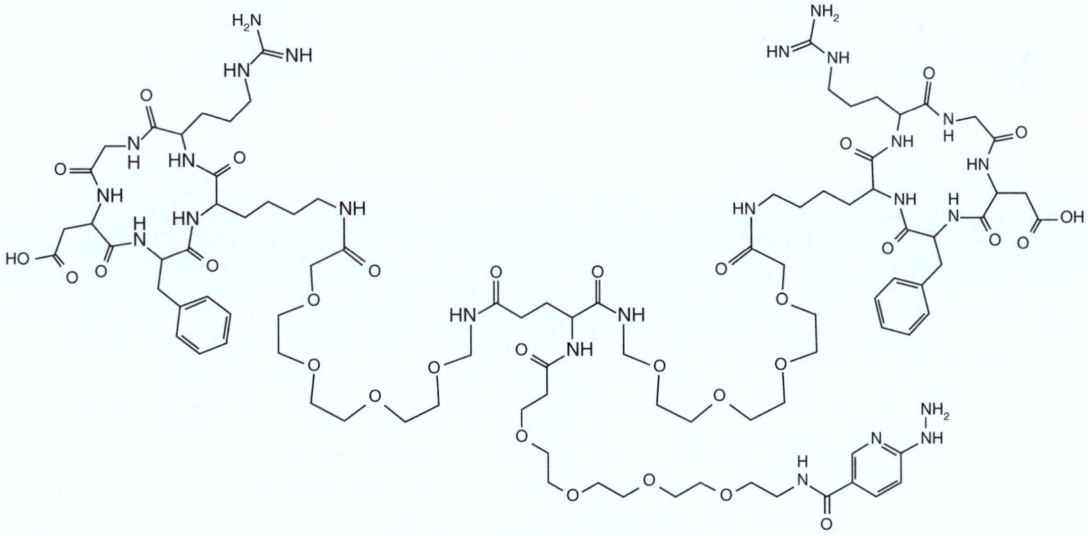

HYNIC-3P-RGD$_2$

Fig. 2.20 Chemical structure of the two RDG analogs NC100692 and HYNIC-3P-RGD$_2$. ^{99m}Tc-labeled versions have reached the stage of clinical studies

Table 2.11 Clinical trials/clinical studies (phases I–II) with ^{99m}Tc-labeled RGD analogs

Aim of the study	Tumor type (number of patients)	Results	References
Comparison of relative performance of ^{99m}Tc-sestamibi and ^{99m}Tc-maraciclatide in patients with suspected BC, using a high-resolution dedicated gamma camera for MBI	BC (39)	^{99m}Tc-maraciclatide offered comparable lesion uptake to ^{99m}Tc sestamibi, in both malignant and benign lesions. There was good correlation between lesion extent and uptake measured from both radiopharmaceuticals. ^{99m}Tc-maraciclatide offered a marginal (but not significant) improvement in sensitivity over ^{99m}Tc-sestamibi. An association between the uptake of either radiopharmaceutical and tumor molecular subtype was not supported	O'Connor et al. [265]
To determine the feasibility of detecting metastatic lesions in the liver, lung, bone, and brain with scintigraphy using the $\alpha_v\beta_3$-avid imaging agent ^{99m}Tc-NC100692 in patients with breast or lung cancer and to assess its safety profile	NSCLC (15), BC (10)	^{99m}Tc-NC100692 scintigraphy metastasis detection, BC patients, 1/7 LvC, 4/5 LC, 8/17 BoC, and 1/1 BrC and for NSCLC were 0/2, 17/18, 2/2, and 7/9. ^{99m}Tc-NC100692 scintigraphy is safe and well tolerated. Detection of lung and brain metastases was feasible, while the detection of liver and bone lesions was poor	Axelsson et al. [266]
Proof-of-concept study to provide an initial indication of the efficacy and safety of imaging malignant breast tumors using ^{99m}Tc-NC100692	BC (20)	^{99m}Tc-NC100692 scintigraphy detected 19/22 lesions (efficacy 86%). 5/20 patients experienced non-serious AEs; all AEs were mild	Bach-Gansmo et al. [267]
Integrin scintimammography with NC100692 and a dedicated gamma camera, LumaGEM, based on semiconductor technology, was performed to investigate the detection ability of this combination in breast cancer	BC (8)	LumaGEM scintigraphy revealed 9/11 malignancies (6–20 mm). Two lesions in patients with multicentric disease were not diagnosed, one of which measured only 2.5 mm. In one patient, the procedure was inconclusive, due to major breast hypertrophy	Bach-Gansmo et al. [268]
[^{99m}Tc]Tc-HYNIC-3P-RGD$_2$ SPECT/CT in LC Patients. A multicenter study was designed to investigate the efficacy of [^{99m}Tc]Tc-HYNIC-3P-RGD$_2$ for the evaluation of patients with LC	LC (70)	[^{99m}Tc]Tc-HYNIC-3P-RGD$_2$ imaging at 1 h was sensitive for the detection of LC. Most lung malignancies were prominent on the 1 h images due to the low [^{99m}Tc]Tc-HYNIC-3P-RGD$_2$ background in the lungs and mediastinum. T/B ratios were significantly lower in the benign lesions ($P < 0.05$). Sensitivity for semiquantitative analysis was 88% and 93–97% for visual analysis when considering the volume effect, necrosis, and metastasis. However, the specificity was only 58–67%. Most lymph node and bone metastases could also be detected	Zhu et al. [269]

Table 2.11 (continued)

Aim of the study	Tumor type (number of patients)	Results	References
Assessing the potential of integrin $\alpha_v\beta_3$ imaging in the detection of RAIR in DTC lesions using [^{99m}Tc]Tc-HYNIC-3P-RGD$_2$, thus providing a feasible antiangiogenetic therapeutic target	DTC (10)	All the target RAIR metastatic lesions were identified as positive on [^{99m}Tc]Tc-HYNIC-3P-RGD$_2$ SPECT images. There was a significant correlation between the mean tumor-to-background ratios and mean growth rates of target lesions ($r = 0.878$, $P = 0.009$). The RAIR (^{131}I-WBS-negative/thyroglobulin-positive) metastatic lesions can be traced using [^{99m}Tc]Tc-HYNIC-3P-RGD$_2$ imaging, meaning these lesions are highly neovascularized. [^{99m}Tc]Tc-HYNIC-3P-RGD$_2$ angiogenesis imaging can be used for the localization and growth evaluation of RAIR lesions, providing a new therapeutic target and a novel imaging modality to monitor the efficacy of certain antiangiogenetic therapy	Zhao et al. [270]
The efficacy of [^{99m}Tc]Tc-HYNIC-3P-RGD$_2$ imaging for evaluating both early treatment response to EGFR-TKIs and prognosis in advanced-stage LaC	LaC (18)	[^{99m}Tc]Tc-HYNIC-3P-RGD$_2$ imaging could evaluate the early response to EGFR-targeted therapy and predict the PFS of LaC patients. After treatment with EGFR-TKIs, for patients with PR (10), SD (6), and PD (2), the mean changes in T/NT ratios on SPECT/CT and planar images were PR 35.8% and 15.0%, SD 8.9% and 0.7%, and PD 76.1% and 18.7%. ROC analysis (cutoff value of 23.8% decrease in T/NT ratio on SPECT/CT images) showed sensitivity 80.0% and specificity 87.5%, in identifying responders. The median PFS for patients with responders and nonresponders (on [^{99m}Tc]Tc-HYNIC-3P-RGD$_2$ SPECT/CT) was 18 months (95% CI 5.8–30.2 months) and 7 months (95% CI 5.2–8.8 months), respectively ($P = 0.006$)	Zhang et al. [271]
Evaluations of an integrin imaging approach based on SPECT/CT by using [^{99m}Tc]Tc-HYNIC-3P-RGD$_2$ as the tracer to target the integrin $\alpha_v\beta_3$ expression in LC and lymph node metastasis	LC (65), NSCLC (53, benign, 12)	[^{99m}Tc]Tc-HYNIC-3P-RGD$_2$ SPECT/CT showed high specificity in the diagnosis of lymph node metastasis from NSCLC. [^{99m}Tc]Tc-HYNIC-3P-RGD$_2$ SPECT/CT was found to be more specific than [^{18}F]FDG PET/CT in the per-region diagnosis of lymph node metastasis (specificity, 94.6% vs. 75.0%; $P = 0.008$) when the sensitivity of the two methods was comparable (88.3% vs. 90.7%; $P = 0.557$). There was no significant difference between the two methods in the per-lesion diagnosis of lung tumor ($z = 0.82$, $P = 0.410$). The accumulation level of [^{99m}Tc]Tc-HYNIC-3P-RGD$_2$ was found in positive correlation with the integrin $\alpha_v\beta_3$ expression ($r = 0.84$, $P = 0.001$) and microvessel density ($r = 0.63$, $P = 0.011$) in the tumors	Jin et al. [272]

(continued)

Table 2.11 (continued)

Aim of the study	Tumor type (number of patients)	Results	References
Comparison of [^{99m}Tc]Tc-HYNIC-3P-RGD_2 integrin receptor imaging with [^{99m}Tc]Tc-MDP bone scan in diagnosis of bone metastasis in patients with LC: a multicenter study	LC (44)	[^{99m}Tc]Tc-MDP bone scan had better contrast in most lesions, whereas the [^{99m}Tc]Tc-HYNIC-3P-RGD_2 imaging seemed to be more effective to exclude pseudo-positive lesions and detect bone metastases without osteogenesis. Eighty-nine bone lesions in 18 patients were diagnosed as metastases, and 23 bone lesions in nine patients were benign. In a lesion-based analysis results, in the same patients, [^{99m}Tc]Tc-HYNIC-3P-RGD_2 imaging/[^{99m}Tc]Tc-MDP bone scan, sensitivity 92.1%/87.6%, specificity 91.3%/60.9%, and accuracy and 92.0%/82.1%	Miao et al. [273]
Detection of aggressive breast tumors using ^{99m}Tc-NC100692 (high-resolution dedicated gamma camera for molecular breast imaging, ^{99m}Tc-maraciclatide vs. [^{99m}Tc]Tc-sestamibi)	BC (39)	^{99m}Tc-maraciclatide offered comparable lesion uptake to [^{99m}Tc]Tc-sestamibi, in both malignant and benign lesions. There was good correlation between lesion extent and uptake measured from both radiopharmaceuticals. ^{99m}Tc-maraciclatide offered a marginal (but not significant) improvement in sensitivity over [^{99m}Tc]Tc-sestamibi	O'Connor et al. [265]
The diagnostic performance of [^{99m}Tc]Tc-HYNIC-3P-RGD_2 scintimammography (SMM) in patients with either palpable or nonpalpable breast lesions and compare SMM to mammography to assess the possible incremental value of SMM in breast cancer detection. Investigation of the $\alpha_v\beta_3$ expression in malignant and benign breast lesions	BC (94)	Histopathology revealed 46 malignant lesions and 64 benign lesions. The diagnostic values of [^{99m}Tc]Tc-HYNIC-3P-RGD_2, SMM were higher than those of mammography in evaluating overall breast lesions. SMM overall sensitivity 73%, specificity 83%, accuracy 77%, positive predictive value 69%, and negative predictive value 85%. The kappa value between the two reviewers was 0.63. A sensitivity of 91% was achieved when SMM and mammography results were combined with 60% of all false-negative mammography findings classified as true-positive results by SMM. Integrin $\alpha_v\beta_3$ expression was positively identified using SMM imaging	Liu et al. [274]

AE adverse effects, *BC* breast cancer, *BoC* bone cancer, *BrC* brain cancer, *DTC* differentiated thyroid cancer, *EGFR-TKIs* epidermal growth factor receptor tyrosine kinase inhibitors, *LaC* lung adenocarcinoma, *LC* lung cancer, *LvC* liver cancer, *NSCLC* non-small cell lung cancer, *MBI* molecular breast imaging, *PD* progressive disease, *PFS* progression-free survival, *PR* partial response, *RAIR* radioactive iodine-refractory, *ROC* receiver operating characteristic, *SD* stable disease, *SMM* scintimammography, *T/NT* tumor to normal tissue ratio

nine patients were benign. In a lesion-based analysis, [^{99m}Tc]Tc-HYNIC-3P-RGD_2 imaging demonstrated a sensitivity, specificity, and accuracy of 92.1%, 91.3%, and 92.0%, respectively. The corresponding diagnostic values for [^{99m}Tc]Tc-MDP bone scans were 87.6%, 60.9%, and 82.1%, respectively, in the same patients. [^{99m}Tc]Tc-MDP bone scans had better contrast in most lesions, whereas the [^{99m}Tc]Tc-HYNIC-3P-RGD_2 imaging seems to be more effective to exclude pseudo-positive lesions and detect bone metastases without osteogenesis [273].

The clinical value of integrin $\alpha_v\beta_3$ as imaging target for the diagnosis of osteolytic bone metastases was assessed with [^{99m}Tc]Tc-HYNIC-3P-RGD$_2$ against [^{99m}Tc]Tc-MDP. The study included 69 patients (LC 59, other cancers 10). Patients were required to receive whole body scan and regional SPECT/CT imaging [^{99m}Tc]Tc-HYNIC-3P-RGD$_2$ and [^{99m}Tc]Tc-MDP successively within 1 week. Final diagnosis was based on the comprehensive assessment of all available data including case history, CT, MRI, SPECT/CT, PET/CT, histopathology and 6–12 months follow-up. The detection sensitivity of RGD tracer whole body scans for osteolytic metastases was significantly higher than that of [^{99m}Tc]Tc-MDP (80.9% vs. 46.6%, $P < 0.01$) and increased to 96.2% (126/131) when it was combined with SPECT/CT. [^{99m}Tc]Tc-HYNIC-3P-RGD$_2$ imaging also promoted the detection of unknown primary tumor and lymph node metastases and offered information for clinical staging. Tumor-to-normal uptake ratio (T/N) for [^{99m}Tc]Tc-HYNIC-3P-RGD$_2$ in lung adenocarcinoma osteolytic metastases showed no statistical difference compared with that in squamous cell carcinoma (6.84 ± 3.46 vs. 7.33 ± 3.22, $t = 0.39$, $P = 0.71$). Whereas it was higher in osteolytic metastases from lung cancer than that from thyroid cancer (7.05 ± 3.01 vs. 4.11 ± 2.67, $P = 0.03$), overall [^{99m}Tc]Tc-HYNIC-3P-RGD$_2$ imaging showed great potential for the detection of osteolytic bone metastasis due to high expression levels of integrin $\alpha_v\beta_3$ on osteoclast and most tumor cells [264].

[^{99m}Tc]Tc-HYNIC-3P-RGD$_2$ has been also assessed for the early identification of response to antiangiogenic treatment with bevacizumab (targeting the vascular endothelial growth factor VEGF) in patients with advanced non-small cell lung cancer (NSCLC). The sensitivity, specificity, and negative predictive value of [^{99m}Tc]Tc-HYNIC-3P-RGD$_2$ SPECT for predicting tumor response were 81.8%, 91.7%, and 84.6%, respectively. Using the cutoff value (T/N ratio 24.4%) defined by receiver operating characteristic ROC analysis of [^{99m}Tc]Tc-HYNIC-3P-RGD$_2$ SPECT, metabolic nonprogressive diseased patients showed prolonged progression-free survival (5.6 months vs. 3.4 months; $P < 0.001$) and overall survival (17.1 months vs. 8.6 months; $P < 0.001$) than metabolic progressive diseased patients. [^{99m}Tc]Tc-HYNIC-3P-RGD$_2$ SPECT scan thus was considered a promising test for predicting tumor response in patients with advanced NSCLC early in the course of bevacizumab therapy [280].

Corresponding receptor-targeted ^{99m}Tc-radiotracers which can be used with radiotracers for radioligand therapy (RLT) or endoradiotherapy are further described in detail in Sect. 2.5 in which the modern theranostic approach in nuclear medicine is discussed.

2.3.2 Indium-111 (^{111}In)

As already mentioned in Sect. 2.2, one example of a successful radiopharmaceutical radiolabeled with ^{111}In is [^{111}In]In-DTPA-(D-Phe^1)-octreotide (^{111}In-pentetreotide, OctreoScan®) for imaging of patients with somatostatin receptor subtype 2 (SSTR2) overexpressing neuroendocrine tumors (NETs). OctreoScan® was approved by the FDA in 1994. It is a derivative of the somatostatin analog octreotide, a cyclic octapeptide containing the physiologically active four-amino acid sequence Phe-D-Trp-Lys-Thr. In order to enable labeling of octreotide with ^{111}In, a DTPA complexing agent has been conjugated to the alpha-NH_2 group of the N-terminal D-Phe residue (Fig. 2.21) [281].

Because ^{111}In-pentetreotide only binds with high binding affinity to the somatostatin receptor subtype SSTR2 and shows only moderate binding affinity to SSTR3 and SSTR5 and no binding affinity to SSTR1 and SSTR4, research has continued to develop other somatostatin analogs, which bind also with high binding affinity to the other receptor subtypes [282–285].

The next generation of modified somatostatin analogs included the macrocyclic chelator DOTA (1,4,7,10-tetraazacyclododecane-1,4,7,10-tetraacetic acid) instead of DTPA, which forms thermodynamically stable and kinetically inert complexes with a variety of radiometals for imaging (e.g., ^{111}In, ^{68}Ga) as well as for peptide receptor radionuclide therapy PRRT (e.g., ^{90}Y and ^{177}Lu).

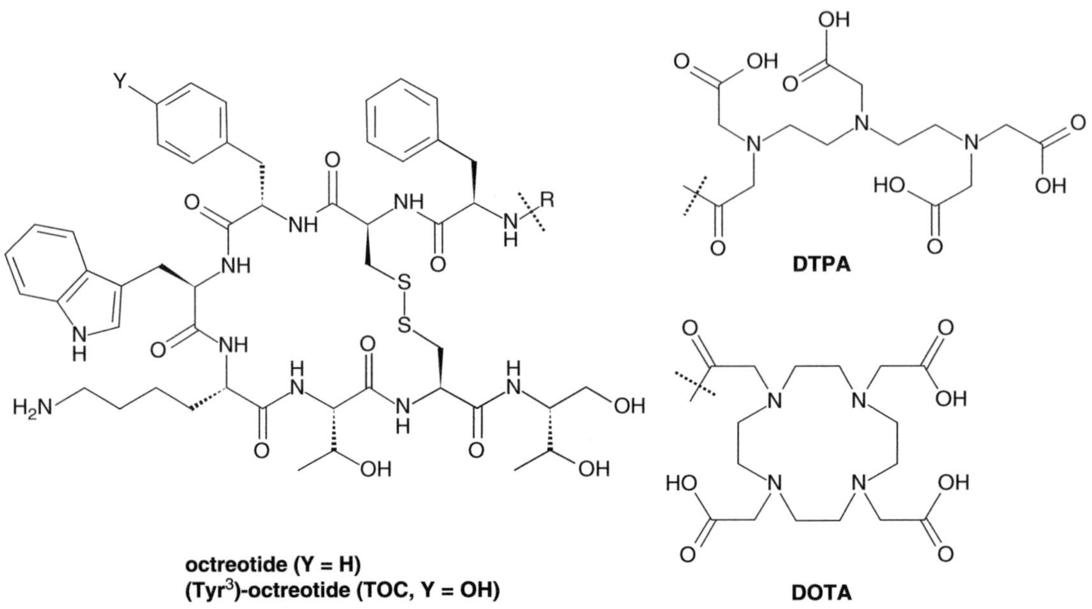

Fig. 2.21 Chemical structures of octreotide derivatives (OctreoScan® and DOTA-TOC)

Table 2.12 Amino acid sequences of the somatostatin analogs discussed in this chapter

Code	Sequence
OC	D-Phe-cyclo(Cys-Phe-D-Trp-Lys-Thr-Cys)-Thr(ol)
TOC	D-Phe-cyclo(Cys-Tyr-D-Trp-Lys-Thr-Cys)-Thr(ol)
TATE	D-Phe-cyclo(Cys-Tyr-D-Trp-Lys-Thr-Cys)-Thr
NOC	D-Phe-cyclo(Cys-1-Nal-D-Trp-Lys-Thr-Cys)-Thr(ol)
Lanreotide	D-2-Nal-cyclo(Cys-Tyr-D-Trp-Lys-Val-Cys)-Thr-NH_2

Currently four ^{111}In-labeled SSTR radiotracers for SPECT/CT imaging are in clinical use: [^{111}In]In-DOTA-lanreotide, [^{111}In]In-DOTA-(D-Phe^1,Tyr^3)-octreotide (DOTA-TOC), [^{111}In]In-DOTA-(D-Phe^1,Tyr^3,Thr^8)-octreotate (DOTA-TATE), and [^{111}In]In-DOTA-NOC. The amino acid sequences of the somatostatin analogs discussed here are shown in Table 2.12.

[^{111}In]In-DOTA-lanreotide is a conjugate of DOTA coupled directly to the N-terminus of lanreotide (D-2-Nal = D-3-(2-naphthyl)alanine). It binds to SSTR2 through SSTR5 with high binding affinity and to SSTR1 with low binding affinity. The high-affinity binding of lanreotide to SSTR3 and SSTR4 enables certain tumors to be visualized such as intestinal adenocarcinomas which are not visualized by ^{111}In-pentetreotide scintigraphy [286–289].

DOTA-TOC is a second-generation somatostatin analog for imaging and PRRT. It has a higher binding affinity for SSTR2. DOTA-TATE differs from DOTA-TOC in that the C-terminal threoninol has been replaced with threonine. In comparison to DOTA-TOC, DOTA-TATE shows considerable improvement in binding to SSTR2-positive tumors [290, 291].

2.3.3 Iodine-123 (^{123}I)

2.3.3.1 Metaiodobenzylguanidine (MIBG)

Metaiodobenzylguanidine (MIBG, iobenguan) was developed in the early 1980s to visualize tumors of the adrenal medulla. It is structurally similar to norepinephrine/noradrenaline (Fig. 2.22) and is taken up by an active mechanism in neuroendocrine cells and stored in neurosecretory granules. Radiolabeled with ^{123}I for SPECT imaging, with ^{124}I for PET imaging, or with ^{131}I for radionuclide therapy of neuroendocrine tumors, MIBG is an impressive example of a theranostic agent. It has been introduced as a molecular nuclear therapeutic in the treatment of neuroendocrine tumors, including neuroblastoma, pheochromocytoma, and paraganglioma [292–298].

MIBG as norepinephrine/noradrenaline analog can also be used as a ^{123}I-labeled radiotracer in nuclear cardiology for the evaluation of sympathetic neuron integrity and function. This allows the evaluation of patients with heart failure which is characterized by activation of the sympathetic cardiac nerves [299]. Apart from the PET tracer [^{11}C] meta-hydroxyephedrine ([^{11}C]mHED) (cf. Sect. 2.4), [^{123}I]MIBG SPECT is the only widely available nuclear imaging method for assessing regional myocardial sympathetic innervation [300, 301].

2.3.3.2 Receptor-Specific Agents for Measurement of Receptor or Transporter Density and Function in the Brain

Fully approved ^{123}I-labeled SPECT radiopharmaceuticals are rare. Most of them were designed to specifically bind neurotransmitter receptors or transporter sites in the central nervous system (CNS) (Fig. 2.23). This mainly results from the necessity of crossing the intact blood-brain barrier (BBB) and the associated requirement to avoid major alterations of the unlabeled lead structures, which would occur by introduction of chelating moieties which are used to bind radiometals [302, 303].

[^{123}I]FP-CIT (ioflupane, DaTScan) is an analog of cocaine which binds to the dopamine transporter (DAT) in the synapses of striatal dopaminergic neurons. This agent has shown efficacy for detecting degeneration of the dopaminergic nigrostriatal pathway, allowing better separation of patients with essential tremor from those with presynaptic Parkinsonian syndromes, as well as differentiating between some causes of parkinsonism [304–307]. Ioflupane has been approved by the European Medicines Agency (EMA) and the Food and Drug Administration (FDA) for clinical use in 2010 and 2011, respectively.

[^{123}I]Iomazenil (Ro16–0154) is an antagonist and partial inverse agonist of benzodiazepine. The compound was introduced in 1989 as ^{123}I-labeled SPECT tracer for imaging benzodiazepine receptors in the brain [308, 309]. The compound is useful in identifying changes of this receptor in various psychiatric disorders such as Huntington's disease [310], schizophrenia [311], and panic disorder [312].

Furthermore, iomazenil was evaluated regarding feasibility of identification of neuronal damage in patients with the chronic phase of thrombotic cerebral ischemia [313], cerebral infarction [314], and traumatic brain injury [315, 316].

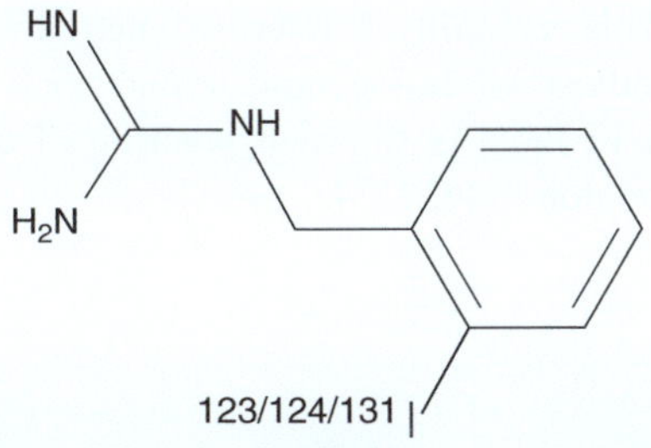

MIBG

Fig. 2.22 Metaiodobenzylguanidine (MIBG) labeled with ^{123}I for SPECT imaging, ^{124}I for PET imaging, and ^{131}I for radionuclide therapy of neuroendocrine tumors

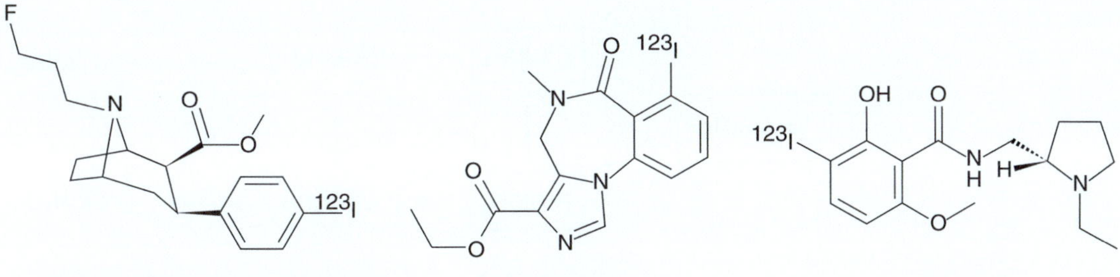

[^{123}I]FP-CIT (Ioflupane, DaTSCAN) **[^{123}I]Iomazenil** **[^{123}I]IBZM**

Fig. 2.23 ^{123}I-labeled agents for imaging of dopamine transporters ([^{123}I]FP-CIT), benzodiazepine receptors ([^{123}I] iomazenil), and D2 receptors ([^{123}I]IBZM)

[^{123}I]IBZM [(*S*)-*N*-[(1-ethyl-2-pyrrolidinyl)] methyl-2-hydroxy-3-iodo-6-methoxybenzamide] was introduced as radiotracer for quantitative imaging of the postsynaptic dopamine D2 receptors, representing the postsynaptic integrity of the nigrostriatal projection system. Biodistribution studies demonstrated that the agent is concentrated in the basal ganglia although some nonspecific binding was noted in cerebral cortex and cerebellum [317].

[^{123}I]IBZM-SPECT is often used to differentiate between idiopathic Parkinson's syndrome and atypical parkinsonian syndromes [318].

In combination with ioflupane, IBZM was used to evaluate the striatal presynaptic dopamine transporter and postsynaptic D2 receptor binding in patients with corticobasal syndrome [319].

2.4 Clinically Relevant Diagnostic Non-radiometal PET Tracers

2.4.1 Carbon-11 (^{11}C)

2.4.1.1 Introduction

Carbon is the essential part of the skeleton of organic, endogenous compounds. Thus, carbon-11 is an attractive positron emitter to study the in vivo behavior of corresponding radiolabeled substances. The ^{11}C-synthesis of endogenous compounds is an important tool to visualize and quantify metabolic pathways allowing mechanistic studies to explore in vivo biochemistry [320]. Carbon-11 is a nearly pure positron emitter (β^+ 99.77%, EC 0.23%) with a physical half-life of 20.3 min (0.3389 h) [321]. The relatively short physical half-life of carbon-11 necessitates fast and reliable chemical methods amenable in remote-controlled synthesis devices, called radiosynthesizers.

2.4.1.2 Basics in ^{11}C-Chemistry

Carbon-11 is produced by the ^{14}N(p,α)^{11}C reaction using nitrogen gas containing either few percent of oxygen or hydrogen. The target chamber is made up of aluminum or aluminum magnesium alloy.

The resulting starting material for all subsequent radiolabeling reactions is either [^{11}C]CO_2 or [^{11}C]CH_4, respectively, which can be converted to different building blocks (Fig. 2.24) [322, 323]. This versatility of intermediates enables the ^{11}C-synthesis of endogenous amino acids with a carbon-11 label in different position of the carbon skeleton [324, 325].

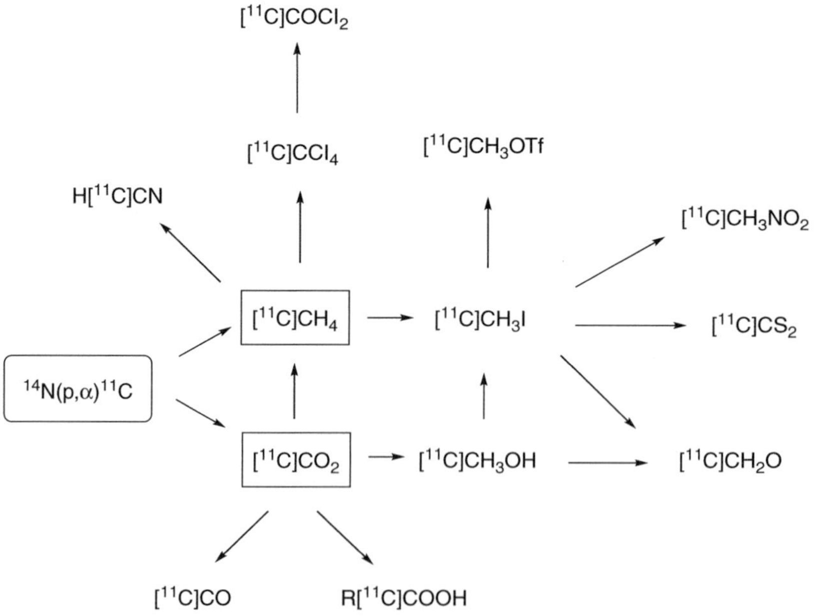

Fig. 2.24 Radiosynthesis of ^{11}C-building blocks [322]

A challenge in ^{11}C-chemistry is the achievement of high molar activities (MA). Carbon is ubiquitous in the environment, thus, the sources of carrier are manifold. Contemplable carrier sources are the target material, tubing, and the chemical process.

2.4.1.3 Reactions with [^{11}C]CO_2

The [^{11}C]CO_2 obtained from the target can directly be converted into ^{11}C-labeled carboxylates by reaction with the organometallic reagents like Grignard or lithium compounds. The most simplest examples is the synthesis of [*carbonyl*-^{11}C]acetate ([1-^{11}C]acetate), where [^{11}C]CO_2 is passed through a solution of methyl magnesium bromide followed by hydrolysis (Fig. 2.25) [326]. The purification of the volatile product can be performed by liquid-liquid extraction [326], distillation [327], or solid phase extraction [328]. The synthesis can be performed in commercially available radiosynthesizers [329].

The resulting [^{11}C]carboxylic acids can be coupled to [^{11}C]amides via their corresponding acid chloride as exemplified for the synthesis of [*carbonyl*-^{11}C]WAY100365, a 5-HT_{1A} receptor antagonist (Fig. 2.26) [330].

2.4.1.4 ^{11}C-Methylation Reactions

One of the most prominent building block in ^{11}C-chemistry is [^{11}C]CH_3I. The most clinical relevant ^{11}C-compounds are synthesized via ^{11}C-methylation reactions. [^{11}C]CH_3I can be obtained either by a "wet" chemical conversion of [^{11}C]CO_2 or by a "dry" gas phase radical reaction starting from [^{11}C]CH_4.

In the "wet" chemistry method, [^{11}C]CO_2 is transferred out of the target, frozen out, and reduced to [^{11}C]methanol by a solution of $LiAlH_4$ in ether. The conversion into [^{11}C]CH_3I can be performed either by heating with hydrogen iodide [331] or by transferring the [^{11}C]methanol, after hydrolysis with phosphoric acid, through a heated glassy cartridge filled with polymer-bonded triphenylphosphine diiodide [332]. A second glassy vial is connected to remove residual water and traces of hydrogen iodide. The advantage of the latter method is the avoidance of corrosive and volatile hydrogen iodide.

The "dry" method for the synthesis of [^{11}C]CH_3I is based on a catalytic conversion of [^{11}C]CH_4 using elemental iodine in the presence of a nickel catalyst at about 700 °C. This reaction can be performed either as single or as multi-pass method [333, 334]. The latter has the advantage that the unchanged [^{11}C]methane is recirculated and therefore enables a continuous production of [^{11}C]CH_3I. The [^{11}C]CH_4 can be obtained either by in-target production [335] or by conversion of [^{11}C]CO_2 in the presence of hydrogen and a NiO catalyst at 410 °C [333, 334].

Both methods for the production of [^{11}C]CH_3I allow the synthesis of ^{11}C-labeled compounds in high molar activities; however, regarding the "wet" method, the use of $LiAlH_4$ is a potential source of carbon and has to be handled carefully in order to avoid the addition of carrier.

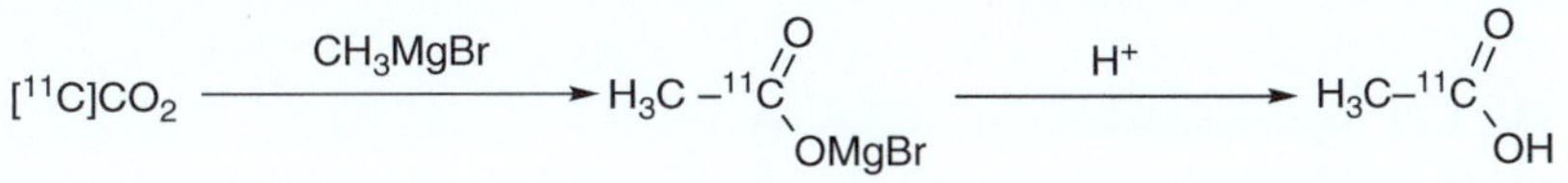

Fig. 2.25 Radiosynthesis of [1-^{11}C]acetate [326]

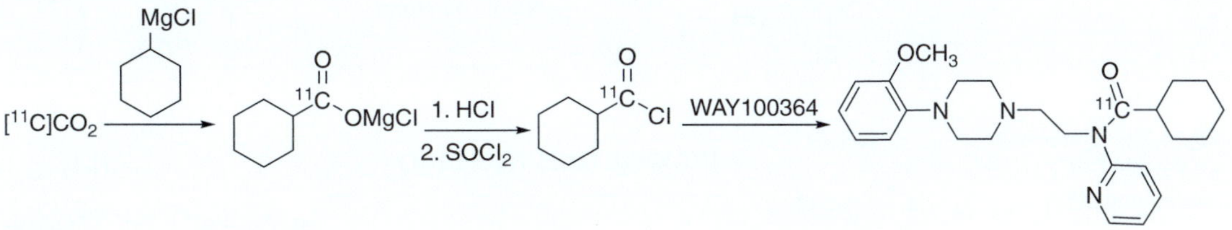

Fig. 2.26 Radiosynthesis of [*carbonyl*-^{11}C]WAY100365 starting from [^{11}C]CO_2 [330]

An alternative to [^{11}C]CH$_3$I is the use of [^{11}C]methyl triflate because of its much higher reactivity. For the preparation of [^{11}C]methyl triflate, gaseous [^{11}C]CH$_3$I is passed through a column of silver triflate bound on Al_2O_3 at 200 °C [336].

The standard route for ^{11}C-methylation reaction is the nucleophilic substitution reaction with free amines, alcohols, or thiol groups to form ^{11}C-labeled *N*-methylamines, ethers, or thioethers. For the preparation of ^{11}C-methylated compounds, a gas stream of [^{11}C]CH$_3$I or [^{11}C]methyl triflate is transferred to the corresponding precursor. The advantage of the low concentration of ^{11}C-methylation reagents is that an over-methylation, often observed in organic reactions, does not occur in ^{11}C-chemistry [322].

Three kinds of reaction methods are available. In the classical approach, the ^{11}C-methylation agent is passed into a vial containing the precursor in the presence of a base. For ^{11}C-methylation reactions with [^{11}C]CH$_3$I typically polar aprotic solvents like acetonitrile, dimethyl sulfoxide (DMSO), or *N,N*-dimethylformamide (DMF) are used. Some reactions needed to be heated to improve the reaction time. In the case of [^{11}C]methyl triflate acetone or polar halogen alkanes, dichloromethane and 1,2-dichloroethane are typically used.

Some important clinically relevant ^{11}C-compounds are obtained by ^{11}C-methylation (cf. Sect. 2.4.5): [^{11}C]choline [337], [^{11}C]flumazenil [338], Pittsburg Compound B ([^{11}C]PIB) [339], *N*-[^{11}C]methylspiperone ([^{11}C]NMSP) [338], [^{11}C]carfentanil [340], and [^{11}C]raclopride [341] (Fig. 2.27).

The most clinically used amino acid is L-[*S*-methyl-^{11}C]methionine (Fig. 2.28). It is synthesized by ^{11}C-methylation of a sulfide anion, which is formed by ring-opening of homocysteine thiolactone with sodium hydroxide directly before the synthesis [342]. The synthesis of L-[*S*-methyl-^{11}C]methionine was optimized in several studies including solid phase supported methods [343] and a loop method to perform a simple and efficient preparation automated radiosynthesizers [344].

To accelerate the reaction and to simplify the reaction, online ^{11}C-methylation reactions using solid phases were developed, where the precursor is coated on the surface [345–347] or captive solvent "loop" methods [348].

To perform the synthesis of [^{11}C]CH$_3$I and [^{11}C]methyl triflate, respectively, and the subsequent ^{11}C-methylation, automated radiosynthesizers are recommended to be used [349] (see Sect. 2.4.4).

Beside the ^{11}C-methylation of heteroatoms, [^{11}C]methyl iodide has also been established in palladium-mediated coupling reactions, that enable the carbon-carbon-bond formation in aromatic or vinylic positions starting from organostannane (Stille coupling: aromatic and vinylic) or aryl boronic acid precursors (Suzuki coupling: only aromatic), respectively. The coupling reaction is possible under one-pot conditions because it is not so sensitive as compared to other functional groups like hydroxyl or amino as demonstrated for the synthesis of 1-(2′-deoxy-2′-fluoro-β-D-arabinofuranosyl [^{11}C]thymine ([^{11}C]FMAU) [350] (Fig. 2.29).

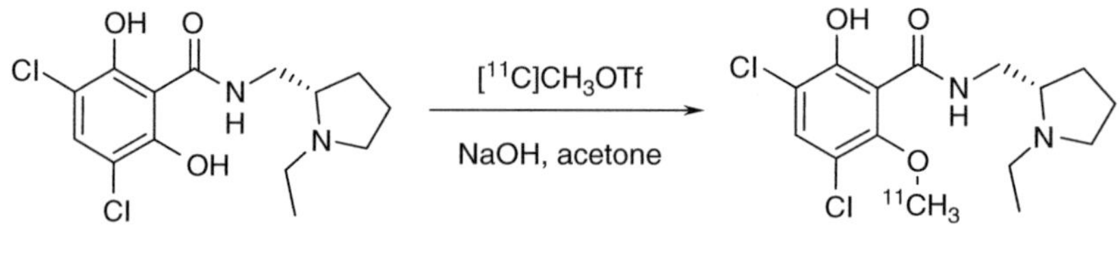

Fig. 2.27 Radiosynthesis of [^{11}C]raclopride by ^{11}C-methylation using [^{11}C]methyl triflate [341]

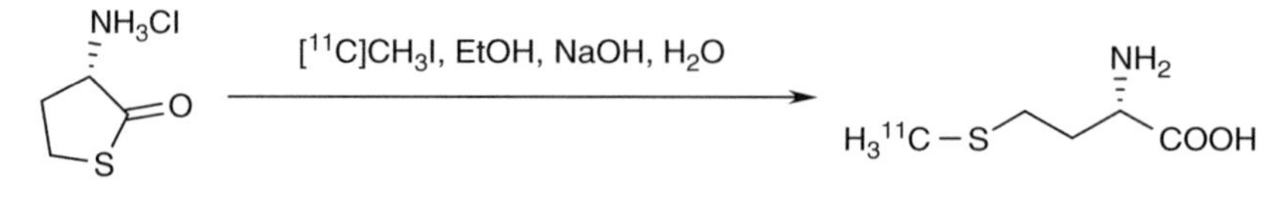

Fig. 2.28 Synthesis of L-[*S*-methyl-^{11}C]methionine [342]

Fig. 2.29 Radiosynthesis of [^{11}C]FMAU via Stille coupling [350]

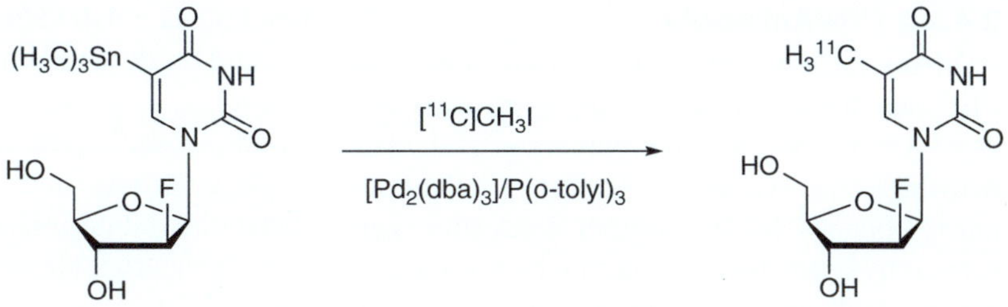

2.4.1.5 Other ^{11}C-Building Blocks

[^{11}C]CH_3I is a starting material for other ^{11}C-building blocks. It can be converted to [^{11}C]CS_2 [351], to [^{11}C]formaldehyde [352], and to [^{11}C]CH_3NO_2 [353] (Fig. 2.24), which are building blocks for conversion into ^{11}C-labeled dithiocarbamates and different kinds of amines, respectively [322].

The ^{11}C-building blocks [^{11}C]$COCl_2$ und [^{11}C]HCN are obtained by high temperature conversion of [^{11}C]CH_4 (Fig. 2.24), that necessitates special technical equipment and is only performed by in-house modified radiosynthesizers [323]. This is also true for the most versatile building block used, [^{11}C]carbon monoxide (Fig. 2.24), that enables the introduction of carbon-11 in carbonyl or amido position of many promising radiotracers [323, 354].

2.4.2 Nitrogen-13 (^{13}N) and Oxygen-15 (^{15}O)

Nitrogen-13 and oxygen-15, both pure positron emitters, are attractive radionuclides for radiolabeling since their stable isotopes are ubiquitous in endogenous compounds [50]. However, their short physical half-lives of 9.97 min (nitrogen-13) and 2.03 min (oxygen-15) limit their application spectrum, and only small number of ^{13}N- or ^{15}O-labeled molecules is in clinical use.

2.4.2.1 Basics in ^{13}N- and ^{15}O-Chemistry

The fast chemistry of the desired radiotracers is performed ideally within one chemical transformation step or directly within the cyclotron target during irradiation.

Different nuclear reactions are available for the production of nitrogen-13. Today, the

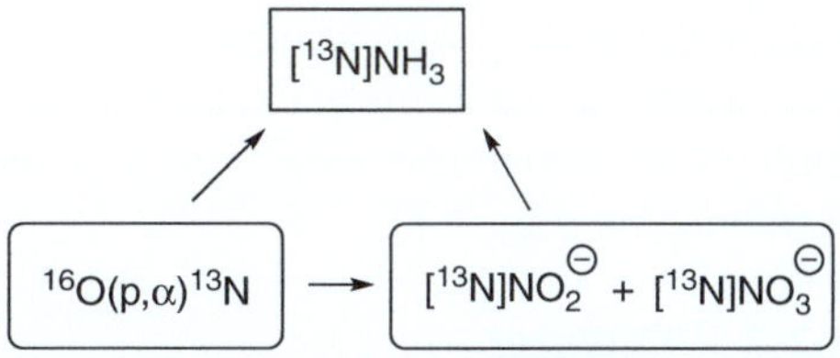

Fig. 2.30 Production of [^{13}N]ammonia [8]

^{16}O(p,α)^{13}N reaction in natural water is the nuclear reaction of choice for routine production of nitrogen-13, which leads to the formation of a mixture of [^{13}N]nitrogen, [^{13}N]nitrite, [^{13}N]nitrate, and [^{13}N]ammonia [1, 41, 50] (Fig. 2.30).

Regarding the production of oxygen-15, three nuclear reactions are predominantly used for the production of oxygen-15 depending on the available cyclotron and the desired product. The ^{14}N(d,n)^{15}O reaction by bombardment of nitrogen gas with deuterons in the presence of an oxygen content (<5%) leads to low molar activities but can be produced with compact cyclotrons that are able to accelerate deuterons. If only low-energy protons and no deuterons are available, then ^{15}O is normally produced via the ^{15}N(p,n)^{15}O reaction in a target of isotopically enriched ^{15}N, which is commercially available as target material but cost-intensive. The ^{16}O(p,pn)^{15}O reaction in an energy range of 26–16 MeV is a method to obtain oxygen-15 in high specific activity and avoids the production of carbon-11. However, it necessitates the use of accelerators with higher proton energies of up to 26 MeV. Despite their short physical half-lives, a lot of different ^{13}N- and ^{15}O-labeled compounds have been developed by fast chemical or biochemical methods, including ^{13}N-labeled amino acids.

2.4.2.2 [^{13}N]Ammonia

[^{13}N]Ammonia is the predominantly used ^{13}N-PET radiotracer for the diagnosis of heart diseases [355, 356] and for exploring glutamate dehydrogenase (GDH) [357]. Pure [^{13}N]ammonia is obtained by an in-target production performed by irradiation of water in the presence of ethanol [358–361] or by reduction of [^{13}N]NO_x using different reducing agents [360, 362, 363]. However, the method using an ethanol solution as liquid target material is one of the best choices in respect of radiochemical yield, molar activity, and automation (Fig. 2.30).

2.4.2.3 [^{15}O]Water

[^{15}O]H_2O is used for measuring regional cerebral blood flow and metabolism [364, 365]. Starting from [^{15}O]O_2, the synthesis of [^{15}O]H_2O is performed by reduction with H_2-gas in the presence of palladium [48, 366, 367] or platinum [368] catalysts at high temperatures. An in-target production of [^{15}O]H_2O using the ^{16}O(p,pn)^{15}O reaction is possible by adding of ca. 5% hydrogen to the nitrogen gas target which leads to high molar activities [49, 369–371] but also to large amounts of *in-target* produced nonradioactive ammonia [335] (Fig. 2.31).

2.4.3 Fluorine-18 (^{18}F)

2.4.3.1 Introduction

Fluorine is a favorable element in medicinal chemistry due to its physical properties including its small van der Waals radius (1.47 Å), high electronegativity, and ability to form a strong bond with carbon (C-F energy bond of 468 kJ/mol), which in comparison to a carbon-hydrogen bond (C–H = 410 kJ/mol) is more thermally stable and oxidant resistant [372]. Fluorine substitution in a bioactive molecule can enhance potency, gain impact regarding biological target binding affinity and selectivity, and increase metabolic stability. Thus, the number of fluorine-containing drugs significantly increased in recent years [373].

In the field of radiochemistry, fluorine-18 also gained high interest due to its favorable nuclear and physical characteristics, including high positron decay ratio (97%) and low positron energy (maximum 0.635 MeV), resulting in a short positron emission range in tissue (<2.4 mm) and thus in a better spatial resolution in PET imaging. With an ideal physical half-life of 109.8 min, ^{18}F permits sufficient time for multi-step synthetic radiolabeling within one to three physical half-lives and transportation of high activity batches to external PET centers several hours away (satellite concept), while offering low overall radiation exposure to a patient [374, 375].

2.4.3.2 Basics in ^{18}F-Chemistry

Optimal radiolabeling yields are obtained by the introduction of the radionuclide into the molecule as late as possible during the multi-step synthesis of a PET radiopharmaceutical. To realize late-stage ^{18}F-fluorination and to prevent unspecific radiolabeling, functional groups in the molecule (such as –OH, –COOH, –NH_2) have to be normally blocked by specific protecting groups. These protecting groups have to be stable during the radiolabeling procedure but also rapidly and easily removable under conditions that maintain the stability of the radiofluorinated target molecule.

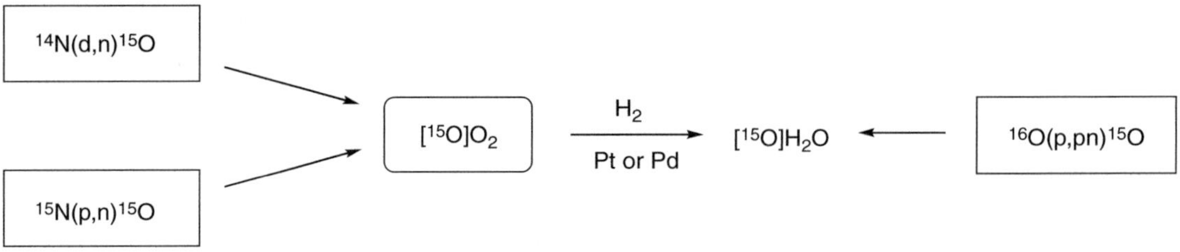

Fig. 2.31 Production routes to [^{15}O]O_2 gas and [^{15}O]H_2O [8]

Generally, there are two different strategies to incorporate ^{18}F into organic molecules: the direct radiofluorination, where the radionuclide is directly introduced into the molecule in the last step of the radiosynthesis, and the indirect radiofluorination, which involves the use of so-called prosthetic groups that require a multi-step radiosynthesis approach. These prosthetic groups are small ^{18}F-labeled alkyl or aryl groups with reactive functional moieties and are often applied for radiolabeling of more complex biomolecules, which do not tolerate direct radiofluorination conditions [376].

Fluorine can react as an electrophile (positively charged) or as a nucleophile (negatively charged). Thus, the direct fluorination strategy can be subdivided into two areas: the electrophilic and the nucleophilic fluorination. Although nucleophilic fluorination is currently the most common synthetic approach for ^{18}F-radiolabeling, electrophilic fluorination has played an important and historic role in the development of ^{18}F-labeled molecules for PET imaging: such as 2-[^{18}F]fluoro-2-deoxyglucose ([^{18}F]FDG) (Fig. 2.32) [377], 6-[^{18}F]fluoro-3,4-dihydroxy-L-phenylalanine ([^{18}F]FDOPA) [379], and 2-[^{18}F]fluoro-L-tyrosine [380].

2.4.3.3 Direct Electrophilic ^{18}F-Fluorination

As discussed in Sect. 2.2, the production of electrophilic [^{18}F]F_2 involves the addition of carrier [^{19}F]F_2 in order to extract the fluorine-18 from the target. Therefore, the maximum radiolabeling yield using [^{18}F]F_2 is limited to 50%, and low molar activities are obtained. In order to improve the molar activity of [^{18}F]F_2, a method for the conversion of [^{18}F]fluoride into [^{18}F]fluorine gas in an electrical discharge chamber was developed (see Sect. 2.2) [55].

Electrophilic [^{18}F]F_2 and its less reactive derivatives, such as xenon [^{18}F]difluoride [381] and O-^{18}F-fluorinated reagents like acetyl [^{18}F] hypofluorite ([^{18}F]CH_3COOF) [382] and [^{18}F] perchloryl fluoride ([^{18}F]FCO_3) [383], (Fig. 2.33) allow radiolabeling of electron-rich aromatic rings and alkenes, but because of high reactivity and low selectivity, a mixture of fluoro isomers is formed, that needs challenging purification (Figs. 2.32 and 2.34, Route a) [381, 388].

Regioselectivity of the radiofluorination reaction can be significantly improved by the introduction of organometallic leaving groups into the molecule (aryltrimethyltin > aryltrimethylgermanium > aryltrimethylsilane). In addition, fewer by-product formation and higher radiochemical yield (RCY) are observed (e.g., Fig. 2.34, Route b) [389]. *N*-[^{18}F]Fluoro compounds, prepared by direct fluorination with [^{18}F]F_2, have been utilized as mild electrophilic and selective fluorination reagents: e.g., *N*-[^{18}F]fluorobenzenesulfonamide ([^{18}F]NFSI) [390], for the labeling of ethers, allylsilanes, and silanols, and *N*-[^{18}F] fluoro-*N*-alkylsulfonamides [391], *N*-[^{18}F]fluoropyridinium triflate [392], and 1-[^{18}F]fluoro-2-pyridone [393] to radiofluorinate electron-rich aryl compounds and alkenes (Fig. 2.33). The mild and efficient ^{18}F-fluorination agent [^{18}F] selectfluor bis(triflate) (1-chloromethyl-4-[^{18}F]fluoro-1,4-diazoniabicyclo[2.2.2]octane bis(triflate)) [394], prepared using [^{18}F]F_2, obtained by electrical discharge with higher molar activity, has been applied to introduce fluorine-18 into a variety of small molecules (e.g.,

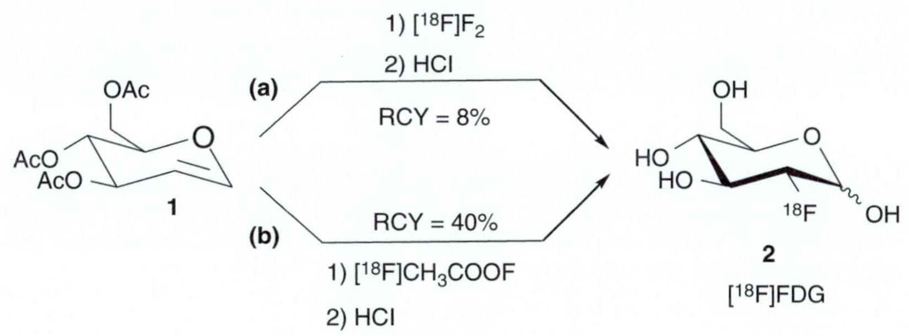

Fig. 2.32 First radiosyntheses of [^{18}F] FDG (**2**) by electrophilic ^{18}F-fluorination of 3,4,6-tri-*O*-acetyl-D-glucal (**1**) using (**a**) [^{18}F] F_2 and (**b**) acetyl [^{18}F] hypofluorite [377, 378]

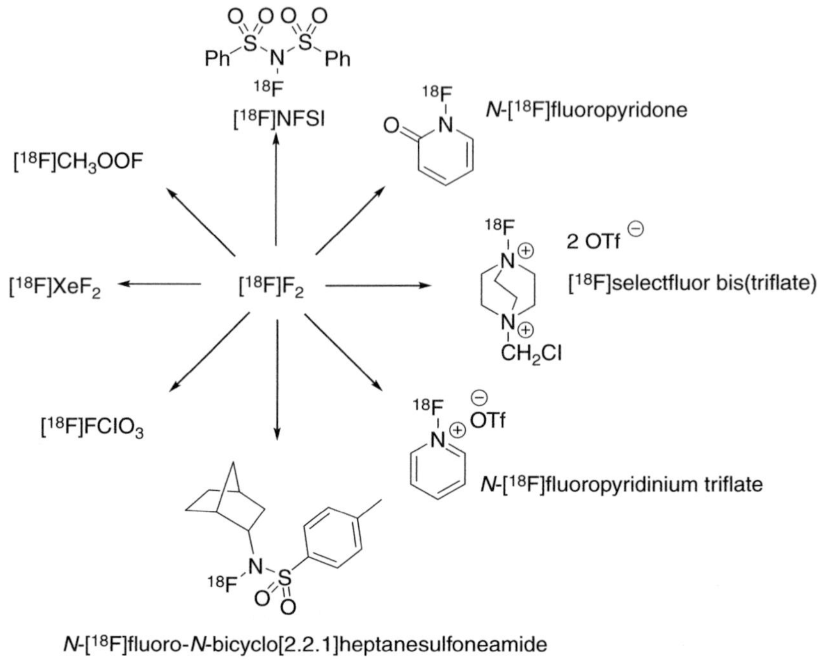

Fig. 2.33 Selection of electrophilic ^{18}F-fluorinating reagents derived from $[^{18}F]F_2$

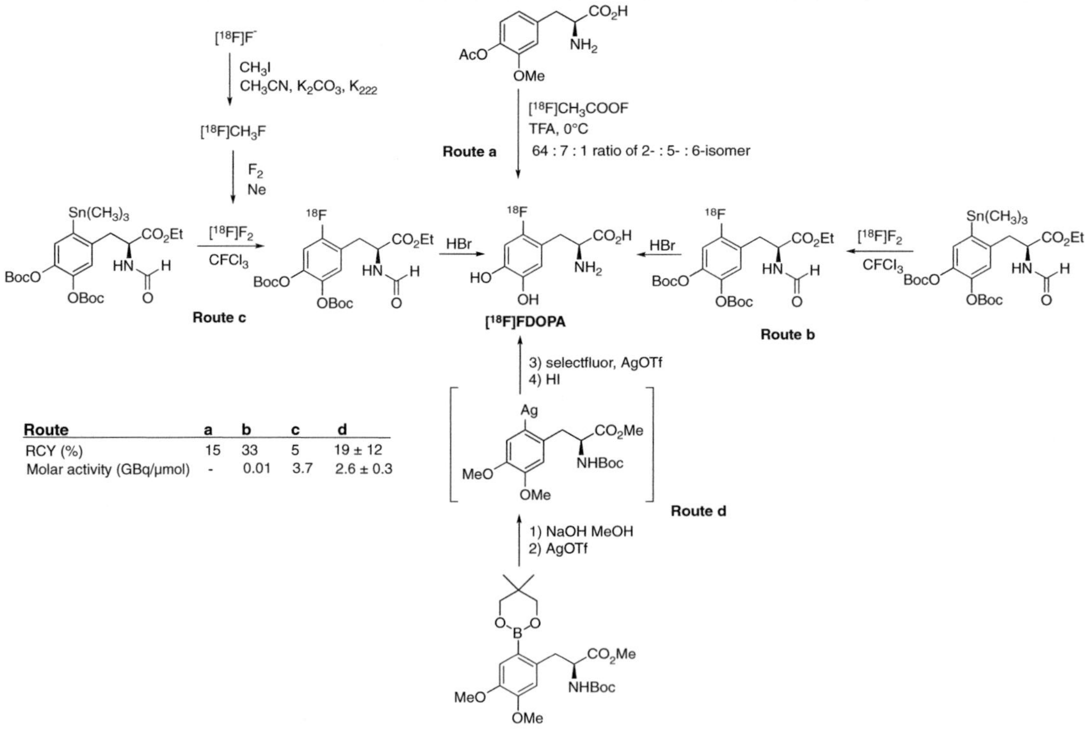

Route	a	b	c	d
RCY (%)	15	33	5	19 ± 12
Molar activity (GBq/μmol)	-	0.01	3.7	2.6 ± 0.3

Fig. 2.34 Electrophilic radiosynthesis of 6-[^{18}F]FDOPA using acetyl [^{18}F]hypofluorite (Route a) [384]; by fluorodestannylation using $[^{18}F]F_2$ (Route b) [385]; by fluorodestannylation using post-targeted produced $[^{18}F]F_2$ (Route c) [386]; silver-mediated using [^{18}F]selectfluor (Route d) [387]

Fig. 2.34, Route d). It proved to be more selective than $[^{18}F]F_2$ and successful when other ^{18}F-fluorination agents were not [387]. Although the utility of $[^{18}F]$selectfluor for mild and selective electrophilic ^{18}F-labeling is very promising, the adoption of this new method is very rare due to challenging preparation of the radiofluorinating agent [394]. Therefore, most of the clinically used radiotracers, such as $[^{18}F]$FDOPA [385], have been prepared by classical electrophilic reaction using low molar activity $[^{18}F]F_2$ and acetyl $[^{18}F]$hypofluorite.

The first electrophilic ^{18}F-fluorination agent derived from nucleophilic $[^{18}F]$fluoride was reported in 2011 by Ritter and coworkers [395]. Reaction of a Pd(IV)-fluoride complex with Pd(II)-aryl compounds results in oxidative fluorine transfer to give a Pd(IV)-fluoride-aryl complex, which undergoes C-F-reductive elimination to yield ^{18}F-aryl products. This method can be applied for ^{18}F-labeling of electron-rich arenes [395].

However, the use of this method is limited due to the need for two separate reaction steps involving two palladium complexes, as well as dry radiofluorination conditions. Therefore, a one-step oxidative ^{18}F-fluorination of aryl-nickel complexes, using aqueous $[^{18}F]$fluoride, 18-crown-6, and the hypervalent iodine oxidant (Fig. 2.35), was developed by the same group [397]. The reaction proceeds in less than 1 min and provides ^{18}F-labeled aryl compounds in high molar activity and good radiochemical yields. 6-$[^{18}F]$FDOPA ($[^{18}F]$**3a**), 6-$[^{18}F]$fluoro-L-*m*-tyrosine ($[^{18}F]$**3b**, $[^{18}F]$FMT), and 6-$[^{18}F]$fluorodopamine ($[^{18}F]$**3c**, $[^{18}F]$FDA) were successfully synthesized with high molar activities using this method (Fig. 2.35) [396].

2.4.3.4 Nucleophilic ^{18}F-Fluorination

Nucleophilic $[^{18}F]$fluoride is commonly produced by bombardment of ^{18}O-enriched water ($[^{18}O]H_2O$ > 95%) with protons using the $^{18}O(p,n)^{18}F$-nuclear reaction using a cyclotron. The aqueous $[^{18}F]$fluoride solution from the target is commonly trapped on an anion exchange column to allow the recovery of $[^{18}O]H_2O$. Eluted from the column with poorly nucleophilic bases (typically potassium carbonate or bicarbonate) in a water/acetonitrile solution, the aqueous $[^{18}F]$fluoride is unreactive and thus cannot be used for nucleophilic substitution, because it forms hydrogen bonds with the surrounding water molecules. Anion activators like the cryptand Kryptofix®2.2.2 in the presence of K_2CO_3 ($(K \subset 2.2.2)_2CO_3$) or the phase transfer catalyst tetrabutylammonium (bi)carbonate are added to the $[^{18}F]$fluoride solution to enhance the nucleophilicity of the $[^{18}F]$fluoride ion. After azeotropic distillation of the water using acetonitrile reactive nucleophilic $[^{18}F]$fluoride is formed, that can be introduced by the S_N2

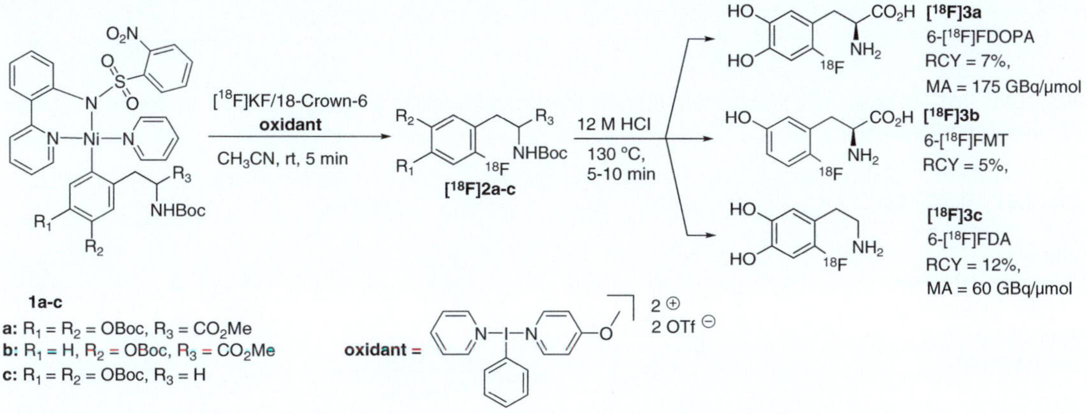

Fig. 2.35 Preparation of 6-$[^{18}F]$FDOPA ($[^{18}F]$**3a**), 6-$[^{18}F]$FMT ($[^{18}F]$**3b**), and 6-$[^{18}F]$FDA ($[^{18}F]$**3c**) via nickel-mediated electrophilic fluorination [396]

reaction into aliphatic positions or by nucleophilic aromatic substitution (S_NAr) into aromatic rings. Polar aprotic solvents such as dimethyl sulfoxide (DMSO), *N,N*-dimethylformamide (DMF), *N,N*-dimethylacetamide, and acetonitrile are preferred solvents for nucleophilic substitution reactions [374].

Recently, a new radiolabeling method called the "minimalist approach" was reported, which eliminates the need not only for a base or other additives but also for time-consuming azeotropic evaporation steps. Direct elution of [^{18}F]fluoride from the anion exchange resin with alcoholic solutions (methanol or ethanol) of precursors bearing a quaternary ammonium, diaryliodonium, diarylsulfonium, or triarylsulfonium functionality followed by heating of the resulting [^{18}F]fluoride salt in suitable solvents (DMSO, acetonitrile, DMF) yielded the ^{18}F-labeled products in good RCY and reduced radiosynthesis times significantly [398].

2.4.3.5 Direct Aliphatic Nucleophilic ^{18}F-Substitution

The direct aliphatic nucleophilic ^{18}F-fluorination involves the S_N2 substitution of [^{18}F]fluoride using precursors that contain a suitable leaving group (such as –Cl < –Br < –I < tosylate < mesylate < nosylate < triflate or cyclic sulfonate) and have been applied to radiolabel a variety of molecules. ^{18}F-Labeled compounds can be obtained in either one or more synthetic steps, depending on the stability of the precursor, the presence of various functional groups, and the reactivity of used leaving group. Usually the first step is the substitution of the leaving group by [^{18}F]fluoride, followed by the second step, the cleavage of the protecting groups, or the conversion of the labeled intermediate into the desired product, if necessary. Many radiopharmaceuticals used for PET imaging are synthesized via aliphatic nucleophilic substitution reaction. Single-step S_N2-radiolabeling has been applied, e.g., for the radiosynthesis of [^{18}F]LBT-999 [399], [^{18}F]fallypride (Fig. 2.36) [400, 401], [^{18}F]fluoropropylcarbomethoxyiodophenylnortropane [^{18}F]FP-CIT (Fig. 2.37) [402], [^{18}F]fluoroethylflumazenil [403], and [^{18}F]Florbetaben (Neuraceq) (Fig. 2.38) [404].

Two-step aliphatic ^{18}F-fluorination reactions involving the cleavage of protecting groups are, e.g., utilized in the radiosynthesis of [^{18}F]FDG (Fig. 2.39) [405], *O*-(2-[^{18}F]fluoroethyl)-L-tyrosine ([^{18}F]FET) [406, 407], 16α-[^{18}F]fluoro-17β-

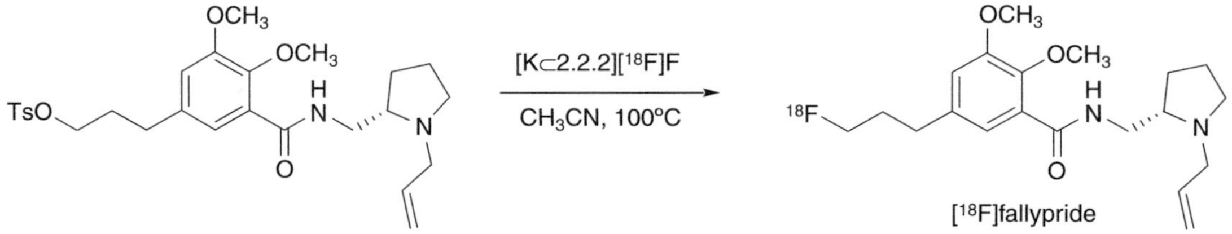

Fig. 2.36 Radiosynthesis of [^{18}F]fallypride from its tosylate precursor in a single-step direct nucleophilic aliphatic ^{18}F-fluorination [400, 401]

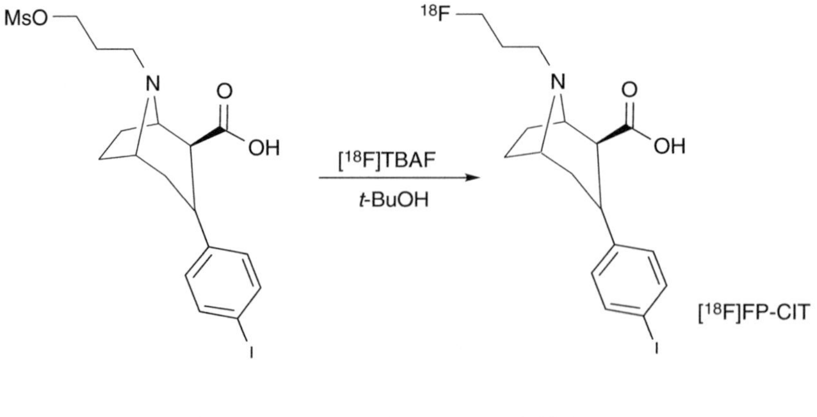

Fig. 2.37 Single-step direct nucleophilic aliphatic ^{18}F-radiosynthesis of [^{18}F]FP-CIT starting from its mesylate precursor [402]

estradiol ([^{18}F]FES) [408, 409], 11β-methoxy-4,16α-[16α-^{18}F]difluoroestradiol (4F-M[^{18}F]FES) (Fig. 2.40) [410], 3′-deoxy-3′-[^{18}F]fluorothymidine ([^{18}F]FLT) (Fig. 2.41) [411–415], [^{18}F]fluoromisonidazole ([^{18}F]FMISO) [416, 417], [^{18}F]fluoromethylcholine [418], [^{18}F]fluoroacetate [419], [^{18}F]fluorofuranyl norprogesterone [420], [^{18}F]fuoroazomycinarabinosidefuranoside ([^{18}F]FAZA) [421], [^{18}F]flortanidazole ([^{18}F]HX4) [422], and [^{18}F]Florbetapir (Amyvid) [423].

2.4.3.6 Direct Aromatic Nucleophilic ^{18}F-Fluorination

Direct nucleophilic aromatic substitution reaction can be applied to synthesize ^{18}F-labeled arenes. Sufficient activation of the phenyl ring by electron withdrawing groups (such as $-NO_2$, $-CN$, $-CF_3$, acyl or carbonyl groups) in *ortho* or *para* position of the leaving group ($-NO_2$, halogen, mesylate, tosylate, triflate, ammoniumtrialkyl) and often harsh reaction conditions

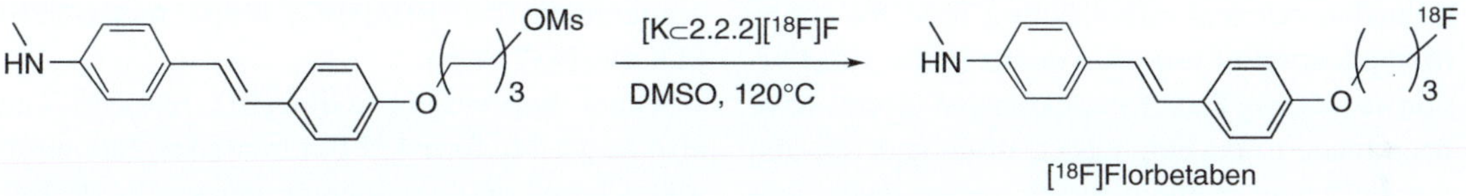

Fig. 2.38 Single-step nucleophilic aliphatic radiosynthesis of [^{18}F]Florbetaben (Neuraceq) [404]

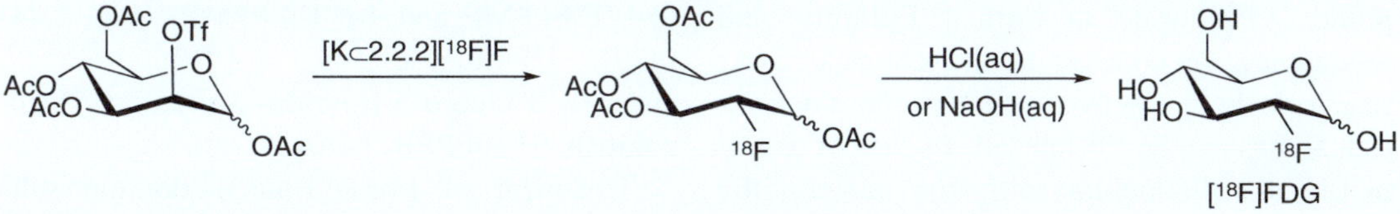

Fig. 2.39 Two-step radiosynthesis of [^{18}F]FDG via nucleophilic aliphatic substitution reaction [405]

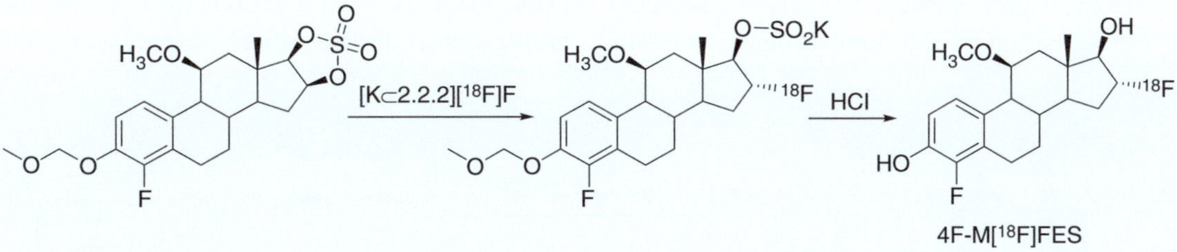

Fig. 2.40 Two-step nucleophilic aliphatic radiosynthesis of the [^{18}F]fluoroestradiol derivative 4F-M[^{18}F]FES from the protected cyclic sulfonate precursor [410]

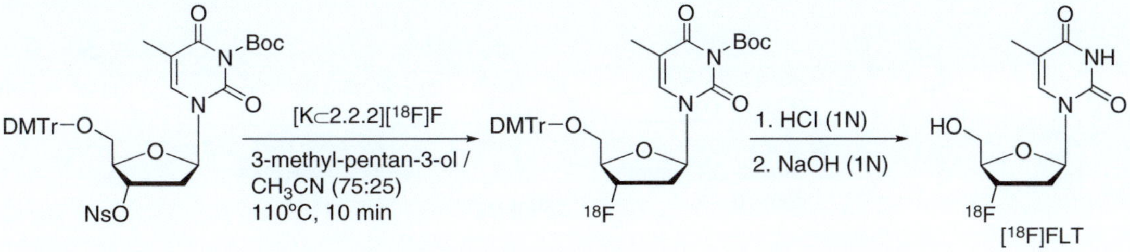

Fig. 2.41 Two-step radiosynthesis of [^{18}F]FLT via nucleophilic aliphatic ^{18}F-fluorination [411]

(temperature > 100 °C, polar aprotic solvents) is required for successful radiofluorination.

Several ^{18}F-labeled radiopharmaceuticals have been synthesized by aromatic nucleophilic substitution including 6-[^{18}F]FDA [424], 4-(2′-methoxyphenyl)-1-[2′-(*N*-2″-pyridinyl)-*p*-[^{18}F]fluorobenzamido]ethylpiperazine ([^{18}F]MPPF) [425], [^{18}F]flutemetamol (Vizamyl) [426], [^{18}F]haloperidol [427], and [^{18}F]altanserin (Fig. 2.42) [428].

However, harsh reaction conditions and the requirement of electron-deficient aromatic rings to enable efficient radiolabeling limit the scope of application of aromatic nucleophilic substitution reactions. Therefore, extensive efforts have been made to develop easier, more general, and more efficient methods to achieve aromatic substitution [429].

Diaryliodonium salts are hypervalent iodine(III) reagents, that also react with nucleophilic [^{18}F]fluoride to form [^{18}F]fluoro- and iodoarenes. In contrast to the classical S_NAr reactions, both electron-deficient and electron-rich arenes can be ^{18}F-labeled. In case of asymmetric diaryliodonium salts, the nucleophilic substitution occurs on the more electron-deficient aromatic component [430]. Asymmetric diaryliodonium salts bearing an electron-rich heteroaromatic substituent allow selective ^{18}F-fluorination of the homoaromatic substituent [431]. Nucleophilic aromatic substitution reaction of asymmetric diaryliodonium precursors has been successfully applied for the syntheses of the following PET tracers: e.g., *N*-(2,5-dimethoxybenzyl)-*N*-(5-[^{18}F]fluoro-2-phenoxyphenyl)-acetamide ([^{18}F]DAA1106) [432], 3-[^{18}F]fluoro-5-((2-(fluoromethyl)thiazol-4-yl)benzonitrile ([^{18}F]SP203B) [433], [^{18}F]flumazenil ([^{18}F]FMZ) (Fig. 2.43) [434], 4-[^{18}F]fluoro-*N*-[4-[6-(isopropylamino)pyrimidin-4-yl]-1,3-thiazol-2-yl]-*N*-methylbenzamide ([^{18}F]FIMX) [435], 4-[^{18}F]fluoro-*m*-hydroxyphenethylguanidine (4-[^{18}F]MHPG) [436], and 6-[^{18}F]FDOPA [437, 438].

Other hypervalent iodine(III) reagents can also be used to form [^{18}F]fluoroarenes. Iodonium ylides based on dimedone or spirocyclic derivatives were used to synthesize radiotracers such as 4-((3-[^{18}F]fluorophenoxy)- and 4-((4-[^{18}F]fluorophenoxy)-phenylmethyl)piperidine (3-[^{18}F]FPPMP and 4-[^{18}F]FPPMP) (Fig. 2.44) [439], [^{18}F]fluoroestrone, 5-[^{18}F]fluorouracil, and 3-[^{18}F]fluoro-5-[(pyridin-3-yl)ethynyl]benzonitrile ([^{18}F]FPEB) [440].

Treatment of (mesityl)(aryl)iodonium salts [441], pinacol arylboronates [442], aryl boronic acids [443], or arylstannanes [444] with [K ⊂ 2.2.2][^{18}F]F and copper catalysts like $(MeCN)_4CuOTf$ and $Cu(OTf)_2(py)_4$ allow the preparation of diverse radiofluorinated arenes via

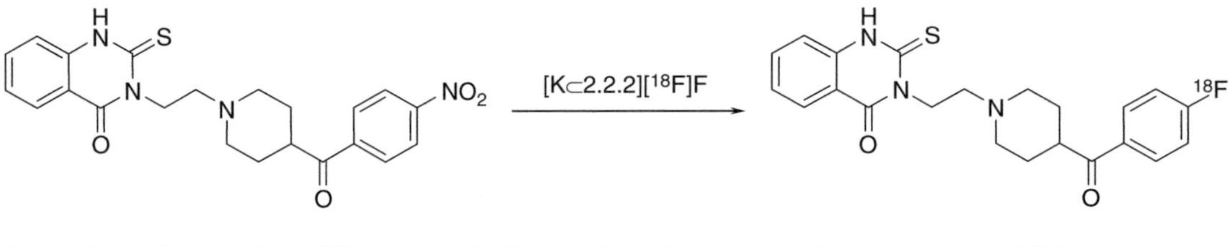

Fig. 2.42 Radiosynthesis of [^{18}F]altanserin via direct nucleophilic aromatic substitution reaction [428]

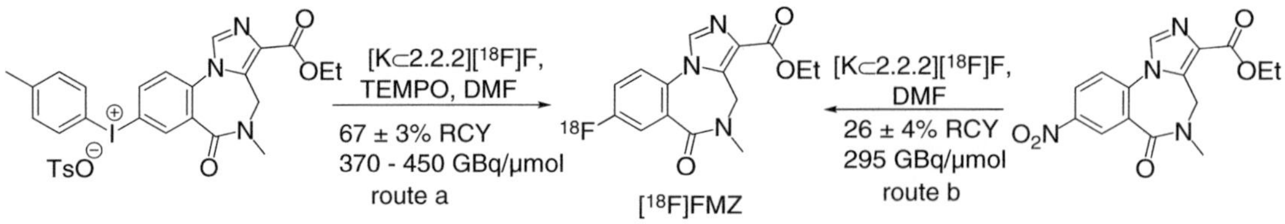

Fig. 2.43 Radiosynthesis of [^{18}F]FMZ starting from asymmetric diaryliodonium salt (route a) and by classical S_NAr (route b) [434]

regioselective Cu-mediated ^{18}F-fluorination. The high-scale production of PET tracers in automated radiosynthesizers using this method is challenging, because of the presence of bases and phase transfer catalysts which are needed for the ^{18}F-preparation. These limitations led to the development of alternative techniques for isolation of [^{18}F]fluoride from the target [445]. Implementation of the minimalist approach to the copper-mediated ^{18}F-fluorination gave rise to ^{18}F-labeled arenes in high RCY [446–448]. Applying this method, automated radiosyntheses of PET tracers like *N*,*N*-diethyl-2-(2-(4-[^{18}F]fluorophenyl)-5,7-dimethylpyrazolo[1,5-a]pyrimidine-3-yl)-acetamide ([^{18}F]FDPA) (Fig. 2.45) [447], [^{18}F]DAA1106, 6-[^{18}F]FMT, 2-[^{18}F]F-Tyr, 6-[^{18}F]FDA, and 6-[^{18}F]FDOPA have been successfully established with good isolated RCYs (Fig. 2.46) [446].

Furthermore, triarylsulfonium [450] and diarylsulfoxide salt [451] proved to be successful precursors for radiolabeling of electron-rich aromatic systems.

Heteroarenes containing nitrogen are more electron-deficient than the corresponding homoarenes and, thus, allow direct ^{18}F-substitution with high RCYs using appropriate leaving groups (like $-NO_2$, trialkylammonium, and halogen) at 2- and 4-positions. This strategy can be applied for the direct ^{18}F-labeling of pyridine- and purine-derived ligands, e.g., the nicotinic acetylcholine receptor agonists 2-([^{18}F]fluoro)-3-[(2*S*)-2-azetidinylmethoxy]pyridine [452] and [^{18}F]flubatine [453] or 6-[^{18}F]fluoropenciclovir (Fig. 2.47) [454], a radiotracer for imaging the reporter gene HSV1-tk, as well as [^{18}F]PSMA-1007, a radiotracer for the detection of prostate cancer (Fig. 2.48) [455, 456].

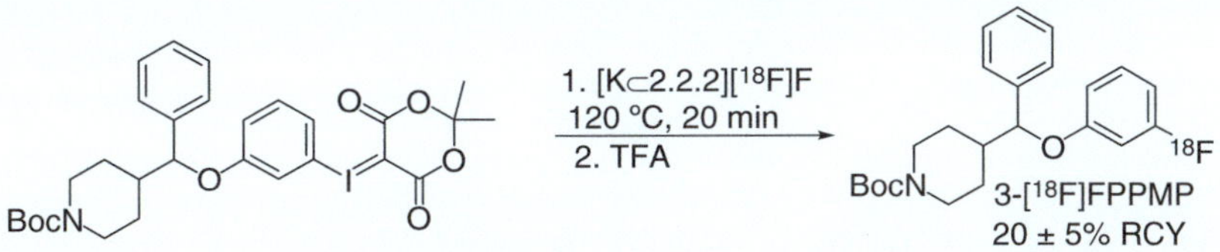

Fig. 2.44 Synthesis of 3-[^{18}F]FPPMP from an aryliodonium ylide precursor with nucleophilic [^{18}F] fluoride [439]

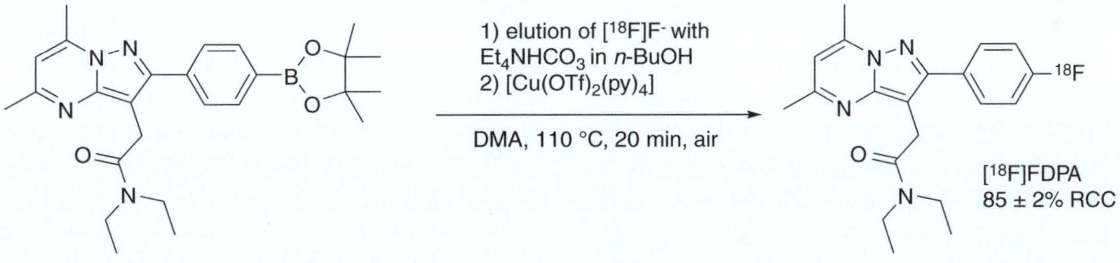

Fig. 2.45 Preparation of [^{18}F]FDPA via *n*BuOH-enhanced Cu-mediated ^{18}F-fluorination starting from a pinacol boronate precursor [449]

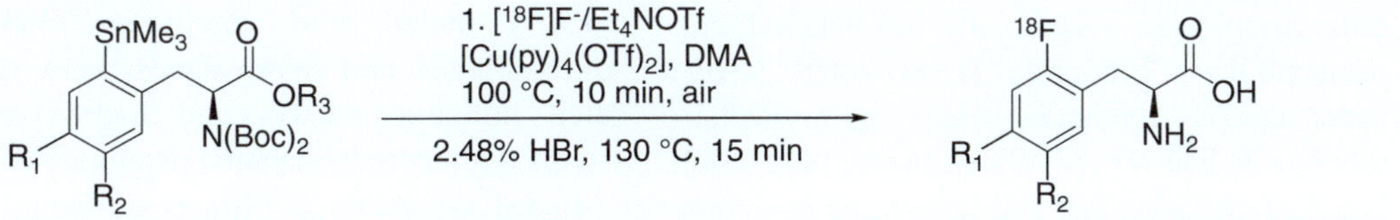

$R_1 = R_2 =$ OBoc, $R_3 =$ Et[Boc$_2$-6-(SnMe$_3$)DOPA(Boc)$_2$-OEt]
$R_1 =$ H, $R_2 =$ OBoc, $R_3 =$ Et[Boc$_2$-6-(SnMe$_3$)mTyr(Boc)-OEt]
$R_1 =$ OBoc, $R_2 =$ H, $R_3 =$ Et[Boc$_2$-6-(SnMe$_3$)Tyr(Boc)-OEt]

$R_1 = R_2 =$ OH, 6-[^{18}F]FDOPA, 54 ± 5%
$R_1 =$ H, $R_2 =$ OH, 6-[^{18}F]FMT, 42 ± 1%
$R_1 =$ OH, $R_2 =$ H, 6-[^{18}F]FTyr, 48 ± 7%

Fig. 2.46 Preparation of 6-[^{18}F]FDOPA, 6-[^{18}F]FMT, and 6-[^{18}F]FTyr via automated Cu-mediated ^{18}F-fluorodestannylation [446]

Fig. 2.47 ^{18}F-Labeling of purine-derived 6-[^{18}F]fluoropenciclovir [454]

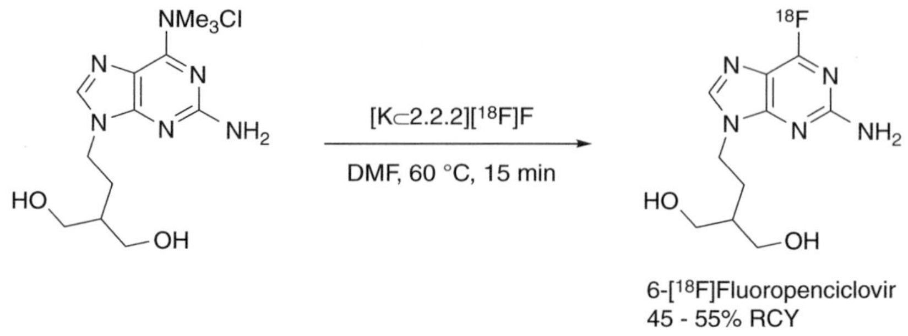

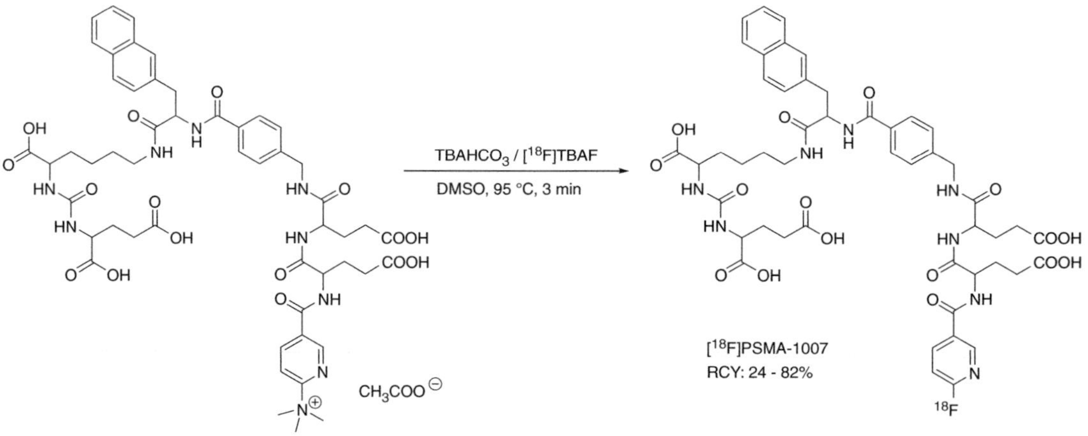

Fig. 2.48 Direct ^{18}F-labeling of [^{18}F]PSMA-1007 [455]

2.4.3.7 Fluoride-Acceptor Chemistry

Beyond classical organic aromatic substitution reaction, nonclassical inorganic approaches utilize fluoride acceptor chemistry to radiofluorinate biomolecules. Several noncarbon elements like aluminum, boron, and silicon also form strong bonds with fluorine. These bonds have strong Lewis acid character, and [^{18}F]fluoride can be introduced under mild ion exchange or chelation conditions [457].

Biomolecules containing aryl boronic acid or ester groups were successfully radiolabeled with nucleophilic [^{18}F]fluoride (most often KHF_2) under aqueous conditions [458], e.g., aryltrifluoroborate derivatives of [^{18}F]marimastat [459, 460]. Practical obstacles that still have to be overcome before routine application are the low molar activities due to [^{19}F]fluoride carrier and low RCY due to slow reaction kinetics. Radiolabeling of 4,4-difluoro-4-bora-3a,4a-diaza-s-indacene (boron-dipyrromethene or BODIPY) derived precursors bearing an aryl and a hydroxyl group on the boron atom revealed higher RCY and molar activities [461]. This method was applied for the synthesis of [^{18}F]BODIPY-trastuzumab (Fig. 2.49) [462] and an isatin based [^{18}F]BODIPY-labeled caspase inhibitor [463].

Organosilicon-based fluoride acceptors, like [^{18}F]fluoro-di-*t*butyldiphenylsilane, were evaluated to successfully radiolabel peptides like cRGD, octreotate (Fig. 2.50), and bombesin analogs, as well as proteins via isotopic exchange reaction under mild conditions [464–466]. Alkoxysilanes and hydrosilanes were radiolabeled utilizing alkoxy- and hydroxy-leaving groups to prepare ^{18}F-labeled peptides [467].

Based on stable [^{18}F]fluoroaluminum complexes folate-PEG-NOTA-[Al[18]F] (Fig. 2.51) [468], [Al[18]F]PSMA-11 [469], [Al[18]F]-NOTA-$PRGD_2$ [470], and other heat-sensitive biomolecules [471] were radiolabeled with fluorine-18 under aqueous conditions.

Fig. 2.49 ^{18}F-Labeling of trastuzumab with [^{18}F]BODIPY [462]

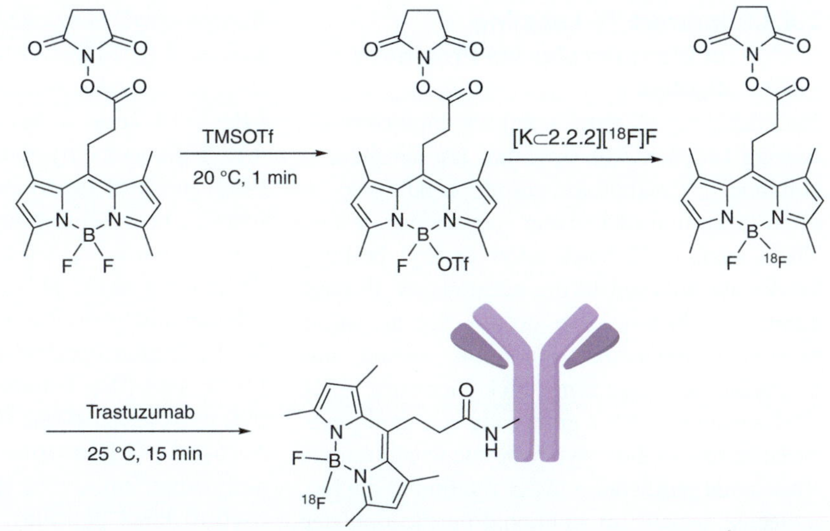

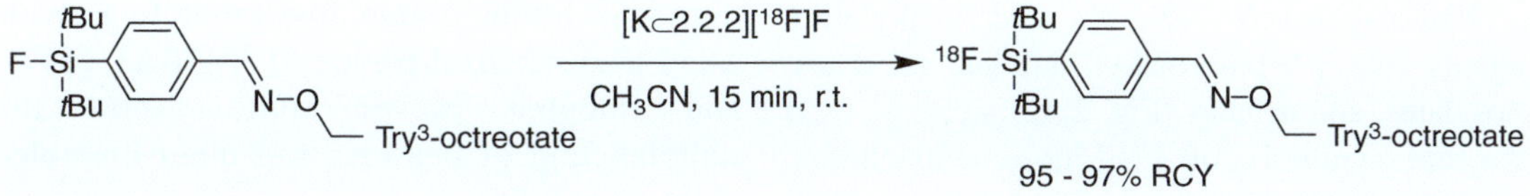

Fig. 2.50 Radiolabeling of Tyr3-octreotate by isotopic $^{19}F/^{18}F$ exchange using [^{18}F]fluoro-di-*t*butyldiphenylsilane [464]

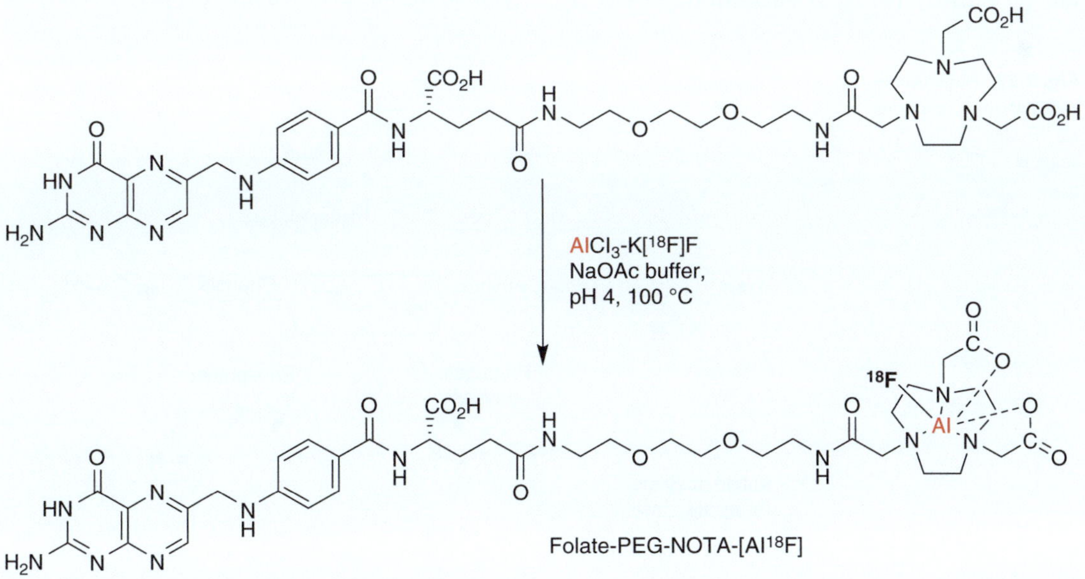

Fig. 2.51 Preparation of folate-PEG-NOTA-[Al^{18}F] [468]

2.4.3.8 Indirect ¹⁸F-Labeling of Biomolecules via Prosthetic Groups

Radiolabeling of more complex biomolecules, bearing functional groups, that are sensitive to common ^{18}F-radiofluorination conditions, is often accomplished using prosthetic groups. These small ^{18}F-labeled alkyl or aryl building blocks are attached to the biomolecule through amine- or thiol-reactive groups via acylation, alkylation, amidation, imidation, oxime, and hydrazine formation using click chemistry [472]. ^{18}F-Labeled prosthetic groups are commonly prepared in one to three synthetic steps and require subsequent purification. After ligation to the biomolecule, usually an additional purification step is needed to obtain the required product.

Radiolabeled *N*-, *O*-, *P*-, and *S*-alkylation agents like [^{18}F]fluoroalkyl halides, tosylates, nosylates, and triflates (Fig. 2.52) are, e.g., used for the synthesis of [^{18}F]fluoromethylcholine [473, 474], [^{18}F]FET (Fig. 2.53) [475], and [^{18}F] fluoroalkyl triphenylphosphonium salts [476].

Amide bond formation using prosthetic groups like *N*-succinimidyl 4-[^{18}F]fluorobenzoate ([^{18}F]SFB) [477], *N*-succinimidyl 4-([^{18}F] fluoromethyl) benzoate [478], 4-[^{18}F]fluorobenzoic acid ([^{18}F]FBzA) [479], 6-[^{18}F]fluoronicotinic acid 2,3,5,6-tetrafluorophenyl ester ([^{18}F] FPy-TFP) (Fig. 2.54) [456, 480, 481], and 4-([^{18}F]fluoromethyl)phenyl isothiocyanate [482], or thiol functionalization applying thiol reactive prosthetic groups like [^{18}F]fluorophenacyl bromide ([^{18}F]FPB) [483], or various ^{18}F-labeled maleimides like *N*-(2-(4-[^{18}F]fluorobenzamido)ethyl)maleimide ([^{18}F]FBEM), *N*-(4-[^{18}F]fluorophenyl)maleimide ([^{18}F]FPM) [484], 1-(3-(2-[^{18}F]fluoropyridine-3-yloxy)propyl) pyrrole-2,5-dione ([^{18}F]FPyME) [485], and *N*-(6-(4-[^{18}F]fluorobenzylidene)aminooxyhexyl)maleimide ([^{18}F]FBAM) [486] are often used to label peptides, proteins, and antibodies. Furthermore other methodologies like formation of imine, oxime, hydrazone (e.g., with 4-[^{18}F]fluorobenzaldehyde ([^{18}F]FBA) [487], and thiourea proved quite useful for radiolabeling of peptides and other biomolecules (Fig. 2.55).

To obtain radiolabeled biomolecules ^{18}F-radiolabeled azides or alkynes can be coupled to PET tracers by Huisgen 1,3-dipolar cycloaddition, also called copper(I)-catalyzed

Fig. 2.52 Selection of radiolabeling reactions of ^{18}F-alkylation reagents [472]

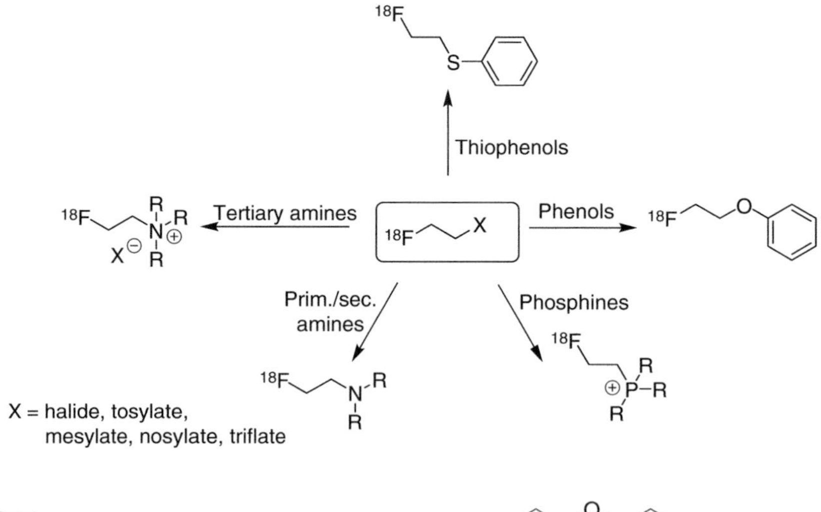

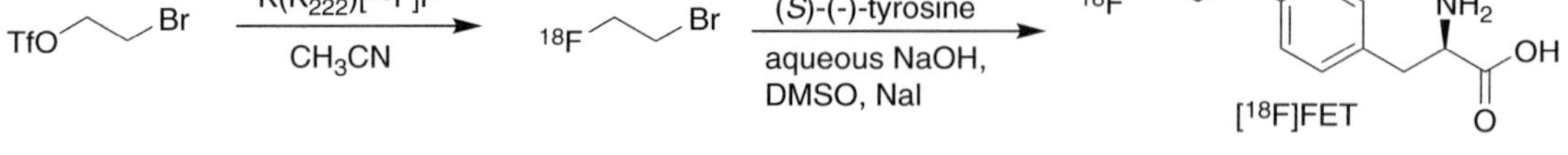

Fig. 2.53 Radiosynthesis of [^{18}F]FET via ^{18}F-fluoroalkylation with [^{18}F]fluoroethyl bromide [475]

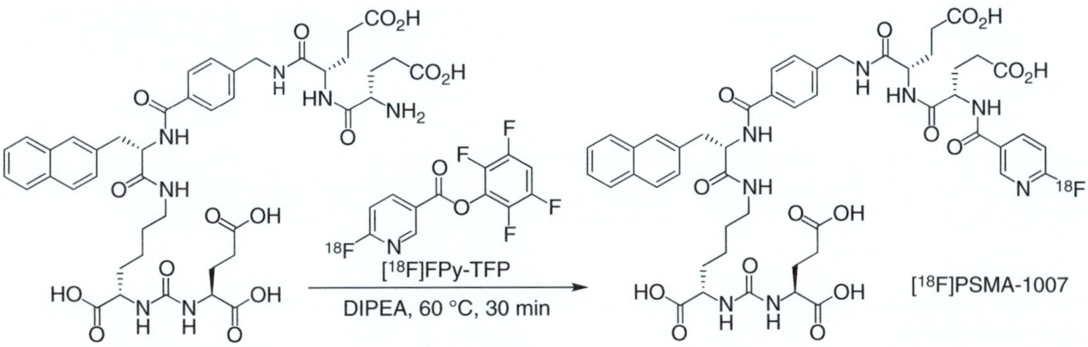

Fig. 2.54 Synthesis of [^{18}F]PSMA-1007 via amide bond formation with the prosthetic group [^{18}F]FPy-TFP. See also direct ^{18}F-labeling strategy for the synthesis of [^{18}F]PSMA-1007 (Fig. 2.44) [456]

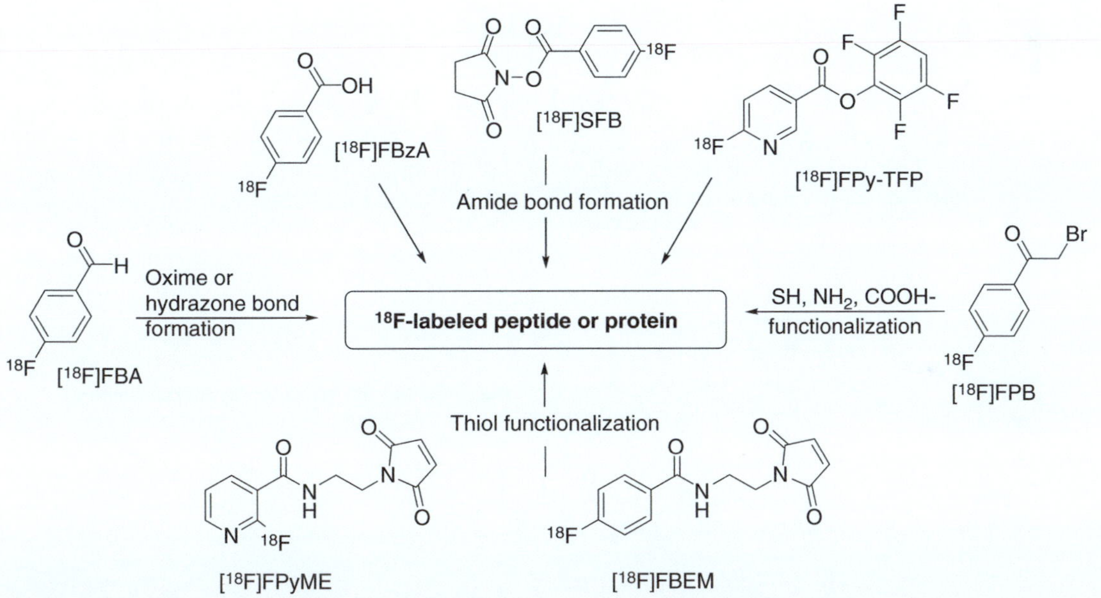

Fig. 2.55 Selection of reagents for the ^{18}F-labeling of proteins, peptides, and oligonucleotides [488]

azide-alkyne cycloaddition (CuAAC) or "click"-reaction. 1,4-Disubstituted triazoles are formed by reaction of an azide group with an alkyne functionality under copper(I) catalysis under mild aqueous reaction conditions and in high RCYs (Fig. 2.56) [490, 491]. An alternative coupling reaction for ^{18}F-labeled azides represents the traceless Staudinger reaction. The reaction of an azide with a phosphine-substituted thioester leads to the formation of an amide bond [492]. Disadvantages of these methods are the in vivo toxicity of copper(I) used in the CuAAC and the instability of the phosphine reagents used in the Staudinger ligation.

The strain relief-promoted alkyne-azide cycloadditon (SPAAC) circumvents the need for a Cu(I) catalyst and involves the reaction of an azide with the bent triple bond of a cyclooctyne, often a dibenzocyclooctyne—to give a triazole (Fig. 2.57) [490, 494].

The inverse electron demand Diels–Alder (IEDDA) [4 + 2] cycloaddition between tetrazine and a ^{18}F-labeled dienophile, most commonly *trans*-cyclooctene (TCO) but also norbornene, also provided fast an efficient radiolabeling using prosthetic groups [495]. Like the SPAAC ligation, the IEDDA reaction is bioorthogonal and proceeds without a catalyst. The principal

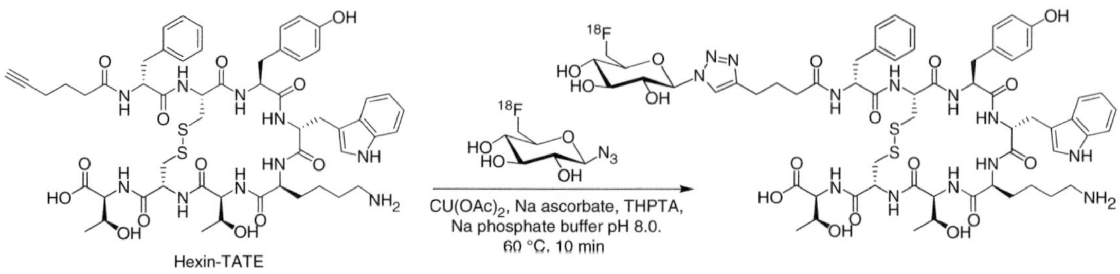

Fig. 2.56 Radiosynthesis of [^{18}F]fluoroglycosylated TATE ([^{18}F]FGlc-TATE) via CuAAC with 6-deoxy-6-[^{18}F]fluoroglucosyl azide [489]

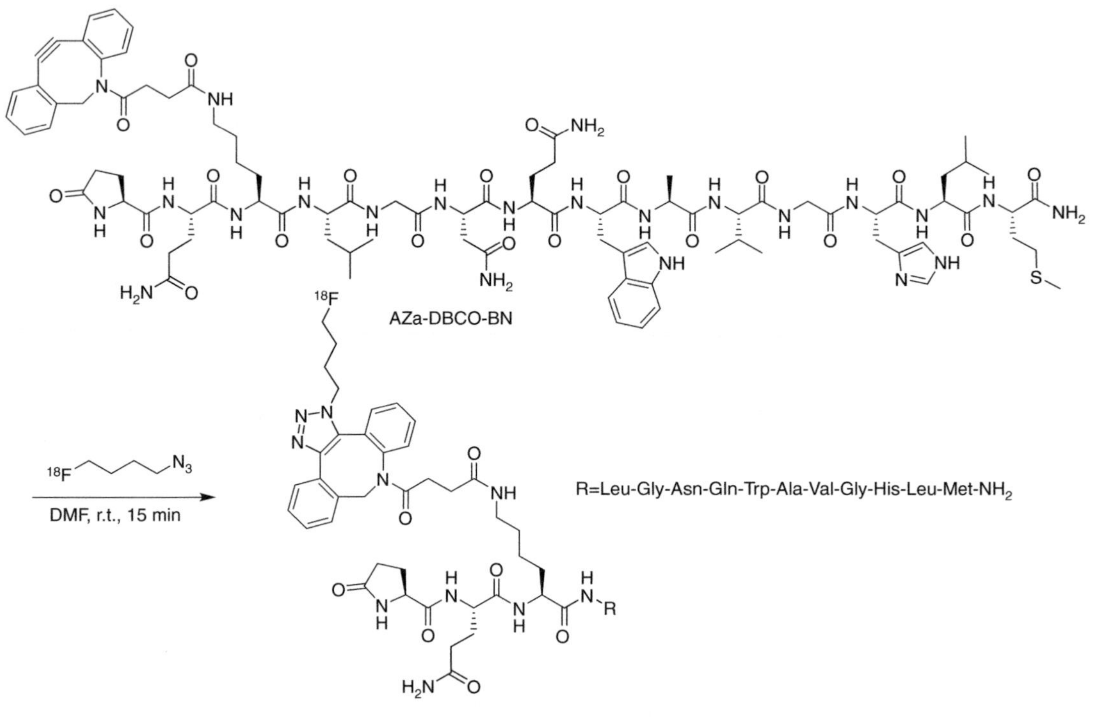

Fig. 2.57 ^{18}F-Labeling of bombesin via strain relief-promoted, copper-free click chemistry (SPAAC) [493]

advantage of the IEDDA ligation is its extraordinary speed, which makes it particularly well suited for applications with short-lived radionuclides [496]. This method was applied, e.g., to radiolabel c(RGDyC) peptide [497], vascular endothelial growth factor (VEGF) protein [498] and poly-ADP-ribose-polymerase 1 inhibitor AZD2281 (Fig. 2.58) [499]. Due to its high selectivity and speed the IEDDA reaction also represents a promising methodology for in vivo pretargeting applications ("biorthogonal reactions"), but until today no application in humans have been reported [491, 500].

Synthesis of ^{18}F-labeled compounds can furthermore be accomplished by palladium-catalyzed cross-coupling reactions. ^{18}F-labeled aryl or vinyl halides can be coupled with terminal alkyne via Sonogashira cross-coupling reaction using Pd(PPh$_3$)$_4$ and CuI as catalyst (Fig. 2.59) [503]. The Suzuki-Miyaura cross-coupling reactions combines aryl or vinyl halides with aryl- or vinyl-boronic acid using Pd(0) and a base or Pd(II) catalysts [501]. The Stille coupling consists of a combination of aryl and vinyl halides with organostannanes by the use of a Pd(0) catalyst [504].

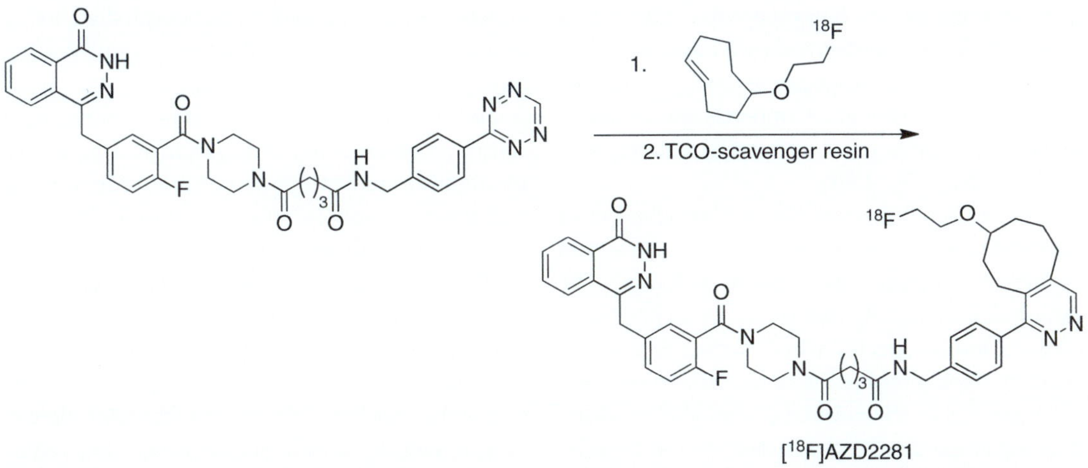

Fig. 2.58 Radiolabeling of poly-ADP-ribose-polymerase 1 inhibitor AZD2281 via inverse electron demand Diels–Alder (IEDDA) cycloaddition [499]

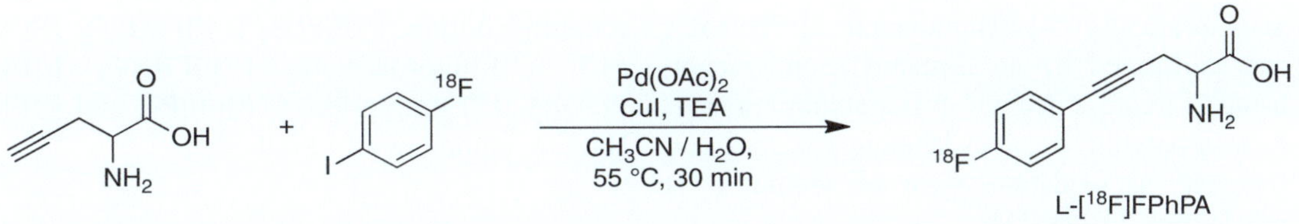

Fig. 2.59 Synthesis of 2-amino-5-(4-[^{18}F]fluorophenyl)pent-4-ynoic acid ([^{18}F]FPhPA) by Sonogashira coupling reaction [501, 502]

2.4.4 Iodine-124 (^{124}I)

2.4.4.1 Introduction

Nonstandard positron emitters with physical half-lives ≥2 h have been developed in order to study predominantly longer biochemical and physiological processes [505]. The most clinically relevant long-lived, non-radiometal positron emitter is iodine-124, which enables quantitative PET imaging over several days with its physical half-life of 4.18 days. The maximum positron energy of 2.13 MeV and the positron intensity of 22% make iodine-124 not an ideal positron emitter; however, several clinical studies showed the principally usefulness of PET studies with this radioisotope of iodine [506, 507]. A first example showing the clinical application of an ^{124}I-labeled compound was a comparison study of L-3-[^{124}I]iodo-α-methyl tyrosine with its ^{123}I-labeled derivative to study brain tumors [508].

The most important production route makes use of the ^{124}Te(p,n)^{124}I nuclear reaction using enriched $^{124}TeO_2$ (cf. Sect. 2.2) [509].

2.4.4.2 Basics in ^{124}I-Chemistry

Radioiodination chemistry with ^{124}I generally employs the same methods with the more commonly used radioisotopes ^{123}I and ^{131}I. These methods can be subdivided into nucleophilic and electrophilic substitution reactions [139].

In general, nucleophilic substitution reactions can be used to introduce radioiodine into aliphatic and aromatic position. The arene ring has to be further activated by an electron withdrawing group. Nucleophilic radioiodination in aromatic positions can be accelerated by the use of copper(I) and copper(II) salts using the corresponding bromo or iodo precursors [506, 507].

The synthesis of ^{124}I-labeled *meta*-iodobenzylguanidine (MIBG), used for diagnosis of neuroblastoama and pheochromacytoma [294] and for imaging the norepinephrine transporter (NET) [510], was performed by a copper(I)-catalyzed, nucleophilic halogen exchange reaction with sodium [^{124}I]iodide. Copper(I) was obtained in situ by reduction of copper(II) sulfate with tin(II) sulfate (Fig. 2.60).

The preferred method for the introduction of radioiodine into arene rings or in vinylic position is the electrophilic substitution reaction. The radioiodide can easily oxidize in situ to positively charged iodine species which serves as electrophile in iododeprotonation or demetallation reactions preferably with aromatic stannyl precursors. The oxidation can be performed by mild oxidation agent including iodomonochloride, peracetic acid, *N*-chlorosuccinimide, chloroamine T, and Iodogen® [506, 507].

The synthesis of 2′-fluoro-2’deoxy-1-β-D-arabinofuranosyl-5-[^{124}I]iodouracil ([^{124}I]FIAU) was performed by an destannylation reaction using 2′-fluoro-2’deoxy-1-β-D-arabinofuranosyl-5-(tri-n-butyltin)-uracil as labeling precursor and Iodogen® as oxidation agent of sodium [^{124}I]iodide (Fig. 2.61) [511].

2.4.5 Automation in ^{18}F- and ^{11}C-Chemistry

Routine production of PET radiopharmaceuticals comprising complex reaction steps involving evaporation, hydrolysis, purification, and sterilization is nowadays accomplished using computer-controlled automated radiosynthesizers, ensuring the realization of the good manufacturing practice (GMP)-compliant radiosynthesis conditions required for human application and at the same time reducing the radiation exposure for personnel involved (Table 2.13). To perform more than one radiosynthesis successively, several radiosynthesizers work with sterile disposable cassettes with ready-to-use reagent vials for each batch production (Table 2.14). Upon completion of the first radiosynthesis, the disposable cassette can be replaced by a new one, and the next radiosynthesis can be performed. Reagent kits and disposable cassettes for the GMP-compliant radiosyntheses of several clinically relevant radiotracers like [^{18}F]FDG, [^{18}F]FET, [^{18}F]fluoromethylcholine, [^{18}F]FES, [^{18}F]FMISO, [^{18}F]FLT, [^{18}F]fluoroacetate, [^{18}F]FHBG, [^{18}F]FDOPA, [^{18}F]fallypride, [^{18}F]MPPF, and [^{18}F]NaF are commercially available.

2.4.6 Important Clinically Relevant ^{11}C-, ^{13}N-, ^{15}O-, and ^{18}F-Radiopharmaceuticals

PET radiopharmaceuticals have found their application in several medical areas: neuroscience, cardiology, and oncology. Several are applied in all three of these areas.

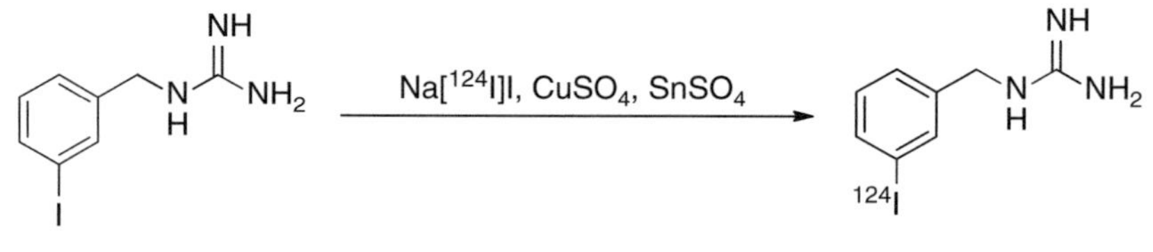

Fig. 2.60 Synthesis of [^{124}I]MIBG (cf. Sect. 2.3)

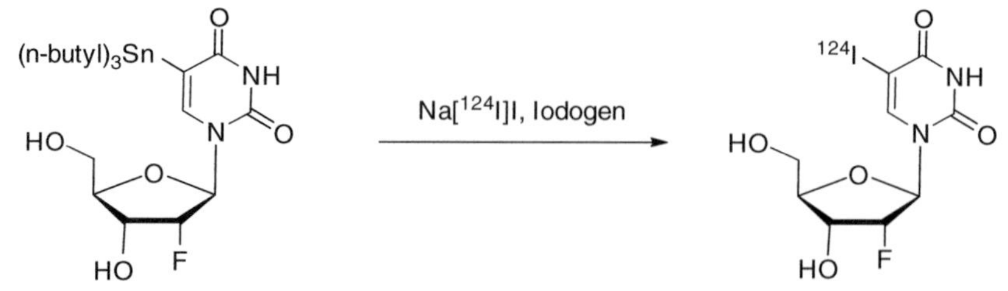

Fig. 2.61 Synthesis of [^{124}I]FIAU

Table 2.13 Automated radiosynthesizers useable with commercially available reagent kits alone

Automated radiosynthesizers		
Synthra RNplus ^{18}F 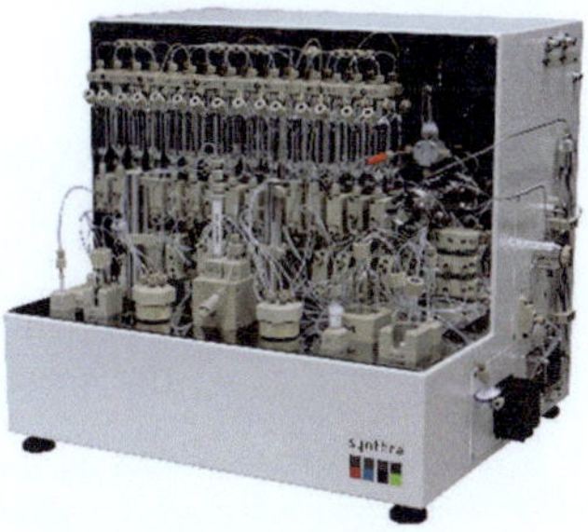	GE TRACERlab FX2 N ^{18}F 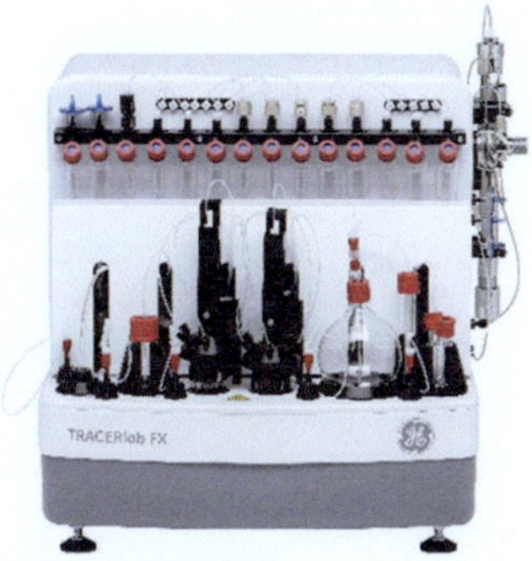	Eckert & Ziegler Modular Lab Standard ^{18}F, ^{11}C 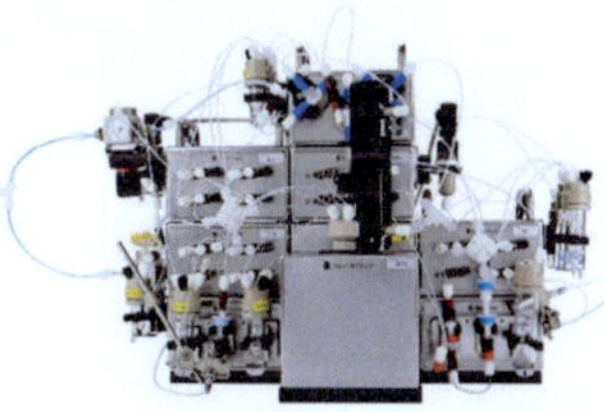
Synthra MeIplus Research ^{11}C 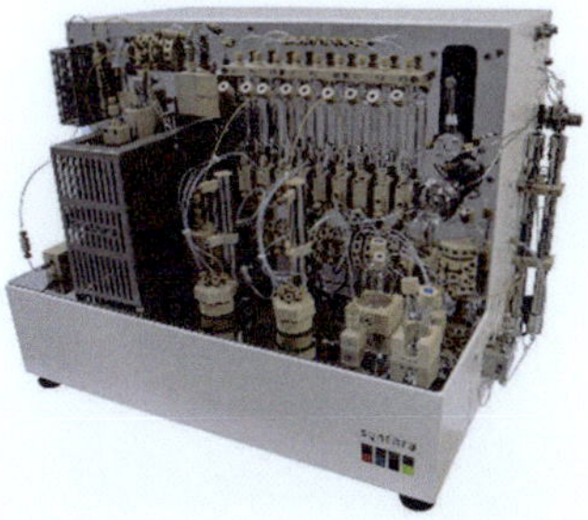	Tracerlab FX2 C ^{11}C 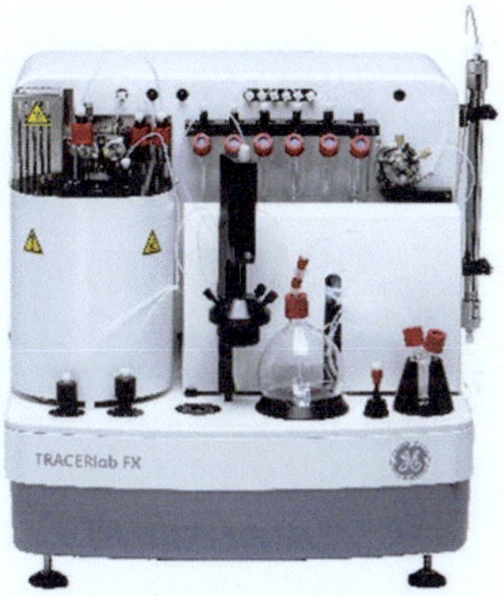	

In general PET radiotracers can be divided according to their specific uptake mechanism or their biological target site; however, each of the classifications does not cover the whole field of PET radiotracers [512]. Thus, in the following, both classifications were used in order to group the different compounds.

2.4.6.1 Tissue/Organ Perfusion/Cerebral Metabolic Rate for Oxygen

Blood flow is the amount or volume of blood supplied to an organ or another specific tissue (e.g., tumor) during a specific time interval. It plays a fundamental role in a wide range of physiological processes and pathologies in the organism. Perfusion is defined as blood flow per unit of mass of tissue. An ideal flow radiotracer accumulates in a tissue or clears from a tissue proportionally linear to the blood flow. Such a linear relationship between blood flow and uptake or clearance of the tracer should be constant and independent of the pathophysiological changes and metabolism of that tissue.

[^{15}O]Water meets most closely the criteria of an ideal tracer for measuring blood flow or tissue perfusion. It is freely diffusible, and the first-pass extraction approaches unity and is independent

Table 2.14 Cassette-based automated radiosynthesizers usable with commercially available disposable cassettes and reagent kits, respectively

Cassette-based automated radiosynthesizers		
Eckert & Ziegler Modular-Lab PharmTracer ^{18}F 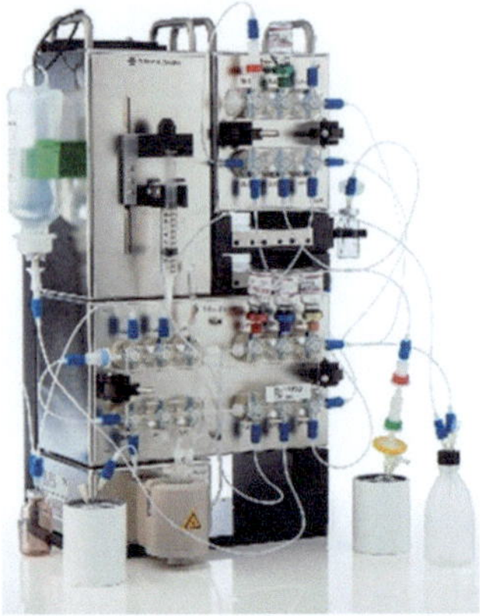	ORA NEPTIS perform and plug ^{18}F 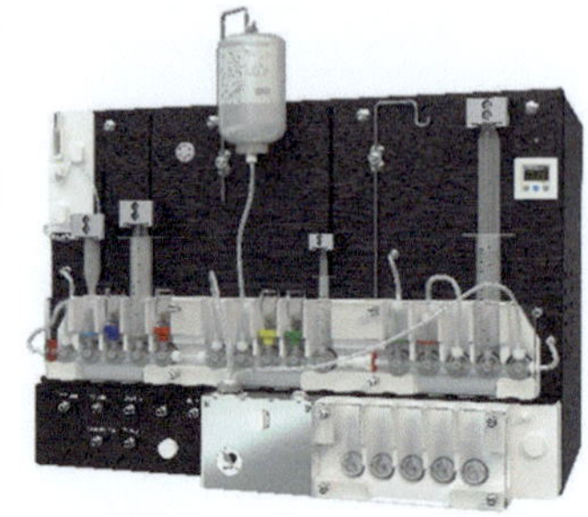	SIEMENS Explora one ^{18}F 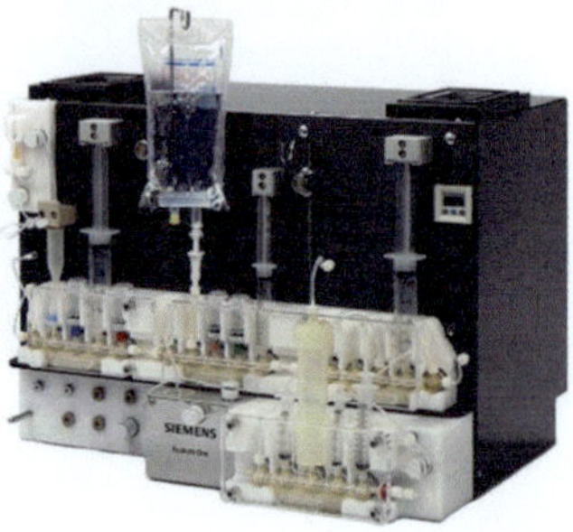
IBA Synthera ^{18}F 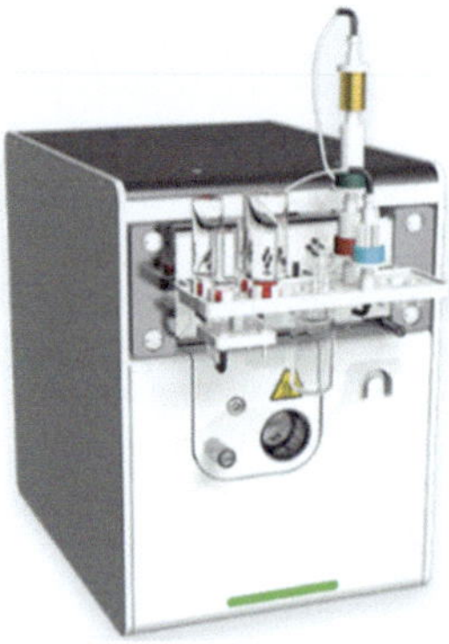	SCINTOMICS GRP ^{18}F, ^{11}C 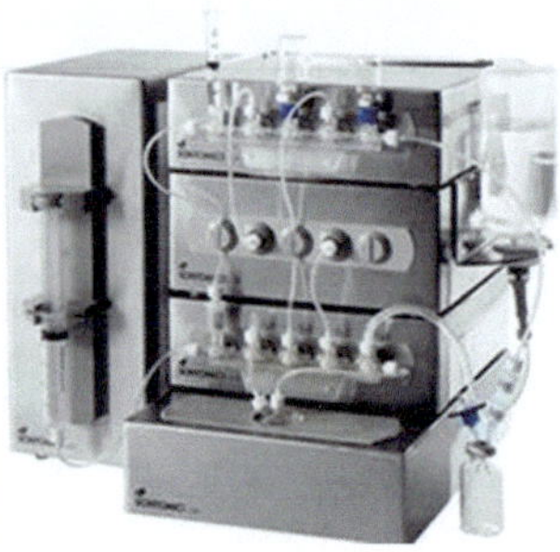	TRASIS AllinONE ^{18}F, ^{11}C 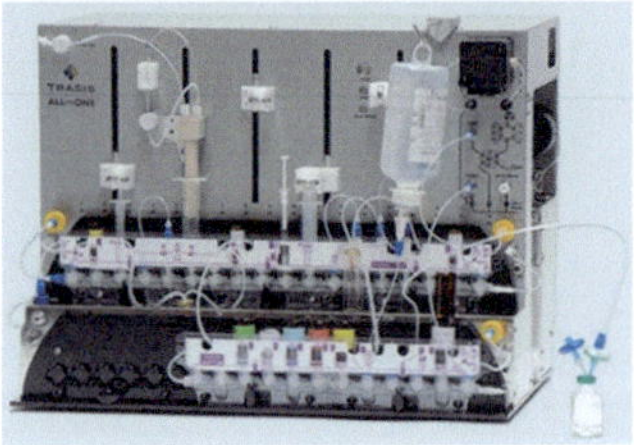
GE FASTlab 2 ^{18}F 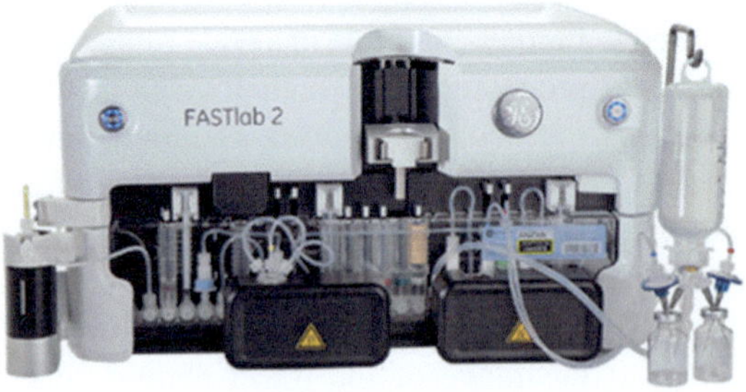 		

of tissue blood flow and metabolic state. It is the most common radiotracer used for cerebral and myocardial blood flow studies as well. PET with ^{15}O-labeled water is considered to be the gold standard for quantifying cerebral blood flow (CBF).

[^{13}N]NH_3 (ammonia) following intravenous administration exists in blood predominantly as NH_4^+ ion, which crosses capillary and cell membranes via passive diffusion. It is effectively trapped in the myocardium following interaction with glutamate to form glutamine. The ammonium ion can substitute for K^+ ion on red blood cells and may, therefore, be actively transported into myocardium and also taken up by myocardium [513]. The first-pass extraction and retention of ammonia is 60–83% [514].

[^{11}C]Acetate has also been used for measuring the relative distribution of myocardial blood flow. Following diffusion into myocardial cells, it is converted to acetyl-CoA in cytosol and then oxidized (metabolized) in the mitochondria by the tricarboxylic acid (TCA) cycle to carbon dioxide and water. The initial uptake in the myocardium serves as a measure of blood flow, while the subsequent clearance may reflect oxidative metabolism [515].

Neuronal activity is primarily supported on oxidative metabolism; thus, cerebral metabolic rate for oxygen ($CMRO_2$) and cerebral oxygen extraction fraction (OEF) are some of the most fundamental parameters to characterize the pathophysiologic status of the brain. The in-target produced [^{15}O]O_2 gas (Fig. 2.31) is used to examine $CMRO_2$ and cerebral oxygen extraction fraction OEF in cerebral tissue [516, 517].

2.4.6.2 Metabolism

Positron-emitting radiotracers have been developed to image metabolism of several biochemicals. The development of an imaging probe involves incorporation of ^{11}C or ^{18}F atom into the molecule of interest (substrate or an analog of the substrate). The enzyme-mediated metabolic transformation of the radiolabeled substrate and subsequent accumulation within the tissue provide a measure of the metabolic rate of the substrate. Since uptake of the probe is based on targeting these specific enzymes (such as *hexokinase*, *thymidine kinase*, etc.), the localization of the radiotracer in the tissue also reflects the level of enzyme expression in the tissue [518, 519].

Glucose Metabolism

The most important molecule to provide energy for various biochemical reactions in the body is adenosine triphosphate (ATP), which is generated in the mitochondria following metabolism of glucose by oxidative phosphorylation to generate the energy needed for cellular processes. In brain, glucose metabolism exclusively generates ATP, while in myocardium, fatty acid metabolism is the major source for the generation of ATP. An accelerated glucose metabolism has been observed in cancer tissue relying on aerobic glycolysis, a phenomenon called "the Warburg effect" even when the oxygen supply is diminished [520]. Glucose is generally transported into the cell by facilitated diffusion through specific glucose transporters on the cell membrane, in case of cancer cells predominantly via the GLUT-1 transporter. In the cytosol, glucose is converted or phosphorylated by the enzyme *hexokinase* to glucose 6-phosphate, which subsequently is metabolized to carbon dioxide and water.

In the 1950s it was shown that the hydroxyl group on carbon-2 of glucose molecule is not necessary for phosphorylation by hexokinase. The deoxyglucose (DG) enters the cell and is converted to deoxyglucose 6-phosphate, which, however, does not undergo further catabolism, however, is trapped in the cell [521]. Therefore, the design of the 2-deoxy-2-fluoro-deoxyglucose (FDG) molecule is based on radiolabeling the carbon-2 atom in DG with ^{18}F [377]. Incidentally the C-F bond, which is more stable than the C-H bond, is chemically unrecognizable by *hexokinase*. As a result, FDG 6-phosphate is also trapped in the cell. In tumor cells, the increased glycolysis and increased uptake of FDG is also associated with increased levels of aforementioned GLUT-1 glucose transporter (insulin independent) and intracellular hexokinase expression [522].

Fatty Acid Metabolism

The ATP production in myocardium is based on a number of substrates (free fatty acids (FFA), glucose, lactate, and ketone bodies) depending on the relative availability of substrates, oxygen, and hormone levels (catecholamines, insulin, glucagons). When plasma glucose levels increase, myocardium shifts to glucose metabolism and, as a result, [^{18}F]FDG can be used to assess myocardial glucose utilization.

In fasting state, when insulin levels are low, FFA levels are high and as much as 70–80% of the ATP production is based on oxidation of FFAs. The enzyme *thiokinase* in cytosol converts FFAs to acetyl-CoA, which subsequently undergo β-oxidation in mitochondria and are broken into two-carbon fragments that are metabolized in the tricarboxylic acid (TCA) cycle. ^{11}C-labeled, 16-carbon FFA chain palmitate (1-[^{11}C]palmitate) is converted to ^{11}C-acyl-CoA in cytosol. Part of this enters the mitochondria and the TCA cycle for oxidation, while the remaining portion is incorporated into the triglycerides and the phospholipid pool in cytosol. Since the metabolism of palmitate is complex, a ^{18}F-labeled FFA analog, known as 14(*R,S*)-[^{18}F]fluoro-6-thiaheptadecanoic acid (FTHA), was developed which shows metabolic trapping in the myocardium with minimal back diffusion of the tracer into blood [523–525].

Choline Metabolism

All cells utilize choline as a precursor for the biosynthesis of phospholipids, which are essential components of all membranes. Within the cell, choline can be phosphorylated, oxidized, or acetylated. The phosphorylation of choline is catalyzed by the enzyme choline kinase [526]. Phosphorylcholine is an intracellular storage pool of choline and is further incorporated into phosphatidylcholine (lecithin), a major phospholipid of all membranes. Carcinogenesis is characterized by enhanced cell proliferation. It has been suggested that malignant transformation of cells is associated with the induction of *choline kinase* activity resulting in increased levels of phosphorylcholine [527]. Furthermore, it is also known that rapidly proliferating tumors contain large amounts of phospholipids, particularly phosphatidylcholine. In 1997–1998, [^{11}C]choline (CH) was introduced as a potential tracer to image brain and prostate cancer. One of the major problems of [^{11}C]choline is the metabolism in blood where it is converted to a major metabolite [^{11}C]betaine [528]. In order to decrease metabolism in the blood, different ^{18}F-labeled choline derivatives like [^{18}F]fluoromethylcholine and [^{18}F]fluoroethylcholine have been developed [529–531], providing high uptake in advanced prostate carcinoma and the detection of osseous and soft tissue metastases [532].

Bone Metabolism

Owing to its high affinity for calcium, sodium [^{18}F]fluoride is ideal for bone imaging which was established in the 1960s [533]. Sodium [^{18}F]fluoride shows high and rapid bone uptake and a good blood clearance that lead to a fast bone-to-background ratio. PET imaging with sodium [^{18}F]fluoride is used for detection of skeletal metastases of breast, head, lung, neck, prostate, and thyroid cancers with high sensitivity [534].

2.4.6.3 DNA Synthesis

Increased mitotic rate, cell proliferation and lack of differentiation were regarded as the main factors responsible for accelerated growth of malignant tissues. Most benign tumors grow slowly over a period of years, but most malignant tumors grow rapidly, sometimes at an erratic pace. The number of cells in the S-phase of the cell cycle is also higher compared to normal cells. As a result, there is an increased requirement of substrates (nucleotides) for DNA synthesis. Intracellularly, thymidine is phosphorylated by thymidine kinase (*TK*) to thymidine phosphate, which subsequently gets incorporated into DNA. Measurement of nucleotide incorporation into DNA in tumor tissue in vitro using [^{3}H]thymidine (thymidine labeling index) is a measure of tumor proliferation.

[^{11}C]Thymidine has been originally developed as a PET tracer to image tumors and measure proliferation rate. Due to rapid metabolism of this tracer in blood, however, the tumor uptake of [^{11}C]thymidine is not optimal for imaging studies and quantitation is difficult. Metabolically stable thymidine analogs, which are substrates for the enzyme TK have been developed [412, 413, 535]. ^{18}F-Labeled 3′-fluoro-3′-deoxythymidine ([^{18}F]FLT) is transported into the cell similar to thymidine and is phosphorylated to [^{18}F]FLT-5′-phosphate by the enzyme thymidine kinase 1 (TK1), which leads to an intracellular trapping of the tracer and accumulation without DNA incorporation [536, 537].

^{18}F-labeled uridine analog, [^{18}F]fluorouridine, also shows accumulation by proliferating cells, but the tracer is incorporated both in DNA and

RNA. Based on this molecule, however, another ^{11}C-tracer known as 2′-fluoro-5-^{11}C-methyl-1-β-D-arabinofuranosyluracil ([^{11}C]FMAU) and the ^{18}F-labeled analogs [^{18}F]fluorouridine and [^{18}F]-2′-fluoro-5-methyl-1-beta-D-arabinofuranosyluracil ([^{18}F]FMAU) were developed, which were also phosphorylated and incorporated into DNA similarly to thymidine [538].

2.4.6.4 Hypoxia

With increasing tumor size, there is a reduced ability of the local vasculature to supply sufficient oxygen to rapidly dividing tumor cells [539]. The resulting hypoxia may inhibit new cell division or even lead to cell death, but it may also lead to adaptive responses that will help cells survive and progress. The presence of hypoxia in tumors has long been established as a key factor in tumor progression and in the resistance of tumors to therapy. Well-oxygenated cells are more sensitive to the cytotoxic effects of ionizing radiation compared to poorly oxygenated cells.

Nitroimidazoles can be used as probes to detect hypoxia. The most extensively studied PET agent in the clinical setting of hypoxia is [^{18}F]fluoromisonidazole ([^{18}F]FMISO) [540, 541]. Several other analogs such as [^{18}F]fluoroerythronitroimidazole ([^{18}F]FETNIM) [542], 1-(5[^{18}F]fluoro-5-deoxy-α-D-arabinofuranosyl)-2-nitroimidazole ([^{18}F]FAZA) [543, 544], 1-[2-[^{18}F]fluoro-1-(hydroxymethyl)ethoxy] methyl-2-nitroimidazole ([^{18}F]FRP170) [545], and 2-(2-nitro-1*H*-imidazol-1-yl)-N-(2,2,3,3,3-pentafluoropropyl)-acetamide ([^{18}F]EF5) [546, 547] have been developed with more favorable pharmacokinetics. Nitroimidazoles enter cells by passive diffusion and undergo a single-electron reduction to form a potentially reactive species. When oxygen is abundant, the molecule is immediately reoxidized, and this futile shuttling takes place for some time, before the molecule diffuses out of the cell. Under hypoxic conditions, further reduction of the nitroimidazole molecule occurs that forms covalent bonds to intracellular macromolecules, in a process of metabolic trapping within the hypoxic cell.

2.4.6.5 Amino Acid Transport and Protein Synthesis

α-Amino acids play an important role in cellular processes including the synthesis of peptides and proteins, energy metabolism, and formation of neurotransmitters and hormones. Furthermore, the sulfur-containing amino acids serves as a methyl donor and source of sulfur in biochemical processes [548]. Therefore, radiolabeled amino acids offer many possibilities as imaging probes for assessing physiological functions [324, 325, 549, 550]. Among all these processes, the use of radiolabeled α-amino acids is mainly focused on cancer diagnostics. It was shown that incorporation of radiolabeled amino acids in proteins has no diagnostic relevance. The cellular uptake and retention is mainly influenced by the amino acid transport process [551].

^{11}C-Labeled amino acids play an important role for the diagnosis with PET. They have been used to track neurotransmitter synthesis, to study metabolic pathways by use of radiolabeling in different positions, or to examine the amino acid transport, which play an important role in diagnosis of tumor tissue [320]. Several methods have been developed in order to radiosynthesize ^{11}C-labeled amino acids in fast and enantiomeric pure ways including biochemical methods [324]. However, up to now only L-[*S*-methyl-^{11}C]methionine is the most applied ^{11}C-labeled amino acid in clinical practice especially for brain tumor imaging.

The short physical half-life of 20 min limits the application of ^{11}C-labeled amino acids. Here, ^{18}F-labeled amino acids serve as a more practical alternative. Several ^{18}F-labeled amino acids are clinically established and ^{18}F-labeled in aliphatic or aromatic positions. The most prominent one is *O*-(2-[^{18}F]fluoroethyl)-L-tyrosine ([^{18}F]FET), a tyrosine derivative, ^{18}F-labeled in aliphatic position and used for localization of brain tumors [552]. [^{18}F]FET is characterized by a high specificity and accumulation in brain tumor tissue and does not accumulate in inflammatory tissues [553, 554].

Other aliphatic ^{18}F-labeled amino acids comprise the different stereoisomers of [^{18}F]fluoroproline [555], and the synthetic, nonnatural [556], non-metabolizable cyclic amino acid analog 1-amino-3-[^{18}F]fluorocyclobutane-1-carboxylic acid ([^{18}F]fluciclovine = Axumin = [^{18}F]FACBC; Blue Earth Diagnostics), a Bracco Company) [557, 558], useful for prostate cancer imaging.

The most prominent representative of amino acids, ^{18}F-labeled in ring position, is 6-[^{18}F]fluoro-L-DOPA ([^{18}F]FDOPA), which is predominantly used for imaging of Parkinson's disease [559] and tumor imaging [560].

Other important [^{18}F]fluorophenylamino acids are 3-[^{18}F]fluoro-α-methyl-L-tyrosine ([^{18}F]FAMT) [561], 2-[^{18}F]fluoro-L-tyrosine [562], and 6-[^{18}F]fluoro-L-*m*-tyrosine (6-[^{18}F]FMT) [563].

2.4.6.6 Gene Expression

Gene therapy holds significant promise in the treatment of human diseases. The main principle of gene therapy is based on achieving a controlled and effective target-specific expression of endogenous genes or transgenes (externally transferred genes into cells) in order to cure or to slow down the progression of a disease. The in vivo method of gene therapy is based on delivering the gene to a specific organ or tissue using a viral or nonviral vector that can be introduced into the patient by inhalation, intravenous, or even local administration. In the ex vivo method, the cells from a tissue (to be treated) are removed from the patient, transfected with the therapeutic gene ex vivo, and then the transgenes readministered into the patient.

One of the common approaches of gene therapy in cancer treatment is suicide gene therapy, in which the genes (like nonmammalian enzymatic genes) make the tumor cells more susceptible to a subsequently introduced prodrug that can be converted to highly toxic active drug. The two most common suicide gene systems are herpes simplex virus type I thymidine kinase (HSV1-tk) [564] and cytosine deaminase (CD) [565]. HSV1-tk is capable of phosphorylating pyrimidine and purine nucleoside derivatives that can be trapped intracellularly [566]. Following treatment, prodrugs like acyclovir, gancyclovir, and pencyclovir are phosphorylated and get incorporated into host DNA in place of thymidine triphosphate. As a result, cellular replication is blocked, leading to a decrease in tumor growth. Similarly, CD, a bacterial gene, converts 5-fluorocytosine into a toxic chemical, 5-fluorouracil (5-FU), which substitutes for uracil in the cellular RNA and prevents translation or protein synthesis [565].

Gene Imaging

The very first stage in gene expression involves transcription of genes into messenger RNA (mRNA), which is responsible for translation of genes into specific proteins (inter alia enzymes and receptors) in the cytosol. PET and SPECT imaging techniques are very important to identify the specific targeting of therapeutic genes, locate the magnitude of gene expression, and finally monitor the response to gene therapy. Two different strategies can be used to image gene expression [567] as follows.

Direct Gene Imaging

In this approach, the endogenous gene expression (mRNA) or transgene expression (therapeutic protein) can be the target for developing radiolabeled probes. A specific sequence of mRNA can be targeted for imaging using a radiolabeled antisense oligonucleotide (RASON) probe such as a ^{18}F-labeled oligonucleotide containing a complementary sequence of mRNA to be imaged. In order to target a specific therapeutic protein, radiolabeled substrates for that protein can be used. But this approach is not necessarily practical since each and every mRNA would require a specific radiolabeled oligonucleotide [568].

Indirect Gene Imaging

The indirect approach involves coupling of the therapeutic gene to a "reporter gene (RG)" and then targeting the reporter gene expression using a PET or SPECT "reporter probe (RP)" [569]. The therapy gene and the RG with a common promoter are administered into a patient using a virus (e.g., adenovirus) vector, which transfers both the therapy gene and RG to the target tumor cell. Subsequently, a radiolabeled RP is used to image the expression of RP gene, which indirectly would provide information about the expression of therapeutic gene. This RG-RP approach can use a gene for the production of a specific enzyme or an intracellular and/or cell-surface receptor in the target cell. When the HSV1-tk gene is used as RG, the protein generated is the HSV1-tk enzyme. Among the pyrimidine analogs, the best radioiodinated (^{123}I, ^{124}I or ^{131}I) substrate for this enzyme is 5-iodo-2′-fluoro-2′-deoxy-1-B-D-arabinofuranosyl-5-iodouracil (FIAU) [570]. The best RP among the acycloguanosine derivatives is 9-(4-[^{18}F]fluoro-3-hydroxy-methylbutyl) guanine (FHBG) [571]. Compared to FIAU, FHBG is a poor substrate for endogenous mammalian thymidine kinase. A mutant HSV1-tk RG was also developed, which generates HSV1-sr39tk enzyme that showed better imaging sensitivity with [^{18}F]fluoroganciclovir (FGCV) and [^{18}F]fluoropenciclovir (FPCV) [572].

Based on the RG-RP approach, a number of other PET probes have been developed to image the expression of genes responsible for dopamine receptors, sodium/iodide symporter (NIS), and somatostatin receptors [573].

2.4.6.7 Aggregated Protein Target

In the human brain, three proteins, β-amyloid (APs), tau, and alpha-synuclein (α-syn), are prone to aggregation and are associated with a variety of neurodegenerative diseases like Alzheimer's disease (AD) or Parkinson disease [574].

One of the common features in the brain of patients with familial or sporadic Alzheimer's disease is the presence of abundant intraneuronal neurofibrils (neurofibrillary tangles, NFTs), extracellular plaques rich in β-amyloid (APs), and neuronal loss [575, 576]. NFTs are aggregates of the hyperphosphorylated tau protein. In contrast, the major components of APs are deposits of a 39- to 43-amino-acid-long β-amyloid peptide generated from a larger β-amyloid precursor protein.

Imaging of β-Amyloid Plaques

The deposition of neuritic plaques is one of the pathological indicators of AD. Thus, the development of PET radiotracers for imaging β-amyloid plaques has been in the focus of research in the last decade [574, 577, 578]. In the last decade, it was shown that the imaging of the density of β-amyloid plaques in brain tissue does not approve the diagnosis of AD, because it does not well correlate with neurodegeneration and cognitive impairment. However, it is a useful method for the exclusion of AD [574, 579].

Probes such as Congo red and chrysamine G known to bind to APs do not appreciably cross the BBB. Therefore, a new generation of radiolabeled highly hydrophobic naphthalene derivatives has been developed for imaging APs in vivo [580]. The investigators at UCLA developed 2-(1-(6-[(2-[^{18}F]fluoroethyl)(methyl)amino]-2-naphthyl)-ethylidene)malononitrile (FDDNP) as a molecular imaging probe using PET, for the localization of NFTs and APs in the brain of living patients suffering from AD. This tracer has the ability to easily diffuse into the brain and bind to both β-APs and NFTs with various degrees of specificity [581].

Modification of the amyloid binding histological dye, thioflavin-T, led to the finding that neutral benzothiazoles bind to amyloid with high affinity and cross the blood-brain barrier very well [339]. The compound 2-(4′-[^{11}C]methylaminophenyl)-6-hydroxybenzothiazole was given the name "Pittsburgh compound B," or simply PIB. The exact form of the amyloid target of PIB binding has not yet been identified with certainty. In vitro studies suggest that PIB binds to aggregated, fibrillar Aβ deposits such as those found in the cortex and striatum, but not to the amorphous Aβ deposits such as those that predominate in the cerebellum. In a human study PIB retention correlated inversely with cerebral glucose metabolism determined with [^{18}F]FDG [582, 583].

The short physical half-life of carbon-11 limits the use of PIB and led to the development of several ^{18}F-labeled derivatives. According to their structure, the amyloid-avid ^{18}F-compounds can be divided according to their structure into stilbene derivatives *trans*-4-(*N*-methylamino)-4′-2-[2-(2-[^{18}F]fluoroethoxy)ethoxy]ethoxy)stilbene ([^{18}F]BAY 94–9172)] [584], [^{18}F]Florbetapir ([^{18}F]AV-45; Amyvid; Avid, Eli Lily) [585], and [^{18}F]Florbetaben (Neuraceq, Piramal Imaging)) [586], a thioflavin T derivative [^{18}F]Flutemetamol

(Vizamyl; GE Healthcare) [426], a benzofurane derivative [^{18}F]AZD 4694 [587], and a benzoxazole derivative [^{18}F]MK3328 [588].

Imaging of Tau/Synuclein

It was shown that the spread and the density of abundant NFTs correlates better with progressive cognitive symptoms of dementia than the presence of Aβ-plaques [589]. Because of the central role of tau in the pathogenesis of AD, the PET imaging of NFTs may enable the early imaging of the disease.

There are four families of compounds which showed high-affinity and selectivity to the tau protein and which were used for first in-human clinical trials. The THK compounds [^{18}F]THK523 [590], [^{18}F]THK5105, and [^{18}F]THK-5117 [591] based on arylquinoline structures; the PBB compounds [^{11}C]PBB3 [592] and [^{18}F]FACT [593], that contain a phenylbutadienylbenzothiazole structure. A series of two lead structures based on carbazole and benzimidazole derivatives led to the development of [^{18}F]T807 [594] and [^{18}F]T808 [595].

2.4.6.8 Apoptosis

Type I programmed cell death, called *apoptosis*, represents a suicide mechanism of cells triggered by a defined energy-dependent genetically controlled program without inflammatory response [596, 597] (cf. Sect. 2.3.1.6). Apoptosis is considered a vital component of various processes including normal cell turnover and the development and functioning of the immune system. On the other side, inappropriate apoptosis is found in many human diseases including neurodegenerative diseases and many types of cancer [598]. Several ^{18}F-labeled derivatives have currently been entered into clinical investigations and prospective phase-I/phase-II or phase-II/phase-III clinical trials for noninvasive imaging of apoptosis: [^{18}F]ML-10, [^{18}F]CP18, and [^{18}F]ICMT-11 [240].

2.4.6.9 Specific Target Interactions

A number of hormones and neurotransmitters bind to specific binding sites or receptors on the cell membrane (such as somatostatin receptors and dopamine receptors) or within the cell (such as estrogen receptors) in order to initiate specific actions. To measure the receptor expression as a function of disease status, radiolabeled receptor ligands (such as peptides and drug molecules) have been developed as PET imaging probes. The binding of these probes to a target site (receptor) is highly specific and depends on the binding affinity (expressed as K_d) of the probe to the receptor and the number of total receptors (expressed as B_{max}) available for binding. Since the number of receptor sites is very limited and low (typically, nmol to fmol), high molar activity (1–10 Ci/μmol) radiotracers are essential to measure the receptor status. In addition, these radiotracers may have either low or high binding affinity to the receptors and are generally trapped in the target tissue following specific binding (reversible or irreversible) of the radiotracer to the receptors. Since agonists are quickly metabolized (or inactivated) following binding to receptors, imaging probes are often developed using receptor binding antagonists ("receptor blockers"). A number of receptor-mediated positron-emitting radiopharmaceuticals have been developed in the last three decades (cf. Table 2.15) [612].

Somatostatin Receptors (SSTR)

Somatostatin (SST), a 14-amino acid cyclic peptide, is secreted throughout the body and has multiple physiological functions including inhibition of secretion of growth hormone, glucagon, insulin, gastrin, and other hormones secreted by the pituitary and gastrointestinal tract. The diverse biological effects of SST are mediated through a family of G protein-coupled receptors of which five subtypes have been identified. Human SST receptors (SSTR) have been identified on most of the neuroendocrine tumors, small cell lung cancers and medullary thyroid carcinoma, and express high densities of SSTRs [628]. The expression of SSTR subtypes in human tumor tissues, however, seems to vary among different tumor types [629]. Octreotide and its analogs (DOTA-TOC, DOTA-NOC,

Table 2.15 Selection of PET radiotracers for imaging neurotransmitter systems

PET radiotracers for neurotransmitter systems that have been advanced for use in human studies			
Neuroreceptor (biological target)	^{11}C-labeled ligand	^{18}F-labeled ligand	References
Adenosine A_1		[^{18}F]CPFPX	Elmenhorst et al. [599]
Adenosine A_{2A}	[^{11}C]SCH442416		
Adrenergic	[*N-methyl*^{11}C]*meta*-hydroxyephedrine		Boschi et al. [600]
Gamma-aminobutyric acid/benzodiazepine ($GABA_A$)	[^{11}C]flumazenil [^{11}C]iomezanil [^{11}C]PK11195 Peripheral BDZ receptor antagonist	[^{18}F]Flumazenil	Andersson and Halldin [601]
Gamma-aminobutyric acid/benzodiazepine ($\alpha 5GABA_A$)	[^{11}C]Ro15 4513		
Cannabinoid (CB_1)	[^{11}C]MePPEP [^{11}C]OMAR [^{11}C]SD5024	[^{18}F]FEMEP-*d2* [^{18}F]MK-9470	Ahamed et al. [602]
Dopamine		6-[^{18}F]FDOPA [^{18}F]FMT	Minn et al. [603], Becker et al. [604]
Dopamine (D_1)	[^{11}C]NNC 112 [^{11}C]Scheme 23390		Prante et al. [605]
Dopamine (D_2/D_3)	[^{11}C]raclopride [^{11}C]FLB 457 [^{11}C]MNPA (agonist) [^{11}C](+)PHNO (agonist) [^{11}C]NPA (agonist)	[^{18}F]fallypride	
Histamine (H_1)	[^{11}C]Doxepin		Funke et al. [606]
Histamine (H_3)	[^{11}C]GSK189254 [^{11}C]GR 103545	[^{18}F]FMH3	
Metabotropic glutamate mGluR1		[^{18}F]FITM	Mu et al. [607], Sobrio [608], Sephton [609]
Metabotropic glutamate mGluR5	[^{11}C]SP 203 [^{11}C]ABP688	[^{18}F]SP 203 [^{18}F]F-FPEB	
Nicotinic ($\alpha 4\beta 2$)		2-[^{18}F]F-A-85380 (2-[^{18}F]FA) 6-[^{18}F]FA [^{18}F]nifene (agonist) [^{18}F]AZAN [^{18}F]flubatine	Horti et al. [610], Sabri et al. [611]
Nicotinic ($\alpha 7$)	[^{11}C]CHIBA-1001	[^{18}F]ASEM	
Neurokinin (NK_1)		[^{18}F]SPA-RQ [^{18}F]MK-0999 ([^{18}F]FE-SPA-RQ)	Pike [612]
N-Methyl-D-aspartate (NMDA)		[^{18}F]GE-179	McGinnity et al. [613]
nociceptin/orphanin FQ peptide NOP	[^{11}C]NOP-1A		Lohith et al. [614]
Opiate (DOR)	[^{11}C]methylnaltrindole		Dannals [615]
Opiate (MOR)	[^{11}C]diprenorphine [^{11}C]carfentanil (agonist)	[^{18}F] fluoroethyl-diprenorphine [^{18}F]cyclofoxy	

(continued)

Table 2.15 (continued)

PET radiotracers for neurotransmitter systems that have been advanced for use in human studies			
Neuroreceptor (biological target)	^{11}C-labeled ligand	^{18}F-labeled ligand	References
Serotonergic (5-HT$_{1A}$)	[*carbonyl*-^{11}C]WAY [*carbonyl*-^{11}C]DWAY [^{11}C]CUMI (agonist)	[^{18}F]FCWAY [^{18}F]FCWAY [^{18}F]MPPF	Zimmer and Le Bars [616]
Serotonergic (5-HT$_{1B}$)	[^{11}C]AZ10419369 [^{11}C]P943		
Serotonergic (5-HT$_{2A}$)	[^{11}C]MDL 1000907	[^{18}F]altanserin [^{18}F]altanserin-*d* [^{18}F]setoperone	
Serotonergic (5-HT$_4$)	[^{11}C]SB-207145		
Serotonergic (5-HT$_6$)	[^{11}C]GSK-215083		
Sigma (σ1)	[^{11}C]SA4503	[^{18}F]fluspidine	Banister et al. [617]
Transporter target			
DAT	[^{11}C]PE2I [^{11}C]Methylphenidate [^{11}C]WIN35,428	[^{18}F^{18}F]FP-CIT [^{18}F]FE-PE2I [^{18}F]FECNT [^{18}F]β-CFT	Riss et al. [618]
Glycine T1	[^{11}C]CFpyPB [^{11}C]GSK 931145 [^{11}C]RO5013853	[^{18}F]CFPyPB	Passchier et al. [619]
NET	[^{11}C]MeNER-d_2	[^{18}F]FMeNER-d_2	Takano et al. [620], Kilbourn [621]
SERT	[^{11}C]DASB [^{11}C]MADAM [^{11}C]AFM [^{11}C]HOHMADAM		Stehouwer and Goodman [622]
Vesicular monoamine transporter (VMAT2)	[^{11}C]DTBZ [^{11}C]MTBZ	[^{18}F]florbenazine ([^{18}F]AV-133) [^{18}F]FP-DTBZ [^{18}F]FEOBV	Kilbourn [623], Aghourian [624]
Channel targets			
Translocator protein 18-kDa (TSPO)	[^{11}C]PK11195 [^{11}C]PBR28	[^{18}F]FBR-06 [^{18}F]DPA-714 [^{18}F]GE180 Flutriciclamide [^{18}F]FEPPA [^{18}F]PBR111 [^{18}F]FEDAA1106	Damont et al. [625], Fan et al. [626], Ghadery et al. [627]

DOTA-TATE) have been labeled with ^{68}Ga and ^{18}F [489, 630, 631], and the potential clinical utility of these tracers to image SSTR-positive tumors has been shown (cf. Sect. 2.3 for ^{111}In-labeled versions and Sect. 2.5 for theranostic radiotracers).

Estrogen Receptors

In breast cancer, the stimulatory effect of estrogen and progesterone is mediated through nuclear estrogen receptors and progesterone receptors. A number of steroidal and nonsteroidal estrogens have been radiolabeled with positron-emitting halogens [632]. The most promising imaging agent for measuring estrogen receptor status in vivo is 16α-[^{18}F]fluoro-17β-estradiol (FES) [633, 634] and for the progesterone receptor status 21-[^{18}F]fluoro-16α,17α-[(R)-(19-α-furylmethylidene)dioxy]-19-norpregn-4-ene-3,20-dione [635].

Integrin $\alpha_v\beta_3$ Receptor

The cellular activation, migration, proliferation, survival, and differentiation are regulated by integrin receptors, which are the dimeric transmembrane glycoproteins located on the cell surface receptors. Especially the integrin $\alpha_v\beta_3$ receptor plays an important role in tumor growth [636]. The noninvasive determination of $\alpha_v\beta_3$ expression is performed by radiolabeling of the tripeptide RGD (*single letter code* for the arginine-glycine-aspartate sequence) with PET and SPECT radionuclides, which led, e.g., to the development of [^{18}F]galacto-RGD [637], [^{18}F]FPPRGD$_2$ [638] (cf. Sect. 2.3), [^{18}F]alfatide [470], and [^{18}F]fluciclatide [639] showing promising results as tumor imaging agents [263, 640–642]. However, the role of radioligands imaging the changes of $\alpha_v\beta_3$ expression in tumor blood vessels (angiogenesis) is controversially discussed [643] (cf. Sect. 2.3).

Metalloproteases

Prostate cancer is a leading cause of cancer-related death in men. A specific biological target for the localization of the primary tumor and its metastases is the prostate-specific membrane antigen (PSMA). PSMA is a zinc metalloenzyme and abundantly expressed on the cell surface of the vast majority of prostate tumors at all stages of the disease and is primarily restricted to the prostate. A specific peptidomimetic inhibitor of PSMA is Glu-ureido derivative Glu-NH-CO-NH-Lys functioning as the a pharmacophore which led to the development of the most promising ^{18}F-labeled PSMA radioligands in the clinics so far, [^{18}F]DCFPyL [644] and [^{18}F]PSMA-1007 [645] (cf. Sect. 2.5).

Matrix metalloproteinases (MMP) are principally targets, i.a., for cell proliferation, tumor invasion, and migration. The radiofluorinated MMP inhibitor (*R*)-2-(*N*-benzyl-4-(2-[^{18}F]fluoroethoxy)phenylsulphonamido)-*N*-hydroxy-3-methylbutanamide ([^{18}F]BR-351) is suggested as a potential candidate for imaging tumor stem cells in glioma [646].

2.4.6.10 Neurotransmitter Systems

Neurons in the human brain communicate with each other by releasing chemical messengers called neurotransmitters, which can be either excitatory or inhibitory in their synaptic signaling effect. The major neurotransmitters in the brain are acetylcholine, dopamine, norepinephrine/noradrenaline, serotonin (5-HT), and histamine. In addition, certain amino acids such as glutamate, aspartate, glycine, and γ-aminobutyric acid/GABA and peptides such as enkephalin, endorphin, substance P, bombesin, and NAAG also act as neurotransmitters in the brain. Each neutransmitter system has three steps in the utility cycle: (1) neurotransmitters are firstly synthesized and packaged into vesicles in the presynaptic neuron; (2) they are released from the presynaptic cell into the synaptic cleft, and then binding to specific receptors occurs on postsynaptic neurons; (3) from the synaptic cleft, they are rapidly removed (into the presynaptic cell through specific "reuptake" transporters) and subsequently stored and/or degraded.

A number of positron-emitting radiotracers have been developed to image neurotransmitter synthesis, neuroreceptor binding on postsynaptic neurons, and specific transporters on the presynaptic neuron (Table 2.15). The rationale of the design and development of PET radiotracers for neuroreceptor systems in general can be explained based on the dopamine system paradigm described below.

Dopamine System

Dopamine plays a major role in the regulation of movement, motivation, and cognition. It is synthesized in the dopaminergic neurons in the substantia nigra, ventral tegmental area, and retrorubral area of the mesencephalon. It is stored within the vesicles and released into the synapse in response to an action potential and binds to specific dopamine receptors (D_1–D_5) that are present on both postsynaptic and presynaptic sites. In Parkinson's disease, there is a significant loss of presynaptic nigrostriatal nerve terminals in the striatum due to the degeneration of dopamine-producing neurons in the substantia nigra in the brain stem. As a result, there is a significant decrease in dopamine terminal density [647]. The synaptic concentration of dopamine is regulated primarily by reuptake. Dopamine is removed or degraded by the enzymes *monoamine oxidase (MAO)* and *catechol O-methyl transferase (COMT)*.

Dopamine Metabolism

Since dopamine does not cross the BBB, it is synthesized from the precursor, the amino acid tyrosine. The first step is the conversion of tyrosine to dihydroxyphenylalanine (DOPA). Subsequently, DOPA decarboxylase/aromatic amino acid decarboxylase (AAAD) converts L-DOPA to dopamine. Since L-DOPA is transported into the brain via the large neutral amino acid carrier (LAT), [^{18}F]6-fluoro-DOPA (6-[^{18}F]FDOPA) was developed to examine the transport of the dopamine precursor from plasma and its decarboxylation by AAAD to fluorodopamine [648]. [^{18}F]Fluoro-*meta*-tyrosine can also be used to image dopamine synthesis [604, 649].

Dopamine Transporters

Dopamine transporters are exclusively localized on dopamine terminals in the striatum. Dopamine is removed into presynaptic terminals by these transporters. Drug molecules that bind specifically to dopamine transporters compete with dopamine thereby increasing intrasynaptic dopamine concentration. Radiotracers that bind selectively to dopamine transporters provide an indirect measure of dopamine terminal density. Since cocaine binds selectively to dopamine transporters, several ^{11}C- and ^{18}F-labeled tropane analogs such as [^{11}C]WIN-35,428, [^{18}F]CFT, and [^{18}F]FP-CIT were developed to image dopamine transporters [618, 621].

In order to prevent dopamine from degradation by *MAO*, vesicular monoamine transporters (VMAT), present on vesicles in the presynaptic nerve terminals, remove dopamine from the cytosol into vesicles. Therefore, VMAT-like dopamine transporters are a potential target to measure dopamine terminal density. A selective tracer for VMAT known as (+)-α-[^{11}C]dihydrotetrabenazine ([^{11}C]DTBZ) was also developed to image dopamine terminal density or dopamine neuronal degeneration in the striatum [623].

Dopamine Receptors

Among the dopamine receptors in the striatum, D_1 and D_2 receptors are relatively high in abundance with lower concentrations occurring in the extrastriatal regions. Striatal D_2 receptor density in schizophrenia has been extensively studied, because these receptors are therapeutic biological targets. In addition, a number of clinical PET studies have measured the D_2 receptor subtype, because of its involvement in psychiatric states, motor disorders, and drug abuse. Several radiotracers have been developed based on receptor antagonists such as neuroleptics. ^{11}C- or ^{18}F-labeled *N*-methylspiroperidol (NMSP) is a high affinity irreversibly binding radiotracer [650], while [^{11}C]raclopride is a reversibly binding radioligand with moderate affinity [651]. High-affinity reversible radiotracers such as [^{18}F]fallypride and [^{11}C]FLB-457 have also been developed. Since reversible ligands have the potential to compete with synaptic dopamine, these tracers may be more optimal for the measurement of quantitative parameters such as K_d, B_{max}, and the binding potential [612].

Monoamine Oxidase (MAO) Inhibitors

Several MAO inhibitor drugs (when given resulting in increased dopamine terminal density) are used in the treatment of depression and Parkinson's disease. PET imaging studies of MAO expression (including MAO-A and MAO-B) in the human brain were studied using the radiolabeled suicide enzyme inactivators, [^{11}C]clorgyline, L-[^{11}C]deprenyl, and *N*-(6-[^{18}F]fluorohexyl)-*N*-methylpropargylamine ([^{18}F]HMP) [652, 653]. These studies demonstrated a significant decrease of MAO levels in smokers, suggesting a neurochemical link, which implies that smokers may have a decreased risk of Parkinson's disease.

In the last two decades, several PET radiotracers were approved by the FDA or the EMA as radiopharmaceuticals, which are summarized in Table 2.16.

Table 2.16 FDA- and/or EMA-approved PET radiopharmaceuticals

Name/brand name	Approved use	Manufacturer
[^{11}C]Choline	Prostate cancer recurrence	Mayo Clinics
[^{18}F]Fluorodeoxy-glucose ([^{18}F]FDG)	*Oncology*: For assessment of abnormal glucose metabolism to assist in the evaluation of malignancy in patients with known or suspected abnormality found by other testing modalities or in patients with an existing diagnosis of cancer *Cardiology*: For the identification of left ventricular myocardium with residual glucose metabolism and reversible loss of systolic function in patients with coronary artery disease and left ventricular dysfunction, when used together with myocardial perfusion imaging *Neurology*: For the identification of regions of abnormal glucose metabolism associated with foci of epileptic seizures	Various manufacturers
[^{18}F]Florbetapir; Amyvid™	Indicated for PET imaging of the brain to estimate β-amyloid neuritic plaque density in adult patients with cognitive impairment who are being evaluated for Alzheimer's disease (AD) and other causes of cognitive decline	Eli Lilly
[^{18}F]Florbetaben; Neuraceq™	Indicated for PET imaging of the brain to estimate β-amyloid neuritic plaque density in adult patients with cognitive impairment who are being evaluated for Alzheimer's disease (AD) and other causes of cognitive decline	Piramal Imaging
[^{18}F]Flutemetamol; Vizamyl™	Indicated for PET imaging of the brain to estimate β-amyloid neuritic plaque density in adult patients with cognitive impairment who are being evaluated for Alzheimer's disease (AD) and other causes of cognitive decline	GE Healthcare
[^{18}F]Fluciclovine; Axumin™	Indicated for PET imaging in men with suspected prostate cancer recurrence based on elevated blood PSA levels following prior treatment	Blue Earth Diagnostics
Sodium [^{18}F] fluoride	Indicated for diagnostic PET imaging of bone to define areas of altered osteogenic activity	Various manufacturers
[^{13}N]Ammonia	Myocardial perfusion imaging	Various manufacturers

2.5 Clinically Relevant Theranostic Radiotracers

2.5.1 Concept of Theranostics and Personalized Medicine

The term "theranostics" (also spelled as "theragnostics") is used for combined diagnosis and therapy. This designation comes from the Greek word *therapeuein*, which means to treat medically, and *gnosis*, indicating knowledge [654]. Theranostics uses in its broader meaning the patient's individual disease state for choosing the optimal treatment. In other words, molecular imaging helps to distinguish cellular phenotype(s) and disease heterogeneity suggesting concrete individuals who will likely respond after a given treatment from those who rather not [655]. Thus, theranostics follows the ideology of targeting rather a "specific tumor of a patient" than a disease in general, meaning the selection of the right treatment for the right patient, at the right dose, and at the right time. On the basis of this strategy, theranostics stands as the opposite to a general "one-size-fits-all" model applying the same treatment for a particular disease [656].

The concept of theranostics was firstly coined by the US consultant and CEO John Funkhouser (PharmaNetics, Inc.) in 1998 [657]. Since then, the field of theranostics has evolved considerably due to the definition of new biological targets, development of various pharmaceuticals (e.g., small low- and high-molecular weight molecules, antibodies, and nanoparticles), broadened availability of relevant diagnostic and therapeutic radionuclides, as well as improvement of imaging techniques [658]. To maximize the likelihood of successful theranostic outcomes, an improved staging of primary as well as recurrent disease, prognostic stratification, therapy follow-up, efficacy monitoring of new radiopharmaceuticals, and guidance of clinical trial enrollment may be obtained in addition to optimal treatment choice [659, 660]. In properly preselected patients, the precision of the theranostic approach has already proven to be highly effective. Moreover, favorable safety profiles obtained with this strategy significantly contrast with the commonly observable cytotoxic effects of standard chemotherapies [661]. Thus, this approach is seen as a powerful tool paving the transition from conventional generalized medicine to a contemporary personalized and precision medicine as the comprehensive treatment management might be tailored to the individual patient [662].

When applied to nuclear medicine, theranostics can be referred to as "radiotheranostics" which is, among others, especially useful in the field of oncology [663]. The basic principle of radiotheranostics has been in practice for almost eight decades, since 1940s. The most prominent and oldest exemplary case of radiotheranostics was pursued by Dr. Hertz in 1941 and describes treatment of a female patient with hyperthyroidism while employing a Na[^{130}I]I/Na[^{131}I]I mixture [664, 665]. Five years later, Seidlin et al. applied Na[^{131}I]I for the successful treatment of metastatic thyroid cancer [666]. In 1951, Na[^{131}I]I gained the first Food and Drug Administration (FDA) approval granted for the use of radioactive material for thyroid cancer endoradiotherapy [667]. Nowadays, the iodine radioisotopes ^{123}I ($T_{1/2}$ = 13.2 h; E_γ = 159 keV, I = 83%) and ^{124}I ($T_{1/2}$ = 4.2 days; $E_{\beta 1,\text{mean}}$ = 687 keV, I = 12% and $E_{\beta 2,\text{mean}}$ = 975 keV, I = 11%) are used for pre-therapeutic nuclear imaging with single-photon emission computed tomography (SPECT) and positron emission tomography (PET), respectively, while ^{131}I ($T_{1/2}$ = 8.0 days; $E_{\beta\text{mean}}$ = 192 keV, I = 89%) is subsequently applied for endoradiotherapy. This concept is particularly employed in the management of thyroid maligancies [668].

To conclude the above discussed approach of radiotheranostics, the combination of targeted molecular imaging and radioligand therapy (RLT) represents a considerable contribution to personalized and precision nuclear medicine. Broader implementation of this concept can significantly enhance efficacy, efficiency, and cost-effectiveness of cancer treatments and hold, thus, a great promise for improved patient outcomes in the future.

2.5.2 Theranostic Radioligands for Peptide Receptor Radionuclide Therapy (PRRT)

Peptide receptor radionuclide therapy (PRRT) is an attractive treatment option in the field of cancer theranostics with the focus on specific targeting of particular tumor types and their environment. In other words, individualized diagnosis may be advantageously applied for the selection of patients suited for PRRT as the assessment of the individual response allows the early termination of an ineffective therapy in favor of alternative treatment options [669, 670].

Both procedures, diagnosis and therapy, may be performed with a single platform, i.e., the same vector molecule, specifically binding to a receptor, antigen, enzyme, or other molecular structures [671]. Such a platform is usually represented by protein-, peptide-, or peptidomimetic-based targeting agents often demonstrating high receptor specificity and selectivity as well as high binding affinity (target accessibility), good tissue penetration, rapid clearance from the blood and the body (resulting in low nonspecific uptake in nontargeted tissues), reduced hepatobiliary excretion, low antigenicity/immunogenicity, common robustness, and resistance against harsh labeling conditions. As a consequence, high tumor-to-background ratios and low toxicity to healthy tissues and organs are achieved [672, 673].

The radiolabeling of the same vector molecule with diagnostic or subsequently therapeutic radionuclides has the potential to overcome undesirable differences in selectivity and in biodistribution behavior that usually exist for distinct imaging and therapeutic agents [674]. In addition, such theranostic radiopharmaceuticals are used in very low substance amounts reducing the probability of side-effect occurrence [675]. On the other hand, renal elimination usually serves as the major excretory pathway of these radiopharmaceuticals from the body which often leads to undesired high renal accumulation and also retention. Thus, the maximum tolerated absorbed dose has to be determined for each individual patient to optimize the therapeutic dose and avoid both undertreatment and undesired nephrotoxicity to the kidneys [676].

Nowadays, the most commonly used metallic radionuclides in combined diagnosis and PPRT are represented by ^{68}Ga ($T_{1/2}$ = 67.8 min; $E_{\beta mean}$ = 836 keV, I = 88%; Fig. 2.62) for pre-therapeutic PET imaging [677] and ^{177}Lu ($T_{1/2}$ = 6.7 days; $E_{\beta mean}$ = 134 keV, I = 100%; Fig. 2.62) for therapeutic purposes.

In addition, ^{177}Lu emits gamma rays ($E_{\gamma 1}$ = 113 keV, I = 6% and $E_{\gamma 2}$ = 208 keV, I = 10%) suitable for an assessment of the dosimetry in individual patients. Such dose estimation can be accomplished by the series of SPECT and whole-body scintigraphy measurements [678]. To highlight other currently used therapeutic radiometals, ^{90}Y ($T_{1/2}$ = 64.1 h; $E_{\beta mean}$ = 934 keV, I = 100%; no gamma), ^{213}Bi ($T_{1/2}$ = 45.6 min; Eα = 5.875 MeV, I = 2%), and ^{225}Ac ($T_{1/2}$ = 9.9 days; E_{α} = 5.830 MeV, I = 51%, and 5.792 MeV, I = 18%) could be mentioned [679, 680].

Radiometals need to be introduced into the patient's body in the form of a stable complex due to the toxicity of their free versions and tendency to be stored in different organs and tissues [681]. These complexes have to demonstrate high in vivo thermodynamic stability and kinetic inertness over the pH range 5.0–7.5 and selectivity for the radiometal as body fluids contain large quantities of various cations (e.g., Na^+, K^+, Ca^{2+}, Zn^{2+}, Mg^{2+}, $Fe^{2+/3+}$) and ligands (e.g., transferrin, amino acids, peptides, proteins) [682]. One of the favorite macrocyclic frameworks for bifunctional chelators are the 9-membered 1,4,7-triazacyclononane (TACN; Fig. 2.63) and the 12-membered 1,4,7,10-tetraazacyclododecane (cyclen; Fig. 2.63). Based on these two concrete frameworks, the most important chelators for the development of theranostic radioligands are attributed to 1,4,7-triazacyclononane-1,4,7-triacetic acid (NOTA; Fig. 2.64) and 1,4,7,10-te traazacyclododecane-1,4,7,10-tetraacetic acid (DOTA; Fig. 2.64) and their derivatives 1,4,7-triazacyclononane, 1-glutaric acid-4,7-acetic acid (NODAGA; Fig. 2.64) and 1,4,7,10-tetraazacyclododececane, 1-glutaric acid-4,7,10-triacetic acid (DOTAGA; Fig. 2.64) [683].

Since many years, several classes of theranostic radioligand platforms are in clinical use for diagnosis and PPRT of various cancer types [684]. The beneficial nature of this con-

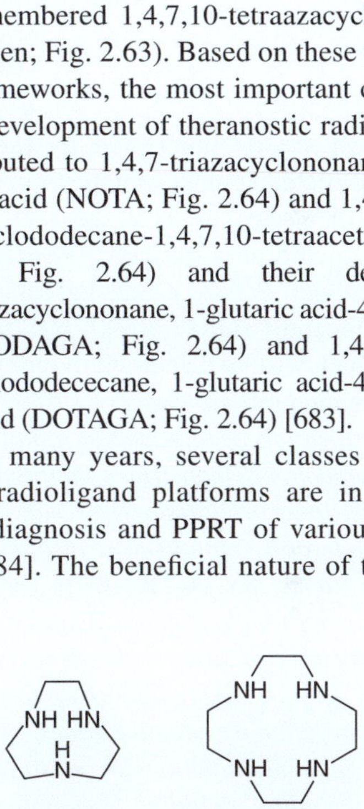

TACN cyclen

Fig. 2.63 Structures of macrocyclic frameworks

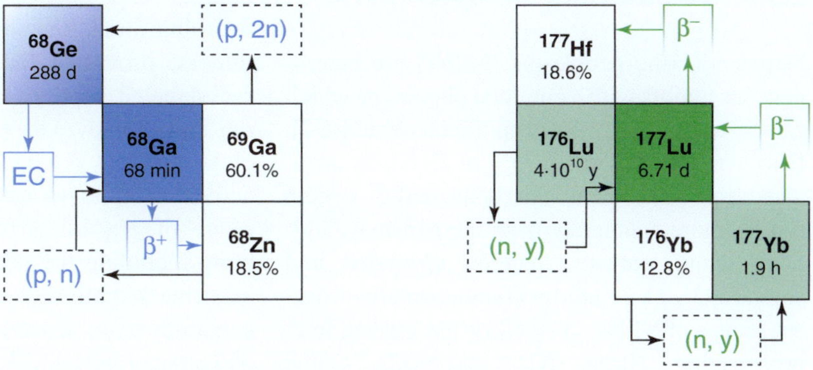

Fig. 2.62 Production routes and decay schemes of ^{68}Ga and ^{177}Lu (*derived from the Karlsruhe Nuclide Chart*)

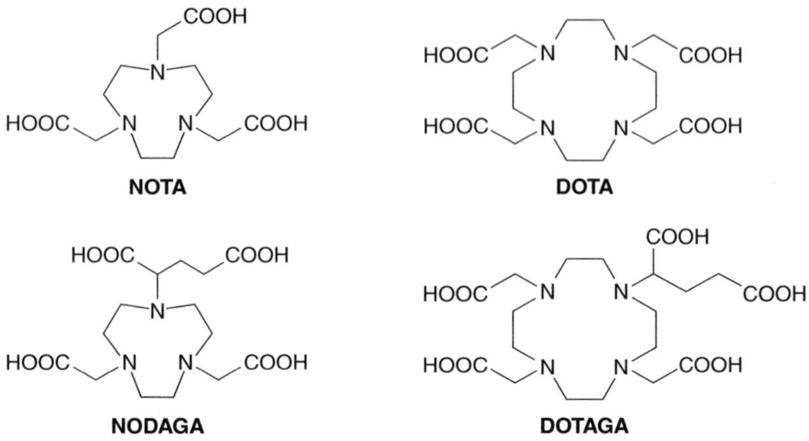

Fig. 2.64 Prominent structures of bifunctional chelators for the utilization in theranostics

cept is especially underlined by the peptide analogs directed against somatostatin receptors (SSTR) [685, 686]; cf. Sect. 2.5.3.1), prostate-specific membrane antigen (PSMA) [687–689]; cf. Sect. 2.5.4.1), and gastrin-releasing peptide receptor (GRPr) [690, 691]; cf. Sect. 2.5.5) which will be discussed in more detail in following chapters.

The utilization of theranostic radioligands in PRRT frequently demonstrates impressive tumor responses, long progression-free survival rates, and considerable improvement in life quality of cancer patients. As this modality represents a systematic approach, it is particularly suited for the treatment of metastatic diseases and serves, thus, as a very promising add-on or even alternative to conventional chemotherapies, or can also be used in combination with existing therapy options, including (cellular) immunotherapy and radiotherapy.

2.5.3 Somatostatin Receptor (SSTR)

Neuroendocrine neoplasms (NENs) are heterogeneous tumors with a common phenotype which can arise in virtually every epithelial organ [692]. However, approximately 75% of all NENs originate from the gastroenteropancreatic system (GEP), more concretely from the pancreas, jejunum, ileum, caecum, rectum, appendix, and colon [693]. There are two fundamentally different groups of NENs: (1) well-differentiated, low-proliferating NENs (G1 and G2), called neuroendocrine tumors (NETs), and (2) poorly differentiated, highly proliferating NENs (G3), called neuroendocrine carcinomas (NECs) [694, 695]. NETs were previously considered as a rare disease, but their incidence and prevalence have significantly increased over the last decade. Moreover, the heterogeneous nature, frequently indolent course, and tumor occurrence in multiple and variable anatomic sites make the diagnosis and treatment of patients with NETs highly challenging [696].

A unique feature of multiple NETs is represented by the expression of all five subtypes of somatostatin receptor (SSTR1–SSTR5), with the dominance of SSTR subtype 2 (SSTR2) [697]. SSTR belongs to the G protein-coupled receptor (GPCR) family and demonstrates a wide expression pattern in both normal and malignant tissues. In addition to neuroendocrine tumors, SSTRs are also expressed in pituitary adenomas, carcinoids, endocrine pancreatic, paraganglioma, medullary thyroid carcinoma, pheochromocytoma, small cell lung carcinoma, neuroblastoma, meningioma, and Merkel cell tumors, providing thus a molecular basis for radiolabeled peptides for tumor receptor imaging and therapy, i.e., peptide receptor radionuclide therapy (PRRT) [697, 698]. Normally, activation of these receptors produces a broad range of physiological effects throughout the body including the inhibition of endocrine and exocrine secretion of many hormones, such as somatothropin, thyrotropin, glucagon, insulin, and others [699]. SSTRs share a common molecular topology: a hydrophobic core of seven transmembrane-spanning α-helices, three intracellular as well as extracellular loops, the NH_2-terminus outside the cell, and the COOH-terminus inside the cell [700]. All five subtypes of SSTR might be divided into two groups, where SSTR2, SSTR3, and SSTR5 are known to differ from SSTR1 and SSTR4 regarding amino acid homology as well as pharmacological profile. The levels of individual receptor subtypes are highly cell specific and vary with the co-expression of different ligand receptors [701].

In 1972, Brazeau et al. incidentally identified the SSTR ligand somatostatin (SST), a growth hormone (GH)-releasing antagonist and a naturally occurring cyclic disulfide peptide, in the sheep hypothalamus. This cyclic oligopeptide have been found in two biologically active forms arising from the C-terminal portion of a single pro-peptide, namely somatostatin-14 (SST-14) and somatostation-28 (SST-28) [702–704]. SST-14 is characterized by high binding affinity to all SSTRs subtypes. SST-28 (octreotide) was originally described in the gut by Pradayrol et al. in 1980 and demonstrates higher binding affinity to SSTR5 (K_i = 0.19 nM), compared to SST-14 (K_i = 2.24 nM) indicating its selectivity toward SSTR5 [705]. The well-known antitumor effect of SST was recognized of practical importance for theranostic applications [706, 707].

The idea of using SSTRs in the diagnosis and treatment of GEP-NETs has become increasingly popular over the last 20 years, and many clinical studies have centered upon the development of new radiolabeled somatostatin analogs (SSA). Proper identification of the exact SSTR subtype and selection of corresponding SSAs is of high importance as the activation of different SSTRs results in diverse biological effects, potentially hampering successful treatment.

2.5.3.1 Somatostatin Analogs (SSA) for Imaging and Treatment of Neuroendocrine Tumors (NETs)

Both natural SSTs have a short plasma half-life (~3 min), thus, synthetic analogs resistant to enzymatic degradation have been developed for clinical applications. Such SST analogs are octreotide and lanreotide (initially developed and clinically used for the treatment of acromegaly and gastroenteropancreatic tumors) (cf. Sect. 2.3) [282, 698, 708, 709]. Radiolabeled SST analogs for imaging and for treatment successfully have been used for more than 20 years in the clinics [282, 708]. Somatostatin analogs (SSA) gained a bigger attention after the introduction of ^{111}In-labeled diethylenetriaminepentaacetic acid DTPA-octreotide (DTPA-(D-Phe^1)-octreotide) (Fig. 2.65) which immediately replaced firstly the radioiodinated somatostatin analog [^{123}I] Iodo-(Tyr^3)-octreotide [710] and since then has been used for GEP-NET imaging since the late 1980s and received FDA approval (OctreoScan®) for imaging SSTR2-expressing malignancies in 1994 [684].

OctreoScan® which includes DTPA as chelator suitable for the complexation of ^{111}In has the following drawbacks: (1) it has moderate binding affinity for SSTR2, and (2) it is unsuitable for binding of beta emitters like ^{90}Y and ^{177}Lu for therapeutic applications [698]. The replacement of DTPA with the macrocyclic chelator DOTA resulted into DOTA-(D-Phe^1,Tyr^3)-octreotide (DOTA-(Tyr^3)-octreotide, DOTA-TOC) and DOTA-(D-Phe^1,Tyr^3,Thr^8)-octreotate (DOTA-TATE) [710], which until now have been extensively used in nuclear medicine clinical practice both for diagnosis and therapy (Fig. 2.65).

The next logical step was to develop radiotracers with both diagnostic as well as therapeutic potential. In the light of this effort, several theranostic SSAs followed, among others, DOTA-conjugated SSTR agonists DOTA-TOC [DOTA-(D-Phe^1,Tyr^3)-octreotide; Fig. 2.65], DOTA-NOC [DOTA-(1-Nal^3)-octreotide; Fig. 2.65], and DOTA-TATE [DOTA-(D-Phe^1,Tyr^3,Thr^8)-octreotate; Fig. 2.65] with variable affinity to SSTR subtypes [708, 711, 712].

All three mentioned DOTA conjugates were used for pre-therapeutic PET imaging (pre-staging) when labeled with ^{68}Ga [630, 713, 714]) and for PRRT with ^{90}Y and ^{177}Lu (beta therapy), i.e., [^{90}Y]Y-DOTA-TOC and [^{177}Lu]Lu-DOTA-TATE [684, 715, 716] or with ^{213}Bi and ^{225}Ac (alpha therapy), i.e., [^{213}Bi]Bi-DOTA-TOC and

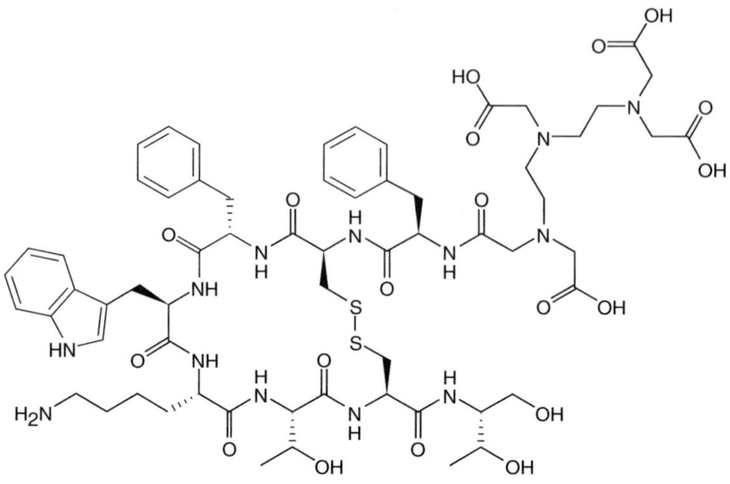

DTPA-octreotide (**OctreoScan®**)
SPECT Diagnostics: ^{111}In

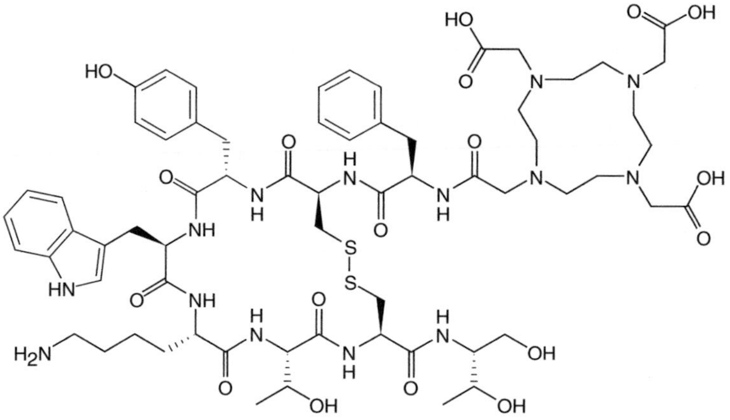

DOTA-(Tyr^{3})-octreotide **(DOTA-TOC; SOMAKIT TOC®)**
Theranostics: ^{44}Sc, ^{68}Ga, ^{90}Y, ^{152}Tb, ^{177}Lu, ^{213}Bi, ^{225}Ac

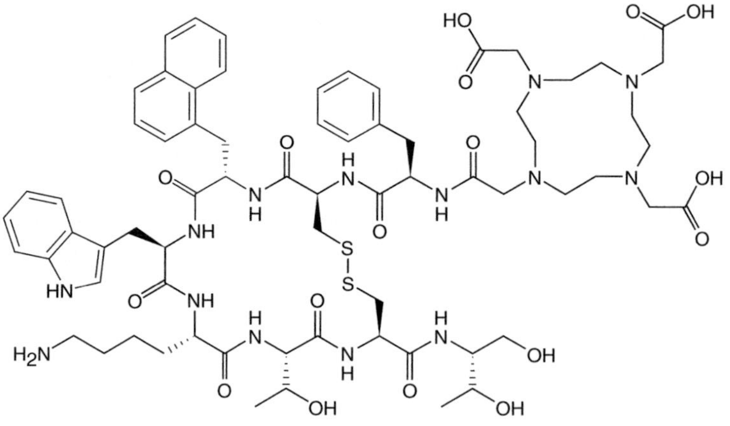

DOTA-(1-Nal^{3})-octreotide (**DOTA-NOC**)
Theranostics: ^{68}Ga, ^{90}Y, ^{177}Lu

Fig. 2.65 Structures of DOTA-conjugated SSTR agonists DTPA-octreotide, DOTA-TOC, DOTA-NOC, and DOTA-TATE

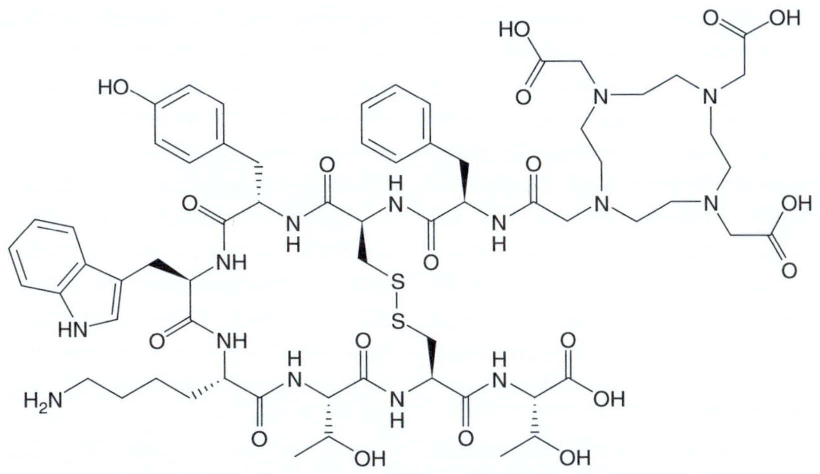

DOTA-(Tyr^3,Thr^8)-octreotate (**DOTA-TATE; NETSPOT®**; **Lutathera®**)
Theranostics: ^{68}Ga, ^{90}Y, ^{177}Lu

Fig. 2.65 (continued)

[^{225}Ac]Ac-DOTA-TOC [717, 718]. Moreover, the possible pre-therapeutic dosimetry with ^{86}Y ($T_{1/2}$ = 14.7 h; $E_{\beta mean}$ = 535 keV, I = 12%) represents an advantageous option in comparison to ^{111}In ($T_{1/2}$ = 2.8 days; $E_{\gamma 1}$ = 245 keV, I = 94% and $E_{\gamma 2}$ = 171 keV, I = 91%) due to its similarity to ^{90}Y used for respective therapies [719]. In addition, DOTA-TOC was the first radiopharmaceutical used for clinical PET/CT imaging with cyclotron-produced ^{44}Sc ($T_{1/2}$ = 4.04 h, $E_{\beta mean}$ = 632 keV, I = 94%) and with the "exotic" radiolanthanide ^{152}Tb ($T_{1/2}$ = 17.5 h; $E_{\beta mean}$ = 1140 keV, I = 20%), both performed at Zentralklinik Bad Berka in Germany [30, 720]. These proof-of-concept studies suggest that PET/CT imaging with ^{44}Sc- and ^{152}Tb-labeled targeting agents could have potential for clinical application in the future, depending on the availability of the radionuclides. This approach may be particularly interesting for the performance of pre-therapeutic dosimetry and offers a great benefit for PET centers without own radiopharmaceutical production sites/radiopharmacies.

Baum et al. and Öberg et al. are considered as pioneers of applied radiotheranostics and personalized medicine with the main focus on NETs [712, 721]. In 1996, the first PRRT employing DOTA-conjugated SSAs was performed for the treatment of metastatic NETs with [^{90}Y]Y-DOTA-TOC [722], followed by other ^{90}Y- and ^{177}Lu-labeled SSAs, i.e., [^{177}Lu]Lu-DOTA-TATE. Many radiolabeled SSAs were subsequently tested in clinical trials in several countries [723–725]. Data from a long follow-up showed an improvement in the quality of life and also a symptomatic improvement in 40–70% of cases [726, 727]. In many centers, ^{177}Lu-labeled analogs are preferred for PRRT in comparison to ^{90}Y-labeled analogs due to the lower probability of resulting nephrotoxicity. ^{177}Lu has a lower energy and shorter range in tissues than ^{90}Y (^{177}Lu: 2 mm vs. ^{90}Y: 11 mm) [728, 729].

The most prominent example is attributed to [^{177}Lu]Lu-DOTA-TATE (Lutathera®), which received FDA approval for the treatment of GEP-NETs in adults, on January 26, 2018, which can be considered as one of the breakthroughs in the twenty-first century for the field of nuclear medicine. The approval of Lutathera® was supported by two studies. The first was the randomized controlled phase-III clinical trial *NETTER-1* in 229 patients, starting in 2012 (ClinicalTrials.gov, NCT01578239). In this clinical trial, PRRT with Lutathera® was compared to standard chemotherapy using Sandostatin® LAR (octreotide long-acting repeatable). The number of patients having disease progression or who died during the trial was 23 in the Lutathera® arm and 68 in the Sandostatin® LAR arm. Thus, endoradiotherapy with Lutathera® was associated with a statistically significant and clinically meaningful reduction of disease progression or death compared to chemotherapy with Sandostatin® LAR. The second study was based on data from 1214 patients who received Lutathera® at a single site in the Netherlands and confirmed markedly longer progression-free survival and a significantly higher response rate than therapy with high-dose Sandostatin® LAR [725].

In addition, the SSTR antagonist DOTA-JR11, both the ^{68}Ga- and ^{177}Lu-labeled versions, was developed and suggested as a more potent radiotracer for the diagnosis and therapy compared to the hitherto used SSTR agonists [730, 731]. This observation might be explained by the ("apparently") higher number of binding sites (B_{max}) recognized by the antagonist [730]. This concept may enable the application of SSTR-based theranostics for other malignancies which express SSTR2 to a lesser extent, for example, breast and renal cell carcinoma or non-Hodgkin's lymphomas (NHLs) [732].

Until today, SSTR-targeted diagnosis and therapy represent the most thoroughly studied radiotheranostic approach in clinical nuclear medicine. Radiolabeled SSAs have demonstrated efficacy in patients harboring SSTR-overexpressing tumors, alleviating symptoms, stabilizing tumor growth, and substantially improving the quality of life with minimal side effects.

2.5.4 Prostate-Specific Membrane Antigen (PSMA) (cf. Sect. 2.4)

Prostate cancer (PC) belongs to the deadliest and most commonly diagnosed tumor disease in men worldwide and varies substantially according to geographic region and ethnicity. The main cause of death is connected with the progression of androgen-independent disease stages [733, 734].

The prostate-specific membrane antigen (PSMA) is a well-recognized biological target for addressing PC, whether for diagnosis or therapy [735]. PSMA plays a significant role in glutamatergic neurotransmission and folate absorption [736] as well as in prostate carcinogenesis and progression [737]. Each of these functions has led to different names; thus, PSMA is also known as glutamate carboxypeptidase II (GCPII), *N*-acetyl-L-aspartyl-L-glutamate peptidase I (NAALADase), or folate hydrolase 1 (FOLH1). High PSMA expression has not only been reported in PC, but also in other cancers, e.g., in tumors of the kidneys [738] and the bladder [739] as well as in the neovasculature of many solid tumors [740, 741]. Due to the presence of PSMA in various tumor types and several healthy organs, this target is no longer considered as entirely prostate specific.

The broader utilization of PSMA was initiated by the identification of the PSMA-positive PC cell line LNCaP by Horoszewicz et al. in 1983 [742] and was followed by the development of a monoclonal mouse antibody (mAb), 7E11-C5, in 1987 [743]. ^{111}In-labeled 7E11-C5 became the first FDA-approved imaging agent for PC known as ProstaScint® [744–746].

In an effort to further improve both the diagnosis and therapy of PC, diverse chemical constructs have been explored as capable PSMA vectors including several peptidomimetic Glu-ureido-based [455, 747–754] (Fig. 2.66) and phosphoramidate-based [755] PSMA inhibitors (Fig. 2.66), multiple generations and variations of PSMA targeted antibodies [756–759], as well as nanocarriers [760] have been designed and are currently designed [761].

In recent years, there has been a greater focus on PSMA as it represents another important approach stepping toward the concept of theranostics and personalized nuclear medicine. In addition, PSMA might expand its utilization in non-prostatic tumor neovasculature of a variety of cancer types in the future.

2.5.4.1 PSMA Inhibitors for Imaging and Treatment of Prostate Cancer (PC)

In recent years, several Glu-ureido-based low-molecular-weight ligands targeting PSMA have been developed and evaluated preclinically [455, 747–754]. The most promising candidates have been introduced as a new class of diagnostic and/or theranostic radiopharmaceuticals for the clinical management of patients suffering from PC [762, 763].

First in-human studies with PSMA radioligands showed highly sensitive and specific imaging of PSMA-positive PC by means of positron emission tomography (PET) and single-photon emission computed tomography (SPECT) as well as significant response after PSMA radioligand therapy (PSMA-RLT) of mCRPC. Such tremendous impact of various low-molecular-weight PSMA radioligands, e.g., MIP-1404, MIP-1095, PSMA-11, PSMA-617, DCFBC, DCFPyL, and PSMA-1007, has led to prospective clinical trials in several countries.

[^{99m}Tc]Tc-MIP-1404 (trofolastat) and ^{123}I-MIP-1072 are used as SPECT PSMA radioligands [764, 765]; [^{68}Ga]Ga-PSMA-11, [^{18}F]DCFBC, [^{18}F]DCFPyL, [^{18}F]CTT-1057, and [^{18}F]

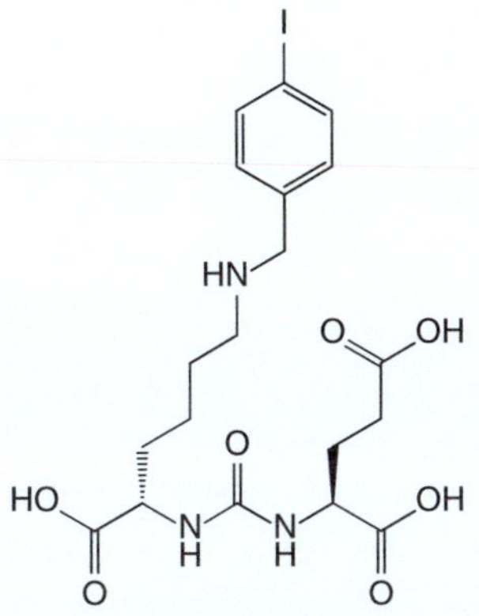

MIP-1072
SPECT Diagnostics: ^{123}I

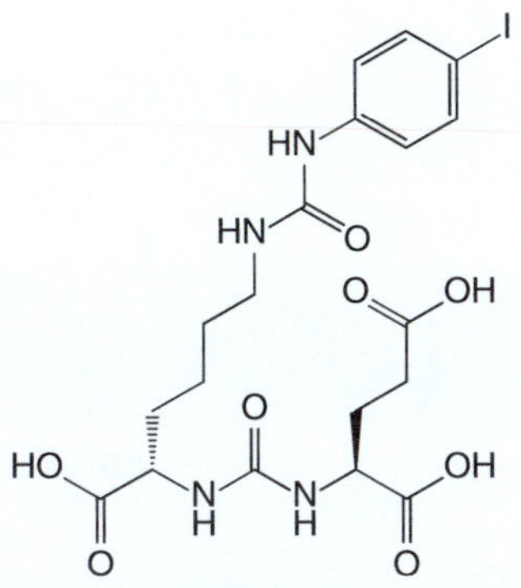

MIP-1095
Theranostics: ^{123}I, ^{124}I, ^{131}I

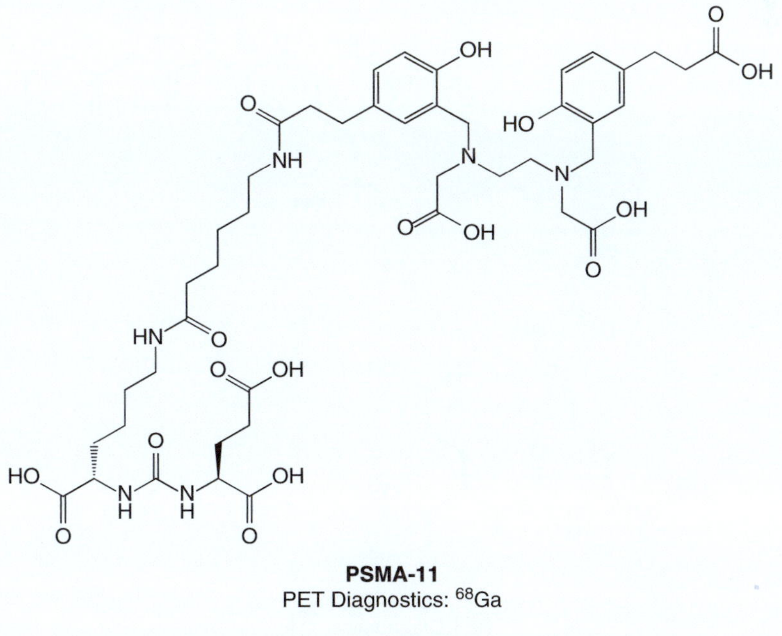

PSMA-11
PET Diagnostics: ^{68}Ga

Fig. 2.66 Structures of the most prominent peptidomimetic Glu-ureido-based PSMA inhibitors MIP-1072, MIP-1095, PSMA-11, PSMA-617, PSMA-1007, PSMA I&T, DCFBC, DCFPyL, and phosphoramidate-based inhibitor CTT1057

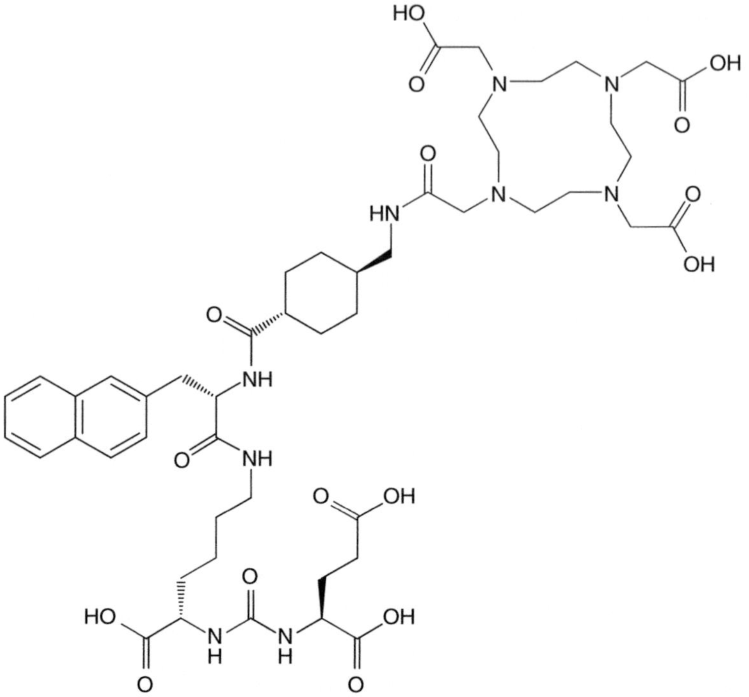

PSMA-617
Theranostics: ^{44}Sc, ^{68}Ga, ^{177}Lu, ^{213}Bi, ^{225}Ac

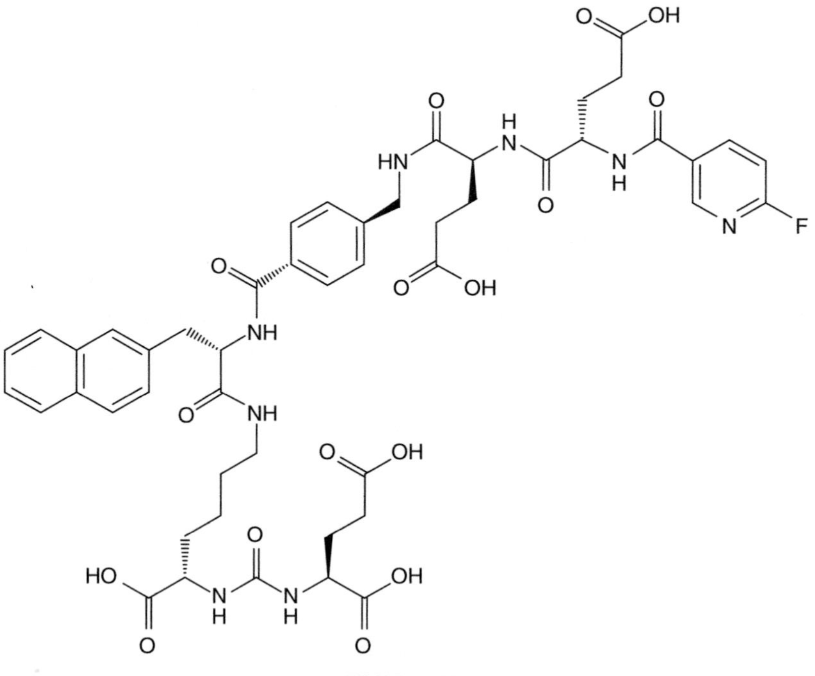

PSMA-1007
PET Diagnostics: ^{18}F

Fig. 2.66 (continued)

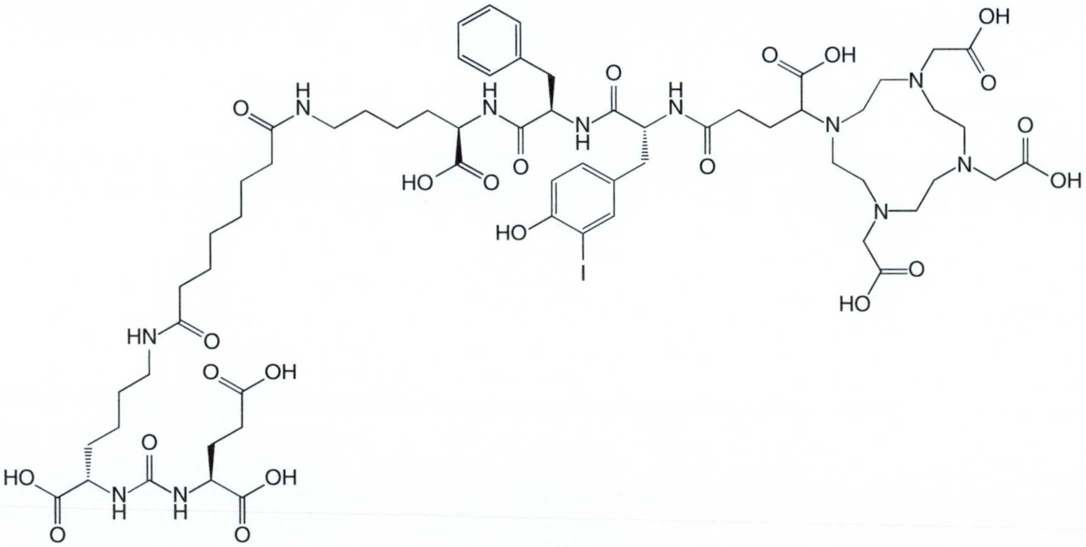

PSMA I&T
Theranostics: ^{68}Ga, ^{111}In, ^{177}Lu

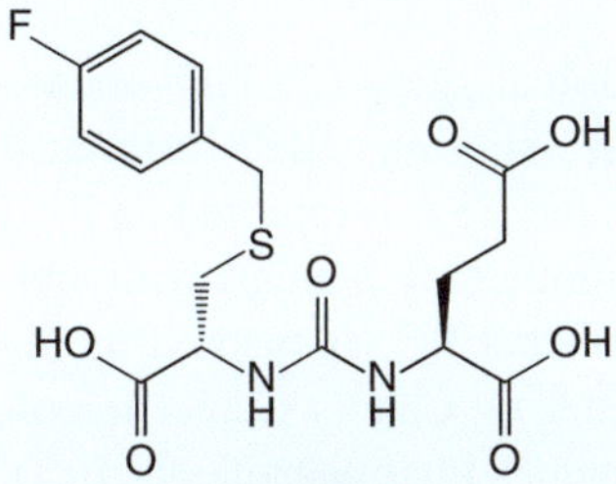

DCFBC
PET Diagnostics: ^{18}F

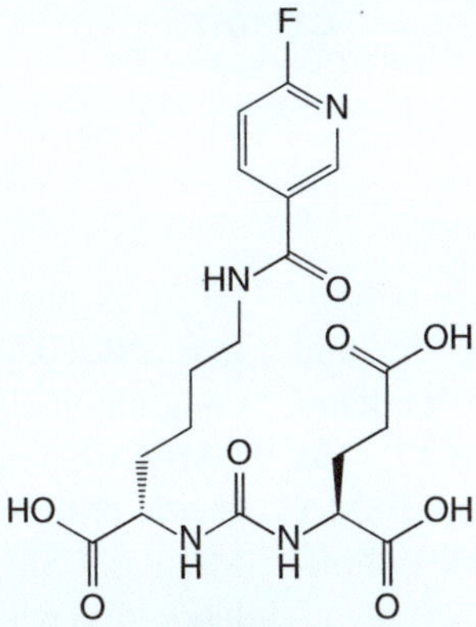

DCFPyL
PET Diagnostics: ^{18}F

Fig. 2.66 (continued)

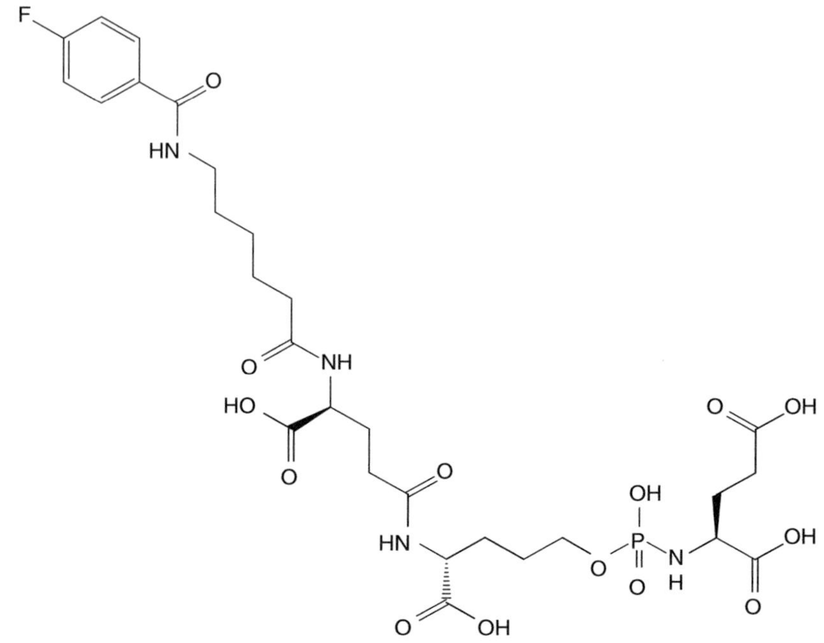

CTT1057
PET Diagnostics: ^{18}F

Fig. 2.66 (continued)

PSMA-1007 are exclusive PET PSMA radioligands [644, 645, 755, 766, 767]. ^{123}I-, ^{124}I-, and ^{131}I-labeled-MIP-1095, [^{44}Sc]Sc-/[^{68}Ga]Ga-/[^{177}Lu]Lu-/[^{213}Bi]Bi-/[^{225}Ac]Ac-PSMA-617, as well as [^{68}Ga]Ga-/[^{111}In]In-/[^{177}Lu]Lu-PSMA I&T are applied as theranostic PSMA radioligands [56, 162, 762, 763, 768–771].

The initial clinical theranostic approach, using the same PSMA ligand for both diagnosis and therapy of PC, is connected with the development of the radioiodinated PSMA inhibitor MIP-1095 firstly described by Hillier et al. in 2009 [751]. This Glu-ureido-based tracer contains aromatic substituents for stable introduction of radioiodine and can be used for SPECT imaging ([^{123}I]I-MIP-1095), PET imaging ([^{124}I]I-MIP-1095), and PSMA-RLT ([^{131}I]I-MIP-1095). The first-in-man evaluation of [^{123}I]I-MIP-1095 for SPECT imaging was originally reported by Barrett et al. in 2013 [769]. One year later, first dosimetry and therapy results using matched pair [^{124}I]I-MIP-1095 PET imaging and [^{131}I]I-MIP-1095 PSMA-RLT were reported by Zechmann et al. [763]. A phase-I clinical study (25.1.17. identifier: NCT03030885, starting 2017 estimated completion 2020) in the USA is reported on [^{131}I]I-MIP-1095 endoradiotherapy patients with metastatic castration-resistant PC (sponsored by the Memorial Sloan Kettering Cancer Center in collaboration with Progenics Pharmaceuticals, Inc.).

Next theranostic approaches emerged from the development of other Glu-ureido-based radiotracers suited for radiometal complexation. More concretely, the diagnostic tracer PSMA-11 for PET imaging was firstly preclinically introduced by Eder et al. in 2011 [750], followed by its transformation into the theranostic variant PSMA-617 by Benešová et al. in 2015 [747] and subsequent alteration of PSMA-617 to another diagnostic tracer PSMA-1007 for PET imaging by Cardinale et al. in 2017 [455]. The preclinical and first clinical evaluation of [^{68}Ga]Ga-PSMA-11 (also known as ^{68}Ga-DKFZ-PSMA-11 or ^{68}Ga-PSMA-HBED-CC) revealed very promising results, and, as a consequence, this radiotracer became the most prominent PSMA radioligand for PET imaging of PSMA-positive PC worldwide so far [772, 773]. The employed chelating agent HBED-CC (*N*,*N*′-bis[2-hydroxy-5-(carboxyethyl)benzyl]-ethylenediamine-*N*,*N*′-diacetic acid) is applicable for the exclusive complexation of gallium and iron [774, 775] and, thus, cannot bind clinically relevant therapeutic radiometals.

Using PSMA-11 as the lead structure, the theranostic variant PSMA-617, employing the chelating agent DOTA (1,4,7,10-tetraazacyclododecane-1,4,7,10-tetraacetic acid), was developed and radiolabeled with diagnostic (^{44}Sc, ^{55}Co, ^{64}Cu, ^{68}Ga) [56, 776–778] and also therapeutic radiometals for both beta therapy (^{177}Lu) [162, 779] as well as alpha therapy (^{213}Bi and ^{225}Ac) [780, 781]. The theranostic tracer PSMA-617 exhibits high PSMA-specific tumor uptake and rapid background clearance resulting in clear visualization of PC lesions with high contrast and fast kidney excretion giving a clear advantage for an efficient endoradiotherapy. Meanwhile, [^{177}Lu]Lu-PSMA-617 [689, 782–784] and [^{225}Ac]Ac-PSMA-617 [780] became the main candidates for PSMA-RLT of PC.

In 2015, the German Society of Nuclear Medicine (DGN) initiated a retrospective multicenter data analysis to evaluate the efficacy and safety of [^{177}Lu]Lu-PSMA-617 in 145 patients from 12 different centers. Finally, RLT with [^{177}Lu]Lu-PSMA-617 demonstrated safety and efficacy which exceeded those of other third-line systemic therapies in mCRPC patients [689]. In general RLT with [^{177}Lu]Lu-PSMA-617 and [^{177}Lu]Lu-PSMA I&T show prolongation of overall survival in patients without any other treatment options [762, 785, 786].

Moreover, Kratochwil et al. initiated the first in-human PSMA-targeted α-therapy (PSMA-TAT) of mCRPC with [^{225}Ac]Ac-PSMA-617 [780]. Patients with a poor prognosis receiving [^{225}Ac]Ac-PSMA-617 (100 kBq/kgBW in three cycles during the two-monthly treatment regime) revealed higher imaging response and tumor marker decrease than those treated with [^{177}Lu]Lu-PSMA-617. Patients treated with α-radiation demonstrated, however, frequent and more severe xerostomia [787].

VISION trial: *The most important prospective clinical trial with the therapeutic PSMA ligand [^{177}Lu]Lu-PSMA-617 for PSMA-targeted beta-endoradiotherapy (single-arm, single-center phase-II trial, the LuPSMA trial) was recently published in Lancet Oncology by scientists of the Peter MacCallum Cancer Centre, Melbourne, VIC, Australia [788]. The VISION trial (phase-III registration trial) with [^{177}Lu]Lu-PSMA-617 for the treatment of patients suffering from progressive PSMA-positive mCRPC started in 2018 in up to ten countries in parallel (https://clinicaltrials.gov/ct2/show/NCT03511664).*

Due to the limited production capacity of [^{68}Ga]Ga-PSMA-11, a strong need for ^{18}F-labeled PSMA ligands occurred recently. For this purpose, PSMA-617 was used as the lead structure, and another PSMA radioligand containing fluoronicotinic acid for the introduction of radiofluorine, [^{18}F]PSMA-1007, was developed for PET imaging of PSMA-positive PC [455]. As PSMA-1007 is derived from PSMA-617, both tracers ([^{18}F]PSMA-1007 and [^{177}Lu]Lu-PSMA-617) can be used as a theranostic tandem for PET imaging and PSMA-RLT of PC. Other tandem combinations (e.g., [^{68}Ga]Ga-PSMA-11 and [^{225}Ac]Ac-PSMA-617) are indeed also possible as the diagnostic component need not be an exact replica of the therapeutic one. Moreover, based on the characteristics of both mentioned PET radiotracers, it appears that [^{18}F]PSMA-1007 is more suited for detection of primary PC and staging of local recurrent disease due to the low accumulation of the tracer into the urinary bladder [645, 789]. In any case [^{68}Ga]Ga-PSMA-11 is currently used predominantly for imaging of mCRPC. A phase-I/phase-II multicenter clinical trial, initiated by the German Cancer Consortium (DKTK), is currently running to elucidate the potential of [^{68}Ga]Ga-PSMA-11 for the initial diagnosis of PC in high-risk PC patients (https://clinicaltrials.gov/ct2/show/NCT03362359).

Based on the clinical need and current evidence, PSMA-targeted diagnosis and therapy is implemented in a growing number of centers worldwide. Combination of PSMA-PET and PSMA-RLT seems to be a highly encouraging option with the potential to extend overall survival while displaying a favorable toxicity profile with less side effects.

2.5.4.2 PSMA-Targeted Antibodies for Imaging and Treatment of Prostate Cancer (PC)

Macromolecules like antibodies have few advantages and some critical disadvantages compared to much smaller molecules. The long circulation time of antibodies in the body can result in high tumor enrichment. On the other hand, penetration into large solid tumors may be limited [790, 791]. The large size ("nanosize") of antibodies prevents renal filtration which decreases toxicity to radiosensitive kidneys. The opposite phenomenon, nephrotoxicity, is often seen in the case of smaller molecules. However, the long circulation time, which is characteristic for antibodies, could cause bone marrow toxicity due to prolonged exposure of the bone marrow to particle radiation [792]. Another concern of radiolabeled antibodies and antibody fragments may be their immunogenicity, when non-humanized antibodies are applied [793].

ProstaScint® is the only commercially available diagnostic imaging agent approved by the FDA so far for noninvasive visualization of PSMA-positive PC [744–746]. The epitope recognized by the ProstaScint® antibody is located inside the cell and consists of 19 amino acids. The intracellular region likely explains the relatively poor performance of ProstaScint® in vivo [794].

The next generation of PSMA-targeted antibodies addresses the extracellular domain of PSMA. Of high interest is especially the deimmunized monoclonal antibody huJ591 [795]. The surface binding and subsequent internalization as well as employment of the DOTA chelator are the fundamental rationales for employing J591 in clinical radiotheranostics [796–798]. J591 has been clinically investigated in a variety of radiolabeled versions for both diagnosis (e.g., [^{89}Zr]Zr-DFO-J591, [^{111}In]In-DOTA-J591, [^{124}I]I-J591) [799–801] as well as therapy (e.g., [^{90}Y]Y-DOTA-J591 and [^{177}Lu]Lu-DOTA-J591) [756, 802]. The imaging studies proved the ability to detect the majority of metastases in the skeleton, lymph nodes, and soft tissues from patients with renal, breast, and colorectal cancer [801]. Phase-I trials with both ^{90}Y- and ^{177}Lu-labeled J591 and a phase-II trial with [^{177}Lu]Lu-DOTA-J591 showed highly promising results for the treatment of patients with mCRPC [756, 758].

Targeted radioligand therapies (RLT), including those employing various antibodies, are becoming increasingly important in cancer theranostics. The crucial limitation is that not every patient benefits from a specific "personalized" therapy. This also urges the need for accurate patients' selection and therapy response monitoring, especially for antibody-based (radioimmuno)therapies.

2.5.5 Gastrin-Releasing Peptide Receptor (GRPr) Ligands for Imaging and Treatment of Cancer

Until now, several radiolabeled GRPr analogs have been studied for imaging and radionuclide therapy of prostate cancer [803, 804] and of breast cancer [691]. However, despite the extensive preclinical reports and numerous applications as PET or SPECT diagnostic agents in clinical studies, only few bombesin analogs have been clinically tested for radiotherapy.

The bombesin analogs that have been investigated so far are either agonists or antagonists for the gastrin-releasing peptide receptor (or BB_2). Agonists are mainly internalized after binding to GRPr, while antagonists remain surface bound. For some scientists BBN agonists, due to their internalization characteristics, are considered advantageous over antagonists for theranostic applications, but on the other side BBN antagonists have shown less acute side effects, i.e., abdominal cramps, emesis, when administered at higher (but still micro)doses, which are needed for radionuclide therapy. In addition antagonists do not have a proliferation effect on cancer cells [805, 806].

The limited clinical data so far are insufficient for a clear conclusion regarding the clinical value of either GRPr agonists or antagonists for radiotherapy. A recent example of a GRPr agonist is represented by the ^{177}Lu-labeled bombesin (7–14) coupled to DOTA via a Gly-4-aminobenzoyl spacer which was studied in seven patients (phase-I trial) with hormone-refractory metastatic prostate cancer. Increasing ^{177}Lu activities (4.17 GBq cumulative) were studied, and the interim analysis showed uptake in the lesions of five out of seven patients. Side effects included abdominal cramps, nausea, and diarrhea but could be controlled by specific drugs. Strong uptake was seen in the pancreas, which is the dose-limiting organ. At 3 months after the end of treatment, all patients showed progression. One problem with this therapeutic agent appeared to be its low plasma stability [807].

The GRPr antagonist ^{68}Ga-RM2, DOTA-4-amino-1-carboxymethyl-piperidine-D-Phe-Gln-Trp-Ala-Val-Gly-His-Sta-Leu-NH_2 (RM2), has been recently tested in pilot studies as a PET diagnostic agent for prostate [808] and breast cancer patients [691]. However, for its therapeutic version, ^{177}Lu-RM2, at present only preclinical data are described [803]. Presently, the bombesin receptor antagonist NeoBOMB1 (DOTA-p-aminomethylaniline-diglycolic acid-D-Phe-Gln-Trp-Ala-Val-Gly-His-Sta-Leu-NH_2) was labeled with ^{67}Ga, ^{68}Ga, ^{111}In, and ^{177}Lu and showed encouraging preclinical results independent from the used radiometal, that is to say high GRPr binding affinity, high in vivo stability, and high PC xenograft tumor targeting potency in mice. The high pancreatic uptake of [^{177}Lu]Lu-DOTA-NeoBOMB1 was an undesirable characteristic that has to be further investigated for its future application in endoradiotherapy. For the first in-human studies of [^{68}Ga]Ga-DOTA-NeoBOMB1 with PET/CT, four patients with PC were included. [^{68}Ga]Ga-DOTA-NeoBOMB1 showed excellent tolerability, while it strongly localized in primary prostate-confined disease and metastatic foci, i.e., in a liver micrometastasis not visible with arterial phase CT, lymph node metastases <5 mm, and osseous metastases. Clinical data gathered with [^{177}Lu]Lu-DOTA-NeoBOMB1 are currently not, but hopefully soon, available. Further clinical studies will prove if [^{68}Ga]Ga- and [^{177}Lu]Lu-DOTA-NeoBOMB1 can be considered as valuable asset for targeting GRPr-expressing tumors in clinical nuclear medicine practice of nuclear medicine [690].

2.5.6 Further Theranostic Concepts and Tracers of Clinical Relevance

The concept of radiotheranostics is predicted to expand significantly in the near future. Except the SSTR-, PSMA-, and GRPr-based concepts, a variety of other examples with a high potential for radiotheranostics in personalized and precision medicine have been evaluated. Some of these approaches include:

- *B-lymphocyte antigen CD20-targeted antibodies* for imaging and treatment of non-Hodgkin's lymphoma (NHL). NHL represents a clinically heterogeneous group of lymphoproliferative disorders with high radiosensitivity [809]. Thus, radioimmunotherapy (RIT) might be applied more advantageously for the treatment of NHL than immunotherapy due to killing the tumor cells instead of solely inhibiting proliferation [810]. The most thoroughly studied CD20 targeted radioimmunoconjugates include rituximab, ibritumomab (Zevalin®,) and tositumomab (Bexxar®) [811, 812]. Patients eligible for (combined) rituximab, Zevalin®, and/or Bexxar® treatment are primarily selected based on CD20 expression levels. Rituximab was the first FDA-approved mAb for therapy of cancer and has been labeled with various radionuclides for imaging and RIT (e.g., ^{123}I, ^{131}I) [813–815]. Zevalin® consists of ibritumomab, derived from the parent mAb rituximab and tiuxetan (DTPA derivative). The RIT with ^{90}Y-labeled Zevalin® received FDA approval in 2003 [816]. SPECT imaging might be performed with ^{111}In-labeled Zevalin® [817]. RIT with ^{90}Y-labeled Zevalin® is combined with the application of unlabeled rituximab to diminish the uptake of the radiolabeled antibodies in the spleen and bone marrow [818, 819]. In randomized control trials in patients with recurrent NHL, ^{90}Y-Zevalin® RIT was proved to be well tolerated with higher rate of overall and complete responses compared to rituximab alone [820]. In addition, combined imaging and RIT with Bexxar® might be performed while employing ^{131}I [821]. Another interesting example describes clinical studies with mouse monoclonal Ab Lym-1 labeled with ^{67}Cu (^{67}Cu-labeled 2IT-BAT-Lym-1) [822, 823].

- *C-X-C chemokine receptor 4 (CXCR4) ligands* for imaging and treatment of multiple myeloma (MM). CXCR4 is a chemokine receptor and a key factor for tumor growth, progression, and metastasis development in several types of human cancer, among others, in MM cells [824]. MM is the second most common malignancy arising from clonally expanding plasma cells in the bone marrow [825]. The CXCR4 ligand Pentixafor was firstly evaluated with ^{68}Ga for PET imaging [826–828]. Endoradiotherapy with ^{90}Y and ^{177}Lu in combination with high-dose chemotherapy and autologous stem cell transplantation for bone marrow rescue followed. First in-human therapeutic experience with [^{177}Lu]Lu-pentixafor in three heavily pretreated patients with MM showed remarkable therapeutic effects without any acute non-hematologic side effects [829]. Later, another group of eight heavily pretreated MM patients underwent endoradiotherapy with [^{177}Lu]Lu-pentixafor. One patient achieved full remission, and five patients (out of eight) showed partial remission [830]. This approach seems to be very promising for radiotheranostics in patients with advanced MM.
- *Carbonic anhydrase IX (CA-IX)* for imaging and treatment of multiple cancer types [831]. Tumor hypoxia is known to possibly trigger tumor progression and metastatic spread [832]. CA-IX is seen as an attractive imaging and therapeutic endogenous biomarker for targeting hypoxia in solid malignancies (e.g., breast, lung, ovarian cancers) [833]. Different classes of targeting molecules such as mAbs, peptides, low-molecular-weight inhibitors, and antibody mimetics have been developed. These constructs have been radiolabeled for both imaging and therapeutic applications using ^{89}Zr, ^{90}Y, ^{111}In, ^{124}I, ^{131}I, and ^{177}Lu. The chimeric monoclonal antibody G250 is the most extensively investigated CA-IX radiopharmaceutical for imaging ([^{124}I]I-G250 and [^{111}In]In-G250) [834, 835] and endoradiotherapy ([^{131}I]I-G250 and [^{177}Lu]Lu-G250) [834, 836]. Other representatives include peptidic CA-IX-P1 radiolabeled with ^{125}I/^{131}I [837] and sulfonamides conjugated with various chelators employing multiple radiometals [838]. This approach holds a great potential for an improved management of different cancer types.
- *Norepinephrine (NE) analogs* for imaging and treatment of neuroblastoma (NB). NB is the most common solid tumor in children expressing the norepinephrine transporter (NET) which transports NE across the cell membrane (NE = noradrenaline = NA) [839]. In 1984, meta-iodobenzylguanidine (mIBG), a synthetic analog of NE, was reported to be readily accumulated in NB [840]. This arylalkylguanidine can be radiolabeled with ^{123}I for SPECT imaging and ^{131}I for endoradiotherapy. This kind of treatment was shown to be safe and gains a therapeutic benefit in patients with early-stage NB as well as with metastatic disease [841–844].

Further examples might be attributed to:

- *Glucagon-like peptide-1 (GLP-1) receptor agonists* such as [^{68}Ga]Ga-NOTA-MAL-(Cys^{40})-exendin-4 and [^{177}Lu]Lu-DO3A-VS-Cys^{40}-exendin-4 for imaging and therapy of insulinoma [845, 846].
- *Cholecystokinin 2 receptor (CCK2R)/gastrin receptor analogs* such as [^{177}Lu]Lu-PP-F11N for imaging and therapy of medullary thyroid carcinomas (MTC) [847, 848]. In the *Lumed* phase-I clinical trial (ClinicalTrials.gov Identifier: NCT02088645), the use of [^{177}Lu]Lu-PP-F11N for imaging and therapy of patients with advanced MTC is being determined.

Moreover, *melanin-binding benzamides* such as [^{123}I]I-BZA2 and [^{131}I]I-BA52 for imaging and treatment of metastatic melanoma [849, 850], radioiodinated *anti-carcinoembryonic antigen (anti-CEA) antibodies* such as ^{131}I-KAb201 or ^{131}I-labetuzumab for radioimmunotherapy of pancreatic and colorectal cancer, respectively [851, 852], *iodometomidate ([^{123}I]IMTO and [^{131}I]IMTO)* targeting adrenocortical CYP11B enzymes 11β-hydroxylase (cytochrome P450c11 enzymes, CYP11B1) and aldosterone synthase (CYP11B2) for imaging and therapy of advanced adrenocortical carcinoma (ACC) [853, 854], and, last but not least, other non-peptide tracers such as the *biphosphonate-based agent BPAMD* ((4-([bis-(phosphonomethyl))carbamoyl] methyl)-7,10 bis(carboxymethyl)-1,4,7,10-tetraazacyclododec-1-yl)acetic acid radiolabeled with ^{68}Ga and ^{177}Lu for diagnosis and treatment of osteoblastic bone metastases [855, 856] are in development.

2.5.7 Peptides and Peptidomimetics for SPECT Imaging with the Option to Be Used in Combination with Radiotracers for Radioligand Therapy RLT

Technetium-99m-labeled peptide for imaging of tumors overexpressing the somatostatin receptors (SSTRs)

With the introduction to the market of [^{111}In]In-DTPA-(D-Phe^1)-octreotide in 1994 somatostatin receptor (SSTR) targeting with radiolabeled peptides has become an integral part in nuclear oncology. Although [^{111}In]In-DTPA-(D-Phe^1)-octreotide proved to be reliable for the detection of neuroendocrine tumors (NET), the potential clinical advantage of ^{99m}Tc-labeling in comparison to radiolabeling with ^{111}In led to the development of ^{99m}Tc-labeled somatostatin analogs. [^{99m}Tc]Tc-EDDA-HYNIC-TOC (^{99m}Tc-Tektrotyd) is a radiopharmaceutical indicated for diagnosis of tumors with overexpression of SSTR, especially subtype 2 (SSTR2) [284, 857–859].

The bifunctional ligand hydrazinonicotinamide (HYNIC) has initially been developed for ^{99m}Tc-labeling of thrombus-binding peptides, chemotactic peptides, somatostatin derivatives, and annexin V. The radiolabeling proceeds well even at very low concentrations. The complex formation requires the use of a coligand such as tricine or ethylenediamine diacetic acid (EDDA). The coordination mode of HYNIC with ^{99m}Tc is not known exactly. Usually, a monodentate "end-on"-N=N-coordination is proposed (Fig. 2.67), but bidentate coordination is also possible [860, 861]. Anyhow, there is also some evidence for a chelating coordination including the pyridine nitrogen. Because of the presence of stereoisomers, it is difficult to determine the exact nature of the formed complexes [861].

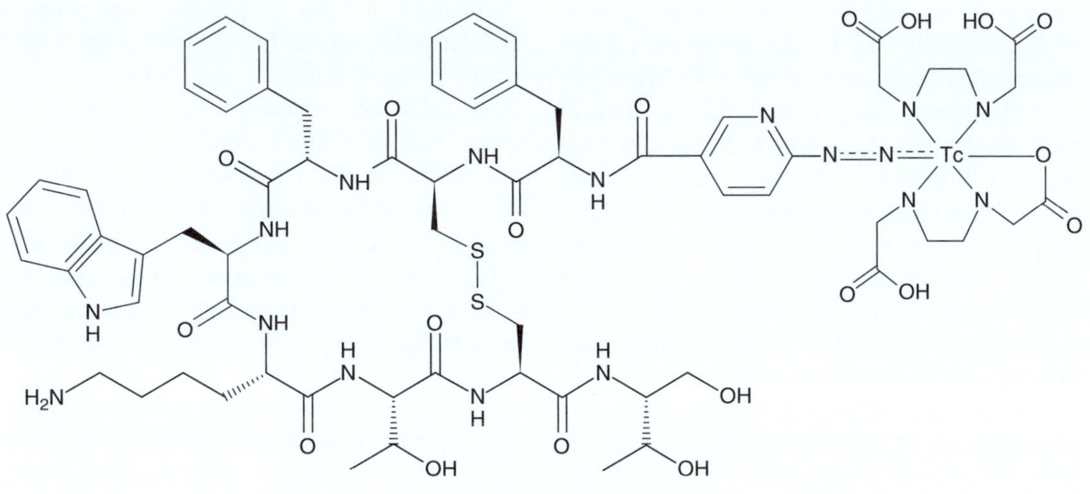

[^{99m}Tc]Tc-Tektrotyd

Fig. 2.67 [^{99m}Tc]Tc-EDDA-HYNIC-TOC (^{99m}Tc-Tektrotyd) for evaluation of neuroendocrine tumors (NET)

2.5.7.1 Somatostatin Receptor SPECT Imaging with ^{99m}Tc Combined with Therapy (cf. Sects. 2.4.5.8.1 and 2.5.3)

As the radionuclidic properties of ^{99m}Tc are superior to ^{111}In based on the octreotide backbone, several radiotracers have subsequently been developed for SPECT imaging of SSTRs, like the FDA-approved ^{99m}Tc-Depreotide (NeoTect), which was withdrawn from the market in 2015, or 6-hydrazinopyridine-3-carboxylic acid coupled to TOC (HYNIC-TOC) or TATE (HYNIC-TATE) [862, 863] and N_4-TATE [864, 865]. Regarding HYNIC the most preferable coligand was EDTA when compared with tricine and tricine-nicotinic acid due to resulting better biodistribution profiles [862], while the TATE derivatives, (Tyr^3,Thr^8)-octreotate, showed preclinical superiority over the corresponding TOC compound, i.e., (Tyr^3)-octreotide, with higher internalization rates and higher tumor-to-normal tissue contrast ratios, indicating that [^{111}In]In-DOTA-TATE and [^{99m}Tc]Tc-EDDA-HYNIC-TATE are suitable candidates for clinical studies [863].

Then, in the 1990s, the first SSTR2 somatostatin antagonists were invented. These analogs (radiolabeled with different radionuclides, i.e., ^{177}Lu, ^{111}In, ^{64}Cu) proved preclinically superior to the agonists. Antagonists showed an improved binding affinity, they recognized a larger number of SSTR binding sites in vitro, and in general they showed improved tumor uptake [282]. These preclinical evidences led to pilot studies for some of these compounds. According to these pilot studies, [^{111}In]In-DOTA-BASS and [^{111}In]In-DOTA-JR11 were superior to [^{111}In]In-DTPA-(D-Phe^1)-octreotide (OctreoScan®) showing higher tumor uptake, higher contrast ratios and a higher number of detectable lesions [866].

Moreover, a phase-I/-II trial for staging well-differentiated to moderately differentiated gastroenteropancreatic NETs was described in which intraindividual PET/CT imaging was conducted with [^{68}Ga]Ga-NODAGA-JR11 (^{68}Ga-OPS202) and [^{68}Ga]Ga-DOTA-TOC, two microdoses each (ClinicalTrials.gov, NCT02162446) [282, 867]. This study indicated an increased image contrast for both doses of [^{68}Ga]Ga-NODAGA-JR11 owing to lower hepatic, intestinal, and pancreatic uptake, which resulted in higher sensitivity and diagnostic accuracy compared to [^{68}Ga]Ga-DOTA-TOC PET/CT. The “theranostic pair” [^{68}Ga]Ga-DOTA-JR11 and [^{177}Lu]Lu-DOTA-JR11 was also investigated in NET patients in a single-center study (ClinicalTrials.gov, NCT02609737). Table 2.17 summarizes the chemical structures and the current clinical status of the most important compounds developed in the field of nuclear medicine.

2.5.7.2 SPECT Imaging with Gastrin/Cholecystokinin 2 (CCK2) Analogs (cf. Sect. 2.5.6)

The gastrin receptor may be an attractive biological target for radiopeptide imaging and therapy since it is overexpressed in several types of human tumors (medullary thyroid carcinoma 92%, small cell lung carcinoma 57%, astrocytoma 65%, stromal ovarian tumors 100%, and gastroenteropancreatic tumors 22%) [710, 873]. These studies are mostly focusing on MTC (metastasized/recurrent medullary thyroid carcinoma), which is another kind of NET, which are known to overexpress CCK2 receptors [874]. Since the proof of concept was established in vivo in patients with various CCK analogs, several human studies have been recorded so far which are summarized in Table 2.18 [880]. However, a marked kidney uptake has made the routine application difficult until now, while the low in vivo stability of these analogs represents an additional challenge [879]. A phase-I clinical trial (GRANT-T-MTC) with [^{111}In]In-DOTA-CP04 (=[^{111}In]In-PP-F11 or [^{111}In]In-DOTA-(D-Glu)$_6$-Ala-Tyr-Gly-Trp-Met-Asp-Phe-NH_2) is ongoing to establish the safety of intravenous injection of a high peptide amount and to assess the radiotracer biodistribution and dosimetry in MTC and normal tissues (ClinicalTrials.gov, NCT03246659).

Table 2.17 Selection of clinical trials and authority approvals for somatostatin-based radiotracers (cf. also Sect. 2.5.3.1 for NETTER-1 phase-III clinical trial with [^{177}Lu]Lu-DOTA-TATE)

Somatostatin analog	Tumor type (number of patients)	Results	References
[^{111}In]In-DTPA-(D-Phe^{1})-octreotide [^{111}In] In-DTPA-D-Phe-cyclo(Cys-Phe-D-Trp-Lys-Thr-Cys)-Thr(ol) (OctreoScan®, Mallinckrodt Pharmaceuticals, FDA approved, agonist)	NET	Diagnosis and workup of NETs	Maxwell and Howe [868]
[^{90}Y]Y-DOTA-TOC [^{90}Y]Y-DOTA-(D-Phe^{1},Tyr^{3})-octreotide (Phase II, agonist)	GEP-NET (38)	Seventeen patients (43.6%) had a partial response, ten patients (25.6%) had stable disease, and 11 patients (28.2%) had progressive disease. A statistically significant difference was observed ($P < 0.001$) between the response to [^{90}Y]Y-DOTA-TOC treatment and the response to biotherapy with somatostatin analogs and chemotherapy and also between the current results and the results from a previous similar study ($P < 0.05$). At the time of the current evaluation with ongoing follow-up for 30 patients, the median progression-free survival was 22.3 months	Savelli et al. [869]
[^{90}Y]Y-DOTA-TATE [^{90}Y]Y-DOTA-(D-Phe^{1},Tyr^{3},Thr^{8}]-octreotate (Phase II, agonist)	GEP-NETs (60)	[^{90}Y]Y-DOTA-TATE therapy is effective and relatively safe in patients with GEP-NET. Standard doses of [^{90}Y]Y-DOTA-TATE result in a relatively low risk of myelotoxicity. However, due to ongoing risk of renal toxicity, careful monitoring of the kidney is recommended	Cwikla et al. [870]
	NET (46)	Out of 46 [^{90}Y]Y-DOTA-TATE-treated patients, one died before completing the therapy and 16 died after completing the therapy, among them one due to myocardial infarction. After 12-month follow-up, stabilization of disease was observed in 47%, partial remission in 31%, and progression in 9% of the 45 patients who completed the therapy. Five patients died before completion of 12 months of follow-up. One of the patients died due to myocardial infarction. In one case, the information after 12 months is incomplete. The progression-free survival was 37.4 months. During 12 months follow-up, transient decrease of PLT, WBC, and hemoglobin values was observed. A transient increase of creatinine level (within normal ranges) and decrease of GFR values were found	
[^{177}Lu]Lu-DOTA-TATE (Lutathera®) [^{177}Lu] Lu-DOTA-(D-Phe^{1},Tyr^{3},Thr^{8})-octreotate (NETTER-1, phase III, agonist)	NET	[^{177}Lu]Lu-DOTA-TATE resulted in markedly longer progression-free survival than high-dose octreotide LAR and was associated with limited acute toxic effects in a population of patients who had progressive neuroendocrine tumors that originated in the midgut	Strosberg et al. [725, 929]

(continued)

Table 2.17 (continued)

Somatostatin analog	Tumor type (number of patients)	Results	References
^{99m}Tc-Tektrotyd [^{99m}Tc] Tc-EDDA-HYNIC-(D-Phe^1,Tyr^3)-octreotide (Polatom, marketing authorization no. 11664, agonist)	bronchial and thymic NET (41)	Somatostatin receptor scintigraphy correctly identified all primary NETs located in the lungs and thymus. SPECT-CT studies with ^{99m}Tc-Tektrotyd resulted in exact pre-surgical and pretreatment N/M staging of bronchial and thymic NETs, except two cases with multiple hepatic metastases and one with massive suprarenal metastasis, sensitivity 81.25% (13/16), specificity 88% (22/25), and accuracy 85.36% (35/41)	Sergieva et al. [871]
[^{99m}Tc]Tc-EDDA-HYNIC-TOC (Phase I, agonist)	NET (16)	[^{99m}Tc]Tc-EDDA-HYNIC-TOC scintigraphy provided additional information in 50% of patients, with impact on patient management in the same percentage of patients. Distant metastases were found in 9 out of 16 patients (56%). [^{99m}Tc]Tc-EDDA-HYNIC-TOC SRS had sensitivity of 100% (75.3–100%), specificity of 66.7% (9.4–99.2%), accuracy of 93.7%, positive predictive value of 92.9% (66.1–99.8%), and negative predictive value of 100% (15.8–100%)	Trogrlic and Tezak [859]
^{99m}Tc-Demotate 1 [^{99m}Tc]Tc-N_4-(D-Phe^1,Tyr^3,Thr^8)-octreotate (N_4 = *N,N′,N″,N′″-tetra-(*tert-*butoxycarbonyl)-6-(carboxy)-1,4,8,11-tetraazaundecane)* (Pilot study, agonist)	6 CT (2) or PT (4)	Blood excretion was very rapid, with <2% ID in plasma after 1 h and urinary excretion <20% ID after 6 h. Two patients complained of mild gastrointestinal problems and paresthesia, but no other adverse reactions were observed. SSTR-positive tumors were rapidly visualized as early as 15 min p.i., with maximum tumor uptake (up to 19% ID) and tumor/organ ratios as early as 1 h p.i. Organs of predominant physiological uptake were the spleen and the kidneys, with no intestinal excretion detectable up to 24 h. ^{99m}Tc-Demotate 1 detected 11 lesions while In-Oct detected 10; differences in uptake behavior were observed in three patients	Decristoforo et al. [872]
[^{111}In]In-DOTA-BASS [^{111}In] In-DOTA-p-NO_2-Phe-cyclo(D-Cys-Tyr-D-Trp-Lys-Thr-Cys)-D-Tyr-NH_2 (Pilot study, antagonist)	MTC/NET (5)	No adverse effects of [^{111}In]In-DOTA-BASS (20 µg) were observed. Twenty-five of 28 lesions were detected, whereas OctreoScan® detected only 17 of 28 lesions. In the same patient, [^{111}In]In-DOTA-BASS showed higher tumor and lower renal uptake than OctreoScan® (3.5 ± 2.8% injected activity [%IA] vs. 1.0 ± 0.99 %IA and 1.5 ± 0.3 %IA vs. 2.3 ± 0.7 %IA) at 4 h after injection	Wild et al. [866]
[^{177}Lu]Lu-DOTA-JR11 (^{177}Lu-OPS201) [^{177}Lu] Lu-DOTA-Cpa-cyclo(D-Cys-Aph(Hor)-D-Aph(Cbm)-Lys-Thr-Cys)-D-Tyr-NH_2 (Pilot study, antagonist)	NET (4)	Reversible minor adverse effects of [^{177}Lu]Lu-DOTA-JR11 were observed. [^{177}Lu]Lu-DOTA-JR11 showed a 1.7–10.6 times higher tumor dose than [^{177}Lu]Lu-DOTA-TATE. At the same time, the tumor-to-kidney and tumor-to-bone marrow dose ratio was 1.1–7.2 times higher. All four patients were treated with [^{177}Lu]Lu-DOTA-JR11, resulting in partial remission in two patients, stable disease in one patient, and mixed response in the other patient	Wild et al. [731]

MTC metastatic thyroid carcinoma, *NET* neuroendocrine tumors, *CT* carcinoid tumors, *PT* endocrine pancreatic tumors, *GEP* gastroenteropancreatic

Table 2.18 Selection of human studies (phase I, pilot) with gastrin analogs radiolabeled with SPECT radionuclides

Aim of the study	Tumor type (number of patients)	Results	References
MTC examined with [^{111}In]In-DTPA-(D-Glu^{1})-minigastrin. All had been staged by ultrasonography, computed tomography, magnetic resonance imaging, and somatostatin receptor and bone scanning (GRS, ^{111}In-labeled DTPA-(D-Glu^{1})-minigastrin)	MTC (45) Healthy volunteers (5)	All tumor manifestations known from conventional imaging were visualized as early as 1 h postinjection, with increasing tumor to background ratios over time; at least one lesion was detected in 20 of 22 patients with occult disease (patient-based sensitivity, 91%). Among them were local recurrences and lymph node, pulmonary, hepatic, splenic, and bone (marrow) metastases. Normal organ uptake was essentially confined to the stomach (and, to a lesser extent, to the gallbladder and, in premenopausal women, to normal breast tissue) as a result of CCK-B receptor-specific binding and to the kidneys as excretory organs	Behr and Béhé [875]
Radiopeptide imaging in the management of patients with NET. The clinical performance of GRS was compared with SRS, CT, and [^{18}F]FDG PET in patients with MTC. (SRS, ^{111}In-OctreoScan®; GRS, [^{111}In]In-DTPA-(D-Glu^{1})-minigastrin)	MTC (27)	Nineteen underwent both GRS and SRS. Tumor detection rates GRS 94.2%, SRS 40.7%. In 26 patients, GRS, CT, and PET were compared. GRS tumor detection rate 87.3% vs. CT 76.1%, PET 67.2%; if GRS and CT were combined, they were able to detect 96.7% of areas of tumor involvement	Gotthardt et al. [876]
Comparison of GRS to SRS in patients with NET. SRS and GRS were performed within 21 days in a series of 60 consecutive patients with NET (SRS, OctreoScan®; GRS, [^{111}In]In-DTPA-(D-Glu^{1})-minigastrin)	Car (51), GS (3), GL (2), IS (1), PRG (3)	The overall tumor detection rates GRS 73.7%, SRS 82.1%. In the 11 patients with negative SRS, GRS was positive in 6 (54.5%). Based on the number of tumor sites detected and the degree of uptake, GRS performed better than SRS in 13 patients (21.7%), equivalent images were obtained in 18 cases (30.0%), and SRS performed better in 24 (40.0%) cases. In six of the SRS-positive patients, 18 additional sites of tumor involvement could be detected. Overall, GRS detected additional tumor sites in 20% of the patients. Localization of the primary tumors or their functional status had no influence on the outcome of imaging	Gotthardt et al. [877]
The clinical value of a new gastrin analog, [^{99m}Tc]Tc-EDDA-HYNIC-D-Glu-octagastrin and a somatostatin analog, [^{99m}Tc]Tc-EDDA-HYNIC-TOC for scintigraphy in patients with MTC to detect recurrences and metastases and select patients for peptide receptor radiotherapy (SRS, [^{99m}Tc]Tc-EDDA-HYNIC-TOC; GRS, [^{99m}Tc]Tc-EDDA-HYNIC-D-Glu-octagastrin)	MTC (30) (with elevated serum calcitonin concentrations)	^{99m}Tc-EDDA/HYNIC-TOC detected somatostatin receptor-positive lesions in 20 patients with MTC, whereas ^{99m}Tc-EDDA/HYNIC-D-Glu-octagastrin displayed gastrin receptors in 11 patients. In nine cases, the scans were positive in both methods, although in two cases different pathologic foci were visualized. In 12 cases, only ^{99m}Tc-EDDA/HYNIC-TOC scintigraphy was positive, whereas in three other cases, only ^{99m}Tc-EDDA/HYNIC-D-Glu-octagastrin revealed pathologic lesions	Kosowicz et al. [878]
Initial clinical aspects of CCK-2 receptor targeting with three radiolabeled peptides (GRS, [^{111}In]In-DOTA-MG11, [^{111}In]In-CCK (DOTA-D-Asp-Tyr-Nle-Gly-Trp-Nle-Asp-Phe-NH_2 or DOTA-CCK), [^{99m}Tc]Tc-Demogastrin 2)	MTC (6)	Radioactivity was cleared rapidly by the kidneys, with no significant differences in the excretion pattern of the three radiotracers. All analogs exhibited low in vivo stability in patients, as revealed during analysis of blood samples, with the respective $T_{1/2}$ found in the order of minutes	Breeman et al. [879]

CCK cholecystokinin, *CT* computed tomography, *Car* carcinoid tumors, *GRS* gastrin receptor scintigraphy, *GS* gastrinoma, *GL* glucagonomas, *IS* insulinoma, *MTC* metastasized/recurrent medullary thyroid carcinoma, *NET* neuroendocrine tumors, *PRG* paraganglioma, *SRS* somatostatin receptor scintigraphy

2.5.7.3 Glucagon-Like Peptide-1 Analogs (cf. Sect. 2.5.6)

Another receptor belonging to the large family of G protein-coupled receptors is the glucagon-like peptide-1 (GLP-1) receptor, which is highly overexpressed on essentially all benign insulinomas and on gastrinomas [708, 881]. Benign insulinomas also may present a diagnostic challenge; they arise from the beta cells of the pancreas and present as small nodules (usually ca. 2 cm). They secrete insulin, leading to potentially life-threatening hypoglycemia. Complete tumor resection is the only way to cure these patients, while standard preoperative noninvasive imaging methods (ultrasound, MRI and CT) have low sensitivity (less than 40%) [708]. The natural ligand GLP-1 consists of 30 amino acids and has a plasma half-life of less than 2 min. Exendin-4 is a 39-amino acid natural peptide originally isolated from saliva of *Heloderma suspectum*, which is metabolically resistant and share nearly 50% homology with the human GLP-1. Initially exendin-4 was radiolabeled with ^{111}In using DTPA coupled to the side chain of Lys^{40} with aminohexanoic acid (Ahx) as a spacer [(Lys^{40}(Ahx-DTPA)NH$_2$)-exendin-4] [882] and this first ^{111}In-labeled exendin-4 was clinically evaluated by a proof-of-concept study [883]. Since then several clinical studies have been conducted which are summarized in Table 2.19. The results from ^{111}In-, ^{99m}Tc-, as well as ^{68}Ga-labeled exendin-4 analogs indicate that this class of radiopeptide is a promising diagnostic tool for the localization of small insulinoma tumors but in best case for benign insulinoma since malignant insulinoma often lack GLP-1 receptors. High kidney uptake of these radiotracers prevents theranostic applications at the moment [708].

Table 2.19 Clinical studies (phase I and pilot) with exendin-4 analogs radiolabeled with SPECT radionuclides

Aim of the study	Tumor type (number of patients)	Results	References
Proof of concept: the diagnostic value of GLP-1–receptor scintigraphy (Lys^{40}(Ahx-DTPA-[^{111}In]In)-NH$_2$]-exendin-4) in two patients with insulinomas	INS (2)	GLP-1 receptor scan can identify barely detectable insulinomas that express GLP-1 receptor	Wild et al. [883]
Insulinoma detection rates with a glucagon-like peptide-1 receptor avid radiotracer ([^{111}In]In-DOTA-exendin-4) using SPECT/CT and comparison with the detection rates of conventional CT/MRI techniques	INS (30)	[^{111}In]In-DTPA-exendin-4 SPECT/CT correctly detected 19 insulinomas and 4 additional positive lesions (two islet cell hyperplasia and two uncharacterized lesions) resulting in a positive predictive value of 83% (95% CI 62–94). One true negative (islet cell hyperplasia) and one false negative (malignant insulinoma) result was identified in separate patients by [^{111}In]In-DTPA-exendin-4 SPECT/CT. Seven patients (23%) were referred to surgery on the basis of [^{111}In]In-DTPA-exendin-4 imaging alone. For 23 assessable patients, [^{111}In]In-DTPA-exendin-4 SPECT/CT had a higher sensitivity (95% [95% CI 74–100]) than did CT/MRI (47% [27–68]; $P = 0.011$)	Christ et al. [884]
[^{111}In]In-DOTA-exendin-4 in localization in insulinomas using SPECT/CT	INS (6)	In all six cases, the GLP-1R scans successfully detected the INS identified using conventional methods in four cases. By using a gamma-probe intraoperatively, GLP-1R detection permitted a successful surgical removal of the tumors in all patients, diagnosed histopathologically as five pancreatic and one extrapancreatic insulinomas. In vitro GLP-1R autoradiography showed a high density of GLP-1R in all tested insulinomas	Christ et al. [885]

Table 2.19 (continued)

Aim of the study	Tumor type (number of patients)	Results	References
The utility of (Lys^{40}(Ahx-HYNIC-[^{99m}Tc]Tc-EDDA) NH_2)-exendin-4 scintigraphy in the management of patients with hypoglycemia, particularly in the detection of occult insulinoma	INS (40)	Positive results of GLP-1 scintigraphy were observed in 28/40. In 18 patients postsurgical histopathological examination confirmed diagnosis of insulinoma. Two patients had contraindications to the surgery, one patient did not want to be operated. One patient, who presented with postprandial hypoglycemia, with positive result of GLP-1 imaging was not qualified for surgery and is in the observational group. Eight patients were lost for follow-up, among them six patients with positive GLP-1 scintigraphy result. One patient with negative scintigraphy was diagnosed with malignant insulinoma. In two patients with negative scintigraphy, Munchausen syndrome was diagnosed (patients were taking insulin). Seven patients with negative results of ^{99m}Tc-GLP-1 scintigraphy and postprandial hypoglycemia with C-peptide and insulin levels within the limits of normal ranges were in the observational group. ^{99m}Tc-GLP-1-SPECT/CT was also performed in three patients with nesidioblastosis (revealing diffuse tracer uptake in 2/3 and a focal lesion in 1/3) and in two patients with malignant insulinoma (with a focal uptake in the localization of a removed pancreatic head in one case and negative GLP-1 1 scintigraphy in the other patient)	Sowa-Staszczak et al. [886]
Diagnosis of insulinoma with the use of [Lys^{40} (Ahx-HYNIC-[^{99m}Tc] Tc-EDDA)NH_2]-exendin-4	INS (11)	Sensitivity and specificity of GLP-1 receptor imaging 100% in patients with benign insulinoma. In all eight cases with suspicion of insulinoma, a focal uptake in the pancreas was found. In six patients surgical excision of the tumor was performed (type G1 tumors were confirmed histopathologically). In one patient surgical treatment is planned. One patient was disqualified from surgery. In one case with malignant insulinoma, pathological accumulation of the tracer was found only in the region of local recurrence. The GLP-1 study was negative in the other malignant insulinoma patient. In one case with suspicion of nesidioblastosis, a focal accumulation of the tracer was observed, and histopathology revealed coexistence of insulinoma and nesidioblastosis	Sowa-Staszczak et al. [887]

GLP-1 glucagon-like peptide-1, *INS* insulinomas

2.5.7.4 Neurotensin Peptide Analogs for SPECT Imaging

Neurotensin (NT) is a tridecapeptide found in the brain and gut with many growth regulatory functions. The pharmacological effects of NT are triggered by the specific interaction of the peptide with three different receptors on the cell surface (NTR1, NTR2, G protein-coupled and NTR3, single transmembrane domain receptor similar to sortilin). Overexpression of NTR1 has been found in several human cancers including Ewing sarcomas, meningiomas, astrocytomas, medulloblastomas, and pancreatic carcinomas. So far only few examples of NT analogs have been used in pilot studies or phase-I clinical trials, the ^{99m}Tc-labeled NT analogs:

1. ^{99m}Tc-NT-XI, [[^{99m}Tc]Tc(CO)$_3$]-(NαHis) Ac-Lys(ψCH_2-NH)-Arg-Pro-Tyr-Tle-Leu, evaluated for its tumor targeting characteristics in ductal pancreatic adenocarcinoma patients ($n = 4$) [888]

2. ^{99m}Tc-Demotensin VI in 14 patients with advanced tumor stages (pancreatic adenocarcinoma, $n = 4$; small cell lung cancer, SCLC, $n = 4$; non-small cell lung cancer, NSCLC, $n = 4$; and colon carcinoma, $n = 2$) [889]

These initial clinical results were not so favorable due to the high nonspecific uptake and rapid metabolism behavior of the radiotracers. More clinical data are required in order to determine the real potential of radiolabeled NT analogs as tumor imaging agents.

2.5.7.5 Bombesin Receptor for Imaging and Therapy

The bombesin (BN) receptor family of receptors, particularly gastrin-releasing peptide receptor (GRPr), has been shown to be one of the most overexpressed or ectopically expressed family of G protein-coupled receptors on small lung cancer, non-small cell lung cancer, pancreatic cancer, prostate cancer, head/neck squamous cell cancers, glioblastomas, neuroblastomas, breast cancer, intestinal carcinoids, and bronchial carcinoids [804].

Until now numerous BN analogs have been preclinically or clinically studied ([804]; *published a detailed review on this subject*). Most of the radiotracers have been radiolabeled with ^{99m}Tc (more than 80 publications exist) or with ^{111}In (more than 40 publications exist) and to a lesser amount with other radionuclides such as ^{18}F, ^{64}Cu, ^{67}Ga, ^{68}Ga, ^{86}Y, ^{90}Y, ^{125}I, ^{177}Lu, ^{186}Re, and ^{188}Re. Despite the numerous preclinical investigations, only a few radiotracers have reached the clinical stage of development so far. Until now approximately a dozen studies have been published of patients studied with suspected and/or confirmed breast, prostate, gastrointestinal, or lung cancer (Table 2.20) [804]. In 83% of the studies, the BN analogs were radiolabeled with ^{99m}Tc, while in more recent studies, the PET radionuclide ^{68}Ga (17%) was used for radiolabeling. The first BN radioligand, RP527, [^{99m}Tc]Tc-N_3S-5-Ava-BN(7–14), a GRPr agonist, was tested in 2001 in patients with breast and prostate cancer. From 2002 to 2004, six studies were published in which the ^{99m}Tc-labeled analog (Cys^0,Aca^1)-BN(2–14), also called (Leu^{13})-BN, again a GRPr agonist, was used for the diagnosis of prostate and breast cancer [891–895, 903, 904]. This initial compound was replaced later by [^{99m}Tc]Tc-EDDA-HYNIC-(Lys^3)-BN for breast cancer imaging, by ^{99m}Tc-labeled N_4-(Pro^1,Tyr^4,Nle^{14})-bombesin (Demobesin 4) for prostate cancer imaging [902, 905], and by [^{99m}Tc]Tc-HYNIC(tricine/TPPTS)-Aca-BN(7–14) (^{99m}Tc-HABBN) again for prostate cancer imaging [901]. Table 2.20 summarizes the BN analogs used in clinical SPECT studies so far.

According to recent literature, most of the studies use BN antagonists for diagnosis (due to their superior pharmacokinetics and higher inherent biosafety) [690, 805, 906] and fewer agonists for therapy applications [907, 908]. Preferably BN analogs [690, 691] for diagnosis and theranostics are radiolabeled with the PET radionuclide like ^{68}Ga or with ^{177}Lu for therapy. Due to recent promising results and success with PSMA-SPECT (e.g., [^{99m}Tc]Tc-MIP-1404) and PSMA-PET radiotracers (e.g., [^{68}Ga]Ga-PSMA-11), preclinical and clinical research on prostate cancer is now more focusing on PSMA as feasible biological target rather than on GRPr.

Anyhow, only one comparative study had been conducted so far in few PC patients (with no conclusive results) comparing imaging of the two prostate cancer-associated biological targets with two PET radiotracers: [^{68}Ga]Ga-RM2 (GRPr-targeted) and [^{68}Ga]Ga-PSMA-11 (PSMA-targeted) [808]. It should also be mentioned that in order to address tumor heterogeneity, bispecific compounds containing both pharmacophores have also been suggested [909, 910]. Currently radiolabeled GRPr radioligands are also investigated toward their potential application in breast cancer patients [691].

2.5.7.6 Small and Low-Molecular-Weight Molecules Targeting Prostate-Specific Membrane Antigen (PSMA)

PSMA is a transmembrane, 750 amino acid type II glycoprotein which is primarily expressed in normal human prostate epithelium and is upreg-

Table 2.20 Clinical studies (phase I, pilot) using ^{99m}Tc-labeled bombesin analogs

Bombesin analog	Tumor type (number of patients)	Results	References
^{99m}Tc-labeled (Cys^{0},Aca^{1})-BN(2–14) (or (Leu^{13})-BN)	NR (3), PC (1), SCLC (1)	No side effects, visualization of both tumors for 3 h, radioactivity accumulation in the liver, kidneys, and thyroid gland. Tumor uptake higher than with [^{99m}Tc]Tc-sestamibi alone (SPECT and planar scintigraphy, biopsy)	De Vincentis et al. [890]
	Biopsies BC (5)	48/48 biopsies high, 19/21 intermediate, and 2/8 low radioactivity uptake positive for cancer (biopsy driven by imaging probe combined with X-ray)	Soluri et al. [891]
	PC (14)	Hundred percentage cancer and lymph nodes visualized. Results confirmed by pathologic evaluation while OctreoScan® only detected 2/3 cases (SPECT and planar scintigraphy)	De Vincentis et al. [892]
	BC (5)	No side effects. Hundred percentage cancer and lymph nodes visualized. Radioactivity accumulated in the liver, kidneys, and thyroid gland. Tumor/breast uptake ratio higher than with [^{99m}Tc]Tc-sestamibi alone (planar scintigraphy)	Scopinaro et al. [893]
	PC (11)	Hundred percentage cancer and lymph nodes visualized. Results confirmed by pathologic evaluation. Detection of the lymph nodes affected better than with MRI (SPECT and planar scintigraphy)	Scopinaro et al. [894]
	(13) (6 suspected + 7 RC)	Cancer detected in 11/13 and two false positives. 5/5 positive lymph nodes detected. Results confirmed by pathologic evaluation. After 60 min all radiopeptide is in the intestine (SPECT and planar scintigraphy)	Scopinaro et al. [895]
^{99m}Tc-Bombesin (no further information are given regarding structure from the authors)	BC (33), women with suspicious palpable breast lesions and no definitive diagnosis with other imaging procedures	Overall sensitivity 100%, specificity 66.1%, negative and positive predictive values 63%, and accuracy of this radiotracer 76% for diagnosis of breast cancer (SPECT and planar scintigraphy)	Shariati et al. [896]
[^{99m}Tc] Tc–EDDA-HYNIC-(Lys^{3})-BN	BC (11), proven cancer (3), possible cancer (8)	No side effects. Predominant renal clearance. Patients with breast cancer showed asymmetrical uptake by breast tissue, with higher accumulation in patients with breast cancer (SPECT and planar scintigraphy)	Santos-Cuevas et al. [897]
[[^{99m}Tc]Tc-N$_3$S]-5-Ava-BN(7–14), (or RP527)	PC (4) with bone metastasis and with androgen resistance BC (6) suspected	No side effects. Hepatic and renal clearance non-blood accumulation. Radiopeptide uptake in 1/4 prostate cancer bone metastases and 4/6 breast cancer metastases and affected lymph nodes (SPECT and planar scintigraphy)	Van de Wiele et al. [898]
	NR (6)	No side effects. Hepatobiliary and renal clearance, non-blood accumulation. Low uptake by the brain, myocardium, lungs, breast, and testes. Possible radiotracer for the supradiaphragmatic region and favorable dosimetry for SPECT	Van de Wiele et al. [899]
	BC (9) suspected, BC (5) tamoxifen resistant and bone metastases	8/9 suspected patients' tumor and lymph nodes were detected. 0/5 resistant patients detected (planar scintigraphy)	[900]

(continued)

Table 2.20 (continued)

Bombesin analog	Tumor type (number of patients)	Results	References
[^{99m}Tc] Tc-HYNIC(tricine/ TPPTS)- Aca-BN(7–14)	PC (8) (patients scheduled for either radical prostatectomy or external beam radiotherapy underwent ^{99m}Tc-HABBN scintigraphy and SPECT/ CT prior to treatment)	No uptake in the prostate was observed at any time point in any patient possibly due to low in vivo stability in man (SPECT/CT)	Ananias et al. [901]
^{99m}Tc-Demobesin 4	PC (8): Group 1 (2 no treatment), Group 2 (six known metastatic disease, previous hormone treatment)	Metastatic disease was not efficiently imaged in group 2 (patients undergone hormone treatment). There was no increased uptake in the prostate bed or in nodal disease. Uptake in skeletal metastases was variable. Tracer effectively imaged newly diagnosed cancer confined to the prostate in group 1. Neither of these patients had received any specific therapy for prostate cancer (SPECT)	Mather et al. [902]

PC prostate cancer, *BC* breast cancer, *SCLC* small cell lung cancer, *RC* rectal cancer, *NR* normal

ulated in prostate cancer, including metastatic disease [911]. PSMA is expressed by the majority of prostate cancers, and its expression is further increased in poorly differentiated, metastatic, and hormone-refractory carcinomas. This exopeptidase reacts with poly γ-glutamated folates removing the poly γ-glutamyl termini and is highly homologous to N-acetylated R-linked acidic dipeptidase (NAALADase), a neuropeptidase that produces the neurotransmitter glutamate and N-acetylaspartate (NAA) through the hydrolysis of N-acetyl-L-aspartyl-L-glutamate (NAAG) [912].

^{123}I- and ^{131}I-Labeled PSMA Radioligands

The first small radioiodinated molecules targeting PSMA comprising MIP-1072 and MIP-1095 were developed by the University of Illinois (USA) and the company Molecular Insight Pharmaceuticals (MIP). MIP-1072 and MIP-1095 are based on urea-linked dipeptides, i.a., Glu-urea-Lys. The first Glu-ureido-derived PSMA inhibitors were initially described by Kozikowski and coworkers [752, 913–915]. One of the first preclinical imaging studies with small-molecule PSMA inhibitor radiotracers in PSMA-positive tumor xenografts were reported in 2005 [916].

The two PSMA ligands, [^{123}I]I-MIP-1072 and [^{123}I]I-MIP-1095, are synthesized in a similar way and have very similar structures (cf. Sect. 2.5.4, Fig. 2.66) and comparable pharmacokinetics [751, 763, 917].

Shortly after their discovery, these two analogs were introduced in the clinics in 2008 [761, 769] by Molecular Insight Pharmaceuticals (ClinicalTrials.gov Identifier: NCT00712829). It was proven for both compounds, that PC imaging is possible early after intravenous injection of the respective radiotracer. In men with metastatic PC, SPECT/CT demonstrated the ability of these radioligands to rapidly detect PC lesions in the soft tissue, bone, and prostate bed as early as 1 h after intravenous injection, although later images, for example, at 4 h after intravenous injection demonstrated even higher contrast of the lesions [769]. In a subsequent evaluation of [^{123}I]I-MIP-1072 using a chemotherapy PC model, tumor uptake of radiotracer was proportional to viable tumor mass; this result provided initial support for the potential of PSMA imaging to track the response to therapy [917]. The impact of successful PC imaging in patients with the ^{123}I-labeled versions and their optimal pharmacokinetics led to the investigation of their potential therapeutic application in a next step with a change of the radioisotope to ^{131}I in the radioligand [^{131}I]I-MIP-1095 [763] (cf. Sect. 2.5.4 and Table 2.21, Sect. 2.5.7).

Table 2.21 Current status of clinical studies with ^{131}I- and ^{99m}Tc-labeled PSMA-targeted low-molecular-weight molecules (cf. Sect. 2.5.4.1 for the VISION phase-III registration trial with [^{177}Lu]Lu-PSMA-617)

Aim of the study	Tumor type (number of patients)	Results	References
Study to evaluate [^{99m}Tc]Tc-MIP-1404 SPECT/CT imaging in men with biopsy-proven low-grade PC ([^{99m}Tc]Tc-MIP-1404 or ^{99m}Tc-trofolastat, phase-III trial)	PC	Ongoing (recruitment of patients completed)	ClinicalTrials.gov NCT02615067 [proSPECT-AS]
First human data in men with metastatic PC and in healthy male subjects for [^{99m}Tc]Tc-MIP-1404 and [^{99m}Tc]Tc-MIP-1405 (phase-I trial)	Healthy volunteers (6), PC (6)	Rapid blood clearance, MIP-1404 lower urinary activity (7%) than MIP-1405 (26%). Both agents showed persistent uptake in the salivary, lacrimal, and parotid glands. Uptake in the liver and kidney was acceptable for imaging at 1–2 h. In men with PC, both agents rapidly localized in bone and lymph node lesions as early as 1 h. SPECT demonstrated excellent lesion contrast. [^{99m}Tc]Tc-MIP-1404 and [^{99m}Tc]Tc-MIP-1405 detected more lesions (bone, soft tissue, including subcentimeter lymph nodes) vs. [^{99m}Tc]Tc-MDP. The high-contrast images exhibited TBR 3:1–9:1 at 4 and 20	Vallabhajosula et al. [918]
First experience using the ^{99m}Tc-labeled PSMA inhibitor MIP-1404 (Progenics Pharmaceuticals, Inc., Tarrytown, NY) in 60 patients with biochemically recurrent PC (pilot study)	PC (60) (biochemical relapse)	42/60 patients positive lesions detected (70%; 95% confidence interval [CI], 0.58–0.82). 20/60 positive lymph nodes suggestive of metastasis, 14/60 pathological uptake in the prostate region indicative of local recurrence, 19/60 tracer accumulation in the skeleton ($n = 18$) or lungs ($n = 1$). Detection rates: 91.4% at PSA > 2 ng/mL and 40.0% at PSA < 2, ($P < 0.01$). Average SUVmax of 82 positive lesions analyzed 16.3 ± 21.6 with a range of 1.7–142.9	Reinfelder et al. [928]
^{99m}Tc-trofolastat SPECT/CT in a phase-II multicenter, multireader prospective study in patients with intermediate- and high-grade PCa, before radical prostatectomy and extended pelvic lymph node (LN) dissection, with histopathology as the gold standard (phase-II trial)	PC (105)	PCa detection (94%). There was a significantly higher VsC and TBR in positive lobes compared with tumor-negative lobes. Receiver-operating characteristic analysis showed that VsC more accurately discriminated lobes with GS ≤ 3 + 3 from ≥3 + 4, whereas TBRs discriminated high-grade disease from normal lobes better. VsC and TBRs correlated significantly with GS. LNI sensitivity 50%, specificity 87%. TBR values significantly predicted LNI, sensitivity 90%. ^{99m}Tc-trofolastat SPECT/CT detects PCa with high sensitivity in patients with intermediate- and high-risk PCa compared with histology, and it has the potential to be used as a surrogate marker for GS and predict LNI	Goffin et al. [925]
Pharmacokinetics and ability to visualize PC (SPECT/CT) in the bone, soft tissue, and the prostate gland using [^{123}I]I-MIP-1072 and [^{123}I]I-MIP-1095, novel radiolabeled small molecules targeting prostate-specific membrane antigen (pilot study)	Healthy volunteers (6), PC (7)	[^{123}I]I-MIP-1072 and [^{123}I]I-MIP-1095 visualized lesions in the soft tissue, bone, and prostate gland within 0.5–1 h after injection, with retention beyond 48 h. TBR from planar images averaged 2:1 at 1 h, 3:1 at 4–24 h, and greater than 10:1 at 4 and 24 h for SPECT/CT. Both agents cleared the blood in a biphasic manner; clearance of [^{123}I]I-MIP-1072 was approximately five times faster. Urine excretion [^{123}I]I-MIP-1072, 54% (24 h) and 74% (72 h), [^{123}I]I-MIP-1095, 7% and 20%, respectively. ARD were [^{123}I]I-MIP-1072 vs. [^{123}I]I-MIP-1095: 0.054 vs. 0.110 (mGy/MBq), kidneys; 0.024 vs. 0.058 mGy/MBq for liver	Barrett et al. [769]

ARD absorbed radiation dose, *GS* Gleason score, *PC* prostate cancer, *PSA* prostate-specific antigen, *LN* lymph node, *LNI* lymph node involvement, *VsC* visual score, *TBR* tumor-to-background ratio

^{99m}Tc-Labeled PSMA Radioligands

Due to widespread use of ^{99m}Tc in diagnostic nuclear medicine and the availability of SPECT scanners in nearly every hospital, several studies have been published so far regarding the preclinical development of ^{99m}Tc-labeled PSMA radiotracers [751, 761, 918–923]. Among all ^{99m}Tc-labeled PSMA radiotracers, those of Molecular Insight Pharmaceuticals (MIP) are the most promising and progress at the drug development forefront [920, 924].

The initial MIP structures contained single-amino-acid chelators (SAACs) with functionalized polar imidazole rings in order to reduce lipophilicity and hepatobiliary excretion, while for their radiolabeling the technetium tricarbonyl chemistry (Fig. 2.68) was used. Of the compounds examined, [^{99m}Tc]Tc-MIP-1404 displayed preclinically the fastest clearance from the kidneys and nontarget tissues while retaining binding to the LNCaP tumor over 4 h. [^{99m}Tc]Tc-MIP-1404 also displayed the highest tumor-to-blood and tumor-to-skeletal muscle ratios [920, 924, 925]. [^{99m}Tc]Tc-MIP-1404 (Trofolastat) is the first PSMA imaging low-molecular-weight molecule that has been used in a phase-III clinical trials for noninvasive imaging of PC (European Union Trials Register EudraCT 2012-001864-30; ClinicalTrials.gov NCT02615067 [proSPECT-AS]). Recruitment of patients is completed.

Recently two additional radiotracers have been introduced, [^{111}In]In-PSMA-I&T ([^{111}In]In-DOTAGA-(3-iodo-y)-f-k-Sub(KuE), where I&T stands for "imaging and therapy," and [^{99m}Tc]Tc-PSMA-I&S ([^{99m}Tc]Tc-mas3-y-nal-k(Sub-KuE), where I&S stands for "imaging and surgery") (Fig. 2.69) [926, 927]. Although only one patient was included in the first in-human

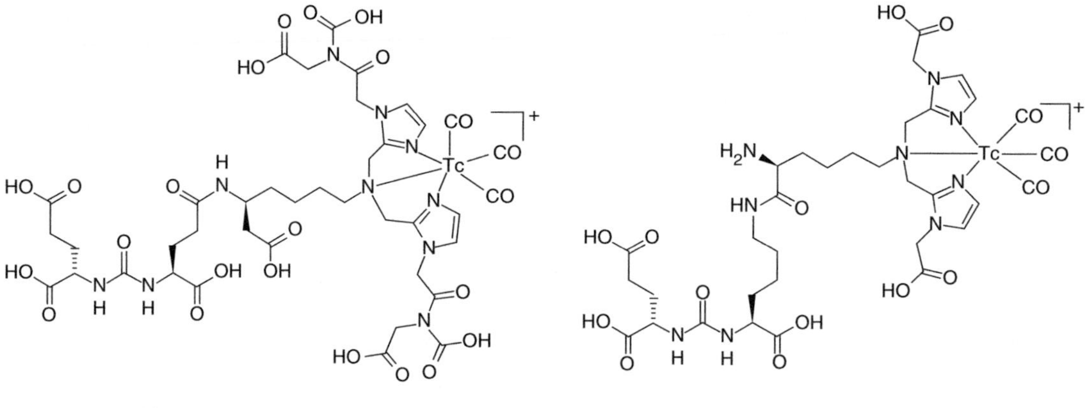

[^{99m}Tc] Tc-MIP-1404 [^{99m}Tc] Tc-MIP-1405

Fig. 2.68 Chemical structures of [^{99m}Tc]Tc-MIP-1404 (Trofolastat) and [^{99m}Tc]Tc-MIP-1405

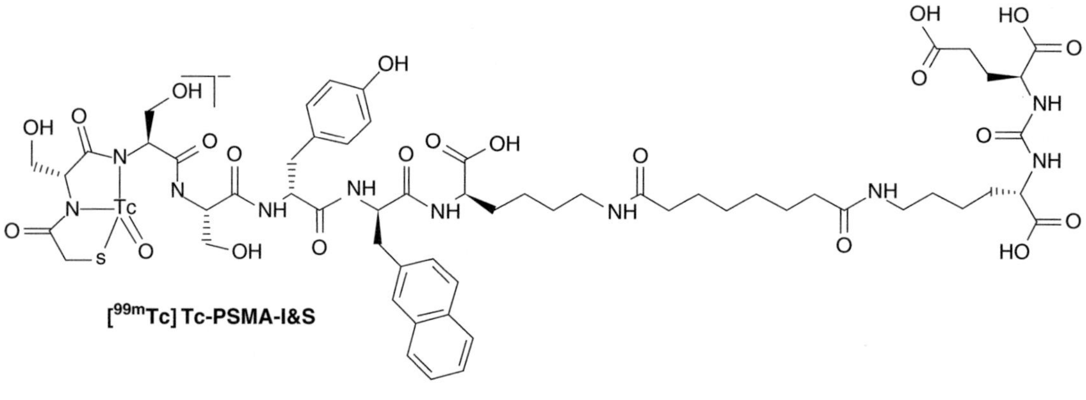

[^{99m}Tc] Tc-PSMA-I&S

Fig. 2.69 Chemical structure of [^{99m}Tc]Tc-PSMA-I&S

study without direct comparison using other radiotracers, the authors claim that [^{99m}Tc]Tc-PSMA-I&S proved superior to [^{99m}Tc]Tc-MIP-1404 due to putative quality of images at early time points [926].

References

1. Stöcklin G, Qaim SM, Rösch F. The impact of radioactivity on medicine. Radiochim Acta. 1995;70-1:249–72.
2. Qaim SM. Nuclear data for production and medical application of radionuclides: present status and future needs. Nucl Med Biol. 2017;44:31–49.
3. Ametamey SM, Honer M, Schubiger PA. Molecular imaging with PET. Chem Rev. 2008;108:1501–16.
4. Krasikova R. PET radiochemistry automation: state of the art and future trends in ^{18}F-nucleophilic fluorination. Curr Org Chem. 2013;17:2097–107.
5. Honer M, Gobbi L, Martarello L, Comley RA. Radioligand development for molecular imaging of the central nervous system with positron emission tomography. Drug Discov Today. 2014;19:1936–44.
6. Coenen HH, Gee AD, Adam M, Antoni G, Cutler CS, Fujibayashi Y, Jeong JM, Mach RH, Mindt TL, Pike VW, Windhorst AD. Consensus nomenclature rules for radiopharmaceutical chemistry – setting the record straight. Nucl Med Biol. 2017;55:v–xi.
7. de Goeij JJM, Bonardi ML. How do we define the concepts specific activity, radioactive concentration, carrier, carrier-free and no-carrier-added? J Radioanal Nucl Chem. 2005;263:13–8.
8. Ermert J. Labelling with positron emitters of pnicogens and chalcogens. J Label Compd Radiopharm. 2018;61:179–95.
9. Piel M, Vernaleken I, Rösch F. Positron emission tomography in CNS drug discovery and drug monitoring. J Med Chem. 2014;57:9232–58.
10. Brust P, van den Hoff J, Steinbach J. Development of ^{18}F-labeled radiotracers for neuroreceptor imaging with positron emission tomography. Neurosci Bull. 2014;30:777–811.
11. Haberkorn U, Mier W, Kopka K, Herold-Mende C, Altmann A, Babich J. Identification of ligands and translation to clinical applications. J Nucl Med. 2017;58:27S–33S.
12. Martić-Kehl MI, Schibli R, Schubiger PA. Can animal data predict human outcome? Problems and pitfalls of translational animal research. Eur J Nucl Med Mol Imaging. 2012;39:1492–6.
13. Rutherford E. LIV. Collision of α particles with light atoms. IV. An anomalous effect in nitrogen. J Sci. 1919;37:581–7.
14. Curie I, Joliot F. Un nouveau type de radioactivité. Comptes Rendus. 1934;198:254–6.
15. IAEA. Research reactors: purposes and future. Technical reports series no. 470. Vienna: International Atomic Energy Agency; 2016.
16. Goethals P, Zimmermann R. A report on cyclotron used in nuclear medicine: world market report & directory. Ottignies-Louvain-la-Neuve: MEDraysintell; 2015.
17. Habs D, Köster U. Production of medical radioisotopes with high specific activity in photonuclear reactions with γ-beams of high intensity and large brilliance. Appl Phys B. 2011;103:501–19.
18. Failla G (1923) System for radium emanation. Patent
19. Stang LGJ, Tucker WD, Doering RF, Weiss AJ, Greene MW, Banks HOJ (1957) Development of methods for the production of certain short-lived radionuclides. In: Proceedings of the First UNESCO conference, 1957, Paris
20. Dash A, Chakravarty R. Pivotal role of separation chemistry in the development of radionuclide enerators to meet clinical demands. RCS Adv. 2014;4:42779–803.
21. Hendee WR, Bednarek DR. The concepts of transient and secular equilibrium are incorrectly described in most textbooks, and incorrectly taught to most physics students and residents. Med Phys. 2004;31:1313–5.
22. Rösch F, Knapp FFR. Radionuclide generators. In: Vertes A, et al., editors. Handbook of nuclear chemistry. Dordrecht: Springer; 2011.
23. Leichner PK. Radiation dosimetry of monoclonal antibodies: practical considerations. In: Henkin RE, et al., editors. Nuclear medicine. St. Louis, MO: Mosby; 1996. p. 558–62.
24. Yang S, Kim K, Zaman M, Naik H, Kim G, Song T-Y, Lee Y-O, Shin SG, Key Y-U, Cho M-H. Isomeric yield ratios for the ^{nat}Nd(γ, xn)$^{1391m,g;141m,g}$Nd reactions in the bremsstrahlung energy region from 45 to 60 MeV. J Radioanal Nucl Chem. 2014;300:367–77.
25. IAEA. Handbook on photonuclear data for applications cross-sections and spectra final report of a co-ordinated research project 1996–1999. IAEA TECDOC series, vol. 1178. Vienna: International Atomic Energy Agency; 2000.
26. Al-Abyad M, Spahn I, Sudár S, Morsy M, Comsan MNH, Csikai J, Qaim SM, Coenen HH. Nuclear data for production of the therapeutic radionuclides ^{32}P, ^{64}Cu, ^{67}Cu, ^{89}Sr, ^{90}Y and ^{153}Sm via the (n,p) reaction: evaluation of excitation function and its validation via integral cross-section measurement using a 14MeV d(Be) neutron source. Appl Radiat Isot. 2006;64:717–24.
27. Spahn I, Coenen HH, Qaim SM. Enhanced production possibility of the therapeutic radionuclides ^{64}Cu, ^{67}Cu and ^{89}Sr via (n,p) reactions induced by fast spectral neutrons. Radiochim Acta. 2004;92:183–6.
28. DeLorme K, Engle J, Kowash B, Nortier F, Birnbaum E, McHale S, Clinton J, John K, Jackman K, Marus L. Production potential of Sc-47 using spallation neutrons at the Los Alamos isotope production facility. J Nucl Med. 2014;55:196.
29. Bauer GS. Physics and technology of spallation neutron sources. Nucl Instrum Methods Phys Res, Sect A. 2001;463:505–43.

30. Baum RP, Singh A, Benešová M, Vermeulen C, Gnesin S, Koster U, Johnston K, Muller D, Senftleben S, Kulkarni HR, Turler A, Schibli R, Prior JO, van der Meulen NP, Muller C. Clinical evaluation of the radiolanthanide terbium-152: first-in-human PET/CT with ^{152}Tb-DOTATOC. Dalton Trans. 2017;46:14638–46.
31. Müller C, Zhernosekov K, Köster U, Johnston K, Dorrer H, Hohn A, van der Walt NT, Türler A, Schibli R. A unique matched quadruplet of terbium radioisotopes for PET and SPECT and for α- and β^--radionuclide therapy: an in vivo proof-of-concept study with a new receptor-targeted folate derivative. J Nucl Med. 2012;53:1951–9.
32. Herzog H, Rösch F, Stöcklin G, Lueders C, Qaim SM, Feinendegen LE. Measurement of pharmacokinetics of yttrium-86 radiopharmaceuticals with PET and radiation dose calculation of analogous yttrium-90 radiotherapeutics. J Nucl Med. 1993;34:2222–6.
33. Rösch F, Herzog H, Qaim S. The beginning and development of the theranostic approach in nuclear medicine, as exemplified by the radionuclide pair ^{86}Y and ^{90}Y. Pharmaceuticals. 2017;10:56.
34. Townsend DW, Beyer T, Kinahan P, Meltzer CC, Brun T, Nutt R. The SMART scanner: a combined PET/CT tomograph for clinical oncology. Radiology. 1998;209P:169–70.
35. Bailey DL, Barthel H, Beuthin-Baumann B, Beyer T, Bisdas S, Boellaard R, Czernin J, Drzezga A, Ernemann U, Franzius C, Guckel B, Handgretinger R, Hartenbach M, Hellwig D, Nadel H, Nekolla SG, Pfluger T, Pichler BJ, Quick HH, Sabri O, Sattler B, Schafer J, Schick F, Siegel BA, Schlemmer HP, Schwenzer NF, van den Hoff J, Veit-Haibach P, Wehrl HF. Combined PET/MR: where are we now? Summary report of the second international workshop on PET/MR imaging, 8-12 Apr 2013, Tubingen, Germany. Mol Imaging Biol. 2014;16:295–310.
36. Schmand M, Burbar Z, Corbeil J, Zhang N, Michael C, Byars L, Eriksson L, Grazioso R, Martin M, Moor A, Camp J, Matschl V, Ladebeck R, Renz W, Fischer H, Jattke K, Schnur G, Rietsch N, Bendriem B, Heiss W-D. BrainPET: first human tomograph for simultaneous (functional) PET and MR imaging. J Nucl Med. 2007;48:45P.
37. Zaidi H, Ojha N, Morich M, Griesmer J, Hu Z, Maniawski P, Ratib O, Izquierdo-Garcia D, Fayad ZA, Shao L. Design and performance evaluation of a whole-body Ingenuity TF PET-MRI system. Phys Med Biol. 2011;56:3091–106.
38. Kiani A, Esquevin A, Lepareur N, Bourguet P, Le Jeune F, Gauvrit JY. Main applications of hybrid PET-MRI contrast agents: a review. Contrast Media Mol Imaging. 2016;11:92–8.
39. Ermert J. ^{18}F-labelled intermediates for radiosynthesis by modular build-up reactions: newer developments. Biomed Res Int. 2014;2014:812973.
40. Miller PW, Long NJ, Vilar R, Gee AD. Synthesis of ^{11}C, ^{18}F, ^{15}O, and ^{13}N radiolabels for positron emission tomography. Angew Chem Int Ed Engl. 2008;47:8998–9033.
41. Qaim SM, Clark JC, Crouzel C, Guillaume M, Helmeke HJ, Nebeling B, Pike VW, Stöcklin G. PET radionuclide production. In: Stöcklin G, Pike VW, editors. Radiopharmaceuticals for positron emission tomography – methodological aspects. Dordrecht: Kluwer; 1993. p. 1–42.
42. Urch DS. Radiochemistry. Annu Rep A. 2013;109:468–83.
43. IAEA. Nuclear data for the production of therapeutic radionuclides. Technical reports series. International Atomic Energy Agency: Vienna; 2011.
44. Vértes A, Nagy S, Klencsár Z, Lovas RG, Rösch F. Handbook of nuclear chemistry. Dordrecht: Kluwer; 2003.
45. Landais P, Crouzel C. A new synthesis of carbon-11 labelled phosgene. Appl Radiat Isot. 1987;38:297–300.
46. Crouzel C, Långström B, Pike VW, Coenen HH. Recommendations for a practical production of [^{11}C]methyl iodide. Appl Radiat Isot. 1987;38:601–3.
47. Suzuki K, Yamazaki T, Sasaki M, Kubodera A. Specific activity of [^{11}C]CO_2generated in a N_2 gas target: effect of irradiation dose, irradiation history, oxygen content and beam energy. Radiochim Acta. 2000;88:211–5.
48. Clark JC, Crouzel C, Meyer GJ, Strijckmans K. Current methodology for oxygen-15 production for clinical use. Int J Appl Radiat Isot. 1987;38:597–600.
49. Powell J, O'Neil JP. Production of [^{15}O]water at low-energy proton cyclotrons. Appl Radiat Isot. 2006;64:755–9.
50. Gómez-Vallejo V, Gaja V, Gona KB, Llop J. Nitrogen-13: historical review and future perspectives. J Label Compd Radiopharm. 2014;57:244–54.
51. Schlyer DJ. Production of radionuclides in accelerators. In: Welch MJ, Redvanly CS, editors. Handbook of radiopharmaceuticals. New York, NY: John Wiley & Sons; 2003. p. 1–70.
52. Bishop A, Satyamurthy N, Bida G, Phelps M, Barrio JR. Identification and quantitation of gaseous compounds of fluorine generated in [^{18}F]F_2 target systems. Nucl Med Biol. 1996;23:391–405.
53. Hess E, Blessing G, Coenen HH, Qaim SM. Improved target system for production of high purity [^{18}F]fluorine via the ^{18}O(p,n)^{18}F reaction. Appl Radiat Isot. 2000;52:1431–40.
54. Roberts AD, Oakes TR, Nickles RJ. Development of an improved target for [^{18}F]F_2 production. Appl Radiat Isot. 1995;46:87–91.
55. Bergman J, Solin O. Fluorine-18-labeled fluorine gas for synthesis of tracer molecules. Nucl Med Biol. 1997;24:677–83.
56. Eppard E, de la Fuente A, Benešová M, Khawar A, Bundschuh RA, Gärtner FC, Kreppel B, Kopka K, Essler M, Rosch F. Clinical translation and first in-human use of [^{44}Sc]Sc-PSMA-617 for PET imaging of metastasized castrate-resistant prostate cancer. Theranostics. 2017;7:4359–69.

57. Hernandez R, Valdovinos HF, Yang Y, Chakravarty R, Hong H, Barnhart TE, Cai W. ^{44}Sc: an attractive isotope for peptide-based PET imaging. Mol Pharm. 2014;11:2954–61.
58. Khawar A, Eppard E, Sinnes JP, Roesch F, Ahmadzadehfar H, Kurpig S, Meisenheimer M, Gaertner FC, Essler M, Bundschuh RA. ^{44}Sc Sc-PSMA-617 biodistribution and dosimetry in patients with metastatic castration-resistant prostate carcinoma. Clin Nucl Med. 2018;43:323–30.
59. Nagy G, Szikra D, Trencsényi G, Fekete A, Garai I, Giani AM, Negri R, Masciocchi N, Maiocchi A, Uggeri F, Tóth I, Aime S, Giovenzana GB, Baranyai Z. AAZTA: an ideal chelating agent for the development of ^{44}Sc PET imaging agents. Angew Chem. 2017;129:2150–4.
60. Carzaniga TS, Auger M, Braccini S, Bunka M, Ereditato A, Nesteruk KP, Scampoli P, Türler A, van der Meulen N. Measurement of ^{43}Sc and ^{44}Sc production cross-section with an 18 MeV medical PET cyclotron. Appl Radiat Isot. 2017;129:96–102.
61. Synowiecki MA, Perk LR, Nijsen JFW. Production of novel diagnostic radionuclides in small medical cyclotrons. EJNMMI Radiopharm Chem. 2018;3:3.
62. Lin Y-J, Koretsky AP. Manganese ion enhances T1-weighted MRI during brain activation: an approach to direct imaging of brain function. Magn Reson Med. 1997;38:378–88.
63. Topping GJ, Schaffer P, Hoehr C, Ruth TJ, Sossi V. Manganese-52 positron emission tomography tracer characterization and initial results in phantoms and in vivo. Med Phys. 2013;40:042502.
64. Abe K, Iizuka A, Hasegawa A, Morozumi S. Induced radioactivity of component materials by 16-MeV protons and 30-MeV alpha particles. J Nucl Mater. 1984;123:972–6.
65. Dmitriev PP. Systematics of nuclear reaction yields for thick target at 22 mev proton energy. Vop At Nauki i Tekhn SerYadernye Konstanty. 1983;2:57.
66. Aslam MN, Qaim SM. Nuclear model analysis of excitation functions of proton, deuteron and α-particle induced reactions on nickel isotopes for production of the medically interesting copper-61. Appl Radiat Isot. 2014;89:65–73.
67. Aslam MN, Sudár S, Hussain M, Malik AA, Shah HA, Qaim SM. Charged particle induced reaction cross section data for production of the emerging medically important positron emitter ^{64}Cu: a comprehensive evaluation. Radiochim Acta. 2009;97:669–86.
68. Szelecsényi F, Blessing G, Qaim SM. Excitation functions of proton induced nuclear reactions on enriched ^{61}Ni and ^{64}Ni: possibility of production of no-carrier-added ^{61}Cu and ^{64}Cu at a small cyclotron. Appl Radiat Isot. 1993;44:575–80.
69. Watanabe S, Iida Y, Suzui N, Katabuchi T, Ishii S, Kawachi N, Hanaoka H, Watanabe S, Matsuhashi S, Endo K, Ishioka NS. Production of no-carrier-added ^{64}Cu and applications to molecular imaging by PET and PETIS as a biomedical tracer. J Radioanal Nucl Chem. 2009;280:199–205.
70. Szelecsényi F, Boothe TE, Takács S, Tárkányi F, Tavano E. Evaluated cross section and thick target yield data bases of Zn+p processes for practical applications. Appl Radiat Isot. 1998;49:1005–32.
71. EXFOR (2018) Experimental nuclear reaction data (EXFOR). https://www-nds.iaea.org/exfor/exfor.htm. Accessed 2018.
72. Takács S, Ditrói F, Szűcs Z, Haba H, Komori Y, Aikawa M, Saito M. Crosschecking of alpha particle monitor reactions up to 50 MeV. Nucl Instrum Methods Phys Res, Sect B. 2017;397:33–8.
73. Tárkányi F, Takács S, Ditrói F, Hermanne A, Sonck M, Shubin Y. Excitation functions of deuteron induced nuclear reactions on natural zinc up to 50 MeV. Nucl Instrum Methods Phys Res, Sect B. 2004;217:531–50.
74. Khandaker MU, Haba H, Murakami M, Otuka N. Production cross-sections of long-lived radionuclides in deuteron-induced reactions on natural zinc up to 23 MeV. Nucl Instrum Methods Phys Res, Sect B. 2015;346:8–16.
75. Isabel M, Prata M. Gallium-68: a new trend in PET radiopharmacy. Curr Radiopharm. 2012;5:142–9.
76. Lambrecht RM, Sajjad M. Accelerator-derived radionuclide generators. Radiochim Acta. 1988;43:171–9.
77. Loc'h C, Mazière B, Comar D. A new generator for ionic gallium-68. J Nucl Med. 1980;21:171–3.
78. Nakayama M, Haratake M, Koiso T, Ishibashi O, Harada K, Nakayama H, Sugii A, Yahara S, Arano Y. Separation of ^{68}Ga from ^{68}Ge using a macroporous organic polymer containing N-methylglucamine groups. Anal Chim Acta. 2002;453:135–41.
79. Zhernosekov KP, Filosofov DV, Baum RP, Aschoff P, Bihl H, Razbash AA, Jahn M, Jennewein M, Rosch F. Processing of generator-produced ^{68}Ga for medical application. J Nucl Med. 2007;48:1741–8.
80. Takács S, Tárkányi F, Hermanne A, Paviotti de Corcuera R. Validation and upgrading of the recommended cross section data of charged particle reactions used for production of PET radioisotopes. Nucl Instrum Methods Phys Res, Sect B. 2003;211:169–89.
81. Basile D, Birattari C, Bonardi M, Goetz L, Sabbioni E, Salomone A. Excitation functions and production of arsenic radioisotopes for environmental toxicology and biomedical purposes. Int J Appl Radiat Isot. 1981;32:403–10.
82. Evans CD, LaDow K, Schumann BL, Savage RE, Caruso J, Vonderheide A, Succop P, Talaska G. Effect of arsenic on benzo a pyrene DNA adduct levels in mouse skin and lung. Carcinogenesis. 2004;25:493–7.
83. Wang Z-Y. Arsenic compounds as anticancer agents. Cancer Chemother Pharmacol. 2001;48:S72–6.
84. Jennewein M, Qaim SM, Kulkarni RV, Mason RP, Hermanne A, Rosch F. A no-carrier-added ^{72}Se/^{72}As radionuclide generator based on solid phase extraction. Radiochim Acta. 2005;93:579–83.
85. Horiguchi T, Kumahora H, Inoue H, Yoshizawa Y. Excitation function of Ge(p,xnyp) reactions

and production of ^{68}Ge. Int J Appl Radiat Isot. 1983;34:1531–5.
86. Spahn I, Steyn GF, Nortier FM, Coenen HH, Qaim SM. Excitation functions of ^{nat}Ge(p,xn)^{71,72,73,74}As reactions up to 100MeV with a focus on the production of ^{72}As for medical and ^{73}As for environmental studies. Appl Radiat Isot. 2007;65:1057–64.
87. Takács S, Takács MP, Hermanne A, Tárkányi F, Adam-Rebeles R. Excitation functions of longer lived radionuclides formed by deuteron irradiation of germanium. Nucl Instrum Methods Phys Res, Sect B. 2014;336:81–95.
88. Didik VA, Malkovich RS, Skoryatina EA, Kozlovskii VV. Experimental determination of the cross sections of nuclear reactions by the method of analysis of the concentration profiles of transmutation nuclides. At Energy. 1994;77:570–2.
89. Takács S, Takács MP, Ditrói F, Aikawa M, Haba H, Komori Y. Activation cross sections of longer-lived radionuclides produced in germanium by alpha particle irradiation. Nucl Instrum Methods Phys Res, Sect B. 2016;383:213–26.
90. Shehata MM, Scholten B, Spahn I, Coenen HH, Qaim SM. Separation of radioarsenic from irradiated germanium oxide targets for the production of ^{71}As and ^{72}As. J Radioanal Nucl Chem. 2011;287:435–42.
91. Mushtaq A, Qaim SM, Stöcklin G. Production of ^{73}Se via (p,3n) and (d,4n) reactions on arsenic. Int J Appl Radiat Isot. 1988;39:1085–91.
92. Faßbender M, de Villiers D, Nortier M, van der Walt N. The ^{nat}Br(p,x)^{73},^{75}Se nuclear processes: a convenient route for the production of radioselenium tracers relevant to amino acid labelling. Appl Radiat Isot. 2001;54:905–13.
93. Mushtaq A, Qaim SM. Excitation functions of α- and ^{3}He-particle induced nuclear reactions on natural germanium: evaluation of production routes for ^{73}Se. Radiochim Acta. 1990;50:27–31.
94. Blessing G, Lavi N, Qaim SM. Production of ^{73}Se via the ^{70}Ge(α, n)-process using high current target materials. Int J Appl Radiat Isot. 1992;43:455–61.
95. Qaim SM, Spahn I, Scholten B, Neumaier B. Uses of alpha particles, especially in nuclear reaction studies and medical radionuclide production. Radiochim Acta. 2016;104:601–24.
96. Qaim SM, Spahn I. Development of novel radionuclides for medical applications. J Label Compd Radiopharm. 2018;61:126–40.
97. Qaim SM, Blessing G, Tárkányi F, Lavi N, Bräutigam W, Scholten B, Stöcklin B. Production of longer-lived positron emitters ^{73}Se, ^{82m}Rb and ^{124}I. In: 14th international conference on cyclotrons and their applications (CYCLOTRONS 95), 1995. Cape Town: Faure; 1995.
98. Qaim SM, Bisinger T, Hilgers K, Nayak D, Coenen HH. Positron emission intensities in the decay of ^{64}Cu-, ^{76}Br and ^{124}I. Radiochim Acta. 2007;95:67–73.
99. Ribeiro MJ, Almeida P, Strul D, Ferreira N, Loc'h C, Brulon V, Trebossen R, Maziere B, Bendriem B. Comparison of fluorine-18 and bromine-76 imaging in positron emission tomography. Eur J Nucl Med. 1999;26:758–66.
100. Rowland DJ, McCarthy TJ, Welch MJ. Radiobromine for imaging and therapy. In: Welch MJ, Redvanly CS, editors. Handbook of radiopharmaceuticals. New York, NY: John Wiley & Sons; 2003. p. 441–65.
101. Qaim SM. Recent developments in the production of ^{18}F, ^{75,76,77}Br and ^{123}I. Appl Radiat Isot. 1986;37:803–10.
102. Spahn I, Steyn GF, Vermeulen C, Kovács Z, Szelecsényi F, Shehata MM, Spellerberg S, Scholten B, Coenen HH, Qaim SM. New cross section measurements for the production of the Auger electron emitters ^{77}Br and ^{80m}Br. Radiochim Acta. 2010;98:749–55.
103. Scholten B, Takács S, Tárkányi F, Coenen Heinz H, Qaim Syed M. Excitation functions of deuteron induced nuclear reactions on enriched ^{78}Kr with particular relevance to the production of ^{76}Br. Radiochim Acta. 2004;92(4–6):203–7.
104. Hassan HE, Qaim SM, Shubin Y, Azzam A, Morsy M, Coenen HH. Experimental studies and nuclear model calculations on proton-induced reactions on ^{nat}Se, ^{76}Se and ^{77}Se with particular reference to the production of the medically interesting radionuclides ^{76}Br and ^{77}Br. Appl Radiat Isot. 2004;60:899–909.
105. Breunig K, Spahn I, Spellerberg S, Coenen HH. Production of no-carrier-added radiobromine: new nickel selenide target and optimized separation by dry distillation. Radiochim Acta. 2015;103:397–402.
106. Hagemann CE, Ghotbi AA, Kjær A, Hasbak P. Quantitative myocardial blood flow with Rubidium-82 PET: a clinical perspective. Am J Nucl Med Mol Imaging. 2015;5:457–68.
107. Chatal J-F, Rouzet F, Haddad F, Bourdeau C, Mathieu C, Le Guludec D. Story of rubidium-82 and advantages for myocardial perfusion PET imaging. Front Med. 2015;2:65.
108. Phillips DR, Peterson EJ, Taylor WA, Jamriska DJ, Hamilton VT, Kitten JJ, Valdez FO, Salazar LL, Pitt LR, Heaton RC, Kolsky KL, Mausner LF, Kurczak S, Zhuikov BL, Kokhanyuk VM, Konyakhin NA, Nortier FM, van der Walt TN, Hanekom J, Sosnowski KM, Carty JS. Production of strontium-82 for the Cardiogen® PET generator: a project of the Department of Energy Virtual Isotope Center. Radiochim Acta. 2000;88:149–55.
109. Tárkányi F, Qaim SM, Stöcklin G. Excitation functions of high-energy ^{3}He and α-particle induced nuclear reactions on natural krypton with special reference to the production of ^{82}Sr. Appl Radiat Isot. 1990;41:91–5.
110. Zaneb H, Hussain M, Amjed N, Qaim SM. Nuclear model analysis of excitation functions of proton induced reactions on ^{86}Sr, ^{88}Sr and ^{nat}Zr: evaluation of production routes of ^{86}Y. Appl Radiat Isot. 2015;104:232–41.
111. Rösch F, Qaim SM, Stöcklin G. Nuclear data relevant to the production of the positron emitting

radioisotope ^{86}Y via the ^{86}Sr(p,n)- and ^{nat}Rb(^{3}He,xn)-processes. Radiochim Acta. 1993;61:1–8.
112. Kettern K, Linse KH, Spellerberg S, Coenen HH, Qaim SM. Radiochemical studies relevant to the production of ^{86}Y and ^{88}Y at a small-sized cyclotron. Radiochim Acta. 2002;90:845–9.
113. Rösch F, Qaim SM, Stöcklin G. Production of the positron emitting radioisotope ^{86}Y for nuclear medical application. Appl Radiat Isot. 1993;44:677–81.
114. Oehlke E, Hoehr C, Hou X, Hanemaayer V, Zeisler S, Adam MJ, Ruth TJ, Celler A, Buckley K, Benard F, Schaffer P. Production of Y-86 and other radiometals for research purposes using a solution target system. Nucl Med Biol. 2015;42:842–9.
115. Kontoghiorghe CN, Kontoghiorghes GJ. Efficacy and safety of iron-chelation therapy with deferoxamine, deferiprone, and deferasirox for the treatment of iron-loaded patients with non-transfusion-dependent thalassemia syndromes. Drug Design Dev Ther. 2016;10:465–81.
116. Fischer G, Seibold U, Schirrmacher R, Wängler B, Wängler C. ^{89}Zr, a radiometal nuclide with high potential for molecular imaging with PET: chemistry, applications and remaining challenges. Molecules. 2013;18:6469–90.
117. Meijs WE, Herscheid JDM, Haisma HJ, Wijbrandts R, van Langevelde F, Van Leuffen PJ, Mooy R, Pinedo HM. Production of highly pure no-carrier added ^{89}Zr for the labelling of antibodies with a positron emitter. Appl Radiat Isot. 1994;45:1143–7.
118. McKnight BN, Viola-Villegas NT. ^{89}Zr-ImmunoPET companion diagnostics and their impact in clinical drug development. J Label Compd Radiopharm. 2018; https://doi.org/10.1002/jlcr.3605.
119. Severin GW, Engle JW, Barnhart TE, Nickles RJ. ^{89}Zr radiochemistry for positron emission tomography. Med Chem. 2011;7:389–94.
120. Omara HM, Hassan KF, Kandil SA, Hegazy FE, Saleh ZA. Proton induced reactions on ^{89}Y with particular reference to the production of the medically interesting radionuclide ^{89}Zr. Radiochim Acta. 2009;97:467–71.
121. Wright CL, Zhang J, Tweedle MF, Knopp MV, Hall NC. Theranostic imaging of yttrium-90. BioMed Res Int. 2015;2015:481279.
122. Minarik D, Sjogreen-Gleisner K, Linden O, Wingardh K, Tennvall J, Strand SE, Ljungberg M. ^{90}Y Bremsstrahlung imaging for absorbed-dose assessment in high-dose radioimmunotherapy. J Nucl Med. 2010;51:1974–8.
123. Elschot M, Nijsen JFW, Dam AJ, de Jong H. Quantitative evaluation of scintillation camera imaging characteristics of isotopes used in liver radioembolization. PLoS One. 2011;6:e26174.
124. IAEA. Therapeutic radionuclide generators: ^{90}Sr/^{90}Y and ^{188}W/^{188}Re generators. Technical reports series. Vienna: International Atomic Energy Agency; 2009.
125. Delaunay-Olkowsky J, Strohal P, Cindro N. Total reaction cross sections of photon induced reactions. Nucl Phys. 1963;47:266–72.
126. Flynn DS, Hershberger RL, Gabbard F. Sub-Coulomb proton absorption for isotopes of zirconium and molybdenum. Phys Rev C. 1979;20:1700–5.
127. Skakun EA, Batij VG, Rakivnenko YN, Rastrepin OA. Excitation functions and isomer ratio for up-to-9 MeV proton interactions with Zr and Mo isotope nuclei. Yad Fiz. 1987;46:28–39.
128. Uddin MS, Hagiwara M, Tarkanyi F, Ditroi F, Baba M. Experimental studies on the proton-induced activation reactions of molybdenum in the energy range 22–67MeV. Appl Radiat Isot. 2004;60:911–20.
129. Eckelman WC. Unparalleled contribution of technetium-99m to medicine over 5 decades. JACC Cardiovasc Imaging. 2009;2:364–8.
130. Einstein AJ. Breaking America's dependence on imported molybdenum. JACC Cardiovasc Imaging. 2009;2:369–71.
131. IAEA. Radiotracer generators for industrial applications. IAEA radiation technology series. Vienna: International Atomic Energy Agency; 2013.
132. Van Noorden R. Radioisotopes: the medical testing crisis. Nature. 2013;504:202–4.
133. Beaver JE, Hupf HB. Production of ^{99m}Tc on a medical cyclotron: a feasibility study. J Nucl Med. 1971;12:739–41.
134. Qaim SM, Sudar S, Scholten B, Koning AJ, Coenen HH. Evaluation of excitation functions of ^{100}Mo(p,d+pn)^{99}Mo and ^{100}Mo(p,2n)^{99m}Tc-reactions: estimation of long-lived Tc-impurity and its implication on the specific activity of cyclotron-produced ^{99m}Tc. Appl Radiat Isot. 2014;85:101–13.
135. Bénard F, Buckley KR, Ruth TJ, Zeisler SK, Klug J, Hanemaayer V, Vuckovic M, Hou X, Celler A, Appiah J-P, Valliant J, Kovacs MS, Schaffer P. Implementation of multi-curie production of ^{99m}Tc by conventional medical cyclotrons. J Nucl Med. 2014;55:1017–22.
136. Schaffer P, Bénard F, Bernstein A, Buckley K, Celler A, Cockburn N, Corsaut J, Dodd M, Economou C, Eriksson T, Frontera M, Hanemaayer V, Hook B, Klug J, Kovacs M, Prato FS, McDiarmid S, Ruth TJ, Shanks C, Valliant JF, Zeisler S, Zetterberg U, Zavodszky PA. Direct production of ^{99m}Tc via ^{100}Mo(p,2n) on small medical cyclotrons. Phys Procedia. 2015;66:383–95.
137. Chen K, Cui M. Recent progress in the development of metal complexes as b-amyloid imaging probes in the brain. Medchemcomm. 2017;8:1393–407.
138. Takács S, Tárkányi F, Hermanne A. Validation and upgrading of the recommended cross-section data of charged particle reactions: gamma emitter radioisotopes. Nucl Instrum Methods Phys Res, Sect B. 2005;240:790–802.
139. Coenen HH, Mertens J, Mazieère B, Bläuenstein P, Emond P, Frangin Y, Guilloteau D, Gysemans M, Holschbach M, Loc'h C, Schubiger AP, Qaim SM. Radioionidation reactions for radio pharmaceuticals: compendium for effective synthesis strategies. New York, NY: Springer; 2006. p. 1–101.

140. IAEA. Final report of a coordinated research project "Charged-particle cross section database for medical radioisotope production": diagnostic radioisotopes and monitor reactions. IAEA-TECDOC-1211. Vienna: International Atomic Energy Agency; 2001.
141. Hassan KF, Qaim SM, Saleh ZA, Coenen HH. Alpha-particle induced reactions on natsb and ^{121}Sb with particular reference to the production of the medically interesting radionuclide ^{124}I. Appl Radiat Isot. 2006;64:101–9.
142. Herzog H, Tellmann L, Scholten B, Coenen HH, Qaim SM. PET imaging problems with the non-standard positron emitters yttrium-86 and iodine-124. Q J Nucl Med Mol Imaging. 2008;52:159–65.
143. Tárkányi F, Takács S, Király B, Szelecsényi F, Andó L, Bergman J, Heselius SJ, Solin O, Hermanne A, Shubin YN, Ignatyuk AV. Excitation functions of ^{3}He- and α-particle induced nuclear reactions on ^{nat}Sb for production of medically relevant ^{123}I and ^{124}I radioisotopes. Appl Radiat Isot. 2009;67:1001–6.
144. Aslam MN, Sudar S, Hussain M, Malik AA, Shah HA, Qaim SM. Evaluation of excitation functions of proton and deuteron induced reactions on enriched tellurium isotopes with special relevance to the production of iodine-124. Appl Radiat Isot. 2010;68:1760–73.
145. IAEA. Nuclear medicine in thyroid cancer management: a practical approach. IAEA, 2009. IAEA TECDOC-1608. Vienna: International Atomic Energy Agency; 2009.
146. Shapiro B, Gross MD. Radiochemistry, biochemistry, and kinetics of ^{131}I-metaiodobenzylguanidine (MIBG) and ^{123}I-MIBG: clinical implications of the use of ^{123}I-MIBG. Med Pediatr Oncol. 1987;15:170–7.
147. Qaim SM. Cyclotron production of medical radionuclides. In: Vertes A, et al., editors. Handbook of nuclear chemsitry. Dordrecht: Kluwer; 2003. p. 47–79.
148. Raleigh DR, Seymour ZA, Tomlin B, Theodosopoulos PV, Berger MS, Aghi MK, Geneser SE, Krishnamurthy D, Fogh SE, Sneed PK, McDermott MW. Resection and brain brachytherapy with permanent iodine-125 sources for brain metastasis. J Neurosurg. 2017;126:1749–55.
149. Huang H, Xu S, Li F, Du Z, Wang L. Clinical application of computed tomography-guided ^{125}I seed interstitial implantation for head and neck cancer patients with unmanageable cervical lymph node metastases. Eur J Med Res. 2016;21:18.
150. Bennett CL, Qureshi ZP, Sartor AO, Norris LB, Murday A, Xirasagar S, Thomsen HS. Gadolinium-induced nephrogenic systemic fibrosis: the rise and fall of an iatrogenic disease. Clin Kidney J. 2012;5:82–8.
151. Denzler FO, Lebedev NA, Novgorodov AF, Rösch F, Qaim SM. Production and radiochemical separation of ^{147}Gd. Appl Radiat Isot. 1997;48:319–26.
152. Nayak D, Lahiri S, Ramaswami A, Manohor SB. Separation of no-carrier added Gd-147,Gd-149 and Eu-147 produced in 70 MeV B-11 irradiated praseodymium foil target. Radiochim Acta. 1999;87:93–6.
153. West HI, Lanier RG, Mustafa MG, Nuckolls RN, Frehaut J, Adam A, Philis CA. Proton and deuteron excitation functions for Eu-151 and Eu-153. Brookhaven Natl Lab Rep. 1989;42382:87–90.
154. Takács S, Tárkányi F, Hermanne A, Adam-Rebeles R, Takács MP. Excitation functions for the formation of longer lived isotopes by deuteron irradiation of Europium. Nucl Instrum Methods Phys Res, Sect B. 2013;310:54–66.
155. Bao ZY, Beer H, Kappeler F, Voss F, Wisshak K, Rauscher T. Neutron cross sections for nucleosynthesis studies. At Data Nucl Data Tables. 2000;76:70–154.
156. IAEA. Optimization of production and quality control of therapeutic radionuclides and radiopharmaceuticals. AEA TECDOC series I. Vienna: International Atomic Energy Agency; 1999.
157. Qaim SM, Spahn I, Kandil SA, Coenen HH. Nuclear data for production of ^{88}Y, ^{140}Nd, ^{153}Sm and ^{169}Yb via novel routes. Radiochim Acta. 2007;95:313–7.
158. Dash A, Chakraborty S, Pillai MRA, Knapp FF. Peptide receptor radionuclide therapy: an overview. Cancer Biother Radiopharm. 2015;30:47–71.
159. Hermanne A, Takacs S, Goldberg MB, Lavie E, Shubin YN, Kovalev S. Deuteron-induced reactions on Yb: measured cross sections and rationale for production pathways of carrier-free, medically relevant radionuclides. Nucl Instrum Methods Phys Res, Sect B. 2006;247:223–31.
160. Manenti S, Bonardi ML, Gini L, Groppi F. Physical optimization of production by deuteron irradiation of high specific activity ^{177g}Lu suitable for radioimmunotherapy. Nucl Med Biol. 2014;41:407–9.
161. Pillai MRA, Venkatesh M, Banerjee S, Samuel G, Kothari K, Dash A, Unni PR, Korde A, Bapat K, Pandey U, Das T, Chakraborty S, Mukherjee A, Sharma HD. Labeling techniques of biomolecules for targeted radiotherapy. IAEA-TECDOC-1359. Vienna: IAEA; 2003. p. 107–22.
162. Kratochwil C, Giesel FL, Stefanova M, Benešová M, Bronzel M, Afshar-Oromieh A, Mier W, Eder M, Kopka K, Haberkorn U. PSMA-targeted radionuclide therapy of metastatic castration-resistant prostate cancer with ^{177}Lu-labeled PSMA-617. J Nucl Med. 2016;57:1170–6.
163. Goyal J, Antonarakis ES. Bone-targeting radiopharmaceuticals for the treatment of prostate cancer with bone metastases. Cancer Lett. 2012;323:135–46.
164. Miyahara H, Wurdiyanto G, Nagata H, Yoshida A, Yanagida K, Mori C. Precise measurements of the gamma-ray emission probabilities of ^{186}Re and ^{188}Re. Appl Radiat Isot. 2000;52:573–9.
165. Mastren T, Radchenko V, Bach HT, Balkin ER, Birnbaum ER, Brugh M, Engle JW, Gott MD, Guthrie J, Hennkens HM, John KD, Ketring AR, Kuchuk M, Maassen JR, Naranjo CM, Nortier FM, Phelps TE, Jurisson SS, Wilbur DS, Fassbender

ME. Bulk production and evaluation of high specific activity ^{186g}Re for cancer therapy using enriched $^{186}WO_3$ targets in a proton beam. Nucl Med Biol. 2017;49:24–9.
166. Guerra Liberal FDC, Tavares AAS, Tavares JMRS. Palliative treatment of metastatic bone pain with radiopharmaceuticals: a perspective beyond Strontium-89 and Samarium-153. Appl Radiat Isot. 2016;110:87–99.
167. Neves M, Kling A, Lambrecht RM. Radionuclide production for therapeutic radiopharmaceuticals. Appl Radiat Isot. 2002;57:657–64.
168. Hussain M, Sudar S, Aslam MN, Malik AA, Ahmad R, Qaim SM. Evaluation of charged particle induced reaction cross section data for production of the important therapeutic radionuclide ^{186}Re. Radiochim Acta. 2010;98:385–95.
169. Lewis RE, Eldridge JS. Production of 70-day Tungsten-188 and development of a 17 hour rhenium-188 radioisotope generator. J Nucl Med. 1966;7:804.
170. Knapp FF, Callahan AP, Beets AL, Mirzadeh S, Hsieh BT. Processing of reactor-produced ^{188}W for fabrication of clinical scale alumina-based ^{188}W/^{188}Re generators. Appl Radiat Isot. 1994;45:1123–8.
171. Uddin MS, Scholten B, Hermanne A, Sudár S, Coenen HH, Qaim SM. Radiochemical determination of cross sections of α-particle induced reactions on ^{192}Os for the production of the therapeutic radionuclide ^{193m}Pt. Appl Radiat Isot. 2010;68:2001–6.
172. Hilgers K, Coenen HH, Qaim SM. Production of the therapeutic radionuclides ^{193m}Pt and ^{195m}Pt with high specific activity via α-particle-induced reactions on ^{192}Os. Appl Radiat Isot. 2008;66:545–51.
173. Takács S, Ditrói F, Szűcs Z, Aikawa M, Haba H, Komori Y, Saito M. Measurement of activation cross sections of alpha particle induced reactions on iridium up to an energy of 50 MeV. Appl Radiat Isot. 2018;136:133–42.
174. Meyer GJ. Astatine. J Label Compd Radiopharm. 2018;61:154–64.
175. Vaidyanathan G, Zalutsky MR. Applications of ^{211}At and ^{223}Ra in targeted alpha-particle radiotherapy. Curr Radiopharm. 2011;4:283–94.
176. Vaidyanathan G, Zalutsky MR. Astatine radiopharmaceuticals: prospects and problems. Curr Radiopharm. 2008;1:177–96.
177. Zalutsky MR, Pruszynski M. Astatine-211: production and availability. Curr Radiopharm. 2011;4:177–85.
178. Hermanne A, Tárkányi F, Takács S, Szücs Z, Shubin YN, Dityuk AI. Experimental study of the cross-sections of α-particle induced reactions on ^{209}Bi. Appl Radiat Isot. 2005;63:1–9.
179. Miederer M, Scheinberg DA, McDevitt MR. Realizing the potential of the actinium-225 radionuclide generator in targeted alpha particle therapy applications. Adv Drug Deliv Rev. 2008;60:1371–82.
180. Kratochwil C, Bruchertseifer F, Rathke H, Hohenfellner M, Giesel FL, Haberkorn U, Morgenstern A. Targeted alpha-therapy of metastatic castration-resistant prostate cancer with ^{225}Ac-PSMA-617: swimmer-plot analysis suggests efficacy regarding duration of tumor control. J Nucl Med. 2018;59:795–802.
181. Alfassi ZB, Bonardi M, Groppi F, Menapace E. A new alpha-emitter for nuclear medicine: ^{230}U. J Radioanal Nucl Chem. 2006;270:483–7.
182. Apostolidis C, Molinet R, Rasmussen G, Morgenstern A. Production of Ac-225 from Th-229 for targeted alpha therapy. Anal Chem. 2005;77:6288–91.
183. Apostolidis C, Molinet R, McGinley J, Abbas K, Mollenbeck J, Morgenstern A. Cyclotron production of Ac-225 for targeted alpha therapy. Appl Radiat Isot. 2005;62:383–7.
184. Weidner JW, Mashnik SG, John KD, Hemez F, Ballard B, Bach H, Birnbaum ER, Bitteker LJ, Couture A, Dry D, Fassbender ME, Gulley MS, Jackman KR, Ullmann JL, Wolfsberg LE, Nortier FM. Proton-induced cross sections relevant to production of ^{225}Ac and ^{223}Ra in natural thorium targets below 200 MeV. Appl Radiat Isot. 2012;70:2602–7.
185. Melville G, Meriarty H, Metcalfe P, Knittel T, Allen BJ. Production of Ac-225 for cancer therapy by photon-induced transmutation of Ra-226. Appl Radiat Isot. 2007;65:1014–22.
186. Chen X, Ji M, Fisher DR, Wai CM. Ionizable calixarene-crown ethers with high selectivity for radium over light alkaline earth metal ions. Inorg Chem. 1999;38:5449–52.
187. Guseva LI. A tandem generator system for production of ^{223}Ra and ^{211}Pb/^{211}Bi in DTPA solutions suitable for potential application in radiotherapy. J Radioanal Nucl Chem. 2009;281:577.
188. Westrøm S, Malenge M, Jorstad Ida S, Napoli E, Bruland Øyvind S, Bønsdorff Tina B, Larsen Roy H. Ra-224 labeling of calcium carbonate microparticles for internal α-therapy: preparation, stability, and biodistribution in mice. J Label Compd Radiopharm. 2018;61:472–86.
189. Abou DS, Pickett J, Mattson JE, Thorek DLJ. A Radium-223 microgenerator from cyclotron-produced trace Actinium-227. Appl Radiat Isot. 2017;119:36–42.
190. Mokhodoeva O, Guseva L, Dogadkin N. Isolation of generator-produced ^{223}Ra in 0.9-% NaCl solutions containing EDTA for direct radiotherapeutic studies. J Radioanal Nucl Chem. 2015;304:449–53.
191. Soderquist CZ, McNamara BK, Fisher DR. Production of high-purity radium-223 from legacy actinium-beryllium neutron sources. Curr Radiopharm. 2012;5:244–52.
192. Larsen R, Bruland O (2006) Thorium-227 for use in radiotherapy of soft tissue disease Patent US 20060228297 A1
193. Transparency Market Research (2018) Radiopharmaceutical market will exhibit a CAGR

of 5.4% between 2017 and 2024. http://www.sbwire.com/press-releases/radiopharmaceutical-market/release-983778.htm
194. Schwochau K. Technetium: chemistry and radiopharmaceutical applications technetium: chemistry and radiopharmaceutical applications. Weinheim: Wiley; 2000.
195. Papagiannopoulou D. Technetium-99m radiochemistry for pharmaceutical applications. J Label Compd Radiopharm. 2017;60:502–20.
196. Blower PJ, Kettle AG, O'Doherty MJ, Coakley AJ, Knapp FF. ^{99m}Tc(V)DMSA quantitatively predicts ^{188}Re(V)DMSA distribution in patients with prostate cancer metastatic to bone. Eur J Nucl Med. 2000;27:1405–9.
197. Alberto R, Schibli R, Egli A, Schubiger AP, Abram U, Kaden TA. A novel organometallic aqua complex of technetium for the labeling of biomolecules: synthesis of $[^{99m}Tc(OH_2)_3(CO)_3]^+$ from $[^{99m}TcO_4]^-$ in aqueous solution and its reaction with a bifunctional ligand. J Am Chem Soc. 1998;120:7987–8.
198. Satpati D, Mallia M, Kothari K, Pillai MRA. Comparative evaluation of ^{99m}Tc-$(H_2O)_3(CO)_3^+$ precursor synthesised by conventional method and by using carbonyl kit. J Label Compd Radiopharm. 2004;47:657–68.
199. Banerjee SR, Maresca KP, Francesconi L, Valliant J, Babich JW, Zubieta J. New directions in the coordination chemistry of ^{99m}Tc: a reflection on technetium core structures and a strategy for new chelate design. Nucl Med Biol. 2005;32:1–20.
200. Piramoon M, Hosseinimehr SJ. The past, current studies and future of organometallic $^{99m}Tc(CO)_3$ labeled peptides and proteins. Curr Pharm Des. 2016;22:4854–67.
201. Schibli R, Schubiger PA. Current use and future potential of organometallic radiopharmaceuticals. Eur J Nucl Med Mol Imaging. 2002;29:1529–42.
202. Mindt TL, Muller C, Stuker F, Salazar JF, Hohn A, Mueggler T, Rudin M, Schibli R. A "click chemistry" approach to the efficient synthesis of multiple imaging probes derived from a single precursor. Bioconjug Chem. 2009;20:1940–9.
203. Mindt TL, Struthers H, Brans L, Anguelov T, Schweinsberg C, Maes V, Tourwe D, Schibli R. "Click to chelate": synthesis and installation of metal chelates into biomolecules in a single step. J Am Chem Soc. 2006;128:15096–7.
204. Andros G, Harper PV, Lathrop KA, McCardle RJ. Pertechnetate-99m localization in man with applications to thyroid scanning and the study of thyroid physiology. J Clin Endocrinol Metab. 1965;25:1067.
205. Cho JY, Leveille R, Kao R, Rousset B, Parlow AF, Burak WE, Mazzaferri EL, Jhiang SM. Hormonal regulation of radioiodide uptake activity and Na+/I– symporter expression in mammary glands. J Clin Endocrinol Metab. 2000;85:2936–43.
206. Jovanovic V, Konstantinovska D, Milivojevic K, Bzenic J. Determination of radiochemical purity and pharmacokinetic parameters of ^{99m}Tc-sulphur colloid and ^{99m}Tc-Tin colloid. Nuklearmedizin. 1981;20:279–82.
207. Suga K. Technical and analytical advances in pulmonary ventilation SPECT with xenon-133 gas and Tc-99m-Technegas. Ann Nucl Med. 2002;16:303–10.
208. Fritzberg AR, Kasina S, Eshima D, Johnson DL. Synthesis and biological evaluation of technetium-99m MAG3 as a Hippuran replacement. J Nucl Med. 1986;27:111–6.
209. Noll B, Johannsen B, May K, Spies H. Preparation of the renal function and imaging agent ^{99m}Tc-MAG3 starting from S-unprotected mercaptoacetyltriglycine. Int J Appl Radiat Isot. 1992;43:899–901.
210. Erbas B, Tuncel M. Renal function assessment during peptide receptor radionuclide therapy. Semin Nucl Med. 2016;46:462–78.
211. Itoh K. ^{99m}Tc-MAG3: review of pharmacokinetics, clinical application to renal diseases and quantification of renal function. Ann Nucl Med. 2001;15:179–90.
212. Taylor RD, MacCoss M, Lawson ADG. Combining molecular scaffolds from FDA approved drugs: application to drug discovery. J Med Chem. 2017;60:1638–47.
213. Dekemp RA, Renaud JM, Klein R, Beanlands RSB. Radionuclide tracers for myocardial perfusion imaging and blood flow quantification. Cardiol Clin. 2016;34:37.
214. Heo J, Iskandrian AS. Technetium-labeled myocardial perfusion agents. Cardiol Clin. 1994;12:187–98.
215. Kailasnath P, Sinusas AJ. Comparison of Tl-201 with Tc-99m-labeled myocardial perfusion agents: technical, physiologic, and clinical issues. J Nucl Cardiol. 2001;8:482–98.
216. Kiat H, Berman DS, Maddahi J. Myocardial perfusion imaging using technetium-99m radiopharmaceuticals. Radiol Clin North Am. 1993;31:795.
217. Berman DS, Kiat H, Van Train K, Garcia E, Friedman J, Maddahi J. Technetium 99m sestamibi in the assessment of chronic coronary artery disease. Semin Nucl Med. 1991;21:190–212.
218. Taillefer R, Laflamme L, Dupras G, Picard M, Phaneuf D-C, Léveillé J. Myocardial perfusion imaging with ^{99m}Tc-methoxy-isobutyl-isonitrile (MIBI): comparison of short and long time intervals between rest and stress injections. Eur J Nucl Med. 1988;13:515–22.
219. Higley B, Smith FW, Smith T, Gemmell HG, Gupta PD, Gvozdanovic DV, Graham D, Hinge D, Davidson J, Lahiri A. Technetium-99m-1,2-bis[bis(2-ethoxyethyl) phosphino]ethane: human biodistribution, dosimetry and safety of a new myocardial perfusion imaging agent. J Nucl Med. 1993;34:30–8.
220. Shanoudy H, Raggi P, Beller GA, Soliman A, Ammermann EG, Kastner RJ, Watson DD. Comparison of technetium-99m tetrofosmin and thallium-201 single-photon emission computed tomographic imaging for detection of myocardial

perfusion defects in patients with coronary artery disease. J Am Coll Cardiol. 1998;31:331–7.
221. Leonard J-P, Nowotnik DP, Neirinckx RD. Technetium-99m-d,1-HM-PAO: a new radiopharmaceutical for imaging regional brain perfusion using SPECT—a comparison with iodine-123 HIPDM. J Nucl Med. 1986;27:1819–23.
222. Léveillé J, Demonceau G, De Roo M, Rigo P, Taillefer R, Morgan RA, Kupranick D, Walovitch RC. Characterization of technetium-99m-l,l-ECD for brain perfusion imaging, part 2: biodistribution and brain imaging in humans. J Nucl Med. 1989;30:1902–10.
223. Vallabhajosula S, Zimmerman RE, Picard M, Stritzke P, Mena I, Hellman RS, Tikofsky RS, Stabin MG, Morgan RA, Goldsmith SJ. Technetium-99m ECD: a new brain imaging agent: in vivo kinetics and biodistribution studies in normal human subjects. J Nucl Med. 1989;30:599–604.
224. Walovitch RC, Hill TC, Garrity ST, Cheesman EH, Burgess BA, O'Leary DH, Watson AD, Ganey MV, Morgan RA, Williams SJ. Characterization of technetium-99m-L,L-ECD for brain perfusion imaging, part 1: pharmacology of technetium-99m ECD in nonhuman primates. J Nucl Med. 1989;30:1892–901.
225. Neirinckx RD, Burke JF, Harrison RC, Forster AM, Andersen AR, Lassen NA. The retention mechanism of technetium-99m-HM-PAO: intracellular reaction with glutathione. J Cereb Blood Flow Metab. 1988;8:S4–S12.
226. Suess E, Malessa S, Ungersböck K, Kitz P, Podreka I, Heimberger K, Hornykiewicz O, Deecke L. Technetium-99m-d, 1-hexamethylpropyleneamine oxime (HMPAO) uptake and glutathione content in brain tumors. J Nucl Med. 1991;32:1675–81.
227. Kung HF, Kung MP, Wey SP, Lin KJ, Yen TC. Clinical acceptance of a molecular imaging agent: a long march with [^{99m}Tc]TRODAT. Nucl Med Biol. 2007;34:787–9.
228. Kung M-P, Stevenson DA, Plössl K, Meegalla SK, Beckwith A, Essman WD, Mu M, Lucki I, Kung HF. [^{99m}Tc]TRODAT-1: a novel technetium-99m complex as a dopamine transporter imaging agent. Eur J Nucl Med. 1997;24:372–80.
229. Meegalla SK, Plössl K, Kung M-P, Stevenson DA, Mu KS, Liable-Sands LM, Rheingold AL, Kung HF. Specificity of diastereomers of [^{99m}Tc] TRODAT-1 as dopamine transporter imaging agents. J Med Chem. 1998;41:428–36.
230. Fallahi B, Esmaeili A, Beiki D, Oveisgharan S, Noorollahi-Moghaddam H, Erfani M, Tafakhori A, Rohani M, Fard-Esfahani A, Emami-Ardekani A, Geramifar P, Eftekhari M. Evaluation of ^{99m}Tc-TRODAT-1 SPECT in the diagnosis of Parkinson's disease versus other progressive movement disorders. Ann Nucl Med. 2016;30:153–62.
231. Hwang WJ, Yao WJ, Wey SP, Ting G. Reproducibility of ^{99m}Tc-TRODAT-1 SPECT measurement of dopamine transporters in Parkinson's disease. J Nucl Med. 2004;45:207–13.
232. Núñez EGF, Faintuch BL, Teodoro R, Wiecek DP, Martinelli JR, NGd S, Castanheira CE, Filho RSO, Pasqualini R. Influence of colloid particle profile on sentinel lymph node uptake. Nucl Med Biol. 2009;36:741–7.
233. van der Poel HG, Buckle T, Brouwer OR, Olmos RAV, van Leeuwen FWB. Intraoperative laparoscopic fluorescence guidance to the sentinel lymph node in prostate cancer patients: clinical proof of concept of an integrated functional imaging approach using a multimodal tracer. Eur Urol. 2011;60:826–33.
234. Azad AK, Rajaram MVS, Metz WL, Cope FO, Blue MS, Vera DR, Schlesinger LS. γ-Tilmanocept, a new radiopharmaceutical tracer for cancer sentinel lymph nodes, binds to the mannose receptor (CD206). J Immunol. 2015;195:2019–29.
235. Baker JL, Pu M, Tokin CA, Hoh CK, Vera DR, Messer K, Wallace AM. Comparison of [^{99m}Tc] tilmanocept and filtered [^{99m}Tc]sulfur colloid for identification of SLNs in breast cancer patients. Ann Surg Oncol. 2015;22:40–5.
236. Surasi DS, O'Malley J, Bhambhvani P. ^{99m}Tc-tilmanocept: a novel molecular agent for lymphatic mapping and sentinel lymph node localization. J Nucl Med Technol. 2015;43:87–91.
237. Vera DR, Wallace AM, Hoh CK, Mattrey RF. A synthetic macromolecule for sentinel node detection: ^{99m}Tc-DTPA-mannosyl-dextran. J Nucl Med. 2001;42:951–9.
238. Chen K, Chen X. Positron emission tomography imaging of cancer biology: current status and future prospects. Semin Oncol. 2011;38:70–86.
239. Hanahan D, Weinberg Robert A. Hallmarks of cancer: the next generation. Cell. 2011;144:646–74.
240. Wang X, Feng H, Zhao S, Xu J, Wu X, Cui J, Zhang Y, Qin Y, Liu Z, Gao T, Gao Y, Zeng W. SPECT and PET radiopharmaceuticals for molecular imaging of apoptosis: from bench to clinic. Oncotarget. 2017;8:20476–95.
241. Adak S, Bhalla R, Vijaya Raj KK, Mandal S, Pickett R, Luthra SK. Radiotracers for SPECT imaging: current scenario and future prospects. Radiochim Acta. 2012;100:95–107.
242. Belhocine TZ, Blankenberg FG, Kartachova MS, Stitt LW, Vanderheyden J-L, Hoebers FJP, Van de Wiele C. ^{99m}Tc-Annexin A5 quantification of apoptotic tumor response: a systematic review and meta-analysis of clinical imaging trials. Eur J Nucl Med Mol Imaging. 2015;42:2083–97.
243. Kemerink GJ, Boersma HH, Thimister PW, Hofstra L, Liem I, Pakbiers M-TW, Janssen D, Reutelingsperger CP, Heidendal GA. Biodistribution and dosimetry of ^{99m}Tc-BTAP-annexin-V in humans. Eur J Nucl Med. 2001;28:1373–8.
244. Belhocine T, Steinmetz N, Green A, Rigo P. In vivo imaging of chemotherapy-induced apoptosis in human cancers. Ann NY Acad Sci. 2006;1010:525–9.
245. Steinmetz N (2004) North American Scientific releases updated observations from European clinical trials of ^{99m}Tc-Hynic-annexin. in 51st. In:

Annual meeting of the society of nuclear medicine, Philadelphia, PA

246. Van de Wiele C, Lahorte C, Vermeersch H, Loose D, Mervillie K, Steinmetz ND, Vanderheyden J-L, Cuvelier CA, Slegers G, Dierck RA. Quantitative tumor apoptosis imaging using technetium-99m–HYNIC annexin V single photon emission computed tomography. J Clin Oncol. 2003;21:3483–7.
247. Vermeersch H, Ham H, Rottey S, Lahorte C, Corsetti F, Dierckx R, Steinmetz N, Van de Wiele C. Intraobserver, interobserver, and day-to-day reproducibility of quantitative ^{99m}Tc-HYNIC annexin-V imaging in head and neck carcinoma. Cancer Biother Radiopharm. 2004;19:205–10.
248. Vermeersch H, Loose D, Lahorte C, Mervillie K, Dierckx R, Steinmetz N, Vanderheyden J-L, Cuvelier C, Slegers G, Van de Wiele C. ^{99m}Tc-HYNIC annexin-V imaging of primary head and neck carcinoma. Nucl Med Commun. 2004;25:259–63.
249. Haas RLM, de Jong D, Valdés Olmos RA, Hoefnagel CA, van Den Heuvel I, Zerp SF, Bartelink H, Verheij M. In vivo imaging of radiation-induced apoptosis in follicular lymphoma patients. Int J Rad Oncol Biol Phys. 2004;59:782–7.
250. Kartachova M, Haas RLM, Valdés Olmos RA, Hoebers FJP, van Zandwijk N, Verheij M. In vivo imaging of apoptosis by ^{99m}Tc-annexin V scintigraphy: visual analysis in relation to treatment response. Radiother Oncol. 2004;72:333–9.
251. Rottey S, Slegers G, Van Belle S, Goethals I, Van De Wiele C. Sequential ^{99m}Tc-hydrazinonicotinamide-annexin V imaging for predicting response to chemotherapy. J Nucl Med. 2006;47:1813–8.
252. Rottey S, Loose D, Vakaet L, Lahorte C, Vermeersch H, Van Belle S, Van De Wiele CV. ^{99m}Tc-HYNIC annexin-V imaging of tumors and its relationship to response to radiotherapy and/or chemotherapy. Q J Nucl Med Mol Imaging. 2007;51:182–8.
253. Kartachova M, van Zandwijk N, Burgers S, van Tinteren H, Verheij M, Olmos RAV. Prognostic significance of ^{99m}Tc Hynic-rh-annexin V scintigraphy during platinum-based chemotherapy in advanced lung cancer. J Clin Oncol. 2007;25:2534–9.
254. Kartachova MS, Olmos RAV, Haas RLM, Hoebers FJR, Herk MV, Verheij M. ^{99m}Tc-HYNIC-rh-annexin-V scintigraphy: visual and quantitative evaluation of early treatment-induced apoptosis to predict treatment outcome. Nucl Med Commun. 2008;29:39–44.
255. Hoebers FJP, Kartachova M, de Bois J, van den Brekel MWM, van Tinteren H, van Herk M, Rasch CRN, Valdés Olmos RA, Verheij M. ^{99m}Tc Hynic-rh-annexin V scintigraphy for in vivo imaging of apoptosis in patients with head and neck cancer treated with chemoradiotherapy. Eur J Nucl Med Mol Imaging. 2008;35:509–18.
256. Loose D, Vermeersch H, De Vos F, Deron P, Slegers G, Van de Wiele C. Prognostic value of ^{99m}Tc-HYNIC annexin-V imaging in squamous cell carcinoma of the head and neck. Eur J Nucl Med Mol Imaging. 2008;35:47–52.
257. Rottey S, Van Den Bossche B, Slegers G, Van Belle S, Van De Wiele C. Influence of chemotherapy on the biodistribution of [^{99m}Tc]hydrazinonicotinamide annexin V in cancer patients. Q J Nucl Med Mol Imaging. 2009;53:127–32.
258. Kurihara H, Yang DJ, Cristofanilli M, Erwin WD, Yu D-F, Kohanim S, Mendez R, Kim EE. Imaging and dosimetry of ^{99m}Tc EC annexin v: preliminary clinical study targeting apoptosis in breast tumors. Appl Radiat Isot. 2008;66:1175–82.
259. Schaper FL, Reutelingsperger CP. ^{99m}Tc-HYNIC-annexin A5 in oncology: evaluating efficacy of anticancer therapies. Cancers. 2013;5:550–68.
260. Cai WB, Rao JH, Gambhir SS, Chen XY. How molecular imaging is speeding up antiangiogenic drug development. Mol Cancer Ther. 2006;5:2624–33.
261. Chen K, Conti PS. Target-specific delivery of peptide-based probes for PET imaging. Adv Drug Deliv Rev. 2010;62:1005–22.
262. Bozon-Petitprin A, Bacot S, Gauchez AS, Ahmadi M, Bourre JC, Marti-Batlle D, Perret P, Broisat A, Riou LM, Claron M, Boturyn D, Fagret D, Ghezzi C, Vuillez JP. Targeted radionuclide therapy with RAFT-RGD radiolabelled with ^{90}Y or ^{177}Lu in a mouse model of $\alpha_v\beta_3$-expressing tumours. Eur J Nucl Med Mol Imaging. 2015;42:252–63.
263. Chen HJ, Niu G, Wu H, Chen XY. Clinical application of radiolabeled RGD peptides for PET imaging of integrin $\alpha_v\beta_3$. Theranostics. 2016;6:78–92.
264. Shao G, Gu W, Guo M, Zang S, Fu J, Liu S, Wang F, Wang Z. Clinical study of ^{99m}Tc-3P-RGD$_2$ peptide imaging in osteolytic bone metastasis. Oncotarget. 2017;8:75587–96.
265. O'Connor MK, Morrow MMB, Hunt KN, Boughey JC, Wahner-Roedler DL, Conners AL, Rhodes DJ, Hruska CB. Comparison of Tc-99m maraciclatide and Tc-99m sestamibi molecular breast imaging in patients with suspected breast cancer. EJNMMI Res. 2017;7:5.
266. Axelsson R, Bach-Gansmo T, Castell-Conesa J, McParland BJ. An open-label, multicenter, phase 2a study to assess the feasibility of imaging metastases in late-stage cancer patients with the a a_vb_3-selective angiogenesis imaging agent ^{99m}Tc-NC100692. Acta Radiol. 2010;51:40–6.
267. Bach-Gansmo T, Danielsson R, Saracco A, Wilczek B, Bogsrud TV, Fangberget A, Tangerud Å, Tobin D. Integrin receptor imaging of breast cancer: a proof-of-concept study to evaluate ^{99m}Tc-NC100692. J Nucl Med. 2006;47:1434–9.
268. Bach-Gansmo T, Bogsrud TV, Skretting A. Integrin scintimammography using a dedicated breast imaging, solid-state gamma-camera and ^{99m}Tc-labelled NC100692. Clin Physiol Funct Imaging. 2008;28:235–9.
269. Zhu Z, Miao W, Li Q, Dai H, Ma Q, Wang F, Yang A, Jia B, Jing X, Liu S, Shi J, Liu Z, Zhao Z, Wang F, Li F. ^{99m}Tc-3PRGD2 for integrin receptor imaging of lung cancer: a multicenter study. J Nucl Med. 2012;53:716–22.

270. Zhao D, Jin X, Li F, Liang J, Lin Y. Integrin $\alpha_v\beta_3$ imaging of radioactive iodine–refractory thyroid cancer using ^{99m}Tc-3PRGD2. J Nucl Med. 2012;53: 1872–7.
271. Zhang Z, Zhao X, Ding C, Wang J, Zhang J, Wang F. ^{99m}Tc-3PRGD$_2$ SPECT/CT imaging for monitoring early response of EGFR-TKIs therapy in patients with advanced-stage lung adenocarcinoma. Cancer Biother Radiopharm. 2016;31:238–45.
272. Jin X, Liang N, Wang M, Meng Y, Jia B, Shi X, Li S, Luo J, Luo Y, Cui Q, Zheng K, Liu Z, Shi J, Li F, Wang F, Zhu Z. Integrin imaging with ^{99m}Tc-3PRGD2 SPECT/CT shows high specificity in the diagnosis of lymph node metastasis from non–small cell lung cancer. Radiology. 2016;281:958–66.
273. Miao W, Zheng S, Dai H, Wang F, Jin X, Zhu Z, Jia B. Comparison of ^{99m}Tc-3PRGD$_2$ integrin receptor imaging with ^{99m}Tc-MDP bone scan in diagnosis of bone metastasis in patients with lung cancer: a multicenter study. PLoS One. 2014;9:e111221.
274. Liu L, Song Y, Gao S, Ji TF, Zhang HS, Ji B, Chen B, Jia B, Wang F, Xu ZL, Ma QJ. ^{99m}Tc-3PRGD$_2$ scintimammography in palpable and nonpalpable breast lesions. Mol Imaging. 2014;13:28650261.
275. Dijkgraaf I, Kruijtzer JAW, Liu S, Soede AC, Oyen WJG, Corstens FHM, Liskamp RMJ, Boerman OC. Improved targeting of the $\alpha_v\beta_3$ integrin by multimerisation of RGD peptides. Eur J Nucl Med Mol Imaging. 2007;34:267–73.
276. Liu Z, Niu G, Shi J, Liu S, Wang F, Liu S, Chen X. ^{68}Ga-labeled cyclic RGD dimers with Gly$_3$ and PEG4 linkers: promising agents for tumor integrin $\alpha_v\beta_3$ PET imaging. Eur J Nucl Med Mol Imaging. 2009;36:947–57.
277. Sancey L, Garanger E, Foillard S, Schoehn G, Hurbin A, Albiges-Rizo C, Boturyn D, Souchier C, Grichine A, Dumy P, Coll J-L. Clustering and internalization of integrin $\alpha_v\beta_3$ with a tetrameric RGD-synthetic peptide. Mol Ther. 2009;17:837–43.
278. Shi J, Kim Y-S, Chakraborty S, Jia B, Wang F, Liu S. 2-Mercaptoacetylglycylglycyl (MAG2) as a bifunctional chelator for ^{99m}Tc-labeling of cyclic RGD dimers: effect of technetium chelate on tumor uptake and pharmacokinetics. Bioconjug Chem. 2009;20:1559–68.
279. Zhou Y, Kim Y-S, Chakraborty S, Shi J, Gao H, Liu S. ^{99m}Tc-Labeled cyclic RGD peptides for noninvasive monitoring of tumor integrin $\alpha_v\beta_3$ expression. Mol Imaging. 2011;10:7290.2011.00006.
280. Chen B, Zhao G, Ma Q, Ji B, Ji T, Xin H, Gao S. ^{99m}Tc-3P-RGD$_2$ SPECT to monitor early response to bevacizumab therapy in patients with advanced non-small cell lung cancer. Int J Clin Exp Pathol. 2015;8:16064–72.
281. Krenning EP, Bakker WH, Kooij PPM, Breeman WAP, Oei HY, de Jong M, Reubi JC, Visser TJ, Bruns C, Kwekkeboom DJ, Reijs AEM, van Hagen PM, Koper JW, Lamberts SWJ. Somatostatin receptor scintigraphy with indium-111-DTPA-D-Phe-1-octreotide in man: metabolism, dosimetry and comparison with iodine-123-Tyr-3-octreotide. J Nucl Med. 1992;33:652–8.
282. Fani M, Nicolas GP, Wild D. Somatostatin receptor antagonists for imaging and therapy. J Nucl Med. 2017;58:61S–6S.
283. Kwekkeboom DJ, Krenning EP. Somatostatin receptor imaging. Semin Nucl Med. 2002;32:84–91.
284. Mikołajczak R, Maecke HR. Radiopharmaceuticals for somatostatin receptor imaging. Nucl Med Rev. 2016;19:126–32.
285. Reubi JC, Schär J-C, Waser B, Wenger S, Heppeler A, Schmitt JS, Mäcke HR. Affinity profiles for human somatostatin receptor subtypes SST1–SST5 of somatostatin radiotracers selected for scintigraphic and radiotherapeutic use. Eur J Nucl Med. 2000;27:273–82.
286. Rodrigues M, Traub-Weidinger T, Leimer M, Li S, Andreae F, Angelberger P, Dudczak R, Virgolini I. Value of ^{111}In-DOTA-lanreotide and ^{111}In-DOTA-DPhe1-Tyr3-octreotide in differentiated thyroid cancer: results of in vitro binding studies and in vivo comparison with ^{18}F-FDG PET. Eur J Nucl Med Mol Imaging. 2005;32:1144–51.
287. Rodrigues M, Traub-Weidinger T, Li S, Ibi B, Virgolini I. Comparison of ^{111}In-DOTA-DPhe1-Tyr3-octreotide and ^{111}In-DOTA-lanreotide scintigraphy and dosimetry in patients with neuroendocrine tumours. Eur J Nucl Med Mol Imaging. 2006;33:532–40.
288. Virgolini I, Britton K, Buscombe J, Moncayo R, Paganelli G, Riva P. ^{111}In- and ^{90}Y-DOTA-lanreotide: results and implications of the MAURITIUS trial. Semin Nucl Med. 2002;32:148–55.
289. Virgolini I, Szilvasi I, Kurtaran A, Angelberger P, Raderer M, Havlik E, Vorbeck F, Bischof C, Leimer M, Dorner G, Kletter K, Niederle B, Scheithauer W, Smith-Jones P. Indium-111-DOTA-lanreotide: biodistribution, safety and radiation absorbed dose in tumor patients. J Nucl Med. 1998;39:1928–36.
290. Forrer F, Uusijärvi H, Waldherr C, Cremonesi M, Bernhardt P, Mueller-Brand J, Maecke HR. A comparison of ^{111}In-DOTATOC and ^{111}In-DOTATATE: biodistribution and dosimetry in the same patients with metastatic neuroendocrine tumours. Eur J Nucl Med Mol Imaging. 2004;31:1257–62.
291. Giovacchini G, Giovannini E, Riondato M, Ciarmiello A. Radiopharmaceuticals for the diagnosis and therapy of neuroendocrine differentiated prostate cancer. Curr Radiopharm. 2017;10:6–15.
292. Carrasquillo JA, Pandit-Taskar N, Chen CC. Radionuclide therapy of adrenal tumors. J Surg Oncol. 2012;106:632–42.
293. Carrasquillo JA, Pandit-Taskar N, Chen CC. I-131 metaiodobenzylguanidine therapy of pheochromocytoma and paraganglioma. Semin Nucl Med. 2016;46:203–14.
294. Cistaro A, Quartuccio N, Caobelli F, Piccardo A, Paratore R, Coppolino P, Sperandeo A, Arnone G, Ficola U. ^{124}I-MIBG: a new promising positron-

emitting radiopharmaceutical for the evaluation of neuroblastoma. Nucl Med Rev. 2015;18:102–6.
295. GrünwaldF,EzziddinS. ^{131}I-Metaiodobenzylguanidine therapy of neuroblastoma and other neuroendocrine tumors. Semin Nucl Med. 2010;40:153–63.
296. Sharp SE, Trout AT, Weiss BD, Gelfand MJ. MIBG in neuroblastoma diagnostic imaging and therapy. Radiographics. 2016;36:258–78.
297. Van Vickle SS, Thompson RC. ^{123}I-MIBG imaging: patient preparation and technologist's role. J Nucl Med Technol. 2015;43:82–6.
298. Vöö S, Bucerius J, Mottaghy FM. I-131-MIBG therapies. Methods. 2011;55:238–45.
299. Verberne HJ, Brewster LM, Somsen GA, van Eck-Smit BLF. Prognostic value of myocardial ^{123}I-metaiodobenzylguanidine (MIBG) parameters in patients with heart failure: a systematic review. Eur Heart J. 2008;29:1147–59.
300. Case J, Courter S, Van Vickle S, Bateman T. Novel approaches to measuring ^{123}I-labeled mIBG heart-to-mediastinal (H/M) ratios in a high efficiency, small field of view cardiac SPECT system. J Nucl Med. 2015;56:407.
301. Dimitriu-Leen AC, Scholte AJHA, Jacobson AF. ^{123}I-MIBG SPECT for evaluation of patients with heart failure. J Nucl Med. 2015;56:25S–30S.
302. Cavina L, van der Born D, Klaren PHM, Feiters MC, Boerman OC, Rutjes FPJT, editors. Design of radioiodinated pharmaceuticals: structural features affecting metabolic stability towards in vivo deiodination. Eur J Org Chem. 2017;2017:3387–414.
303. Kung HF, Kung M-P, Choi SR. Radiopharmaceuticals for single-photon emission computed tomography brain imaging. Semin Nucl Med. 2003;33:2–13.
304. Bajaj N, Hauser RA, Grachev ID. Clinical utility of dopamine transporter single photon emission CT (DaT-SPECT) with (^{123}I) ioflupane in diagnosis of parkinsonian syndromes. J Neurol Neurosurg Psychiatry. 2013;84:1288–95.
305. Djang DSW, Janssen MJR, Bohnen N, Booij J, Henderson TA, Herholz K, Minoshima S, Rowe CC, Sabri O, Seibyl J, Van Berckel BNM, Wanner M. SNM practice guideline for dopamine transporter imaging with ^{123}I-ioflupane SPECT 1.0. J Nucl Med. 2012;53:154–63.
306. Tatsch K, Asenbaum S, Bartenstein P, Catafau A, Halldin C, Pilowsky LS, Pupi A. European association of nuclear medicine procedure guidelines for brain neurotransmission SPET using I-123-labelled dopamine transporter ligands. Eur J Nucl Med Mol Imaging. 2002;29:BP30–5.
307. Wu X, Cai H, Ge R, Li L, Jia Z. Recent progress of imaging agents for Parkinson's disease. Curr Neuropharmacol. 2014;12:551–63.
308. Innis R, Zoghbi S, Johnson E, Woods S, Al-Tikriti M, Baldwin R, Seibyl J, Malison R, Zubal G, Charney D, Heninger G, Hoffer P. SPECT imaging of the benzodiazepine receptor in non-human primate brain with [^{123}I]Ro 16-0154. Eur J Pharmacol. 1991;193:249–52.
309. Zoghbi SS, Baldwin RM, Seibyl JP, Al-Tikriti MS, Zea-Ponce Y, Laruelle M, Sybirska EH, Woods SW, Goddard AW, Malison RT, Zimmerman R, Charney DS, Smith EO, Hoffer PB, Innis RB. Pharmacokinetics of the SPECT benzodiazepine receptor radioligand [^{123}I]iomazenil in human and non-human primates. Nucl Med Biol. 1992;19:881–8.
310. Pinborg LH, Videbaek C, Hasselbalch SG, Sorensen SA, Wagner A, Paulson OB, Knudsen GM. Benzodiazepine receptor quantification in Huntington's disease with [^{123}I]iomazenil and SPECT. J Neurol Neurosurg Psychiatry. 2001;70:657–61.
311. Verhoeff N, Soares JC, D'Souza CD, Gil R, Degen K, Abi-Dargham A, Zoghbi SS, Fujita M, Rajeevan N, Seibyl JP, Krystal JH, van Dyck CH, Charney DS, Innis RB. [^{123}I]Iomazenil SPECT benzodiazepine receptor imaging in schizophrenia. Psychiatry Res Neuroimaging. 1999;91:163–73.
312. Bremner JD, Innis RB, White T, Fujita M, Silbersweig D, Goddard AW, Staib L, Stern E, Cappiello A, Woods S, Baldwin R, Charney DS. SPECT [I-123]iomazenil measurement of the benzodiazepine receptor in panic disorder. Biol Psychiatry. 2000;47:96–106.
313. Moriwaki H, Matsumoto M, Hashikawa K, Oku N, Ishida M, Seike Y, Fukuchi K, Hori M, Nishimura T. Iodine-123-iomazenil and iodine-123-iodoamphetamine SPECT in major cerebral artery occlusive disease. J Nucl Med. 1998;39:1348–53.
314. Hatazawa J, Satoh T, Shimosegawa E, Okudera T, Inugami A, Ogawa T, Fujita H, Noguchi K, Kanno I, Miura S, Murakami M, Iida H, Miura Y, Uemura K. Evaluation of cerebral infarction with iodine 123-iomazenil SPECT. J Nucl Med. 1995;36:2154–61.
315. Abiko K, Ikoma K, Shiga T, Katoh C, Hirata K, Kuge Y, Kobayashi K, Tamaki N. I-123 iomazenil single photon emission computed tomography for detecting loss of neuronal integrity in patients with traumatic brain injury. EJNMMI Res. 2017;7:28.
316. Koizumi H, Fujisawa H, Kurokawa T, Suehiro E, Iwanaga H, Nakagawara J, Suzuki M. Recovered neuronal viability revealed by Iodine-123-iomazenil SPECT following traumatic brain injury. J Cereb Blood Flow Metab. 2010;30:1673–81.
317. Kung HF, Pan S, Kung M-P, Billings J, Kasliwal R, Reilley J, Alavi A. In vitro and in vivo evaluation of [^{123}I]IBZM: a potential CNS D-2 dopamine receptor imaging agent. J Nucl Med. 1989;30:88–92.
318. Heinzel A, Mohammadkhani Shali S, Dafotakis M, Verburg FA, Mottaghy FM, Winz OH. Comparison of automatic versus manual procedures for the quantification of dopamine D2 receptor availability using I-123-IBZM-SPECT. Nucl Med Commun. 2015;36:1120–6.
319. Hammesfahr S, Antke C, Mamlins E, Beu M, Wojtecki L, Ferrea S, Dinkelbach L, Moldovan AS, Schnitzler A, Müller HW, Südmeyer M. FP-CIT-

and IBZM-SPECT in corticobasal syndrome: results from a clinical follow-up study. Neurodegener Dis. 2016;16:342–7.
320. Långström B, Karimi F, Watanabe Y. Endogenous compounds labeled with radionuclides of short half-life—some perspectives. J Label Compd Radiopharm. 2013;56:251–62.
321. Woods DH, Baker MI, Keightley JD, Keightley LJ, Makepeace JL, Pearce AK, Woodman AP, Woods MJ, Woods SA, Waters S. Standardisation of ^{11}C. Appl Radiat Isot. 2002;56:327–30.
322. Miller PW, Kato K, Långström B. Carbon-11, nitrogen-13, and oxygen-15 chemistry: an introduction to chemistry with short-lived radioisotopes. In: Long NJ, Wong W-T, editors. The chemistry of molecular imaging. Hoboken, NJ: Wiley; 2014. p. 79–103.
323. Allard M, Fouquet E, James D, Szlosek-Pinaud M. State of art in ^{11}C labelled radiotracers synthesis. Curr Med Chem. 2008;15:235–77.
324. Ermert J, Coenen HH. Methods for ^{11}C- and ^{18}F-labelling of amino acids and derivatives for positron emission tomography imaging. J Label Compd Radiopharm. 2013;56:225–36.
325. Pekošak A, Filp U, Poot AJ, Windhorst AD. From carbon-11-labeled amino acids to peptides in positron emission tomography: the synthesis and clinical application. Mol Imaging Biol. 2018;20(4):510–32.
326. Pike VW, Eakins MN, Allan RM, Selwyn AP. Preparation of [1–^{11}C]acetate—an agent for the study of myocardial metabolism by positron emission tomography. Int J Appl Radiat Isot. 1982;33:505–12.
327. Norenberg JP, Simpson NR, Dunn BB, Kiesewetter DO. Remote synthesis of [^{11}C]acetate. Int J Appl Radiat Isot. 1992;43:943–5.
328. Mock BH, Brown-Proctor C, Green MA, Steele B, Glick-Wilson BE, Zheng Q-H. An automated SPE-based high-yield synthesis of [^{11}C]acetate and [^{11}C]palmitate: no liquid–liquid extraction, solvent evaporation or distillation required. Nucl Med Biol. 2011;38:1135–42.
329. Le Helleix S, Dollé F, Kuhnast B. Easy upgrade of the TRACERLab FX C Pro for [^{11}C]carboxylation reactions: application to the routine production of [1-^{11}C]acetate. Appl Radiat Isot. 2013;82:7–11.
330. McCarron JA, Turton DR, Pike VW, Poole KG. Remotely-controlled production of the 5-HT_{1A} receptor radioligand, carbonyl-^{11}C WAY-100635, via ^{11}C-carboxylation of an immobilized Grignard reagent. J Label Compd Radiopharm. 1996;38:941–53.
331. Långström B, Lundqvist H. The preparation of ^{11}C-methyl iodide and its use in the synthesis of ^{11}C-methyl-L-methionine. Int J Appl Radiat Isot. 1976;27:357–63.
332. Holschbach M, Schüller M. A new and simple on-line method for the preparation of n.c.a. [^{11}C]methyl iodide. Appl Radiat Isot. 1993;44:779–80.
333. Larsen P, Ulin J, Dahlstrøm K, Jensen M. Synthesis of [^{11}C]iodomethane by iodination of [^{11}C]methane. Appl Radiat Isot. 1997;48:153–7.
334. Link JM, Krohn KA, Clark JC. Production of [^{11}C]CH_3I by single pass reaction of [^{11}C]CH_4 with I_2. Nucl Med Biol. 1997;24:93–7.
335. Buckley KR, Huser JM, Jivan S, Chun KS, Ruth TJ. ^{11}C-methane production in small volume, high pressure gas targets. Radiochim Acta. 2000;88:201.
336. Holschbach M, Schüller M. An on-line method for the preparation of n.c.a. [$^{11}CH_3$]trifluoromethanesulfonic acid methyl ester. Appl Radiat Isot. 1993;44:897–8.
337. Hara T, Yuasa M. Automated synthesis of [^{11}C]choline, a positron-emitting tracer for tumor imaging. Appl Radiat Isot. 1999;50:531–3.
338. Någren K, Halldin C. Methylation of amide and thiol functions with [^{11}C]methyl triflate, as exemplified by [^{11}C]NMSP, [^{11}C]flumazenil and [^{11}C]methionine. J Label Compd Radiopharm. 1998;41:831–41.
339. Mathis CA, Wang Y, Holt DP, Huang G-F, Debnath ML, Klunk WE. Synthesis and evaluation of ^{11}C-labeled 6-substituted 2-arylbenzothiazoles as amyloid imaging agents. J Med Chem. 2003;46:2740–54.
340. Dannals RF, Ravert HT, James Frost J, Wilson AA, Donald Burns H, Wagner HN. Radiosynthesis of an opiate receptor binding radiotracer: [^{11}C]carfentanil. Int J Appl Radiat Isot. 1985;36:303–6.
341. Langer O, Nagren K, Dolle F, Lundkvist C, Sandell J, Swahn CG, Vaufrey F, Crouzel C, Maziere B, Halldin C. Precursor synthesis and radiolabelling of the dopamine D_2 receptor ligand [^{11}C]raclopride from [^{11}C]methyl triflate. J Label Compd Radiopharm. 1999;42:1183–93.
342. Comar D, Cartron JC, Maziere M, Marazano C. Labelling and metabolism of methionine methyl-^{11}C. Eur J Nucl Med. 1976;1:11–4.
343. Mitterhauser M, Wadsak W, Krcal A, Schmaljohann J, Eidherr H, Schmid A, Viernstein H, Dudczak R, Kletter K. New aspects on the preparation of [^{11}C]methionine—a simple and fast online approach without preparative HPLC. Appl Radiat Isot. 2005;62:441–5.
344. Gómez V, Gispert JD, Amador V, Llop J. New method for routine production of L-[methyl-^{11}C]methionine: in loop synthesis. J Label Compd Radiopharm. 2008;51:83–6.
345. Iwata R, Pascali C, Yuasa M, Yanai K, Takahashi T, Ido T. On-line [^{11}C]methylation using [^{11}C]methyl iodide for the automated preparation of ^{11}C-radiopharmaceuticals. Int J Appl Radiat Isot. 1992;43:1083–8.
346. Studenov AR, Jivan S, Adam MJ, Ruth TJ, Buckley KR. Studies of the mechanism of the in-loop synthesis of radiopharmaceuticals. Appl Radiat Isot. 2004;61:1195–201.
347. Watkins GL, Jewett DM, Keith Mulholland G, Kilbourn MR, Toorongian SA. A captive solvent method for rapid N-[^{11}C]methylation of secondary amides: application to the benzodiazepine, 4′-chlorodiazepam (RO5-4864). Int J Appl Radiat Isot. 1988;39:441–4.
348. Wilson AA, Garcia A, Jin L, Houle S. Radiotracer synthesis from [^{11}C]-iodomethane: a remarkably

simple captive solvent method. Nucl Med Biol. 2000;27:529–32.
349. Shao X, Hoareau R, Runkle AC, Tluczek LJM, Hockley BG, Henderson BD, Scott PJH. Highlighting the versatility of the Tracerlab synthesis modules. Part 2: fully automated production of [^{11}C]-labeled radiopharmaceuticals using a Tracerlab FXC-Pro. J Label Compd Radiopharm. 2011;54:819–38.
350. Samuelsson L, Långström B. Synthesis of 1-(2′-deoxy-2′-fluoro-beta-D-arabinofuranosyl)-[*methyl*-^{11}C]thymine ([^{11}C]FMAU) via a Stille cross-coupling reaction with [^{11}C]methyl iodide. J Label Compd Radiopharm. 2003;46:263–72.
351. Miller PW, Bender D. [^{11}C]carbon disulfide: a versatile reagent for PET radiolabelling. Chem Eur J. 2012;18:433–6.
352. Roeda D, Crouzel C. [^{11}C]Formaldehyde revisited: considerable concurrent [^{11}C]formic acid formation in the low-temperature conversion of [^{11}C]carbon dioxide into [^{11}C]formaldehyde. Appl Radiat Isot. 2001;54:935–9.
353. Kato K, Zhang M-R, Suzuki K. Rapid C-carboxylation of nitro[^{11}C]methane for the synthesis of ethyl nitro[2-^{11}C]acetate. Mol BioSyst. 2008;4:53–5.
354. Långström B, Itsenko O, Rahman O. [^{11}C]Carbon monoxide, a versatile and useful precursor in labelling chemistry for PET-ligand development. J Label Compd Radiopharm. 2007;50:794–810.
355. Schelbert HR, Phelps ME, Huang SC, Macdonald NS, Hansen H, Kuhl DE. N-13 ammonia as an indicator of myocardial blood-flow. Circulation. 1981;63:1259–72.
356. Suda M, Onoguchi M, Tomiyama T, Ishihara K, Takahashi N, Sakurai M, Matsumoto K, Kumita S-i. The reproducibility of time-of-flight PET and conventional PET for the quantification of myocardial blood flow and coronary flow reserve with ^{13}N-ammonia. J Nucl Cardiol. 2016;23:457–72.
357. Cooper AJL. ^{13}N as a tracer for studying glutamate metabolism. Neurochem Int. 2011;59:456–64.
358. Bormans G, Langendries W, Mortelmans L, Verbruggen A. On-line anion exchange purification of [^{13}N]NH_3 produced by 10 MeV proton irradiation of dilute aqueous ethanol. Appl Radiat Isot. 1995;46:83–6.
359. Statuto M, Galli E, Bertagna F, Migliorati E, Zanella I, Di Lorenzo D, De Agostini A, Rodella C, Apostoli P, Caimi L, Giubbini R, Biasiotto G. The strange case of the [^{13}N]NH_3: validation of the production process for human use. Nucl Med Commun. 2016;37:412–21.
360. Suzuki K, Yoshida Y. Production of [^{13}N]NH_3 with ultra-high specific activity. Appl Radiat Isot. 1999;50:497–503.
361. Wieland B, Bida G, Padgett H, Hendry G, Zippi E, Kabalka G, Morelle J-L, Verbruggen R, Ghyoot M. In-target production of [^{13}N]ammonia via proton irradiation of dilute aqueous ethanol and acetic acid mixtures. Int J Appl Radiat Isot. 1991;42:1095–8.
362. Berridge MS, Landmeier BJ. In-target production of [^{13}N]ammonia: target design, products, and operating parameters. Appl Radiat Isot. 1993;44:1433–41.
363. Vaalburg W, Kamphuis JAA, Beerling-van der Molen HD, Reiffers S, Rijskamp A, Woldring MG. An improved method for the cyclotron production of ^{13}N-labelled ammonia. Int J Appl Radiat Isot. 1975;26:316–8.
364. Baron J-C, Jones T. Oxygen metabolism, oxygen extraction and positron emission tomography: historical perspective and impact on basic and clinical neuroscience. NeuroImage. 2012;61:492–504.
365. Zhang K, Herzog H, Mauler J, Filss C, Okell TW, Kops ER, Tellmann L, Fischer T, Brocke B, Sturm W, Coenen HH, Shah NJ. Comparison of cerebral blood flow acquired by simultaneous [^{15}O]water positron emission tomography and arterial spin labeling magnetic resonance imaging. J Cereb Blood Flow Metab. 2014;34:1373–80.
366. Palmer BM, Sajjad M, Rottenberg DA. An automated [^{15}O]H_2O production and injection system for PET imaging. Nucl Med Biol. 1995;22:241–9.
367. Sajjad M, Liow J-S, Moreno-Cantu J. A system for continuous production and infusion of [^{15}O]H_2O for PET activation studies. Appl Radiat Isot. 2000;52:205–10.
368. Berridge MS, Kjellström R. Designs and use of silver [^{18}O]water targets for [^{18}F]fluoride production. Appl Radiat Isot. 1999;50:699–705.
369. Ferrieri RA, Alexoff DL, Schlyer DJ, Wolf AP. Remote processing, delivery and injection of H_2[^{15}O] produced from a N_2/H_2 gas target using a simple and compact apparatus. Appl Radiat Isot. 1994;45:1149–54.
370. Mulholland GK, Kilbourn MR, Moskwa JJ. Direct simultaneous production of [^{15}O]water and [^{13}N]ammonia or [^{18}F]fluoride ion by 26 MeV proton irradiation of a double chamber water target. Int J Appl Radiat Isot. 1990;41:1193–9.
371. Van Naemen J, Monclus M, Damhaut P, Luxen A, Goldman S. Production, automatic delivery and bolus injection of [^{15}O]water for positron emission tomography studies. Nucl Med Biol. 1996;23:413–6.
372. Park BK, Kitteringham NR. Effects of fluorine substitution on drug metabolism: pharmacological and toxicological implications. Drug Metab Rev. 1994;26:605–43.
373. Gillis EP, Eastman KJ, Hill MD, Donnelly DJ, Meanwell NA. Applications of fluorine in medicinal chemistry. J Med Chem. 2015;58:8315–59.
374. Coenen HH. Fluorine-18 labeling methods: features and possibilities of basic reactions. In: Schubiger PA, Lehmann L, Friebe M, editors. PET chemistry: the driving force in molecular imaging. Ernst Schering Research Foundation workshop, vol. 62. Berlin: Springer-Verlag; 2007. p. 15–50.
375. Coenen HH, Ermert J. ^{18}F-labelling innovations and their potential for clinical application. Clin Transl Imaging. 2018;6:169–93.

376. Ermert J, Coenen HH. No-carrier-added [^{18}F]fluorobenzene derivatives as intermediates for built-up radiosyntheses. Curr Radiopharm. 2010;3:127–60.
377. Ido T, Wan CN, Casella V, Fowler JS, Wolf AP, Reivich M, Kuhl DE. Labeled 2-deoxy-D-glucose analogs. ^{18}F-labeled 2-deoxy-2-fluoro-D-glucose, 2-deoxy-2-fluoro-D-mannose and 14C-2-deoxy-2-fluoro-D-glucose. J Label Compd Radiopharm. 1978;14:175–83.
378. Shiue C-Y, Salvadori PA, Wolf AP, Fowler JS, MacGregor RR. A new improved synthesis of 2-deoxy-2-[^{18}F]fluoro-D-glucose from ^{18}F-labeled acetyl hypofluorite. J Nucl Med. 1982;23:899–903.
379. Firnau G, Chirakal R, Sood S, Garnett S. Aromatic fluorination with xenon difluoride: L-3,4-dihydroxy-6-fluorophenylalanine. Can J Chem. 1980;58:1449–50.
380. Coenen HH, Franken K, Kling P, Stöcklin G. Direct electrophilic radiofluorination of phenylalanine, tyrosine and dopa. Int J Appl Radiat Isot. 1988;39:1243–50.
381. Chirakal R, Firnau G, Couse J, Garnett ES. Radiofluorination with ^{18}F-labelled acetyl hypofluorite: [^{18}F]L-6-fluorodopa. Int J Appl Radiat Isot. 1984;35:651–3.
382. Fowler JS, Shiue CY, Wolf AP, Salvadori PA, MacGregor RR. ^{18}F-labeled acetyl hypofluorite for radiotracer synthesis. J Label Compd Radiopharm. 1982;19:1634–6.
383. Hiller A, Fischer C, Jordanova A, Patt JT, Steinbach J. Investigations to the synthesis of n.c.a. [^{18}F]FClO3 as electrophilic fluorinating agent. Appl Radiat Isot. 2008;66:152–7.
384. Adam MJ, Ruth TJ, Grierson JR, Abeysekera B, Pate BD. Routine synthesis of L-[^{18}F]6-fluorodopa with fluorine-18 acetyl hypofluorite. J Nucl Med. 1986;27:1462–6.
385. de Vries EFJ, Luurtsema G, Brüssermann M, Elsinga PH, Vaalburg W. Fully automated synthesis module for the high yield one-pot preparation of 6-[^{18}F]fluoro-l-DOPA. Appl Radiat Isot. 1999;51:389–94.
386. Forsback S, Eskola O, Haaparanta M, Bergmann J, Solin O. Electrophilic synthesis of 6-[^{18}F]fluoro-L-DOPA using post-target produced [^{18}F]F_2. Radiochim Acta. 2008;96:845–8.
387. Stenhagen ISR, Kirjavainen AK, Forsback SJ, Jørgensen CG, Robins EG, Luthra SK, Solin O, Gouverneur V. Fluorination of an arylboronic ester using [^{18}F]selectfluor bis(triflate): application to 6-[^{18}F]fluoro-L-DOPA. Chem Commun. 2013;49:1386–8.
388. Murali D, Flores LG, Roberts AD, Nickles RJ, DeJesus OT. Aromatic l-amino acid decarboxylase (AAAD) inhibitors as carcinoid tumor-imaging agents: synthesis of ^{18}F-labeled α-fluoromethyl-6-fluoro-m-tyrosine (FM-6-FmT). Appl Radiat Isot. 2003;59:237–43.
389. Coenen HH, Moerlein SM. Regiospecific aromatic fluorodemetallation of group IVb metalloarenes using elemental fluorine or acetyl hypofluorite. J Fluor Chem. 1987;36:63–75.
390. Teare H, Robins EG, Årstad E, Luthra SK, Gouverneur V. Synthesis and reactivity of [^{18}F]-N-fluorobenzenesulfonimide. Chem Commun. 2007;23:2330–2.
391. Satyamurthy N, Bida GT, Phelps ME, Barrio JR. N-[^{18}F]fluoro-N-alkylsulfonamides: novel reagents for mild and regioselective radiofluorination. Appl Radiat Isot. 1990;41:733–8.
392. Oberdorfer F, Hofmann E, Maier-Borst W. Preparation of ^{18}F-labelled N-fluoropyridinium triflate. J Label Compd Radiopharm. 1988;25:999–1005.
393. Purrington ST, Jones WA. 1-Fluoro-2-pyridone: a useful fluorinating reagent. J Org Chem. 1983;48:761–2.
394. Teare H, Robins EG, Kirjavainen A, Forsback S, Sandford G, Solin O, Luthra SK, Gouverneur V. Radiosynthesis and evaluation of [^{18}F]selectfluor bis(triflate). Angew Chem Int Ed Engl. 2010;49:6821–4.
395. Lee E, Kamlet AS, Powers DC, Neumann CN, Boursalian GB, Furuya T, Choi DC, Hooker JM, Ritter T. A fluoride-derived electrophilic late-stage fluorination reagent for PET imaging. Science. 2011;334:639–42.
396. Zlatopolskiy BD, Zischler J, Urusova EA, Endepols H, Kordys E, Frauendorf H, Mottaghy FM, Neumaier B. A practical one-pot synthesis of positron emission tomography (PET) tracers via nickel-mediated radiofluorination. Chem Open. 2015;4:457–62.
397. Lee E, Hooker JM, Ritter T. Nickel-mediated oxidative fluorination for PET with aqueous [^{18}F]fluoride. J Am Chem Soc. 2012;134:17456–8.
398. Richarz R, Krapf P, Zarrad F, Urusova EA, Neumaier B, Zlatopolskiy BD. Neither azeotropic drying, nor base nor other additives: a minimalist approach to ^{18}F-labeling. Org Biomol Chem. 2014;12:8094–9.
399. Dollé F, Helfenbein J, Hinnen F, Mavel S, Mincheva Z, Saba W, Schollhorn-Peyronneau MA, Valette H, Garreau L, Chalon S, Halldin C, Madelmont JC, Deloye JB, Bottlaender M, Le Gailliard J, Guilloteau D, Emond P. One-step radiosynthesis of [^{18}F]LBT-999: a selective radioligand for the visualization of the dopamine transporter with PET. J Label Compd Radiopharm. 2007;50:716–23.
400. Mukherjee J, Christian BT, Dunigan KA, Shi BZ, Narayanan TK, Satter M, Mantil J. Brain imaging of ^{18}F-fallypride in normal volunteers: blood analysis, distribution, test-retest studies, and preliminary assessment of sensitivity to aging effects on dopamine D-2/D-3 receptors. Synapse. 2002;46:170–88.
401. Mukherjee J, Yang Z-Y, Brown T, Lew R, Wernick M, Ouyang X, Yasillo N, Chen C-T, Mintzer R, Cooper M. Preliminary assessment of extrastriatal dopamine d-2 receptor binding in the rodent and nonhuman primate brains using the high affinity radioligand, ^{18}F-fallypride. Nucl Med Biol. 1999;26:519–27.

402. Lee SJ, Oh SJ, Moon WY, Choi MS, Kim JS, Chi DY, Moon DH, Ryu JS. New automated synthesis of [^{18}F]FP-CIT with base amount control affording high and stable radiochemical yield: a 1.5-year production report. Nucl Med Biol. 2011;38:593–7.
403. Gründer G, Siessmeier T, Lange-Asschenfeldt C, Vernaleken I, Buchholz H-G, Stoeter P, Drzezga A, Lüddens H, Rösch F, Bartenstein P. [^{18}F] Fluoroethylflumazenil: a novel tracer for PET imaging of human benzodiazepine receptors. Eur J Nucl Med. 2001;28:1463–70.
404. Wang HL, Guo XY, Jiang SD, Tang GH. Automated synthesis of [^{18}F]Florbetaben as Alzheimer's disease imaging agent based on a synthesis module system. Appl Radiat Isot. 2013;71:41–6.
405. Hamacher K, Coenen HH, Stöcklin G. Efficient stereospecific synthesis of no-carrier-added 2-[^{18}F] fluoro-2-deoxy-D-glucose using aminopolyether supported nucleophilic substitution. J Nucl Med. 1986;27:235–8.
406. Bourdier T, Greguric I, Roselt P, Jackson T, Faragalla J, Katsifis A. Fully automated one-pot radiosynthesis of O-(2-[^{18}F]fluoroethyl)-L-tyrosine on the TracerLab FXFN module. Nucl Med Biol. 2011;38:645–51.
407. Hamacher K, Coenen HH. Efficient routine production of the ^{18}F-labelled amino acid O-(2-[^{18}F]fluoroethyl)-l-tyrosine. Appl Radiat Isot. 2002;57:853–6.
408. Kiesewetter DO, Kilbourn MR, Landvatter SW, Heiman DF, Katzenellenbogen JA, Welch MJ. Preparation of four fluorine-18-labeled estrogens and their selective uptakes in target tissues of immature rats. J Nucl Med. 1984;25:1212–21.
409. Römer J, Steinbach J, Kasch H. Studies on the synthesis of 16α-[^{18}F]fluoroestradiol. Appl Radiat Isot. 1996;47:395–9.
410. Ahmed N, Langlois R, Rodrigue S, Bénard F, van Lier JE. Automated synthesis of 11b-methoxy-4,16a-[16a-^{18}F]difluoroestradiol (4F-M[^{18}F]FES) for estrogen receptor imaging by positron emission tomography. Nucl Med Biol. 2007;34:459–64.
411. Marchand P, Ouadi A, Pellicioli M, Schuler J, Laquerriere P, Boisson F, Brasse D. Automated and efficient radiosynthesis of [^{18}F]FLT using a low amount of precursor. Nucl Med Biol. 2016;43:520–7.
412. Been LB, Suurmeijer AJH, Cobben DCP, Jager PL, Hoekstra HJ, Elsinga PH. [^{18}F]FLT-PET in oncology: current status and opportunities. Eur J Nucl Med Mol Imaging. 2004;31:1659–72.
413. Grierson JR, Shields AF. Radiosynthesis of 3′-deoxy-3′-[^{18}F]fluorothymidine: [^{18}F]FLT for imaging of cellular proliferation in vivo. Nucl Med Biol. 2000;27:143–56.
414. Machulla H-J, Blocher A, Kuntzsch M, Piert M, Wei R, Grierson JR. Simplified labeling approach for synthesizing 3′-deoxy-3′-[^{18}F]fluorothymidine ([^{18}F] FLT). J Radioanal Nucl Chem. 2000;243:843–6.
415. Shields AF, Grierson JR, Dohmen BM, Machulla HJ, Stayanoff JC, Lawhorn-Crews JM, Obradovich JE, Muzik O, Mangner TJ. Imaging proliferation in vivo with F-18 FLT and positron emission tomography. Nat Med. 1998;4:1334–6.
416. Chang CW, Chou TK, Liu RS, Wang SJ, Lin WJ, Chen CH, Wang HE. A robotic synthesis of [^{18}F] fluoromisonidazole ([^{18}F]FMISO). Appl Radiat Isot. 2007;65:682–6.
417. Grierson JR, Link JM, Mathis CA, Rasey JS, Krohn KA. A radiosynthesis of fluorine-18 fluoromisonidazole. J Nucl Med. 1989;30:343–50.
418. Bauman G, Belhocine T, Kovacs M, Ward A, Beheshti M, Rachinsky I. ^{18}F-fluorocholine for prostate cancer imaging: a systematic review of the literature. Prostate Cancer Prostatic Dis. 2012;15:45–55.
419. Ponde DE, Dence CS, Oyama N, Kim J, Tai Y-C, Laforest R, Siegel BA, Welch MJ. ^{18}F-fluoroacetate: a potential acetate analog for prostate tumor imaging—in vivo evaluation of ^{18}F-fluoroacetate versus ^{11}C-acetate. J Nucl Med. 2007;48:420–8.
420. Zhou D, Lin M, Yasui N, Al-Qahtani MH, Dence CS, Schwarz S, Katzenellenbogen JA. Optimization of the preparation of fluorine-18-labeled steroid receptor ligands 16alpha-^{18}F-fluoroestradiol (FES), ^{18}F-fluoro furanyl norprogesterone (FFNP), and 16beta-^{18}F-fluoro-5alpha-dihydrotestosterone (FDHT) as radiopharmaceuticals. J Label Compd Radiopharm. 2014;57:371–7.
421. Piert M, Machulla HJ, Picchio M, Reischl G, Ziegler S, Kumar P, Wester HJ, Beck R, McEwan AJB, Wiebe LI, Schwaiger M. Hypoxia-specific tumor imaging with ^{18}F-fluoroazomycin arabinoside. J Nucl Med. 2005;46:106–13.
422. Turton DR, Betts HM, Dutton D, Perkins AC. Automated radiosynthesis of GMP quality [^{18}F] HX4 for PET imaging of hypoxia. Nucl Med Biol. 2015;42:494–8.
423. Liu YJ, Zhu L, Plossl K, Choi SR, Qiao HW, Sun XT, Li S, Zha ZH, Kung HF. Optimization of automated radiosynthesis of [^{18}F]AV-45: a new PET imaging agent for Alzheimer's disease. Nucl Med Biol. 2010;37:917–25.
424. Ding YS, Fowler JS, Gatley SJ, Dewey SL, Wolf AP, Schlyer DJ. Synthesis of high specific activity 6-[^{18}F]fluorodopamine for positron emission tomography studies of sympathetic nervous tissue. J Med Chem. 1991;34:861–3.
425. Shiue CY, Shiue GG, Mozley PD, Kung MP, Zhuang ZP, Kim HJ, Kung HF. p-[^{18}F]-MPPF: a potential radioligand for PET studies of 5-HT_{1A} receptors in humans. Synapse. 1997;25:147–54.
426. Martinez G, Vernooij RWM, Padilla PF, Zamora J, Flicker L, Cosp XB. ^{18}F PET with flutemetamol for the early diagnosis of Alzheimer's disease dementia and other dementias in people with mild cognitive impairment (MCI). Cochrane Database Syst Rev. 2017;11:CD012884.
427. Kilbourn MR, Welch MJ, Dence CS. Carrier-added and no-carrier-added syntheses of [^{18}F]spiroperidol and [^{18}F]haloperidol. Int J Appl Radiat Isot. 1984;35:591–8.

428. Lemaire C, Cantineau R, Guillaume M, Plenevaux A, Christiaens L. Fluorine-18-altanserin: a radioligand for the study of serotonin receptors with PET: radiolabeling and in vivo biologic behavior in rats. J Nucl Med. 1991;32:2266–72.
429. Preshlock S, Tredwell M, Gouverneur V. ^{18}F-labeling of arenes and heteroarenes for applications in positron emission tomography. Chem Rev. 2016;116:719–66.
430. Pike VW. Hypervalent aryliodine compounds as precursors for radiofluorination. J Label Compd Radiopharm. 2018;61:196–227.
431. Ross TL, Ermert J, Hocke C, Coenen HH. Nucleophilic ^{18}F-fluorination of heteroaromatic iodonium salts with no-carrier-added [^{18}F]fluoride. J Am Chem Soc. 2007;129:8018–25.
432. Zhang MR, Kumata K, Suzuki K. A practical route for synthesizing a PET ligand containing [^{18}F]fluorobenzene using reaction of diphenyliodonium salt with [^{18}F]F–. Tetrahedron Lett. 2007;48:8632–5.
433. Telu S, Chun J-H, Simeon FG, Lu S, Pike VW. Syntheses of mGluR5 PET radioligands through the radiofluorination of diaryliodonium tosylates. Org Biomol Chem. 2011;9(19):6629–38.
434. Moon B, Park J, Lee H, Lee B, Kim S. Routine production of [^{18}F]flumazenil from iodonium tosylate using a sample pretreatment method: a 2.5-year production report. Mol Imaging Biol. 2014;16:619–25.
435. Xu R, Zanotti-Fregonara P, Zoghbi SS, Gladding RL, Woock AE, Innis RB, Pike VW. Synthesis and evaluation in monkey of [^{18}F]4-fluoro-N-methyl-N-(4-(6-(methylamino)pyrimidin-4-yl)thiazol-2-yl) benzamide ([^{18}F]FIMX): a promising radioligand for PET imaging of brain metabotropic glutamate receptor 1 (mGluR1). J Med Chem. 2013;56:9146–55.
436. Jung Y-W, Jang KS, Gu G, Koeppe RA, Sherman PS, Quesada CA, Raffel DM. [^{18}F]Fluorohydroxyphenethylguanidines: efficient synthesis and comparison of two structural isomers as radiotracers of cardiac sympathetic innervation. ACS Chem Neurosci. 2017;8:1530–42.
437. Edwards R, Westwell AD, Daniels S, Wirth T. Convenient synthesis of diaryliodonium salts for the production of [^{18}F]F-DOPA. Eur J Org Chem. 2015;2015:625–30.
438. Libert LC, Franci X, Plenevaux AR, Ooi T, Maruoka K, Luxen AJ, Lemaire CF. Production at the curie level of no-carrier-added 6-^{18}F-fluoro-L-dopa. J Nucl Med. 2013;54:1154–61.
439. Cardinale J, Ermert J, Humpert S, Coenen HH. Iodonium ylides for one-step, no-carrier-added radiofluorination of electron rich arenes, exemplified with 4-(([^{18}F]fluorophenoxy)-phenylmethyl) piperidine NET and SERT ligands. RSC Adv. 2014;4:17293–9.
440. Rotstein BH, Stephenson NA, Vasdev N, Liang SH. Spirocyclic hypervalent iodine(III)-mediated radiofluorination of non-activated and hindered aromatics. Nat Commun. 2014;5:4365.
441. Ichiishi N, Brooks AF, Topczewski JJ, Rodnick ME, Sanford MS, Scott PJH. Copper-catalyzed [^{18}F]fluorination of (Mesityl)(aryl)iodonium salts. Org Lett. 2014;16:3224–7.
442. Tredwell M, Preshlock SM, Taylor NJ, Gruber S, Huiban M, Passchier J, Mercier J, Génicot C, Gouverneur V. A general copper-mediated nucleophilic ^{18}F fluorination of arenes. Angew Chem Int Ed Engl. 2014;53:7751–5.
443. Mossine AV, Brooks AF, Makaravage KJ, Miller JM, Ichiishi N, Sanford MS, Scott PJH. Synthesis of [^{18}F]arenes via the copper-mediated [^{18}F]fluorination of boronic acids. Org Lett. 2015;17:5780–3.
444. Makaravage KJ, Brooks AF, Mossine AV, Sanford MS, Scott PJH. Copper-mediated radiofluorination of arylstannanes with [^{18}F]KF. Org Lett. 2016;18:5440–3.
445. Mossine AV, Brooks AF, Ichiishi N, Makaravage KJ, Sanford MS, Scott PJH. Development of customized [^{18}F]fluoride elution techniques for the enhancement of copper-mediated late-stage radiofluorination. Sci Rep. 2017;7:233.
446. Zarrad F, Zlatopolskiy B, Krapf P, Zischler J, Neumaier B. A practical method for the preparation of ^{18}F-labeled aromatic amino acids from nucleophilic [^{18}F]fluoride and stannyl precursors for electrophilic radiohalogenation. Molecules. 2017;22:2231.
447. Zischler J, Kolks N, Modemann D, Neumaier B, Zlatopolskiy BD. Alcohol-enhanced Cu-mediated radiofluorination. Chem Eur J. 2017;23:3251–6.
448. Zlatopolskiy BD, Zischler J, Krapf P, Zarrad F, Urusova EA, Kordys E, Endepols H, Neumaier B. Copper-mediated aromatic radiofluorination revisited: efficient production of PET tracers on a preparative scale. Chem Eur J. 2015;21:5972–9.
449. Zischler J, Krapf P, Richarz R, Zlatopolskiy BD, Neumaier B. Automated synthesis of 4-[^{18}F]fluoroanisole, [^{18}F]DAA1106 and 4-[^{18}F]FPhe using Cu-mediated radiofluorination under "minimalist" conditions. Appl Radiat Isot. 2016;115:133–7.
450. Mu L, Fischer CR, Holland JP, Becaud J, Schubiger PA, Schibli R, Ametamey SM, Graham K, Stellfeld T, Dinkelborg LM, Lehmann L. ^{18}F-radiolabeling of aromatic compounds using triarylsulfonium salts. Eur J Org Chem. 2012;2012:889–92.
451. Chun J-H, Morse CL, Chin FT, Pike VW. No-carrier-added [^{18}F]fluoroarenes from the radiofluorination of diaryl sulfoxides. Chem Commun. 2013;49:2151–3.
452. Ravert HT, Holt DP, Dannals RF. Synthesis of 2-([^{18}F]fluoro)-3-[(2S)-2-azetidinylmethoxy]pyridine ([^{18}F]2FA). In: Scott PJH, Hockley BG, editors. Radiochemical syntheses. Hoboken, NJ: John Wiley and Sons; 2012.
453. Fischer S, Hiller A, Smits R, Hoepping A, Funke U, Wenzel B, Cumming P, Sabri O, Steinbach J, Brust P. Radiosynthesis of racemic and enantiomerically pure (−)-[^{18}F]flubatine—a promising PET radiotracer for neuroimaging of $\alpha_4\beta_2$ nicotinic acetylcholine receptors. Appl Radiat Isot. 2013;74:128–36.
454. Cai H, Yin DZ, Zhang L, Wang YX. The synthesis of a new probe for PET imaging reporter gene HSV1-tk: 2-amino-6-[^{18}F]fluoro-9-(4-hydroxy-3-hydroxy-

methylbutyl) purine (6-[^{18}F]fluoropenciclovir). J Label Compd Radiopharm. 2006;49:653–61.
455. Cardinale J, Schäfer M, Benešová M, Bauder-Wüst U, Leotta K, Eder M, Neels OC, Haberkorn U, Giesel FL, Kopka K. Preclinical evaluation of ^{18}F-PSMA-1007, a new prostate-specific membrane antigen ligand for prostate cancer imaging. J Nucl Med. 2017;58:425–31.
456. Cardinale J, Martin R, Remde Y, Schäfer M, Hienzsch A, Hübner S, Zerges A-M, Marx H, Hesse R, Weber K, Smits R, Hoepping A, Müller M, Neels O, Kopka K. Procedures for the GMP-compliant production and quality control of [^{18}F]PSMA-1007: a next generation radiofluorinated tracer for the detection of prostate cancer. Pharmaceuticals. 2017;10:77.
457. Smith GE, Sladen HL, Biagini SCG, Blower PJ. Inorganic approaches for radiolabelling biomolecules with fluorine-18 for imaging with positron emission tomography. Dalton Trans. 2011;40:6196–205.
458. Burke BP, Clemente GS, Archibald SJ. Boron-^{18}F containing positron emission tomography radiotracers: advances and opportunities. Contrast Media Mol Imaging. 2015;10:96–110.
459. Keller UAD, Bellac CL, Li Y, Lou YM, Lange PF, Ting R, Harwig C, Kappelhoff R, Dedhar S, Adam MJ, Ruth TJ, Benard F, Perrin DM, Overall CM. Novel matrix metalloproteinase inhibitor [^{18}F] marimastat-aryltrifluoroborate as a probe for in vivo positron emission tomography imaging in cancer. Cancer Res. 2010;70:7562–9.
460. Li Y, Ting R, Harwig CW, Auf Dem Keller U, Bellac CL, Lange PF, Inkster JAH, Schaffer P, Adam MJ, Ruth TJ, Overall CM, Perrin DM. Towards kit-like ^{18}F-labeling of marimastat, a noncovalent inhibitor drug for in vivo PET imaging cancer associated matrix metalloproteases. Medchemcomm. 2011;2:942–9.
461. Li Z, Lin T-P, Liu S, Huang C-W, Hudnall TW, Gabbai FP, Conti PS. Rapid aqueous [^{18}F]-labeling of a bodipy dye for positron emission tomography/fluorescence dual modality imaging. Chem Commun. 2011;47:9324–6.
462. Hendricks JA, Keliher EJ, Wan D, Hilderbrand SA, Weissleder R, Mazitschek R. Synthesis of [^{18}F] BODIPY: bifunctional reporter for hybrid optical/positron emission tomography imaging. Angew Chem. 2012;124:4681–4.
463. Ortmeyer CP, Haufe G, Schwegmann K, Hermann S, Schafers M, Borgel F, Wunsch B, Wagner S, Hugenberg V. Synthesis and evaluation of a [^{18}F] BODIPY-labeled caspase-inhibitor. Bioorg Med Chem. 2017;25:2167–76.
464. Schirrmacher R, Bradtmöller G, Schirrmacher E, Thews O, Tillmanns J, Siessmeier T, Buchholz HG, Bartenstein P, Wängler B, Niemeyer CM, Jurkschat K. ^{18}F-labeling of peptides by means of an organosilicon-based fluoride acceptor. Angew Chem Int Ed Engl. 2006;45:6047–50.
465. Bernard-Gauthier V, Bailey JJ, Liu Z, Wängler B, Wängler C, Jurkschat K, Perrin DM, Schirrmacher R. From unorthodox to established: the current status of ^{18}F-trifluoroborate- and ^{18}F-SiFA-based radiopharmaceuticals in PET nuclear imaging. Bioconjug Chem. 2016;27:267–79.
466. Lindner S, Michler C, Leidner S, Rensch C, Wängler C, Schirrmacher R, Bartenstein P, Wängler B. Synthesis and in vitro and in vivo evaluation of SiFA-tagged bombesin and RGD peptides as tumor imaging probes for positron emission tomography. Bioconjug Chem. 2014;25:738–49.
467. Höhne A, Mu L, Honer M, Schubiger PA, Ametamey SM, Graham K, Stellfeld T, Borkowski S, Berndorff D, Klar U, Voigtmann U, Cyr JE, Friebe M, Dinkelborg L, Srinivasan A. Synthesis, ^{18}F-labeling, and in vitro and in vivo studies of bombesin peptides modified with silicon-based building blocks. Bioconjug Chem. 2008;19:1871–9.
468. Chen QS, Meng XJ, McQuade P, Rubins D, Lin SA, Zeng ZZ, Haley H, Miller P, Trotter DG, Low PS. Folate-PEG-NOTA-Al^{18}F: a new folate based radiotracer for PET imaging of folate receptor-positive tumors. Mol Pharm. 2017;14:4353–61.
469. Al-Momani E, Israel I, Samnick S. Validation of a [Al^{18}F]PSMA-11 preparation for clinical applications. Appl Radiat Isot. 2017;130:102–8.
470. Wan WX, Guo N, Pan DH, Yu CJ, Weng Y, Luo SN, Ding H, Xu YP, Wang LZ, Lang LX, Xie QG, Yang M, Chen XY. First experience of ^{18}F-alfatide in lung cancer patients using a new lyophilized kit for rapid radiofluorination. J Nucl Med. 2013;54:691–8.
471. Cleeren F, Lecina J, Ahamed M, Raes G, Devoogdt N, Caveliers V, McQuade P, Rubins DJ, Li WP, Verbruggen A, Xavier C, Bormans G. Al^{18}F-labeling of heat-sensitive biomolecules for positron emission tomography imaging. Theranostics. 2017;7:2924–39.
472. van der Born D, Pees A, Poot AJ, Orru RVA, Windhorst AD, Vugts DJ. Fluorine-18 labelled building blocks for PET tracer synthesis. Chem Soc Rev. 2017;46:4709–73.
473. Rodnick ME, Brooks AF, Hockley BG, Henderson BD, Scott PJH. A fully-automated one-pot synthesis of [^{18}F]fluoromethylcholine with reduced dimethylaminoethanol contamination via [^{18}F]fluoromethyl tosylate. Appl Radiat Isot. 2013;78:26–32.
474. Shao X, Hockley BG, Hoareau R, Schnau PL, Scott PJH. Fully automated preparation of [^{11}C]choline and [^{18}F]fluoromethylcholine using TracerLab synthesis modules and facilitated quality control using analytical HPLC. Appl Radiat Isot. 2011;69:403–9.
475. Zuhayra M, Alfteimi A, Forstner CV, Lützen U, Meller B, Henze E. New approach for the synthesis of [^{18}F]fluoroethyltyrosine for cancer imaging: simple, fast, and high yielding automated synthesis. Bioorg Med Chem. 2009;17:7441–8.
476. Kim D-Y, Kim H-J, Yu K-H, Min J-J. Synthesis of [^{18}F]-labeled (2-(2-fluoroethoxy)ethyl)tris(4-methoxyphenyl)phosphonium cation as a potential

agent for positron emission tomography myocardial imaging. Nucl Med Biol. 2012;39:1093–8.
477. Tang G, Zeng W, Yu M, Kabalka G. Facile synthesis ofN-succinimidyl 4-[^{18}F]fluorobenzoate ([^{18}F]SFB) for protein labeling. J Label Compd Radiopharm. 2008;51:68–71.
478. Lang L, Eckelman WC. Labeling proteins at high specific activity using N-succinidyl 4-[^{18}F](fluoromethyl) benzoate. Appl Radiat Isot. 1997;48:169–73.
479. Marik J, Sutcliffe JL. Fully automated preparation of n.c.a. 4-[^{18}F]fluorobenzoic acid and N-succinimidyl 4-[^{18}F]fluorobenzoate using a Siemens/CTI chemistry process control unit (CPCU). Appl Radiat Isot. 2007;65:199–203.
480. Basuli F, Zhang X, Woodroofe CC, Jagoda EM, Choyke PL, Swenson RE. Fast indirect fluorine-18 labeling of protein/peptide using the useful 6-fluoronicotinic acid-2,3,5,6-tetrafluorophenyl prosthetic group: a method comparable to direct fluorination. J Label Compd Radiopharm. 2017;60:168–75.
481. Olberg DE, Arukwe JM, Grace D, Hjelstuen OK, Solbakken M, Kindberg GM, Cuthbertson A. One step radiosynthesis of 6-[^{18}F]fluoronicotinic acid 2,3,5,6-tetrafluorophenyl ester ([^{18}F]F-Py-TFP): a new prosthetic group for efficient labeling of biomolecules with fluorine-18. J Med Chem. 2010;53:1732–40.
482. Hedberg E, Langström B. Synthesis of 4-([^{18}F] fluoromethyl)phenyl isothiocyanate and its use in labelling oligonucleotides. Acta Chem Scand. 1997;51:1236–40.
483. Downer JB, McCarthy TJ, Edwards WB, Anderson CJ, Welch MJ. Reactivity of p-[^{18}F]fluorophenacyl bromide for radiolabeling of proteins and peptides. Appl Radiat Isot. 1997;48:907–16.
484. Cai W, Zhang X, Wu Y, Chen X. A thiol-reactive ^{18}F-labeling agent, N-[2-(4-^{18}F-fluorobenzamido) ethyl]maleimide, and synthesis of RGD peptide-based tracer for PET imaging of $\alpha_v\beta_3$ integrin expression. J Nucl Med. 2006;47:1172–80.
485. de Bruin B, Kuhnast B, Hinnen F, Yaouancq L, Amessou M, Johannes L, Samson A, Boisgard R, Tavitian B, Dolle F. 1-3-(2-[^{18}F]fluoropyridin-3-yloxy)propyl pyrrole-2,5-dione: design, synthesis, and radiosynthesis of a new [^{18}F]fluoropyridine-based maleimide reagent for the labeling of peptides and proteins. Bioconjug Chem. 2005;16:406–20.
486. Berndt M, Pietzsch J, Wuest F. Labeling of low-density lipoproteins using the ^{18}F-labeled thiol-reactive reagent N-[6-(4-[18]fluorobenzylidene)aminooxyhexyl]maleimide. Nucl Med Biol. 2007;34:5–15.
487. Speranza A, Ortosecco G, Castaldi E, Nardelli A, Pace L, Salvatore M. Fully automated synthesis procedure of 4-[^{18}F]fluorobenzaldehyde by commercial synthesizer: amino-oxi peptide labelling prosthetic group. Appl Radiat Isot. 2009;67:1664–9.
488. Kuhnast B, Dollé F. The challenge of labeling macromolecules with fluorine-18: three decades of research. Curr Radiopharm. 2010;3:174–201.
489. Maschauer S, Heilmann M, Wängler C, Schirrmacher R, Prante O. Radiosynthesis and preclinical evaluation of ^{18}F-fluoroglycosylated octreotate for somatostatin receptor imaging. Bioconjug Chem. 2016;27:2707–14.
490. Choi JY, Lee BC. Click reaction: an applicable radiolabeling method for molecular imaging. Nucl Med Mol Imaging. 2015;49:258–67.
491. Meyer J-P, Adumeau P, Lewis JS, Zeglis BM. Click chemistry and radiochemistry: the first 10 years. Bioconjug Chem. 2016;27:2791–807.
492. Mamat C, Gott M, Steinbach J. Recent progress using the Staudinger ligation for radiolabeling applications. J Label Compd Radiopharm. 2018;61:165–78.
493. Campbell-Verduyn LS, Mirfeizi L, Schoonen AK, Dierckx RA, Elsinga PH, Feringa BL. Strain-promoted copper-free "click" chemistry for ^{18}F radiolabeling of bombesin. Angew Chem Int Ed Engl. 2011;50:11117–20.
494. Agard NJ, Prescher JA, Bertozzi CR. A strain-promoted 3+2 azide-alkyne cycloaddition for covalent modification of blomolecules in living systems. J Am Chem Soc. 2004;126:15046–7.
495. Zeng DX, Zeglis BM, Lewis JS, Anderson CJ. The growing impact of bioorthogonal click chemistry on the development of radiopharmaceuticals. J Nucl Med. 2013;54:829–32.
496. Blackman ML, Royzen M, Fox JM. Tetrazine ligation: fast bioconjugation based on inverse-electron-demand Diels-Alder reactivity. J Am Chem Soc. 2008;130:13518.
497. Selvaraj R, Liu SL, Hassink M, Huang CW, Yap LP, Park R, Fox JM, Li ZB, Conti PS. Tetrazine-trans-cyclooctene ligation for the rapid construction of integrin $\alpha_v\beta_3$ targeted PET tracer based on a cyclic RGD peptide. Bioorg Med Chem Lett. 2011;21:5011–4.
498. Liu SL, Hassink M, Selvaraj R, Yap LP, Park R, Wang H, Chen XY, Fox JM, Li ZB, Conti PS. Efficient ^{18}F labeling of cysteine-containing peptides and proteins using tetrazine-trans-cyclooctene ligation. Mol Imaging. 2013;12:121–8.
499. Reiner T, Keliher EJ, Earley S, Marinelli B, Weissleder R. Synthesis and in vivo imaging of a ^{18}F-labeled PARP1 inhibitor using a chemically orthogonal scavenger-assisted high-performance method. Angew Chem Int Ed Engl. 2011;50:1922–5.
500. Keinanen O, Fung K, Pourat J, Jallinoja V, Vivier D, Pillarsetty NK, Airaksinen AJ, Lewis JS, Zeglis BM, Sarparanta M. Pretargeting of internalizing trastuzumab and cetuximab with a ^{18}F-tetrazine tracer in xenograft models. EJNMMI Res. 2017;7(1):95.
501. Gao Z, Gouverneur V, Davis BG. Enhanced aqueous Suzuki–Miyaura coupling allows site-specific polypeptide ^{18}F-labeling. J Am Chem Soc. 2013;135:13612–5.
502. Way JD, Wang M, Hamann I, Wuest M, Wuest F. Synthesis and evaluation of 2-amino-5-(4-[^{18}F]fluorophenyl)pent-4-ynoic acid ([^{18}F]FPhPA): a novel

^{18}F-labeled amino acid for oncologic PET imaging. Nucl Med Biol. 2014;41:660–9.
503. Wüst FR, Kniess T. Synthesis of 4-[^{18}F]fluoroiodobenzene and its application in Sonogashira cross-coupling reactions. J Label Compd Radiopharm. 2003;46:699–713.
504. Wüst FR, Höhne A, Metz P. Synthesis of ^{18}F-labelled cyclooxygenase-2 (COX-2) inhibitors via Stille reaction with 4-[^{18}F]fluoroiodobenzene as radiotracers for positron emission tomography (PET). Org Biomol Chem. 2005;3:503–7.
505. Qaim SM. Development of novel positron emitters for medical applications: nuclear and radiochemical aspects. Radiochim Acta. 2011;99:611–25.
506. Cascini GL, Niccoli Asabella A, Notaristefano A, Restuccia A, Ferrari C, Rubini D, Altini C, Rubini G. ^{124}Iodine: a longer-life positron emitter isotope – new opportunities in molecular imaging. Biomed Res Int. 2014;2014:672094.
507. Koehler L, Gagnon K, McQuarrie S, Wuest F. Iodine-124: a promising positron emitter for organic PET chemistry. Molecules. 2010;15:2686–718.
508. Langen KJ, Coenen HH, Roosen N, Kling P, Muzik O, Herzog H, Kuwert T, Stöcklin G, Feinendegen LE. SPECT studies of brain tumors with L-3-[^{123}I] iodo-α-methyl tyrosine: comparison with PET, ^{124}IMT and first clinical results. J Nucl Med. 1990;31:281–6.
509. Qaim SM, Hohn A, Bastian T, El-Azoney KM, Blessing G, Spellerberg S, Scholten B, Coenen HH. Some optimisation studies relevant to the production of high-purity ^{124}I and ^{124}I at a small-sized cyclotron. Appl Radiat Isot. 2003;58:69–78.
510. Moroz MA, Serganova I, Zanzonico P, Ageyeva L, Beresten T, Dyomina E, Burnazi E, Finn RD, Doubrovin M, Blasberg RG. Imaging hNET reporter gene expression with ^{124}I-MIBG. J Nucl Med. 2007;48:827–36.
511. Doubrovin M, Ponomarev V, Beresten T, Balatoni J, Bornmann W, Finn R, Humm J, Larson S, Sadelain M, Blasberg R, Tjuvajev JG. Imaging transcriptional regulation of p53-dependent genes with positron emission tomography in vivo. Proc Natl Acad Sci U S A. 2001;98:9300–5.
512. Wadsak W, Mitterhauser M. Basics and principles of radiopharmaceuticals for PET/CT. Eur J Radiol. 2010;73:461–9.
513. Post RL, Jolly PC. The linkage of sodium, potassium, and ammonium active transport across the human erythrocyte membrane. Biochim Biophys Acta. 1957;25:118–28.
514. Yoshida K, Mullani N, Gould KL. Coronary flow and flow reserve by PET simplified for clinical applications using rubidium-82 or nitrogen-13-ammonia. J Nucl Med. 1996;37:1701–12.
515. Sciacca RR, Akinboboye O, Ling Chou R, Epstein S, Bergmann SR. Measurement of myocardial blood flow with PET using 1-^{11}C-acetate. J Nucl Med. 2001;42:63–70.
516. Magata Y, Temma T, Iida H, Ogawa M, Mukai T, Iida Y, Morimoto T, Konishi J, Saji H. Development of injectable O-15 oxygen and estimation of rat OEF. J Cereb Blood Flow Metab. 2003;23:671–6.
517. Yamauchi H, Higashi T, Kagawa S, Nishii R, Kudo T, Sugimoto K, Okazawa H, Fukuyama H. Is misery perfusion still a predictor of stroke in symptomatic major cerebral artery disease? Brain. 2012;135:2515–26.
518. Holland JP, Cumming P, Vasdev N. PET radiopharmaceuticals for probing enzymes in the brain. Am J Nucl Med Mol Imaging. 2013;3:194–216.
519. Rempel BP, Price EW, Phenix CP. Molecular imaging of hydrolytic enzymes using PET and SPECT. Mol Imaging. 2017;16:1536012117717852.
520. Vander Heiden MG, Cantley LC, Thompson CB. Understanding the Warburg effect: the metabolic requirements of cell proliferation. Science. 2009;324:1029–33.
521. Sols A, Crane RK. Substrate specificity of brain hexokinase. J Biol Chem. 1954;210:581–95.
522. Brown RS, Wahl RL. Over expression of glut-1 glucose transporter in human breast cancer: an immunohistochemical study. Cancer. 1993;72:2979–85.
523. DeGrado TR, Wang SY, Holden JE, Nickles RJ, Taylor M, Stone CK. Synthesis and preliminary evaluation of ^{18}F-labeled 4-thia palmitate as a PET tracer of myocardial fatty acid oxidation. Nucl Med Biol. 2000;27:221–31.
524. Noll C, Carpentier AC. Dietary fatty acid metabolism in prediabetes. Curr Opin Lipidol. 2017;28:1–10.
525. Takala TO, Nuutila P, Pulkki K, Oikonen V, Gronroos T, Savunen T, Vahasilta T, Luotolahti M, Kallajoki M, Bergman J, Forsback S, Knuuti J. 14(R,S)-[^{18}F]fluoro-6-thia-heptadecanoic acid as a tracer of free fatty acid uptake and oxidation in myocardium and skeletal muscle. Eur J Nucl Med Mol Imaging. 2002;29:1617–22.
526. Clary GL, Tsai C-F, Guynn RW. Substrate specificity of choline kinase. Arch Biochem Biophys. 1987;254:214–21.
527. Awwad HM, Geisel J, Obeid R. The role of choline in prostate cancer. Clin Biochem. 2012;45:1548–53.
528. Calabria F, Gallo G, Schillaci O, Cascini GL. Biodistribution, imaging protocols and diagnostic accuracy of PET with tracers of lipogenesis in imaging prostate cancer: a comparison between ^{11}C-choline, ^{18}F-fluoroethylcholine and ^{18}F-methylcholine. Curr Pharm Des. 2015;21:4738–47.
529. DeGrado TR, Baldwin SW, Wang S, Orr MD, Liao RP, Friedman HS, Reiman R, Price DT, Coleman RE. Synthesis and evaluation of ^{18}F-labeled choline analogs as oncologic PET tracers. J Nucl Med. 2001;42:1805–14.
530. Hara T. ^{18}F-Fluorocholine: a new oncologic PET tracer. J Nucl Med. 2001;42:1815–7.
531. Oprea-Lager DE, van Kanten MP, van Moorselaar RJA, van den Eertwegh AJM, van de Ven PM, Bijnsdorp IV, Hoekstra OS, Geldof AA. [^{18}F]Fluoromethylcholine as a chemotherapy response

read-out in prostate cancer cells. Mol Imaging Biol. 2015;17:319–27.
532. Hodolič M. Imaging of prostate cancer using ^{18}F-choline PET/computed tomography. PET Clin. 2017;12:173–84.
533. Blau M, Nagler W, Bender MA. Fluorine-18: a new isotope for bone scanning. J Nucl Med. 1962;3:332–4.
534. Grant FD, Fahey FH, Packard AB, Davis RT, Alavi A, Treves ST. Skeletal PET with ^{18}F-fluoride: applying new technology to an old tracer. J Nucl Med. 2008;49:68–78.
535. Shields AF, Grierson JR, Kozawa SM, Zheng M. Development of labeled thymidine analogs for imaging tumor proliferation. Nucl Med Biol. 1996;23:17–22.
536. McKinley ET, Ayers GD, Smith RA, Saleh SA, Zhao P, Washington MK, Coffey RJ, Manning HC. Limits of [^{18}F]-FLT PET as a biomarker of proliferation in oncology. PLoS One. 2013;8:e58938.
537. Schelhaas S, Heinzmann K, Bollineni VR, Kramer GM, Liu Y, Waterton JC, Aboagye EO, Shields AF, Soloviev D, Jacobs AH. Preclinical applications of 3′-deoxy-3′-[^{18}F]fluoro-thymidine in oncology – a systematic review. Theranostics. 2017;7:40–50.
538. Alauddin MM. Nucleoside-based probes for imaging tumor proliferation using positron emission tomography. J Label Compd Radiopharm. 2013;56:237–43.
539. Krohn KA, Link JM, Mason RP. Molecular imaging of hypoxia. J Nucl Med. 2008;49:129S–48S.
540. Bell C, Dowson N, Fay M, Thomas P, Puttick S, Gal Y, Rose S. Hypoxia imaging in gliomas with ^{18}F-fluoromisonidazole PET: toward clinical translation. Semin Nucl Med. 2015;45:136–50.
541. Wuest M, Wuest F. Positron emission tomography radiotracers for imaging hypoxia. J Label Compd Radiopharm. 2013;56:244–50.
542. Grönroos T, Eskola O, Lehtiö K, Minn H, Marjamäki P, Bergman J, Haaparanta M, Forsback S, Solin O. Pharmacokinetics of [^{18}F]FETNIM: a potential hypoxia marker for PET. J Nucl Med. 2001;42:1397–404.
543. Hayashi K, Furutsuka K, Takei M, Muto M, Nakao R, Aki H, Suzuki K, Fukumura T. High-yield automated synthesis of [^{18}F]fluoroazomycin arabinoside ([^{18}F]FAZA) for hypoxia-specific tumor imaging. Appl Radiat Isot. 2011;69:1007–13.
544. Reischl G, Ehrlichmann W, Bieg C, Solbach C, Kumar P, Wiebe LI, Machulla HJ. Preparation of the hypoxia imaging PET tracer [^{18}F]FAZA: reaction parameters and automation. Appl Radiat Isot. 2005;62:897–901.
545. Kaneta T, Takai Y, Iwata R, Hakamatsuka T, Yasuda H, Nakayama K, Ishikawa Y, Watanuki S, Furumoto S, Funaki Y, Nakata E, Jingu K, Tsujitani M, Ito M, Fukuda H, Takahashi S, Yamada S. Initial evaluation of dynamic human imaging using ^{18}F-FRP170 as a new PET tracer for imaging hypoxia. Ann Nucl Med. 2007;21:101–7.
546. Eskola O, Grönroos TJ, Forsback S, Tuomela J, Komar G, Bergman J, Härkönen P, Haaparanta M, Minn H, Solin O. Tracer level electrophilic synthesis and pharmacokinetics of the hypoxia tracer [^{18}F]EF5. Mol Imaging Biol. 2012;14:205–12.
547. Silvoniemi A, Suilamo S, Laitinen T, Forsback S, Löyttyniemi E, Vaittinen S, Saunavaara V, Solin O, Grönroos TJ, Minn H. Repeatability of tumour hypoxia imaging using [^{18}F]EF5 PET/CT in head and neck cancer. Eur J Nucl Med Mol Imaging. 2018;45:161–9.
548. Brosnan JT, Brosnan ME. The sulfur-containing amino acids: an overview. J Nutr. 2006;136:1636S–40S.
549. Huang C, McConathy J. Fluorine-18 labeled amino acids for oncologic imaging with positron emission tomography. Curr Top Med Chem. 2013;13:871–91.
550. Jager PL, Vaalburg W, Pruim J, de Vries EGE, Langen K-J, Piers DA. Radiolabeled amino acids: basic aspects and clinical applications in oncology. J Nucl Med. 2001;42:432–45.
551. Gulyás B, Halldin C. New PET radiopharmaceuticals beyond FDG for brain tumor imaging. Q J Nucl Med Mol Imaging. 2012;56:173–90.
552. Wester HJ, Herz M, Weber W, Heiss P, Senekowitsch-Schmidtke R, Schwaiger M, Stöcklin G. Synthesis and radiopharmacology of O-(2-[^{18}F]fluoroethyl)-L-tyrosine for tumor imaging. J Nucl Med. 1999;40:205–12.
553. Langen K-J, Galldiks N, Hattingen E, Shah NJ. Advances in neuro-oncology imaging. Nat Rev Neurol. 2017;13:279–89.
554. Langen K-J, Hamacher K, Weckesser M, Floeth F, Stoffels G, Bauer D, Coenen HH, Pauleit D. O-(2-[^{18}F]fluoroethyl)-l-tyrosine: uptake mechanisms and clinical applications. Nucl Med Biol. 2006;33:287–94.
555. Geisler S, Ermert J, Stoffels G, Willuweit A, Galldiks N, Filss CP, Shah NJ, Coenen HH, Langen KJ. Isomers of 4-[^{18}F]fluoroproline: radiosynthesis, biological evaluation and results in humans using PET. Curr Radiopharm. 2014;7:123–32.
556. Goodman MM, Yu W, Jarkas N. Synthesis and biological properties of radiohalogenated α,α-disubstituted amino acids for PET and SPECT imaging of amino acid transporters (AATs). J Label Compd Radiopharm. 2018;61:272–90.
557. Shoup TM, Olson J, Hoffman JM, Votaw J, Eshima D, Eshima L, Camp VM, Stabin M, Votaw D, Goodman MM. Synthesis and evaluation of [^{18}F]1-amino-3-fluorocyclobutane-1-carboxylic acid to image brain tumors. J Nucl Med. 1999;40:331–8.
558. Wallitt KL, Khan SR, Dubash S, Tam HH, Khan S, Barwick TD. Clinical PET imaging in prostate cancer. Radiographics. 2017;37:1512–36.
559. Politis M. Neuroimaging in Parkinson disease: from research setting to clinical practice. Nat Rev Neurol. 2014;10:708–22.
560. Lussey-Lepoutre C, Hindié E, Montravers F, Detour J, Ribeiro MJS, Taïeb D, Imperiale A. The current

role of ^{18}F-FDOPA PET for neuroendocrine tumor imaging. Med Nucl. 2016;40:20–30.
561. Inoue T, Shibasaki T, Oriuchi N, Aoyagi K, Tomiyoshi K, Amano S, Mikuni M, Itsurou I, Aoki J, Endo K. [18]F α-methyl tyrosine PET studies in patients with brain tumors. J Nucl Med. 1999;40:399–405.
562. Wienhard K, Herholz K, Coenen HH, Rudolf J, Kling P, Stöcklin G, Heiss W-D. Increased amino acid transport into brain tumors measured by PET of L-(2-^{18}F)fluorotyrosine. J Nucl Med. 1991;32:1338–46.
563. Wahl LM, Chen JJ, Thompson M, Chirakal R, Nahmias C. The time course of metabolites in human plasma after 6-[^{18}F]fluoro-L-m-tyrosine administration. Eur J Nucl Med. 1999;26:1407–12.
564. Moolten FL. Tumor chemosensitivity conferred by inserted herpes thymidine kinase genes: paradigm for a prospective cancer control strategy. Cancer Res. 1986;46:5276–81.
565. Haberkorn U, Oberdorfer F, Gebert J, Morr I, Haack K, Weber K, Lindauer M, vanKaick G, Schackert HK. Monitoring gene therapy with cytosine deaminase: in vitro studies using tritiated-5-fluorocytosine. J Nucl Med. 1996;37:87–94.
566. Alrabiah FA, Sacks SL. New antiherpesvirus agents – their targets and therapeutic potential. Drugs. 1996;52:17–32.
567. Gambhir SS, Barrio JR, Herschman HR, Phelps ME. Imaging gene expression: principles and assays. J Nucl Cardiol. 1999;6:219–33.
568. Yaghoubi SS, Campbell DO, Radu CG, Czernin J. Positron emission tomography reporter genes and reporter probes: gene and cell therapy applications. Theranostics. 2012;2:374–91.
569. Ray P, Bauer E, Lyer M, Barrio JR, Satyamurthy N, Phelps ME, Herschman HR, Gambhir SS. Monitoring gene therapy with reporter gene imaging. Semin Nucl Med. 2001;31:312–20.
570. Tjuvajev JG, Avril N, Oku T, Sasajima T, Miyagawa T, Joshi R, Safer M, Beattie B, DiResta G, Daghighian F, Augensen F, Koutcher J, Zweit J, Humm J, Larson SM, Finn R, Blasberg R. Imaging Herpes virus thymidine kinase gene transfer and expression by positron emission tomography. Cancer Res. 1998;58:4333–41.
571. Alauddin MM, Conti PS. Synthesis and preliminary evaluation of 9-(4-[^{18}F]-fluoro-3-hydroxymethylbutyl)guanine ([^{18}F]FHBG): a new potential imaging agent for viral infection and gene therapy using PET. Nucl Med Biol. 1998;25:175–80.
572. Iyer M, Barrio JR, Namavari M, Bauer E, Satyamurthy N, Nguyen K, Toyokuni T, Phelps ME, Herschman HR, Gambhir SS. 8-[^{18}F]fluoropenciclovir: an improved reporter probe for imaging HSV1-tk reporter gene expression in vivo using PET. J Nucl Med. 2001;42:96–105.
573. Alauddin MM, Gelovani JG. Radiolabeled nucleoside analogues for PET imaging of HSV1-tk gene expression. Curr Top Med Chem. 2010;10:1617–32.
574. Mathis CA, Lopresti BJ, Ikonomovic MD, Klunk WE. Small-molecule PET tracers for Imaging Proteinopathies. Semin Nucl Med. 2017;47:553–75.
575. Spencer B, Rockenstein E, Crews L, Marr R, Masliah E. Novel strategies for Alzheimer's disease treatment. Expert Opin Biol Ther. 2007;7:1853–67.
576. Trojanowski JQ, Shin RW, Schmidt ML, Lee VMY. Relationship between plaques, tangles, and dystrophic processes in Alzheimer's disease. Neurobiol Aging. 1995;16:335–40.
577. George N, Gean E, Nandi A, Brašić JR, Wong DF. Radiotracers used to image the brains of patients with Alzheimer's disease imaging of the human brain in health and disease. Boston, MA: Academic; 2014. p. 407–16.
578. Oukoloff K, Cieslikiewicz-Bouet M, Chao S, Branquinho ED, Bouteiller C, Jean L, Renard PY. PET and SPECT radiotracers for Alzheimer's disease. Curr Med Chem. 2015;22:3278–304.
579. Villemagne VL, Furumoto S, Fodero-Tavoletti M, Harada R, Mulligan RS, Kudo Y, Masters CL, Yanai K, Rowe CC, Okamura N. The challenges of tau imaging. Future Neurol. 2012;7:409–21.
580. Agdeppa ED, Kepe V, Liu J, Flores-Torres S, Satyamurthy N, Petric A, Cole GM, Small GW, Huang SC, Barrio JR. Binding characteristics of radiofluorinated 6-dialkylamino-2-naphthylethylidene derivatives as positron emission tomography imaging probes for beta-amyloid plaques in Alzheimer's disease. J Neurosci. 2001;21:Article no. RC189.
581. Shoghi-Jadid K, Small GW, Agdeppa ED, Kepe V, Ercoli LM, Siddarth P, Read S, Satyamurthy N, Petric A, Huang S-C. Localization of neurofibrillary tangles and beta-amyloid plaques in the brains of living patients with Alzheimer disease. Am J Geriatr Psychiatry. 2002;10:24–35.
582. Klunk WE, Engler H, Nordberg A, Wang YM, Blomqvist G, Holt DP, Bergstrom M, Savitcheva I, Huang GF, Estrada S, Ausen B, Debnath ML, Barletta J, Price JC, Sandell J, Lopresti BJ, Wall A, Koivisto P, Antoni G, Mathis CA, Langstrom B. Imaging brain amyloid in Alzheimer's disease with Pittsburgh compound-B. Ann Neurol. 2004;55:306–19.
583. Zhang S, Han D, Tan X, Feng J, Guo Y, Ding Y. Diagnostic accuracy of ^{18}F-FDG and ^{11}C-PIB-PET for prediction of short-term conversion to Alzheimer's disease in subjects with mild cognitive impairment. Int J Clin Pract. 2012;66:185–98.
584. Rowe CC, Ackerman U, Browne W, Mulligan R, Pike KL, O'Keefe G, Tochon-Danguy H, Chan G, Berlangieri SU, Jones G, Dickinson-Rowe KL, Kung HP, Zhang W, Kung MP, Skovronsky D, Dyrks T, Holl G, Krause S, Friebe M, Lehman L, Lindemann S, Dinkelborg LM, Masters CL, Villemagne VL. Imaging of amyloid b in Alzheimer's disease with ^{18}F-BAY94-9172 a novel PET tracer: proof of mechanism. Lancet Neurol. 2008;7:129–35.

585. Martinez G, Vernooij RWM, Padilla PF, Zamora J, Cosp XB, Flicker L. ^{18}F PET with florbetapir for the early diagnosis of Alzheimer's disease dementia and other dementias in people with mild cognitive impairment (MCI). Cochrane Database Syst Rev. 2017;11:CD012216.
586. Martinez G, Vernooij RWM, Padilla PF, Zamora J, Flicker L, Cosp XB. ^{18}F PET with florbetaben for the early diagnosis of Alzheimer's disease dementia and other dementias in people with mild cognitive impairment (MCI). Cochrane Database Syst Rev. 2017;11:CD012883.
587. Cselényi Z, Jönhagen ME, Forsberg A, Halldin C, Julin P, Schou M, Johnström P, Varnäs K, Svensson S, Farde L. Clinical validation of ^{18}F-AZD4694, an amyloid-beta-specific PET radioligand. J Nucl Med. 2012;53:415–24.
588. Hostetler ED, Sanabria-Bohorquez S, Fan H, Zeng ZZ, Gammage L, Miller P, O'Malley S, Connolly B, Mulhearn J, Harrison ST, Wolkenberg SE, Barrow JC, Williams DL, Hargreaves RJ, Sur C, Cook JJ. [^{18}F] Fluoroazabenzoxazoles as potential amyloid plaque PET tracers: synthesis and in vivo evaluation in rhesus monkey. Nucl Med Biol. 2011;38:1193–203.
589. Ariza M, Kolb HC, Moechars D, Rombouts F, Andrés JI. Tau positron emission tomography (PET) imaging: past, present, and future. J Med Chem. 2015;58:4365–82.
590. Fodero-Tavoletti MT, Okamura N, Furumoto S, Mulligan RS, Connor AR, McLean CA, Cao DN, Rigopoulos A, Cartwright GA, O'Keefe G, Gong S, Adlard PA, Barnham KJ, Rowe CC, Masters CL, Kudo Y, Cappai R, Yanai K, Villemagne VL. ^{18}F-THK523: a novel in vivo tau imaging ligand for Alzheimer's disease. Brain. 2011;134:1089–100.
591. Okamura N, Furumoto S, Harada R, Tago T, Yoshikawa T, Fodero-Tavoletti M, Mulligan RS, Villemagne VL, Akatsu H, Yamamoto T, Arai H, Iwata R, Yanai K, Kudo Y. Novel ^{18}F-labeled arylquinoline derivatives for noninvasive imaging of tau pathology in Alzheimer disease. J Nucl Med. 2013;54:1420–7.
592. Hashimoto H, Kawamura K, Igarashi N, Takei M, Fujishiro T, Aihara Y, Shiomi S, Muto M, Ito T, Furutsuka K, Yamasaki T, Yui JJ, Xie L, Ono M, Hatori A, Nemoto K, Suhara T, Higuchi M, Zhang MR. Radiosynthesis, photoisomerization, biodistribution, and metabolite analysis of ^{11}C-PBB3 as a clinically useful PET probe for imaging of tau pathology. J Nucl Med. 2014;55:1532–8.
593. Shidahara M, Watabe H, Tashiro M, Okamura N, Furumoto S, Watanuki S, Furukawa K, Arakawa Y, Funaki Y, Iwata R, Gonda K, Kudo Y, Arai H, Ishiwata K, Yanai K. Quantitative kinetic analysis of PET amyloid imaging agents [^{11}C]BF227 and [^{18}F]FACT in human brain. Nucl Med Biol. 2015;42:734–44.
594. Wooten DW, Guehl NJ, Verwer EE, Shoup TM, Yokell DL, Zubcevik N, Vasdev N, Zafonte RD, Johnson KA, Fakhri GE, Normandin MD. Pharmacokinetic evaluation of the tau PET radiotracer ^{18}F-T807 (^{18}F-AV-1451) in human subjects. J Nucl Med. 2017;58:484–91.
595. Declercq L, Celen S, Lecina J, Ahamed M, Tousseyn T, Moechars D, Alcazar J, Ariza M, Fierens K, Bottelbergs A, Mariën J, Vandenberghe R, Andres IJ, Van Laere K, Verbruggen A, Bormans G. Comparison of new tau PET-tracer candidates with [^{18}F]T808 and [^{18}F]T807. Mol Imaging. 2016;15:1–15.
596. Bredesen DE. Genetic control of neural cell apoptosis. Perspect Dev Neurobiol. 1996;3:101–9.
597. Faust A, Hermann S, Wagner S, Haufe G, Schober O, Schäfers M, Kopka K. Molecular imaging of apoptosis in vivo with scintigraphic and optical biomarkers – a status report. Anti Cancer Agents Med Chem. 2009;9:968–85.
598. Elmore S. Apoptosis: a review of programmed cell death. Toxicol Pathol. 2007;35:495–516.
599. Elmenhorst D, Bier D, Holschbach M, Bauer A. Imaging of adenosine receptors PET and SPECT of neurobiological systems. New York, NY: Springer; 2014. p. 181–98.
600. Boschi S, Lodi F, Boschi L, Nanni C, Chondrogiannis S, Colletti PM, Rubello D, Fanti S. ^{11}C-meta-hydroxyephedrine a promising PET radiopharmaceutical for imaging the sympathetic nervous system. Clin Nucl Med. 2015;40:E96–E103.
601. Andersson JD, Halldin C. PET radioligands targeting the brain GABAA/benzodiazepine receptor complex. J Label Compd Radiopharm. 2013;56:196–206.
602. Ahamed M, Verbruggen A, Bormans G. Synthetic strategies for radioligands for in vivo imaging of brain cannabinoid type-1 receptors. J Label Compd Radiopharm. 2013;56:207–14.
603. Minn H, Kauhanen S, Seppanen M, Nuutila P. ^{18}F-FDOPA: a multiple-target molecule. J Nucl Med. 2009;50:1915–8.
604. Becker G, Bahri MA, Michel A, Hustadt F, Garraux G, Luxen A, Lemaire C, Plenevaux A. Comparative assessment of 6-[^{18}F]fluoro-L-m-tyrosine and 6-[^{18}F] fluoro-L-dopa to evaluate dopaminergic presynaptic integrity in a Parkinson's disease rat model. J Neurochem. 2017;141:626–35.
605. Prante O, Maschauer S, Banerjee A. Radioligands for the dopamine receptor subtypes. J Label Compd Radiopharm. 2013;56:130–48.
606. Funke U, Vugts DJ, Janssen B, Spaans A, Kruijer PS, Lammertsma AA, Perk LR, Windhorst AD. ^{11}C-labeled and ^{18}F-labeled PET ligands for subtype-specific imaging of histamine receptors in the brain. J Label Compd Radiopharm. 2013;56:120–9.
607. Mu L, Schubiger PA, Ametamey SM. Radioligands for the PET imaging of metabotropic glutamate receptor subtype 5 (mGluR5). Curr Top Med Chem. 2010;10:1558–68.
608. Sobrio F. Radiosynthesis of carbon-11 and fluorine-18 labelled radiotracers to image the ionotropic and metabotropic glutamate receptors. J Label Compd Radiopharm. 2013;56:180–6.

609. Sephton SM. Positron emission tomography of metabotropic glutamate receptors. In: Parrot S, Denoroy L, editors. Biochemical approaches for glutamatergic neurotransmission. New York, NY: Springer; 2018. p. 51–82.
610. Horti AG, Kuwabara H, Holt DP, Dannals RF, Wong DF. Recent PET radioligands with optimal brain kinetics for imaging nicotinic acetylcholine receptors. J Label Compd Radiopharm. 2013;56:159–66.
611. Sabri O, Meyer PM, Gräf S, Hesse S, Wilke S, Becker G-A, Rullmann M, Patt M, Luthardt J, Wagenknecht G, Hoepping A, Smits R, Franke A, Sattler B, Tiepolt S, Fischer S, Deuther-Conrad W, Hegerl U, Barthel H, Schönknecht P, Brust P. Cognitive correlates of α4β2 nicotinic acetylcholine receptors in mild Alzheimer's dementia. Brain. 2018;141:1840–54.
612. Pike VW. Considerations in the development of reversibly binding PET radioligands for brain imaging. Curr Med Chem. 2016;23:1818–69.
613. McGinnity CJ, Hammers A, Riaño Barros DA, Luthra SK, Jones PA, Trigg W, Micallef C, Symms MR, Brooks DJ, Koepp MJ, Duncan JS. Initial evaluation of ^{18}F-GE-179, a putative PET tracer for activated N-methyl d-aspartate receptors. J Nucl Med. 2014;55:423–30.
614. Lohith TG, Zoghbi SS, Morse CL, Araneta MDF, Barth VN, Goebl NA, Tauscher JT, Pike VW, Innis RB, Fujita M. Retest imaging of [^{11}C]NOP-1A binding to nociceptin/orphanin FQ peptide (NOP) receptors in the brain of healthy humans. NeuroImage. 2014;87:89–95.
615. Dannals RF. Positron emission tomography radioligands for the opioid system. J Label Compd Radiopharm. 2013;56:187–95.
616. Zimmer L, Le Bars D. Current status of positron emission tomography radiotracers for serotonin receptors in humans. J Label Compd Radiopharm. 2013;56:105–13.
617. Banister SD, Manoli M, Kassiou M. The development of radiotracers for imaging sigma (σ) receptors in the central nervous system (CNS) using positron emission tomography (PET). J Label Compd Radiopharm. 2013;56:215–24.
618. Riss PJ, Stockhofe K, Roesch F. Tropane-derived ^{11}C-labelled and ^{18}F-labelled DAT ligands. J Label Compd Radiopharm. 2013;56:149–58.
619. Passchier J, Gunn RN, Van Waarde A. Imaging type 1 glycine transporters in the CNS using positron emission tomography. In: de Vries EFJ, Luiten PGM, Otte A, editors. PET and SPECT of neurobiological systems. New York, NY: Springer; 2014. p. 321–30.
620. Takano A, Gulyás B, Varrone A, Halldin C. Comparative evaluations of norepinephrine transporter radioligands with reference tissue models in rhesus monkeys: (S,S)-[^{18}F]FMeNER-D_2 and (S,S)-[^{11}C]MeNER. Eur J Nucl Med Mol Imaging. 2009;36:1885.
621. Kilbourn MR. Small molecule PET tracers for transporter imaging. Semin Nucl Med. 2017;47:536–52.
622. Stehouwer JS, Goodman MM. ^{11}C and ^{18}F PET radioligands for the serotonin transporter (SERT). J Label Compd Radiopharm. 2013;56:114–9.
623. Kilbourn MR. Radioligands for imaging vesicular monoamine transporters. In: Dierckx RAJO, et al., editors. PET and SPECT of neurobiological systems. Berlin: Springer; 2014. p. 765–90.
624. Aghourian M, Legault-Denis C, Soucy JP, Rosa-Neto P, Gauthier S, Kostikov A, Gravel P, Bedard MA. Quantification of brain cholinergic denervation in Alzheimer's disease using PET imaging with [^{18}F]-FEOBV. Mol Psychiatry. 2017;22:1531–8.
625. Damont A, Roeda D, Dollé F. The potential of carbon-11 and fluorine-18 chemistry: illustration through the development of positron emission tomography radioligands targeting the translocator protein 18 kDa. J Label Compd Radiopharm. 2013;56:96–104.
626. Fan Z, Calsolaro V, Atkinson RA, Femminella GD, Waldman A, Buckley C, Trigg W, Brooks DJ, Hinz R, Edison P. Flutriciclamide (^{18}F-GE180) PET: first-in-human PET study of novel third-generation in vivo marker of human translocator protein. J Nucl Med. 2016;57:1753–9.
627. Ghadery C, Koshimori Y, Coakeley S, Harris M, Rusjan P, Kim J, Houle S, Strafella AP. Microglial activation in Parkinson's disease using [^{18}F]-FEPPA. J Neuroinflammation. 2017;14:8.
628. Reubi JC, Laissue J, Krenning E, Lamberts SWJ. Somatostatin receptors in human cancer: incidence, characteristics, functional correlates and clinical implications. J Steroid Biochem Mol Biol. 1992;43:27–35.
629. Virgolini I, Pangerl T, Bischof C, Smith-Jones P, Peck-Radosavljevic M. Somatostatin receptor subtype expression in human tissues: a prediction for diagnosis and treatment of cancer? Eur J Clin Investig. 1997;27:645–7.
630. Breeman WAP, de Blois E, Sze Chan H, Konijnenberg M, Kwekkeboom DJ, Krenning EP. ^{68}Ga-labeled DOTA-peptides and ^{68}Ga-labeled radiopharmaceuticals for positron emission tomography: current status of research, clinical applications, and future perspectives. Semin Nucl Med. 2011;41:314–21.
631. Schottelius M, Wester H-J. Molecular imaging targeting peptide receptors. Methods. 2009;48:161–77.
632. Mintun MA, Welch MJ, Siegel BA, Mathias CJ, Brodack JW, McGuire AH, Katzenellenbogen JA. Breast cancer: PET imaging of estrogen receptors. Radiology. 1988;169:45–8.
633. Hostetler ED, Jonson SD, Welch MJ, Katzenellenbogen JA. Synthesis of 2-[^{18}F]fluoroestradiol, a potential diagnostic imaging agent for breast cancer: strategies to achieve nucleophilic substitution of an electron-rich aromatic ring with [^{18}F]F–. J Org Chem. 1999;64:178–85.
634. Kumar P, Mercer J, Doerkson C, Tonkin K, McEwan AJB. Clinical production, stability studies and PET imaging with 16-α-[^{18}F]fluoroestradiol ([^{18}F]FES) in ER positive breast cancer patients. J Pharm Pharm Sci. 2007;10:256s–65s.

635. Dehdashti F, Laforest R, Gao F, Aft RL, Dence CS, Zhou D, Shoghi KI, Siegel BA, Katzenellenbogen JA, Welch MJ. Assessment of progesterone receptors in breast carcinoma by PET with 21-^{18}F-fluoro-16α,17α-[(R)-(1′-α-furylmethylidene) dioxy]-19-norpregn-4-ene-3,20-dione. J Nucl Med. 2012;53:363–70.
636. Hood JD, Cheresh DA. Role of integrins in cell invasion and migration. Nat Rev Cancer. 2002;2:91.
637. Beer AJ, Haubner R, Sarbia M, Goebel M, Luderschmidt S, Grosu AL, Schnell O, Niemeyer M, Kessler H, Wester HJ, Weber WA, Schwaiger M. Positron emission tomography using [^{18}F]Galacto-RGD identifies the level of integrin a_vb_3 expression in man. Clin Cancer Res. 2006;12:3942–9.
638. Mittra ES, Goris ML, Iagaru AH, Kardan A, Burton L, Berganos R, Chang E, Liu SL, Shen B, Chin FT, Chen XY, Gambhir SS. Pilot pharmacokinetic and dosimetric studies of ^{18}F-FPPRGD$_2$: a PET radiopharmaceutical agent for imaging $\alpha_v\beta_3$ integrin levels. Radiology. 2011;260:182–91.
639. Mena E, Owenius R, Turkbey B, Sherry R, Bratslavsky G, Macholl S, Miller MP, Somer EJ, Lindenberg L, Adler S, Shih J, Choyke P, Kurdziel K. [^{18}F]Fluciclatide in the in vivo evaluation of human melanoma and renal tumors expressing $\alpha_v\beta_3$ and $\alpha_v\beta_5$ integrins. Eur J Nucl Med Mol Imaging. 2014;41:1879–88.
640. Backer MV, Backer JM. Imaging key biomarkers of tumor angiogenesis. Theranostics. 2012;2:502–15.
641. Cai H, Conti PS. RGD-based PET tracers for imaging receptor integrin $\alpha_v\beta_3$ expression. J Label Compd Radiopharm. 2013;56:264–79.
642. Sun X, Li Y, Liu T, Li Z, Zhang X, Chen X. Peptide-based imaging agents for cancer detection. Adv Drug Deliv Rev. 2017;110-111:38–51.
643. Rylova SN, Barnucz E, Fani M, Braun F, Werner M, Lassmann S, Maecke HR, Weber WA. Does imaging $\alpha_v\beta_3$ integrin expression with PET detect changes in angiogenesis during bevacizumab therapy? J Nucl Med. 2014;55:1878–84.
644. Rowe SP, Macura KJ, Mena E, Blackford AL, Nadal R, Antonarakis ES, Eisenberger M, Carducci M, Fan H, Dannals RF, Chen Y, Mease RC, Szabo Z, Pomper MG, Cho SY. PSMA-based [^{18}F]DCFPyL PET/CT is superior to conventional imaging for lesion detection in patients with metastatic prostate cancer. Mol Imaging Biol. 2016;18:411–9.
645. Giesel FL, Hadaschik B, Cardinale J, Radtke J, Vinsensia M, Lehnert W, Kesch C, Tolstov Y, Singer S, Grabe N, Duensing S, Schafer M, Neels OC, Mier W, Haberkorn U, Kopka K, Kratochwil C. F-18 labelled PSMA-1007: biodistribution, radiation dosimetry and histopathological validation of tumor lesions in prostate cancer patients. Eur J Nucl Med Mol Imaging. 2017;44:678–88.
646. Zinnhardt B, Pigeon H, Thézé B, Viel T, Wachsmuth L, Fricke IB, Schelhaas S, Honold L, Schwegmann K, Wagner S, Faust A, Faber C, Kuhlmann MT, Hermann S, Schäfers M, Winkeler A, Jacobs AH. Combined PET imaging of the inflammatory tumor microenvironment identifies margins of unique radiotracer uptake. Cancer Res. 2017;77:1831–41.
647. Hughes AJ. Clinicopathological aspects of Parkinson's disease. Eur Neurol. 1997;38:13–20.
648. Firnau G, Sood S, Chirakal R, Nahmias C, Garnett ES. Cerebral metabolism of 6-[^{18}F]fluoro-l-3,4-dihydroxyphenylalanine in the primate. J Neurochem. 1987;48:1077–82.
649. DeJesus OT, Endres CJ, Shelton SE, Nickles RJ, Holden JE. Evaluation of fluorinated m-tyrosine analogs as PET imaging agents of dopamine nerve terminals: comparison with 6-fluorodopa. J Nucl Med. 1997;38:630–6.
650. Wong D, Wagner H, Tune L, Dannals R, Pearlson G, Links J, Tamminga C, Broussolle E, Ravert H, Wilson A, et al. Positron emission tomography reveals elevated D2 dopamine receptors in drug-naive schizophrenics. Science. 1986;234:1558–63.
651. Farde L, Ehrin E, Eriksson L, Greitz T, Hall H, Hedstrom CG, Litton JE, Sedvall G. Substituted benzamides as ligands for visualization of dopamine receptor binding in the human brain by positron emission tomography. Proc Natl Acad Sci U S A. 1985;82:3863–7.
652. Albrecht DS, Granziera C, Hooker JM, Loggia ML. In vivo imaging of human neuroinflammation. ACS Chem Neurosci. 2016;7:470–83.
653. Kersemans K, Van Laeken N, De Vos F. Radiochemistry devoted to the production of monoamine oxidase (MAO-A and MAO-B) ligands for brain imaging with positron emission tomography. J Label Compd Radiopharm. 2013;56:78–88.
654. Bentzen SM. Theragnostic imaging for radiation oncology: dose-painting by numbers. Lancet Oncol. 2005;6:112–7.
655. Verburg FA, Heinzel A, Hänscheid H, Mottaghy FM, Luster M, Giovanella L. Nothing new under the nuclear sun: towards 80 years of theranostics in nuclear medicine. Eur J Nucl Med Mol Imaging. 2014;41:199–201.
656. Vogenberg FR, Isaacson Barash C, Pursel M. Personalized medicine: part 1: evolution and development into theranostics. P T. 2010;35:560–76.
657. Funkhouser J. Reinventing pharma: the theranostic revolution. Curr Drug Discov. 2002;2002:17–9.
658. Jeelani S, Jagat Reddy R, Maheswaran T, Asokan G, Dany A, Anand B. Theranostics: a treasured tailor for tomorrow. J Pharm Bioallied Sci. 2014;6:6–8.
659. Liao S, Penney BC, Wroblewski K, Zhang H, Simon CA, Kampalath R, Shih M-C, Shimada N, Chen S, Salgia R, Appelbaum DE, Suzuki K, Chen C-T, Pu Y. Prognostic value of metabolic tumor burden on ^{18}F-FDG PET in nonsurgical patients with non-small cell lung cancer. Eur J Nucl Med Mol Imaging. 2012;39:27–38.
660. Velikyan I. Molecular imaging and radiotherapy: theranostics for personalized patient management. Theranostics. 2012;2:424–6.

661. Teng F-F, Meng X, Sun X-D, Yu J-M. New strategy for monitoring targeted therapy: molecular imaging. Int J Nanomedicine. 2013;8:3703–13.
662. Gerber DE. Targeted therapies: a new generation of cancer treatments. Am Fam Physician. 2008;77:311–9.
663. Jadvar H, Chen X, Cai W, Mahmood U. Radiotheranostics in cancer diagnosis and management. Radiology. 2018;286:388–400.
664. Fahey FH, Grant FD, Thrall JH. Saul Hertz, MD, and the birth of radionuclide therapy. EJNMMI Phys. 2017;4:15.
665. Hertz B. Dr. Saul Hertz (1905–1950) discovers the medical uses of radioactive iodine: the first targeted cancer therapy thyroid cancer – advances in diagnosis and therapy. London: IntechOpen; 2016.
666. Seidlin SM, Marinelli LD, Oshry E. Radioactive iodine therapy: effect on functioning metastases of adenocarcinoma of the thyroid. J Am Med Assoc. 1946;132:838–47.
667. Volkert WA, Huffman TJ. Therapeutic radiopharmaceuticals. Chem Rev. 1999;99:2269–92.
668. Luster M, Clarke SE, Dietlein M, Lassmann M, Lind P, Oyen WJG, Tennvall J, Bombardieri E. Guidelines for radioiodine therapy of differentiated thyroid cancer. Eur J Nucl Med Mol Imaging. 2008;35:1941.
669. Okarvi SM. Peptide-based radiopharmaceuticals: future tools for diagnostic imaging of cancers and other diseases. Med Res Rev. 2004;24:357–97.
670. Zukotynski K, Jadvar H, Capala J, Fahey F. Targeted radionuclide therapy: practical applications and future prospects. Biomark Cancer. 2016;8:35–8.
671. Dash A, Pillai MRA, Knapp FF. Production of ^{177}Lu for targeted radionuclide therapy: available options. Nucl Med Mol Imaging. 2015;49:85–107.
672. Fani M, Maecke HR, Okarvi SM. Radiolabeled peptides: valuable tools for the detection and treatment of cancer. Theranostics. 2012;2:481–501.
673. Srinivasarao M, Galliford CV, Low PS. Principles in the design of ligand-targeted cancer therapeutics and imaging agents. Nat Rev Drug Discov. 2015;14:203.
674. Ding H, Wu F. Image guided biodistribution and pharmacokinetic studies of theranostics. Theranostics. 2012;2:1040–53.
675. Santos-Oliveira R, Smith SW, Carneiro-Leão AMA. Radiopharmaceuticals drug interactions: a critical review. An Acad Bras Cienc. 2008;80:665–75.
676. Brans B, Bodei L, Giammarile F, Linden O, Luster M, Oyen WJG, Tennvall J. Clinical radionuclide therapy dosimetry: the quest for the "Holy Gray". Eur J Nucl Med Mol Imaging. 2007;34:772–86.
677. Banerjee SR, Pomper MG. Clinical applications of gallium-68. Appl Radiat Isot. 2013;76:2–13.
678. Das T, Banerjee S. Theranostic applications of lutetium-177 in radionuclide therapy. Curr Radiopharm. 2016;9:94–101.
679. Elgqvist J, Frost S, Pouget J-P, Albertsson P. The potential and hurdles of targeted alpha therapy – clinical trials and beyond. Front Oncol. 2013;3:324.
680. Goffredo V, Paradiso A, Ranieri G, Gadaleta CD. Yttrium-90 (^{90}Y) in the principal radionuclide therapies: an efficacy correlation between peptide receptor radionuclide therapy, radioimmunotherapy and transarterial radioembolization therapy. Ten years of experience (1999–2009). Crit Rev Oncol Hematol. 2011;80:393–410.
681. Liu S. Bifunctional coupling agents for radiolabeling of biomolecules and target-specific delivery of metallic radionuclides. Adv Drug Deliv Rev. 2008;60:1347–70.
682. Brechbiel MW. Bifunctional chelates for metal nuclides. Q J Nucl Med Mol Imaging. 2008;52:166–73.
683. Milenic DE, Baidoo KE, Kim Y-S, Barkley R, Brechbiel MW. Comparative studies on the therapeutic benefit of targeted [small alpha]-particle radiation therapy for the treatment of disseminated intraperitoneal disease. Dalton Trans. 2017;46:14591–601.
684. Pool SE, Krenning EP, Koning GA, van Eijck CHJ, Teunissen JJM, Kam B, Valkema R, Kwekkeboom DJ, de Jong M. Preclinical and clinical studies of peptide receptor radionuclide therapy. Semin Nucl Med. 2010;40:209–18.
685. Bison SM, Konijnenberg MW, Melis M, Pool SE, Bernsen MR, Teunissen JJM, Kwekkeboom DJ, de Jong M. Peptide receptor radionuclide therapy using radiolabeled somatostatin analogs: focus on future developments. Clin Transl Imaging. 2014;2:55–66.
686. Keskin O, Yalcin S. A review of the use of somatostatin analogs in oncology. OncoTargets Ther. 2013;6:471–83.
687. Heck MM, Schwaiger S, Knorr K, Retz M, Maurer T, Janssen F, D'Alessandria C, Wester H-J, Gschwend JE, Schwaiger M, Tauber R, Eiber M. Clinical experience with 100 consecutive patients treated with ^{177}Lu-labeled PSMA-I&T radioligand therapy for metastatic castration-resistant prostate cancer. J Clin Oncol. 2018;36:206.
688. Lütje S, Heskamp S, Cornelissen AS, Poeppel TD, van den Broek SAMW, Rosenbaum-Krumme S, Bockisch A, Gotthardt M, Rijpkema M, Boerman OC. PSMA ligands for radionuclide imaging and therapy of prostate cancer: clinical status. Theranostics. 2015;5:1388–401.
689. Rahbar K, Ahmadzadehfar H, Kratochwil C, Haberkorn U, Schäfers M, Essler M, Baum RP, Kulkarni HR, Schmidt M, Drzezga A, Bartenstein P, Pfestroff A, Luster M, Lützen U, Marx M, Prasad V, Brenner W, Heinzel A, Mottaghy FM, Ruf J, Meyer PT, Heuschkel M, Eveslage M, Bögemann M, Fendler WP, Krause BJ. German multicenter study investigating ^{177}Lu-PSMA-617 radioligand therapy in advanced prostate cancer patients. J Nucl Med. 2017;58:85–90.
690. Nock BA, Kaloudi A, Lymperis E, Giarika A, Kulkarni HR, Klette I, Singh A, Krenning EP, de Jong M, Maina T, Baum RP. Theranostic perspectives in prostate cancer with the gastrin-releasing

peptide receptor antagonist NeoBOMB1: preclinical and first clinical results. J Nucl Med. 2017;58:75–80.
691. Stoykow C, Erbes T, Maecke HR, Bulla S, Bartholoma M, Mayer S, Drendel V, Bronsert P, Werner M, Gitsch G, Weber WA, Stickeler E, Meyer PT. Gastrin-releasing peptide receptor imaging in breast cancer using the receptor antagonist ^{68}Ga-RM2 and PET. Theranostics. 2016;6:1641–50.
692. Kruljac I, Pape UF. "Neuroendocrine carcinomas" revisited – a 2017 update and future perspectives. Endocr Oncol Metab. 2017;3:37–42.
693. Klöppel G. Neuroendocrine neoplasms: dichotomy, origin and classifications. Visc Med. 2017;33:324–30.
694. Jann H, Roll S, Couvelard A, Hentic O, Pavel M, Müller-Nordhorn J, Koch M, Röcken C, Rindi G, Ruszniewski P, Wiedenmann B, Pape U-F. Neuroendocrine tumors of midgut and hindgut origin: tumor-node-metastasis classification determines clinical outcome. Cancer. 2011;117:3332–41.
695. Klöppel G. Classification and pathology of gastroenteropancreatic neuroendocrine neoplasms. Endocr Relat Cancer. 2011;18:S1–S16.
696. Dasari A, Shen C, Halperin D, Zhao B, Zhou S, Xu Y, Shih T, Yao JC. Trends in the incidence, prevalence, and survival outcomes in patients with neuroendocrine tumors in the United States. JAMA Oncol. 2017;3:1335–42.
697. Reubi J, Waser B, Schaer J-C, Laissue JA. Somatostatin receptor sst1–sst5 expression in normal and neoplastic human tissues using receptor autoradiography with subtype-selective ligands. Eur J Nucl Med. 2001;28:836–46.
698. Reubi JC, Maecke HR. Peptide-based probes for cancer imaging. J Nucl Med. 2008;49:1735–8.
699. Hoyer D, Bell GI, Berelowitz M, Epelbaum J, Feniuk W, Humphrey PPA, O'Carroll AM, Patel YC, Schonbrunn A, Taylor JE, Reisine T. Classification and nomenclature of somatostatin receptors. Trends Pharmacol Sci. 1995;16:86–8.
700. Csaba Z, Peineau S, Dournaud P. Molecular mechanisms of somatostatin receptor trafficking. J Mol Endocrinol. 2012;48:R1–R12.
701. Nilsson O, Kölby L, Wängberg B, Wigander A, Billig H, William-Olsson L, Fjälling M, Forssell-Aronsson E, Ahlman H. Comparative studies on the expression of somatostatin receptor subtypes, outcome of octreotide scintigraphy and response to octreotide treatment in patients with carcinoid tumours. Br J Cancer. 1998;77:632–7.
702. Brazeau P, Vale W, Burgus R, Ling N, Butcher M, Rivier J, Guillemin R. Hypothalamic polypeptide that inhibits the secretion of immunoreactive pituitary growth hormone. Science. 1973;179:77–9.
703. Burgus R, Ling N, Butcher M, Guillemin R. Primary structure of somatostatin, a hypothalamic peptide that inhibits the secretion of pituitary growth hormone. Proc Natl Acad Sci U S A. 1973;70:684–8.
704. Reisine T, Bell GI. Molecular biology of somatostatin receptors. Endocr Rev. 1995;16:427–42.
705. Panetta R, Greenwood MT, Warszynska A, Demchyshyn LL, Day R, Niznik HB, Srikant CB, Patel YC. Molecular cloning, functional characterization, and chromosomal localization of a human somatostatin receptor (somatostatin receptor type 5) with preferential affinity for somatostatin-28. Mol Pharmacol. 1994;45:417–27.
706. Patel YC. Somatostatin and its receptor family. Front Neuroendocrinol. 1999;20:157–98.
707. Reubi JC, Schaer J-C, Laissue JA, Waser B. Somatostatin receptors and their subtypes in human tumors and in peritumoral vessels. Metabolism. 1996;45:39–41.
708. Ambrosini V, Fani M, Fanti S, Forrer F, Maecke HR. Radiopeptide imaging and therapy in Europe. J Nucl Med. 2011;52:42S–55S.
709. Theodoropoulou M, Stalla GK. Somatostatin receptors: from signaling to clinical practice. Front Neuroendocrinol. 2013;34:228–52.
710. Reubi JC. Peptide receptors as molecular targets for cancer diagnosis and therapy. Endocr Rev. 2003;24:389–427.
711. Antunes P, Ginj M, Zhang H, Waser B, Baum RP, Reubi JC, Maecke H. Are radiogallium-labelled DOTA-conjugated somatostatin analogues superior to those labelled with other radiometals? Eur J Nucl Med Mol Imaging. 2007;34:982–93.
712. Öberg K. Molecular imaging radiotherapy: theranostics for personalized patient management of neuroendocrine tumors (NETs). Theranostics. 2012;2:448–58.
713. Virgolini I, Ambrosini V, Bomanji JB, Baum RP, Fanti S, Gabriel M, Papathanasiou ND, Pepe G, Oyen W, De Cristoforo C, Chiti A. Procedure guidelines for PET/CT tumour imaging with ^{68}Ga-DOTA-conjugated peptides: ^{68}Ga-DOTA-TOC, ^{68}Ga-DOTA-NOC, ^{68}Ga-DOTA-TATE. Eur J Nucl Med Mol Imaging. 2010;37:2004–10.
714. Wild D, Bomanji JB, Benkert P, Maecke H, Ell PJ, Reubi JC, Caplin ME. Comparison of ^{68}Ga-DOTANOC and ^{68}Ga-DOTATATE PET/CT within patients with gastroenteropancreatic neuroendocrine tumors. J Nucl Med. 2013;54:364–72.
715. Kam BLR, Teunissen JJM, Krenning EP, de Herder WW, Khan S, van Vliet EI, Kwekkeboom DJ. Lutetium-labelled peptides for therapy of neuroendocrine tumours. Eur J Nucl Med Mol Imaging. 2012;39:103–12.
716. Marincek N, Jörg A-C, Brunner P, Schindler C, Koller MT, Rochlitz C, Müller-Brand J, Maecke HR, Briel M, Walter MA. Somatostatin-based radiotherapy with [^{90}Y-DOTA]-TOC in neuroendocrine tumors: long-term outcome of a phase I dose escalation study. J Transl Med. 2013;11:17.
717. Kratochwil C, Bruchertseifer F, Giesel F, Apostolidis C, Haberkorn U, Morgenstern A. Ac-225-DOTATOC – an empiric dose finding for alpha particle emitter based radionuclide therapy of neuroendocrine tumors. J Nucl Med. 2015;56:1232.

718. Kratochwil C, Giesel FL, Bruchertseifer F, Mier W, Apostolidis C, Boll R, Murphy K, Haberkorn U, Morgenstern A. ^{213}Bi-DOTATOC receptor-targeted alpha-radionuclide therapy induces remission in neuroendocrine tumours refractory to beta radiation: a first-in-human experience. Eur J Nucl Med Mol Imaging. 2014;41:2106–19.
719. Helisch A, Förster GJ, Reber H, Buchholz H-G, Arnold R, Göke B, Weber MM, Wiedenmann B, Pauwels S, Haus U, Bouterfa H, Bartenstein P. Pre-therapeutic dosimetry and biodistribution of ^{86}Y-DOTA-Phe1-Tyr3-octreotide versus ^{111}In-pentetreotide in patients with advanced neuroendocrine tumours. Eur J Nucl Med Mol Imaging. 2004;31:1386–92.
720. Singh A, van der Meulen NP, Müller C, Klette I, Kulkarni HR, Türler A, Schibli R, Baum RP. First-in-human PET/CT imaging of metastatic neuroendocrine neoplasms with cyclotron-produced ^{44}Sc-DOTATOC: a proof-of-concept study. Cancer Biother Radiopharm. 2017;32:124–32.
721. Baum RP, Kulkarni HR. THERANOSTICS: from molecular imaging using Ga-68 labeled tracers and PET/CT to personalized radionuclide therapy – the bad Berka experience. Theranostics. 2012;2:437–47.
722. Zaknun JJ, Bodei L, Mueller-Brand J, Pavel ME, Baum RP, Hörsch D, O'Dorisio MS, O'Dorisiol TM, Howe JR, Cremonesi M, Kwekkeboom DJ. The joint IAEA, EANM, and SNMMI practical guidance on peptide receptor radionuclide therapy (PRRNT) in neuroendocrine tumours. Eur J Nucl Med Mol Imaging. 2013;40:800–16.
723. Bodei L, Cremonesi M, Grana CM, Fazio N, Iodice S, Baio SM, Bartolomei M, Lombardo D, Ferrari ME, Sansovini M, Chinol M, Paganelli G. Peptide receptor radionuclide therapy with ^{177}Lu-DOTATATE: the IEO phase I-II study. Eur J Nucl Med Mol Imaging. 2011;38:2125–35.
724. Kwekkeboom DJ, Mueller-Brand J, Paganelli G, Anthony LB, Pauwels S, Kvols LK, O'Dorisio TM, Valkema R, Bodei L, Chinol M, Maecke HR, Krenning EP. Overview of results of peptide receptor radionuclide therapy with 3 radiolabeled somatostatin analogs. J Nucl Med. 2005;46:62S–6S.
725. Strosberg JR, El-Haddad G, Wolin E, Hendifar A, Yao J, Chasen B, Mittra E, Kunz PL, Kulke MH, Jacene H, Bushnell D, O'Dorisio TM, Baum RP, Kulkarni HR, Caplin M, Lebtahi R, Hobday T, Delpassand E, Van Cutsem E, Benson A, Srirajaskanthan R, Pavel M, Mora J, Berlin J, Grande E, Reed N, Seregni E, Öberg K, Lopera Sierra M, Santoro P, Thevenet T, Erion JL, Ruszniewski P, Kwekkeboom D, Krenning E. Phase 3 trial of ^{177}Lu-dotatate for midgut neuroendocrine tumors. N Engl J Med. 2017;376:125–35.
726. Bodei L, Kidd M, Paganelli G, Grana CM, Drozdov I, Cremonesi M, Lepensky C, Kwekkeboom DJ, Baum RP, Krenning EP, Modlin IM. Long-term tolerability of PRRT in 807 patients with neuroendocrine tumours: the value and limitations of clinical factors. Eur J Nucl Med Mol Imaging. 2015;42:5–19.
727. Kwekkeboom DJ, Krenning EP. Peptide receptor radionuclide therapy in the treatment of neuroendocrine tumors. Hematol Oncol Clin North Am. 2016;30:179–91.
728. Imhof A, Brunner P, Marincek N, Briel M, Schindler C, Rasch H, Mäcke HR, Rochlitz C, Müller-Brand J, Walter MA. Response, survival, and long-term toxicity after therapy with the radiolabeled somatostatin analogue [^{90}Y-DOTA]-TOC in metastasized neuroendocrine cancers. J Clin Oncol. 2011;29:2416–23.
729. Sabet A, Ezziddin K, Pape U-F, Reichman K, Haslerud T, Ahmadzadehfar H, Biersack H-J, Nagarajah J, Ezziddin S. Accurate assessment of long-term nephrotoxicity after peptide receptor radionuclide therapy with ^{177}Lu-octreotate. Eur J Nucl Med Mol Imaging. 2014;41:505–10.
730. Ginj M, Zhang H, Waser B, Cescato R, Wild D, Wang X, Erchegyi J, Rivier J, Mäcke HR, Reubi JC. Radiolabeled somatostatin receptor antagonists are preferable to agonists for in vivo peptide receptor targeting of tumors. Proc Natl Acad Sci U S A. 2006;103:16436–41.
731. Wild D, Fani M, Fischer R, Del Pozzo L, Kaul F, Krebs S, Fischer R, Rivier JEF, Reubi JC, Maecke HR, Weber WA. Comparison of somatostatin receptor agonist and antagonist for peptide receptor radionuclide therapy: a pilot study. J Nucl Med. 2014;55:1248–52.
732. Fani M, Kolenc Peitl P, Velikyan I. Current status of radiopharmaceuticals for the theranostics of neuroendocrine neoplasms. Pharmaceuticals. 2017;10:30.
733. Ahmadzadehfar H. Targeted therapy for metastatic prostate cancer with radionuclides prostate cancer. London: IntechOpen; 2016.
734. Ferlay J, Soerjomataram I, Dikshit R, Eser S, Mathers C, Rebelo M, Parkin Donald M, Forman D, Bray F. Cancer incidence and mortality worldwide: sources, methods and major patterns in GLOBOCAN 2012. Int J Cancer. 2014;136:E359–86.
735. Kiess AP, Banerjee SR, Mease RC, Rowe SP, Rao A, Foss CA, Chen Y, Yang X, Cho SY, Nimmagadda S, Pomper MG. Prostate-specific membrane antigen as a target for cancer imaging and therapy. Q J Nucl Med Mol Imaging. 2015;59:241–68.
736. O'Keefe DS, Bacich DJ, Heston WDW. Prostate specific membrane antigen. In: Chung L, Issacs W, Simons J, editors. Prostate cancer, biology, genetics, and the new therapeutics. Totowa, NJ: Humana; 2001. p. 307–26.
737. Silver DA, Pellicer I, Fair WR, Heston WD, Cordon-Cardo C. Prostate-specific membrane antigen expression in normal and malignant human tissues. Clin Cancer Res. 1997;3:81–5.
738. Dumas F, Gala Jean L, Berteau P, Brasseur F, Eschwège P, Paradis V, Lacour B, Philippe M, Loric S. Molecular expression of PSMA mRNA and protein in primary renal tumors. Int J Cancer. 1999;80:799–803.
739. Gala J-L, Loric S, Guiot Y, Denmeade SR, Gady A, Brasseur F, Heusterspreute M, Eschwège P, De

Nayer P, Van Cangh P, Tombal B. Expression of prostate-specific membrane antigen in transitional cell carcinoma of the bladder: prognostic value? Clin Cancer Res. 2000;6:4049–54.
740. Chang SS, Reuter VE, Heston WDW, Bander NH, Grauer LS, Gaudin PB. Five different anti-prostate-specific membrane antigen (PSMA) antibodies confirm PSMA expression in tumor-associated neovasculature. Cancer Res. 1999;59:3192–8.
741. Haffner MC, Kronberger IE, Ross JS, Sheehan CE, Zitt M, Mühlmann G, Öfner D, Zelger B, Ensinger C, Yang XJ, Geley S, Margreiter R, Bander NH. Prostate-specific membrane antigen expression in the neovasculature of gastric and colorectal cancers. Hum Pathol. 2009;40:1754–61.
742. Horoszewicz JS, Leong SS, Kawinski E, Karr JP, Rosenthal H, Chu TM, Mirand EA, Murphy GP. LNCaP model of human prostatic carcinoma. Cancer Res. 1983;43:1809–18.
743. Horoszewicz JS, Kawinski E, Murphy GP. Monoclonal antibodies to a new antigenic marker in epithelial prostatic cells and serum of prostatic cancer patients. Anticancer Res. 1987;7:927–35.
744. Ellis RJ, Kaminsky DA, Zhou EH, Fu P, Chen W-D, Brelin A, Faulhaber PF, Bodner D. Ten-year outcomes: the clinical utility of single photon emission computed tomography/computed tomography capromab pendetide (prostascint) in a cohort diagnosed with localized prostate cancer. Int J Radiat Oncol Biol Phys. 2011;81:29–34.
745. Sodee DB, Malguria N, Faulhaber P, Resnick MI, Albert J, Bakale G. Multicenter ProstaScint imaging findings in 2154 patients with prostate cancer11A complete list of the ProstaScint imaging centers is provided in the appendix. Urology. 2000;56:988–93.
746. Taneja SS. ProstaScint® scan: contemporary use in clinical practice. Rev Urol. 2004;6:S19–28.
747. Benešová M, Schäfer M, Bauder-Wüst U, Afshar-Oromieh A, Kratochwil C, Mier W, Haberkorn U, Kopka K, Eder M. Preclinical evaluation of a tailor-made DOTA-conjugated PSMA inhibitor with optimized linker moiety for imaging and endoradiotherapy of prostate cancer. J Nucl Med. 2015;56:914–20.
748. Chen Y, Pullambhatla M, Foss CA, Byun Y, Nimmagadda S, Senthamizhchelvan S, Sgouros G, Mease RC, Pomper MG. 2-(3-(1-Carboxy-5-(6-[^{18}F]fluoro-pyridine-3-carbonyl)-amino-pentyl)-U reido)-pentanedioic acid, [^{18}F] DCFPyL, a PSMA-based PET imaging agent for prostate cancer. Clin Cancer Res. 2011;17:7645–53.
749. Cho SY, Gage KL, Mease RC, Senthamizhchelvan S, Holt DP, Jeffrey-Kwanisai A, Endres CJ, Dannals RF, Sgouros G, Lodge M, Eisenberger MA, Rodriguez R, Carducci MA, Rojas C, Slusher BS, Kozikowski AP, Pomper MG. Biodistribution, tumor detection, and radiation dosimetry of ^{18}F-DCFBC, a low-molecular-weight inhibitor of prostate-specific membrane antigen, in patients with metastatic prostate cancer. J Nucl Med. 2012;53:1883–91.
750. Eder M, Schäfer M, Bauder-Wüst U, Hull W-E, Wängler C, Mier W, Haberkorn U, Eisenhut M. ^{68}Ga-complex lipophilicity and the targeting property of a urea-based PSMA inhibitor for PET imaging. Bioconjug Chem. 2012;23:688–97.
751. Hillier SM, Maresca KP, Femia FJ, Marquis JC, Foss CA, Nguyen N, Zimmerman CN, Barrett JA, Eckelman WC, Pomper MG, Joyal JL, Babich JW. Preclinical evaluation of novel glutamate-urea-lysine analogues that target prostate-specific membrane antigen as molecular imaging pharmaceuticals for prostate cancer. Cancer Res. 2009;69:6932–40.
752. Maresca KP, Hillier SM, Femia FJ, Keith D, Barone C, Joyal JL, Zimmerman CN, Kozikowski AP, Barrett JA, Eckelman WC, Babich JW. A series of halogenated heterodimeric inhibitors of prostate specific membrane antigen (PSMA) as radiolabeled probes for targeting prostate cancer. J Med Chem. 2009;52:347–57.
753. Szabo Z, Mena E, Rowe SP, Plyku D, Nidal R, Eisenberger MA, Antonarakis ES, Fan H, Dannals RF, Chen Y, Mease RC, Vranesic M, Bhatnagar A, Sgouros G, Cho SY, Pomper MG. Initial evaluation of [^{18}F]DCFPyL for prostate-specific membrane antigen (PSMA)-targeted PET imaging of prostate cancer. Mol Imaging Biol. 2015;17:565–74.
754. Weineisen M, Schottelius M, Simecek J, Baum RP, Yildiz A, Beykan S, Kulkarni HR, Lassmann M, Klette I, Eiber M, Schwaiger M, Wester H-J. ^{68}Ga- and ^{177}Lu-labeled PSMA I&T: optimization of a PSMA-targeted theranostic concept and first proof-of-concept human studies. J Nucl Med. 2015;56:1169–76.
755. Langton-Webster B, Berkman C, Slater J, Jivan S, Neumann K, Whalley E, Ketteridge P, Behr S, Aggarwal R, VanBrocklin H. Development of a novel PSMA-targeted PET imaging agent, CTT1057, for use in prostate cancer. J Nucl Med. 2016;57:467.
756. Bander NH, Milowsky MI, Nanus DM, Kostakoglu L, Vallabhajosula S, Goldsmith SJ. Phase I trial of ^{177}lutetium-labeled J591, a monoclonal antibody to prostate-specific membrane antigen, in patients with androgen-independent prostate cancer. J Clin Oncol. 2005;23:4591–601.
757. Kampmeier F, Williams JD, Maher J, Mullen GE, Blower PJ. Design and preclinical evaluation of a ^{99m}Tc-labelled diabody of mAb J591 for SPECT imaging of prostate-specific membrane antigen (PSMA). EJNMMI Res. 2014;4:13.
758. Milowsky MI, Nanus DM, Kostakoglu L, Vallabhajosula S, Goldsmith SJ, Bander NH. Phase I trial of yttrium-90-labeled anti-prostate-specific membrane antigen monoclonal antibody J591 for androgen-independent prostate cancer. J Clin Oncol. 2004;22:2522–31.
759. Olafsen T, Bartlett D, Ho D, Zhang G, Torgov M, Keppler J, Behrenbruch C, Wu A, Pandit-Taskar N, Morris MJ, Lewis JS, Lyashchenko SK, Gudas JMJ. Minibody imaging of prostate-specific mem-

brane antigen (PSMA): from concept to clinic. Clin Oncol. 2014;32:e16057.
760. Flores O, Santra S, Kaittanis C, Bassiouni R, Khaled AS, Khaled AR, Grimm J, Perez JM. PSMA-targeted theranostic nanocarrier for prostate cancer. Theranostics. 2017;7:2477–94.
761. Kopka K, Benešová M, Bařinka C, Haberkorn U, Babich J. Glu-Ureido-based inhibitors of prostate-specific membrane antigen: lessons learned during the development of a novel class of low-molecular-weight theranostic radiotracers. J Nucl Med. 2017;58:17S–26S.
762. von Eyben FE, Roviello G, Kiljunen T, Uprimny C, Virgolini I, Kairemo K, Joensuu T. Third-line treatment and ^{177}Lu-PSMA radioligand therapy of metastatic castration-resistant prostate cancer: a systematic review. Eur J Nucl Med Mol Imaging. 2018;45:496–508.
763. Zechmann CM, Afshar-Oromieh A, Armor T, Stubbs JB, Mier W, Hadaschik B, Joyal J, Kopka K, Debus J, Babich JW, Haberkorn U. Radiation dosimetry and first therapy results with a ^{124}I/^{131}I-labeled small molecule (MIP-1095) targeting PSMA for prostate cancer therapy. Eur J Nucl Med Mol Imaging. 2014;41:1280–92.
764. Coleman RE, Barrett JA, Hussain A, Slawin KM, Armor T, LaFrance ND, Babich JW. Prostate-specific membrane antigen (PSMA)-targeted imaging of metastatic prostate cancer (PCa) via small molecule inhibitors: comparison to bone scan, CT/MRI, and ^{111}In capromab. J Clin Oncol. 2011;29:4658.
765. Schmidkonz C, Cordes M, Beck M, Goetz TI, Schmidt D, Prante O, Bäuerle T, Uder M, Wullich B, Goebell P, Kuwert T, Ritt P. SPECT/CT with the PSMA ligand ^{99m}Tc-MIP-1404 for whole-body primary staging of patients with prostate cancer. Clin Nucl Med. 2018;43:225–31.
766. Afshar-Oromieh A, Haberkorn U, Hadaschik B, Habl G, Eder M, Eisenhut M, Schlemmer HP, Roethke MC. PET/MRI with a ^{68}Ga-PSMA ligand for the detection of prostate cancer. Eur J Nucl Med Mol Imaging. 2013;40:1629–30.
767. Rowe SP, Gage KL, Faraj SF, Macura KJ, Cornish TC, Gonzalez-Roibon N, Guner G, Munari E, Partin AW, Pavlovich CP, Han M, Carter HB, Bivalacqua TJ, Blackford A, Holt D, Dannals RF, Netto GJ, Lodge MA, Mease RC, Pomper MG, Cho SY. ^{18}F-DCFBC PET/CT for PSMA-based detection and characterization of primary prostate cancer. J Nucl Med. 2015;56:1003–10.
768. Afshar-Oromieh A, Hetzheim H, Kratochwil C, Benešová M, Eder M, Neels OC, Eisenhut M, Kübler W, Holland-Letz T, Giesel FL, Mier W, Kopka K, Haberkorn U. The theranostic PSMA ligand PSMA-617 in the diagnosis of prostate cancer by PET/CT: biodistribution in humans, radiation dosimetry, and first evaluation of tumor lesions. J Nucl Med. 2015;56:1697–705.
769. Barrett JA, Coleman RE, Goldsmith SJ, Vallabhajosula S, Petry NA, Cho S, Armor T, Stubbs JB, Maresca KP, Stabin MG, Joyal JL, Eckelman WC, Babich JW. First-in-man evaluation of 2 high-affinity PSMA-avid small molecules for imaging prostate cancer. J Nucl Med. 2013;54:380–7.
770. Meyrick DP, Asokendaran M, Skelly LA, Lenzo NP, Henderson A. The role of ^{68}Ga-PSMA-I&T PET/CT in the pretreatment staging of primary prostate cancer. Nucl Med Commun. 2017;38:956–63.
771. Schottelius M, Wirtz M, Eiber M, Maurer T, Wester H-J. [^{111}In]PSMA-I&T: expanding the spectrum of PSMA-I&T applications towards SPECT and radioguided surgery. EJNMMI Res. 2015;5:68.
772. Afshar-Oromieh A, Haberkorn U, Eder M, Eisenhut M, Zechmann C. [^{68}Ga]Gallium-labelled PSMA ligand as superior PET tracer for the diagnosis of prostate cancer: comparison with ^{18}F-FECH. Eur J Nucl Med Mol Imaging. 2012;39:1085–6.
773. Afshar-Oromieh A, Malcher A, Eder M, Eisenhut M, Linhart HG, Hadaschik BA, Holland-Letz T, Giesel FL, Kratochwil C, Haufe S, Haberkorn U, Zechmann CM. PET imaging with a [^{68}Ga]gallium-labelled PSMA ligand for the diagnosis of prostate cancer: biodistribution in humans and first evaluation of tumour lesions. Eur J Nucl Med Mol Imaging. 2013;40:486–95.
774. Schuhmacher J, Matys R, Hauser H, Maier-Borst W, Matzku S. Labeling of monoclonal antibodies with a ^{67}Ga-phenolic aminocarboxylic acid chelate. Eur J Nucl Med. 1986;12:397–404.
775. Zöller M, Schuhmacher J, Reed J, Maier-Borst W, Matzku S. Establishment and characterization of monoclonal antibodies against an octahedral gallium chelate suitable for immunoscintigraphy with PET. J Nucl Med. 1992;33:1366–72.
776. Dam JH, Olsen BB, Baun C, Høilund-Carlsen PF, Thisgaard H. A PSMA ligand labeled with cobalt-55 for PET imaging of prostate cancer. Mol Imaging Biol. 2017;19:915–22.
777. Han X-D, Liu C, Liu F, Xie Q-H, Liu T-L, Guo X-Y, Xu X-X, Yang X, Zhu H, Yang Z. ^{64}Cu-PSMA-617: a novel PSMA-targeted radio-tracer for PET imaging in gastric adenocarcinoma xenografted mice model. Oncotarget. 2017;8:74159–69.
778. Umbricht CA, Benešová M, Schmid RM, Türler A, Schibli R, van der Meulen NP, Müller C. ^{44}Sc-PSMA-617 for radiotheragnostics in tandem with ^{177}Lu-PSMA-617—preclinical investigations in comparison with ^{68}Ga-PSMA-11 and ^{68}Ga-PSMA-617. EJNMMI Res. 2017;7:9.
779. Delker A, Fendler WP, Kratochwil C, Brunegraf A, Gosewisch A, Gildehaus FJ, Tritschler S, Stief CG, Kopka K, Haberkorn U, Bartenstein P, Böning G. Dosimetry for ^{177}Lu-DKFZ-PSMA-617: a new radiopharmaceutical for the treatment of metastatic prostate cancer. Eur J Nucl Med Mol Imaging. 2016;43:42–51.
780. Kratochwil C, Bruchertseifer F, Giesel FL, Weis M, Verburg FA, Mottaghy F, Kopka K, Apostolidis C, Haberkorn U, Morgenstern A. ^{225}Ac-PSMA-617 for PSMA-targeted α-radiation therapy of metastatic

castration-resistant prostate cancer. J Nucl Med. 2016;57:1941–4.
781. Sathekge M, Knoesen O, Meckel M, Modiselle M, Vorster M, Marx S. ^{213}Bi-PSMA-617 targeted alpha-radionuclide therapy in metastatic castration-resistant prostate cancer. Eur J Nucl Med Mol Imaging. 2017;44:1099–100.
782. Bräuer A, Grubert LS, Roll W, Schrader AJ, Schäfers M, Bögemann M, Rahbar K. ^{177}Lu-PSMA-617 radioligand therapy and outcome in patients with metastasized castration-resistant prostate cancer. Eur J Nucl Med Mol Imaging. 2017;44:1663–70.
783. von Eyben FE, Kiljunen T, Joensuu T, Kairemo K, Uprimny C, Virgolini I. ^{177}Lu-PSMA-617 radioligand therapy for a patient with lymph node metastatic prostate cancer. Oncotarget. 2017;8:66112–6.
784. Yadav MP, Ballal S, Tripathi M, Damle NA, Sahoo RK, Seth A, Bal C. ^{177}Lu-DKFZ-PSMA-617 therapy in metastatic castration resistant prostate cancer: safety, efficacy, and quality of life assessment. Eur J Nucl Med Mol Imaging. 2017;44:81–91.
785. Ahmadzadehfar H, Wegen S, Yordanova A, Fimmers R, Kürpig S, Eppard E, Wei X, Schlenkhoff C, Hauser S, Essler M. Overall survival and response pattern of castration-resistant metastatic prostate cancer to multiple cycles of radioligand therapy using [^{177}Lu]Lu-PSMA-617. Eur J Nucl Med Mol Imaging. 2017;44:1448–54.
786. Yordanova A, Becker A, Eppard E, Kürpig S, Fisang C, Feldmann G, Essler M, Ahmadzadehfar H. The impact of repeated cycles of radioligand therapy using [^{177}Lu]Lu-PSMA-617 on renal function in patients with hormone refractory metastatic prostate cancer. Eur J Nucl Med Mol Imaging. 2017;44:1473–9.
787. Kratochwil C, Bruchertseifer F, Giesel FL, Apostolidis C, Haberkorn U, Morgenstern A. Ac-225-PSMA-617 for PSMA targeting alpha-radiation therapy of 28 patients with mCRPC. Eur J Nucl Med Mol Imaging. 2016;43:S137.
788. Hofman MS, Violet J, Hicks RJ, Ferdinandus J, Thang SP, Akhurst T, Iravani A, Kong G, Ravi Kumar A, Murphy DG, Eu P, Jackson P, Scalzo M, Williams SG, Sandhu S. [^{177}Lu]-PSMA-617 radionuclide treatment in patients with metastatic castration-resistant prostate cancer (LuPSMA trial): a single-centre, single-arm, phase 2 study. Lancet Oncol. 2018;19:825–33.
789. Giesel FL, Kesch C, Yun M, Cardinale J, Haberkorn U, Kopka K, Kratochwil C, Hadaschik BA. ^{18}F-PSMA-1007 PET/CT detects micrometastases in a patient with biochemically recurrent prostate cancer. Clin Genitourin Cancer. 2017;15:e497–9.
790. Lee CM, Tannock IF. The distribution of the therapeutic monoclonal antibodies cetuximab and trastuzumab within solid tumors. BMC Cancer. 2010;10:255.
791. Rudnick SI, Adams GP. Affinity and avidity in antibody-based tumor targeting. Cancer Biother Radiopharm. 2009;24:155–61.
792. Goldenberg DM. Targeted therapy of cancer with radiolabeled antibodies. J Nucl Med. 2002;43:693–713.
793. Schellekens H. Immunogenicity of therapeutic proteins: clinical implications and future prospects. Clin Ther. 2002;24:1720–40.
794. Troyer JK, Beckett ML, Wright GL. Location of prostate-specific membrane antigen in the LNCaP prostate carcinoma cell line. Prostate. 1997;30:232–42.
795. Bander NH, Trabulsi EJ, Kostakoglu L, Yao D, Vallabhajosula S, Smith-Jones P, Joyce MA, Milowsky M, Nanus DM, Goldsmith SJ. Targeting metastatic prostate cancer with radiolabeled monoclonal antibody J591 to the extracellular domain of prostate specific membrane antigen. J Urol. 2003;170:1717–21.
796. DiPippo VA, Olson WC, Nguyen HM, Brown LG, Vessella RL, Corey E. Efficacy studies of an antibody-drug conjugate PSMA-ADC in patient-derived prostate cancer xenografts. Prostate. 2015;75:303–13.
797. Fleuren EDG, Versleijen-Jonkers YMH, Heskamp S, van Herpen CML, Oyen WJG, van der Graaf WTA, Boerman Otto C. Theranostic applications of antibodies in oncology. Mol Oncol. 2014;8:799–812.
798. Olson WC, Israel RJ. Antibody-drug conjugates targeting prostate-specific membrane antigen. Front Biosci. 2014;19:12–33.
799. Fung EK, Cheal SM, Fareedy SB, Punzalan B, Beylergil V, Amir J, Chalasani S, Weber WA, Spratt DE, Veach DR, Bander NH, Larson SM, Zanzonico PB, Osborne JR. Targeting of radiolabeled J591 antibody to PSMA-expressing tumors: optimization of imaging and therapy based on non-linear compartmental modeling. EJNMMI Res. 2016;6:7.
800. Pandit-Taskar N, O'Donoghue JA, Beylergil V, Lyashchenko S, Ruan S, Solomon SB, Durack JC, Carrasquillo JA, Lefkowitz RA, Gonen M, Lewis JS, Holland JP, Cheal SM, Reuter VE, Osborne JR, Loda MF, Smith-Jones PM, Weber WA, Bander NH, Scher HI, Morris MJ, Larson SM. Zr-huJ591 immuno-PET imaging in patients with advanced metastatic prostate cancer. Eur J Nucl Med Mol Imaging. 2014;41:2093–105.
801. Pandit-Taskar N, O'Donoghue JA, Divgi CR, Wills EA, Schwartz L, Gönen M, Smith-Jones P, Bander NH, Scher HI, Larson SM, Morris MJ. Indium 111-labeled J591 anti-PSMA antibody for vascular targeted imaging in progressive solid tumors. EJNMMI Res. 2015;5:28.
802. Tagawa ST, Milowsky MI, Morris M, Vallabhajosula S, Christos P, Akhtar NH, Osborne J, Goldsmith SJ, Larson S, Taskar NP, Scher HI, Bander NH, Nanus DM. Phase II study of lutetium-177-labeled anti-prostate-specific membrane antigen monoclonal antibody J591 for metastatic castration-resistant prostate cancer. Clin Cancer Res. 2013;19:5182–91.
803. Dumont RA, Tamma M, Braun F, Borkowski S, Reubi JC, Maecke H, Weber WA, Mansi R. Targeted radiotherapy of prostate cancer with a gastrin-releas-

ing peptide receptor antagonist is effective as monotherapy and in combination with rapamycin. J Nucl Med. 2013;54:762–9.
804. Sancho V, Florio AD, Moody TW, Jensen RT. Bombesin receptor-mediated imaging and cytotoxicity. Rev Curr Stat Curr Drug Deliv. 2011;8:79–134.
805. Cescato R, Maina T, Nock B, Nikolopoulou A, Charalambidis D, Piccand V, Reubi JC. Bombesin receptor antagonists may be preferable to agonists for tumor targeting. J Nucl Med. 2008;49:318–26.
806. Wieser G, Mansi R, Grosu AL, Schultze-Seemann W, Dumont-Walter RA, Meyer PT, Maecke HR, Reubi JC, Weber WA. Positron emission tomography (PET) imaging of prostate cancer with a gastrin releasing peptide receptor antagonist – from mice to men. Theranostics. 2014;4:412–9.
807. Bodei L, Ferrari M, Nunn A, Llull J, Cremonesi M, Martano L, Laurora G, Scardino E, Tiberini S, Bufi G, Eaton S, de Cobelli O, Paganelli G. ^{177}Lu-AMBA bombesin analogue in hormone refractory prostate cancer patients: a phase I escalation study with single-cycle administrations. Eur J Nucl Med Mol Imaging. 2007;34:S221.
808. Minamimoto R, Hancock S, Schneider B, Chin FT, Jamali M, Loening A, Vasanawala S, Gambhir SS, Iagaru A. Pilot comparison of ^{68}Ga-RM2 PET and ^{68}Ga-PSMA-11 PET in patients with biochemically recurrent prostate cancer. J Nucl Med. 2016;57:557–62.
809. Armitage JO, Gascoyne RD, Lunning MA, Cavalli F. Non-Hodgkin lymphoma. Lancet. 2017;390:298–310.
810. Kosmas C, Stamatopoulos K, Stavroyianni N, Tsavaris N, Papadaki T. Anti-CD20-based therapy of B cell lymphoma: state of the art. Leukemia. 2002;16:2004.
811. Dotan E, Aggarwal C, Smith MR. Impact of rituximab (rituxan) on the treatment of B-cell non-Hodgkin's lymphoma. P T. 2010;35:148–57.
812. Goldsmith SJ. Radioimmunotherapy of lymphoma: bexxar and zevalin. Semin Nucl Med. 2010;40:122–35.
813. Boucek JA, Turner JH. Validation of prospective whole-body bone marrow dosimetry by SPECT/CT multimodality imaging in ^{131}I-anti-CD20 rituximab radioimmunotherapy of non-Hodgkin's lymphoma. Eur J Nucl Med Mol Imaging. 2005;32:458–69.
814. Dietlein M, Pels H, Schulz H, Staak O, Borchmann P, Schomäcker K, Fischer T, Eschner W, Strandmann Elke P, Schicha H, Engert A, Schnell R. Imaging of central nervous system lymphomas with iodine-123 labeled rituximab. Eur J Haematol. 2005;74:348–52.
815. Leahy MF, Seymour JF, Hicks RJ, Turner JH. Multicenter phase II clinical study of iodine-131-rituximab radioimmunotherapy in relapsed or refractory indolent non-Hodgkin's lymphoma. J Clin Oncol. 2006;24:4418–25.
816. Rizzieri D. Zevalin® (ibritumomab tiuxetan): after more than a decade of treatment experience, what have we learned? Crit Rev Oncol Hematol. 2016;105:5–17.
817. Spies SM. Imaging and dosing in radioimmunotherapy with Yttrium 90 ibritumomab tiuxetan (Zevalin). Semin Nucl Med. 2004;34:10–3.
818. Evens AM, Gordon LI. Radioimmunotherapy in non-Hodgkin's lymphoma: trials of yttrium 90-labeled ibritumomab tiuxetan and beyond. Clin Lymphoma. 2004;5:S11–5.
819. Scholz CW, Pinto A, Linkesch W, Lindén O, Viardot A, Keller U, Hess G, Lastoria S, Lerch K, Frigeri F, Arcamone M, Stroux A, Frericks B, Pott C, Pezzutto A. ^{90}Yttrium-ibritumomab-tiuxetan as first-line treatment for follicular lymphoma: 30 months of follow-up data from an international multicenter phase II clinical trial. J Clin Oncol. 2013;31:308–13.
820. Witzig TE, Gordon LI, Cabanillas F, Czuczman MS, Emmanouilides C, Joyce R, Pohlman BL, Bartlett NL, Wiseman GA, Padre N, Grillo-López AJ, Multani P, White CA. Randomized controlled trial of yttrium-90-labeled ibritumomab tiuxetan radioimmunotherapy versus rituximab immunotherapy for patients with relapsed or refractory low-grade, follicular, or transformed B-cell non-Hodgkin's lymphoma. J Clin Oncol. 2002;20:2453–63.
821. Iagaru A, Mittra ES, Ganjoo K, Knox SJ, Goris ML. ^{131}I-tositumomab (Bexxar®) vs. ^{90}Y-ibritumomab (Zevalin®) therapy of low-grade refractory/relapsed non-Hodgkin lymphoma. Mol Imaging Biol. 2010;12:198–203.
822. DeNardo GL, Kukis DL, Shen S, DeNardo DA, Meares CF, DeNardo SJ. ^{67}Cu-*versus* ^{131}I-labeled Lym-1 antibody: comparative pharmacokinetics and dosimetry in patients with non-Hodgkin's lymphoma. Clin Cancer Res. 1999;5:533–41.
823. O'Donnell RT, DeNardo GL, Kukis DL, Lamborn KR, Shen S, Yuan A, Goldstein DS, Carr CE, Mirick GR, DeNardo SJ. A clinical trial of radioimmunotherapy with ^{67}Cu-21T-BAT-Lym-1 for non-Hodgkin's lymphoma. J Nucl Med. 1999;40:2014–20.
824. Peled A, Tavor S. Role of CXCR4 in the pathogenesis of acute myeloid leukemia. Theranostics. 2013;3:34–9.
825. Röllig C, Knop S, Bornhäuser M. Multiple myeloma. Lancet. 2015;385:2197–208.
826. Gourni E, Demmer O, Schottelius M, D'Alessandria C, Schulz S, Dijkgraaf I, Schumacher U, Schwaiger M, Kessler H, Wester H-J. PET of CXCR4 expression by a ^{68}Ga-labeled highly specific targeted contrast agent. J Nucl Med. 2011;52:1803–10.
827. Lapa C, Schreder M, Schirbel A, Samnick S, Kortüm KM, Herrmann K, Kropf S, Einsele H, Buck AK, Wester H-J, Knop S, Lückerath K. [^{68}Ga]Pentixafor-PET/CT for imaging of chemokine receptor CXCR4 expression in multiple myeloma – comparison to [^{18}F]FDG and laboratory values. Theranostics. 2017;7:205–12.
828. Vag T, Gerngross C, Herhaus P, Eiber M, Philipp-Abbrederis K, Graner F-P, Ettl J, Keller U, Wester H-J, Schwaiger M. First experience with chemokine

receptor CXCR4-targeted PET imaging of patients with solid cancers. J Nucl Med. 2016;57:741–6.
829. Herrmann K, Schottelius M, Lapa C, Osl T, Poschenrieder A, Hänscheid H, Lückerath K, Schreder M, Bluemel C, Knott M, Keller U, Schirbel A, Samnick S, Lassmann M, Kropf S, Buck AK, Einsele H, Wester H-J, Knop S. First-in-human experience of CXCR4-directed endoradiotherapy with ^{177}Lu- and ^{90}Y-labeled pentixather in advanced-stage multiple myeloma with extensive intra- and extramedullary disease. J Nucl Med. 2016;57:248–51.
830. Lapa C, Herrmann K, Schirbel A, Hänscheid H, Lückerath K, Schottelius M, Kircher M, Werner RA, Schreder M, Samnick S, Kropf S, Knop S, Buck AK, Einsele H, Wester H-J, Kortüm KM. CXCR4-directed endoradiotherapy induces high response rates in extramedullary relapsed multiple myeloma. Theranostics. 2017;7:1589–97.
831. Lau J, Lin KS, Benard F. Past, present, and future: development of theranostic agents targeting carbonic anhydrase IX. Theranostics. 2017;7:4322–39.
832. Harris AL. Hypoxia – a key regulatory factor in tumour growth. Nat Rev Cancer. 2002;2:38.
833. Supuran CT. Carbonic anhydrases: novel therapeutic applications for inhibitors and activators. Nat Rev Drug Discov. 2008;7:168.
834. Divgi CR, Uzzo RG, Gatsonis C, Bartz R, Treutner S, Yu JQ, Chen D, Carrasquillo JA, Larson S, Bevan P, Russo P. Positron emission tomography/computed tomography identification of clear cell renal cell carcinoma: results from the REDECT trial. J Clin Oncol. 2013;31:187–94.
835. Muselaers CHJ, Boerman OC, Oosterwijk E, Langenhuijsen JF, Oyen WJG, Mulders PFA. Indium-111-labeled girentuximab immuno-SPECT as a diagnostic tool in clear cell renal cell carcinoma. Eur Urol. 2013;63:1101–6.
836. Stillebroer AB, Boerman OC, Desar IME, Boers-Sonderen MJ, van Herpen CML, Langenhuijsen JF, Smith-Jones PM, Oosterwijk E, Oyen WJG, Mulders PFA. Phase 1 radioimmunotherapy study with lutetium 177-labeled anti-carbonic anhydrase IX monoclonal antibody girentuximab in patients with advanced renal cell carcinoma. Eur Urol. 2013;64:478–85.
837. Askoxylakis V, Garcia-Boy R, Rana S, Krämer S, Hebling U, Mier W, Altmann A, Markert A, Debus J, Haberkorn U. A new peptide ligand for targeting human carbonic anhydrase IX, identified through the phage display technology. PLoS One. 2011;5:e15962.
838. Rami M, Cecchi A, Montero J-L, Innocenti A, Vullo D, Scozzafava A, Winum J-Y, Supuran Claudiu T. Carbonic anhydrase inhibitors: design of membrane-impermeant copper(II) complexes of DTPA-, DOTA-, and TETA-tailed sulfonamides targeting the tumor-associated transmembrane isoform IX. ChemMedChem. 2008;3:1780–8.
839. Davidoff AM. Neuroblastoma. Semin Pediatr Surg. 2012;21:2–14.
840. Pashankar FD, O'Dorisio MS, Menda Y. MIBG and somatostatin receptor analogs in children: current concepts on diagnostic and therapeutic use. J Nucl Med. 2005;46:55S–61S.
841. DuBois SG, Matthay KK. Radiolabeled metaiodobenzylguanidine for the treatment of neuroblastoma. Nucl Med Biol. 2008;35:S35–48.
842. El-Maghraby T. ^{131}I-MIBG in the diagnosis of primary and metastatic neuroblastoma. Gulf J Oncolog. 2007;2007:33–41.
843. Kraal KCJM, Bleeker GM, van Eck-Smit BLF, van Eijkelenburg NKA, Berthold F, van Noesel MM, Caron HN, Tytgat GAM. Feasibility, toxicity and response of upfront metaiodobenzylguanidine therapy therapy followed by German Pediatric Oncology Group Neuroblastoma 2004 protocol in newly diagnosed stage 4 neuroblastoma patients. Eur J Cancer. 2017;76:188–96.
844. Streby KA, Shah N, Ranalli MA, Kunkler A, Cripe TP. Nothing but NET: a review of norepinephrine transporter expression and efficacy of ^{131}I-mIBG therapy. Pediatr Blood Cancer. 2015;62:5–11.
845. Luo Y, Pan Q, Yao S, Yu M, Wu W, Xue H, Kiesewetter DO, Zhu Z, Li F, Zhao Y, Chen X. Glucagon-like peptide-1 receptor PET/CT with ^{68}Ga-NOTA-exendin-4 for detecting localized insulinoma: a prospective cohort study. J Nucl Med. 2016;57:715–20.
846. Velikyan I, Bulenga TN, Selvaraju R, Lubberink M, Espes D, Rosenström U, Eriksson O. Dosimetry of [^{177}Lu]-DO3A-VS-Cys40-Exendin-4 – impact on the feasibility of insulinoma internal radiotherapy. Am J Nucl Med Mol Imaging. 2015;5:109–26.
847. Roosenburg S, Laverman P, van Delft FL, Boerman OC. Radiolabeled CCK/gastrin peptides for imaging and therapy of CCK2 receptor-expressing tumors. Amino Acids. 2011;41:1049–58.
848. Rottenburger C, Nicolas G, McDougall L, Kaul F, Cachovan M, Schibli R, Geistlich S, Béhé M, Wild D, Christ E. Evaluation of the CCK-2-receptor agonist ^{177}Lu-PP-F11N for peptide receptor radionuclide therapy (PRRT) of medullary thyroid carcinoma – first results of a phase 0 'Lumed' study. Endocr Abstr. 2018;56:GP234.
849. Cachin F, Miot-Noirault E, Gillet B, Isnardi V, Labeille B, Payoux P, Meyer N, Cammilleri S, Gaudy C, Razzouk-Cadet M, Lacour JP, Granel-Brocard F, Tychyj C, Benbouzid F, Grange JD, Baulieu F, Kelly A, Merlin C, Mestas D, Gachon F, Chezal JM, Degoul F, D'Incan M. ^{123}I-BZA2 as a melanin-targeted radiotracer for the identification of melanoma metastases: results and perspectives of a multicenter phase III clinical trial. J Nucl Med. 2014;55:15–22.
850. Mier W, Kratochwil C, Hassel JC, Giesel FL, Beijer B, Babich JW, Friebe M, Eisenhut M, Enk A, Haberkorn U. Radiopharmaceutical therapy of patients with metastasized melanoma with the melanin-binding benzamide ^{131}I-BA52. J Nucl Med. 2014;55:9–14.

851. Sahlmann Carsten O, Homayounfar K, Niessner M, Dyczkowski J, Conradi L-C, Braulke F, Meller B, Beißbarth T, Ghadimi BM, Meller J, Goldenberg David M, Liersch T. Repeated adjuvant anti-CEA radioimmunotherapy after resection of colorectal liver metastases: safety, feasibility, and long-term efficacy results of a prospective phase 2 study. Cancer. 2016;123:638–49.
852. Sultana A, Shore S, Raraty MGT, Vinjamuri S, Evans JE, Smith CT, Lane S, Chauhan S, Bosonnet L, Garvey C, Sutton R, Neoptolemos JP, Ghaneh P. Randomised phase I/II trial assessing the safety and efficacy of radiolabelled anti-carcinoembryonic antigen (^{131}I)KAb201 antibodies given intra-arterially or intravenously in patients with unresectable pancreatic adenocarcinoma. BMC Cancer. 2009;9:66.
853. Hahner S, Kreissl MC, Fassnacht M, Haenscheid H, Knoedler P, Lang K, Buck AK, Reiners C, Allolio B, Schirbel A. [^{131}I]Iodometomidate for targeted radionuclide therapy of advanced adrenocortical carcinoma. J Clin Endocrinol Metabol. 2012;97:914–22.
854. Kreissl MC, Schirbel A, Fassnacht M, Haenscheid H, Verburg FA, Bock S, Saeger W, Knoedler P, Reiners C, Buck AK, Allolio B, Hahner S. [^{123}I] Iodometomidate imaging in adrenocortical carcinoma. J Clin Endocrinol Metabol. 2013;98:2755–64.
855. Bergmann R, Meckel M, Kubíček V, Pietzsch J, Steinbach J, Hermann P, Rösch F. ^{177}Lu-labelled macrocyclic bisphosphonates for targeting bone metastasis in cancer treatment. EJNMMI Res. 2016;6:5.
856. Fellner M, Baum RP, Kubíček V, Hermann P, Lukeš I, Prasad V, Rösch F. PET/CT imaging of osteoblastic bone metastases with ^{68}Ga-bisphosphonates: first human study. Eur J Nucl Med Mol Imaging. 2010;37:834.
857. Artiko V, Afgan A, Petrović J, Radović B, Petrović N, Vlajković M, Šobic-Šaranović D, Obradović V. Evaluation of neuroendocrine tumors with ^{99m}Tc-EDDA/HYNIC TOC. Nucl Med Rev. 2016;19:99–103.
858. Hankus J, Tomaszewska R. Neuroendocrine neoplasms and somatostatin receptor subtypes expression. Nucl Med Rev. 2016;19:111–7.
859. Trogrlic M, Tezak S. ^{99m}Tc-EDDA/HYNIC-TOC in management of patients with head and neck somatostatin receptor positive tumors. Nucl Med Rev. 2016;19:74–80.
860. King RC, Surfraz MB-U, Biagini SCG, Blower PJ, Mather SJ. How do HYNIC-conjugated peptides bind technetium? Insights from LC-MS and stability studies. Cambridge: Dalton Transactions; 2007. p. 4998–5007.
861. Meszaros LK, Dose A, Biagini SCG, Blower PJ. Hydrazinonicotinic acid (HYNIC) – coordination chemistry and applications in radiopharmaceutical chemistry. Inorg Chim Acta. 2010;363:1059–69.
862. Decristoforo C, Mather SJ. Preparation, ^{99m}Tc-labeling, and in vitro characterization of HYNIC and N_3S modified RC-160 and [Tyr3]octreotide. Bioconjug Chem. 1999;10:431–8.
863. Storch D, Béhé M, Walter MA, Chen J, Powell P, Mikolajczak R, Mäcke HR. Evaluation of [^{99m}Tc/EDDA/HYNIC0]octreotide derivatives compared with [^{111}In-DOTA0,Tyr3, Thr8]octreotide and [^{111}In-DTPA0]octreotide: does tumor or pancreas uptake correlate with the rate of internalization? J Nucl Med. 2005;46:1561–9.
864. Maina T, Nock B, Nikolopoulou A, Sotiriou P, Loudos G, Maintas D, Cordopatis P, Chiotellis E. [^{99m}Tc]demotate, a new ^{99m}Tc-based [Tyr3]octreotate analogue for the detection of somatostatin receptor-positive tumours: synthesis and preclinical results. Eur J Nucl Med Mol Imaging. 2002;29:742–53.
865. Maina T, Nock BA, Cordopatis P, Bernard BF, Breeman WAP, van Gameren A, van den Berg R, Reubi J-C, Krenning EP, de Jong M. [^{99m}Tc] Demotate 2 in the detection of sst_2-positive tumours: a preclinical comparison with [^{111}In]DOTA-tate. Eur J Nucl Med Mol Imaging. 2006;33:831–40.
866. Wild D, Fani M, Behe M, Brink I, Rivier JEF, Reubi JC, Maecke HR, Weber WA. First clinical evidence that imaging with somatostatin receptor antagonists is feasible. J Nucl Med. 2011;52:1412–7.
867. Morgat C, Mishra AK, Varshney R, Allard M, Fernandez P, Hindié E. Targeting neuropeptide receptors for cancer imaging and therapy: perspectives with bombesin, neurotensin, and neuropeptide-Y receptors. J Nucl Med. 2014;55:1650–7.
868. Maxwell JE, Howe JR. Imaging in neuroendocrine tumors: an update for the clinician. Int J Endocr Oncol. 2015;2:159–68.
869. Savelli G, Bertagna F, Franco F, Dognini L, Bosio G, Migliorati E, Rodella C, Biasiotto G, Bettinsoli G, Minari C, Zaniboni A, Ferrari C, Tomassetti P, Ferrari V, Giubbini R. Final results of a phase 2A study for the treatment of metastatic neuroendocrine tumors with a fixed activity of ^{90}Y-DOTA-D-Phe1-Tyr3 octreotide. Cancer. 2012;118:2915–24.
870. Cwikla JB, Sankowski A, Seklecka N, Buscombe JR, Nasierowska-Guttmejer A, Jeziorski KG, Mikolajczak R, Pawlak D, Stepien K, Walecki J. Efficacy of radionuclide treatment DOTATATE Y-90 in patients with progressive metastatic gastroenteropancreatic neuroendocrine carcinomas (GEP-NETs): a phase II study. Ann Oncol. 2010;21:787–94.
871. Sergieva S, Robev B, Dimcheva M, Fakirova A, Hristoskova R. Clinical application of SPECT-CT with ^{99m}Tc-Tektrotyd in bronchial and thymic neuroendocrine tumors (NETs). Nucl Med Rev. 2016;19(2):81–7.
872. Decristoforo C, Maina T, Nock B, Gabriel M, Cordopatis P, Moncayo R. ^{99m}Tc-Demotate 1: first data in tumour patients—results of a pilot/phase I study. Eur J Nucl Med Mol Imaging. 2003;30:1211–9.
873. Reubi JC, Schaer J-C, Waser B. Cholecystokinin(CCK)-A and CCK-B/gas-

trin receptors in human tumors. Cancer Res. 1997;57:1377–86.
874. Reubi JC. Targeting CCK receptors in human cancers. Curr Top Med Chem. 2007;7:1239–42.
875. Behr TM, Béhé MP. Cholecystokinin-B/gastrin receptor-targeting peptides for staging and therapy of medullary thyroid cancer and other cholecystokinin-B receptor-expressing malignancies. Semin Nucl Med. 2002;32:97–109.
876. Gotthardt M, Béhé MP, Grass J, Bauhofer A, Rinke A, Schipper ML, Kalinowski M, Arnold R, Oyen WJG, Behr TM. Added value of gastrin receptor scintigraphy in comparison to somatostatin receptor scintigraphy in patients with carcinoids and other neuroendocrine tumours. Endocr Relat Cancer. 2006;13:1203–11.
877. Gotthardt M, Béhé P, Beuter D, Battmann A, Bauhofer A, Schurrat T, Schipper M, Pollum H, Oyen WJG, Behr TM. Improved tumour detection by gastrin receptor scintigraphy in patients with metastasised medullary thyroid carcinoma. Eur J Nucl Med Mol Imaging. 2006;33:1273–9.
878. Kosowicz J, Mikołajczak R, Czepczyński R, Ziemnicka K, Gryczyńska M, Sowiński J. Two peptide receptor ligands ^{99m}Tc-EDDA/HYNIC-Tyr3-octreotide and ^{99m}Tc-EDDA/HYNIC-DGlu-octagastrin for scintigraphy of medullary thyroid carcinoma. Cancer Biother Radiopharm. 2007;22:613–28.
879. Breeman WAP, Fröberg AC, de Blois E, van Gameren A, Melis M, de Jong M, Maina T, Nock BA, Erion JL, Mäcke HR, Krenning EP. Optimised labeling, preclinical and initial clinical aspects of CCK-2 receptor-targeting with 3 radiolabeled peptides. Nucl Med Biol. 2008;35:839–49.
880. Reubi JC, Maecke HR. Approaches to multireceptor targeting: hybrid radioligands, radioligand cocktails, and sequential radioligand applications. J Nucl Med. 2017;58:10S–6S.
881. Körner M, Stöckli M, Waser B, Reubi JC. GLP-1 receptor expression in human tumors and human normal tissues: potential for in vivo targeting. J Nucl Med. 2007;48:736–43.
882. Wild D, Béhé M, Wicki A, Storch D, Waser B, Gotthardt M, Keil B, Christofori G, Reubi JC, Mäcke HR. [Lys40(Ahx-DTPA-^{111}In)NH_2]exendin-4, a very promising ligand for glucagon-like peptide-1 (GLP-1) receptor targeting. J Nucl Med. 2006;47:2025–33.
883. Wild D, Mäcke H, Christ E, Gloor B, Reubi JC. Glucagon-like peptide 1-receptor scans to localize occult insulinomas. N Engl J Med. 2008;359:766–8.
884. Christ E, Wild D, Ederer S, Béhé M, Nicolas G, Caplin ME, Brändle M, Clerici T, Fischli S, Stettler C, Ell PJ, Seufert J, Gloor B, Perren A, Reubi JC, Forrer F. Glucagon-like peptide-1 receptor imaging for the localisation of insulinomas: a prospective multicentre imaging study. The Lancet Diabetes & Endocrinology. 2013;1:115–22.
885. Christ E, Wild D, Forrer F, Brändle M, Sahli R, Clerici T, Gloor B, Martius F, Maecke H, Reubi JC. Glucagon-like peptide-1 receptor imaging for localization of insulinomas. J Clin Endocrinol Metabol. 2009;94:4398–405.
886. Sowa-Staszczak A, Trofimiuk-Müldner M, Stefańska A, Tomaszuk M, Buziak-Bereza M, Gilis-Januszewska A, Jabrocka-Hybel A, Głowa B, Małecki M, Bednarczuk T, Kamiński G, Kowalska A, Mikołajczak R, Janota B, Hubalewska-Dydejczyk A. ^{99m}Tc labeled glucagon-like peptide-1-analogue (^{99m}Tc-GLP1) scintigraphy in the management of patients with occult insulinoma. PLoS One. 2016;11:e0160714.
887. Sowa-Staszczak A, Pach D, Mikołajczak R, Mäcke H, Jabrocka-Hybel A, Stefańska A, Tomaszuk M, Janota B, Gilis-Januszewska A, Małecki M, Kamiński G, Kowalska A, Kulig J, Matyja A, Osuch C, Hubalewska-Dydejczyk A. Glucagon-like peptide-1 receptor imaging with [Lys40(Ahx-HYNIC-^{99m}Tc/EDDA)NH_2]-exendin-4 for the detection of insulinoma. Eur J Nucl Med Mol Imaging. 2013;40:524–31.
888. Buchegger F, Bonvin F, Kosinski M, Schaffland AO, Prior J, Reubi JC, Bläuenstein P, Tourwé D, García Garayoa E, Bischof Delaloye A. Radiolabeled neurotensin analog, ^{99m}Tc-NT-XI, evaluated in ductal pancreatic adenocarcinoma patients. J Nucl Med. 2003;44:1649–54.
889. Gabriel M, Decristoforo C, Woll E, Eisterer W, Nock B, Maina T, Moncayo R, Virgolini I. [^{99m}Tc] Demotensin VI: biodistribution and initial clinical results in tumor patients of a pilot/phase I study. Cancer Biother Radiopharm. 2011;26:557–63.
890. De Vincentis G, Scopinaro F, Varvarigou A, Ussof W, Schillaci O, Archimandritis S, Corleto V, Longo F, Fave GD. Phase I trial of technetium [Leu13] bombesin as cancer seeking agent: possible scintigraphic guide for surgery? Tumori. 2002;88:S28–30.
891. Soluri A, Scopinaro F, De Vincentis G, Varvarigou A, Scafé R, Massa R, Schillaci O, Spanu A, David V. ^{99m}Tc [13LEU] bombesin and a new gamma camera, the imaging probe, are able to guide mammotome breast biopsy. Anticancer Res. 2003;23:2139–42.
892. De Vincentis G, Remediani S, Varvarigou AD, Di Santo G, Iori F, Laurenti C, Scopinaro F. Role of ^{99m}Tc-bombesin scan in diagnosis and staging of prostate cancer. Cancer Biother Radiopharm. 2004;19:81–4.
893. Scopinaro F, Varvarigou AD, Ussof W, De Vincentis G, Sourlingas TG, Evangelatos GP, Datsteris J, Archimandritis SC. Technetium labeled bombesin-like peptide: preliminary report on breast cancer uptake in patients. Cancer Biother Radiopharm. 2002;17:327–35.
894. Scopinaro F, De Vincentis G, Varvarigou AD, Laurenti C, Iori F, Remediani S, Chiarini S, Stella S. ^{99m}Tc-bombesin detects prostate cancer and invasion of pelvic lymph nodes. Eur J Nucl Med Mol Imaging. 2003;30:1378–82.

895. Scopinaro F, De Vincentis G, Corazziari E, Massa R, Osti M, Pallotta N, Covotta A, Remediani S, Di Paolo M, Monteleone F, Varvarigou A. Detection of colon cancer with ^{99m}Tc-labeled bombesin derivative (^{99m}Tc-leu13-BN1). Cancer Biother Radiopharm. 2004;19:245–52.
896. Shariati F, Aryana K, Fattahi A, Forghani MN, Azarian A, Zakavi SR, Sadeghi R, Ayati N, Sadri K. Diagnostic value of ^{99m}Tc-bombesin scintigraphy for differentiation of malignant from benign breast lesions. Nucl Med Commun. 2014;35:620–5.
897. Santos-Cuevas CL, Ferro-Flores G, de Murphy CA, Pichardo-Romero PA. Targeted imaging of gastrin-releasing peptide receptors with ^{99m}Tc-EDDA/HYNIC-Lys3-bombesin: biokinetics and dosimetry in women. Nucl Med Commun. 2008;29:741–7.
898. Van de Wiele C, Dumont F, Vanden Broecke R, Oosterlinck W, Cocquyt V, Serreyn R, Peers S, Thornback J, Slegers G, Dierckx RA. Technetium-99m RP527, a GRP analogue for visualisation of GRP receptor-expressing malignancies: a feasibility study. Eur J Nucl Med. 2000;27:1694–9.
899. Van de Wiele CV, Dumont F, Dierckx RA, Peers SH, Thornback JR, Slegers G, Thierens H. Biodistribution and dosimetry of ^{99m}Tc-RP527, a gastrin-releasing peptide (GRP) agonist for the visualization of GRP receptor-expressing malignancies. J Nucl Med. 2001;42:1722–7.
900. Van de Wiele C, Phonteyne P, Pauwels P, Goethals I, Van den Broecke R, Cocquyt V, Dierckx RA. Gastrin-releasing peptide receptor imaging in human breast carcinoma versus immunohistochemistry. J Nucl Med. 2008;49:260–4.
901. Ananias HJK, Yu Z, Dierckx RA, van der Wiele C, Helfrich W, Wang F, Yan Y, Chen X, de Jong IJ, Elsinga PH. Technetium-HYNIC(tricine/TPPTS)-Aca-bombesin(7–14) as a targeted imaging agent with MicroSPECT in a PC-3 prostate cancer xenograft model. Mol Pharm. 2011;8:1165–73.
902. Mather SJ, Nock BA, Maina T, Gibson V, Ellison D, Murray I, Sobnack R, Colebrook S, Wan S, Halberrt G, Szysko T, Powles T, Avril N. GRP receptor imaging of prostate cancer using [^{99m}Tc] Demobesin 4: a First-in-Man Study. Mol Imaging Biol. 2014;16:888–95.
903. Scopinaro F, De Vincentis G, Varvarigou AD. Use of radiolabeled bombesin in humans. J Clin Oncol. 2005;23:3170–1.
904. Varvarigou A, Bouziotis P, Zikos C, Scopinaro F, De Vincentis G. Gastrin-releasing peptide (GRP) analogues for cancer imaging. Cancer Biother Radiopharm. 2004;19:219–29.
905. Nock BA, Nikolopoulou A, Galanis A, Cordopatis P, Waser B, Reubi J-C, Maina T. Potent bombesin-like peptides for GRP-receptor targeting of tumors with ^{99m}Tc: a preclinical study. J Med Chem. 2005;48:100–10.
906. Abiraj K, Mansi R, Tamma M-L, Fani M, Forrer F, Nicolas G, Cescato R, Reubi JC, Maecke HR. Bombesin antagonist-based radioligands for translational nuclear imaging of gastrin-releasing peptide receptor–positive tumors. J Nucl Med. 2011;52:1970–8.
907. Maddalena ME, Fox J, Chen J, Feng W, Cagnolini A, Linder KE, Tweedle MF, Nunn AD, Lantry LE. ^{177}Lu-AMBA biodistribution, radiotherapeutic efficacy, imaging, and autoradiography in prostate cancer models with low GRP-R expression. J Nucl Med. 2009;50:2017–24.
908. Thomas R, Chen J, Roudier MM, Vessella RL, Lantry LE, Nunn AD. In vitro binding evaluation of ^{177}Lu-AMBA, a novel ^{177}Lu-labeled GRP-R agonist for systemic radiotherapy in human tissues. Clin Exp Metastasis. 2009;26:105–19.
909. Eder M, Schäfer M, Bauder-Wüst U, Haberkorn U, Eisenhut M, Kopka K. Preclinical evaluation of a bispecific low-molecular heterodimer targeting both PSMA and GRPR for improved PET imaging and therapy of prostate cancer. Prostate. 2014;74:659–68.
910. Liolios C, Schäfer M, Haberkorn U, Eder M, Kopka K. Novel bispecific PSMA/GRPr targeting radioligands with optimized pharmacokinetics for improved PET imaging of prostate cancer. Bioconjug Chem. 2016;27:737–51.
911. Yao CH, Lin KJ, Weng CC, Hsiao IT, Ting YS, Yen TC, Jan TR, Skovronsky D, Kung MP, Wey SP. GMP-compliant automated synthesis of [^{18}F] AV-45 (Florbetapir F 18) for imaging beta-amyloid plaques in human brain. Appl Radiat Isot. 2010;68:2293–7.
912. Davis MI, Bennett MJ, Thomas LM, Bjorkman PJ. Crystal structure of prostate-specific membrane antigen, a tumor marker and peptidase. Proc Natl Acad Sci. 2005;102:5981–6.
913. Bařinka C, Rojas C, Slusher B, Pomper M. Glutamate carboxypeptidase II in diagnosis and treatment of neurologic disorders and prostate cancer. Curr Med Chem. 2012;19:856–70.
914. Kozikowski AP, Nan F, Conti P, Zhang J, Ramadan E, Bzdega T, Wroblewska B, Neale JH, Pshenichkin S, Wroblewski JT. Design of remarkably simple, yet potent urea-based inhibitors of glutamate carboxypeptidase II (NAALADase). J Med Chem. 2001;44:298–301.
915. Zhou J, Neale JH, Pomper MG, Kozikowski AP. NAAG peptidase inhibitors and their potential for diagnosis and therapy. Nat Rev Drug Discov. 2005;4:1015–26.
916. Foss CA, Mease RC, Fan H, Wang Y, Ravert HT, Dannals RF, Olszewski RT, Heston WD, Kozikowski AP, Pomper MG. Radiolabeled small-molecule ligands for prostate-specific membrane antigen: in vivo imaging in experimental models of prostate cancer. Clin Cancer Res. 2005;11:4022–8.
917. Hillier SM, Kern AM, Maresca KP, Marquis JC, Eckelman WC, Joyal JL, Babich JW. ^{123}I-MIP-1072, a small-molecule inhibitor of prostate-specific membrane antigen, is effective at monitoring tumor response to taxane therapy. J Nucl Med. 2011;52:1087–93.

918. Vallabhajosula S, Nikolopoulou A, Babich JW, Osborne JR, Tagawa ST, Lipai I, Solnes L, Maresca KP, Armor T, Joyal JL, Crummet R, Stubbs JB, Goldsmith SJ. ^{99m}Tc-labeled small-molecule inhibitors of prostate-specific membrane antigen: pharmacokinetics and biodistribution studies in healthy subjects and patients with metastatic prostate cancer. J Nucl Med. 2014;55:1791–8.
919. Bartholomä M, Valliant J, Maresca KP, Babich J, Zubieta J. Single amino acid chelates (SAAC): a strategy for the design of technetium and rhenium radiopharmaceuticals. Chem Commun. 2009;5:493–512.
920. Hillier SM, Maresca KP, Lu G, Merkin RD, Marquis JC, Zimmerman CN, Eckelman WC, Joyal JL, Babich JW. ^{99m}Tc-labeled small-molecule inhibitors of prostate-specific membrane antigen for molecular imaging of prostate cancer. J Nucl Med. 2013;54:1369–76.
921. Kimura H, Okuda H, Ishiguro M, Arimitsu K, Makino A, Nishii R, Miyazaki A, Yagi Y, Watanabe H, Kawasaki I, Ono M, Saji H. ^{18}F-labeled pyrido[3,4-*d*]pyrimidine as an effective probe for imaging of L858R mutant epidermal growth factor receptor. ACS Med Chem Lett. 2017;8:418–22.
922. Lu G, Maresca KP, Hillier SM, Zimmerman CN, Eckelman WC, Joyal JL, Babich JW. Synthesis and SAR of ^{99m}Tc/Re-labeled small molecule prostate specific membrane antigen inhibitors with novel polar chelates. Bioorg Med Chem Lett. 2013;23:1557–63.
923. Misra P, Humblet V, Pannier N, Maison W, Frangioni JV. Production of multimeric prostate-specific membrane antigen small-molecule radiotracers using a solid-phase ^{99m}Tc preloading strategy. J Nucl Med. 2007;48:1379–89.
924. Maresca KP, Hillier SM, Lu G, Marquis JC, Zimmerman CN, Eckelman WC, Joyal JL, Babich JW. Small molecule inhibitors of PSMA incorporating technetium-99m for imaging prostate cancer: effects of chelate design on pharmacokinetics. Inorg Chim Acta. 2012;389:168–75.
925. Goffin KE, Joniau S, Tenke P, Slawin K, Klein EA, Stambler N, Strack T, Babich J, Armor T, Wong V. Phase 2 study of ^{99m}Tc-trofolastat SPECT/CT to identify and localize prostate cancer in intermediate- and high-risk patients undergoing radical prostatectomy and extended pelvic LN dissection. J Nucl Med. 2017;58:1408–13.
926. Robu S, Schottelius M, Eiber M, Maurer T, Gschwend J, Schwaiger M, Wester H-J. Preclinical evaluation and first patient application of ^{99m}Tc-PSMA-I&S for SPECT imaging and radioguided surgery in prostate cancer. J Nucl Med. 2017;58:235–42.
927. Weineisen M, Šimeček J, Schottelius M, Schwaiger M, Wester H-J. Synthesis and preclinical evaluation of DOTAGA-conjugated PSMA ligands for functional imaging and endoradiotherapy of prostate cancer. EJNMMI Res. 2014;4:63.
928. Reinfelder J, Kuwert T, Beck M, Sanders JC, Ritt P, Schmidkonz C, Hennig P, Prante O, Uder M, Wullich B, Goebell P. First experience with SPECT/CT using a ^{99m}Tc-labeled inhibitor for prostate-specific membrane antigen in patients with biochemical recurrence of prostate cancer. Clin Nucl Med. 2017;42:26–33.
929. Strosberg JR, Halfdanarson TR, Bellizzi AM, Chan JA, Dillon J, Heaney AP, Kunz PL, O'Dorisio TM, Salem R, Segelov E, Howe J, Pommier R, Brendtro K, Bashir M, Singh S, Soulen MC, Tang L, Zacks JS, Yao J, Bergsland E. The North American Neuroendocrine Society (NANETS) consensus guidelines for surveillance and medical management of midgut neuroendocrine tumors. Pancreas. 2017;46:707–14.

3 Radiomics as Applied in Precision Medicine

Faiq Shaikh, Benjamin Franc,
and Francisca Mulero

3.1 Introduction

Radiomics can be defined as the extraction and analysis of large amounts of advanced quantitative imaging features with high throughput from medical images obtained with various modalities. We describe it as the process of transferring the nuclear medicine interpretation knowledge and skill set from humans to machines in a way that they can see more, process more information, and have deeper insights into what the disease is and how it behaves and might respond to therapeutic intervention. Radiomics methods can be applied across various cancers to identify tumor phenotype characteristics in the images that correlate with their likelihood of survival, as well as their association with the underlying driving biology. Identifying this characteristic set of features called tumor signature holds tremendous value in predicting cancer behavior and progression, which in turn has the potential to predict cancer's response to various therapeutic options (Fig. 3.1). Moreover, we are beginning to see the application of radiomics principles in non-oncologic indications as well, such as cardiovascular disease. In allowing us to have this capacity, radiomics holds the promise of driving the engine of precision medicine. However, there are numerous challenges in the validation methods needed to establish radiomics as a clinically viable solution.

In the context of nuclear medicine, radiomics imaging features may consist of metabolic features, shape features, and textural features of multiple orders. In many imaging applications, radiomics analyses may simply allow greater access to tissue-specific data that cannot be appreciated visually by an imaging clinician or as differences in levels of contrast enhancement on CT, differences in radiopharmaceutical uptake on PET, or using various MR (magnetic resonance) sequences, but nevertheless exists within the imaging dataset itself. For example, the addition of shape and textural features on PET to metabolic parameters and histology can improve prediction of tumor response to therapy in some cases [1].

The practical implementation of radiomics in nuclear medicine typically consists of some level of image preprocessing, segmentation of the volumes of interest using manual or semiautomated means, feature extraction, selection of discriminant features, and, potentially, implementation of features within a model created using statistical analyses or machine learning algorithms.

F. Shaikh (✉)
IAG, Philadelphia, PA, USA

B. Franc
Stanford University, Palo Alto, CA, USA

F. Mulero
CNIO, Madrid, Spain

H. Ahmadzadehfar et al. (eds.), *Clinical Nuclear Medicine*,
https://doi.org/10.1007/978-3-030-39457-8_3

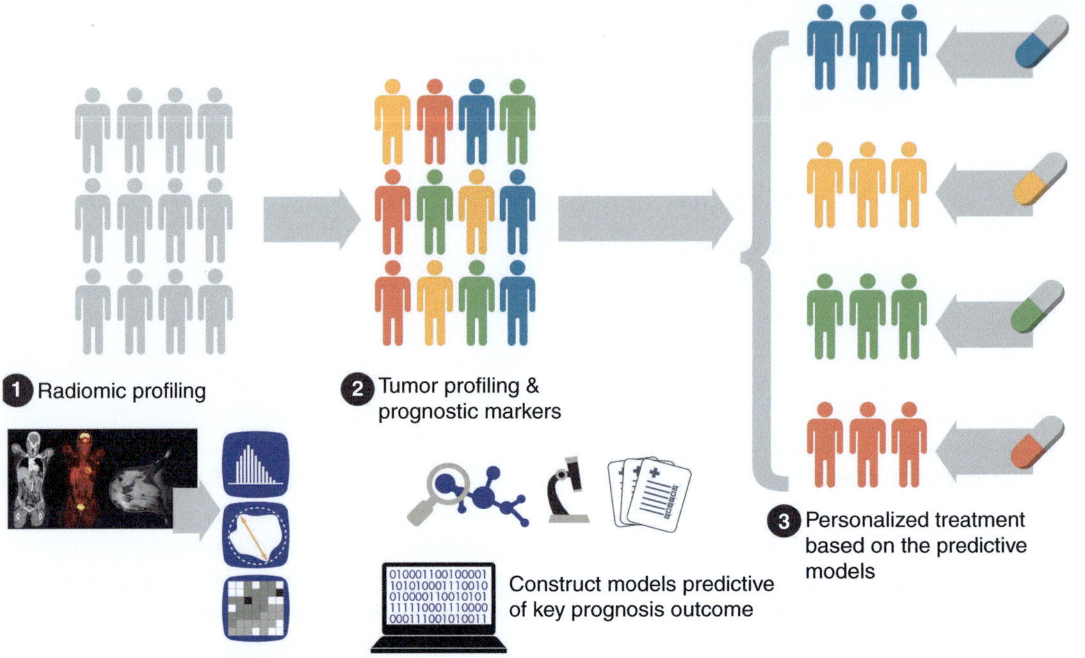

Fig. 3.1 Overview of combining radiomics data with tumor-specific and outcomes data to create predictive models that may be used to identify patient-specific optimized treatment regimens in precision medicine

3.2 Scientific Background

- *Tumor biology—microstructure and microenvironment*: Besides hosting carcinoma cells, the tumor microenvironment encompasses other various components who play a major role in influencing the aggressiveness and outcome of the malignancy. Broad classification of tumor microenvironment results into three main groups: cells of hematopoietic origin (T cells, B cells, NK cells, macrophages, etc.), cells of mesenchymal origin (fibroblasts, mesenchymal stem cells, endothelial cells, pericytes, etc.), and noncellular components found in the extracellular and interstitial matrices (collagen, fibronectin, glycoproteins, etc.). Tumors of different origins and at different stages of progression will inevitably contain varying proportions of these components [2].
  Vascularization is another important component of the tumor microenvironment. Tumors possess an abnormal organization of both blood vessels and tissue structure which results in heterogeneous perfusion and extravasation, together with a hostile microenvironment with increased interstitial pressure. These tumor regions are often hypoxic and resistant to chemo- and radiation therapy. The knowledge of the value of the partial pressure of oxygen concentration (pO_2) in hypoxic areas, in conjunction with data regarding tissue organization, can predict the health status of the tissue of interest and may thus be eventually used to plan program different therapies such as intensity-modulated radiation therapy (IMRT) aimed to the targeted destruction of radiation-resistant areas, while sparing healthy tissues [2, 3].
  There is considerable evidence that the tumor microenvironment contributes actively to tumor heterogeneity through its different components [3]. Right from the moment of niche formation at the pre-metastatic stage, the tumor microenvironment commences on the one hand establishing those appropriate surrounding conditions that would promote local tumor

growth, and, on the other hand, it also begins planning dissemination to other organs, each cancer strategizing differently depending on the specific microenvironment. Through the secretion of cytokines, chemokines, and growth factors, primary tumors "prime" a distal site to become an ideal target organ, favorable to future metastatic colonization [4]. For a given primary tumor, in most of the cases, the eventual metastasis can locate to either always the same destination or to different ones depending on the primary microenvironment being or not being favorable [5]. A better understanding of the tumor microenvironment and its involvement in cancer aggressiveness and prognosis demands an effort from researchers to establish and comprehend local changes within distant organs and their major drivers.

The stroma, another pivotal component of the microenvironment, is found abnormal in most malignancies, and it is characterized by exhibiting an aberrant activation of endothelial cells, leukocytes, pericytes, and fibroblasts. An abnormal stroma is thought to induce chemoresistance [6, 7]. Agents targeting the stroma that can renormalize it would also be capable of re-sensitizing the tumor to chemotherapy through various mechanisms, including increased chemotherapy delivery to the interstitium, decreased hypoxia, and recovery of the antitumor immune response [8]. There is heterogeneity in the treatment of the stromal response and of the vascularization and hypoxia normalization; it should therefore be assessed on an individual basis. Molecular imaging can help to describe in a 3D fashion what is happening in the stroma and in the tumoral vascularization, offering thus the capability to screen in patients that would be good candidates for a certain treatment due to their specific tumor microstructure and microenvironment [9].

- *Tumor heterogeneity and signature*: Different tumor cells show distinct morphological and phenotypic profiles, including cellular morphology, gene expression, metabolism, motility, proliferation, and metastatic potential. This heterogeneity occurs both among tumors (inter-tumor heterogeneity) and within tumors (intratumor heterogeneity). Minimal degrees of intratumor heterogeneity are expected, as a direct consequence of the imperfection of the DNA replication process: whenever a cell (normal or cancerous) divides, mutations are acquired and expressed in different intensity, resulting in a diverse population of cancer cells. The heterogeneity of cancer cells introduces significant challenges to the design of effective treatment strategies. There are two models used to explain the heterogeneity of tumor cells, the cancer stem cell model and the clonal evolution model. The former two models are not mutually exclusive, and it is believed that they both contribute to heterogeneity in varying extents across different tumor types [10]. But, as stated earlier, the tumor microenvironment does play an important role in heterogeneity. The vascular abnormalities, the stroma compartment, etc., can be very different among tumors, and it also is a dynamic process that can change over time.

  Tumor heterogeneity has come to play a vital role in how we understand and treat cancers; many efforts in cancer research currently focus in trying to explain tumoral heterogeneity and the different responses to treatment within different tumors. Although some significant advancements in oncological management have already been achieved, personalized care, however, remains yet an elusive goal. This tumor heterogeneity provides a powerful internal mechanism through which cancer cells can ultimately escape environmental stresses, including oncological therapies, posing a considerable challenge for translational researchers. Research into the understanding and characterization of heterogeneity would allow for a better comprehension of the causes and progression of disease. In turn, this has the potential to guide the design of more refined treatment strategies that incorporate an educated knowledge of heterogeneity to yield higher efficacy. Inter- and intratumor heterogeneity, particularly in the clinical setting, has been difficult to identify, quantify, and, therefore, treat. For most tumors, biopsies remain the standard of care for assessing cancer biology, but they cannot be expected to represent the entirety of a tumor in this tumor heterogenic era [11]. Many physicians advocate the re-biopsy of metastatic disease at re-presentation to further histological analysis and comparison with the archived primary biopsies, attempting to improve the choice of therapy upon relapse, having considered, for instance, inter-tumoral heterogeneity between the primary and the metastatic disease. Repeated biopsy of tumor tissue is invasive, may be difficult in practical terms, has resource implications to ponder about, and is clearly affected by intratumoral heterogeneity. The histological quantification of heterogeneity of tumors can become a logistical and clinical challenge. With the currently available histological techniques, it is difficult to examine in a patient not just the whole tumor but also all the molecular variations of metastatic disease. Advances in molecular imaging techniques and novel applications can surely enhance our understanding of tumor heterogeneity and will bring about a plethora of noninvasive, 3D biomarkers with potential for examining tumors, studying their heterogeneity, and predicting the evolution and the treatment response [12].

This chapter will focus on how the various imaging methods together with the quantification tools currently under development will improve our approach when facing individualized tumor heterogeneity, helping us thus to select the best personalized treatment that meets the constraints imposed by the different behaviors arising from metastatic tumor heterogeneity. The integration into the imaging methods of other in vitro diagnostic approaches such as genomics and exosome analyses will allow to design patient-customized algorithms, which have incorporated the individual variability that emerges from metastatic tumor heterogeneity [11, 12].

Current radiological practice in cancer is mainly qualitative, describing tumor morphology and measuring tumor size according to established standards, for the follow-up of cancer evolution employing the anatomic criteria provided by RECIST (Response Evaluation Criteria In Solid Tumors) or WHO (World Health Organization). The quantification of tumoral evolution is based on short-axis dimensional measurements, which do not reflect the complexity of tumor morphology nor its behavior. Changes in those length parameters often do not reflect or predict a therapeutic benefit. When additional quantitative measurements are obtained, they are generally average values over an entire region of interest (ROI) [13]. PERCIST (Positron Emission Tomography (PET) Response Criteria in Solid Tumors) take into account the SUV (standardized uptake values) of PET, and in doing so it considers information additional to the purely anatomic one, i.e., tumor size measurements, being SUV a measurement of glucose metabolism in cancer cells. PERCIST is useful in the assessment of the efficacy of those therapies that achieve cancer stabilization without a clear decrease in the size of the lesions, often due to intrinsic cancer heterogeneity [14].

Recent advances in molecular imaging allow the visualization and, more importantly, the quantification of the heterogeneity of tumor receptor expression, metabolism, apoptosis, blood flow, or structure, in a noninvasively fashion over time, i.e., at baseline and to assess response to treatment [12, 13].

- *Textural image analysis of PET/CT*: Early radiomics studies explored the use of PET imaging first-order statistics, such as the maximum standardized uptake value (SUVmax) of a voxel within a volume of interest, for their association with other biological and genomic information and value in predicting overall survival and/or progression-free survival outcomes. More recent studies have incorporated multi-order textural analyses to predict these and additional outcomes, such as locoregional recurrence, distant metastasis, or response to therapy from an imaging study early in the treatment course. Textural analyses often employ statistical-based texture features calculated from gray-level co-occurrence matrices (GLCM) which measure the gray-level distribution of neighboring pairs of voxels in multiple orientations and directions.

Most of the PET radiomics work to date has focused on PET using ^{18}F-fluorodeoxyglucose (^{18}F-FDG) thus far.

Calculated radiomics features can number in the tens to thousands, and separating the important features from those less valuable in their predictive capability can be challenging. Often the association of features with an outcome can be assessed with univariate and multivariate analyses. Supervised or unsupervised clustering techniques can be used to explore groups of features that, together, have some association with a biological value (such as histology) or outcome, and heat maps are often employed as a tool to assist in visualizing such analyses [15]. If using hypothesis testing to demonstrate the significance of associations between features and outcomes, the multiple testing problem, whereby statistically significant findings are identified due to random chance because of the sheer number of repeated tests, must be accounted for without crippling the power of the statistical test [16]. A number of means of dealing with this issue in the context of this type of discovery research exist [17–20].

The predictive value of any single feature can be evaluated using the outcome data itself to separate features using one of many methods including supervised classification by decision tree analyses such as random forest analysis, support vector machines (SVM) analysis, neural network classification, or logistic regression [21, 22]. The predictive capability of models used for feature selection may be enhanced using various methods that balance the local structure that can be detected by increasing a model's number of terms and the variance introduced by this increase in terms [23–26]. A set of predictive radiomics features can also be included in a larger disease prediction model that may also include other clinical, histologic, or biochemical factor [27].

Care must be taken to validate the results of any radiomics investigation as steps in the process of achieving the final feature values, such as the method of segmentation of the organ or tumor of interest, may have significant effects on the robustness of the derived radiomics feature associations [28]. Tests of the stability and reproducibility of features must be incorporated into any radiomics study [29]. The application of radiomics to nuclear medicine modalities is further complicated by several variables that do not exist in its application to other imaging modalities. For example, the values of textural features can depend on the time between initial administration of the radiopharmaceutical and acquisition of the emission image [30] as well as the parameters used in reconstructing the PET image [31]. PET, PET-CT, and now PET-MRI technologies are also advancing quickly, and textural features can vary greatly between images acquired on different scanners [32]. Approaches to de-noise and homogenize data from differing sources may potentially be employed, but some parameters cannot be accounted for despite their significant potential effects on the resulting images [33–35]. Relationships between radiomics features calculated from different imaging modalities, such as PET and MR, have also been explored, and optimal image acquisition parameters developed for these multi-modality radiomics pursuits [36, 37].

- *Textural image analysis of SPECT/CT*: The concept of using textural features of a SPECT image to assist in a clinical diagnosis dates back at least two decades [38, 39]. However, the number of applications of radiomics in SPECT is growing less rapidly than in PET. Differences in textural features of ventilation SPECT-CT data have been explored in patients with asthma, chronic obstructive pulmonary disease (COPD), or the combination of COPD and lung cancer [40]. Textural feature analysis has been applied in a computer-aided detection capacity in evaluating ^{123}I-ioflupane SPECT images for evidence of Parkinsonism [41], as well as to classify the severity of Parkinson's disease [42]. Radiomics analyses of SPECT in oncology have explored differences between imaging features of highly and less-differentiated malignancies possibly reflecting variations of intratumoral distribution of antibodies targeting various cancer markers [43].

3.3 Methodology

Radiomics focuses on improvements of image analysis, using an automated high-throughput extraction of large amounts of quantitative features of medical images, and belongs to the last category of innovations in medical imaging analysis. The hypothesis is that quantitative analysis of medical image data through automatic or semiautomatic software of a given imaging modality can provide more and better information than that of a physician. This is supported by the fact that patients exhibit differences in tumor shape and texture measurable by different imaging modalities.

Following are the steps involved in the radiomics methodology (Fig. 3.2):

- *Imaging data acquisition and reconstruction*: A radiomics-compatible system requires mechanisms in place that accommodate high levels of data collection, transfer, and process-

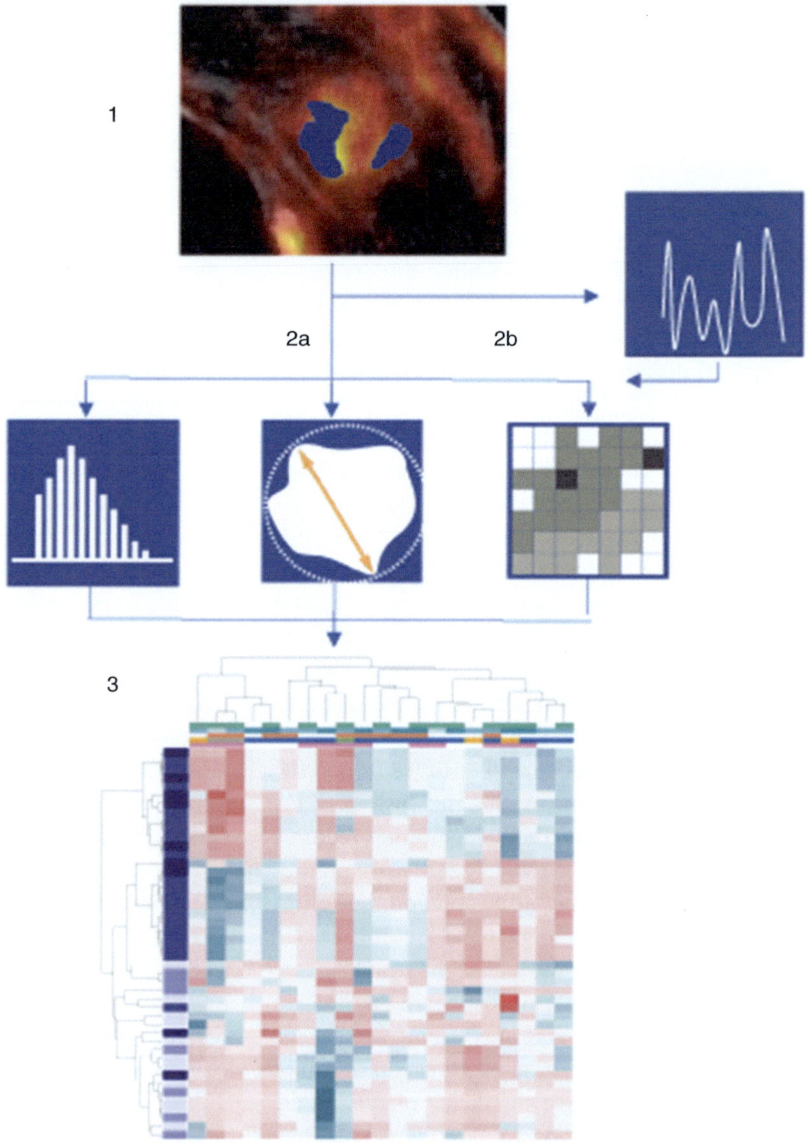

Fig. 3.2 Overview of feature extraction steps—(1) The image volume is segmented. (2) First-order, shape, textural, and higher-order features are calculated on the volume (2a). Wavelet analysis may also be included (2b). (3) Data on multiple features is explored for associations and correlations, aided by machine learning methods

ing/analysis. This begins with collection of raw imaging data. This dataset is conventionally sequestered for standard clinical use; however, tremendous amounts of valuable information can be extracted from that preprocessed data for radiomics assessment, and architectural framework (RIS) and protocols need to be customized to accommodate that process prior to further sequestration. Having said that, radiomics methodologies can be applied to DICOM datasets of images that have been conventionally acquired and have been processed through post-acquisition reconstruction models, such as PET time-of-flight (TOF).

Even when using raw imaging data, preprocessing filters are needed to discriminate the signal from the noise, which is determined by the imaging modality and tumor histology. Discretization techniques to resample signal intensities to partition continuous voxel values to finite/nominal intervals can be performed, which can be either absolute (using a fixed bin size) or relative (using a fixed number of bins whose size depends on the minimum and maximum values within the tumor). Of the two, absolute discretization leads to better repeatability and lower sensitivity to changes and is also less volume-dependent [44].

- *Image segmentation, lesion detection, and ROIs*: These imaging datasets are then subjected to a segmentation process (Fig. 3.3). There are various algorithms for modality-specific lesion detection, such as lung cancer screening CAD for CT. Once detected, an ROI is drawn that contains either the whole tumor or subregions within the tumor using an automated or semiautomated process. Radiomics techniques quantitatively explore the distribution of signal intensities within the ROI. It is

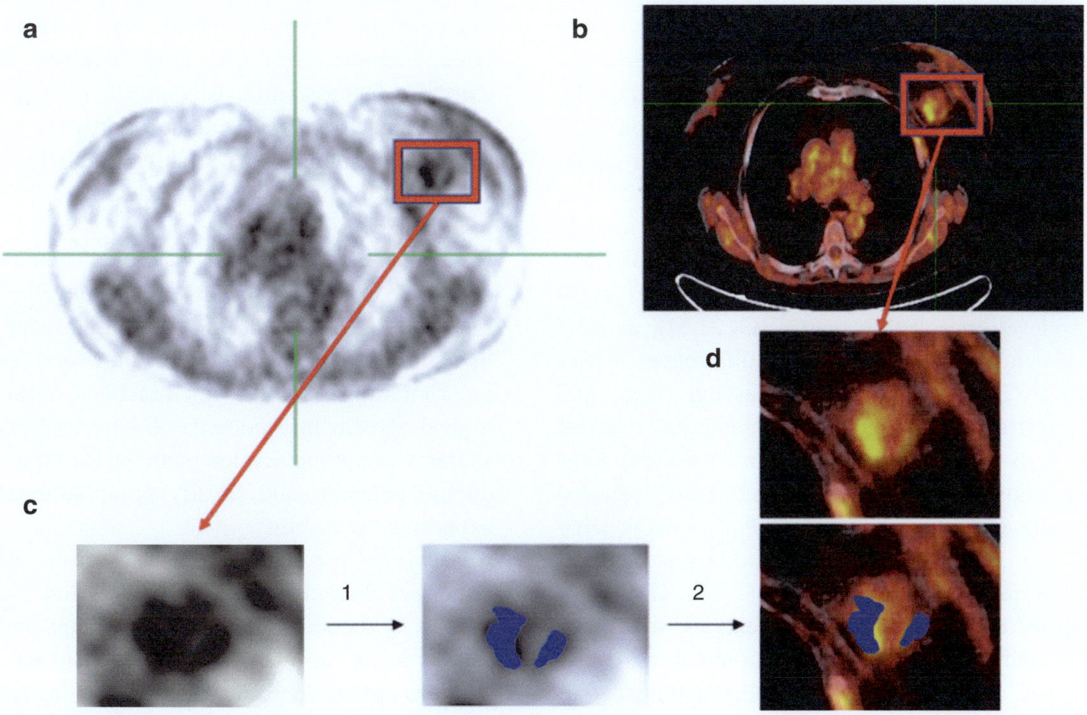

Fig. 3.3 Segmentation of hypoxic volume of primary breast tumor on ^{18}F-MISO PET-CT images—transaxial PET (**a**) and co-registered PET-CT (**b**) images through the chest, with magnified images of the region containing the primary breast tumor (**c**, **d**, respectively). A threshold uptake value was used to segment the hypoxic volume on PET (1), and this volume was transferred to the co-registered CT image allowing both PET and CT radiomics features to be calculated on the hypoxic volume

crucial to correctly delineate the ROIs to be analyzed, as the segmentations must be reproducible and reliable. Automatic methods improve precision and efficiency with reduced inter- and intraobserver variabilities, and there is a need for robust and operator-independent systems to standardize this process, especially keeping in mind the aims of the radiomics methodology (detecting hypoxia, fibrosis, etc.). Conversely, semiautomatic delineation can be necessary where an experienced radiologist is required to correct contours initially defined by CAD [44].

At this time, there is no universal segmentation algorithm available to work with all modalities, and there are no agreed-upon metrics to evaluate them. However, there are open-source platforms equipped with automatic and semiautomatic contouring functions, such as 3D Slicer, NIfTI, etc.

- *Feature extraction and classification*: Radiomics features are quantitatively extracted descriptors of size, shape, and other traits that characterize the tumor microstructure. First-order statistics are used to study the distribution of voxel values without considering spatial relationships. Second-order statistics characterize spatial relationships between voxels (Haralick features), which include gray-level co-occurrence matrix (GLCM), gray-level run length matrix (GLRLM), gray-level zone length matrix (GLZLM), and the neighborhood gray-level difference matrix (NGLDM). The preprocessing step and extracting spatial or spatiotemporal features can be performed by Gabor or Fourier filter grids. The extracted features can be global (one value for the whole ROI) or local (a value per image patch) when inhomogeneous patterns are present in the image [44]. The stability and the accuracy of features should be confirmed through the use of test-retest datasets. A wide range of algorithms are needed to build classifiers. It is important to reduce redundancy of variables in the covariance matrices (too much noise) and also need to reduce feature dimensionality (currently combining ad hoc algorithms).
- *Statistical analysis and developing insights for CDS*: When quantitative features are extracted from the rendered volumes, the resulting dataset undergoes statistical analysis to generate inferences that lead to clinical decision support, especially when it is correlated with clinical and genomic data (Fig. 3.4). This process includes the analysis of the extracted and classified data to develop diagnostic, predictive, and prognostic models for outcomes of interest. There is a need for creating annotated databases with integrated clinical, research (from trials), and genomic data in a PACS-ready easy workflow stream, which is also easily exportable. There are multiple testing issues, issues with supervised and unsupervised analysis and with validating biomarker classifiers. There is also a need to synergize biostatistics, epidemiology, and bioinformatics approaches to build robust, clinically relevant predictive models relating image features to phenotypes/endpoints or gene-protein signatures. With few patients (small sample size) and large number of extracted features, dimensionality is an additional concern, which can be addressed by reducing the number of variables for analysis by exploiting statistical correlations and data redundancy [44].

  Beyond the development of novel feature extraction methods, success in the development and sharing of machine learning models in radiomics (Fig. 3.5) may be improved by incorporating the following practices: ontological agreement, standard software toolsets shared via containerization methods for reproducible research, and, ideally, computational experiment reusability.
- *Informatics considerations*: Integration of radiomics datasets into clinical workflows is limited by the ability of existing systems and standards to accept nonstandard datasets. While mapping these new datasets to legacy (e.g., DICOM, HL7) or emerging (HL7 FHIR) standards might provide a bridge solution, it is more likely to be limiting in data resolution (amount of data stored) and utility (access to the user through existing software packages)

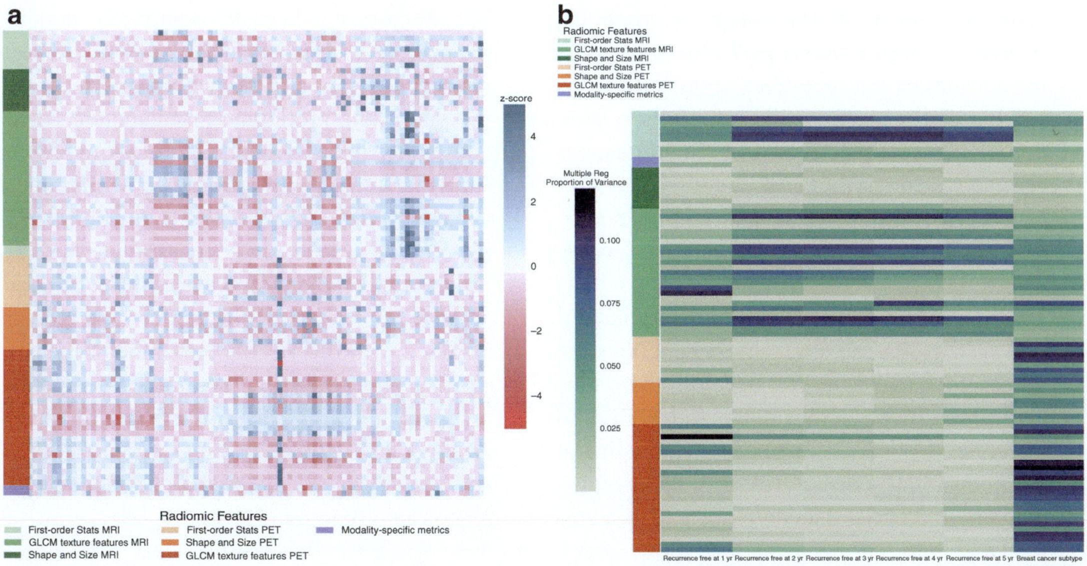

Fig. 3.4 Methods of radiomics data exploration—When visualized as a heat map, clustering analyses (**a**) enable identification of feature groups that tend to cluster. In this example, each column contains features associated with a primary breast tumor segmented from ^{18}F FDG whole-body PET-MR images. Each row in the heat map corresponds to a different feature with the general groups of features organized by the imaging modality and feature order. Hierarchical clustering, where the distances between each datapoint are used in an iterative algorithm to define clusters, was performed on both the feature and histology of the imaged tumors (cluster dendrogram is omitted due to space limitations). The *z*-score statistic, denoted by the color associated with each feature-tumor pair, enables identification of those statistics and tumor histologies that may be associated (positively or negatively) beyond what might be expected by pure chance. The black rectangle surrounds a cluster of feature-tumor pairs that are negatively associated. This cluster suggests a group of features that are commonly low in value when a specific type of tumor histology is present, to define features that group significantly in a similar direction. A heat map generated from univariate correlation (**b**) enables visual display of potential associations of features grouped in rows in a manner similar to that displayed in (**a**). Columns in this graphic represent clinical outcomes of the patients whose primary tumors were imaged with PET-MRI, enabling visual identification of those features or feature orders that may provide outcome prediction

Supervised learning		Unsupervised learning		Deep learning	
Regression	Classification	Clustering	Factor Analysis	Time series	Unstructured
e.g. Lasso	e.g. Random forest	e.g. K-means	e.g. Principal component analysis	e.g. Convolutional Neural networks	

Fig. 3.5 Machine learning techniques—each learning category can be further divided into two classes of methods. One of a number of examples of each method is included

to the end user. Standards like HL7 FHIR are the most promising, because they adopt newer Web architecture conventions and more easily support microservice architectures. The DICOM QUERY supports a finite set of search criteria mostly modeled around the patient, study, series, and instance (or image) attributes. While it has evolved over time to support interchange of data between DICOM archives, it was not designed to support big data analytic use cases [45].

From the IT architectural point of view, there are two models of feature extraction: on demand and static. Feature extraction is presumably computationally intensive because of both the amount of imaging data being processed and the time to retrieve imaging data from the archives. Caching of features statically at a point in time, such as when the patient is scanned, has a performance benefit for consumers but may have significant overhead in data storage for the information technology management team. Caching thousands of features for millions of examinations will be extremely cumbersome and will need revisions as feature extraction techniques evolve over time [45].

Traditional picture archiving and communication system (PACS) platforms do not have the necessary capabilities to develop radiomics algorithms, nor do they have the ability to integrate the radiomics outputs into clinical workflows [44]. Once developed, these multimodality radiomics data outputs need to seamlessly tie into the physician workflow, which requires deep integration into examination worklists, imaging viewers, and electronic medical record (EMR) systems. Radiomics data are stored in a mineable form that can be used to build descriptive and predictive models, relating image features to phenotypes or gene-protein signatures. Cloud computing is a modern paradigm used to reduce the barrier to entry for cancer scientists to participate in challenges of rigorous validation of new algorithms [45].

3.4 Clinical Application and Impact of Radiomics

- *Cancer detection and prognosis*: Perhaps the most direct application of radiomics from an imaging physician's standpoint is for the classification of lesions that are identified on imaging. Feature analysis has been employed to improve classification of pulmonary nodules and bone tumors as malignant or benign on PET-CT and metabolically active lesions as lymphoma versus inflammation on PET [46].

  However, the opportunities to bring imaging directly into precision medicine—in a way similar to genomics and proteomics and other "omics"-related fields—is one of the most intriguing areas of radiomics' utilization. One of the most aggressively pursued applications of radiomics has been in identifying imaging phenotypes of various cancers [47–49]. These phenotypes may or may not have corresponding detectable proteomic and genomic correlates and may be used independently to predict survival, select patients for specific therapies, assess response to systemic or targeted therapies, or otherwise guide therapy [1, 50–58]. By identifying the noninvasive means to characterize the whole tumor, rather than rely on results of a single needle core biopsy, the disease prognosis may be more accurately assessed, allowing selection of a more appropriate course of neoadjuvant or adjuvant therapy as well as improved assessment of response to therapy [33, 48, 59–63].
- *New frontiers for SPECT- and PET-based radiomics within and outside of oncology*: There are a significant number of cardiac SPECT and PET imaging studies performed annually, providing opportunity to employ radiomics techniques to better understand the more intricate processes of cardiovascular disease. For example, different textural features may inform underlying differences in tissue (e.g., scarred myocardium) that indicates an elevated risk for a poor patient outcome [64, 65]. Textural analysis of ultrasound images has been used to monitor the risk of atherosclerotic plaques over time and predict patient outcomes following intervention [66–69]. Similarly, CT-based feature analysis has been explored as a means to assess rupture risk of abdominal aortic aneurysms [70].

  Extracting multi-organ anatomic and metabolic phenotypic data from molecular imaging studies to identify as-of-yet unknown connections between specific therapeutics and changes in organ health is another potential area of radiomics application. The whole-body nature of many nuclear imaging exams facilitate interrogation of multiple systems interactions whereby alterations of imaging features in one organ system may portend subtle anatomic, functional, or molecular changes in another [71].

  Another interesting area of radiomics application may be in the field image-guided therapy.

The use of feature analysis for more precise delineation of anatomic boundaries in cardiology or vascular images has potential to improve the segmentation process for quantitative volumetric analyses themselves or to delineate boundaries or track them for treatment purposes [72–74]. Feature-based tumor boundary delineation has applications in staging as well as radiation oncology treatment planning [75–78].

- *Clinical validation of radiomics*: Performing radiomics clinically requires a multispecialty approach. In addition to imaging specialists, each analysis benefits from input of those most knowledgeable of the disease process and its natural evolution (e.g., cardiologist, neurologist, or oncologist) and those most familiar with its physical manifestations on pathology (e.g., a pathologist with specialization in cardiovascular, neurologic, or oncologic processes). Input should be sought from a medical physicist with expertise in PET/SPECT to fine-tune the preacquisiton and acquisition image acquisition, as well as post-acquisition reiteration for optimal clinical application of radiomics. Imaging physicians should be versed in proper interpretation of radiomics-based biomarkers within the context of the clinical question at hand. All results and their interpretations should undergo robust internal cross-validation and a rigorous external statistical analysis. The focus should be on the inter-reader as well as inter-center reproducibility of these results, which can lead to a higher confidence on part of the order physician as well as the radiologist to rely on these interpretations.
- *Clinical workflow considerations for Radiomics*: The power of radiomics rests on the ability to associate imaging features with physiologic, anatomic, genomic, proteomic, or clinical outcome variables. Clinical outcome is often not a single predefined number. Seemingly straightforward concepts, such as overall survival (OS) or progression-free survival (PFS), are at times difficult to extract from electronic medical records or other sources. Other outcome variables might include more complex concepts such as significant cardiac events, the performance of one or more specified procedures, reported pain or discomfort, the development of a new symptom (e.g., chest pain) or new defined medical condition, altered mentation, memory loss, or even general well-being. Free-text fields within the medical record, such as the physician progress note or nursing notes, are rich with information, but making sense of that information without manual review of each chart is challenging. To address the need for standardization of clinical context in the electronic health record (EHR) in a manner that can be processed in a meaningful way using information technology tools, many clinical and biomedical ontologies have been developed over decades [79–83]. Such ontologies can assist in the extraction of both structured and unstructured data from the EHR. Structured information provides specific events or therapies (e.g., drug names/administration dates, primary endpoints such as hospitalization, or secondary endpoints such as abnormal coronary angiography ± percutaneous coronary) to be placed on clinical timelines relative to the imaging event on which radiomics is being performed. The unstructured information in free-text fields (e.g., physician's notes) requires a sophisticated review of clinical notes and other free-text entries potentially aided by natural language processing (NLP)- or artificial intelligence (AI)-based methodologies [84–91]. Open-source NLP tools have been developed specifically for application in medical contexts, such as the clinical Text Analysis Knowledge Extraction System (cTAKES) and Python Natural Language Toolkit (PyNLTK) [92–94]. Of course, as these techniques evolve, manual chart review on random subsamples of the record pool is required to ensure the robustness of the NLP-based outcomes extraction.
- *Clinical comprehension of radiomics-based insights*: The realization that diseases and their relationships cannot be understood or treated effectively using traditional disease

classifiers has led to the concept of precision medicine [95, 96]. Precision medicine seeks to provide highly targeted approaches for disease diagnosis and treatment at the individual level that intergrate large datasets from numerous sources to develop a complete description of the components and contributors to the disease, and predict how an individual will respond to a particular therapy. The role of radiomics in precision medicine is to collect, connect, and apply data from anatomic and molecular imaging sources to identify disease pathways, specific effects of therapies on normal and diseased tissues, and organ-organ interactions at the anatomic and biochemical levels. Clinical implementation of radiomics has and underlying methodology for personalized medicine is most evident in the field of radiation oncology [97]. Numerous labs and enterprises have developed radiomics models that tackle various clinical challenges [98–100]. However, there is a increasing need to have a standardize system to deliver accurate and reproducible radiomics results. This will be key to usher translational radiomics into the precision medicine mainstream.

References

1. Cook GJ, et al. Are pretreatment 18F-FDG PET tumor textural features in non-small cell lung cancer associated with response and survival after chemoradiotherapy? J Nucl Med. 2013;54(1):19–26.
2. Pattabiraman DR, Weinberg RA. Tackling the cancer stem cells – what challenges do they pose? Nat Rev Drug Discov. 2014;13(7):497–512.
3. Quail DF, Joyce JA. Microenvironmental regulation of tumor progression and metastasis. Nat Med. 2013;19(11):1423–37.
4. Psaila B, Lyden D. The metastatic niche: adapting the foreign soil. Nat Rev Cancer. 2009;9(4):285–93.
5. Husemann Y, et al. Systemic spread is an early step in breast cancer. Cancer Cell. 2008;13(1):58–68.
6. Goubran HA, et al. Regulation of tumor growth and metastasis: the role of tumor microenvironment. Cancer Growth Metastasis. 2014;7:9–18.
7. Jain RK. Normalizing tumor microenvironment to treat cancer: bench to bedside to biomarkers. J Clin Oncol. 2013;31(17):2205–18.
8. Funahashi Y, et al. Eribulin mesylate reduces tumor microenvironment abnormality by vascular remodeling in preclinical human breast cancer models. Cancer Sci. 2014;105(10):1334–42.
9. Quintela-Fandino M, et al. (18)F-fluoromisonidazole PET and activity of neoadjuvant Nintedanib in early HER2-negative breast cancer: a window-of-opportunity randomized trial. Clin Cancer Res. 2017;23(6):1432–41.
10. Shackleton M, et al. Heterogeneity in cancer: cancer stem cells versus clonal evolution. Cell. 2009;138(5):822–9.
11. Gerlinger M, et al. Intratumor heterogeneity and branched evolution revealed by multiregion sequencing. N Engl J Med. 2012;366(10):883–92.
12. Chowdhury R, et al. The use of molecular imaging combined with genomic techniques to understand the heterogeneity in cancer metastasis. Br J Radiol. 2014;87(1038):20140065.
13. Kumar V, et al. Radiomics: the process and the challenges. Magn Reson Imaging. 2012;30(9):1234–48.
14. Wahl RL, et al. From RECIST to PERCIST: evolving considerations for PET response criteria in solid tumors. J Nucl Med. 2009;50(Suppl 1):122S–50S.
15. Tsujikawa T, et al. (18)F-FDG PET radiomics approaches: comparing and clustering features in cervical cancer. Ann Nucl Med. 2017;31(9):678–85.
16. Chalkidou A, O'Doherty MJ, Marsden PK. False discovery rates in PET and CT studies with texture features: a systematic review. PLoS One. 2015;10(5):e0124165.
17. Armstrong RA. When to use the Bonferroni correction. Ophthalmic Physiol Opt. 2014;34(5):502–8.
18. Benjamini Y, Hochberg Y. Controlling the false discovery rate: a practical and powerful approach to multiple testing. J R Stat Soc Ser B. 1995;57(1):289–300.
19. Benjamini Y, Yekutieli D. Quantitative trait loci analysis using the false discovery rate. Genetics. 2005;171(2):783–90.
20. Storey JD. A direct approach to false discovery rates. J R Stat Soc Ser B Stat Methodol. 2002;64:479–98.
21. Desbordes P, et al. Predictive value of initial FDG-PET features for treatment response and survival in esophageal cancer patients treated with chemo-radiation therapy using a random forest classifier. PLoS One. 2017;12(3):e0173208.
22. Vidyasagar M. Machine learning methods in the computational biology of cancer. Proc Math Phys Eng Sci. 2014;470(2167):20140081.
23. Bunea F, et al. Penalized least squares regression methods and applications to neuroimaging. NeuroImage. 2011;55(4):1519–27.
24. de Vlaming R, Groenen PJ. The current and future use of ridge regression for prediction in quantitative genetics. Biomed Res Int. 2015;2015:143712.
25. Fort G, Lambert-Lacroix S. Classification using partial least squares with penalized logistic regression. Bioinformatics. 2005;21(7):1104–11.

26. Li Z, Sillanpaa MJ. Overview of LASSO-related penalized regression methods for quantitative trait mapping and genomic selection. Theor Appl Genet. 2012;125(3):419–35.
27. Foley KG, et al. Development and validation of a prognostic model incorporating texture analysis derived from standardised segmentation of PET in patients with oesophageal cancer. Eur Radiol. 2017;28(1):428–36.
28. Bashir U, et al. The effects of segmentation algorithms on the measurement of 18F-FDG PET texture parameters in non-small cell lung cancer. EJNMMI Res. 2017;7(1):60.
29. Leijenaar RT, et al. Stability of FDG-PET radiomics features: an integrated analysis of test-retest and inter-observer variability. Acta Oncol. 2013;52(7):1391–7.
30. Lovat E, et al. The effect of post-injection 18F-FDG PET scanning time on texture analysis of peripheral nerve sheath tumours in neurofibromatosis-1. EJNMMI Res. 2017;7(1):35.
31. Shiri I, et al. The impact of image reconstruction settings on 18F-FDG PET radiomic features: multi-scanner phantom and patient studies. Eur Radiol. 2017;27:4498.
32. Reuze S, et al. Prediction of cervical cancer recurrence using textural features extracted from 18F-FDG PET images acquired with different scanners. Oncotarget. 2017;8(26):43169–79.
33. Galavis PE, et al. Variability of textural features in FDG PET images due to different acquisition modes and reconstruction parameters. Acta Oncol. 2010;49(7):1012–6.
34. Le Pogam A, et al. Denoising of PET images by combining wavelets and curvelets for improved preservation of resolution and quantitation. Med Image Anal. 2013;17(8):877–91.
35. Teo BK, et al. Partial-volume correction in PET: validation of an iterative postreconstruction method with phantom and patient data. J Nucl Med. 2007;48(5):802–10.
36. Bolouri MS, et al. Triple-negative and non-triple-negative invasive breast cancer: association between MR and fluorine 18 fluorodeoxyglucose PET imaging. Radiology. 2013;269(2):354–61.
37. Vallieres M, et al. Enhancement of multimodality texture-based prediction models via optimization of PET and MR image acquisition protocols: a proof of concept. Phys Med Biol. 2017;62:8536.
38. Staff RT, et al. Texture analysis of divers' brains using 99Tcm-HMPAO SPET. Nucl Med Commun. 1995;16(6):438–42.
39. Staff, R.T, et al. Decompression illness in sports divers detected with technetium-99m-HMPAO SPECT and texture analysis. J Nucl Med. 1996;37(7):1154–8.
40. Meier A, et al. Application of texture analysis to ventilation SPECT/CT data. Comput Med Imaging Graph. 2011;35(6):438–50.
41. Martinez-Murcia FJ, et al. Parametrization of textural patterns in 123I-ioflupane imaging for the automatic detection of Parkinsonism. Med Phys. 2014;41(1):012502.
42. Rahmim A, et al. Application of texture analysis to DAT SPECT imaging: relationship to clinical assessments. Neuroimage Clin. 2016;12:e1–9.
43. Rajkumar V, et al. Texture analysis of (125) I-A5B7 anti-CEA antibody SPECT differentiates metastatic colorectal cancer model phenotypes and anti-vascular therapy response. Br J Cancer. 2015;112(12):1882–7.
44. Limkin EJ, et al. Promises and challenges for the implementation of computational medical imaging (radiomics) in oncology. Ann Oncol. 2017;28(6):1191–206.
45. Shaikh F, et al. Technical challenges in clinical applications of radiomics. J Clin Oncol Clin Cancer Informat. 2017;1:1–8.
46. Lartizien C, et al. Computer-aided staging of lymphoma patients with FDG PET/CT imaging based on textural information. IEEE J Biomed Health Inform. 2014;18(3):946–55.
47. Aerts HJ, et al. Decoding tumour phenotype by noninvasive imaging using a quantitative radiomics approach. Nat Commun. 2014;5:4006.
48. Ha S, et al. Metabolic Radiomics for pretreatment 18F-FDG PET/CT to characterize locally advanced breast cancer: histopathologic characteristics, response to neoadjuvant chemotherapy, and prognosis. Sci Rep. 2017;7(1):1556.
49. Lambin P, et al. Radiomics: extracting more information from medical images using advanced feature analysis. Eur J Cancer. 2012;48(4):441–6.
50. Cheng NM, et al. Zone-size nonuniformity of 18F-FDG PET regional textural features predicts survival in patients with oropharyngeal cancer. Eur J Nucl Med Mol Imaging. 2015;42(3):419–28.
51. Cheng NM, Fang YH, Yen TC. The promise and limits of PET texture analysis. Ann Nucl Med. 2013;27(9):867–9.
52. Cook GJ, et al. Non-small cell lung cancer treated with Erlotinib: heterogeneity of (18)F-FDG uptake at PET-association with treatment response and prognosis. Radiology. 2015;276(3):883–93.
53. Knogler T, et al. Three-dimensional texture analysis of contrast enhanced CT images for treatment response assessment in Hodgkin lymphoma: comparison with F-18-FDG PET. Med Phys. 2014;41(12):121904.
54. Panth KM, et al. Is there a causal relationship between genetic changes and radiomics-based image features? An in vivo preclinical experiment with doxycycline inducible GADD34 tumor cells. Radiother Oncol. 2015;116(3):462–6.
55. Pyka T, et al. Textural features in pre-treatment [F18]-FDG-PET/CT are correlated with risk of local recurrence and disease-specific survival in early stage NSCLC patients receiving primary stereotactic radiation therapy. Radiat Oncol. 2015;10:100.
56. Pyka T, et al. Textural analysis of pre-therapeutic [18F]-FET-PET and its correlation with tumor grade

and patient survival in high-grade gliomas. Eur J Nucl Med Mol Imaging. 2016;43(1):133–41.
57. Tixier F, et al. Intratumor heterogeneity characterized by textural features on baseline 18F-FDG PET images predicts response to concomitant radiochemotherapy in esophageal cancer. J Nucl Med. 2011;52(3):369–78.
58. Vaidya M, et al. Combined PET/CT image characteristics for radiotherapy tumor response in lung cancer. Radiother Oncol. 2012;102(2):239–45.
59. Al-Kadi OS, Watson D. Texture analysis of aggressive and nonaggressive lung tumor CE CT images. IEEE Trans Biomed Eng. 2008;55(7):1822–30.
60. Chicklore S, et al. Quantifying tumour heterogeneity in 18F-FDG PET/CT imaging by texture analysis. Eur J Nucl Med Mol Imaging. 2013;40(1):133–40.
61. de Jong EE, et al. [18F]FDG PET/CT-based response assessment of stage IV non-small cell lung cancer treated with paclitaxel-carboplatin-bevacizumab with or without nitroglycerin patches. Eur J Nucl Med Mol Imaging. 2017;44(1):8–16.
62. Ganeshan B, et al. Tumour heterogeneity in non-small cell lung carcinoma assessed by CT texture analysis: a potential marker of survival. Eur Radiol. 2012;22(4):796–802.
63. Hatt M, et al. 18F-FDG PET uptake characterization through texture analysis: investigating the complementary nature of heterogeneity and functional tumor volume in a multi-cancer site patient cohort. J Nucl Med. 2015;56(1):38–44.
64. Engan K, et al. Exploratory data analysis of image texture and statistical features on myocardium and infarction areas in cardiac magnetic resonance images. Conf Proc IEEE Eng Med Biol Soc. 2010;2010:5728–31.
65. Kotu LP, et al. Probability mapping of scarred myocardium using texture and intensity features in CMR images. Biomed Eng Online. 2013;12:91.
66. Awad J, et al. Texture analysis of carotid artery atherosclerosis from three-dimensional ultrasound images. Med Phys. 2010;37(4):1382–91.
67. Coleman DP, et al. Development and validation of an in vivo analysis tool to identify changes in carotid plaque tissue types in serial 3-D ultrasound scans. Ultrasound Med Biol. 2005;31(3):329–35.
68. Madycki G, Staszkiewicz W, Gabrusiewicz A. Carotid plaque texture analysis can predict the incidence of silent brain infarcts among patients undergoing carotid endarterectomy. Eur J Vasc Endovasc Surg. 2006;31(4):373–80.
69. Niu L, et al. Surface roughness detection of arteries via texture analysis of ultrasound images for early diagnosis of atherosclerosis. PLoS One. 2013;8(10):e76880.
70. Kotze CW, et al. CT signal heterogeneity of abdominal aortic aneurysm as a possible predictive biomarker for expansion. Atherosclerosis. 2014;233(2):510–7.
71. Aghini-Lombardi F, et al. Early textural and functional alterations of left ventricular myocardium in mild hypothyroidism. Eur J Endocrinol. 2006;155(1):3–9.
72. Adjeroh DA, Kandaswamy U, Odom JV. Texton-based segmentation of retinal vessels. J Opt Soc Am A Opt Image Sci Vis. 2007;24(5):1384–93.
73. Histace A, Matuszewski B, Zhang Y. Segmentation of myocardial boundaries in tagged cardiac MRI using active contours: a gradient-based approach integrating texture analysis. Int J Biomed Imaging. 2009;2009:983794.
74. Noce A, Triboulet J, Poignet P. Efficient tracking of the heart using texture. Conf Proc IEEE Eng Med Biol Soc. 2007;2007:4480–3.
75. Bagci U, et al. Predicting future morphological changes of lesions from radiotracer uptake in 18F-FDG-PET images. PLoS One. 2013;8(2):e57105.
76. Mu W, et al. Staging of cervical cancer based on tumor heterogeneity characterized by texture features on (18)F-FDG PET images. Phys Med Biol. 2015;60(13):5123–39.
77. Shiradkar R, et al. Radiomics based targeted radiotherapy planning (rad-TRaP): a computational framework for prostate cancer treatment planning with MRI. Radiat Oncol. 2016;11(1):148.
78. Yu H, et al. Automated radiation targeting in head-and-neck cancer using region-based texture analysis of PET and CT images. Int J Radiat Oncol Biol Phys. 2009;75(2):618–25.
79. https://www.nlm.nih.gov/healthit/snomedct/. Accessed 12 Jun 2017.
80. Bodenreider O, Stevens R. Bio-ontologies: current trends and future directions. Brief Bioinform. 2006;7(3):256–74.
81. Schulz S, Marko K, Suntisrivaraporn B. Formal representation of complex SNOMED CT expressions. BMC Med Inform Decis Mak. 2008;8(Suppl 1):S9.
82. Schulz S, Suntisrivaraporn B, Baader F. SNOMED CT's problem list: ontologists' and logicians' therapy suggestions. Stud Health Technol Inform. 2007;129(Pt 1):802–6.
83. Schulz S, et al. SNOMED reaching its adolescence: ontologists' and logicians' health check. Int J Med Inform. 2009;78(Suppl 1):S86–94.
84. Bromuri S, et al. Multi-label classification of chronically ill patients with bag of words and supervised dimensionality reduction algorithms. J Biomed Inform. 2014;51:165–75.
85. Friedman C, Hripcsak G. Natural language processing and its future in medicine. Acad Med. 1999;74(8):890–5.
86. Friedman C, et al. Representing information in patient reports using natural language processing and the extensible markup language. J Am Med Inform Assoc. 1999;6(1):76–87.
87. Ohno-Machado L, Nadkarni P, Johnson K. Natural language processing: algorithms and tools to extract computable information from EHRs and from the biomedical literature. J Am Med Inform Assoc. 2013;20(5):805.

88. Powell RT, et al. Identification of histological correlates of overall survival in lower grade gliomas using a bag-of-words paradigm: a preliminary analysis based on Hematoxylin & Eosin Stained Slides from the lower grade glioma cohort of the Cancer genome atlas. J Pathol Inform. 2017;8:9.
89. Soguero-Ruiz C, et al. Support vector feature selection for early detection of anastomosis leakage from bag-of-words in electronic health records. IEEE J Biomed Health Inform. 2016;20(5):1404–15.
90. Hripcsak G, et al. Unlocking clinical data from narrative reports: a study of natural language processing. Ann Intern Med. 1995;122(9):681–8.
91. Nadkarni PM, Ohno-Machado L, Chapman WW. Natural language processing: an introduction. J Am Med Inform Assoc. 2011;18(5):544–51.
92. Bird S, Klein E, Loper E. Natural language processing with Python – analyzing text with the natural language toolkit. Sebastopol, CA: O'Reilly Media; 2009.
93. Garla V, et al. The Yale cTAKES extensions for document classification: architecture and application. J Am Med Inform Assoc. 2011;18(5):614–20.
94. Savova GK, et al. Mayo clinical text analysis and knowledge extraction system (cTAKES): architecture, component evaluation and applications. J Am Med Inform Assoc. 2010;17(5):507–13.
95. Moving toward precision medicine. Lancet. 2011;378(9804):1678.
96. National Research Council. D.o.E.a.L.S., Committee on a framework for developing a new taxonomy of disease, toward precision medicine: building a knowledge network for biomedical research and a new taxonomy of disease. Washington, DC: National Academies Press; 2011.
97. Jin JY, Kong FM. Personalized radiation therapy (PRT) for lung cancer. Adv Exp Med Biol. 2016;890:175–202.
98. http://www.healthmyne.com. Accessed 9 Jun 2017.
99. Szczypinski PM, et al. MaZda—a software package for image texture analysis. Comput Methods Prog Biomed. 2009;94(1):66–76.
100. http://www.oncoradiomics.com. Accessed 9 Jun 2017.

Part II

Diagnostic Nuclear Medicine

SPECT and PET of the Brain

4

Yasuyuki Kimura, Takashi Kato, Kengo Ito, and Masanori Ichise

4.1 SPECT and PET Brain Imaging in the Evaluation of Dementia

There has been an explosion of developments in nuclear medicine imaging in the evaluation of dementia disorders since the first edition of the current textbook over a decade ago. Great efforts have been made to image two neuropathological hallmarks of Alzheimer's disease (AD), namely, β-amyloid and hyperphosphorylated tau protein accumulations in the brain. A number of selective PET radiopharmaceuticals for β-amyloid imaging have recently been approved for clinical use in the USA, Europe, and Japan; and several other PET radiopharmaceuticals for tau imaging are expected to follow a similar path toward clinical use.

PET brain imaging with these radiopharmaceuticals are aimed to visualize and quantify accumulations of β-amyloid and abnormal tau proteins in neurodegenerative disorders. Amyloid and tau PET scans are, therefore, not only useful as a clinical diagnostic tool, but also, they can be used as imaging biomarkers in clinical therapeutic trials, allowing for the selection of appropriate subjects and monitoring of therapeutic efficacy of disease-modifying drugs that target these proteins. In addition, PET brain research studies using these radiopharmaceuticals are contributing to furthering our understanding of the pathophysiology of neurodegenerative disorders, leading to refinement of clinical diagnosis and differential diagnosis as well as improvements in the strategy to treat these disorders.

Y. Kimura
Department of Clinical and Experimental Neuroimaging, Center for Development of Advanced Medicine for Dementia, National Center for Geriatrics and Gerontology, Obu, Aichi, Japan
e-mail: yazkim@ncgg.go.jp

T. Kato
Department of Clinical and Experimental Neuroimaging, Center for Development of Advanced Medicine for Dementia, National Center for Geriatrics and Gerontology, Obu, Aichi, Japan

Department of Radiology, National Center for Geriatrics and Gerontology, Obu, Aichi, Japan
e-mail: tkato@ncgg.go.jp

K. Ito
Department of Clinical and Experimental Neuroimaging, Center for Development of Advanced Medicine for Dementia, National Center for Geriatrics and Gerontology, Obu, Aichi, Japan
e-mail: kito@ncgg.go.jp

M. Ichise (✉)
Department of Clinical and Experimental Neuroimaging, Center for Development of Advanced Medicine for Dementia, National Center for Geriatrics and Gerontology, Obu, Aichi, Japan

Department of Functional Brain Imaging Research, National Institute of Radiological Sciences, National Institutes for Quantum and Radiological Science and Technology, Chiba, Chiba, Japan

Department of Radiology, Fujita Health University, Toyoake, Aichi, Japan

H. Ahmadzadehfar et al. (eds.), *Clinical Nuclear Medicine*,
https://doi.org/10.1007/978-3-030-39457-8_4

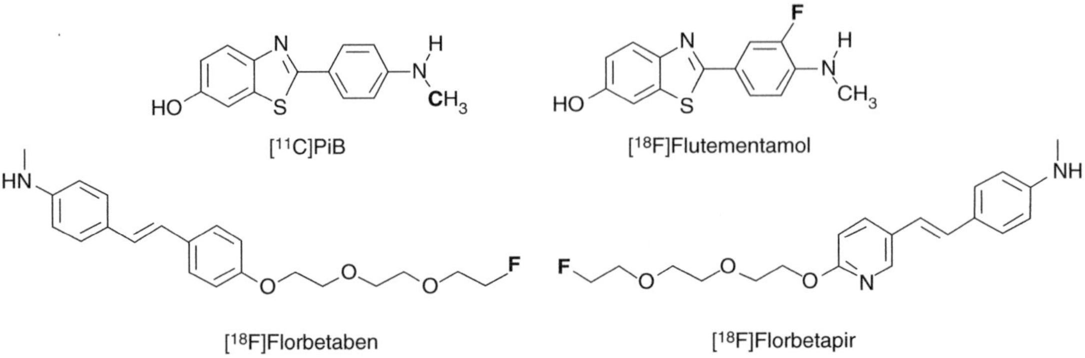

Fig. 4.1 Chemical structures of [^{11}C]PIB and three ^{18}F-labeled compounds for imaging β-amyloid. Note the similarity of the chemical structure between [^{11}C]PIB and [^{18}F]flutemetamol and between [^{18}F]florbetapir and [^{18}F]florbetaben

PET radiopharmaceuticals for β-amyloid have been developed from a modification of the amyloid-binding staining thioflavin-T. Following the successful imaging studies of AD using [^{11}C]PIB [1] (full chemical names of all radiopharmaceuticals in the text are listed in Appendix), several ^{18}F-labeled compounds have been available for clinical use (Fig. 4.1). Labeling with ^{18}F compared with ^{11}C enables much wider accessibility to β-amyloid imaging because ^{18}F radiopharmaceuticals can be delivered conveniently from nearby radiopharmaceutical production centers to imaging centers that do not have cyclotron facility. Among the ^{18}F-labeled compounds, [^{18}F]flutemetamol and [^{18}F]NAV4694 are derivatives of [^{11}C]PIB [1]. On the other hand, [^{18}F]florbetapir and [^{18}F]florbetaben share a similar structure originated from another ^{11}C-labeled amyloid ligand, [^{11}C]SB-13 [2]. Among these radiopharmaceuticals, [^{18}F]flutemetamol, [^{18}F]florbetapir, and [^{18}F]florbetaben have been approved by the regulatory agencies in the USA, Europe, and Japan and are becoming widely used for clinical workup and research purposes as well in clinical therapeutic trials of AD.

On the other hand, development of tau PET radiopharmaceuticals has taken a somewhat tortuous path. [^{18}F]FDDNP is the first PET radiopharmaceutical, which was originally claimed to be a tau imaging radiopharmaceutical, but it lacks selectivity for tau over β-amyloid [3]. [^{11}C]PBB3 was introduced in 2013 as a highly selective radiopharmaceutical for tau imaging [4], and two other tau radiopharmaceuticals, [^{18}F]flortaucipir (a.k.a. T-807 or AV1451) and [^{18}F]THK5351, were developed shortly thereafter [5, 6]. Hyperphosphorylated tau proteins are found not only in AD but also in other tauopathies such as progressive supranuclear palsy, corticobasal degeneration, etc.

These abnormal tau proteins exist in six pathological isoforms, and the tau isoform profile differs among various tau pathologies. PET tau radiopharmaceuticals can have different binding affinities for each of the six isoforms depending on their chemical formulations. Of the first-generation tau radiopharmaceuticals, [^{11}C]PBB3 binds to all six isoforms of tau with significant affinity, allowing imaging of diverse tau pathologies. [^{11}C]PBB3 PET affords accurate quantification of tau burden despite radiopharmaceutical's fast metabolism and complex in vivo kinetics and suited for longitudinal research studies where accurate quantification of tau binding is essential [7]. However, this radiopharmaceutical is limited in its wide availability due to ^{11}C labeling.

[^{18}F]flortaucipir and [^{18}F]THK5351 are potentially available widely because of ^{18}F labeling and have been used in many clinical research studies [8, 9]. These two radiopharmaceuticals do not bind to all six isoforms; instead they bind to a mixture of three- and four-repeat tau isoforms with less ability to bind to three- or four-repeat tau isoforms, allowing imaging of only certain types of tauopathies [10]. In addition, recent studies found that these two radiopharmaceuticals show binding to other non-tau proteins (off-target binding), including monoamine oxidase and melanin, thus compromising PET scan interpretations. Second generations of tau PET radiopharmaceuticals that do not possess off-target binding are currently under development supported by pharmaceutical companies. Promising radiopharmaceuticals include [^{18}F]PI-2620, [^{18}F]MK-6240, and [^{18}F]PM-PBB3 [11]. While [^{18}F]PI-2620 and [^{18}F]PM-PBB3 can bind to all isoforms of tau, [^{18}F]MK-6240 appears to bind only to the mixture of three- and four-repeat tau isoforms.

PET and SPECT are clinically used for early detection and differential diagnosis of neurodegenerative disorders. The most common cause of dementing disorders is AD, which is pathologically characterized by formation of neuritic plaques due to accumulation of β-amyloid and neurofibrillary tangles as a result of hyperphosphorylated tau proteins. Accumulation of these proteins causes synaptic dysfunction and loss of neurons, leading to cognitive dysfunction and eventually to dementia. In AD, the time course of β-amyloid deposition has traditionally been investigated by examining postmortem AD brains. The advent of β-amyloid PET now provides visualization of β-amyloid deposition in living patients with AD (Fig. 4.2). The β-amyloid deposition begins in temporobasal and frontomedial areas and then spreads to the remaining associative neocortex, primary sensory-motor areas and the medial temporal lobe, and finally the striatum [12]. β-Amyloid PET studies in patients with a genetic variant of AD with autosomal dominant transmission and their cognitively normal family members have shown that accumulation of β-amyloid begins decades earlier than the development of cognitive decline [13]. Although β-amyloid deposition is one of the two pathological features of AD, the other being tau deposition, cognitively healthy aged subjects can have β-amyloid depositions with increasing frequencies with advancing age (12% of subjects in the 60s and 30% of subjects in the 70s [14]. Therefore, positive β-amyloid PET scans alone do not constitute a diagnosis of AD. However, negative β-amyloid PET scans virtually exclude the possibility of AD in demented patients and other types of neurodegenerative disorders than AD need to be considered in the differential diagnosis.

β-Amyloid PET imaging has also proven to be useful for predicting the outcome of subjects with mild cognitive impairment (MCI). In MCI, approximately 70% of subjects have high amyloid accumulation, and 70% of them progress to clinically diagnosed AD in 3 years, whereas under 5% of those with low amyloid accumulation progress to clinically diagnosed AD, and 20% of those with low amyloid accumulation progress to other dementia in the same time interval [15].

As a clinical aid to the differential diagnosis of neurodegenerative disorders, β-amyloid PET imaging can be useful, where patients with the frontotemporal dementia are β-amyloid negative, whereas patients with AD and ~60% of patients with dementia with Lewy bodies (DLB) are β-amyloid positive [16]. The interim analysis of the US Imaging Dementia—Evidence for

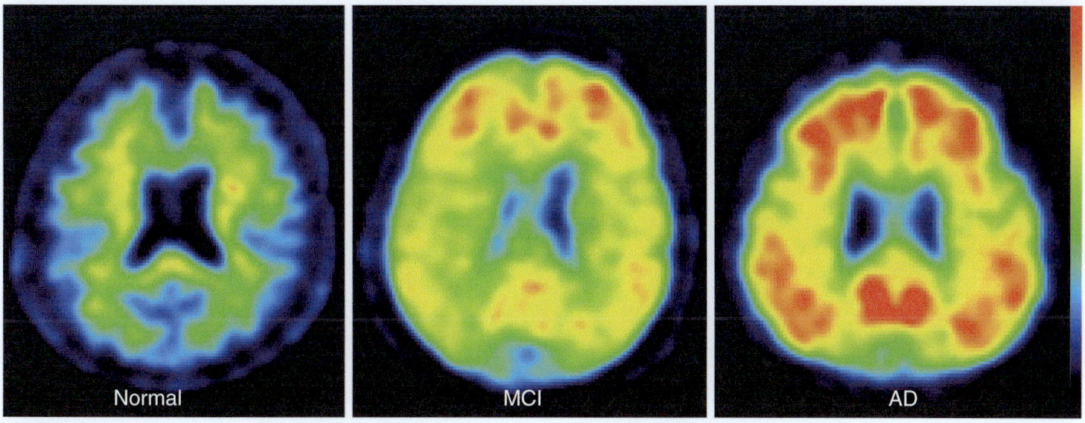

Fig. 4.2 β-Amyloid imaging in a cognitively normal subject, patient with mild cognitive impairment (MCI), and patient with Alzheimer's disease (AD). Trans-axial [^{11}C]PIB PET images show a mild tracer uptake throughout the white matter of a cognitively normal subject (left); a high tracer uptake in the frontal, parietal, and cingulate cortices of a patient with MCI (middle); and a high tracer uptake homogenously in the gray matter of a patient with AD (right)

Amyloid Scanning (IDEAS) study showed that β-amyloid PET findings prompted changes in treatment recommendations for two-thirds of participants and changes in diagnosis for the remaining one-third (https://www.ideas-study.org).

Neurofibrillary tangles as a result of hyperphosphorylation of tau proteins reflect loss of functioning neurons, whereas neuritic plaques represent extraneuronal accumulation of β-amyloid proteins. Thus, tau imaging is expected to be a more suitable biomarker for disease progression in clinical trials for AD (Fig. 4.3) compared with β-amyloid imaging, where β-amyloid accumulation may not correlate with progression of AD symptoms once the disease has been established [13]. Tau accumulations are also seen in other neurodegenerative disorders. The clinical value of tau imaging in non-AD tauopathies like frontotemporal dementia (Fig. 4.4), progressive supranuclear palsy, and traumatic brain injury is to be determined [10, 17]. In addition, tau accumulation is also detected in β-amyloid-negative healthy subjects especially in the medial temporal cortex. These age-related findings are summarized as a new clinical concept called primary age-related tauopathy (PART) [18].

Although the new PET imaging of β-amyloid and tau protein is opening a door into an exciting field of molecular imaging of pathology of dementia, conventional PET/SPECT imaging in dementia is still playing an important role in the evaluation of patients with dementia. [^{18}F]FDG-PET and perfusion SPECT using [^{123}I]IMP, [^{99m}Tc]ECD, and [^{99m}Tc]HMPAO have been used

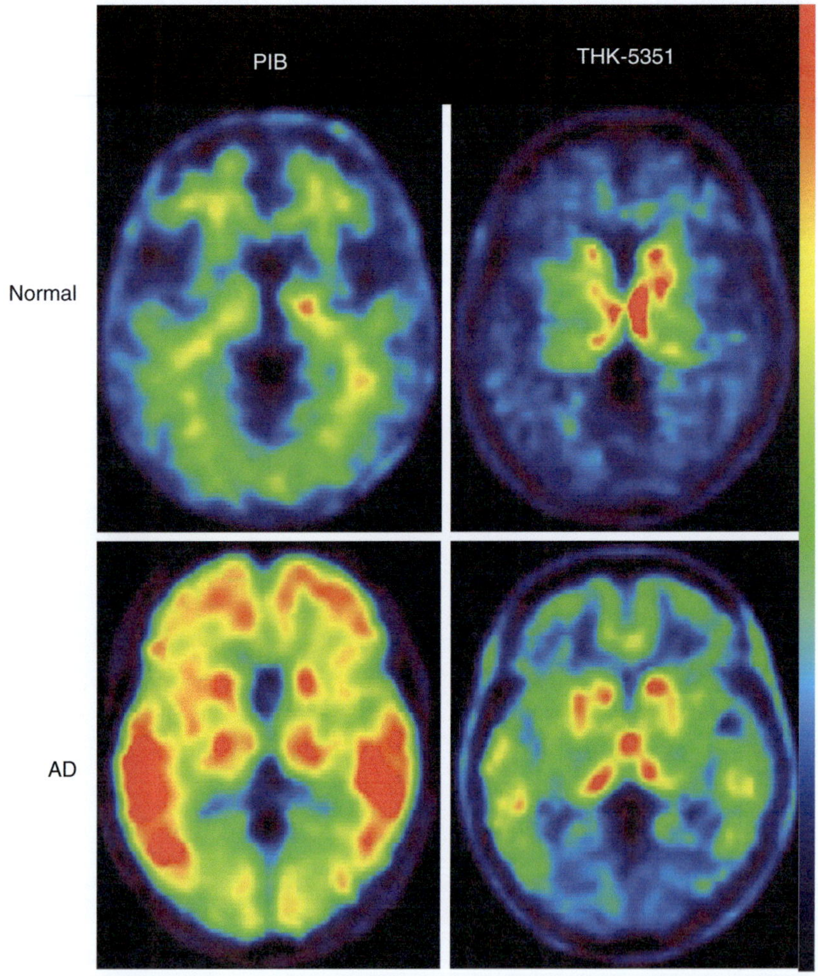

Fig. 4.3 Assessment of β-amyloid and tau accumulation in the brain of a cognitively normal subject (top row) and patient with Alzheimer's disease (AD) (bottom row). PET scans reveal accumulation of ligands due to off-target binding in the white matter with [^{11}C]PIB (top left) and in the striatum and choroid plexus with [^{18}F]THK-5351 (top right) in a cognitively normal subject. Patient with AD shows a high tracer uptake in the cortical and subcortical gray matters for both [^{11}C]PIB indicating accumulation of β-amyloid (bottom left) and [^{18}F]THK-5351 indicating accumulation of tau and increased monoamine oxidase density due to gliosis (bottom right)

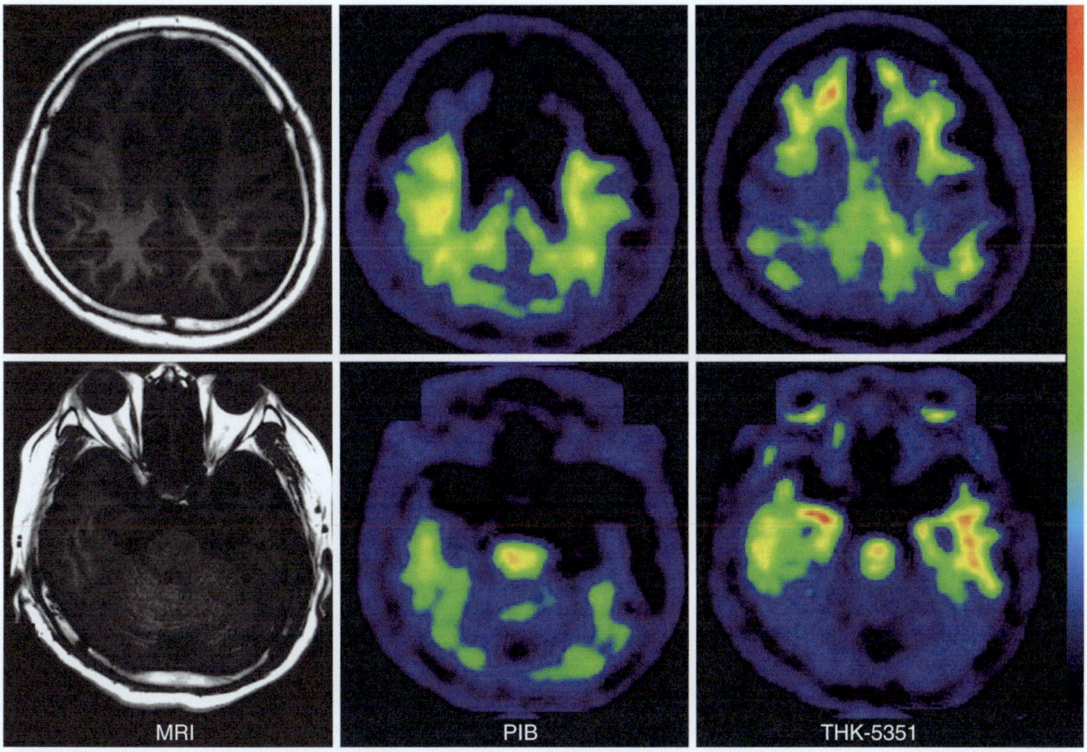

Fig. 4.4 PET imaging of a patient with behavioral variant frontotemporal dementia. T1-weighted MRI shows severe atrophy in the bilateral frontotemporal cortex. [^{11}C] PIB PET shows no accumulation of β-amyloid in the cerebral cortices. [^{18}F]THK-5351 PET shows high uptake in the bilateral frontotemporal cortex indicating combination of high tau accumulation and monoamine oxidase density due to gliosis

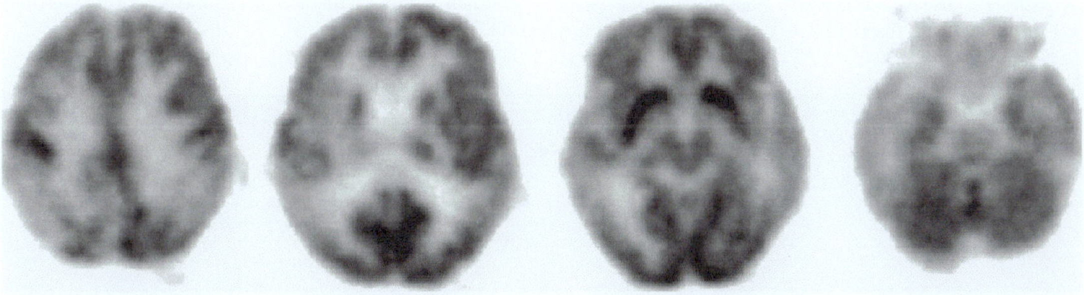

Fig. 4.5 Early dementia. A 57-year-old man who presented with "difficulty processing information" was referred for a FDG-PET scan to assess for cognitive dysfunction. Transverse plane FDG-PET images (vertex to cerebellum) reveal hypometabolism in the posterior parietal-temporal lobe (right greater than left) and the posterior cingulum. The findings when combined with the history are most compatible with early dementia of the Alzheimer type

for early detection and differential diagnosis of the diseases. These imaging techniques detect functional metabolic and flow changes in the brain legions. [^{18}F]FDG-PET has a nearly 100% sensitivity and specificity to diagnose probable AD patients from normal subjects [19]. [^{18}F] FDG-PET also predicts conversion to AD in patients with MCI [20–22] (Figs. 4.5 and 4.6). Although many studies showed superiority of FDG-PET over SPECT, SPECT is widely used in clinical examinations because of its low cost and better accessibility. Perfusion SPECT can also be used to detect early AD and predict conversion to AD in patients with MCI [23, 24].

There is sometimes a discrepancy between the conventional imaging results and amyloid imaging. The new clinical concept called suspected non-Alzheimer's pathology (SNAP) is defined by negative amyloid PET but abnormal neuronal injury biomarkers such as FDG or magnetic resonance imaging (MRI) [25]. The patients with SNAP are believed to be in the preclinical stage of non-AD pathophysiological processes.

The diagnostic criteria for DLB, the second common cause of dementia, which also shows parkinsonism, are recently updated. It includes SPECT/PET imaging of reduced dopamine transporter in basal ganglia (see the next section) and low uptake in [123I]MIBG myocardial scintigraphy as indicative biomarkers [26]. MIBG is a physiologic analogue of norepinephrine and decreased uptake of which reflects local myocardial sympathetic nerve damage caused by the disease [27]. Low perfusion and metabolism in the occipital lobe observed by perfusion SPECT or FDG-PET as well as "cingulate island sign" on FDG-PET are also included in the guideline as supportive biomarkers (Fig. 4.7).

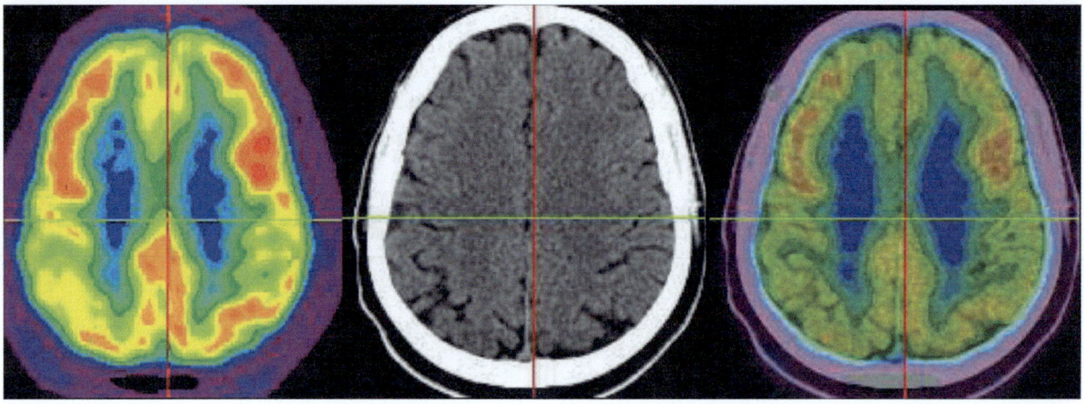

Fig. 4.6 The value of PET/CT in the evaluation of Alzheimer's disease—transverse plane FDG-PET (left), CT (middle), and fused PET/CT (right) images. Study reveals evidence of bilateral posterior parietal hypometabolism without evidence of significant cortical atrophy on CT

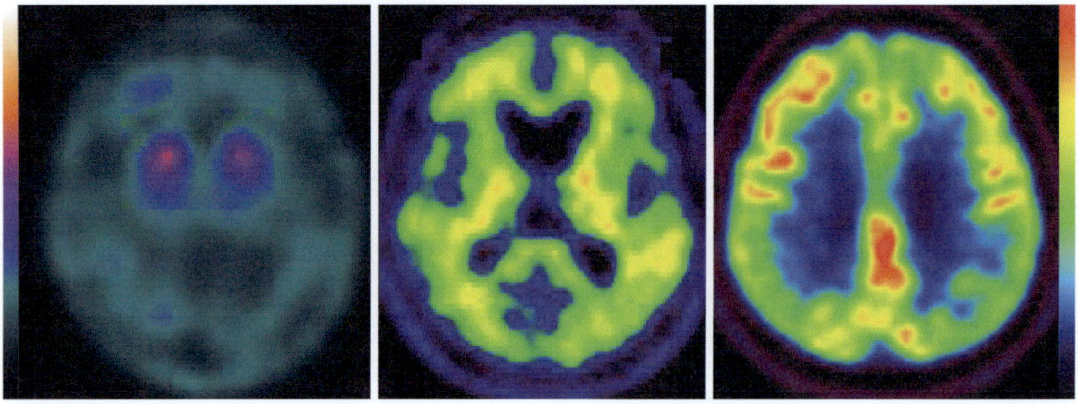

Fig. 4.7 PET and SPECT imaging of a patient with dementia with Lewy bodies. Reduced uptake of [123I] FP-CIT reveals reduced density of dopamine transporter (DAT) in the striatum (top left). Increased [11C] PIB uptake indicates localized accumulation of β-amyloid in the temporal cortex (top middle). [18F] FDG uptake is decreased in the parieto-occipital cortex showing an island of preserved uptake in the cingulate ("cingulate island sign") (top right). [123I]MIBG myocardial scintigraphy shows reduced uptake in the heart indicating local myocardial sympathetic nerve damage (bottom)

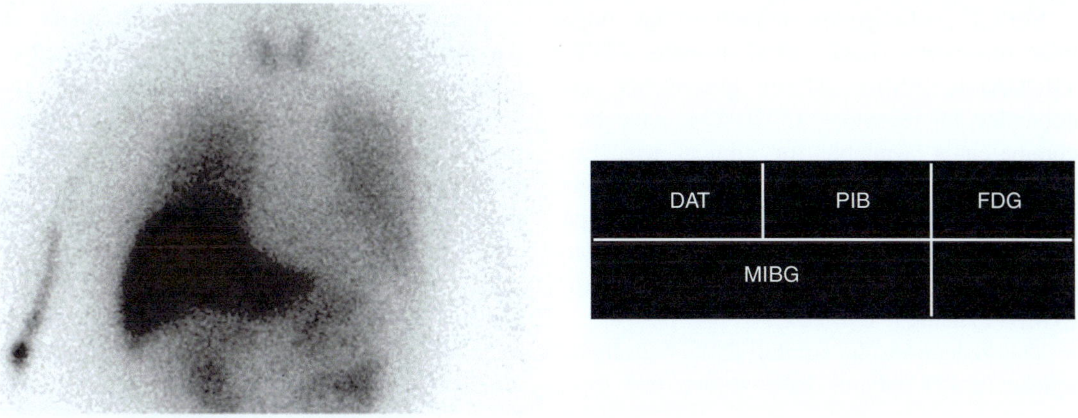

Fig. 4.7 (continued)

4.2 SPECT and PET Imaging of the Dopamine System in Movement Disorders

The dopamine system is one of the important neurotransmission systems of the central nervous system. There are three major dopaminergic projections in the brain (Fig. 4.8).

The nigrostriatal pathway originates from the substantia nigra in the midbrain and projects onto the striatum that consists of the caudate and putamen; the mesolimbic pathway originates from the ventral tegmentum and projects onto the limbic system including the nucleus accumbens, hippocampus, amygdala, and limbic cortex; and the tuberoinfundibular pathway originates from the retrobulbar midbrain to the hypothalamus and pituitary gland. These three pathways are involved in the control of movement, emotional behavior, and endocrine function, respectively.

PET and SPECT allow quantitative imaging of the dopamine system. They have been used extensively in clinical research to evaluate patients with Parkinson's disease (PD) and other movement disorders such as progressive supranuclear palsy (PSP) and multiple system atrophy (MSA) (Fig. 4.9).

These conditions are characterized pathologically by progressive degeneration of the dopamine neurons that originate in the substantia nigra and project to the striatum (Fig. 4.8).

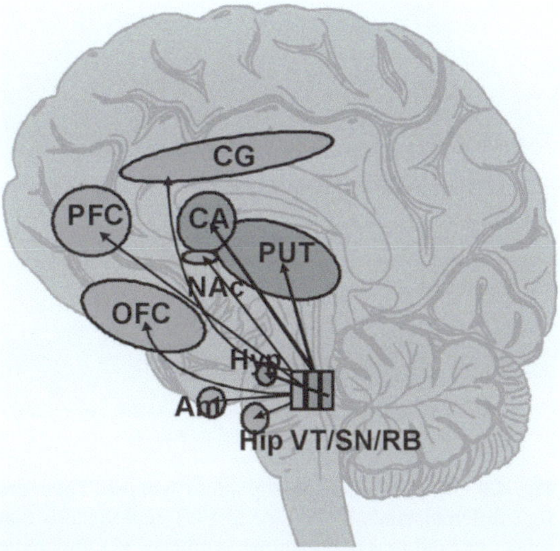

Fig. 4.8 Three major dopaminergic projections, namely, the nigrostriatal, mesolimbic, and tuberoinfundibular pathways. *SN* substantia nigra, *VT* ventral tegmentum, *RB* retrobulbar area, *CA* caudate, *PUT* putamen, *NAc* nucleus accumbens, *Hip* hippocampus, *Am* amygdala, *CG* cingulate gyrus, *PFC* prefrontal cortex, *OFC* orbitofrontal cortex, *Hyp* hypothalamus

PET and SPECT imaging using radioligands targeting the dopamine system is a useful tool for the early diagnosis and differential diagnosis of movement disorders, measuring disease progression and monitoring the efficacy of neuroprotective therapy in PD (Table 4.1).

SPECT radioligands targeting the dopamine transporter (DAT), [^{123}I]altropane, [^{99m}Tc] TRODAT-1, [^{123}I]FP-CIT or DATSCAN, and dopamine D_2 receptors, [^{123}I]IBZM, have been commercially available for clinical use. PET radioligands are used to evaluate additional presynaptic functions by investigating dopamine synthesis using [^{18}F]FDOPA and density of the type 2 vesicular monoamine transporter (VMAT2) using [^{11}C]DTBZ.

The reductions in striatal DAT radioligand uptake in PD patients have shown two topographic characteristics: radioligand uptake in the striatum contralateral to the clinically more affected side is reduced more compared with the ipsilateral side, and radioligand uptake is reduced more in the putamen than in the caudate [28–31]. Reductions in putamen DAT binding show an inverse correlation with limb bradykinesia and rigidity in PD but not with rest tremor severity [32]. Also, dopamine transporter SPECT may be sensitive enough to detect subclinical involvement of dopamine projections in PD [30] because 40–50% losses of these projections are said to have occurred before PD patients develop parkinsonian symptoms [33]. The presynaptic imaging differentiates clinically probable early PD from normal subjects or essential tremor patients with approximately 100% sensitivity (for recent reviews see Felicio et al. [34]). A positive presynaptic scan thus supports a diagnosis of PD when there is diagnostic doubt clinically (Fig. 4.10).

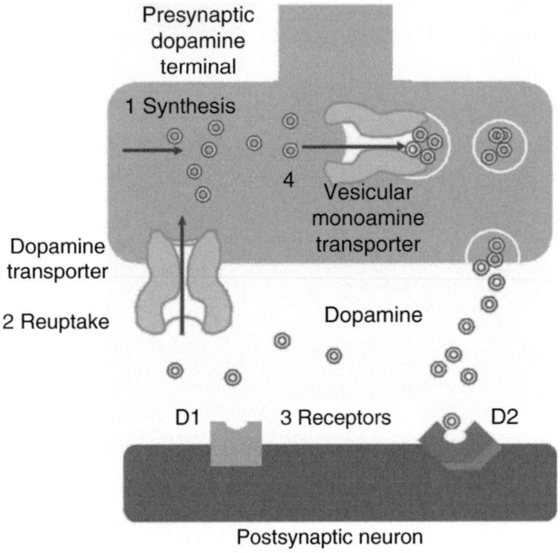

Fig. 4.9 Illustration of the dopamine synapse. There are four different kinds of PET or SPECT radioligands that reflect or bind to: (1) dopamine synthesis, (2) dopamine reuptake sites (dopamine transporter), (3) dopamine receptors and (4) monoamine reuptake or transporter sites

Dopamine neurons also degenerate in other parkinsonian syndromes such as MSA and PSP. Here, PET and SPECT imaging studies designed to evaluate the postsynaptic dopamine D_2 receptor have shown that striatal dopamine D_2 receptor binding is intact in PD, but it can be reduced in MSA and PSP and other movement disorders such as Huntington's disease [28, 35–39] (Figs. 4.11 and 4.12). However, a normal SPECT or PET scan for dopamine D_2 receptors cannot exclude an atypical parkinsonian syndrome because of a large overlap [40]. PET studies with [^{18}F]FDOPA show a pattern of extensive nigrostriatal involvement, which can discrimi-

Table 4.1 Radioligands for PET and SPECT imaging of the dopamine system

	Target site	PET	SPECT
Presynaptic	1. Synthesis	[^{18}F]FDOPA	–
	2. Dopamine transporter	[^{11}C]cocaine	[^{123}I] β-CIT
		[^{11}C]methylphenidate	[^{123}I]FP-CIT
		[^{11}C]WIN-35, 428	[^{123}I]altropane
		[^{11}C]PE2I	
		[^{18}F]FE-PE2I	
	4. Monoamine transporter	[^{11}C]DTBZ	[[99]mTc]TRODAT-l
Postsynaptic	3. Receptors	–	–
	D_1	[^{11}C]Scheme 23390	–
		[^{11}C]NNC 112	
	$D_{2/3}$	[^{11}C]raclopride	[^{123}I]IBZM
		[^{11}C]FLB 457, [^{18}F]fallypride	[^{123}I]IBF, [^{123}I]epidepride
		[^{11}C](+)-PHNO	

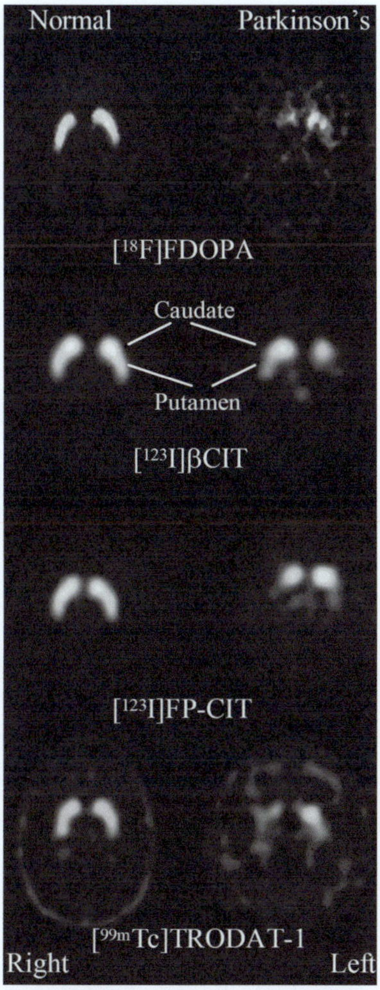

Fig. 4.10 [18F]FDOPA PET images (parametric images of influx rate constant, K_i) and dopamine transporter (DAT) SPECT images using [123I] ß-CIT (24 h postinjection), [123I]FP-CIT (4 h postinjection), and [99mTc] TRODAT-1 (3 h postinjection) of normal controls (left column row) and Parkinson's disease patients (right column). In both columns, scans shown are from different normal individuals and Parkinson's disease patients

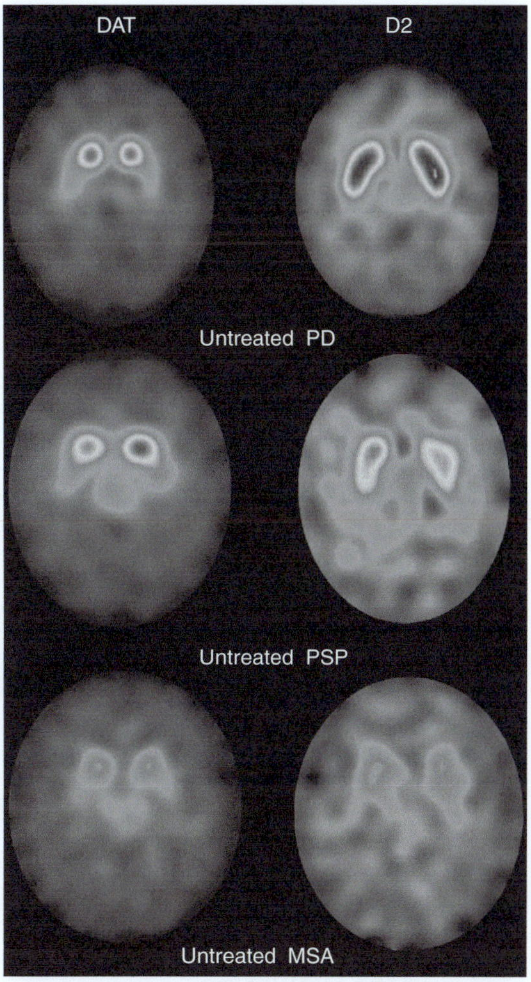

Fig. 4.11 Presynaptic dopamine transporter (DAT) images with [123I] ß-CIT (left column) and postsynaptic dopamine D2 receptor images with [123I]IBF (right column) in patients with untreated Parkinson's disease (PD) (top row), progressive supranuclear palsy (PSP) (middle row), and multiple system atrophy (MSA) (bottom row), respectively

nate patients with PD from patients with PSP, but is less reliable to discriminate patients with PD from patients with MSA [41].

PET and SPECT imaging of the presynaptic nigrostriatal dopamine system as a "state" marker of PD may have then the potential to be used in clinical trials of putative neuroprotective therapy to monitor its efficacy. There is a distinction between imaging as a surrogate marker or primary endpoint in clinical trials and biomarkers as adjunctive endpoints [42]. It is sometimes useful to stress the fact that imaging data may be best seen as complementary to the clinical data, interrogating the system at a different point than a clinical assessment and hence providing different information.

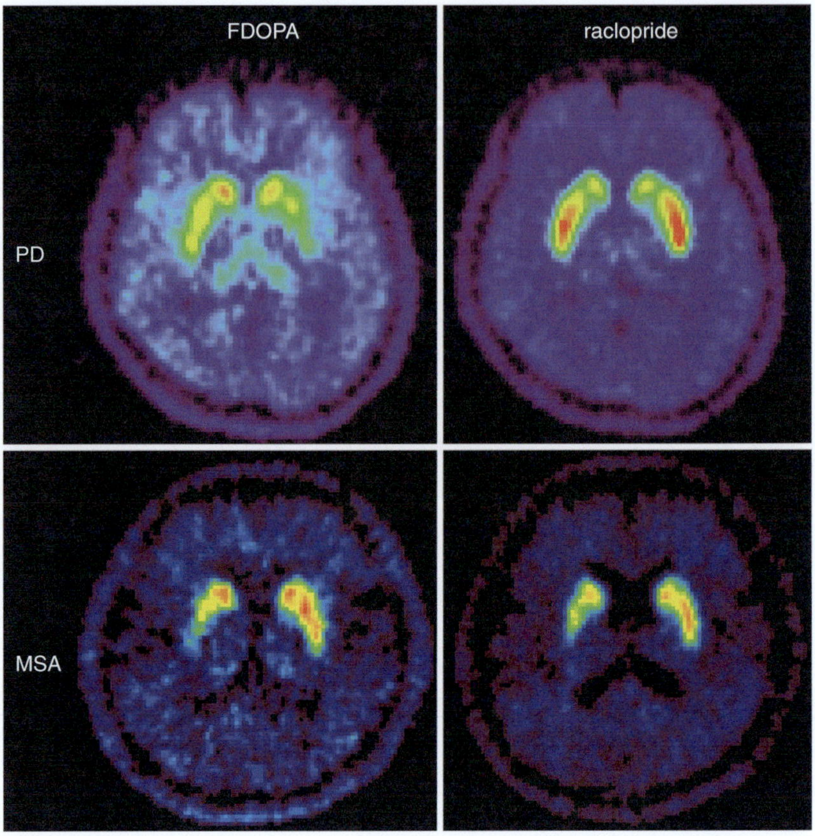

Fig. 4.12 Pre- and postsynaptic assessment of dopaminergic neurons in the striatum of patients with Parkinson disease and multiple system atrophy. [^{18}F] FDOPA PET reveals asymmetric presynaptic damage in the putamen of a patient with Parkinson disease (top left) and multiple system atrophy (bottom left). [^{11}C]raclopride PET shows intact postsynaptic D_2 receptors in a patient with Parkinson disease (top right), while reduced postsynaptic D_2 receptor density in a patient with multiple system atrophy (bottom right)

4.3 SPECT and PET Imaging in the Evaluation of Cerebrovascular Diseases

Cerebrovascular diseases (CVD) affect the blood supply to the brain and cause brain tissue damage by a shortage of oxygen and glucose required for survival of the tissue. Measurement of cerebral blood flow and glucose metabolism using radioligand with PET and SPECT used to be essential for understanding pathophysiology of the diseases. However, the role of brain SPECT and PET in the assessment of CVD has changed dramatically. These changes have largely occurred as a result of continuing advances in computed tomography (CT) and more importantly MRI and functional magnetic resonance (fMR) imaging technology. Also, there has been a declining interest in the use of SPECT and PET imaging for CVD.

As a result, CT and MRI have largely replaced SPECT and PET, for the detection, differential diagnosis, and prognosis assessment and follow-up of patients with acute stroke. At present, brain SPECT is still, however, used in the assessment of complex cases and also for the evaluation of cerebrovascular reserve with and without an acetazolamide challenge [43]. PET imaging is additionally utilized in the determination of the oxygen extraction fraction (OEF) in patients being considered for corrective carotid artery obstructive disease surgery [44]. Although superficial temporal artery-middle cerebral artery (STA-MCA) bypass was expected to reduce subsequent ipsilateral stroke in patients with complete internal carotid artery (ICA) occlusion and an elevated OEF, the Carotid Occlusion Surgery Study revealed no benefit of the surgery over medical therapy regarding ipsilateral

2-year stroke recurrence [45]. This unexpected result was mainly because of a much better than expected stroke recurrence rate in the medical group, but also because of a significant postoperative stroke rate.

4.4 SPECT and PET Brain Imaging in the Evaluation of Brain Tumors

A wide variety of neuroimaging procedures are used in the evaluation of brain tumors. CT and MR are, in large part, used as anatomic imaging techniques. Overall the accuracy of CT and MRI for detecting the presence of brain tumors is approximately 95%; however, CT and MRI are less helpful in defining cell type and degree of malignancy [46]. Magnetic resonance spectroscopy and nuclear medicine techniques are often useful adjunctive techniques when this type of cellular biochemical distinction becomes important to ascertain.

SPECT imaging is widely available using more cost-effective available SPECT radioligands compared to PET. However, the inferior spatial resolution is a disadvantage of SPECT. Among SPECT ligands, cationic compounds (thallium-201, [^{99m}Tc]MIBI) and labeled amino acids [^{123}I] IMT are often used for brain tumor imaging. Thallium-201 is a chemical analog of potassium, and its uptake reflects multiple factors including blood-brain barrier breakdown, NA^+/K^+ ATP pump activity, and blood flow, which correlates with tumor grade. [^{99m}Tc]MIBI is a cationic compound that accumulates in cytoplasm and mitochondria. The normal distribution of [^{99m}Tc]MIBI uptake is not in brain parenchyma, but choroid plexus, scalp, and pituitary grand. The uptake of [^{99m}Tc]MIBI can be a marker of recurrent glioma and chemotherapy response. [^{123}I]IMT is a less expensive analog of PET ligand, [^{11}C]MET, in which uptake reflects cellular proliferation. Uptake of [^{123}I]IMT can be a biomarker for brain tumor detection, diagnosis of recurrence, and differentiation of tumors from inflammation.

PET brain imaging is most commonly performed with [^{18}F]FDG, which is a glucose analog transported into cells, phosphorylated by hexokinase to form fluorodeoxyglucose-6-phosphate that is eventually trapped in the cell. FDG-PET is of value for tumor detection and defining tumor extent and degree of malignancy, as well as in the assessment of tumor response and differentiation of viable tumor versus radiation necrosis in cases where MRI cannot make the distinction or the MRI results are equivocal [47] (Fig. 4.13).

Since the first introduction of FDG-PET imaging, it has been recognized that the technique is very sensitive for detecting high-grade gliomas with an overall accuracy in the range of 90–95% but less accurate for the detection of histologic low-grade tumors [48]. In part, this lower accuracy rate is due to the high cortical gray matter of FDG uptake often surrounding the actual tumor. The absolute uptake of labeled glucose is also confounded by uptake in areas of inflammation and infection including the tumor itself during and immediately after treatment. Delaying the initial scan 6–8 weeks after completion of treatment and the performance of serial imaging at a number of time points post FDG administration is of some value for improving the accuracy of tumor detection [49].

In addition, the degree of uptake in tumors cells has been shown to correlate directly with the degree of malignancy noted on histopathology. Some investigators [50] have reported that the level of FDG uptake is a better measure of the malignancy potential of individual brain tumors than actual histopathology. Specifically, patients with histological low-grade brain tumors and markedly elevated glucose metabolism have a shorter survival time than patients with low-grade tumors and lower glucose metabolism [51]. The ability of FDG to assess tumor glucose metabolism is a very important aspect of brain tumor evaluation, particularly in the follow-up assessment of patients posttreatment. FDG-PET is also a very useful technique for distinguishing radiation necrosis posttreatment from viable residual or recurrent tumor in those cases where MRI is unable to make the distinction or is equivocal [52].

[^{11}C]MET and [^{18}F]FET, amino acid analogs, which are transported via amino acid transporters across the cell membrane and incorporated into

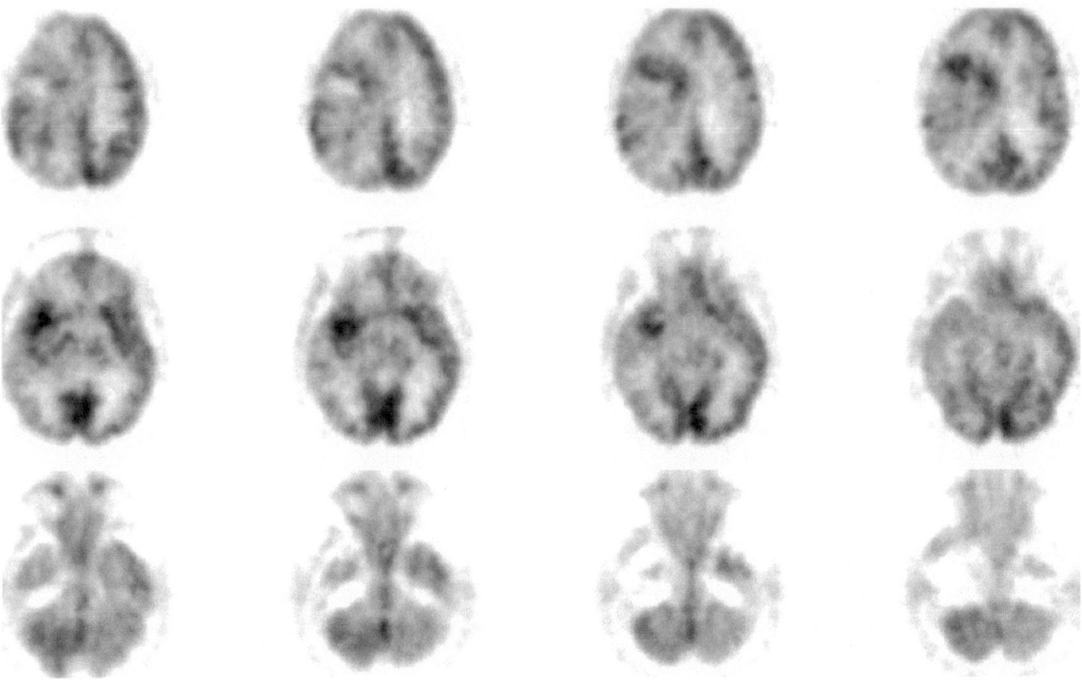

Fig. 4.13 Recurrent right frontotemporal astrocytoma grade IV posttreatment—FDG-PET images in the transverse plane (superior to inferior) reveal evidence of a large area of mixed hypo- and hypermetabolic foci involving the right posterior frontal lobe and the right anterior to mid-temporal lobe consistent with residual viable tumor posttreatment

proteins, are very useful for detection of brain tumors. An important characteristic of MET is that it is more accurate for detecting low-grade brain tumors than FDG [53]. [^{18}F]FLT is a thymidine nucleoside analog, in which uptake reflects the activity of thymidine kinase-1, an enzyme expressed during the DNA synthesis phase of cell cycle and useful to evaluate brain tumors particularly chemotherapeutic responses.

4.5 SPECT and PET Brain Imaging in the Evaluation of Seizure Disorders

The standard epilepsy workup includes a variety of procedures and tests including video electroencephalogram (EEG) monitoring, neuroimaging, preferably MRI, and where necessary depth electrode measurements. While there are a significant number of patients that can be diagnosed when there is concordance of the clinical findings with video EEG and MRI results [54], there are, however, also many patients with disparate findings that require additional procedures including neuroimaging with SPECT and PET imaging and, in some instances, magnetic resonance spectroscopy or depth electrode analysis. The patients that benefit the most from surgery are individuals with medically intractable partial-onset seizures arising in the temporal lobe although on occasion extra temporal seizures are amenable to surgical treatment [55].

The optimum brain SPECT method for localizing a seizure focus is to perform ictal and interictal perfusion imaging studies, on separate days, followed by subtraction of the co-registered images. SPECT imaging in patients with temporal lobe epilepsy (TLE) has a sensitivity as 44% (interictal), 75% (postictal), and 97% (ictal) [56]. The sensitivity to extra-TLE was much lower than TLE as 40% (interictal) and 66% (ictal) [57, 58]. [^{123}I]iomazenil is also used to detect epileptic foci as a decreased density of γ-aminobutyric acid (GABA) receptors.

FDG-PET brain studies are also utilized to evaluate seizure disorder patients in the interictal

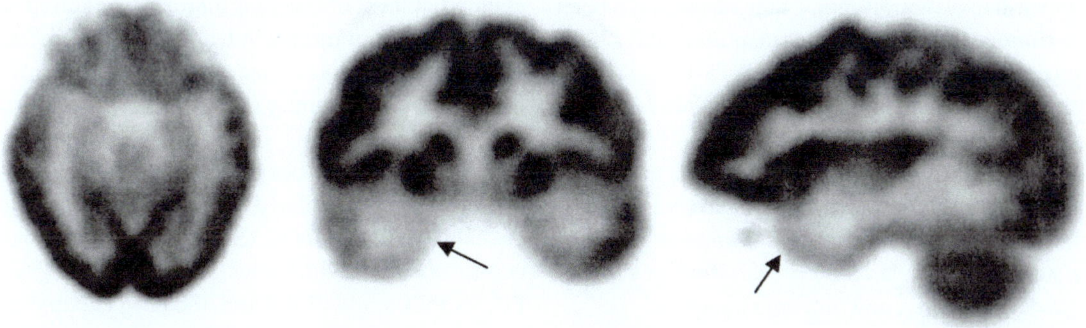

Fig. 4.14 Interictal FDG-PET brain image of a patient with partial complex seizure disorder. The axial, coronal, and sagittal image planes reveal localized glucose hypometabolism involving the anterior and mesial right temporal lobe (arrows)

state. Similar to interictal SPECT, this technique identifies a seizure focus as an area of focal hypometabolism (Fig. 4.14). The sensitivities of FDG-PET in TLE and extra-TLE were reported as 84% and 33%, respectively [57]. In addition to FDG-PET, [^{11}C]flumazenil is used to image GABA receptors, in which [^{11}C]flumazenil uptake is reduced in seizure foci [59].

4.6 SPECT and PET Imaging of the Dopamine System in Psychiatric Disorders

Despite being of limited diagnostic utility in psychiatric disorders, PET imaging techniques of neurotransmission systems have been shown to be a valuable research tool to further our understanding of the pathophysiological mechanisms of important psychiatric disorders such as schizophrenia, depression, and substance abuse. Furthermore, these techniques can play an essential role in understanding drug action and new drug development in psychiatry.

The dopamine system has been closely linked to the pathophysiology of schizophrenia. Here, the mesolimbic dopamine pathway, as opposed to the nigrostriatal pathway, plays an important role in psychiatric disorders. PET and SPECT imaging studies of the dopamine system in schizophrenia have been performed on dopamine $D_{2/3}$ and D_1 receptors and DAT availability and dopamine synthesis and release in the striatum and extrastriatal cortices [60].

Striatal $D_{2/3}$ receptor densities appear to be increased in patients with schizophrenia [60]. The radioligands used to image striatal $D_{2/3}$ receptors are [^{11}C]raclopride and [^{123}I]IBZM, both of which show D_3 receptor binding in addition to D_2 binding. For extrastriatal $D_{2/3}$ receptors, which can be assessed using high-affinity ligands such as [^{11}C] FLB 457 and [^{18}F]fallypride, no significant differences were found in a meta-analysis study in patients with schizophrenia [61]. Similarly, studies for measuring D_1 receptor densities showed inconsistent results [62–66]. These inconsistent findings may be partially explained by the fact that the radioligands used for imaging D_1 receptors, [^{11}C]NNC112 and [^{11}C]SCH23390, also bind to serotonin 2A (5-HT_{2A}) receptors [67, 68]. Studies for measuring striatal DAT densities in patients with schizophrenia also showed inconsistent results, and a meta-analysis found no evidence for DAT alterations in schizophrenia patients [60, 69].

On the other hand, dopamine synthesis in patients with schizophrenia is elevated as measured with [^{18}F]F-DOPA uptake in the striatum [60]. Dopamine release is also increased, which can be measured using [^{11}C]raclopride competing with endogenous dopamine released in response to pharmacological challenges [70]. These findings support the hypothesis that there is dysregulation of dopamine synthesis and release in schizophrenia.

In major depression, the abnormal serotonin transmission has been linked to its pathophysiology. PET and SPECT imaging studies of the dopamine system in major depression have been performed on serotonin transporter and 5-HT receptors [71]. The serotonin 1A (5-HT_{1A}) receptors have been studied with [^{11}C]WAY-100635 and its analogs, the serotonin 2A (5-HT_{2A}) with [^{18}F]altanserin and [^{11}C]MDL100907, and serotonin transporters with [^{11}C](+)McN5652 and [^{11}C]DASB. However, the findings are inconsistent probably because of variation in radioligands, modeling, and outcome measures.

In substance abuse research, many PET and SPECT imaging studies, particularly those conducted by Volkow and colleagues at the Brookhaven National Laboratory and National Institute on Drug Abuse, have made an enormous contribution to our understanding of the pathophysiological brain mechanisms of substance abuse [72]. These investigators have focused on imaging of the dopamine and opioid system because drugs of abuse such as cocaine, methamphetamine, nicotine, and methylenediomethamphetamine (MDMA, ecstasy) all directly or indirectly increase brain dopamine and opioid. PET studies using [^{11}C]cocaine and [^{11}C]methylphenidate revealed that the "high" is associated with the initial fast rate of uptake of methylphenidate in the brain and fast dopamine increases as measured with the decreased uptake of [^{11}C]cocaine. PET studies in cocaine abusers also show significant reductions in dopamine release in response to a stimulant challenge. [^{11}C]carfentanil is used to assess mu opioid receptor and their occupancy by enkephalin. Both acute alcohol and cigarette smoking increase endogenous enkephalin as measured with [^{11}C]carfentanil. Mu opioid receptor availability is also increased in alcoholics and cocaine abusers showing a reduced level of endogenous enkephalin. This led to the hypothesis that decreases in dopamine and enkephalin releases result in an understimulation of reward circuits, whereby subjects are at a greater risk for seeking drugs of abuse to temporarily stimulate reward circuits.

PET and SPECT imaging of neuroreceptors and transporters has been used to study antipsychotic or antidepressant drug action by examining the relationship between neuroreceptor or transporter occupancy of psychiatric drugs and clinical response. Although it is still not fully clear what level of receptor binding is required to achieve the minimum clinically effective therapeutic response, occupancy of over 70% is recommended for D_2 antagonists. However, atypical neuroleptics, such as clozapine, are clinically effective when only occupying 50% of D_2 receptors [73, 74]. Similarly, minimum therapeutic doses of antidepressants (SSRIs) occupy 80% of central SERT binding sites according to a [^{11}C]DASB PET study [75]. Here, the drug occupancy refers to the percentage of receptor sites occupied by a drug with a particular dosing regimen.

In the development of novel drugs for psychiatric illnesses, pharmaceutical companies have frequently been employing PET and SPECT imaging techniques. One such way is to determine the dose-occupancy profiles of novel drugs using existing radioligands and so help guide dose selection for phase I and II trials. Another way of making use of PET imaging in drug development involves microdosing techniques where multiple candidate drugs are prepared as radioligands (by usually [^{11}C]-labeling) and tested simultaneously. Because subpharmacological doses are being administered (<20 μg) on only one or two occasions, the toxicology requirements for administration of these novel radiotracers in man are less stringent than for pharmacological drugs. PET can then assess the plasma, regional brain, and other organ pharmacokinetics in human ahead of therapeutic trials. Thus, phase I studies in drug development allow for the assessment of the penetration of investigational agents across the blood-brain barrier in humans and determination of the selectivity of binding to the appropriate target. Also, it is important to stress that screening out of candidate agents is important from a financial perspective, that is, killing a drug in phase I prior to initiation of costly phase II studies is a useful outcome of phase I microdosing studies.

4.7 Radionuclide Cerebrospinal Fluid Flow Studies

Radionuclide cisternography involves the injection of a radiotracer into the intrathecal space usually at the level of the lumbar spine. [^{111}In]DTPA is the most commonly used radiopharmaceutical (Fig. 4.15). Under normal circumstances, there is no evidence of retrograde cerebrospinal fluid (CSF) flow into the ventricles [76]. In communicating hydrocephalus (normal pressure hydrocephalus), the lateral ventricles are visualized early in the study ("ventricular penetration"), and the radiotracer remains in the ventricular system beyond 24 h ("ventricular stasis"). Another aspect of the altered CSF flow pattern, observed in communicating hydrocephalus, is delayed or even complete obstruction of CSF movement, around the brain (Fig. 4.16). The observed impediment to CSF flow may occur at any level all the way up

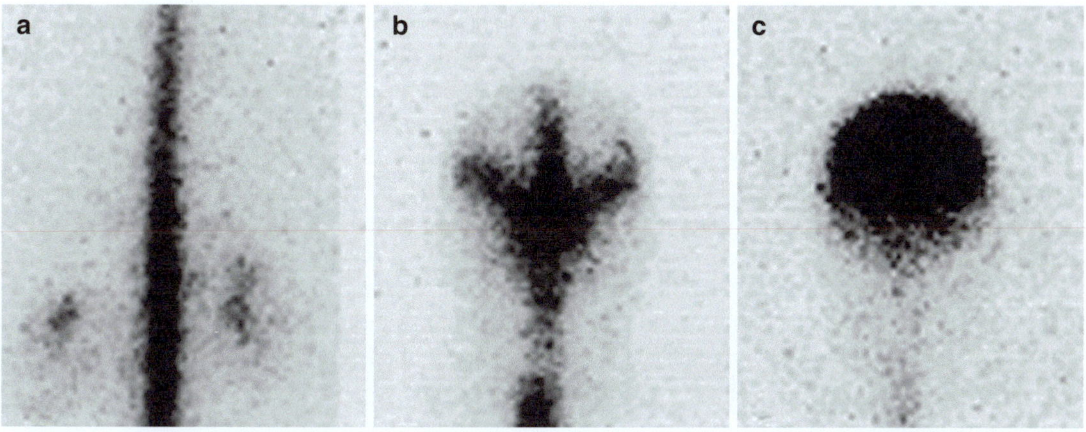

Fig. 4.15 Normal CSF flow pattern: Images at 2 h (**a**) reveal radiotracer, in CSF, ascending up the thoracolumbar spinal canal; at 6 h (**b**) the radiotracer is in the basilar cisterns; and at 24 h (**c**) the radiotracer is being reabsorbed in the arachnoid villi at the convexity of the brain

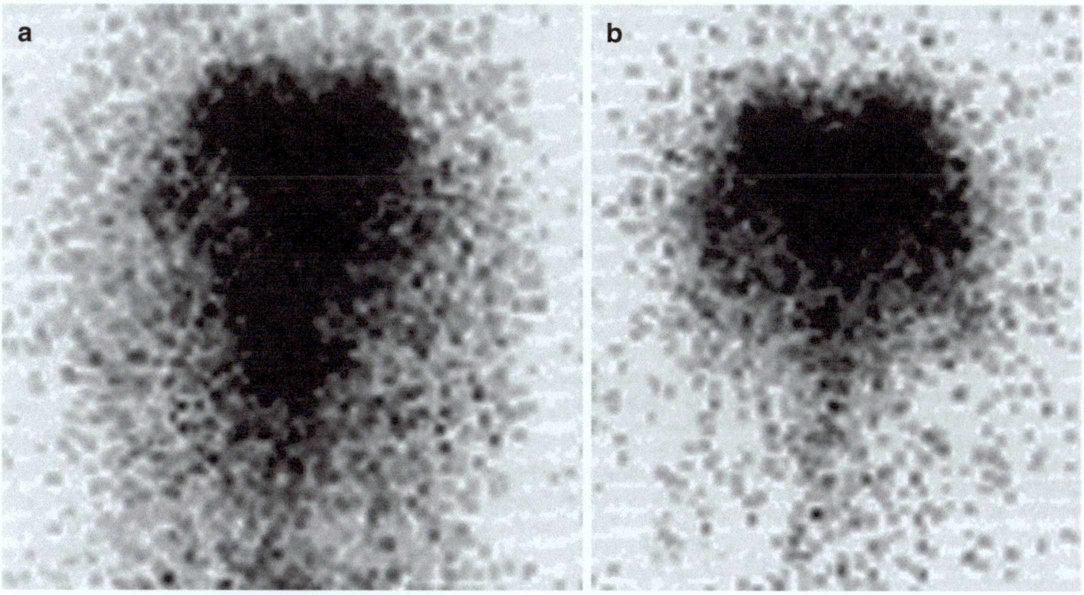

Fig. 4.16 Normal pressure hydrocephalus pattern: Images at 24 h (**a**) demonstrate radiotracer in the lateral ventricles, "ventricular penetration," and at 48 h (**b**) persistence of radiotracer in the lateral ventricles, "ventricular stasis" and no movement of the radiotracer beyond the basilar cisterns consistent with extra-ventricular obstruction to CSF flow

to the parasagittal arachnoid villa [77]. Unilateral or bilateral delayed, but typically not obstructed, CSF flow, without ventricular penetration or stasis, may be seen in cortical atrophy or prior cerebral infarction without communicating hydrocephalus. The type of information that is available from radionuclide cisternography in the communicating hydrocephalic patient is useful to the neurosurgeon in helping to decide on the type of shunting procedure to be performed. In particular, radionuclide cisternography is very informative in normal pressure hydrocephalus, a form of communicating hydrocephalus, where the opening CSF spinal tap pressure level is within the normal range (for review, see Thut et al. [78]). In this respect, SPECT/CT can complement the anatomic information on the radionuclide cisternography. However, new MR techniques are being developed to image CSF flow and anatomic details. Therefore, the nuclear imaging approach may be less frequently used for the assessment of CSF flow dynamics.

Radionuclide cisternography, when combined with surgical packing, is also, on occasion, very helpful in identifying the presence and site of a CSF leak [79]. The imaging is especially useful when combined SPECT imaging and measures of the amount of radioactivity present in surgical gauze pledgets [80].

The second technique used for the assessment of CSF dynamics is radionuclide ventriculography. This procedure is used to check the patency of the afferent and efferent limbs of a ventricular shunt as well as the function of the shunt pump. [^{99m}Tc]DTPA is the radiotracer typically used for this procedure. For assessment of the distal limb of the shunt, the radiotracer is injected directly into the shunt reservoir, using a low-pressure injection technique, and follow-up drainage from the reservoir and distal limb is monitored over time. Under normal circumstances, clearance from the reservoir and distal limb is less than 10 min. The drainage from the distal ventriculoperitoneal (V-P) limb should be unimpeded and without evidence of holdup at the distal drainage point into the peritoneum. The distal limb may be kinked, partially or even completely obstructed. These types of observed changes will, in general, require neurosurgical intervention, including possible shunt revision or shunt replacement.

Radionuclide ventriculography can also be used to assess the function of the proximal limb of the shunt. This approach requires a higher-pressure injection of the radiotracer into the shunt reservoir. The higher-pressure injection should result in a retrograde flow of the radiotracer out of the patent proximal shunt limb into the ventricle, which is then monitored for clearance over. Although an individual experienced with shunts should perform all types of injections into the shunt reservoir, particular care should be exercised when employing the high-pressure injection technique to achieve backflow from the shunt reservoir into the proximal limb of the shunt and the lateral ventricle.

4.8 Brain Death Scintigraphy

Brain death is defined as the irreversible loss of all brain and brainstem functions including the capacity to breathe, even though the heart continues to beat and spinal functions may persist. The diagnosis of brain death is primarily clinical and needs to establish the irreversible cessation of all function of the cerebrum and brainstem [81]. Brain scintigraphy is an important confirmatory test of brain death that can be used to shorten an observation time in the presence of confounding factors especially when the clinical history is unknown [82]. Brain scintigraphy with [^{99m}Tc]HMPAO or [^{99m}Tc]ECD is used for the assessment of brain blood flow in patients suspected of brain death [83, 84]. Flow images will help to confirm lack of brain blood flow when the brain is not visualized on delayed images (Fig. 4.17). For details on the methodology of brain death scintigraphy, the reader is referred to the procedure guideline published by the Society of Nuclear Medicine [85].

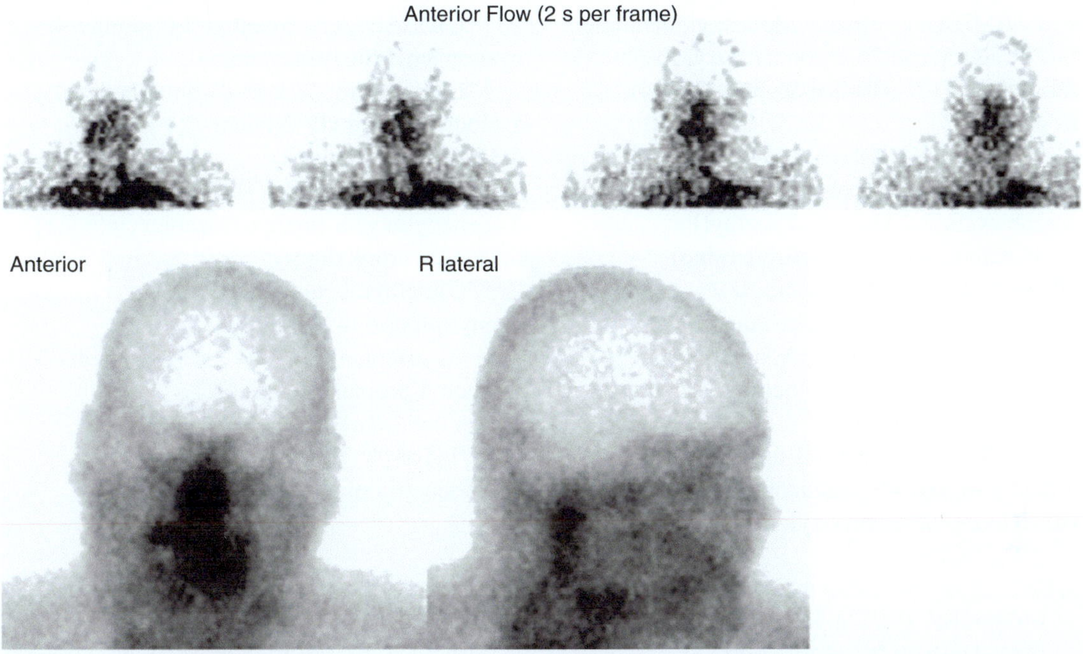

Fig. 4.17 A 41-year-old man with a history of massive cerebral hemorrhage. Dynamic cerebral angiograms after bolus injection of 740 MBq of [^{99m}Tc]HMPAO (top row) show flow in the common and external carotid regions but not in the anterior or middle cerebral artery distribution. Static planar images (bottom row) show no tracer retention within the cerebrum and cerebellum ("hollow skull sign"), which is confirmatory of brain death

Appendix

Radiopharmaceutical Abbreviations

[^{11}C]PIB (Pittsburg Compound B): 2-(4′-[^{11}C]methylaminophenyl)-6-hydroxybenzothiazole

[^{18}F]flutemetamol: 2-[3-(^{18}F)fluoranyl-4-(methylamino)phenyl]-1,3-benzothiazol-6-ol

[^{18}F]NAV4694: 2-[2-(^{18}F)fluoro-6-(methylamino)-3-pyridinyl]-1-benzofuran-5-ol

[^{18}F]florbetapir: 4-{(E)-2-[6-(2-{2-[2-(^{18}F)fluoroethoxy]ethoxy}ethoxy)-3-pyridinyl]vinyl}-*N*-methylaniline

[^{18}F]florbetaben: 4-{(E)-2-[4-(2-{2-[2-(^{18}F)fluoroethoxy]ethoxy}ethoxy)phenyl]vinyl}-*N*-methylaniline

[^{11}C]SB-13: 4-[(E)-2-{4-[(^{11}C)methylamino]phenyl}vinyl]phenol

[^{18}F]FDDNP: 2-(1-{6-[(2-[^{18}F]fluoroethyl)(methyl)amino]-2-naphthyl}-ethylidene)malononitrile

[^{11}C]PBB3: 2-[(1E,3E)-4-[6-([^{11}C]methylamino)pyridin-3-yl]buta-1,3-dienyl]-1,3-benzothiazol-6-ol

[^{18}F]flortaucipir: 7-[6-(^{18}F)fluoro-3-pyridinyl]-5H-pyrido[4,3-b]indole

[^{18}F]THK5351: (2S)-1-(^{18}F)fluoro-3-[2-[6-(methylamino)pyridin-3-yl]quinolin-6-yl]oxypropan-2-ol

[^{18}F]PI-2620: not disclosed

[^{18}F]MK-6240: 6-(^{18}F)fluoro-3-pyrrolo[2,3-c]pyridin-1-ylisoquinolin-5-amine

[^{18}F]PM-PBB3: not disclosed

[^{18}F]FDG: [^{18}F]fludeoxyglucose

[^{123}I]IMP: [^{123}I]iodoamphetamine

[^{99m}Tc]ECD: [^{99m}Tc]ethylcysteinate dimer

[^{99m}Tc]HMPAO: [^{99m}Tc]hexamethylpropyleneamine oxime

$[^{123}I]$MIBG: $[^{123}I]$metaiodobenzylguanidine

$[^{123}I]$altropane: 2β-carbomethoxy-3β-(4-fluorophenyl)-*N*-((E)-3-iodo-prop-2-enyl) tropane

$[^{99m}Tc]$TRODAT-1: ([2-[[2-[[[3-(4-chlorophenyl)-8-methyl-8-azabicyclo[3,2,1]oct-2-yl]methyl](2-mercaptoethyl)amino]ethyl]amino] ethanethiolato(3-)-N2,N2′,S2,S2′] oxo-[1R-(exo-exo)]-^{99m}Tc-technetium)

$[^{123}I]$FP-CIT or DATSCAN: ^{123}I-N-omega-fluoropropyl- 2beta-carbomethoxy-3beta-(4-iodoph enyl)nortropane

$[^{11}C]$flumazenil: ethyl 8-fluoro-5,6-dihydro-5-methyl-6-oxo-4*H*-imidazo[1,5-a][1,4] benzodiazepine-3-carboxylate

$[^{18}F]$FDOPA: 3,4-dihydroxy-6-^{18}F-fluoro-l-phenylalanine

$[^{11}C]$DTBZ: $[^{11}C]$dihydrotetrabenazine

$[^{99m}Tc]$MIBI: $[^{99m}Tc]$sestamibi

$[^{123}I]$IMT: $[^{123}I]$iodo-α-methyltyrosine

$[^{11}C]$MET: $[^{11}C]$methionine (MET)

$[^{18}F]$FET: $[^{18}F]$fluoroethyl-L-tyrosine

$[^{18}F]$FLT: $[^{18}F]$fluoro-thymidine

$[^{11}C]$raclopride: 3,5-dichloro-N-[[(2S)-1-ethylpyrrolidin-2-yl] methyl]-2-hydroxy-6-methoxybenzamide

$[^{123}I]$IBZM: $[^{123}I]$iodobenzamide

$[^{11}C]$FLB 457: ((S)-*N*-((1-ethyl-2-pyrrolidinyl) methyl)-5-bromo-2,3-dimethoxybenzamide)

$[^{18}F]$fallypride: *N*-{[(2S)-1-allyl-2-pyrrolidinyl]methyl}-5-(3-$[^{18}F]$ fluoropropyl)-2,3-dimethoxybenzamide

$[^{11}C]$NNC112: ((+)-8-chloro-5-(7-benzofuranyl)-7-hydroxy-3-methyl-2,3,4,5-tetra-hydro-lH-3-benzazepine

$[^{11}C]$SCH23390: R-(+)-8-chIoro-2,3,4,5-tetrahydro-3-methyI-5-phe-nyl-1H-3-benzazepine-7-ol

$[^{11}C]$WAY-100635: *N*-(2-(4-(2-methoxyphenyl)-1-piperazi-nyl)ethyl)-*N*-(2-pyridinyl) cyclohexanecarboxamide

$[^{11}C]$MDL100,907: (R)-(+)-4-(1-hydroxy-1-(2,3-dimethoxyphenyl)methy1)-*N*-2-(4-fluorophenylethyl) piperidine

$[^{11}C]$(+)McN5652: (+)*trans*-l,2,3,5,6,10β-hexahydro-6-14-(methylthio)phenyl] pyrrolo-[2,1-a]-isoquinoline

$[^{11}C]$DASB: *N*,*N*-dimethyl-2-(2-amino-4-cyanophenylthio)benzylamine

$[^{18}F]$altanserin: 3-{2-[4-(4-fluorobenzoyl)-1-piperidinyl]ethyl}-2-thioxo-2,3-dihydro-4(1H)-quinazolinone

$[^{11}C]$cocaine: methyl(1R,2R,3S,5S)-3-(benzoyloxy)-8-methyl-8-azabicyclo[3.2.1] octane-2-carboxylate

$[^{11}C]$methylphenidate: methyl phenyl(piperidin-2-yl)acetate

$[^{11}C]$carfentanil: methyl 1-(2-phenylethyl)-4-[phenyl(propanoyl)amino] piperidine-4-carboxylate

$[^{111}In]$ or $[^{99m}Tc]$DTPA: ^{111}In- or ^{99m}Tc-diethylenetriamine pentaacetic acid

References

1. Mathis CA, Bacskai BJ, Kajdasz ST, McLellan ME, Frosch MP, Hyman BT, et al. A lipophilic thioflavin-T derivative for positron emission tomography (PET) imaging of amyloid in brain. Bioorg Med Chem Lett. 2002;12(3):295–8.
2. Verhoeff NPLG, Wilson AA, Takeshita S, Trop L, Hussey D, Singh K, et al. In-vivo imaging of Alzheimer disease beta-amyloid with $[^{11}C]$SB-13 PET. Am J Geriatr Psychiatry. 2004;12(6):584–95.
3. Shin J, Lee S-Y, Kim S-H, Kim Y-B, Cho S-J. Multitracer PET imaging of amyloid plaques and neurofibrillary tangles in Alzheimer's disease. NeuroImage. 2008;43(2):236–44.
4. Maruyama M, Shimada H, Suhara T, Shinotoh H, Ji B, Maeda J, et al. Imaging of tau pathology in a tauopathy mouse model and in Alzheimer patients compared to normal controls. Neuron. 2013;79(6):1094–108.
5. Xia C-F, Arteaga J, Chen G, Gangadharmath U, Gomez LF, Kasi D, et al. $[^{18}F]$T807, a novel tau positron emission tomography imaging agent for Alzheimer's disease. Alzheimers Dement. 2013;9(6):666–76.
6. Harada R, Okamura N, Furumoto S, Furukawa K, Ishiki A, Tomita N, et al. 18F-THK5351: a novel PET radiotracer for imaging neurofibrillary pathology in alzheimer disease. J Nucl Med. 2016;57(2):208–14.
7. Kimura Y, Ichise M, Ito H, Shimada H, Ikoma Y, Seki C, et al. PET quantification of tau pathology in human brain with ^{11}C-PBB3. J Nucl Med. 2015;56(9):1359–65. http://jnm.snmjournals.org/cgi/doi/10.2967/jnumed.115.160127doi/10.2967/jnumed.115.160127
8. Pontecorvo MJ, Devous MD, Navitsky M, Lu M, Salloway S, Schaerf FW, et al. Relationships between flortaucipir PET tau binding and amyloid

burden, clinical diagnosis, age and cognition. Brain. 2017;140(3):aww334–763.
9. Sepulcre J, Grothe MJ, Sabuncu M, Chhatwal J, Schultz AP, Hanseeuw B, et al. Hierarchical organization of tau and amyloid deposits in the cerebral cortex. JAMA Neurol. 2017;74(7):813–20.
10. Saint-Aubert L, Lemoine L, Chiotis K, Leuzy A, Rodriguez-Vieitez E, Nordberg A. Tau PET imaging: present and future directions. Mol Neurodegeneration. 2017;12(1):652–21. http://molecularneurodegeneration.biomedcentral.com/articles/10.1186/s13024-017-0162-3
11. Drzezga A. 2017 SNMMI highlights lecture: neuroscience. J Nucl Med. 2017;58(10):9N–15N.
12. Thal DR, Rüb U, Orantes M, Braak H. Phases of a beta-deposition in the human brain and its relevance for the development of AD. Neurology. 2002;58(12):1791–800.
13. Bateman RJ, Xiong C, Benzinger TLS, Fagan AM, Goate A, Fox NC, et al. Clinical and biomarker changes in dominantly inherited Alzheimer's disease. N Engl J Med. 2012;367(9):795–804.
14. Rowe CC, Villemagne VL. Brain amyloid imaging. J Nucl Med Technol. 2013;41(1):11–8.
15. Villemagne VL, Pike KE, Chételat G, Ellis KA, Mulligan RS, Bourgeat P, et al. Longitudinal assessment of Aβ and cognition in aging and Alzheimer disease. Ann. Neurol. 2011;69(1):181–92.
16. Frey KA, Petrou M. Imaging amyloidopathy in Parkinson disease and parkinsonian dementia syndromes. Clin Transl Imaging. 2015;3(1):57–64.
17. Hall B, Mak E, Cervenka S, Aigbirhio FI, Rowe JB, O'Brien JT. In vivo tau PET imaging in dementia: pathophysiology, radiotracer quantification, and a systematic review of clinical findings. Ageing Res Rev. 2017;36:50–63.
18. Crary JF, Trojanowski JQ, Schneider JA, Abisambra JF, Abner EL, Alafuzoff I, et al. Primary age-related tauopathy (PART): a common pathology associated with human aging. Acta Neuropathol. 2014;128(6):755–66.
19. Minoshima S, Frey KA, Koeppe RA, Foster NL, Kuhl DE. A diagnostic approach in Alzheimer's disease using three-dimensional stereotactic surface projections of fluorine-^{18}-FDG PET. J Nucl Med. 1995;36(7):1238–48.
20. Drzezga A, Grimmer T, Riemenschneider M, Lautenschlager N, Siebner H, Alexopoulus P, et al. Prediction of individual clinical outcome in MCI by means of genetic assessment and (18) F-FDG PET. J Nucl Med. 2005;46(10):1625–32.
21. Inui Y, Ito K, Kato T, SEAD-J Study Group. Longer-term investigation of the value of ^{18}F-FDG-PET and magnetic resonance imaging for predicting the conversion of mild cognitive impairment to Alzheimer's disease: a multicenter study. J Alzheimers Dis. 2017;60(3):877–87.
22. Ito K, Fukuyama H, Senda M, Ishii K, Maeda K, Yamamoto Y, et al. Prediction of outcomes in mild cognitive impairment by using ^{18}F-FDG-PET: a multicenter study. J Alzheimers Dis. 2015;45(2):543–52.
23. Encinas M, de Juan R, Marcos A, Gil P, Barabash A, Fernández C, et al. Regional cerebral blood flow assessed with ^{99m}Tc-ECD SPET as a marker of progression of mild cognitive impairment to Alzheimer's disease. Eur J Nucl Med Mol Imaging. 2003;30(11):1473–80.
24. Huang C, Wahlund L-O, Svensson L, Winblad B, Julin P. Cingulate cortex hypoperfusion predicts Alzheimer's disease in mild cognitive impairment. BMC Neurol. 2002;2(1):9.
25. Jack CR, Knopman DS, Wiste HJ, Vemuri P, Gunter JL, Ivnik RJ, et al. An operational approach to National Institute on Aging-Alzheimer's Association criteria for preclinical Alzheimer disease. Ann Neurol. 2012;71(6):765–75.
26. McKeith IG, Boeve BF, Dickson DW, Halliday G, Taylor J-P, Weintraub D, et al. Diagnosis and management of dementia with Lewy bodies. Neurology. 2017;89(1):88–100.
27. Yoshita M, Taki J, Yokoyama K, Noguchi-Shinohara M, Matsumoto Y, Nakajima K, et al. Value of ^{123}I-MIBG radioactivity in the differential diagnosis of DLB from AD. Neurology. 2006;66(12):1850–4.
28. Ichise M, Kim YJ, Ballinger JR, Vines D, Erami SS, Tanaka F, et al. SPECT imaging of pre- and postsynaptic dopaminergic alterations in L-dopa-untreated PD. Neurology. 1999a;52(6):1206–14.
29. Ichise M, Kim YJ, Erami SS, Ballinger JR, Vines D, Tanaka F, et al. Functional morphometry of the striatum in Parkinson's disease on three-dimensional surface display of ^{123}I-beta-CIT SPECT data. J Nucl Med. 1999b;40(4):530–8.
30. Marek KL, Seibyl JP, Zoghbi SS, Zea-Ponce Y, Baldwin RM, Fussell B, et al. [^{123}I] Beta-CIT/SPECT imaging demonstrates bilateral loss of dopamine transporters in hemi-Parkinson's disease. Neurology. 1996;46(1):231–7.
31. Seibyl JP, Marek KL, Quinlan D, Sheff K, Zoghbi S, Zea-Ponce Y, et al. Decreased single-photon emission computed tomographic [^{123}I]beta-CIT striatal uptake correlates with symptom severity in Parkinson's disease. Ann Neurol. 1995;38(4):589–98.
32. Benamer TS, Patterson J, Grosset DG, Booij J, de Bruin K, van Royen E, et al. Accurate differentiation of parkinsonism and essential tremor using visual assessment of [^{123}I]-FP-CIT SPECT imaging: the [^{123}I]-FP-CIT study group. Mov Disord. 2000;15(3):503–10.
33. Fearnley JM, Lees AJ. Ageing and Parkinson's disease: substantia nigra regional selectivity. Brain. 1991;114(Pt 5):2283–301.
34. Felicio AC, Shih MC, Godeiro-Junior C, Andrade LAF, Bressan RA, Ferraz HB. Molecular imaging studies in Parkinson disease. Neurologist. 2009;15(1):6–16.
35. Brooks DJ, Ibanez V, Sawle GV, Playford ED, Quinn N, Mathias CJ, et al. Striatal D_2 receptor status in patients with Parkinson's disease, striatonigral degeneration, and progressive supranuclear palsy, measured with ^{11}C-raclopride and positron emission tomography. Ann Neurol. 1992;31(2):184–92.

36. Buck A, Westera G, Sutter M, Albani C, Kung HF, vonSchulthess GK. Iodine-123-IBF SPECT evaluation of extrapyramidal diseases. J Nucl Med. 1995;36(7):1196–200.
37. Ichise M, Toyama H, Fornazzari L, Ballinger JR, Kirsh JC. Iodine-^{123}-IBZM dopamine D2 receptor and technetium-99m-HMPAO brain perfusion SPECT in the evaluation of patients with and subjects at risk for Huntington's disease. J Nucl Med. 1993;34(8):1274–81.
38. Schwarz J, Tatsch K, Arnold G, Gasser T, Trenkwalder C, Kirsch CM, et al. ^{123}I-iodobenzamide-SPECT predicts dopaminergic responsiveness in patients with de novo parkinsonism. Neurology. 1992;42(3 Pt 1):556–61.
39. van Royen E, Verhoeff NF, Speelman JD, Wolters EC, Kuiper MA, Janssen AG. Multiple system atrophy and progressive supranuclear palsy. Diminished striatal D_2 dopamine receptor activity demonstrated by 123I-IBZM single photon emission computed tomography. Arch Neurol. 1993;50(5):513–6.
40. Plotkin M, Amthauer H, Klaffke S, Kühn A, Lüdemann L, Arnold G, et al. Combined ^{123}I-FP-CIT and ^{123}I-IBZM SPECT for the diagnosis of parkinsonian syndromes: study on 72 patients. J Neural Transm Gen Sect. 2005;112(5):677–92.
41. Brooks DJ, Ibanez V, Sawle GV, Quinn N, Lees AJ, Mathias CJ, et al. Differing patterns of striatal ^{18}F-dopa uptake in Parkinson's disease, multiple system atrophy, and progressive supranuclear palsy. Ann Neurol. 1990;28(4):547–55.
42. Ravina B, Eidelberg D, Ahlskog JE, Albin RL, Brooks DJ, Carbon M, et al. The role of radiotracer imaging in Parkinson disease. Neurology. 2005;64(2):208–15.
43. Van Heertum RL, Drocea C, Ichise M, Lobotesis K, Fawwaz RA. Single photon emission CT and positron emission tomography in the evaluation of neurologic disease. Radiol Clin N Am. 2001;39(5):1007–33.
44. Grubb RL, Powers WJ, Derdeyn CP, Adams HP, Clarke WR. The carotid occlusion surgery study. Neurosurg Focus. 2003;14(3):e9.
45. Grubb RL, Powers WJ, Clarke WR, Videena TO, Adams HP, Derdeyn CP, et al. Surgical results of the carotid occlusion surgery study. J Neurosurg. 2013;118(1):25–33.
46. Ricci PE. Imaging of adult brain tumors. Neuroimaging Clin N Am. 1999;9(4):651–69.
47. van Heertum RL, Greenstein EA, Tikofsky RS. 2-Deoxy-fluorglucose-positron emission tomography imaging of the brain: current clinical applications with emphasis on the dementias. Semin Nucl Med. 2004;34(4):300–12.
48. Di Chiro G, DeLaPaz RL, Brooks RA, Sokoloff L, Kornblith PL, Smith BH, et al. Glucose utilization of cerebral gliomas measured by [^{18}F]fluorodeoxyglucose and positron emission tomography. Neurology. 1982;32(12):1323–9.
49. Spence AM, Muzi M, Mankoff DA, O'Sullivan SF, Link JM, Lewellen TK, et al. ^{18}F-FDG PET of gliomas at delayed intervals: improved distinction between tumor and normal gray matter. J Nucl Med. 2004;45(10):1653–9.
50. Alavi JB, Alavi A, Chawluk J, Kushner M, Powe J, Hickey W, et al. Positron emission tomography in patients with glioma. A predictor of prognosis. Cancer. 1988;62(6):1074–8.
51. Di Chiro G. Positron emission tomography using [^{18}F]fluorodeoxyglucose in brain tumors. A powerful diagnostic and prognostic tool. Investig Radiol. 1987;22(5):360–71.
52. Kim EE, Chung SK, Haynie TP, Kim CG, Cho BJ, Podoloff DA, et al. Differentiation of residual or recurrent tumors from post-treatment changes with F-18 FDG PET. Radiographics. 1992;12(2):269–79.
53. Pirotte B, Goldman S, Massager N, David P, Wikler D, Vandesteene A, et al. Comparison of ^{18}F-FDG and ^{11}C-methionine for PET-guided stereotactic brain biopsy of gliomas. J Nucl Med. 2004;45(8):1293–8.
54. Lee DH, Gao FQ, Rogers JM, Gulka I, Mackenzie IR, Parrent AG, et al. MR in temporal lobe epilepsy: analysis with pathologic confirmation. Am J Neuroradiol. 1998;19(1):19–27.
55. Duncan JS. Imaging and epilepsy. Brain. 1997;120(Pt 2):339–77.
56. Devous MD, Thisted RA, Morgan GF, Leroy RF, Rowe CC. SPECT brain imaging in epilepsy: a meta-analysis. J Nucl Med. 1998;39(2):285–93.
57. Spencer SS. The relative contributions of MRI, SPECT, and PET imaging in epilepsy. Epilepsia. 1994;35(Suppl 6):S72–89.
58. Weil S, Noachtar S, Arnold S, Yousry TA, Winkler PA, Tatsch K. Ictal ECD-SPECT differentiates between temporal and extratemporal epilepsy: confirmation by excellent postoperative seizure control. Nucl Med Commun. 2001;22(2):233–7.
59. Sarikaya I. PET studies in epilepsy. Am J Nucl Med Mol Imaging. 2015;5(5):416–30.
60. Howes OD, Kambeitz J, Kim E, Stahl D, Slifstein M, Abi-Dargham A, et al. The nature of dopamine dysfunction in schizophrenia and what this means for treatment. Arch Gen Psychiatry. 2012;69(8):776–86.
61. Kambeitz J, Abi-Dargham A, Kapur S, Howes OD. Alterations in cortical and extrastriatal subcortical dopamine function in schizophrenia: systematic review and meta-analysis of imaging studies. Br J Psychiatry. 2014;204(6):420–9.
62. Abi-Dargham A, Mawlawi O, Lombardo I, Gil R, Martinez D, Huang Y, et al. Prefrontal dopamine D_1 receptors and working memory in schizophrenia. J Neurosci. 2002;22(9):3708–19.
63. Hirvonen J, van Erp TGM, Huttunen J, Aalto S, Någren K, Huttunen M, et al. Brain dopamine D_1 receptors in twins discordant for schizophrenia. Am J Psychiatry. 2006;163(10):1747–53.
64. Karlsson P, Farde L, Halldin C, Sedvall G. PET study of D_1 dopamine receptor binding in neuroleptic-naive patients with schizophrenia. Am J Psychiatry. 2002;159(5):761–7.
65. Kosaka J, Takahashi H, Ito H, Takano A, Fujimura Y, Matsumoto R, et al. Decreased binding of [^{11}C]

NNC112 and [^{11}C]SCH23390 in patients with chronic schizophrenia. Life Sci. 2010;86(21–22):814–8.
66. Okubo Y, Suhara T, Suhara T, Suzuki K, Kobayashi K, Inoue O, et al. Decreased prefrontal dopamine D_1 receptors in schizophrenia revealed by PET. Nature. 1997;385(6617):634–6.
67. Catafau AM, Searle GE, Bullich S, Gunn RN, Rabiner EA, Herance R, et al. Imaging cortical dopamine D_1 receptors using [^{11}C]NNC112 and ketanserin blockade of the 5-HT2A receptors. J Cerebr Blood Flow Metab. 2010;30(5):985–93.
68. Ekelund J, Slifstein M, Narendran R, Guillin O, Belani H, Guo N-N, et al. In vivo DA D_1 receptor selectivity of NNC 112 and SCH 23390. Mol Imaging Biol. 2007;9(3):117–25.
69. Chen KC, Yang YK, Howes O, Lee IH, Landau S, Yeh TL, et al. Striatal dopamine transporter availability in drug-naive patients with schizophrenia: a case-control SPECT study with [^{99m}Tc]-TRODAT-1 and a meta-analysis. Schizophr Bull. 2013;39(2):378–86.
70. Laruelle MA, Frankle WG, Narendran R, Kegeles LS, Abi-Dargham A. Mechanism of action of antipsychotic drugs: from dopamine D_2 receptor antagonism to glutamate NMDA facilitation. Clin Ther. 2005;27(Suppl A):S16–24.
71. Savitz JB, Drevets WC. Neuroreceptor imaging in depression. Neurobiol Dis. 2013;52:49–65.
72. Volkow ND, Morales M. The brain on drugs: from reward to addiction. Cell. 2015;162(4):712–25.
73. Brooks DJ. Positron emission tomography and single-photon emission computed tomography in central nervous system drug development. NeuroRX. 2005;2(2):226–36.
74. Talbot PS, Laruelle MA. The role of in vivo molecular imaging with PET and SPECT in the elucidation of psychiatric drug action and new drug development. Eur Neuropsychopharmacol. 2002;12(6):503–11.
75. Meyer JH, Wilson AA, Sagrati S, Hussey D, Carella A, Potter WZ, et al. Serotonin transporter occupancy of five selective serotonin reuptake inhibitors at different doses: an [^{11}C]DASB positron emission tomography study. Am J Psychiatry. 2004;161(5):826–35.
76. Schossberger PF, Touya JJ. Dynamic cisternography in normal dogs and in human beings. Neurology. 1976;26(3):254–60.
77. Bartelt D, Jordan CE, Strecker EP, James AE. Comparison of ventricular enlargement and radiopharmaceutical retention: a cisternographic-pneumoencephalographic comparison. Radiology. 1975;116(1):111–5.
78. Thut DP, Kreychman A, Obando JA. ^{111}In-DTPA cisternography with SPECT/CT for the evaluation of normal pressure hydrocephalus. J Nucl Med Technol. 2014;42(1):70–4.
79. Primeau M, Carrier L, Milette PC, Chartrand R, Picard D, Picard M. Spinal cerebrospinal fluid leak demonstrated by radioisotopic cisternography. Clin Nucl Med. 1988;13(10):701–3.
80. Servadei F, Moscatelli G, Giuliani G, Cremonini AM, Piazza G, Agostini M, et al. Cisternography in combination with single photon emission tomography for the detection of the leakage site in patients with cerebrospinal fluid rhinorrhea: preliminary report. Acta Neurochir. 1998;140(11):1183–9.
81. Hoch DB. Brain death: a diagnostic dilemma. J Nucl Med. 1992;33(12):2211–3.
82. Wijdicks EFM, Varelas PN, Gronseth GS, Greer DM. American Academy of Neurology. Evidence-based guideline update: determining brain death in adults: report of the quality standards Subcommittee of the American Academy of neurology. Neurology. 2010;74(23):1911–8.
83. Bertagna F, Barozzi O, Puta E, Lucchini S, Paghera B, Savelli G, et al. Residual brain viability, evaluated by ^{99m}Tc-ECD SPECT, in patients with suspected brain death and with confounding clinical factors. Nucl Med Commun. 2009;30(10):815–21.
84. Larar GN, Nagel JS. Technetium-99m-HMPAO cerebral perfusion scintigraphy: considerations for timely brain death declaration. J Nucl Med. 1992;33(12):2209–11.
85. Donohoe KJ, Agrawal G, Frey KA, Gerbaudo VH, Mariani G, Nagel JS, et al. SNM practice guideline for brain death scintigraphy 2.0. J Nucl Med Technol. 2012;40:198–203.

5 Clinical Applications of Nuclear Cardiology

Maria João Vidigal Ferreira
and Manuel D. Cerqueira

5.1 Introduction

Radionuclide techniques are used for cardiovascular imaging to assess perfusion, function, metabolism, innervation, and infarction [1–3]. Single-photon emission computed tomographic (SPECT) techniques prevail relative to the use of planar or positron emission tomography (PET). With SPECT there is an extensive body of literature supporting efficacy and prognostic value in a wide variety of clinical scenarios. As practiced in the United States and Europe, myocardial perfusion imaging (MPI) using SPECT or PET predominates and accounts for the majority of nuclear cardiology procedures. This concise clinical overview will mainly focus on the assessment of myocardial perfusion, viability, and left ventricular function. Imaging of myocardial sympathetic innervation, infection, inflammation, and infiltrative diseases that involve the myocardium will also be addressed.

M. J. V. Ferreira
Faculty of Medicine, Coimbra Hospital and University Center, University of Coimbra, Coimbra, Portugal

M. D. Cerqueira (✉)
Department of Nuclear Medicine, Cleveland Clinic, Cleveland, OH, USA

Cleveland Clinic Lerner College of Medicine, Of Case Western Reserve University, Cleveland, OH, USA
e-mail: cerquem@ccf.org

5.2 Historical Perspective of Nuclear Cardiology

MPI has evolved over more than 50 years to the point where it can now provide diagnostic and prognostic information in nearly all patient groups. Early studies were performed with K-43 in animal models and in man, but it was only with the availability of thallium-201 (Tl-201) in the mid-1970s that the technique using planar imaging became widely utilized for detecting the presence and extent of coronary artery disease (CAD). A decade later single-photon emission computed tomography, SPECT, was introduced and rapidly became the predominate method of acquisition. Since not all patients were capable of exercising, the use of pharmacologic stress, either with vasodilators or inotropic positive agents, allowed perfusion studies to be performed in nearly all patients. It also became evident that Tl-201 was not the ideal perfusion tracer and the availability of technetium-99m (Tc-99m)-labeled perfusion tracers, sestamibi (late 1980s) and tetrofosmin (late 1990s), improved image quality and reduced radiation exposure. These two tracers now account for the majority of perfusion studies. Perfusion imaging was shown not only to be capable of diagnosing the presence or absence of CAD but also to provide accurate information on risk assessment and prognosis. By the late 1980s, ECG-gated acquisition of perfusion images was developed and the

H. Ahmadzadehfar et al. (eds.), *Clinical Nuclear Medicine*,
https://doi.org/10.1007/978-3-030-39457-8_5

simultaneous assessment of perfusion and left ventricular global and regional function became an important tool in the diagnosis and management of CAD.

PET cardiac applications have been available since the early 1980s but were performed at a limited number of tertiary referral centers. With the development of PET/CT systems and greater availability of Rb-82 generators and on-site cyclotrons to produce N-13 for ammonia synthesis, cardiac PET achieved greater clinical penetration. PET tracers and imaging systems show clear advantages over SPECT. The high-energy emitted photons and the shorter half-life of the different tracers provide higher-quality images with reduced radiation exposure. Evaluation of perfusion and myocyte metabolism using F-18 fluorodeoxyglucose (FDG) are important features in the detection and risk stratification of CAD, and in the last decades, PET has been increasingly used for these purposes.

There have also been significant advances in SPECT systems with high-sensitivity detectors and hybrid CT systems for attenuation correction becoming available for improved image quality. Despite the higher cost of such systems, the advantages related to lower radiation exposure and better image quality offer significant advantages over older systems. Nuclear cardiology has advanced beyond perfusion imaging, assessment of function, and viability and is now providing clinical valuable information on the cardiac sympathetic nervous system, myocardial inflammation, and infiltrative diseases and infection. The future looks very promising for an established modality that has continued to be innovative in answering today's clinical needs for the evaluation and management of all types of cardiac patients.

5.3 Perfusion Imaging

5.3.1 Basic Concepts

Myocardial blood flow to the myocardium is through large epicardial conduit vessels, which offer almost no resistance to blood flow, intermediate arterioles that regulate resistance, and the extensive intramyocardial microcirculation which deliver nutrients and oxygen to the myocytes. Increases in myocardial work and, thus, in energy demands are accompanied by an increase in myocardial blood flow facilitated by a decrease in small vessel resistance due to the vasodilation mediated by several endothelium-dependent factors.

In the presence of dynamically significant large epicardial coronary vessel stenosis (≥50–80%), the site of resistance moves from the small vessels to the stenotic vessel. As long as there is adequate compensatory downstream vasodilation and decreased resistance, resting blood flow will be enough to meet myocardial energy demand. With progression of a coronary stenosis, the small vessel dilation capacity increases to maintain myocardial perfusion. Following exercise or pharmacologic stress, blood flow increases in the myocardium with normal coronary arteries, but in those perfused by arteries with a critical luminal stenosis (50–90% lumen stenosis) or endothelial dysfunction, a failure to increase or even a decrease of blood flow may occur resulting in symptoms of ischemia and a heterogeneity in myocardial blood flow that can be measured by flow tracers [4].

Given the above framework, MPI requires the comparison of images acquired in the resting state and after dynamic exercise or pharmacologic stress. Heterogeneous radiotracer uptake reflects abnormal blood flow caused by a coronary anatomic or functional abnormality. Ischemia is characterized by areas of reduced or absent uptake of the perfusion tracer on stress images with normal uptake on rest images (reversible defect), while myocardial scar has diminished uptake on both stress and rest images (fixed defect). Areas of normal myocardium have a homogeneous distribution of the perfusion tracer on both sets of images (stress and rest).

5.3.2 Radiopharmaceuticals and Imaging Protocols

The following sections will describe the characteristic of each of the cardiac radiopharmaceuticals and how they are used in the most commonly performed imaging protocols. The recommendations are based on the published guidelines [2, 3, 5].

5.3.2.1 Thallium-201

Tl-201 is a K+ analog that is transported across cell membranes by the Na/K ATPase system [6]. Initial myocardial uptake is proportional to blood flow over a wide physiological range and is dependent on the presence of viable myocardial cells. Following the rapid high initial myocardial uptake, Tl-201 re-equilibrates with the lower concentration in the blood in a time-dependent fashion. This is called redistribution and like the initial uptake is directly proportional to blood flow to the area and the presence of functioning myocytes. Tl-201 can also be used to identify viable myocardium through delayed uptake representing eventual K+ concentrations in the myocytes [7]. The high and nearly linear initial myocardial uptake following stress makes Tl-201 a better marker of myocardial blood flow and then the Tc-99m tracers which have a lower extraction fraction across the coronary bed and plateau at lower flow rates. Tl-201 uptake and redistribution over time is a marker of the K+ blood pool and of viable myocardium. In areas where blood flow is severely reduced following stress, there may be very low uptake of Tl-201, initially, despite the presence of living myocytes. Even the 3–4 h redistribution images may still be abnormal in areas with living and viable myocytes. However, over 18–24 h or following reinjection of an additional dose to boost blood levels, if there are viable myocytes, with an intact Na/K ATPase system, Tl-201 is eventually taken up, and these areas will be clearly identified as hibernating myocardium and not infarction. The major disadvantages of Tl-201 are the low energy of the photons (69–83 KeV), easily attenuated by the tissues around the heart, and the long half-life (72 h) which give a high radiation exposure [6]. The effective radiation dose for this radiotracer is approximately 4.4 mSv per 37 MBq (1 mCi), and for these reasons, the routine use of Tl-201 to assess perfusion is no longer advised [2].

Figure 5.1 has four rows that identify all the possible combinations for identification of ischemia, infarction, and hibernating myocardium using Tl-201. In the typical imaging sequence using Tl-201, shown in the top row of Fig. 5.1, the patient is stressed with dynamic exercise or pharmacologic stress and 111–148 MBq (3–4 mCi) of Tl-201 injected at peak stress. The patient must be imaged within 10–15 min of completion of stress to avoid early redistribution and a resulting decrease in sensitivity. If the post-stress images are completely normal after physician review, the rest study is optional. If the stress images are not reviewed or are abnormal, this is followed 2.5–4 h later by a redistribution set of images. If the stress and redistribution images are normal, there is no ischemia or infarction, and there is no need to look for hibernation. If the stress images are abnormal and the redistribution images are normal, there is ischemia. When perfusion defects are present on the redistribution images, most likely this is scarred myocardium. However, if a clinical question of hibernating myocardium remains, there are several options for using Tl-201 as a marker of viable myocardium (Rows 2, 3, and 4, Fig. 5.1). The major disadvantages of Tl-201 are the low energy of the photons (69–83 KeV), easily attenuated by the tissues around the heart, and the long half-life (72 h) which gives a high radiation exposure [6] [2].

Assessment of viability is especially important in patients with congestive heart failure, known cardiomyopathies, or myocardial infarction [8]. In patients where myocardial viability assessment is of critical clinical importance and PET or cardiac MRI are not available, several approaches using Tl-201 can be used to further improve on the accuracy of the regular 4-h stress/redistribution sequence. These approaches include delayed imaging at 24 h (Row 1, Fig. 5.1). The patient may also be reinjection with 37 MBq of Tl-201 immediately following the redistribution images with imaging 15 min later (Row 2, Fig. 5.1) or imaging at 24 h (Row 3, Fig. 5.1). Both of these approaches result in three separate sets of images. Alternatively, Row 4, Fig. 5.1, four sets of images may be acquired. A rest/3–4-h

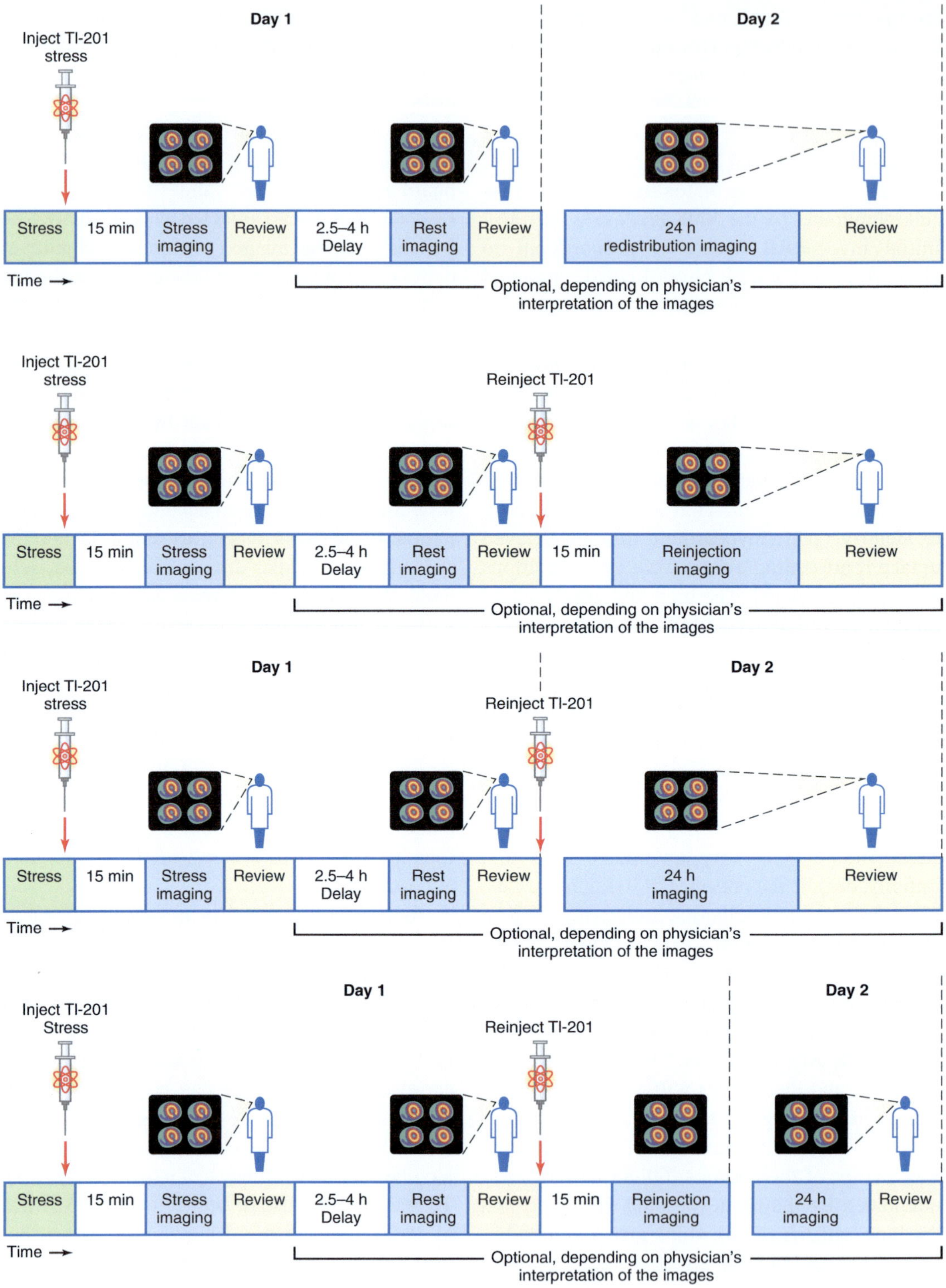

Fig. 5.1 Tl-201 protocols for detection of ischemia and viable myocardium

redistribution Tl-201 protocol can also be used for viability assessment, but this does not provide information on ischemia.

With the dual isotope approach, both ischemia and hibernation can be identified, but this procedure is no longer recommended, due to higher radiation exposure and increase rate of false-positive results for ischemia, as rest and stress images are obtained with different tracers, unless there is a clear indication to assess perfusion and viability in elderly patients that require shorter protocols or in the case that alternative methods are not available [2].

5.3.2.2 Technetium-99m Radiotracers

Tc-99m tracers were developed to overcome the limitations of Tl-201. Only two Tc-99m tracers are in clinical use: Tc-99m sestamibi (Cardiolite™) and Tc-99m tetrofosmin (Myoview™) [6]. The monoenergetic 140 keV higher energy of Tc-99m versus the 69–83 keV range of Tl-201 results in improved image resolution with less overall attenuation and scatter during imaging. Tc-99m has a half-life of 6 h in comparison to the 72 h of Tl-201. The shorter half-life allows administration of a higher Tc-99m dose resulting in high-count images. As an example, 148 MBq (4 mCi) f Tl-201 is administered compared to 444–1110 MBq (12–30 mCi) of the Tc-99m radiotracers. The higher counts obtained with a Tc-99m radiopharmaceutical and the lack of redistribution allows ECG-triggered gated acquisition for assessment of function. The minimal redistribution of Tc-99m tracers following injection allows greater flexibility as to when acquisition can be performed, as soon as 10 min or as far out as 4 h following stress. The whole-body effective dose is approximately 0.3 mSv per 37 MBq (1 mCi) of Tc-99m [2].

5.3.2.3 Tc-99m Sestamibi and Tetrofosmin

Both are monovalent cations which make them very lipophilic and facilitate entry into cells. Uptake is dependent on blood flow, plasma- and mitochondrial-derived membrane electrochemical gradients, cellular pH, and intact energy pathways [6]. Chemical or structural conversion of the molecule is not required, and unlike Tl-201 inhibitors of Na+, K+ and Ca2+ transport do not prevent uptake or retention in myocytes. Once inside the myocyte, they remain trapped with the greatest concentration in the mitochondria, and there is minimal washout. Following intravenous injection, they are cleared from blood by the liver, concentrated in the gall bladder, and excreted through the common bile duct into the GI tract. The initial high liver uptake does not allow the inferior wall to be seen clearly early post-injection and requires waiting 15–45 min following resting or pharmacologic stress injection to get adequate visualization. Clearance post-dynamic exercise is faster, and image acquisition can be started as soon as 10–20 min following injection [2, 6]. Tetrofosmin has the advantage to allow earlier scanning because of its lower hepatic uptake.

5.3.2.4 Tc-99m Radiotracer Imaging Protocol Options

The uptake and clearance characteristics of Tc-99m sestamibi and tetrofosmin are sufficiently similar that recommendations for imaging are identical with minor variation between injection time and when to image due to differences in liver clearance between the two tracers. In general Tc-99m tetrofosmin can be imaged sooner after injection.

Protocol options include a 2-day protocol, a 1-day split dose protocol (rest/stress, Fig. 5.2, or stress/rest sequence, Fig. 5.3),s and a dual isotope approach (Fig. 5.4) using Tl-201 at rest. The diagnostic accuracy results in the literature did not report significant differences between the various protocols or between these agents and Tl-201 [1, 2].

In the 2-day protocol (bottom rows of Figs. 5.2 and 5.3) the maximal dose of Tc-99m, 740–1110 MBq (20-30 mCi), is used for both images and provides high counts and better image quality. This protocol is optimal in obese patients and allows higher counts and accurate rest EF to be calculated as well a post-stress measurement which provides additional value. Due to time delays in getting test results and patient inconvenience, this protocol is not used widely. When

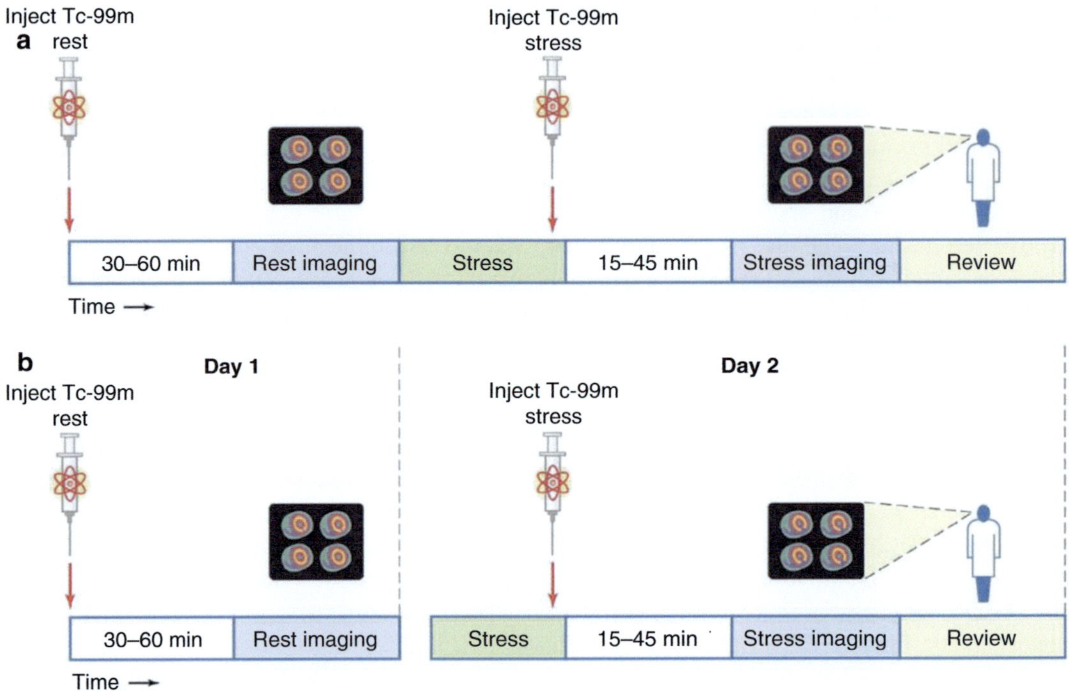

Fig. 5.2 Tc-99m 1- and 2-day stress/rest protocols

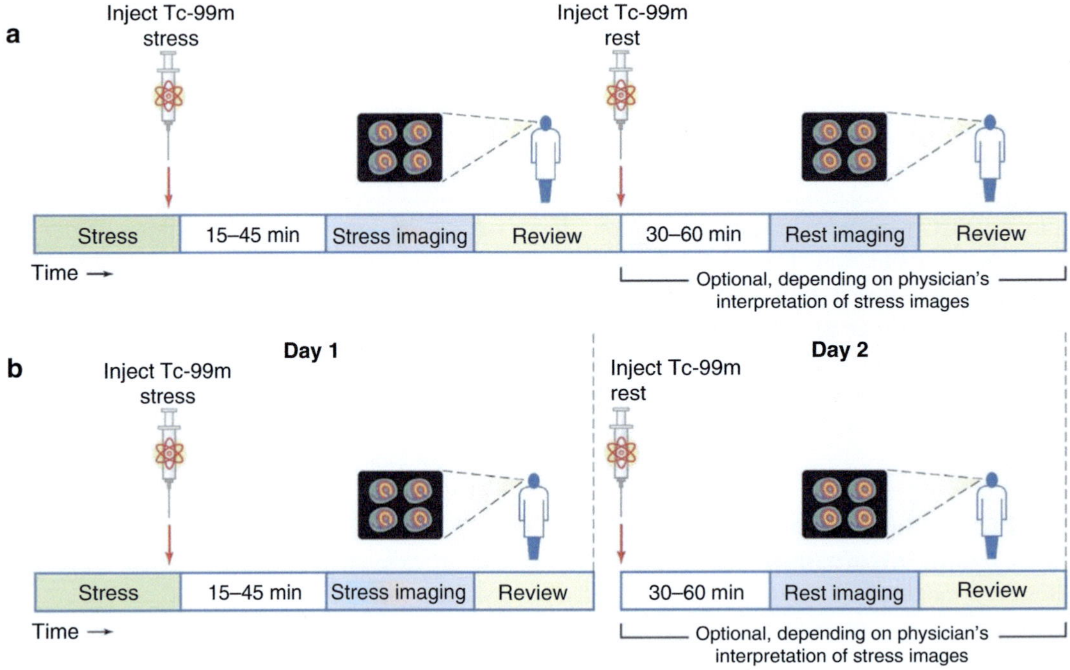

Fig. 5.3 Tc-99m 1- and 2-day rest/stress protocols

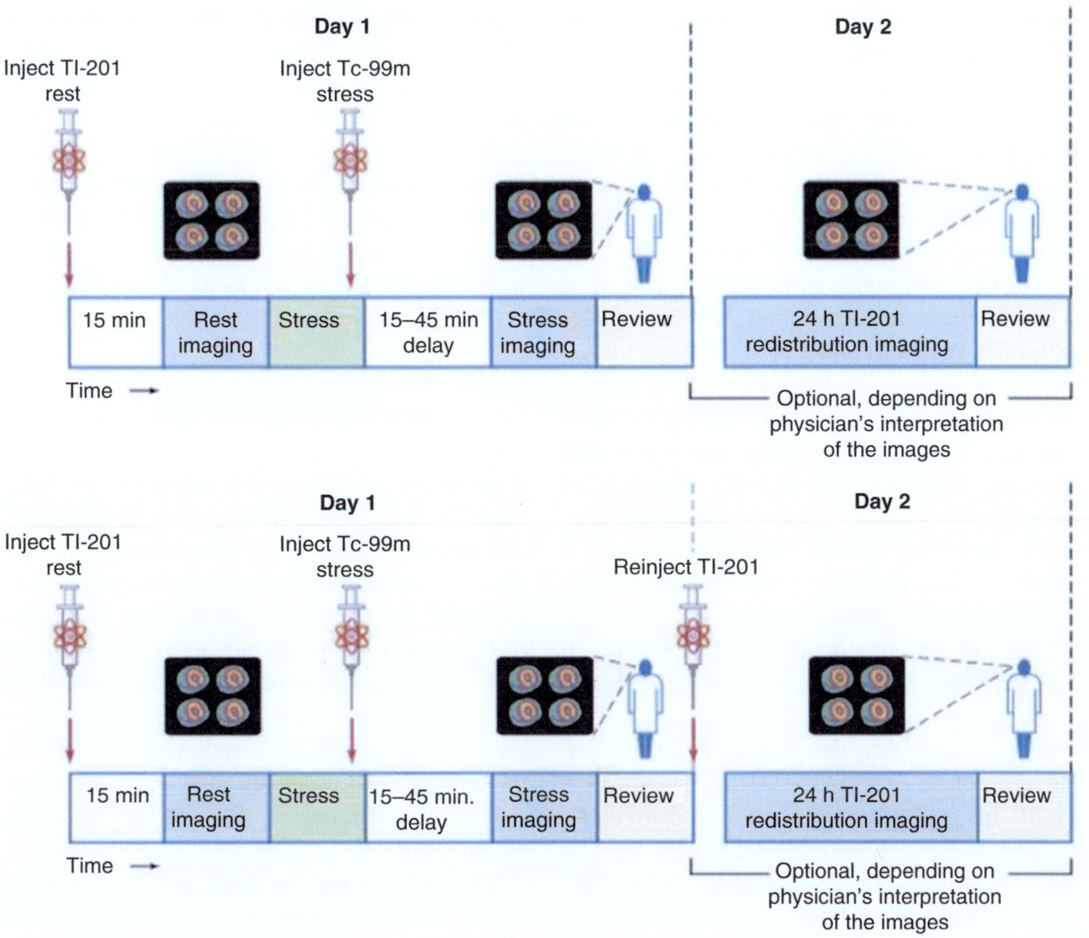

Fig. 5.4 Dual isotope rest Tl-201 and stress Tc-99m stress protocols with optional delayed redistribution and reinjection of Tl-201 for 24-h viability assessment

doing a 2-day protocol, the stress study should be done first, and if normal the resting study is not needed. Stress first provides results sooner and has a lower radiation exposure, especially if the stress is normal and the rest portion is not performed. In obese patients with soft tissue attenuation and low counts, gating and attenuation correction improves specificity and decreases the number of patients needing to return for a rest study [9].

For logistical reasons, 1-day stress and rest studies are usually performed as shown in top rows of Figs. 5.2 and 5.3. This requires administration of a low dose, 1/3 of the total dose or 296–444 MBq (8–12 mCi) for the first study, and a larger dose, 2/3 of the total dose or 740–1110 MBq (20–30 mCi), for the second study and waiting as long as possible between studies, usually 1.5–2.5 h, to allow for physical decay of Tc-99m. Using this approach, when the second set of images is acquired there is relatively little contamination from the first injection. The 1-day rest/stress sequence, shown in Fig. 5.2, is the most frequently performed protocol in the United States. The disadvantage of this sequence is that the low dose is given at rest when blood flow is lowest and there will be less myocardial tracer uptake. The higher stress dose, administered when blood flow is maximal, will give higher counts and better quality images. The gated post-stress image in patients with extensive ischemia may give a lower EF, due to residual myocardial stunning, and then a true resting ejection fraction [10]. In patients with ischemia, a lower post-stress EF is a better predictor of higher cardiac death and infarction rate and then the size and severity of the defect alone [11]. The 1-day stress/rest protocol in upper row of Fig. 5.3 gives the lower dose when myocardial blood flow is the highest, during stress, and background activity in the subdiaphragmatic area is low due to a decrease in mesenteric blood flow associated with stress. With this protocol, if the stress images are normal, the rest study is not needed, improving laboratory efficiency and reducing radiation exposure [12–14]. Stress-first and stress-only protocols, whether in a 1- or 2-day sequence, are efficient and reduce radiation exposure. They require physician review of the stress images in order to make a decision on the need for a resting study the same or the following day.

The timing and sequence for a Tl-201/Tc-99m radiotracer dual isotope separate acquisition protocol is displayed in Fig. 5.4. For the resting Tl-201 study, the patient should be fasting and a dose of 111–148 MBq (3–4 mCi) of Tl-201 injected. Imaging should be delayed for 10–15 min. For stress, the patient is injected with 240–1110 MBq 740–1110 MBq (20–30 mCi) of a Tc-99m tracer. The separate acquisition approach takes advantage of the two distinct and separate energy levels of Tl-201 and Tc-99m. During the second acquisition, the gamma camera selectively acquires data centering on the higher energy Tc-99m window. Although, there is residual Tl-201 present from the resting study, the lower energy Tl-201 photons are excluded by using the higher Tc-99m window. When using the dual isotope approach and myocardial viability is in question, a rest-4-h redistribution Tl-201 study may be performed prior to performing the stress study [15]. Patients can also be injected with Tl-201 the evening before to give an approximate 12-h Tl-201 acquisition the following morning. This is an alternative method for the identification of myocardial viability, as mentioned above [2]. When the Tc-99m stress study has already been performed and questions of viability remain, delayed Tl-201 imaging cannot be performed on the same day due to the down scatter of the Tc-99m into the Tl-201 energy window. If both the rest and stress images have fixed perfusion defects, viability assessment can be performed with reinjection of 37 MBq (1 mCi) of Tl-201. In such situations, the patient may return at 24 h for Tl-201 viability imaging by which time there has been sufficient decay of the Tc-99m to allow uptake of the K+ properties of Tl-2-1 (Fig. 5.4).

5.3.3 Perfusion Tracers and Protocols for PET

Assessment of myocardial perfusion has been established as an important tool in the diagnosis and prognosis of coronary artery disease. SPECT has been one of the most used techniques for this purpose. PET improves the functional evaluation of CAD as it shows higher diagnostic accuracy and it allows measurements of myocardial blood flow (MBF) in absolute terms (milliliters per gram per minute). Quantification of MBF extends the conventional perfusion imaging to the detection of microvascular disease and balanced ischemia [3, 16].

PET tracers use positron emitting radionuclides, such as oxygen-15 (O-15), nitrogen-13 (N-13), rubidium-82 (Rb-82), or fluoride-18 (Fl-18). Due to their short half-lives, oxygen-15 water and N-13 ammonia studies are limited or best performed in centers with an on-site cyclotron. All PET tracers can be used with pharmacologic stress. Only N-13 ammonia and F-18 flurpiridaz can be used with dynamic exercise stress. Positrons are positively charged particles, emitted by the nuclei of unstable isotopes during radioactive decay. They interact with electrons, and annihilation occurs with the emission of two 511 KeV photons that travel in exactly 180° opposite directions. As PET detectors are placed in a ring surrounding the patient, events with temporal coincidence photons are located by opposing detectors. This result in an improved spatial and temporal resolution compared to SPECT, offering lower radiation exposure due to the very short half-lives of the radioisotopes with higher diagnostic accuracy.

Table 5.1 compares PET with SPECT MPI, pointing out the advantages and disadvantages of each technique [3, 17, 18].

5.3.3.1 O-15 Water

This tracer requires an on-site cyclotron and is often considered the ideal tracer for quantifying MBF in absolute terms. With no barrier effect from cellular membranes, the activity of O-15 water in an area of interest can be described by a one-compartment tracer kinetic model. Its use is limited due to a very short half-life (2 min) and poor contrast images between blood pool and the immediately adjacent myocardium [3, 6, 19].

Table 5.1 Advantages and disadvantages of SPECT and PET cardiac imaging

Advantages of SPECT	*Advantages of PET*
Widely available Standardized protocols Familiar procedure to healthcare providers Large evidence supporting efficacy and prognostic value	Superior image quality Higher diagnostic accuracy Lower radiation exposure Possibility of myocardial blood flow quantification (advantage in multivessel disease and microvascular disease) All studies done with attenuation correction
Disadvantages of SPECT	*Disadvantages of PET*
Higher radiation exposure Higher prevalence of equivocal studies Suboptimal identification of multivessel disease or balanced Unpredictable supply of Tc-99m tracers	Higher cost Limited availability for cardiac studies Less familiar to healthcare providers

5.3.3.2 N-13 Ammonia

N-13 ammonia is used to assess myocardial perfusion visually and with absolute quantification of MBF using dynamic acquisition from time of injection and a compartment kinetic model that incorporates extraction and rate constants. At physiologic pH, N-13 ammonia is in its cationic form and has a physical half-life of 10 min. The first-pass extraction is related to blood flow for low flow rates. It crosses myocardial cell membranes through passive diffusion or active transport. In the cell, N13 ammonia is incorporated into the amino acid pool as N13-glutamine or back diffuses into the blood. A 740 MBq (20 mCi) dose of N13 ammonia results in an effective dose of 1.48 mSv [3, 6, 19]. A typical imaging protocol for N-13 ammonia using regadenoson is shown in Fig. 5.5.

Typically 370–740 MBq (10–20 mCi) of N-13 ammonia is injected over 20–30 s. Dynamic images should be acquired immediately during infusion, and static images should be started 1.5–3 min after the end of infusion. Imaging duration is usually 10–15 min [3, 6].

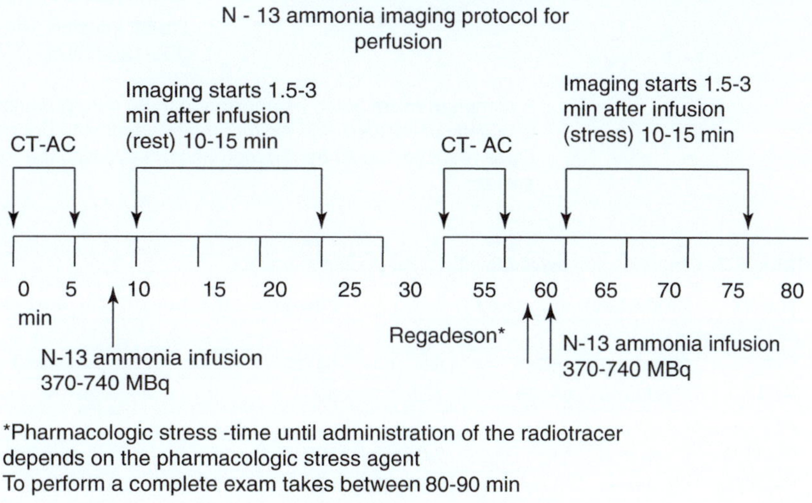

Fig. 5.5 N-13 ammonia rest and stress PET perfusion imaging protocol with regadenoson stress

5.3.3.3 Rubidium-82

Rb-82 is a monovalent cationic analog to potassium. It is produced by a generator system through decay from strontium-82 (Sr-82). It decays to rubidium-82, by emission of several high-energy positrons, and has a half-life of 75 s. It enters the myocyte via sodium/potassium adenosine triphosphate transporter. First-pass extraction is less than ammonia and decreases or plateaus with higher blood flow rates. The total effective dose for a maximal allowable activity of 2220 MBq (60 mCi) vary from 1.1 to 3.5 mSv [3, 6, 19]. A typical imaging protocol for Rb-82 rest and stress is shown in Fig. 5.6.

Perfusion imaging with Rb-82 can be acquired using 740–1850 MBq (20–50 mCi) of the tracer for each study with the type of detectors and acquisition parameters determining the exact dose. Rest images are acquired first to reduce contamination by stress effects. The tracer is infused during a maximum of 30 s and imaging started 70–90 s after injection if left ventricle ejection fraction is over 50% and 90–130 s if under that value [3].

Table 5.2 compares the differences between available SPECT and PET MPI tracers [18–20].

5.3.3.4 F-18 Flurpiridaz

This is a novel PET mitochondrial complex-1 inhibitor, structurally an analog to pyridaben. With the longer half-life of F-18 (120 min), there is no need for on-site cyclotron production. Image quality, compared with N-13 ammonia or Rb-82, is higher. Protocols can be performed with dynamic exercise or pharmacologic stress. A sustained higher extraction rate with high flow

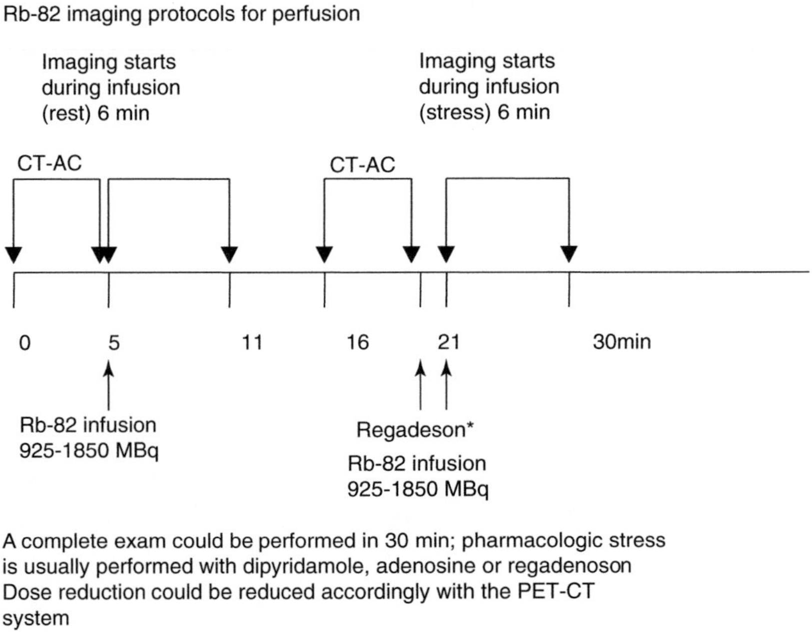

Fig. 5.6 Rb-82 rest and stress PET perfusion imaging protocol with regadenoson stress

Table 5.2 Comparison between the different perfusion tracers

Tracers	Production	$E_{\gamma\ \text{rays}}$ (KeV)	$T_{1/2}$	First-pass extraction, %	Inj. dose (MBq)	Total dose/study (mSv)
SPECT tracers						
^{99m}Tc	Generator	140	6 h	54–65	740–1480	3–16.3
^{201}Tl	Cyclotron	69–70	72 h	85	74–148	10.9–15.3
PET tracers						
$^{15}O\text{-}H_2O$	Cyclotron	511	2.06 min	100	No guidelines	No guidelines
$^{13}N\text{-}NH_3$	Cyclotron	511	9.96 min	80	370–740	1.5
^{82}Rb	Generator	511	1.25 min	65	370–2220	1.75–7.5

rates enables enhanced absolute quantification of blood flow. This tracer is not yet approved for clinical use [6, 19].

5.3.4 Pharmacologic Stress Agents and Protocols

All myocardial perfusion imaging studies should be performed using dynamic exercise stress whenever possible to obtain exercise duration, heart rate and blood pressure response, and variables that are important for CAD diagnosis and management and not available from pharmacologic stress [21]. Pharmacologic stress is reserved for patients who are unable to exercise, unable to achieve at least 85% of the maximal age-adjusted heart rate, or unable to reach an ischemic end-point on the bases of symptoms or ECG changes. Sensitivity of MPI decreases in patients who achieve <85% of the predicted heart rate [22]. If the myocardial perfusion images are normal, it cannot be certain if they are truly normal or due to an inadequate level of stress achieved during submaximal exercise. Alternatively, if there is ischemia, it is never certain if the full extent of ischemia was detected.

The pharmacologic agents in common use include the vasodilators, adenosine, dipyridamole, and regadenoson, and the adrenergic stimulant dobutamine. The properties of these agents are shown in Table 5.3. The vasodilators produce maximal coronary hyperemia creating blood flow heterogeneity by causing a greater increase in

Table 5.3 Comparison between pharmacological stress agents

	Adenosine	Regadenoson	Dipyridamole	Dobutamine
Mechanism of action	Vasodilation through activation A_{2A} Also activates A_1 A_{2B} and A_3 receptors	A_{2A} adenosine receptor agonist	Prevents the intracellular reuptake and deamination of adenosine	Stimulation of b1 and b2 receptors (effect similar to exercise)
Increase in MBF	3.5–4	3.5–4	3.5–7	–
Peak effect	1–2 min	1–4 min	6.5 min	> 10 min
Half-life	10 s	First phase: 2–4 min Second phase: 30 min Third phase: 2 h	30–45 min	2 min
Administration	Continuous infusion 140 μg/kg/min over 4–6 min	Intravenous dose of 0.4 mg	0.56 mg/kg over 4 min	Given incrementally starting at 5–10 μg/kg/min, increasing every 3 min until 40 μg/kg/min or 85% of the predicted heart rate
Side effects	AV block, peripheral vasodilation and bronchospasm	Shortness of breath, headache, and flushing	Chest pain; headache; dizziness; extrasystoles; nausea; hypotension; flushing	Palpitation; chest pain; headache; flushing; dyspnea; supraventricular and ventricular arrhythmias
Absolute contraindications	COPD High-degree AV block or sinus node disease Hypotension or severe hypertension Unstable CAD Hypersensitivity to adenosine or regadenoson	COPD with ongoing wheezing High-degree AV block or sinus node disease Hypotension or severe hypertension Unstable CAD Hypersensitivity to adenosine or regadenoson	COPD Hypotension or severe hypertension Unstable CAD Hypersensitivity	Unstable CAD Hemodynamically significant left ventricular outflow tract obstruction Atrial tachyarrhythmias with uncontrolled ventricular response History of ventricular tachycardia Uncontrolled hypertension Aortic dissection Hypersensitivity

blood flow in territories perfused by normal coronary arteries and then in those perfused by arteries with flow-limiting stenosis. Dobutamine increases not only blood flow but heart rate and blood pressure, and this increase in myocardial work and oxygen demand may create true ischemia.

5.3.4.1 Vasodilators

Mechanism of Action, Safety, and Efficacy

Adenosine and regadenoson stimulate A_{2a} receptors directly producing coronary vasodilation. Adenosine is produced inside many cell types, and inside the cell, it has no effect on blood flow. It is actively transported into the extracellular space where it is capable of binding and stimulating a series of adenosine (A) receptors [23]. The A_{2a} receptors, present on vascular smooth muscle and endothelial cells, enhance arterial wall smooth muscle dilation and increase coronary blood flow. Adenosine also stimulates the A_1, A_{2b}, and A_3 receptors, which cause peripheral vasodilation, nonischemic cardiac chest pain, atrioventricular nodal block, and bronchospasm which are undesirable side effects in the context of perfusion imaging. Inactivation of extracellular adenosine, whether endogenously produced or exogenously administered, is under 10 s due to reuptake by all types of cells using the same cell membrane transport system and active metabolism [2].

Regadenoson is an A_{2a} agonist with a lower affinity for A_1 and almost no affinity to A_{2b} and A_3 adenosine receptors. The coronary vasodilatory effects are achieved during the first pass through the heart with a doubling of coronary blood flow by 30 s, and maximal plasma concentration is achieved in 2–4 min after injection. The loss of its pharmacodynamic effect on coronary blood flow occurs in approximately 30 min. The most common side effects of regadenoson are shortness of breath, headache, and flushing [2, 5].

Dipyridamole blocks the reuptake mechanism of adenosine and increases coronary blood flow by rising extracellular concentration of endogenously produced adenosine. Dipyridamole hyperemia lasts for more than 50 min, peak action occurs 6.5 min after the start of infusion, and the half-life is between 30 and 45 min [2].

Caffeine-containing beverages and foods and methylxanthine-containing medications, such as aminophylline, block adenosine receptors and thereby antagonize its effects; flow heterogeneity is not created with ingestion of these compounds and in patients with CAD; this may result in a false-negative test. This antagonist action, however, is helpful when side effects are present and administration of aminophylline blocks the adenosine receptors and reverses the side effects [2].

Side effects have been reported to occur in 50% of patients receiving dipyridamole with reversal required in 12%. Side effects occur in 80% of patients receiving adenosine with <1% receiving aminophylline reversal [24, 25]. Vasodilators cause, on average, a 10 mmHg decrease in systolic and diastolic blood pressure with a compensatory 12–15 beats per minute increase in heart rate [24]. The most common cardiac side effects with dipyridamole include chest pain (20%), ECG changes (16%), and ST depression (7.5%). With adenosine, the cardiac side effects included chest pain (35%), transient A-V nodal block (7.6%), and ST-T wave changes (5.7%). The majority of reported chest pain is not ischemic but due to nonselective stimulation of bradykinin pain receptors by adenosine. Patients with ECG changes consistent with ischemia are felt to have a higher dependence on collateral vessel blood flow which may be decreased due to coronary steal associated with a marked increase in coronary flow in normal vessels during vasodilation and a resultant decrease in collateral flow. At some institutions, it is standard practice to reverse the effects of dipyridamole in all patients using aminophylline. The effective half-life of dipyridamole is 30 min, which is longer than the half-life of aminophylline, and this means additional doses maybe required to prevent recurrence of side effects. Adenosine can be reversed by stopping the infusion. With regadenoson a lower incidence of chest pain, flushing, and throat, neck, and jaw pain are experienced, and a higher incidence of headache and gastrointestinal discomfort are reported. A rare but important side effect of regadenoson is an increase incidence of seizures. Patients having seizures associated with regadenoson use should not receive aminophylline for reversal as this has the potential to increase seizure activity (see product package insert). Patients with unstable angina or decompensated COPD should not receive dipyridamole, adenosine, or regadenoson. As regadenoson is a more selective A_{2a} receptor agonist, it can be used in patients with mild to moderate asthma and moderate to severe COPD [2, 5].

Dipyridamole and adenosine have been used extensively and have an excellent overall safety record. More recently, regadenoson has also proved to have a good safety profile [26–28]. Although general side effects are common, cardiac and severe adverse events are rare. When considering that patients referred for pharmacologic stress testing are generally more debilitated, overall safety is comparable to that reported for conventional dynamic exercise stress testing [24]. Severe adverse complications such as death and myocardial infarction in association with pharmacologic stress testing are uncommon. In a retrospective review of 73,806 patients from 59 centers in 19 countries, there were 9 reported cardiac deaths and 13 nonfatal myocardial infarctions using intravenous dipyridamole [29]. In a prospective registry that included 9256 patients receiving intravenous adenosine, there were no deaths and one patient had a myocardial infarction [24]. The reported diagnostic accuracy using adenosine, regadenoson, or dipyridamole has been shown to be comparable to exercise. In early studies performed mostly using planar Tl-201 imaging in which each patient was studied twice with exercise and dipyridamole, sensitivity was in the 80% range and specificity in the range of 90%. There were no differences between the two forms of stress [30]. The published studies looking at the accuracy of adenosine stress did not in general perform stress twice and used predominately SPECT imaging with Tl-201 or the Tc-99m tracers. The average sensitivity for pharmacologic stress with vasodilators was 87%, and the specificity was 74% [30]. Regadenoson and adenosine were compared in the ADVANCE MPI trials, and regadenoson proved to induce similar perfusion defects as those observed with adenosine, irrespective to age, gender, diabetic status, body mass index, or prior cardiovascular history [26]. Based on extensive publications and practical clinical experience in everyday use, the accuracy of vasodilator pharmacologic stress is accepted as being equivalent to exercise stress.

Pharmacologic Stress Protocols

The vasodilator stress protocols using adenosine, dipyridamole, or regadenoson can be performed using low-level exercise stress prior to and during infusion to improve image quality, by decreasing background activity and lowering patient side effects. Figure 5.7 demonstrates the imaging protocol for adenosine pharmacologic stress.

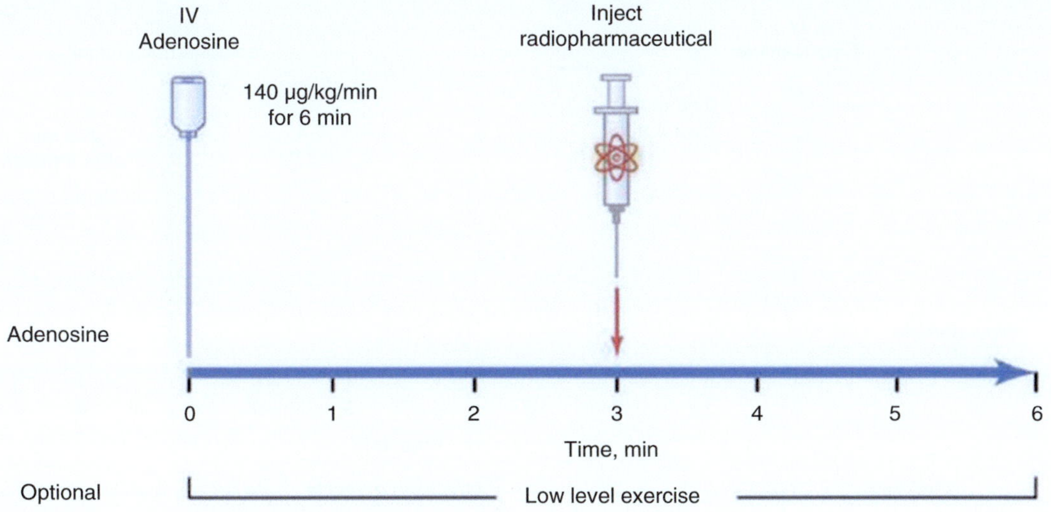

Fig. 5.7 Protocol for pharmacologic stress with adenosine

Patients should fast a minimum of 8 h and medications and foods containing caffeine stopped for 24 h. Methylxanthines and dipyridamole need to be stopped for 48 h prior to testing as they inhibit the vasodilatory effects of the adenosine and dipyridamole. Patients with 2° A-V nodal block (Mobitz Type II) or 3° A-V nodal block without a functioning pacemaker should not receive adenosine, regadenoson, or dipyridamole due to the potential A-V node blocking effects. Patients with a prolonged PR interval or Wenckebach can be tested safely. The use of vasodilator stress is recommended in all patients with a LBBB as the use of exercise leads to a higher rate of false-positive studies due to septal defects [31].

Adenosine is infused at a rate of 140 μg/kg/min for 4 or 6 min with the radiotracer injected at minutes 2 or 3 and the infusion continued a minimum of 1 min to allow maximal extraction, especially of the Tc-99m tracers which have a lower extraction fraction and then Tl-201 across the coronary bed. If the patient has evidence of ischemia by symptoms or profound ECG changes, the radiotracer can be administered earlier, but the infusion must be maintained a minimum of 1 min to allow radiotracer extraction at the high coronary blood flow rates. Performing low-level exercise during adenosine infusion decreases side effects and improves image quality and is recommended in all patients capable of walking on a treadmill [2].

Dipyridamole stress protocol is shown in Fig. 5.8. It is infused at a rate of 0.56 mg/kg of body weight over 4 min to a maximum total dose of 60 mg. Tl-201 or a Tc-99m radiotracer can be administered by bolus injection 3–5 min following completion of the infusion or earlier if the patient has evidence of ischemia by symptoms or profound ECG changes. Maximal coronary hyperemia is delayed due to the need to allow endogenous adenosine levels to increase following the inhibition of the adenosine reuptake mechanism by dipyridamole. Aminophylline administration is required more often due to the longer half-life, and side effects may recur due to the shorter half-life of aminophylline [2].

Unlike the other pharmacologic stress agents, regadenoson is given at a fixed dose of 0.4 mg, regardless of body weight, as a 10 s bolus. This is shown in Fig. 5.9. Since there is a very rapid increase in coronary blood flow, the radiotracer is administered 30 s after starting the regadenoson bolus [2, 5]. Since regadenoson is given as a bolus at a fixed dose, this allow it to be administered more efficiently to those patients who attempt dynamic exercise stress but are not able to achieve the target heart rate. In such patients, a bolus of regadenoson can be given while the patient is still on the treadmill or immediately in recovery. All the other stress agents require weight-based dosing and continuous infusion over several minutes to get the desired increase in

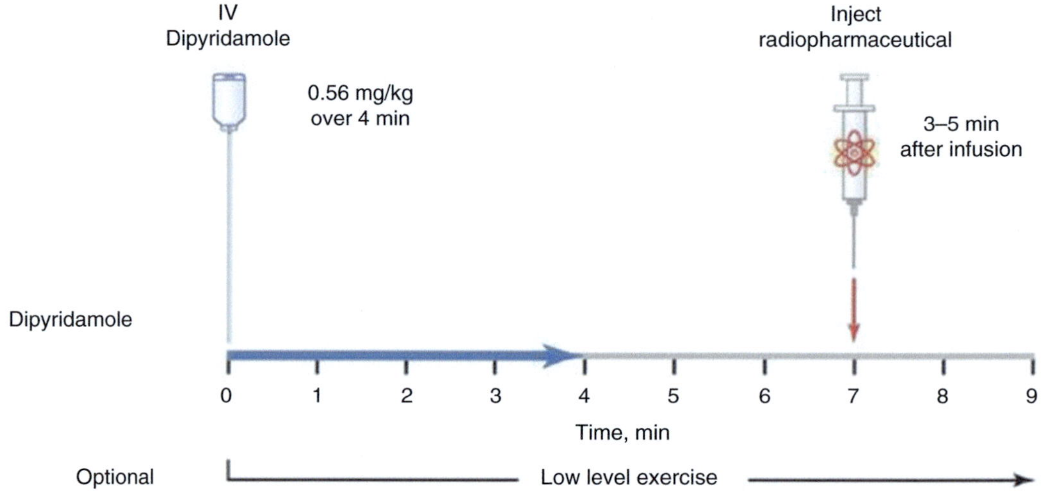

Fig. 5.8 Protocol for pharmacologic stress with dipyridamole

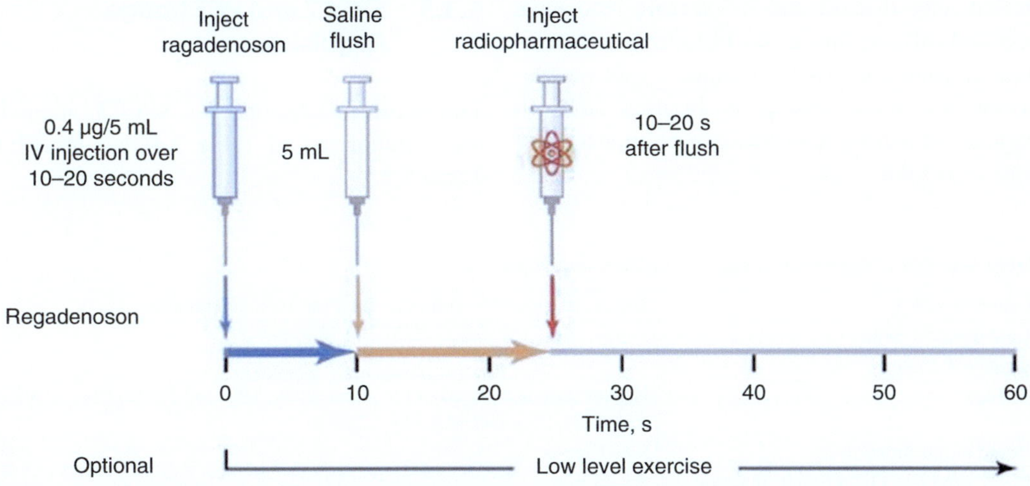

Fig. 5.9 Protocol for pharmacologic stress with regadenoson

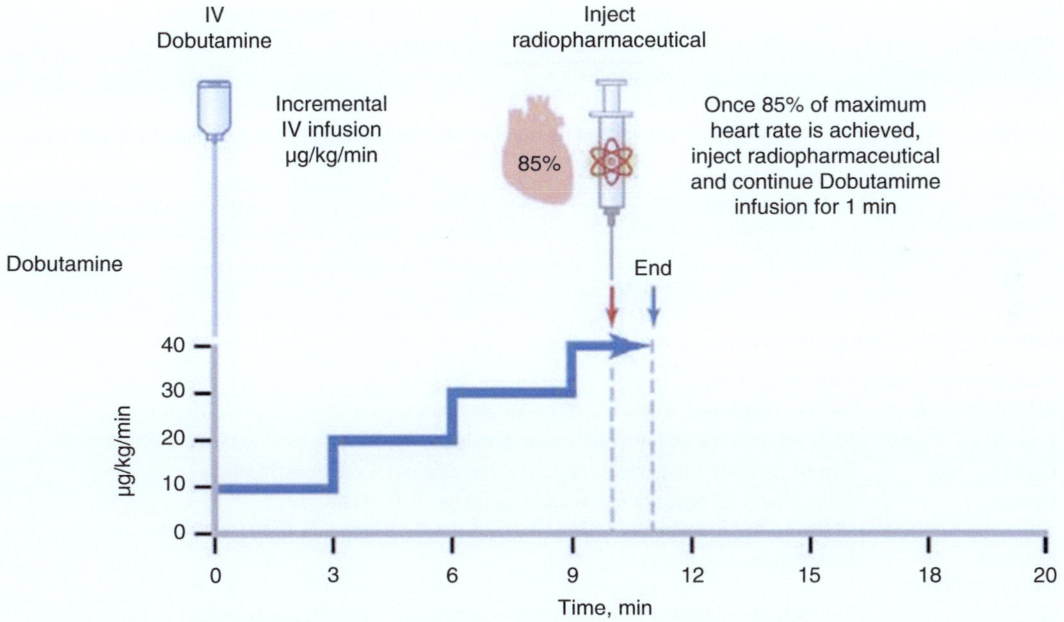

Fig. 5.10 Protocol for pharmacologic stress with dobutamine

coronary blood flow. This protocol has been shown to be safe but should not be used in patients who have achieved an ischemic endpoint even if they have not reached the target heart rate.

5.3.4.2 Catecholamines

Dobutamine is used infrequently for myocardial perfusion imaging. As shown in Fig. 5.10, the protocol requires 3 min stepwise infusion stages of increasing doses of dobutamine until an ischemic endpoint is reached or the patient achieves 85% of the maximal age-predicted heart rate. Protocols typically take much longer then vasodilator stress [32]. Patients with hypertension, abdominal aortic aneurysms, poorly controlled supraventricular arrhythmias, or ventricular arrhythmias should not be studied. Although some nuclear cardiology laboratories use it exclusively, at most centers it is used predominately in patients with severe and poorly controlled lung disease and in patients who have ingested caffeine on the day of testing, and vasodilators cannot be used [2]. Studies with regadenoson have shown that it can be used safely in patients with chronic obstructive pulmonary disease or asthma.

5.3.5 SPECT and PET Image Acquisition

The recommendations for SPECT acquisition are summarized in Table 5.4 and for PET in Table 5.5.

Table 5.4 SPECT perfusion imaging with Tc-99m tracers

Patient position	Supine or prone to minimize diaphragmatic attenuation
Low-dose CT scan	
Gated CT scan	
Dosage	Higher dose is advised in the stress study, 890–1332 MBq (24–36 mCi); rest study, 296–444 MBq (8–12 mCi)
Route of administration	Intravenous
Delay time from injection to imaging	30–45 min
Delay time of the two sets of images	3–4 h
Energy window	140 KeV ± 15%
Collimators	Low-energy high-resolution (LEHR)
Orbit	180° from 45° RAO to 45° LPO (circular or noncircular)
Pixel size	6.4 ± 0.4 mm (64 × 64 matrix)
Acquisition type	Step-and-shot
Number of projections	64
Total time	Dependent on number of detectors but should get adequate number of counts in under 20 min to avoid patient motion
ECG gated	Standard in at least one of the acquisitions (stress)
Frames/cycle	8–16
Attenuation correction with CT	Optional

Table 5.5 PET-CT perfusion imaging

Radiopharmaceutical	^{82}Rb or ^{13}N-NH_3
Patient position	Supine, performed with a CT scout image or topogram
Low-dose CT scan	Slow rotation speed; high pitch; non-gated; acquired during tidal expiration breath-hold
Gated CT scan	Can be used for attenuation correction and calcium score quantification
Dosage[a]	^{82}Rb: 1.48–2.22 GBq for stress and rest images (40–60 mCi) ^{13}N-NH_3: rest images 0.37 GBq (10 mCi); stress images 1.11 GBq (30 mCi)
Route of administration	Intravenous
ECG gating image	For ^{82}Rb image begins 90–120 s after injection; for ^{13}N-NH_3 image begins 3–5 min after injection; the scan time is of 5 min for ^{82}Rb and 20 min for ^{13}N-NH_3
Dynamic imaging	Allows quantification of myocardial blood flow and for that purpose after injection imaging begins and continues for 7–8 min for ^{82}Rb or 20 min for ^{13}N-NH_3; to acquire dynamic and gated images, two separate injections of 82Rb are required; only one with ^{13}N-NH_3
List mode imaging	Ideal approach as a single injection allows multiple reconstructions but requires significant computer power
Stress	Pharmacological/exercise
Image reconstruction	Filtered back projection or iterative reconstruction
Attenuation correction	CT-based attenuation correction in almost all the cases; rotating rod sources

[a]3D imaging requires less dosage than 2D imaging

High-quality imaging and optimal diagnostic accuracy can be achieved through the selection of equipment and a well-designed quality assurance program.

The majority of SPECT systems are based on Anger camera technology where one or more camera heads rotate around the patient's body. Anger cameras consist of a collimator that selects photons traveling parallel to the collimator and a single NaI crystal that absorbs and amplifies incident gamma photons. The photomultiplier tubes (PMTs) further amplify the signal and spatially locate the scintillation events within the crystal.

New dedicated cardiac cameras are characterized by increased photon sensitivity. This is achieved by different collimator methods which include multiple pinhole collimators and ultrahigh-sensitivity detectors focusing on the heart. Sensitivity is also improved by the scanner geometry surrounding the patient. Solid detectors replace the combination of scintillation crystals with photomultiplier tubes, and this result in an improved energy resolution. These new scanners can reduce acquisition time or lower patient radiation exposure by allowing administration of a lower dose (Table 5.6) [33, 34].

Positrons are positively charged particles with the same mass as electrons. Annihilation occurs when a positron collides with an electron with the emission of two 511 KeV gamma rays, traveling in opposite directions. PET detectors fitted with various crystal materials are placed in a ring gantry surrounding the patient and configured to register only coincident photon pairs. Compared to SPECT, PET exhibits higher spatial and temporal resolution [3].

Table 5.6 Advantages and disadvantages of the cardiac dedicated ultrafast SPECT cameras

Advantages
Images may be acquired in reduced time without compromising quality
Images may be acquired with lower injected dose without compromising quality
More convenient for patients
The information provided has similar diagnostic quality
Disadvantages
Expensive
Limited availability
Lack of evidence due to their limited use

5.3.5.1 ECG Gating

Since being introduced in the early 1990s, it is now a critical element of all cardiac SPECT and PET studies [35]. ECG-gated perfusion studies allow the simultaneous acquisition of information regarding perfusion and global and regional left ventricular function and volumes. During gated acquisition, the ECG signal allows usually 8 or 16 intervals or time frames to be acquired for each beat with counts for each subsequent beat being added to the frames in the first beat. This is done for each beat in all the projections. The increasing number of frames gives higher count rates that allow more accurate assessment of the ejection fraction. Ejection fraction measured using 8 frames will give values that are approximately 3 ejection fraction units lower than when 16-frame acquisition is performed. Sixteen-frame acquisition allows analysis of filling and ejection rates that can be used for assessment of diastolic function [36].

For arrhythmia rejection, it is best to avoid selection of parameters that will compromise the perfusion information or prolong the acquisition. Thus, accepting all beats will guarantee high-count perfusion images without increasing the imaging time, but this may compromise the results of the ejection fraction calculation. To guarantee optimal perfusion information, a ±50% acceptance window around the pre-study sampled heart rate will give the most counts. Newer systems allow simultaneous and separate windows for static perfusion, keeping all beats, and ECG-gated windows, applying a narrower acceptance window. This allows getting the most accurate ejection fraction without compromising the perfusion data. Patients in atrial fibrillation with a narrow RR interval have accurate EF measurements. If more than one out of every six beats is an APC or PVC, EF measurements are not reliable. With increase in heart rate variability, the accuracy of the EF decreases. Review of the beat length histogram is advised as a quality control step for EF measurements.

Areas that have normal wall motion and thickening on the gated images may be associated with normal or ischemic myocardium. Apical thinning and areas with breast or diaphragm attenuation are also associated with normal wall motion. Since gated Tc-99m studies are acquired a minimum of 10–15 min following peak exercise stress, regional wall motion in most patients with ischemia usually returns to normal by the time of imaging. Severe ischemia induces persistent wall motion abnormalities that are detected during gated acquisition in as many as 1/3 of cases [10]. One of the most important benefits of gated SPECT acquisition is helping to differentiate attenuation due to the diaphragm or breast from areas of old myocardial infarction or scar [37]. Areas of scar have absent or diminished motion and thickening, while areas with decreased activity due to attenuation will show normal motion and thickening. Patients with prior heart surgery will show akinesis or hypokinesis of the septum because of the surgery in the absence of ischemia or infarction. Such areas will have normal thickening. Patients with LBBB or a paced rhythm will also demonstrate abnormal septal motion. In addition to improving diagnostic accuracy during subjective visual image interpretation, gated measurements of global ejection fraction and regional wall thickening have been validated using equilibrium blood pool imaging, cardiac catheterization, and cardiac MRI [38–41]. These studies found excellent agreement across EF values ranging from 12% to 88%. Small hearts gave very high EF values due to the poor spatial resolution of the SPECT systems.

The availability of automated methods for measuring ischemic or scar burden, LVEF, ventricular volumes, transient ischemic dilatation, and phase analysis have been attractive though, until now, underutilized [42]. The assessment of left ventricle mechanical dyssynchrony using phase analysis of gated SPECT or PET myocardial perfusion imaging has been shown to be related to the severity of heart failure and could potentially expand the indications of gated perfusion imaging. Compared with other techniques used for the same purpose, phase analysis offers simplicity and reproducibility. It can be applied retrospectively and combined with myocardial scar detection, and it can be used to optimize cardiac resynchronization therapy [43].

5.3.5.2 Attenuation Correction

Attenuation correction removes soft tissue artifacts from myocardial perfusion images. It can be performed using either a sealed source such as Gd-153 or an X-ray or CT-based method for acquiring the transmission maps. Gd-153 line source methods are only available on older systems. The size of the patient and the amount of tissue between the heart and the detector lead to attenuation artifacts that adversely affect image quality. Not only SPECT but also PET images are prone to attenuation due to the loss of true coincidence events either by absorption or scattering. All PET images are acquired with attenuation correction. It is well recognized that the ability to correct cardiac emission data for the effects of attenuation may improve significantly the interpretation of the reconstructed images [2, 5, 44].

5.3.5.3 Hybrid Imaging

Hybrid imaging combines different imaging modalities in a way where both contribute to the final information. Hybrid whole-body PET-CT and PET-MR in oncology allowed, for the first time, to associate anatomy with a functional radiopharmaceutical. Initially thoracic CT data was used only for attenuation correction of MPI, as mentioned above, but incorporating the information of the CT or MRI to SPECT or PET gives an additional input by providing morphology and functional assessment of the cardiovascular system [44–46]. Calcium scoring derived from these images may also prove useful for diagnosis and management.

5.3.6 Quality Control (QC) of the Images and Reporting

Once the SPECT or PET acquisition is completed, the results need to be reviewed to determine whether the patient can leave the laboratory or additional acquisition is required. Rotating projection images should be reviewed to unmask potential sources of errors such as patient motion, low count density, extra cardiac activity, soft tissue uptake, or sources of attenuation. Processing can by performed by technologists or physicians but requires careful review by both the technologists before the patient leaves to see if re-imaging is required and the physician at the time of interpretation in order to see if technical factors will influence the perfusion images. Communication between the two is important in order to get the most accurate results. Orientation and segmentation should be in accordance with published guidelines [47]. Technical advances in computer processing are providing more options that should result in better image quality [2, 3, 5].

5.3.6.1 Quantitative Analysis of MPI

Visual analysis is the most common method of interpretation [47], but automated methods may be useful to provide over reads. For performing quantitative analysis, the limits for automated delimitation of the epicardial and endocardial borders should be manually defined and the generated images reviewed to make certain there is no tracking into hot areas outside the heart. Once the epicardial and endocardial borders and mitral valve plane have been visually verified, a polar plot is generated by comparison with a normal database. Polar maps reduce the three-dimensional information to a simple plot giving the severity and reversibility of perfusion abnormalities. All the above described steps are critical to get good results. Poor definition of the borders is likely to result in errors [48]. Sometimes the most difficult problem of using quantitative analysis is overcoming the fear of not calling abnormalities when they are identified as abnormal by the automated reading. This fear may be related to concerns about liability or an over eager need for high sensitivity to not miss any disease. In either case, it is important to reach a decision based on visual interpretation before reviewing the automated analysis. Some suggest that automated methods have a performance, if not superior, at least equivalent to visual scoring [49]. In fact they seem sensitive but less specific, and areas identified as abnormal by automated analysis are given a second look just in case something was missed. Problems with scaling, boundary definitions, inappropriate alignment, and scatter lead to erroneous quantitative results that should not lead to patients being inappropriately labeled as having CAD [50].

5.3.6.2 Absolute Quantification of Perfusion

Absolute quantification of myocardial blood flow is a potentially more objective and reliable analysis of the functional significance of a coronary stenosis. Although there are reports of such measurements using SPECT acquisition, PET remains the main method used to derive these measurements. It reduces false-negative results of perfusion due to balanced or subendocardial ischemia. Myocardial blood flow is measured in ml/min/g and assessed in hyperemic and rest conditions by dynamic acquisition with measurements of myocardial and blood pool time-activity curves. Absolute quantification potentially increases the value of PET perfusion imaging [3, 20, 51].

5.3.6.3 Image Interpretation

As mentioned above, accurate interpretation of MPI studies involves a systematic approach that starts with technical QC performed on the rotating projection images, rest/stress perfusion and function comparison, reaching a conclusion based on the imaging information, reviewing the clinical history and the stress test results, and reconciling all this data to reach a final conclusion. An important part of this process is the initial quality control that must be done on an interactive workstation that allows image manipulation and modification. The items mentioned in QC must be systematically examined on every study to identify technical factors that may influence the perfusion data seen on the aligned slices. False-positive SPECT MPI studies very often are due to poor-quality acquisition data that in the process of filtering, reconstruction, and display, perfusion defects are created and not recognized as artifact. Once this initial QC has been performed, the matched stress and rest slices must be aligned and reviewed ideally using at one or two color scales. The first one used should be linear, preferably gray scale, which displays the data spectrum in a continuous manner. Color scales have different characteristics that require careful correlation with coronary angiography or patient outcomes to determine the accuracy of diagnosis for each individual laboratory.

5.3.6.4 Generating a Report

The final product of all the above steps is a report for the referring physician that includes an accurate, unambiguous, and clinically relevant assessment of the probability that the patient has abnormal myocardial blood flow. It is beyond the scope of this concise review to cover this most important detail [52–55]. Good communication is encouraged between the referring physician and the nuclear cardiologist not only to report the results but, even before the performance of the test, to discuss its appropriateness. In summary the report should contain information about the laboratory where the study is performed and details about patient demographics; the clinical indication should be stated; tracer administration protocol and image acquisition details are technical aspects that should be described; and finally the report of the findings should lead to a concise, unambiguous conclusion. Putting too many qualifiers in the conclusion negates the value of the test results for the referring clinicians.

5.3.7 Clinical Indications

5.3.7.1 Diagnosis and Risk Stratification of CAD

Sensitivity and specificity for MPI have been extensively reported; initially using planar Tl-201 to more recent publications using the Tc-99m tracers with SPECT, quantitative analysis, ECG gating, and PET [56, 57]. The accuracy is heavily influenced by the populations being studied and the type of stress and posttest referral bias. In a meta-analysis using primarily planar Tl-201 studies weighted by sample size, a sensitivity of 87% and a specificity of 64% were reported [58]. In an analysis including more contemporary studies with Tc-99m SPECT and gating, the sensitivity was found to be 87% and the specificity was 73% [1]. Tc-99m radiotracers provide the best quality gated images and are the most commonly used. PET has been compared with SPECT, and PET has a better diagnostic. In a meta-analysis with 11,862 patients, a sensitivity of 92.6% was achieved by PET compared to 88.3% with SPECT to diagnose CAD. No significant differences in specificity were reported [59]. Besides an improved accuracy to detect disease, PET allows the absolute quantification of myocardial blood flow which seems to unmask clinically significant CAD and offers an objective interpretation that is more reproducible than visual analysis. Quantitative PET measures when integrated with qualitative myocardial perfusion assessment provide superior diagnostic accuracy and improve the capacity to detect functionally significant coronary artery stenosis [60]. Despite the growing evidence that quantitative perfusion PET can play a major role in the clinical setting, there are not yet clear indications for its clinical use [61]. In addition PET exposes patients to lower radiation doses. Its limitations are mainly due to the high costs, cyclotron dependency when using N-13 ammonia or O-15 water, and limited availability of PET camera systems.

According to guidelines and appropriate use criteria, MPI is recommended when there is an intermediate pretest probability of disease or when risk stratification is mandatory after an established diagnosis [62, 63]. It is recommended that an exercise ECG test should be used first in a stepwise approach for patients with an intermediate risk for CAD who have a normal baseline ECG and are capable of performing dynamic exercise [64]. For patients who are unable to exercise, SPECT or PET MPI are capable of providing diagnostic and prognostic information that cannot be gotten from treadmill testing alone. However, such patients have more risk factors, and even if the perfusion study is normal, the occurrence of cardiac death is higher than in patients who are capable of exercising [65]. In patients who have positive ECG changes of ischemia, MPI provides additional information for management, especially in the intermediate risk category [66]. In a study with 4649 intermediate Duke treadmill score patients who had normal perfusion, the 7-year cardiac mortality was very low at 1.5%, and the cumulative frequency of catheterization was 17% [67].

MPI is recommended in patients with abnormal ST segments, LBBB, ventricular paced rhythms, pre-excitation, LVH, or prior revascularization [64, 68]. The effects of referral bias, testing in patients with prior revascularization, and the documented occurrence of abnormal perfusion in patients without obstructive CAD but functionally abnormal flow reserve all influence the accuracy of testing when comparing it to the "gold standard" coronary angiography. For that reason, accuracy of testing for the detection of disease and assessment of prognosis will be discussed in the context of recognized specific patient populations that can influence the results of SPECT or PET testing.

5.3.7.2 Special Populations

Ethnic and Racial Differences

Most of the published data on SPECT is in Caucasian males capable of performing dynamic exercise. SPECT accuracy and prognosis results vary and usually loose accuracy and prognostic value when tests are performed in other groups [69, 70]. Many of these groups have a higher cardiovascular risk factor profile and other potential factors influencing test performance. African Americans have overall lower test accuracy and worse prognosis across the range of ischemia [70]. Whereas the death and MI rate in Caucasians is <1% with a normal SPECT MPI, two studies have shown it to be 2%/year in African Americans [69, 71].

Women

Ischemic heart disease is the leading cause of death in women in Western countries. The SPECT diagnostic and prognostic accuracy in women is influenced by gender differences in the prevalence of obstructive CAD and technical limitations due to breast attenuation and smaller left ventricular size. Low specificity was a major limitation in the early studies using planar Tl-201 that was overcome with the availability of SPECT and ECG gating and the use of attenuation correction. Using these techniques, gender differences in the performance of testing for diagnosis have been minimized, but not totally eliminated [72, 73]. It is known that the traditional approach to ischemic heart disease detection based on the identification of obstructive CAD is less effective when factors such as abnormal coronary reactivity, microvascular dysfunction, and plaque erosion with distal microembolization seemed to be related to chest pain in women. PET imaging could help to understand the mechanisms of CAD in women due to its ability to provide measures of blood flow and of coronary flow reserve [74–76].

Patients with LBBB/Pacemakers, Left Ventricular Hypertrophy, Nonspecific ST-T Wave Changes

For patients in these categories, treadmill testing does not provide accurate diagnostic or prognostic information, and SPECT MPI is indicated for evaluation. Patients with LBBB with exercise MPI have a low specificity in the LAD distribution due to a septal defect caused by diminished septal blood flow at high heart rates in the absence of obstructive CAD [77]. If there are associated defects in the apex or anterior wall, specificity is improved, but the use of vasodilator stress improves diagnostic accuracy and gives prognostic information. Overall prognosis is worse in such patients, but imaging is predictive of events. In 245 patients, the 3-year survival was 27% in high-risk scans and 87% in low-risk scans [77]. Less well documented is the effect of pacemakers on SPECT accuracy and prognosis, but such patients are treated in the same way as those with LBBB, and the prognostic value of SPECT is retained [78]. In the presence of LVH, hypertension, or nonspecific ST-T wave changes on the resting ECG, SPECT retains diagnostic and prognostic value [79, 80]. Well-trained athletes with LVH by echocardiography have been reported to have a higher incidence of false-positive studies due to "hot spot" scaling problems [81].

Asymptomatic Patients

Although testing is not recommended in asymptomatic patients, SPECT can detect the presence of disease and give prognostic information [82, 83]. Testing may be appropriate in high-risk occupations such as aviators, fireman, and policeman with multiple risk factors [64], but computed tomography coronary angiography with calcium score assessment seems to be the first approach for high-risk asymptomatic populations [63] .

Patients with Diabetes

Patients with diabetes are at a very high risk for having critical coronary stenosis and cardiovascular events [84]. Despite the diffuse nature of vessel involvement with a higher occurrence of balanced disease, SPECT has diagnostic and prognostic value [85–88]. In a retrospective analysis, event-free survival was found to be lower in diabetics across all categories of ischemia [87]. In a prospective study involving 1123 carefully screened asymptomatic diabetics, half were randomized to SPECT imaging, and 118 (22%) were found to have silent ischemia on SPECT of which 33 (6%) had moderate or large perfusion defects. The prevalence of silent ischemia was higher than expected. All patients in this study were prospectively followed to determine if the imaging results, which were not blinded, influenced management and long-term survival. It was found that among randomized patients, the event rates were low and not significantly reduced by perfusion imaging screening over 4.8 years. These results could reflect, partially, the impact of aggressive guideline-driven management of risk factors which improve outcomes regardless of the presence or absence of ischemia [89].

Patients with Chest Pain in ED

Patients presenting to an emergency department within several hours of chest pain and a nondiagnostic ECG and normal or equivocal troponins can be risk stratified based on acute injection at rest of a Tc-99m perfusion tracer [90]. Patients with a perfusion abnormality are at higher risk for having infarction or unstable angina and deserve very aggressive medical and interventional management. Such patients can have abnormal perfusion due to occlusion or spasm of an unstable vessel, and the perfusion abnormalities can be detected prior to elevation of serum enzyme markers [91–93]. The sensitivity of the procedure improves if the tracer administration occurs during or immediately after the chest pain episode. Studies performed in this context have shown a high-sensitivity and high-negative predictive value, and patients with a normal study who are discharged have a very low likelihood of having cardiac events. If the acute study is normal, it can be used as the resting image for comparison following exercise or pharmacologic stress to exclude underlying CAD in such patients. In a prospective randomized controlled study comparing resting SPECT imaging to conventional ED care, imaging significantly lowered hospitalization rates from 52% to 42% [93]. Several limitations are recognized to this approach, namely, the difficulty to distinguish a perfusion abnormality due to an old infarction from that due to an acute coronary syndrome and the availability of nuclear medicine laboratories working 24 h/day.

Patients Before and After Revascularization

Before revascularization, myocardial perfusion imaging either with SPECT or PET is used to assess the highly variable physiological relationship between coronary lesion severity and coronary flow reserve. Even in the presence of flow-limiting stenosis, if exercise or pharmacologic stress perfusion is normal or mildly abnormal, patients are at low risk for cardiac events [94]. Using SPECT as a gatekeeper for referral to coronary angiography has been shown to not only be cost-effective but in no circumstance does it place patients at a higher risk for cardiac death or nonfatal myocardial infarction in comparison to the more expensive and invasive approach of performing coronary angiography on all patients [95]. It also has a role in determining the sequence and number of grafted vessels in high-risk CABG patients and for identification of the culprit lesion at the time of PCI. According to the guidelines, in a symptomatic patient, an area of ischemia equal or above 10% is a recommendation to perform revascularization whenever possible [63].

In asymptomatic patients after percutaneous coronary intervention (PCI), routine myocardial perfusion imaging is not indicated at any time in the first 2 years following a procedure [96]. In the first few months after a procedure, it has been shown that <30% of symptomatic patients have documented stenosis [97]. In addition, periprocedural changes in the treated area may result in perfusion defects even in the absence of restenosis, and testing in the first 4–6 weeks following a procedure is not recommended due to the occurrence of false positives [98]. If ischemia is detected beyond the immediate period of the procedure, the prognostic value of SPECT persists, and the occurrence of cardiac death and MI is increased in patients with large amounts of ischemia [99]. With the placement of drug-eluting stents to prevent restenosis, delayed healing, prolonged inflammation, and exercise-induced paradoxical coronary vasoconstriction of the adjacent segment have been reported [100, 101].

Even with the altered anatomy following CABG, myocardial perfusion imaging retains diagnostic and prognostic accuracy early and late for detection of stenosis in grafts as well as progression in the native vessel [102–104]. Routine testing in asymptomatic patients is not recommended [96]. The extent and severity of perfusion abnormalities detected by SPECT is predictive of death in both symptomatic and asymptomatic patients in the first 5 years after surgical revascularization [104]. Beyond 5 years, it has been shown that the presence of ischemia is the strongest predictor of mortality [103, 105, 106]. In 9000 asymptomatic patients, the presence of ischemia predicted a 3% annual mortality [105].

Risk Assessment of Patients Before Noncardiac Surgery

Risk assessment prior to noncardiac surgery requires a thorough review of the clinical, demographic, and surgical indications of risk rather than nonselective use of MPI [107]. Major predictors of increased perioperative risk include recent acute MI, unstable angina pectoris, decompensated congestive heart failure, significant arrhythmias, high degree of atrioventricular block, and severe valvular heart disease. Such patients are already high risk, and SPECT is not indicated as it is unlikely to further stratify such high-risk patients [1, 108]. Perfusion markers of high risk include a large area of ischemia, perfusion defects in multiple vascular territories and transient left ventricular dilatation. The ACC/AHA guidelines recommend coronary angiography in patients in whom the results of the noninvasive testing indicate a high risk of cardiac events or in those with angina unresponsive to medical therapy. In low-risk patients with a low-risk surgery, myocardial perfusion imaging is not indicated [109]. In the last published ESC guidelines, MPI testing is advised before high-risk surgery in patients with two or more clinical risk factors and when functional capacity is poor (<4 Mets) and may be considered in those undergoing intermediate risk procedures [110].

5.4 Myocardial Viability

5.4.1 Basic Concepts

Viable myocardium refers to myocardial tissue that is still alive but hypokinetic due to persistent but low blood flow to living myocytes that decrease contractility to remain alive. This is the concept of hibernation initially identified by Rahimtoola [111]. The blood flow must be adequate to deliver enough glucose to maintain anaerobic glycolysis with a lower production of adenosine triphosphate (ATP) that is able to maintain transmembrane gradients and lactic acid washout but not enough to maintain contractility. Revascularization, by improving blood flow, would enhance oxygen delivery and beta-oxidation of fatty acids which allow a more efficient way of getting ATP and regain contractile function. Contractile dysfunction could also arise from a transient severe ischemia episode, with spontaneous recovery with time, called myocardial stunning. Although theoretically distinct, an overlap between the two could occur as repetitive episodes of ischemia, and stunning could lead to a state of chronic dysfunction and hibernation [112].

5.4.2 Nuclear Cardiology to Assess Viability

Viable myocardium could be identified by several techniques among which cardiac SPECT and PET have an important role.

SPECT is widely available and uses perfusion tracers such as Tl-201 or Tc-99m tracers to evaluate cellular integrity. Evaluation of viability with Tl-201 has been described in a previous section of this chapter. Resting uptake of Tl-201 or Tc-99m tracers is capable of identifying areas of myocardium that will show functional recovery after revascularization, but SPECT accuracy is best when a threshold of 60% of maximal myocardial tracer uptake is used for Tl-201 and 55% for the Tc-99m tracers [113]. There were no differences in predicting wall motion recovery between the three tracers using these thresholds.

PET is capable of evaluating metabolism either with a glucose analog, F18-fluorodeoxyglucose (F-18 FDG), or with C11-palmitic acid or C11-acetate. We will focus on F-18 FDG as it is the most used PET tracer for viability assessment. Areas of reduced resting myocardial perfusion and enhanced uptake of F-18 FDG are regarded as viable.

5.4.2.1 F18-Fluorodeoxyglucose (F-18 FDG)

F-18 FDG competes with glucose for transport and phosphorylation by hexokinase. As opposed to glucose, it doesn't proceed into glycogen synthesis and stays trapped in the tissue. It is a cyclotron-produced tracer with a half-life of 110 min. The administration of 10 mCi, intravenously, exposes to an effective dose of 7 mSv [3].

Viability Protocol

Figure 5.11 shows a frequently used protocol for viability assessment that can be used in both diabetic and nondiabetic patients. Myocardial perfusion at rest and stress or rest alone should be evaluated using Rb-82 or N-13 ammonia. The use of Tc-99m SPECT perfusion images for comparison to F-18 FDG PET should be discouraged due to the differences in image quality between the perfusion and metabolic images. For the F-18 FDG images, patient preparation is different whether identification of viability or inflammation is required. For viability, the goal is to enhance tracer uptake by the myocardium. Patients are fasted for at least 6 h; serum glucose is measured. A protocol of glucose loading and insulin is required (Fig. 5.11) prior to F-18 FDG administration. An initial glucose is measured, if

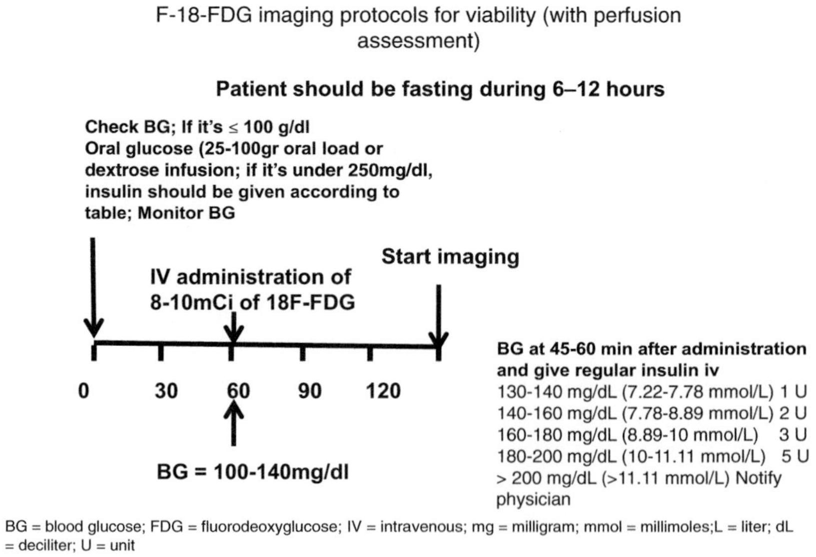

Fig. 5.11 F-18 FDG imaging protocol for viability assessment

<100 mg/dl 25–100 g oral load or dextrose infusion is administered. When the initial glucose is ≤250 mg/dl, insulin is administered in the units shown in Fig. 5.11. Patients with glucose values >250 mg/cl should be canceled and a better preparation implemented. Diabetic patients are challenging due to their limited ability to produce or respond to insulin stimulation [3].

In a viability study, myocardial areas that have a perfusion/metabolism mismatch, consisting of severely diminished or absent perfusion but preserved or enhanced metabolic activity, have a high probability of regaining function after revascularization, and are hibernating but viable. Fig. 5.12 is an example of a rest/stress Rb-82 perfusion and F-18 FDG study showing myocardial ischemia and viability in three views. The stress images on the top row show extensive areas of abnormal perfusion involving the anterior, lateral, inferolateral, and inferior walls. The rest images in the middle row show marked improvement in the apical, midcavity, and basal areas, but they are not completely normal. There is enhanced right ventricular uptake in an enlarged and hypertrophied right ventricle on stress as well as dilation of the left ventricle with transient ischemia dilation (TID) giving a ratio of 1.27. On the F-18 FDG images, bottom row, there is enhanced FDG uptake throughout the anterior, lateral, inferolateral, and inferior walls. In this situation there was enhanced F-18 FDG uptake in areas with decreased perfusion identifying areas of hibernation. The areas that were ischemic have enhanced FDG uptake on the basis of memory of ischemia whereby the transient ischemic areas switched from fatty acids to the use of FDG. Only the basal anterior wall had diminished uptake on stress, rest, and FDG indicating that this areas was scarred.

5.4.3 Clinical Indications

5.4.3.1 Ischemic Cardiomyopathy

The presence of viable myocardium favors revascularization in the management of ischemic heart failure. Several observational studies seemed to support this notion, but until now prospective studies designed with this purpose failed to prove completely the concept [114]. The benefits of

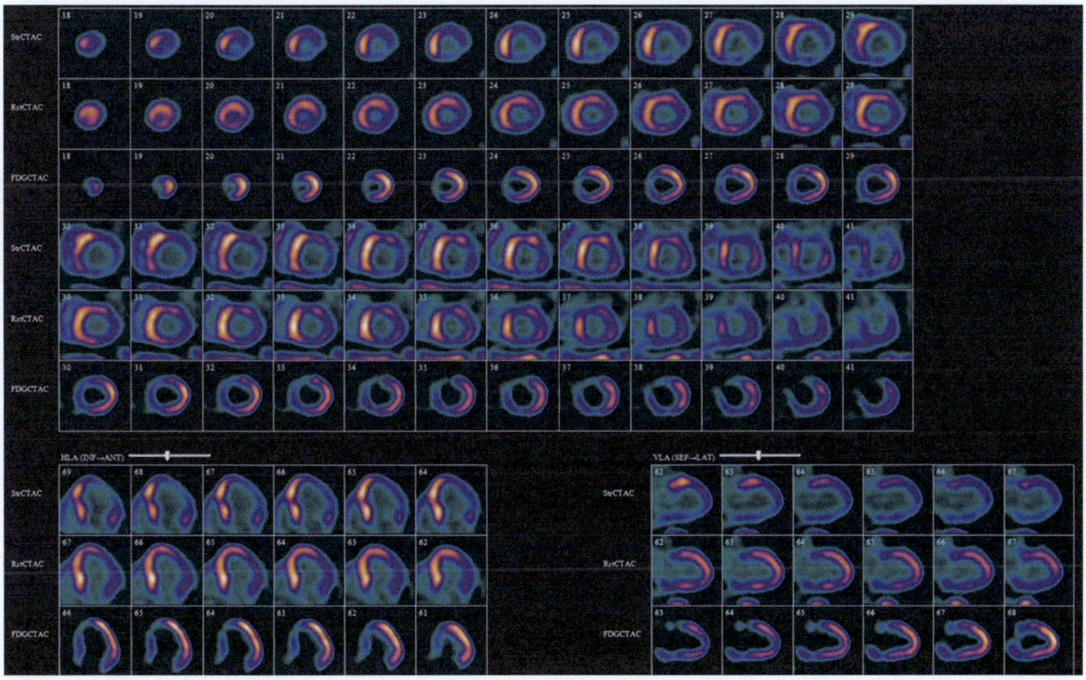

Fig. 5.12 Rest and stress Rb-82 perfusion and F-18 FDG viability PET study showing extensive ischemia and viability in the anterior and lateral walls

revascularization in terms of survival and symptoms seemed to be positively related to the amount of viable tissue and inversely related to the extension of scar [115–119]. Detection of myocardial viability is still a matter of debate, and more evidence is necessary to emphasize its role in the management of ischemic heart failure.

5.5 Assessment of Ventricular Function by Radionuclide Ventriculography

Assessment of ventricular function and volumes is essential to risk stratify cardiac disease. Equilibrium radionuclide angiography (ERNA) and first-pass radionuclide angiography (FPRNA) are reliable and robust methods to assess ventricular function. In the past, they were used widely but have declined due to the use of methods, such as echocardiography and cardiac MRI, that could provide more extensive information without radiation exposure and with ECG-gated SPECT MPI. These factors in combination with the declining availability of small field view cameras, that are optimal for high-quality studies, have resulted in resting ERNA studies being performed almost exclusively for monitoring chemotherapy-induced cardiotoxicity and heart failure. It is not likely that the use of these techniques will increase in the future.

5.5.1 Equilibrium Radionuclide Angiocardiography (ERNA)

The nomenclature for this technique includes MUGA (name of an early software program) and equilibrium-gated blood pool imaging and radionuclide ventriculography. It can be used to determine global and regional left ventricular (LV) and right ventricular (RV) function at rest and following exercise or pharmacologic stress. Analysis of the time activity curve provides information on systolic and diastolic function. Both planar and tomographic methods have been used for acquisition, but planar predominates due to ease of use and extensive experience [120].

5.5.1.1 Technique

Radiopharmaceuticals and Red Blood Cell Labeling

The basic technique uses stannous pyrophosphate to create a favorable oxidation/reduction environment inside red blood cells (RBC) so that when 10–30 min after Tc-99m pertechnetate is administered, it binds to hemoglobin and remains attached. Labeling can be accomplished in three ways: in vivo, modified in vivo/in vitro, and in vitro. There are differences in the efficiency of labeling, defined as the percentage of total radioactivity attached to RBCs versus the time and expense required to perform the technique. The amount of the stannous agent required for optimal labeling is in the range of 0.03–0.15 mg/ml of blood or 10–20 mg/kg of body weight. The usual administered activity is 800 MBq (23 mCi) for adult patients. The effective dose is of 5.6 mSv.

Labeling Techniques

In Vivo: This is the simplest, fastest, and least expensive labeling method but gives the lowest labeling efficiency. The stannous pyrophosphate is given intravenously followed 15 min later by Tc-99m which can be given as a rapid bolus for first-pass radionuclide angiography (FPRNA). This method achieves only 80–90% RBC labeling and the background activity is higher due to labeling of structures outside the vascular space such as the stomach and thyroid.

Modified In Vivo/In Vitro: The stannous pyrophosphate is given intravenously, and 20–30 min later, an aliquot of blood is withdrawn into a syringe containing the Tc-99m pertechnetate, and this is gently shaken for 10 min before being injected back into the patient. The labeling efficiency approaches 95%.

In Vitro: This should be performed under strictly aseptic conditions, in a laminar airflow unit dedicated to cell labeling. An aliquot of blood is withdrawn and centrifuged and the RBC pellet washed and incubated first with stannous pyrophosphate followed by the Tc-99m before being reinjected into the patient. There are commercial kits available which give a labeling efficiency of >97% [120].

Instrumentation and Procedure

Rest studies allow longer acquisition times and can be performed with a high-resolution collimator (parallel hole or slant hole). A collimator with 30° angulation allows optimal separation of the left atrium from the LV especially in patients with a horizontally positioned heart. Stress studies are limited to a 2 min acquisition at rest and peak stress, and in such situations a low energy all-purpose collimator gives a higher count rate. Cameras should be peaked at 140 ± 10 keV. The heart rate is sampled prior to acquisition to establish the time interval for each frame, and a ±10–15% arrhythmia rejection window should be used with elimination of the early beat as well as the next beat which has a longer filling period. List mode acquisition allows 10 ms temporal resolution and maximal flexibility in image processing but is memory intensive, and many of the current programs do not make it easy to acquire or process studies. Buffered beat techniques with forward and backward reconstruction of the time activity curve to eliminate drop-off in counts provide greater flexibility when diastolic function analysis is required. In order to measure the minimum volume in the time activity curve at end systole, a minimum of 16 frames is required to get an accurate ejection fraction (EF) in patients with fast heart rates or rest or during exercise stress. Rest studies with very slow heart rates require up to 32 frames to get accurate EF measurements.

Acquisition can be set up based on acquiring a fixed number of beats, time, or counts. Whichever method is used, it is necessary to acquire a minimum of 20,000 cm^{-1} over the center of the LV to get sufficient information density for an accurate EF calculation. The patient is positioned, and three views are acquired. The most important view for calculating the EF is the left anterior oblique (LAO) which provides the best septal separation between the two ventricles. Once this view has been acquired, the camera head is rotated 45° in the anterior direction and 45° toward the left lateral to get orthogonal views [120]. An example of the three acquired views at end systole and end diastole is shown in Fig. 5.13.

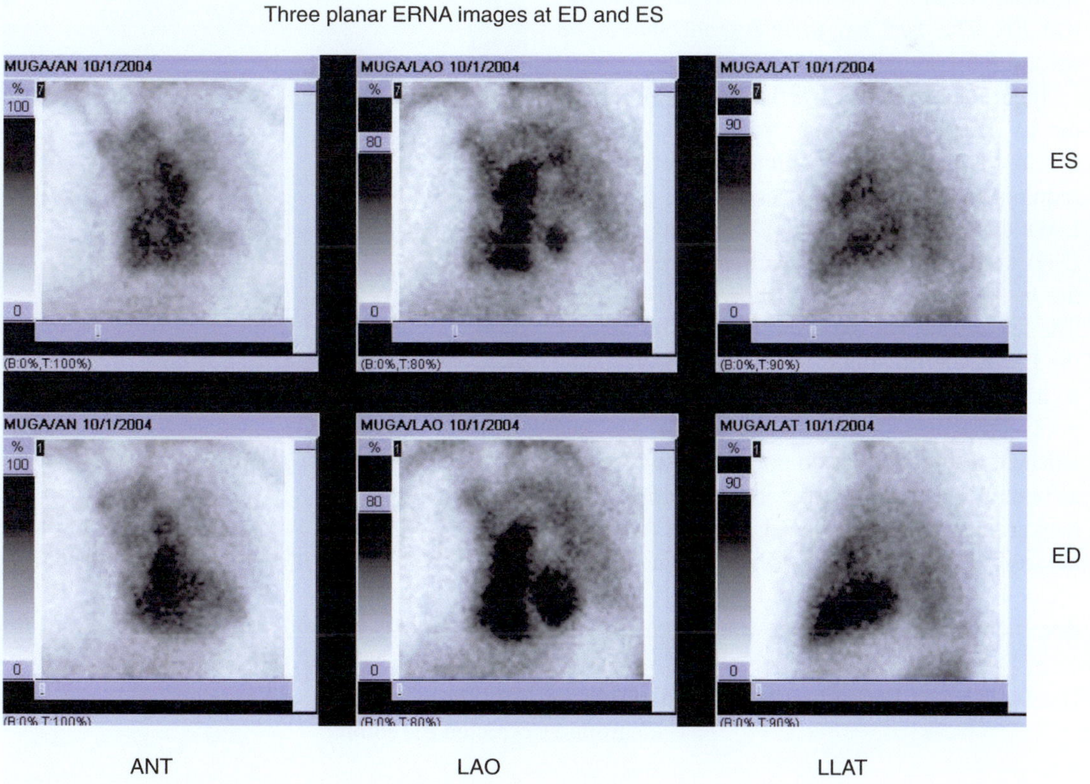

Fig. 5.13 Three planar ERNA views at end systole and end diastole

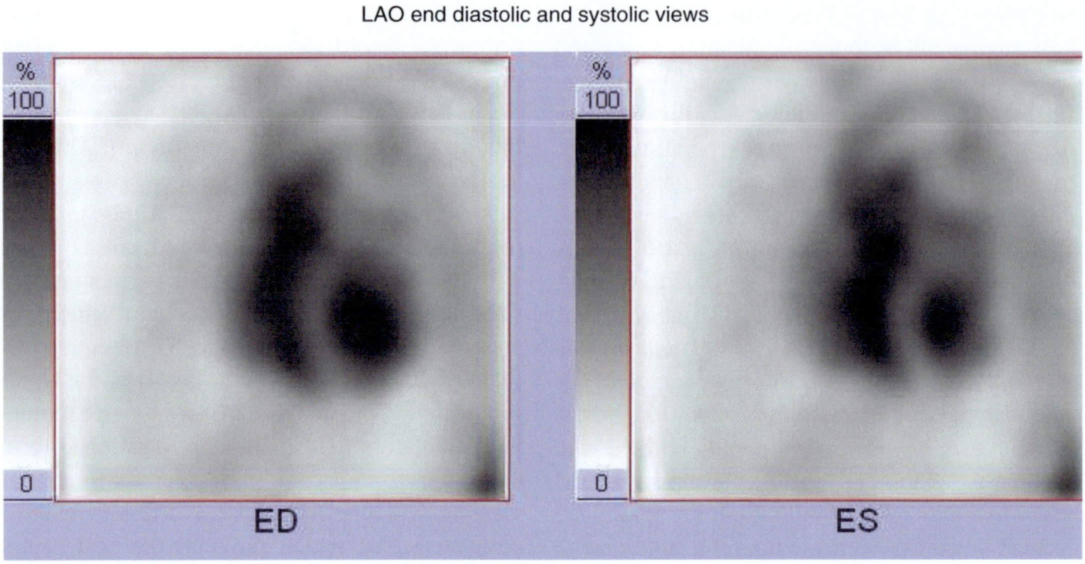

Fig. 5.14 ERNA LAO views at end diastole and end systole

Once acquisition is completed, the images are temporally and spatially smoothed, and three views in a cine loop should be reviewed in gray scale for a visual assessment of global and regional function to correlate with the quantitative EF. The beat-length histogram should be reviewed for adequacy of ECG gating.

Figure 5.14 shows how the septum separates the LV from surrounding structures at ED and ES in the LAO view. Calculation of the EF requires measuring counts or volume from the LAO view in the isolated LV at end diastole (ED) and end systole (ES) after correcting for the background activity as shown in Fig. 5.15. The left atrium can be seen popping up behind the LV on the ES frame. Background correction is necessary to eliminate the effects of blood pool activity in the structures overlaying and adjacent to the LV that do not change cyclically as in the LV function during its contraction. This background region is placed in the LAO view adjacent to the heart anywhere from 2 to 5 o'clock with care to avoid the left atrium, descending thoracic aorta, gastric, or spleen free Tc-99m pertechnetate uptake. Putting the background area in any of these regions will lead to erroneous results. To estimate the EF, the following formula is currently used.

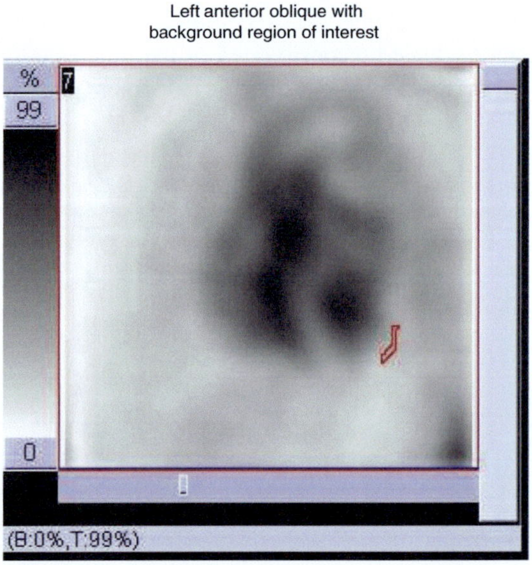

Fig. 5.15 LAO view with background region of interest

$$\mathrm{LVEF} = \left[\left(\frac{\text{Background Corrected ED counts} - \text{Background Corrected ES counts}}{\text{Background Corrected ED counts}}\right)\right] \times 100.$$

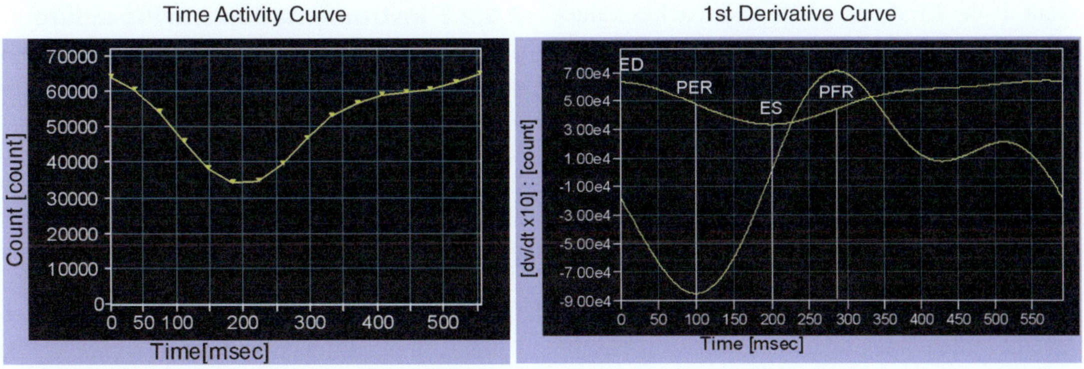

Fig. 5.16 Time activity curve and first derivative curve on LAO ERNA

Analysis of systolic and diastolic function using emptying and filling rates can be performed on the time activity curves as shown in Fig. 5.16.

Exercise Studies

To detect CAD, dynamic exercise can be performed using upright or supine bicycle exercise following RBC labeling. The patient is positioned on the bicycle with the camera in the LAO position, and a 2 min acquisition is performed for a baseline measurement. Incremental exercise is performed in 3 min stages during which the patient exercise for 1 min before a 2 min acquisition until the patient reaches symptom limited maximal exercise. In patients without CAD or other forms of heart disease, with peak exercise there is a minimum augmentation in global EF by at least 5 EF units from the baseline measurement. In patients with critical flow-limiting stenosis, EF may drop, stay the same, or fail to augment by at least 5 EF units. Attempts to look at regional wall motion rather than the global EF response to improve sensitivity have not been successful due to the limited regional wall motion assessment available from the single LAO planar view.

5.5.1.2 Clinical Indications

Assessment of LV Function

ERNA is capable of providing accurate and consistent measurements of LV global and regional function. Although RV EF can be measured, overlap of the right atrium does not allow complete isolation of counts or volume in the RV, and this introduces errors depending on the position of the two chambers. Assessment of diastolic and systolic filling and emptying rates requires accurate time activity curves for analysis which conventional frame mode acquisition does not provide [120].

Detection of CAD

With the availability of SPECT MPI, this technique is not used widely. Since the EF response to exercise may be abnormal in patients with nonischemic cardiomyopathies and other forms of cardiac muscle disease, specificity was low. In a composite of the published literature, a sensitivity of 86% and a specificity of 79% have been reported [121]. For patients unable to exercise, vasodilator stress does not provide sufficient accuracy in the ability to induce global or regional functional changes.

Monitoring Cardiotoxicity

ERNA continues to have a role in the serial monitoring of adults receiving anthracyclines or trastuzumab for the treatment of cancer [122]. This approach allows patients to receive the highest possible doses of these drugs for effective tumor treatment at the lowest possible risk of developing cardiotoxicity which in early studies could be as deadly as the tumor being treated. A baseline EF is measured prior to treatment. If normal, monitoring should be performed when doses of 250–300 mg/m^2 are achieved and then repeat the assessment at 450 mg/m^2 and afterward before every treatment. If the EF drops ≥10% and reaches values below 50%, consider therapy discontinuation. If the EF is less than 50%, treatment could proceed with EF evaluations before each session, and a EF drop of ≥10% (EF units) or an EF ≤ 30% therapy discontinuation should be considered. If the EF is ≤30% at baseline, alternative methods should be used [123]. According to the position paper published by the ESC, ERNA can be used for monitoring cardiotoxicity. Since there are several cardiac imaging modalities available, the choice depends on local availability and expertise. The same modality should be used throughout the treatment. In this setting, ERNA has the great advantage of reproducibility, but radiation exposure and limited structural and functional information on cardiac structures should be considered [124]. Attempts to develop less toxic drugs or to pretreat patients with agents to lower or prevent cardiotoxicity have been under development, and serial monitoring is still required [125, 126].

5.5.2 First-Pass Radionuclide Angiography (FPRNA)

FPRNA can be used to assess left and right ventricular function at rest or during stress. It provides information on wall motion, ejection fraction, and assessment of systolic and diastolic parameters. It is best performed with a dedicated multicrystal or digital system, capable of delivering a minimum of 150,000 counts/s, to provide sufficient information density. A bolus of radioactivity is injected into the venous system, and multiple serial images are acquired at a 25–100 ms frame rate that allows the radioactivity to be tracked from when it enters the RV to when it exits from the LV. Using individual or summed time frames, measurements of global and regional RV and LV function can be performed. If there are atrial or ventricular shunts present, these may be detected and measured. Despite these unique features, the lack of adequate equipment, and payer reimbursement for performing studies, it is seldom performed in current clinical practice.

5.5.2.1 Instrumentation and Procedure

Studies are best performed using Tc-99m DTPA as the radiopharmaceutical which is cleared by the kidneys which is sufficiently far from the heart to not cause interference in case a second bolus injection is required. The injection site should be in a large vein to allow rapid, compact bolus administration. Injection rate should be slower if RV function is required or more rapid if LV function or shunt detection are the issues. Patients are positioned upright or supine in the anterior or a shallow RAO position for rest or exercise studies. The choice of collimators and the window time frame depends on what is the main purpose of the study. For patients performing exercise, motion correction methods should be used [120].

5.6 Neurocardiac Imaging

5.6.1 Basic Concepts of Neurocardiac Imaging

Cardiac autonomic control depends on the circulating neurotransmitters, norepinephrine and acetylcholine, and local innervation by the sympathetic and parasympathetic systems.

Myocardial sympathetic fibers are relatively abundant in the ventricles, especially in the left ventricular anterior and lateral walls. They run adjacent to the coronary arteries, in the epicardium, before penetrating into the myocardium. Central nervous system control of the sympathetic output depends on signals by the brain itself or by peripheral receptors. The descending pathway involves the spinal cord and the paravertebral stellate ganglia.

There are few parasympathetic fibers in the heart, especially in the ventricles. They are involved in the innervation of the atria and the inferior wall of the left ventricle, and they also modulate the atrioventricular nodal function. They begin in the medulla and run along the vagus nerves.

Norepinephrine is produced in the presynaptic terminal, stored in vesicles, and released in response to a stimulus into the synaptic space where it binds to postsynaptic receptors. The sympathetic response depends on two processes: norepinephrine transport I uptake, which is the most important regulator, that controls the uptake, storage, and/or the catabolic disposal of norepinephrine, and the uptake 2 referring to the nonneuronal postsynaptic uptake of the neurotransmitter.

SPECT and PET autonomic radiotracers were first used to detect adrenal neoplasms. I123-metaiodobenzylguanidine (MIBG) is a physiologic analog of guanidine. It shares the transport pathway of norepinephrine and accumulates and displaces the neurotransmitter from the storage granules. Besides the use of I123-MIBG with SPECT, other radiotracers are used to assess myocardial sympathetic innervation. PET tracers, such as C11-hydroxyephedrine or C11-ephedrine, more similar to noradrenaline, with better image properties due to their higher uptake 1 selectivity, have been used. Their clinical application is limited by the short half-life of C11 [2, 3].

5.6.2 Imaging Myocardium Sympathetic Innervation

I-123-MIBG emits 159 KeV photons and has a half-life of 13.2 h. Radiation exposure after an administered dose of 370 MBq (10 mCi) is 5 mSv with the highest exposure in the bladder, liver, spleen, gall bladder, heart, and adrenals [2, 5].

Imaging, as shown in Fig. 5.17, is performed at rest and requires discontinuation of medications and substances known to interfere with the mechanisms of noradrenaline uptake (opioids, cocaine, tricyclic antidepressants, sympathicomimetics, antipsychotics, and some antihypertensive drugs). Prior to administration of I-123 MIBG, iodine may be given to block uptake by the thyroid. Intravenous administration of 370 MBq (10 mCi) over 1–2 min followed by saline flush is usually performed with the patient already positioned under the camera. Planar imaging is performed at 15 min and 4 h with SPECT imaging optional at 4 h. A standard Anger gamma camera with a low-energy high-resolution collimator is used, and almost all the published work used data from planar imaging. The use of a medium-energy collimator may result in better image quality. Analysis of the anterior planar image is used to calculate the ratio between heart and mediastinum uptake of the tracer, heart/mediastinum ratio (H/M), and in the difference of tracer uptake and retention in early and late images – washout rate (WR). Regions of interest (ROI) are drawn around the heart and in the mediastinum, and values of H/M from 1.9 to 2.8 are considered normal. Four examples are shown in Fig. 5.18 with the anterior images on the left column and the regions for the ratios on the right for a range of ratios. With the highest ratio, the

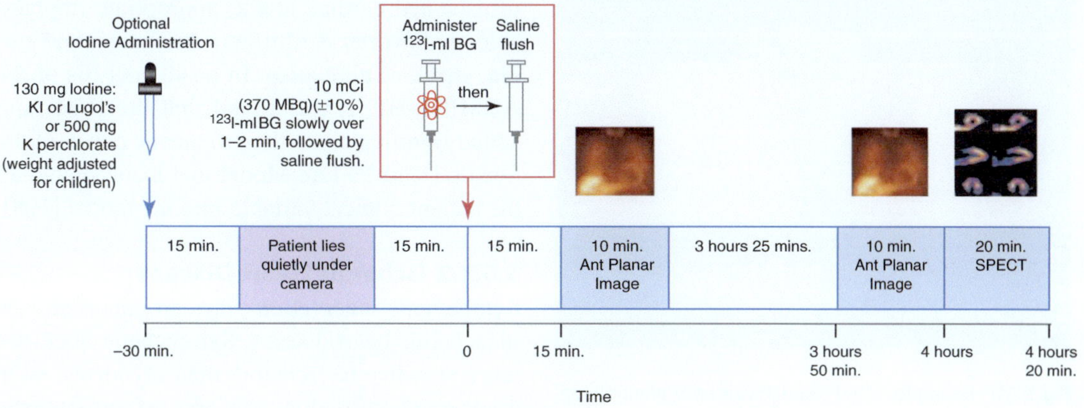

Fig. 5.17 Imaging protocol for I-123 mIBG cardiac imaging

heart can be visualized with uptake, but with the lowest ratio, the heart is barely visible and the lung up is markedly increased. For the WR a formula is used considering the uptake in early and late images [2].

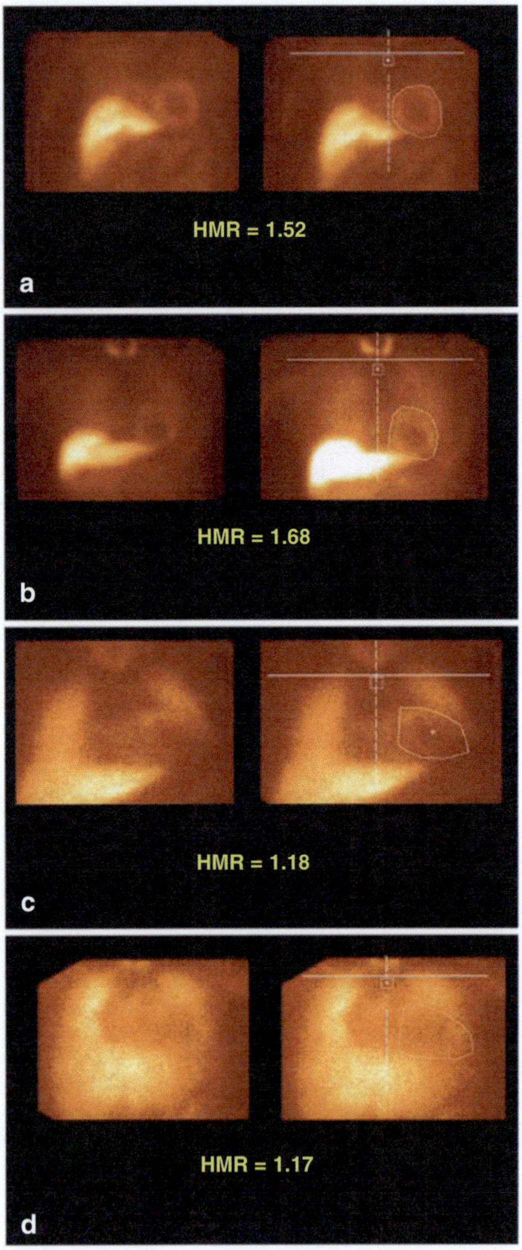

Fig. 5.18 Examples of I-123 mIBG anterior planar imaging in a variety of myocardial innervation

5.6.3 Clinical Indications

5.6.3.1 Heart Failure

The most investigated use of I-123 MIBG sympathetic imaging is in heart failure. In fact this condition involves disruption of the neurohumoral equilibrium, activating the renin-angiotensin-aldosterone system and the sympathetic system. In the initial stages of the disease, there is an increased response of the SNS in patients with low cardiac output which leads to increased norepinephrine release and transport. Eventually there is downregulation of the postsynaptic receptor number. With disease progression, the NET 1 transport system becomes overwhelmed leading to downregulation and spillover of the norepinephrine resulting in an increased washout ratio of MIBG. Presynaptic function decreases with time due to a loss of neurons and downregulation transport, and this leads to decreased cardiac uptake in advanced disease (low H/M ratio).

Several observational studies related the uptake of MIBG with the prognosis of heart failure with decreased ejection fraction [127]. The AdreView Myocardial Imaging for Risk Evaluation in Heart Failure (ADMIRE-HF) trial was a prospective, multicenter international study enrolling 961 patients with an ejection fraction equal or below 35% and in NYHA class II–III. The results showed that during the 17 months of follow-up, an H/M $\leq$ 1.6 was related to worsening NYHA class, life-threatening arrhythmias, resuscitated cardiac arrest, appropriate implantable cardioverter defibrillator discharge, and cardiac death of all causes. In a sub-analysis of the ADMIRE-HF, it was found that the H/M ratio added significantly to the prognostic power of the Seattle Heart Failure Model that incorporated all the patient clinical variable into the model [128].

5.6.3.2 Ischemic Heart Disease

Sympathetic innervation plays an important role in ischemic heart disease. Sympathetic fibers are more sensitive to ischemia than myocytes, so in myocardial infarction, the area of sympathetic denervation is more extensive than the infarct area. The PAREPET trial (Prediction of ARrhythmic Events with Positron Emission Tomography) examined the utility of autonomic, perfusion, and viability imaging in patients with ischemia cardiomyopathy (NYHA I–III and LVEF ≤35%). Perfusion images were obtained with N13 ammonia, and viability was identified by F-18 FDG and innervation with C11-HED. In a 4-year follow-up, the occurrence of sudden cardiac arrest increased in relation to the severity and extent of C-HED autonomic image abnormalities [129]. Autonomic nervous system imaging has a promising role in heart failure.

5.7 Nuclear Techniques in the Management of Inflammatory, Infectious, and Infiltrative Heart Diseases

Nuclear cardiology techniques have an increasing and important role in management of systemic inflammatory diseases involving the heart. Inflammatory diseases such as sarcoidosis and infiltrative disease such as amyloidosis are among those where radiotracer techniques can contribute to an early diagnosis and monitor therapeutic approaches [130, 131].

5.7.1 Sarcoidosis

Sarcoidosis is a systemic granulomatous disease, where cardiac involvement is a major cause of death. In patients with systemic sarcoidosis, cardiac involvement is present in approximately 25–30%. Typical presentations of cardiac involvement include heart block, ventricular arrhythmias, myocardial thickening, diastolic dysfunction, fibrosis, dilatation, and systolic dysfunction [130].

Early detection is important in order to make therapeutic decisions such as aggressive anti-inflammatory therapy, implantation of a cardioverter-defibrillator, and eventual heart transplantation in some patients [132, 133]. There may also be a role for serial monitoring of the response to therapy, but at this time there is insufficient data to know the true role this will play in the future.

The inflammatory nature of sarcoidosis leads to a potential role for PET perfusion and F-18 FDG imaging as granulomas have increased metabolic activity due to increased use of glucose by inflammatory cells. There may also be a noncoronary distribution interference in myocardial blood flow due to arterial compression and dilation as well as eventual myocardial scaring. The major limitation of F-18 FDG is the nonspecificity of glucose uptake. Normal myocardium derives a portion of its energy production through glucose even though there is a preference for the use of fatty acids. Thus, the suppression of myocyte glucose uptake is critical to improving the specificity of FDG PET imaging. Despite these limitations, the use of PET is superior to other nuclear techniques such as SPECT with gallium-67 [134].

A typical protocol for the F-18 FDG PET evaluation of cardiac sarcoid is shown in Fig. 5.19. The best patient preparation involves a 24–48 h diet low in carbohydrates and sugar and high in protein and fat. In addition to this diet, patients should fast for a minimum of 12–18 h. The use of low-dose intravenous unfractionated heparin, 50 IU/kg, is recommended. Heparin causes the liver to release fatty acids that become available as myocardial substrate and thus decrease glucose utilization by myocytes. Diabetics present unique problems, and the recommendations are to use a high fat/low carbohydrate diet and hold oral medications the morning of the study. Diabetics on insulin should hold their long-acting insulin for 48 h and fast-acting insulin the morning of the examination. Getting dietary compliance is difficult, and there is no way to adequately monitor compliance.

It is recommended that whole-body imaging be performed, or at a minimum the chest, to look

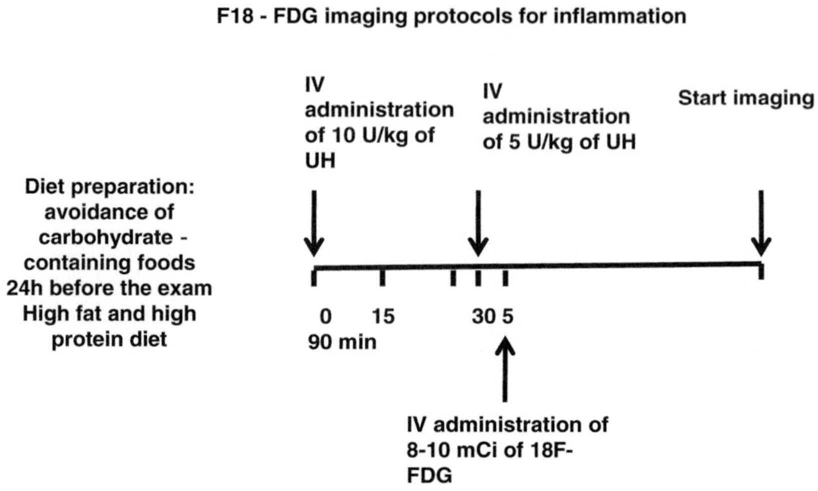

Fig. 5.19 Patient preparation and F-18 FDG imaging for myocardial inflammation

for noncardiac sarcoid involvement. Visual image interpretation is performed looking at reoriented serial slices in three views and comparing the resting perfusion Rb-82 or N-13 ammonia to F-18 FDG. This means that the images are normalized individually for the perfusion and FDG which is not optimal for interpretation as very low myocardial uptake when normalized may display images of homogenous or focal uptake. For this reason, it is recommended that quantitative measures such as standardized uptake values (SUVs) be used to avoid the issues associated with normalization.

Figure 5.20 shows serial resting Rb-82 perfusion and F-18 FDG slices in three views. On the perfusion images, there is a septal perfusion defect extending from the apical to basal slices, and the remainder of the myocardium has normal perfusion. On the FDG images, there is enhanced FGD uptake in the lateral wall starting at the apex and extending all the way to the base and involving the adjacent anterior and inferior walls. Although the basal lateral wall, especially when adjacent to a papillary muscle with marked uptake, can be a normal variant, the extent of the uptake observed is greater than would be expected as a variant. Since this patient does not have coronary artery disease, the perfusion defect in the septum is most consistent with scarring of the septum.

Although PET perfusion/metabolism imaging in patients with suspected or known sarcoid is promising, the lack of specificity for glucose uptake is a major problem that will need to be overcome by developing granuloma-specific tracers. Even with the continued use of FDG for inflammation, quantitative methods of analysis are needed.

5.7.2 Amyloidosis

Amyloidosis encompasses a broad spectrum of diseases that have in common the multisystem deposition of insoluble fibrillary proteins, known as amyloid fibrils, which ultimately lead to increased local oxidative stress, mechanical disruption, and tissue damage. Cardiac amyloidosis involvement is recognized but is probably underdiagnosed.

All types of amyloid are characterized by extracellular deposition of misfolded genetically abnormal or genetically normal transthyretin or light chain proteins manufactured in the bone marrow or liver. Several forms of cardiac involvement have been identified with important differences in diagnosis, prognosis, and treatment. Defined by their precursor proteins, the common types are:

1. Amyloid light chain (AL), due to deposition of immunoglobulin light chains, which is the most aggressive form, and where cardiac involvement, present in 50% of the cases, shortens life

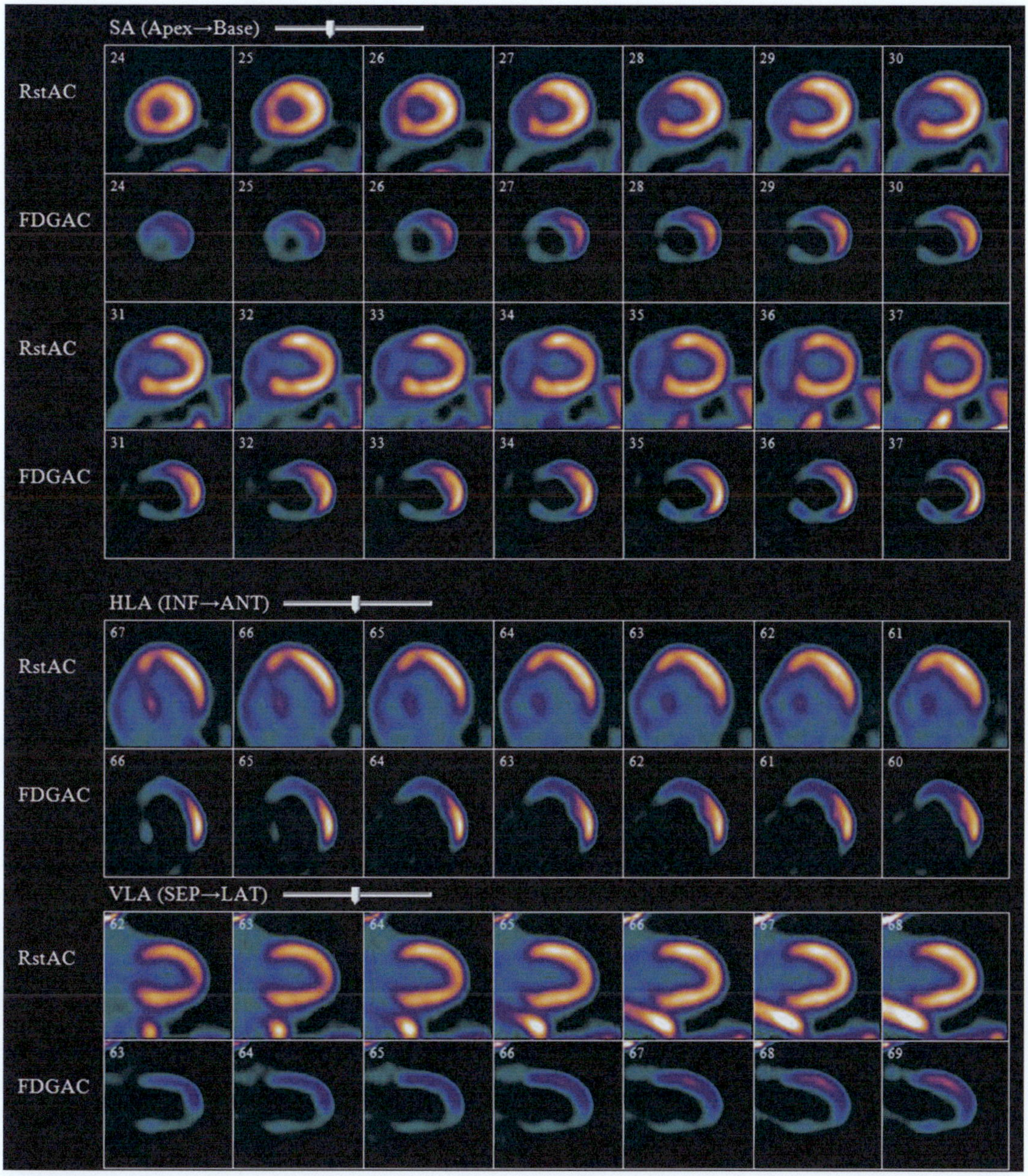

Fig. 5.20 Example of Rb-82 perfusion and active inflammation using F-18 FDG in suspected sarcoid

expectancy significantly. Frequently seen in patients with multiple myeloma.

2. Hereditary transthyretin-derived amyloidosis (ATTRm), an autosomal dominant disease, caused by more than 80 mutations of the protein transthyretin with a significant involvement of the peripheral nervous system and the myocardium.
3. Wild-type or senile transthyretin (ATTRwt). Probably the most common form and estimated to be present in 5–18% of patients over age 65 with heart failure with preserved EF. High prevalence in patients with aortic stenosis.

ATTR is also used to define presence of transthyretin amyloid without designation of wild or mutant type. The extracellular deposition of amyloid fibrils leads to abnormalities in cardiac contractility, conduction, and perfusion. Patients develop symptoms of a restrictive cardiomyopathy. The involvement of the conduction system leads to various degrees of atrioventricular node block and ventricular arrhythmias. Microvascular disease is also common, giving rise to ischemia [130].

The final diagnosis is based on several procedures that culminate with endomyocardial biopsy as it is crucial in the identification of the specific type of amyloidosis for management. Given the invasive nature of myocardial biopsy and the need for immunohistochemistry or mass spectroscopy in inconclusive cases, readily available imaging techniques have been sought. With the pending approval of several drugs for treatment, the diagnosis is needed to select patients who will benefit. Echocardiography and cardiac MR have evolving roles.

Radioisotope imaging techniques, initially developed for detection of remote infarcts or bone imaging, identify the presence of transthyretin deposits in the myocardium. The two most commonly used radiotracers are Tc 99m-DPD (diphosphonate), available in Europe, or Tc 99m PYP (pyrophosphate) used exclusively in the United States. Studies using I123-MIBG have also performed to characterize the involvement of the peripheral nervous system of the heart by the ATTRm [135].

5.7.2.1 Imaging Protocols for Transthyretin Cardiac Amyloidosis

Imaging Procedures: There is no specific patient preparation required prior to the study. Patients are injected with 370–740 MBq (10–20 mCi) of Tc99m PYP or DPD. A variable period of time is required to get the tracer out of the blood pool and into the bone and myocardium. A 1-h wait is the most convenient for patients but is limited by persistent blood pool activity and mild uptake in bone. A 3-h delay allows blood pool clearance and higher concentration in the myocardium and bone but is inconvenient for patients. There is no consensus on which of the two time points is optimal for imaging. Both planar and SPECT supine images of the chest to include the heart and adjacent lung fields are acquired using small or large field of view cameras. When using small field of view cameras, it is essential to make certain that the contralateral lung filed is in the field of view to calculate a ratio. Whole-body imaging to look at other boney structures is optional but recommended.

Image Interpretation: Both the planar and SPECT images need to be reviewed for visual semiquantitative and quantitative interpretation. Depending on whether images are acquired at 1 or 3 h postinjection, there may be differences in visual scoring and quantitative analysis. Visual interpretation involves scoring the activity in the myocardium relative to bone uptake using the following system: Grade 0, no myocardial uptake and normal bone uptake; Grade 1, myocardial uptake <rib uptake; Grade 2, myocardial uptake equal to rib uptake; and Grade 3, myocardial uptake >rib uptake. At 3 h on planar or SPECT, a score $\geq$2 is considered positive for transthyretin amyloid.

Quantitative analysis can be performed on the planar anterior image using a region of interest that includes the myocardium but excludes the ribs and sternum. The total counts in the heart (H) are calculated. This same region should be moved to the contralateral lung field (CL), again being careful to avoid the sternum and ribs. The counts in the heart should be divided by the counts in the contralateral lung to get the H/CL ratio. When imaging at 1 h, a H/CL ratio $\geq$1.5 is considered ATTR positive and ratios <1.5 as ATTR negative. For 3-h images, a ratio $\geq$1.25 is considered ATTR positive and ratios <1.15 as ATTR negative.

Figure 5.21 is an anterior Tc-99m PYP whole-body image at 3 h in an 85-year-old male with severe dyspnea that worsens when he goes into atrial fibrillation. He had recurring right pleural effusions, and on echocardiography his EF is 60%. The image shows diffuse, marked uptake in the left chest with a H/CL ratio of 2.1. Also seen

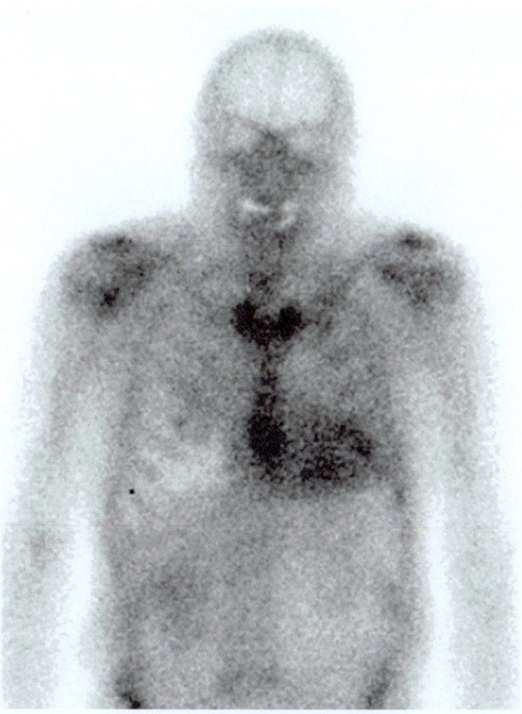

Fig. 5.21 Anterior Tc-99m pyrophosphate amyloid scan at 3 h in a patient with heart failure and preserved ejection fraction showing diffuse myocardial uptake in the heart

is a low count area in the right lung field corresponding to an existing pleural effusion. Fig. 5.22 shows serial slices in three views on the reoriented SPECT images in the same patient. There is very homogenous amyloid uptake throughout the myocardium that looks almost like a perfusion study.

5.7.3 Myocardial Infections and Endocarditis

Radionuclide techniques using both SPECT and PET may be used for diagnosis of infections in the heart caused by endocarditis, abscess formation, or infected devices such as pacemaker leads. Currently F-18 FDG PET imaging has the greatest interest and utilization but is limited by uptake in normal myocardium that requires aggressive measures to suppress normal uptake in order to differentiate between areas of normal myocardium and pathologic inflammation. Agents that specifically target components of inflammation are needed but not widely available.

The diagnosis of endocarditis using the Duke modified criteria is suboptimal in general and even lower when prosthetic materials such as heart valves and pacer/defibrillator leads are present. Echocardiography has a pivotal role in the management of this condition, but other imaging modalities have been used with good results. Cardiac computed tomography and magnetic resonance imaging are excellent in providing high-quality anatomical information. Radionuclide techniques provide physical/functional information that is increasingly important in the diagnoses and therapy monitoring of the disease.

The guidelines of the ESC include the use of nuclear techniques, namely, PET-CT with F-18 FDG and SPECT with Tc 99m-HMPAO (hexamethylpropyleneamine oxime)-labeled leucocytes in specific conditions of endocarditis [136]. A statement from the AHA mentioned the use of other imaging techniques, namely, PET-CT with FDG, although more data is required to define accuracy. Enhanced metabolism due to inflammation results in FDG uptake, and leucocytes are recruited to sites of active inflammation [137]. As was mentioned for the diagnosis of sarcoid with F-18 FDG, myocytes also take up FDG so meticulous patient preparation to suppress myocyte FDG uptake is required to improve specificity.

The advantages of using these imaging techniques are due to the ability to provide excellent functional information as opposed to just anatomic findings which can be nonspecific, especially in the postoperative setting. Both techniques demonstrated added diagnostic value in difficult cases involving prosthetic material (prosthetic valves, pacemakers, implantable cardioverter defibrillators, or ventricular assist devices) as well as demonstrating extracardiac foci of the disease [138].

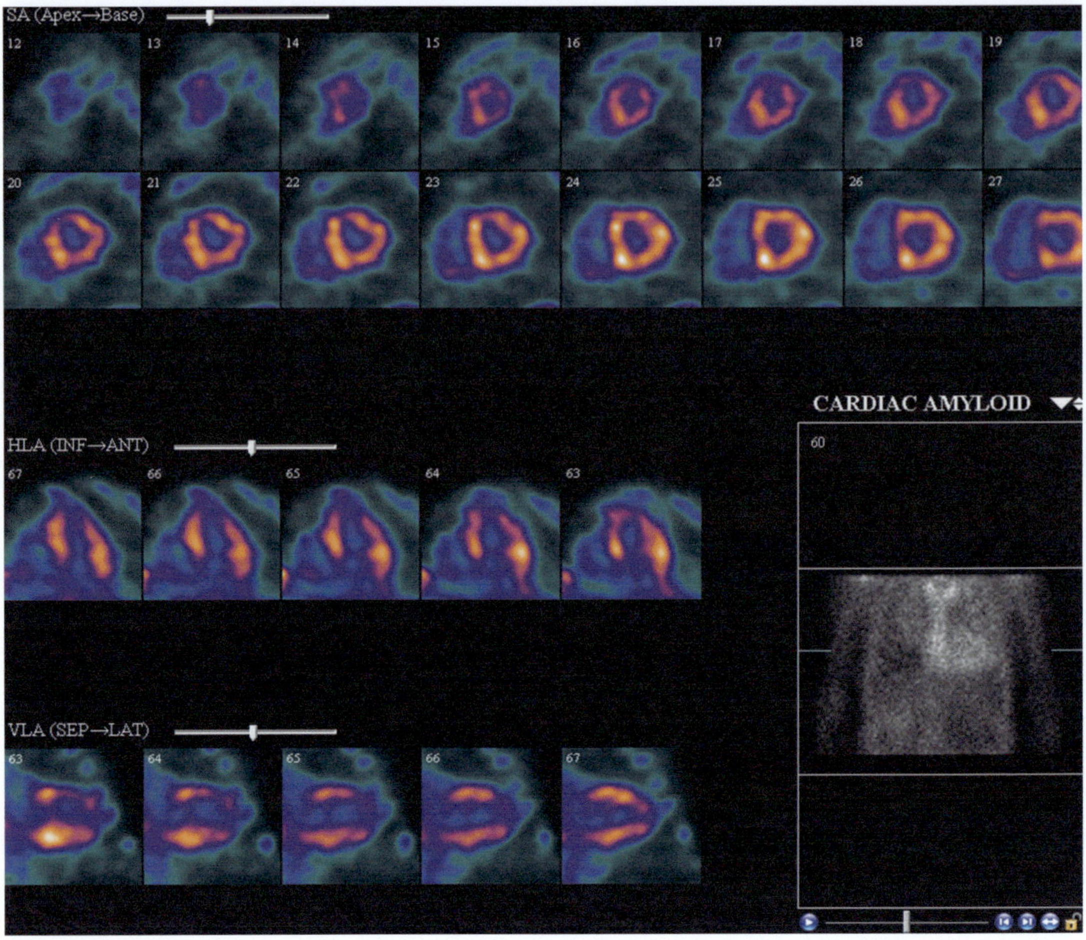

Fig. 5.22 Serial three-view Tc-99m pyrophosphate amyloid scan and anterior projection showing very homogenous uptake in the myocardium

References

1. Klocke FJ, Baird MG, Lorell BH, Bateman TM, Messer JV, Berman DS, et al. ACC/AHA/ASNC guidelines for the clinical use of cardiac radionuclide imaging--executive summary: a report of the American College of Cardiology/American Heart Association Task Force on practice guidelines (ACC/AHA/ASNC Committee to revise the 1995 guidelines for the clinical use of cardiac radionuclide imaging). J Am Coll Cardiol. 2003;42(7):1318–33.
2. Henzlova MJ, Duvall WL, Einstein AJ, Travin MI, Verberne HJ. ASNC imaging guidelines for SPECT nuclear cardiology procedures: stress, protocols, and tracers. J Nucl Cardiol. 2016;23(3):606–39.
3. Dilsizian V, Bacharach SL, Beanlands RS, Bergmann SR, Delbeke D, Dorbala S, et al. ASNC imaging guidelines/SNMMI procedure standard for positron emission tomography (PET) nuclear cardiology procedures. J Nucl Cardiol. 2016;23(5):1187–226.
4. Schelbert HR. Anatomy and physiology of coronary blood flow. J Nucl Cardiol. 2010;17(4):545–54.
5. Verberne HJ, Acampa W, Anagnostopoulos C, Ballinger J, Bengel F, De Bondt P, et al. EANM procedural guidelines for radionuclide myocardial perfusion imaging with SPECT and SPECT/CT: 2015 revision. Eur J Nucl Med Mol Imaging. 2015;42(12):1929–40.
6. Sogbein OO, Pelletier-Galarneau M, Schindler TH, Wei L, Wells RG, Ruddy TD. New SPECT and PET radiopharmaceuticals for imaging cardiovascular disease. Biomed Res Int. 2014;2014:942960.
7. Udelson JE, Bonow RO, Dilsizian V. The historical and conceptual evolution of radionuclide assessment of myocardial viability. J Nucl Cardiol. 2004;11(3):318–34.

8. Camici PG, Prasad SK, Rimoldi OE. Stunning, hibernation, and assessment of myocardial viability. Circulation. 2008;117(1):103–14.
9. Thompson RC, Heller GV, Johnson LL, Case JA, Cullom SJ, Garcia EV, et al. Value of attenuation correction on ECG-gated SPECT myocardial perfusion imaging related to body mass index. J Nucl Cardiol. 2005;12(2):195–202.
10. Johnson LL, Verdesca SA, Aude WY, Xavier RC, Nott LT, Campanella MW, et al. Postischemic stunning can affect left ventricular ejection fraction and regional wall motion on post-stress gated sestamibi tomograms. J Am Coll Cardiol. 1997;30(7):1641–8.
11. Sharir T, Germano G, Kang X, Lewin HC, Miranda R, Cohen I, et al. Prediction of myocardial infarction versus cardiac death by gated myocardial perfusion SPECT: risk stratification by the amount of stress-induced ischemia and the poststress ejection fraction. J Nucl Med. 2001;42(6):831–7.
12. Mathur S, Heller GV, Bateman TM, Ruffin R, Yekta A, Katten D, et al. Clinical value of stress-only Tc-99m SPECT imaging: importance of attenuation correction. J Nucl Cardiol. 2013;20(1):27–37.
13. Ferreira MJ, Cunha MJ, Albuquerque A, Moreira AP, Ramos D, Costa G, et al. Prognosis of normal stress-only gated-SPECT myocardial perfusion imaging: a single center study. Int J Cardiovasc Imaging. 2013;29(7):1639–44.
14. Gowd BM, Heller GV, Parker MW. Stress-only SPECT myocardial perfusion imaging: a review. J Nucl Cardiol. 2014;21(6):1200–12.
15. Dilsizian V, Bonow RO. Current diagnostic techniques of assessing myocardial viability in patients with hibernating and stunned myocardium. Circulation. 1993;87(1):1–20.
16. Dilsizian V. Transition from SPECT to PET myocardial perfusion imaging: a desirable change in nuclear cardiology to approach perfection. J Nucl Cardiol. 2016;23(3):337–8.
17. Bateman TM. Advantages and disadvantages of PET and SPECT in a busy clinical practice. J Nucl Cardiol. 2012;19(Suppl 1):S3–11.
18. Stabin MG. Radiopharmaceuticals for nuclear cardiology: radiation dosimetry, uncertainties, and risk. J Nucl Med. 2008;49(9):1555–63.
19. Maddahi J, Packard RR. Cardiac PET perfusion tracers: current status and future directions. Semin Nucl Med. 2014;44(5):333–43.
20. Nakazato R, Berman DS, Alexanderson E, Slomka P. Myocardial perfusion imaging with PET. Imaging Med. 2013;5(1):35–46.
21. Cerqueira MD. Pharmacologic stress versus maximal-exercise stress for perfusion imaging: which, when, and why? J Nucl Cardiol. 1996;3(6 Pt 2):S10–4.
22. Iskandrian AS, Heo J, Kong B, Lyons E. Effect of exercise level on the ability of thallium-201 tomographic imaging in detecting coronary artery disease: analysis of 461 patients. J Am Coll Cardiol. 1989;14(6):1477–86.
23. Cerqueira MD. The future of pharmacologic stress: selective A2A adenosine receptor agonists. Am J Cardiol. 2004;94(2A):33D–40D. discussion D-2D
24. Cerqueira MD, Verani MS, Schwaiger M, Heo J, Iskandrian AS. Safety profile of adenosine stress perfusion imaging: results from the Adenoscan multicenter trial registry. J Am Coll Cardiol. 1994;23(2):384–9.
25. Ranhosky A, Kempthorne-Rawson J. The safety of intravenous dipyridamole thallium myocardial perfusion imaging. Intravenous dipyridamole thallium imaging study group. Circulation. 1990;81(4):1205–9.
26. Mahmarian JJ, Cerqueira MD, Iskandrian AE, Bateman TM, Thomas GS, Hendel RC, et al. Regadenoson induces comparable left ventricular perfusion defects as adenosine: a quantitative analysis from the ADVANCE MPI 2 trial. J Am Coll Cardiol Img. 2009;2(8):959–68.
27. Hendel RC, Bateman TM, Cerqueira MD, Iskandrian AE, Leppo JA, Blackburn B, et al. Initial clinical experience with regadenoson, a novel selective A2A agonist for pharmacologic stress single-photon emission computed tomography myocardial perfusion imaging. J Am Coll Cardiol. 2005;46(11):2069–75.
28. Al Jaroudi W, Iskandrian AE. Regadenoson: a new myocardial stress agent. J Am Coll Cardiol. 2009;54(13):1123–30.
29. Lette J, Tatum J, Fraser S, Miller D, Waters D, Heller G, et al. Safety of dipyridamole testing in 73,806 patients: the multicenter dipyridamole safety study. J Nucl Cardiol. 1995;2(1):3–17.
30. Leppo JA. Comparison of pharmacologic stress agents. J Nucl Cardiol. 1996;3(6 Pt 2):S22–6.
31. American Society of Nuclear Cardiology. Updated imaging guidelines for nuclear cardiology procedures, part 1. J Nucl Cardiol. 2001;8(1):G5–G58.
32. Hays JT, Mahmarian JJ, Cochran AJ, Verani MS. Dobutamine thallium-201 tomography for evaluating patients with suspected coronary artery disease unable to undergo exercise or vasodilator pharmacologic stress testing. J Am Coll Cardiol. 1993;21(7):1583–90.
33. Agostini D, Marie PY, Ben-Haim S, Rouzet F, Songy B, Giordano A, et al. Performance of cardiac cadmium-zinc-telluride gamma camera imaging in coronary artery disease: a review from the cardiovascular committee of the European Association of Nuclear Medicine (EANM). Eur J Nucl Med Mol Imaging. 2016;43(13):2423–32.
34. Nudi F, Iskandrian AE, Schillaci O, Peruzzi M, Frati G, Biondi-Zoccai G. Diagnostic accuracy of myocardial perfusion imaging with CZT technology: systemic review and meta-analysis of comparison with invasive coronary angiography. J Am Coll Cardiol Img. 2017;10(7):787–94.
35. Germano G, Kiat H, Kavanagh PB, Moriel M, Mazzanti M, Su HT, et al. Automatic quantification of ejection fraction from gated myocardial perfusion SPECT. J Nucl Med. 1995;36(11):2138–47.

36. Akincioglu C, Berman DS, Nishina H, Kavanagh PB, Slomka PJ, Abidov A, et al. Assessment of diastolic function using 16-frame 99mTc-sestamibi gated myocardial perfusion SPECT: normal values. J Nucl Med. 2005;46(7):1102–8.
37. Choi JY, Lee KH, Kim SJ, Kim SE, Kim BT, Lee SH, et al. Gating provides improved accuracy for differentiating artifacts from true lesions in equivocal fixed defects on technetium 99m tetrofosmin perfusion SPECT. J Nucl Cardiol. 1998;5(4):395–401.
38. Everaert H, Franken PR, Flamen P, Goris M, Momen A, Bossuyt A. Left ventricular ejection fraction from gated SPET myocardial perfusion studies: a method based on the radial distribution of count rate density across the myocardial wall. Eur J Nucl Med. 1996;23(12):1628–33.
39. Everaert H, Vanhove C, Franken PR. Gated SPET myocardial perfusion acquisition within 5 minutes using focussing collimators and a three-head gamma camera. Eur J Nucl Med. 1998;25(6):587–93.
40. Gunning MG, Anagnostopoulos C, Davies G, Forbat SM, Ell PJ, Underwood SR. Gated technetium-99m-tetrofosmin SPECT and cine MRI to assess left ventricular contraction. J Nucl Med. 1997;38(3):438–42.
41. Mochizuki T, Murase K, Tanaka H, Kondoh T, Hamamoto K, Tauxe WN. Assessment of left ventricular volume using ECG-gated SPECT with technetium-99m-MIBI and technetium-99m-tetrofosmin. J Nucl Med. 1997;38(1):53–7.
42. Slomka PJ, Berman DS, Xu Y, Kavanagh P, Hayes SW, Dorbala S, et al. Fully automated wall motion and thickening scoring system for myocardial perfusion SPECT: method development and validation in large population. J Nucl Cardiol. 2012;19(2):291–302.
43. Abidov A, Germano G, Hachamovitch R, Slomka P, Berman DS. Gated SPECT in assessment of regional and global left ventricular function: an update. J Nucl Cardiol. 2013;20(6):1118–43. quiz 44-6
44. Dorbala S, Di Carli MF, Delbeke D, Abbara S, DePuey EG, Dilsizian V, et al. SNMMI/ASNC/SCCT guideline for cardiac SPECT/CT and PET/CT 1.0. J Nucl Med. 2013;54(8):1485–507.
45. Gaemperli O, Kaufmann PA, Alkadhi H. Cardiac hybrid imaging. Eur J Nucl Med Mol Imaging. 2014;41(Suppl 1):S91–103.
46. Schaap J, de Groot JA, Nieman K, Meijboom WB, Boekholdt SM, Kauling RM, et al. Added value of hybrid myocardial perfusion SPECT and CT coronary angiography in the diagnosis of coronary artery disease. Eur Heart J Cardiovasc Imaging. 2014;15(11):1281–8.
47. Cerqueira MD, Weissman NJ, Dilsizian V, Jacobs AK, Kaul S, Laskey WK, et al. Standardized myocardial segmentation and nomenclature for tomographic imaging of the heart. A statement for healthcare professionals from the cardiac imaging Committee of the Council on clinical cardiology of the American Heart Association. Int J Cardiovasc Imaging. 2002;18(1):539–42.
48. Xu Y, Kavanagh P, Fish M, Gerlach J, Ramesh A, Lemley M, et al. Automated quality control for segmentation of myocardial perfusion SPECT. J Nucl Med. 2009;50(9):1418–26.
49. Slomka PJ, Nishina H, Berman DS, Akincioglu C, Abidov A, Friedman JD, et al. Automated quantification of myocardial perfusion SPECT using simplified normal limits. J Nucl Cardiol. 2005;12(1):66–77.
50. Slomka P, Xu Y, Berman D, Germano G. Quantitative analysis of perfusion studies: strengths and pitfalls. J Nucl Cardiol. 2012;19(2):338–46.
51. Ziadi MC. Myocardial flow reserve (MFR) with positron emission tomography (PET)/computed tomography (CT): clinical impact in diagnosis and prognosis. Cardiovasc diagn Ther. 2017;7(2):206–18.
52. Cerqueira MD. The user-friendly nuclear cardiology report: what needs to be considered and what is included. J Nucl Cardiol. 1996;3(4):350–5.
53. Hendel RC, Wackers FJ, Berman DS, Ficaro E, Depuey EG, Klein L, et al. American society of nuclear cardiology consensus statement: reporting of radionuclide myocardial perfusion imaging studies. J Nucl Cardiol. 2003;10(6):705–8.
54. Tragardh E, Hesse B, Knuuti J, Flotats A, Kaufmann PA, Kitsiou A, et al. Reporting nuclear cardiology: a joint position paper by the European Association of Nuclear Medicine (EANM) and the European Association of Cardiovascular Imaging (EACVI). Eur Heart J Cardiovasc Imaging. 2015;16(3):272–9.
55. Tilkemeier PL, Bourque J, Doukky R, Sanghani R, Weinberg RL. ASNC imaging guidelines for nuclear cardiology procedures : standardized reporting of nuclear cardiology procedures. J Nucl Cardiol. 2017;24:2064.
56. Iskandrian AE, Heo J, Nallamothu N. Detection of coronary artery disease in women with use of stress single-photon emission computed tomography myocardial perfusion imaging. J Nucl Cardiol. 1997;4(4):329–35.
57. Mahmarian JJ, Boyce TM, Goldberg RK, Cocanougher MK, Roberts R, Verani MS. Quantitative exercise thallium-201 single photon emission computed tomography for the enhanced diagnosis of ischemic heart disease. J Am Coll Cardiol. 1990;15(2):318–29.
58. Fleischmann KE, Hunink MG, Kuntz KM, Douglas PS. Exercise echocardiography or exercise SPECT imaging? A meta-analysis of diagnostic test performance. JAMA. 1998;280(10):913–20.
59. Parker MW, Iskandar A, Limone B, Perugini A, Kim H, Jones C, et al. Diagnostic accuracy of cardiac positron emission tomography versus single photon emission computed tomography for coronary artery disease: a bivariate meta-analysis. Circ Cardiovasc Imaging. 2012;5(6):700–7.
60. Lee JM, Kim CH, Koo BK, Hwang D, Park J, Zhang J, et al. Integrated myocardial perfusion imaging diagnostics improve detection of functionally significant coronary artery stenosis by 13N-ammonia

positron emission tomography. Circ Cardiovasc Imaging. 2016;9(9):pii: e004768.
61. Sciagra R, Passeri A, Bucerius J, Verberne HJ, Slart RH, Lindner O, et al. Clinical use of quantitative cardiac perfusion PET: rationale, modalities and possible indications. Position paper of the cardiovascular Committee of the European Association of nuclear medicine (EANM). Eur J Nucl Med Mol Imaging. 2016;43(8):1530–45.
62. Hendel RC, Berman DS, Di Carli MF, Heidenreich PA, Henkin RE, Pellikka PA, et al. ACCF/ASNC/ACR/AHA/ASE/SCCT/SCMR/SNM 2009 appropriate use criteria for cardiac radionuclide imaging: a report of the American College of Cardiology Foundation appropriate use criteria task force, the American Society of Nuclear Cardiology, the American College of Radiology, the American Heart Association, the American Society of Echocardiography, the Society of Cardiovascular Computed Tomography, the Society for Cardiovascular Magnetic Resonance, and the Society of Nuclear Medicine. J Am Coll Cardiol. 2009;53(23):2201–29.
63. Task Force M, Montalescot G, Sechtem U, Achenbach S, Andreotti F, Arden C, et al. 2013 ESC guidelines on the management of stable coronary artery disease: the Task Force on the management of stable coronary artery disease of the European Society of Cardiology. Eur Heart J. 2013;34(38):2949–3003.
64. Gibbons RJ, Balady GJ, Bricker JT, Chaitman BR, Fletcher GF, Froelicher VF, et al. ACC/AHA 2002 guideline update for exercise testing: summary article. A report of the American College of Cardiology/American Heart Association Task Force on practice guidelines (committee to update the 1997 exercise testing guidelines). J Am Coll Cardiol. 2002;40(8):1531–40.
65. Hachamovitch R, Berman DS, Shaw LJ, Kiat H, Cohen I, Cabico JA, et al. Incremental prognostic value of myocardial perfusion single photon emission computed tomography for the prediction of cardiac death: differential stratification for risk of cardiac death and myocardial infarction. Circulation. 1998;97(6):535–43.
66. Shaw LJ, Hachamovitch R, Peterson ED, Lewin HC, Iskandrian AE, Miller DD, et al. Using an outcomes-based approach to identify candidates for risk stratification after exercise treadmill testing. J Gen Intern Med. 1999;14(1):1–9.
67. Gibbons RJ, Hodge DO, Berman DS, Akinboboye OO, Heo J, Hachamovitch R, et al. Long-term outcome of patients with intermediate-risk exercise electrocardiograms who do not have myocardial perfusion defects on radionuclide imaging. Circulation. 1999;100(21):2140–5.
68. Gibbons RJ, Abrams J, Chatterjee K, Daley J, Deedwania PC, Douglas JS, et al. ACC/AHA 2002 guideline update for the management of patients with chronic stable angina--summary article: a report of the American College of Cardiology/American Heart Association Task Force on practice guidelines (committee on the Management of Patients with Chronic Stable Angina). J Am Coll Cardiol. 2003;41(1):159–68.
69. Akinboboye OO, Idris O, Onwuanyi A, Berekashvili K, Bergmann SR. Incidence of major cardiovascular events in black patients with normal myocardial stress perfusion study results. J Nucl Cardiol. 2001;8(5):541–7.
70. Shaw LJ, Hendel RC, Cerquiera M, Mieres JH, Alazraki N, Krawczynska E, et al. Ethnic differences in the prognostic value of stress technetium-99m tetrofosmin gated single-photon emission computed tomography myocardial perfusion imaging. J Am Coll Cardiol. 2005;45(9):1494–504.
71. Alkeylani A, Miller DD, Shaw LJ, Travin MI, Stratmann HG, Jenkins R, et al. Influence of race on the prediction of cardiac events with stress technetium-99m sestamibi tomographic imaging in patients with stable angina pectoris. Am J Cardiol. 1998;81(3):293–7.
72. Shaw LJ, Bairey Merz CN, Pepine CJ, Reis SE, Bittner V, Kelsey SF, et al. Insights from the NHLBI-sponsored Women's ischemia syndrome evaluation (WISE) study: part I: gender differences in traditional and novel risk factors, symptom evaluation, and gender-optimized diagnostic strategies. J Am Coll Cardiol. 2006;47(3 Suppl):S4–S20.
73. Iskandar A, Limone B, Parker MW, Perugini A, Kim H, Jones C, et al. Gender differences in the diagnostic accuracy of SPECT myocardial perfusion imaging: a bivariate meta-analysis. J Nucl Cardiol. 2013;20(1):53–63.
74. Phillips LM, Mieres JH. Noninvasive assessment of coronary artery disease in women: what's next? Curr Cardiol Rep. 2010;12(2):147–54.
75. Patel MB, Bui LP, Kirkeeide RL, Gould KL. Imaging microvascular dysfunction and mechanisms for female-male differences in CAD. J Am Coll Cardiol Img. 2016;9(4):465–82.
76. Campisi R, Marengo FD. Coronary microvascular dysfunction in women with nonobstructive ischemic heart disease as assessed by positron emission tomography. Cardiovasc Diagn Ther. 2017;7(2):196–205.
77. Wagdy HM, Hodge D, Christian TF, Miller TD, Gibbons RJ. Prognostic value of vasodilator myocardial perfusion imaging in patients with left bundle-branch block. Circulation. 1998;97(16):1563–70.
78. Gioia G, Bagheri B, Gottlieb CD, Schwartzman DS, Callans DJ, Marchlinski FE, et al. Prediction of outcome of patients with life-threatening ventricular arrhythmias treated with automatic implantable cardioverter-defibrillators using SPECT perfusion imaging. Circulation. 1997;95(2):390–4.
79. Amanullah AM, Berman DS, Kang X, Cohen I, Germano G, Friedman JD. Enhanced prognostic stratification of patients with left ventricular hypertrophy with the use of single-photon emission computed tomography. Am Heart J. 2000;140(3):456–62.

80. Elhendy A, van Domburg RT, Sozzi FB, Poldermans D, Bax JJ, Roelandt JR. Impact of hypertension on the accuracy of exercise stress myocardial perfusion imaging for the diagnosis of coronary artery disease. Heart. 2001;85(6):655–61.
81. Bartram P, Toft J, Hanel B, Ali S, Gustafsson F, Mortensen J, et al. False-positive defects in technetium-99m sestamibi myocardial single-photon emission tomography in healthy athletes with left ventricular hypertrophy. Eur J Nucl Med. 1998;25(9):1308–12.
82. Blumenthal RS, Becker DM, Moy TF, Coresh J, Wilder LB, Becker LC. Exercise thallium tomography predicts future clinically manifest coronary heart disease in a high-risk asymptomatic population. Circulation. 1996;93(5):915–23.
83. Blumenthal RS, Becker DM, Yanek LR, Aversano TR, Moy TF, Kral BG, et al. Detecting occult coronary disease in a high-risk asymptomatic population. Circulation. 2003;107(5):702–7.
84. American Diabetes Association. Diabetes mellitus: a major risk factor for cardiovascular disease. A joint editorial statement by the American Diabetes Association; The National Heart, Lung, and Blood Institute; The Juvenile Diabetes Foundation International; The National Institute of Diabetes and Digestive and Kidney Diseases; and The American Heart Association. Circulation. 1999;100(10):1132–3.
85. Giri S, Shaw LJ, Murthy DR, Travin MI, Miller DD, Hachamovitch R, et al. Impact of diabetes on the risk stratification using stress single-photon emission computed tomography myocardial perfusion imaging in patients with symptoms suggestive of coronary artery disease. Circulation. 2002;105(1):32–40.
86. Kang X, Berman DS, Lewin H, Miranda R, Erel J, Friedman JD, et al. Comparative ability of myocardial perfusion single-photon emission computed tomography to detect coronary artery disease in patients with and without diabetes mellitus. Am Heart J. 1999;137(5):949–57.
87. Kang X, Berman DS, Lewin HC, Cohen I, Friedman JD, Germano G, et al. Incremental prognostic value of myocardial perfusion single photon emission computed tomography in patients with diabetes mellitus. Am Heart J. 1999;138(6 Pt 1):1025–32.
88. Wackers FJ, Young LH, Inzucchi SE, Chyun DA, Davey JA, Barrett EJ, et al. Detection of silent myocardial ischemia in asymptomatic diabetic subjects: the DIAD study. Diabetes Care. 2004;27(8):1954–61.
89. Young LH, Wackers FJ, Chyun DA, Davey JA, Barrett EJ, Taillefer R, et al. Cardiac outcomes after screening for asymptomatic coronary artery disease in patients with type 2 diabetes: the DIAD study: a randomized controlled trial. JAMA. 2009;301(15):1547–55.
90. Amsterdam EA, Kirk JD, Bluemke DA, Diercks D, Farkouh ME, Garvey JL, et al. Testing of low-risk patients presenting to the emergency department with chest pain: a scientific statement from the American Heart Association. Circulation. 2010;122(17):1756–76.
91. Tatum JL, Jesse RL, Kontos MC, Nicholson CS, Schmidt KL, Roberts CS, et al. Comprehensive strategy for the evaluation and triage of the chest pain patient. Ann Emerg Med. 1997;29(1):116–25.
92. Heller GV, Stowers SA, Hendel RC, Herman SD, Daher E, Ahlberg AW, et al. Clinical value of acute rest technetium-99m tetrofosmin tomographic myocardial perfusion imaging in patients with acute chest pain and nondiagnostic electrocardiograms. J Am Coll Cardiol. 1998;31(5):1011–7.
93. Udelson JE, Beshansky JR, Ballin DS, Feldman JA, Griffith JL, Handler J, et al. Myocardial perfusion imaging for evaluation and triage of patients with suspected acute cardiac ischemia: a randomized controlled trial. JAMA. 2002;288(21):2693–700.
94. Brown KA, Rowen M. Prognostic value of a normal exercise myocardial perfusion imaging study in patients with angiographically significant coronary artery disease. Am J Cardiol. 1993;71(10):865–7.
95. Shaw LJ, Hachamovitch R, Berman DS, Marwick TH, Lauer MS, Heller GV, et al. The economic consequences of available diagnostic and prognostic strategies for the evaluation of stable angina patients: an observational assessment of the value of precatheterization ischemia. Economics of noninvasive diagnosis (END) multicenter study group. J Am Coll Cardiol. 1999;33(3):661–9.
96. Brindis RG, Douglas PS, Hendel RC, Peterson ED, Wolk MJ, Allen JM, et al. ACCF/ASNC appropriateness criteria for single-photon emission computed tomography myocardial perfusion imaging (SPECT MPI): a report of the American College of Cardiology Foundation quality strategic directions committee appropriateness criteria working group and the American Society of Nuclear Cardiology endorsed by the American Heart Association. J Am Coll Cardiol. 2005;46(8):1587–605.
97. McPherson JA, Robinson PS, Powers ER, Sarembock IJ, Gimple LW, Ragosta M. Angiographic findings in patients undergoing catheterization for recurrent symptoms within 30 days of successful coronary intervention. Am J Cardiol. 1999;84(5):589–92. A8
98. Jain A, Mahmarian JJ, Borges-Neto S, Johnston DL, Cashion WR, Lewis JM, et al. Clinical significance of perfusion defects by thallium-201 single photon emission tomography following oral dipyridamole early after coronary angioplasty. J Am Coll Cardiol. 1988;11(5):970–6.
99. Ho KT, Miller TD, Holmes DR, Hodge DO, Gibbons RJ. Long-term prognostic value of Duke treadmill score and exercise thallium-201 imaging performed one to three years after percutaneous transluminal coronary angioplasty. Am J Cardiol. 1999;84(11):1323–7.
100. Hamilos MI, Ostojic M, Beleslin B, Sagic D, Mangovski L, Stojkovic S, et al. Differential effects of drug-eluting stents on local endothelium-

dependent coronary vasomotion. J Am Coll Cardiol. 2008;51(22):2123–9.
101. Ertas G, van Beusekom HM, van der Giessen WJ. Late stent thrombosis, endothelialisation and drug-eluting stents. Netherlands Jeart J. 2009;17(4):177–80.
102. Miller TD, Christian TF, Hodge DO, Mullan BP, Gibbons RJ. Prognostic value of exercise thallium-201 imaging performed within 2 years of coronary artery bypass graft surgery. J Am Coll Cardiol. 1998;31(4):848–54.
103. Palmas W, Bingham S, Diamond GA, Denton TA, Kiat H, Friedman JD, et al. Incremental prognostic value of exercise thallium-201 myocardial single-photon emission computed tomography late after coronary artery bypass surgery. J Am Coll Cardiol. 1995;25(2):403–9.
104. Zellweger MJ, Lewin HC, Lai S, Dubois EA, Friedman JD, Germano G, et al. When to stress patients after coronary artery bypass surgery? Risk stratification in patients early and late post-CABG using stress myocardial perfusion SPECT: implications of appropriate clinical strategies. J Am Coll Cardiol. 2001;37(1):144–52.
105. Lauer MS, Lytle B, Pashkow F, Snader CE, Marwick TH. Prediction of death and myocardial infarction by screening with exercise-thallium testing after coronary-artery-bypass grafting. Lancet. 1998;351(9103):615–22.
106. Nallamothu N, Johnson JH, Bagheri B, Heo J, Iskandrian AE. Utility of stress single-photon emission computed tomography (SPECT) perfusion imaging in predicting outcome after coronary artery bypass grafting. Am J Cardiol. 1997;80(12):1517–21.
107. Eagle KA, Berger PB, Calkins H, Chaitman BR, Ewy GA, Fleischmann KE, et al. ACC/AHA guideline update for perioperative cardiovascular evaluation for noncardiac surgery--executive summary: a report of the American College of Cardiology/American Heart Association Task Force on practice guidelines (committee to update the 1996 guidelines on perioperative cardiovascular evaluation for noncardiac surgery). J Am Coll Cardiol. 2002;39(3):542–53.
108. Mangano DT, Goldman L. Preoperative assessment of patients with known or suspected coronary disease. N Engl J Med. 1995;333(26):1750–6.
109. Fleisher LA, Fleischmann KE, Auerbach AD, Barnason SA, Beckman JA, Bozkurt B, et al. 2014 ACC/AHA guideline on perioperative cardiovascular evaluation and management of patients undergoing noncardiac surgery: executive summary: a report of the American College of Cardiology/American Heart Association Task Force on practice guidelines. Developed in collaboration with the American College of Surgeons, American Society of Anesthesiologists, American Society of Echocardiography, American Society of Nuclear Cardiology, Heart Rhythm Society, Society for Cardiovascular Angiography and Interventions, Society of Cardiovascular Anesthesiologists, and Society of Vascular Medicine Endorsed by the Society of Hospital Medicine. J Nucl Cardiol. 2015;22(1):162–215.
110. Kristensen SD, Knuuti J, Saraste A, Anker S, Botker HE, Hert SD, et al. 2014 ESC/ESA guidelines on non-cardiac surgery: cardiovascular assessment and management: the joint Task Force on non-cardiac surgery: cardiovascular assessment and management of the European Society of Cardiology (ESC) and the European Society of Anaesthesiology (ESA). Eur Heart J. 2014;35(35):2383–431.
111. Rahimtoola SH. Chronic myocardial hibernation. Circulation. 1994;89(4):1907–8.
112. Patel H, Mazur W, Williams KA Sr, Kalra DK. Myocardial viability-state of the art: is it still relevant and how to best assess it with imaging? Trends Cardiovasc Med. 2018;28(1):24–37.
113. Acampa W, Cuocolo A, Petretta M, Bruno A, Castellani M, Finzi A, et al. Tetrofosmin imaging in the detection of myocardial viability in patients with previous myocardial infarction: comparison with sestamibi and Tl-201 scintigraphy. J Nucl Cardiol. 2002;9(1):33–40.
114. Orlandini A, Castellana N, Pascual A, Botto F, Cecilia Bahit M, Chacon C, et al. Myocardial viability for decision-making concerning revascularization in patients with left ventricular dysfunction and coronary artery disease: a meta-analysis of non-randomized and randomized studies. Int J Cardiol. 2015;182:494–9.
115. Di Carli MF, Davidson M, Little R, Khanna S, Mody FV, Brunken RC, et al. Value of metabolic imaging with positron emission tomography for evaluating prognosis in patients with coronary artery disease and left ventricular dysfunction. Am J Cardiol. 1994;73(8):527–33.
116. Di Carli MF, Asgarzadie F, Schelbert HR, Brunken RC, Laks H, Phelps ME, et al. Quantitative relation between myocardial viability and improvement in heart failure symptoms after revascularization in patients with ischemic cardiomyopathy. Circulation. 1995;92(12):3436–44.
117. Allman KC, Shaw LJ, Hachamovitch R, Udelson JE. Myocardial viability testing and impact of revascularization on prognosis in patients with coronary artery disease and left ventricular dysfunction: a meta-analysis. J Am Coll Cardiol. 2002;39(7):1151–8.
118. Beanlands RS, Ruddy TD, de Kemp RA, Iwanochko RM, Coates G, Freeman M, et al. Positron emission tomography and recovery following revascularization (PARR-1): the importance of scar and the development of a prediction rule for the degree of recovery of left ventricular function. J Am Coll Cardiol. 2002;40(10):1735–43.
119. D'Egidio G, Nichol G, Williams KA, Guo A, Garrard L, de Kemp RA, et al. Increasing benefit from revascularization is associated with increasing amounts of myocardial hibernation: a substudy of the PARR-2 trial. J Am Coll Cardiol Img. 2009;2(9):1060–8.

120. Hesse B, Lindhardt TB, Acampa W, Anagnostopoulos C, Ballinger J, Bax JJ, et al. EANM/ESC guidelines for radionuclide imaging of cardiac function. Eur J Nucl Med Mol Imaging. 2008;35(4):851–85.
121. Gibbons RJ. Rest and exercise radionuclide angiography for diagnosis in chronic ischemic heart disease. Circulation. 1991;84(3 Suppl):I93–9.
122. Schwartz RG, McKenzie WB, Alexander J, Sager P, D'Souza A, Manatunga A, et al. Congestive heart failure and left ventricular dysfunction complicating doxorubicin therapy. Seven-year experience using serial radionuclide angiocardiography. Am J Med. 1987;82(6):1109–18.
123. Schwartz RG, Jain D, Storozynsky E. Traditional and novel methods to assess and prevent chemotherapy-related cardiac dysfunction noninvasively. J Nucl Cardiol. 2013;20(3):443–64.
124. Zamorano JL, Lancellotti P, Rodriguez Munoz D, Aboyans V, Asteggiano R, Galderisi M, et al. 2016 ESC position paper on cancer treatments and cardiovascular toxicity developed under the auspices of the ESC Committee for practice guidelines: the Task Force for cancer treatments and cardiovascular toxicity of the European Society of Cardiology (ESC). Eur Heart J. 2016;37(36):2768–801.
125. Bloom MW, Hamo CE, Cardinale D, Ky B, Nohria A, Baer L, et al. Cancer therapy-related cardiac dysfunction and heart failure: part 1: definitions, pathophysiology, risk factors, and imaging. Circ Heart Fail. 2016;9(1):e002661.
126. Hamo CE, Bloom MW, Cardinale D, Ky B, Nohria A, Baer L, et al. Cancer therapy-related cardiac dysfunction and heart failure: part 2: prevention, treatment, guidelines, and future directions. Circ Heart Fail. 2016;9(2):e002843.
127. Verberne HJ, Brewster LM, Somsen GA, van Eck-Smit BL. Prognostic value of myocardial 123I-metaiodobenzylguanidine (MIBG) parameters in patients with heart failure: a systematic review. Eur Heart J. 2008;29(9):1147–59.
128. Jacobson AF, Senior R, Cerqueira MD, Wong ND, Thomas GS, Lopez VA, et al. Myocardial iodine-123 meta-iodobenzylguanidine imaging and cardiac events in heart failure. Results of the prospective ADMIRE-HF (AdreView myocardial imaging for risk evaluation in heart failure) study. J Am Coll Cardiol. 2010;55(20):2212–21.
129. Fallavollita JA, Heavey BM, Luisi AJ Jr, Michalek SM, Baldwa S, Mashtare TL Jr, et al. Regional myocardial sympathetic denervation predicts the risk of sudden cardiac arrest in ischemic cardiomyopathy. J Am Coll Cardiol. 2014;63(2):141–9.
130. Bejar D, Colombo PC, Latif F, Yuzefpolskaya M. Infiltrative cardiomyopathies. Clin Med Insights Cardiol. 2015;9(Suppl 2):29–38.
131. Juneau D, Erthal F, Alzahrani A, Alenazy A, Nery PB, Beanlands RS, et al. Systemic and inflammatory disorders involving the heart: the role of PET imaging. Q J Nucl Med Mol Imaging. 2016;60(4):383–96.
132. Erthal F, Juneau D, Lim SP, Dwivedi G, Nery PB, Birnie D, et al. Imaging of cardiac sarcoidosis. Q J Nucl Med Mol Imaging. 2016;60(3):252–63.
133. Ahmadian A, Pawar S, Govender P, Berman J, Ruberg FL, Miller EJ. The response of FDG uptake to immunosuppressive treatment on FDG PET/CT imaging for cardiac sarcoidosis. J Nucl Cardiol. 2017;24(2):413–24.
134. Chareonthaitawee P, Beanlands RS, Chen W, Dorbala S, Miller EJ, Murthy VL, et al. Joint SNMMI-ASNC expert consensus document on the role of 18F-FDG PET/CT in cardiac sarcoid detection and therapy monitoring. J Nucl Cardiol. 2017;24:1741.
135. Bokhari S, Shahzad R, Castano A, Maurer MS. Nuclear imaging modalities for cardiac amyloidosis. J Nucl Cardiol. 2014;21(1):175–84.
136. Habib G, Lancellotti P, Antunes MJ, Bongiorni MG, Casalta JP, Del Zotti F, et al. 2015 ESC guidelines for the management of infective endocarditis: the Task Force for the Management of Infective Endocarditis of the European Society of Cardiology (ESC). Endorsed by: European Association for Cardio-Thoracic Surgery (EACTS), the European Association of Nuclear Medicine (EANM). Eur Heart J. 2015;36(44):3075–128.
137. Baddour LM, Wilson WR, Bayer AS, Fowler VG Jr, Tleyjeh IM, Rybak MJ, et al. Infective endocarditis in adults: diagnosis, antimicrobial therapy, and Management of Complications: a scientific statement for healthcare professionals from the American Heart Association. Circulation. 2015;132(15):1435–86.
138. Gomes A, Glaudemans A, Touw DJ, van Melle JP, Willems TP, Maass AH, et al. Diagnostic value of imaging in infective endocarditis: a systematic review. Lancet Infect Dis. 2017;17(1):e1–e14.

6 Ventilation/Perfusion SPECT Imaging Diagnosing PE and Other Cardiopulmonary Diseases

Marika Bajc and Ari Lindqvist

6.1 Introduction

Scintigraphic pulmonary studies are designed to demonstrate patterns of ventilation and perfusion. In the healthy individuals, there is a balance between regional ventilation and perfusion to achieve optimal gas exchange. When pulmonary diseases cause deficiency in ventilation and perfusion, they cause "matched" defect. Mismatch implies an imbalance between perfusion and ventilation. The single most important application for pulmonary scintigraphy is the evaluation of patients with suspected pulmonary embolism (PE). In patients with pulmonary embolism, characteristic finding is segmental perfusion defect with preserved ventilation. In 1964, Wagner recognized and first demonstrated the value of pulmonary scintigraphy by using I131—human serum albumin (HSA) and rectilinear scanner [1, 2]. Scanners were further replaced with gamma camera and mainly planar technique was used for imaging. Planar imaging is still used technique in majority hospitals in the USA. On the other hand, in Europe, Australia, Japan, China and Canada, the planar technique is replaced with a single photon emission tomography (V/P SPECT). V/P SPECT was endorsed by EANM as recommended scintigraphic technique for the diagnosis of pulmonary embolism (PE) in 2009. Since then many studies have confirmed its value.

M. Bajc (✉)
Skåne University Hospital, Department of Clinical Sciences, University Hospital Lund, Lund, Sweden
e-mail: marika.bajc@med.lu.se

A. Lindqvist
Research Unit of Pulmonary Diseases, Clinical Research Institute, HUS Helsinki University Hospital and Helsinki University, Helsinki, Finland

6.2 Diagnosing Pulmonary Embolism

Pulmonary embolism (PE) is a common disease with about 250,000 patients diagnosed each year in the USA. In spite of advanced technology, it remains a big diagnostic challenge because the clinical symptoms and signs that are frequently observed in pulmonary embolism are also a feature of other conditions. Accordingly, the initial clinical suspicion needs to be confirmed or negated using a conclusive imaging test. Routinely, computed tomography pulmonary angiography (CTPA) is suggested as the initial imaging study. However, the latest evidence shows that the optimal imaging procedure is V/P SPECT. Before imaging tests, it is recommended to estimate clinical probability that might be performed empirically or by clinical probability tests. Wells score is most frequently applied [3].

H. Ahmadzadehfar et al. (eds.), *Clinical Nuclear Medicine*,
https://doi.org/10.1007/978-3-030-39457-8_6

The measurement of D-dimer—a breakdown product of cross-linked fibrin clot—is widely used in the investigative workup of patients with suspected venous thromboembolism. However, D-dimer has a low specificity (40%) because a number of conditions, other than venous thromboembolism, may cause it to be elevated, e.g. acute myocardial infarction, stroke, inflammation, active cancer and pregnancy. The specificity declines even further with age and, in the elderly, may reach only 10%. Due to the low predictive value, a positive quantitative D-dimer test does not modify the pretest probability. A negative quantitative D-dimer test combined with a low clinical probability is associated with a low risk of thromboembolic disease [4]. At moderate to high pretest clinical probability, D-dimer has no incremental value.

6.3 Basic Principles of Pulmonary Embolism Diagnosis with V/P SPECT

The lung circulation has a distinct architecture where each bronchopulmonary segment and sub-segment is supplied by a single end-artery. Emboli are usually multiple, occluding the arteries causing segmental or sub-segmental perfusion defects within still ventilated regions, causing so-called mismatch (Fig. 6.1). PE is often a recurring process giving rise to multiple emboli in various stages of resolution (Fig. 6.2).

In clinical practice, it is essential to have a procedure that is both fast and conclusive to avoid the risks associated with untreated disease. Therefore it is recommended that imaging tests

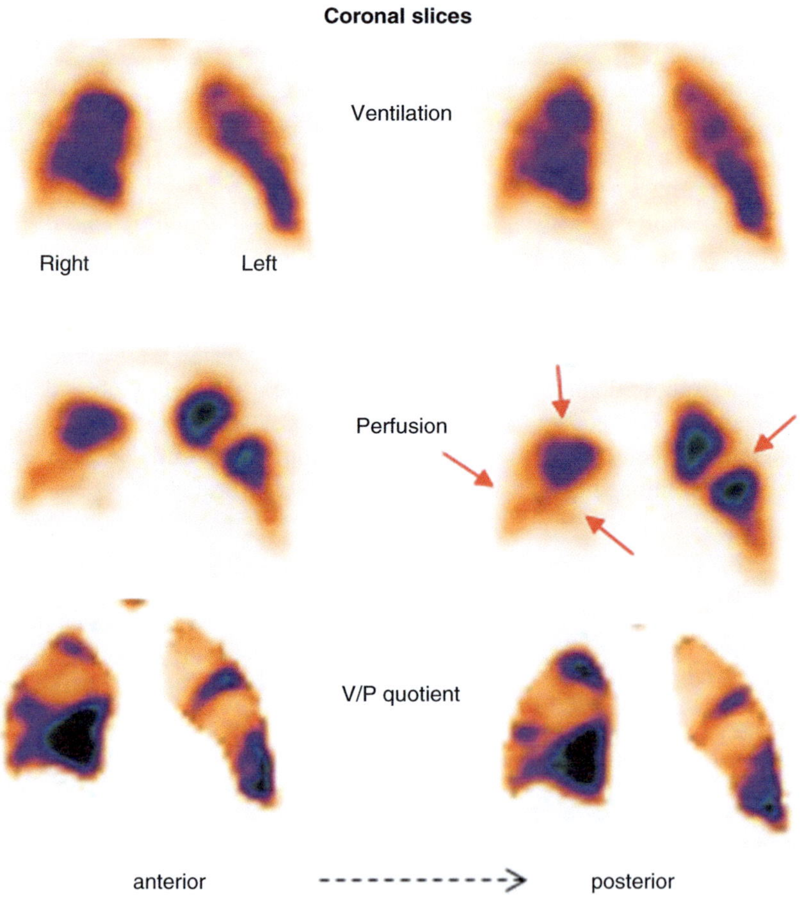

Fig. 6.1 Patient with PE. Coronal slices; multiple bilateral segmental perfusion defects (PE, red arrows) in areas with normal ventilation. These are delineated on V/P quotient images which facilitate interpretation

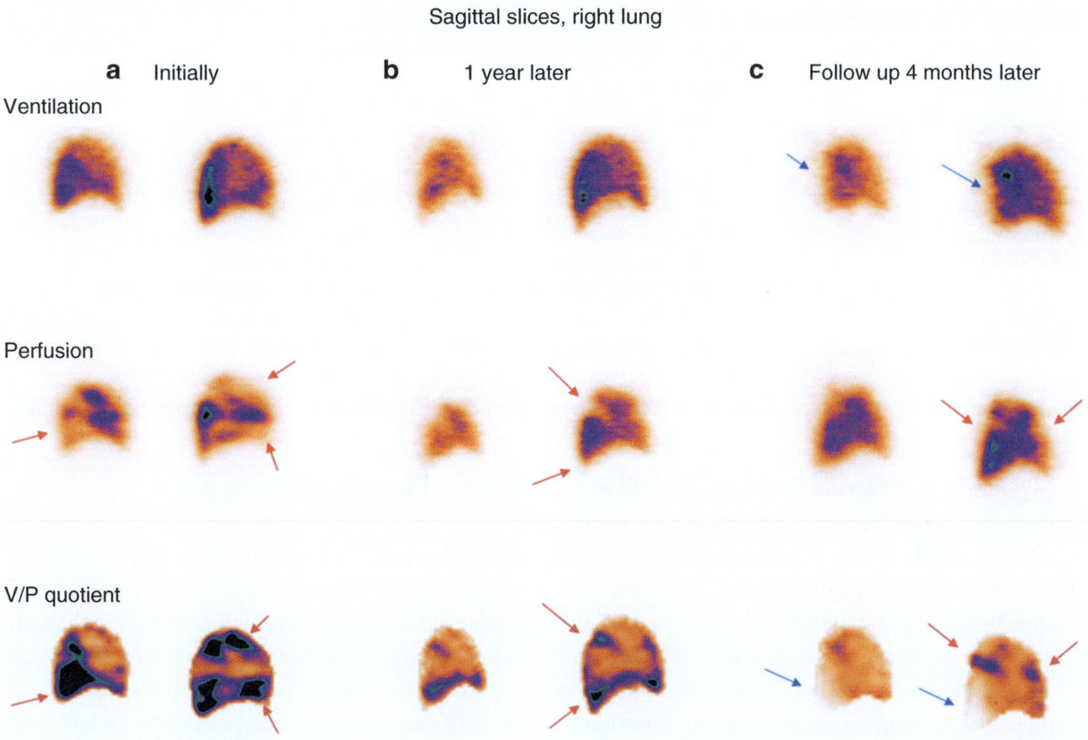

Fig. 6.2 Patient with recurrent PE and evolving comorbidity. Sagittal slices, right lung; (**a**) initially multiple perfusion segmental defects were observed (PE, red arrows); (**b**) 1 year after discontinuing therapy, patient experienced new symptoms. Perfusion defects were observed (red arrows). Hard to assess whether there were new defects or they represent rest after earlier PE. Patient started treatment again; (**c**) on follow-up 4 months later (under treatment), patient experienced new symptoms. The follow-up scan showed evolving ventilation defect (blue arrows) and improved perfusion defects (red arrows). Patient had developed pneumonia (blue arrows)

for PE diagnosis should be carried out as soon as possible, preferably within 24 h of the onset of symptoms.

6.4 Radiopharmaceuticals for V/P SPECT

6.4.1 Ventilation

Ventilation can be measured with the ^{99m}Tc-labelled aerosols, DTPA and Technegas®, or krypton gas (^{81m}Kr) (Table 6.1).

^{99m}Tc-DTPA (^{99m}Tc-diethylen-tetraamino-pentaacetate) is aerosolized from a water solution with a particle size of 1.2–2 μm. ^{99m}Tc-DTPA allows studies of alveolo-capillary permeability [5].

Technegas® is an aerosol of ^{99m}Tc-labelled solid graphite hydrophobic particles, with a diameter of about 0.005–0.09 μm [6]. The particles tend to grow by aggregation and should, therefore, be used within 10 min after generation [7]. The particle size is so small that the aerosol behaves nearly like a gas until it arrives at the periphery of the lung where the particles are deposited in bronchioli and alveoli, mostly by diffusion. For the ventilation imaging, Technegas® particles show advantages over radiolabelled liquid aerosols and are not restricted by the presence of obstructive lung disease [8]. Hotspots are nevertheless seen in patients with severe airway obstruction. The penetration index for Technegas® may be used for grading of COPD severity [9–11].

Table 6.1 Ventilation/perfusion protocol for lung tomography (V/P SPECT)

	Ventilation	Perfusion
Administration	Inhalation	i.v. injection
Radiopharmaceutical and administered activity	*Technegas®* 25–30 MBq to reach the lung	*^{99m}Tc-MAA* 120–160 MBq
Particle size	0.09 μm	15–100 μm
Time of imaging	Ca 11 min	Ca 5 min
Acquisition protocol	General-purpose collimator: 64 × 64 matrix 60–64 steps for each head 10 s/step	General-purpose collimator: 64 × 64 matrix 60–64 steps for each head 5 s/step
Reconstruction	Iterative reconstruction—Eight subsets and four iterations	Iterative reconstruction—Eight subsets and four iterations

Patient preparation is not needed. Patient is in the supine position during inhalation, i.v. injection and the acquisition

Krypton gas (^{81m}Kr) is an inert radioactive gas delivered from an ^{81}Rb/^{81m}Kr generator. ^{81m}Kr has a half-life of 13 s. ^{81m}Kr is inhaled until it reaches a steady-state activity in the alveoli and then continuously during the whole imaging procedure. Due to the higher gamma energy (190 keV) of ^{81m}Kr compared to ^{99m}Tc (140 keV), ventilation and perfusion images can be acquired simultaneously. Because elimination of ^{81m}Kr from the alveoli is largely due to decay of the isotope rather than by expiration, regional activity at steady state accurately represents regional ventilation. In COPD the inhalation time to reach steady state may, however, be too long to reach steady state. As the half-life of ^{81}Rb is only 4.6 h, the need for daily delivery of the expensive cyclotron-produced generator limits the clinical use of ^{81m}Kr.

6.4.2 Perfusion

For perfusion scintigraphy intravenously injected macroaggregates of ^{99m}Tc-labelled human albumin (MAA) with a diameter of 15–100 μm are nearly universally used. Intravenous injection of MAA leads to microembolization of pulmonary precapillary arterioles and capillaries. Whilst 60,000 particles may suffice to reflect regional perfusion [12], about 400,000 labelled particles are usually injected. This leads to obstruction of a very small fraction of pulmonary vessels. Injection of no more than 100,000–200,000 particles is recommended for children and for patients with known pulmonary hypertension and right-to-left heart shunt, and after single-lung transplantation.

6.5 Imaging Protocols

Administration of ventilation and perfusion agents should be performed with patients in a supine position to minimize gravitational gradients. During inhalation, activity over the lungs should be monitored to ensure adequacy of pulmonary deposition. The procedure starts with ventilation scintigraphy that is usually based upon inhalation of a radio-aerosol (Table 6.1).

Large particles (>2 μm) are deposited mainly by impaction in large airways. Very fine particles, <1 μm, are mainly deposited in alveoli by diffusion. In comparison with liquid aerosols, Technegas® shows significantly reduced problems of central airway deposition and peripheral hotspot formation in patients with obstructive lung disease. Therefore the use of Technegas® is recommended in COPD.

Perfusion tomography follows immediately after ventilation SPECT without changing the patient position. The nearly universally used agent for perfusion scintigraphy is technetium-labelled particles of macroaggregates of human albumin (^{99m}Tc-MAA). After i.v. injection, the particles of size 15–100 μm are lodged in the pulmonary capillaries and in the precapillary arterioles in proportion to perfusion.

To achieve adequate imaging quality with a low radiation exposure and in a short time, relationships between activities, acquisition times, collimators and matrices for SPECT imaging must be optimized. This problem was systematically analysed by Palmer et al. [13] in the context of a dual head gamma camera.

Doses of 25–30 MBq for ventilation studies and 120–160 MBq for perfusion studies were found optimal by using a general-purpose collimator and 64 × 64 matrix. A total acquisition time is about 20 min. If a matrix of 128 × 128 is used, then a higher dose and/or longer acquisition time is required. This is not promoted as it did not yield images of significantly higher quality.

Many centres are using much higher doses. To follow a good medical practice, radiation exposure should be minimized to the lowest level consistent with satisfactory image quality. For V/P SPECT it is essential to use iterative reconstruction.

For quality control and fast orientation, an overview of ventilation and perfusion in coronal and sagittal slices is useful. It is important to present the images so that ventilation and perfusion are carefully aligned to each other (Fig. 6.3). This is greatly facilitated by the one-session protocol with the patient in unchanged position. The option to triangulate between coronal, sagittal and transverse slices is valuable for identification of matching and non-matching ventilation and perfusion changes. Proper alignment is also a prerequisite for V/P quotient images. These facilitate the interpretation and quantification of PE extension and all ventilation and perfusion defects. However, quotient images are not prerequisite for high-quality V/P SPECT.

6.6 Reporting Findings

6.6.1 Ventilation/Perfusion Patterns

For V/P SPECT, interpretation criteria are as important as the imaging technique itself. According to European guideline, all patterns of V and P as well as numbers of defects are described, and clinical probability is taken into account [14]. This holistic principle for reporting gives also a clear answer: yes or no for pulmonary embolism. This goal was not achieved with previous probabilistic reporting methods according to PIOPED (Prospective Investigation of Pulmonary Embolism Diagnosis) study or modified PIOPED. Large V/P SPECT studies have shown that interpretation of all patterns representing ventilation together with perfusion achieves this result. Conclusive reports were given in 97–99% of cases [15–19].

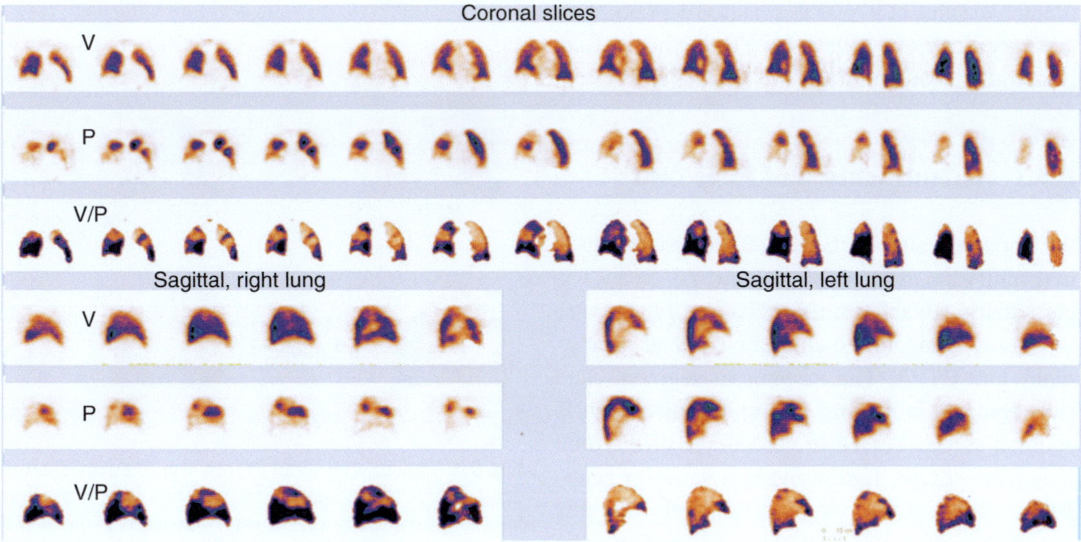

Fig. 6.3 Overview image of ventilation and perfusion in coronal and sagittal slices. Ventilation and perfusion are carefully aligned to each other

6.6.2 Criteria for Acute Pulmonary Embolism

Recommended criteria for reading V/P SPECT with respect to acute pulmonary embolism are the following:

- *Pulmonary embolism* is reported if there is V/P mismatch of at least one segment or two sub-segments that conforms to the pulmonary vascular anatomy.
- *No pulmonary embolism* is reported if there is (a) normal perfusion pattern conforming to the anatomic boundaries of the lungs matched or reversed mismatch V/P defects of any size, shape or number in the absence of mismatch and (b) mismatch that does not have a lobar, segmental or sub-segmental pattern.
- *Non-diagnostic for pulmonary embolism* is reported if there are multiple V/P abnormalities not typical of specific diseases.

It is important to report that with pulmonary embolism, a mismatch has its base along the pleura and conforms to known sub-segmental and segmental vascular anatomy. Applying these principles of interpretation, recent V/P SPECT studies amounting to over 5000 cases reported a negative predictive value of 97–99%, sensitivity of 96–99% and specificity of 91–98% for PE diagnosis. Rate of non-diagnostic findings was 1–3% [20].

6.6.3 Quantification of PE Extent

An important step in the diagnostic procedure is to quantify the extent of embolism. V/P SPECT is particularly suitable for this because of its greater sensitivity compared to alternative planar scintigraphy and CTPA. The number of segments and sub-segments indicating PE typical mismatch is counted and expressed in percentage of the total lung parenchyma. Furthermore, areas with ventilation abnormalities were recognized, and this allowed the degree of total lung malfunction to be estimated. The study showed that patients with up to 40% pulmonary embolism could be safely treated at home if ventilation abnormalities engaged not more that 20% of the lung [21]. Outpatient management in haemodynamically stable patients with pulmonary embolism is safe provided that the embolic burden, quantified using V/P SPECT, is included in the treatment decision algorithm. The extent of PE is an independent risk factor for PE recurrence [22–24]. In haemodynamically stable patients with PE, outpatient management is safe provided that the embolic burden, quantified using V/P SPECT, is included in the treatment decision algorithm [25].

6.7 Follow-Up

Knowledge about the natural history of PE is limited. There is a need to study alternative strategies for PE therapy, with respect to therapy duration and choice of drugs in different categories of patients. The issue of small emboli is particularly important, particularly regarding the treatment. Figure 6.4 presents a patient with untreated small

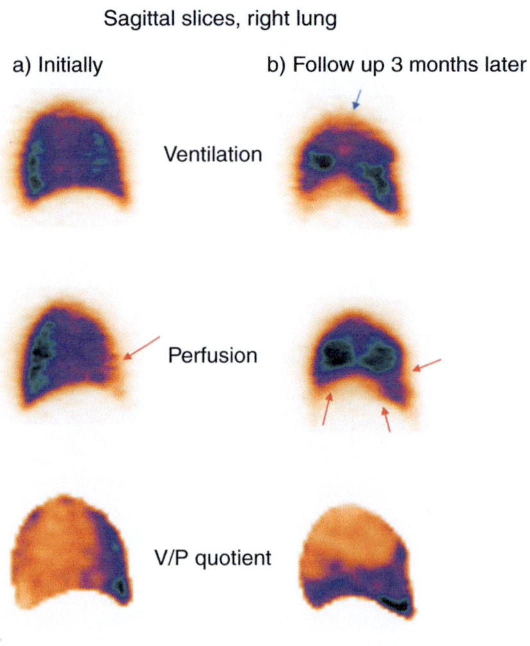

Fig. 6.4 Patient with small PE that was not treated developed chronic PE and pneumonia. Sagittal slice of the right lung showed initially a small perfusion defect in the medial lobe (PE, red arrow). This patient was not treated but was examined again 3 months later. On follow-up, the initial perfusion defect was more prominent, and perfusion defects were extended into the whole lower lobe. In addition, deterioration in the ventilation appeared apical segment. The patient also developed pneumonia (blue arrow)

PE who developed chronic PE after 3-month follow-up.

Follow-up of PE using imaging is essential to:

- Assess the effect of therapy.
- Differentiate between new and old PE when there is a suspicion of PE recurrence.
- Explain physical incapacity after PE.

Some patients have a tendency to develop recurrent episodes of PE. Figure 6.2 presents a patient with recurrent PE, shown by follow-up scans. Patient was treated initially for 6 months. One year after discontinuing therapy, patient experienced new symptoms. Perfusion defects were observed (Fig. 6.2b). Without the control scan after therapy was discontinued, it was hard to assess whether these defects were new or they represented rest after earlier PE. Patient started treatment again. Four months later, during the treatment, patient experienced new symptoms. The follow-up scan shows new ventilation defect (blue arrow) and improved perfusion. Reason for the patient's new symptoms was a pneumonia (Fig. 6.2c). Without initial and follow-up images, it is often impossible to differentiate between old and new PE. Immediate imaging control gives objective information about the further therapy decisions. Symptomatic patients with small emboli are diagnosed with sensitive methods, particularly V/P SPECT. Figure 6.5 presents a case with a PE in lingula and a pneumonia in the posterior part of the left lung. PE could not have been identified without SPECT and ventilation images. The natural history and the value of treatment in this group of patients is rather unknown. Follow-up is indicated to personalize therapy [21, 26–28].

Requirements on a method used for follow-up are:

- Applicability to all patients.
- Low radiation dose.
- High sensitivity to allow estimation of resolution of even small emboli and occurrence of new ones.

V/P SPECT seems ideally suited for use in the follow-up of PE because small and large emboli are recognized so that regression or progression of thrombotic disease can be studied in detail [21, 26–28]. Furthermore, the low radiation exposure enables repeated studies. Obviously, using the same method for diagnosis and follow-up is advantageous. Research in this area is particularly indicated.

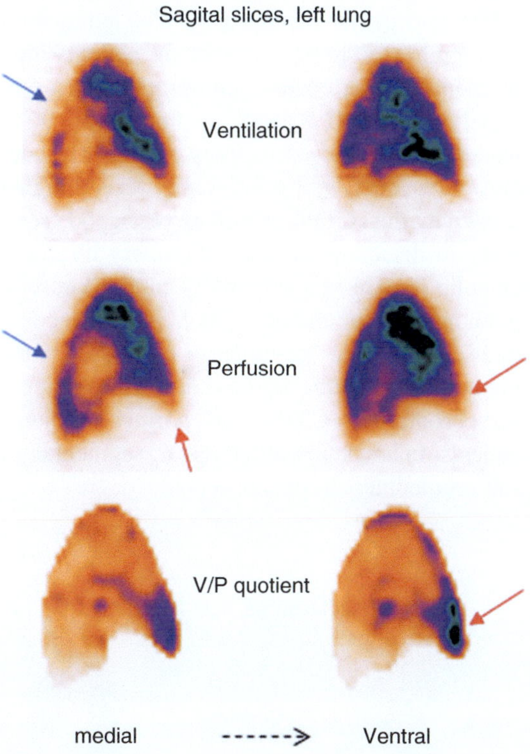

Fig. 6.5 Patient with PE and pneumonia. Sagittal slices of the left lung in a patient with perfusion defect in the lingula (red arrow). Stripe sign posteriorly seen on both ventilation and perfusion image (pneumonia, blue arrow)

6.8 Chronic Pulmonary Embolism

Chronic pulmonary embolism is a progressive disease that develops in about 1–5% after an acute episode of PE, even in treated patients. It might lead to pulmonary hypertension, right heart failure and arrhythmia, which are frequent causes of death. The value of V/P scintigraphy in this situation is well established. This has been confirmed in a head-to-head comparison between

CTPA and planar scintigraphy with pulmonary angiography as reference. Among patients with pulmonary hypertension, scintigraphy had a sensitivity of 96–97% and specificity of 90%, whereas CTPA had a sensitivity of 51%. The conclusion was that V/P scintigraphy "has a higher sensitivity than CTPA as well as very good specificity in detecting chronic pulmonary thromboembolic disease as a potentially curable cause of pulmonary hypertension" [29]. Scintigraphic features of chronic pulmonary embolism vary. Figure 6.6 illustrates one case of a typical pattern for chronic PE. CTPA was normal. In some patients mismatch without clear segmental or sub-segmental pattern is observed.

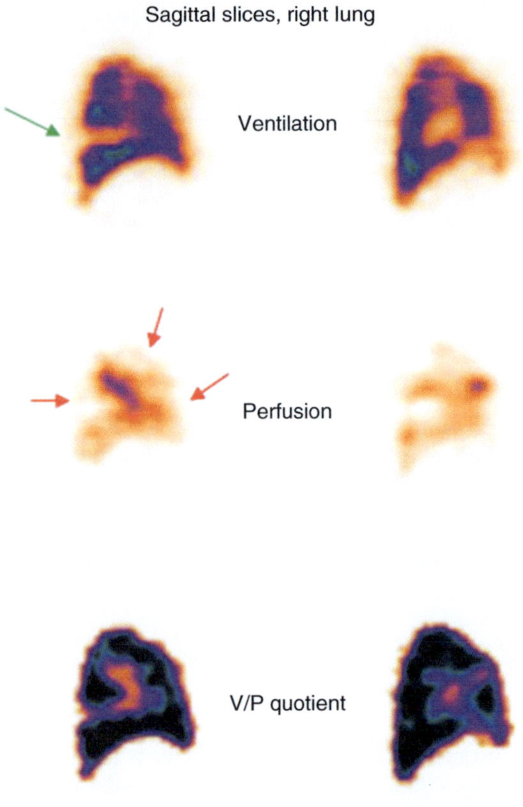

Fig. 6.6 Patient with chronic pulmonary embolism. Sagittal slices of the right lung: uneven ventilation with ventilation/perfusion defect posterior (lung infarct, green arrow). Perfusion images show preserved perfusion only in the central part of the lung. Perfusion defects (red arrows) around the lung, well delineated on quotient images

6.9 CTPA

Computed tomography angiography of the pulmonary artery (CTPA) is imaging of the pulmonary arteries during the passage of intravenously injected iodinated contrast material. Pulmonary emboli are visualized as so-called filling defects caused by emboli within otherwise homogenously contrast-filled pulmonary arteries. CTPA is easy to perform in a few minutes. CTPA needs to be embedded in decision strategies that are based on the assessment of clinical PE likelihood [30]. CTPA confirms the diagnosis of PE in clinically high probability patients (PPV > 95%). In case of high pretest probability of PE and a negative CTPA, current data on diagnostic accuracy are inconsistent [31–33]; CTPA is overused in a great number of patients with low prevalence of PE [34, 35]. A PE located centrally in the pulmonary circulation can be detected by CTPA with a high positive predictive value. The positive predictive value decreases at segmental and subsegmental levels [33]. When clinical probability of PE is low or intermediate, CTPA may overdiagnose PE, leading to a low negative predictive value [33].

CTPA has the potential to visualize additional pathologies other than PE such as pneumothorax, pneumonia, interstitial lung disease, pleural disease, aortic dissection and pathologies of the spine and rib cage [36–38].

6.10 Sensitivity and Specificity of V/P SPECT and CT in Diagnosis of PE

CTPA is often recommended as the first-line test for PE diagnosis. However, the principal study evaluating the use of CTPA as an imaging tool for PE diagnosis shows that sensitivity is not more than 78% and that there is a high number of false-positive results when clinical probability is not high [33]. The positive predictive value for a PE within a lobar pulmonary artery was 97% but fell to 68% and 25% in segmental and sub-segmental pulmonary vessels, respectively [33]. PIOPED II confirmed that CT has important limitations with respect to applicability: sensitivity and specificity are low in large number of patients, even if pretest probability is taken into account. The authors concluded: "The false negative rate for CTA alone indicates the need for additional information to rule out PE". The absolute gain by adding venous-phase imaging combination was also modest. The authors concluded "the false negative rate for CTA alone indicates the need for additional information to rule out PE" [39].

The sensitivity of V/P SPECT was tested in a porcine model using latex emboli, labelled with ^{201}Tl to enable precise localization of the emboli that were 2.2–3.7 mm in diameter and caused only sub-segmental defects. For the planar technique, sensitivity and specificity were 67% and 80% and for SPECT 93% and 94%, respectively [40]. Angiography and CTPA had sensitivities of 87% and 82%, respectively, for emboli sized about 4 mm when a methacrylate cast of the porcine pulmonary vessels was used as the independent standard and when CTPA was performed under apnoea that is often not possible in the clinic [41]. Therefore angiography as the gold standard can be misleading. In summary, animal studies indicate that V/P SPECT has a sensitivity superior to scintigraphic planar technique, angiography and CTPA.

6.11 Pregnancy

Pregnancy poses unique circumstances in diagnosing PE: The incidence of PE in pregnancy is about fivefold higher than in nonpregnant females of a similar age and is the leading non-obstetric cause of death during pregnancy in developed countries.

V/P SPECT is a recommended method by EANM and SNM guidelines [42–44, 14].

To minimize radiation, a 2-day protocol is recommended. Perfusion-only SPECT is performed on day 1, with only 50 MBq 99mTc-MAA. Because of the low incidence of pulmonary disorders in pregnant women, PE is usually excluded based on a normal perfusion pattern. In case of an abnormal perfusion pattern, anticoagulation therapy can be started until a ventilation study is performed on day 2, using a lung deposited activity of 20–30 MBq. This strategy leads to a high sensitivity and specificity of the examination [9, 10] [45]. After the first trimester, the standard 1-day V/P SPECT protocol may be considered.

D-dimer is not useful because it is elevated during pregnancy [46]. CTPA has a high rate of non-diagnostic tests due to changed haemodynamics; increased blood volume and cardiac output shortens the arrival time of intravenous contrast in the pulmonary vessels, necessitating adjustments in triggered scan delays. Non-diagnostic CTPA scans occur in 6–36% of patients, whilst alternative diagnoses were identified in 2–13% [9, 10, 45, 47].

CTPA leads to unique radiation hazards to the maternal breast.

6.12 Radiation Doses

Following the good clinical practice, it is important to minimize radiation exposure without sacrificing image quality and diagnostic accuracy.

Based upon data from ICRP reports [48], the effective dose for V/P SPECT with the recommended protocol is 2 mSv. In a systematic review and meta-analysis of literature, radiation exposure was 2.12 mSv for V/P SPECT per correct diagnosis compared with 4.96 mSv for CTPA [49]. In clinical routine, radiation doses between 3.5 and 13.2 mSv have been reported for CTPA [50–52]. In general, higher effective doses (>5 mSv) are reported from automatically collected data [53–55].

The most critical organ in CTPA is the female breast. Absorbed radiation doses to the female breast ranging from 8.6 to 44 mSv have been reported [56–58]. Tube current modulation is able to decrease the breast dose from 51.5 mSv to 8.6 mSv [58], whilst shielding is less effective [59]. Absorbed radiation dose to the female breast from V/P SPECT is <1 mSv [56]. Fetal-absorbed doses for V/P SPECT and CTPA are similar and so small that they are unlikely to be clinically significant [45, 56, 57].

6.13 Clinical Use of Hybrid V/P SPECT/CT

The Hybrid SPECT/CT System Is a Dual Imaging Modality Technique. Its Clinical Application Is Particularly Relevant in Oncological Diseases as it Leads to Improved Sensitivity and Specificity, Combining Co-Registration of Anatomical and Functional Data. It May Lead to Improved Staging and Treatment Monitoring. As Nuclear Medicine Procedures Have the Ability to Visualize Early Functional Changes Much sooner than Structural Changes Occur, Additional CT Procedure May Improve Correction for Photon Attenuation and Allow Co-Registration of Morphology and Function. However, SPECT/CT Acquisition of the Chest Constitutes a Challenge Due to Respiratory Movements, which Can Cause Image Artefacts and Thus Decrease Diagnostic Accuracy

The procedure starts with CT overview image and continues with diagnostic low-dose CT, (120 kV, 20 mAs/slice, 16 × 1.5 collimator, 0.5-s rotation time and pitch of 0.813) not used for attenuation correction but to exactly co-localize the morphological and functional changes visualized in either of the two modalities (Table 6.2). Thereafter follows the protocol for V/P SPECT as described above and according to the European guideline [42, 43 14]. Low-dose CT delivers approximately 1 mSv when used for alignment and attenuation correction. However, as a diagnostic tool in this hybrid system, it delivers 2–3 mSv and V/P SPECT 2 mSv.

Some authors have recently recommended V/P SPECT/low-dose CT as a first-line procedure in patients with suspected PE. This was based on their prospective study performing V/P SPECT and low-dose CT and making head-to-head comparison with CTPA [60]. In a total of 81 simultaneous studies, 38% of patients had PE. They showed 97% sensitivity and 88% specificity when only V/P SPECT was used. However, adding low-dose CT, the sensitivity was unchanged but specificity increased to 100%. Interestingly 18% of patients had false-positive PE diagnosis when V/P SPECT alone was interpreted [60]. A reason for this may be that they were interpreting every mismatch as PE and not only mismatches that conform to segmental lung circulation as recommended by European guideline [42, 43 14].

In our opinion, V/P SPECT is a primary tool in patients with suspected PE. Since 2003, more than 20,000 examinations have been performed. Based on our experience, we do not recommend hybrid V/P SPECT/CT as a first-line procedure for all patients with suspected PE. We recognize an ethical problem in advocating higher radiation dose (2–3 mSv) CT study in addition to V/P SPECT for every patient with suspected PE when prevalence of PE is about 30% in our experience and might be as low as 10% [61]. Following the good clinical practice recommendation to use a hybrid system for PE diagnosis is premature [62]. CT utilization has increased dramatically in the evaluation of patients with suspected PE without improving rate of PE or other clinically significant diagnoses [63]. Therefore, it is important to validate the V/P SPECT/CT system and to assess the benefits and risks [63–65]

We consider, however, that the dual modality will have impact in some groups of patients.

SPECT/CT may provide adding value to COPD patients showing morphological changes in addition to functional defects, particularly in visualizing small tumours. Figure 6.7 presents a patient with COPD, small tumour and LHF [66].

Pitfalls exist both with respect to imaging technique and scan interpretation.

Table 6.2 V/P SPECT/CT Protocol

CT overview image				
	Tube potential	Tube current	Collimation/slice width	Pitch
Low-dose CT	120 kV	20 mAs	16 × 1.5–0.5 s rotation	0.813

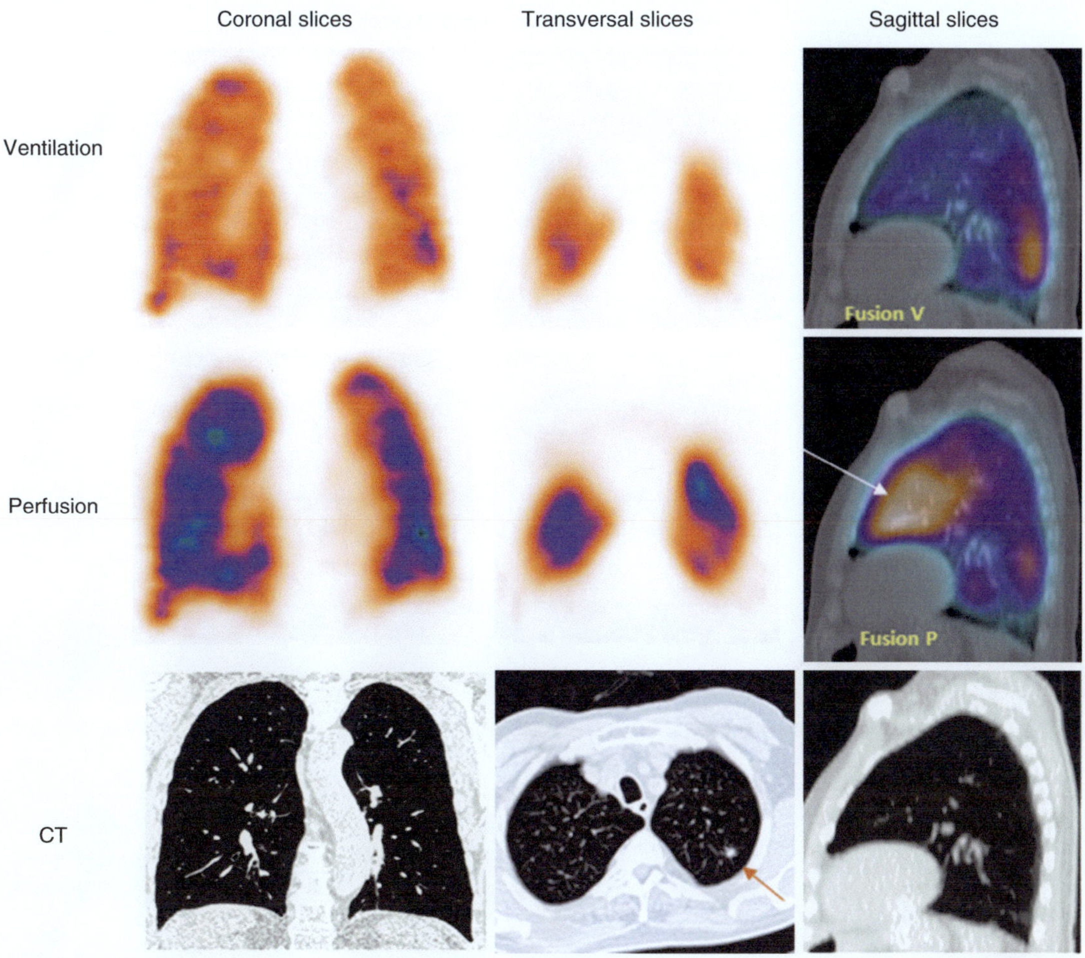

Fig. 6.7 Patient with COPD, small tumour and left heart failure. Coronal and transversal slices of ventilation and perfusion SPECT image: On the right, corresponding sagittal V/P SPECT/CT fusion images. In the lower row, corresponding CT images. On CT image small tumour (1 cm) is visualized (red arrow). Aligning both modalities small perfusion defect is observed in this area. On perfusion SPECT antigravitational redistribution of perfusion is visualized, representing LHF (white arrow) not visible on CT nor on ventilation (non-segmental mismatch)

6.14 Role of Ventilation SPECT in Diagnosis of Other Lung Diseases

6.14.1 Chronic Obstructive Pulmonary Disease (COPD)

COPD is frequently observed in patients suspected for PE, because COPD patients are at high risk of pulmonary embolism [15, 27, 28, 67]. The rate of PE in patients hospitalized for acute exacerbation of COPD may be as high as 25%. Pulmonary embolism accounts for up to 10% of deaths in stable COPD patients. Different from PIOPED study, PE can be diagnosed even in the presence of COPD with V/P SPECT [67].

The characteristic of COPD is a general unevenness of ventilation. Focal deposition of aerosol in central or peripheral airways may even locate sites of airway obstruction [68]. The degree of unevenness of aerosol distribution correlates with lung function tests [9, 10, 69, 70]. In healthy subjects, even distribution of Technegas® with good peripheral penetration and without accumulation in large or small airways is observed (Fig. 6.8). The grading of obstruction in

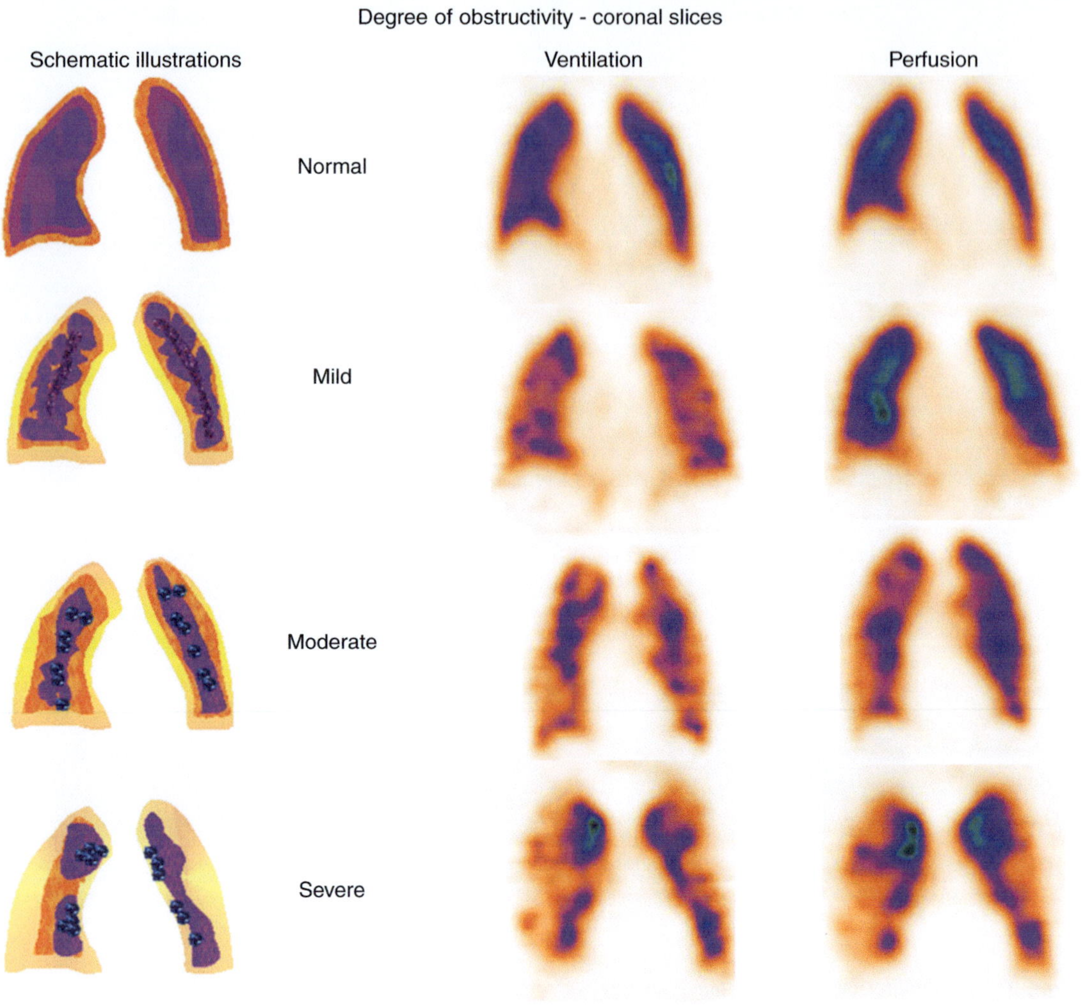

Fig. 6.8 Degree of airway obstruction. Coronal slices: schematic presentation of the obstructive lung disease grading system in the left column. In the middle and the right column, typical V/P SPECT images that show different degrees of airway obstruction

ventilation SPECT has been standardized using Technegas® VSPECT [9, 10]:

- Grade 1: Mild airway obstruction, slightly uneven distribution with some deposition of Technegas® in small and intermediate airways. Only minor areas with reduced peripheral penetration are observed.
- Grade 2: Moderate airway obstruction, deposition of Technegas® in intermediate and large airways, diminished peripheral penetration with maximum accumulation in the central half of the lung.
- Grade 3: Severe airway obstruction, central deposition in large airways with severely impaired penetration of Technegas® and major areas with reduced or abolished function.

V/P SPECT has a high sensitivity to show an obstructive pattern in the lungs of many apparently healthy smokers (work in progress).

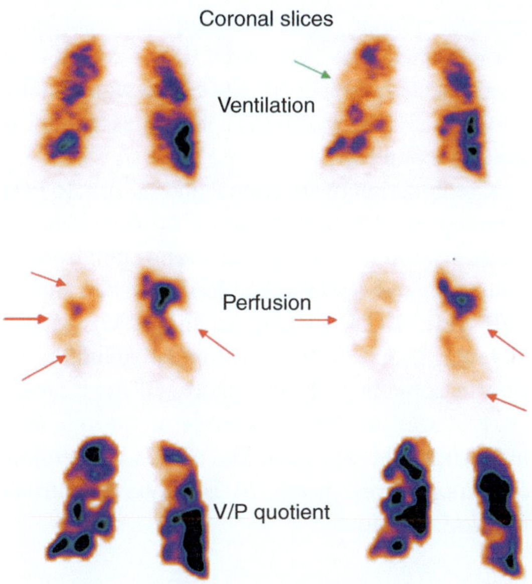

Fig. 6.9 Patient with severe COPD, massive PE and emphysema. Coronal slices: uneven distribution of ventilation with central deposition of aerosols indicating severe degree of airway obstruction. In the right upper lobe is area with reduced/absent ventilation and perfusion (emphysema, green arrow). Corresponding perfusion images (middle row) show multiple segmental perfusion defects in the ventilated areas (PE, red arrows) well delineated on V/P quotient image

V/P SPECT gives the possibility to localize ventilation and perfusion impairment and also estimate the total lung function [71]. It is noteworthy that there are no contraindications to V/P SPECT and that even very sick and breathless patients can be studied. Figure 6.9 shows coronal slices in a patient with a severe COPD, massive PE and emphysema.

6.14.2 Pneumonia

Pneumonia is also a frequent finding in patients investigated for suspected PE (Figs. 6.2, 6.4, and 6.5). Pneumonia is here a general term for conditions of lung inflammation, often caused by a bacterial, viral or fungal infection, where blood biomarkers are not sufficient for diagnosing pneumonia and unspecific clinical symptoms can lead to diagnostic problems [72, 73].

In pneumonia, V/P SPECT shows ventilation defects that usually exceed perfusion defects known as reverse mismatch (reversed V/P mismatch) [74, 75]. Preserved perfusion along the pleural border peripheral to a central matched defect recognized as the "stripe sign" is a specific sign of pneumonia (Fig. 6.5) [76]. In a recent study, following patients with PE and pneumonia clinically and with V/P SPECT, reversed mismatched or matched V/P defects typical for pneumonia were confirmed [27, 28]. Dyspnoea was a common symptom in these patients. It can be caused by pneumonia as well as by PE or COPD. In some patients, V/P defects typical for pneumonia reduce the total lung function in the absence of any morphological CT changes. Frequently, pneumonia is comorbid with PE (Figs. 6.2, 6.4, and 6.5). In these clinical scenarios, PE is frequently missed by CT [9, 10, 77]. This is important information because in general, current clinical and nuclear medicine practices do not recognize nor use V/P SPECT as a potential imaging method to diagnose or manage pneumonia.

6.14.3 Left Heart Failure

Antigravitational perfusion distribution from posterior to anterior region indicates pulmonary congestion. The pattern was described already in 1966 [78] and studied later [27, 28, 79–82]. As ventilation is usually less affected, the typical pattern is antigravitational redistribution of perfusion and V/P mismatch in dorsal regions of the lung. This V/P mismatch has a non-segmental pattern (does not conform pulmonary vascular architecture) and should not be misinterpreted as pulmonary embolism (Fig. 6.10). The positive predictive value ≥88% for heart failure has been observed [81]. The power of V/P SPECT for diagnosis of heart failure was recently confirmed against right heart catheterization [80].

6.14.4 Preoperative Evaluation of Lung Function

The assessment of lung function is essential for planning and predicting the outcomes of surgery such as lung volume reduction surgery and in

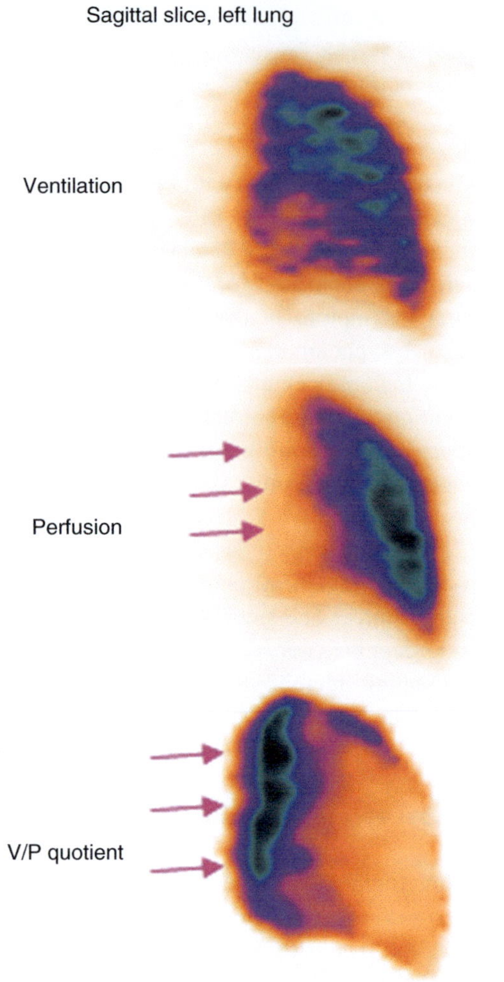

Fig. 6.10 Patient with left heart failure. Sagittal slices from the left lung show antigravitational redistribution of perfusion (purple arrows). Ventilation is less affected causing mismatch. Mind the pattern; it is not of segmental character

patients with lung tumour or lung transplantation.

Previously, planar lung scintigraphy was applied for this purpose measuring ventilation and perfusion from geometrical mean of anterior and posterior projection using the whole lung and upper middle and lower zone. Today, V/P SPECT is recommended because it allows quantitative measurement of ventilation and perfusion and a better evaluation of the regional lung function reserve. Planar and tomographic techniques allow comparable assessment of the whole lung function. However, V/P SPECT is significantly better than planar scintigraphy to assess lobar lung function [83].

Combination of functional and morphological imaging by V/P SPECT and CT offers a better identification of malignancy and emphysema than using only one method [66]. The new hybrid V/P SPECT/CT imaging technique has shown advantages in predicting postoperative lung function in patients with non-small cell lung cancer [84] as well as the assessment of the outcome after chemotherapy [85]. The area is challenging and more work needs to be done to further develop techniques.

6.15 Conclusion

Ventilation/perfusion SPECT (V/P SPECT) is the recommended scintigraphic technique for the diagnosis of pulmonary embolism (PE) and many other disorders that affect lung function. Moreover, according to European Association of Nuclear Medicine guideline, it should be the preferred modality whenever possible for the diagnosis of PE because it has the highest sensitivity and accuracy and neither contraindications nor complications. It produces very few non-diagnostic reports, and radiation doses are low. This is particularly important for women in the reproductive period and during pregnancy [9, 10]. Furthermore, full use should be made of display options, which are integrated in modern camera systems. Holistic interpretation is the most important strategy for V/P SPECT, giving a clear report with respect to PE, its extension as well as other diagnoses based on V/P patterns typical for various diseases. Interpretation is based upon all relevant clinical information about the patient and all V/P patterns. The abovementioned advantages of V/P SPECT for studying PE imply that it may be the most suitable technique both for follow-up in patients with PE and for research regarding treatment and pathophysiology of PE.

References

1. Wagner HN, Sabiston DC, McAfee JG, et al. Diagnosis of massive pulmonary embolism in man by radioisotope scanning. N Engl J Med. 1964;271(8):377–84.
2. Tow DE, Wagner HN, Lopez- Majano V. Validity of measuring regional pulmonarya arterial blood flow With macroaggregates Of human serum albumin. Am J Roentgenol. 1966;96(3):664–76.
3. Lucassen W, Geersing GJ, Erkens PM, et al. Clinical decision rules for excluding pulmonary embolism: a meta-analysis. Ann Intern Med. 2011;155(7):448–60.
4. Konstantinides S, Torbicki A. Management of venous thrombo-embolism: an update. Eur Heart J. 2014;35:2855.
5. Evander E, Wollmer P, Valind S, et al. Biexponential pulmonary clearance of 99mTc-DTPA induced by detergent aerosol. J Appl Physiol (1985). 1994;77(1):190–6.
6. Burch WM, Tetley IJ, Gras JL. Technetium-99m 'pseudogas' for diagnostic studies in the lung. Clin Phys Physiol Meas. 1984;5(2):79–85.
7. Lemb M, Oei TH, Eifert H, Gunther B. Technegas: a study of particle structure, size and distribution. Eur J Nucl Med. 1993;20(7):576–9.
8. Jogi J, Jonson B, Ekberg M, Bajc M. Ventilation-perfusion SPECT with 99mTc-DTPA versus Technegas: a head-to-head study in obstructive and nonobstructive disease. J Nucl Med. 2010;51:735.
9. Bajc M, Markstad H, Jarenback L, et al. Grading obstructive lung disease using tomographic pulmonary scintigraphy in patients with chronic obstructive pulmonary disease (COPD) and long-term smokers. Ann Nucl Med. 2015a;29(1):91–9.
10. Bajc M, Olsson B, Gottsater A, et al. V/P SPECT as a diagnostic tool for pregnant women with suspected pulmonary embolism. Eur J Nucl Med Mol Imaging. 2015b;42(8):1325–30.
11. Jögi J, Ekberg M, Jonson B, et al. Ventilation/perfusion SPECT in chronic obstructive pulmonary disease: an evaluation by reference to symptoms, spirometric lung function and emphysema, as assessed with HRCT. Eur J Nucl Med Mol Imaging. 2011;38(7):1344–52.
12. Heck LL, Duley JW Jr. Statistical considerations in lung imaging with 99mTc albumin particles. Radiology. 1974;113(3):675–9.
13. Palmer J, Bitzen U, Jonson B, Bajc M. Comprehensive ventilation/perfusion SPECT. J Nucl Med. 2001;42(8):1288–94.
14. Bajc M, Schümichen C, Grüning T, et al. EANM guideline for ventilation/perfusion single-photon emission computed tomography (SPECT) for diagnosis of pulmonary embolism and beyond. European Eur J Nucl Med Mol Imag. 2019;46(12):2429–51.
15. Bajc M, Olsson B, Palmer J, Jonson B. Ventilation/perfusion SPECT for diagnostics of pulmonary embolism in clinical practice. J Intern Med. 2008;264(4):379–87.
16. Gruning T, Drake BE, Farrell SL, Nokes T. Three-year clinical experience with VQ SPECT for diagnosing pulmonary embolism: diagnostic performance. Clin Imaging. 2014;38:831–5.
17. Le Duc-Pennec A, Le Roux PY, Cornily JC, et al. Diagnostic accuracy of single-photon emission tomography ventilation/perfusion lung scan in the diagnosis of pulmonary embolism. Chest. 2012;141(2):381–7.
18. Le Roux PY, Palard X, Robin P, et al. Safety of ventilation/perfusion single photon emission computed tomography for pulmonary embolism diagnosis. Eur J Nucl Med Mol Imaging. 2014;41(10):1957–64.
19. Leblanc M, Leveillee F, Turcotte E. Prospective evaluation of the negative predictive value of V/Q SPECT using 99mTc-Technegas. Nucl Med Commun. 2007;28(8):667–72.
20. Kan Y, Yuan L, Meeks JK, et al. The accuracy of V/Q SPECT in the diagnosis of pulmonary embolism: a meta-analysis. Acta Radiol. 2015;56(5):565–72.
21. Olsson CG, Bitzen U, Olsson B, et al. Outpatient tinzaparin therapy in pulmonary embolism quantified with ventilation/perfusion scintigraphy. Med Sci Monit. 2006;12(2):PI9–13.
22. Alhadad A, Miniati M, Alhadad H, et al. The value of tomographic ventilation/perfusion scintigraphy (V/PSPECT) for follow-up and prediction of recurrence in pulmonary embolism. Thromb Res. 2012;130(6):877–81.
23. Couturaud F. Guided duration of anticoagulation after unprovoked venous thromboembolism using D-dimer testing. Eur Respir J. 2016;47(5):1313–4.
24. Couturaud F, Sanchez O, Pernod G, et al. Six months vs extended oral anticoagulation after a first episode of pulmonary embolism: the PADIS-PE randomized clinical trial. JAMA. 2015;314(1):31–40.
25. Elf JE, Jogi J, Bajc M. Home treatment of patients with small to medium sized acute pulmonary embolism. J Thromb Thrombolysis. 2015;39(2):166–72.
26. Begic A, Jogi J, Hadziredzepovic A, et al. Tomographic ventilation/perfusion lung scintigraphy in the monitoring of the effect of treatment in pulmonary embolism: serial follow-up over a 6-month period. Nucl Med Commun. 2011;32(6):508–14.
27. Begic A, Opankovic E, Cukic V, et al. Ancillary findings assessed by ventilation/perfusion tomography. Impact and clinical outcome in patients with suspected pulmonary embolism. Nuklearmedizin. 2015a;54(5):223–30.
28. Begic A, Opankovic E, Cukic V, et al. Impact of ventilation/perfusion single-photon emission computed tomography on treatment duration of pulmonary embolism. Nucl Med Commun. 2015b;36(2):162–7.
29. Tunariu N, Gibbs SJ, Win Z, et al. Ventilation-perfusion scintigraphy is more sensitive than multidetector CTPA in detecting chronic thromboembolic pulmonary disease as a treatable cause of pulmonary hypertension. J Nucl Med. 2007;48(5):680–4.

30. Konstantinides SV, Torbicki A, Agnelli G, et al. 2014 ESC guidelines on the diagnosis and management of acute pulmonary embolism. Eur Heart J. 2014;35(43):3033–69. 3069a–k
31. Moores L, Kline J, Portillo AK, et al. Multidetector computed tomographic pulmonary angiography in patients with a high clinical probability of pulmonary embolism. J Thromb Haemost. 2016;14(1):114–20.
32. Robert-Ebadi H, Glauser F, Planquette B, et al. Safety of multidetector computed tomography pulmonary angiography to exclude pulmonary embolism in patients with a likely pretest clinical probability. J Thromb Haemost. 2017;15(8):1584–90.
33. Stein PD, Fowler SE, Goodman LR, et al. Multidetector computed tomography for acute pulmonary embolism. N Engl J Med. 2006;354(22):2317–27.
34. Feng LB, Pines JM, Yusuf HR, Grosse SD. U.S. trends in computed tomography use and diagnoses in emergency department visits by patients with symptoms suggestive of pulmonary embolism, 2001–2009. Acad Emerg Med. 2013;20(10):1033–40.
35. Hutchinson BD, Navin P, Marom EM, et al. Overdiagnosis of pulmonary embolism by pulmonary CT angiography. AJR Am J Roentgenol. 2015;205(2):271–7.
36. Becattini C, Agnelli G, Germini F, Vedovati MC. Computed tomography to assess risk of death in acute pulmonary embolism: a meta-analysis. Eur Respir J. 2014;43(6):1678–90.
37. Meinel FG, Nance JW Jr, Schoepf UJ, et al. Predictive value of computed tomography in acute pulmonary embolism: systematic review and meta-analysis. Am J Med. 2015;128(7):747–59.e2.
38. Stein PD, Matta F, Sedrick JA, et al. Ancillary findings on CT pulmonary angiograms and abnormalities on chest radiographs in patients in whom pulmonary embolism was excluded. Clin Appl Thromb Hemost. 2012;18(2):201–5.
39. Perrier A, Bounameaux H. Accuracy or outcome in suspected pulmonary embolism. N Engl J Med. 2006;354(22):2383–5.
40. Bajc M, Bitzen U, Olsson B, et al. Lung ventilation/perfusion SPECT in the artificially embolized pig. J Nucl Med. 2002;43(5):640–7.
41. Baile EM, King GG, Muller NL, et al. Spiral computed tomography is comparable to angiography for the diagnosis of pulmonary embolism. Non-invasive diagnosis of venous thromboembolism in outpatients. Am J Respir Crit Care Med. 2000;161(3 Pt 1):1010–5.
42. Bajc M, Neilly JB, Miniati M, et al. EANM guidelines for ventilation/perfusion scintigraphy: part 1. Pulmonary imaging with ventilation/perfusion single photon emission tomography. Eur J Nucl Med Mol Imaging. 2009a;36(8):1356–70.
43. Bajc M, Neilly JB, Miniati M, et al. EANM guidelines for ventilation/perfusion scintigraphy: part 2. Algorithms and clinical considerations for diagnosis of pulmonary emboli with V/P(SPECT) and MDCT. Eur J Nucl Med Mol Imaging. 2009b;36(9):1528–38.
44. Waxman AD, Bajc M, Brown M, et al. Appropriate use criteria for ventilation-perfusion imaging in pulmonary embolism: summary and excerpts. J Nucl Med. 2017;58(5):13N–5N.
45. Gruning T, Mingo RE, Gosling MG, et al. Diagnosing venous thromboembolism in pregnancy. Br J Radiol. 2016;89(1062):20160021.
46. Sivandarajah S. Towards evidence-based emergency medicine: best BETs from the Manchester Royal Infirmary. BET 4: current evidence does not support the use of a negative D-dimer to rule out suspected pulmonary embolism in pregnancy. Emerg Med J. 2011;28(3):245–6.
47. Ridge CA, McDermott S, Freyne BJ, et al. Pulmonary embolism in pregnancy: comparison of pulmonary CT angiography and lung scintigraphy. AJR Am J Roentgenol. 2009;193(5):1223–7.
48. ICRP. Radiation dose to patients from radiopharmaceuticals, vol. 121. Oxford, NY: ICRP; 1988. publication 53
49. Phillips JJ, Straiton J, R. T. Staff. Planar and SPECT ventilation/perfusion imaging and computed tomography for the diagnosis of pulmonary embolism: a systematic review and meta-analysis of the literature, and cost and dose comparison. Eur J Radiol. 2015;84(7):1392–400.
50. Bucher AM, Kerl MJ, Albrecht MH, et al. Systematic comparison of reduced tube current protocols for high-pitch and standard-pitch pulmonary CT angiography in a large single-center population. Acad Radiol. 2016;23(5):619–27.
51. De Zordo T, von Lutterotti K, Dejaco C, et al. Comparison of image quality and radiation dose of different pulmonary CTA protocols on a 128-slice CT: high-pitch dual source CT, dual energy CT and conventional spiral CT. Eur Radiol. 2012;22(2):279–86.
52. Elbakri IA, Kirkpatrick IDC. Survey of clinical doses from computed tomography examinations in the Canadian province of Manitoba. Radiat Prot Dosim. 2013;157(4):525–35.
53. Liang CR, Chen PXH, Kapur J, et al. Establishment of institutional diagnostic reference level for computed tomography with automated dose-tracking software. J Med Radiat Sci. 2017;64(2):82–9.
54. MacGregor K, Li I, Dowdell T, Gray BG. Identifying institutional diagnostic reference levels for CT with radiation dose index monitoring software. Radiology. 2015;276(2):507–17.
55. Smith-Bindman R, Wang Y, Yellen-Nelson TR, et al. Predictors of CT radiation dose and their effect on patient care: a comprehensive analysis using automated data. Radiology. 2017;282(1):182–93.
56. Astani SA, Davis LC, Harkness BA, et al. Detection of pulmonary embolism during pregnancy: comparing radiation doses of CTPA and pulmonary scintigraphy. Nucl Med Commun. 2014;35(7):704–11.
57. Isidoro J, Gil P, Costa G, et al. Radiation dose comparison between V/P-SPECT and CT-angiography in the diagnosis of pulmonary embolism. Phys Med. 2017;41:93–6.

58. Sabarudin A, Mustafa Z, Nassir KM, et al. Radiation dose reduction in thoracic and abdomen-pelvic CT using tube current modulation: a phantom study. J Appl Clin Med Phys. 2014;16(1):5135.
59. Revel MP, Fitton I, Audureau E, et al. Breast dose reduction options during thoracic CT: influence of breast thickness. AJR Am J Roentgenol. 2015;204(4):W421–8.
60. Gutte H, Mortensen J, Jensen CV, et al. Detection of pulmonary embolism with combined ventilation-perfusion SPECT and low-dose CT: head-to-head comparison with multidetector CT angiography. J Nucl Med. 2009;50(12):1987–92.
61. Mamlouk MD, vanSonnenberg E, Gosalia R, et al. Pulmonary embolism at CT angiography: implications for appropriateness, cost, and radiation exposure in 2003 patients. Radiology. 2010;256(2):625–32.
62. Bajc M, Maffioli L, Miniati M. Good clinical practice in pulmonary embolism diagnosis: where do we stand today? Eur J Nucl Med Mol Imaging. 2014;41(2):333–6.
63. Coco AS, O'Gurek DT. Increased emergency department computed tomography use for common chest symptoms without clear patient benefits. J Am Board Fam Med. 2012;25(1):33–41.
64. Einstein AJ, Moser KW, Thompson RC, et al. Radiation dose to patients from cardiac diagnostic imaging. Circulation. 2007;116(11):1290–305.
65. Roche LM, Niu X, Pawlish KS, Henry KA. Thyroid cancer incidence in New Jersey: time trend, birth cohort and socioeconomic status analysis (1979–2006). J Environ Public Health. 2011;2011:850105.
66. Jogi J, Markstad H, Tufvesson E, et al. The added value of hybrid ventilation/perfusion SPECT/CT in patients with stable COPD or apparently healthy smokers. Cancer-suspected CT findings in the lungs are common when hybrid imaging is used. Int J Chron Obstruct Pulmon Dis. 2015;10:25–30.
67. Nasr A, A L, M B. Ventilation defect typical for COPD is frequent among patients suspected for pulmonary embolism but does not prevent the diagnosis of PE by V/P SPECT. EC Pulmanol Respir Med. 2017;4(3):85–91.
68. Jobse BN, Rhem RG, McCurry CA, et al. Imaging lung function in mice using SPECT/CT and per-voxel analysis. PLoS One. 2012;7(8):e42187.
69. Jogi J, Ekberg M, Jonson B, et al. Ventilation/perfusion SPECT in chronic obstructive pulmonary disease: an evaluation by reference to symptoms, spirometric lung function and emphysema, as assessed with HRCT. Eur J Nucl Med Mol Imaging. 2011;93:1344–52.
70. Norberg P, Persson HL, Schmekel B, et al. Does quantitative lung SPECT detect lung abnormalities earlier than lung function tests? Results of a pilot study. EJNMMI Res. 2014;4(1):39.
71. Bajc M, Chen Y, Wang J, et al. Identifying the heterogeneity of COPD by V/P SPECT: a new tool for improving the diagnosis of parenchymal defects and grading the severity of small airways disease. Int J Chron Obstruct Pulmon Dis. 2017;12:1579–87.
72. Ewig S, Birkner N, Strauss R, et al. New perspectives on community-acquired pneumonia in 388 406 patients. Results from a nationwide mandatory performance measurement programme in healthcare quality. Thorax. 2009;64(12):1062–9.
73. Scherer PM, Chen DL. Imaging pulmonary inflammation. J Nucl Med. 2016;57(11):1764–70.
74. Carvalho P, Lavender JP. The incidence and etiology of the ventilation/perfusion reverse mismatch defect. Clin Nucl Med. 1989;14(8):571–6.
75. Li DJ, Stewart I, Miles KA, Wraight EP. Scintigraphic appearances in patients with pulmonary infection and lung scintigrams of intermediate or low probability for pulmonary embolism. Clin Nucl Med. 1994;19(12):1091–3.
76. Sostman HD, Gottschalk A. The stripe sign: a new sign for diagnosis of nonembolic defects on pulmonary perfusion scintigraphy. Radiology. 1982;142(3):737–41.
77. Bajc M. Value of ventilation/perfusion SPECT detecting extensive pulmonary embolism in a patient with pneumonia. Thromb Haemost. 2005;93(5):993–4.
78. Friedman WF, Braunwald E. Alterations in regional pulmonary blood flow in mitral valve disease studied by radioisotope scanning. A simple nontraumatic technique for estimation of left atrial pressure. Circulation. 1966;34(3):363–76.
79. Freeman LM, Krynyckyi B, Zuckier LS. Enhanced lung scan diagnosis of pulmonary embolism with the use of ancillary scintigraphic findings and clinical correlation. Semin Nucl Med. 2001;31(2):143–57.
80. Jogi J, Al-Mashat M, Radegran G, et al. Diagnosing and grading heart failure with tomographic perfusion lung scintigraphy: validation with right heart catheterization. In: ESC heart fail, vol. 5; 2018. p. 902.
81. Jogi J, Palmer J, Jonson B, Bajc M. Heart failure diagnostics based on ventilation/perfusion single photon emission computed tomography pattern and quantitative perfusion gradients. Nucl Med Commun. 2008;29(8):666–73.
82. Pistolesi M, Miniati M, Bonsignore M, et al. Factors affecting regional pulmonary blood flow in chronic ischemic heart disease. J Thorac Imaging. 1988;3(3):65–72.
83. Wechalekar K, Garner J, Gregg S. Pre-surgical evaluation of lung function. Semin Nucl Med. 2019;49(1):22–30.
84. Ohno Y, Koyama H, Nogami M, et al. State-of-the-art radiological techniques improve the assessment of postoperative lung function in patients with non-small cell lung cancer. Eur J Radiol. 2011;77(1):97–104.
85. Ma Q, Min K, Wang T, et al. (99m)Tc-3PRGD 2 SPECT/CT predicts the outcome of advanced non-squamous non-small cell lung cancer receiving chemoradiotherapy plus bevacizumab. Ann Nucl Med. 2015;29(6):519–27.

Scintigraphy of the Liver, Spleen, and Biliary Tree

7

Lionel S. Zuckier and Leonard M. Freeman

7.1 Brief Introduction and Historical Perspective

Nuclear medicine occupies a unique niche among various imaging modalities by virtue of its ability to probe functional and physiologic parameters in a noninvasive and quantitative manner. Although at one time scintigraphic studies were used as primary modalities to address anatomic questions, these tasks are currently performed by higher-resolution modalities such as ultrasound (US), computed tomography (CT), and magnetic resonance (MR) imaging. In current practice, nuclear medicine retains a more limited though unique role in the functional and physiologic characterization of tissue [1].

Within the solid gastrointestinal (GI) tract, colloid imaging of the liver visualizes the distribution of reticuloendothelial (RE) system cells which phagocytize intravascular particulate material from the blood, while hepatobiliary scintigraphy evaluates the uptake and excretion of bile-like radiopharmaceuticals by hepatocytes. Specific radiopharmaceuticals such as ^{18}F-FDG, ^{123}I- or ^{131}I-MIBG, ^{67}Ga-gallium citrate, ^{111}In-octreotide, and ^{68}Ga-DOTATATE are used to evaluate metabolic and receptor characteristics of tissues relevant to various pathological processes that affect the liver and spleen. Radiolabeled red blood cells (RBCs) are used to quantitate the blood flow and intravascular blood pool within the liver, helpful when confirming the diagnosis of intrahepatic hemangioma. These applications are summarized in Table 7.1 and will be featured in the chapter below. The role of nuclear medicine tests in evaluating of malignant processes in the liver will be covered elsewhere in this book.

7.2 Biliary Excretion

The initial indication for biliary scintigraphy, to evaluate the etiology of acute right upper quadrant pain, remains current today. A second indication for this technique is the noninvasive evaluation of bile flow to assess extravasation or obstruction in the postsurgical and post-traumatic patient. A third application, which has seen increasing use, is the functional assessment of the gall bladder and biliary tree, so-called biliary kinetics.

L. S. Zuckier (✉) · L. M. Freeman
Division of Nuclear Medicine, Department of Radiology, Montefiore Medical Center, Bronx, NY, USA

Albert Einstein College of Medicine, Bronx, NY, USA
e-mail: Lzuckier@montefiore.org; Lfreeman@montefiore.org

H. Ahmadzadehfar et al. (eds.), *Clinical Nuclear Medicine*,
https://doi.org/10.1007/978-3-030-39457-8_7

Table 7.1 Physiological correlates of radiopharmaceutical behavior in the liver

Radiopharmaceutical	Parameter	Physiologic correlate
^{99m}Tc-sulfur colloid	Uptake	Kupffer cell function
^{99m}Tc-HIDA	Uptake	Hepatocyte function
^{99m}Tc-HIDA	Liver washout	Presence of biliary radicals
^{99m}Tc-red blood cells	Visualization on flow images	Hepatic artery supply
^{99m}Tc-red blood cells	Visualization on delayed images	Intravascular volume
^{133}Xe gas	Uptake	Lipid solubility
^{67}Ga-citrate	Uptake	Transferrin binding
^{111}In-Octreoscan	Uptake	Somatostatin (sstr2) receptor
^{123}I- or ^{131}I-MIBG	Uptake	Catecholamine-producing cells
^{68}Ga-DOTATATE[a]	Uptake	Somatostatin (sstr2) receptor
^{18}F-FDG[a]	Uptake	(glut) transporter

[a]PET based

7.2.1 Radiopharmaceuticals

Attributes of an ideal radiopharmaceutical for evaluation of bile flow include labeling with a radionuclide of favorable imaging and dosimetry characteristics, rapid liver extraction and transit into the biliary system, little or no absorption from the intestine, and minimal renal excretion [2]. ^{99m}Tc-labeled iminodiacetic acid (IDA) derivatives approach these ideal criteria. Typically, 111–185 MBq (3–5 mCi) of ^{99m}Tc-disofenin (2,6-diisopropylacetanilido-iminodiacetic acid) or ^{99m}Tc-mebrofenin (bromo-2,4,6-trimethylacetanilido-iminodiacetic acid) analogs are used for biliary scintigraphy in an adult; the latter has an advantage of superior liver extraction and is therefore favored in patients with more severe hepatic dysfunction. While the IDA analogs generally resemble bilirubin in their uptake and excretion, they are not conjugated as is bilirubin.

7.2.2 Methodology

Clinical information of relevance prior to a hepatobiliary study includes history of previous surgeries, recent bilirubin and liver enzyme levels, and current medications, with special attention to opioids which increase the sphincter of Oddi tone and thereby alter biliary kinetics. Time of most-recent food ingestion is also important as eating profoundly alters biliary kinetics and the pattern of gallbladder (GB) filling.

For evaluation of right upper quadrant pain, patients are generally imaged after a preferably 6-h period of fasting, designed to avoid postprandial contraction of the GB. Patients who are on total parenteral nutrition or have not eaten for over 24 h may have tumefactive bile ("sludge") in the GB which also impedes GB filling. In this situation, a 15-min IV injection of 20 ng/kg of sincalide (CCK-8, the terminal octapeptide of cholecystokinin) given 30 min prior to radiopharmaceutical (Table 7.2) will serve to contract and empty the GB, allowing for subsequent filling with IDA [5]. Interference by opioids can be minimized by delaying the study for a time corresponding to four half-lives of the medication following prior administration [6].

Radiopharmaceutical is injected intravenously, and anterior images over the liver and upper abdomen are obtained at intervals of 5 min or less using a large-field-of-view gamma-camera. Wherever possible, continuous computer acquisition, at approximately one frame per minute, is obtained for subsequent presentation of the data in cine mode. In traditional protocols, imaging is continued for up to 4 h postinjection, until the bowel and GB are visualized or no significant activity remains within the liver (Fig. 7.1). On rare occasions, such as when hepatic uptake is impaired, delayed imaging, up to 24 h, may be helpful.

Table 7.2 Pharmacologic interventions in biliary scintigraphy (after [3] and [4])

Drug	Dose, route	Mechanism	Use
Cholecystokinin-8	20 ng/kg, IV	Stimulates contraction of the GB and relaxes sphincter of Oddi	1. Evacuation of sludge from the GB prior to study, given over 15 min, 30 min prior to radiopharmaceutical 2. Evaluation of percent GB emptying poststimulus (ejection fraction), given over 60 min concurrent with imaging
Morphine sulfate	40 μg/kg or a 2 mg dose slowly over 2–3 min, IV	Constricts sphincter of Oddi	Diverts IDA from the CBD into GB, thereby reducing period of biliary scintigraphy
Phenobarbital	5 mg/kg daily in two divided doses × 5 days, PO	Induces hepatic enzymes	Used to promote liver excretion of IDA in differentiation of neonatal hepatitis from biliary atresia

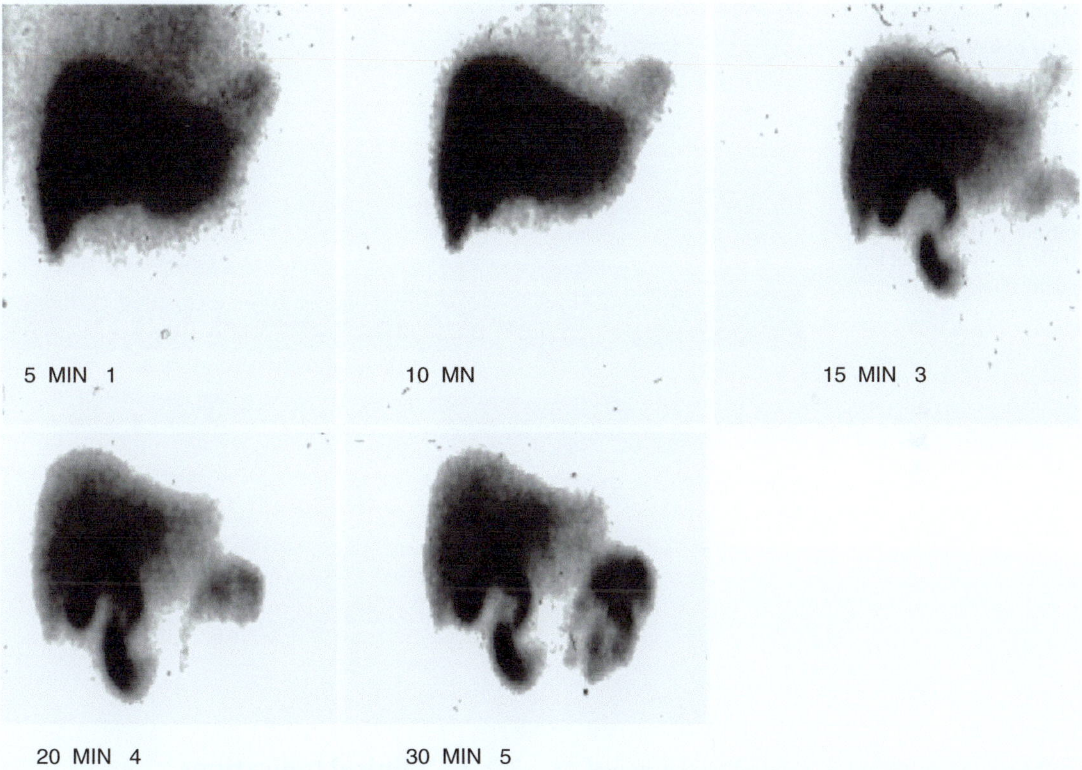

Fig. 7.1 Normal biliary excretion study in a 43-year-old man with acute abdominal pain. Prompt uptake and excretion of radiotracer into the bowel is noted. The gallbladder also fills promptly establishing cystic duct patency, ruling out acute cholecystitis with a greater than 90% accuracy

Rather than continuing the study through 4 h, an alternate accelerated method of biliary scintigraphy can be performed if by 1 h activity is noted within the duodenum but no GB is evident. A quantity of 40 μg/kg or a standard 2 mg dose of morphine sulfate is administered intravenously over 2–3 min (Table 7.2) [6]. This serves to constrict the sphincter of Oddi, thereby shunting bile into the GB (Fig. 7.2). Imaging is terminated 30–60 min following morphine administration, which is functionally equivalent to continuing through the standard 4-h period.

At times it may be difficult to ascertain if a collection of activity medially placed in the

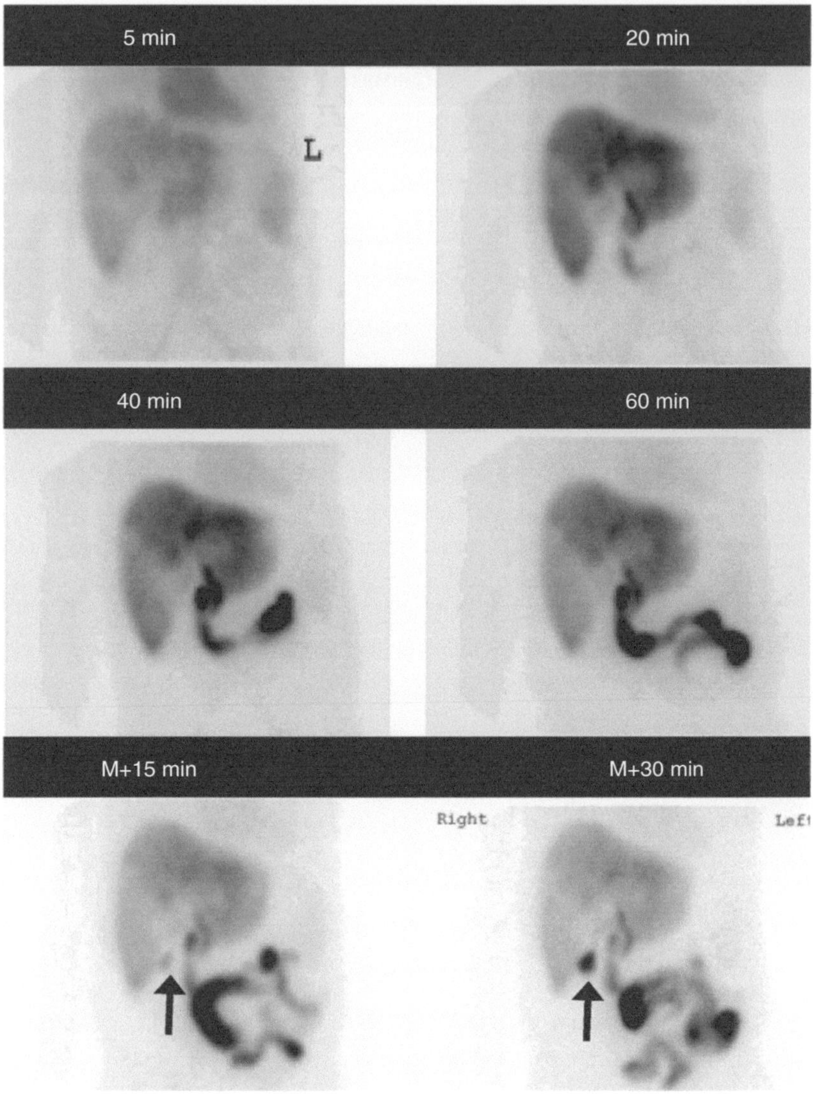

Fig. 7.2 Morphine-augmented cholescintigraphy in a 53-year-old male with history of gallstones and right upper quadrant pain. Imaging through 1 h demonstrated prolonged cardiac blood pool activity and slightly inhomogeneous uptake within the liver, consistent with a known history of liver dysfunction. Increasing activity is noted in the bowel between 20 min and 1 h. At this juncture, 2 mg of morphine sulfate was administrated intravenously, and additional images were obtained, demonstrating filling of the GB (arrows). These findings indicate chronic (but not acute) cholecystitis

right upper quadrant is related to the bowel or in fact is contained within the GB. In addition to obtaining oblique views which may be helpful, patients can be imaged following ingestion of a small amount of water. This serves to wash out the activity within the duodenum but would not affect activity in the GB (Fig. 7.3). SPECT and especially SPECT-CT can also be used to accurately localize ambiguous collections of activity.

7.2.3 Clinical Indications and Interpretation

In the normal patient, hepatic uptake of a ^{99m}Tc-labeled iminodiacetic acid derivative is prompt, with observable blood pool activity in the heart clearing by 5 min postinjection. There is likewise rapid excretion of radiopharmaceutical by the liver, through the biliary tree, and into the duodenum and GB, both of which visualize

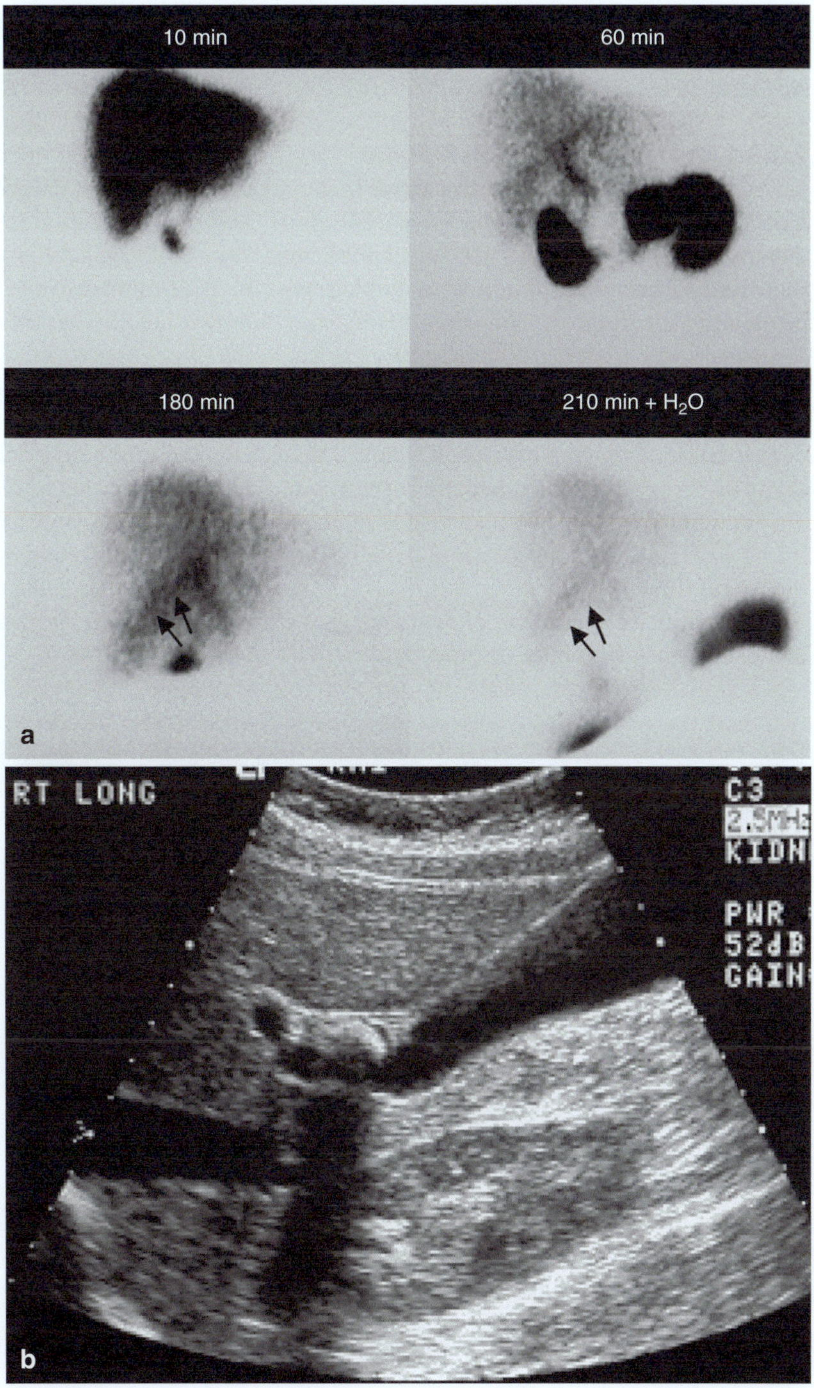

Fig. 7.3 Acute cholecystitis in a 27-year-old woman who presented with right upper quadrant pain. Biliary excretion study (**a**) reveals prompt uptake by the liver and rapid excretion into the small bowel with no visualization of the GB through 3½ h. Of note, there is a suggestion of a faint "stripe" of activity in the region of the GB fossa (arrows), suggesting acute gangrenous cholecystitis. To eliminate the confounding possibility of duodenal activity adjacent to the GB fossa, water was given to the patient following the 3-h view. Additionally, the bowel is shielded by a lead cape on the 3½-h view. Ultrasound study (**b**) demonstrates stones in the region of the neck of the GB (Reprinted from Zuckier and Freeman 2003 with permission)

within the first hour (Fig. 7.1). Transient reflux of activity into the stomach may be seen and a small amount of activity is frequently noted in the urinary tract. Over time, activity proceeds distally into the small and large bowel, while the liver activity diminishes to background levels. Criteria of evaluation include the rate of uptake and excretion of the radiotracer by the liver, the timing of visualization of the bowel and GB, and the appearance of abnormal collections of activity within the abdomen. Deviations from the norm are associated with various disease states, as described below.

7.2.3.1 Disorders of Hepatic Uptake and Excretion into the Bowel

Uptake by the liver may be impaired, evidenced by slow clearance of the blood pool and increased vicarious excretion of radiopharmaceutical by the kidneys. This abnormality may be primary, due to parenchymal disease such as hepatitis, or secondary, due to obstruction at the level of the common hepatic or common bile duct (CBD). At times it may be difficult to distinguish between intrinsic hepatic disease and obstruction as in both cases activity is retained in the liver and does not proceed distally into the bowel (Fig. 7.4).

In hepatitis, impairment of hepatic uptake and excretion is variable. In mild dysfunction, decreased liver extraction may be evidenced by prolongation of blood pool activity (typically beyond 5 min) and an increase in vicarious excretion by the kidneys. In patients with severe dysfunction, liver uptake may be diminished to the point where the liver is poorly defined, and no biliary excretion is noted. Generally, performance of hepatobiliary studies in patients with total bilirubin above 15–20 mg/dl is of little value in that insufficient activity will be excreted into the biliary tree to yield information regarding its patency. Instances where uptake of radiopharmaceutical by the liver is relatively preserved in contrast to severely decreased hepatic excretion may be rarely seen as an idiosyncratic reaction to medications such as isoniazid and halothane. This unusual combination is termed "intrahepatic cholestasis" and can be confused with relatively acute high-grade mechanical obstruction of the biliary tree.

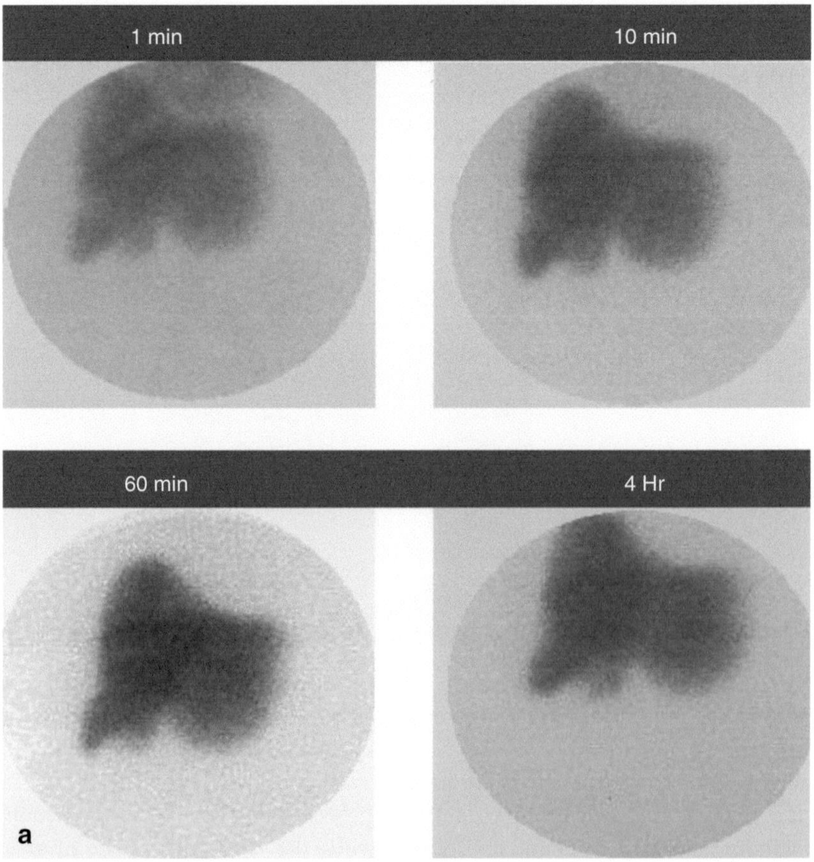

Fig. 7.4 Common bile duct obstruction in a woman who presented with right upper quadrant pain and with suspicion of acute cholecystitis. A fixed "hepatogram" pattern is present through 4 h (**a**), consistent with the diagnosis of CBD obstruction. Correlative ultrasound performed the following day (**b**) demonstrates mild dilation of the CBD to a diameter of 10.7 mm (Reprinted from Zuckier and Freeman 2003 with permission)

Fig. 7.4 (continued)

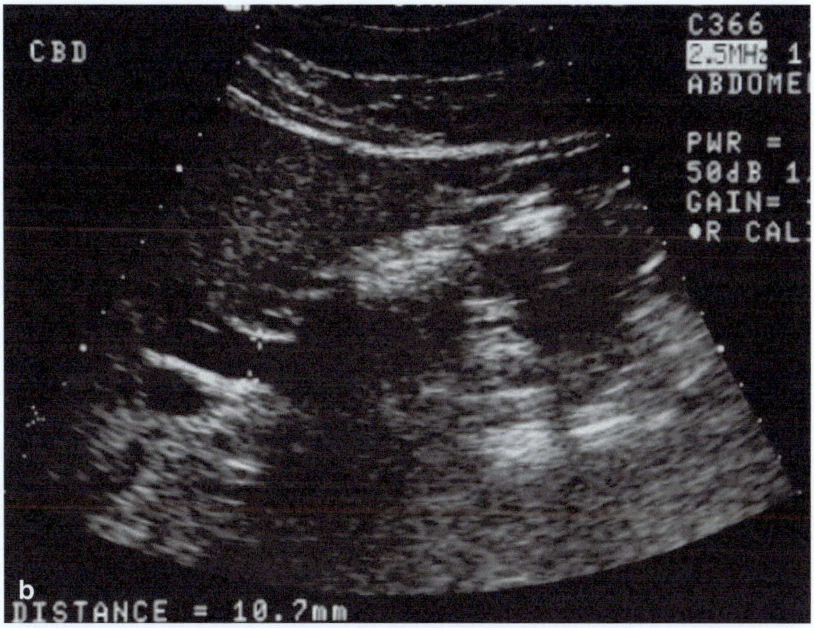

In very early mechanical obstruction of the biliary tree, liver uptake and excretion remain intact, and excreted activity may be observed within the dilated biliary tree to the level of obstruction. As high-grade obstruction of the biliary tree progresses over hours to days, from acute to subacute and chronic, liver uptake and excretion of radiopharmaceutical become increasingly impaired to the point where no activity is observed in the bile ducts, which can even appear as linear photon deficiencies. With prolonged obstruction, the degree of hepatic dysfunction becomes profound, no activity is excreted into the ducts, and it is impossible to differentiate mechanical obstruction from hepatitis.

When partial CBD obstruction is present, ductal prominence and stasis as well as delayed biliary to bile transit may occur, with appearance of activity with the bowel delayed to beyond 60 min. This latter finding is nonspecific and can be seen with a variety of intra-abdominal pathologies as well as following opioid administration or in patients administered CCK-8 prior to scintigraphy [7]. Chronic cholecystitis may also be associated with this finding in some cases.

7.2.3.2 Disorders of Gallbladder Visualization

The primary parameter evaluated on IDA scanning in patients with right upper quadrant pain and suspected cholecystitis is filling of the GB. Assuming sufficient radiotracer reaches the bowel, the GB normally fills between 10 min and 1 h postinjection of radiopharmaceutical. Delayed visualization, between 1 and 4 h, is most commonly ascribed to chronic cholecystitis. Complete non-visualization through 4 h in an acutely ill patient is both highly sensitive and specific for acute cholecystitis, reflecting cystic duct obstruction [8]. This is usually caused by impaction of a stone in the cystic duct; however, acute acalculous cholecystitis will also cause non-visualization of the GB [9]. A recent systematic review and meta-analysis has indicated that cholescintigraphy has the highest diagnostic accuracy of all imaging modalities in the detection of acute cholecystitis [10]. It should be cautioned that in the presence of CBD obstruction or severe hepatic dysfunction, non-visualization of the GB is not diagnostic as there is insufficient flow of activity into the bowel to make any determination of cystic duct patency.

The morphine-enhanced IDA study, as discussed above, shortens the total examination time to 1.5 h instead of the 4 h needed to reliably differentiate acute from chronic cholecystitis. Filling of the GB within 30 min following morphine is analogous to delayed visualization on a 4-h study and suggests chronic cholecystitis (Fig. 7.2). If no filling of the GB occurs by 30 min post-administration of morphine, the cystic duct is demonstrated to be obstructed, consistent with the diagnosis of acute cholecystitis [11, 12].

An important finding, suggestive of complicated acute cholecystitis, is the "rim" or "stripe" sign which consists of a band of increased activity at the lower margin of the liver in the region of the GB fossa (Fig. 7.3). This finding is postulated as being due to adjacent cholestasis in inflamed regional hepatocytes or to actual leakage from a GB perforation. When present, the rim sign has high specificity for complicated acute cholecystitis and predicts increased morbidity [13, 14].

7.2.3.3 Functional Disorders of the Gallbladder [15]

In patients with biliary colic and biliary dyskinesia, routine biliary scintigraphy may be normal. In these cases, an additional provocative test may be necessary to confirm suspected pathology. In one such technique, radiopharmaceutical is administered, and the GB is allowed to fill for 60 min at which point CCK-8 is administered intravenously (Table 7.2) to elicit GB emptying. While various protocols for gallbladder emptying had previously been employed, a multicenter trial conclusively established superiority of a 60-min infusion of 0.02 mg of sincalide per kilogram, with emptying quantified at 60 min [16] (Fig. 7.5). In normal patients, a decrease of activity within the GB of greater than 38% is observed, while in patients with biliary dyskinesia, the GB ejection fraction (EF) remains lower. In instances where CCK-8 is not available, a situation which has occurred periodically, standardized fatty meals have been used to stimulate GB contraction [17, 18]. It must be remembered that physiologic quantitative studies are complicated and must be interpreted within the entire clinical context including pharmacologic effects of other medications [19].

Occasionally, right upper quadrant pain persists following cholecystectomy. In these circumstances, quantitative scintigraphy may be used to assess the physiologic transit of radiotracer from the liver to the bowel, thereby evaluating function of the sphincter of Oddi. Scoring systems have been proposed as a means of objectively and noninvasively predicting which patients would benefit from sphincterotomy (Fig. 7.6) [20].

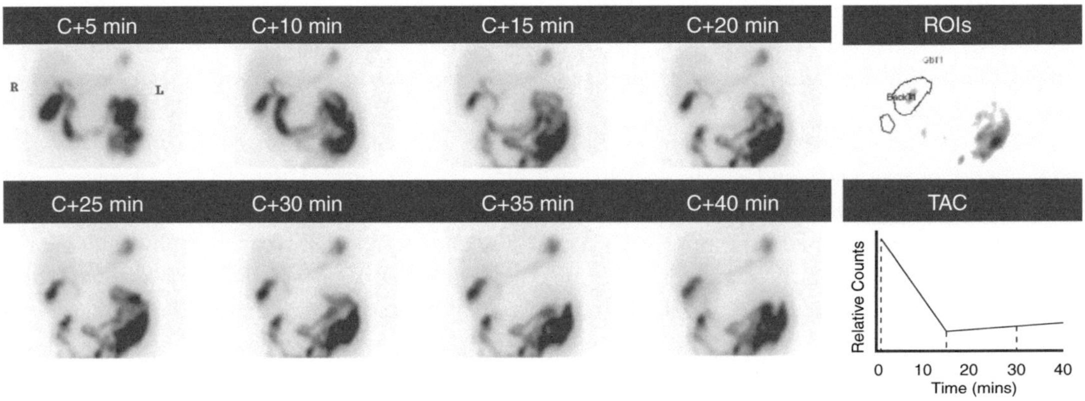

Fig. 7.5 Normal GB ejection fraction. Two micrograms of CCK-8 was administrated a 1 h by slow infusion and images were obtained over 40 min. There is prompt and excellent emptying of the GB. Time-activity curve (TAC) demonstrates an ejection fraction of 85%, which peaks at 12 min post-infusion

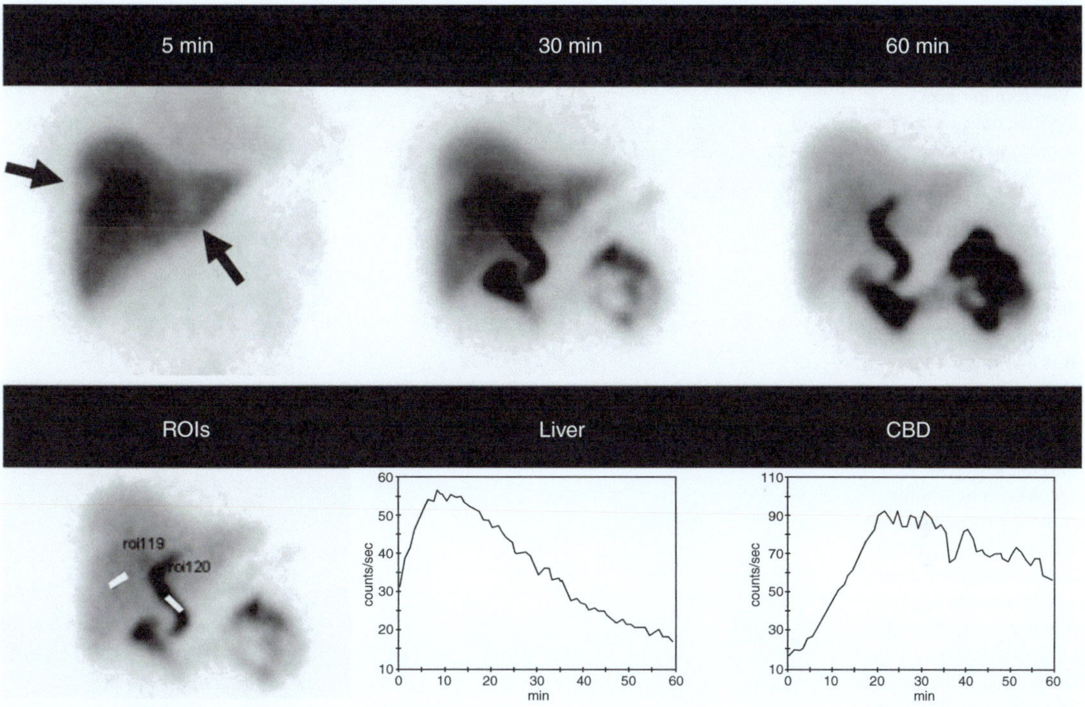

Fig. 7.6 A 28-year-old female with recurrent right-sided abdominal pain following cholecystectomy. Representative images at 5, 30, and 60 min are displayed (top row). Regions of interest (ROIs) were applied as per the method of Sostre et al. [20] in order to generate a quantitative score. TACs of indicated regions over the liver and common bile duct are displayed. For this patient, analysis does not support the diagnosis of sphincter of Oddi dysfunction. Incidentally noted are focal detects within the liver parenchyma due to two known hemangiomas (arrows)

7.2.3.4 Postoperative and Post-traumatic Patients

Because of the ability to track bile flow, biliary scintigraphy is effective in monitoring extravasation of bile following surgery [21, 22] or trauma [23]. Biliary scintigraphy is therefore used in symptomatic post-laparoscopic cholecystectomy patients, where reduced surgical exposure may lead to complications such as retained stones, transection, or ligation of the CBD [24] (Fig. 7.7). Scintigraphy is performed to visualize the expected flow of radiopharmaceutical from the liver into the bowel. Delayed images are helpful in identifying extravasated activity and can visualize loculated collections and free intraperitoneal leaks (Fig. 7.7), while decubitus views can be used to demonstrate free flow of intraperitoneal activity. In the current era, SPECT-CT is a powerful tool to enable precise anatomic localization of extravasated activity within a particular fluid collection.

Following trauma, collections may be observed on CT or US; however, their etiology may be unclear. Cholescintigraphy can help define a collection in relationship to biliary excretion in this context as well (Fig. 7.8). Flow of activity into a biloma is typically slow, and visualization may only appear on delayed images following gradual accumulation of radiopharmaceutical within the collection and maximal washout of activity from the normal liver [1]. Scintigraphy can be used to quantitate the degree of bile leak and thereby assess significance of injury [25] (Fig. 7.9). If the majority of bile flow progresses through the biliary tree into the duodenum, conservative management, rather than surgical repair, is usually attempted.

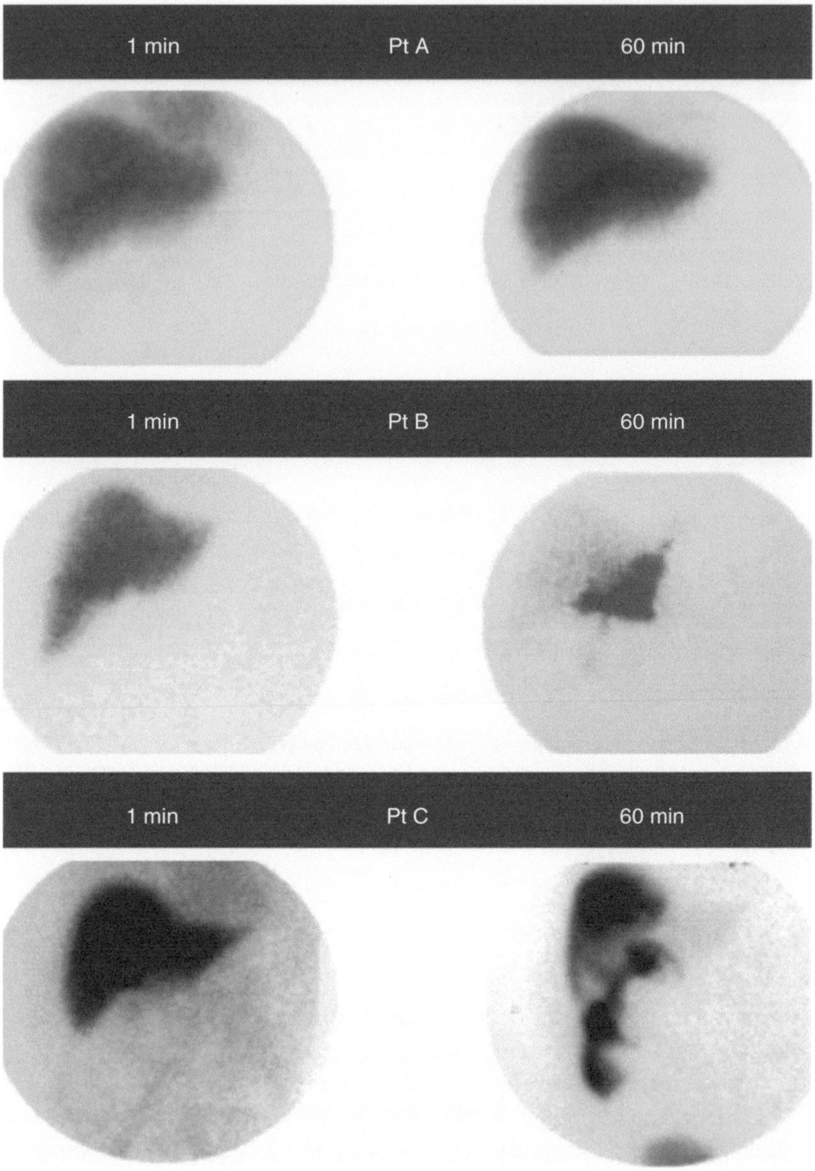

Fig. 7.7 Representative biliary scintigraphic images in three symptomatic post-laparoscopic cholecystectomy patients. Patient A is a 23-year-old female, 6 days post-procedure, who has increasing nausea, vomiting, and pain. A CBD obstructive pattern is noted. Patient B is a young female studied 10 days post-procedure. A relatively confined leak into the lesser sac is noted with negligible activity proceeding into the small bowel. Patient C also evidences a leak, which appears freely flowing down the right paracolic gutter (Reprinted from Zuckier and Freeman 2003 with permission)

7.2.3.5 Biliary Atresia

A specialized use of biliary scintigraphy is in differentiating biliary atresia from neonatal hepatitis. Infants are typically prepared by pretreatment with 5 mg/kg/day of phenobarbital, given orally in two divided doses, over a minimum of 3–5 days, designed to induce hepatic enzymes and maximize excretion of radiopharmaceutical [11, 26] (Table 7.2). For infants and children, 1.8 MBq/kg (0.05 mCi/kg) of radiopharmaceutical is typically administered with a minimum of 18.5 MBq (0.5 mCi) [6]. BRIDA is preferred to DISIDA due to its higher liver extraction. Imaging begins immediately postinjection and extends intermittently through several hours. If no bowel activity is observed, patients return for delayed imaging through 24 h. Any activity noted within the bowel or GB indicates patency

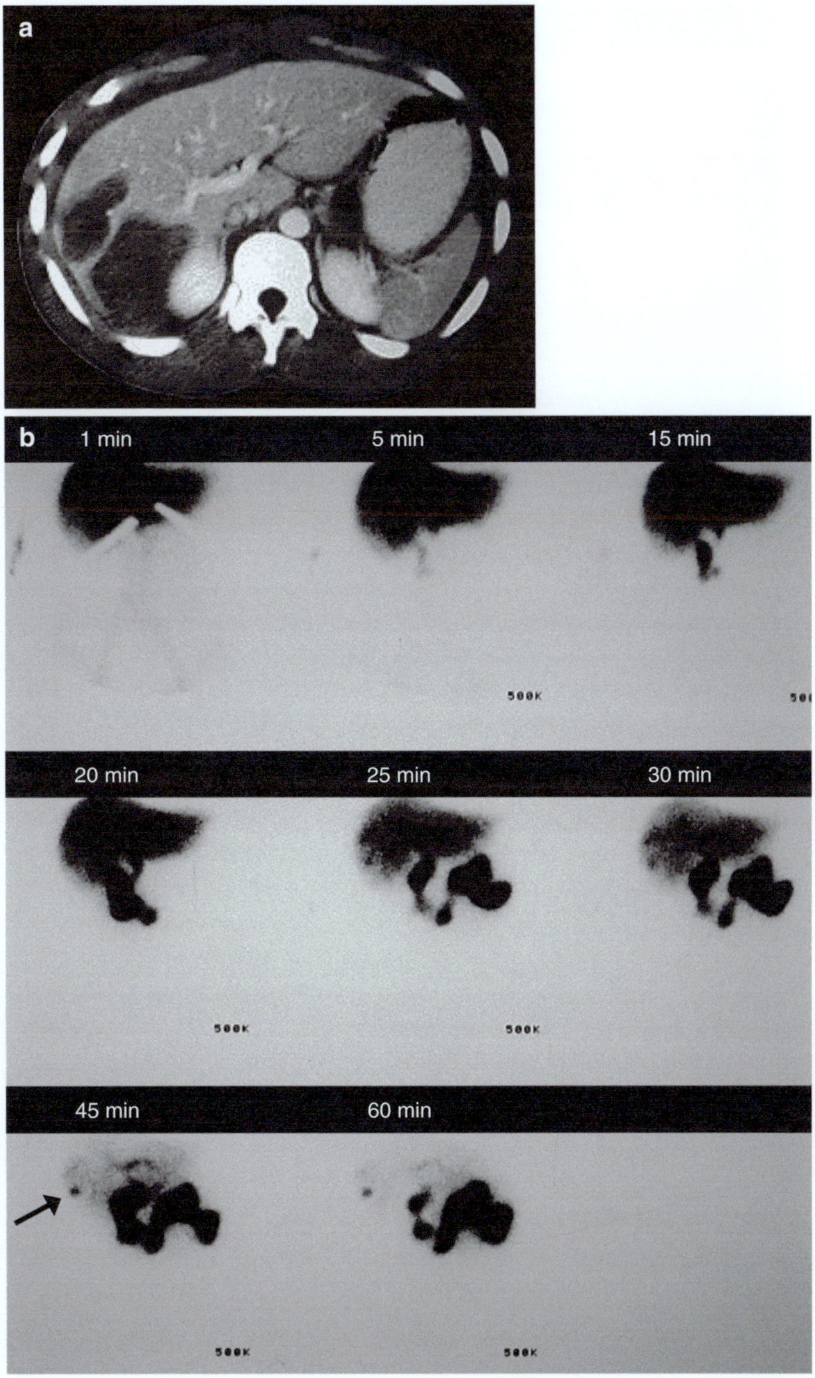

Fig. 7.8 Biloma following penetrating injury to the abdomen in an 18-year-old male who sustained a stab wound to his right flank. CT (**a**) demonstrates a large hemoperitoneum, laceration of the anterior and posterior segments of the right lobe of the liver, and a hematoma in Morrison's pouch. Biliary scintigraphy performed the following day (**b**) initially demonstrates presence of a photon-poor collection in the lateral aspect of the right lobe; however, over the hour course of imaging, a small focus of bile extravasation within the region of the collection is noted (arrow). The majority of the bile is excreted into the small bowel (Reprinted from Zuckier and Freeman 2003 with permission)

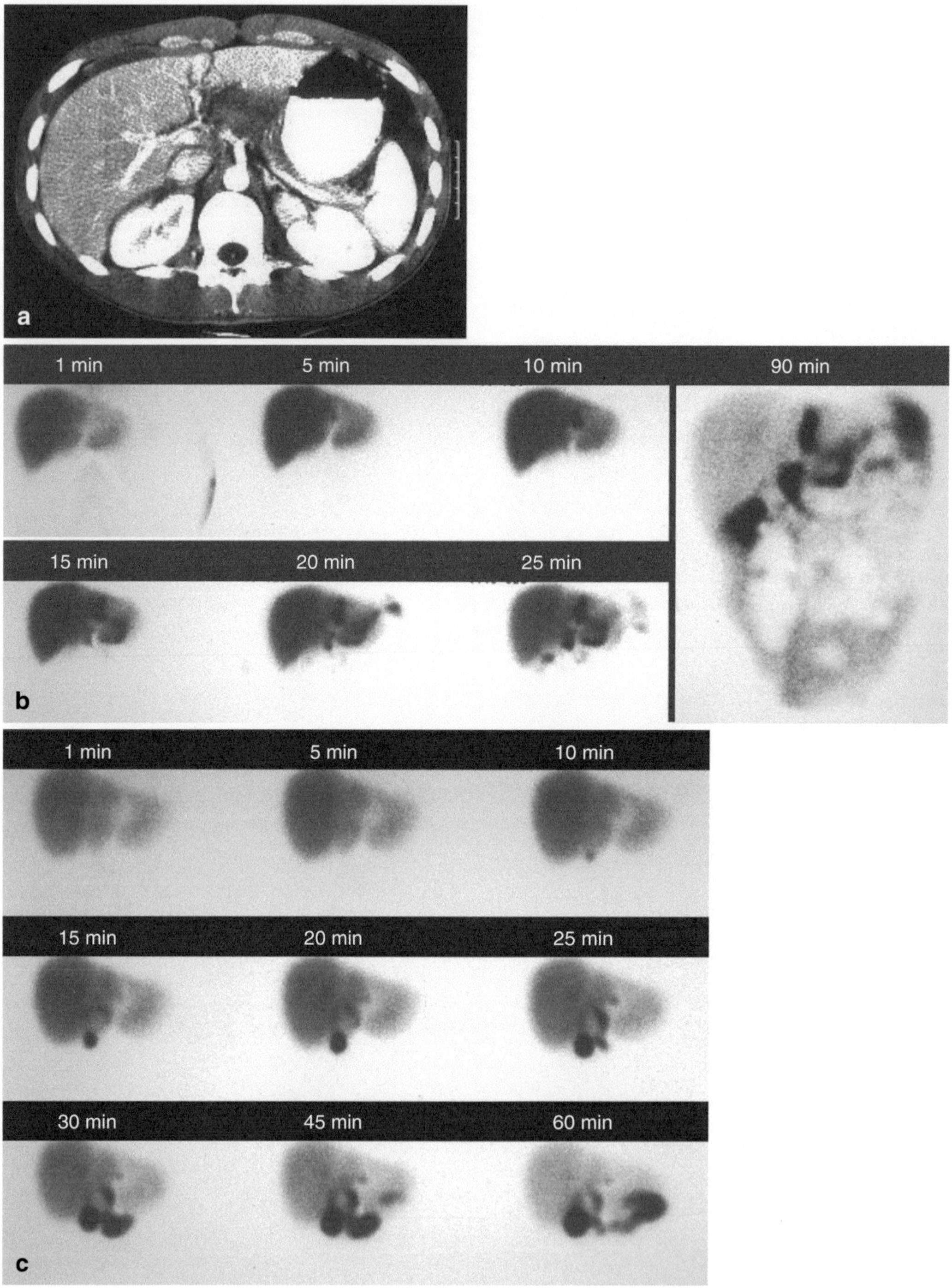

Fig. 7.9 Utility of biliary scintigraphy in evaluating traumatic injury to the liver and biliary structures in a 25-year-old male who was ejected from a car during a motor vehicle accident. A large liver laceration was noted on CT (**a**) with collection of fluid behind the left lobe of the liver. Initial biliary scintigraphy (**b**) demonstrates a large leak with spread of radiotracer throughout the peritoneal cavity by 90 min. Bowel loops are visualized as photon deficiencies. Follow-up scintigraphy performed after 5 days of conservative management (**c**) demonstrates near-complete resolution of the leak with progression of activity into the small bowel (Reprinted from Zuckier and Freeman 2003 with permission)

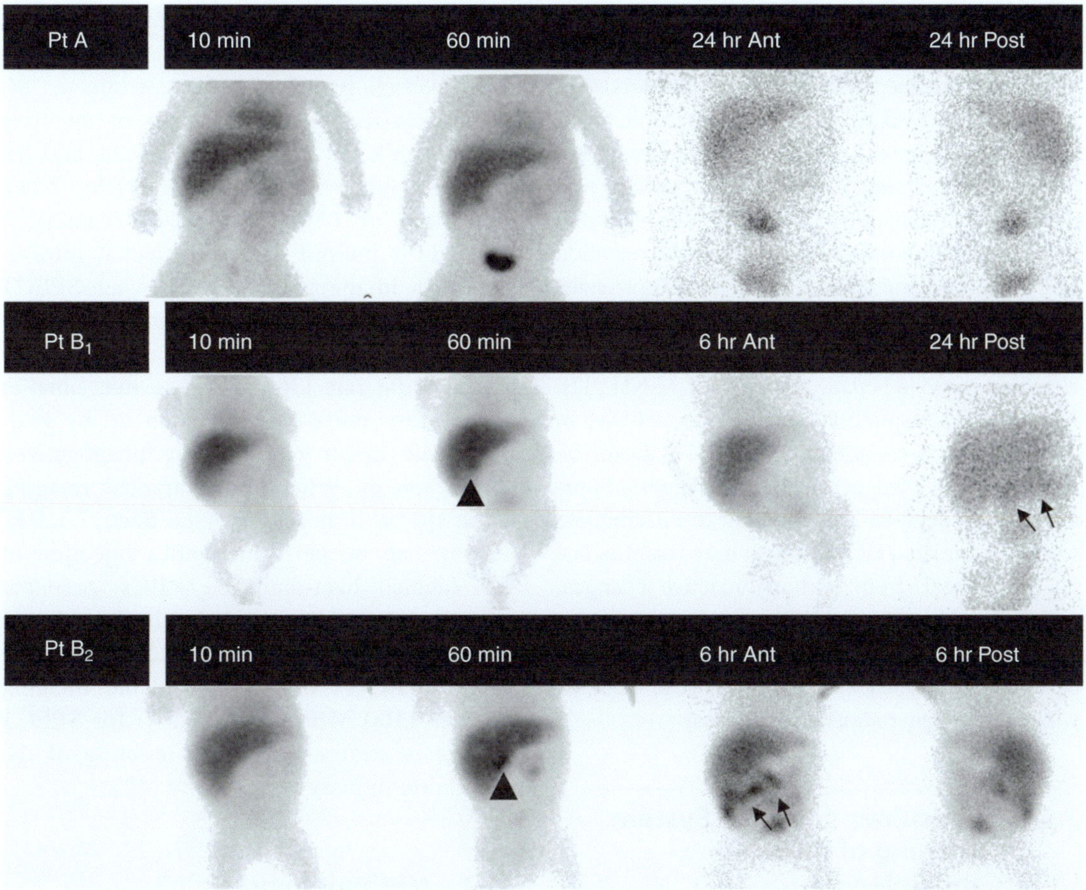

Fig. 7.10 Three separate studies performed on two infants to exclude biliary atresia. Patients were all administered phenobarbital prior to imaging in order to enhance excretion (see text and Table 7.2). Patient A: 4-month-old baby boy, delivered at a gestational age of 26 weeks, who presented with cholestatic jaundice. Persistent cardiac blood pool activity is noted up to 60 min of imaging, suggestive of hepatocellular dysfunction. Absence of gastrointestinal excretion of radiotracer in both early and 24-h delayed images is consistent with either biliary atresia or severe hepatocellular dysfunction. Activity within the kidneys and urinary system and diaper should not be confused with bowel excretion. Patient B is a 41-day-old baby girl who presented with increased bilirubin. Initial study (B_1) demonstrates relatively prompt uptake of radiotracer by the liver. The cardiac blood pool activity has cleared by 5 min. There is no evidence of radiotracer excretion into the GI system at the end of 1 h although the GB is faintly observed (arrowhead). Delayed images obtained at 6 h demonstrate vague activity into the intestine, while further delayed images obtained at 24 h confirm gastrointestinal excretion (arrows). Biliary atresia can therefore be excluded. Study was repeated 6 weeks thereafter (B_2). At this juncture, the GB is better visualized on the 60-min image (arrowhead), and bowel excretion is clearly noted on 6-h delayed images (arrows). These findings exclude biliary atresia

of the CBD and excludes the diagnosis of biliary atresia [27] (Fig. 7.10). When no bowel excretion is visualized, findings are ambiguous, as lack of excretion may be due to either severe neonatal hepatitis or biliary atresia [28]. In this instance, liver biopsy will be necessary to establish the diagnosis.

7.2.3.6 Characterization of Liver Masses

Biliary scintigraphy can contribute to the characterization of liver lesions (Table 7.1). Uptake of hepatobiliary radiopharmaceutical within a mass indicates presence of functioning hepatocytes and thereby excludes masses of non-hepatic origin. If within a mass of hepatic origin the biliary radicals are not well developed, excretion of activity will be impaired, evidenced by slow washout and persistent activity on delayed imaging. For this reason, hepatocellular carcinoma (HCC) typically is best seen on delayed imaging several hours postinjection due to the combination of relatively reduced initial uptake by the tumor and slow washout and retention [29, 30]. In general, uptake within HCC correlates strongly with degree of tumor differentiation [31]. Slow washout of biliary radiopharmaceutical has also been noted in hepatic adenoma and FNH [32]. In cases where aspiration biopsy is inconclusive in differentiating well-differentiated HCCs from cirrhotic reactive changes, some have suggested utility in using delayed IDA imaging to differentiate well-differentiated HCCs, which may retain radiopharmaceutical, from cirrhotic reactive changes, which should not [29, 33, 34]. Unfortunately, no such distinction can be made scintigraphically between hepatic adenomas and HCCs, both of which may retain radiopharmaceutical.

7.3 Reticuloendothelial System Imaging of the Liver and Spleen

7.3.1 Radiopharmaceuticals

The distribution of the RE system is visualized following intravenous administration of radiolabeled colloids. Particles of SC range in size from 100 nm to approximately 1.0 μm. In the average patient, 80–90% of injected SC is phagocytized by the RE cells of the liver (Kupffer cells), 5–10% by the spleen, and the remainder by the bone marrow [35] (Fig. 7.11). A quantity of 111–222 MBq (3–6 mCi) of ^{99m}Tc-sulfur colloid (SC) is injected intravenously for imaging of the liver; when SPECT imaging is performed, the amount used is typically raised to 370 MBq (10 mCi) to provide a greater count rate [36, 37]. As a rule, smaller particles are preferentially taken up by marrow, while larger particles are phagocytized by the spleen. When more-targeted imaging of the spleen is necessary (see Sect. 7.3.3.3), imaging can be performed after injection of ^{99m}Tc-labeled heat-damaged RBCs, prepared by incubation of the labeled cells for 15 min in a water bath at 49–50 °C [36, 37]. Typically 37–222 MBQ (1–6 mCi) for planar imaging and 555–1100 MBq (15–20 mCi) for SPECT imaging is administered after cooling of the preparation to body temperature [37].

7.3.2 Methodology [36, 37]

Imaging of the liver and spleen commences approximately 10–20 min following SC injection. Flow studies obtained during injection are occasionally useful [37]. Planar views of the

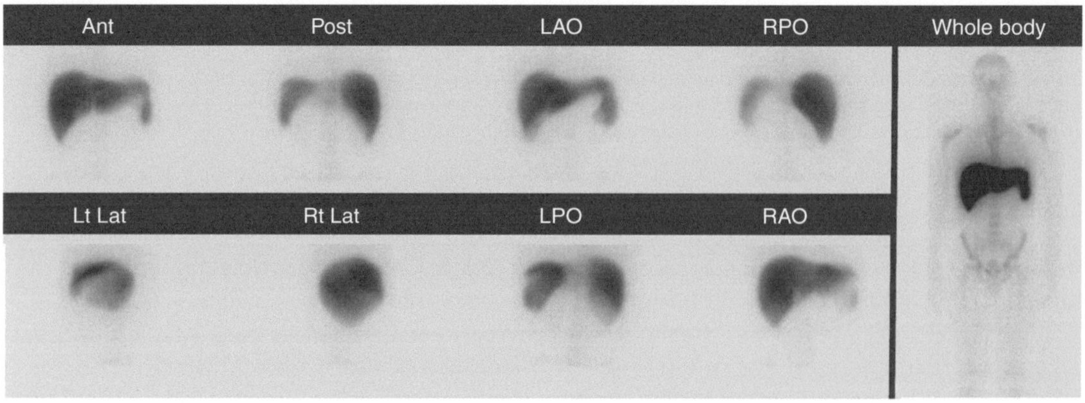

Fig. 7.11 Normal appearance of liver-spleen sulfur colloid scan in a 15-year-old boy. Standard planar views are shown in the left panel. Anterior whole-body view at increased intensity (right panel) illustrates the relative distribution of activity

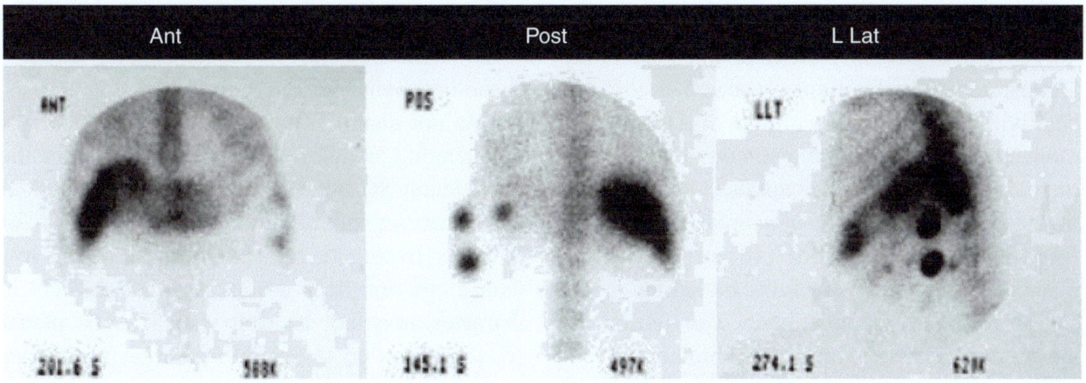

Fig. 7.12 Splenosis noted on a ^{99m}Tc-sulfur colloid study in a patient with cirrhosis and a remote history of abdominal trauma and splenectomy. In place of the spleen, three intense foci of activity are noted in the left upper quadrant of the abdomen, representing areas of functioning splenic tissue. Size and function of the spleen cannot be used to assess diffuse hepatic disease in the patient with splenectomy; however other signs may be observed. Uptake of colloid within the marrow is markedly increased and tertiary uptake in the lung is also noted. The liver appears small and there is separation of the lateral aspect of the liver from the rib margin (Helman's sign), suggesting ascites (Reprinted from Zuckier and Freeman 2003 with permission)

liver and spleen are taken in multiple obliquities (anterior, posterior, right lateral, right anterior oblique, right posterior oblique), or a tomographic SPECT image can be obtained. An image which includes a lead marker of standardized size placed on the costal margin is usually obtained in the planar technique. The left anterior oblique view, helpful in separating the left lobe of the liver from the spleen, and left posterior oblique and left lateral views are often added for imaging of the spleen. If ectopic splenic tissue is being evaluated, more extensive views of the entire abdomen, and possibly of the thorax as well [38], should be obtained (Fig. 7.12). On a large-field-of-view camera, the anterior image is usually acquired for approximately 500,000 to one million counts; other views are acquired for the same amount of time to facilitate comparison. SPECT imaging is especially helpful in resolving three-dimensional distributions of activity and in enabling comparison with findings on anatomic modalities, such as CT, US, and MRI. Current imaging on SPECT-CT cameras provides the optimum registration of nuclear medicine and CT images and has challenged the nuclear medicine physician to become proficient in the detection and diagnosis of liver incidentalomas [39].

7.3.3 Clinical Indications and Interpretation

Colloid studies of the liver are currently performed to assess diffuse hepatic disease and less frequently to evaluate focal processes within the liver. Colloid or ^{99m}Tc-labeled heat-damaged RBC splenic imaging is primarily performed to identify functional splenic tissue. These applications are discussed below.

7.3.3.1 Diffuse Parenchymal Disease of the Liver

Phagocytosis of particulate matter in the blood is an intrinsic function of the Kupffer cells of the liver [40]. The distribution of RE activity normally appears more intense in the liver than in the spleen, and marrow activity is generally only faintly appreciated. Variations in distribution of SC can therefore be used as a measure of hepatic function. In this sense, colloid scintigraphy yields information regarding physiologic function in addition to anatomy [41]. For evaluation of diffuse parenchymal liver disease, criteria of interpretation include hepatic size, splenic size, and the relative distribution of colloid between the various sites within the RES. Standardized technique is important as size of the colloid particles, and the prandial state of the patient, affects quantitative parameters including the ratio of counts in the liver and spleen [42].

Features of the liver-spleen scan that correlate best with diffuse hepatocellular disease include moderate to severe inhomogeneous liver uptake, increased bone marrow uptake, and reversal of the normal liver-to-spleen uptake ratios [43] (Fig. 7.12). Colloid "shift" is not specific for hepatic dysfunction; factors including portal hypertension, hypersplenism, stimulation of the marrow as a response to chemotherapy, and malignant melanoma may also result in this finding. Splenomegaly is not a specific finding in hepatic disease, because other pathology, such as lymphoma, can alter splenic size [43, 44].

7.3.3.2 Focal Processes within the Liver

At one time, colloid scintigraphy had a role in identifying space-occupying lesions of the liver; today its use in identifying and characterizing focal processes within the liver is uncommon. Most true space-occupying processes within the liver, such as metastases and abscesses, are devoid of Kupffer cells, with resultant defects noted on SC imaging (Fig. 7.13). In contrast, processes that simulate space-occupying lesions on radiographic studies, but do not disturb Kupffer cell function, such as regenerating nodules or fatty change within the liver, retain SC uptake [45, 46]. Many investigators report sensitivity on the order of 80–85% for detecting liver metastases [47]; surface lesions less than 2 cm, and deep lesions less than 3–4 cm in diameter, may not be well visualized on planar scintigraphy due to spatial-resolution limitations of the gamma-camera [48]. At low disease prevalence, SPECT has been shown to offer only a marginal benefit over planar scintigraphy [49]. SPECT slightly improves the detection of small lesions, but may cause a concomitant decrease in specificity, as small normal structures, such as vessels or ducts, may become visible and simulate lesions [48]. Advent of SPECT-CT systems may obviate this confusion and improve tomographic colloid studies by combining physiology and anatomic detail.

Primary masses originating within the liver include HCC, focal nodular hyperplasia (FNH),

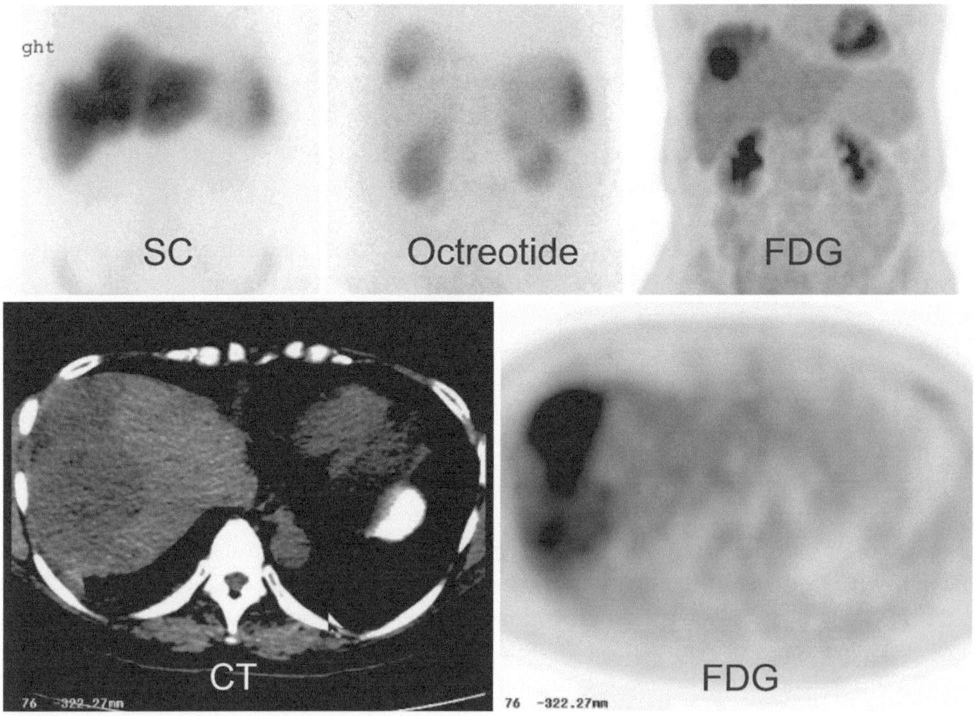

Fig. 7.13 A 48-year-old female with history of pancreatic carcinoid tumor metastatic to the liver. Anterior ^{99m}Tc-sulfur colloid image demonstrates a defect in the superior aspect of the liver. Focal uptake is noted on ^{111}In-octreotide anterior planar image and ^{18}F-FDG anterior MIP image, consistent with metastatic carcinoid tumor. On the lower panels, transaxial PET-CT images illustrate FDG uptake corresponding to a low-density liver metastasis

and hepatic adenoma. HCC is devoid of uptake on SC studies. In FNH, lesions have variable degrees of Kupffer cell function, and consequently variable colloid uptake has been described in these lesions ranging from decreased (in 30% of lesions) to normal (30%), to supranormal (30%), and even to intense (10%) [50]. Recent scintigraphic and pathologic literature has also documented possible presence of Kupffer cells in hepatic adenomas [51, 52], with moderate uptake in up to one-quarter of the patients studied. Masses with uptake above normal are believed to be relatively pathognomonic for FNH, Table 7.3 (Fig. 7.14).

In addition to FNH, several vascular derangements may lead to focal regions of increased SC uptake within the liver (Table 7.4). In superior

Table 7.3 Variable Colloid and IDA uptake patterns as a function of hepatic space-occupying lesions[a]

Space-occupying lesion	^{99m}Tc-sulfur colloid	^{99m}Tc-HIDA
Hepatoma	Cold (↓↓)	Cold (↓↓). May show slow uptake without washout
Hepatic adenoma	Variable reduced (↓↓ to ↓)	Uptake with slow washout
Focal nodular hyperplasia	Variable (↓↓ to ↑↑)	Uptake with slow washout
Liver metastases	Cold (↓↓)	Cold (↓↓)

↓ mildly decreased, ↓↓ markedly decreased, ↑↑ markedly increased

[a]After Drane [32]

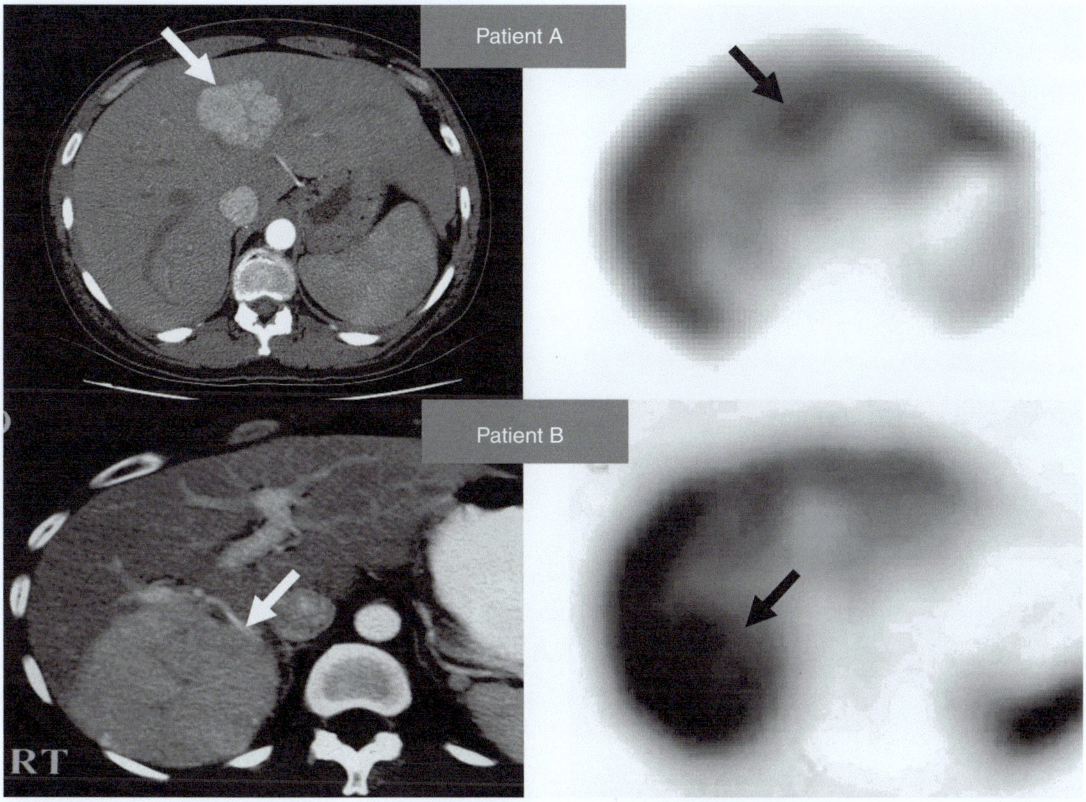

Fig. 7.14 Two examples of relatively intense uptake of SC in FNH. On non-AC corrected SPECT imaging, the center of the liver normally appears less intense than the periphery due to the effect of photon attenuation. Patient A is a 38-year-old woman with abdominal discomfort noted to have an enhancing lesion within the right lobe of the liver (arrow) on CT scan. Tomographic image from a liver-spleen colloid scan shows an area of increased colloid uptake relative to the surrounding liver, pathognomonic of FNH. Patient B is a 42-year-old woman with a liver mass incidentally detected on sonography. An area of relatively intense SC uptake is seen corresponding to the enhancing mass seen on arterial phase CT (arrow)

vena cava (SVC) obstruction, a venous injection of SC into the upper extremities must bypass the occluded SVC and reach the heart via porto-systemic collaterals, typically through the internal mammary vein that connects to the para-umbilical and left portal vein [53, 54]. Adjacent regions of the liver, specifically the medial segment of the left lobe, receive relatively enriched amounts of colloid and consequently appear intense on subsequent imaging (Fig. 7.15). In obstruction of the inferior vena cava (IVC), a similar finding has been noted following injection of radiotracer via the lower extremities though in this case injection via the upper extremities will result in a normal distribution of activity [55].

In Budd-Chiari syndrome, hepatic venous drainage into the SVC is obstructed, thereby impairing overall liver function. In contrast, the liver parenchyma in the region of the caudate lobe often drains directly into the adjacent SVC via accessory veins. This segment thereby exhibits relatively intact uptake of colloid in comparison

Table 7.4 Vascular causes of relative "hot spots" in the liver

Disorder	Region	Mechanism
Budd-Chiari syndrome	Caudate lobe	Direct drainage by accessory vein
SVC or IVC obstruction	Quadrate lobe	Collateral pathway to the left portal vein
Ethanol abuse	Left lobe	"Streamlining" of toxins to the right lobe

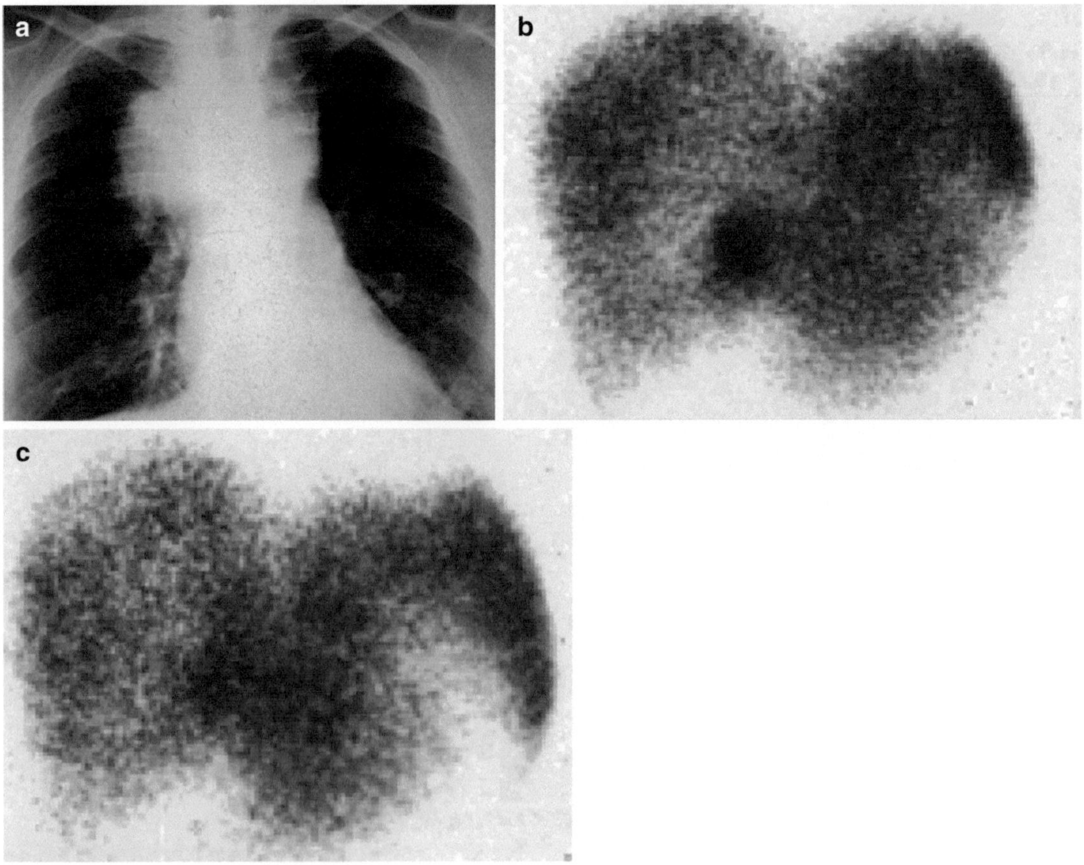

Fig. 7.15 Adult male with obstruction of the SVC caused by mediastinal malignancy (**a**). Anterior view from liver-spleen colloid scan (**b**) shows presence of a hot region in the medial aspect of the right lobe ("quadrate lobe"), due to collateralization of blood flow through the umbilical vein. Following radiotherapy to the mediastinum, the area of increased hepatic uptake resolves (**c**)

to the remainder of the affected liver, a finding coined the "bullseye" sign [56].

An additional cause of relatively increased uptake within the liver may be seen in alcoholic liver disease, which preferentially affects the right lobe of the liver resulting in an "intrahepatic colloid shift" from the severely affected right lobe to the relatively preserved left lobe. This phenomenon is believed to be due to asymmetric "streamlining" of toxic portal venous blood within the lobes of the liver [57].

7.3.3.3 Splenic Imaging

Utility of colloid imaging of the spleen derives from a relatively high degree of tissue specificity based on the functional nature of the examination. Because larger particles preferentially localize in the spleen, denatured RBCs are superior to SC for splenic imaging [58, 59], although this more-complicated procedure is currently only selectively employed.

Splenic imaging may be performed in children to rule out congenital asplenia or polysplenia. SPECT imaging is especially valuable for this purpose because of the ability to resolve splenic uptake adjacent to the liver as distinct from the liver itself [60]. Other indications for splenic imaging include confirming presence of functional splenic tissue in cases of splenic autotransplantation following splenic trauma (Fig. 7.12) or absence of such tissue in patients who have been treated previously with splenectomy for conditions such as idiopathic thrombocytopenic purpura (ITP) [59]. Splenic imaging can also be performed in order to characterize incidentally noted abdominal masses, which may represent accessory spleens or splenic tissue rather than malignant deposits (Fig. 7.16).

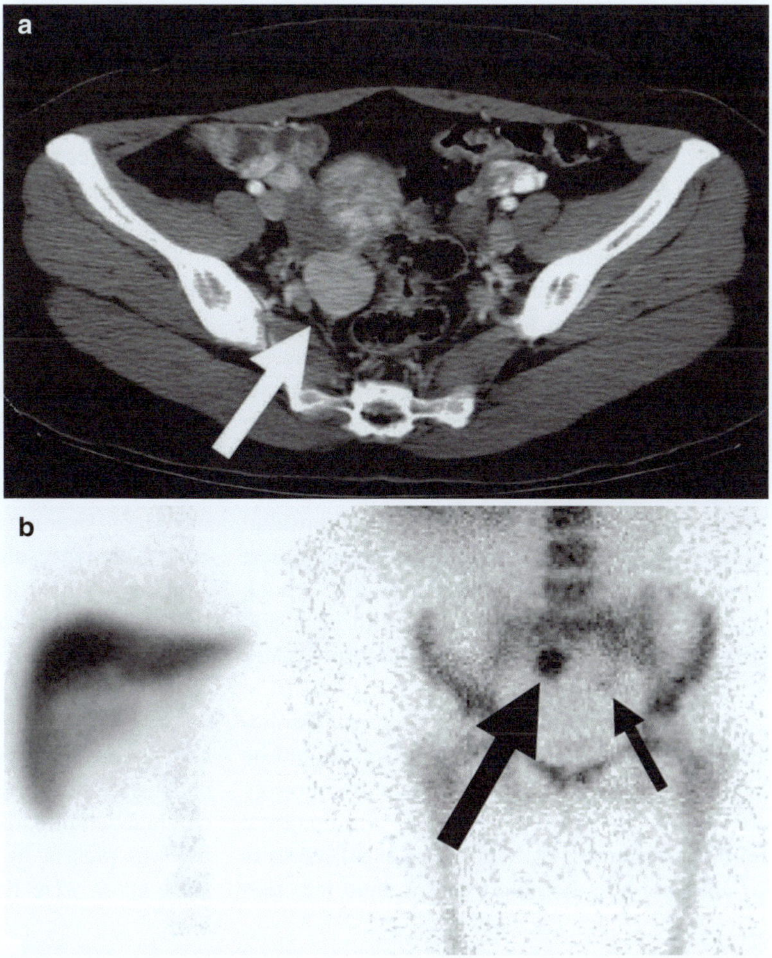

Fig. 7.16 Contrast-enhanced CT scan (**a**) in this 36-year-old Hispanic female demonstrates several enhancing masses within the abdomen and pelvis (one such pelvic mass is illustrated by arrow). History was significant for a motor vehicle accident several years earlier with probable splenectomy. Colloid study demonstrates absence of orthotopic spleen (**b**). When viewed at increased intensity, a prominent focus of colloid accumulation is noted anterior to the right SI joint corresponding to the region of the enhancing mass (large arrow) with a smaller focus noted inferior to the left SI joint (small arrow), both of which are caused by splenosis

7.4 Hemangioma Imaging

The most common benign lesion of the liver is hemangioma, occurring in up to 7% of the population and therefore representing a frequent incidental finding in the course of imaging of the abdomen [61]. Hemangiomas are typically less than 3 cm in diameter; when larger than 4 cm, they bear the designation "giant" [62]. As a rule, hemangiomas do not require any medical intervention or treatment, and a noninvasive and specific means of characterizing these lesions would serve to obviate further concern. Imaging of the liver with ^{99m}Tc-labeled RBCs fulfills this role.

7.4.1 Radiopharmaceuticals

For identification of hemangioma, 740–925 MBq (20–25 mCi) of ^{99m}Tc-RBCs is used [36, 37], optimally labeled by the in vitro method. Methods of RBC labeling are common to other scintigraphic applications, such as GI bleeding studies, and are discussed elsewhere in this book.

7.4.2 Methodology [36, 37]

Prior to hemangioma imaging, it is important to identify location of the suspect lesion, most commonly by reference to the previously obtained CT, US, or MRI study. Where no prior images are available for consultation, a low-dose SC study can be performed immediately preceding RBC imaging to define the defect; however, this procedure is usually unnecessary where other cross-sectional images are available for consultation. Generally, imaging consists of three phases: arterial perfusion (flow), immediate blood pool, and delayed blood pool [63]. Arterial perfusion imaging, typically obtained at one to three frames per second during injection of the labeled RBCs, reveals useful information about regional distribution of hepatic arterial blood flow and should be performed in the view best-predicted to portray the lesion while avoiding overlap with normal vascular structures. Care should be exercised so as to not hemolyze the blood with a rapid injection through a narrow catheter. Immediate blood pool images are then acquired for 1–2 million counts each, in this optimal projection as well as in standard anterior, posterior, and right lateral views. Delayed blood pool images, designed to portray the maximal washin of RBCs into the hemangioma, are acquired approximately 1–2 h following injection in similar projections to the immediate blood pool images. SPECT (possibly in combination with CT) will often be necessary to visualize small lesions, especially when deep within the liver parenchyma or not detected on planar views [64], and is useful for comparison to other cross-sectional imaging modalities.

7.4.3 Clinical Indications and Interpretation

Classic findings in hemangioma are absent visualization during arterial perfusion imaging, while on blood pool imaging, the lesion becomes more intense than surrounding normal liver, a phenomenon termed the "perfusion-blood pool mismatch" [52] (Fig. 7.17). Activity greater than adjacent liver is observed on the 2- to 3-h delayed image but may even be evident on the immediate blood pool images.

Overall imaging accuracy for detecting hemangiomas is reported to be 90%, especially if SPECT is used for smaller lesions. Sensitivity for characterizing hemangiomas greater than 2–3 cm in diameter is high; smaller lesions can be best detected when peripheral and SPECT is performed [64, 65]. In giant cavernous hemangiomas, RBC SPECT has been shown to be useful in differentiation from other large liver masses and is superior to US [66]. False-negative results have been rarely seen in hemangiomas with extensive fibrosis and thrombosis [67] or when attempting to visualize lesions below the effective resolution. False-positive studies demonstrating increased blood pool have been rarely described in patients with hemangiosarcoma [68] and very rarely in HCC. In a meta-analysis of 365 patients with 254 hemangiomas [63], the unusual combination of early flow and delayed intense filling was present in 16 lesions (4.4%). Twelve of these cases were determined to be hemangioma,

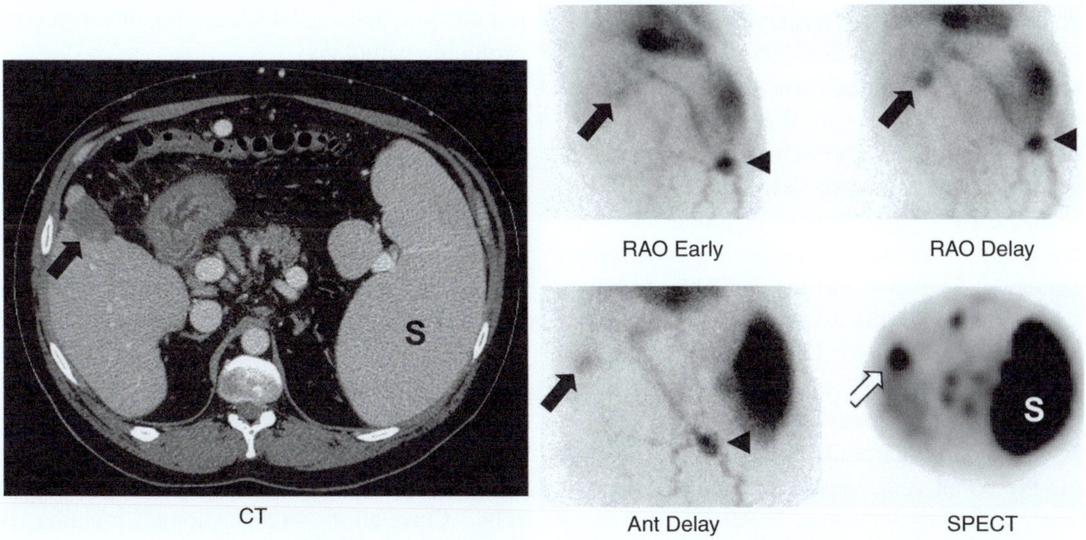

Fig. 7.17 A 50-year-old male with hepatitis C and alcoholic cirrhosis. CT scan of the abdomen (left panel) suggests hemangioma of the liver (arrow). Multiple venous collaterals are noted throughout the abdomen. Images from RBC hemangioma study (right panels) demonstrate presence of intense blood pool in the region of the lesion, increasing between the early and delayed images. The spleen (*S*) is enlarged and multiple venous anastomoses over the abdomen are noted (arrowhead, *caput medusae*)

while four were diagnosed as HCC. In an effort to increase specificity, these authors recommended restricting the diagnosis of hemangioma to lesions that do not evidence increased arterial perfusion, even though sensitivity will be slightly reduced. When increased arterial flow is present, as in the 4.4% of examinations in their meta-analysis, additional diagnostic studies and biopsy are then needed to make a definitive diagnosis.

7.5 Other Ancillary Techniques

7.5.1 ^{18}F-Fluorodeoxyglucose PET

^{18}F-Fluorodeoxyglucose (FDG) PET has become a mainstay of oncologic imaging [69], discussed elsewhere in this text. It is therefore not surprising that this modality has been successfully used in evaluating tumors of the liver and GI tract (Fig. 7.13). Liver tissue normally exhibits moderate FDG uptake with standardized uptake values (SUVs) typically on the order of 2.0. Increased FDG uptake in tumor cells has been shown to be due to increased expression of glucose transporter (GLUT) molecules on the cell surface, increased activity of hexokinase, and reduced levels of glucose-6-phosphatase [70].

Uptake of FDG is not restricted to malignancy, and various inflammatory and infectious states can lead to increased FDG uptake, by virtue of the collection of cells and organisms that utilize glucose and its analogs. This can include tuberculous [71], mycotic, and pyogenic abscesses.

7.5.2 Hepatic Arterial Perfusion Scintigraphy [37, 72]

Hepatic arterial perfusion scintigraphy (HAPS) was initially developed and is still used as a means of confirming proper placement of hepatic artery chemotherapy infusion catheters prior to delivery of arterial chemotherapy to intrahepatic tumors [73, 74]. A quantity of 37–185 MBq (1–5 mCi) of ^{99m}Tc-macroaggregated albumin (MAA), particle size 10–90 μm, is injected through an infusion catheter placed in the hepatic artery, resulting in trapping of radiopharmaceutical within the downstream perfused capillary bed [37]. The rate of injection should be less than 1 ml/min to avoid creating artifactual perfusion patterns and should optimally be similar to that of the proposed therapeutic agent. The distribution of activity is subsequently imaged using planar, SPECT, or SPECT-CT scintigraphy, including views of the lungs to identify intrahepatic arteriovenous fistulas. If SPECT-CT is not available, comparison to imaging of the liver following injection of colloid may be helpful [37]. This technique has been adopted as a sensitive means of detecting intrahepatic metastases based on the differences in perfusion of normal liver parenchyma, largely via the portal vein, versus intrahepatic metastases, via the hepatic artery. Metastatic lesions as small as 0.5–1.0 cm in size may be detected as "hot spots" [75]. Small lesions have been identified that were not seen by CT or CT arterial portography and which could only be confirmed at blind resection or biopsy [76]. While effective, HAPS is not commonly performed for detection of intrahepatic malignancy due to the invasiveness of placing an injection catheter into the hepatic artery.

Based on similar physiologic principles, treatment with ^{90}Y-containing microspheres has been introduced as a means of delivering localized radiation to sites of hepatocellular carcinoma and metastatic lesions [72, 77, 78]. Prior to treatment, hepatopulmonary shunting secondary to tumor-related pathologic arteriovenous channels, as well as reflux toward the gastrointestinal region, should be evaluated at scintigraphy following injection of 5–6 mCi (185–222 MBq) of ^{99m}Tc-labeled MAA as a microsphere surrogate into the hepatic arterial territory (see also Chap. 38) [79–81].

7.5.3 ^{133}Xenon Gas

Though not commonly performed today, radioactive xenon has historically been used to identify focal fatty changes in the liver, based on retention of the radioactive gas within the liver on delayed washout studies [82–84]. When the liver exhibits only a moderate degree of hepatic steatosis, a normal SC examination appears to be a more reliable [45] and available scintigraphic means of excluding pathology.

7.5.4 ^{123}I- and ^{131}I-Metaiodobenzylg uanadine

^{123}I- and ^{131}I-metaiodobenzylguanadine (MIBG) is used in the imaging of pheochromocytomas, paragangliomas, neuroblastoma, carcinoid, and medullary thyroid tumors and can be helpful in evaluating lesions metastatic to the liver [85–87]. MIBG is a guanidine derivative, structurally similar to norepinephrine, that concentrates within secretory granules of catecholamine-producing cells. Correlation with anatomic imaging is important in achieving accuracy [88].

The ^{123}I-labeled analog has superior imaging and dosimetry characteristics and is preferred if available. Some authors have reported relatively higher concentration of MIBG in normal parenchyma of the left lobe of the liver as compared to the right, possibly due to a greater presence of catecholamines and a higher sympathetic nerve density [89]. MIBG imaging may be useful in selecting patients slated for therapy with therapeutic amounts of ^{131}I-MIBG (s. also Chaps. 13 and 35) [90].

7.5.5 ^{111}In-Octreotide (Octreoscan) and ^{68}Ga-DOTATATE

^{111}In-octreotide represents a receptor binding radiopharmaceutical that is used in the staging of various endocrinologic tumors and can detect presence of liver metastases (Figs. 7.13, 7.18). This ^{111}In-labeled somatostatin analog binds to the sstr2 receptor that is present on the extracellular membrane of numerous neuroendocrine tumor (NET) types [70]. Overall, reported sensitivity of ^{111}In-octreotide is 80–90% for gastrinomas, 70% for carcinoids, 40% for insulinomas, and 30% for glucagonoma [91]. Somatostatin receptor scintigraphy has been shown to be superior to FDG PET for diagnosing and staging carcinoid tumors; the latter should be reserved for patients with negative results on octreotide

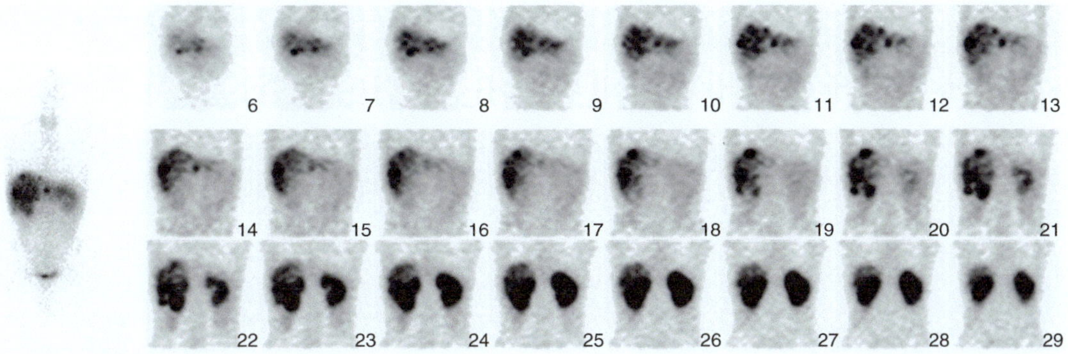

Fig. 7.18 A 42-year-old male with history of carcinoid tumor. Whole-body image (left panel) and sequential coronal SPECT images (right panel) were obtained 24 h following injection of ^{111}In-octreotide. Numerous foci of radiopharmaceutical uptake are noted which stud the liver. Physiologic excretion of octreotide is noted on posterior tomographic images through the kidneys (*frames 22–29*)

scintigraphy [92]. In the current era, analogous PET tracers have enjoyed considerable success in the imaging of NET-type tumors, especially ^{68}Ga-DOTATATE [93]. The uncinate process of the pancreas may physiologically exhibit increased radiopharmaceutical uptake; this pattern should be recognized as a normal variant [93, 94]. These applications will be discussed in Chaps. 13 and 34.

7.5.6 ^{67}Ga-Citrate

Since the 1970s, ^{67}Ga-citrate has been known to accumulate in both malignant and infectious processes that affect the liver [95]. More recently, the mechanism of localization of ^{67}Ga-citrate in tumors has been understood to be receptor based, reflecting increased presence of transferrin receptors to which circulating ^{67}Ga-transferrin complexes bind [96]. Comparison to SC imaging is recommended [48], as a gallium-avid tumor may appear isointense to normal liver and would therefore be difficult to diagnose on gallium scan alone though it would be readily identifiable when compared to the defect on a SC or other anatomic studies.

Approximately 90–95% of HCCs are reported to have ^{67}Ga-citrate uptake, and this radiopharmaceutical has historically served an important ancillary role in making this diagnosis [95, 97, 98] (Fig. 7.19) though today gallium imaging is not usually employed in this diagnosis. In addition to HCC, other tumor types that are frequently ^{67}Ga-citrate avid include lymphoma and metastases from lung carcinoma, melanoma, colorectal carcinoma, sarcoma, and testicular neoplasms. A variety of abscesses concentrate gallium citrate, and this application is discussed elsewhere in this book under the topic of infection imaging (Chap. 16).

7.6 Summary and Future Developments

Scintigraphic imaging retains a role in the functional and noninvasive evaluation of the solid GI tract. In the near future, the area of greatest growth which will likely impact on this modality is the continued development of novel PET radiopharmaceuticals that target those tumors presently not well localized by the currently available radiopharmaceutical ^{18}F-FDG [99]. Increasing experience and knowledge will also lead to consolidation of radionuclide studies into diagnostic and treatment algorithms. Through fusion of scintigraphic images with CT, hybrid imaging seeks to combine the functional strength of scintigraphic imaging with the superior resolution of anatomic radiologic modalities.

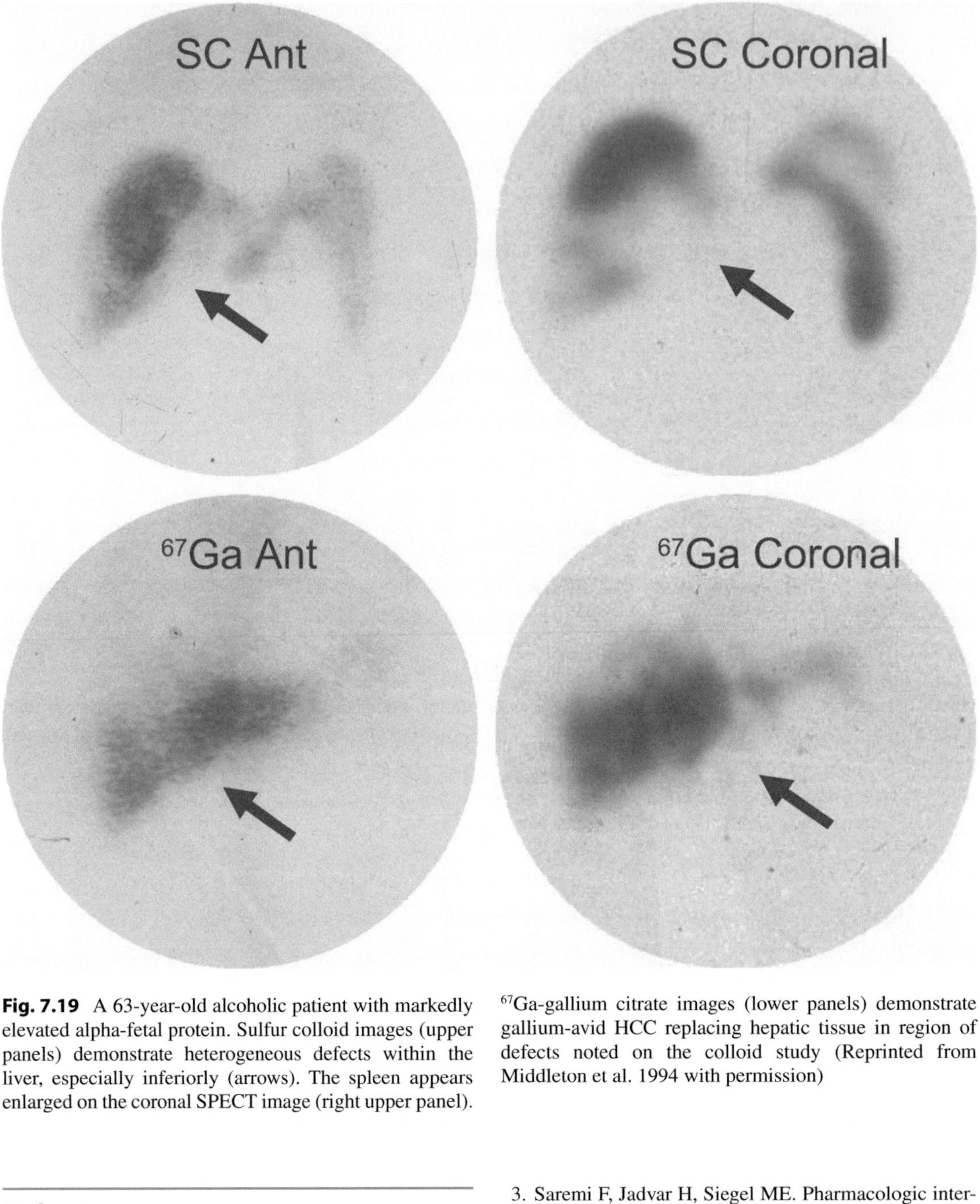

Fig. 7.19 A 63-year-old alcoholic patient with markedly elevated alpha-fetal protein. Sulfur colloid images (upper panels) demonstrate heterogeneous defects within the liver, especially inferiorly (arrows). The spleen appears enlarged on the coronal SPECT image (right upper panel). ^{67}Ga-gallium citrate images (lower panels) demonstrate gallium-avid HCC replacing hepatic tissue in region of defects noted on the colloid study (Reprinted from Middleton et al. 1994 with permission)

References

1. Zuckier LS, Freeman LM. Selective role of nuclear medicine in evaluating the acute abdomen. Radiol Clin North Am. 2003;41:1275–88.
2. Wistow BW, Subramanian G, Heertum RL, Henderson RW, Gagne GM, Hall RC, McAfee JG. An evaluation of 99mTc-labeled hepatobiliary agents. J Nucl Med. 1977;18:455–61.
3. Saremi F, Jadvar H, Siegel ME. Pharmacologic interventions in nuclear radiology: indications, imaging protocols, and clinical results. Radiographics. 2002;22:477–90.
4. Ziessman HA. Interventions used with cholescintigraphy for the diagnosis of hepatobiliary disease. Semin Nucl Med. 2009;39:174–85.
5. Gerard PS, Brown RKJ, Parisi MT, Tulchinsky M, Biyyam DR, Servaes S, Treves ST. ACR–SPR practice parameter for the performance of hepatobiliary scintigraphy. ACR–SPR. 2017;2017:1–8.

6. Tulchinsky M, Ciak BW, Delbeke D, Hilson A, Holes-Lewis KA, Stabin MG, Ziessman HA. SNM practice guideline for hepatobiliary scintigraphy 4.0. J Nucl Med Technol. 2010;38:210–8.
7. Kim CK, Palestro CJ, Solomon RW, Molinari DS, Lee SO, Goldsmith SJ. Delayed biliary-to-bowel transit in cholescintigraphy after cholecystokinin treatment. Radiology. 1990;176:553–6.
8. Weissmann HS, Frank MS, Bernstein LH, Freeman LM. Rapid and accurate diagnosis of acute cholecystitis with 99mTc-HIDA cholescintigraphy. AJR. 1979;132:523–8.
9. Weissmann HS, Berkowitz D, Fox MS, Gliedman ML, Rosenblatt R, Sugarman LA, Freeman LM. The role of technetium-99m iminodiacetic acid (IDA) cholescintigraphy in acute acalculous cholecystitis. Radiology. 1983;146:177–80.
10. Kiewiet JJ, Leeuwenburgh MM, Bipat S, Bossuyt PM, Stoker J, Boermeester MA. A systematic review and meta-analysis of diagnostic performance of imaging in acute cholecystitis. Radiology. 2012;264:708–20.
11. Fink-Bennett D, Balon H, Robbins T, Tsai D. Morphine-augmented cholescintigraphy: its efficacy in detecting acute cholecystitis. J Nucl Med. 1991;32:1231–3.
12. Kim CK, Juweid M, Woda A, Rothstein RD, Alavi A. Hepatobiliary scintigraphy: morphine-augmented versus delayed imaging in patients with suspected acute cholecystitis. J Nucl Med. 1993;34:506–9.
13. Meekin GK, Ziessman HA, Klappenbach RS. Prognostic value and pathophysiologic significance of the rim sign in cholescintigraphy. J Nucl Med. 1987;28:1679–82.
14. Smith R, Rosen JM, Gallo LN, Alderson PO. Pericholecystic hepatic activity in cholescintigraphy. Radiology. 1985;156:797–800.
15. DiBaise JK, Richmond BK, Ziessman HA, Everson GT, Fanelli RD, Maurer AH, Ouyang A, Shamamian P, Simons RJ, Wall LA, Weida TJ, Tulchinsky M. Cholecystokinin-cholescintigraphy in adults: consensus recommendations of an interdisciplinary panel. Clin Nucl Med. 2012;37:63–70.
16. Ziessman HA, Tulchinsky M, Lavely WC, Gaughan JP, Allen TW, Maru A, Parkman HP, Maurer AH. Sincalide-stimulated cholescintigraphy: a multicenter investigation to determine optimal infusion methodology and gallbladder ejection fraction normal values. J Nucl Med. 2010;51:277–81.
17. Krishnamurthy GT, Brown PH. Comparison of fatty meal and intravenous cholecystokinin infusion for gallbladder ejection fraction. J Nucl Med. 2002;43:1603–10.
18. Ziessman HA, Jones DA, Muenz LR, Agarval AK. Cholecystokinin cholescintigraphy: methodology and normal values using a lactose-free fatty-meal food supplement. J Nucl Med. 2003;44:1263–6.
19. Ziessman HA. Cholecystokinin cholescintigraphy: victim of its own success? J Nucl Med. 1999;40:2038–42.
20. Sostre S, Kalloo AN, Spiegler EJ, Camargo EE, Wagner HN Jr. A noninvasive test of sphincter of Oddi dysfunction in postcholecystectomy patients: the scintigraphic score. J Nucl Med. 1992;33:1216–22.
21. Matesan M, Bermo M, Cruite I, Shih CH, Elojeimy S, Behnia F, Lewis D, Vesselle H. Biliary leak in the postsurgical abdomen: a primer to HIDA scan interpretation. Semin Nucl Med. 2017;47:618–29.
22. Trerotola SO, Savader SJ, Lund GB, Venbrux AC, Sostre S, Lillemoe KD, Cameron JL, Osterman FA Jr. Biliary tract complications following laparoscopic cholecystectomy: imaging and intervention. Radiology. 1992;184:195–200.
23. Zeman RK, Lee CH, Stahl R, Viscomi GN, Baker C, Cahow CE, Dobbins J, Neumann R, Burrell MI. Strategy for the use of biliary scintigraphy in non-iatrogenic biliary trauma. Radiology. 1984;151:771–7.
24. Estrada WN, Zanzi I, Ward R, Negrin JA, Margouleff D. Scintigraphic evaluation of postoperative complications of laparoscopic cholecystectomy. J Nucl Med. 1991;32:1910–1.
25. Weissmann HS, Byun KJ, Freeman LM. Role of Tc-99m IDA scintigraphy in the evaluation of hepatobiliary trauma. Semin Nucl Med. 1983;13:199–222.
26. Majd M, Reba RC, Altman RP. Effect of phenobarbital on 99mTc-IDA scintigraphy in the evaluation of neonatal jaundice. Semin Nucl Med. 1981;11:194–204.
27. Lee CH, Wang PW, Lee TT, Tiao MM, Huang FC, Chuang JH, Shieh CS, Cheng YF. The significance of functioning gallbladder visualization on hepatobiliary scintigraphy in infants with persistent jaundice. J Nucl Med. 2000;41:1209–13.
28. Kianifar HR, Tehranian S, Shojaei P, Adinehpoor Z, Sadeghi R, Kakhki VR, Keshtgar AS. Accuracy of hepatobiliary scintigraphy for differentiation of neonatal hepatitis from biliary atresia: systematic review and meta-analysis of the literature. Pediatr Radiol. 2013;43:905–19.
29. Hasegawa Y, Nakano S, Ibuka K, Hashizume T, Noguchi A, Sasaki Y, Imaoka S, Fujita M, Kawamoto S, Kasugai H, et al. Specific diagnosis of hepatocellular carcinoma by delayed hepatobiliary imaging. Cancer. 1986;57:230–6.
30. Lee VW, O'Brien MJ, Devereux DF, Morris PM, Shapiro JH. Hepatocellular carcinoma: uptake of 99mTc-IDA in primary tumor and metastasis. AJR. 1984;143:57–61.
31. Calvet X, Pons F, Bruix J, Bru C, Lomena F, Herranz R, Brugera M, Faus R, Rodes J. Technetium-99m DISIDA hepatobiliary agent in diagnosis of hepatocellular carcinoma: relationship between detectability and tumor differentiation. J Nucl Med. 1988;29:1916–20.
32. Drane WE, Krasicky GA, Johnson DA. Radionuclide imaging of primary tumors and tumor-like conditions of the liver. Clin Nucl Med. 1987;12:569–82.
33. Lee VW, O'Brien MJ, Morris PM, Devereux DF, Shapiro JH. The specific diagnosis of hepatocellular carcinoma by scintigraphy. Multiple radiotracer approach. Cancer. 1985;56:25–36.
34. Middleton ML. Scintigraphic evaluation of hepatic mass lesions: emphasis on hemangioma detection. Semin Nucl Med. 1996;26:4–15.

35. Chilton HM, Brown ML, Swanson DP, Chilton HM, Thrall JH. Radiopharmaceuticals for abdominal and gastrointestinal imaging: reticuloendothelial, hepatobiliary, and intestinal. In: Pharmaceuticals in Medical Imaging. New York, NY: Macmillan Publishing Co., Inc.; 1990. p. 462–500.
36. Metter DF, Elman S, Shreve PD, Majd M, Servaes S, Shore RM, Williams JL. ACR–SPR practice parameter for the performance of liver and spleen scintigraphy. ACR–SPR. 2015;2015:1–8.
37. Metter DF, Fig LM, Gelfand MJ, Shreve PD, Binkovitz LA, Majd M, Parisi MT, Spottswood SE, Balon HR, Powsner RA. ACR–SNM–SPR practice guideline for the performance of liver and spleen scintigraphy. ACR–SNM–SPR. 2010;2010:1–5.
38. Yammine JN, Yatim A, Barbari A. Radionuclide imaging in thoracic splenosis and a review of the literature. Clin Nucl Med. 2003;28:121–3.
39. Gore RM, Newmark GM, Thakrar KH, Mehta UK, Berlin JW. Hepatic incidentalomas. Radiol Clin North Am. 2011;49:291–322.
40. Waxman AD. Scintigraphic evaluation of diffuse hepatic disease. Semin Nucl Med. 1982;12:75–88.
41. McClees EC, Gedgaudas-McClees RK. Screening for diffuse and focal liver disease: the case for hepatic scintigraphy. J Clin Ultrasound. 1984;12:75–81.
42. Hoefs JC, Sheikh MY, Guerrero H, Milne N. Factors affecting the quantitative liver-spleen scan in normal individuals. Dig Dis Sci. 2005;50:283–9.
43. Geslien GE, Pinsky SM, Poth RK, Johnson MC. The sensitivity and specificity of 99mTc-sulfur colloid liver imaging in diffuse hepatocellular disease. Radiology. 1976;118:115–9.
44. Kim EE. Focal splenic defect. Semin Nucl Med. 1979;9:320–1.
45. Baker MK, Schauwecker DS, Wenker JC, Kopecky KK. Nuclear medicine evaluation of focal fatty infiltration of the liver. Clin Nucl Med. 1986;11:503–6.
46. Lisbona R, Rush CL, Derbekyan V, Novales-Diaz JA. Radiocolloid liver imaging in hepatic steatosis. Clin Nucl Med. 1986;11:183–7.
47. Alderson PO, Adams DF, McNeil BJ, Sanders R, Siegelman SS, Finberg HJ, Hessel SJ, Abrams HL. Computed tomography, ultrasound, and scintigraphy of the liver in patients with colon or breast carcinoma: a prospective comparison. Radiology. 1983;149:225–30.
48. Davis LP, McCarroll K. Correlative imaging of the liver and hepatobiliary system. Semin Nucl Med. 1994;24:208–18.
49. Fawcett HD, Sayle BA. SPECT versus planar liver scintigraphy: is SPECT worth it? J Nucl Med. 1989;30:57–9.
50. Welch TJ, Sheedy PF 2nd, Johnson CM, Stephens DH, Charboneau JW, Brown ML, May GR, Adson MA, McGill DB. Focal nodular hyperplasia and hepatic adenoma: comparison of angiography, CT, US, and scintigraphy. Radiology. 1985;156:593–5.
51. Lubbers PR, Ros PR, Goodman ZD, Ishak KG. Accumulation of technetium-99m sulfur colloid by hepatocellular adenoma: scintigraphic-pathologic correlation. AJR. 1987;148:1105–8.
52. Rubin RA, Lichtenstein GR. Hepatic scintigraphy in the evaluation of solitary solid liver masses. J Nucl Med. 1993;34:697–705.
53. Dickson AM. The focal hepatic hot spot sign. Radiology. 2005;237:647–8.
54. Tetalman MR, Kusumi R, Gaughran G, Baba N. Radionuclide liver spots: indicator of liver disease or a blood flow phenomenon. AJR. 1978;130:291–6.
55. Muramatsu T, Miyamae T, Mashimo M, Suzuki K, Kinoshita S, Dohi Y. Hot spots on liver scans associated with superior or inferior vena caval obstruction. Clin Nucl Med. 1994;19:622–9.
56. Meindok H, Langer B. Liver scan in Budd-Chiari syndrome. J Nucl Med. 1976;17:365–8.
57. Shreiner DP, Barlai-Kovach M. Diagnosis of alcoholic cirrhosis with the right-to-left hepatic lobe ratio: concise communication. J Nucl Med. 1981;22:116–20.
58. Armas RR. Clinical studies with spleen-specific radiolabeled agents. Semin Nucl Med. 1985;15:260–75.
59. Massey MD, Stevens JS. Residual spleen found on denatured red blood cell scan following negative colloid scans. J Nucl Med. 1991;32:2286–7.
60. Oates E, Austin JM, Becker JL. Technetium-99m-sulfur colloid SPECT imaging in infants with suspected heterotaxy syndrome. J Nucl Med. 1995;36:1368–71.
61. Ishak KG, Rabin L. Benign tumors of the liver. Med Clin North Am. 1975;59:995–1013.
62. Nelson RC, Chezmar JL. Diagnostic approach to hepatic hemangiomas. Radiology. 1990;176:11–3.
63. Middleton ML, Milstein DM, Freeman LM, Freeman LM. Hepatic mass lesions: scintigraphic update with emphasis on hemangioma detection. In: Nuclear medicine annual 1994. New York, NY: Raven Press, Ltd.; 1994. p. 55–90.
64. Kudo M, Ikekubo K, Yamamoto K, Ibuki Y, Hino M, Tomita S, Komori H, Orino A, Todo A. Distinction between hemangioma of the liver and hepatocellular carcinoma: value of labeled RBC-SPECT scanning. AJR Am J Roentgenol. 1989;152:977–83.
65. Ziessman HA, Silverman PM, Patterson J, Harkness B, Fahey FH, Zeman RK, Keyes JW Jr. Improved detection of small cavernous hemangiomas of the liver with high-resolution three-headed SPECT. J Nucl Med. 1991;32:2086–91.
66. Tsai CC, Yen TC, Tzen KY. The value of Tc-99m red blood cell SPECT in differentiating giant cavernous hemangioma of the liver from other liver solid masses. Clin Nucl Med. 2002;27:578–81.
67. Rabinowitz SA, McKusick KA, Strauss HW. 99mTc red blood cell scintigraphy in evaluating focal liver lesions. AJR. 1984;143:63–8.
68. Ginsberg F, Slavin JD Jr, Spencer RP. Hepatic angiosarcoma: mimicking of angioma on three-phase technetium-99m red blood cell scintigraphy. J Nucl Med. 1986;27:1861–3.
69. Khandani AH, Wahl RL. Applications of PET in liver imaging. Radiol Clin North Am. 2005;43:849–60.

70. Bombardieri E, Aliberti G, de Graaf C, Pauwels E, Crippa F. Positron emission tomography (PET) and other nuclear medicine modalities in staging gastrointestinal cancer. Semin Surg Oncol. 2001;20:134–46.
71. Pelletier-Galarneau M, Martineau P, Zuckier LS, Pham X, Lambert R, Turpin S. (18)F-FDG-PET/CT imaging of thoracic and extrathoracic tuberculosis in children. Semin Nucl Med. 2017;47:304–18.
72. Rosenthal SA, Yung EY-K, Zaki BI, Salem R, Coldwell DM, Murthy R, Nutting CW. ACR–SIR practice parameter for radioembolization with microsphere brachytherapy device (RMBD) for treatment of liver malignancies. edited by American College of Radiology (ACR), and SIR; 2014.
73. Civelek AC, Sitzmann JV, Chin BB, Venbrux A, Wagner HN Jr, Grochow LB. Misperfusion of the liver during hepatic artery infusion chemotherapy: value of preoperative angiography and postoperative pump scintigraphy. AJR. 1993;160:865–70.
74. Thrall JH. Hepatic arterial chemotherapy: pharmacokinetic rationale and radionuclide perfusion imaging. Nucl Med Annu. 1984;1984:211–26.
75. Drane WE. Nuclear medicine techniques for the liver and biliary system. Update for the 1990s. Radiol Clin North Am. 1991;29:1129–50.
76. Vogel SB, Drane WE, Ros PR, Kerns SR, Bland KI. Prediction of surgical resectability in patients with hepatic colorectal metastases. Ann Surg. 1994;219:508–14; discussion 514–506.
77. Bozkurt MF, Salanci BV, Ugur O. Intra-arterial radionuclide therapies for liver tumors. Semin Nucl Med. 2016;46:324–39.
78. Salem R, Lewandowski RJ, Atassi B, Gordon SC, Gates VL, Barakat O, Sergie Z, Wong CY, Thurston KG. Treatment of unresectable hepatocellular carcinoma with use of 90Y microspheres (TheraSphere): safety, tumor response, and survival. J Vasc Interv Radiol. 2005;16:1627–39.
79. Biocompatibles UK Limited. TheraSphere® Yttrium-90 glass microspheres; 2014.
80. Murthy R, Nunez R, Szklaruk J, Erwin W, Madoff DC, Gupta S, Ahrar K, Wallace MJ, Cohen A, Coldwell DM, Kennedy AS, Hicks ME. Yttrium-90 microsphere therapy for hepatic malignancy: devices, indications, technical considerations, and potential complications. Radiographics. 2005;25(Suppl 1):S41–55.
81. Sirtex Medical Limited. SIR-Spheres® microspheres (Yttrium-90 Microspheres); 2014.
82. Ahmad M, Witztum KF, Fletcher JW, Hendershott LR, Klos D, George EA, Donati RM. Xenon-133 accumulation in hepatic steatosis. J Nucl Med. 1977;18:881–5.
83. Lisbona R, Mishkin S, Derbekyan V, Novales-Diaz JA, Roy A, Sanders L. Role of scintigraphy in focally abnormal sonograms of fatty livers. J Nucl Med. 1988;29:1050–6.
84. Shih WJ, Shih GL, Milan PP. Xenon 133 ventilation studies as an alternative for detecting and quantifying fatty infiltration of the liver. Radiographics. 2010;30:958–9; author reply 959–960
85. Kaltsas G, Rockall A, Papadogias D, Reznek R, Grossman AB. Recent advances in radiological and radionuclide imaging and therapy of neuroendocrine tumours. Eur J Endocrinol. 2004;151:15–27.
86. Pashankar FD, O'Dorisio MS, Menda Y. MIBG and somatostatin receptor analogs in children: current concepts on diagnostic and therapeutic use. J Nucl Med. 2005;46(Suppl 1):55S–61S.
87. Pfluger T, Piccardo A. Neuroblastoma: MIBG imaging and new tracers. Semin Nucl Med. 2017;47:143–57.
88. Pfannenberg AC, Eschmann SM, Horger M, Lamberts R, Vonthein R, Claussen CD, Bares R. Benefit of anatomical-functional image fusion in the diagnostic work-up of neuroendocrine neoplasms. Eur J Nucl Med Mol Imaging. 2003;30:835–43.
89. Jacobsson H, Jonas E, Hellstrom PM, Larsson SA. Different concentrations of various radiopharmaceuticals in the two main liver lobes: a preliminary study in clinical patients. Journal of gastroenterology. 2005;40:733–8.
90. Ezuddin S, Fragkaki C. MIBG and FDG PET findings in a patient with malignant pheochromocytoma: a significant discrepancy. Clin Nucl Med. 2005;30:579–81.
91. Drane WE. Scintigraphic techniques for hepatic imaging. Update for 2000. Radiol Clin North Am. 1998;36:309–18.
92. Belhocine T, Foidart J, Rigo P, Najjar F, Thiry A, Quatresooz P, Hustinx R. Fluorodeoxyglucose positron emission tomography and somatostatin receptor scintigraphy for diagnosing and staging carcinoid tumours: correlations with the pathological indexes p53 and Ki-67. Nucl Med Commun. 2002;23:727–34.
93. Hofman MS, Lau WF, Hicks RJ. Somatostatin receptor imaging with 68Ga DOTATATE PET/CT: clinical utility, normal patterns, pearls, and pitfalls in interpretation. Radiographics. 2015;35:500–16.
94. Agrawal K, Esmail AA, Gnanasegaran G, Navalkissoor S, Mittal BR, Fogelman I. Pitfalls and limitations of radionuclide imaging in endocrinology. Semin Nucl Med. 2015;45:440–57.
95. Lomas F, Dibos PE, Wagner HN Jr. Increased specificity of liver scanning with the use of 67 gallium citrate. N Engl J Med. 1972;286:1323–9.
96. Larson SM, Rasey JS, Allen DR, Nelson NJ, Grunbaum Z, Harp GD, Williams DL. Common pathway for tumor cell uptake of gallium-67 and iron-59 via a transferrin receptor. J Natl Cancer Inst. 1980;64:41–53.
97. Hauser MF, Alderson PO. Gallium-67 imaging in abdominal disease. Semin Nucl Med. 1978;8:251–70.
98. Suzuki T, Matsumoto Y, Manabe T, Honjo I, Proceedings HK. Serum alpha-fetoprotein and Ga67 citrate uptake in hepatoma. AJR. 1974;120:627–33.
99. Rosenbaum SJ, Stergar H, Antoch G, Veit P, Bockisch A, Kuhl H. Staging and follow-up of gastrointestinal tumors with PET/CT. Abdom Imaging. 2006;31:25–35.

Nuclear Medicine Imaging Techniques of the Kidney

8

Andrew T. Taylor

8.1 Radiopharmaceuticals

The radiopharmaceuticals available for assessment of renal function and anatomy can be grouped into three broad categories: those excreted by glomerular filtration, those primarily excreted by tubular secretion, and those retained in the renal tubules for long periods of time.

8.1.1 ^{99m}Tc-DTPA (Glomerular Filtration)

Glomerular filtration is an important measure of renal function; each day the glomeruli filter about 160 l of water and a kilogram of salt. Technetium-99m diethylenetriaminepentaacetic acid (DTPA) is the only renal radiopharmaceutical available for routine imaging that is purely filtered by the glomerulus and can be used to measure GFR. In normal subjects, the extraction fraction of DTPA (the percentage of the tracer extracted with each pass through the kidney) is approximately 20%; this extraction fraction is relatively low compared to the extraction fraction of tubular tracers (40–80%), and this difference has important clinical implications particularly in selecting a radiopharmaceutical for patients with azotemia or suspected obstruction.

8.1.2 ^{51}Cr-EDTA (Glomerular Filtration)

^{51}Cr-EDTA (ethylenediaminetetraacetic acid) is cleared by glomerular filtration and is used to measure GFR using plasma sample techniques (see clearances below).

8.1.3 ^{123}I- and ^{131}I-OIH (Tubular Secretion)

^{123}I- and ^{131}I-orthoiodohippurate (OIH) are cleared primarily by the proximal tubules although a small component is filtered by the glomeruli. The clearance of OIH is approximately 500–600 ml/min in subjects with normal kidneys; this clearance is often described as the effective renal plasma flow (ERPF) [1]. There is a common misconception that the ERPF (OIH clearance) is equivalent to renal plasma flow or, at least, proportional to renal plasma flow. The clearance of OIH is usually proportional to renal plasma flow, but OIH clearance (and the clearance of other Tc-99m tubular tracers) has two components: (1) renal plasma flow (the tracer must be delivered to the kidney) and (2) tubular

A. T. Taylor (✉)
Department of Radiology and Imaging Sciences, Emory University School of Medicine, Atlanta, GA, USA
e-mail: ataylor@emory.edu

H. Ahmadzadehfar et al. (eds.), *Clinical Nuclear Medicine*, https://doi.org/10.1007/978-3-030-39457-8_8

extraction (the tracer must be removed from the plasma by the proximal tubules). These two components do not always change in a parallel fashion. The main disadvantages of ^{131}I-OIH are the suboptimal imaging characteristics of many cameras for the high-energy 364-keV photon of ^{131}I- and the ^{131}I-beta emission which can result in radiation doses as high as one Sv (100 rems) to the kidneys of patients with impaired renal function following the administration of only 11.1 MBq (300 μCi) [2, 3]. For these reasons, ^{131}I-OIH is not recommended for routine use. ^{123}I-OIH is an excellent renal radiopharmaceutical, but it is limited by the logistics associated with the 13 h half-life of ^{123}I and lack of availability in many countries.

8.1.4 ^{99m}Tc-MAG3 (Tubular Secretion)

The clearance of ^{99m}Tc-mercaptoacetyltriglycine (MAG3) is highly correlated with the clearance of OIH, and the ^{99m}Tc-MAG3 clearance can be used as an independent measure of renal function. ^{99m}Tc-MAG3 is highly protein bound and is cleared almost exclusively by the proximal renal tubules [1, 4]. The extraction fraction is 40–50% [4, 5], more than twice that of ^{99m}Tc-DTPA. Because of its more efficient extraction, ^{99m}Tc-MAG3 is preferred over ^{99m}Tc-DTPA in patients with suspected obstruction and impaired renal function [6–14].

The ^{99m}Tc-MAG3 clearance averages about 300 ml/min/1.73 m^2 in adults under age 40 and tends to decrease at a rate of about 3–4 ml/year after age 40 [15]. The clearance of ^{99m}Tc-MAG3 is only 50–60% that of OIH, but ^{99m}Tc-MAG3 is more highly protein bound than OIH and tends to remain in the intravascular compartment; for this reason, blood pool activity in the heart, spleen, and liver is often prominent on the early images, especially in patients with impaired function. In contrast to OIH, however, ^{99m}Tc-MAG3 does not enter the red cells to any significant degree [1, 4, 16]. For these two reasons, a greater proportion of ^{99m}Tc-MAG3 remains in the plasma, and the increased plasma concentration compensates for the lower extraction fraction so that MAG3 is excreted from the body at essentially the same rate as OIH. Because of the similar rates of excretion, the renogram curves of ^{99m}Tc-MAG3 and OIH are almost identical.

The reproducibility of the MAG3 clearance has been a focus of debate. ^{99m}Tc-MAG3 clearance measurements based on blood samples have shown mixed results [17–19]; however, in one study of a large series of patients, the coefficient of variation was only 8.5% which is certainly adequate for most clinical uses [20]. Although plasma sample techniques are considered to have greater accuracy than camera-based clearance measurements [21], clearances that rely on blood samples have sources of error (timing of plasma samples, correction for radioactive decay, dilution of standards, pipetting errors) that are largely avoided by camera-based techniques (see below for a discussion of clearances). Camera-based clearances appear to be reproducible and superior to the creatinine clearance for monitoring changes in renal function [22–24].

In normal subjects, approximately 0.5% of the injected dose of ^{99m}Tc-MAG3 accumulates in the gallbladder by 30–60 min postinjection, and 1% of the dose is present in the GI tract by 3 h [25]. Elimination of ^{99m}Tc-MAG3 via the gallbladder can increase when patients have impaired renal function, and it can be accentuated by kit impurities [25–27]. The gallbladder is not a problem on early images but on rare occasions can simulate pelvic or calyceal activity on delayed images; if this question arises, it can be resolved by a lateral image. Bowel activity can also be observed and can present a problem in interpretation if delayed images are obtained to search for a urine leak [25].

8.1.5 ^{99m}Tc-L,L and D,D-EC (Tubular Secretion)

^{99m}Tc-L,L and D,D-ethylenedicysteine (EC) are both excellent renal radiopharmaceuticals with clearances slightly higher than MAG3 [28–30].

^{99m}Tc-LL-EC is available in several countries as a kit formulation and is clinically comparable to ^{99m}Tc-MAG3.

8.1.6 ^{99m}Tc-(CO_3) NTA (Tubular Secretion)

^{99m}Tc-(CO_3) NTA, tricarbonyl nitrilotriacetic acid, is a new ^{99m}Tc renal tracer with a more rapid clearance than ^{99m}Tc-MAG3; unlike ^{99m}Tc-MAG3, however, there was no evidence of gallbladder or gut activity in patients with chronic kidney disease [25, 27, 31]. In fact, the clearance of ^{99m}Tc-(CO_3) NTA is equivalent to that of OIH but, at present, ^{99m}Tc-(CO_3) NTA is not commercially available [31, 32].

8.1.7 Tc-99m DMSA (Cortical Retention)

^{99m}Tc-DMSA (dimercaptosuccinic acid) is an excellent cortical imaging agent. Approximately 40% of the injected dose binds to the renal tubules within 1 h after injection; the remainder is slowly excreted in the urine over the subsequent 24 h. ^{99m}Tc-DMSA is used when high-resolution anatomic images are required, such as the detection of pyelonephritis. Cortical scans can also confirm a suspected column of Bertin, measure relative function, and identify functioning renal tissue in patients with congenital abnormalities.

8.1.8 Tc-99m GH (Cortical Retention and GFR)

^{99m}Tc-GH (glucoheptonate) is cleared both by GFR and the renal tubules. In patients with normal renal function, most of the dose is rapidly excreted; however, 10–15% of the injected dose remains bound to the renal tubules, and high-resolution delayed static images can be obtained. ^{99m}Tc-GH tends to be used when ^{99m}Tc-DMSA is unavailable. Because of retention in the renal tubules, ^{99m}Tc-GH should not be used to evaluate suspected renal obstruction.

8.1.9 ^{99m}Tc-MDP (GFR)

^{99m}Tc-MDP (methylene diphosphonate) is not usually considered a renal imaging agent; however, it is cleared by GFR, and measurements of relative renal uptake (relative GFR) can be obtained at the time of a bone scan injection using standard renal software.

8.2 Technical Issues and Quality Control

8.2.1 Patient Information

Adequate patient information is not always provided. A simple and focused questionnaire given to the patient on arrival in the department can potentially generate useful information to help the nuclear medicine physician place the scan results in an appropriate clinical context. Useful information might include current medications, a description of any known kidney abnormality, renal function if known, and any history of heart disease, diabetes, atherosclerosis, hypertension, kidney infection, renal trauma, renal surgery, or prior radiation therapy to the area of the kidney.

8.2.2 Administered Dose

Renal scans are frequently performed following the intravenous injection of ≈370 MBq (10 mCi) of ^{99m}Tc-MAG3 or ^{99m}Tc-DTPA. Administration of activities in the range of 370 MBq may be required to obtain sufficient counts to visualize the initial bolus as it transits the aorta and kidneys or to calculate quantitative flow indices; however, except for the evaluation of renal transplants, neither 2 s flow images nor quantitative flow calculations obtained in the first few seconds following injection have been clearly demonstrated to contribute to the evaluation of relative function, suspected obstruction, or renovascular hypertension [33–36]. An administered dose of 370 MBq is unnecessarily high for almost all applications, and a range from 37 to 185 MBq is much more appropriate [8, 10, 36–39].

8.2.3 Hydration

For routine renography, patients should be well hydrated. Dehydration can lead to calyceal or pelvic retention and prolong the excretory phase of the renogram curve. Outpatients should be instructed to drink plenty of fluids prior to coming for the test, and the nursing staff should be requested to hydrate inpatients. To facilitate hydration, patients can also be given 5–10 ml of water/kg immediately on arrival in the nuclear medicine department, preferably 30–60 min before the exam. If a two-stage angiotensin-converting enzyme inhibition (ACEI) renography examination is scheduled, it is important to continue hydration between the studies. Despite these efforts, hydration may still be suboptimal [40]. The state of hydration can be evaluated when the patient arrives by collecting a urine sample and measuring the specific gravity. A specific gravity greater than 1.015 suggests dehydration.

8.2.4 Image Over the Injection Site

If part of the dose is infiltrated, the effect is variable depending on the rapidity of reabsorption of the infiltrated dose; however, single sample clearances are apt to be incorrect, and the excretory phase of the renogram curve may be prolonged [41] (Fig. 8.1). A spurious increase in the grade of the renogram curve from 0 to 2 or from 1 to 2 (Fig. 8.2) due to infiltration could result in an erroneous interpretation of an ACEI renogram (see below). A quantitative estimate of infiltration can be obtained if the decay-corrected counts in the injection site are divided by the injected counts. If the infiltration exceeds 0.5%, plasma sample clearances may be erroneous, and caution should be exercised before reporting the value. Infiltration can also be evaluated qualitatively by imaging the injection site. Finally, the likelihood of infiltration appears to be reduced if the

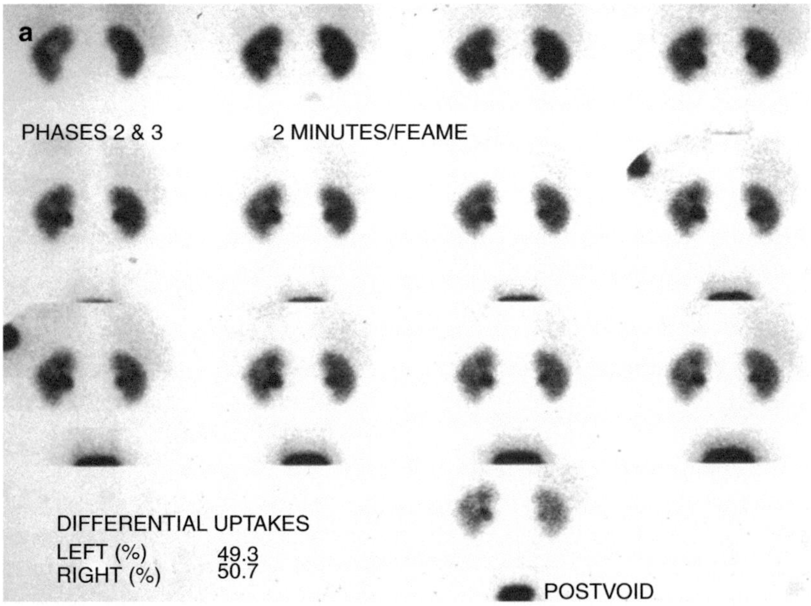

Fig. 8.1 (**a**) Two minute sequential renal images and a postvoid image were obtained following the intravenous injection of approximately 370 MBq of ^{99m}Tc-MAG3. There is marked infiltration of the dose noted in the left arm at 16–18 and 18–20 min postinjection. An estimated 18% of the dose was infiltrated based on placing an ROI over the infiltration site and dividing the decay-corrected infiltration counts at the completion of the study by the counts injected. (**b**) The renogram curves appear to show slow washout of the tracer with cortical 20 min/maximum count ratios of 0.57 and 0.73 (normal is less than 0.35). The apparent slow washout was due to the gradual absorption of infiltrated ^{99m}Tc-MAG3 from the infiltrated site. A repeat study was normal

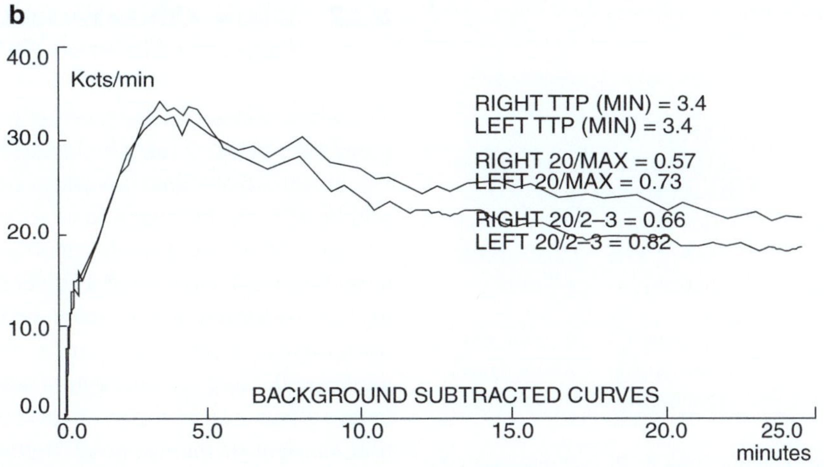

Fig. 8.1 (continued)

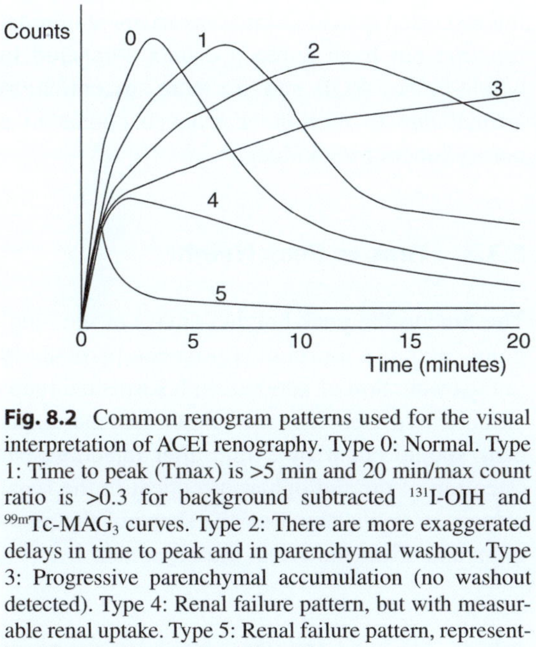

Fig. 8.2 Common renogram patterns used for the visual interpretation of ACEI renography. Type 0: Normal. Type 1: Time to peak (Tmax) is >5 min and 20 min/max count ratio is >0.3 for background subtracted ^{131}I-OIH and ^{99m}Tc-MAG$_3$ curves. Type 2: There are more exaggerated delays in time to peak and in parenchymal washout. Type 3: Progressive parenchymal accumulation (no washout detected). Type 4: Renal failure pattern, but with measurable renal uptake. Type 5: Renal failure pattern, representing blood background activity only

radiopharmaceutical is injected through a small indwelling catheter versus direct venipuncture.

8.2.5 Minimizing the Radiation Dose to the Patient

The patient should always be instructed to void at the conclusion of the study. In normal well-hydrated subjects, approximately 70% of the injected dose of ^{131}I-OIH and ^{99m}Tc-MAG3 reaches the bladder by 30 min postinjection [25]. Although the radiation dose from ^{99m}Tc-MAG3 and ^{99m}Tc-DTPA is quite low (Table 8.1), voiding at the conclusion of a ^{99m}Tc-MAG3 study and continuing to void at 30–60 min intervals for 3 h after the study can further reduce the radiation dose to the whole body, bladder, and ovaries by more than 50% compared to voiding 4 h after tracer injection [3, 8, 36].

8.2.6 Postvoid Images of the Kidneys

A postvoid image of the kidneys can be a useful adjunct to the standard renogram and can be particularly useful in evaluating the adult and pediatric patient with suspected obstruction (see below) [7–9, 42–45].

8.3 Quantitative Measurements

8.3.1 Relative Uptake

The relative renal uptake of each radiopharmaceutical provides a measure of relative function and is an important parameter in the interpreta-

Table 8.1 Radiation dose estimates for Tc-99m DTPA and MAG3[a]

Organ	DTPA, mSv (rem)	MAG3, mSv (rem)
Kidneys	0.14 (0.014)	0.14 (0.014)
Ovaries	0.13 (0.013)	0.086 (0.009)
Red marrow	0.045 (0.005)	0.018 (0.002)
Bone surfaces	0.068 (0.007)	0.025 (0.003)
Testes	0.088 (0.009)	0.050 (0.006)
Urinary bladder wall	1.9 (0.19)	1.7 (0.17)
Uterus	0.24 (0.024)	0.109 (0.011)
Total body	0.049 (0.005)	0.024 (0.002)
Effective dose equivalent	0.20 (0.020)	0.15 (0.015)

Bladder voided at 30 min, then at 4h, and then every 4 h thereafter

[a]37 MBq of Tc-99m DTPA or MAG3

tion of most studies. The measurement is usually made in the 1–2, 1–2.5, or 2–3 min period postinjection and needs to be completed prior to any drainage from the renal pelvis. Background subtraction using a C-shaped, elliptical, or perirenal region of interest appears to be superior to no background or inferior background regions of interest [8, 13, 14, 38, 46, 47], and an automated background subtraction probably improves reproducibility [48, 49]. Differences in the renal depth of the two kidneys can affect the relative uptake due to differences in attenuation, but this is rarely a clinically important problem. In a recent study where renal depth was determined by CT in 201 patients without abdominal pathology, the average difference in renal depth between the two kidneys was 0.61 cm. If the two kidneys have equal function and lie at a depth of 7 cm and the effective attenuation coefficient is 0.12, a 0.6 cm difference in renal depth would change the relative uptake from 50/50 to 52/48. The difference in renal depth was less than 2.0 cm in 99% of the patients, and a difference in 2.0 cm would change the relative uptake from 50/50 to 56/44. A recent study using ^{99m}Tc-MAG3 with automated C-shaped perirenal background regions of interest to measure relative function in 106 potential renal donors showed that all values fell between 40% and 60% [50].

8.3.2 Whole-Kidney Versus Cortical Regions of Interest (ROIs)

The whole-kidney ROI consists of an ROI placed around the whole kidney including the renal pelvis. Quantitative values generated using this ROI will be affected by retention of tracer in the kidney and collecting system; retention may be due to pathological states such as diabetic nephropathy or obstruction or may occur in nonpathological states such as a nonobstructed dilated collecting system or mild dehydration. To obtain a better assessment of parenchymal function, cortical or parenchymal regions of interest may be assigned over the renal cortex (parenchyma) that exclude any activity retained in the pelvis or calyces (Fig. 8.3). Cortical regions of interest often provide a better assessment of renal function but have reduced counts compared to whole-kidney ROIs and are more susceptible to artifact due to motion or reduced counts in a poorly functioning kidney.

8.3.3 Time to Peak Height

The time to the peak height (Tmax) of the renogram curve is a useful measurement, particularly in the evaluation of patients with suspected renovascular hypertension (see below). In general, the peak should occur by 5 min after injection, but retention of the radiopharmaceutical in the renal calyces or pelvis can alter the shape of the renogram and affect the Tmax measurement.

8.3.4 Twenty Min/Maximum Count Ratios

As renal function deteriorates, there is often a flattening of the renogram curve with a prolonged time to peak and delayed washout (Fig. 8.2). The degree of abnormality can be quantitated by a measurement of residual cortical activity using the ratio of the counts at 20 or 30 min to the maximum (peak) counts. These or similar ratios may also prove to be useful in monitoring patients

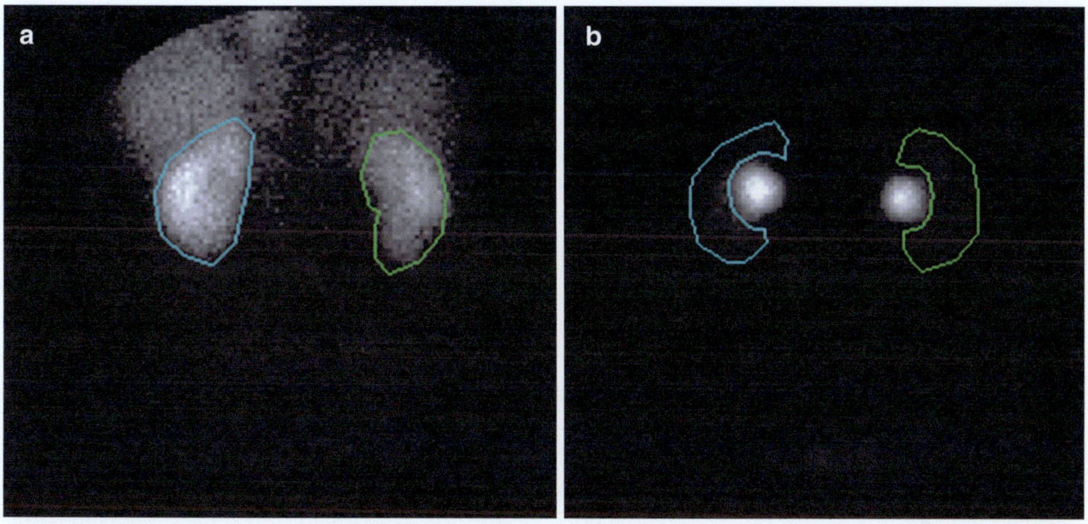

Fig. 8.3 (**a**) The whole-kidney ROI is illustrated using an image obtained 2–3 min after ^{99m}Tc-MAG3 injection. (**b**) The parenchymal (cortical) ROI is illustrated using the 19–20 min image to ensure that the parenchymal ROI would exclude the collecting system; assigning the parenchymal ROI on the early 2–3 min image is problematic since the collecting system is rarely visualized early in the study

with suspected urinary tract obstruction or renovascular hypertension [42, 51, 52]. Using background subtracted parenchymal regions of interest (activity within the collecting system excluded from the parenchymal ROI) (Fig. 8.3), the 20 min/max count ratio in a series of potential renal donors studied with ^{99m}Tc-MAG3 was 0.19 ± 0.07 for the right kidney and 0.19 ± 0.04 for the left kidney [50]. If the patient is not dehydrated and the 20 min/max count ratio for the cortical ROI exceeds 0.35 (greater than 2 standard deviations above the mean), the kidney is likely to be abnormal.

8.3.5 Prevoid/Maximum, Postvoid/Maximum, Prevoid/1–2 Min, and Postvoid/1–2 Min Count Ratios

These simple indices correlate with the more computational-intensive measurement of output efficiency to evaluate obstruction and can provide a useful adjunct to the interpretation of diuresis renography [43, 44, 53]. They can be easily derived from the renogram curve and/or a postvoid image of the kidneys; the postvoid image should be obtained after the patient assumes an upright posture so that gravity can assist drainage from the collecting system. Infants should be held in an erect position for 5 min before the postvoid image is obtained.

8.3.6 Residual Urine Volume

The patient population referred for renography often includes older males and patients with diabetes. Patients with prostatic hypertrophy may have substantial postvoid residuals, and patients with diabetes may present with a diabetic cystopathy, bladder distention, and an increased risk of reflux and pyelonephritis. Residual urine volume can be measured based on the counts in pre- and postvoid ROIs over the bladder and a measurement of the voided volume using the following formula: residual urine volume = (voided volume) (postvoid counts)/(prevoid counts − postvoid counts) [54]. Calculation of residual urine volume is a routine measurement at some institutions and can provide additional information for the referring clinician.

8.4 Renal Function

An assessment of renal function is often a critical element in the management of patients with renal disease. The most common measure of renal function in clinical practice is the serum creatinine, and it can be used to estimate the glomerular filtration rate (GFR); however, a number of factors (muscle mass, diet, age, certain drugs, illness, tubular secretion) can affect the serum creatinine, and the serum creatinine is not a sensitive measurement for detecting early renal disease [55–57]. In fact, there is a wide range of values for serum creatinine for all levels of GFR, and the serum creatinine can remain within the normal range despite a GFR 60–80% below normal [56]. The creatinine clearance provides a more sensitive method for monitoring renal function, but formal measurement of creatinine clearance with blood and 24 h urine samples is cumbersome, inconvenient for patients, and often unreliable [58, 59]. Moreover, repeated measurements of creatinine clearance in stable patients have been shown to have a disappointingly high 25% coefficient of variation (standard deviation/mean) [60]. The GFR can be estimated from the serum creatinine using the Modification of Diet in Renal Disease (MDRD), but there are clinical settings when a confirmatory test is needed [56, 57, 61, 62].

Measurement of renal function at the time of the scan can aid in the interpretation of a radionuclide study and provide a baseline for monitoring changes. From a clinical point of view, it is often more important to know if the renal function is stable, improving, or deteriorating than to know a precise clearance measurement; depending on the clinical question, reproducibility may be much more important than accuracy. A ^{99m}Tc-DTPA scan can be combined with a measurement of GFR, an ^{131}I-OIH scan can be combined with a measurement of ERPF, and a ^{99m}Tc-MAG3 scan can be combined with a measurement of the ^{99m}Tc-MAG3 clearance. Since the ^{99m}Tc-MAG3 and OIH clearances are highly correlated over a wide range of renal function, some institutions use a conversion factor to convert the ^{99m}Tc-MAG3 clearance into an ^{131}I-OIH equivalent. The two most widely used techniques to measure clearances are plasma sample and camera-based techniques.

8.4.1 Plasma Sample Clearances

The clearances of ^{131}I-OIH and ^{99m}Tc-MAG3 can be estimated from the dose injected and the amount of radioactivity in a single blood sample obtained approximately 45 min after injection [15, 21, 63]. Since ^{99m}Tc-DTPA is cleared more slowly than ^{131}I-OIH or ^{99m}Tc-MAG3, its clearance (GFR) must be estimated from the dose injected and the activity in one or more plasma samples obtained 1–4 h after injection [21, 64]. If carefully performed, clearance measurements based on plasma samples are more accurate than camera-based clearances, but plasma sample clearances require meticulous technique and attention to detail. Standards must be accurately prepared, dilutions carefully made, and the Tc-99m samples corrected for decay. In addition, the time of injection and the time of drawing the blood must be accurately recorded, and plasma samples must be carefully obtained without contamination by saline, heparin, or plasma from an earlier time. If the measurement is performed by a poorly trained or inexperienced individual, technical errors are often made and the results are spurious. The Radionuclides in Nephrourology Consensus Report and British Nuclear Medicine Society provide specific details regarding the recommended methodology for plasma sample clearances [21, 61].

8.4.2 Camera-Based Clearances

With nuclear medicine evolving toward increasing camera and computer sophistication and with pressures to increase the procedure volume, many technologists and physicians no longer have adequate training and/or time to obtain reliable plasma sample clearances. To address this need, camera clearance methods that do not require blood samples have been developed for ^{99m}Tc-DTPA, ^{131}I-OIH, and ^{99m}Tc-MAG3 [65–68]. Camera-based approaches to measure the renal uptake of ^{99m}Tc-DTPA, ^{131}I-OIH, and ^{99m}Tc-MAG3 have been reviewed in a recent consensus report [38]. The integral method has an accuracy comparable to the other camera-based methods, is simpler to perform [38, 69], and requires a measurement of the injected counts and counts in the kidney in an interval from 1–2, 1–2.5, or 2–3 min postinjection.

The methodology underlying the camera-based approach is illustrated using a current method for calculating the ^{99m}Tc-MAG3 clearance; briefly, processing software determines the percent injected dose in each kidney from 1 to 2.5 min postinjection and uses an algorithm derived from a multicenter trial to convert the percent injected dose in the left and right kidneys to a global ^{99m}Tc-MAG3 clearance (ml/min/1.73 m^2) [68, 70]. This is accomplished by counting the preinjection and postinjection syringes on the camera; counts in the postinjection syringe are corrected for decay and subtracted from the counts in the preinjection syringe to determine counts injected. To obtain percent injected dose in each kidney, regions of interest are assigned over each kidney; kidney counts from 1 to 2.5 min postinjection are corrected for background, infiltration, attenuation, and renal depth and divided by the counts injected to obtain the percent injected dose in the kidney at 1–2.5 min postinjection. If a large dose such as 370 MBq (10 mCi) is to be given, there is a risk of dead-time losses if the syringe containing 370 MBq is counted on the camera. The injected counts can be determined without dead-time losses by use of an attenuator [70] or by counting a small dose (37 MBq) on the camera and multiplying the counts in the small dose by the ratio of the injected dose to the small dose, both measured in a dose calibrator.

Not surprisingly, camera clearance methods have problems of their own. Two common sources of error are the estimation of renal depth for attenuation correction and background subtraction. In regard to background subtraction errors, ^{131}I-OIH and ^{99m}Tc-^{99m}Tc-MAG3 have an inherent advantage over ^{99m}Tc-DTPA because they are extracted more than twice as efficiently as ^{99m}Tc-DTPA. Because of the more efficient extraction, the kidney-to-background ratio is much higher for ^{131}I-OIH and ^{99m}Tc-MAG3 than ^{99m}Tc-DTPA, and any potential error introduced by over- or under-subtraction of background is substantially reduced. Renal depth is usually estimated from a nomogram based on height and weight [71, 72]. To the degree that a population-derived nomogram fails to fit a particular individual, the clearance measurement will vary from the true clearance. An alternative approach is to measure the renal depth based on a lateral image, but this requires extra steps, and defining an accurate renal outline on a lateral view 30 min following the injection of ^{131}I-OIH or ^{99m}Tc-MAG3 can be problematic, particularly in patients with good renal function. The sources of error due to background, self-attenuation, and renal depth tend to be reflected in a wider confidence interval associated with the accuracy of camera-based clearance compared to plasma sample clearances. Preliminary results suggest that the accuracy of gamma-camera clearance methods can be improved using software adapted to a dual-acquisition protocol [73].

Commercial camera-based techniques are currently available for measuring GFR (^{99m}Tc-DTPA), effective renal plasma flow (^{131}I-OIH), and the ^{99m}Tc-MAG3 clearance. In evaluating commercial software, it is important to confirm that the vendor has (1) incorporated the appropriate quality control features (a check for dose infiltration, avoidance of dead-time losses, preferably automated and reproducible perirenal background regions of interest, and a standardized time zero that is constant between studies) and (2) provided citable validation studies to confirm that there have been no coding errors and that the software is performing as claimed.

8.5 Renal Transplantation

Renal transplantation is the preferred treatment for end-stage renal disease, but the use of renal scintigraphy to evaluate the potential donor and the transplant recipient varies from center to center. Some centers use a renal scan to screen potential donors to ensure that both kidneys are functioning normally; other centers rely primarily on other imaging procedures. A normal renal scan in the immediate posttransplant period reliably excludes clinically important complications such as vascular occlusion, urine leak, and obstruction [74]. In cadaveric transplants, a scan in the immediate postoperative period can assess the presence of acute transplant nephropathy (ATN, acute tubular necrosis) which is related to ischemic damage that occurs before the donor's death and/or during the preservation period prior to transplantation. The kidney with ATN typically shows relatively preserved perfusion with reduced function, but perfusion can be also decreased in severe cases; the functional impairment usually resolves without therapy [74].

Scan interpretation requires knowledge of the clinical course and a review of prior scans, if available. Sequential scans with monitoring of renal function can identify early graft failure, and ACEI renography can detect renovascular hypertension as a late cause of deteriorating renal function; however, an isolated scan demonstrating prolonged transit and reduced function cannot reliably distinguish between rejection, ATN, or calcineurin inhibitor (cyclosporine and tacrolimus) toxicity [74, 75]. Chronic transplant nephropathy represents cumulative and incremental damage to nephrons from both immunologic and non-immunologic causes; calcineurin inhibitor nephrotoxicity appears to be the chief cause of late histologic injury associated with a continuing decline in renal function [76]. When transplant patients present with a decline in renal function, imaging studies are obtained if the clinician suspects complications relating to renal blood flow, urine leak, urinoma, obstruction, abscess, hematoma, or lymphoma, whereas renal biopsy is usually obtained to distinguish between rejection and calcineurin inhibitor nephrotoxicity.

8.6 Diuresis Renography

Obstruction to urinary outflow may lead to obstructive uropathy (dilation of the calices, pelvis or ureters) and obstructive nephropathy (damage to the kidney itself). Urine outflow obstruction may be suspected based on clinical findings, the incidental detection of a dilated renal collecting system, or diagnosis of previous obstruction in a patient referred for follow-up. Diuresis renography is the only widely available study that can evaluate renal function and urodynamics in a single test and is the subject of a recent procedure guideline [8]. This noninvasive test is based on a high endogenous rate of urine flow stimulated by the administration of furosemide. Interpretation of the test is based on the rate of washout of the radiopharmaceutical from the collecting system in the upper urinary tract.

8.6.1 Technical Issues Relating to Diuresis Renography

8.6.1.1 Pretest Voiding

The patient should void immediately prior to the examination. A full bladder may affect upper tract emptying and give false-positive results [10, 77].

8.6.1.2 Choice of Radiopharmaceutical

Adult and pediatric consensus groups recommend tubular agents for diuresis renography because tubular tracers are extracted much more efficiently by the kidney than ^{99m}Tc-DTPA, and, therefore, washout is easier to evaluate [7, 8, 10, 39, 78, 79]. Tubular agents such as ^{99m}Tc-MAG3 are particularly useful in infants and patients with impaired renal function, and their advantages compared to DTPA are illustrated in Fig. 8.4 [14].

8.6.1.3 Hydration

The patient should arrive for the study well hydrated and should receive an additional oral fluid load of 5–10 ml/kg of body weight 30–60 min before the procedure [8, 38]. If intravenous hydration is clinically indicated, it can be accomplished with a volume of fluid comparable to the amount of water recommended for oral hydration.

8.6.1.4 Dose of Furosemide

The recommended dose of furosemide is 0.5 mg/kg or 40 mg in an adult and 1.0 mg/kg in a child with a maximum dose of 20 mg [7, 8, 10, 79]. Furosemide is secreted by the proximal tubule and reaches its site of action in the tubular lumen of the thick ascending loop of Henle via the tubular fluid. In patients with impaired renal function, secretion of furosemide is proportionally reduced because of the underlying kidney disease; in addition,

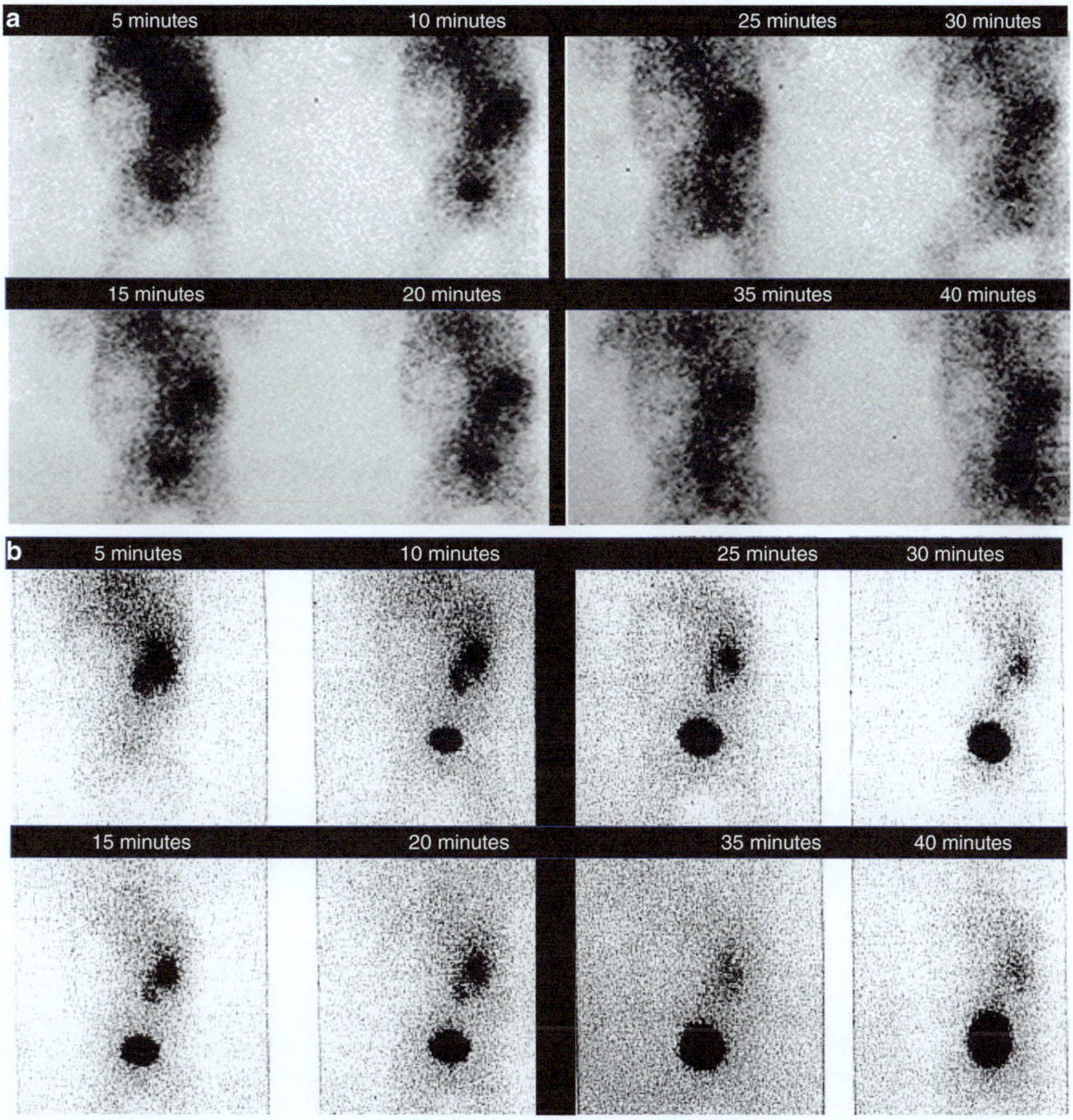

Fig. 8.4 A female infant underwent ultrasonography at age 3 days because of a rising creatinine. Renal ultrasonography showed a large, multicystic, dysplastic left kidney with marked dysplastic changes, peripheral cysts, and mild hydronephrosis of the right kidney and a dilated right ureter. Voiding cystourethrography showed no evidence of reflux. A ^{99m}Tc-DTPA scan (74 MBq) was obtained 4 days after birth (Fig. 8.4a). Sequential posterior 5 min images for 20 min are displayed in the left panel. The patient then received 1 mg of furosemide, and sequential 5 min images from 25 to 40 min are shown in the right panel. There is poor kidney definition, and the study was repeated with 74 MBq of ^{99m}Tc-MAG3 3 days later (Fig. 8.4b). Sequential posterior 5 min images for 20 min are displayed in the left panel. Furosemide was then administered, and sequential 5 min images from 25 to 40 min are shown in the right panel. ^{99m}Tc-MAG3 is already in the renal pelvis and upper ureter by 5 min; there is an excellent kidney-to-background ratio, and the tracer washes out rapidly following furosemide, thus excluding obstruction. The higher extraction fraction of ^{99m}Tc-MAG3 contributed to the superior image quality and led to greater diagnostic certainty (Reproduced with permission, Taylor et al. [14])

endogenous organic acids accumulate in chronic renal insufficiency and competitively inhibit the organic transport system of the proximal tubule further reducing the secretion of furosemide. To counteract these effects, a larger dose of furosemide must often be given to attain an effective level of diuretic in the tubular fluid (Fig. 8.5) [8, 80, 81]. A reasonable approach is to double the

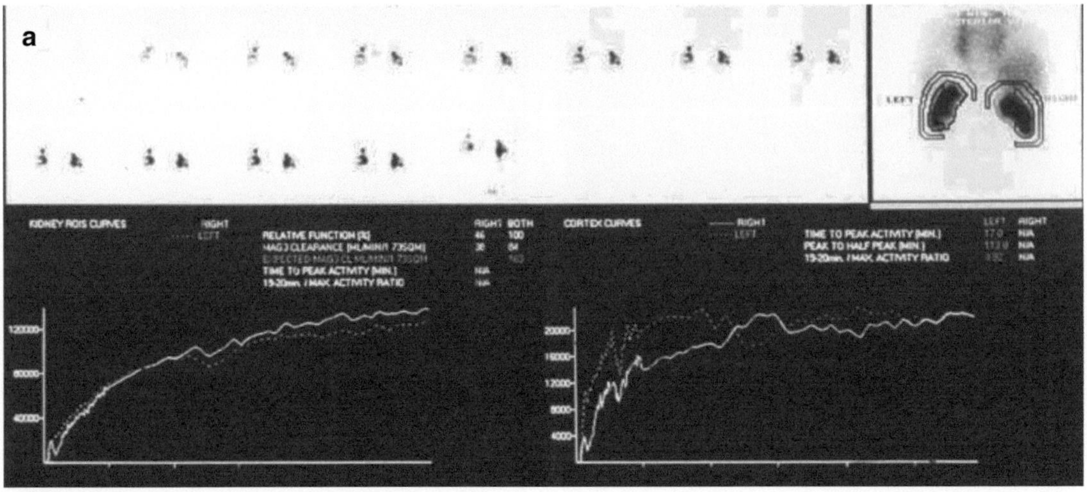

Fig. 8.5 A 77-year-old man with a complicated medical history had bilateral obstruction and bilateral nephrostomies placed in 1995. Four years later, he was observed to be voiding normally as well as draining from his nephrostomy tubes, and he was referred for diuresis ^{99m}Tc-MAG3 renography to determine if obstruction was still present or if the nephrostomy tubes could be removed. His creatinine had been stable at 2.0 mg/dl. (**a**) Following the injection of 280 MBq of ^{99m}Tc-MAG3, sequential 2 min images were obtained for 24 min (upper left panel); the last image in the sequence is a postvoid image. The upper right panel shows a 1–2.5 min image with whole-kidney, cortical, and background regions of interest. Whole-kidney renogram (lower left panel) shows a prolonged time to peak activity bilaterally ("N/A" indicates that the time to peak and the 19/20 to max ratio were not reached during the period of the examination on the left). On the right, the time to peak and the 19/20 to max ratio were 18.7 and 0.97 min, respectively. The relative function was 53% on the left and 47% on the right. The camera-based ^{99m}Tc-MAG3 clearance was 113 ml/min/1.73 m^2, compared with an expected ^{99m}Tc-MAG3 clearance value of 163 ml/min/1.73 m^2. The renogram obtained with a cortical region of interest (lower right) shows a prolonged time to peak activity bilaterally ("N/A" indicates that the time to peak, the peak to half peak, and the 19/20 to max ratio were 7.7, 14.8, and 0.6 min, respectively). (**b**) Forty milligram of furosemide were administered and sequential 2 min images were obtained for 20 min after furosemide administration (upper left panel). The kidneys show prominent pelvic retention. The time activity curve (lower panel) shows minimal excretion with prolonged half-times of 98 min on the left and 54 min on the right, consistent with obstruction. (**c**) By increasing the intensity, the percutaneous nephrostomy tubes (arrows) and the ureters could be visualized, although they were not apparent on the standard image display. The nephrostomy tubes had not been clamped; consequently, the patient was still in his baseline state and could not have been obstructed even though the scan appearance was that of obstruction. (**d**) The study was repeated with 366 MBq of ^{99m}Tc-MAG3, and the nephrostomy tubes were clamped. Sequential 2 min ^{99m}Tc-MAG3 images were obtained for 24 min (upper left panel); the last image in the sequence is a postvoid image. The upper right panel shows a 1–2.5 min image with whole-kidney, cortical, and background regions of interest. Whole-kidney renogram (lower left panel) shows a prolonged time to peak activity bilaterally ("N/A" indicates that the time to peak and the 19/20 to max ratio were not reached during the period of the examination on both sides). The relative function was 54% on the left and 46% on the right. The camera-based ^{99m}Tc-MAG3 clearance was 84 ml/min/1.73 m^2, compared with an expected ^{99m}Tc-MAG3 clearance value of 163 ml/min/1.73 m^2 based on the patient's gender and age. The renogram obtained with a cortical region of interest (lower right) shows a prolonged time to peak activity bilaterally ("N/A" indicates that the time to peak, the peak to half peak, and the 19/20 to max ratio were 17, 113, and 0.92 min, respectively). (**e**) Forty milligram of furosemide was not sufficient to cause an adequate diuresis to exclude obstruction in the initial study, and because the patient had an elevated creatinine of 2.0 mg/dl, 80 mg of furosemide were administered. The upper panel (sequential 2 min images obtained for 20 min after furosemide administration) and the time activity curves (lower panel) show no signs of obstruction with prompt washout of the tracer from the right kidney; the left kidney had largely emptied before furosemide administration. The $T_{1/2}$ was 12 min for the left kidney and 13 min for the right kidney. The nephrostomies were removed, and the patient's renal function has remained stable for 3 years (Reproduced with permission Hunsche et al. [80])

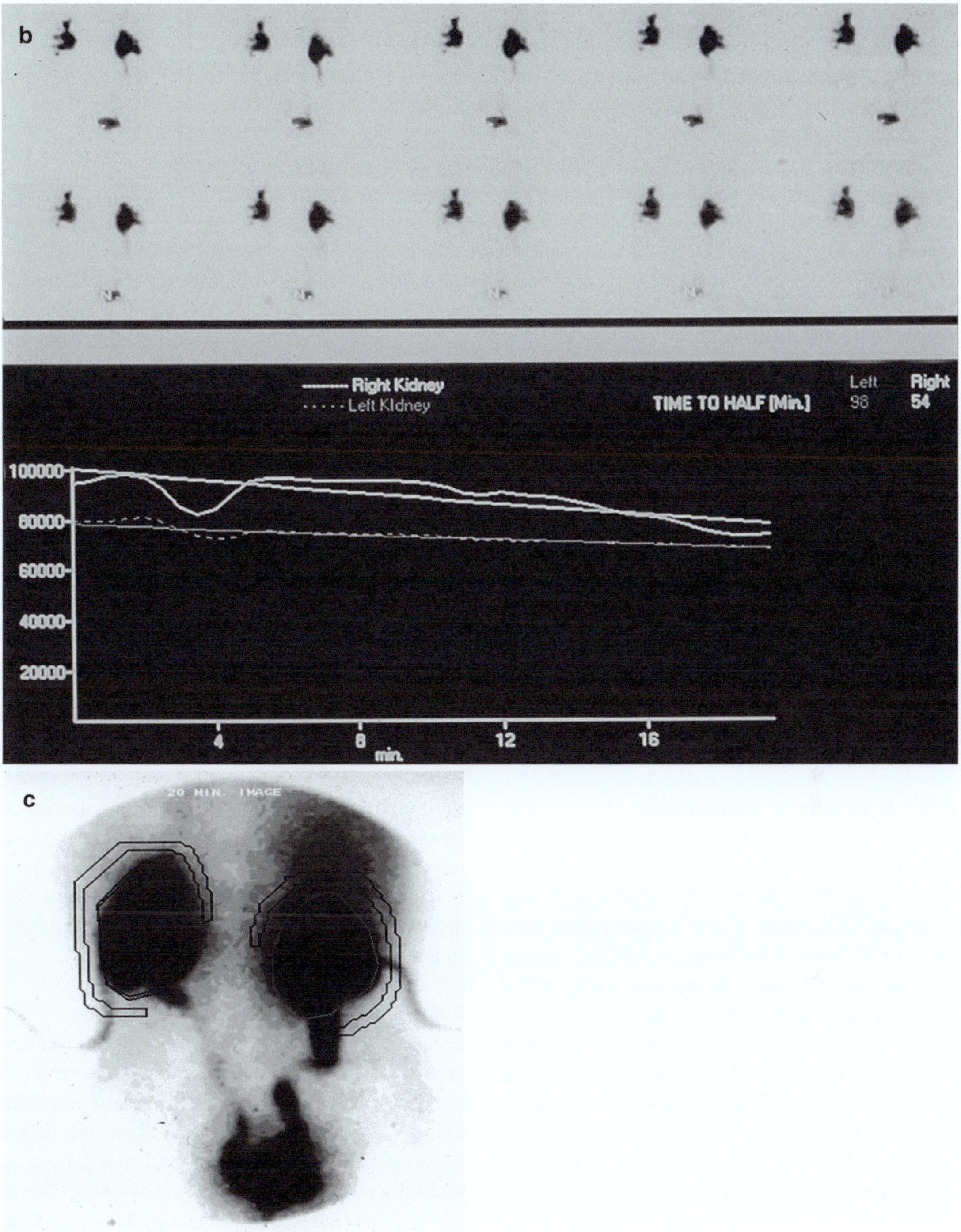

Fig. 8.5 (continued)

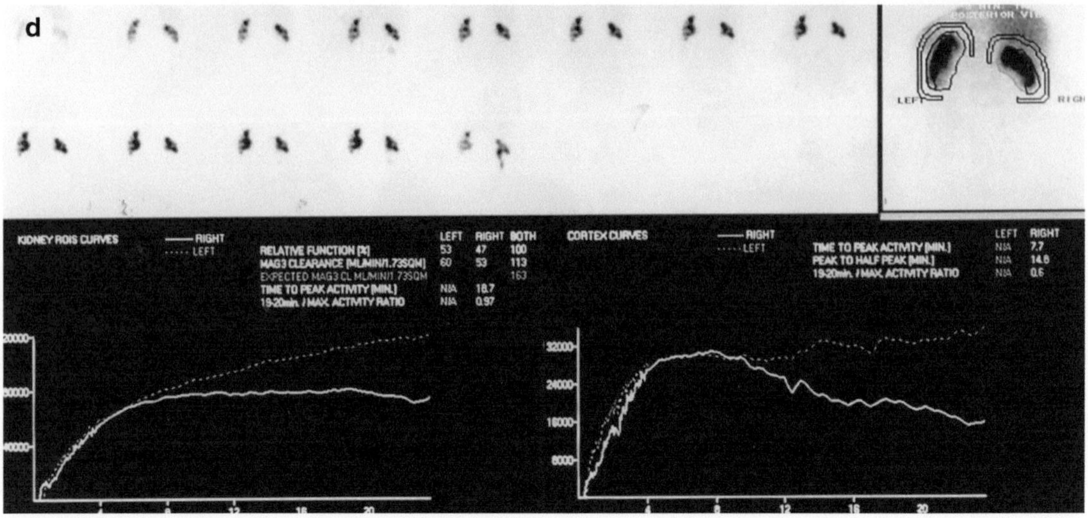

Fig. 8.5 (continued)

dose of furosemide to 80 mg for patients with a creatinine level that is elevated or for a MAG3 clearance that is reduced by 50% or more [8]. Most prescribers do not consider the use of sulfonamide nonantibiotics (such as furosemide) as problematic in the sulfonamide-allergic patients; furosemide is typically administered as a bolus over a few seconds [8, 82].

8.6.1.5 Timing of Furosemide Administration

Multiple protocols have been used for diuretic renography; they differ in the timing of furosemide and in the use of one or two acquisitions. The 1996 Santa Fe Consensus Report recommended that the time of furosemide be specified; typical times for furosemide administration are the $F - 15$, $F = 0$, and $F + 20$ protocols where the furosemide is administered 15 min before, simultaneously with or 20 min after the tracer administration. The Santa Fe Consensus Report recommended a 35 min acquisition with furosemide administered 20 min into the study [10]. A disadvantage of this protocol is that a percentage of patients (30% in one series) will not complete the acquisition because of a need to void [83]. The study can be divided into two separate acquisitions, a 20–25 min baseline acquisition followed by patient voiding and then a second 15–20 min acquisition following furosemide administration. If the baseline study is normal, obstruction can be excluded, and the furosemide acquisition can be omitted [84]. Since the test is based on the washout of the tracer from the collecting system, some physicians prefer to see retention of the radiopharmaceutical clearly visible in the collecting system (calyces, pelvis, or ureters) at the time of furosemide administration. If there is no radiopharmaceutical retention in the collecting system, the activity entering the kidney from the blood may largely replace the activity leaving the kidney resulting in a prolonged T½ even if the kidney is completely normal. All three protocols are acceptable and appear to give comparable results in the majority of patients [8, 85, 86].

8.6.1.6 Patient Position

Imaging is usually performed with the patient supine. The supine position allows a more accurate estimate of relative renal function since the kidneys are more likely to lie at the same depth. If the patient is initially imaged in a sitting or reclining position, one of the kidneys may change position leading to a difference in relative uptake which is due to differences in attenuation rather than differences in relative function. Gravity-assisted drainage is important for the interpretation of selected studies, and routine acquisition of postvoid images (see below) is a recommended component of the acquisition protocol [8, 39].

8.6.1.7 Postvoid Images

If a large proportion of the radiopharmaceutical remains in the collecting system at the end of the study, the patient should be asked to get off the table, stand up, go to the toilet, and void. After the patient voids, the postvoid image of the kidney should be obtained with the patient in the original supine position to maintain a consistent geometry; if the postvoid image is obtained with the patient upright, a ptotic kidney may give a false impression of adequate emptying. Infants should be held in an upright position for about 5 min to allow gravity to assist drainage, and then another image of the kidney should be obtained [7, 86]. Measurements to quantitate postvoid emptying or gravity-assisted drainage may facilitate interpretation of the study [8, 44, 85, 86]. In adults or infants who cannot empty their bladders, use of a catheter will minimize false-positive or indeterminate findings. Prompt drainage of radiopharmaceutical from the collecting system excludes obstruction and obviates administration of furosemide in a dual-acquisition protocol (Fig. 8.6).

8.6.1.8 Region of Interest (ROI) Selection for the Diuretic Portion of the Study

For the diuretic portion of the study, some experts assign a ROI over the whole kidney; others recommend placing the ROI only around the retained activity in the collecting system [8, 10, 78, 86, 87]. Placement of the ROI around retained activity in the collecting system rather than placing the ROI around the whole kidney provides a better assessment of the response to furosemide, particularly in poorly functioning kidneys with slow parenchymal transit [88].

8.6.1.9 Calculating the T½

Measurement of the T½ has not been standardized, and the T½ will vary depending on the placement of the ROI (whole kidney or dilated collecting system), and it will also vary depending on whether the measurement begins at the start of the data acquisition, the time the diuretic is injected, or at the beginning of the diuretic response. The T½ will also be affected by the algorithm (linear or exponential) used to fit the washout curve.

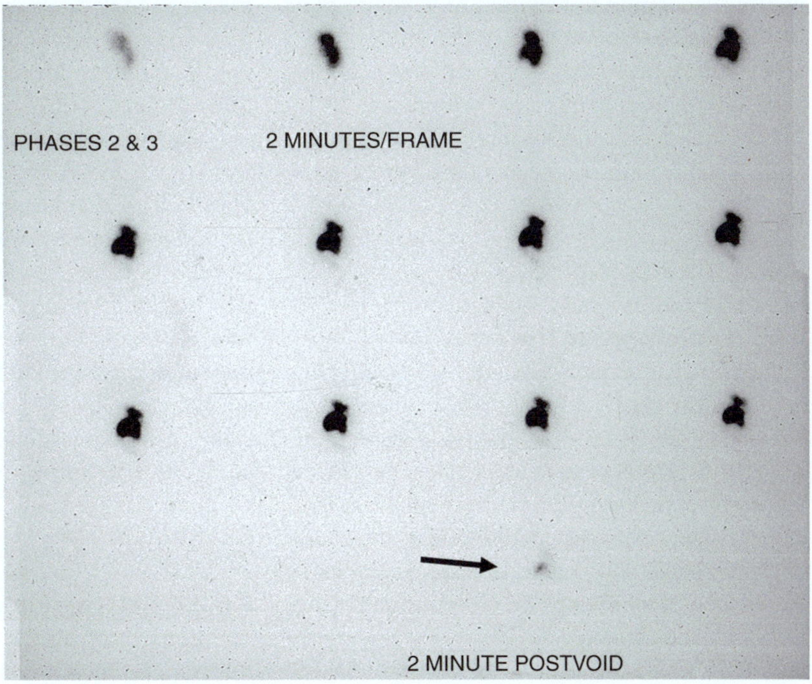

Fig. 8.6 A CT scan obtained in a middle-aged male with abdominal pain showed congenital absence of the left kidney and a dilated right renal pelvis. A ^{99m}Tc-MAG3 renal scan was performed with approximately 185 MBq of ^{99m}Tc-MAG3 and 2 min posterior images were obtained by a postvoid image (arrow). Following the patient's assumption of an upright posture and voiding, urine rapidly drained from the kidney excluding obstruction, obviating the need for furosemide and illustrating the value of the post-micturition image

8.6.1.10 Adequacy of Diuresis

The patient should void at the beginning and end of the diuretic acquisition. Dividing the volume of urine voided at the conclusion of the diuretic acquisition by the time in minutes between the two voiding periods gives an estimate of the urine flow rate. If the patient has normal renal function and 40 mg of furosemide are administered at the time of radiopharmaceutical injection, the patient should produce 200–300 ml of urine by the end of the 20–30 min [89]. A poor diuretic response may indicate dehydration or impaired renal function and result in false-positive or indeterminate findings. Measuring the voided volume alerts the nuclear medicine physician to an inadequate diuresis.

The rate of urine flow will decrease as renal function decreases, but urine flow rates as high as 4 ml/min have been reported for kidneys with creatinine clearances reduced to 20% of normal [90, 91]. A flow rate of 4 ml/min may be sufficient to wash the tracer out of the kidney allowing obstruction to be excluded even in kidneys with poor renal function, particularly if the renal pelvis is not excessively dilated. As renal function further deteriorates, an abnormal response cannot be used to distinguish obstruction from a poorly functioning kidney that failed to respond to furosemide. Conversely, if the kidney has a near-normal clearance, it should have a good diuretic response; in this case, retention of ^{99m}Tc-MAG3 in the collecting system following furosemide is much more suspicious for obstruction.

8.6.2 Interpretation

8.6.2.1 Interpreting the T½

Some experts interpret the study by visually analyzing of the washout curve, while others prefer to evaluate the rate of washout by measuring the T½ [10]. It is important to emphasize that normal values for T½ depend on the radiopharmaceutical, the delay between administering the radiopharmaceutical and administering furosemide, the method of hydration, the presence or absence of a bladder catheter, the dose of furosemide, region of interest selection, the interval used to make the measurement, and the method of calculating the T½. For these reasons, normal values for the T½ tend to be institution specific; nevertheless, there is general agreement that prompt clearance of the radiopharmaceutical from the renal collecting system with a T½ under 10 min is a normal response. Depending on the technique, a T½ between 10 and 20 min is often considered indeterminate, and a T½ greater than 20 min is suspicious for obstruction. However, the T½ value alone should never be the sole criterion for determining the presence or absence of obstruction; the T½ must always be interpreted in the context of the whole set of images, curves, and quantitative indices including total function, relative function, and the voided volume as well as any clinical information or diagnostic studies that may be available.

8.6.2.2 Alternatives to the T½

Some experts recommend that the T½ not even be used to assess drainage in asymptomatic children with unilateral ureteropelvic junction dilation. Instead, techniques which consider renal function, gravity, and an empty bladder are recommended. These include more complex measurements such as output efficiency and simpler measurements such as normalized residual activity (NORA), prevoid/maximum, postvoid/maximum, prevoid/1–2 min and postvoid/1–2 min count ratios, and the pelvic excretion efficiency (PEE) [44, 53, 92]. Simple ratios that incorporate gravity-facilitated drainage from the kidneys, such as the count in the postvoid kidney divided by the maximum count in the kidney, appear to provide more robust measurements of drainage than the T½ [8, 86, 93, 94]. In a study using the two-stage dual-acquisition protocol, the mean baseline postvoid-to-maximum ratio for kidneys interpreted as having normal drainage was 0.18 ± 0.16 [94]. In the same dual-acquisition study, the ratio of count at 20 min after furosemide to maximum count at baseline was 0.11 ± 0.12 for nonobstructed kidneys [94].

8.6.2.3 Relative Function

The purpose of intervention is to preserve renal function. Unless it is acute, obstruction usually causes a loss of function in the affected kidney. If the relative renal function is 50/50 in a patient with suspected unilateral obstruction, it may be appropriate to observe the patient and repeat the study even if the quantitative data such as the T½ are abnormal or equivocal.

8.6.2.4 Nondiagnostic Studies

Despite optimal technique, a certain number of studies (approximately 10–15%) will be difficult to interpret because of underlying poor function and/or an intermediate diuretic response. From a clinical point of view, it is important to decrease the number of tests that are nondiagnostic and to recognize the conditions other than obstruction that may lead to an abnormal diuretic response. Equivocal or false-positive results can occur due to a distended bladder [77], an insufficient dose of furosemide, the failure of a poorly functioning kidney to respond to furosemide, or slow washout of the radiopharmaceutical due to the reservoir effect of a grossly dilated collecting system [8, 89, 90].

The response to furosemide usually begins 2–4 min after injection, but the maximum diuresis is usually not reached until 15–18 min after injection. In equivocal cases, some investigators recommend repeating the study with the $F - 15$ renogram so that the patient will be in a state of maximum diuresis at the time the radiopharmaceutical is administered [93]. In selected cases, an equivocal $F + 20$ study will become normal or obstructed following an $F - 15$ renogram [93].

8.6.3 Diuresis Renography in Acute Renal Colic

Unenhanced (non-contrast) helical CT is a valuable test in the management of the patient presenting with acute renal colic; the test can detect a ureteral stone with a high degree of accuracy, but unenhanced helical CT cannot predict the presence or absence of obstruction. The addition of a diuretic renal scan can determine the presence or absence of obstruction and direct patient management [95–97]. If additional data show that a renal scan leads to better patient outcomes and/or reduces medical costs, then diuresis renography may develop an increasingly important role in the management of patients presenting with an acute renal colic.

8.7 Renovascular Hypertension and ACE Inhibition Renography

Renovascular hypertension (RVH) is estimated to affect <0.5–3% of the unselected hypertension population and up to 15–30% of patients referred to a subspecialty center because of refractory hypertension [98]. Renovascular hypertension is part of the spectrum of renovascular disease which also includes renal artery stenosis and azotemic renal vascular disease (ARVD). Renovascular hypertension is defined as a functionally significant renal artery stenosis that leads to an elevated blood pressure due to a reduction of perfusion pressure distal to the stenosis and activation of the renin-angiotensin system. ARVD refers to the gradual loss of kidney function associated with severe occlusive disease of the renal artery. Pathological findings associated with ARVD include intrarenal vascular lesions, glomerulosclerosis, and atrophy, while clinical findings may include hypertension and azotemia. Patients with ARVD may or may not have coexisting renovascular hypertension; however, revascularization is sometimes undertaken in these patients in an attempt to improve or stabilize renal function although the long-term utility of this approach versus current medical therapy is debated.

Renal artery stenosis is common in the aging population; as many as 30–50% of normotensive patients with advancing age may have moderate or even severe RAS [99, 100]; similarly, renal artery stenosis may be an associated but non-etiologic finding in patients with essential hypertension. Consequently, it comes as no surprise that revascularization of a stenotic artery in a hypertensive patient does not always result in amelioration of the hypertension. In fact, three randomized studies comparing revascularization with medical therapy suggest that angioplasty appears to have little advantage over antihypertensive drug therapy [101–103]. Alternatively, however, the data in these three studies can also be interpreted as demonstrating the need to determine the hemodynamic significance of a renal artery stenosis prior to revascularization [104]. The goals of ACEI renography are twofold: (1) to detect those patients with hypertension who have a functionally significant renal artery stenosis as the cause of their hypertension and who would benefit from revascularization and (2) to determine which hypertensive patients do not have RVH and obviate the expense and risk of a revascularization procedure.

ACE inhibition renography has been shown to be cost-effective in a carefully selected population with a prevalence of RVH of 11.6%, but it is probably most cost-effective in patients with a moderate to high risk of renovascular hypertension [105, 106]. Clinical features which indicate patients with a moderate or high risk of renovascular hypertension include abrupt onset of hypertension in patients under age 30 or over age 55, severe hypertension resistant to medical therapy in a compliant patient, bruits in the abdomen or flank, occlusive disease in other vascular beds, and unexplained azotemia or worsening renal function during therapy with angiotensin-converting enzyme (ACE) inhibitors. To best utilize the test and maximize the congruence between the performance of the test and the expectations of the referring physicians, it is important to distinguish between renal artery stenosis, renovascular hypertension, and ARVD.

The protocols and the criteria for findings indicative of renovascular hypertension have tended to vary from center to center. The lack of standardization coupled with the fact that many reported studies use stenosis of the renal artery, not blood pressure response to revascularization (i.e., true renovascular hypertension), as the end point, makes it more difficult to draw definitive conclusions. In an attempt to address these issues, an International Consensus Committee on ACE inhibitor renography was established by the Ninth International Symposium of Radionuclides in Nephrourology. The 1996 guidelines published by the Consensus Committee and updated in 2003 form the basis for the following recommendations [52, 107].

8.7.1 Pathophysiology of Renovascular Hypertension and ACE Inhibition

A functionally significant renal artery stenosis causes a decrease in the perfusion pressure to the afferent arterioles of the glomeruli resulting in a decrease in the transglomerular pressure gradient; the fall in the transglomerular pressure gradient leads to a decrease in glomerular filtration and a decrease in sodium delivery to the distal tubule. The decrease in perfusion pressure and the reduction in distal tubule sodium delivery stimulate the juxtaglomerular apparatus to release renin which cleaves angiotensin I from angiotensinogen; angiotensin I is then converted to angiotensin II by angiotensin-converting enzyme. Angiotensin II is a potent vasoconstrictor and acts preferentially on the efferent glomerular arteriole. Constriction of the efferent arteriole raises the transglomerular pressure gradient and can maintain GFR even in the face of a moderate reduction in perfusion pressure resulting from a functionally significant renal artery stenosis.

In patients with renovascular hypertension, ACE inhibitors have two important mechanisms of action: (1) ACE inhibitors block the conversion of angiotensin I to angiotensin II and thereby interfere with the angiotensin II-mediated constriction of the efferent arteriole. (2) ACE inhibitors also inhibit kininase II, a dipeptidylcarboxypeptidase that inactivates bradykinin; consequently, bradykinin accumulates following ACE inhibition. Bradykinin is a potent vasodilator and causes selective efferent arteriolar dilation [108–110]. This second mechanism is probably quite important since only 60% of angiotensin II is synthesized by ACE-dependent pathways in the human renal cortex, and neither acute nor chronic ACE inhibition completely eliminates angiotensin II from the plasma [110, 111].

The reduction in GFR induced by ACE inhibition can be detected by renography. For ^{99m}Tc-DTPA, the primary effect is a reduction in renal uptake of ^{99m}Tc-DTPA by the affected kidney. For tubular tracers such as ^{99m}Tc-MAG3 or ^{131}I-OIH, renovascular hypertension is best detected by cortical retention following ACE inhibition (Fig. 8.7) although a change in relative uptake or a decrease in absolute uptake of the ^{131}I-OIH or ^{99m}Tc-MAG3 by the affected kidney is an important finding when it occurs [51, 52, 112, 113]. The cortical retention of ^{99m}Tc-MAG3 and ^{131}I-OIH is secondary to the decrease in glomerular filtration induced by ACE inhibition; with the decrease in GFR, there is decreased flow in the renal tubules and

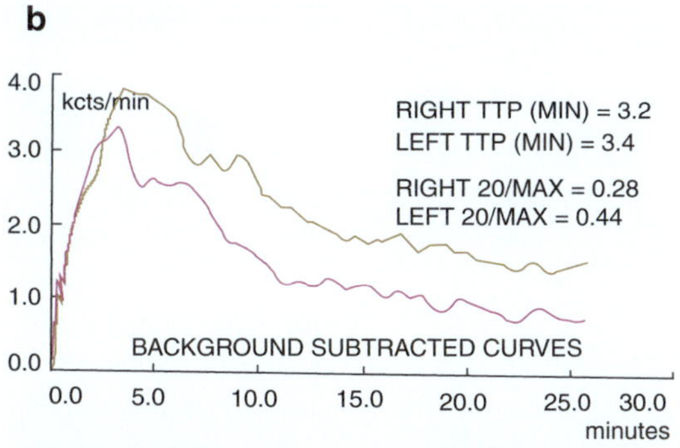

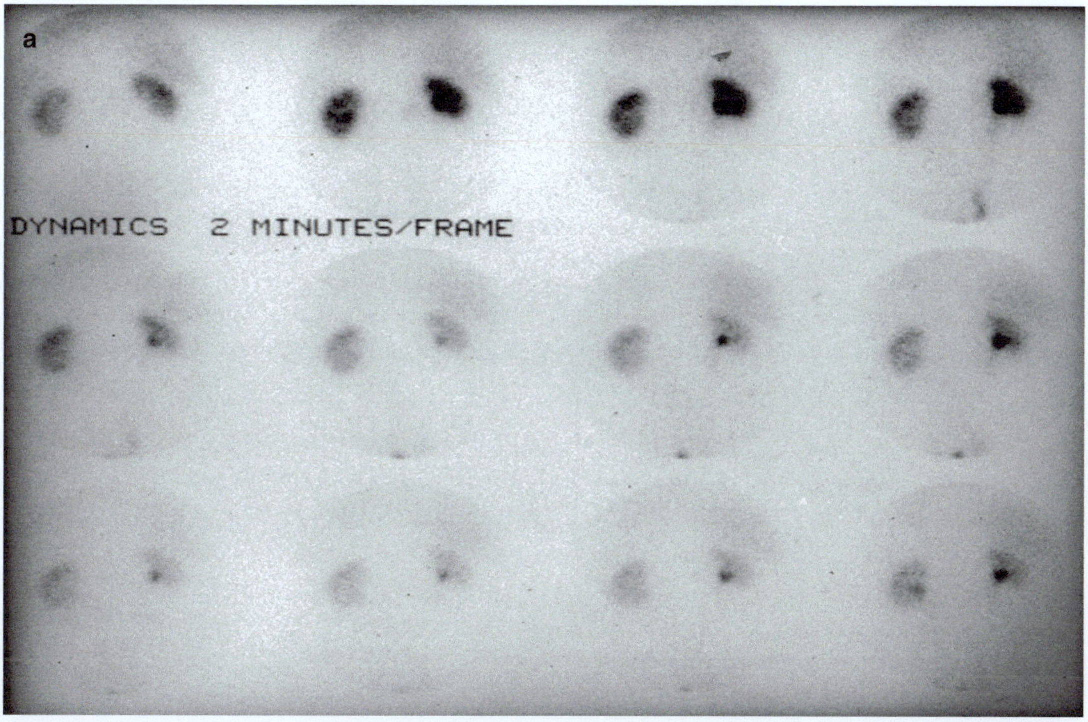

Fig. 8.7 A 78-year-old man who presented with dizziness, a creatinine of 1.7 mg/dl, and blood pressure of 230/120 was referred for ACEI renography. (**a**) A baseline scintigram was obtained with 44 MBq (1.2 mCi) of ^{99m}Tc-MAG3. Images obtained at 2 min intervals for 24 min show prompt uptake and washout of the tracer. (**b**) The relative uptake was 52% in the right kidney and 48% in the left kidney. The background subtracted cortical renogram curves show a normal Tmax for both kidneys; however, there is an abnormal 20 min/max ratio of 0.44 (normal <0.35). (**c**) Following completion of the baseline study, the patient was given 50 mg of captopril, and a second ^{99m}Tc-MAG3 scintigram was obtained with 344 MBq (9.3 mCi), approximately 1.5 h later. The sequential 2 min images show cortical retention in the left kidney; however, the right kidney appears normal. (**d**) Following captopril, the left cortical renogram curve has become markedly abnormal; the time to peak has increased to 11.7 min, and the 20 min/max ratio has increased from 0.44 to 0.93. Although the cortical renogram curves are noisier than whole-kidney renogram curves, the 20 min/max ratio for the right cortical ROI has increased from a baseline high normal value of 0.28 to an elevated value of 0.37 although this is not considered to be a significant change. Angiography demonstrated bilateral renal artery stenosis. A revascularization procedure was not performed

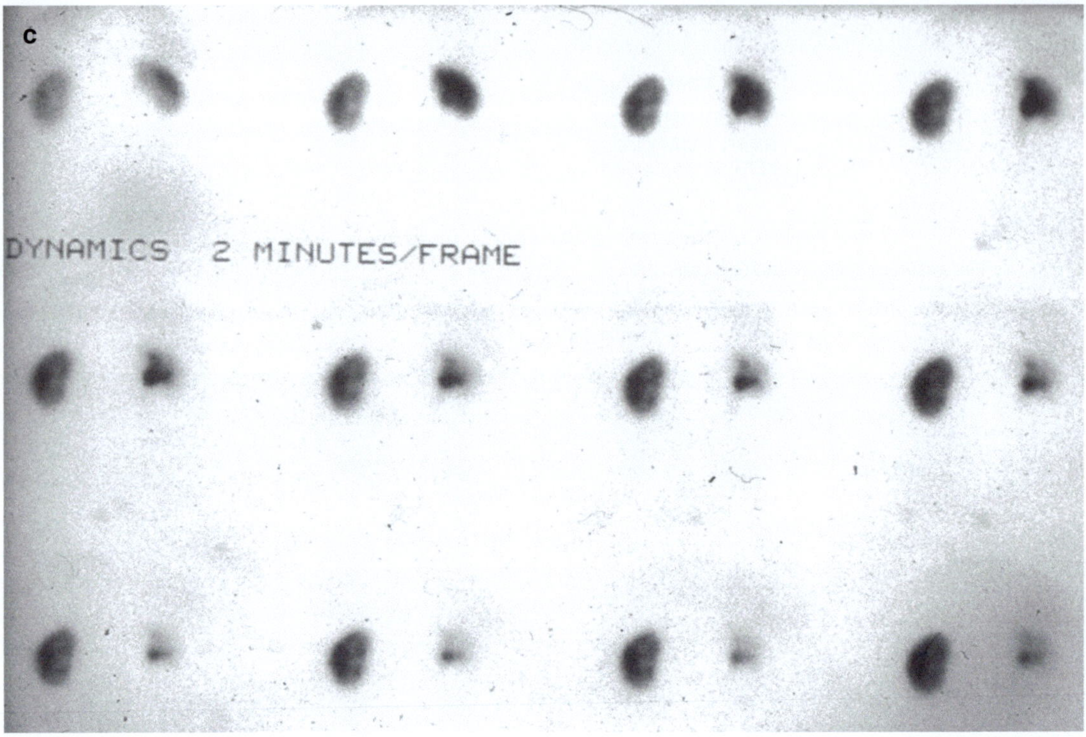

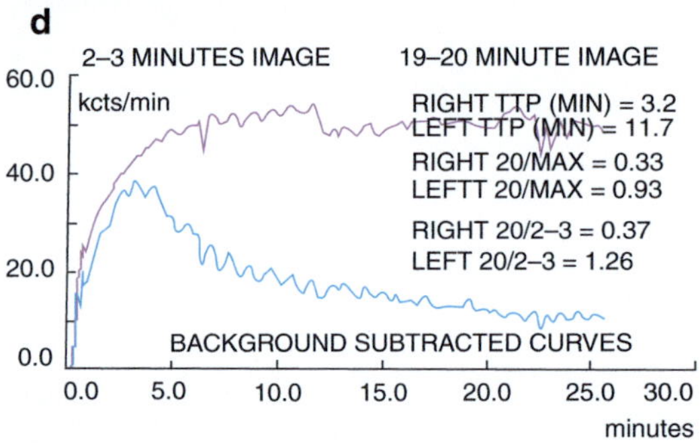

Fig. 8.7 (continued)

delayed washout of the radionuclide from the tubules and tubular lumen [114]. Cortical retention can be quantitated by measuring the Tmax and the 20 or 30 min/maximum ratio [51, 52].

8.7.2 Technical Issues Relating to ACE Inhibition Renography

8.7.2.1 Diet and Hydration

Ideally, patients should be instructed to arrive well hydrated and receive 5–10 ml/kg of water on arrival in the department, preferably 30–60 min before the study. If baseline and ACEI studies are to be performed on the same day, hydration should be continued between studies.

Food may delay gastric emptying and interfere with the absorption of captopril. If captopril is to be given as the ACE inhibitor, the patient should be instructed not to eat any solids after midnight before the exam; however, instructions should clearly distinguish between avoiding solid food and the importance of hydration. Low-sodium diets need to be avoided for several days prior to the test to avoid extracellular volume depletion which might accentuate a hypotensive response following ACE inhibitor administration.

8.7.2.2 Medications

The following drugs may impact the interpretation of ACE inhibition studies:

ACE Inhibitors and Angiotensin II Receptor Blockers (ARBs): The majority of ACE inhibition studies have been performed with captopril, but enalaprilat is an acceptable alternative [52, 107, 115]. Limited data suggest that chronic ACE inhibition may reduce the sensitivity of the test [116, 117] and the consensus recommendation is to discontinue captopril for 4 days prior to the study and discontinue the longer half-life ACE inhibitors for 7 days [52, 107]. Since ACE inhibitors and ARBs both block the vasoconstrictive effect of angiotensin II on the efferent vessels in patients with RVH, it was thought that chronic ARB administration might also reduce the sensitivity of the ACE inhibition renography. Recent data, however, indicate that it is probably not necessary to discontinue the ARB class of drugs [109]. Captopril renograms were obtained in 26 hypertensive patients with normal or near-normal renal function who were receiving angiotensin II receptor blockers; in this patient population, the sensitivity of ACE inhibition renography for renovascular hypertension was 92% and specificity was 100%, values comparable to those obtained in patients not taking ARBs [109, 118]. Finally, a recent study showed that ARB renography is considerably less sensitive than captopril renography for detecting RAS in hypertensive patients or for detecting RVH [119]. The superiority of ACE inhibitors over the ARBs in detecting renovascular hypertension probably derives from the action of ACE inhibitors on kininase II (see above).

Diuretics: Chronic diuretic administration increases the likelihood of volume depletion which may reduce the specificity of the test and increase the risk of a hypotensive response. These concerns can be minimized if diuretics are discontinued for 2–3 days prior to the study.

Calcium Channel Blockers: Calcium channel blockers have been associated with a bilaterally symmetrical abnormal renogram curves in the absence of renal artery stenosis [120, 121]. As an alternative to discontinuing another drug, a reasonable option is to ensure adequate hydration and to note the use of a calcium channel blocker. In the rare setting where bilateral symmetrical abnormalities occur in the absence of dehydration, hypotension, or infiltration, the ACEI component of the test could be repeated after discontinuation of calcium channel blockers.

8.7.2.3 Choice of Radiopharmaceutical

In patients with azotemia, tubular agents such as ^{99m}Tc-MAG3 or ^{123}I-OIH are agents of choice [51, 52, 122]. In patients with normal renal function, ^{99m}Tc-MAG3 and ^{99m}Tc-DTPA appear to give comparable results.

8.7.2.4 Choice of ACE Inhibitor

Captopril (25–50 mg crushed and administered orally with 250 ml of water) has been used in most published studies. A 25 mg tablet is sufficient unless the patient has delayed gastric emptying or poor absorption from the gastrointestinal tract. Food can interfere with the absorption of captopril, and patients should not eat before captopril scintigraphy. The peak activity of captopril does not occur until approximately 60 min after ingestion; for this reason, the radiopharmaceutical should be given an hour after captopril. A second approach is to inject enalaprilat (Vasotec, 40 μg/kg IV over 3–5 min, maximum dose of 2.5 mg), wait a minimum of 15 min, and then inject the radiopharmaceutical [115, 123, 124]. Intravenous injection of enalaprilat avoids the possibility of a false-negative test due to delayed gastric emptying in a diabetic patient or poor absorption, and the patient is usually under continuous observation after enalaprilat injection as the technologist prepares for the study. A potential disadvantage is possibly a greater risk of a hypotensive response and the need for venous access. Both ACE inhibitors are acceptable [52, 107].

8.7.2.5 Blood Pressure

Blood pressure must be monitored. Asymptomatic hypotension secondary to ACE inhibition can result in bilateral symmetrical abnormalities in the renogram curves (Fig. 8.8). This phenomenon may occur in 1–3% of patients referred for ACEI renog-

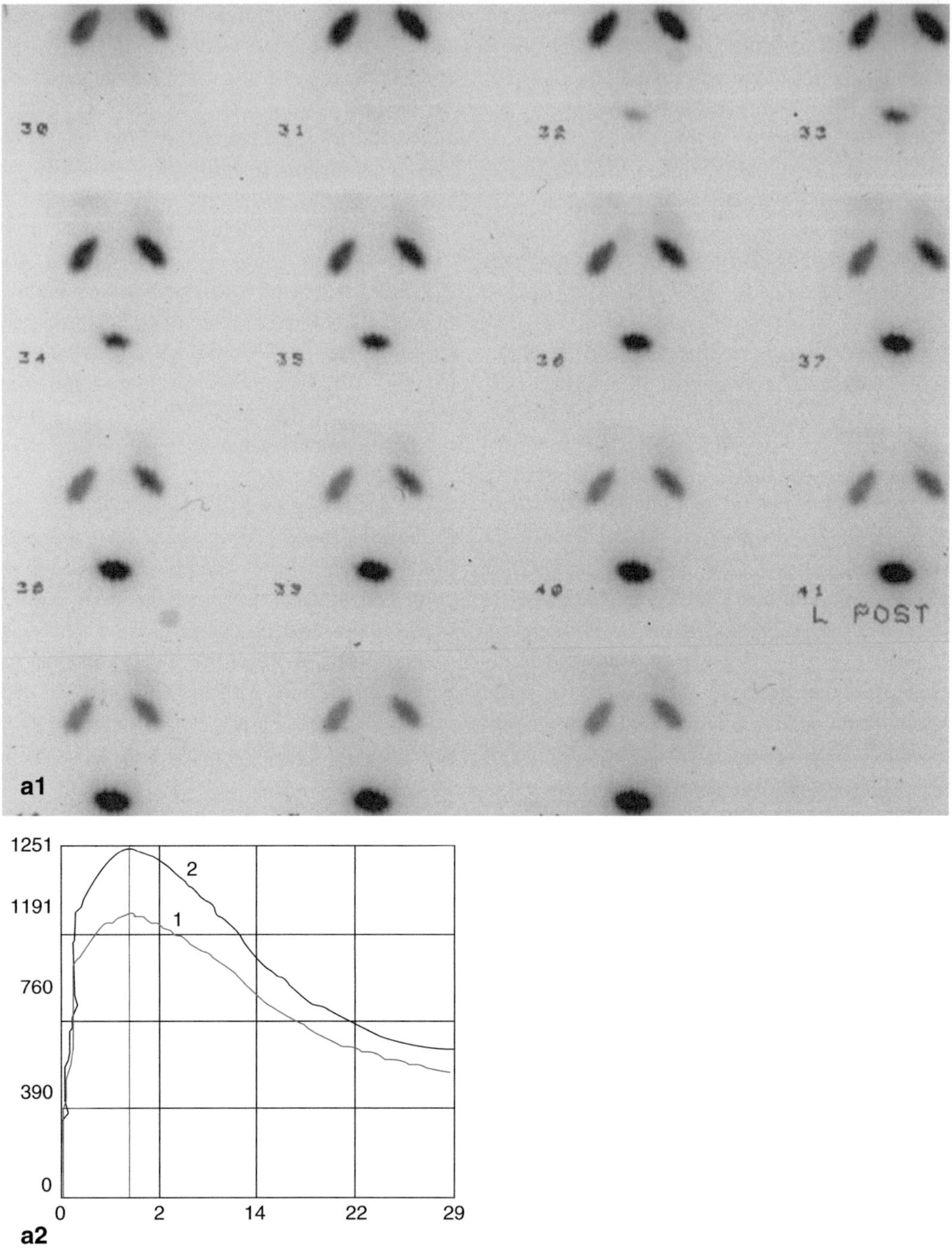

Fig. 8.8 A middle-aged male with refractory hypertension was referred for ACE inhibition renography. Sequential 2 min images (**a1**) and whole-kidney renogram curves (**a2**) were obtained following a baseline injection of approximately 1.0 (37 MBq) of ^{99m}Tc-MAG3. The patient received 50 mg of captopril and 10 mCi (370 MBq) were injected an hour later. The 2 min images (**b1**) demonstrate parenchymal retention with bilateral rising whole-kidney renogram curves (**b2**). Usually, renovascular hypertension produces asymmetrical abnormalities. On further review, the patient's pre-captopril blood pressure was 165/71, but it fell to 102/41 during the study even though the patient remained asymptomatic. Several days later the study was repeated with 50 mg of captopril and intravenous hydration to maintain blood pressure. The 2 min sequential images (**c1**) and renogram curves (**c2**) are normal. Bilateral symmetrical abnormality following ACE inhibition is a non-specific finding, often due to volume depletion and hypotension

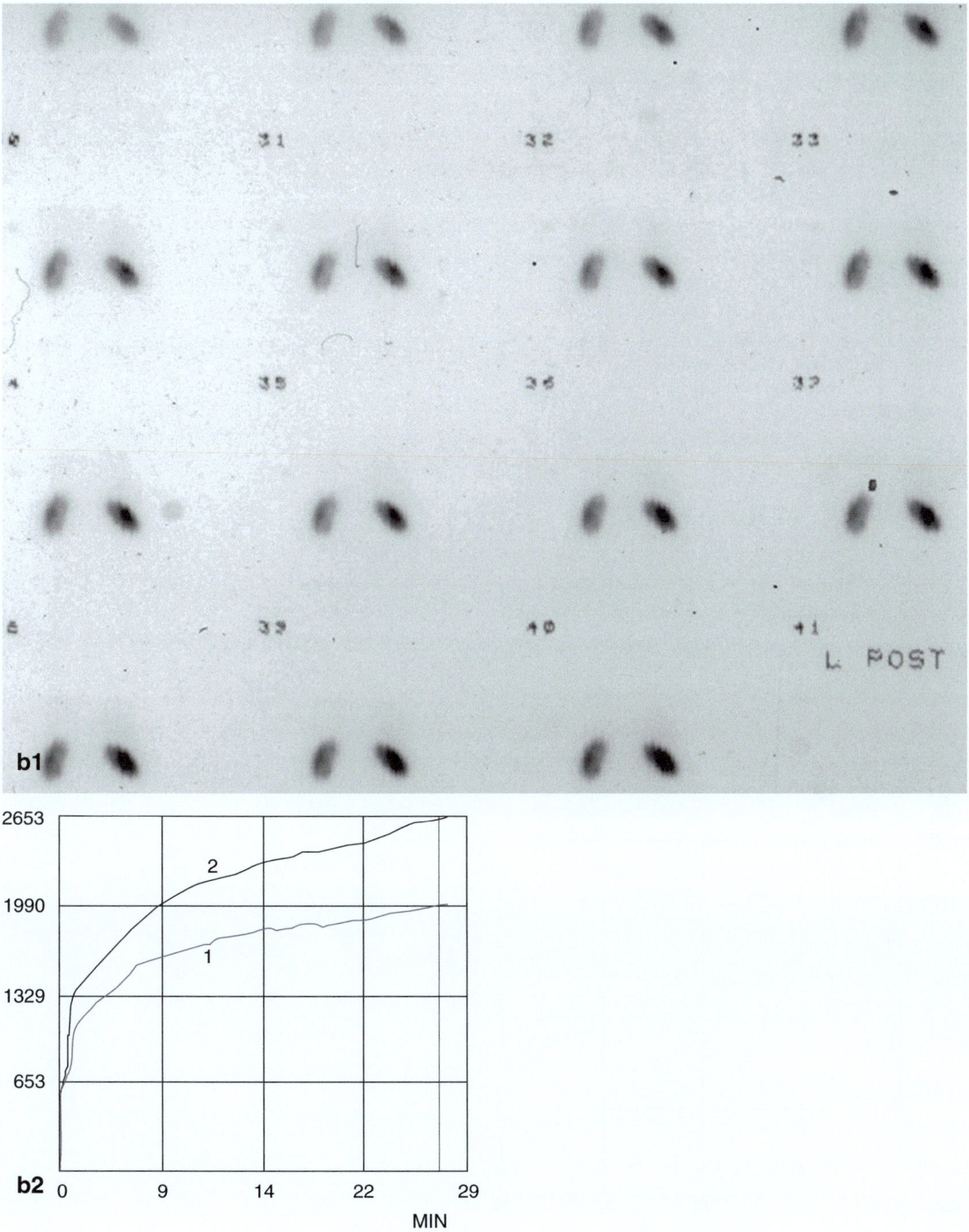

Fig. 8.8 (continued)

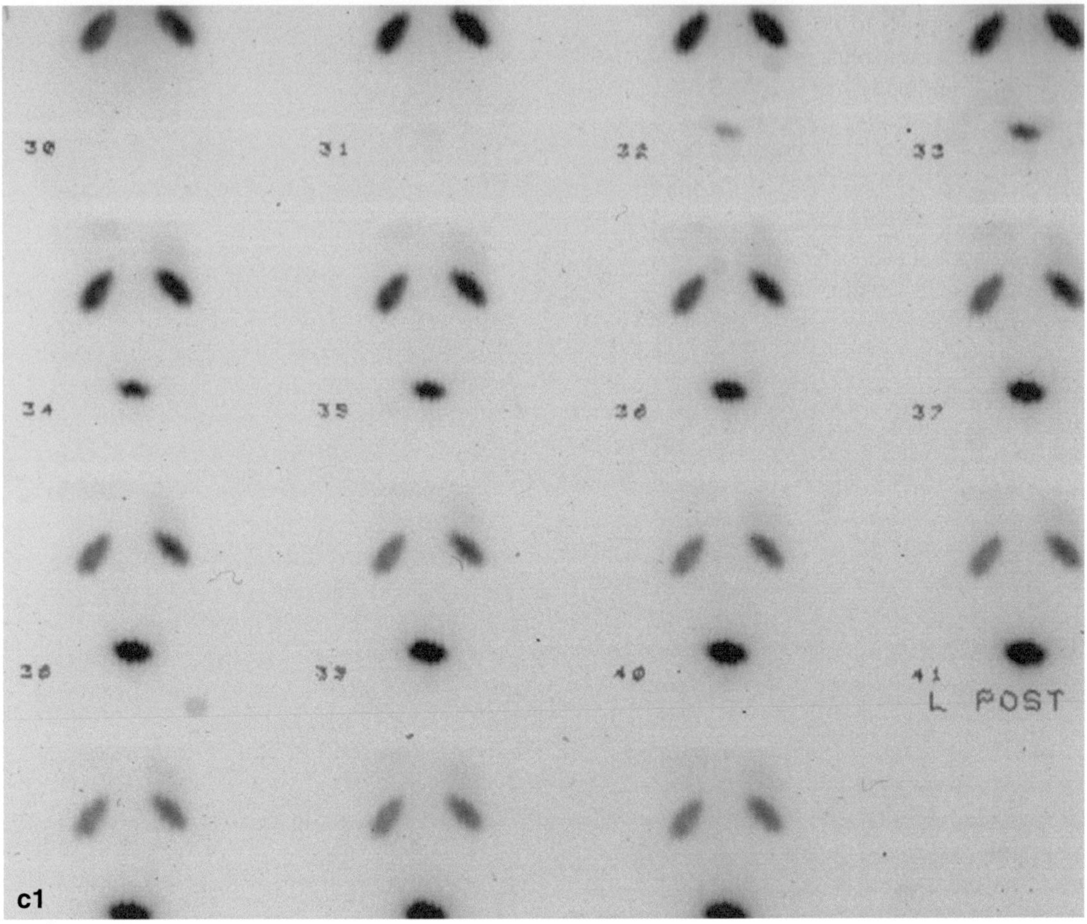

c1

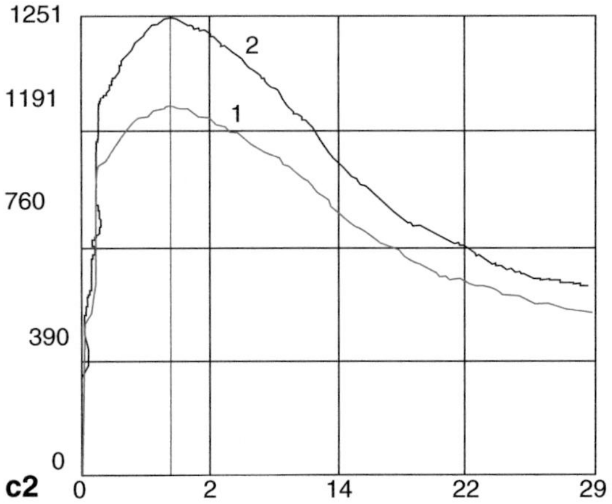

c2

Fig. 8.8 (continued)

raphy and appears to be most likely to occur in patients who are volume or salt depleted [125, 126]. ACE inhibitors can also cause in a major hypotensive episode, although the prevalence appears to be quite low in well-hydrated patients. The hypotension can usually be reversed by placing the patient supine, raising the patient's legs, and infusing normal saline. Some centers establish an IV line before scintigraphy; this precaution is important for high-risk patients such as those with angina, recent myocardial infarction, a history of transient ischemic attacks, recent stroke and patients receiving enalaprilat or furosemide. Before the patient leaves the department, it is probably wise to document that the standing blood pressure is greater than 70% of the baseline blood pressure and that the patient is asymptomatic. A statement to this effect can be included in the report.

8.7.2.6 1- Versus a 2-Day Protocol

Some centers begin with a captopril or enalaprilat renography because a normal study following ACE inhibition renography obviates the need for a baseline study. If the ACE inhibition study is abnormal, the specificity can be improved by obtaining a baseline renogram; however, because of the administration of the ACE inhibitor, the patient will have to return for the baseline study on another day. In some centers an abnormal ACEI study coupled with a high clinical probability for renovascular hypertension is justification for angiography.

A second approach is to use a low dose (37 MBq or 1 mCi) of ^{99m}Tc-MAG3 or ^{99m}Tc-DTPA for the baseline study, administer the ACE inhibitor, and then obtain a second study with a significantly higher dose (approximately 370 MBq or 10 mCi). This protocol requires two studies on the same day and requires the patient to spend a longer time in the department, but the complete study is finished in a single day. The first approach is less costly if the time required for the patient to return on a second day for a baseline test is not factored into the calculation.

8.7.2.7 Furosemide-Augmented ACEI Renography

With ^{99m}Tc-MAG3 or ^{131}I-OIH, the diagnosis of renovascular hypertension is primarily based on cortical retention of the radiopharmaceutical; physiologic retention of these radioactive agents in the calices can distort both the visual and quantitative analysis (Tmax and the 20–30 min/maximum ratio). To minimize retention of tracer in the collecting system, some centers advocate furosemide-augmented captopril or enalaprilat renography for the detection of renovascular hypertension [115, 122, 127]. Furosemide is a loop diuretic and acts distal to the proximal tubules, where ^{99m}Tc-MAG3 and ^{131}I-OIH are secreted. Consequently, furosemide can wash the radiopharmaceutical out of the calices and pelvis, but it does not affect cortical retention [122]. A disadvantage of furosemide is volume depletion and a greater risk of significant hypotension. The Consensus Committee considered the use of furosemide to be a local option but not a necessary component of ACEI renography; if furosemide is administered, an IV line should be placed in case supplemental hydration is necessary [52, 106].

8.7.3 Diagnostic Criteria

Two recent consensus panels have recommended that the test be interpreted as high, low, or intermediate probability for renovascular hypertension [52, 128].

High Probability: Unilateral deterioration of the renogram curve and/or change in relative function following ACE inhibition compared to the baseline study

Intermediate (Indeterminate) Probability: Small poorly functioning kidney or kidneys with abnormal baseline renograms (Grades III–V) (Fig. 8.2) which are unchanged following ACE inhibition

Low Probability: A normal ACE inhibition renogram or Grade II renogram which is unchanged or improves following ACE inhibition.

A change in the shape of the renogram curve may be evaluated quantitatively by a prolongation of the 20 or 30 min/max ratio and/or a prolongation of the time to peak. For tubular tracers, a *unilateral* increase in the 20 min/max ratio of 0.15 (0.30 to 0.45) or greater for parenchymal (cortical) ROIs represents the 90% confidence limit for a significant change [51, 52]. A bilateral symmetrical increase in the 20 min/max ratio is more likely to be salt or volume depletion rather than renovascular hypertension [125, 126]. A unilateral prolongation of the time to peak of 120 s for a cortical ROI is significant at the 90–95% confidence limit. It is important to note, however, that a change from 5 to 7 min is much more significant than a change from 15 to 17 min. Renogram curves derived from the cortical ROIs minimize the error or diagnostic difficulty that can be introduced by retention of the tracer in the collecting system. A change in the relative uptake of ^{99m}Tc-MAG3 or ^{131}I-OIH by 10% points (50/50–40/60) is uncommon even in a patient with RVH but it is highly significant when it occurs.

The principal diagnostic criterion for ^{99m}Tc-DTPA is a change in the relative uptake. A reduction in the relative uptake greater than 10% points (50/50–60/40) is a highly significant change, and 5–9% points is considered to be an intermediate response, although a recent study performed under carefully controlled conditions suggests that smaller changes in relative uptake may be significant [51, 52, 129, 130]. Parenchymal retention of ^{99m}Tc-DTPA following ACE inhibition can also be an important diagnostic finding and can be quantitated by a delay in the time to peak or an increase in the 20–30 min/max ratios although, in general, changes have to be much more pronounced than with ^{99m}Tc-MAG3 and ^{131}I-OIH to be significant [52, 122].

8.7.4 Sensitivity and Specificity

The sensitivity and specificity depend on the patient selection (see below), the analysis of the patient with an indeterminate scan, and the difficulty in determining the response to revascularization; the response to revascularization may be affected by restenosis, a change in medications, and the lack of a systematic approach to determining the blood pressure response. Most studies report sensitivities and specificities in the range of 80–90% although many studies use an inappropriate gold standard and compare the results of ACE inhibition renography to the presence or absence of renal artery stenosis rather than the blood pressure response to revascularization. Different diagnostic criteria as well as different populations of patients probably explain some of the variation in results. Better results are often obtained when the end point is normalization or reduction in blood pressure following revascularization rather than the presence or absence of renal artery stenosis [52, 118, 131–135].

Intermediate probability results present a problem for analysis; they can be included with the positive studies, in which case sensitivity is increased at the expense of specificity; they can be included with the low probability studies, increasing specificity at the expense of sensitivity, or they can all be counted as incorrect. The sensitivities and specificities will vary depending on the frequency of intermediate probability studies in the study population and how these results are handled in the data analysis.

Results are improved by appropriate patient selection. In selecting patients for ACE inhibition renography and in communicating with the referring physician, *it is essential to distinguish between the hypertensive patient with azotemic renovascular disease (ARVD) and hypertensive patient without ARVD because results differ in these two patient populations (see below).*

8.7.4.1 Hypertensive Patients with Azotemic Renovascular Disease (ARVD)

Current data indicate that the test is not as accurate in patients with ARVD and is likely to be nondiagnostic. Fortunately, these patients are not difficult to identify. The likelihood that a patient has severe atherosclerotic vascular disease involving one or both kidneys is substantially increased if the patient is azotemic or if the patient is already known to have a small kidney. These patients will have a high percentage of intermediate (nondiagnostic) probability test results. This is not necessarily a problem if the referring physician understands the relatively high likelihood of an intermediate nondiagnostic result when such a patient is referred for ACEI renography. An intermediate test result in the appropriate clinical setting may be sufficient to refer a patient for angiography. False-negative results are uncommon, but when they occur, they appear to be more likely in azotemic patients with bilateral disease, probably due to suppression of the renin-angiotensin system.

8.7.4.2 Hypertensive Patients Without Azotemic Renovascular Disease (ARVD)

The probability of RVH is considered high (greater than 90%) when marked unilateral deterioration of the renogram curve occurs after ACE inhibition, compared to baseline findings [51, 52, 118]. Normal findings on ACE inhibition renography indicate a low probability (less than 10%) for renovascular hypertension. Abnormal baseline findings that improve after ACE inhibition also indicate low probability for renovascular hypertension. In the patient population that does not have a small poorly functioning kidney and that has normal or near-normal renal function, the sensitivity, specificity, and positive and negative predictive value of ACE inhibition renography probably exceed 90%. A proposed algorithm for investigating suspected RVH is shown in Fig. 8.9 [104].

8.8 The Role of Positron Emission Tomography in Renal Imaging

Renal blood flow can be determined with O-15 water ($H_2{}^{15}O$), N-13 ammonia, rubidium-82, and copper-64 or copper-62 pyruvaldehyde bis (N4-methyl)thiosemicarbazone (PTSM) [136] The use of PET tracers to monitor renal blood flow has the potential to serve as a useful measurement in the study of renal physiology and pharmacology. Carbon-11 acetate is a marker of oxidative metabolism, and it is efficiently extracted by the kidney. Carbon-11 acetate is converted to carbon-11 acetyl-CoA and enters the Krebs cycle where it is metabolized, releasing the carbon-11 as carbon-11 CO^2. Although carbon-11 acetate is not excreted into the urine, its role in imaging renal metabolism or renal pathology has so far been limited. Work is also underway to develop PET tubular tracers with pharmacokinetics similar to ^{131}I-OIH or ^{99m}Tc-MAG3 [137, 138].

The angiotensin receptor subtype, AT1R, mediates most of the physiological effects of angiotensin II including renal blood flow, glomerular filtration, sodium and water reabsorption, myocardial contractility, and aldosterone secretion, and studies have been conducted to monitor AT1R expression using positron-labeled

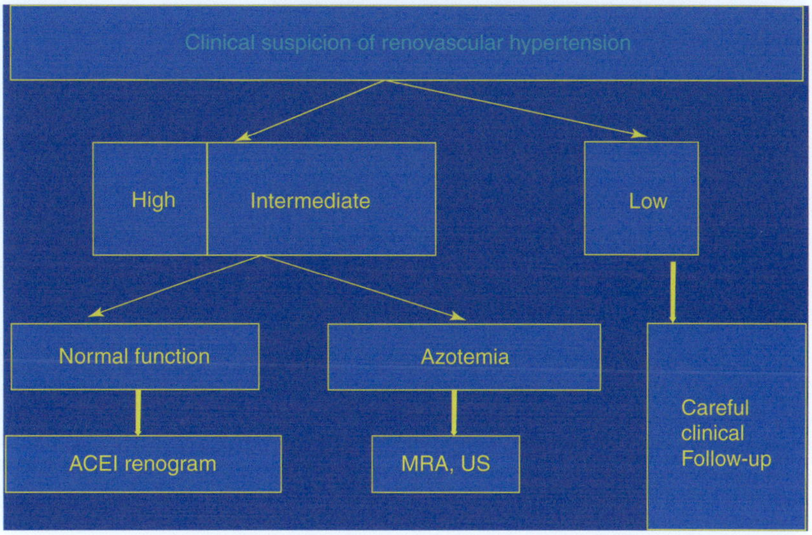

Fig. 8.9 Algorithm for the evaluation of suspected renovascular hypertension

drugs with a high selectivity and affinity for the receptor [136]. The use of PET to monitor AT1R expression in humans may provide a window for investigating the mechanisms of human hypertension and other AT1R-modulated diseases in vivo.

Fluorine-18 fluorodeoxyglucose (FDG) is an increasingly important PET imaging agent in oncology, but it is not optimal for imaging renal pathology because it is filtered by the glomerulus and, unlike glucose, it is not reabsorbed from the tubular lumen; consequently, fluorine-18 FDG accumulates in the renal pelvis and bladder potentially obscuring ^{18}F-FDG avid pathology in the kidney or region of the bladder.

8.8.1 PET Applications in Renal Cell Carcinoma (RCC)

Renal cell carcinoma (RCC) accounts for 2–3% of all adult malignancies. Although patients may present with local signs and symptoms such as hematuria, flank pain, or a palpable abdominal mass, most presentations are incidental and result from imaging procedures that include the kidney in the field of view. The initial assessment of a renal mass is best performed with sonography, CT, or MRI. Purely cystic lesions are benign; more complex cystic renal masses require observation or removal depending on the characteristics of the cystic mass. The majority of patients with localized RCC who receive treatment have a favorable prognosis, but 20–40% later develop metastases with a 5-year survival below 10%. ^{18}F-FDG PET and ^{18}F-FDG PET/CT are not appropriate for the initial assessment of a renal mass because the normal ^{18}F-FDG in the kidney may mask uptake by a renal cell carcinoma. In contrast, FDG PET/CT has shown good performance in detecting recurrent disease and predicting survival and progression (Fig. 8.10), and a recent study demonstrated an effect on treatment decision-making in more than 40% of subjects with recurrent RCC [139, 140]. Studies are also underway to develop and evaluate new PET tracers that

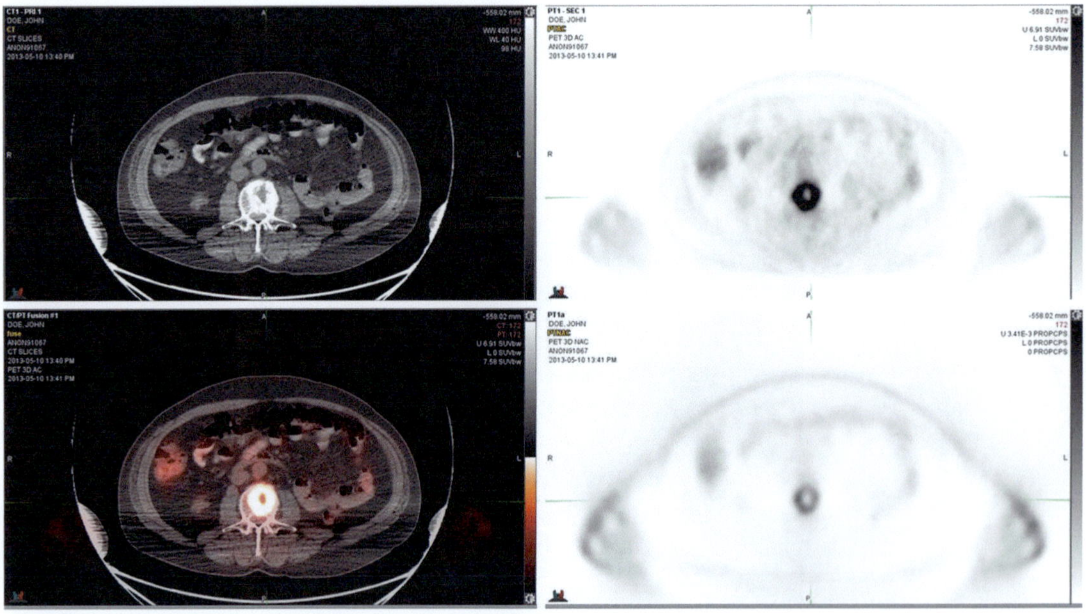

Fig. 8.10 A 67-year-old man with a history of metastatic renal cell carcinoma was referred for a PET/CT scan to assist in treatment planning. Following an intravenous injection of 662 MBq (17.9 mCi) of ^{18}F-FDG, noncontrast images were obtained after a delay of 60–90 min. The PET images (right panels) show a hypermetabolic focus that corresponds to the mixed density bone metastasis almost completely involving the L3 vertebral body (*CT,* upper left panel*; fused PET/CT image* lower left panel)

may have a greater sensitivity and specificity for evaluation of RCC than ^{18}F-FDG [141]. Contribution of PET imaging to the management of renal oncologic patients is discussed in Chap. 26 of this text.

References

1. Eshima D, Taylor A Jr. Technetium-99m (99mTc) mercaptoacetyltriglycine: update on the new 99m Tc renal tubular function agent. Semin Nucl Med. 1992;22:61–73.
2. Marcus CS, Kuperus JH. Pediatric renal I-123 orthoiodohippurate dosimetry. J Nucl Med. 1985;26:1211–4.
3. Stabin M, Taylor A, Eshima D, Wooten W. Radiation dosimetry for technetium-99m-MAG3, technetium-99m-DTPA, and iodine-131-OIH based on human biodistribution studies. J Nucl Med. 1992;33:33–40.
4. Bubeck B, Brandau W, Weber E, et al. Pharmacokinetics of technetium-99m-MAG3 in humans. J Nucl Med. 1990;31:1285–93.
5. Schaap GH, Alferink THR, deJong RBJ, et al. Tc-99m MAG3: dynamic studies in patients with renal diseases. Eur J Nucl Med. 1988;14:28–31.
6. Al-Nahhas AA, Jafri RA, Britton KE, et al. Clinical experience with 99m Tc-MAG3, mercaptoacetyltriglycine, and a comparison with 99mTc-DTPA. Eur J Nucl Med. 1988;14:453–62.
7. Gordon I, Colarinha P, Fettich J, Fischer S, Frøkiær J, Hahn K, Kabasakal L, Mitjavila M, Olivier P, Piepsz A, Porn U, Sixt R, van Velzen J. Guidelines for standard and diuretic renogram in children. Eur J Nucl Med. 2001;28:BP31–6.
8. Taylor AT, Blaufox MD, Brandon DC, et al. SNMMI procedure standard/EANM practice guideline for diuretic renal scintigraphy in adults with suspected upper urinary tract obstruction 1.0. Semin Nucl Med. 2018;48(4):377–90.
9. Gordon I, Colarinha P, Fettich J, Fischer S, Frøkiær J, Hahn K, Kabasakal L, Mitjavila M, Olivier P, Piepsz A, Porn U, Sixt R, van Velzen J. Guidelines for standard and diuretic renogram in children. EANM Web J. http://www.eanm.org/. Auspices of the Paediatric Committee of the European Association of Nuclear Medicine; 2000.
10. O'Reilly P, Aurell M, Britton K, et al. Consensus on diuresis renography for investigating the dilated upper urinary tract. J Nucl Med. 1996;37:1872–6.
11. Taylor A, Eshima D, Christian P, Milton W. Evaluation of Tc-99m mercaptoacetyltriglycine in patients with impaired renal function. Radiology. 1987;162:365–70.
12. Taylor A Jr, Ziffer JA, Eshima D. Comparison of Tc-99m MAG3 and Tc-99m DTPA in renal transplant patients with impaired renal function. Clin Nucl Med. 1990;15:371–8.
13. Taylor A, Thakore K, Folks R, Halkar R, Manatunga A. Background subtraction in Tc-99m-MAG3 renography. J Nucl Med. 1994;35:2054–5.
14. Taylor A, Clark S, Ball T. Comparison of Tc-99m MAG3 and Tc-99m DTPA scintigraphy in neonates. Clin Nucl Med. 1994;19:575–80.
15. Russell CD, Taylor AT, Dubovsky EV. Measurement of renal function with technetium-99m-MAG3 in children and adults. J Nucl Med. 1996;37:588–93.
16. Russell CD, Thorstad B, Yester MV, et al. Comparison of technetium-99m MAG3 with iodine-131 hippuran by a simultaneous dual channel technique. J Nucl Med. 1988;29:1189–93.
17. Kanazawa T, Shimizu M, Seto H, et al. Reproducibility of ^{99}Tc^{m}-MAG3 clearance in normal volunteers with the two-sample method: comparison with OIH. Nucl Med Commun. 1998;19:899–903.
18. Kotzerke J, Glatz S, Grillenberger K, et al. Reproducibility of a single-sample method for ^{99}Tc^{m}-MAG3 clearance under clinical conditions. Nucl Med Commun. 1997;18:352–7.
19. Piepsz A, Tondeur M, Kinthaert J, et al. Reproducibility of technetium-99m-mercaptoacetylglycine clearance. Eur J Nucl Med. 1988;23:195–8.
20. Russell CD, Dubovsky EV. Reproducibility of single-sample clearance of 99mTc-mercaptoacetyltriglycine and 131I-orthohippurate. J Nucl Med. 1999;40:1122–4.
21. Blaufox MD, Aurell M, Bubeck B, et al. Report of the radionuclides in nephrourology committee on renal clearance. J Nucl Med. 1996;37:1883–90.
22. Klingensmith WC, Briggss DE, Smith WI. Technetium-99m-MAG3 renal studies: normal range and reproducibility of physiologic parameters as a function of age and sex. J Nucl Med. 1994;35:1612–7.
23. Taylor A, Myrick S, Grant S, Issa M, Halkar R, Alazraki NP. A prospective study to compare the reproducibility of camera based MAG3 and creatinine clearance measurements. J Nucl Med. 1999;40:52P.
24. Halkar R, Taylor A, Manatunga A, Issa MM, Myrick SE, Grant S, Shenvi NV. Monitoring renal function: a prospective study comparing camera-based Tc-99m mercaptoacetyltriglycine clearance and creatinine clearance. Urology. 2007;69:426–30.
25. Taylor A, Eshima D, Christian PE, et al. A technetium-99m MAG3 kit formulation: preliminary results in normal volunteers and patients with renal failure. J Nucl Med. 1988;29:616–22.
26. Sanchez J, Friedman S, Kempf J, Abdel-Dayem H. Gallbladder activity appearing 6 minutes after the intravenous injection of Tc99m MAG3 simulating a picture of obstructive uropathy of the right kidney. Clin Nucl Med. 1993;18:30–4.
27. Shattuck LA, Eshima D, Taylor AT, Anderson T, Graham DL, Latino FA, Payne SE. Evaluation of the hepatobiliary excretion of Tc-99m MAG3 and reconstitution factors affecting the radiochemical purity. J Nucl Med. 1994;35:349–55.

28. Kabasakal L, Atay S, Vural AV, et al. Evaluation of Tc-99m-L,L-ethylenedicysteine in renal disorders and determination of extraction ratio. J Nucl Med. 1995;36:1398–403.
29. Taylor A, Hansen L, Eshima D, et al. Comparison of technetium-99m-L,L-EC isomers in rats and humans. J Nucl Med. 1997;38:821–82.
30. Van Nerom CG, Bormans GM, De Roo MF, Verbruggen AM. First experience in healthy volunteers with Tc-99m-L,L-ethylenedicysteine: a new renal imaging agent. Eur J Nucl Med. 1993;20:738–46.
31. Taylor AT, Lipowska M, Cai H. $^{99m}Tc(CO)_3(NTA)$ and ^{131}I-OIH: comparable plasma clearances in patients with chronic kidney disease. J Nucl Med. 2013;54:578–84.
32. Taylor AT, Lipowska M, Marzilli LG. $^{99m}Tc(CO)_3(NTA)$: a ^{99m}Tc renal tracer with pharmacokinetic properties comparable to those of ^{131}I-OIH in healthy volunteers. J Nucl Med. 2010;51:391–6.
33. El-Maghraby TA, van Eck-Smit BL, de Fijter JW, Pauwels EK. Quantitative scintigraphic parameters for the assessment of renal transplant patients. Eur J Radiol. 1998;28:256–69.
34. Hilson AJW, Maisey MN, Brown CB, Ogg CS, Bewick MS. Dynamic renal transplant imaging with Tc-99m DTPA (Sn) supplemented by a transplant perfusion index in the management of renal transplants. J Nucl Med. 1978;19:994–1000.
35. Peters AM, Brown J, Crossman D, et al. Noninvasive measurement of renal blood flow with technetium-99m-DTPA in the evaluation of patients with suspected renovascular hypertension. J Nucl Med. 1990;31:1980–5.
36. Taylor AT, Folks RD, Rahman AKMF, et al. ^{99m}Tc-MAG3: image wisely. Radiology. 2017;284:200–9.
37. O'Reilly PH. Upper urinary tract: standardization of the renogram technique for investigating the dilated upper urinary tract and assessing the results of surgery. BJU Int. 2003;91:239–43.
38. Prigent A, Cosgriff P, Gates GF, et al. Consensus report on quality control of quantitative measurements of renal function obtained from renogram. Semin Nucl Med. 1999;29:146–59.
39. Taylor AT, Blaufox MD, De Palma D, et al. Guidance document for structured reporting of diuresis renography. Semin Nucl Med. 2012;42:41–8.
40. Lindh A, Malmgren M, Ekberg S, Stenstrom M, Granerus G. Analysis of the diuretic response to 7ml/kg hydration prior to captopril renography. Eur J Nucl Med. 1998;25:1190.
41. Slavin JD, Jung WK, Spencer RP. False-positive study with Tc-99m DTPA caused by infiltration of dose. Clin Nucl Med. 1996;21:978–80.
42. Anderson PJ, Rangarajan V, Gordon I. Assessment of drainage in PUJ obstruction: pelvic excretion efficiency as an index of renal function. Nucl Med Commun. 1997;18:823–6.
43. Donoso G, Kuyvenhoven JD, Ham H, Piepsz A. 99mTc-MAG3 diuretic renography in children: a comparison between F0 and F = 20. Nucl Med Commun. 2003;24:1189–93.
44. Piepsz A, Kuyvenhoven JD, Tondeur M, Ham H. Normalized residual activity: usual values and robustness of the method. J Nucl Med. 2002;43:33–8.
45. Wong DC, Rossleigh MA, Farnsworth RH. Diuretic renography with the addition of quantitative gravity-assisted drainage in infants and children. J Nucl Med. 2000;41:1030–6.
46. Eskild-Jensen A, Gordon I, Piepsz A, Frokier J. Interpretation of the renogram: problems and pitfalls in hydronephrosis in children. BJU Int. 2004;94:887–92.
47. Peters AM, George P, Ballardie F, et al. Appropriate selection of background for 99mTc-DTPA. Nucl Med Commun. 1988;9:973–85.
48. Halkar RK, Chrem Y, Galt JR, et al. Interoperator variability in quantitating the MAG3 renal uptake based on semiautomated and manual regions of interest. J Nucl Med. 1996;37:293P.
49. Garcia EV, Taylor A, Halkar RK, et al. RENEX: an expert system for the interpretation of 99mTc-MAG3 scans to detect renal obstruction. J Nucl Med. 2006;47:320–9.
50. Esteves FP, Taylor A, Manatunga A, et al. Normal values for camera-based ^{99m}Tc-MAG3 clearance, MAG3 curve parameters, excretory parameters and residual urine volume. AJR. 2006;187:W610–7.
51. Blaufox MD, Fine EJ, Heller S, et al. Prospective study of simultaneous orthoiodohipurate and diethylenetriaminepentaacetic acid captopril renography. J Nucl Med. 1998;39:522–8.
52. Taylor AT, Nally J, Aurell M, et al. Consensus report on ACE inhibitor renography for detecting renovascular hypertension. J Nucl Med. 1996;37:1876–82.
53. Chaiwatanarat T, Padhy AK, Bomanji JB. Validation of renal output efficiency as an objective parameter in the evaluation of upper urineary tract obstruction. J Nucl Med. 1993;34:845–8.
54. Strauss BS, Blaufox MD. Estimation of residual urine and urine flow rates without ureteral catherization. J Nucl Med. 1970;11:81–4.
55. Manjunath G, Sarnak MJ, Levey AS. Estimating the glomerular filtration rate; dos and don't's for assessing kidney function. Postgrad Med. 2001;110(6):55–62.
56. Prigent A. Monitoring renal function and limitations of renal function tests. Semin Nucl Med. 2008;38:32–46.
57. Stevens LA, Coresh J, Green T, Levey AS. Assessing kidney function—measured and estimated glomerular filtration rate. N Engl J Med. 2006;354:2473–83.
58. Brown SCW, O'Reilly PH. Glomerular filtration rate measurement: a neglected test in urological practice. Brit J Urol. 1995;75:296–300.
59. Rosenbaum JL. Evaluation of clearance studies in chronic kidney disease. J Chron Dis. 1970;22:507–14.
60. Brochner-Mortensen J, Rodbro P. Selection of routine method for determination of glomerular filtration rate in adult patients. Scand J Clin Lab Invest. 1976;36:35–43.

61. Fleming JS, Zivanovic MA, Blake GM, Burniston M, Cosgriff P. Guidelines for the measurement of glomerular filtration rate using plasma sampling. Nucl Med Commun. 2004;25:759–69.
62. Stevens LA, Levey AS. Measured GFR as a confirmatory test for estimated GFR. J Am Soc Nephrol. 2009;20:2305–13.
63. Bubeck B. Renal clearance determination with one blood sample: improved accuracy and universal applicability by a new calculation principle. Semin Nucl Med. 1993;23:73–86.
64. Russell CD. Optimum sample times for single-injection, multi-sample renal clearance methods. J Nucl Med. 1993;10:1761–5.
65. Gates GF. Glomerular filtration rate: estimation from fractional renal accumulation of Tc-99m DTPA (stannous). AJR. 1982;138:565–70.
66. Inoue Y, Ohtake T, Yokoyama I, Yoshikawa K, Asai S, Ohtomo K. Evaluation of renal function from 99mTc-MAG3 renography without blood sampling. J Nucl Med. 1999;40:793–8.
67. Schlegel JU, Hamway SA. Individual renal plasma flow determination in 2 minutes. J Urol. 1976;116:2882–285.
68. Taylor A, Manatunga A, Morton K, et al. Multicenter trial validation of a camera based method to measure Tc-99m mercaptoacetyltriglycine or Tc-99m MAG3, clearance. Radiology. 1997;204:47–54.
69. Bocher M, Shrem Y, Tappiser A, Klein M, Schecter D, Taylor A Jr, Chisin R. Technetium-99m-MAG3 clearance: comparison of camera based methods. Clin Nucl Med. 2001;26:745–50.
70. Taylor A, Corrigan PL, Galt J, et al. Measuring technetium-99m-MAG3 clearance with an improved camera-based method. J Nucl Med. 1995;36:1689–95.
71. Taylor A, Lewis C, Giacometti A, et al. Improved formulas for the estimation of renal depth in adults. J Nucl Med. 1993;34:1766–9.
72. Tonnesen KH, Munck O, Hald T, et al. Influence on the radiorenogram of variation in skin to kidney distance and the clinical importance hereof. In: Zum Winkel K, Mlaufox MD, Funck-Bretano JL, editors. Proceedings of the international symposium on radionuclides in nephrourology. Stuttgart: Thieme; 1974. p. 79–86.
73. Samal M, Ptacnik V, Skibova D, Jiskrova H, Kubinyi J. Simple model-based method for gamma-camera measurement of 99m-MAG3 plasma clearance. J Nucl Med Mol Image. 2013;54:170–1.
74. Dubovsky EV, Russell CD, Bischof-Delaoye A, et al. Report of the radionuclides in nephrourology committee for evaluation of transplanted kidney (review of techniques). Sem Nucl Med. 1999;29:175–88.
75. Dubovsky EV, Russell CD. Diagnosis of renovascular hypertension after renal transplantation (suppl). Am J Hypertens. 1991;4:724–30.
76. Nankivell BJ, Borrows RJ, Fung CL, O'Connell PJ, Allen RDM, Chapman JR. The natural history of chronic allograft nephropathy. N Engl J Med. 2003;349:2326–33.
77. Hvistendahl JJ, Pedersen TS, Schmidt F, et al. Renal function is modulated by a vesico-renal relflex mechanism during elevated bladder pressure in the pig. Nucl Med Commun. 1998;19:502.
78. Shulkin BL, Mandell GA, Cooper JA, et al. Procedure guideline for diuretic renography in children 3.0. J Nucl Med Tech. 2008;36:162–8.
79. Members of the Society for Fetal Urology and Pediatric Nuclear Medicine Council Members, Society of Nuclear Medicine. The "well tempered" diuretic renogram: a standard method to examine the asymptomatic neonate with hydronephrosis or hydroureteronephrosis. J Nucl Med. 1992;33:2047–51.
80. Hunsche A, Press H, Taylor A. Increasing the dose of furosemide in patients with azotemia and suspected obstruction. Clin Nucl Med. 2004;26:149–53.
81. Brater CD. Diuretic therapy. N Engl J Med. 1998;339:387–95.
82. Hemstreet BA, Page RL. Sulfonamide allergies and outcomes related to use of potentially cross-reactive drugs in hospitalized patients. Pharmacotherapy. 2006;26:551–7.
83. Liu Y, Ghesani NV, Skurnick JH, Zukier LS. The F + 0 protocol for diuretic renography results in fewer interrupted studies due to voiding than the F – 15 protocol. J Nucl Med. 2005;46:317–20.
84. Kuyvenhoven J, Piepsz M, Ham H. When could the administration of furosemide be avoided? Clin Nucl Med. 2003;28:732–7.
85. Adeyoju AA, Burke D, Atkinson C, et al. The choice of timing for diuresis renography for the assessment of equivocal pelviureteric obstruction. Br J Urol Int. 2001;88:1–5.
86. Wong DC, Rossleigh MA, Farnsworth RH. F+0 diuresis renography in infants and children. J Nucl Med. 1999;40:1805–11.
87. Kass EJ, Majd M. Evaluation and management of upper urinary tract obstruction in infancy and childhood. Urol Clin North Am. 1985;12(1):133–41.
88. Connolly LP, Zurakowski D, Peters CA, et al. Variability of diuresis renography interpretation due to method of post-diuretic renal pelvic clearance half-time determination. J Urol. 2000;164:467–71.
89. Brown SCW, Upsdell SM, O'Reilly PH. The importance of renal function for the interpretation of diuresis renography. Br J Urol. 1992;69:121–5.
90. Kletter K, Nurnberger N. Diagnostic potential of diuresis renography: limitation by the severity of hydronephrosis and by impairment of renal function. Nucl Med Comm. 1989;10:51–61.
91. Upsdell SM, Leeson SM, Brooman PJC, et al. Diuretic-induced urinary flow rates at varying clearances and their relevance to the performance and interpretation of diuresis renography. Br J Urol. 1988;61:14–8.
92. Piepsz A, Tondeur M, Ham HR. NORA: a simple and reliable parameter for estiming renal output with or without frusemide challenge. Nucl Med Commun. 2000;21:317–23.

93. Upsdell SM, Testa HJ, Lawson RS. The F-15 diuresis renogram in suspected obstruction of the upper urinary tract. Br J Urol. 1992;69:126–31.
94. Bao J, Manatunga A, Binongo JN, et al. Key variables for interpreting 99mTc-mercaptoacetyltriglycine diuretic scans: development and validation of a predictive model. AJR Am J Roentgenol. 2011;197:325–33.
95. Bird VG, Gomez-Martin O, Leveillee RJ, Sfakianakis GN, Rivas LA, Amendola MA. A comparison of unenhanced helical computerized tomography findings and renal obstruction determined by furosemide ^{99m}technetium mercaptoacetyltriglycine diuretic scintirenography for patients with acute renal colic. J Urol. 2000;167:1597–160395.
96. Lorberboym M, Kapustin Z, Elias S, Nikolov G, Katz R. The role of renal scintigraphy and unenhanced helical computerized tomography in patients with ureterolithiasis. Eur J Nucl Med. 2000;27:441–6.
97. Sfakianakis GN, Cohen DJ, Braunstein RH, et al. MAG3-F0 scintigraphy in decision making for emergency intervention in renal colic after helical CT positive for a urolith. J Nucl Med. 2000;41:1813–22.
98. Prigent A. The diagnosis of renovascular hypertension: the role of captopril renal scintigraphy and related issues. Eur J Nucl Med. 1993;20:625–44.
99. Eyler WR, Clark MD, Garman JE, Rian RL, Meininger DE. Angiography of the renal areas including a comparative study of renal arterial stenosis in patients with and without hypertension. Radiology. 1962;78:879–92.
100. Holley KE, Hunt JC, Brown AL Jr, et al. Renal artery stenosis: a clinical pathologic study in normotensive and hypertensive patients. Am J Med. 1964;37:14–22.
101. Plouin PF, Chatellier G, Darne B, Raynaud A. Blood pressure outcome of angioplasty in atherosclerotic renal artery stenosis: a randomized trial. Essai Multicentrique Medicaments vs Angioplastie (EMMA) Study Group. Hypertension. 1998;31(3):823–9.
102. van Jaarsveld BC, Krijnen P, Pieterman H, Derkx FH, Deinum J, Postma CT, Dees A, Woittiez AJ, Bartelink AK, Man in 't Veld AJ, Schalekamp MA. The effect of balloon angioplasty on hypertension in atherosclerotic renal-artery stenosis. Dutch Renal Artery Stenosis Intervention Cooperative Study Group. N Engl J Med. 2000;342(14):1007–14.
103. Webster J, Marshall F, Abdalla M, Dominiczak A, Edwards R, Isles CG, Loose H, Main J, Padfield P, Russell IT, Walker B, Watson M, Wilkinson R. Randomised comparison of percutaneous angioplasty vs continued medical therapy for hypertensive patients with atheromatous renal artery stenosis. Scottish and Newcastle Renal Artery Stenosis Collaborative Group. J Hum Hypertens. 1998;12(5):329–35.
104. Taylor A. ACE inhibition renography in the evaluation of suspected renovascular hypertension. In: Prigent A, Peipsz A, editors. Functional imaging in nephrourology. London: Taylor and Francis; 2006. p. 149–64.
105. Helin KH, Tikkanen I, von Knorring JE, et al. Screening for renovascular hypertension in a population with relatively low prevalence. J Hypertens. 1998;16:1523–9.
106. Blaufox MD, Middleton ML, Bongiovanni J, Davis BR. Cost efficacy of the diagnosis and therapy of renovascular hypertension. J Nucl Med. 1996;37:171–7.
107. Taylor AT, Blaufox MD, Dubovsky EV et al (2003) Society of Nuclear Medicine procedure guideline for diagnosis of renovascular hypertension. http://snmmi.files.cms-plus.com/docs/Renovascular_Hypertention.pdf
108. Gainer JV, Morrow JD, Loveland A, King DJ, Brown NJ. Effect of bradykinin-receptor blockade on the response to angiotensin-converting-enzyme inhibitor in normotensive and hypertensive subjects. N Eng J Med. 1998;339:1285–92.
109. Karanikas G, Becherer A, Wiesner K, Dudczak R, Kletter K. ACE inhibition is superior to angiotensin receptor blockade for renography in renal artery stenosis. Eur J Nucl Med. 2002;29:312–8.
110. Kon V, Fogo A, Ichikawa I, et al. Bradykinin causes selective efferent arteriolar dilation during angiotensin I converting enzyme inhibition. Kidney Int. 1993;44:545–50.
111. Sandberg K, Hong J. Kidney angeiotensin receptors and their role in renal pathophysiology. Sem Nephrol. 2000;20:402–16.
112. Müller-Suur R, Tidgren B, Lundberg HJ. Effect of captopril on MAG3 clearance in patients with and without renal artery stenosis and after PTRA. Eur J Nucl Med. 1998;25:845.
113. Taylor A, Eshima D. Renal artery stenosis and ischemia: effect on renal blood flow and extraction fraction. Hypertension. 1994;23:96–103.
114. Visscher CA, de Zeeuw D, de Jong PE, et al. Angiotensin-converting enzyme inhibition-induced changes in hippurate renography and renal function in renovascular hypertension. J Nucl Med. 1996;37:482–8.
115. Erbslöh-Möller B, Dumas A, Roth D, Sfakianakis G, Bourgoignie JJ. Furosemide I-131 hippuran renography after angiotensin-converting enzyme inhibition for the diagnosis of renovascular hypertension. Am J Med. 1991;90:23–9.
116. Setaro JF, Saddler MC, Chen CC, et al. Simplified captopril renography in diagnosis and treatment of renal artery stenosis. Hypertension. 1991;18:289–98.
117. Visscher CA, de Zeeuw D, Huisman RM. Effect of chronic ACE inhibition on the diagnostic value of renography for renovascular hypertension:

a preliminary report. Nephrol Dial Transplant. 1995;10:263–5.
118. Taylor A. Functional testing: ACEI renography. Semin Nephrol. 2000;20:437–44.
119. Picciotto G, Sargiotto A, Petrarulo M, Rabbia C, De Filippi PG, Roccatello D. Reliability of captopril renography in patients under chronic therapy with angiotensin II (AT1) receptor antagonists. J Nucl Med. 2003;44:1574–81.
120. Claveau-Tremblay R, Turpin S, Debraekeleer M, et al. False-positive captopril renography in patients taking calcium antagonists. J Nucl Med. 1998;39:1621–6.
121. Ludwig V, Martin WH, Delbeke D. Calcium channel blockers: a potential cause of false-positive captopril renography. Clin Nucl Med. 2003;28:108–12.
122. Sfakianakis GM, Bourgoignie JJ, Georgiou M, et al. Diagnosis of renovascular hypertension with ACE inhibition scintigraphy. Radiol Clin North Am. 1993;31:831–48.
123. Black HR, Bourgoignie JJ, Pickering T, Svetkey L, Saddler MC, et al. Report of the working party group for patient selection and preparation. Am J Hypertens. 1991;4:745S–456S.
124. Kopecky RT, McAfee JG, Thomas FD, et al. Enalaprilat-enhanced renography in a rat model of renovascular hypertension. J Nucl Med. 1990;31:501–7.
125. Fanti S, Dondi M, Guidalotti PL, et al. Bilateral symmetrical induced changes in captopril scintigraphy. J Nucl Med. 1998;39:86P.
126. Stavropoulos SW, Sevigny SA, Ende JF, Drane WE. Hypotensive response to captopril: a potential pitfall of scintigraphic assessment for renal artery stenosis. J Nucl Med. 1999;40:406–11.
127. Caglar M, Moretti JL, Buchet P, et al. Enalapril plus frusemide MAG3 scintigraphy in hypertensive patients with atherosclerosis and moderate renal insufficiency. Nucl Med Commun. 1998;19:1135–40.
128. Nally JW Jr, Chen C, Fine E, et al. Diagnostic criteria of renovascular hypertension with captopril renography. Am J Hypertens. 1991;4:749S–52S.
129. Dey HM, Hoffer PB, Lerner E, et al. Quantitative analysis of the technetium-99m-DTPA captopril renogram: contribution of washout parameters to the diagnosis of renal artery stenosis. J Nucl Med. 1993;34:1416–9.
130. Fommei E, Ghione S, Hilson AJW, et al. Captopril radionuclide test in renovascular hypertension: a European multicentre study. Eur J Nucl Med. 1993;20:625–44.
131. Dondi M, Fanti S, De Fabritiis A, et al. Prognostic value of captopril renal scintigraphy in renovascular hypertension. J Nucl Med. 1992;33:2040–4.
132. Fommei E, Ghione S, Hilson AJW, et al. Captopril radionuclide test in renovascular hypertension: European multicenter study. In: O'Reilly PH, Taylor A, Nally JV, editors. Radionuclides in nephrourology, vol. 1. Field and Wood: Blue Bell, PA; 1994.
133. Geyskes GG, deBruyn AJG. Captopril renography and the effect of percutaneous transluminal angioplasty on blood pressure in 94 patients with renal artery stenosis. Am J Hypertens. 1991;4:685S–9S.
134. Kahn D, Ben-Haim S, Bushnell DL, et al. Captopril-enhanced Tc-99m MAG3 renal scintigraphy in subjects with suspected renovascular hypertension. Nucl Med Commun. 1994;15:515–28.
135. Mittal BR, Kumar P, Arora P, et al. Role of captopril renography in the diagnosis of renovascular hypertension. Am J Kidney Dis. 1996;28:209–13.
136. Szabo Z, Xia J, Mathews WB. Radiopharmaceuticals for renal positron emission tomography imaging. Semin Nucl Med. 2008;38:20–31.
137. Awasthi V, Pathuri G, Agashe HB, Gali H. Synthesis and in vivo evaluation of *p*-^{18}F-fluorohippurate as a new radiopharmaceutical for assessment of renal function by PET. J Nucl Med. 2011;52:147–53.
138. Lipowska M, Jarkas N, Voll RJ, Nye JA, Klenc J, Goodman MM, Taylor AT. $Re(CO)_3$([^{18}F]FEDA), a novel ^{18}F PET renal tracer: radiosynthesis and preclinical evaluation. Nucl Med Biol. 2018;58:42–50.
139. Alongi P, Picchio M, Zattoni F, Spallino M, Gianolli L, Saladini G, Evangelista L. Recurrent renal cell carcinoma: clinical and prognostic value of FDG PET/CT. Eur J Nucl Med Mol Imaging. 2016;42:464–73.
140. Wang H, Ding H, Chen J, Chao C, Lu Y, Lin W, Kao C. Meta-analysis of the diagnostic performance of [^{18}F]FDG-PET and PET/CT in renal cell carcinoma. Cancer Imaging. 2012;12:464–74.
141. Divgi CR, Uzzo RG, Gatsonis C, et al. Positron emission tomography/computed tomography identification of clear cell renal cell carcinoma: results from the REDECT trial. J Clin Oncol. 2012;31:187–94.

9 Nuclear Medicine Imaging Techniques of the Gastrointestinal System

Harvey A. Ziessman

9.1 Introduction

Gastrointestinal scintigraphy takes advantage of the physiologic basis of radionuclide imaging and makes effective use of its quantitative potential. This chapter discusses the importance and clinical use of older, tried, and true scintigraphic studies of the gastrointestinal system, as well as newer techniques that are increasing in clinical importance. They are discussed not in the more common aboral order, from mouth to rectum, but according to a logical progression. All topics will be covered, beginning with solid gastric emptying, then liquid gastric emptying, gastric accommodation, small and large bowel intestinal transit, esophageal transit, gastroesophageal reflux, gastrointestinal bleeding, and the Meckel's scan.

H. A. Ziessman (✉)
Division of Nuclear Medicine and Molecular Imaging, Department of Radiology and Radiological Sciences, Johns Hopkins University, Baltimore, MD, USA
e-mail: Hziessm1@jhmi.edu

9.2 Gastric Emptying

Gastric motility is the result of a complex interaction between the smooth muscle of the stomach, the central and peripheral nervous system, and neurohormonal feedback. From a functional standpoint, the stomach has two compartments. After ingestion of a meal, the proximal stomach, or *fundus*, undergoes receptive relaxation and accommodation of the meal. The fundus has tonic contraction producing a constant pressure gradient from proximal to distal, responsible for liquid emptying and also for moving the ingested food into the distal stomach. Liquids empty in an exponential pattern: clear liquids, monoexponentially, and full liquids, multiexponentially. The distal stomach or *antrum* has intermittent phasic contractions initiated by a rhythmic depolarization of smooth muscle cells along the greater curvature, acting like a pacemaker. These phasic contractions are responsible for mixing, grinding, and trituration of the food into 1–2 mm particles small enough to pass through the pylorus. The antrum is responsible for solid gastric emptying. Solids usually empty in a linear pattern after an initial delay or lag phase of 5–25 min, the time required for breaking down the food into small-enough particles that can pass through the pylorus [1, 2]. The lag phase may not be appreciated with infrequent intermittent imaging, acquired at intervals of 15 min or longer. The smooth muscle of the pylorus acts as a physiologic sieve to regu-

H. Ahmadzadehfar et al. (eds.), *Clinical Nuclear Medicine*,
https://doi.org/10.1007/978-3-030-39457-8_9

Table 9.1 Medications that delay gastric emptying

Nifedipine
Beta-adrenergic agonists
Isoproterenol
Theophylline
Sulfcralate
Anticholinergics
Tegaserod
Diazepam, Librium
Tricyclic antidepressants
Phenothiazine
Levodopa
Progesterone, oral contraceptives
Opiates
Alcohol and nicotine

late outflow. A variety of external factors, particularly many therapeutic drugs, can alter the rate of gastric emptying (Table 9.1).

9.3 Clinical Presentation

Symptoms of gastroparesis include postprandial nausea, vomiting, abdominal discomfort, and early satiety. Insulin-dependent diabetes is a common cause of delayed gastric emptying, due to an autonomic gastroenteropathy. Delayed emptying can lead to poor insulin control of the blood sugar. Because hyperglycemia per se, without underlying disease, may cause a delay in gastric emptying, a fasting blood sugar should be confirmed in diabetics prior to the radionuclide gastric emptying study to be <250 mg/dL. Approximately 30–60% of patients with symptoms of dyspeptic syndrome (defined by gastroenterologists as pain or discomfort originating from the upper abdomen) have delayed gastric emptying [3, 4]. Gastroparesis has been associated with a variety of other diseases; however, the pathophysiologic basis for delayed emptying is not understood. Most causes, other than insulin-dependent diabetes, are called *functional* because there is no known pathophysiologic basis [5]. Biopsy is not informative.

The diagnosis of functional gastroparesis should be made with caution until an anatomic cause has been excluded. Some patients with predominantly upper abdominal symptoms may actually have small or large bowel transit abnormalities, and it is not uncommon for patients to have both gastric and intestinal transit abnormalities. Although most gastroparesis is chronic, it sometimes presents as an acute self-resolving process, e.g., due to viral infection or metabolic derangement. Indications for gastric emptying studies are numerous, and common ones are listed in Table 9.2, including gastroesophageal reflux unresponsive to usual therapy and insulin-dependent diabetics with poor glycemic control.

Table 9.2 Clinical indications for radionuclide gastric emptying

Unexplained recurrent postprandial nausea, vomiting, abdominal pain
Insulin-dependent diabetics with recurrent postprandial symptoms or poor blood sugar control
Severe reflux esophagitis not well-controlled with usual therapy
Assessment of response to a motility drug

Rapid gastric emptying is most commonly seen in patients after pyloroplasty or gastrectomy or in those with Zollinger-Ellison syndrome (gastrinoma); however, it sometimes occurs in diabetics with symptoms mimicking gastroparesis and in other patients without any known underlying illness [6]. Most commonly, patients with rapid emptying have symptoms referred to as “gastric dumping syndrome,” which consists of diaphoresis, palpitations, and diarrhea after eating.

9.4 Standardized Gastric Emptying Scintigraphy

The first publication of a human radionuclide gastric emptying study dates back to 1966 [7]. Radionuclide gastric emptying has been the standard method for evaluating gastric motility for decades. However, many different methodologies have been used, including meal content, length of the study, and frequency of image acquisition; use of attenuation and decay correction; methods of quantification; and normal values [8]. There is no convincing evidence that quantitative parameters described by frequent image acquisition, such as characterization of the lag phase, have any clinical relevance. Gastroenterologists wanted a standardized solid gastric emptying methodology with normal values so that patient results could be compared across imaging clinics. In 2007, a standardized methodology was agreed upon by expert gastroenterologists and nuclear medicine physicians and was published in both nuclear medicine and gastroenterology literature [9]. The recommended methodology had originally been published by Tougas et al. [10] and is described in detail in Table 9.3. Their data, as well as others', have demonstrated that the results of infrequent imaging, e.g., once each hour, did not differ significantly from more frequent imaging, e.g., every 10 min [10, 11]. Normal values were established from their large database of 123 volunteer subjects. The methodology is a simplified protocol that can be performed in any laboratory with a gamma camera and computer workstation. The standardized meal is an egg-white sandwich with jam and water. One-minute images are required at only four time points: after ingestion at time 0 and at 1, 2, and 4 h (Fig. 9.1).

Correction for attenuation and radioactive decay is necessary for accurate quantification and is required by the standardized methodology. Anterior-only imaging results in an underestimation of gastric emptying by as much as 20–30% or greater [12, 13]. Although attenuation is invariably an issue in obese patients, it is by no means limited to them, and the degree is not predictable in others. Attenuation varies as the stomach contents move from the relatively posterior fundus to the more anterior antrum. Correction for attenuation is best performed by acquiring anterior and posterior images, then calculating the geometric mean (GM) (square root of the product of anterior and posterior counts) at each time point [12]. Acquiring the study in the left anterior oblique (LAO) view approximates the geometric mean attenuation correction [14, 15]. It compensates for attenuation because in that projection, the stomach contents move approximately parallel to the head of the gamma camera. However, the GM is preferable and is more reliably

Table 9.3 Standardized gastric emptying scintigraphy protocol

Patient preparation
Discontinuation of medications should be decided beforehand by the referring physician
Diabetics should have a fasting blood sugar <250 mg/dL prior to the study
Perform the study in the morning after an overnight fast, NPO for at least 6 h
Radiopharmaceutical and meal
Tc-99m sulfur colloid 1 mCi (37 MBq) should be bound to 4 oz. egg substitute (generic egg white equivalent) by microwaving or scrambling after mixing the egg with Tc-99m sulfur colloid. Stir once or twice while cooking until the mixture reaches a consistency of omelet. Meal also consists of two slices of white bread, strawberry jam (30 g), and water (120 mL)
Meal should be ingested within 10–15 min
Instrumentation
Gamma camera: Large field of view, dual detector camera
Collimator: Low energy, parallel hole, high resolution, or general purpose
Tc-99m photopeak with a 20% window around 140 keV photopeak
Computer setup: 1-min static images (128 × 128 word mode matrix)
Patient position
Position patient either standing upright or lying supine, with camera heads anterior and posterior. A single-head camera can be used, acquiring an image first anteriorly, then posteriorly
Imaging procedure
Acquire images at time 0 (immediately after ingestion) and 1, 2, and 4 h. Three hours is optional
Processing
Draw ROI for anterior and posterior stomach views
The geometric mean of the anterior and posterior views is calculated at each time point, and percent retention or gastric emptying is calculated
Decay correction is mandatory
Interpretation
Delayed gastric emptying
1 h < 10% emptying (>90% retention)
2 h < 40% emptying (>60% retention)
3 h < 70% emptying (>30% retention)
4 h < 90% emptying (>10% retention)
Rapid gastric emptying
>70% emptying at 1 h
>90% emptying at 2 h
These values apply to the entire meal and are not valid for different meals or incomplete ingestion of the standard meal

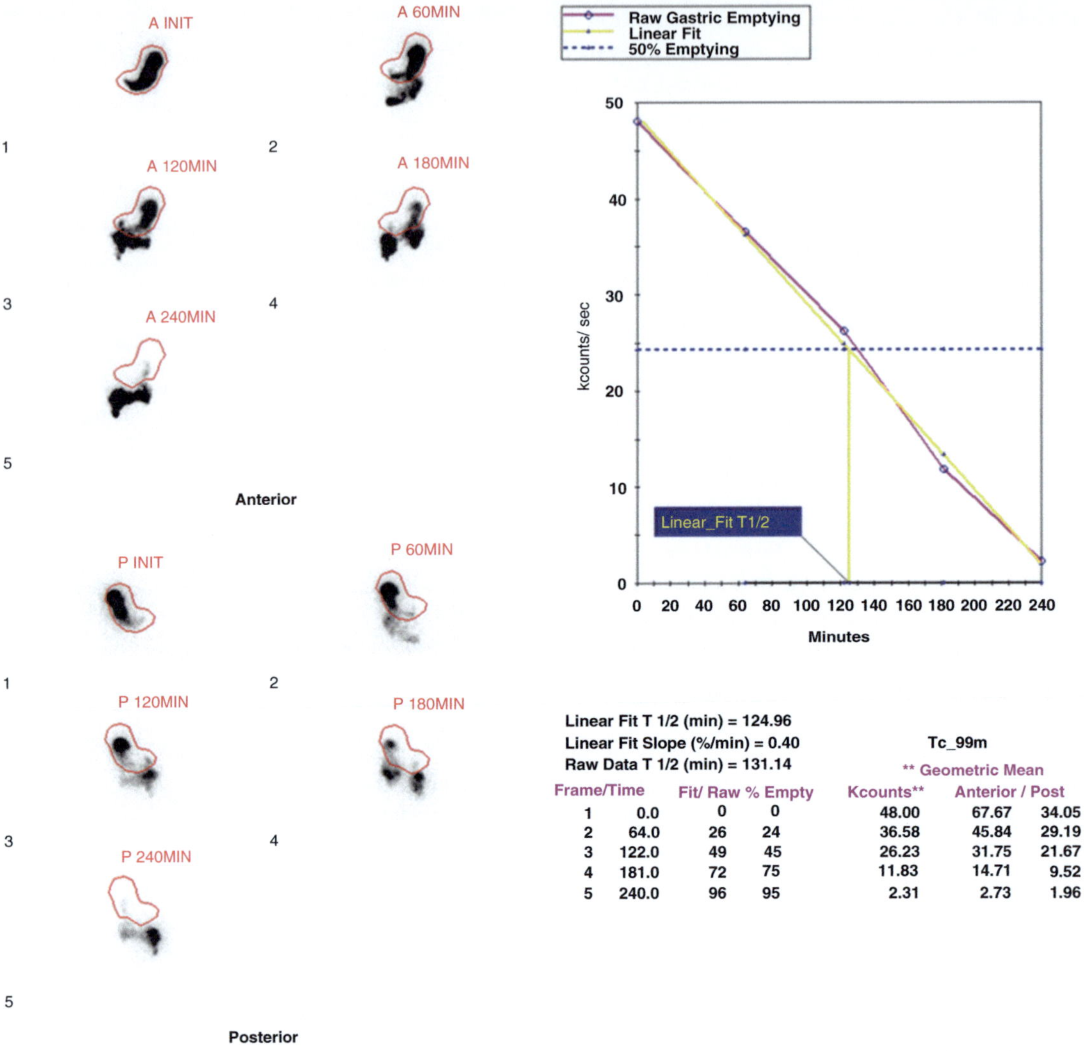

Frame/Time		Fit/ Raw % Empty		Kcounts**	Anterior / Post	
1	0.0	0	0	48.00	67.67	34.05
2	64.0	26	24	36.58	45.84	29.19
3	122.0	49	45	26.23	31.75	21.67
4	181.0	72	75	11.83	14.71	9.52
5	240.0	96	95	2.31	2.73	1.96

Fig. 9.1 Standardized solid gastric emptying study—normal. Anterior images are above; posterior images are below. The first image is acquired immediately after meal ingestion (left upper row image, quantification: frame 1, time 0), then at 64 min (right upper row, frame 2), 122 min (second row left, frame 3), 181 min (second row right, frame 4), and 240 min (third row, frame 5). Images at 180 min are not required by the standardized protocol and thus optional. Gastric ROIs are drawn around the stomach in anterior and posterior images. Geometric mean percent emptying values are calculated and listed in the fourth column (lower right), 45% at 2 h (normal >40%) and 95% at 4 h (frame 5) (normal >90%)

accurate. Liquid studies do not require attenuation correction due to the rapid transit.

A 4-h solid gastric emptying study length has been shown to detect a greater number of patients with gastroparesis than does a 2-h study, as many as 30% more (Fig. 9.2) [16–18]. In the past, studies were often 60–120 min in length. Although 4-h imaging may seem like a potential logistical problem, 1-min images at four time points actually allow for more patients to be imaged in a single morning than most prior methods do. Some clinics image at 3 h as well so that if the patient has reached the 4-h normal values, the study can be stopped (Fig. 9.3). Normal 3-h val-

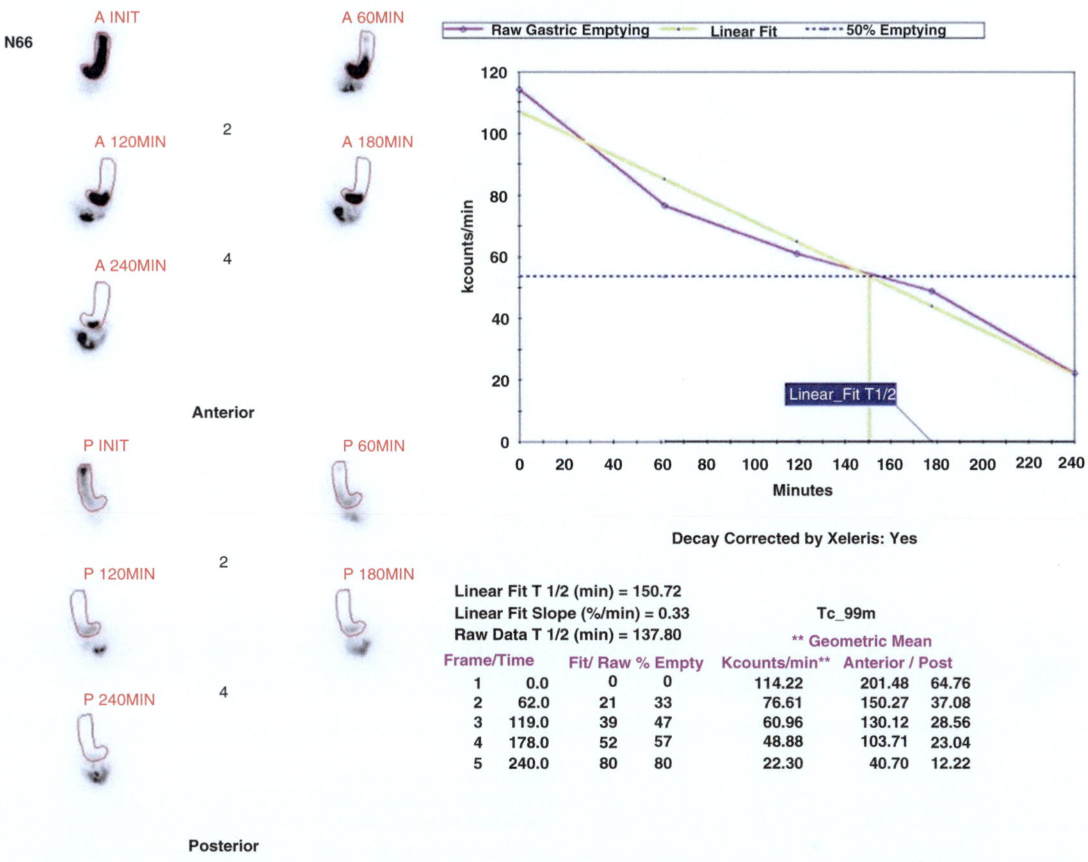

Fig. 9.2 Normal solid gastric emptying at 2 h (47%) but delayed emptying at 4 h (80%). This demonstrates the advantage of a 4-h study over a 2-h study. The 4-h study diagnoses an additional 30% of patients with gastroparesis

ues are >70% gastric emptying [18]. A study should be read as abnormal if the patient has delayed emptying at either 2 h (<40% emptying or > 60% retention) or 4 h (<90% emptying or >10% retention) (Fig. 9.4). Although Tougas et al. described gastric retention, this chapter will primarily use the reverse terminology, gastric emptying. Two publications have now shown that in approximately 50% of patients referred for suspected gastroparesis, the study can be interpreted as positive or negative at 2 h with good accuracy, specifically patients with <35% emptying at 2 h (abnormal) or >55% at 2 h (normal) [19, 20]. One should be aware that a number of therapeutic drugs will delay emptying (Table 9.2), and this should be considered during patient preparation and at the time of interpreting the study. It is often left to the clinician to decide whether the patient should continue to take medications that may affect emptying.

Rapid gastric emptying occurs in 10–30% of patients referred for suspected delayed gastric emptying [6, 21]. The standardized protocol has defined rapid emptying as >70% emptying at 1 h. Greater than 90 percent emptying at 2 h should also be considered rapid. Established normal values assume that the patient ate the entire meal. Ingestion of smaller volume or content of the meal will result in more rapid emptying, and normal values have not been adjusted for reduced ingested content. The study report should therefore state the approximate percentage of the meal ingested and its implication, if incompletely ingested. The results may overestimate gastric emptying.

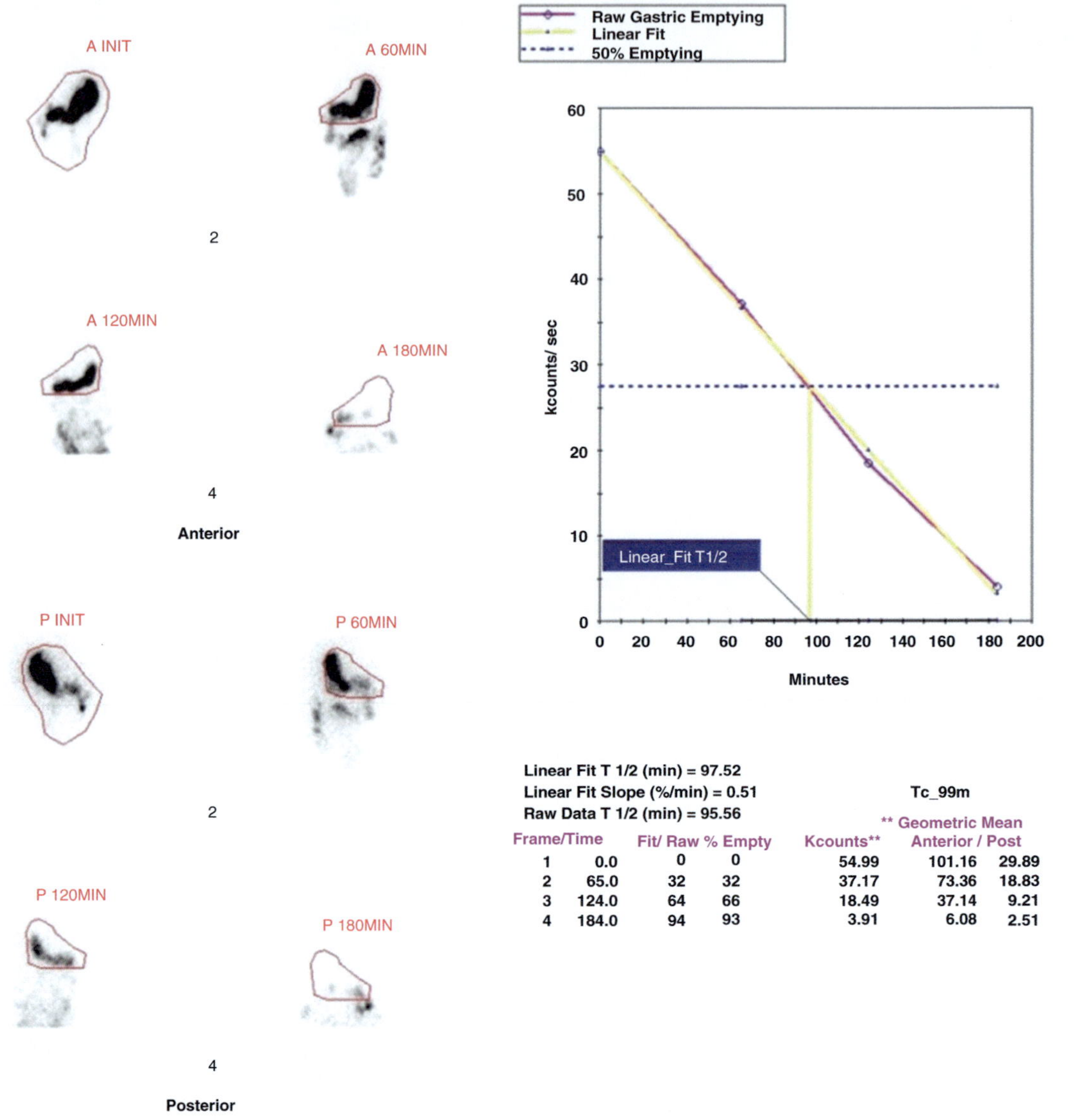

Fig. 9.3 Solid gastric emptying—normal (93%) at 3 h (frame 4). The study was thus stopped at this time point. Note that a larger ROI was drawn around the first image anteriorly and posteriorly than in the other frames. The reason is that some intestinal activity was seen in the first frame. In order for the quantification to be accurate, all the ingested activity must be included in the first frame ROI

Some patients are allergic to eggs or for other reasons cannot eat them. Thus, an alternative meal is necessary. Although various alternative meals have been used, normal values are limited, often for performed for less than 4 h, and the meals are often specific to the country of origin. A meal that has been directly compared to the standardized meal is EnsurePlus® (Abbott Laboratories) [22]. In spite of being an 8-oz. full liquid meal with 11 g of fat (the standardized meal is low fat, 2%), the normal values are, surprisingly, not significantly different.

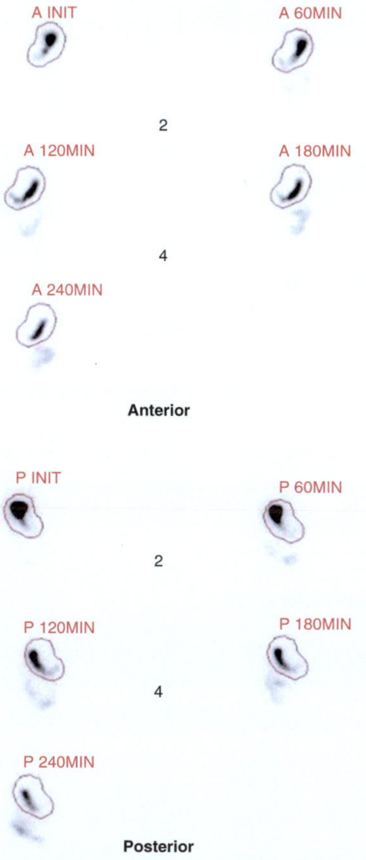

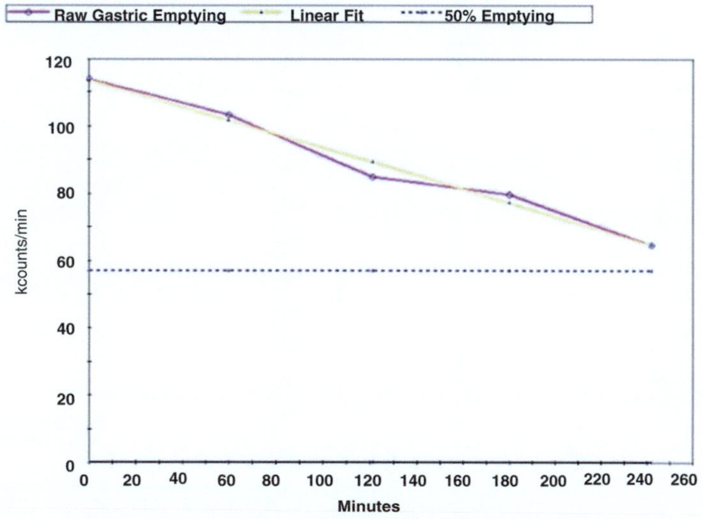

Decay Corrected by Xeleris: Yes

Linear Fit T 1/2 (min) = 280.49
Linear Fit Slope (%/min) = 0.18
Raw Data T 1/2 (min) = None

Tc_99m

** Geometric Mean

Frame	Time	Fit	Raw % Empty	Kcounts/min**	Anterior	Post
1	0.0	0	0	114.00	136.06	95.52
2	60.0	11	10	103.15	147.92	71.94
3	121.0	22	25	84.96	159.42	45.29
4	180.0	32	30	79.73	150.36	42.28
5	242.0	43	43	64.53	123.66	33.67

Fig. 9.4 Solid gastric emptying—delayed at 2 h (frame 3) (25%) and 4 h (frame 5) (43%). Normal is >40% at 2 h and >90% at 4 h

9.5 Liquid Gastric Emptying

It had been a common teaching that liquid gastric emptying is less sensitive for the detection of gastroparesis than a solid study is, that it is never abnormal when the solid study is normal and becomes abnormal only when solid gastroparesis is severe, and that only solid gastric emptying is necessary for clinical purposes. However, there have been no published investigations that have proven this, and three studies have now shown that this is in fact incorrect [23–25]. There is a poor correlation between the solid and clear liquid emptying studies. They may both be normal, both abnormal, or one normal and the other abnormal. The most clinically important finding of these studies is that in patients referred with symptoms suggestive of gastroparesis, who have a normal solid emptying study, over 25% will have delayed liquid emptying. Why this occurs physiologically is uncertain at present; however, it may explain the patient's symptoms.

Clear liquid studies can be performed alone (if patients cannot tolerate solids or full liquids), simultaneously with the solid meal, or sequentially, e.g., liquid then solid. A clear liquid study alone requires only 30 min. Normal halftime is <25 min (Figs. 9.5 and 9.6). The emptying values of a simultaneously ingested solid-liquid study are slower than those of liquid-only studies. There

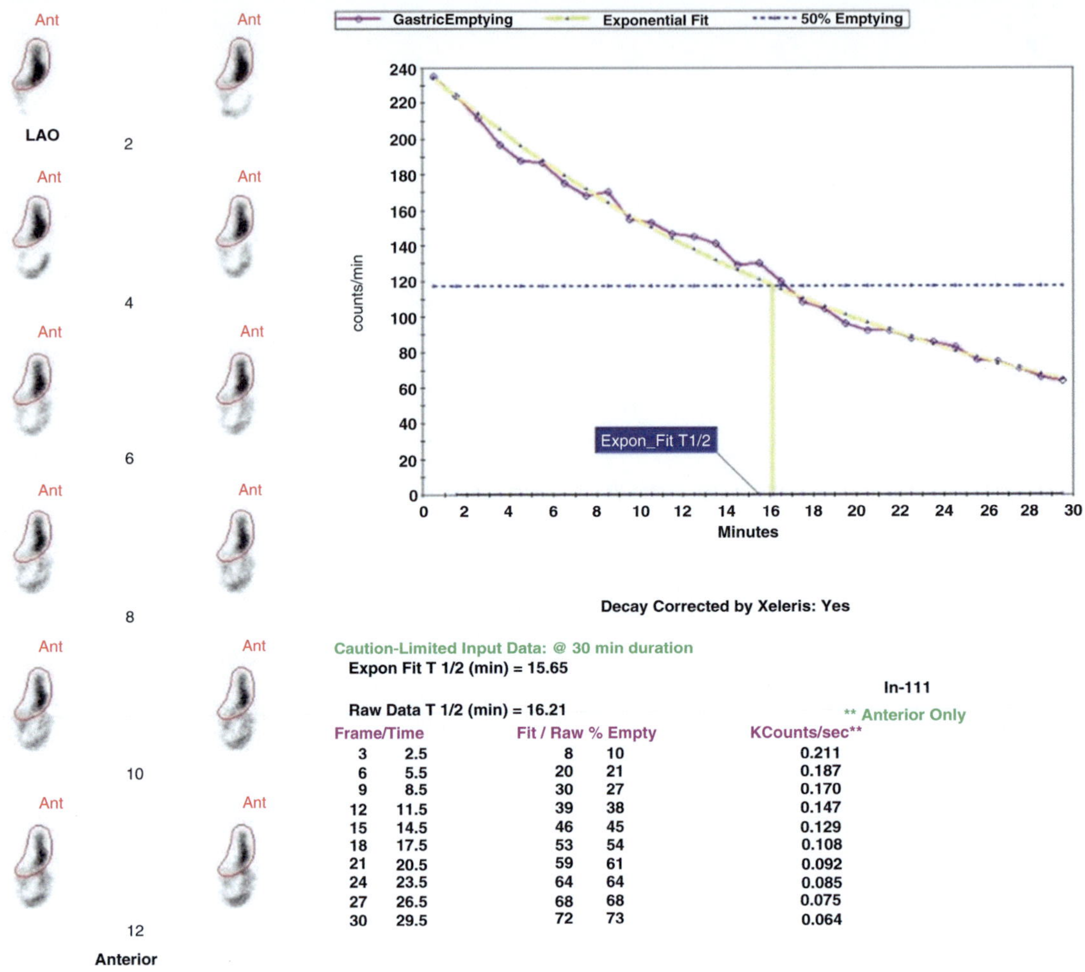

Fig. 9.5 Clear liquid (water) gastric emptying—normal. The study is performed in the LAO projection. Only the first 12 of 30 one-minute imaging frames are shown here. Note that the time-activity curve of the clear liquid emptying has an exponential clearance pattern into the small bowel. The purple curve is the actual raw data; the yellow curve is the fitted exponential data. In this case, they overlap. The halftime of emptying is approximately16 min (normal is less than 25 min)

is no correlation between the results of liquid only or liquid combined with solid, which suggests different pathophysiologies [26]. Tc-99m diethylenetriamine pentaacetic acid (DTPA) is adequate for liquid-only studies, but sequential or simultaneous studies require a medium-energy collimator for the In-111 DTPA liquid radiolabel.

Clear liquids disperse rapidly throughout the stomach and empty uniformly throughout. Thus, a halftime of emptying is a reliable parameter to quantifying the emptying rate. Occasionally, when there is an overlap of intestinal activity with the stomach, a half-emptying time or T-1/2 may suggest an apparent delay. In these cases, the region of interest (ROI) must be modified to eliminate overlapping small bowels from the stomach ROI. Since the stomach usually empties clear liquids at the same rate throughout its volume, it is not critical that some of the stomach is outside of the ROI, and this correction method is very useful. This is in contrast to solids that first localize in the fundus, then move into the antrum,

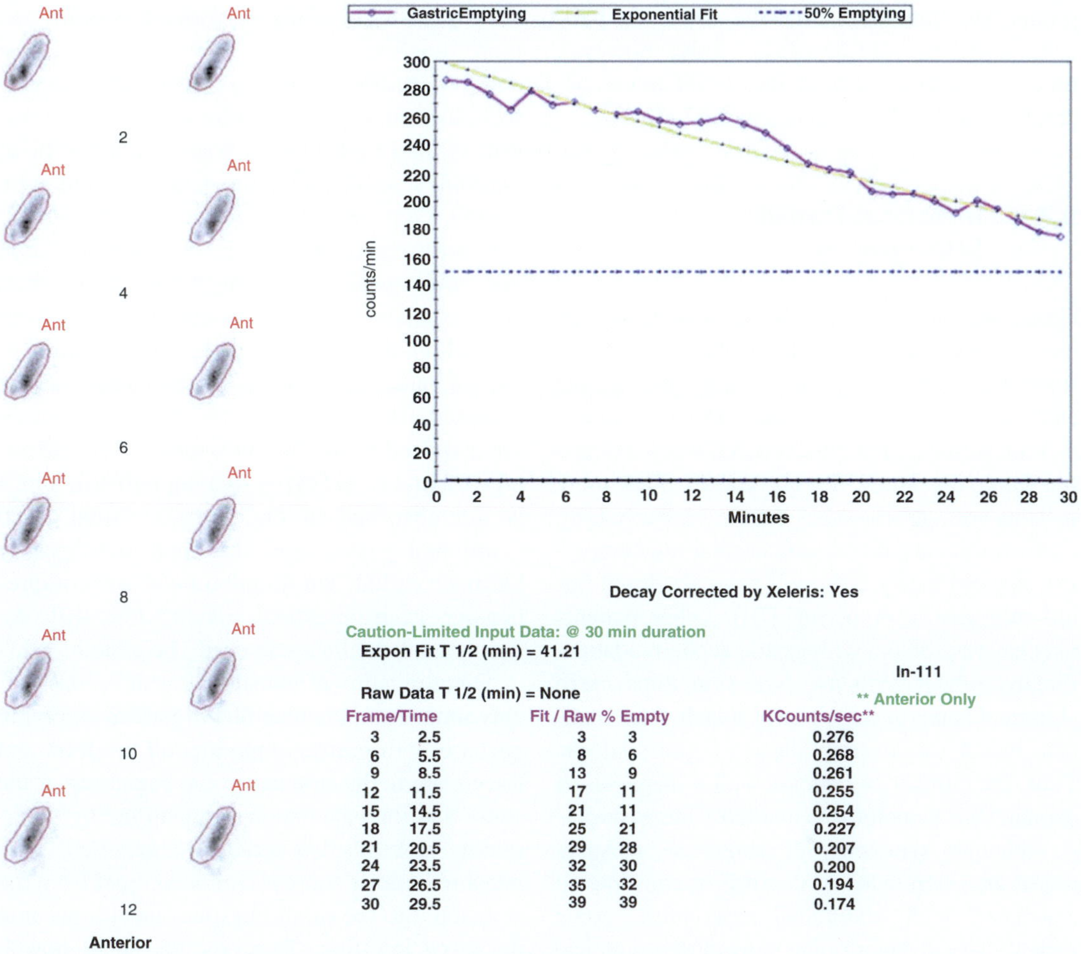

Fig. 9.6 Clear liquid (water) gastric emptying—abnormal, delayed. Halftime with the exponential fitted *T*1/2 is 40 min (normal, <25 min). The raw data did not reach a half-time value

and finally empty through the pylorus. Excluding some of the stomach in solid-meal studies may result in a quantification error when using percent emptying.

9.6 Gastric Accommodation Scintigraphy

Some patients with upper gastrointestinal symptoms have normal gastric emptying but have a problem with gastric accommodation, that is, the stomach does not relax and accommodate an ingested meal, and this results in pain and early satiety. A gastric barostat has been the diagnostic gold standard for this diagnosis, but it is invasive, is poorly tolerated by patients, and is usually reserved for research. Fluid loading protocols have also been used, but patients also do not find this desirable, and they involve more than one methodology. Ultrasonography and magnetic resonance (MR) methods have been published, but they need further validation. An attractive radionuclide alternative is a Tc-99m pertechnetate gastric SPECT study prior to and after ingestion of a meal to determine if the stomach dilates normally by calculating volumes at the two time points. The Mayo clinic has the greatest experience with this radionuclide study; however, other institutions around the world have successfully utilized this technique [27–30].

9.7 Intestinal Transit Scintigraphy

Gastroenterologists have been concerned that only approximately 40% of patients referred with suspected gastroparesis have abnormal gastric emptying studies [31]. This can now be explained, at least partially. The standardized 4-h solid gastric emptying study detects almost 30% more patients with gastroparesis than a 2-h study [18]. Furthermore, in patients with normal solid emptying, approximately 25% will have abnormal liquid-only gastric emptying [24]. Other patients may have a problem with gastric accommodation. Finally, some patients may have symptoms due to abnormal small or large bowel transit abnormalities, which can overlap those of gastroparesis. Thus, the number of patients with a diagnosis to explain their symptoms is markedly increasing.

Although symptoms of abnormal intestinal transit are often those of diarrhea or constipation associated with abdominal discomfort, some patients have symptoms that more closely simulate those of gastric dysmotility, but will have a normal gastric emptying study. Tests often used to evaluate intestinal transit, e.g., the lactulose breath test, radiopaque markers, and the newer wireless motility capsules, are not always reliable, may be expensive, can expose the patient to relatively high radiation, and are not really physiologic, that is, they are not food and the intestinal tract may treat them differently. Radionuclide methods allow for qualitative and quantitative physiologic assessment of food transit through the intestinal tract [32].

Since 1976, publications have described various radionuclide intestinal transit studies; however, the methodologies used have varied considerably [33–38]. There is no standard methodology or generalizable normal values. Many different foods and radiotracers have been used. Regardless, intestinal transit studies are increasingly being performed at more and more nuclear medicine facilities. The most common radionuclide and method used to perform intestinal transit scintigraphy is the ingestion of In-111 DTPA in water, either with or without a solid meal, the latter labeled with Tc-99m, e.g., standardized meal. A convenient and informative method is to combine liquid and solid gastric emptying study with small bowel transit study by extending the study from 4 to 6 h on day 1. If images are also acquired at 24, 48, and 72 h, large bowel transit can be assessed. The small and large intestinal images are acquired in the In-111 window. The advantage of In-111 DTPA is its long half-life and it is not absorbed in the gastrointestinal tract. Combined gastric and intestinal scintigraphy has been called "whole-gut transit" or "comprehensive gastrointestinal transit" [39, 40]. An esophageal swallow can easily be added [39].

Quantification of intestinal transit is considerably more complex than that of gastric emptying because with gastric emptying, all the food and tracers are in the stomach at the beginning of the study and the calculation is quantified by determining how much is retained or emptied. With intestinal transit, there is continual input from the stomach into the small intestines and output into the large intestine. Thus, for the small bowel, indices of transit have been used, such as the time required for 10% of the administered radiotracer to reach the ileocecal valve or the percent that reaches the ileocecal valve at 5 or 6 h (Figs. 9.7 and 9.8). Preliminary data suggest that Tc-99m hepatobiliary iminodiacetic acid (HIDA) can be used to estimate small bowel transit and Ga-67 can be used to quantify large bowel transit [41].

Large bowel transit can be even more challenging because it occurs over days. One needs a radiopharmaceutical that can withstand the acid environment of the stomach and transit through the small intestines to the higher pH environment of the large bowel. Various radiopharmaceuticals have been used, including radiolabeled fiber, cellulose, polystyrene resin, and bran. One method that is not currently FDA approved uses an ingested methacrylate-coated

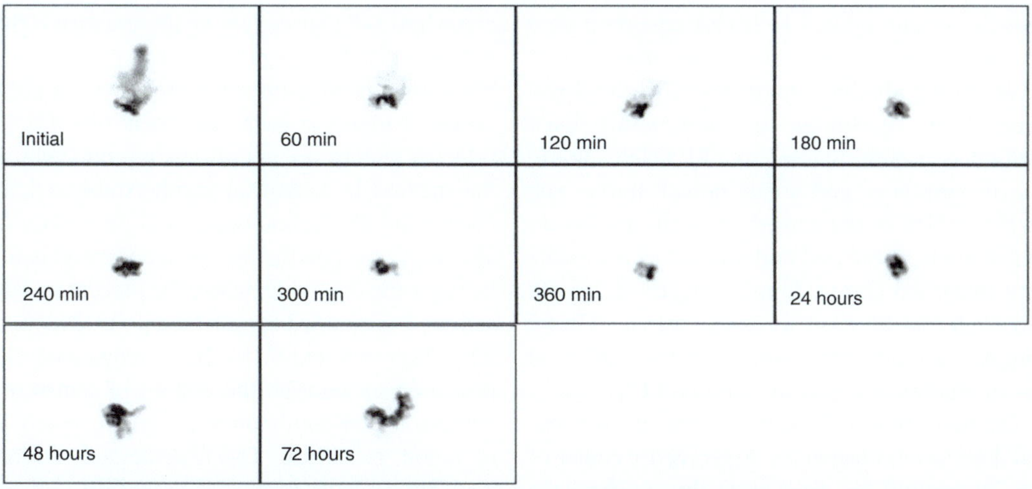

Fig. 9.7 Intestinal transit—normal small intestinal transit, delayed colonic transit. Only the anterior In-111 DTPA images are shown, although posterior views were also acquired and used for the calculation of the geometric mean. The initial image shows the stomach after ingestion of the liquid starting to empty into the small bowel. There is rapid transit through the small intestines (underestimated on these images due to somewhat low-intensity setting). However, most all the activity reaches the region of the ileocecal valve by 300–360 min. A ROI was drawn around all the activity that has reached the ileocecal valve or that has passed distally into the colon at 360 min. In this case, it is normal small bowel transit. However, the activity is still in the region of the ileocecal valve at 24 h (it should be in the transverse colon), is at the hepatic flexure at 48 h (it should be in the descending colon), and is in the transverse colon at 72 h (normally most is cleared at this time point). Colonic transit is very delayed

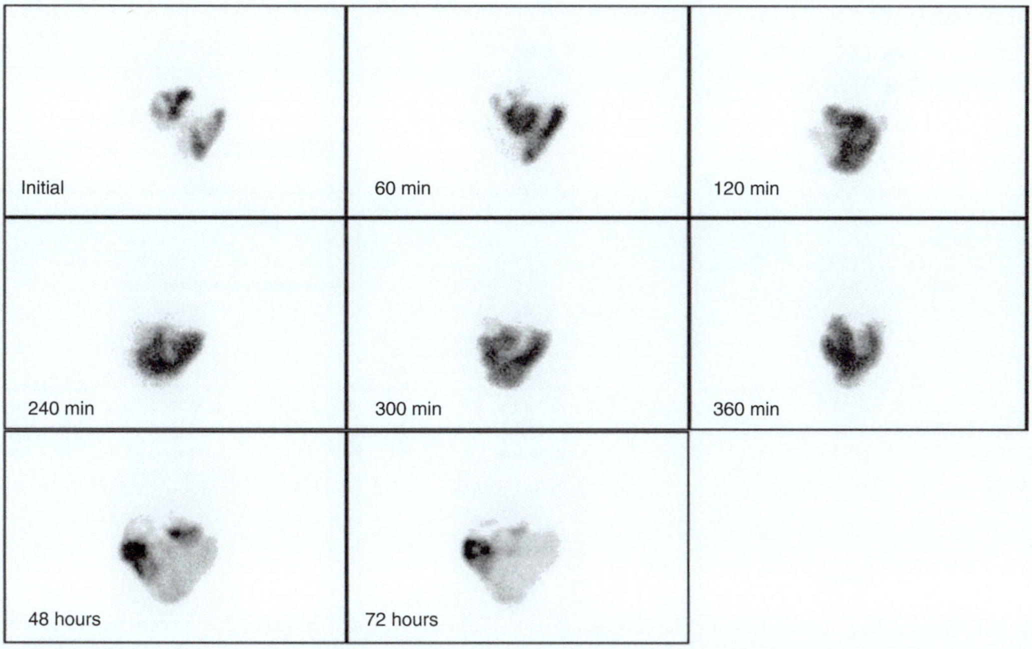

Fig. 9.8 Delayed small and large intestinal transit. The initial and 60-min images show that the In-111 DTPA liquid has mostly rapidly emptied from the stomach and what is left overlaps with the small bowel. On subsequent images, there is very slow transit within the small bowel so that by 360 min, it still has not reached the ileocecal valve, or ascending colon. At 72 h, there is little change. Thus, small intestinal transit is very slow, and large intestinal transit is also very poor. Delayed small bowel transit can impact the apparent transit of the large bowel, making the latter less reliable

capsule containing In-111 DTPA adsorbed onto activated charcoal particles. The coating dissolves in the alkaline environment of the distal ileum [40]. A simpler and commonly used method is a continuation In-111 DTPA liquid gastric emptying and small bowel study. The In-111 DTPA is not absorbed in the intestines and remains stable and undamaged as it transits with intestinal chime. Single images at 24, 48, and 72 h can be used to assess transit. Ga-67 complexes have also been used for intestinal transit studies, but data are limited [42].

Quantification of large bowel transit over several days has its challenges. A geometric center of activity method has been used, by dividing the colon into 5–7 regions, giving increasing weight to the more distal segments of the colon, thus providing a quantitative estimate of the movement of the center of transit at each time point [40, 43]. The selected regions are not always reproducible, and the method is somewhat cumbersome and time consuming for technologists and physicians. An alternative method that has been described is similar to gastric emptying, where the percent transit of activity is quantified at each time point, 24, 48, and 72 h (Figs. 9.9 and 9.10). Here image analysis is also used to describe the pattern of transit, e.g., whether it is primarily proximal colon, mostly distal colon, or diffuse. The two methods correlate well, but the latter is much simpler [39].

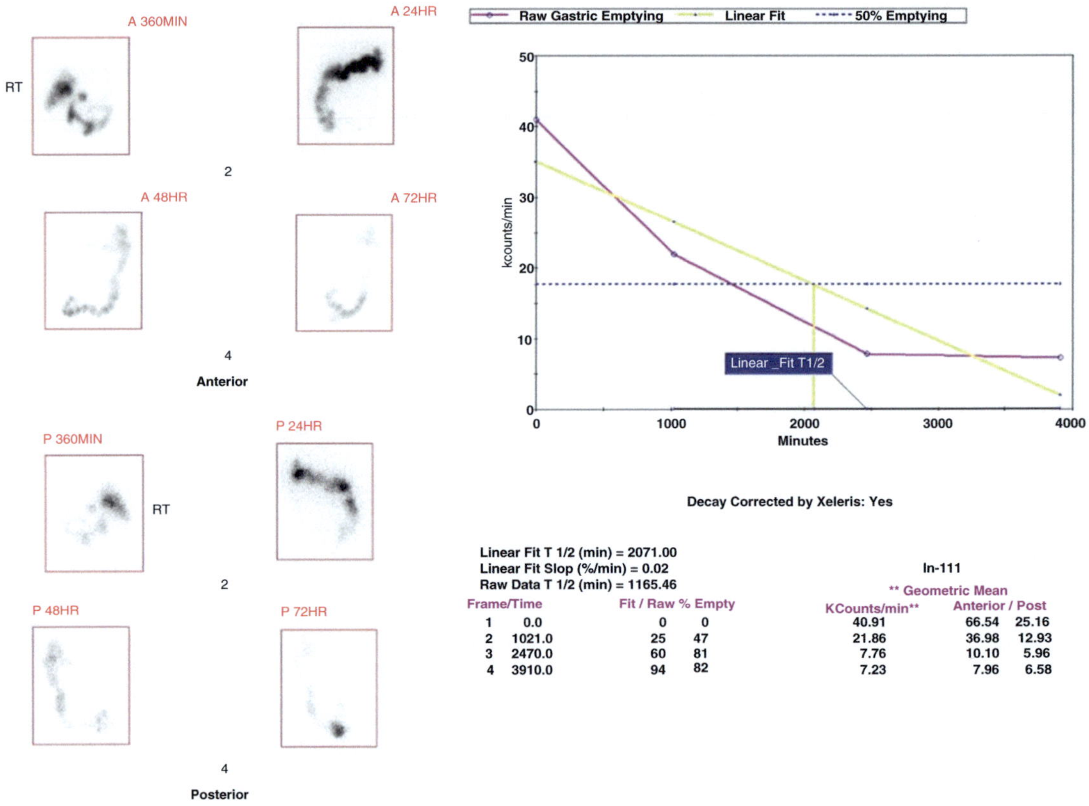

Fig. 9.9 Normal large bowel transit. The processing is shown using modified gastric emptying software. Activity is seen in the transverse colon at 24 h, in the descending colon and rectosigmoid at 48 h, and mostly in the rectosigmoid at 72 h. The calculated percent transit is 47% at 24 h (normal >14%), 81% at 48 h (normal >41%), and 82% (normal >67%) at 72 h. The 360-min image is used as the baseline activity for quantification

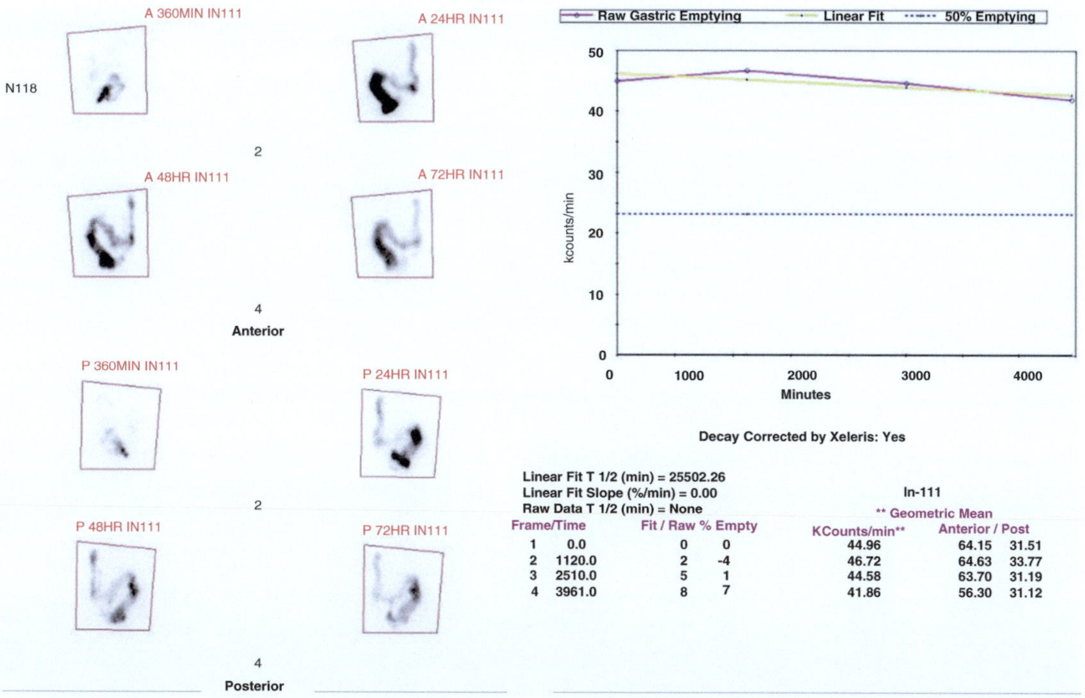

Fig. 9.10 Delayed colonic transit. This study is processed using gastric emptying software. The whole field of view at 360 min (upper left) is used as the denominator for transit. At 24 h (upper right), most of the activity should be in the transverse colon; however, although it has reached the splenic flexure, most resides within the ascending colon. The distribution does not change much over 72 h, although a small amount of activity can be seen in the descending colon. Quantification shows essentially no significant transit. It is hard to fully evaluate the descending colon because most of the activity is still in the proximal colon. Some patients with quantitatively delayed colonic transit will have activity seen throughout, to the descending colon and rectosigmoid. However, it has not significantly left the body

9.8 Esophageal Transit Scintigraphy

Since the early 1970s, esophageal transit studies have been performed in nuclear medicine clinics; however, at most centers today, they are not commonly requested. Gastroenterologists have other diagnostic methods available for evaluating patients with symptoms of painful swallowing (dysphagia), including barium swallow esophagrams, endoscopy, and manometry. The most common etiologies of dysphagia include achalasia, scleroderma, diffuse esophageal spasm, and various other smooth muscle and striated muscle diseases. The nuclear medicine study is most commonly performed today to screen patients with a low suspicion of a motility disorder, to avoid invasive manometry, or to evaluate patient response to therapy [4]. The study is quite straightforward and simple to perform.

As the patient swallows Tc-99m DTPA or Tc-99m sulfur colloid (100–250 μCi) in 5 ml of water, images are acquired in a rapid dynamic mode (0.25–0.5 s per frame). Limited data suggest that semisolid meals may be more sensitive to detect dysmotility (Fig. 9.11) [44]. For a follow-up of achalasia after treatment, a 1-min framing rate is adequate (Fig. 9.12). Supine position eliminates the effect of gravity and thus is more sensitive for the detection of delayed transit. However, for patients with achalasia, gravity is the only emptying mechanism, and thus upright positioning is required. There are various acquisition and quantification variations reported, e.g., the framing rate, the number of swallows, patient's position, and the method of qualitative evaluation

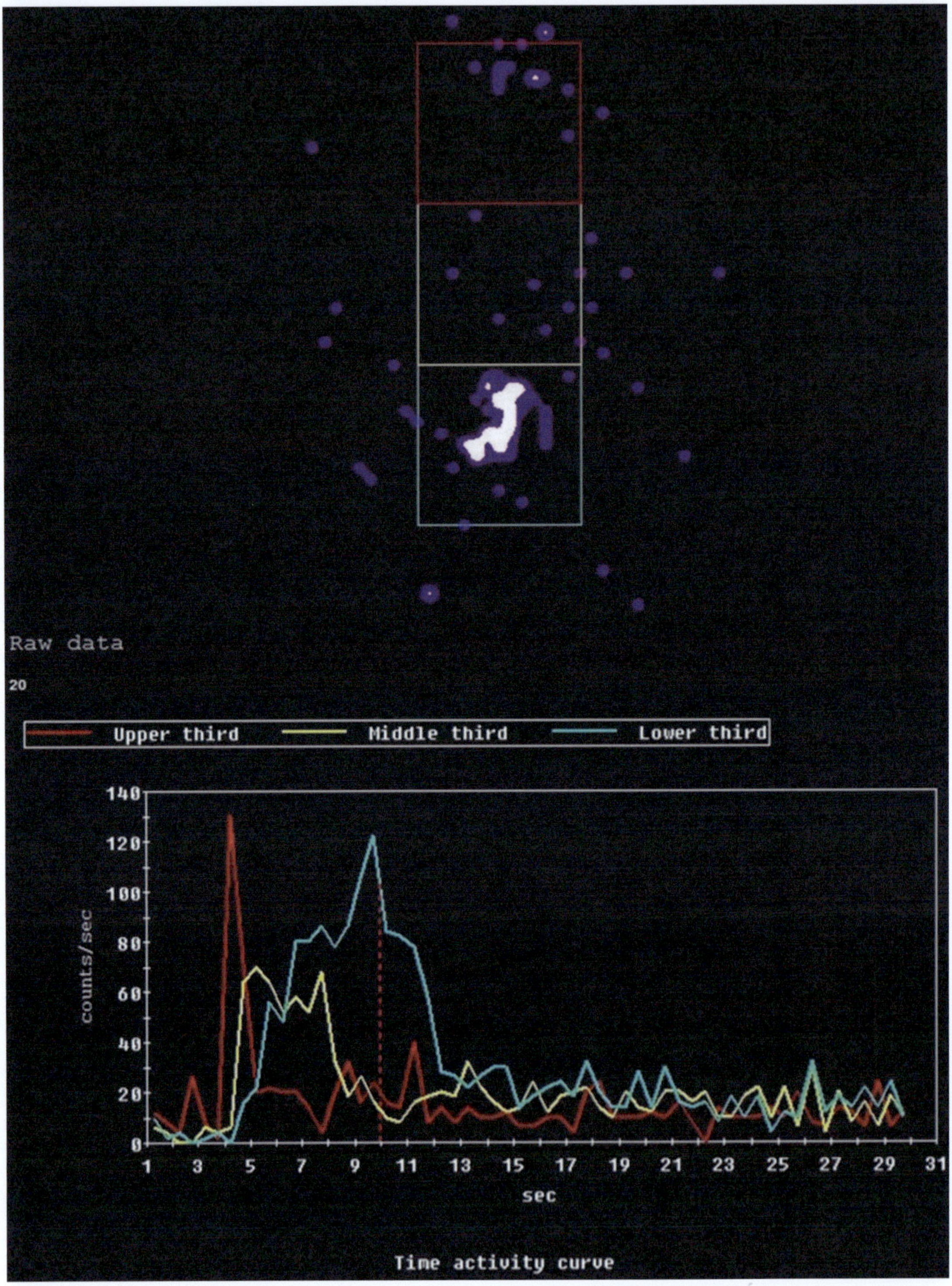

Fig. 9.11 Esophageal transit—In-111 DTPA in 5 cc water swallowed as a bolus. This patient has scleroderma. Transit was slow in the distal esophagus. The lower third ROI shows delayed transit (turquoise ROI). Quantitatively, the percent total esophageal emptying was 60% (normal is greater than a 75% decrease from peak over 10 s)

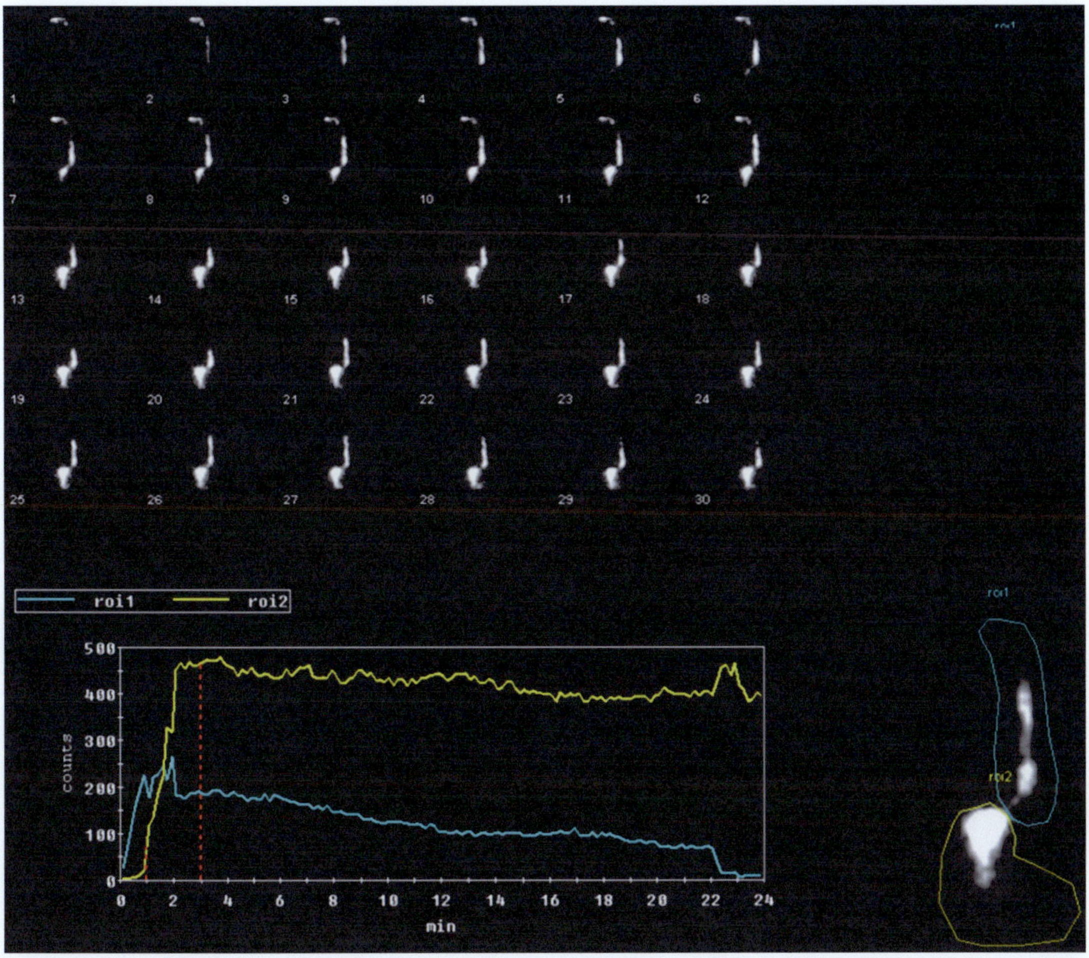

Fig. 9.12 Esophageal transit—semisolid meal of cornflakes and milk. This is a follow-up study (1-min frames) after therapy for achalasia. The study shows that there is still considerable retention in the esophagus (turquoise ROI); however, the meal is getting into the stomach (yellow ROI) over the 30 min

and quantification (transit time, percent emptying) [45–47]. Some studies have shown that up to five swallows are needed to maximize sensitivity [48, 49]. Dry practice swallows are also recommended. The overall accuracy reported has varied but generally is high, particularly for achalasia and scleroderma [50].

The studies are evaluated qualitatively and quantitatively. Watching the bolus swallow dynamically can be informative, but time-activity curves and quantitative data are of definite added value. Typically, three regions of interest are drawn over the esophagus with which to derive time-activity curves. Either a transit time or percent emptying at a designated time is commonly used for the quantification.

9.9 Gastroesophageal Reflux Disease (GERD)

Because there are many tests available to confirm the diagnosis of gastroesophageal reflux, including barium esophagography, endoscopy, the Bernstein acid infusion test, and Tuttle acid reflux test, scintigraphy is not commonly requested for adults; however, at many centers, it is not an uncommon test requested for neonates.

Symptoms of reflux in neonates are quite different than those in adults. For adults, heartburn is the most common symptom with an uncomplicated disease. However, young children often present with respiratory symptoms, iron deficiency anemia, and failure to thrive. Reflux occurs normally in infants, although it usually resolves by 18 months of age. Delayed gastric emptying may exacerbate the symptoms of reflux and make it more difficult to treat.

Scintigraphic "milk" study is a common methodology for neonates and young children, but a variation of this can be used with adults, for example, utilizing orange juice [51, 52]. Children ingest their normal formula feeding or milk. The acquisition framing rate is 5–10 s frames for 60 min (Fig. 9.13). This can be combined with a gastric emptying study with images acquired immediately after ingestion and at 1 and 2 h. Normal gastric emptying is approximately 40–50% at 1 h and 60–75% at 2 h.

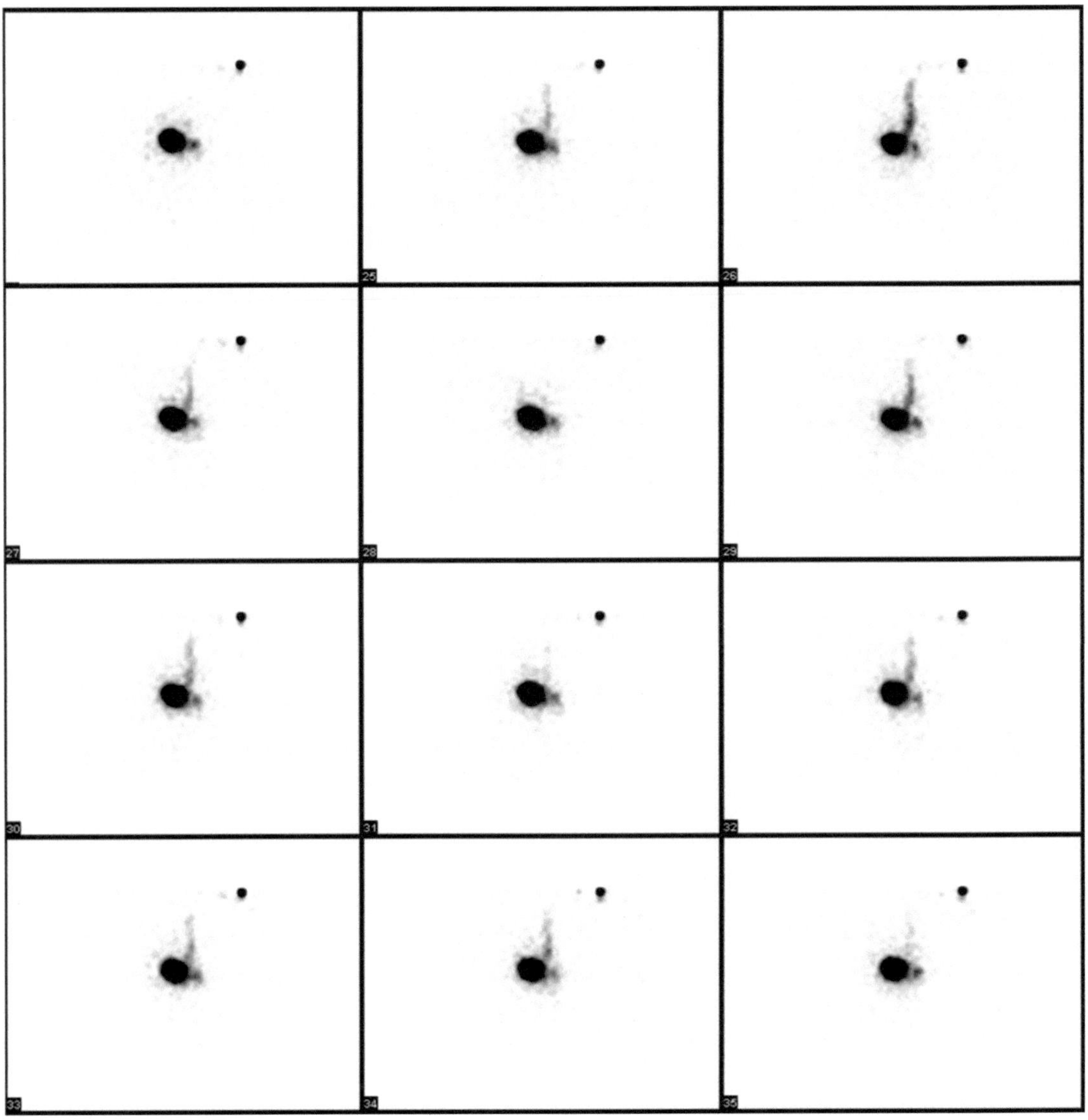

Fig. 9.13 Gastroesophageal reflux. Neonate with symptoms of failure to thrive and anemia. Note recurrent reflux events, some of which are long and high (framing rate 0.5 s/frame). Marker in the left upper corner of each image is at the level of the mouth

Since all neonates have some reflux, the question becomes how much and how frequent is abnormal. The more prolonged, proximal, and frequent the events are, the greater is the likelihood of a clinically significant disease. The milk study is quite sensitive for reflux. However, this study is not very sensitive for aspiration. A "salivagram," which is a variation of an esophageal swallow study, is more sensitive for the diagnosis of aspiration [53].

9.10 Gastrointestinal Bleeding Scintigraphy

Radionuclide gastrointestinal (GI) bleeding studies have a long history of use in nuclear medicine. Although there is some disagreement among clinicians regarding the value of the study, many publications confirm its utility [54]. The fact that many angiographers request this study prior to performing visceral angiography is evidence of its value. A negative radionuclide bleeding test almost invariably predicts a negative angiography. A positive bleeding test significantly increases the likelihood that subsequent angiography will detect the site of bleeding and thus be able to treat the bleeding site.

The purpose of radionuclide study is (1) to determine whether bleeding is active and (2) to localize the approximate origin of the bleed. Computed tomography angiography (CTA) is used as an alternative to radionuclide study at some hospitals because of its superior resolution and more ready availability (weekend and evening radionuclide studies are not available at some institutions). However, CTA has limitations: mainly, bleeding is intermittent, and there is no way to be certain clinically whether the patient is actively bleeding at the time of the procedure and there is only one opportunity for success with CTA. In contrast, GI bleeding study is performed over time, initially 60 or 90 min, and intermittent dynamic imaging is potentially possible for up to 24 h. If positive, the patient should be promptly sent to interventional radiology.

Several methods have been used to radiolabel the patient's red blood cells (RBCs). A simple in vivo method was first described. Stannous pyrophosphate was injected intravenously (IV), then Tc-99m pertechnetate 10 min later. The stannous ion reduces the Tc-99m, allowing it to bind to the beta-globulin chains of hemoglobin. However, the efficiency of RBC labeling is only 75%. The only use for this method today is for patients who cannot have blood infusions for religious reasons. Subsequently, a *modified* in vivo method was described. Stannous pyrophosphate is injected into an IV line. After 15 min, 3–5 mL of blood is withdrawn through the line into a lead-shielded syringe containing Tc-99m pertechnetate and a small amount of anticoagulant. The syringe is left attached during the procedure so that the system is closed. The syringe is agitated gently for about 10 min, then its contents are reinjected into the patient. Labeling efficiency is approximately 85%. This is quite adequate for most bleeding studies. However, both of these methods are susceptible to poor labeling due to therapeutic drug interactions and other factors.

A superior method is now available, the in vitro kit method. The patient's blood is withdrawn into a syringe, then injected into a reaction vial contacting stannous chloride. The stannous ion diffuses across the RBC membrane. Tc-99m pertechnetate is added, also crossing the RBC membrane. The RBC is then reduced by the stannous ion, allowing the Tc-99m pertechnetate to bind to hemoglobin. Sodium hypochlorite is added to oxidize any extracellular stannous ion and thus prevent extracellular reduction of Tc-99m pertechnetate, ensuring only RBC cellular radiolabeling. Binding is >97%. The only downside of this method is that it is more costly than the modified in vivo method.

Strict diagnostic interpretive scintigraphic criteria should be applied to radionuclide study for it to be interpreted as positive. The radiotracer must first appear where there was no activity before, then increase over time, and finally move in a pattern consistent with intestinal anatomy (Figs. 9.14 and 9.15) (Table 9.4). Fixed, nonmoving activity should not be interpreted as an active

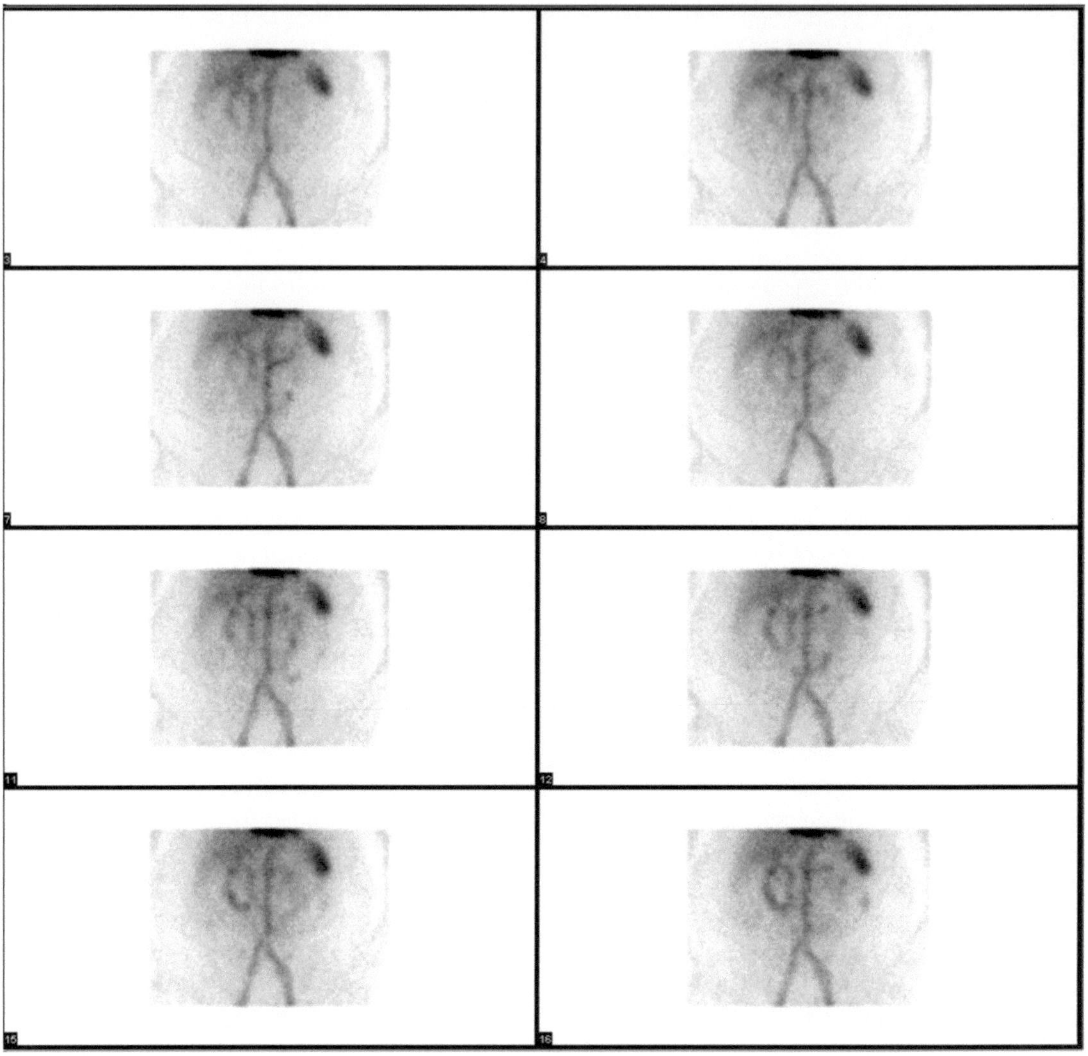

Fig. 9.14 Tc-99m RBC bleeding study—positive in small bowel. The first image shows activity in the duodenal C loop, the origin of the bleed. Subsequent images show progression of bleeding activity moving through the small intestines

bleed. It is likely due to a vascular structure, e.g., cavernous hemangioma, accessory spleen, ectopic kidney, etc. Bleeding can usually be localized to the region of the bowel actively bleeding, whether the cecum, ascending colon, hepatic flexure, transverse or descending colon, sigmoid, or rectum, and from this determine which is the likely vascular supply, e.g., celiac, superior, or inferior mesenteric. A 1-min flow study (1–2 s frames) is often initially performed. It can reveal a suspected site of bleeding by showing increased flow in the absence of active bleeding, as seen with angiodysplasia, A-V malformation, or tumors. Typically, bleeding studies are acquired for 60–90 min (1-min frames). A left lateral or LAO view can help differentiate rectal activity from bladder or genital activity. Although drug interference and other labeling problems can

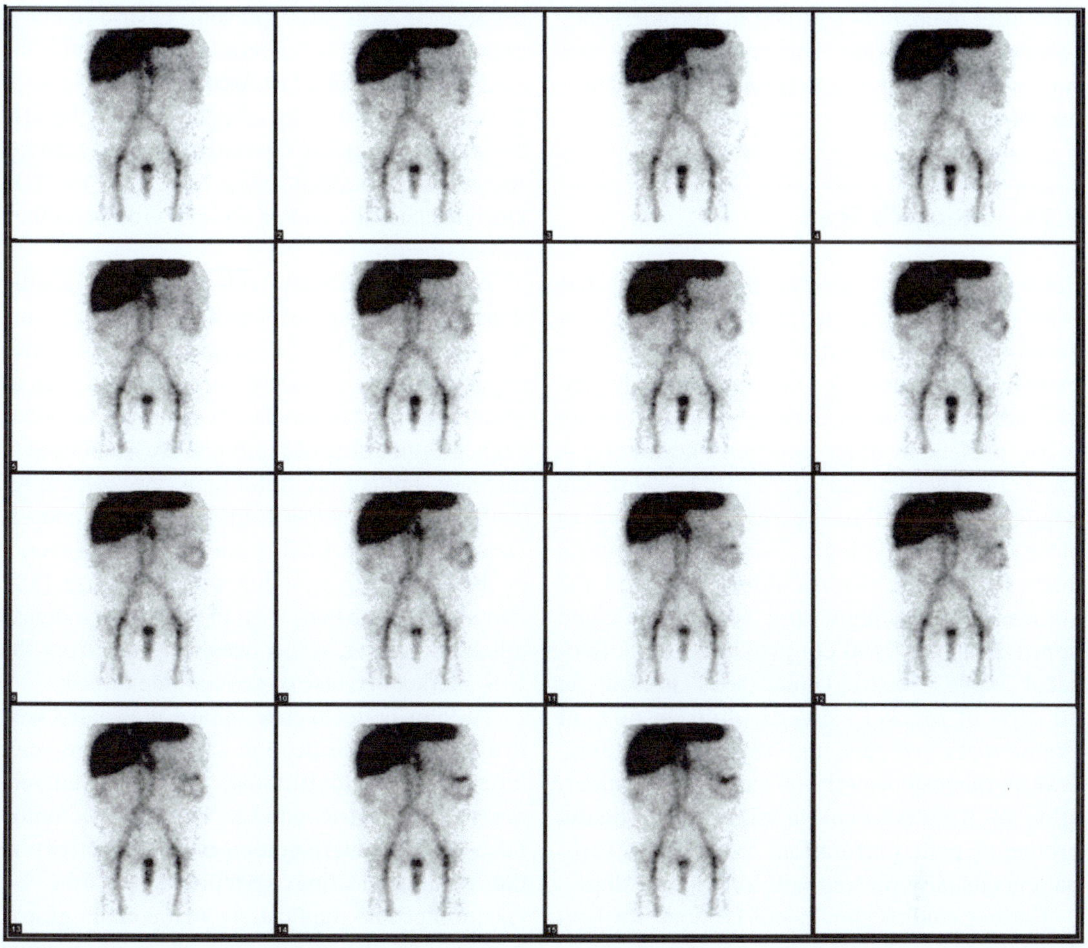

Fig. 9.15 Gastrointestinal bleeding study (Tc-99m RBCs)—large bowel. Increasing focal activity seen in the left upper quadrant and accumulating just distal to the splenic flexure, consistent with active bleed. However, simultanously activity is seen in the right upper quadrant transiting to the transverse colon. This is the actual bleeding site. Activity between the iliac vessels is normal penile blood pool and does not represent a bleeding site

Table 9.4 Diagnostic criteria to determine bleeding site with Tc-99m RBC scintigraphy

Focal activity appears where none was seen initially
Radiotracer activity increases over time
Movement of activity, antegrade or retrograde, conforms to intestinal anatomy

occur when using the in vivo and modified in vivo methods of radiolabeling, this is rarely a problem with the use of the in vitro kit method. Delayed imaging should always be performed in a dynamic mode.

There are potential pitfalls in the diagnosis of active bleeding. One is that of transiting genitourinary tract activity, which can be misinterpreted as GI bleeding. Another is free Tc-99m pertechnetate, which can also be misinterpreted as bleeding. Fixed activity that does not move is not due to bleeding but rather caused by varices, hemangiomas, accessary spleens, etc. Sticking to the criteria described in Table 9.4 is therefore quite important. Bleeding studies should be performed as early as after the patient presents clinically. Studies are more likely to be positive soon after the patient's arrival in the emergency room or on admission. This study is rarely useful for finding a cause of chronic anemia or suspected slow bleed.

9.11 Meckel's Scan

Since the 1970s, Tc-99m pertechnetate has been successfully used for diagnosing a suspected Meckel's diverticulum as a cause of the patient's symptoms. The majority of symptomatic patients are under 2 years of age, although it can present in older children and adults. A Meckel's diverticulum occurs in 1–3% of the population, and it is the result of failure to close the embryologic omphalomesenteric duct. It is a true diverticulum arising on the antimesenteric foregut and typically located approximately 80–90 cm proximal to the ileocecal valve. Gastric mucosa is present in 10–30% of Meckel's diverticulum, in 60% of symptomatic patients, and 98% with bleeding. Gastric mucosal secretions cause peptic ulceration of the diverticulum or adjacent ileum, producing pain, perforation, or bleeding. Thus, patients usually present with rectal bleeding.

Barium studies should not be done for several days prior to scintigraphy because of potential attenuation. Colonoscopy and laxatives should be avoided to prevent artifactual uptake due to irritation. Potassium perchlorate should not be administered to avoid thyroid uptake because it will also prevent gastric mucosa uptake; however, it can be administered after the study. Patients must fast for 4–6 h and void prior to the study. A urinary catheter may be helpful at times to minimize overlap of urinary activity. Images are obtained every 5–10 min for 1 h. Upright, laterals, and/or oblique views can then be obtained.

Although parietal cells were originally thought to be responsible for gastric uptake and the secretion of Tc-99m pertechnetate, evidence suggests that mucin-secreting cells are at least as important. Histamine H2 receptor antagonists such as cimetidine or ranitidine are often used to increase uptake by inhibiting the release of Tc-99m pertechnetate from the gastric mucosa. Data on its clinical utility are limited; however, it is deemed quite safe for short-term use [55]. Pentagastrin has been used in the past to increase uptake; however, it has been removed from the U.S. market because of serious side effects.

Tc-99m pertechnetate uptake is usually seen in a Meckel's diverticulum within 5–10 min after intravenous administration, usually simultaneously with gastric uptake. The most common false positive interpretation is due to activity in the renal collecting system (Fig. 9.16a, b). Gastrointestinal duplications that contain gastric mucosa are also a potential cause of imaging ectopic activity. Inflammatory or obstructive lesions of the intestines and tumors have been reported to cause false positive interpretations. Overall accuracy is high [56, 57].

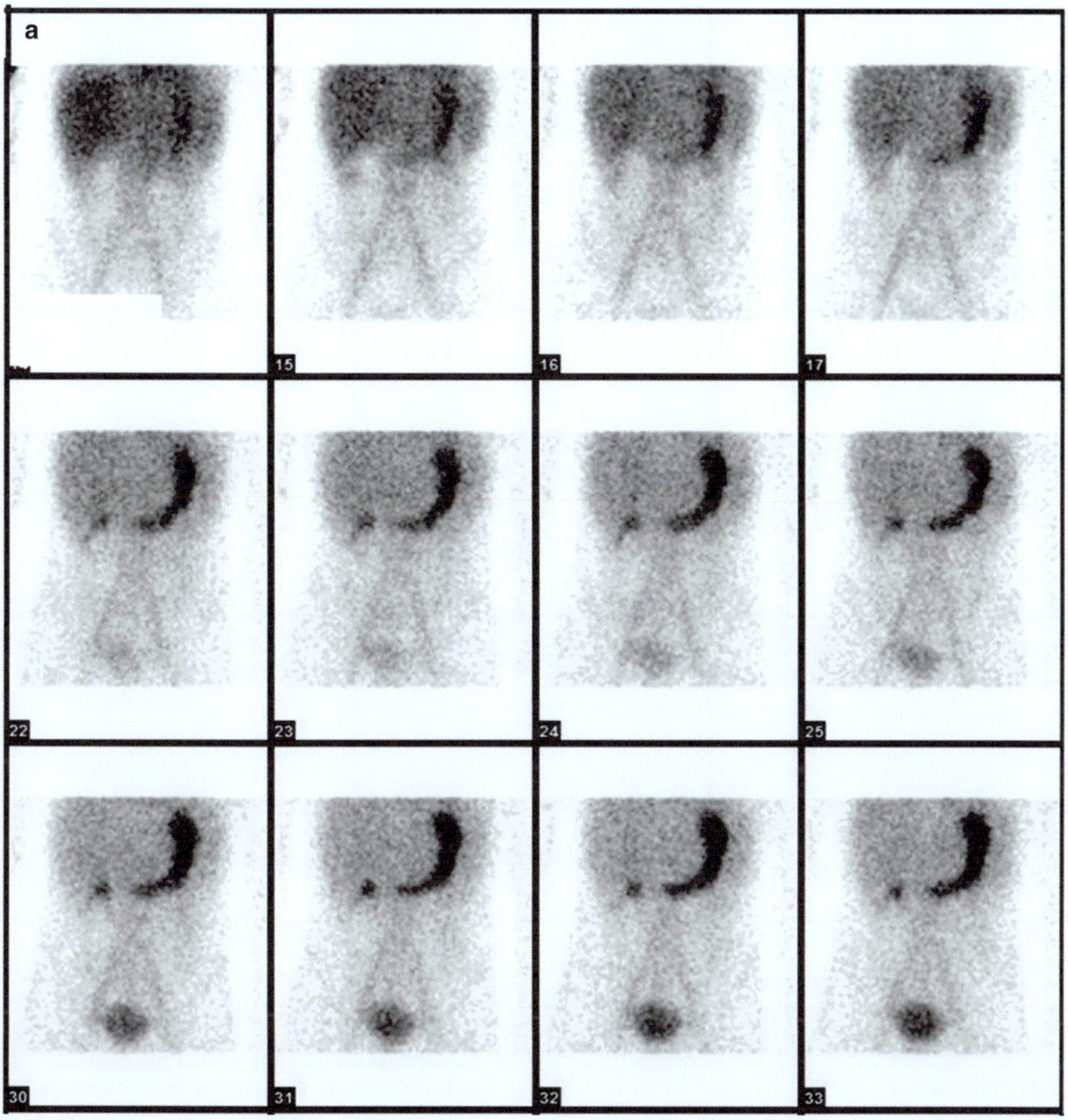

Fig. 9.16 (**a**) Meckel's scan shows that in addition to expected gastric activity, there is focal uptake in the right upper quadrant at the lower margin of the liver. This would be an atypical location for a Meckel's diverticulum, which is usually seen in the right lower quadrant, though the location can vary. (**b**) Renal scan (Tc-99m MAG3) (posterior view) performed the next day shows prominent accumulation in the right renal pelvis, which corresponds to the location of the uptake on the Meckel's scan. Thus this is a false positive Meckel's study

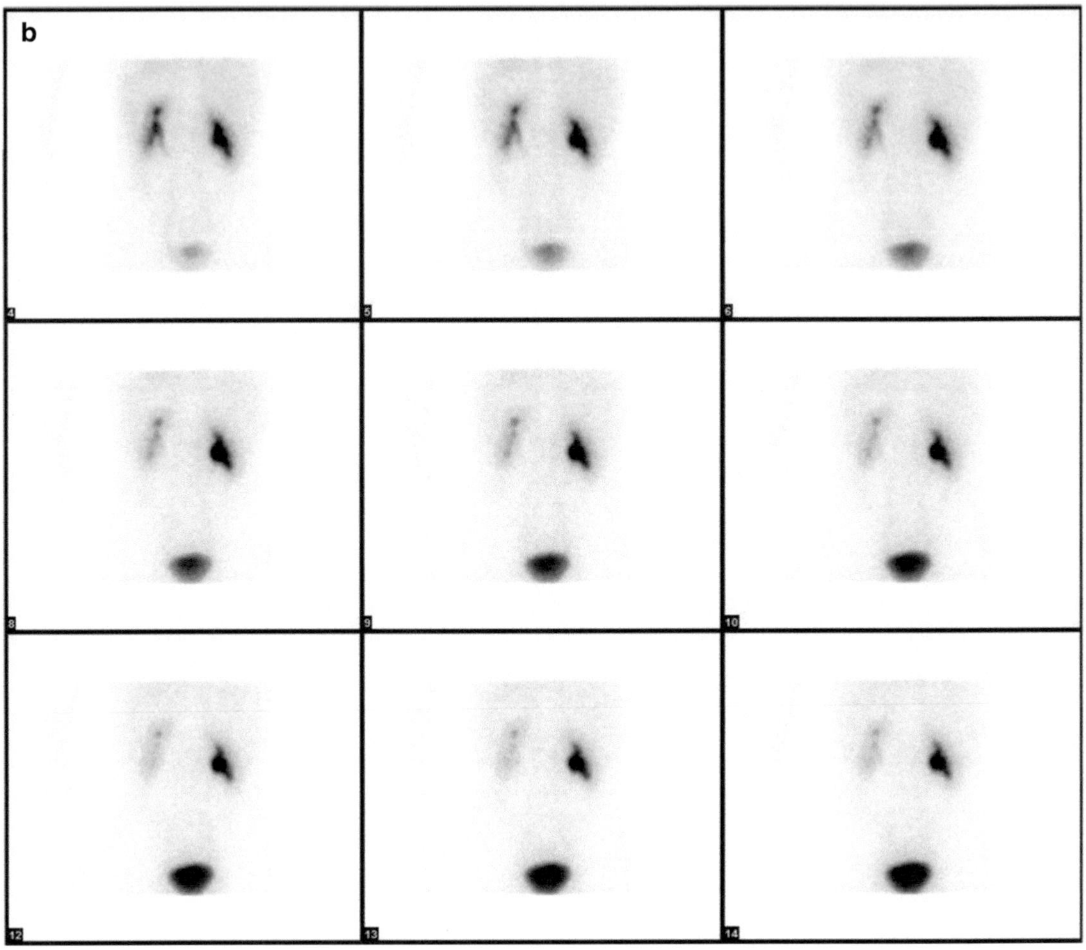

Fig. 9.16 (continued)

References

1. Collins PJ, Horowitz M, Chatterton BE. Attenuation correction and lag period in gastric emptying studies. J Nucl Med. 1986;27:867–8.
2. Ziessman HA, Atkins FB, Vemulakonda US, Tall J, Harkness B, Fahey FH. Lag phase quantification for solid gastric emptying studies. J Nucl Med. 1996;21:602–8.
3. Fisher RS, Parkman H. Current concepts: management of nonulcer dyspepsia. N Engl J Med. 1998;339:1376–81.
4. Parkman HP, Miller MA, Fisher RS. Role of nuclear medicine in evaluating patients with suspected gastrointestinal motility disorders. Semin Nucl Med. 1995;25:289–305.
5. Drossman DA. Functional gastrointestinal disorders: history, pathophysiology, clinical features, and Rome IV. Gastroenterology. 2016;150:1262–79.
6. Ziessman HA, Fahey FH, Collen MJ. Biphasic solid and liquid gastric emptying in normal controls and diabetics using continuous acquisition in the LAO view. Dig Dis Sci. 1992;37:744–50.
7. Griffith GH, Owen GM, Kirkman S, Shields R. Measurement of the rate of gastric emptying using chromium-51. Lancet. 1966;1:1244.
8. Ziessman HA, Fahey FH, Atkins FB, Tall J. Standardization and quantification of radionuclide solid gastric-emptying studies. J Nucl Med. 2004;45:760–4.
9. Abell TL, Camilleri M, Donohoe K, Hasler HL, Lin HC, Maurer AH, McCallum RW, Nowak T, Nusynowitz ML, Parkman HP, Shreve P, Szarka LA, Snape WJ Jr, Ziessman HA. Consensus recommendations for gastric emptying scintigraphy: a joint report of the American Neurogastroenterology and motility society and the Society of Nuclear Medicine. J Nucl Med Technol. 2008;36:44–54.
10. Tougas G, Coates G, Patterson W, Dallaire C, Pare P, Bolvin M, Watier A, Daniels S, Diamant

N. Standardization of a simplified scintigraphic methodology for the assessment of gastric emptying in a multicenter setting. Am J Gastroenterol. 2000;95:78–86.
11. Camilleri M, Zinmeister AR, Greydanus MP, Brown ML, Proano M (1991) Towards a less costly but accurate test of gastric emptying and small bowel transit. Dig Dis Sci. 36(5):609-615.
12. Christian PE, Moore JG, Sorenson JA, Coleman RE, Welch DM. Effects of meal size and correction technique on gastric emptying times. J Nucl Med. 1980;21:883–5.
13. Tothill P, Mclojughlin GP, Hading RC. Techniques and errors in scintigraphic measurements of gastric emptying. J Nucl Med. 1978;19:256–61.
14. Fahey FH, Ziessman HA, Collen MJ, Eggli DF. Left anterior oblique projection and peak-to-scatter ratio for attenuation compensation of gastric emptying studies. J Nucl Med. 1989;30:233–9.
15. Maurer AH, Knight LC, Charkes ND, Vitti RA, Krevsky B, Fisher RS, Siegel JA. Comparison of left anterior oblique and geometric mean gastric emptying. J Nucl Med. 1991;32:2176–80.
16. Guo J-P, Maurer AH, Fisher RS, Parkman HP. Extending gastric emptying scintigraphy from 2 to 4 hours detects more patients with gastroparesis. Dig Dis Sci. 2001;46:24–9.
17. Thomford GM, Camilleri M, Phillips SF, Forstrom LA. Evaluation of an inexpensive screening scintigraphic test of gastric empting. J Nucl Med. 1995;36:93–6.
18. Ziessman HA, Goetze S, Bonta D, Ravich W. Experience with a new standardized 4-hr gastric emptying protocol. J Nucl Med. 2007;48:568–72.
19. Bonta DV, Lee HY, Ziessman HA. Shortening the four-hour gastric emptying protocol. Clin Nucl Med. 2011;36:283–5.
20. Pelletier-Galarneau M, Sogbein OO, Pham X, Hao J, Le J, Strober MD, Middleton ML, Kikut J, Freeman LM, Zuckier LS. Multicenter validation of a shortened gastric-emptying protocol. J Nucl Med. 2015;56:873–6.
21. Nowak TV, Johnson CP, Kableisch JH. Highly variable gastric emptying in patients with insulin dependent diabetes mellitus. Gut. 1995;37:23–9.
22. Sachdeva P, Kantor S, Knight LC, Maurer AH, Fisher RS, Parkman HP. Use of a high caloric liquid meal as an alternative to a solid meal for gastric emptying scintigraphy. Dig Dis Sci. 2013;58:2002–20006.
23. Horowitz M, Maddox A, Wishart J, Harding P, Chatterton B, Shearman D. Relationships between oesophageal transit and solid and liquid gastric emptying in diabetes mellitus. Eur J Nucl Med. 1991;18:229–34.
24. Ziessman HA, Chander A, Ramos A, Wahl RL, Clark JO. The added value of liquid gastric emptying compared to solid emptying alone. J Nucl Med. 2009a;50:726–31.
25. Ziessman HA, Okolo PI, Mullin GE, Chander A. Liquid gastric emptying is often abnormal when solid emptying is normal. J Clin Gastroenterol. 2009b;43:639–43.
26. Ziessman HA. Gastrointestinal transit assessment: role of scintigraphy: where are we now? Where are we going? Curr Treat Options Gastroenterol. 2016;14:452–60.
27. Ang D. Measurement of gastric accommodation: a reappraisal of conventional and emerging modalities. Neurogastroenterol Motil. 2011;23:287–91.
28. Simmonian HP, Maurer AH, Knight LC, Kantor S, Kontos D, Megalooikonomou V, Fisher RS, Parkman HP. Simultaneous assessment of gastric accommodation and emptying studies with liquid and solid meals. J Nucl Med. 2004;45:760–4.
29. Vasavid P, Chalwatanarata T, Gonlachanvit S. The reproducibility of Tc-pertechnetate single photon emission computed tomography (SPECT) for measurement of gastric accommodation in healthy humans: evaluation of the test results performed at the same time and different time of day. J Neurgastroenterol Motil. 2010;16:401–6.
30. Vijayvargiya P, Camilleri M, Shin A, Breen M, Burton D. Simplifying the measurement of gastric accommodation using SPECT. Neurogastroenterol Motil. 2013;25:542–6.
31. Quartero AO, deWit N, Lodder A, Numans ME, Smout AJ, Hoes AW. Disturbed solid-phase gastric emptying in functional dyspepsia: a met-analysis. Dig Dis Sci. 1998;43:2028–33.
32. Maurer AH. Gastrointestinal motility, part 2: small-bowel and colon transit. J Nucl Med. 2015b;56:1395–400.
33. Caride VJ, Prokop E, Troncale FJ, Buddoura W, Winchenbach K, McCallum RW. Scintigraphic determination of small intestinal transit time: comparison with a hydrogen breath test. Gastroenterology. 1984;86:714–20.
34. Carryer PW, Brown MI, Malagelada JR, Carlson GL, McCall JT. Quantification of the fate of dietary fiber in humans by a newly developed radiolabeled fiber marker. Gastroenterology. 1982;82:1389–94.
35. Krevsky B, Malmud LS, D'Ercole F, Maurer AH, Fisher RS. Colonic transit scintigraphy. A physiologic approach to the quantitative measurement of colonic transit in humans. Gastroenterology. 1986;91:1102–12.
36. Nielsen OH, Gjorup T, Christensen FN. Gastric emptying rate and small bowel transit time in patients with irritable bowel syndrome determined with 99mTc-labeled pellets and scintigraphy. Dig Dis Sci. 1986;31:1287–91.
37. Read NW, Al-janabi MN, Holgate AM, Barber DC, Edwards CA. Simultaneous measurement of gastric emptying, small bowel residence and colonic filling of a solid meal by the use of the gamma camera. Gut. 1986;27:300–8.
38. Waller SL. Differential measurement of small and large bowel transit times in constipation and diarrhoea: a new approach. Gut. 1975;16:372–8.

39. Antoniou AJ, Raja S, El-Khouli R, Mena E, Lodge MA, Wahl RL, Clarke JO, Pasricha P, Ziessman HA. Comprehensive radionuclide esophago-gastro-intestinal transit: methodology, normal values, and initial clinical experience. J Nucl Med. 2015;56:721–7.
40. Francois C, Camilleri M, Phillips SF, Thomforde GM, Forstrom LA. Scintigraphy of the whole gut: clinical evaluation of transit disorders. May Clin Proc. 1995;70:113–8.
41. Gryback P, Jacobsson H, Blomquist L, Schnell PO, Hellstrom PM. Scintigraphy of the small intestine: a simplified standard for study of transit with reference to normal values. Eur J Nucl Med Mol Imaging. 2002;29:39–45.
42. Bellen JC, Chatterton B, Penglis S, Tsopelas C. Gallium-67 complexes as radioactive markers to assess gastric and colonic transit. J Nucl Med. 1995;36:513–7.
43. Bonapace ES, Maurer AH, Davidoff S, Krevsky B, Fisher RS, Parkman HP. Whole gut transit scintigraphy in the clinical evaluation of patients with upper and lower gastrointestinal symptoms. Am J Gastroenterol. 2000;95:2838–47.
44. Tatsch K. Multiple swallow test for quantitative and qualitative evaluation of esophageal motility disorders. J Nucl Med. 1991;32:1365–70.
45. Jorgensen F, Hesse B, Tromholt N, Hojgaarde L, Stubgaard M. Esophageal scintigraphy: reproducibility and normal ranges. J Nucl Med. 1992;33:2106–9.
46. Mariani G, Boni G, Barreca M, Bellini M, Bruno F, AlSharif A, Grosso M, Stasi C, Costa F, Anselmino M, Marchi S, Rubello D, Strauss HW. Radionuclide gastroesophageal motor studies. J Nucl Med. 2004;45:1004–28.
47. Maurer AH. Gastrointestinal motility, part 1: esophageal transit and gastric emptying. J Nucl Med. 2015a;56:1229–38.
48. Klein HA, Wald A. Computer analysis of radionuclide esophageal transit studies. J Nucl Med. 1984;25:957–64.
49. Ott DJ, Chen YM, Hewson EG, Richter JE, Dalton CB, Gelfand DW, Wu WC. Esophageal motility: assessment with synchronous video tape fluoroscopy and manometry. Radiology. 1989;173:419–22.
50. Tatsch K, Voderholzer WA, Weiss MJ, Schrottle W, Hahn K. Re-appraisal of quantitative esophageal scintigraphy by optimizing results with ROC analyses. J Nucl Med. 1996;37:1799–805.
51. Heyman S, Kirkpatrick JA, Winter S, Treves S. An improved radionuclide method for the diagnosis of gastroesophageal reflux and aspiration in children (milk scan). Radiology. 1979;131:479–82.
52. Shay SS, Eggli D, Johnson LF. Simultaneous esophageal pH monitoring and scintigraphy during the postprandial period in patients with severe reflux esophagitis. Dig Dis Sci. 1991;36:558–64.
53. Yang J, Codreanu I, Servaes S, Zhuang H. Radionuclide salivagram and gastroesophageal reflux scintigraphy in pediatric patients: targeting different types of pulmonary aspiration. Clin Nucl Med. 2015;40:559–63.
54. Gralnek IM, Neeman Z, Strate LL. Acute lower gastrointestinal bleeding. NEJM. 2017;376:1054–63.
55. Diamond RH, Rothstein RD, Alavi A. The role of cimetidine-enhanced Tc-99m pertechnetate imaging for visualizing Meckel's diverticulum (1991). J Nucl Med. 2011;32:1422–4.
56. Irvine I, Doherty A, Hayes R. Bleeding meckel's diverticulum: a study of the accuracy of pertechnetate scintigraphy as a diagnostic tool. Eur J Radiol. 2017;96:27–30.
57. Sfakianakis GN, Haase GM. Abdominal scintigraphy for ectopic gastric mucosa: a retrospective analysis of 143 studies. AJR Am J Roentgenol. 1982;138:7–12.

10 Nuclear Medicine Imaging Techniques of the Musculoskeletal System

Gopinath Gnanasegaran and Gary Cook

10.1 Introduction

Bone scintigraphy is used as a common screening test for suspected bone metastases because of its high sensitivity, availability, low cost and ability to scan the entire skeleton. Historical data and clinical experience has established bone scintigraphy as the reference standard in the search for skeletal metastatic disease, and many indications have become established for benign skeletal disorders (Table 10.1). Chiewitz and Hevesy first described the use of radionuclides to study the skeleton in 1935 [1] where ^{32}phosphorus (^{32}P) activity was measured in rat organs with a Geiger Muller counter and where uptake of ^{32}P from blood to bone was noted suggesting that skeletal metabolism is a dynamic process. Fleming and colleagues produced the first radionuclide skeletal images in 1961 using ^{85}Sr [2], and this radioisotope was commonly used for bone scanning and the study of skeletal kinetics. Although ^{87m}Sr was introduced as an alternative bone scanning agent with a more suitable gamma ray for imaging of 388 KeV and half-life of 2.8 h, the introduction of ^{18}F-fluoride and then ^{99m}Tc-labeled compounds superseded this. In 1971 Subramanian and McAfee successfully prepared technetium-99m-polyphosphates. However, it was later found that the bone localizing properties were due to pyrophosphate [3, 4]. Since then there have been many developments in both radiopharmaceuticals and scanning techniques to aid evaluation of metastatic bone disease. In recent years technetium-99m (^{99m}Tc)-labeled diphosphonates have become the most widely used radiopharmaceuticals, particularly ^{99m}Tc-methylene diphosphonate (MDP). Improvements in gamma camera design, including the increased availability of tomographic scintigraphy (single photon emission computed tomography, SPECT), have also helped nuclear medicine techniques which provide functional information and maintain their clinical utility in spite of the major advances in cross-sectional anatomical imaging techniques such as computed tomography (CT) and magnetic resonance imaging (MRI). In recent years, there has been increasing interest in the use of positron emission tomography (PET) tracers in the investigation of various aspects of skeletal disease but especially in the diagnosis of bone metastases.

The positron emitting ion, ^{18}F-fluoride, was first described as a scanning agent in 1962 by Blau [5]. Its rapid blood clearance, high skeletal uptake and convenient half-life (~110 min) showed advantages over previous scanning agents. The 511 KeV annihilation photons are

G. Gnanasegaran (✉)
Department of Nuclear Medicine, Royal Free London NHS Foundation Trust, London, UK

G. Cook
Department of Nuclear Medicine and PET, Guys & St. Thomas' NHS Foundation Trust, London, UK
e-mail: Gook@icr.ac.uk

H. Ahmadzadehfar et al. (eds.), *Clinical Nuclear Medicine*,
https://doi.org/10.1007/978-3-030-39457-8_10

Table 10.1 Indications for bone scintigraphy

Oncology (suspected or presence of presence of skeletal disease) 1. Solid tumours (e.g. prostate, breast, lung and renal cancer, etc.) 2. Malignant haematological conditions limited to the bone, e.g. Hodgkin's disease and non-Hodgkin's lymphoma) 3. Bone tumours 4. Soft tissue sarcomas 5. Assessment of therapy response (e.g. $^{223}Ra\text{-}Cl_2$, $^{89}Sr\text{-}Cl_2$, etc.)	*Sports and orthopaedics* 1. Periostitis (e.g. shin splints and thigh splints) 2. Enthesopathies, (e.g. plantar fasciitis, Achilles tendinitis and bursitis) 3. Radiological occult stress-related fractures (e.g. scaphoid, tarsals) or nonspecific symptoms 4. Insufficiency fractures 5. Spondylolisthesis 6. Septic loosening, and synovitis of internal fixation or prosthesis 7. Mechanical complication of internal fixation or prosthesis (hardware complications) 8. Pseudoarthrosis
Rheumatology 1. Chronic inflammatory arthritis (e.g. rheumatoid arthritis, spondyloarthropathies ankylosing spondylitis, psoriatic arthritis, sacroiliitis, etc.) 2. Osteoarthritis of the lumbar facet joints, hip, femorotibial and femoropatellar osteoarthritis 3. Enthesopathies, including plantar fasciitis, Achilles tendinitis and bursitis 4. Avascular/ osteonecrosis (e.g. femoral head, femoral condyle and tibial plateau) and osteonecrosis of the jaw 5. Complex regional pain syndrome type I of the hand, hip, knee and foot 6. Tietze's syndrome (costochondritis) 7. Paget's disease	*Bone and joint infections* 1. Osteomyelitis (e.g. acute, subacute or chronic) 2. Septic arthritis 3. Spondylodiscitis or spondylitis 4. Prosthetic infection and hardware complications 5. Malignant (necrotizing) external otitis
Metabolic bone disease 1. Primary and secondary hyperparathyroidism 2. Osteomalacia 3. Renal osteodystrophy 4. Vitamin D deficiency	*Paediatrics* 1. Osteochondritis of the hip (Legg-Calvé-Perthes disease) 2. Transient synovitis of the hip 3. Battered child syndrome 4. Mandibular condylar hyperplasia 5. Bone infarction (e.g. sickle cell disease, thalassaemia)
Exploration of unexplained symptoms Subacute or chronic musculoskeletal or bone pain localized or multifocal bone pain and backache Unexplained bone pain (to localize pain generator)	*Pretreatment assessment and monitoring* 1. Evaluation of active synovitis prior to radiation synovectomy 2. Evaluation of metabolic activity within facet joints before infiltration with corticosteroids 3. Evaluation of osteoblast activity (Paget's disease before treatment with bisphosphonate) 4. Assessment of vertebral compression fractures (prior to vertebroplasty or kyphoplasty)

Adapted from Van den Wyngaert T et al. 2016, EANM Bone Scintigraphy Guidelines – Eur J Nucl Med Mol Imaging (2016) 43:1723–1738

not ideal for conventional gamma cameras which are optimized for ^{99m}Tc (140 keV), and although the use of ^{99m}Tc bone seeking agents has taken over in the last two decades, ^{18}F-fluoride was an important bone-scanning agent in the early days of clinical nuclear medicine. Recently both ^{18}F-fluorodeoxyglucose (^{18}FDG), as a tumour-specific tracer, and ^{18}F-fluoride ion, as a non-specific bone tracer, have been assessed and early results suggest that both agents may have a role to play in clinical management of patients.

10.2 Radiopharmaceuticals and Mechanisms of Uptake

Initially ^{99m}Tc polyphosphates and pyrophosphates were employed, but subsequently diphosphonates such as hydroxyethylidene diphosphonate (HEDP) and methylene diphosphonate (MDP) were introduced [4, 6]. Uptake of diphosphonates depends on local blood flow, osteoblastic activity and extraction efficiency. The actual mechanism of uptake is still not fully understood, but diphosphonates are probably incorporated into the hydroxyapatite crystal on the bone surface. ^{99m}Tc-Methylene diphosphonate (MDP) is the most widely used bone agent, giving optimal contrast between normal and diseased bone, but similar, alternative ^{99m}Tc diphosphonate tracers exist [7]. Excretion of ^{99m}Tc-MDP is primarily renal, and 70% of the administered dose is eliminated by 6 h.

Other single photon radiopharmaceuticals have been used in the assessment of both primary and metastatic bone tumours and are most commonly non-specific tumour agents rather than acting as bone tracers [8, 9]. Thallium-201 (^{201}Tl), an analogue of potassium, enters tumour cells via the Na^+/K^+ ATPase pump but as well as reflecting the metabolic status of the cell, uptake also depends on blood flow. ^{99m}Tc-labeled sestamibi shows a similar distribution to ^{201}Tl, but has a different mechanism of accumulation and is thought to reflect cell viability being mainly associated with mitochondria intracellularly. ^{99m}Tc-pentavalent dimercaptosuccinic acid (^{99m}Tc(V) DMSA) uptake has also been described in bone metastases, the exact mechanism of uptake being uncertain [10]. However, compared to the diphosphonates and tumour-specific tracers, these are rarely used in clinical practice to specifically evaluate the skeleton.

Positron emission tomography (PET) tracers that are currently available and have potential roles for assessing skeletal metastases include ^{18}F-sodium fluoride ion (18F-NaF) and fluorine-18-labeled deoxyglucose (^{18}F-FDG). The mechanism of uptake of ^{18}F-fluoride is similar to other bone tracers used in nuclear medicine and depends on both regional blood flow and osteoblastic activity. It is preferentially deposited at sites of high bone turnover and remodelling by chemisorption onto bone surfaces, exchanging with hydroxyl groups in hydroxyapatite crystal of bone to form fluoroapatite [11].

As tumour uptake of ^{18}FDG depends on glycolysis and membrane glucose transporters, both of which are known to be increased in malignant tissue [12, 13], the mechanism of uptake and hence the information available from this tracer in the skeleton, are significantly different to ^{18}F-fluoride. The uptake of ^{18}FDG is relatively tumour specific but obviously not restricted to tumour involving the skeleton and has the advantage of demonstrating all metastatic sites in a cancer patient, whether they are in soft tissue or bone.

In addition to non-specific skeletal tracers, there are a number of radiopharmaceuticals, which exist for specific types, or groups of tumours and which in addition to evaluating soft tissue metastases can be helpful in assessing the skeleton. Examples include iodine-131 (^{131}I) for differentiated thyroid cancer metastases (see also Chap. 29), ^{123}I or ^{131}I-metaiodobenzylguanidine (mIBG) (see also Chap. 34), ^{111}In-pentetreotide and ^{68}Ga-DOTATATE for neuroendocrine tumours (see also Chap. 13) and ^{68}Ga or ^{18}F-prostate specific membrane antigen (PSMA) and ^{18}F-fluciclovine for prostate cancer (see also Chap. 26).

10.3 Scintigraphy Techniques

In practice bone scans with diphosphonates are obtained between 2 and 4 h after injection (and with ^{18}F-NaF at 1–2 h), but if renal function is significantly impaired (without concomitant renal osteodystrophy and associated skeletal remodeling), then scans may be performed at a later time to allow further clearance of ECF and vascular activity. Although in the past, many ^{99m}Tc-MDP bone scans have been acquired as multiple overlapping spot views of the skeleton, modern dual-headed gamma cameras allow high-resolution, whole-body images of the entire skeleton in a short acquisition time, including both anterior and posterior images. Most modern gamma camera systems also have the ability to acquire additional tomographic images (single photon emission computed tomography, SPECT), allowing an increased sensitivity for lesion detection because of the resultant improvement in contrast compared to planar imaging and a better three-dimensional localization of abnormalities, which aids specificity. It has been suggested that SPECT imaging not only increases sensitivity in the detection of vertebral metastases in cancer patients but by being able to examine the pattern and position of lesions tomographically that it may be possible to improve differentiation between metastases and coincidental benign lesion [14, 15]. A three-phase bone scan is primarily used to evaluate patients with suspected bone infections. Phase 1 involves intravenous (IV) injection of a radiolabeled tracer and short sequential imaging of the blood flow at the region of concern or interest. In the second phase (2–5 min postinjection), an image of the blood pool is obtained followed by the third phase, which includes delayed skeletal images 3 or 4 h later of the specific area (Tables 10.2 and 10.3). In general, for ^{99m}Tc-bisphosphonates bone scintigraphy, the average administered activity is approximately 500 MBq (300–740 MBq, 8–20 mCi) in adults. The administered activity usually ranges between 8 and 10 MBq/kg in adult patients, and use of increased activity is suggested in obese patients and might be increased to 11–13 MBq/kg [17]. The administered activity in children are based according to the factors recommended by the EANM/SNMMI Paediatric Dosage Harmonization Working Group, and the EANM recommends a baseline activity of 35 MBq for ^{99m}Tc-bisphosphonates (with a minimum activity of 40 MBq) [18, 19].

Table 10.2 Common Types of bone scintigraphy

Three-phase bone scan	Phase 1: blood flow/vascular images (as the radiopharmaceutical is injected) Phase 2: immediate blood pool/ soft-tissue images (within 10 min after injection of the tracer) Phase 3: delayed bone images (acquired 2–4 h after injection)
Two-phase bone scan	Phase 1: Immediate blood pool/ soft-tissue images (within 10 min after injection of the tracer) Phase 2: Delayed bone images (usually acquired 2–4 h after injection)
Four-phase bone scan (rare)	Phase 1: Blood flow/vascular images (as the radiopharmaceutical is injected) Phase 2: Immediate blood pool/ soft-tissue images (within 10 min after injection of the tracer) Phase 3: Delayed bone images (acquired 2–4 h after injection) Phase 4: Acquired after an additional delay up to 24 h later
Whole-body planar bone scan	Planar anterior and posterior static images of the skeleton
Limited planar imaging (spot view imaging)	Additional views after whole-body imaging or as initial imaging over a specific area of interest
SPECT imaging	Delayed tomographic images of a portion of the skeleton or specific region of interest
SPECT-CT (SPECT imaging with integrated CT)	Delayed SPECT-CT (tomographic images of specific region of interest)
PET-CT	Whole body bone PET-CT with 18F-NaF (acquired 1–2 h postinjection)

Bartel TB, Kuruva M, Gnanasegaran G et al. SNMMI Procedure Standard for Bone Scintigraphy 4.0. J Nucl Med Technol. 2018;46(4):398–404 [16]

PET imaging depends on the detection of two coincident 511 keV gamma rays, which are emitted at 180° from one another following the annihilation of a positron (a positively charged, antimatter equivalent of an electron from an unstable nucleus). The synchronous detection of the two photons allows accurate placement of the point of emission and with standard image reconstruction algorithms, tomographic images can be acquired and displayed. There are a number of advantages over conventional nuclear medicine techniques. PET shows higher spatial resolution and accurate, absolute quantitation, the latter because of the ability to accurately correct for the effects of attenuation of photons within the body. The dual-imaging modality PET/CT is a relatively new investigation method that has not been extensively studied in the context of the skeleton. ^{18}F-Sodium fluoride is a specific PET bone tracer which is injected intravenously and the administered activ-

Table 10.3 Planar and SPECT bone scintigraphy acquisition

Protocol	Image acquisition
Phase 1 images	30–60 images at 1–3 s/frame Blood flow images may be obtained in a 64 × 64 or greater matrix (digital images)
Phase 2 images	3–5 min/image immediately after the flow phase and within 10 min after injection Usually obtained in a 128 × 128 or greater matrix Count density of approximately 300,000 counts per image (150,000–200,000 counts per image may be adequate for the extremities)
Phase 3 images	Routine delayed images are usually obtained from 2 to 4 h after injection Whole-body scanning: More than 1.5 million total counts Anterior and posterior views are usually obtained in a 256 × 1024 or greater matrix
Spot views Common: Anterior, posterior lateral, oblique or tangential views special views: Frog-leg views of the hips or sitting-on-detector [caudal] views of the pelvis	The recommended counts per region are: 500,000–one million for the thorax and abdomen 250,000–400,000 for the skull and large joints 150,000–250,000 for distal extremities More counts should be obtained when the field of view is larger 128 × 128 or 256 × 256 matrix can be used
Pelvic views (technically difficult to interpret when there is overlying bladder activity)	Images repeated immediately post voiding (sitting-on-detector/caudal or oblique images, lateral images) 24-h delayed images After bladder catheterization (very rare)
SPECT Corrections are made for attenuation, scatter and resolution recovery	Dual-head gamma camera: 180° detector head orientation, a 360° circular orbit, 60–120 stops, a 64 × 64 or greater matrix and 10–40 s/stop Three-dimensional iterative ordered-subsets expectation maximization (OSEM) is the typical reconstruction algorithm (3–5 iterations and 8–10 subsets) Post-processing usually includes application of a Gaussian filter (width at half maximum, 4–10 mm) or a Butterworth filter (conventional parameters of 10.0.5)

Bartel TB, Kuruva M, Gnanasegaran G et al. SNMMI Procedure Standard for Bone Scintigraphy 4.0. J Nucl Med Technol. 2018;46(4):398–404 [16]

ity for adults is in the range of 185–370 MBq (5–10 mCi), and use of higher activity (370 MBq [10 mCi]) is suggested in obese patients. In children, the injected activity should be weight-based (2.22 MBq/kg [0.06 mCi/kg]), using a range of 18.5–185 MBq (0.5–5 mCi) [20].

10.4 Scintigraphic Patterns, Variants and Artefacts

A normal bone scan will show higher activity concentration in the parts of the skeleton predominated by trabecular bone, e.g. spine, compared to the shafts of long bones that are predominantly cortical bone. Urinary bladder activity, renal activity and minimal soft tissue activity are also normally present (Fig. 10.1). To obtain optimum contrast in all areas of the skeleton, this variation in activity may necessitate viewing images at different intensity settings to optimize contrast at different skeletal sites. Although uptake of labeled diphosphonate on a bone scan is not specific for metastases, by studying the pattern and distribution of lesions, it is often possible to infer the aetiology of abnormalities without requiring further correlative imaging, although a number of cases will remain problematic.

The majority of bone metastases are distributed irregularly in the axial skeleton and ribs, and

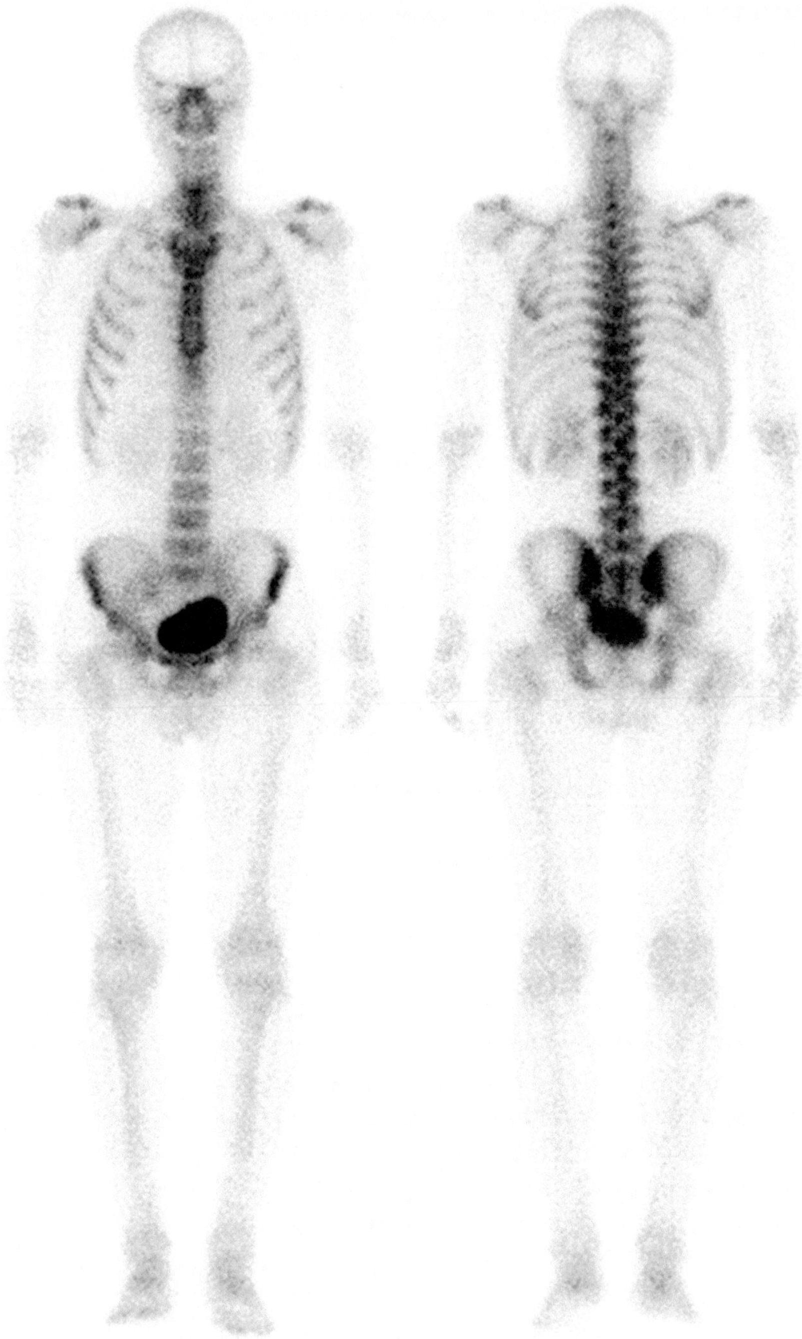

Fig. 10.1 Normal whole-body 99mTc-MDP bone scan showing symmetrical distribution of tracer throughout the skeleton. Urinary bladder activity, renal activity, is also normally observed

there is seldom any confusion in this situation. A small proportion (<10%) affect the appendicular skeleton, and this is most commonly seen in clinical practice in carcinoma of the lung, prostate and breast [21]. An unexpected finding from scanning the peripheries, particularly in patients with bronchogenic carcinoma, may be the observation of hypertrophic pulmonary osteoarthropathy (HPOA) (Fig. 10.2). This typically appears as symmetrical increased uptake of tracer in the cortices ('tram lines'), generally seen in the femora and tibiae.

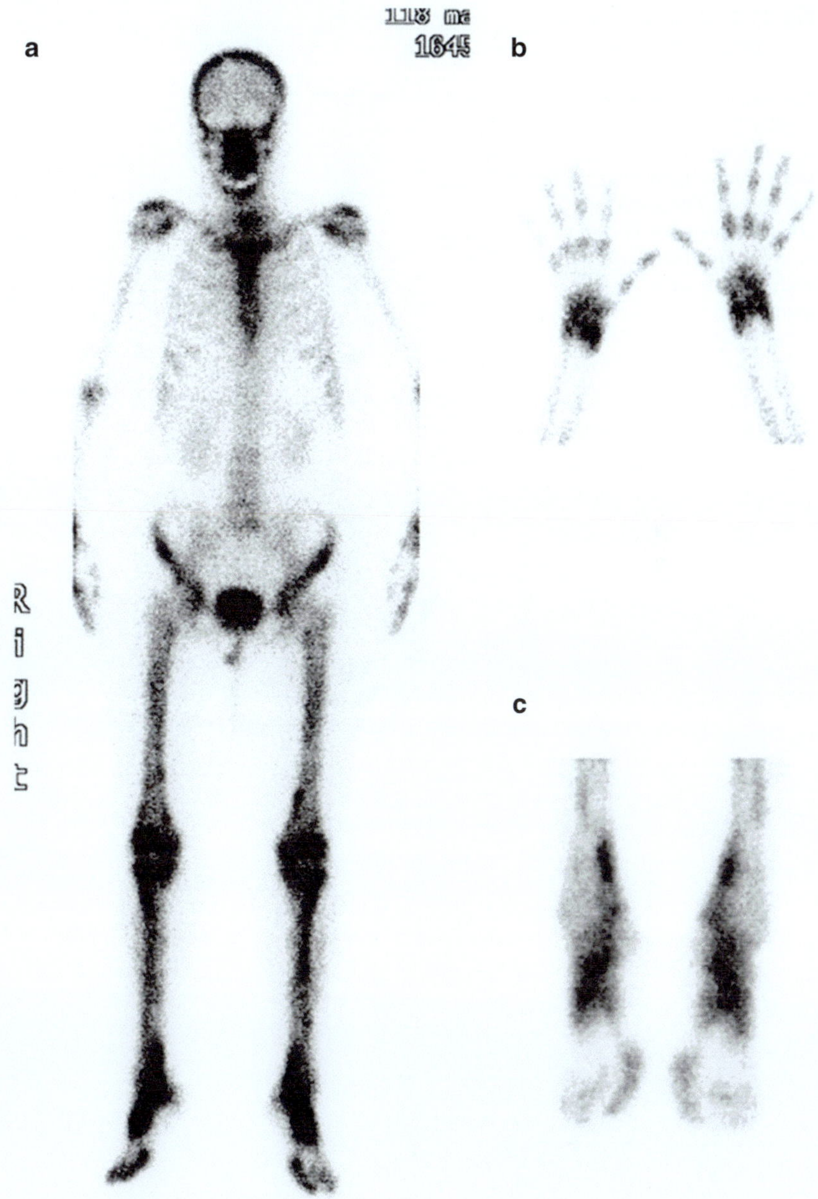

Fig. 10.2 Hypertrophic pulmonary osteoarthropathy (HPOA). Characteristic pericortical uptake involving the long bones of the lower limbs

Rarely, when bone metastases are very extensive, a bone scan on first inspection may appear normal due to the confluent nature of the lesions. However, the superscan, so-called because of the apparent good quality of the scan due to diffusely increased skeletal uptake, has a number of distinguishing features (Fig. 10.3). In addition to the apparent high quality of the scan, the soft tissues, particularly the kidneys, may be inconspicuous or invisible due to the increased ratio between skeletal and soft tissue accumulation. Metabolic bone diseases may also cause a superscan, but that caused by malignancy may be differentiated on close inspection where some irregularity of uptake and indeed more focal abnormality is usually visible. This is more apparent in the ribs or the ends of the long bones.

To increase the specificity of bone scan interpretation, it is necessary to have knowledge of normal variants, which may mimic metastases, and of

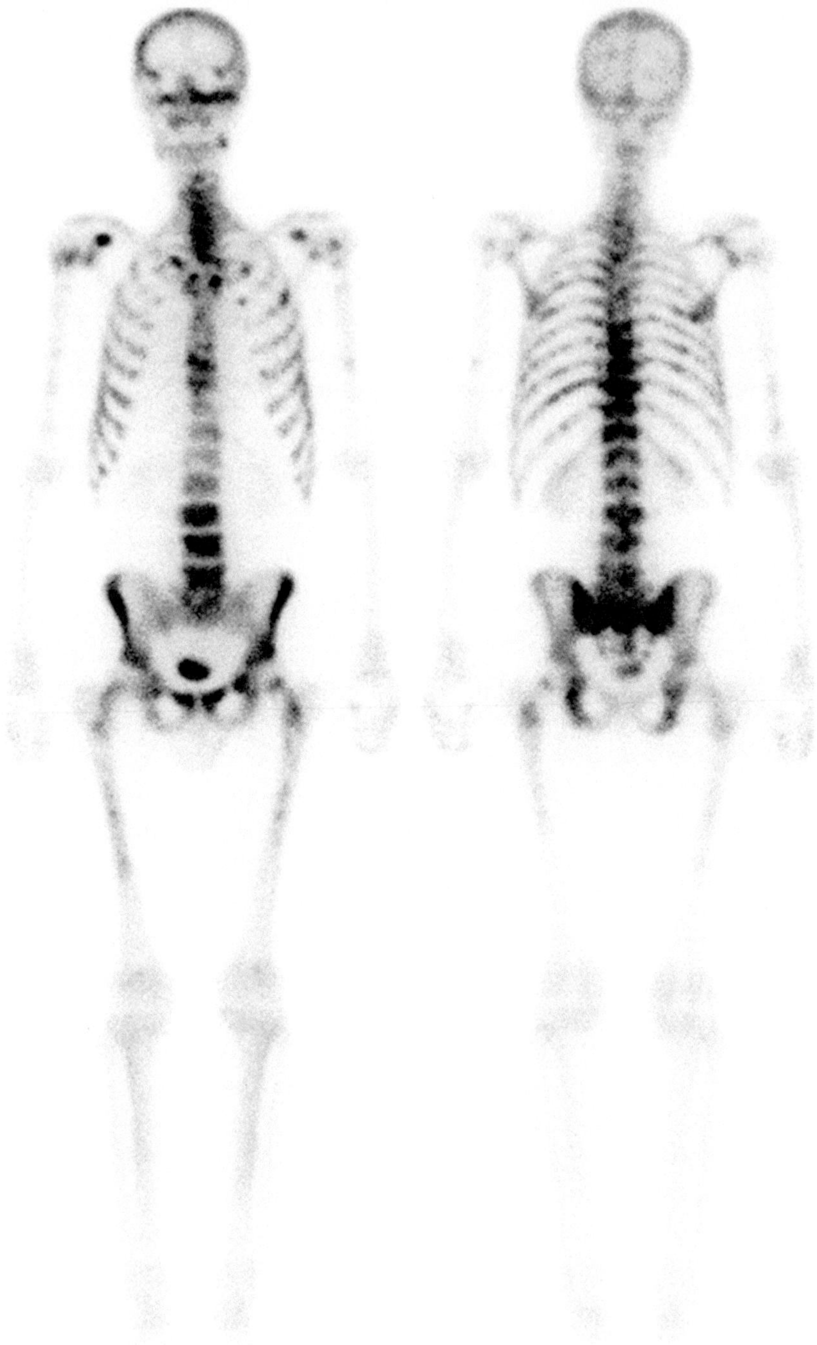

Fig. 10.3 Disseminated metastatic involvement from underlying breast cancer, showing diffuse involvement of multiple ribs and spine, with some patchy uptake in the femora. The kidneys are not visualized. The scan pattern consistent with 'superscan' of malignancy

other skeletal disorders which may cause confusion. One example is of increased tracer accumulation at the manubriosternal junction. This is a relatively common normal variant but may cause difficulty in patients with carcinoma of the breast, as the sternum is a common site for early metastatic disease. Clues that a lesion at this site is not benign are asymmetry and/or lack of linearity. When doubtful or if there are local symptoms or signs then further, imaging may be required. The sternum is often difficult to adequately visualize with radiography, and localized CT or MRI is often more helpful in this circumstance.

Other variants, which should be recognized, include activity at the confluence of sutures at the pterion in the skull, the deltoid muscle insertion on the humerus and symmetrical muscle insertion in the posterior ribs of paraspinal muscles causing a stippled appearance. On occasion, the tip of the scapula overlying a rib may mimic a focal abnormality. It is useful to take an extra view with the arms raised, thereby moving the tip of the scapula outside the line of the ribs. Bladder and renal collecting system activity is usually appreciated even if patients void prior to scanning.

The appearance of a lesion may aid interpretation. A single focal rib lesion is often the result of trauma, which may not even be recalled by the patient, but a lesion extending along the length of a rib is usually malignant in nature. However, Baxter et al. [22] have suggested that a single rib hot spot in a patient with a known malignancy may turn out to have a malignant aetiology in a surprisingly large number of patients (41%). Even focal abnormalities at the anterior ends of ribs, a position where abnormalities are often considered benign in the majority of cases, showed a large number of confirmed metastases (36%). However, these findings differ from those previously reported by Tumeh et al. in a similar retrospective study, where only 10% of solitary rib lesions proved to be malignant [23] and indeed seems a gross overestimate based on our personal experience. A linear array of rib lesions in adjacent ribs remains a situation where one may be confident of a traumatic aetiology (Figs. 10.4 and 10.5).

The interpretation of hot spots, whether solitary or multiple, may be especially problematic in the spine as there is a high prevalence of benign abnormalities such as degenerative disease, which may be indistinguishable without further investigation. In the scenario of a single spinal hot spot in patients with a known primary tumour, Coakley et al. found that just over one half (57%) turned out to be benign on subsequent clinical and imaging follow-up [24].

Vertebral body fractures have a characteristic appearance on bone scintigraphy showing a linear pattern of increased tracer accumulation. However, it is not possible to differentiate fractures due to benign diseases such as osteoporosis from malignant collapse (Fig. 10.6). MRI is probably the best current method for differentiating benign from malignant causes. A follow-up bone scan after a few months that shows reducing activity at a vertebral fracture site suggests a benign cause.

10.5 Clinical Application of Bone Scans in Specific Cancers

10.5.1 Breast Cancer

The skeleton is the most common distant site to which breast cancer spreads, 8% of patients being affected, rising to between 50% and 85% in those with advanced disease [25, 26]. The majority of bone metastases from breast cancer are either lytic or of a mixed pattern with a smaller proportion being purely sclerotic (Fig. 10.7). Bone scintigraphy is very sensitive with a false-negative rate of 2% [27]. However, some controversy has existed as to the precise role of bone scanning in patients at different stages of disease and the use of bone scintigraphy still varies between institutions. The positive bone scan is a poor prognostic factor [28]. The median survival of patients with bone metastases is only 24 months [27]. In breast cancer, the role of bone scintigraphy has been evaluated in the initial staging, routine/symptomatic follow-up and evaluation of effectiveness of treatment [27, 29, 30] (Fig. 10.8).

10.5.2 Prostate Cancer

Prostate cancer is one of the commonest cancers in men, and 85% of patients dying from this cancer have bone metastases [31]. Knowledge of the presence of bone metastases has a huge impact on the treatment of prostate cancer. The majority of bone metastases is osteoblastic and appears sclerotic on X-ray. Because of the osteoblastic nature of the

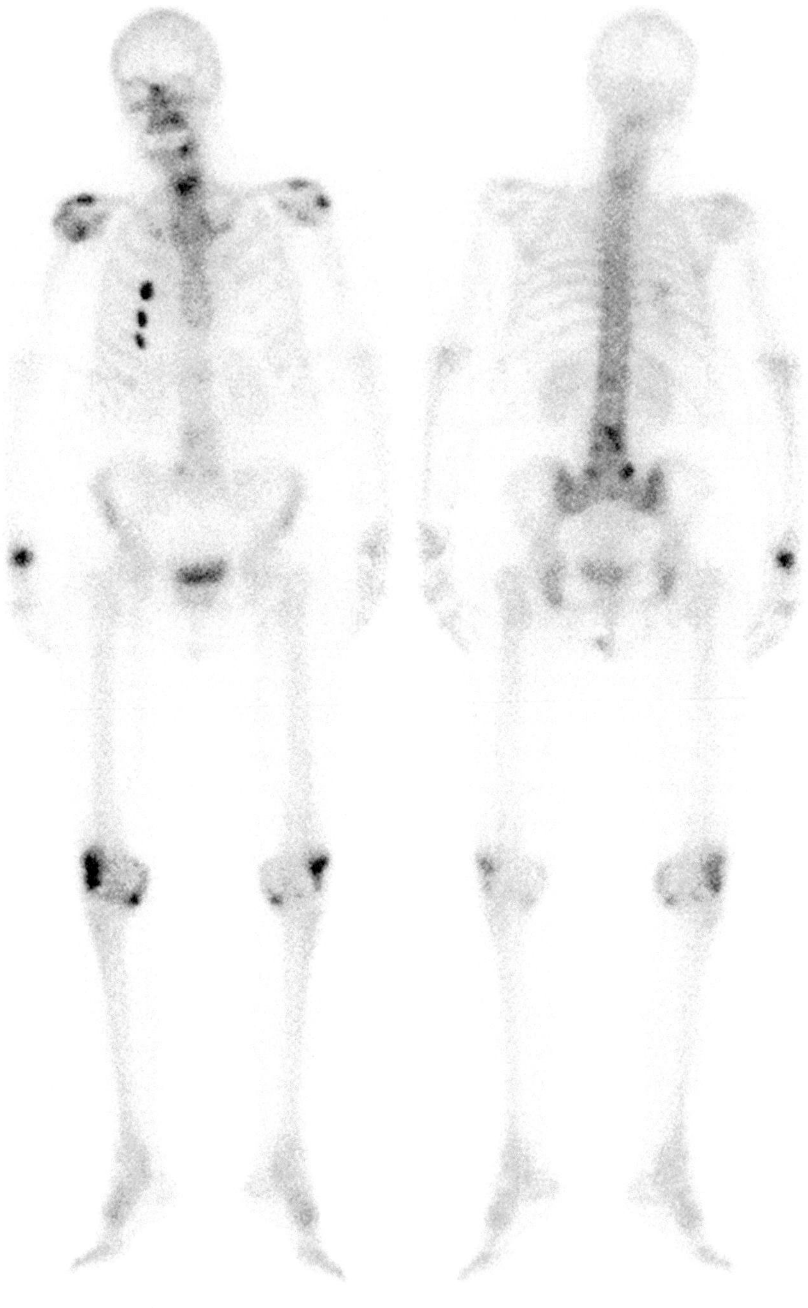

Fig. 10.4 Rib fractures: the whole body bone scan shows intense uptake in the right 4-sixth ribs anteriorly typical for rib fractures. Elsewhere there are degenerative changes

majority of prostate metastases, the bone scan is exquisitely sensitive. Prostate cancer most commonly involves well-vascularized areas of the skeleton such as the vertebral column, pelvis, skull and long bones (Fig. 10.9). Debate exists with regard to the mechanism of spread. Some authors suggest that the low-pressure Batson's venous plexus is involved, while others dispute this [32, 33]. Metastatic carcinoma of the prostate is one of the commonest causes of a malignant superscan seen in bone scintigraphy. As with breast cancer, the areas where bone scintigraphy has been evaluated include initial staging, both routine and symptomatic follow-up and the evaluation of the effectiveness of treatment (Fig. 10.10). There has been ongoing debate and investigation into the

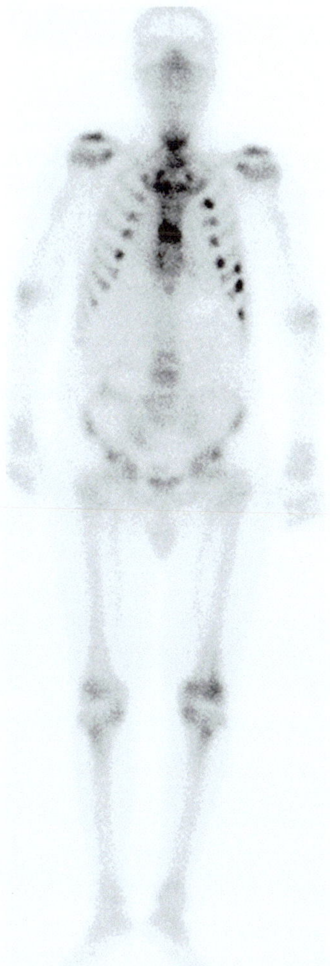

Fig. 10.5 Traumatic fracture: whole body bone scan shows increased uptake involving multiple ribs bilaterally and linear intense uptake in the body of the sternum in a patient who received CPR following a cardiac arrest

need for staging bone scans in prostate cancer [34]. Using PSA (prostate-specific antigen), Gleason score and clinical stage, it is possible to place patients into three risk categories such as low, medium and high. This information can help decide which patients require a bone scan for staging and also in the interpretation of equivocal lesions [34, 35]. As an independent factor, PSA also provides a readily available tool for risk assessment in these patients. Although there is some uncertainty whether a level of PSA of 10 or 20 ng/ml should be used as an upper threshold for performing scintigraphy, a level of less than 10 ng/ml is very rarely associated with bone metastases at presentation [36].

10.5.3 Other Genitourinary Tumours

Renal cell carcinoma metastasizes to bone relatively frequently. At presentation the incidence of bone metastases varies in reported series from 7.5% to 32% [37], but the majority of patients have either clinical or biochemical evidence of metastases. There would not therefore seem to be a need for routine scintigraphy of asymptomatic patients at presentation. If patients are symptomatic and have bone disease, the bone scan may not alter surgical management of the primary tumour but may be valuable in confirming and localizing lesions and assessing the extent prior to local or systemic palliative therapy. Metastases from renal carcinoma are mostly lytic and frequently do not excite much in the way of an osteoblastic response. Lesions may therefore be inconspicuous on bone scan, and a careful review for cold lesions should be made [38]. Tumours such as bladder and cervical, ovarian and uterine carcinomas have a low incidence of bone metastases at presentation, and therefore the routine scanning of asymptomatic patients is not justified. The role of bone scintigraphy in these tumours would seem to be in the assessment and treatment follow-up of patients with clinical suspicion of bone involvement.

10.5.4 Lung Cancer

The reported rates of positive bone scans in patients presenting with lung cancer varies widely (2–19%) [37], and this may reflect differences in the proportion of tumour types in the populations studied. Certainly, small cell carcinoma, which is seldom treated surgically, appears to have a higher incidence of bone involvement at presentation approaching 50% [39, 40] (Fig. 10.11). The prognosis of those with a positive bone scan at presentation is extremely poor where nearly all patients are dead by 12 months [41]. Practice may change as clinical PET scanning becomes more widely

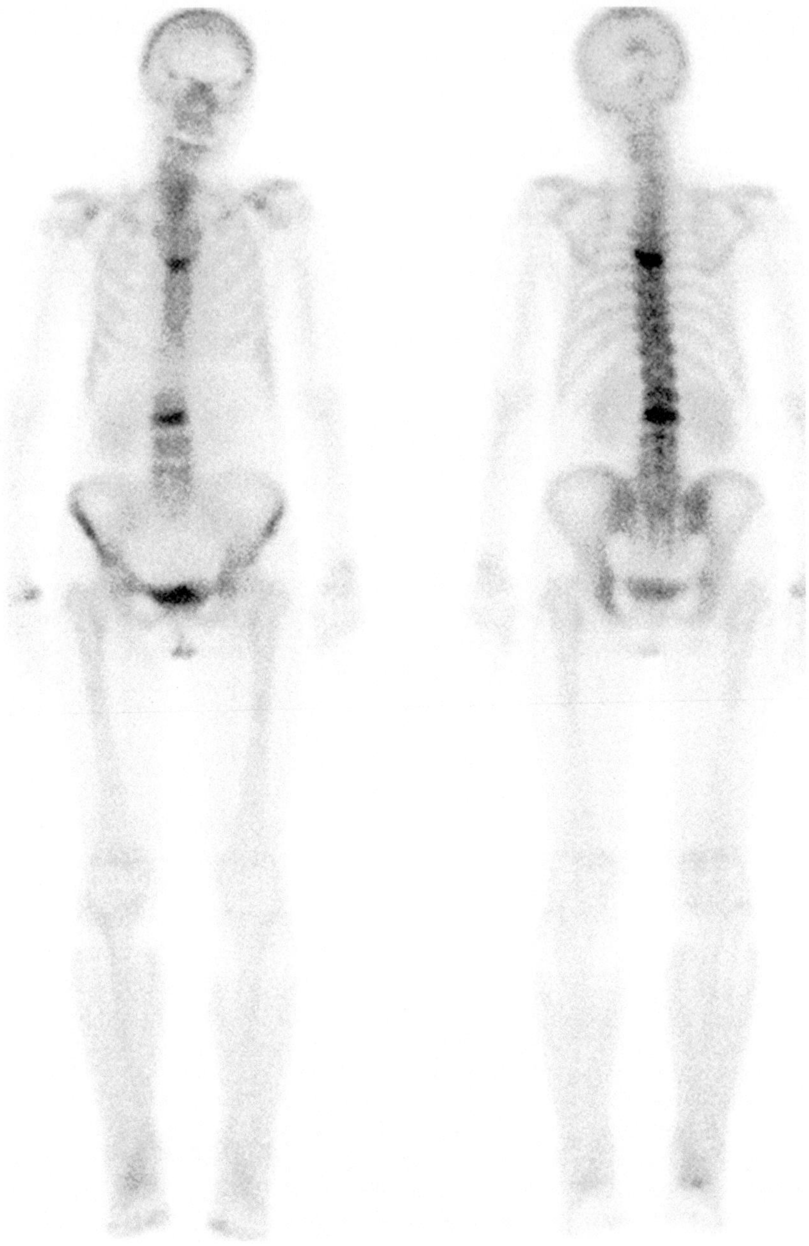

Fig. 10.6 Compression fractures/collapse: whole-body bone scan of an elderly male showing linear intense uptake in the T7 thoracic and L3 vertebrae with loss of vertebral contour. The scan appearances are compatible with vertebral fracture/collapse, which is likely to be benign. However, in patients with known malignancy, pathological fracture cannot absolutely be excluded

available as whole body imaging with ^{18}FDG can assess local and distant metastatic spread to soft tissues and bone. This technique is also more sensitive than current staging techniques with CT alone, demonstrated in a series of 35 non-small cell lung cancers, which were otherwise operable, where 18% had management changed to a non-surgical regime because of the detection of previously unsuspected metastases [42].

10.5.5 Neuroblastoma

This solid, childhood tumour frequently metastasizes to the skeleton, and bone scintigraphy has been demonstrated as a sensitive method for assessment of the skeletal involvement. Obtaining very good-quality studies is important in this disease if false-negative interpretations are to be avoided. Photopoenic lesions may occur which

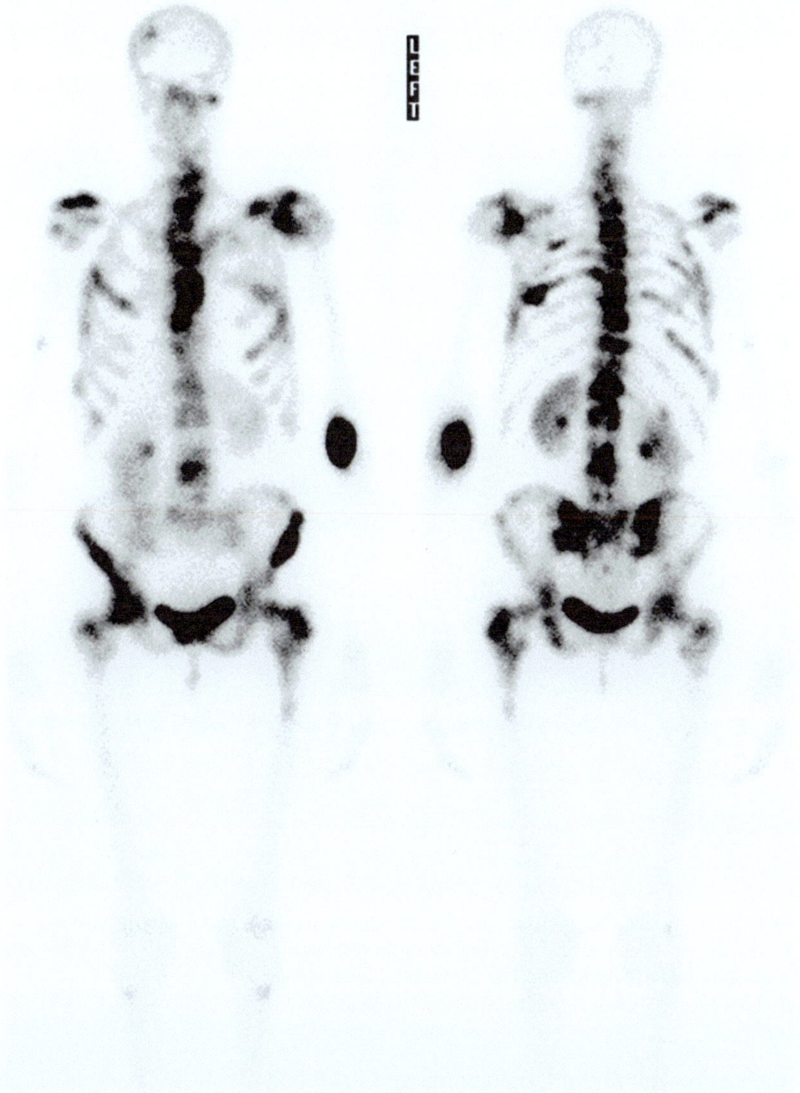

Fig. 10.7 Breast cancer metastases: whole-body bone scan showing disseminated metastatic involvement of skeleton involving, skull, multiple ribs bilaterally, multiple vertebrae, pelvis and long bones

can be difficult to resolve in the smaller paediatric skeleton [43], and symmetrical, diffuse uptake of tracer next to the joints, seen as blurring of the borders of epiphyseal activity, requires high-resolution images for detection. Uptake of ^{99m}Tc-MDP is often noted in the primary tumour and soft tissue metastases [44, 45]. Although ^{123}I MIBG is a specific tracer for staging and follow-up of neuroblastoma, false negatives have been noted in relation to the skeleton, and full assessment with both ^{99m}Tc-MDP and ^{123}I MIBG is recommended [46].

10.5.6 Miscellaneous Tumours

Due to the low incidence of bone involvement at presentation in many of the commoner cancers

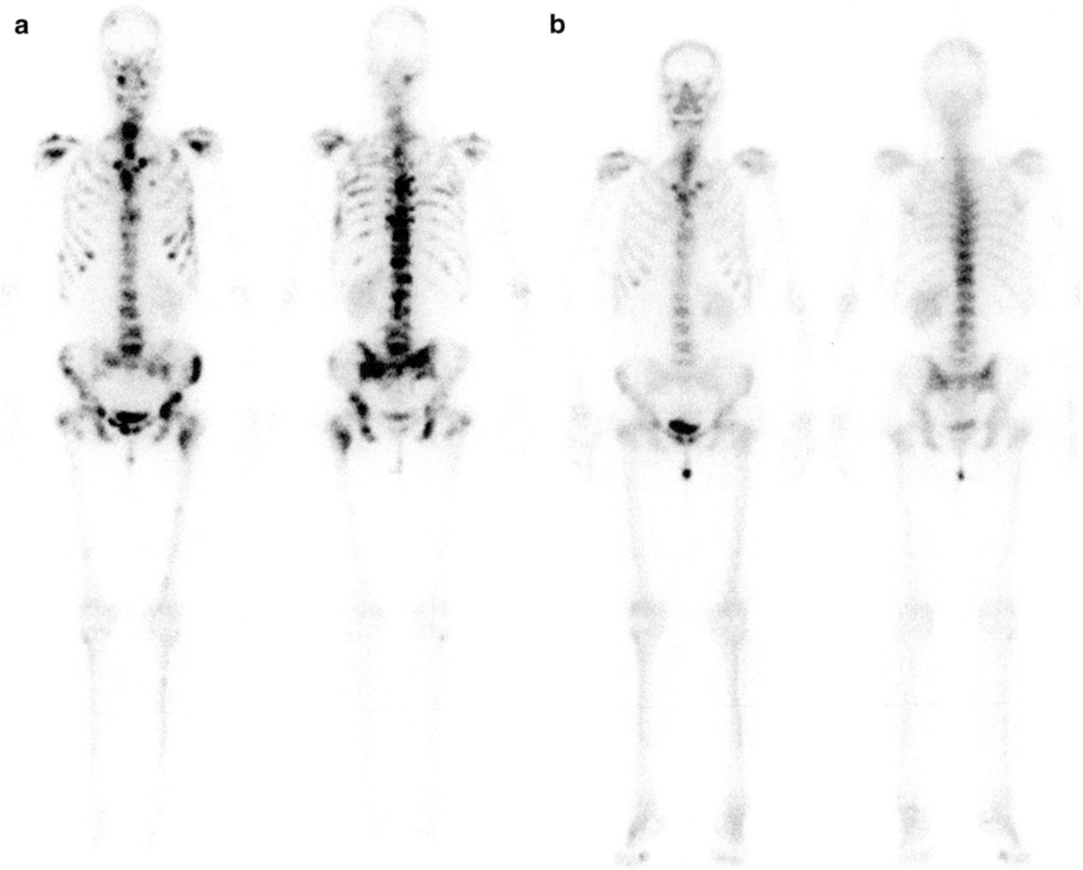

Fig. 10.8 Disease regression. (**a**) Disseminated metastatic disease from cancer involving multiple ribs, spine, sacroiliac joints, femora and (**b**) 18 months later shows significant improvement with resolution of lesions in the spine, pelvis and ribs following treatment

such as bowel, thyroid, melanoma and head and neck tumours, bone scintigraphy is usually only performed in those with suspicion of bone involvement and in the treatment assessment of those with proven bone metastases.

10.6 Clinical Applications of Bone Scan in Metabolic Bone Disease

10.6.1 Osteoporosis

In clinical management of the metabolic bone diseases, the isotope bone scan is most useful in osteoporotic patients, in whom it has a valuable role in evaluation and management [47]. The bone scan has no role in the diagnosis of osteoporosis per se but may be used in established osteoporosis to confirm or exclude recent vertebral fractures. The characteristic appearance of this type of fracture is of intense, linearly increased tracer uptake at the affected level (Fig. 10.12). It should be noted that although the bone scan may become positive immediately after a fracture, it could take up to 2 weeks for the scan to become abnormal, especially in the elderly. Subsequently there is a gradual reduction in tracer uptake, with the scan normalizing between 3 and 18 months after the incident, the average being between 9 and 12 months [48, 49]. Because of this, the bone scan also is

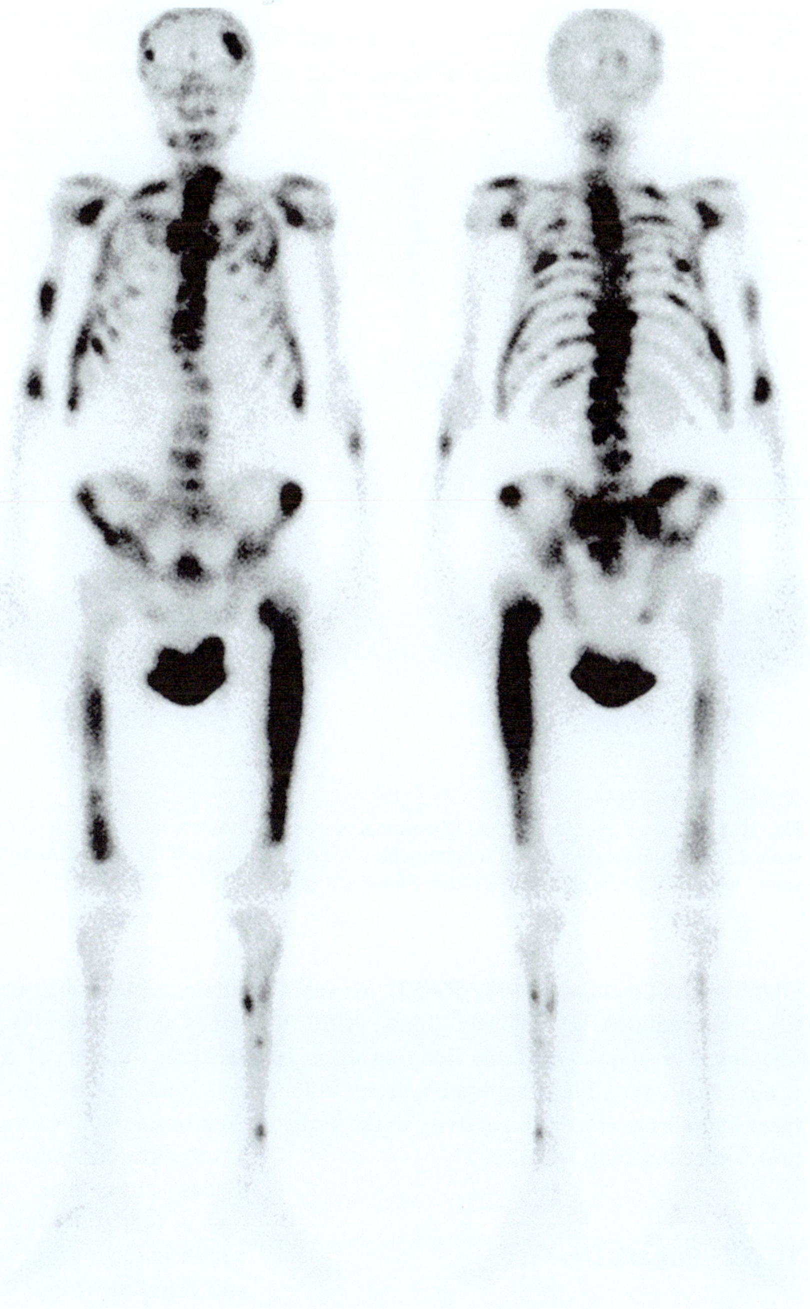

Fig. 10.9 Prostate cancer: disseminated metastatic involvement of the skull, multiple ribs, vertebrae, humeri, femora, left tibia, sacroiliac joints and pelvis

extremely useful in assessing the age of fractures. If a patient complains of back pain with multiple vertebral fractures on radiographs, and the bone scan is normal, then this essentially excludes recent fracture as a cause of symptoms. An isotope bone scan also may be valuable in patients in whom back pain persists for longer than one would expect after vertebral fracture. It is common to find that there has been an additional unsuspected vertebral or sacral fracture or a rib fracture in close proximity to spine. In addition, we are increasingly becoming aware that osteoporotic patients with chronic back pain may have unsuspected abnormalities

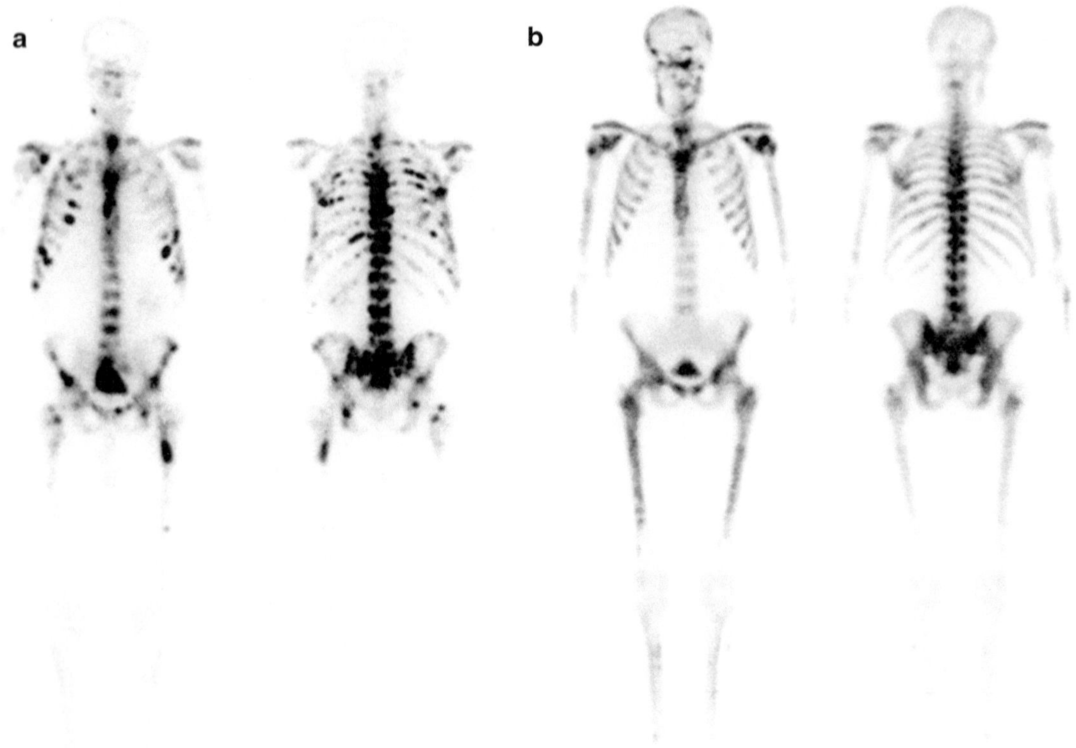

Fig. 10.10 Disease progression. (**a**) Disseminated metastatic disease from prostate cancer involving multiple ribs, spine, sacroiliac joints, humeri, femora which has progressed into a superscan of malignancy in 15 months (**b**) with diffuse involvement of the skeleton

affecting the facet joints [47, 50–53]. To identify abnormalities in the facet joints, SPECT imaging is essential. On planar imaging alone, it is not usually possible to separate activity in the facet joints from associated activity in the vertebral body caused by fracture.

10.6.2 Paget's Disease

The isotope bone scan is invaluable in the assessment of patients with suspected Paget's disease, both for diagnosis and to define the extent of skeletal involvement. The majority of patients with Paget's disease have polyostotic disease (80–90%) (Fig. 10.13). The bone scan is a convenient way to evaluate the whole skeleton and has shown a greater sensitivity for detecting affected sites than having radiographic skeletal surveys [48, 49]. Characteristically, affected bones show intensely increased activity, which starts at the end of a bone and spreads either proximally or distally, often showing a "V" or "flame-shaped" leading edge. Another clue that a scintigraphic abnormality is due to Paget's disease rather than other focal skeletal pathology is that the whole bone is often involved, which is most often seen in the pelvis, scapula and vertebrae (Figs. 10.14, 10.15, and 10.16). In the vertebrae, the characteristic finding is of abnormal tracer accumulation throughout the vertebra, affecting the body and posterior elements, including the spinous and transverse processes. The radionuclide bone scan is useful for the evaluation of the extent of the disease and response to the treatment. The radionuclide bone scan may occasionally identify complications of Paget's disease.

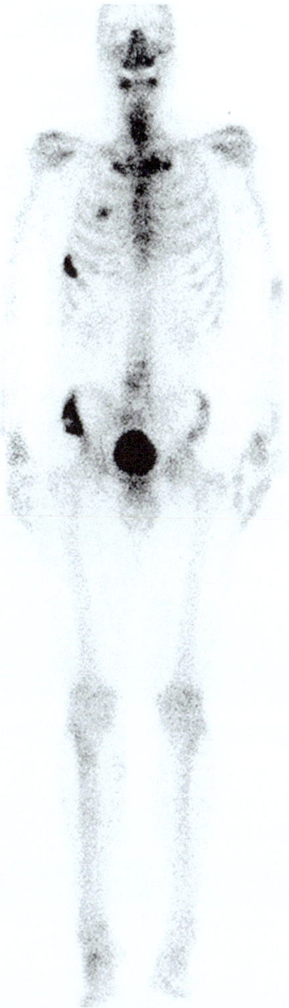

Fig. 10.11 Lung cancer. Whole-body scan shows abnormal uptake in the ribs and right iliac crest (note the photopoenic area in the centre due to an osteolytic lesion) suggestive of multiple metastases. Some patchy uptake is also present in the left strenoclavicular joint due to degenerative disease at that site

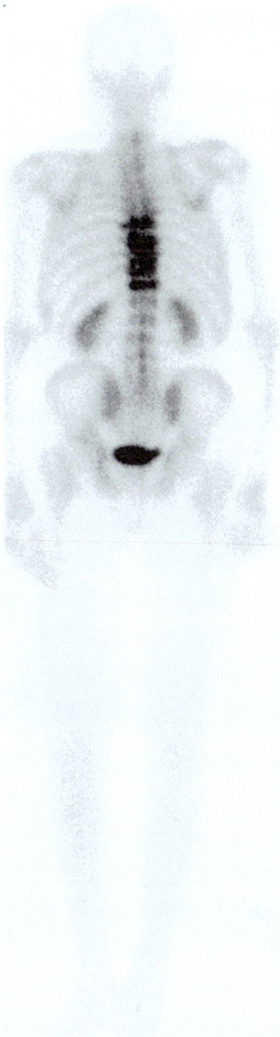

Fig. 10.12 Multiple osteoporotic fractures: whole-body bone scan of an elderly male with osteoporosis showing multiple foci of linear, intense uptake in the thoracic vertebrae with loss of vertebral contour

10.6.3 Hyperparathyroidism

Most cases of primary hyperparathyroidism are asymptomatic and are unlikely to be associated with changes on bone scintigraphy. The diagnosis is a biochemical one, and the bone scan therefore has no routine role in diagnosis. Bone scans are often used to help differentiate the causes of hypercalcaemia; in particular, hyperparathyroidism versus malignancy (although hypercalcaemia in the later may also be due to humoral factors related to PTH, etc.) and so typical features of metabolic bone disorders should be recognized. In hyperparathyroidism, there is increased skeletal turnover, and in the more severe cases, commonly seen as part of renal osteodystrophy, this will be evident scintigraphically. A bone scan may show a number of features in hyperparathyroidism, but the most important is the generalized increased uptake throughout the skeleton, that may be identified because of increased contrast between bone and soft tissues. Other typical metabolic features that have been described in bone scans in metabolic bone diseases include a prominent calvarium and mandible, beading of the costochondral junctions and a 'tie' sternum.

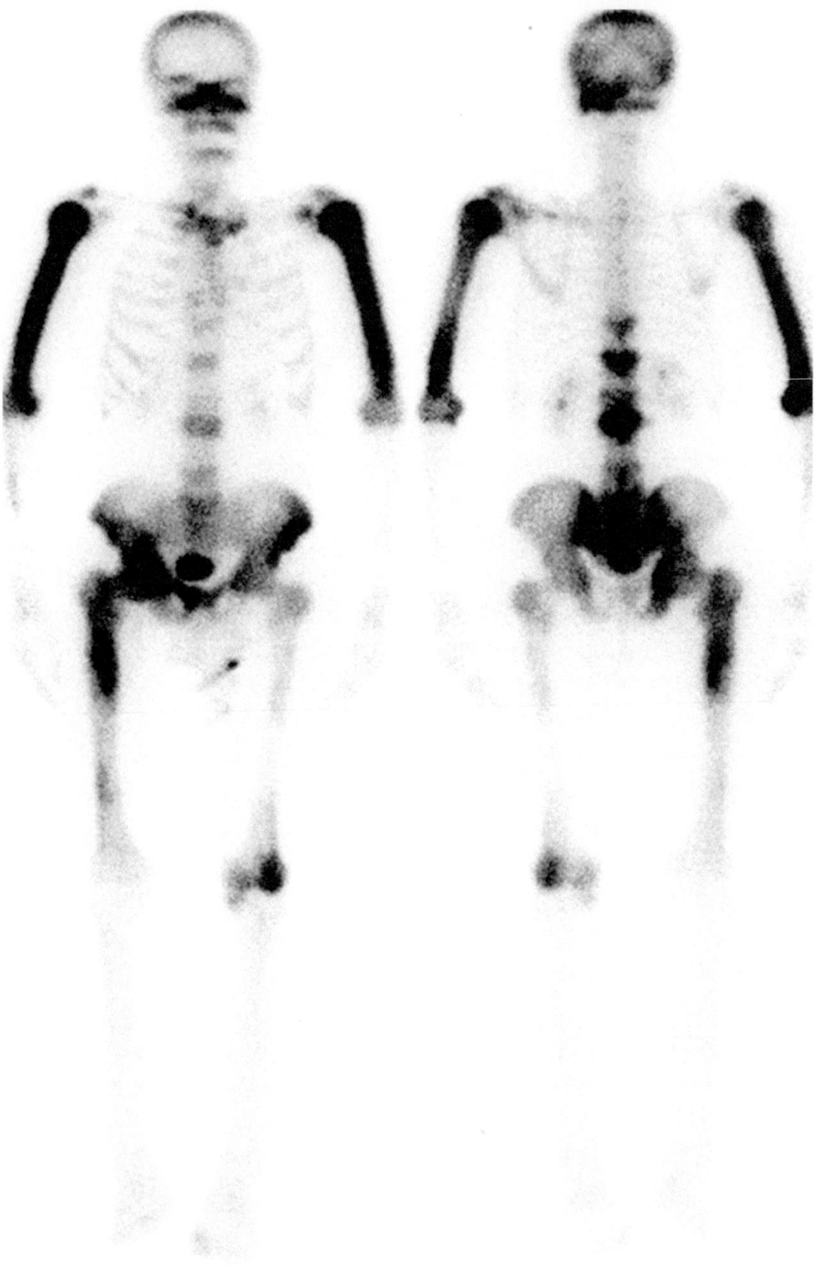

Fig. 10.13 Polyostotic Paget's disease: whole-body bone scan showing multiple areas of intense increased uptake in the skull, humeri, right femur, lumbar spine and pelvis

10.6.4 Renal Osteodystrophy

Renal osteodystrophy is due to a combination of bone disorders as a consequence of chronic renal dysfunction and often demonstrates the most severe cases of metabolic bone disease. It may comprise osteoporosis, osteomalacia, adynamic bone and secondary hyperparathyroidism in varying degrees. The bone scan appearance generally reflects the degree of hyperparathyroidism and in severe cases leads to a 'metabolic' super scan, and uptake of diphosphonate in areas of ectopic calcification also may be seen although it is now relatively uncommon. A clue in differentiating this type of scintigraphic pattern from others is that there may be a lack of bladder activity in view of renal failure.

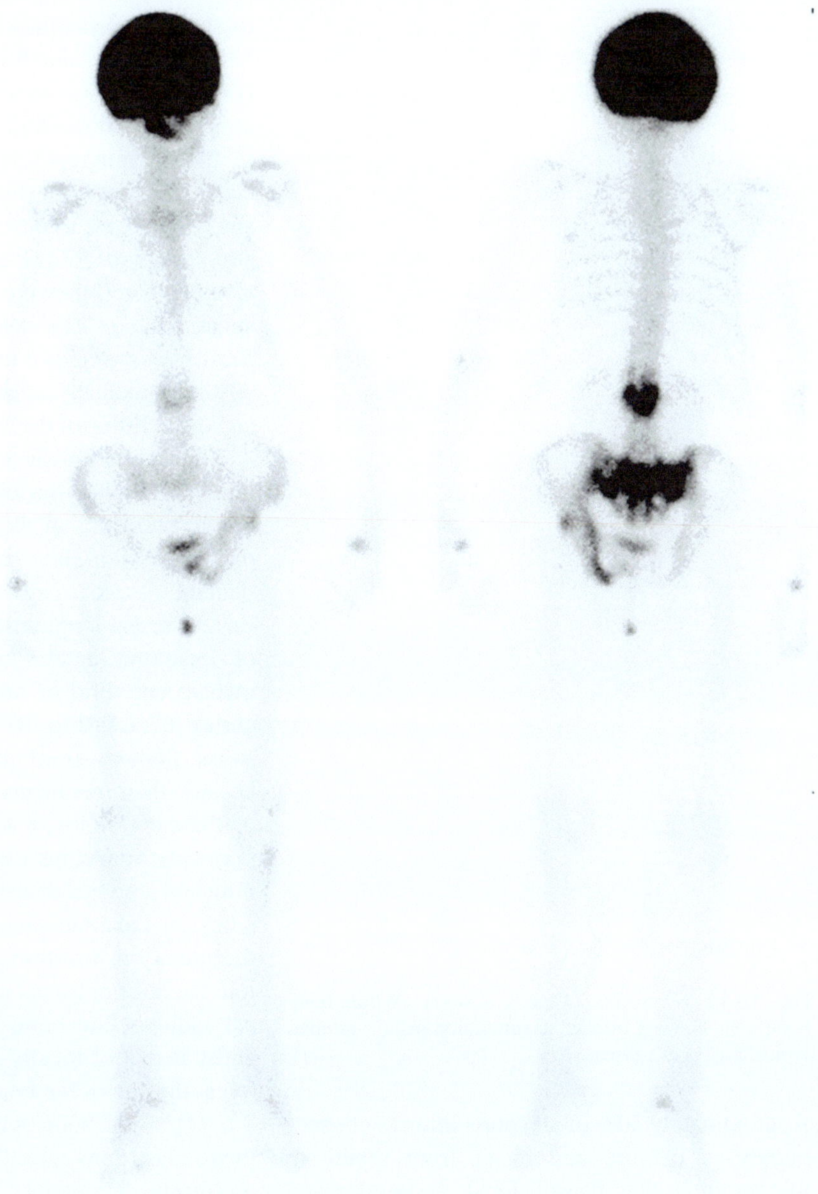

Fig. 10.14 Polyostotic Paget's disease. Whole-body bone scan showing intense accumulation in the skull, L3 lumbar vertebra, sacrum and less prominently in the left hemi-pelvis

10.6.5 Osteomalacia

Patients with osteomalacia usually demonstrate similar features on a bone scan as described in hyperparathyroidism, although in the early stages of the disease, it may appear normal [58]. Tc-99m MDP can detect Looser's zones or pseudofractures with high sensitivity, especially in ribs where X-ray may not be helpful [59, 60]. The pseudofractures are often noted in the ribs, which is the most common site seen on the bone scan. The distribution is usually symmetrical and perpendicular to the bone surface [59].

10.7 Clinical Application of Bone Scans in Sports-/Exercise-Related Injuries

Sports-induced injuries include a host of musculotendinous abnormalities, such as stress fractures, shin splints, arthritis, muscle injuries, etc.

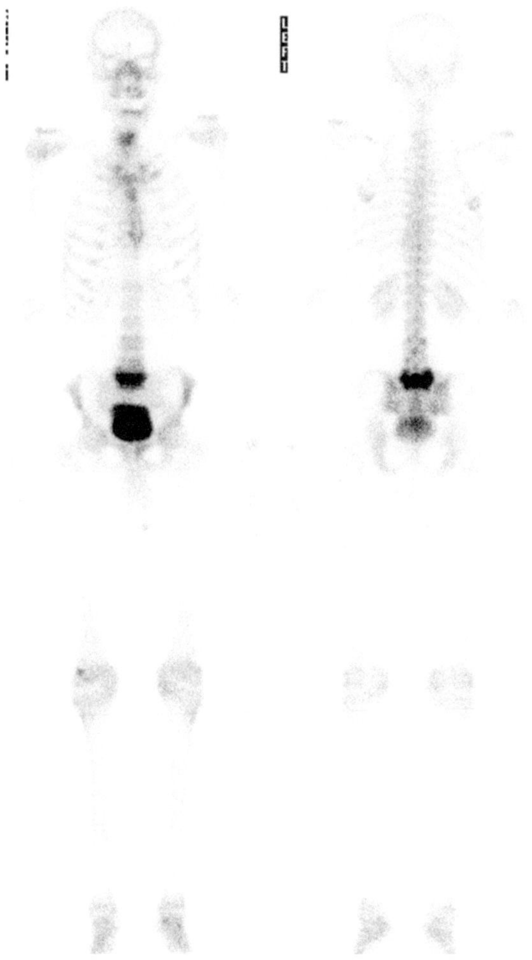

Fig. 10.15 Monostotic Paget's disease. Whole-body bone scan showing intense accumulation in L5 vertebra, typical for Paget's disease

Approximately 50% of all sports injuries are secondary to overuse and result from repetitive microtrauma that causes local tissue damage [61–63]. Sports-induced injuries are generally due to biomechanical abnormalities (malalignments, muscle imbalance/weakness, inflexibility/instability), poor technique, improper equipment, and changes in duration or frequency of activity [63]. The pathogenesis of stress fracture is multifactorial and usually involves repetitive submaximal stress [64].

Bone scintigraphy with Tc-99m MDP has been used with increasing frequency in detecting sports-induced injuries especially stress fractures, because of its high sensitivity and its ability to show abnormalities in bone metabolism well before they are manifested radiographically [65] (Fig. 10.17). Its sensitivity for this diagnosis approaches 100% [65].

Bone scintigraphy is also used to differentiate stress fractures from shin splints in the tibia. Tibial stress fractures accounts for half of all reported stress fractures [66] (Fig. 10.18). Increased perfusion and blood flow are typically present in acute stress fracture. The delayed images often reveal focal fusiform uptake in the lesion, which is usually seen medially at the junction of the middle and distal thirds of the tibia [67, 68].

Shin splints are due to excessive exertion of the tibialis and soleus muscles of the legs, which gives rise to periostitis at the tibial insertions of these muscles [67]. In shin splints, blood flow and blood pool images are usually normal. However, delayed images reveal longitudinally oriented linear areas of increased uptake of varying intensity that involve one third or more of the posterior tibial cortex [67, 69] (Fig. 10.19). The differentiation of stress fracture from shin splints is important because their treatments are different [67].

Plantar fasciitis, a form of localized reactive periostitis, develops during events such as running and aerobics that involve extensive foot dorsiflexion. Pain and tenderness are concentrated at the site of the insertion of the long plantar tendon into the inferior aspect of the calcaneus. The typical radionuclide bone scan appearance of this entity is that of focally increased (intense) activity, at the site of the tendon insertion [61, 62, 67, 70, 71]. With bone scintigraphy, reflex sympathetic dystrophy usually manifests as diffuse, uniformly increased uptake throughout the affected region. In childhood cases and occasionally in adults the uptake can be reduced [72, 73].

10.8 Clinical Applications of Bone Scan in Infection and Evaluation of Joint Prostheses

^{99m}Tc-MDP bone scintigraphy is used as a complementary imaging procedure in evaluation of infection. It is routinely used in the evaluation for

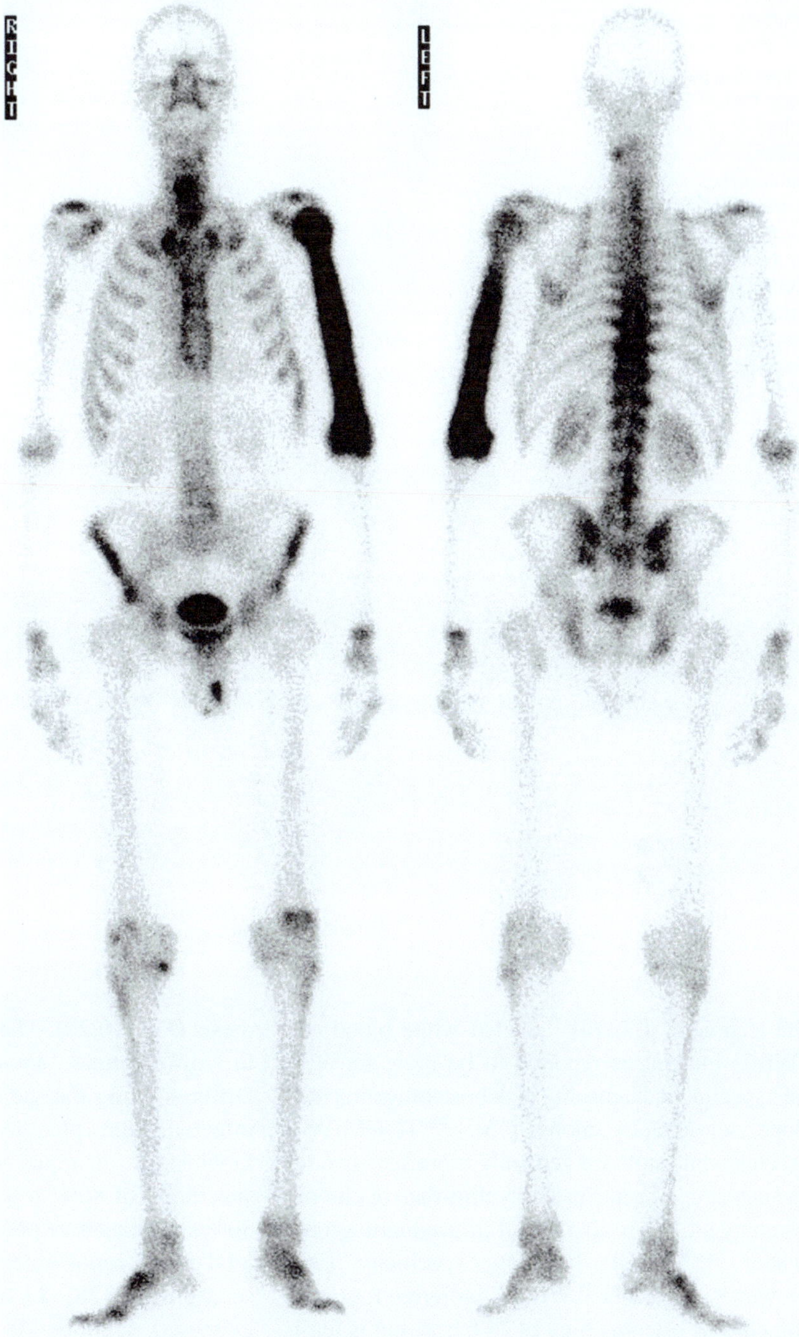

Fig. 10.16 Monostotic Paget's disease. Whole-body bone scan showing intense accumulation in the left humerus due to Paget's disease

osteomyelitis in a diabetic patient. Early diagnosis and treatment of the condition can reduce the likelihood of complications. Three-phase bone scan is reported to have an accuracy of over 90% [74]. The classic appearance of osteomyelitis on three-phase bone scans consists of focal hyperperfusion, focal hyperaemia and focally increased bone uptake [67, 74]. However, fractures, tumours and joint neuropathy may also mimic osteomyelitis on a three-phase bone scan, thus reducing the specificity of

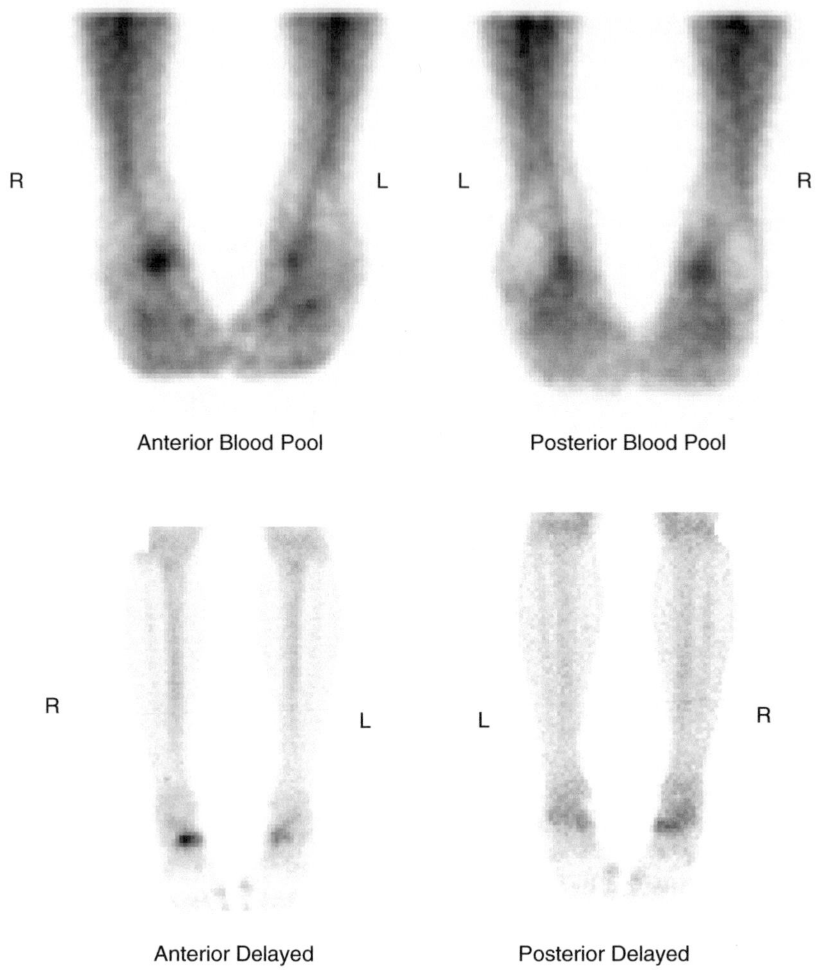

Fig. 10.17 Stress fractures: 28-year-old footballer with increasing pain in the right foot. No previous injury or problems with lower limbs. (**a**) Blood pool images shows increased vascularity over the medial aspect of the right foot and (**b**) the delayed images show intense uptake at this site due to a navicular fracture

the technique [67, 74]. Labeled white blood cell (WBC) imaging is reported to be more sensitive and specific in diagnosing pedal osteomyelitis than bone scintigraphy alone [75]. ^{99m}Tc-HMPAO-labeled white cells are generally more sensitive for the detection of acute osteomyelitis than of chronic osteomyelitis. It is also useful in paediatric group, where ^{99m}Tc-MDP has low specificity [76]. However, ^{111}In-labeled WBC is preferred for imaging chronic osteomyelitis as 24 h imaging is feasible [74, 77], which is important in the presence of low-grade infection. But false-positive WBC scans have occurred in Charcot's (neuropathic) joints, probably attributable to inflammation and hematopoietically active bone marrow [74].

^{99m}Tc-MDP bone scintigraphy is used to evaluate patients with painful joint replacement/prosthesis (Fig. 10.20). The commonest indication is to differentiate loosening from infection. Differentiating the aseptically loosened from the infected joint prosthesis is not always easy. Lewinski et al. reported a sensitivity of 33%, a specificity of 86%, a positive predictive value of 30% and a negative predictive value of 88% in 72 total joint replacements examined with bone scintigraphy [78]. In bone scintigraphy, focally increased radionuclide uptake around the prosthesis is commonly considered to represent loosening (Figs. 10.21 and 10.22), while diffusely increased uptake in blood pool and delayed phase is commonly considered to represent infection [74, 79, 80]. However, infection may also be present in prostheses with focal uptake patterns [81, 82]. Bone scintigraphy within 12 months of

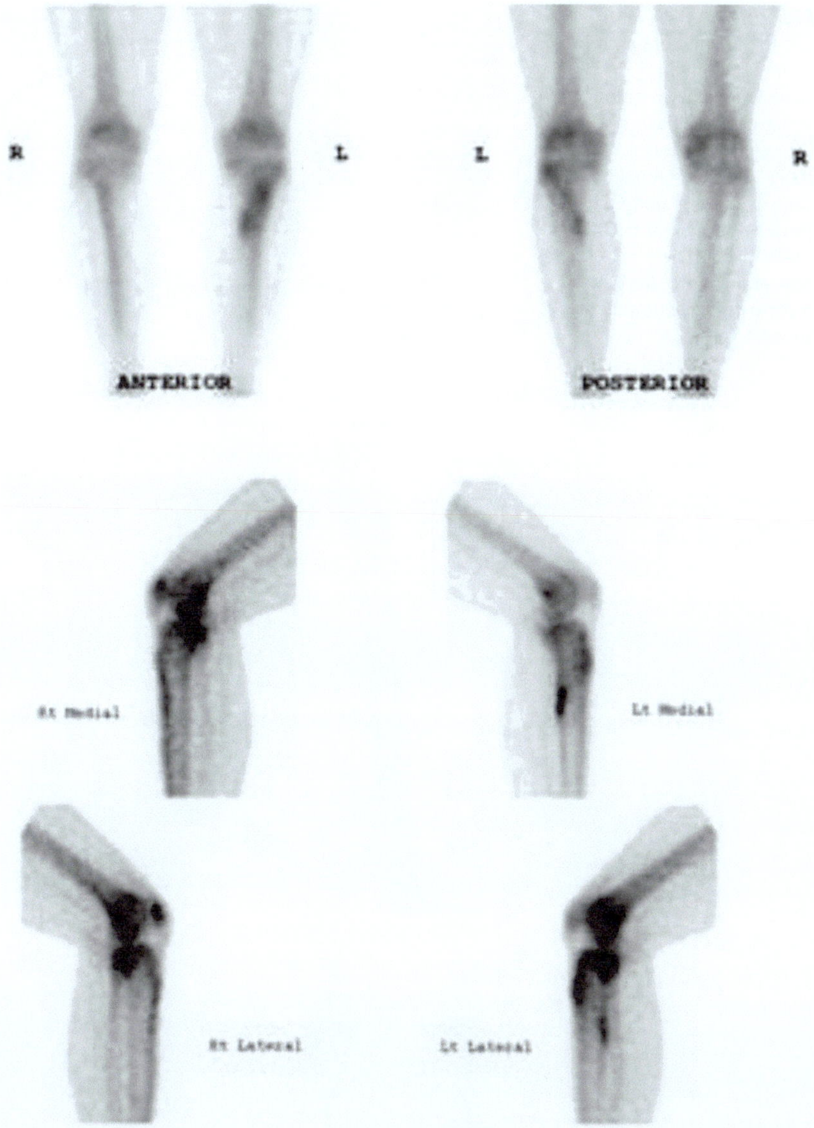

Fig. 10.18 Stress fracture. Stress fracture: 32-year-old male (Triathlete), complaining of pain in left tibia over past 2 months. The delayed images show focal intense uptake at the medial aspect of the upper left tibia. The appearances are typical of a stress fracture

an arthroplasty procedure may be of limited value in ruling out loosening and infection due to existent inflammatory changes following surgery [79]. Type, location of the prosthesis and the amount of time elapsed between implantation and imaging must be taken into account during interpretation [83]. Hip and knee replacements can be a cemented or cementless. In patients with a cemented hip prosthesis, the majority of the asymptomatic patients will have a normal bone scan beyond 1 year, and about 10% will have persistent increased uptake beyond this period [84]. In patients with a cementless hip prosthesis, the persistent uptake is more prevalent beyond 1-year post-replacement [85, 86]. In patients with knee replacements persistent periprosthetic uptake beyond 1-year post-implantation is also noted (89% of tibial components and 63% of femoral components) [87, 88]. Hofmann et al. found that a single post-operative bone scan could not differentiate loosening from early bone remodelling [87].

^{111}In-labeled WBC scintigraphy in general is a good agent for diagnosing infection in prosthesis. However, diagnostic accuracy of labeled white cell imaging can be limited as it accumulates in

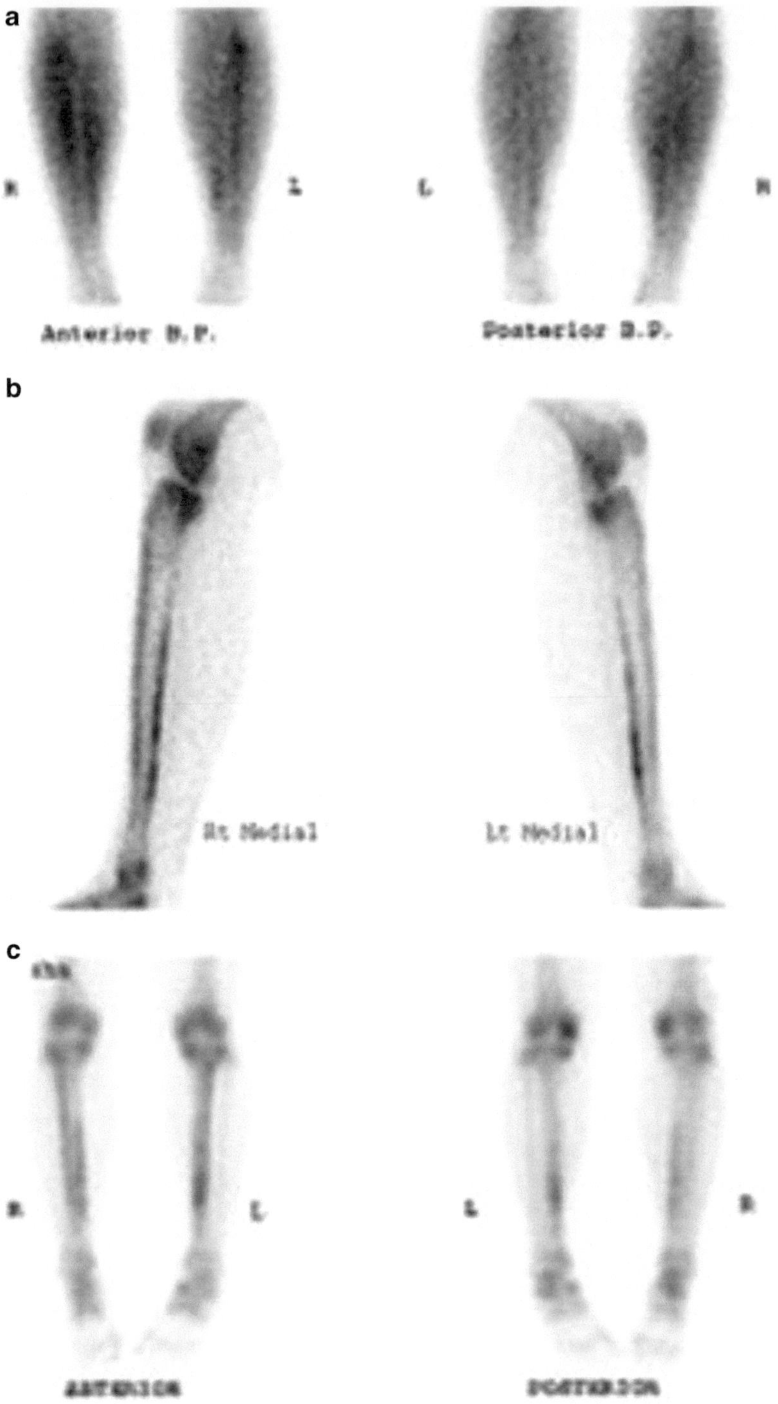

Fig. 10.19 A 29-year-old female marathon runner complaining of increasing pain in both tibiae over the past 3 months. There is increased tracer uptake seen extending along the posterior aspect of both tibiae (**b**, **c**). The appearances are those of a periosteal reaction due to 'shin splints'

normal reticuloendothelial bone marrow [74, 76]. Implantation of prosthesis may alter the bone marrow distribution at the site of intervention. However, inability to distinguish labeled leukocyte uptake in infection from uptake in bone marrow is a problem. This issue can be overcome by performing additional bone marrow imaging with ^{99m}Tc-sulphur colloid. Both labeled leukocytes and sulphur colloid accumulate in the bone marrow, whereas there is mismatch in infection

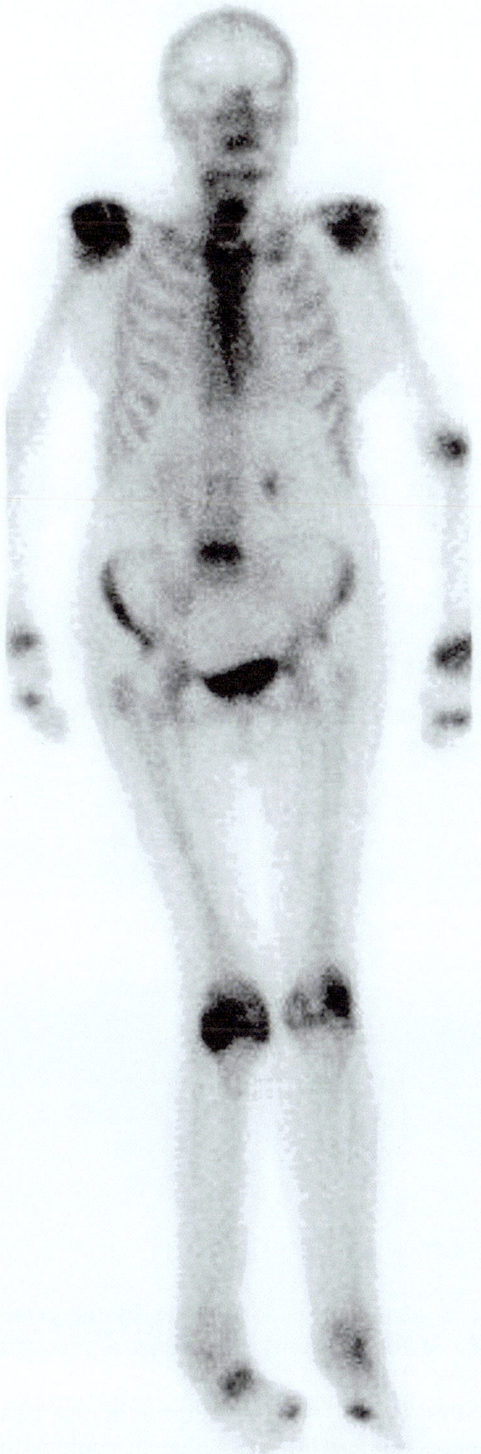

Fig. 10.20 Severe osteoarthritis with bilateral total hip replacement (THR). Whole-body bone scan shows abnormal uptake involving multiple joints (shoulders, knees and L5 vertebra and small joints in the feet). Bilateral hip replacements are also noted

when leukocytes accumulate but sulphur colloid does not [89, 90]. The reported sensitivity, specificity, and accuracy of labeled leukocytes plus sulphur colloid bone marrow imaging is 96%, 97%, and 97%, respectively [89].

10.9 Clinical Application of Bone SPECT

In patients with chronic low back pain, the addition of SPECT to bone scintigraphy is a useful adjunct that some departments perform routinely. SPECT has been shown to be more sensitive that plain film radiology, with most SPECT lesions corresponding to identifiable disease on computed tomography (CT) [50–53, 54–57]. One third of lesions may not be visible on planar scintigraphy [50–53] (Fig. 10.23). Lesions can be accurately located to the vertebral bodies or posterior vertebral elements [50–53]. It was noted that the main benefit occurred in lesions localized to the posterior aspect of the vertebra where radiographs failed to detect abnormalities in the majority of cases, even when additional oblique views were available.

SPECT has been found to be particularly valuable in the investigation of facet syndrome as a cause of low back pain [91, 92] (Fig. 10.24). Not only is it a sensitive method for detecting facet joint related pain compared to planar imaging, but also it can predict those patients who are more likely to benefit from local facet joint injections or denervation [91]. As clinical features are often non-specific in facet joint-related pain, bone SPECT is also helpful in identifying the cause of pain in those without a facetal aetiology [92]. Pars interarticularis defects, thought to be due to a repeated stress phenomenon causing spondylolysis, are a significant cause of back pain, particularly in young people actively participating in sport. Bone SPECT is able to identify more lesions than radiographs [93–99], and a normal SPECT scan makes spondylolysis an unlikely cause of back pain. SPECT scans may be helpful in guiding management, by correlating the presence or absence of abnormal metabolic activity with pars defects identified on CT.

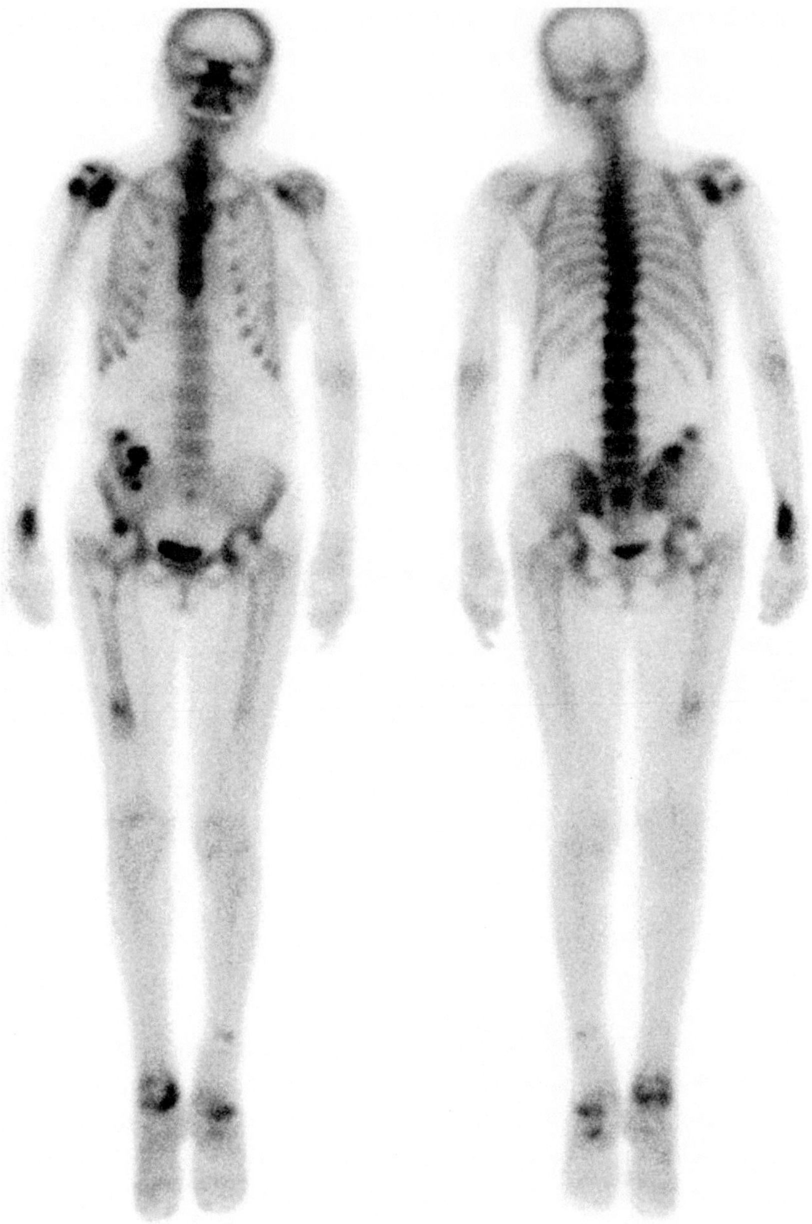

Fig. 10.21 Loosening of hip prostheses. Patient presented with right-sided hip pain 2 years after total hip replacement (THR). The delayed whole body images show bilateral THR's, right shoulder replacement and a right ankle prosthesis. Increased metabolic activity with normal blood pool (not shown) in the acetabular components bilaterally and at the tip of right femoral component is consistent with loosening. The uptake noted in the right shoulder and ankle is consistent with degenerative changes. A right transplant kidney is also noted, and the patient has been treated for avascular necrosis

Bone SPECT of the lumbar spine may contribute to the evaluation of symptomatic patients following spinal surgery. SPECT is more sensitive than planar imaging alone [100] and is valuable in precisely locating the level of maximum instability or cause of symptoms distal from the operative site [101, 102]. Bone scintigraphy with SPECT is not hampered by artefacts caused by surgical metalwork as are CT and MRI. It is able to identify pseudoarthroses by the persistence of focal activity more than a year after surgery.

SPECT may also be helpful in the early diagnosis of sacroiliitis, where in conjunction with MRI, objective and complementary evidence for inflammatory activity may be gained before radiographic changes [103]. It is likely that the addition of a SPECT acquisition may

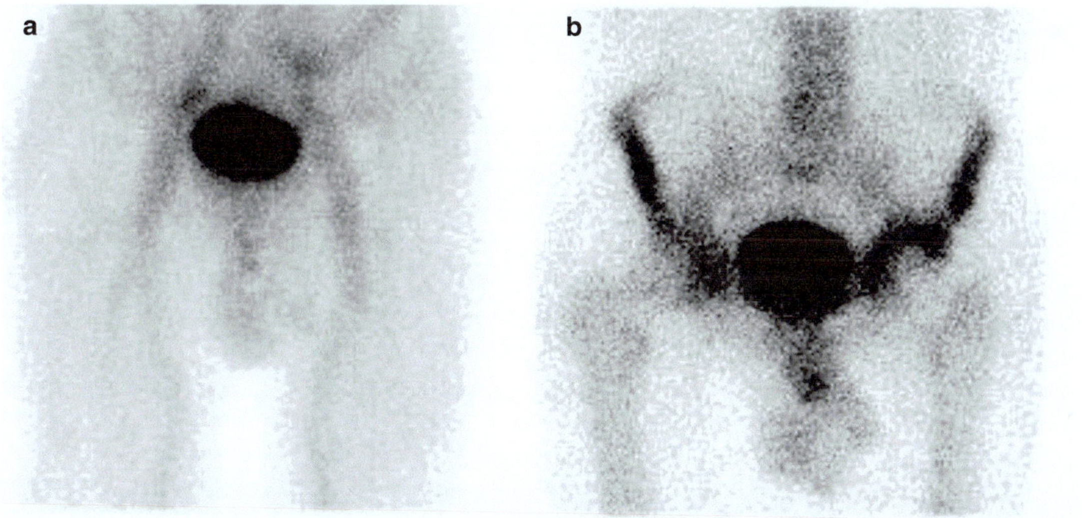

Fig. 10.22 Loosening of left THR. Patient with left THR (performed 4 years ago) with pain in the left hip. The delayed images (**b**) on the right shows increased accumulation in the acetabular component of the prosthesis with normal blood pool (**a**), which is compatible with loosening of the acetabular component

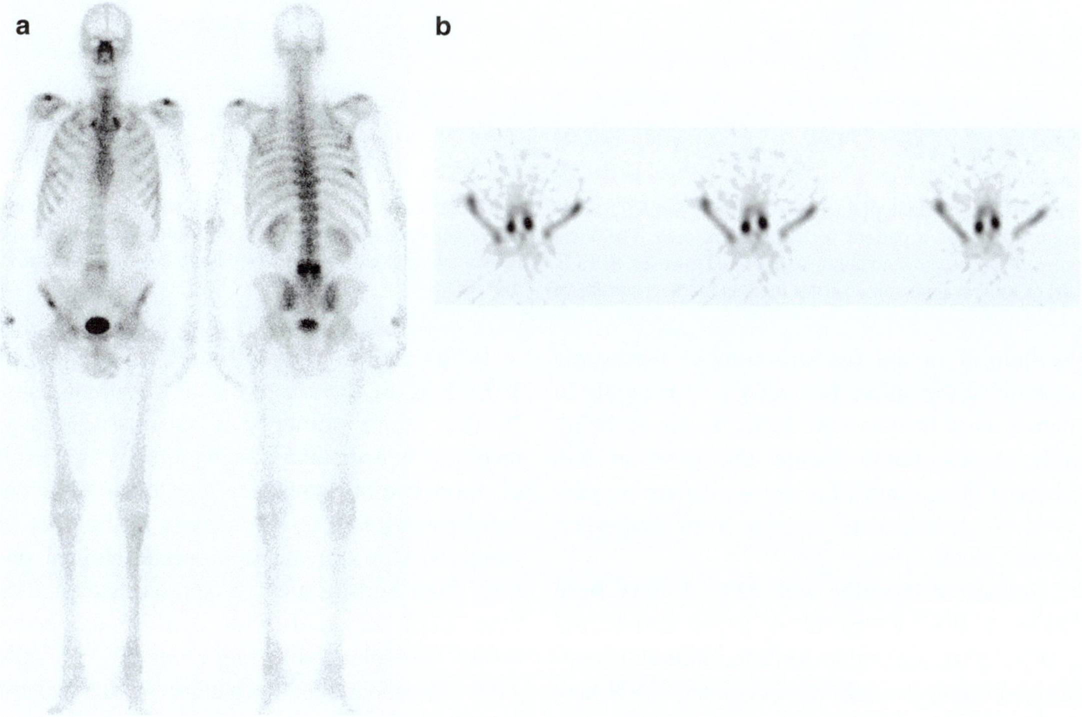

Fig. 10.23 Facet joint disease in a patient with low back pain. (**a**) Whole-body bone scan and SPECT (**b**) of lumbosacral spine show intense uptake in the facet joints of L5/S1. Increased uptake of tracer is also seen in the right ninth rib posteriorly, which was traumatic in nature

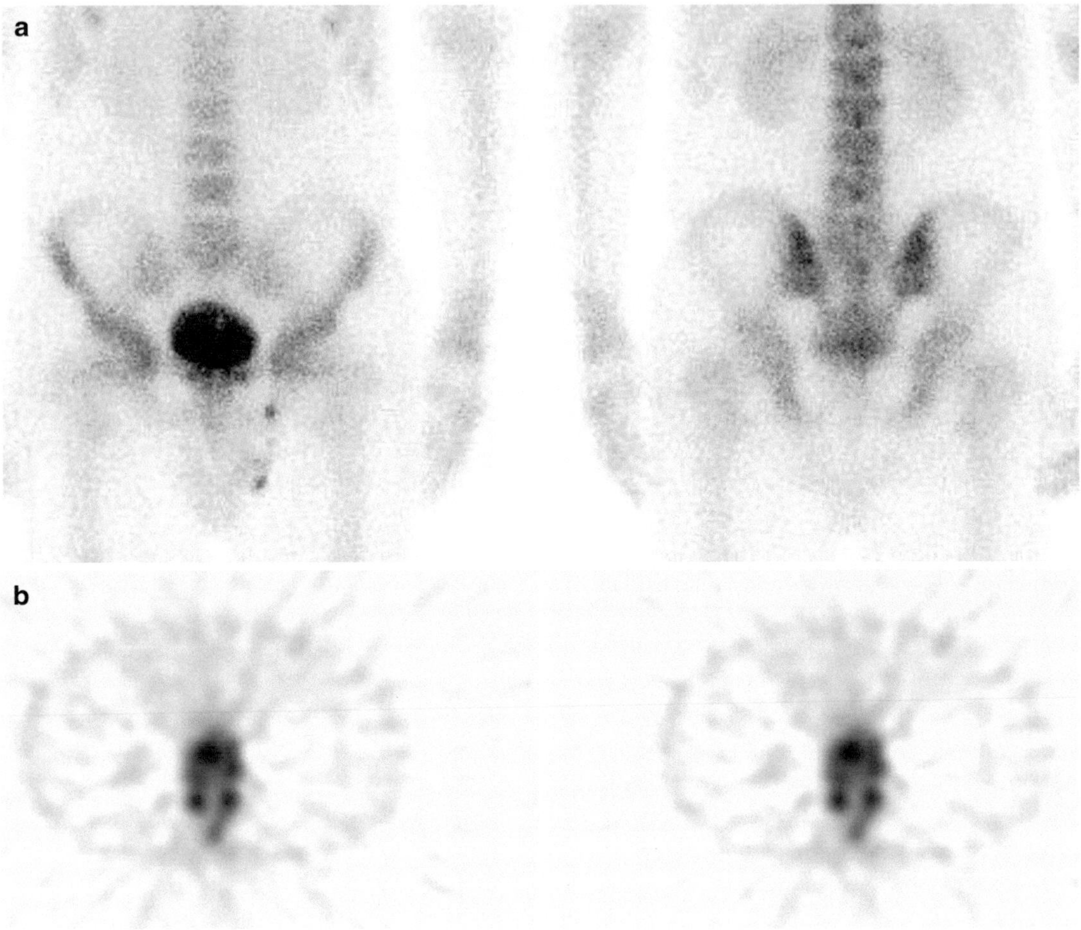

Fig. 10.24 Normal planar and positive SPECT. Facet joint disease in a patient with low back pain. The local views of spine show no abnormality (**a**). However, SPECT (**b**) of lumbosacral spine shows increased tracer uptake in the facet joints at the level of L5 vertebra, suggesting active inflammatory disease at this site. Note also some increased uptake in the vertebral body due to degenerative disease

be helpful in the investigation of metastatic disease in the spine. Not only is it possible to detect more lesions with SPECT, but by being able to accurately locate the position and observe the pattern of a lesion, it may be possible to differentiate benign from malignant lesions in the spine.

Studies of the hips with SPECT have been related to the investigation of avascular necrosis (AVN). Both idiopathic AVN in children (Legg-Calve-Perthes disease) and secondary AVN may be identified by SPECT bone scanning, with sensitivities approaching 90% being reported [95–97, 104–106, 107, 108].

In the knees the major interest in the use of SPECT is in the diagnosis of meniscal tears. Despite being primarily a soft tissue injury, increased bone uptake is seen probably as a result of altered joint mechanics due to the deficient meniscus with increased activity at the sites of increased stress. In the appropriate clinical setting, high sensitivities of approximately 90% have been reported with consistently better results than planar imaging alone [95–97, 109, 110]. The most specific pattern for a meniscal tear is an increase in vascularity on equilibrium images, abutting femoral and tibial condyle activity on delayed tomographic slices and a crescentic region of uptake on transaxial tibial slices corresponding to the injured meniscus [111]. Specific patterns have also been described in other ligamentous knee injuries including anterior cruciate ligament tears [110, 112] and lateral collateral ligament injury [113].

Temporomandibular joint (TMJ) dysfunction has a high prevalence, and bone SPECT has been proposed as a method to evaluate patients with this disorder. SPECT has been reported as being more sensitive than planar scintigraphy [114] as well as X-ray tomography [115].

Skull SPECT is helpful in malignant otitis externa in diabetic patients. Not only does SPECT appear to be more sensitive than CT [116], but also it may be possible to differentiate those with bone involvement from the less serious type where only soft tissues are affected [117].

The addition of tomography to bone scintigraphy allows accurate calculation of tracer uptake per volume of bone. By expressing regional activity in units of MBq/ml, it is possible to quantify bone turnover in different skeletal regions conceptually. This is still primarily a research application rarely carried out in clinical practice.

There is now clear evidence that SPECT adds to the diagnostic utility of bone scans, especially in the lumbar spine. Now that most departments with modern gamma cameras are able to make SPECT acquisitions, it should be possible to make use of the extra information available to improve accuracy in interpretation.

10.10 Bone SPECT/CT in Skeletal Disease

10.10.1 Orthopaedics: Pre- and Postoperative Scenario

Radiological imaging techniques such as ultrasound, CT and MRI are routinely used in the assessment of patients with bone pain in both pre- and postoperative clinical scenarios. CT provides cortical bone and MRI provides useful soft tissue details. In addition, ultrasound is often used to assess effusions and superficial structures. In general, the radiological techniques are prone to artefacts such as magnetic susceptibility artefacts and beam-hardening artefacts in MRI and CT, respectively. There are several hardware- and software-based artefact reduction algorithms available to overcome these limitations. 99mTc-MDP bone SPECT/CT is reported to be useful in the assessment of musculoskeletal conditions and is shown to be most useful in chronic scenarios with inconclusive results on radiological imaging techniques [118]. 99mTc-MDP bone SPECT/CT offers a useful combination of a high sensitivity (bone scan) and high specificity (CT) for bone pathology [118].

A significant number of patients complain of recurring or persistent pain after operative procedures, and it is often challenging to localize the cause of pain in postsurgical setting. Bone SPECT/CT imaging often provides useful information by accurately localizing and characterizing potential sites of pain or pain generators [118] (Figs. 10.25, 10.26, 10.27, 10.28, 10.29, 10.30, 10.31, 10.32, and 10.33). Recurrent back pain after lumbar spine surgery is due to multiple causes, and identifying the source of pain is often challenging. Bone SPECT/CT is useful to assess complications related to spinal surgery such as pseudoarthrosis, cage subsidence, hardware failure, facet joint degeneration, Instability, spondylolysis/spondylolisthesis, postoperative spondylodiskitis, etc. and should be used routinely in an appropriate clinical setting [119]. Bone SPECT/CT imaging is often used in the assessment of patients with recurrent pain after hip or knee arthroplasties and reported to be useful in the assessment of complications such as lysis/aseptic loosening, septic loosening, heterotopic ossification, periprosthetic fracture and tendinopathies [120–123]. Bone SPECT/CT can often contribute in the assessment of overloading or biodegradation problems [120, 122–124]. Due to complicated anatomy, assessment, and accurate localization of pain after foot and ankle surgery is challenging. Bone SPECT/CT is reported to be useful in the evaluation of ankle and foot pathologies in both pre- and postopera-

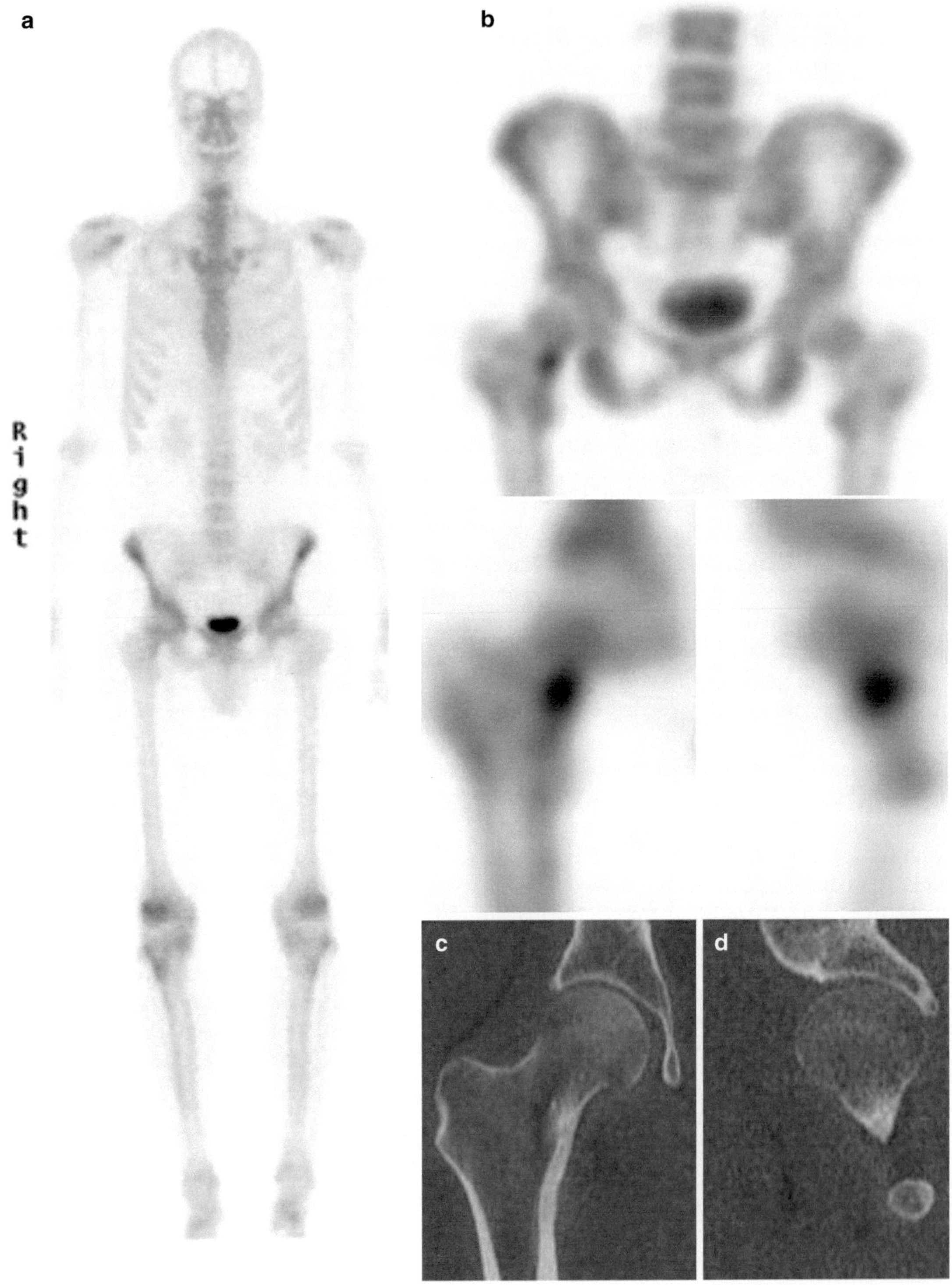

Fig. 10.25 Stress fracture: pain in the right hip,? Stress fracture or any other pain generators. There was normal blood flow and blood pool phase activity in both hips (not shown). (**a**) Whole-body planar imaging is unremarkable. (**b**) SPECT and (**c**, **d**) SPECT-CT through the hips reveals focal intense increased uptake within the inferior aspect of the right femoral neck. There is a subtle linear lucency through the cortex in this location, in keeping with a stress fracture

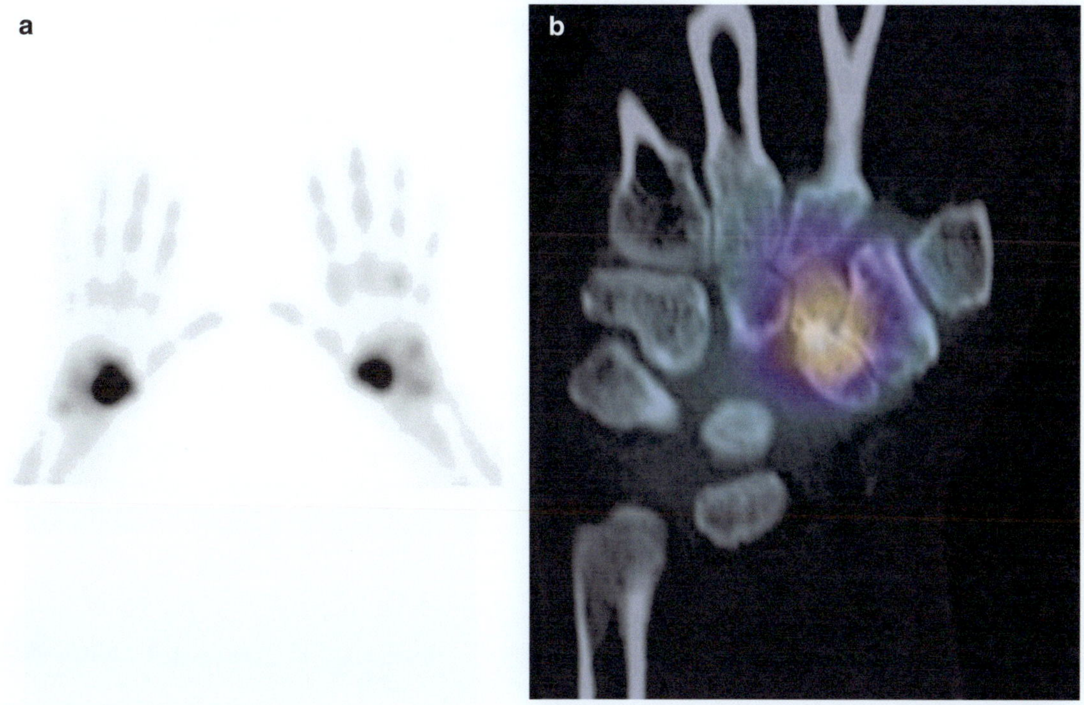

Fig. 10.26 Scaphotrapeziotrapezoidal (STT) arthropathy: patient presented with right base of thumb pain. (**a**) SPECT image shows increased tracer uptake at the radial aspect of the distal carpal row bilaterally. (**b**) On the SPECT-CT (right hand), the epicentre of intense tracer uptake localizes to the ulnar aspect of the trapezium, extending to involve the palmar aspect of the STT joint. Degenerative changes are seen at the STT joint, most severe in the trapezium

tive setting [118, 125]. In general, hand and wrist surgery is often performed in traumatic, degenerative, malformed, neoplastic or inflammatory/infectious diseases, and persistent pain can be caused by non-union, malposition, secondary osteoarthritis (OA) and infection [126], and bone SPECT/CT can help in assessment of persistent pain after hand and wrist surgery. Overall, current literature regarding SPECT/CT of in orthopaedics both in pre- and postoperative scenario is limited, but it is evolving and there is significant potential to expand application of SPECT/CT in the future (Tables 10.4 and 10.5).

10.10.2 Bone SPECT/CT in Oncology

In general, conventional whole body bone scan has relatively reduced specificity as previously discussed, and several studies have shown addition of bone SPECT/CT reduces the rate of indeterminate lesions when compared to planar whole body or SPECT alone [142–145]. Bone SPECT/CT is useful in differentiating metastatic lesions from benign lesions (e.g. osteophytes, facet joint disease and endplate degenerative and fractures) and helps in accurate localization and making a definite diagnosis in most cases. Currently in most of nuclear medicine departments, a whole-body planar scan is followed, by a localized SPECT/CT to characterize indeterminate lesions as seen on planar whole-body scans (Figs. 10.32, 10.33, and 10.34). Further, several centres in Europe are moving towards whole-body bone SPECT/CT imaging, and in the near future, it may replace conventional planar whole-body bone scans [149, 150].

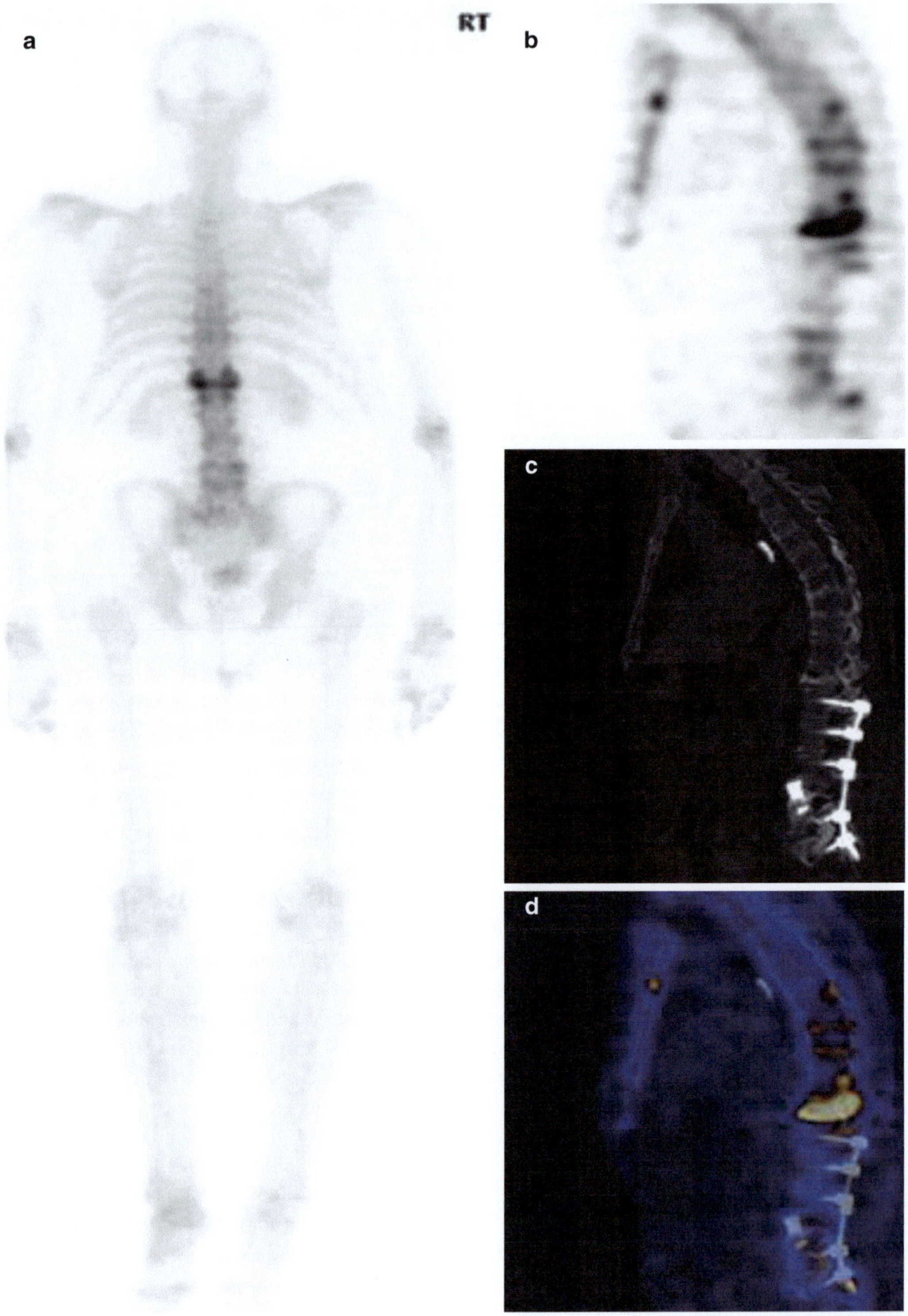

Fig. 10.27 Adjacent segment degeneration: patient with previous lumbar spine surgery and back pain. (**a**) Whole-body bone scan shows inhomogeneous tracer uptake in the spine with more linear increased tracer uptake at T12 vertebra. (**b–d**) On SPECT/CT, the linear increased tracer uptake is seen above and adjacent to the cage reconstruction site at T12 vertebra and is compatible with a recent fracture. There is no significant abnormal tracer activity in the lumbar spine

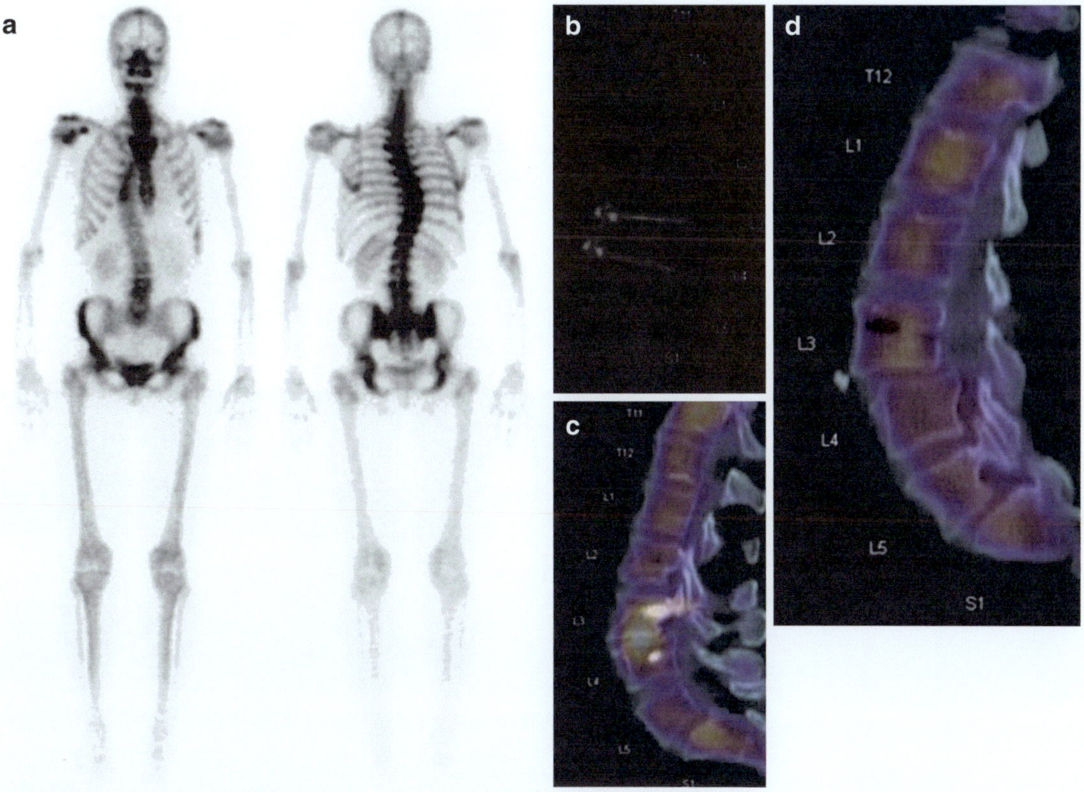

Fig. 10.28 Fracture of the pedicle screw: patient with back pain after L3–4 decompression surgery 5 years ago. (**a**) Whole-body bone scan shows scoliosis of the lumbar spine convex to the left centred on L3, with a thoracic scoliosis convex to the right. (**b**) On the CT scan, note is made of a previous right sided posterolateral stabilisation of L3–4. The L4 pedicle screw has fractured. (**c**) On the fused SPECT/CT, there is intense increased uptake in the right side of the L3–4 intervertebral joint, where there is loss of joint space, osteophyte formation and endplate sclerosis. (**d**) Grade 1 spondylolisthesis noted at L3–4

10.11 Positron Emission Tomography (PET) in Skeletal Disease

^{18}FDG is the most widely used oncological PET tracer, but to date there has been little work on the use of pet specifically in bone. ^{18}FDG PET has the advantage of better spatial resolution than conventional bone scans, and even if one is primarily interested in the bone, it does provide additional information regarding soft tissue disease (Fig. 10.35).

In breast carcinoma, the literature is far from clear as to whether ^{18}FDG PET is more sensitive than the conventional bone scan in identification of bone metastases [151]. However, early observations in the use of this technique in women with metastatic breast cancer showed that significantly more bone metastases are detected compared to ^{99m}Tc-MDP scintigraphy. This may be due to a combination of the physical advantages of PET and because ^{18}FDG localizes in tumour rather than bone and so may detect metastases before they are large enough to cause a bone reaction [151].

Lonneux et al. studied women with breast cancer who were treated with surgery, both with and without chemotherapy and radiotherapy. They concluded ^{18}FDG PET was more sensitive than the bone scan in detecting skeletal metastases [152]. A study from ohta in patients with breast

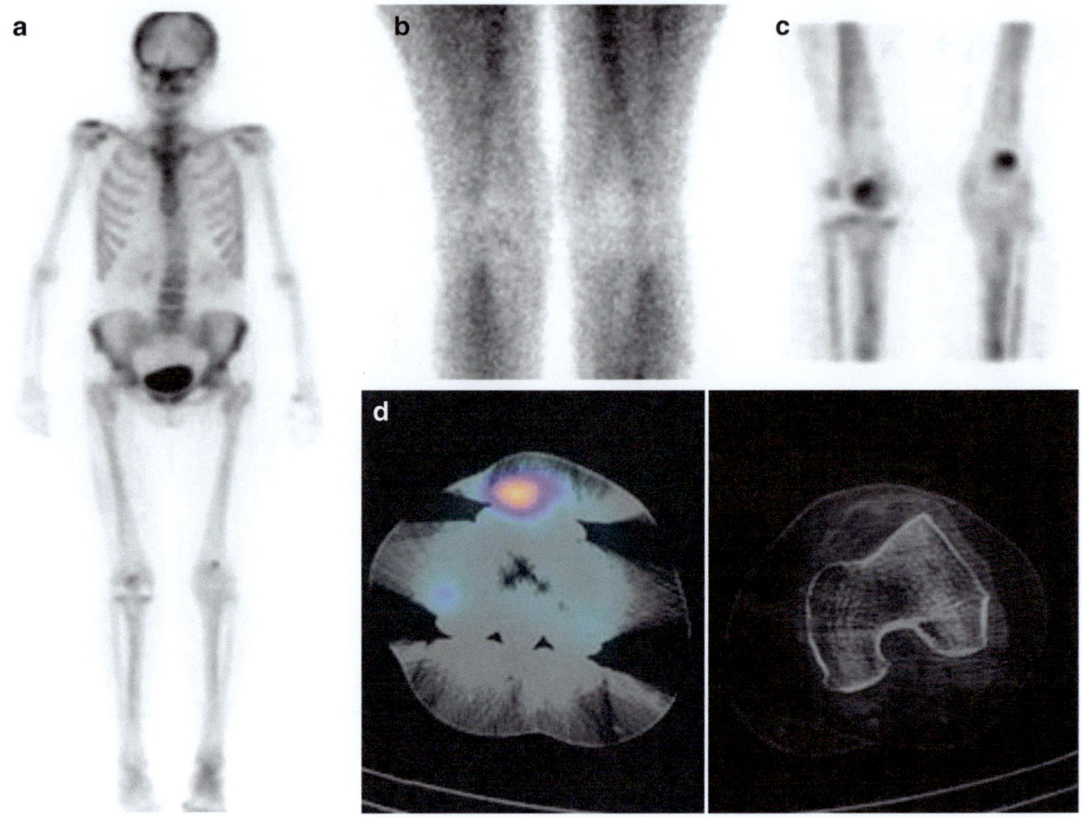

Fig. 10.29 Patellofemoral degeneration: painful right total knee replacement,? Evidence of infection/loosening. (**a**) Whole-body planar imaging reveals a scoliosis of the lumbar spine convex to the left. There is physiological uptake throughout the rest the skeleton except for minor increased tracer uptake in the patellofemoral joints bilaterally. (**b**) Blood pool phase shows normal activity in the right knee. (**c**) On the SPECT image (coronal), there is increased tracer uptake in the patellofemoral joints. (**d**) SPECT CT of the right knee replacement reveals normal tracer uptake surrounding both femoral and tibial components. Most intense uptake is within the lateral aspect of the right patella, adjacent to the articular surface, suggestive of patellofemoral degeneration. No evidence of loosening or infection of the right knee replacement

cancer found that both ^{18}FDG PET and the bone scan had identical sensitivity (77.7%) but that ^{18}FDG PET was more specific (97.6% vs. 80.9%) [153]. Cook et al. found that patients who had either lytic or a mixed pattern of disease had a higher number of lesions identified on ^{18}FDG PET than on the isotope bone scan, but for the subgroup with sclerotic lesions, a lower number was seen [154]. It has been suggested that while there may be differences in the glycolytic rate between these types of metastases, sclerotic lesions have much smaller tumour volume relative to the size of the whole skeletal lesion and may therefore simply be less likely to be identified.

Prostate cancer is now established as the "classic" cancer with false-negative results on ^{18}FDG PET. These observations concur with those of Shreve et al. who noted only 65% sensitivity for the detection of skeletal metastases from prostate cancer, which is predominantly osteoblastic, when using ^{18}FDG compared to

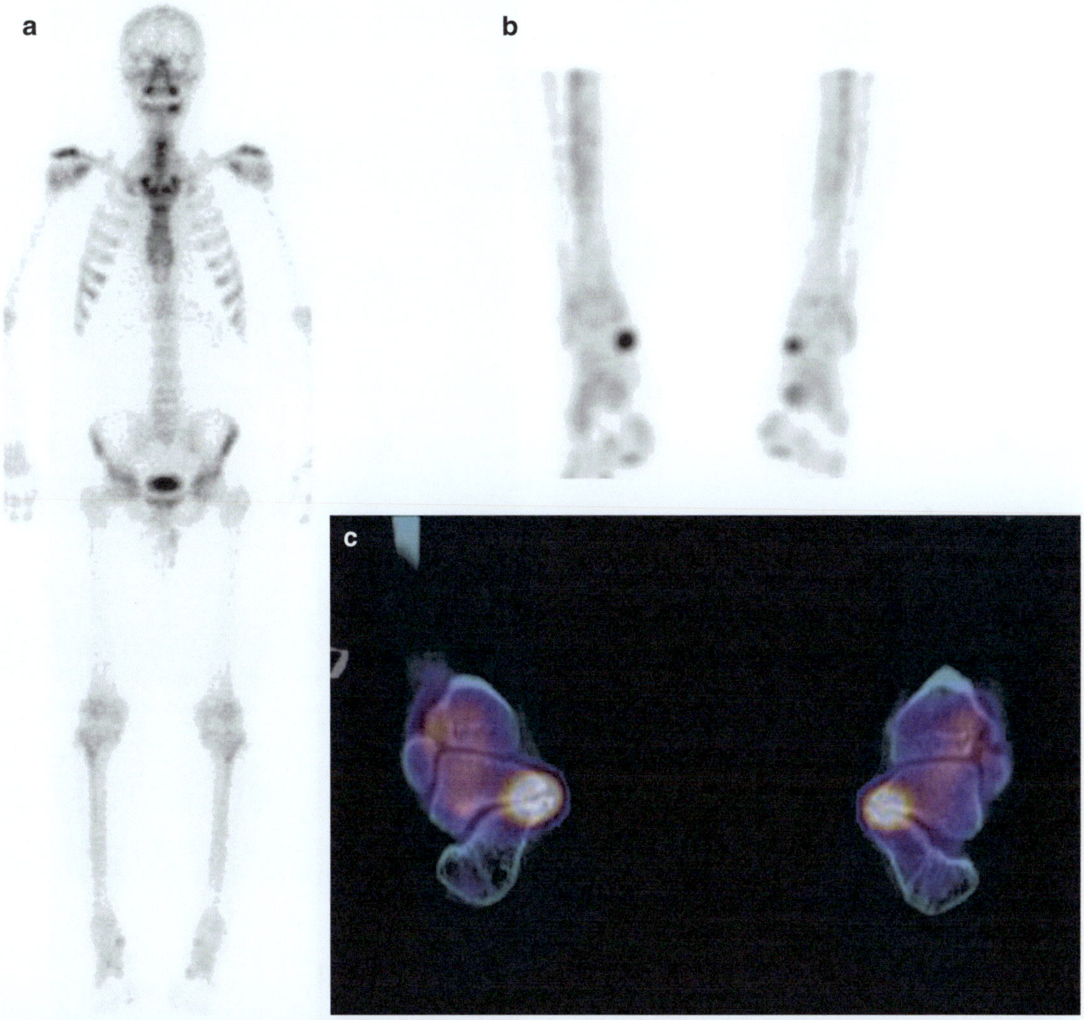

Fig. 10.30 Bilateral fibrous talocalcaneal coalition. Patient with left hindfoot pain, MRI showing subtalar joint arthropathy, but no effect from subtalar injection. (**a**) Whole-body planar imaging reveals low-grade foci in the mid- and hindfeet medially. (**b**) Coronal SPECT shows focal increased tracer uptake in the ankles medially. (**c**) On delayed SPECT CT imaging of the feet and ankles, there is focal intense tracer uptake associated with the talocalcaneal fibrous coalition bilaterally suggesting a symptomatic pseudoarthrosis

^{99m}Tc-MDP [155]. However, Morris et al. in their study in patients with progressive metastatic prostate cancer concluded that ^{18}FDG PET could discriminate active osseous disease from scintigraphically quiescent lesions [156]. In patients with lung cancer, both the Bury and Gayed studies reached essentially identical conclusions, i.e. that both techniques had similar sensitivity for the detection of bone metastases but that ^{18}FDG PET was more specific [157, 158].

There is relatively little in the literature relating to lymphoma (Fig. 10.35) and the skeleton, but ^{18}FDG PET seems to perform better than the bone scan [159], and there is an increasing body of evidence relating to the

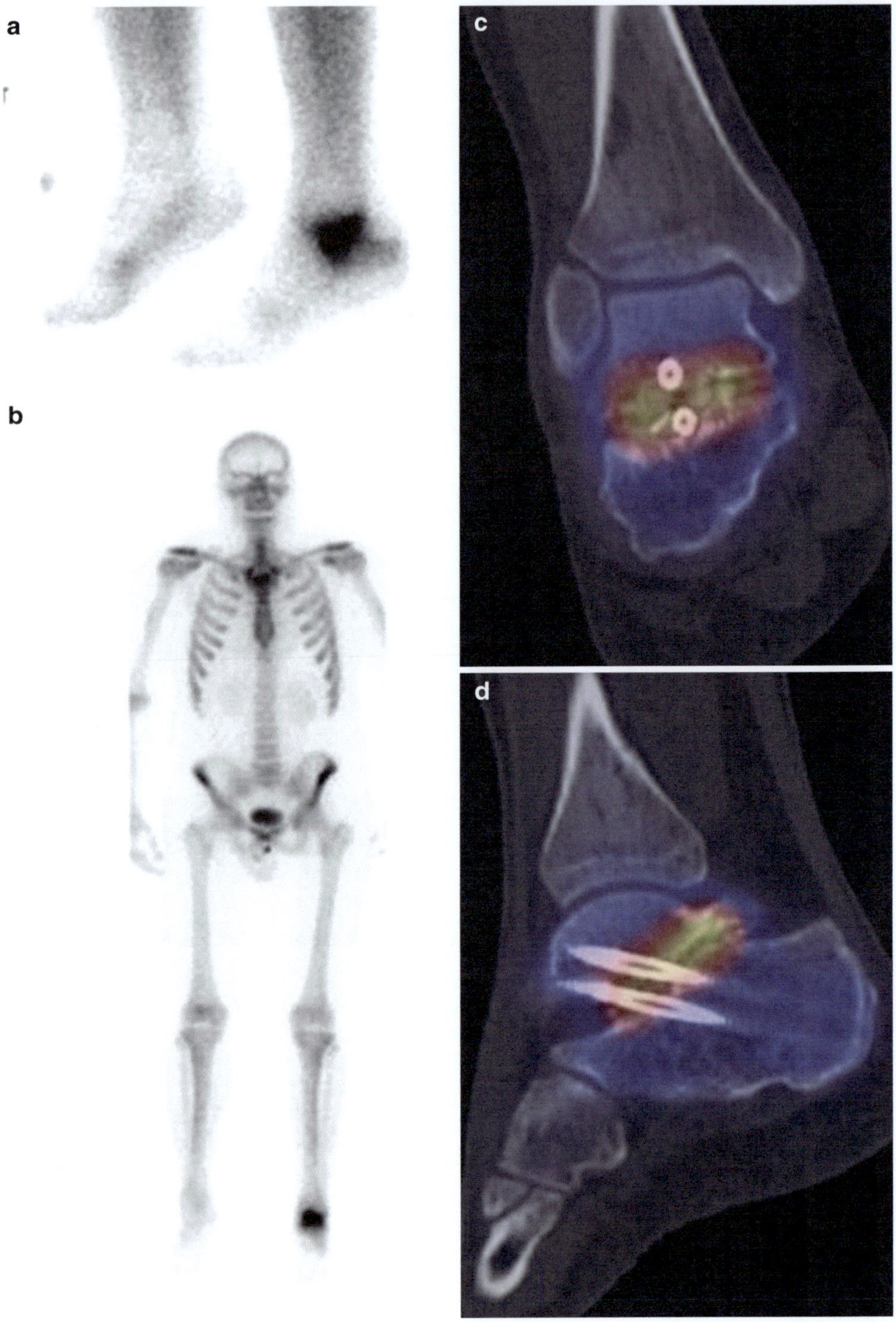

Fig. 10.31 Non-union: left subtalar joint fusion with allograft? Non-union. (**a**) On blood pool image and (**b**) on delayed whole-body image, there is marked increased tracer activity in the left hindfoot. (**c**, **d**) On delayed SPECT CT imaging, there is intense tracer uptake within the posterior facet of the subtalar joint. Note is made of an attempted fusion, but there is a persistent pseudoarthrosis at this level with no evidence of cross-trabeculation seen on CT. The appearances in the left hindfoot are consistent with a non-union of the attempted subtalar joint fusion. There were no features to suggest infection or metalwork failure

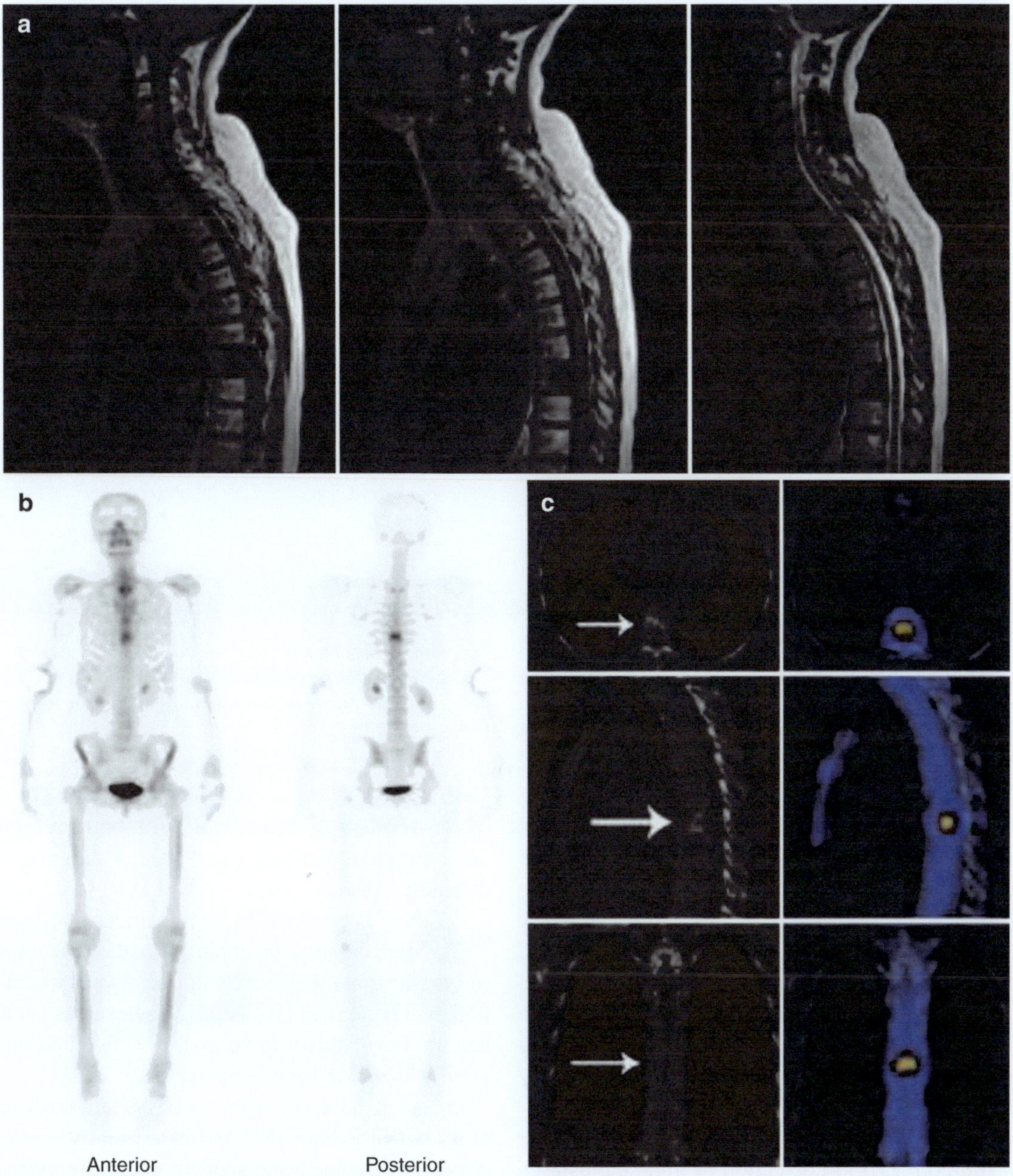

Fig. 10.32 Bone metastasis. (**a–c**) A 51-year-old lady with known breast carcinoma, status postmastectomy, presented with pain in the thoracic and lumbar vertebrae, worse at night. (**a**) MR images of spine (T1, T2 and STIR sagittal sequences) show low signal intensity lesion in the D8 vertebral body, which raises possibility of a metastasis. (**b**) Whole-body bone scan shows focal increased tracer uptake in the D8 vertebra. (**c**) SPECT-CT of thoracic spine localizes the abnormal tracer uptake seen in whole body study to a sclerotic lesion in the D8 vertebral body (arrows), compatible with solitary bone metastasis

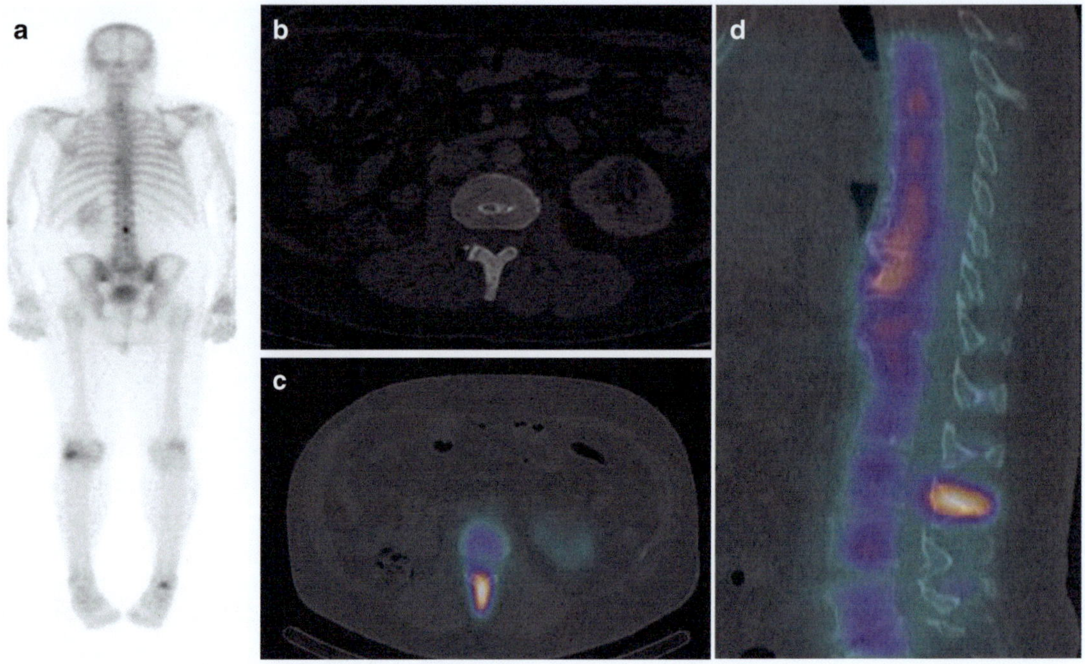

Fig. 10.33 Bone metastasis: right nephrectomy for renal cancer (**a**) whole-body bone scan shows a focal area of increased tracer uptake in the mid lumbar spine. (**c**, **d**) On the fused SPECT-CT images, the epicentre of intense tracer uptake localizes to the spinous process of L2 vertebra with corresponding sclerosis on the CT scan (**b**). Degenerative disease at left T8 costovertebral joint, left knee joint lateral compartment and right hindfoot on the whole-body study

valuable role of FDG PET in myeloma [160, 162], where it is clearly better than the bone scan (although this is hardly an area where the bone scan shines), and this is presumably because ^{18}FDG is identifying marrow-based disease at an early stage (Fig. 10.36).

There is very little data in the literature regarding the use of ^{18}FDG PET in monitoring the response of bone metastases to therapy (Fig. 10.37).

Recent report on use of 18F-labeled NaF (18F-NaF PET) in detection of bone metastases is encouraging and has been shown to be significantly more accurate in detecting bone metastases than ^{99m}Tc-MDP scans [161, 163]. Uptake of the fluoride ion (^{18}F) is twofold higher than that of ^{99m}Tc-polyphosphonates [164]. However, it is difficult to differentiate benign from malignant ^{18}F-fluoride uptake [165]. The high sensitivity of ^{18}F-sodium fluoride (NaF) for both benign and malignant lesions may pose a diagnostic dilemma [164].

^{18}F-NaF is reported to be more sensitive than ^{99m}Tc-MDP bone scan, mainly for the detection of lytic lesions, which may not be always identified on a bone scan [160–163]. However, as yet it has not been shown to be cost effective and not readily available for routine use.

A lesion-based comparison by Schirrmeister et al. with ^{18}F-NaF PET indicated that the sensitivity of planar bone scan in detecting vertebral bone metastases was as low as 40%. However, the sensitivity ranged from 80% to 90% in the skull, thorax and extremities [161, 163]. It is suggested that the sensitivity of ^{99m}Tc-MDP could be improved by additional SPECT imaging [166] However, in the assessment of the entire vertebral column, two

Table 10.4 Common clinical applications and advantages of bone SPECT/CT

Clinical application	Advantages/current evidence
Low back pain: Pre- and postoperative 1. Localizing metabolically active facet joints 2. Localizing alternate metabolically active pain generators 3. Assessment of complications related to postoperative spine 4. Mechanical/hardware complications	Precise localization Identifies other potential causes of recurrent low back pain Compliment's clinical diagnosis Guides therapy Procedure of choice for patients with low back pain after lumbar fusion surgery Highly sensitive and specific tool for the exclusion of screw loosening ([127]; [128]; [129]. [130]; [131]; [132]; [133])
Hand and wrist pain: Pre- and postoperative 1. Localizing abnormal metabolic active sites 2. Detecting post-traumatic bone remodeling 3. Detecting occult fractures which are often missed in other modalities	High lesion detection rates compared to standard X-rays and planar bone scan Good inter-observer agreement Significant impact on patient management Beneficial to integrate into the diagnostic imaging algorithm ([134]; [135])
Foot and ankle pain: Pre and postoperative 1. Localization and characterization of abnormal increased tracer uptake in the foot and ankle joints 2. Localizing alternate metabolically active pain generators 3. Assessment of postoperative complications 4. Mechanical/hardware complications	Complementary and comparable diagnostic performance with MRI Useful in localizing And characterizing impingement syndrome and soft tissue pathology ([136]; [137])
Pelvis and hip pain: Pre- and postoperative 1. Evaluation of painful joint prostheses evaluating aseptic and septic loosening of hip prosthesis 2. Identifying potential pain generators 3. Evaluation of bone viability 4. Mechanical/hardware complications	Increased diagnostic accuracy in the evaluation of aseptic and septic loosening in hip prostheses Significantly better than planar scanning for the acetabular cup loosening but not for the femoral stem ([138], [139])
Knee pain: Pre- and postoperative 1. Evaluation of painful joint prostheses evaluating aseptic and septic loosening of hip prostheses 2. Identifying potential pain generators 3. Mechanical/hardware complications	Increased diagnostic accuracy in the evaluation of aseptic and septic loosening in hip Significantly better than planar scanning in assessment femoral component with superior results in assessment of tibial component Ideal imaging modality for evaluation of patellofemoral disorders after knee replacements ([140]; [141]; [139]; [120], [123])
Indeterminate lesions in oncology patients	Accurate localization and characterization Improved sensitivity, specificity and accuracy Outperforms SPECT alone for the interpretation of skeletal lesions Definitive diagnosis and reduction of equivocal lesions Accurately differentiates benign from malignant lesions Increases diagnostic confidence ([142]; [143], [144]; [145]; [146]; [147]; [148] [149] [150])

SPECT acquisitions might be necessary, and this increases the acquisition time and also the risk of movement during acquisition. These factors can reduce spatial localization with SPECT when compared with ^{18}F-NaF PET [166]. Overall the problem seems to be more technical than biological; hence, ^{18}F-NaF PET will become more attractive in the future, though the reported accuracies of ^{18}F-NaF PET and of SPECT were not statistically significant [166]. But this was a small study, and it is probable that future studies will confirm the advantages of ^{18}F-NaF PET (Figs. 10.38, 10.39, 10.40, and 10.41).

Table 10.5 Suggested indications and acquisition parameters for skeletal scintigraphy of major joints using multimodality SPECT/CT equipment

Region	SPECT/CT indication	SPECT acquisition	Attenuation correction or localization CT	Diagnostic CT
Spine	If planar imaging is non-diagnostic, usually late-phase SPECT/CT To help identify patients with low back pain who would benefit from facet joint infiltration In the postsurgery setting (with or without implants)	LEHR collimators matrix 128 × 128 60–128 angles 15–20 s/angle step mode noncircular rotation	2.5–40 mA 80–130 keV 1–5 mm slice thickness	40–335 mA 80–130 keV 0.33–2.0 mm slice thickness
Hand and wrist	If planar imaging is non-diagnostic, usually late-phase SPECT/CT	LEHR collimators matrix 128 × 128,128 angles 20 s/angle step mode noncircular rotation	2.5–40 mA 80–130 keV 1–5 mm slice thickness	40–335 mA 80–130 keV 0.33–2.0 mm slice thickness
Hips	If planar imaging is non-diagnostic, usually late-phase SPECT/CT particularly useful for evaluation of hip prosthesis	LEHR collimators matrix 128 × 128,128 angles 20 s/angle step mode noncircular rotation	2.5–40 mA 80–130 keV 1–5 mm slice thickness	40–335 mA 80–130 keV 0.33–2.0 mm slice thickness
Knee	If planar imaging is non-diagnostic, usually late-phase SPECT/CT Particularly useful for the evaluation of knee prosthesis	LEHR collimators matrix 128 × 128,128 angles 20 s/angle step mode noncircular rotation	2.5–40 mA 80–130 keV 1–5 mm slice thickness	40–335 mA 80–130 keV 0.33–2.0 mm slice thickness

Modified from The EANM practice guidelines for bone scintigraphy-T. Van den Wyngaert et al. Eur J Nucl Med Mol Imaging. 2016; 43: 1723–1738

Note: (a) Whole-body image acquisition should be considered in patients with suspected malignancy (metastatic, primary), rheumatoid arthritis, elevated alkaline phosphatase level, metabolic bone disorders, hyperparathyroidism (brown tumours, superscan, soft tissue uptake in lung, stomach, kidneys, heart or pancreas), infectious disease. (b) Routine early blood pool and delayed static images of region is recommended for the aforementioned joints in postoperative indications if the clinical question is infection/inflammation, and (c) CT settings are variable depending on local requirements/protocols/cameras

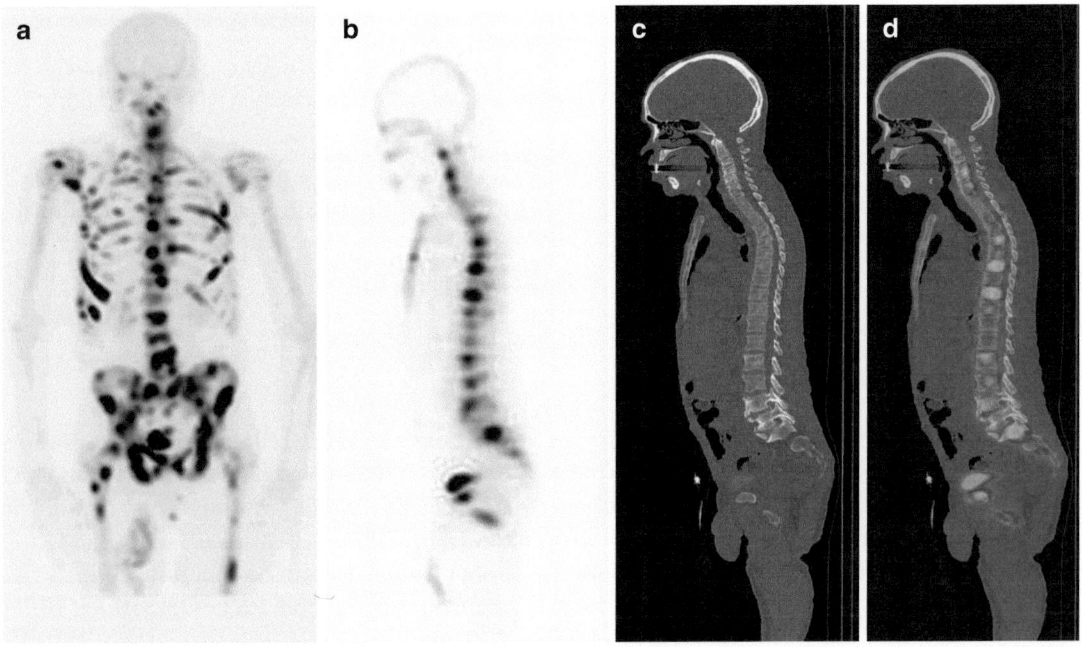

Fig. 10.34 Bone metastases: 99mTc-MDP SPECT-CT (vertex to thighs). (**a**) MIP images show widespread multifocal increased tracer uptake within the axial and appendicular skeleton. (**b**) The sagittal SPECT image shows multifoci increased tracer uptake in the spine which correspond to bone metastases in multiple vertebrae (**c**, **d**) (Image Courtesy Dr. A. Parthipun)

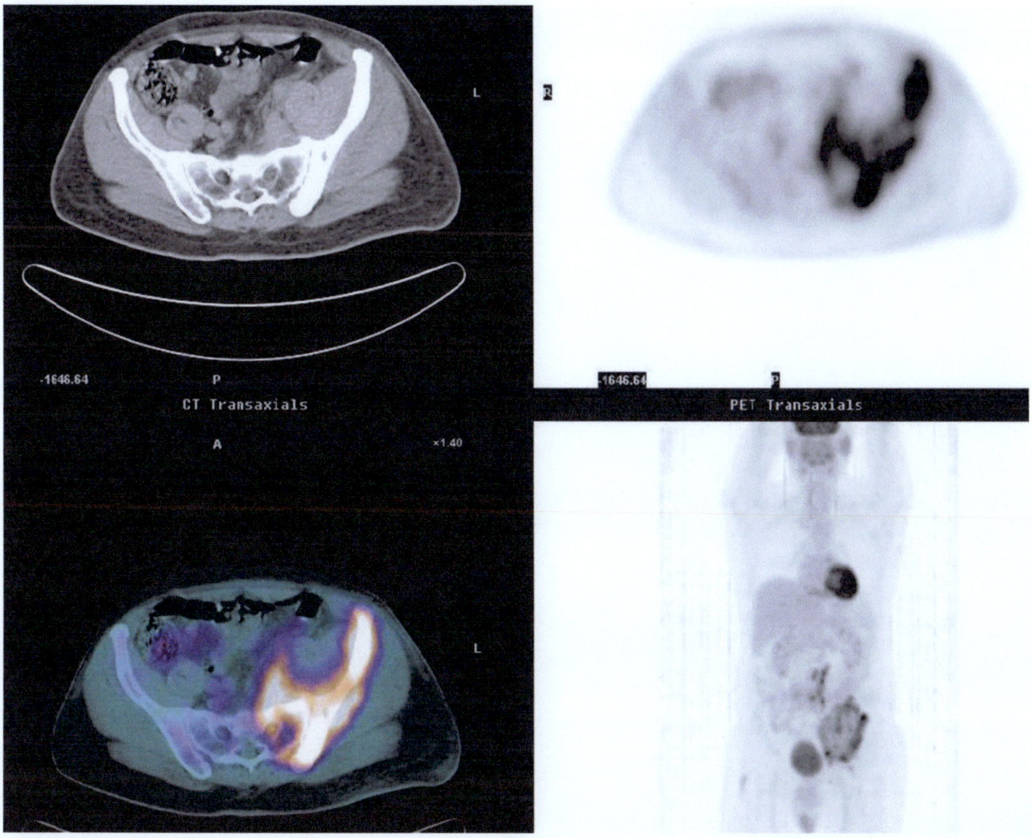

Fig. 10.35 Bone lymphoma: 18F-FDG PET/CT scan in a patient with lymphoma involving the left hemipelvis and adjacent soft tissue

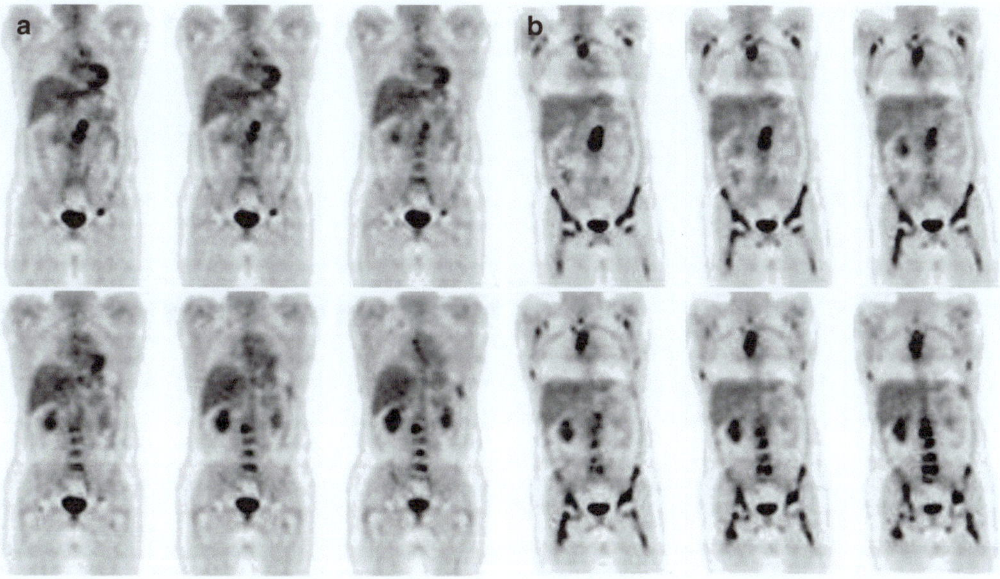

Fig. 10.36 (**a**) Bone marrow: 18F-FDG PET scan in NHL with bone marrow and nodal involvement. (**b**) Progression with widespread intense focal FDG uptake in bone marrow and nodes after transformation into a high-grade lymphoma

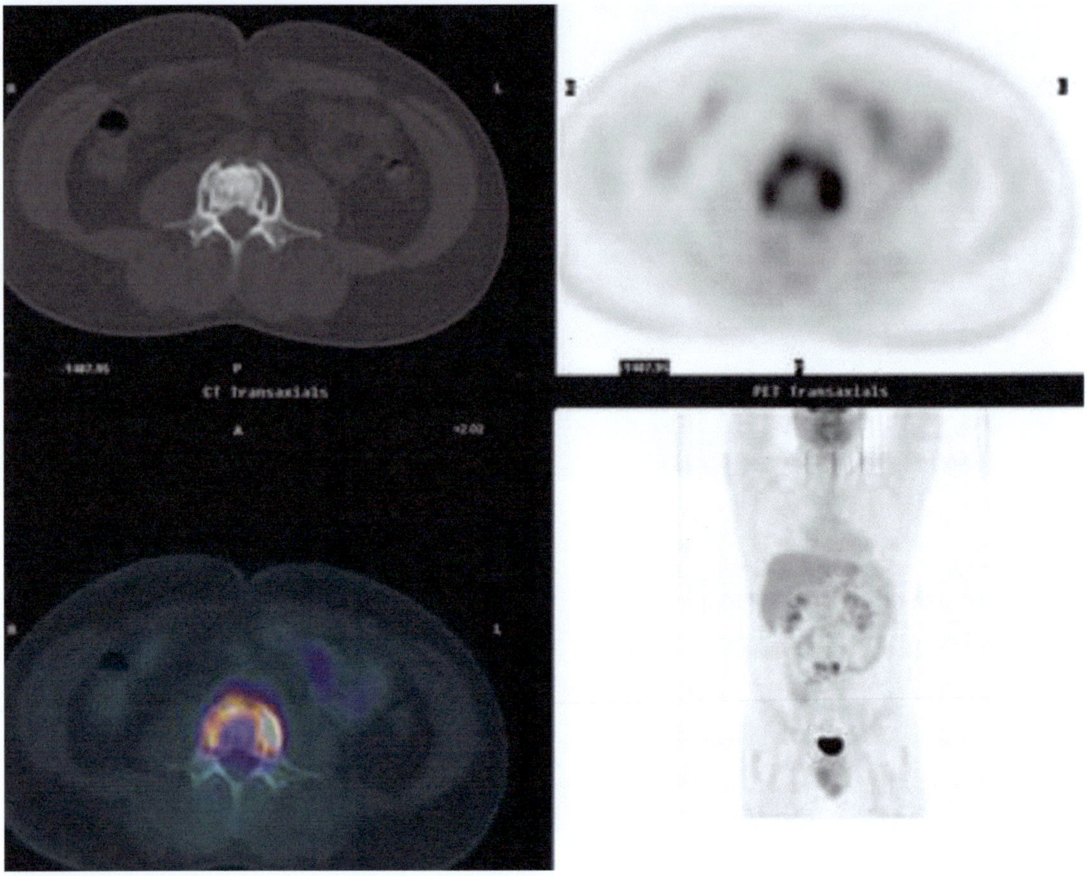

Fig. 10.37 Plasmacytoma: 18F-FDG PET/CT scan in a patient with a treated plasmacytoma (with radiotherapy) in the lumbar spine with rising tumour markers. CT shows sclerotic changes due to previous treatment and PET reveals new disease in the surrounding marrow

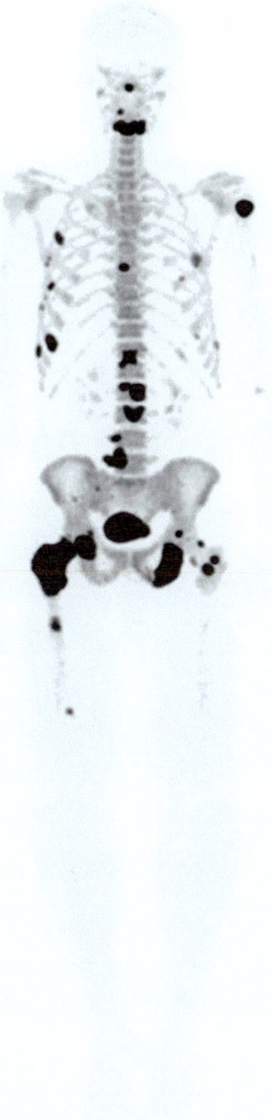

Fig. 10.38 Prostate cancer. 18F-NaF PET scan shows multiple foci of abnormal increased tracer uptake in multiple ribs, multiple vertebrae, left humerus, pelvis and femora bilaterally consistent with multiple bone metastases (Image Courtesy Dr. S. Usmani)

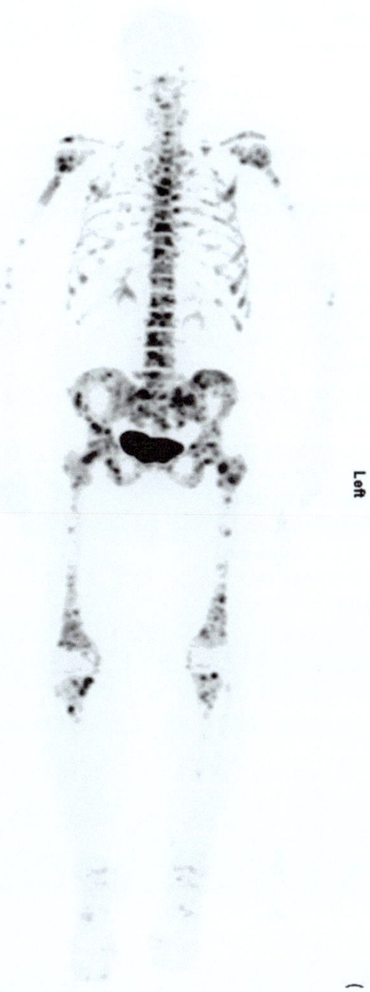

Fig. 10.39 Breast cancer. 18F-NaF PET scan shows multiple foci of abnormal increased tracer uptake in the axial and appendicular skeleton consistent with widespread bone metastases (Image Courtesy Dr. S. Usmani)

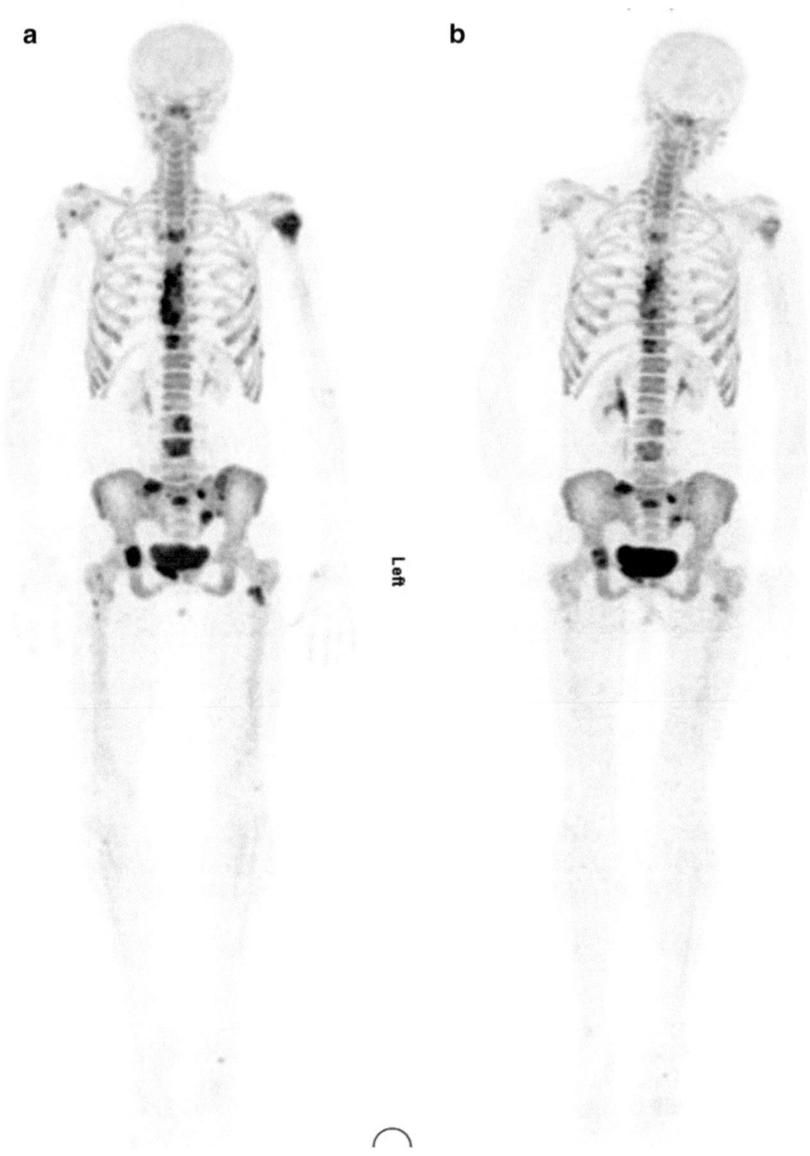

Fig. 10.40 Breast cancer treatment response: 18F-NaF PET scan (**a**) shows multiple foci of abnormal increased tracer uptake in the sternum, multiple ribs, multiple vertebrae, left humerus, pelvis and femora bilaterally consistent with multiple bone metastases, and following chemotherapy there is relatively reduced tracer uptake at these sites (**b**) suggesting of ongoing metabolic response to treatment with no new sites of abnormal increased tracer uptake (Image Courtesy Dr. S. Usmani)

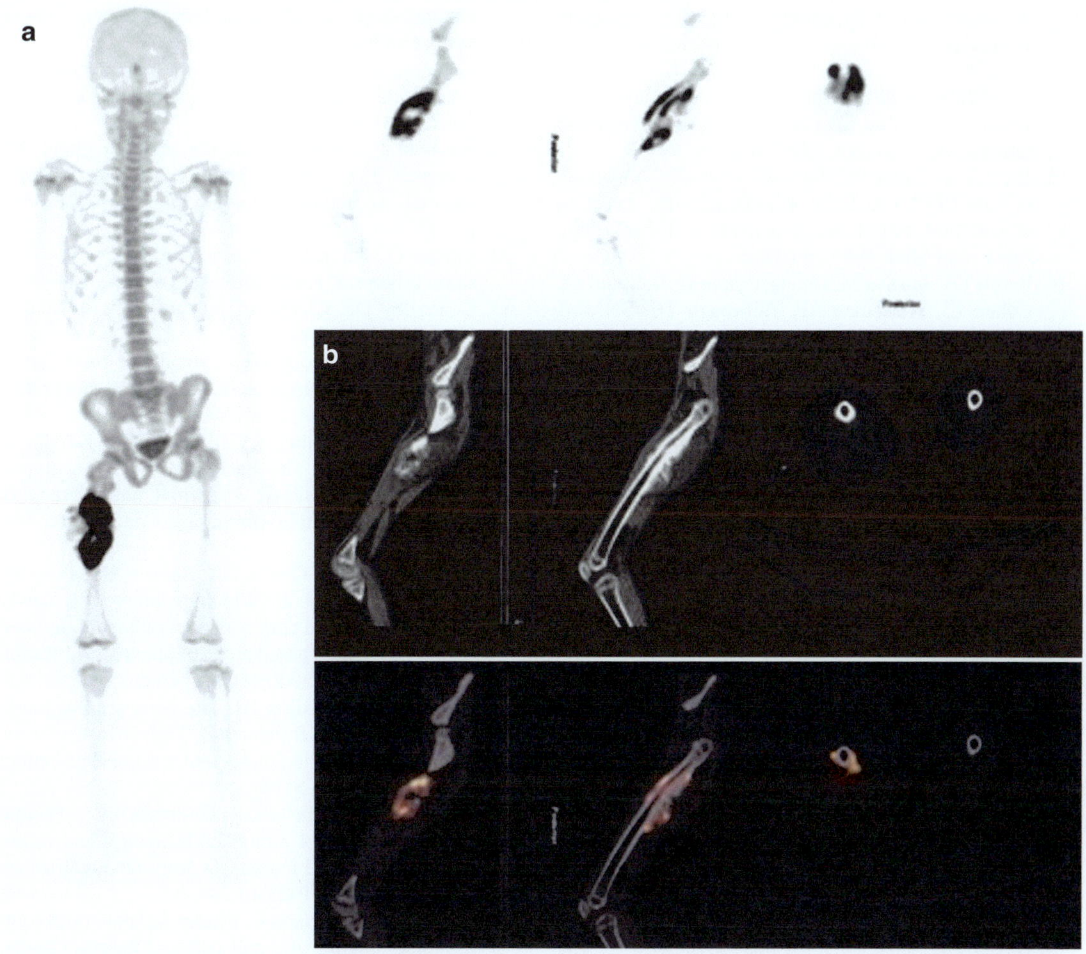

Fig. 10.41 Bone tumour: an 8-year-old female with chondroblastic osteosarcoma of right femur. 18F-NaF-PET-CT. (**a**) MIP images and (**b**) fused PET-CT images show increase tracer uptake at right mid femur with no abnormal foci of increased tracer uptake elsewhere (Image Courtesy Dr. S. Usmani)

References

1. Chiewitz P, Hevesy G. Radioactive indicators in the study of phosphorus metabolism in rats. Nature. 1935;136:754–5.
2. Fleming WH, McIraith JD, King ER. Photoscanning of bone lesions utilising strontium-85. Radiology. 1961;77:635–6.
3. Davis MA, Jones AL. Comparison of 99mTc-labeled phosphate and phosphonate agents for skeletal imaging. Semin Nucl Med. 1976;6:19–31.
4. Subramanian G, McAfee JG. A new complex of Tc-99m for skeletal imaging. Radiology. 1971;99:192–6.
5. Blau M, Nagler W, Bender MA. Fluorine-18: a new isotope for bone scanning. J Nucl Med. 1962;3:332–4.
6. Subramanian G, McAfee JG, Bell EG, et al. 99m Tc-labeled polyphosphate as a skeletal imaging agent. Radiology. 1972;102:701–4.
7. Fogelman I. Diphosphonate bone scanning agents – current concepts. Eur J Nucl Med. 1982;7:506–9.
8. Caner B, Kitapcl M, Unlu M, Erbengi G, Calikoglu T, Gogus T, Bekdik C. Technetium-99m-MIBI uptake in benign and malignant bone lesions: a comparative study with technetium-99m-MDP. J Nucl Med. 1992;33:319–24.
9. Elgazzar AH, Malki AA, Abdel-Dayem HM, Sahweil A, Razzak S, Jahan S, El-Sayed M, Omar YT. Role of thallium-201 in the diagnosis of solitary bone lesions. Nucl Med Commun. 1989;10:477–85.
10. Lam AS, Kettle AG, O'Doherty MJ, et al. Pentavalent 99Tcm-DMSA imaging in patients with bone metastases. Nucl Med Commun. 1997;18:907–14.
11. Blau M, Ganatra R, Bender MA. 18 F-fluoride for bone imaging. Semin Nucl Med. 1972;2:31–7.
12. Warburg O. On the origin of cancer cells. Science. 1954;123:306–14.
13. Yamamoto T, Seino Y, Fukumoto H, et al. Over-expression of facilitative glucose transporter genes

in human cancer. Biochem Biophys Res Commun. 1990;170:223–30.
14. Bushnell DL, Kahn D, Huston B, Bevering CG. Utility of SPECT imaging for determination of vertebral metastases in patients with known primary tumors. Skelet Radiol. 1995;24:13–6.
15. Han LJ, Au-Yong TK, Tong WCM, et al. Comparison of bone SPECT and planar imaging in the detection of vertebral metastases in patients with back pain. Eur J Nucl Med. 1998;25:635–8.
16. Bartel TB, Kuruva M, Gnanasegaran G, Beheshti M, Cohen EJ, Weissman AF, Yarbrough TL. SNMMI procedure standard for bone scintigraphy 4.0. J Nucl Med Technol. 2018;46(4):398–404.
17. Van den Wyngaert T, Strobel K, Kampen WU, Kuwert T, et al. The EANM practice guidelines for bone scintigraphy. Eur J Nucl Med Mol Imaging. 2016;43(9):1723–38.
18. Lassmann M, Treves ST. Paediatric radiopharmaceutical administration: harmonization of the 2007 EANM paediatric dosage card (version 1.5.2008) and the 2010 North American consensus guidelines. Eur J Nucl Med Mol Imaging. 2014;41:1036–41.
19. Stauss J, Hahn K, Mann M, De Palma D. Guidelines for paediatric bone scanning with 99mTc-labelled radiopharmaceuticals and 18F-fluoride. Eur J Nucl Med Mol Imaging. 2010;37:1621–8.
20. Segall G, Delbeke D, Stabin MG, Even-Sapir E, Fair J, Sajdak R, Smith GT. SNM practice guideline for sodium 18F-fluoride PET/CT bone scans 1.0. J Nucl Med. 2010;51(11):1813–20.
21. Tofe AJ, Francis MD, Harvey WJ. Correlation of neoplasms with incidence and localisation of skeletal metastases. An analysis Of 1355 diphosphonate bone scans. J Nucl Med. 1975;16:986–9.
22. Baxter AD, Coakley FV, Finlay DB, West C. The aetiology of solitary hot spots in the ribs on planar bone scans. Nucl Med Commun. 1995;16:834–7.
23. Tumeh SS, Beadle G, Kaplan WD. Clinical significance of solitary rib lesions in patients with extraskeletal malignancy. J Nucl Med. 1985;26:1140–3.
24. Coakley FV, Jones AR, Finlay DB, Belton IP. The aetiology and distinguishing features of solitary spinal hot spots on planar bone scans. Clin Radiol. 1995;50:327–30.
25. Coleman RE, Rubens RD, Fogelman I. A reappraisal of the baseline bone scan in breast cancer. J Nucl Med. 1988;29:1045–9.
26. Galasko CSB. Skeletal metastases, vol. 1986. London: Butterworth; 1986.
27. Coleman RE, Mashiter G, Whitaker KB, Moss DW, Rubens RD, Fogelman I. Bone scan flare predicts successful systemic therapy for bone metastases. J Nucl Med. 1988;29:1354–9.
28. McKillop JH, Blumgart LH, Wood CB, et al. The prognostic and therapeutic implications of the positive radionuclide bone scan in clinically early breast cancer. Br J Surg. 1978;65:649–52.
29. Bitran JD, Bekerman C, Desser RK. The predictive value of serial bone scans in assessing response to chemotherapy in advanced breast cancer. Cancer. 1980;45:1562–8.
30. Coleman RE, Rubens RD. The clinical course of bone metastases from breast cancer. Br J Cancer. 1987;55:61–6.
31. Narayan P. Neoplasms of the prostate gland. In: Tanagho EA, editor. Smith's general urology. 14th ed. Appleton and Lange: Norwalk, CT; 1995. p. 392.
32. Batson O. The role of the vertebral veins in metastatic processes. Ann Intern Med. 1942;16:38–45.
33. Dearnaley DP. Cancer of the prostate. Br Med J. 1994;308(6931):780–4.
34. O'Sullivan JM, Cook GJ. A review of the efficacy of bone scanning in prostate and breast cancer. Q J Nucl Med. 2002;46(2):152–9.
35. Zelefsky MJ, Leibel SA, Kutcher GJ, Kelson S, Ling CC, Fuks Z. The feasibility of dose escalation with three-dimensional conformal radiotherapy in patients with prostatic carcinoma. Cancer J Sci Am. 1995;1(2):142.
36. Lee N, Fawaaz R, Olsson CA, Benson MC, Petrylak DP, Schiff PB, et al. Which patients with newly diagnosed prostate cancer need a radionuclide bone scan? An analysis based on 631 patients. Int J Radiat Oncol Biol Phys. 2000;48(5):1443–6.
37. Fogelman I, McKillop JH. The bone scan in metastatic disease. In: Rubens RD, Fogelman I, editors. Bone metastases: diagnosis and treatment. London: Springer; 1991. p. 31–5.
38. Kim EE, Bledin AG, Gutierrez C, Haynie TP. Comparison of radionuclide images and radiographs for skeletal metastases from renal cell carcinoma. Oncology. 1983;40:284–6.
39. Bitran JD, Beckerman C, Pinsky S. Sequential scintigraphic staging of small cell carcinoma. Cancer. 1981;47:1971–5.
40. Levenson RM, Sauerbrunn FJL, Ihde DC, Bunn PA, Cohen MH, Minna JD. Small cell lung cancer: radionuclide bone scans for assessment of tumour extent and response. AJR. 1981;137:31–5.
41. Gravenstein S, Peltz MA, Poreis W. How ominous is an abnormal scan in bronchogenic carcinoma. JAMA. 1979;241:2523–4.
42. Lewis P, Griffin S, Marsden P, et al. Whole body ^{18}F-fluorodeoxyglucose positron emission tomography in preoperative evaluation of lung cancer. Lancet. 1994;344:1265–6.
43. Fawcett HD, McDougall IR. Bone scan in extraskeletal neuroblastoma with hot primary and cold skeletal metastases. Clin Nucl Med. 1980;5:49–50.
44. Howman-Giles R, Gilday DL, Ash JM. Radionuclide skeletal survey in neuroblastoma. Radiology. 1979;131:497–502.
45. Podrasky AER, Stark DD, Hattner RS, Gooding GA, Moss AA. Radionuclide bone scanning in neuroblastoma: skeletal metastases and primary tumour localisation of 99m-Tc MDP. AJR. 1983;141:469–72.
46. Gordon I, Peters AM, Gutman A, Morony S, Dicks-Mireaux C, Pritchard J. Skeletal assessment in neu-

roblastoma – the pitfalls of iodine-123-MIBG scans. J Nucl Med. 1990;31:129–34.
47. Cook GJR, Hannaford E, Lee M, Clarke SEM, Fogelman I. The value of bone scintigraphy in the evaluation of osteoporotic patients with back pain. Scand J Rheumatol. 2002;31:245–8.
48. Fogelman I, Carr D. A comparison of bone scanning and radiology in the assessment of patients with symptomatic Paget's disease. Eur J Nucl Med. 1980;5:417–21.
49. Fogelman I, Carr D. A comparison of bone scanning and radiology in the evaluation of patients with metabolic bone disease. Clin Radiol. 1980;31: 321–6.
50. Ryan PJ, Evans P, Gibson T, Fogelman I. Osteoporosis and chronic back pain: a study with SPECT bone scintigraphy. J Bone Miner Res. 1992;7:1455–60.
51. Ryan PJ, Evans PA, Gibson T, et al. Osteoporosis and chronic back pain: a study with single photon emission computed bone scintigraphy. J Bone Min Res. 1992;7(12):1455–60.
52. Ryan PJ, Evans PA, Gibson T, Fogelman I. Chronic low back pain: comparison of bone SPECT with radiography and CT. Radiology. 1992;182:849–54.
53. Ryan PJ, Gibson T, Fogelman I. The identification of spinal pathology in chronic low back pain using SPECT. Nucl Med Commun. 1992;13:497–502.
54. Kosuda S, Tatsumi K, Yokoyama H, et al. Does bone SPECT actually have lower sensitivity for detecting vertebral metastases than MRI? J Nucl Med. 1996;37:975–8.
55. McKillop JH. Bone scanning in metastatic disease. In: Fogelman I, editor. Bone scanning in clinical practice. Berlin: Springer; 1987. p. 41–60.
56. Roland J, van den Weygaert D, Krug B, Brans B, Scalliet P, Vandevivere J. Metastases seen on SPECT imaging despite a normal planar bone scan. Clin Nucl Med. 1995;20:1052–4.
57. Sedonja I, Budihna NV. The benefit of SPECT when added to planar scintigraphy in patients with bone metastases in the spine. Clin Nucl Med. 1999;24:407–13.
58. Fogelman I, McKillop JH, Bessent RG, et al. The role of bone scanning in osteomalacia. J Nucl Med. 1978;19:245–8.
59. Mari C, Catafau A, Carrio I. Bone scintigraphy and metabolic bone disease. Semin Nucl Med. 1999;27:291–305.
60. Ryan PJ, Fogelman I. Bone scintigraphy in metabolic bone disease. Semin Nucl Med. 1997;27: 291–305.
61. Murray IPC. Bone scintigraphy in trauma. In: IPC M, Ell PJ, editors. Nuclear medicine in clinical diagnosis and treatment. 2nd ed. Edinburgh: Churchill Livingstone; 1998. p. 1241–67.
62. Murray IPC. Vascular manifestations. In: Murray IPC, Ell PJ, editors. Nuclear medicine in clinical diagnosis and treatment. 2nd ed. Edinburgh: Churchill Livingstone; 1998. p. 1223–40.
63. Wilder RP, Sethi S. Overuse injuries: tendinopathies, stress fractures, compartment syndrome, and shin splints. Clin Sports Med. 2004;23:55–81.
64. Boden BP, Osbahr DC. High-risk stress fractures: evaluation and treatment. J Am Acad Orthop Surg. 2000;8:344–53.
65. Drubach LA, Connolly LP, D'Hemecourt PA, Treves ST. Assessment of the clinical significance of asymptomatic lower extremity uptake abnormality in young athletes. J Nucl Med. 2001;42:209–12.
66. McBryde AM Jr. Stress fractures in athletes. Clin Sports Med. 1985;4:737–52.
67. Love C, Din AS, Tomas MB, Kalapparambath TP, Palestro CJ. Radionuclide bone imaging: an illustrative review. Radiographics. 2003;23:341–58.
68. Rupani HD, Holder LE, Espinola DA, Engin SI. Three-phase radionuclide bone imaging in sports medicine. Radiology. 1985;156:187–96.
69. Holder LE, Michael RH. The specific scintigraphic pattern of "shin splints in the lower leg": concise communication. J Nucl Med. 1984;25:865–9.
70. Aburano T, Yokoyama K, Taki J, Nakajima K, Tonami N, Hisada K. Tc-99m MDP bone imaging in inflammatory enthesopathy. Clin Nucl Med. 1990;15:105–6.
71. Intenzo CM, Wapner KL, Park CH, Kim SM. Evaluation of plantar fasciitis by three-phase bone scintigraphy. Clin Nucl Med. 1991;16:325–8.
72. Goldsmith DP, Vivino FB, Eichenfield AH, et al. (1989) nuclear imaging and clinical features of childhood reflex neurovascular dystrophy: comparison with adults. Arthritis Rheum. 1989;32(4):480–5.
73. Turpin S, Taillefer R, Lambert R, Leveille J. "Cold" reflex sympathetic dystrophy in an adult. Clin Nucl Med. 1996;21(2):94–7.
74. Palestro CJ, Torres MA. Radionuclide imaging in orthopedic infections. Semin Nucl Med. 1997;27:334–45.
75. Palestro CJ. Musculoskeletal infection. In: Freeman LM, editor. Nuclear medicine annual. New York, NY: Raven Press; 1994. p. 91–119.
76. Peters AM. The utility of 99mTc-HMPAO-leukocytes for imaging infection. Semin Nucl Med. 1994;24(2):110–27.
77. Seabold JE, Nepola JV. Imaging techniques for evaluation of postoperative orthopedic infections. Q J Nucl Med. 1999;43(1):21–8.
78. Levitsky KA, Hozack WJ, Balderston RA, et al. Evaluation of the painful prosthetic joint: relative value of bone scan, sedimentation rate, and joint aspiration. J Arthroplasty. 1991;6:237–44.
79. Stumpe KDM, Notzli HP, Zanetti M, Kamel EM, Hany TF, von Gorres GW, Schulthess GK, Hodler J. FDG PET for differentiation of infection and aseptic loosening in total hip replacements: comparison with conventional radiography and three-phase Bone scintigraphy. Radiology. 2004;231:333–41.
80. Williamson BR, McLaughlin RE, Wang GW, Miller CW, Teates CD, Bray ST. Radionuclide bone imaging as a means of differentiating loosening and

infection in patients with a painful total hip prosthesis. Radiology. 1979;133:723–5.
81. Aliabadi P, Tumeh SS, Weissman BN, McNeil BJ. Cemented total hip prosthesis: radiographic and scintigraphic evaluation. Radiology. 1989;173:203–6.
82. Mountford PJ, Coakley AJ. Role of technetium-99m phosphonate bone and indium-111 leukocyte scanning for detecting the infected hip prosthesis. J Nucl Med. 1989;30:562–3.
83. Love C, Tomas MB, Marwin SE, Pugliese PV, Palestro CJ. Role of nuclear medicine in diagnosis of the infected joint replacement. Radiographics. 2001;21:1229–38.
84. Utz JA, Lull RJ, Galvin EG. Asymptomatic total hip prosthesis: natural history determined using Tc-MDP bone scans. Radiology. 1986;161:509–12.
85. Oswald SG, Van Nostrand D, Savory CG, Anderson JH, Callaghan JJ. Three-phase bone scan and indium white cell scintigraphy following porous coated hip arthroplasty: a prospective study of the prosthetic tip. J Nucl Med. 1989;30:1321–31.
86. Oswald SG, Van Nostrand D, Savory CG, Anderson JH, Callaghan JJ. The acetabulum: a prospective study of three-phase bone and indium white blood cell scintigraphy following porous-coated hip arthroplasty. J Nucl Med. 1990;31:274–80.
87. Hofmann AA, Wyatt RWB, Daniels AU, Armstrong L, Alazraki N, Taylor A Jr. Bone scan after total knee arthroplasty in asymptomatic patients. Clin Orthop. 1990;251:183–8.
88. Rosenthal L, Lepanto L, Raymond F. Radiophosphate uptake in asymptomatic knee arthroplasty. J Nucl Med. 1987;28:1546–9.
89. Palestro CJ, Kim CK, Swyer AJ, Capozzi JD, Solomon RW, Goldsmith SJ. Total-hip arthroplasty: periprosthetic indium-111-labelled leukocyte activity and complementary technetium-99-m sulfur colloid imaging in suspected infection. J Nucl Med. 1990;31:1950–5.
90. Palestro CJ, Swyer AJ, Kim CK, Goldsmith SJ. Infected knee prostheses: diagnosis with in-111 leukocyte, Tc-99m sulfur colloid, and Tc-99m MDP imaging. Radiology. 1991;179:645–8.
91. Dolan AL, Ryan PJ, Arden NK, et al. The value of SPECT scans in identifying back pain likely to benefit from facet joint injection. Br J Rheumatol. 1996;35:1269–73.
92. Holder LE, Machin JL, Asdourian PL, et al. Planar and high resolution SPECT bone imaging in the diagnosis of facet syndrome. J Nucl Med. 1995;36:37–44.
93. Bellah RD, Summerville DA, Treves ST, et al. Low back pain in adolescent athletes: detection of stress injury to the pars interarticularis with SPECT. Radiology. 1991;180:509–12.
94. Bodner RJ, Heyman S, Drummond DS, et al. The use of SPECT in the diagnosis of low back pain in young patients. Spine. 1988;13:1155–60.
95. Collier BD, Carerra GF, Johnson RP, et al. Detection of femoral head avascular necrosis in adults by SPECT. J Nucl Med. 1985;26:979–87.
96. Collier BD, Johnson RP, Carrera GF, et al. Chronic knee pain assessed by SPECT: comparison with other modalities. Radiology. 1985;157:795–802.
97. Collier BD, Johnson RP, Carrera GF, et al. Painful spondylolysis or spondylolisthesis studies by radiography and SPECT. Radiology. 1985;154:207–11.
98. Dutton JA, Hughes SP, Peters AM. SPECT in the management of patients with back pain and spondylolysis. Clin Nucl Med. 2000;25:93–6.
99. Read MT. SPECT scanning for adolescent back pain. A sine qua non? Br J Sports Med. 1994;28:56–7.
100. Slizofski WJ, Collier BD, Flately TJ, et al. Painful pseudoarthrosis following lumbar spine fusion: detection by combined SPECT and planar bone scintigraphy. Skel Radiol. 1987;16:136–41.
101. Lusins JO, Danielski EF, Goldsmith SJ. Bone SPECT in patients with persistent back pain after lumbar spine surgery. J Nucl Med. 1989;30:490–6.
102. Gates GF, McDonald RJ. Bone SPECT of the back after lumbar surgery. Clin Nucl Med. 1999;24(6):395–403.
103. Hanly JG, Mitchell MJ, Barnes DC, MacMillan L. Early recognition of sacroiliitis by MRI and SPECT. J Rheumatol. 1994;21:2088–95.
104. Kim KY, Lee SH, Moon DH, et al. The diagnostic value of triple head SPECT in avascular necrosis of the femoral head. Int Orthop. 1993;17:132–8.
105. Siddiqui AR, Kopecky KK, Wellman HN, et al. Prospective study of MRI and SPECT bone scans in renal allograft recipients: evidence for self-limited subclinical abnormality of the hips. J Nucl Med. 1993;34:381–6.
106. Stulberg BN, Levine M, Bauer TW, et al. Multimodality approach to osteonecrosis of the femoral head. Clin Orthop Rel Res. 1989;240:181–93.
107. Desmet AA, Dalinka MK, Alazraki N, et al. Diagnostic imaging of avascular necrosis of the hip. Radiology. 2000;215:247–54.
108. Galasko CSB, Weber DA. Avascular necrosis. In: Galasko CSB, Weber DA, editors. Radionuclide scintigraphy in orthopaedics. Edinburgh: Churchill Livingstone; 1984. p. 200–9.
109. Fajman WA, Diehl M, Dunaway E. SPECT for acute knee pain. J Nucl Med. 1985;26:77.
110. Murray IPC, Dixon J, Kohan L. SPECT for acute knee pain. Clin Nucl Med. 1990;15:828–40.
111. Ryan PJ, Taylor M, Grevitt M, et al. Bone single-photon emission tomography in recent meniscal tears: an assessment of diagnostic criteria. Eur J Nucl Med. 1993;20:703–7.
112. Cook GJR, Ryan PJ, Clarke SEM, Fogelman I. Anterior cruciate ligament tear: findings on SPECT bone scintigraphy of the knee. J Nucl Med. 1996;37:1353–6.
113. Cook GJR, Fogelman I. Lateral collateral ligament tear of the knee: appearances on bone scintigraphy with SPECT. Eur J Nucl Med. 1996;23:720–2.
114. Kraznow AZ, Collier BD, Kneeland JB, et al. Comparison of high resolution MRI and SPECT

bone scintigraphy for non-invasive imaging of the temporomandibular joint. J Nucl Med. 1987; 28:1268–74.
115. Toni MG, Calderazzi A, Battolia L, et al. SPECT in the study of pathology of the temporomandibular joint. Radiol Med. 1992;84:549–52. The authors personal experience.
116. Strashun AM, Nejatheim M, Goldsmith SJ. Malignant otitis externa; early scintigraphic detection. Radiology. 1984;150:541–5.
117. Hardoff R, Gips S, Uri N, Front A, Tamir A. Semiquantitative skull planar and SPECT bone scintigraphy in diabetic patients: differentiation of necrotizing (malignant) external otitis from severe external otitis. J Nucl Med. 1994;35:411–5.
118. Saha S, Burke C, Desai A, et al. SPECT-CT: applications in musculoskeletal radiology. Br J Radiol. 2013;86:20120519.
119. Gnanasegaran G, Paycha F, Strobel K, et al. Bone SPECT/CT in postoperative spine. Semin Nucl Med. 2018;48(5):410–24.
120. Hirschmann MT, Amsler F, Rasch H. Clinical value of SPECT/CT in the painful total knee arthroplasty (TKA): a prospective study in a consecutive series of 100 TKA. Eur J Nucl Med Mol Imaging. 2015;42(12):1869–82.
121. Van den Wyngaert T, Paycha F, Strobel K, et al. SPECT/CT in postoperative painful hip arthroplasty. Semin Nucl Med. 2018;48(5):425–38.
122. Van der Bruggen W, Hirschmann MT, Strobel K, et al. SPECT/CT in the postoperative painful knee. Semin Nucl Med. 2018;48(5):439–53.
123. Hirschmann A, Hirschmann MT. Chronic knee pain: clinical value of MRI versus SPECT/CT. Semin Musculoskelet Radiol. 2016;20(1):3–11.
124. Huellner MW, Strobel K. Clinical applications of SPECT/CT in imaging the extremities. Eur J Nucl Med Mol Imaging. 2014;41(Suppl 1):S50–8.
125. Kampen WU, Westphal F, Van den Wyngaert T, et al. SPECT/CT in postoperative foot and ankle pain. Semin Nucl Med. 2018;48(5):454–68.
126. Strobel K, van der Bruggen W, Hug U, et al. Bone SPECT/CT in postoperative hand and wrist pain. Semin Nucl Med. 2018;48(5):396–409.
127. Russo VM, Dhawan RT, Baudracco I, Dharmarajah N, Lazzarino AI, Casey AT. Hybrid bone SPECT/CT imaging in evaluation of chronic low back pain: correlation with facet joint arthropathy. World Neurosurg. 2017;107:732–8.
128. Jain A, Jain S, Agarwal A, Gambhir S, Shamshery C, Agarwal A. Evaluation of efficacy of bone scan with SPECT/CT in the Management of low back pain: a study supported by differential diagnostic local anesthetic blocks. Clin J Pain. 2015;31(12):1054–9.
129. Lee I, Budiawan H, Moon JY, Cheon GJ, Kim YC, Paeng JC, Kang KW, Chung JK, Lee DS. The value of SPECT/CT in localizing pain site and prediction of treatment response in patients with chronic low back pain. J Korean Med Sci. 2014;29(12):1711–6.
130. Al-Riyami K, Gnanasegaran G, Van den Wyngaert T, Bomanji J. Bone SPECT/CT in the postoperative spine: a focus on spinal fusion. Eur J Nucl Med Mol Imaging. 2017;44(12):2094–104.
131. Rager O, Schaller K, Payer M, Tchernin D, Ratib O, Tessitore E. SPECT/CT in differentiation of pseudarthrosis from other causes of back pain in lumbar spinal fusion: report on 10 consecutive cases. Clin Nucl Med. 2012;37(4):339–43.
132. Sumer J, Schmidt D, Ritt P, Lell M, Forst R, Kuwert T, Richter R. SPECT/CT in patients with lower back pain after lumbar fusion surgery. Nucl Med Commun. 2013;34(10):964–70.
133. Hudyana H, Maes A, Vandenberghe T, Fidlers L, Sathekge M, Nicolai D, Van de Wiele C. Accuracy of bone SPECT/CT for identifying hardware loosening in patients who underwent lumbar fusion with pedicle screws. Eur J Nucl Med Mol Imaging. 2016;43(2):349–54.
134. Schleich FS, Schürch M, Huellner MW, Hug U, von Wartburg U, Strobel K, Veit-Haibach P. Diagnostic and therapeutic impact of SPECT/CT in patients with unspecific pain of the hand and wrist. EJNMMI Res. 2012;2(1):53.
135. Huellner MW, Bürkert A, Schleich FS, Schürch M, Hug U, von Wartburg U, Strobel K, Veit-Haibach P. SPECT/CT versus MRI in patients with nonspecific pain of the hand and wrist – a pilot study. Eur J Nucl Med Mol Imaging. 2012;39(5):750–9.
136. Biersack HJ, Wingenfeld C, Hinterthaner B, Frank D, Sabet A. SPECT-CT of the foot. Nuklearmedizin. 2012;51(1):26–31.
137. Singh VK, Javed S, Parthipun A, Sott AH. The diagnostic value of single photon-emission computed tomography bone scans combined with CT (SPECT-CT) in diseases of the foot and ankle. Foot Ankle Surg. 2013;19(2):80–3.
138. Barthassat E, Afifi F, Konala P, Rasch H, Hirschmann MT. Evaluation of patients with painful total hip arthroplasty using combined single photon emission tomography and conventional computerized tomography (SPECT/CT) – a comparison of semi-quantitative versus 3D volumetric quantitative measurements. BMC Med Imaging. 2017;17(1):31.
139. Cew CG, Lewis P, Middleton F, van den Wijngaard R, Deshaies A. Radionuclide arthrogram with SPECT/CT for the evaluation of mechanical loosening of hip and knee prostheses. Ann Nucl Med. 2010;24(10):735–43.
140. Slevin O, Schmid FA, Schiapparelli F, Rasch H, Hirschmann MT. Increased in vivo patellofemoral loading after total knee arthroplasty in resurfaced patellae. Knee Surg Sports Traumatol Arthrosc. 2018;26:1805–10.
141. Al-Nabhani K, Michopoulou S, Allie R, Alkalbani J, Saad Z, Sajjan R, Syed R, Bomanji J. Painful knee prosthesis: can we help with bone SPECT/CT? Nucl Med Commun. 2014;35(2):182–8.
142. Helyar V, Mohan HK, Barwick T, Livieratos L, Gnanasegaran G, Clarke SE, et al. The added value

of multislice SPECT/CT in patients with equivocal bony metastasis from carcinoma of the prostate. Eur J Nucl Med Mol Imaging. 2010;37:706–13.
143. Romer W, Nomayr A, Uder M, Bautz W, Kuwert T. SPECT-guided CT for evaluating foci of increased bone metabolism classified as indeterminate on SPECT in cancer patients. J Nucl Med. 2006;47:1102–6.
144. Sharma P, Singh H, Kumar R, Bal C, Thulkar S, Seenu V, et al. Bone scintigraphy in breast cancer: added value of hybrid SPECT-CT and its impact on patient management. Nucl Med Commun. 2012;33:139–47.
145. Utsunomiya D, Shiraishi S, Imuta M, Tomiguchi S, Kawanaka K, Morishita S, et al. Added value of SPECT/CT fusion in assessing suspected bone metastasis: comparison with scintigraphy alone and nonfused scintigraphy and CT. Radiology. 2006;238:264–71.
146. Ndlovu X, George R, Ellmann A, Warwick J. Should SPECT-CT replace SPECT for the evaluation of equivocal bone scan lesions in patients with underlying malignancies? Nucl Med Commun. 2010;31:659–65.
147. Horger M, Eschmann SM, Pfannenberg C, Vonthein R, Besenfelder H, Claussen CD, et al. Evaluation of combined transmission and emission tomography for classification of skeletal lesions. AJR Am J Roentgenol. 2004;183:655–61.
148. Strobel K, Burger C, Seifert B, Husarik DB, Soyka JD, Hany TF. Characterization of focal bone lesions in the axial skeleton: performance of planar bone scintigraphy compared with SPECT and SPECT fused with CT. AJR Am J Roentgenol. 2007;188:W467–74.
149. Guezennec C, Keromnes N, Robin P, et al. Incremental diagnostic utility of systematic double-bed SPECT/CT for bone scintigraphy in initial staging of cancer patients. Cancer Imaging. 2017;17:16.
150. Rager O, Nkoulou R, Exquis N, et al. Whole-body SPECT/CT versus planar bone scan with targeted SPECT/CT for metastatic workup. Biomed Res Int. 2017;2017:1–8.
151. Cook GJR, Fogelman I. The role of positron emission tomography in skeletal disease. Semin Nucl Med. 2001;31:50–61.
152. Lonneux M, Borbath II, Berliere M, et al. The place of whole-body PET FDG for the diagnosis of distant recurrence of breast cancer. Clin Positron Imaging. 2000;3:45–9.
153. Ohta M, Tokuda Y, Suzuki Y, et al. Whole body PET for the evaluation of bony metastases in patients with breast cancer: comparison with 99Tcm-MDP bone scintigraphy. Nucl Med Commun. 2001;22:875–9.
154. Cook GJ, Houston S, Rubens R, et al. Detection of bone metastases in breast cancer by 18FDG PET: differing metabolic activity in osteoblastic and osteolytic lesions. J Clin Oncol. 1998;16:3375–9.
155. Shreve PD, Grossman HB, Gross MD, et al. Metastatic prostate cancer: initial findings of PET with 2-deoxy-2-[F-18]fluoro-D-glucose. Radiology. 1996;199:751–6.
156. Morris MJ, Akhurst T, Osman I, et al. Fluorinated deoxyglucose positron emission tomography imaging in progressive metastatic prostate cancer. Urology. 2002;59:913–8.
157. Bury T, Barreto A, Daenen F, et al. Fluorine-18 deoxyglucose positron emission tomography for the detection of bone metastases in patients with non-small cell lung cancer. Eur J Nucl Med. 1998;25:1244–7.
158. Gayed I, Vu T, Johnson M, et al. Comparison of bone and 2-deoxy-2-[18F]fluoro-D-glucose positron emission tomography in the evaluation of bony metastases in lung cancer. Mol Imaging Biol. 2003;5:26–31.
159. Moog F, Kotzerke J, Reske SN. FDG PET can replace bone scintigraphy in primary staging of malignant lymphoma. J Nucl Med. 1999;40:1407–13.
160. Schirrmeister H, Bommer M, Buck AK, et al. Initial results in the assessment of multiple myeloma using 18F-FDG PET. Eur J Nucl Med Mol Imaging. 2002;29:361–6.
161. Schirrmeister H, Guhlmann A, Elsner K, et al. Sensitivity in detecting osseous lesions depends on anatomic localization: planar bone scintigraphy versus 18F PET. J Nucl Med. 1999;40:1623–9.
162. Durie BG, Waxman AD, D'Agnolo A, et al. Whole-body (18)F-FDG PET identifies high-risk myeloma. J Nucl Med. 2002;43:1457–63.
163. Schirrmeister H, Guhlnamm A, Kotzerke J, et al. Early detection and accurate description of extent of metastatic bone disease in breast cancer with fluoride ion and positron emission tomography. J Clin Oncol. 1999;17:2381–9.
164. Even-Sapir E, Metser U, Flusser G. Assessment of malignant skeletal disease: initial experience with 18F-fluoride PET/CT and comparison between 18F-fluoride PET and 18F-fluoride PET/CT. J Nucl Med. 2004;45(2):272–8.
165. Cook GJR, Fogelman I. The role of positron emission tomography in the management of bone metastases. Cancer. 2000;88:2927–33.
166. Schirrmeister H, Glatting G, Hetzel J, et al. Prospective evaluation of clinical value of planar bone scan, SPECT and ^{18}F-labeled NaF PET in newly diagnosed lung cancer. J Nucl Med. 2001;42:1800–4.

11 Application of Lymphatic Mapping and Sentinel Node Biopsy in Surgical Oncology

Ramin Sadeghi and Leili Zarifmahmoudi

11.1 Brief Introduction and Historical Perspective

The first nodes receiving lymphatic drainage of a tumor are known as the sentinel or guarding nodes. The concept of sentinel node mapping suggests that lymphatic basin involvement starts from the sentinel nodes, and if sentinel nodes are pathologically clear from tumor cells, the other lymph nodes of the basin are clear either [1, 2].

The concept of sentinel node was primarily introduced through lymphangiographic studies conducted in 1977 by Cabanas, who performed lymphangiography on the dorsal lymphatic of the penis, at the anterior or medial aspect of the superficial epigastric vein [3]. More studies on lymphatic drainage of testicular tumors revealed the primary metastatic site and the existence of sentinel lymph nodes (SLNs) [4].

Intraoperative detection of SLNs via the injection of blue dye at primary tumor sites by Morton et al. was a real milestone in the general acceptance of sentinel lymph node biopsy (SLNB), which led to the rejection of lymph node dissection for patients with clinical stage I melanomas who had negative SLNs [5]. Patent blue and isosulfan blue were also examined for SLN mapping in melanomas by Morton's group [6].

SLNB was then performed on breast cancer patients using blue dye, and it showed high accuracy in the detection of SLNs and the staging of the disease [7]. To improve the accuracy and sensitivity of SLN detection, radiolabeled colloid was used as a tracer and gamma-ray detection probe was applied for intraoperative SLN mapping in melanoma and breast cancers [8–10]. Preoperative lymphoscintigraphy also increased the sensitivity of SLN mapping procedure in future studies.

The prognostic or predictive value of SLNs in determining the metastatic status of the disease and the staging of the axillary lymph nodes increased the multidisciplinary interest in lymphoscintigraphy and led to the conduct of large clinical trials on patients with different types of tumors so as to obtain a gold standard method. Sentinel node mapping has become an integral part of management in many malignancies with lower comorbidities compared to the traditional lymph node staging methods.

The main problem in sentinel node mapping is the identification of sentinel nodes among numerous lymph nodes in each lymphatic basins, which take up the lymphatic flow of a tumor. This is done by injecting mapping materials around the tumor to find out the location of sentinel nodes. Several mapping materials are available that can be used for sentinel node mapping in different tumors. The most widely used materials are visually assisted (vital dyes or coal par-

R. Sadeghi (✉) · L. Zarifmahmoudi
Nuclear Medicine Research Center, Mashhad University of Medical Sciences, Mashhad, Iran
e-mail: sadeghir@mums.ac.ir

H. Ahmadzadehfar et al. (eds.), *Clinical Nuclear Medicine*,
https://doi.org/10.1007/978-3-030-39457-8_11

ticles for the naked eyes and fluorescent materials, which are usually near infrared assisted), probe assisted (radiocolloids with intraoperative gamma probes and magnetic particles with intraoperative magnetic probes), and contrast materials for ultrasonography-assisted sentinel node mapping [11–13].

Vital dyes have long been used in sentinel node mapping with acceptable success. These dyes include patent blue V, methylene blue, isosulfan blue, etc. The major problems with vital dyes are low success rate, as compared with probe-assisted methods, and adverse reactions, which can be life threatening. Usually a combination of vital dyes and probe-assisted methods is used to optimize the success of lymphatic mapping [14–16]. Figure 11.1 shows an example of the use of blue dye in an endometrial cancer patient.

Fluorescent materials are being increasingly used for sentinel node mapping, especially in their hybrid form as radiotracer/fluorescent. The most commonly used mapping material of this kind is indocyanine green, which is labeled with Tc-99m too [17]. The sentinel nodes and lymphatic vessels can be identified visually with the

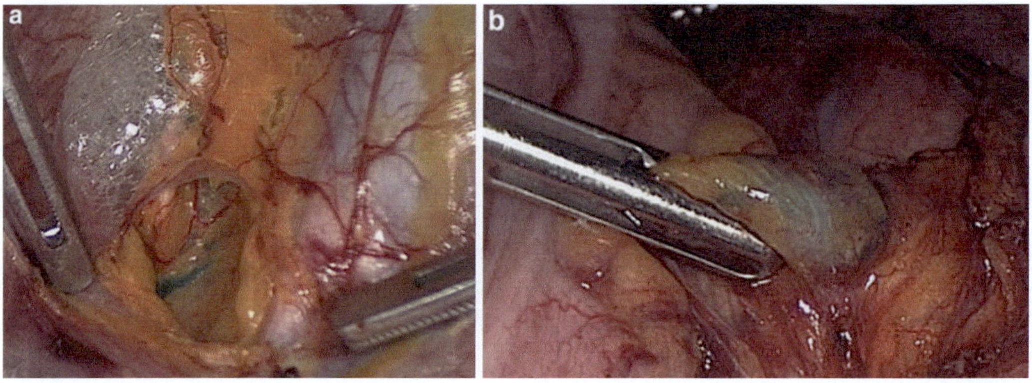

Fig. 11.1 Sentinel node mapping using a blue dye in an endometrial cancer patient. (**a**) After injection in the cervix, the dye is moving in the lymphatic vessels. (**b**) The blue-stained sentinel nodes can be easily found visually (Reproduced with permission from https://doi.org/10.1007/s00432-017-2501-8)

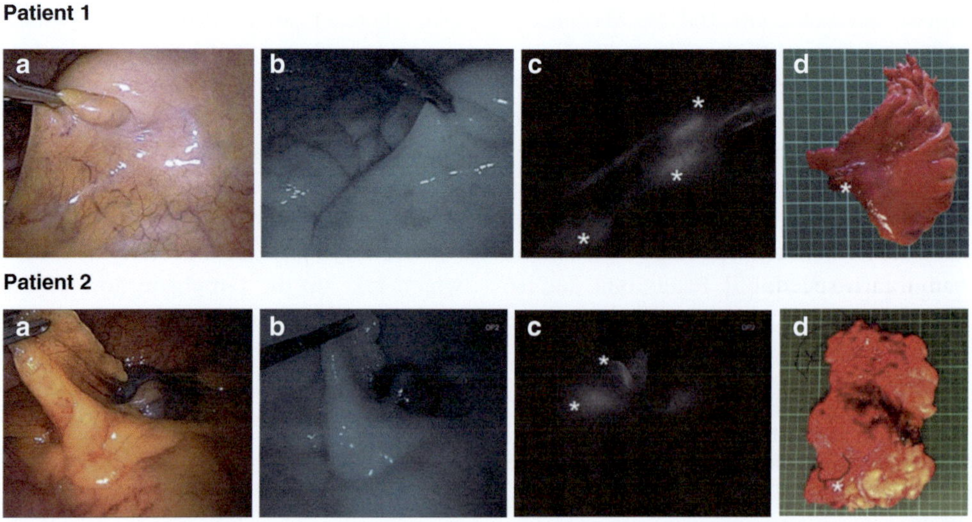

Fig. 11.2 (**a**) Operative theater with white light, (**b**) with near infrared without filter, (**c**) with filter that shows mesocolic sentinel nodes, and (**d**) harvested specimen with sentinel nodes (identified by asterisk). Patient 1: with sigmoid colon cancer, patient 2: with caecal cancer (Reproduced with permission from https://doi.org/10.1016/j.ejso.2017.05.026)

aim of a near-infrared source. Figure 11.2 shows an example of sentinel node mapping using this technique in a colon cancer patient.

Magnetic materials and contrast-enhanced ultrasonography are being used less frequently in sentinel node mapping and are still under development.

In the rest of this chapter, we will focus on sentinel node mapping using radiocolloids, which is thus far the most commonly used technique for sentinel node identification.

11.2 General Aspects of Sentinel Node Mapping in Surgical Oncology

11.2.1 Radiopharmaceuticals

Injected tracers should be absorbed by lymphatic vessels, have fast and predictable transition to SLN, and have marked retention. The kinetics of the tracer clearance, the rate of tracer transport through the lymphatic channel, and the detection of SLNs are directly dependent on the particle size of the applied tracer, which can be determined by electron microscopy, photon correlation spectroscopy, and ultracentrifugation (membrane filtration). Although small-size particles lead to the rapid detection of SLNs, particles smaller than 4–5 nm might penetrate the capillary membrane and prevent SLN detection the next day, and particles larger than 500 nm slowly transit through the interstitial space and might be retained at the injection site for a long time [18, 19]. So tracers with particle size between 100 and 200 nm in diameter are the ideal radiopharmaceuticals, which do not penetrate the capillaries membrane and have optimum transit speed, lymphatic drainage, and retention in SLNs.

Table 11.1 shows the most commonly used radiotracers with their particle size ranges. It is worth mentioning that all of these radiotracers work surprisingly well for sentinel node mapping, and the tracers on the list can be used interchangeably [20].

Table 11.1 The most frequently used Tc-99m-labeled radiopharmaceuticals for sentinel node mapping

Radiopharmaceutical	Particle size (nm)
Antimony sulfide colloid	<30
Nanocolloid	<80
Sulfur colloid	Mostly 100–600
Filtered sulfur colloid	10 nm
Phytate	150–1000

11.2.2 Injection Site, Time, Dose, and Volume

Logically, the best injection site for sentinel node mapping is in the peri-tumoral location. This can be achieved for many tumors, such as melanoma, penile tumor, vulvar tumor, uterine cervix tumor, etc. [21]. Although intratumoral injection can be successful, the detection rate is usually suboptimal, so intratumoral injections should be discouraged.

For some tumors, the injection site can be modified in order to increase the convenience and success of the procedure. Injection site modification is mostly done in breast cancer and endometrial cancer patients, which will be discussed in detail in the specific sections of these tumors.

Injection time has been a matter of controversy in sentinel node mapping. Although some surgeons prefer a same-day protocol (injection and surgery in the same day), two-day protocol (injection the day before surgery) has several advantages. In a two-day protocol, lymphoscintigraphy can be done without any interference with regard to operating room schedule. In addition, decay of radioactivity in the injection site can simplify the detection of sentinel nodes by gamma probes by decreasing the interfering counts [22]. Several studies showed that the sentinel nodes identified via a two-day protocol are the same as those identified via a one-day protocol, and success rate are comparable in both techniques [23–26].

The time frame for the success of sentinel node detection is also an important aspect of sentinel node mapping. Tracer movement in the lymphatic system is very rapid, especially in lymphatic-rich areas, such as peri-areolar regions of the breast. However, several factors can change the speed of tracer movement in the lymphatic system, namely, patient age, body mass index (BMI), previous manipulation of the tumor, injection site, and radiotracer particle size. As a rule of thumb, most of the sentinel nodes are visible in 30 min following radiotracer injections, even in intraoperative injections in gastrointestinal tumors [27–30]. This means that even intraoperative injections are successful enough and surgeons have a wide margin of time for radiotracer injections from the day before to a couple of minutes before surgery or even intraoperative injections. Figure 11.3 shows the rapid movement of a radiotracer in the lymphatic system of the breast on dynamic lymphoscintigraphy images.

The best injection dose and number of injections are also controversial. However, there is a consensus that for a two-day protocol, higher doses of radiotracer should be used. Usually, 0.5 mCi (18.5 MBq)/injection for a single day and 1 mCi (37 MBq)/injection for a two-day protocol is sufficient. In tumors with bilateral or unpredictable drainage (midline tumors, head and neck tumors, melanoma, etc.), at least two injections around the tumor are needed [24, 31].

The volume of injection can be of importance, especially in places with low volume of interstitial tissue, which can hamper the injection. In addition, in some tumors such as breast cancer, the higher is the volume, the more severe is the pain felt by the patient. The volume of each injected dose varies in different studies, and all were successful. Some studies evaluated the effect of injection volume on the success of sentinel node mapping in breast cancer, and all showed good results with 0.1–0.5 mL per injection [32–34].

Caution should be exerted during radiotracer injections. A very simple technique to prevent radiotracer contamination and ensure receiving all doses of the tracer is to draw air behind the injected material in the syringe.

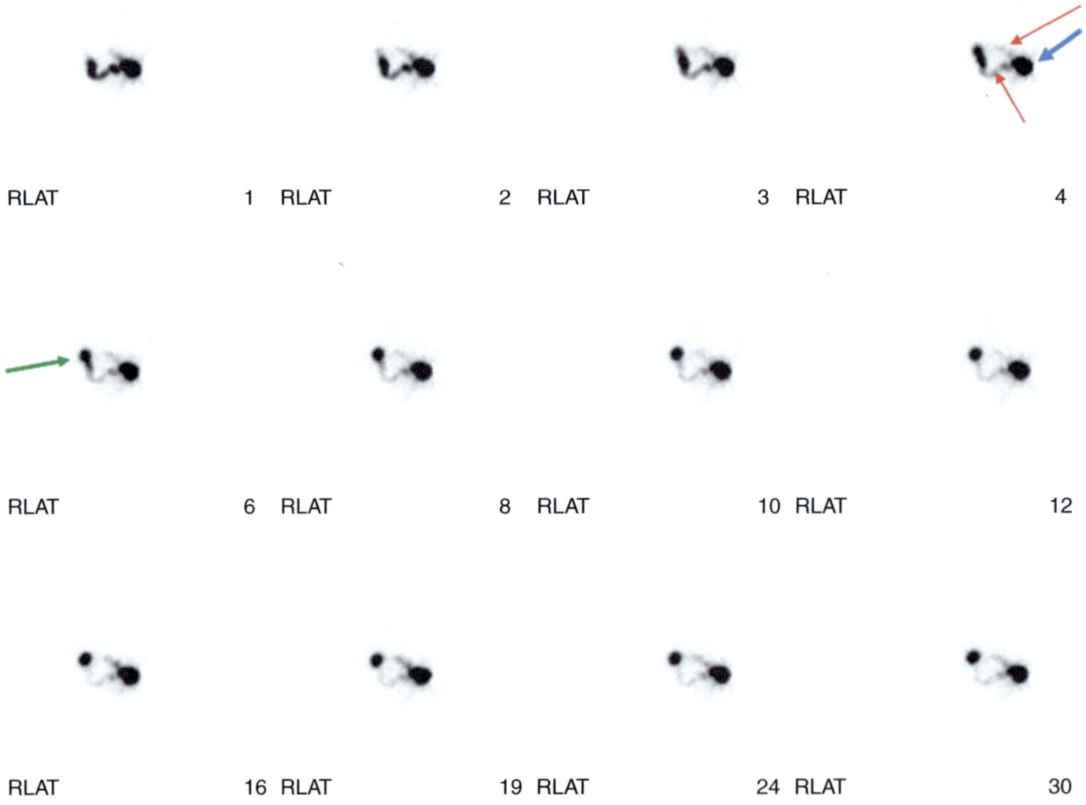

Fig. 11.3 Dynamic lymphoscintigraphy of a breast cancer patient immediately after intradermal injection of the radiotracer in the right breast. Note immediate movement of the tracer in the lymphatics (red arrows) from the injection site (blue arrow). Note axillary sentinel node visualization as early as 6 min throughout the study (green arrow)

11.2.3 Lymphoscintigraphy

Lymphoscintigraphy is an integral part of sentinel node biopsy in surgical oncology. It can provide surgeons with very useful information and guide them with the location and number of sentinel nodes before surgery. In addition, aberrant sentinel nodes can be identified, which are of utmost importance in tumors with multidirectional lymph flow such as trunk melanomas [35–39].

Currently there are three forms of imaging in sentinel node mapping using radiotracers: planar, SPECT, and intraoperative imaging.

Planar lymphoscintigraphy is a simple imaging that can show the location and number of sentinel nodes. A 300-s image using a large field of view gamma camera equipped with a low-energy high-resolution collimator is sufficient for a quality image. At least two perpendicular views are needed for a better evaluation of the depth of the sentinel nodes. For tumors with multidirectional lymph flow, all possible draining basins should be imaged. For example, for melanoma of the trunk, both axillae and inguinal areas should be included in the imaging field. Figure 11.4 shows a planar lymphoscintigraphy of a breast cancer patient with two visible sentinel nodes in the axilla. Figure 11.5 is an example of a head and neck melanoma with bilateral lymphatic drainage detected by lymphoscintigraphy.

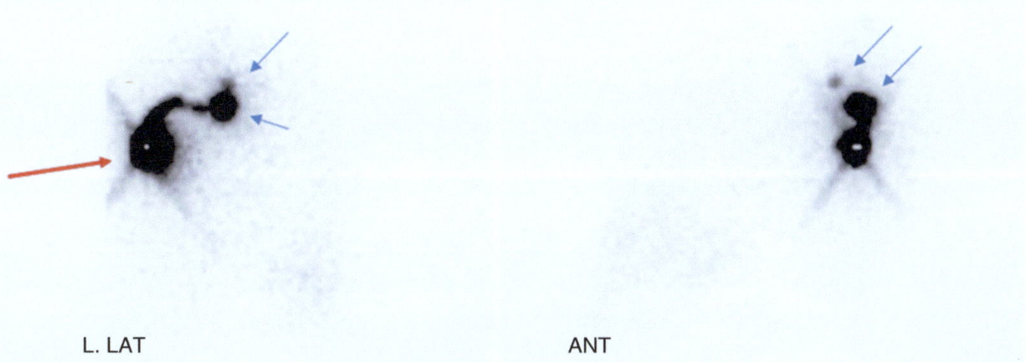

Fig. 11.4 Planar lymphoscintigraphy images of a breast cancer patient with two visible sentinel nodes in the axilla (blue arrows). Injection site is shown by a red arrow

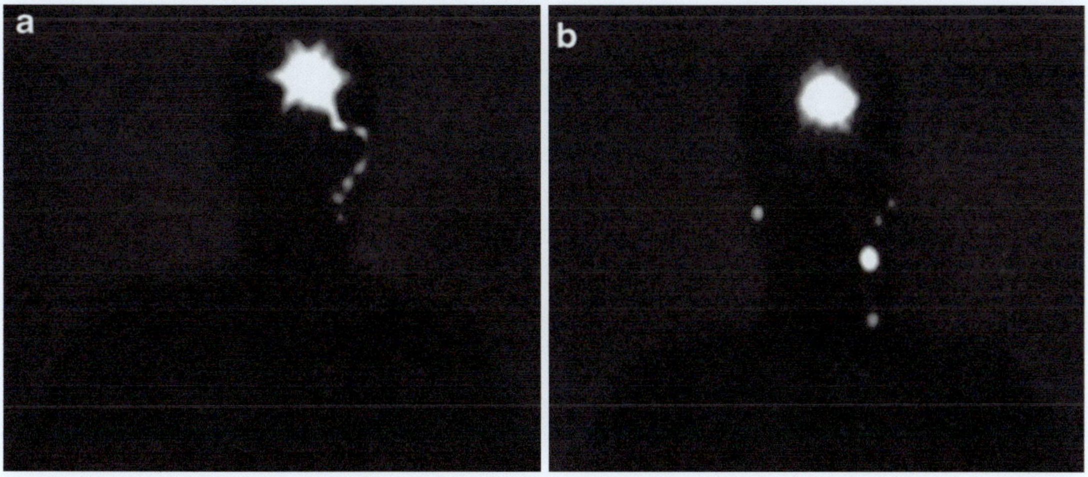

Fig. 11.5 Early (**a**) and delayed (**b**) lymphoscintigraphy of the patient with forehead melanoma. Note bilateral sentinel nodes in the peri-auricular area (Reproduced with permission from https://doi.org/10.1007/s00259-015-3256-6)

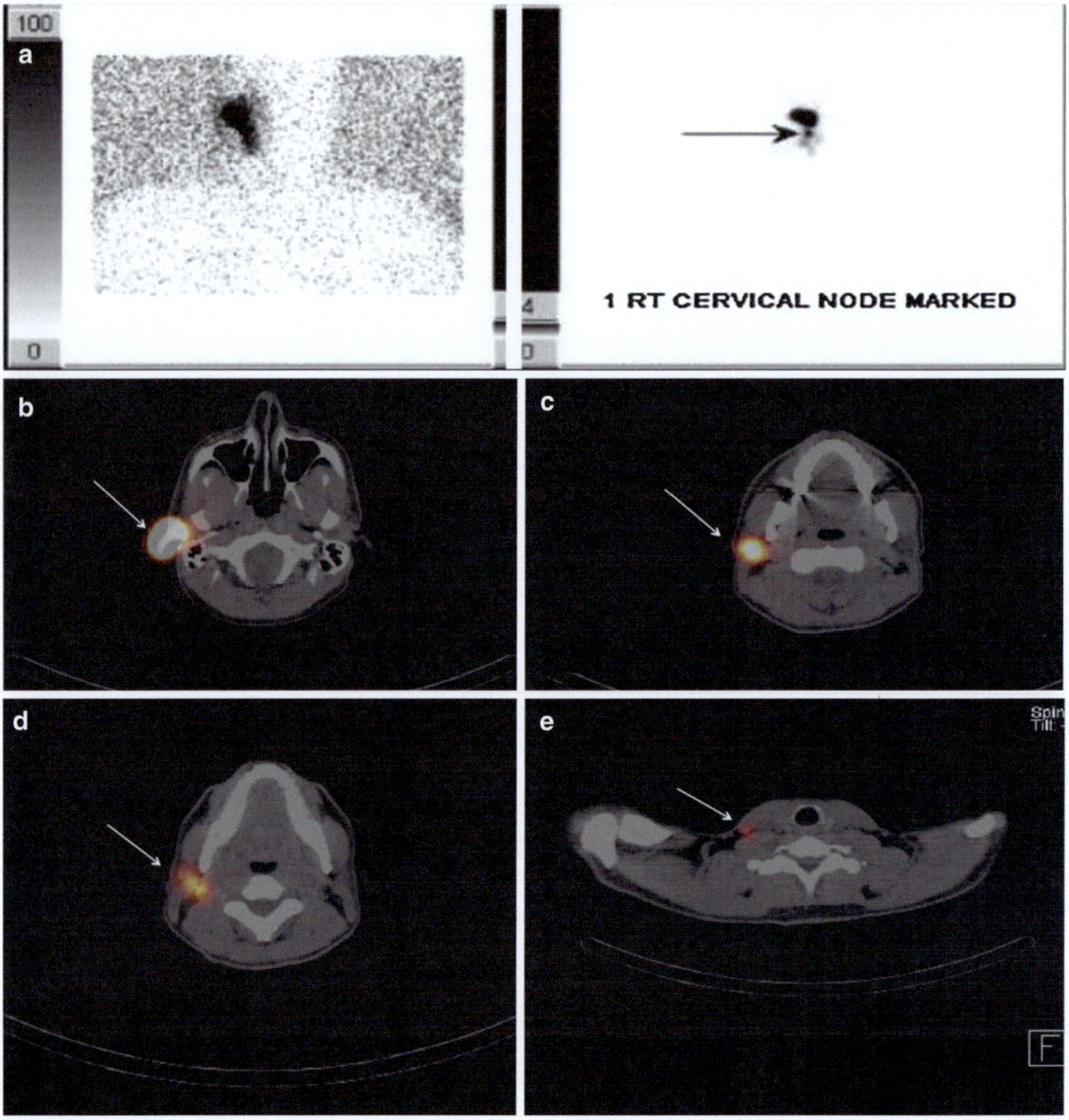

Fig. 11.6 Planar lymphoscintigraphy of a patient with right ear malignancy (**a**) that showed a cervical sentinel node. SPECT/CT demonstrated the injection site (**b**) and a parotid sentinel lymph node inferior to the injection site (**c**) (white arrows). SPECT/CT also showed nodes in the right IIB (**d**) and IV (**e**) (white arrows) neck levels (Reproduced with permission from https://doi.org/10.1245/s10434-016-5590-8)

Hybrid scintigraphy using SPECT/CT lymphoscintigraphy has increased the localization accuracy of sentinel nodes before surgery and is considered indispensable by many surgeons. SPECT/CT is definitely more informative than planar imaging. SPECT imaging parameters can be set at 64 views of 20–40 s (matrix 128 × 128). Figures 11.6 and 11.7 show the added value of SPECT/CT over planar imaging in sentinel node mapping.

Intraoperative gamma cameras are small gamma cameras with the ability to perform easy and rapid intraoperative imaging [40, 41]. Portable intraoperative gamma cameras have

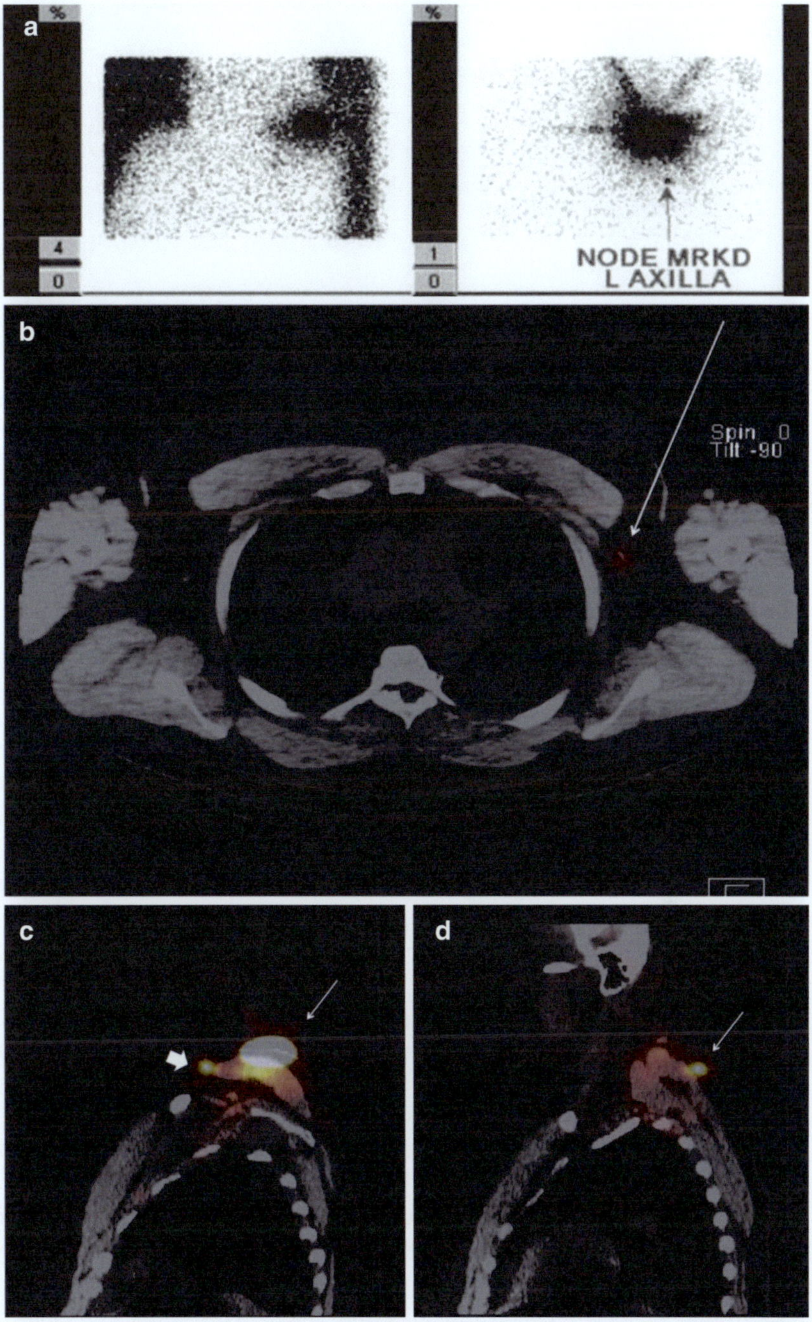

Fig. 11.7 Planar lymphoscintigraphy showed the primary malignancy on the left shoulder with an axillary sentinel node (**a**). SPECT/CT showed an axillary sentinel node (white arrow) (**b**), injection site (white arrow), along with left supraclavicular node (arrowhead) (**c**) and left posterior superficial subcutaneous node (white arrow) (**d**) (Reproduced with permission from https://doi.org/10.1245/s10434-016-5590-8)

shown to be of value in sentinel node mapping, especially in conditions of intraoperative injections of the radiotracer. Intraoperative radiotracer injections virtually preclude the ability to perform preoperative lymphoscintigraphy, and intraoperative gamma cameras are the only option for imaging [42–44]. The added value of portable intraoperative gamma cameras over preoperative lymphoscintigraphy has also been shown in several studies (Fig. 11.8).

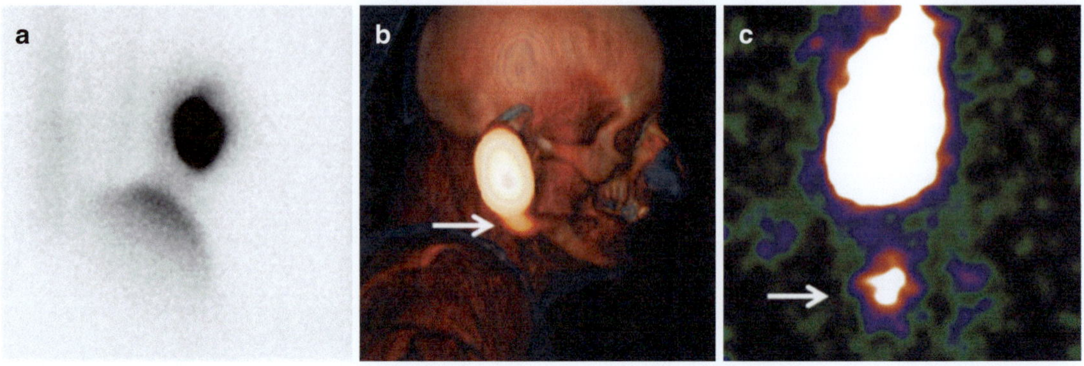

Fig. 11.8 Lymphoscintigraphy of a melanoma patient in the head and neck area. Planar lymphoscintigraphy (**a**) did not show any sentinel nodes. SPECT/CT (**b**) showed a faint activity inferior to the injected site (white arrow). Portable gamma camera image (**c**) revealed the exact location of the sentinel node (white arrow) (Reproduced with permission from https://doi.org/10.1097/RLU.0000000000000370)

11.2.4 Intraoperative Gamma Probes and Issues to Be Considered during Surgery

Intraoperative gamma probes are an integral part of sentinel node mapping by radiotracers. There are various gamma probes available for different tracers and for different purposes. However, for sentinel node mapping, gamma probes with the ability to detect Tc-99m would be sufficient. The size of gamma probe is also of importance as small gamma probes are needed for head and neck or pediatric patients.

The definition of sentinel node is of utmost importance. Not all active nodes in the draining basin should be harvested, and no highly active lymph node should be left behind. Two methods are available for sentinel node definitions both based on count rate of the nodes: background related and hottest sentinel node related. Background-related definition asserts that any node with an "*n*" times count rate higher than background (a location far from injection site, such as thigh in breast cancer) should be harvested. The number of "*n*" is highly controversial, although it is usually set at 10 [45]. Hottest sentinel node related defines sentinel nodes as all nodes with more than "*n*%" count of the hottest sentinel node. Again, the best "*n*" is controversial despite using 10%, as recommended by many studies [46]. It is worth mentioning that the count used in sentinel node harvesting is "ex vivo" counts, which means that the sentinel node is positioned on the gamma probe head and is pointing to the nonactive area (preferably the ceiling).

Using a liberal definition for harvesting sentinel nodes results in a high number of sentinel nodes, which increases the invasiveness of the procedure and actually defeats the purpose of sentinel node mapping in the first place. Using stringent criteria on the other hand increases the false negative rate. Figure 11.9 shows an example of a breast cancer patient with two hot axillary sentinel nodes; the less hot sentinel node was actually pathologically involved.

Another important consideration during surgery that can decrease the false negative rate of sentinel node mapping is harvesting cold but large and suspicious lymph nodes. It has been shown that the replacement of sentinel nodes with tumor cells can result in bypassing of the real sentinel nodes and the detection of "false" sentinel nodes (Fig. 11.10). Harvesting the enlarged suspicious cold nodes (for example, by palpation through the incision of the axilla in breast cancer) would obviate this problem [47].

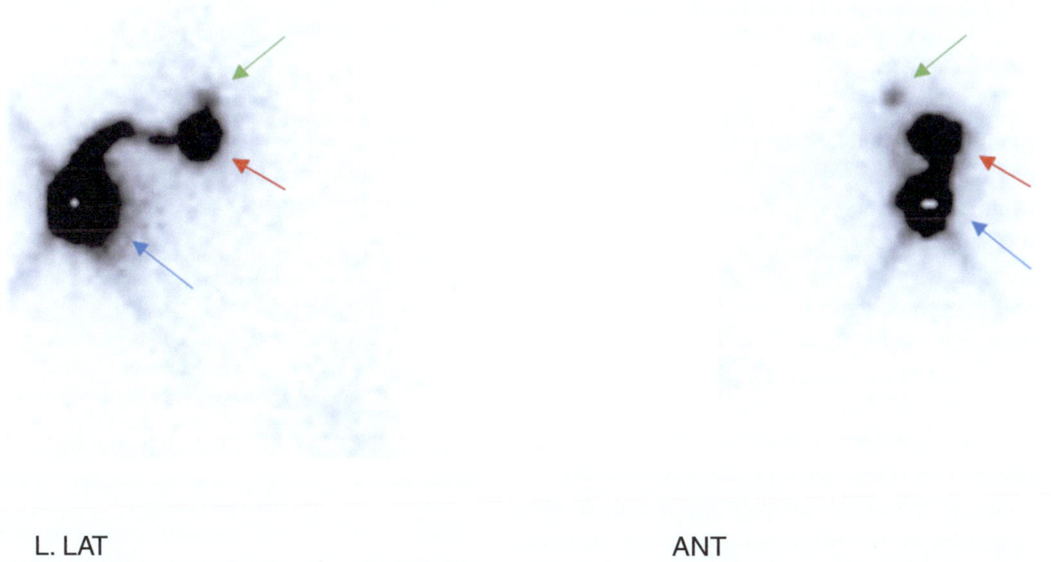

Fig. 11.9 Anterior and lateral lymphoscintigraphy images of a breast cancer patient. Injection site (blue arrow) and the hottest sentinel node (red arrow) are easily visible. Another hot sentinel node (green arrow) is visible in the axilla with remarkably less count. During surgery, only the latter was pathologically involved

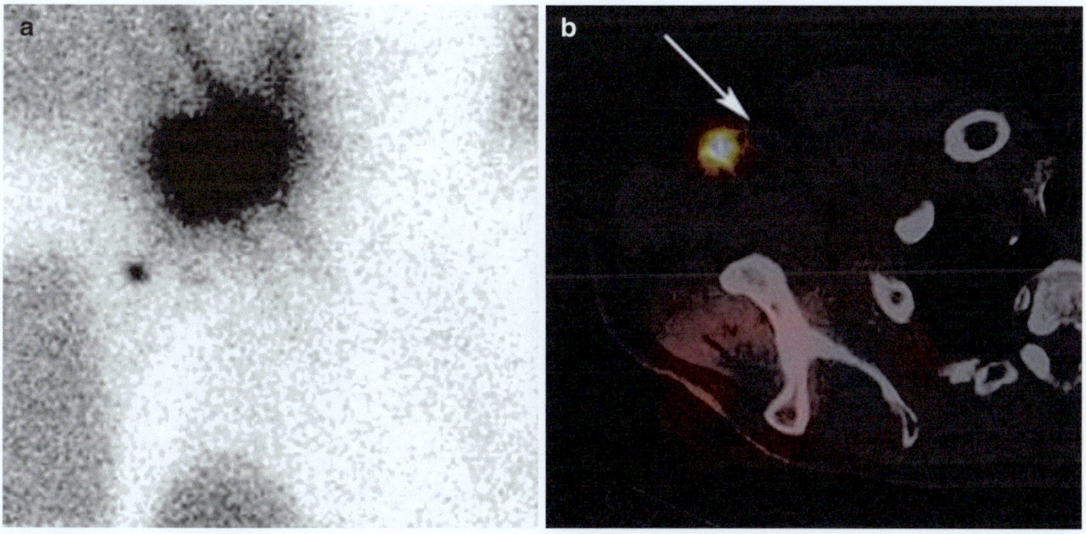

Fig. 11.10 An example of a false negative sentinel node due to tumoral infiltration in a melanoma on the right shoulder area. (**a**) Anterior planar view with a right axillary sentinel node. (**b**) Axial SPECT/CT image shows an enlarged metastatic node (arrow) without tracer uptake next to the sentinel node (Reproduced with permission from https://doi.org/10.1097/RLU.0000000000001407)

11.2.5 Sentinel Node Algorithm and Problem of Midline Tumors

Many organs in the body are midline organs with bilateral drainage of the lymph, such as endometrium, uterine cervix, penis, etc. For sentinel node mapping of these organs, the consensus is to consider each side of the patient as a separate entity, and in case of sentinel node detection failure on each side, lymph node dissection should be done regardless of the contralateral sentinel node condition [31, 48–50]. This approach is called sentinel node algorithm in midline tumors, which can decrease the false negative rate considerably.

In the rest of this chapter, sentinel node mapping in different malignancies would be explained in more detail.

11.3 Breast Cancer

SLN mapping and resection is routinely performed as the preferred axillary staging approach for patients with breast cancer who are clinically node negative at the time of diagnosis (clinical stages I and II). Except for clinically involved axillary lymph nodes, no absolute contraindication is known for sentinel node mapping in breast cancer patients (Table 11.2) [51–54]. Multiple studies showed excellent detection rate (DR) and low false negative rate (FNR) for sentinel node mapping in breast cancer patients. Using a combination of radiotracer/blue dye and superficial injections optimizes the procedure with lowest FNR and highest DR [55, 56].

Injection methods are a matter of controversy in breast cancer. Deep and superficial injections have been shown to be concordant for axillary sentinel node mapping [57]. The peri-areolar intradermal injection of the radiotracer leads to the highest detection rate of the SLN (Fig. 11.11). However, with superficial injections, drainage to the internal mammary nodes is minimal and internal mammary sentinel node visualization is very rare (Fig. 11.12). This is not considered as a drawback for superficial injections as isolated internal mammary node involvement is very rare in breast cancer and most centers in the world do not harvest internal mammary sentinel node [58, 59].

The metastasis of the resected SLN should be assessed by hematoxylin and eosin (H&E) (using a multilevel sectioning) or immunohistochemistry (IHC) staining methods (for equivocal cases

Table 11.2 Sentinel node mapping in breast cancer: special considerations

Condition	Consideration
Clinical involvement of the axilla	Absolute contraindication
Previous surgery of the axilla	Although sentinel node mapping can be done, it is better to be avoided
Previous excisional biopsy of the breast cancer lesion	No contraindication. If the excision line is extended to the axilla, it is better to inject the radiotracer at the ends of the excision line to bypass the excision
Pregnancy	No contraindication. Radiation to the fetus is minimal, especially with the one-day protocol of the procedure
Inflammatory breast cancer	Not recommended. Axillary lymph node dissection is still the standard of care
History of neoadjuvant chemotherapy	No contraindication. However, for patients with axillary involvement before chemotherapy, still axillary lymph node dissection is recommended
Male breast cancer	Sentinel node mapping is the standard of care in clinically N0 patients
Ductal carcinoma in situ	Sentinel node mapping is indicated only in patients scheduled to undergo total mastectomy
Multifocality and multicenterity	No contraindication. However, multiple injections may be more appropriate
History of neoadjuvant chemotherapy	If the axilla was not clinically involved before neoadjuvant therapy, sentinel node mapping can be done successfully
Local recurrence	Sentinel node mapping is possible for patients with local recurrence after breast-conserving surgery who had undergone sentinel node mapping. However, its accuracy is not well documented and is not routinely recommended
Paget's disease of the breast	Sentinel node mapping should be done alongside surgery
Phyllodes tumor	Sentinel node mapping is not needed

on H&E). Routine cytokeratin immunohistochemistry is not recommended. Before ACOSOG Z11 trial, level I/II axillary lymph node dissection was recommended in all cases of pathologically involved sentinel lymph nodes. However, the results of ACOSOG Z11 trial showed that axillary dissection can be omitted in selected cases with positive sentinel node due to minimal chance of nonsentinel involvement. Currently, if all the following criteria are met, axillary dissection can be omitted despite pathologically involved axillary sentinel nodes: T1/T1, less than three involved sentinel nodes, no history of neoadjuvant chemotherapy, and planned breast conserving surgery in addition to breast radiation therapy [60].

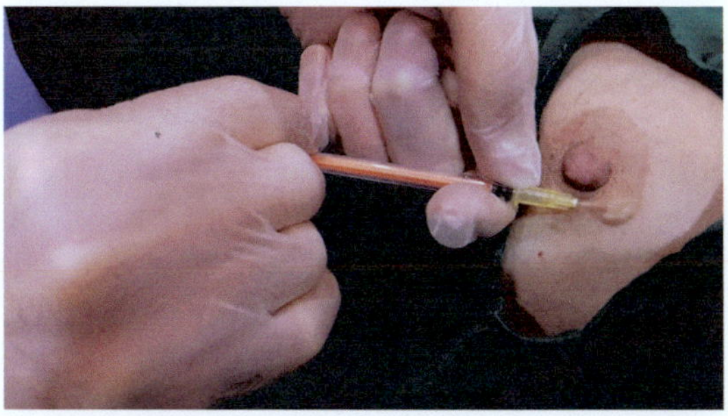

Fig. 11.11 Intradermal injection of the radiotracer in a breast cancer patient. Note the raised weal, which is the hallmark of intradermal injection

11.4 Melanoma

Sentinel lymph node biopsy is a well-established method for regional lymph node staging of melanoma. The concept of sentinel node mapping in melanoma has been supported by very important clinical trials thus far [61]. Table 11.3 summarizes the important aspects of sentinel node mapping indication in melanoma patients [62, 63].

A large number of studies have evaluated sentinel node mapping in melanoma. Despite accumulating experience in sentinel node mapping of

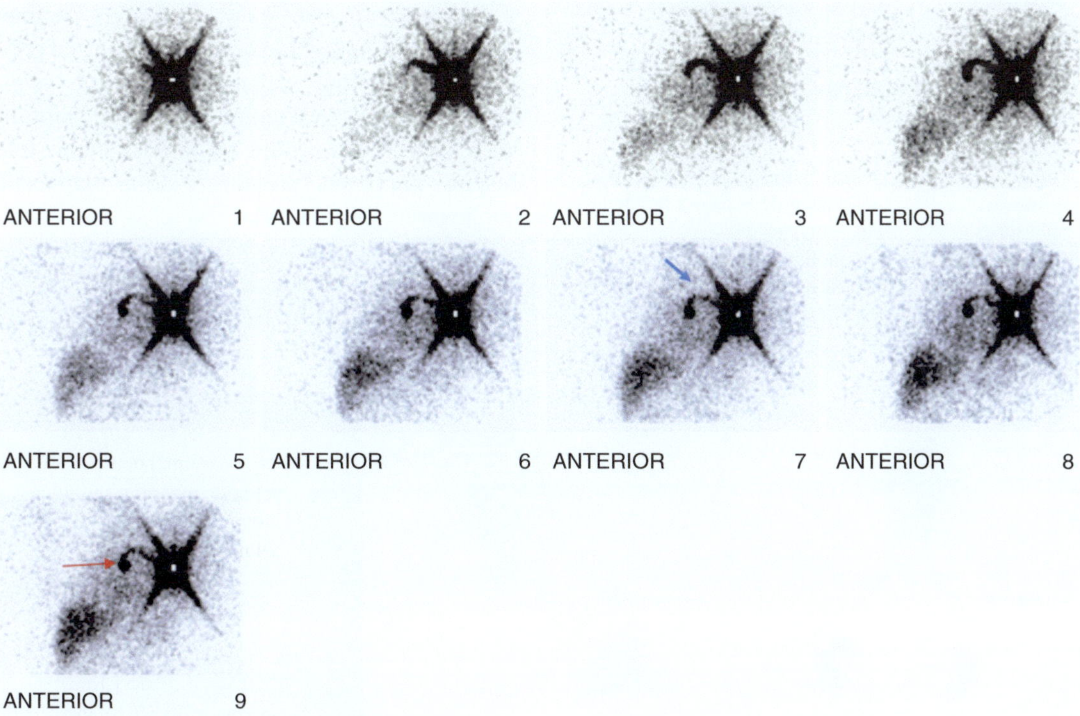

Fig. 11.12 Anterior view dynamic lymphoscintigraphy of a breast cancer patient after intradermal injection of the radiotracer. Note the lymphatic (blue arrow) and internal mammary sentinel nodes (red arrow). This finding is extremely rare in superficial injections

melanoma, high FNR of about 15% is still encountered. Several aspects of sentinel lymph node mapping in melanoma are associated with higher FNR, including old age at diagnosis, deeper lesions, ulceration, and location in the head and neck region [64, 65]. Techniques that can decrease FNR and increase DR are lymphoscintigraphy (especially SPECT/CT) and a combination of blue dye and radiotracer [66]. Overall, it is shown that regional nodal recurrence in melanoma patients with pathologically negative sentinel nodes is acceptable (<5%) and sentinel node mapping with a correct technique is a safe and practical method for regional lymph node staging in melanoma [67].

Table 11.3 Sentinel node mapping in melanoma: special considerations

Condition	Consideration
Patients with less than 5–10% probability of positive sentinel node	Sentinel node mapping is not recommended. These patients include T1a melanoma (Breslow <0.8 mm without ulceration)
Pure desmoplastic melanoma	Sentinel node mapping is not recommended due to the very low possibility of lymph node involvement
Early-stage patients (I/II) with more than 5–10% probability of positive sentinel node	It is a major indication for sentinel node mapping. These patients include T1b (Breslow <0.8 mm with ulceration or 0.8–1 mm with or without ulceration), T1a with adverse features (including very high mitotic index ($\geq 2/mm^2$), lymphovascular invasion), and all other patients with >1 mm thickness without clinically lymph node involvement
History of wide local excision or skin graft of the primary lesion	Sentinel node mapping can be done despite lower accuracy
Isolated in-transit metastasis	Despite being stage III, sentinel node mapping is recommended unless unresectable
Local recurrence of a primary melanoma	If without regional node metastasis, sentinel node mapping can be considered

Injection of the radiotracer is done in a peritumoral fashion (intradermal or subcutaneous), and both same-day and 2-day protocols worked well [68]. Imaging using planar and SPECT/CT is mandatory in sentinel node mapping of melanoma as lymphatic drainage of melanoma can be unpredictable and into multiple basins, especially in the trunk or head and neck melanomas [69, 70] (Fig. 11.13). Imaging should cover all potentially relevant lymphatic basins: for example, for limb melanomas, the entire limb, including intercalary nodes, and for trunk melanoma, bilateral axillary and inguinal areas should be imaged.

Imaging can also show intercalary sentinel nodes such as epitrochlear in upper limb and popliteal in lower limb melanomas. Without preoperative lymphoscintigraphy, the identification of intercalary nodes would be almost impossible despite important prognostic and diagnostic implications (Fig. 11.14).

Frozen section analysis is not useful for melanoma sentinel nodes, and all sentinel nodes should be analyzed by H&E and step sectioning.

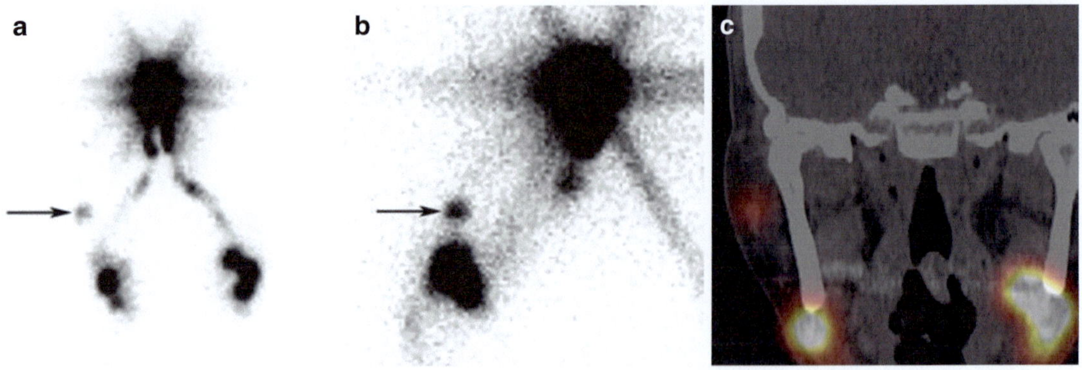

Fig. 11.13 Importance of SPECT/CT lymphoscintigraphy for sentinel node mapping of a forehead melanoma. Anterior planar (**a**), right lateral (**b**), and SPECT/CT image (**c**) showing an intraparotid sentinel node (arrow) (Reproduced with permission from https://doi.org/10.1097/RLU.0000000000001407)

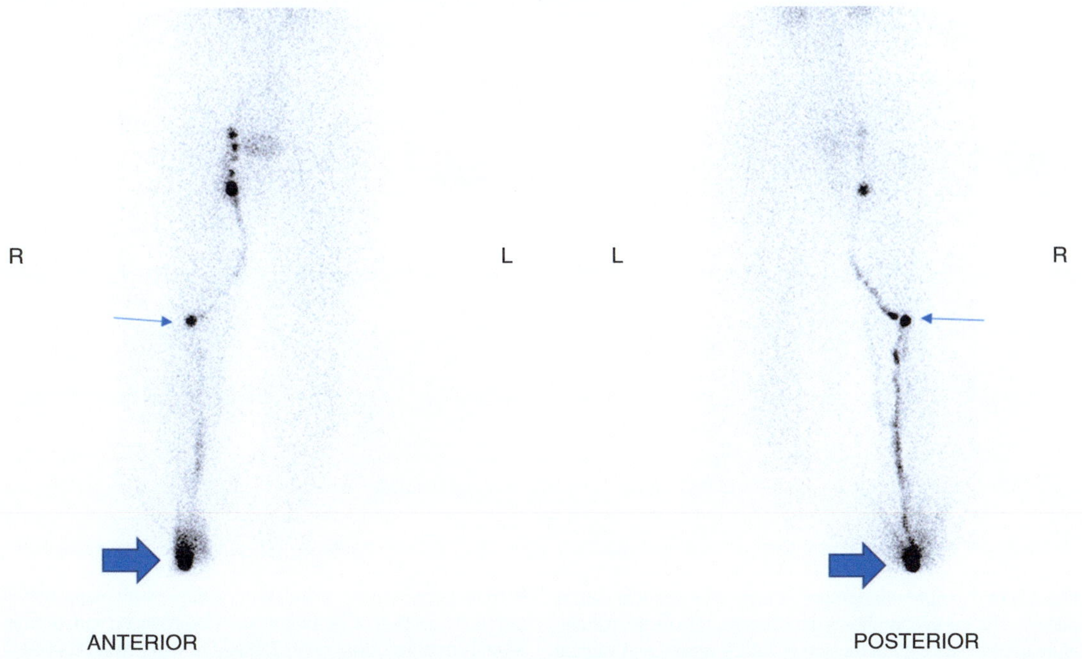

Fig. 11.14 Intercalary popliteal sentinel node on a planar lymphoscintigraphy of a melanoma patient. The sentinel node was harvested intraoperatively and was pathologically involved

IHC should also be done using HMB45, S100, MELAN-A, or SOX-10 stains.

A pathologically involved sentinel node is an important prognostic factor in melanoma patients. However, the best approach following a positive sentinel node results is very controversial. Sentinel node tumor burden and T stage of primary tumor are important factors that determine the probability of nonsentinel node involvement. Regional lymph node dissection did not show any improvement of disease-free survival or overall survival in patients with positive sentinel nodes [71]. On the other hand, regional lymph node dissection can improve the rate of regional disease control and provide prognostic information at the expense of higher complications such as lymphedema [72].

11.5 Uterine Cervix Cancer

Sentinel node mapping is considered the standard of care for pelvic lymph node staging of early uterine cervix cancer [73, 74]. The procedure is done by intracervical injections of mapping materials. Radiotracers can be injected the day before or the same day of the surgery with comparable results [75]. Multiple studies showed that sentinel node mapping in uterine cervix cancer is practical with high DR and low FNR. Using both radiotracer and blue dye and sentinel node algorithm consideration can optimize the procedure (FNR lower than 5%). This procedure is best suited for patients with lower stage (<2 cm diameter confined to the cervix showed the best results) [48].

Preoperative lymphoscintigraphy (especially with SPECT/CT) is of utmost importance in cervical cancer patients. It can show technical failures such as inappropriate injections [76] or unusual locations of the sentinel nodes [77, 78] (Fig. 11.15).

Special considerations for sentinel node mapping in uterine cervix cancer are summarized in Table 11.4 [48, 79].

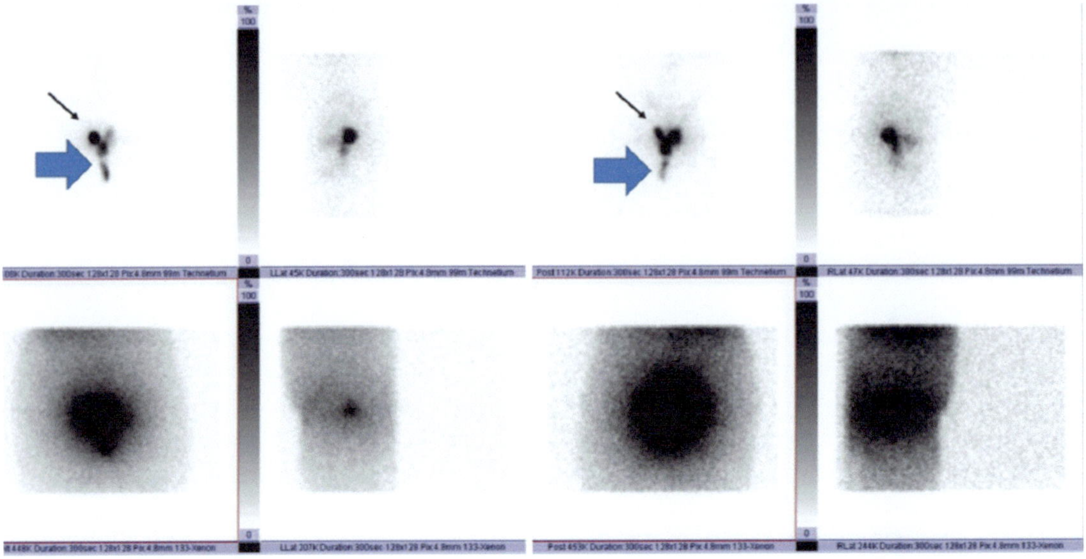

Fig. 11.15 Lymphoscintigraphy images of a cervical cancer patient. The lower row shows the scatterogram of the patient. Note minimal activity in the cervix (black arrow) and vaginal activity (large arrow), which is compatible with inappropriate cervical injection of the radiotracer (Reproduced with permission from https://doi.org/10.7508/AOJNMB.2014.02.009)

Table 11.4 Sentinel node mapping in uterine cervix cancer: special considerations

Condition	Consideration
Cervical lesions confined to cervix with less than 4 cm in greatest diameter (stage IB1 or less)	It is a major indication for sentinel node mapping in cervical cancer. The best results have been achieved in tumors less than 2 cm in greater diameter
History of conization	It is not a contraindication for sentinel node mapping. However, tracer injection can be difficult and needs special expertise to ensure proper injection
History of neoadjuvant chemotherapy	It is not an absolute contraindication for sentinel node mapping. However, detection rate can be low and evidence regarding false negative rate is sparse
Unilateral sentinel lymph node identification	The concept of sentinel lymph node algorithm should be used in all midline tumors, including cervical cancer. In case of unilateral sentinel node detection failure, side-specific lymph node dissection should be performed to decrease the false negative rate

11.6 Endometrial Cancer

In contrast to many solid tumors, regional lymph node dissection is not widely accepted as a standard procedure in the treatment of endometrial cancer. Many experts recommend external beam radiotherapy for high-risk patients. On the other hand, other experts still recommend pelvic and/or para-aortic lymph node dissection even in low-risk endometrial cancer patients [80]. However, the risk of lymph node involvement in low-risk endometrial cancer patients is very low, and many surgeons omit lymph node dissection from the surgical procedure of these patients. Sentinel lymph node mapping is considered as a viable compromise between these two extremes and can be considered for select low-risk patients (endometrioid pathology, especially GI and GII) with uterine-confined malignancy [81–84].

Injection site is a major controversial issue in sentinel node mapping of endometrial cancer patients. Cervical and fundal injections both have been used for this purpose. Cervical injection site is readily available and very easy to reach. In addition, it has been shown that both cervical and fundal injections show same pelvic sentinel nodes with minimal discordance between these two injection cites [85]. However, lymphatic drainage to the para-aortic lymph nodes is only possible with fundal injections. On the other hand, fundal injections need laparoscopic (submucosal injections) or hysteroscopic (subserosal injections) procedures, which make it less feasible [85, 86]. As isolated para-aortic lymph node involvement is extremely rare in low-risk endometrial cancer patients, cervical injections seem to be enough and the best method for delivering mapping materials [87]. Two to four cervical injections have been used with one-day or two-day protocols with comparable success.

Same as other malignancies, lymphoscintigraphy, especially SPECT/CT, can provide useful information regarding sentinel node locations and is strongly recommended preoperatively [88] (Figs. 11.16 and 11.17).

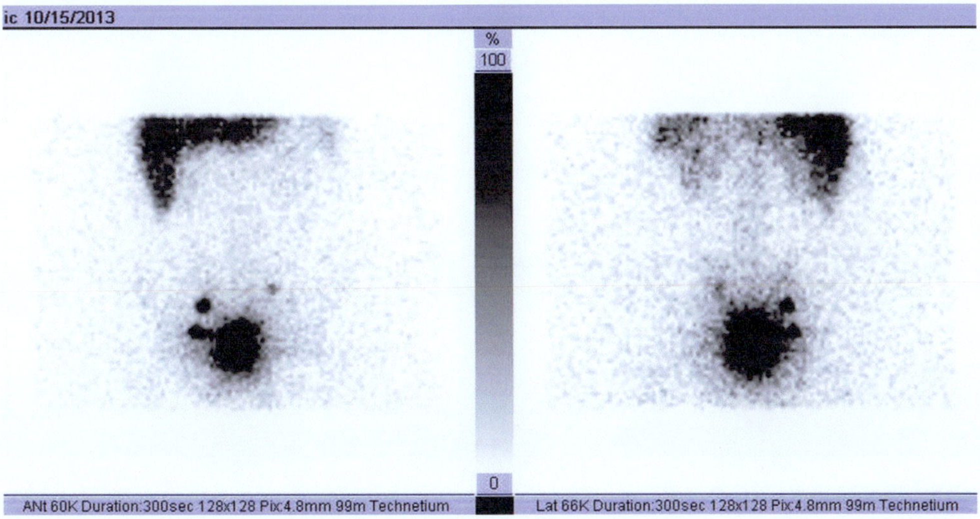

Fig. 11.16 Anterior and posterior planar lymphoscintigraphy images of an endometrial cancer patient following cervical injection of the radiotracer. Note bilateral sentinel node visualization in the pelvic area without any para-aortic sentinel node

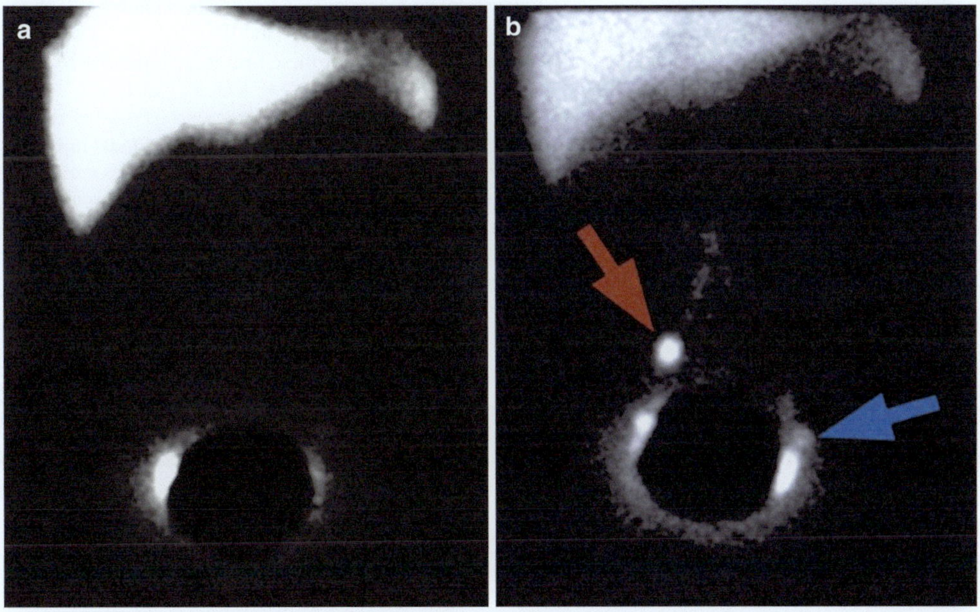

Fig. 11.17 Lymphoscintigraphy images of an endometrial cancer patient. Planar image showed a faint left pelvic sentinel node (**a**). Note the shield used to cover the injection site. Delayed planar image shows a right pelvic sentinel node (red arrow), as well as a left sentinel node (blue arrow) (**b**). 3D volume-rendering image shows two posterior and caudal nodes (dotted circle) corresponding to external iliac nodes during surgery (arrow) (**c**, **d**) (Reproduced with permission from https://doi.org/10.1007/s40336-016-0187-6)

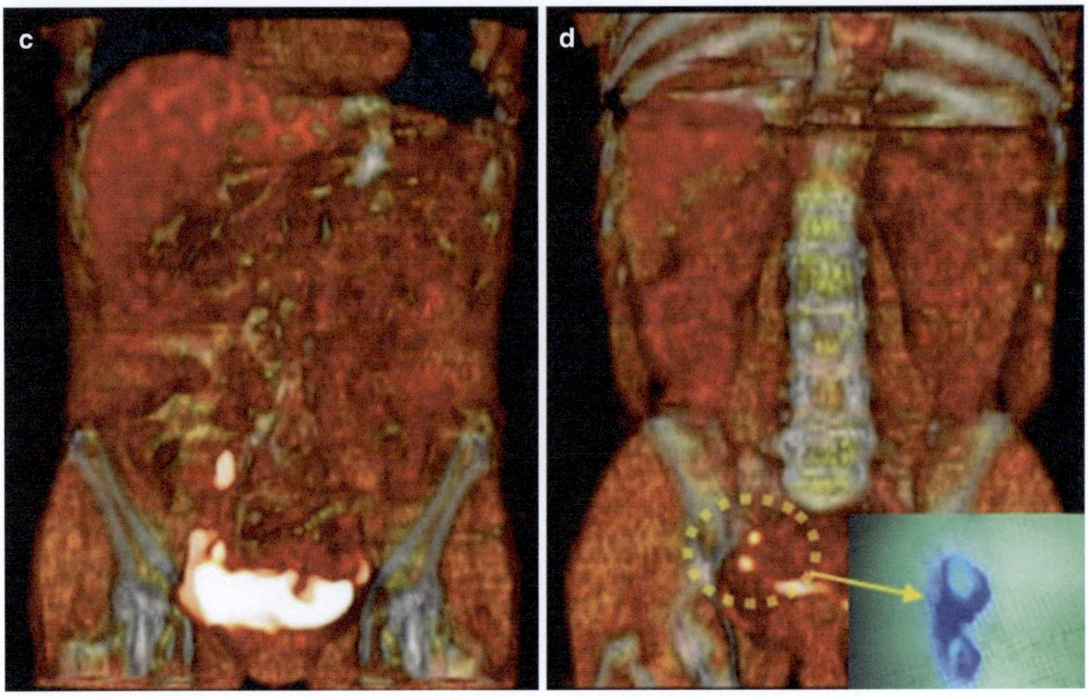

Fig. 11.17 (continued)

Table 11.5 Sentinel node mapping in endometrial cancer: special considerations

Condition	Consideration
Low-risk uterine-confined cancers	It is a major indication for sentinel node mapping in endometrial cancer, which includes endometrioid histology, especially grades I and II
Serous carcinoma, clear cell carcinoma, and carcinosarcoma	Sentinel node mapping is not recommended for these histologic types due to suboptimal accuracy
Para-aortic sentinel node harvesting	Para-aortic sentinel nodes can only be expected to be found using fundal injections of the mapping materials. In cervical injections, Para-aortic sentinel nodes are very rare but should be harvested in case of visualization on preoperative lymphoscintigraphy
Unilateral sentinel lymph node identification	The concept of sentinel lymph node algorithm should be used in all midline tumors, including endometrial cancer. In case of unilateral sentinel node detection failure, side-specific lymph node dissection should be performed to decrease the false negative rate

Overall, using a combination of blue dye and radiotracer, intracervical injection of the mapping material, and considering the concept of sentinel node algorithm can optimize the sentinel node mapping procedure in endometrial cancer with highest DR and lowest FNR. This is especially true for low-risk patients, including patients with grade I or II endometrioid cancers without lymphovascular invasion or <50% myometrial invasion [84].

Table 11.5 shows special considerations regarding the indications of sentinel node mapping in endometrial cancer patients.

11.7 Vulvar Cancer

The feasibility, safety, and validity of sentinel lymph node biopsy of inguinofemoral lymph node basins have been proven through different studies [89–91], and SLNB is widely accepted as a standard alternative to lymphadenectomy in selected women with squamous cell carcinoma (SCC) of the vulva. This technique is associated with less morbidity and low risk of groin recurrences compared with lymphadenectomy, which might lead to lymphedema or wound complications. Multiple studies showed the feasibility and accuracy of sentinel node mapping in vulvar cancer. A combination of blue dye and radiotracer, limiting patients to unifocal tumors <4 cm, and considering sentinel node algorithm in midline tumors (<2 cm distance from midline) can optimize DR and FNR (87% DR and 6.4% FNR and 2.8% recurrence rate) [49, 92].

For vulvar cancer, two to four preoperative injections of radiotracer are performed with a total dose depending on the same-day or previous-day protocol [49, 93]. Patients with positive SNs are a candidate for inguinofemoral lymphadenectomy and/or adjuvant radiotherapy; however, negative SNs are proposed to be followed by future observations.

Preoperative lymphoscintigraphy and SPECT/CT can provide very useful information and should be done preoperatively if possible [49] (Fig. 11.18).

Table 11.6 shows the special considerations regarding sentinel node mapping in vulvar SCC.

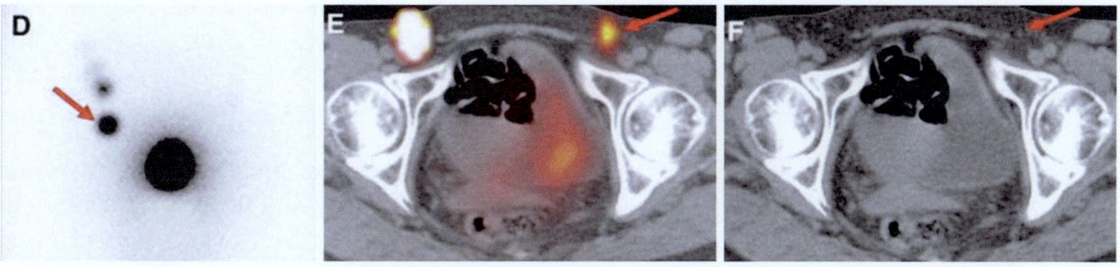

Fig. 11.18 Planar and SPECT/CT images of a vulvar cancer patient. Note unilateral drainage on planar but bilateral drainage on SPECT/CT images (Reproduced with permission from https://doi.org/10.1007/s40336-016-0187-6)

Table 11.6 Sentinel node mapping in vulvar cancer: special considerations

Condition	Consideration
Tumors confined to the vulva without clinical or radiological groin involvement	It is a major indication for sentinel node mapping in vulvar cancer
History of excisional biopsy of the primary lesion	Sentinel node mapping can be done in this setting. Injections should be done with special attention to possible distorted anatomy
Clinically or radiologically involved groins	It is an absolute contraindication for sentinel node mapping
Unilateral sentinel lymph node identification	The concept of sentinel lymph node algorithm should be used in all midline tumors, including vulvar cancer However, vulvar cancers can be divided into lateral (≥2 cm from midline) and midline lesions. Only midline lesions should be considered for sentinel node algorithm (Fig. 11.19), and in case of unilateral sentinel node detection failure in midline lesions, side-specific lymph node dissection should be performed to decrease the false negative rate

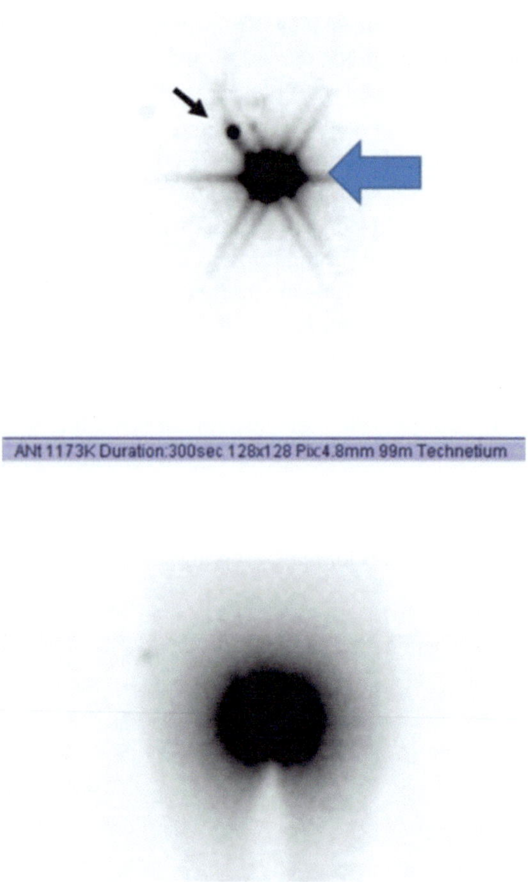

Fig. 11.19 Planar lymphoscintigraphy of a patient with a vulvar SCC in the right labia major area. Note unilateral sentinel node visualization. The lower image is the corresponding scatterogram (Reproduced with permission from http://irjnm.tums.ac.ir/article_4071_828.html)

Table 11.7 Sentinel node mapping in penile SCC: special considerations

Condition	Consideration
Tumors without palpable inguinal lymph nodes	It is a major indication for sentinel node mapping in penile cancer. Any T stage, as long as there is no palpable inguinal lymph node
Preoperative ultrasound	In order to decrease the false negative rate, inguinal ultrasound with FNA of the suspicious lymph nodes is mandatory. This approach can decrease false negative rate up to 10%
Clinically involved groins	It is an absolute contraindication for sentinel node mapping
Unilateral sentinel lymph node identification	The concept of sentinel lymph node algorithm should be used in all midline tumors, including penile cancer. In case of unilateral sentinel node detection failure, side-specific lymph node dissection should be performed to decrease the false negative rate

11.8 Penile Cancer

Historically, penile SCC was the first solid tumor for which the concept of sentinel node was used [3]. The concept of sentinel node mapping is now the standard of care for regional lymph node staging in penile SCC [94–97]. However, the technique should be standardized to avoid false negative results. Special considerations for sentinel node mapping in penile cancer are shown in Table 11.7 [96, 98]. Injection of the tracer is usually done in an intradermal fashion around the tumor. Step sectioning and IHC of the harvested sentinel nodes can also contribute to a successful lymph node staging.

Preoperative lymphoscintigraphy and SPECT/CT can also show unusual locations of the sentinel nodes, as well as false sentinels, such as contaminations or tracer holdup in the lymphatics [99, 100] (Figs. 11.20 and 11.21).

Best results of sentinel node mapping can be achieved in cN0 patients using a combination of blue dye and radiotracer (90% DR and 8% FNR). In patients with palpable inguinal nodes, preoperative lymph node sampling can decrease FNR. Following the sentinel node algorithm concept can also decrease FNR [96, 101].

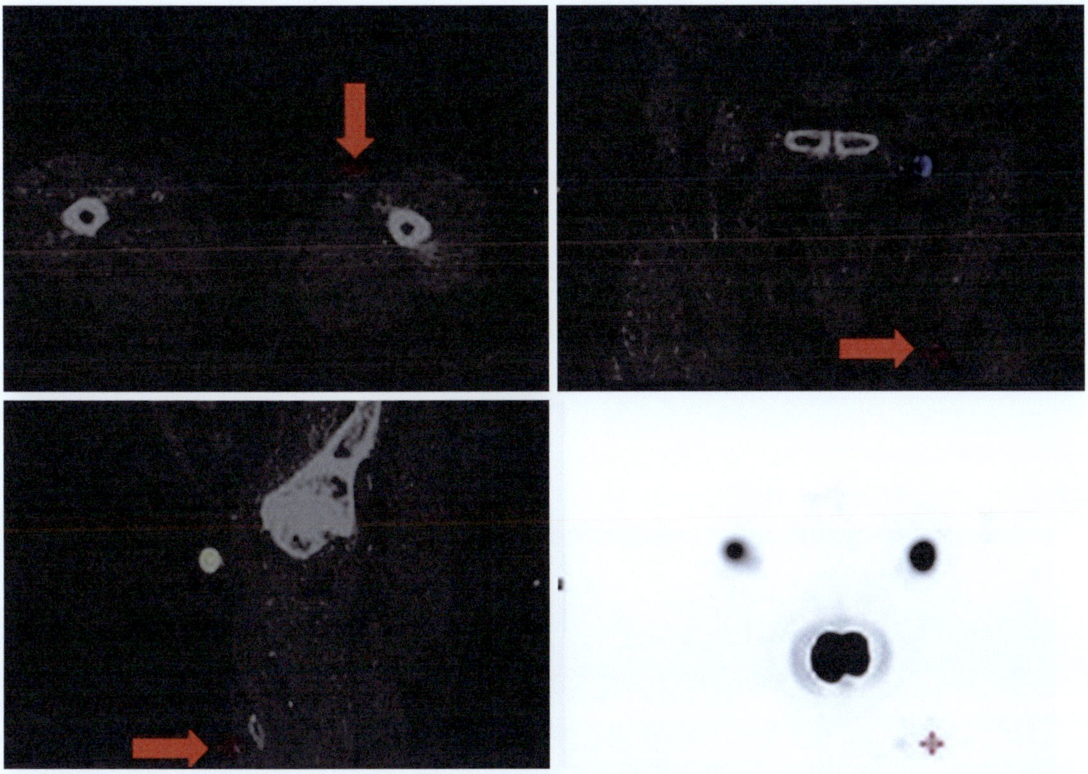

Fig. 11.20 An unusual location of a sentinel node in a penile SCC shown by SPECT/CT in the left mid-thigh (red arrows) (Reproduced with permission from https://doi.org/10.1007/s00259-017-3636-1)

11.9 Colorectal Cancer

In colorectal cancer, the number of lymph nodes to be evaluated by the pathologists is a major problem in staging. At least 12 lymph nodes should be evaluated for complete lymph node staging. This is not always possible, and many specimens have less than 12 lymph nodes suitable for pathological evaluation, especially in rectal cancer patients with a history of neoadjuvant radiotherapy. Sentinel node mapping in colorectal cancer has shown excellent sensitivity for the detection of lymph node involvement [102, 103]. However, a major benefit of sentinel node mapping in colorectal cancer resides in the possibility of IHC and the detection of micrometastases in the sentinel nodes, which would result in upstaging in apparently stage II patients. Prognostic significance of sentinel node involvement has been shown in multiple studies, and sentinel node mapping may change the management of certain patients with colorectal cancer [104–108]. Table 11.8 shows special considerations in colorectal cancer sentinel node mapping.

The injection techniques for colorectal cancers are very diverse: in vivo injections (submucosal or subserosal, intraoperatively or preoperatively using endoscopy) and ex vivo technique (injections following removal of the tumor) have both done well [109–111]. In in vivo techniques, the mapping material is injected in the submucosal or subserosal areas around the tumor. Lymphoscintigraphy can be done if available. In ex vivo technique, the mapping material is injected in a subserosal fashion around the resected tumor (Fig. 11.22). A certain amount of

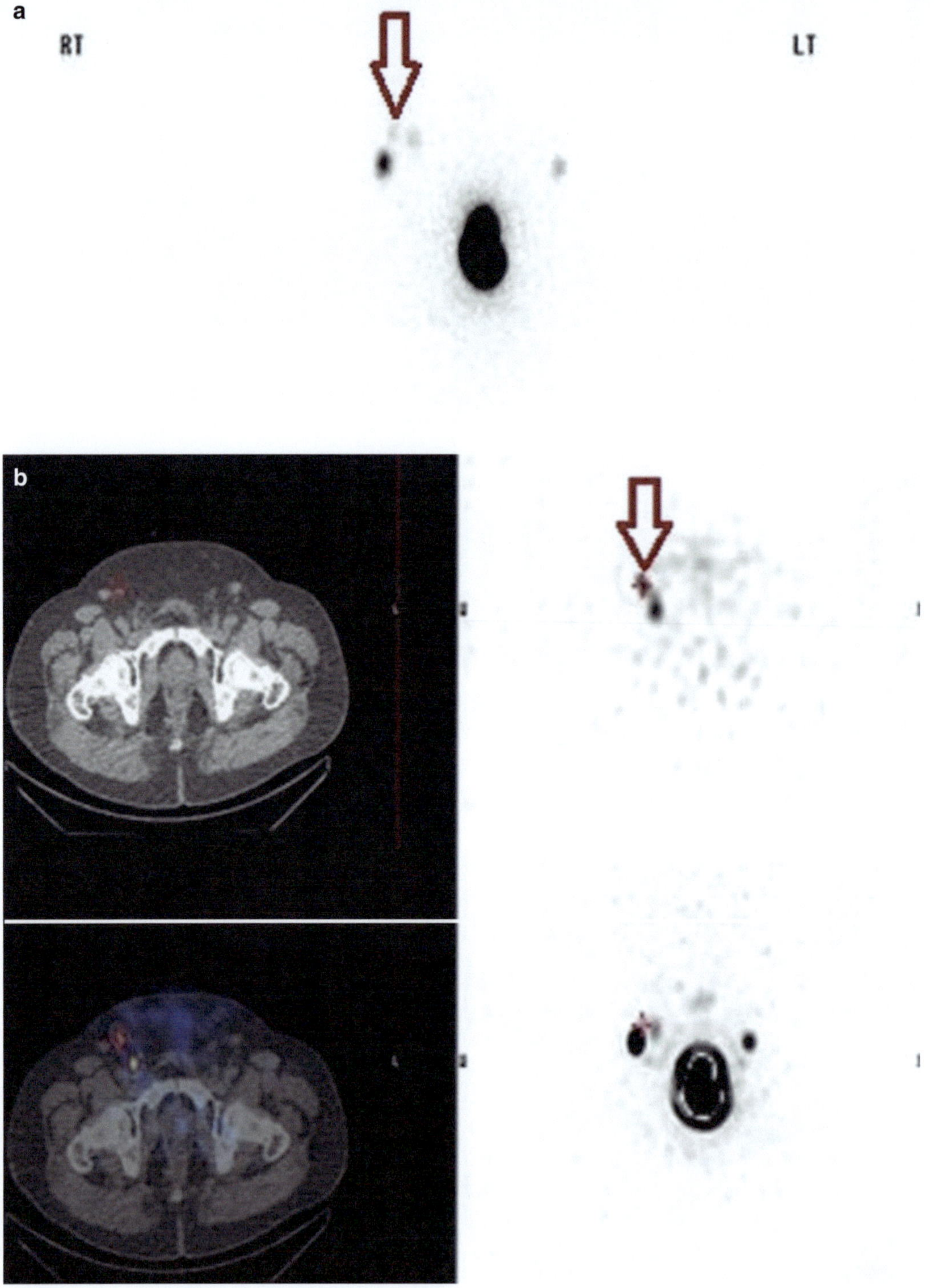

Fig. 11.21 Planar and SPECT/CT lymphoscintigraphy of a penile cancer patient. Planar image shows three hot areas (red arrow) presuming to be sentinel nodes in the right groin (**a**). SPECT/CT images shows one of the foci in holdup of the tracer in the lymphatic channel (red arrow) (**b**) (Reproduced with permission from https://doi.org/10.1007/s00259-017-3636-1)

Table 11.8 Sentinel node mapping in colorectal cancer: special considerations

Condition	Consideration
Tumors in surgically stage II or lower stage cancers	Major indication of sentinel node mapping in colorectal cancer
Clinically or radiologically involved lymph nodes	Absolute contraindication for sentinel node mapping
History of neoadjuvant radiotherapy in rectal cancers	Not recommended. Detection rate and sensitivity have shown to be low

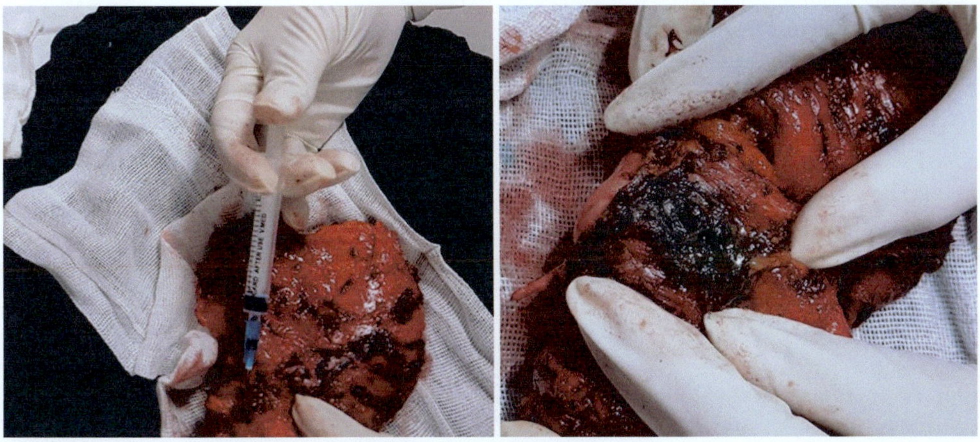

Fig. 11.22 Ex vivo Injection of a radiolabeled blue dye in the peri-tumoral subserosal region of a colon cancer (left image). Note sentinel node visualization after 5 min (right image)

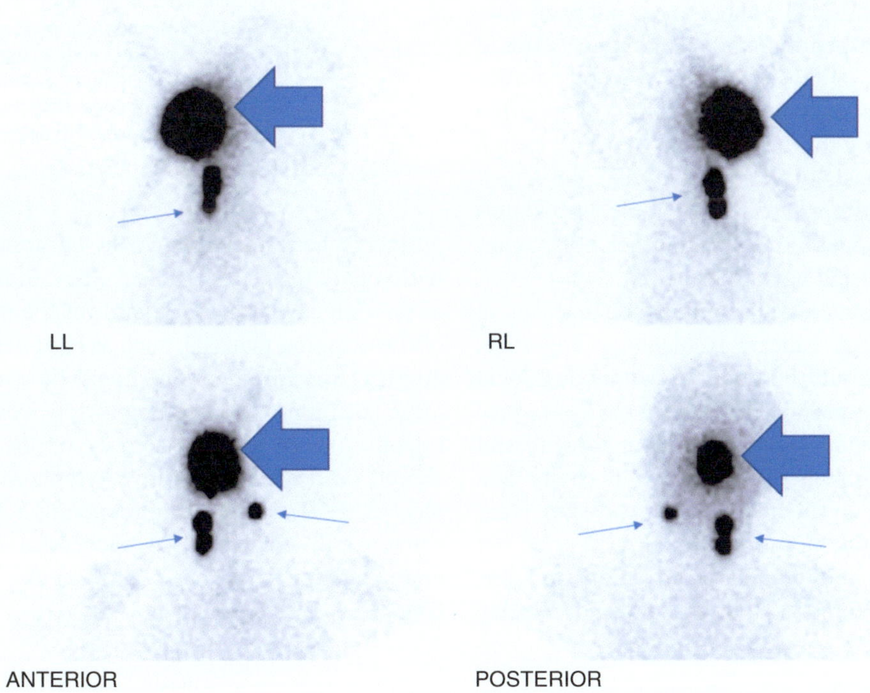

Fig. 11.23 Bilateral lymph node drainage in a midline tongue SCC. Note bilateral cervical sentinel node visualization (arrows). Bilateral sentinel nodes were harvested during surgery (two on the right and one on the left side). The large arrows are injection sites

time should pass (at least 5–15 min) for the mapping material to reach the sentinel nodes. All harvested sentinel nodes should be subjected to step sectioning and IHC to identify micrometastases.

The detection rate of sentinel node mapping is high (>90%). The overall FNR of sentinel node biopsy in colorectal cancer is about 20–30% without any difference for different T stages or tumor location. Despite a relatively high FNR, upstaging has been reported in up to 32% of colon cancer and 17% of rectal cancer patients [112]. History of neoadjuvant radiotherapy is associated with low DR, and sentinel node mapping should be discouraged in this group of rectal cancer patients [113].

11.10 Head and Neck Cancers

Sentinel node mapping has been used with great success for SCC of the head and neck area. The overall FNR for sentinel node mapping in head and neck SCC is reported to be 4.7% [114]. The accuracy of sentinel node mapping for tumors >4 cm or with >10 mm depth of invasion (T3 and T4) has not been documented, and sentinel node mapping is better to be avoided in these tumors. Several studies have shown excellent sensitivity of sentinel node mapping for the detection of occult lymph node metastasis in SCC of the oral cavity, oropharynx, and lips [115, 116]. Table 11.9 shows special considerations for sentinel node mapping in head and neck SCC [114].

Table 11.9 Sentinel node mapping in head and neck SCC: special considerations

Condition	Consideration
Clinically and radiologically N0 patients	It is a major indication for sentinel node mapping in head and neck SCC. Only tumors of the oral cavity and lips have been studied enough and validated for sentinel node mapping. Tumors of the larynx and pharyngeal areas should not be considered for sentinel node mapping yet (only for research purposes)
Clinically involved cervical nodes	It is an absolute contraindication for sentinel node mapping
Large or locally advanced tumors	Accuracy of sentinel node mapping for tumors >4 cm or with >10 mm depth of invasion (T3 and T4) has not been documented, and sentinel node mapping is better to be avoided in these tumors
Unilateral sentinel lymph node identification	The concept of sentinel lymph node algorithm should be used in all midline tumors, including head and neck cancers However, not all head and neck cancers are in midline locations. Only lesions involving midline locations should be considered for sentinel node algorithm (Fig. 11.23), and in case of unilateral sentinel node detection failure in these tumors, side-specific cervical lymph node dissection should be performed to decrease the false negative rate

A key to successful sentinel node mapping in head and neck cancers is technical expertise. Injections should be done after applying local anesthesia (especially in the oral cavity) to prevent patient movement. Two to four peri-tumoral injections (submucosal in the oral cavity and intradermal or subcutaneous in the skin area) should be done. Caution should be exerted not to cross the midline area by injections in laterally located tumors. Both one-day and two-day protocols have been shown to be comparable with regard to success and accuracy. Some parts of the oral cavity are very hard for the injection of the mapping material, such as hard palate and gingiva. Special attention should be exerted in these locations, and preferably low volume of injection (high specific activity of the tracer) should be used. Preoperative lymphoscintigraphy, SPECT/CT, and intraoperative gamma cameras all contribute to successful sentinel node mapping in head and neck cancers (Fig. 11.24).

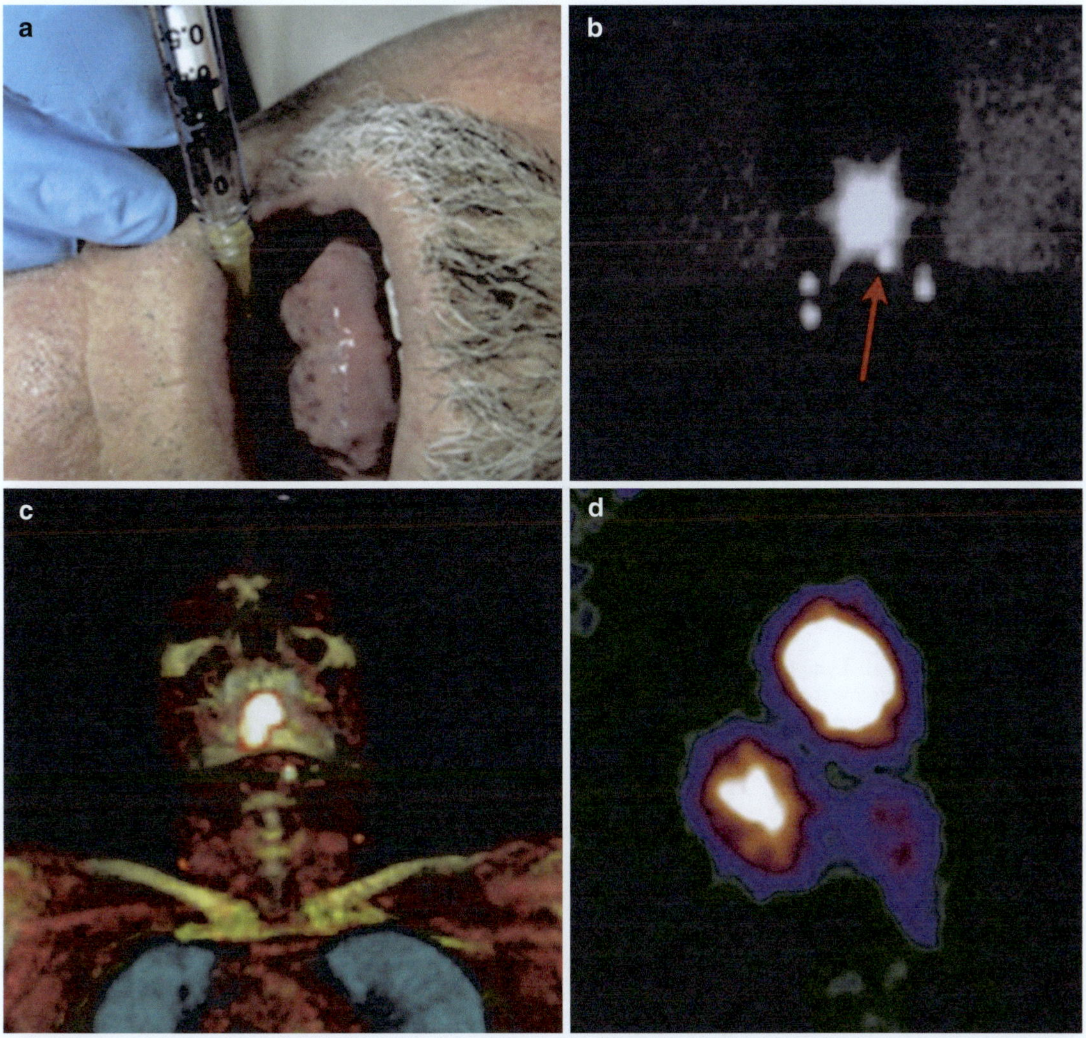

Fig. 11.24 Sentinel node mapping in a floor of a floor of the mouth SCC that involved midline. Injection of radiotracer (**a**). Anterior planar lymphoscintigraphy 2 h post injection, which shows bilateral drainage and a level I node (red arrow) (**b**). SPECT/CT 3D reconstruction shows the sentinel node in the left level I (**c**). Portable gamma camera image also shows the same node in level 1 (**d**) (Reproduced with permission from https://doi.org/10.1016/j.jcms.2015.10.006)

11.11 Other Solid Tumors

Sentinel node mapping has been used for lymph node staging of other cancers, such as gastric cancer [117, 118], esophageal cancer [119, 120], laryngeal SCC [121], Merkel cell carcinoma [122, 123], thyroid cancer [124], prostate cancer [125], Marjolin's ulcer [126], non-small cell lung cancers [127, 128], ovarian malignancies [129], anal canal cancers [50, 130], bladder and kidney malignancies [131], and soft tissue sarcomas [132, 133]. However, its clinical utility has yet to be determined in future studies. Routine clinical use in these malignancies is not recommended.

References

1. KleinJan GH, et al. Multimodal hybrid imaging agents for sentinel node mapping as a means to (re) connect nuclear medicine to advances made in robot-assisted surgery. Eur J Nucl Med Mol Imaging. 2016;43(7):1278–87.
2. Sadeghi R. Sentinel node mapping diagnostic studies warrant a unique reporting criteria: comment on Xiong et al. systematic review. Eur J Surg Oncol. 2014;40(8):1025–6.
3. Cabanas RM. An approach for the treatment of penile carcinoma. Cancer. 1977;39(2):456–66.
4. Weissbach L, Boedefeld E. Localization of solitary and multiple metastases in stage II nonseminomatous testis tumor as basis for a modified staging lymph node dissection in stage I. J Urol. 1987;138(1):77–82.
5. Morton DL, et al. Technical details of intraoperative lymphatic mapping for early stage melanoma. Arch Surg. 1992;127(4):392–9.
6. Morton DL, et al. Intraoperative lymphatic mapping and selective cervical lymphadenectomy for early-stage melanomas of the head and neck. J Clin Oncol. 1993;11(9):1751–6.
7. Giuliano AE, et al. Lymphatic mapping and sentinel lymphadenectomy for breast cancer. Ann Surg. 1994;220(3):391.
8. Krag D, et al. Surgical resection and radiolocalization of the sentinel lymph node in breast cancer using a gamma probe. Surg Oncol. 1993;2(6):335–40.
9. Alex J, Krag D. Gamma-probe guided localization of lymph nodes. Surg Oncol. 1993;2(3):137–43.
10. Alex J, et al. Gamma-probe-guided lymph node localization in malignant melanoma. Surg Oncol. 1993;2(5):303–8.
11. Scherer K, Bircher AJ, Figueiredo V. Blue dyes in medicine—a confusing terminology. Contact Dermatitis. 2006;54(4):231–2.
12. Howard JD, Moo V, Sivalingam P. Anaphylaxis and other adverse reactions to blue dyes: a case series. Anaesth Intensive Care. 2011;39(2):287–92.
13. Uhara H, et al. Applicability of radiocolloids, blue dyes and fluorescent indocyanine green to sentinel node biopsy in melanoma. J Dermatol. 2012;39(4):336–8.
14. Fattahi AS, et al. Can methylene blue dye be used as an alternative to patent blue dye to find the sentinel lymph node in breast cancer surgery? J Res Med Sci. 2014;19(10):918–22.
15. Sadeghi R, et al. Added value of blue dye injection in sentinel node biopsy of breast cancer patients: do all patients need blue dye? Int J Surg. 2014;12(4):325–8.
16. Jangjoo A, et al. Anaphylaxis reaction of a breast cancer patient to methylene blue during breast surgery with sentinel node mapping. Acta Oncol. 2010;49(6):877–8.
17. Xiong L, et al. Indocyanine green fluorescence-guided sentinel node biopsy: a meta-analysis on detection rate and diagnostic performance. Eur J Surg Oncol. 2014;40(7):843–9.
18. Gulec S, et al. Gamma probe guided sentinel node biopsy in breast cancer. Q J Nucl Med. 1997;41(3):251–61.
19. Henze E, et al. Lymphoscintigraphy with Tc-99m-labeled dextran. J Nucl Med. 1982;23(10):923–9.
20. Czerniecki BJ, et al. Revolutionary impact of lymphoscintigraphy and intraoperative sentinel node mapping in the clinical practice of oncology. Semin Nucl Med. 2001;31(2):158–64.
21. Kaleya RN, et al. Lymphatic mapping and sentinel node biopsy: a surgical perspective. Semin Nucl Med. 2005;35(2):129–34.
22. Mount MG, et al. Evaluating one day versus two days preoperative lymphoscintigraphy protocols for sentinel lymph node biopsy in breast cancer. Am Surg. 2015;81(5):454–7.
23. Ali J, et al. Comparison between one day and two days protocols for sentinel node mapping of breast cancer patients. Hell J Nucl Med. 2011;14(3):313–5.
24. Koizumi M, et al. Sentinel node detection using 99mTc-rhenium sulphide colloid in breast cancer patients: evaluation of 1 day and 2 day protocols, and a dose-finding study. Nucl Med Commun. 2003;24(6):663–70.
25. Unkart JT, Proudfoot J, Wallace AM. Outcomes of "one-day" vs "two-day" injection protocols using Tc-99m tilmanocept for sentinel lymph node biopsy in breast cancer. Breast J. 2018;24:526.
26. Jangjoo A, et al. Comparison of early and delayed lymphoscintigraphy images of early breast cancer patients undergoing sentinel node mapping. Nucl Med Commun. 2010;31(6):521–5.
27. Aliakbarian M, et al. Factors influencing the time of sentinel node visualization in breast cancer patients using intradermal injection of the radiotracer. Am J Surg. 2011;202(2):199–202.
28. Sadeghi R, et al. How long the lymphoscintigraphy imaging should be continued for sentinel lymph node mapping? Ann Nucl Med. 2009;23(6):507–10.
29. Abdollahi A, et al. Factors affecting sentinel lymph node detection failure in breast cancer patients using intradermal injection of the tracer. Rev Esp Med Nucl. 2010;29(2):73–7.
30. Zarifmahmoudi L, et al. Dynamic lymphoscintigraphy in breast cancer patients: feasibility and added value. Iran J Nucl Med. 2016;24(2):130–5.
31. Sadeghi R, Hasanzadeh M. Sentinel lymph node biopsy algorithm: can it be a universal method for midline tumors? Gynecol Oncol. 2014;132(2):273–4.
32. Lloyd LR, Wesen CA, McCallum S. An analysis of filtration and volume of radionucleotide in sentinel lymph node biopsy in breast cancer patients. Am Surg. 2002;68(4):373–5. discussion 375–6
33. Nunez EG, et al. Combining dose and injection volume for good performance of a specific radiopharmaceutical for sentinel node detection. Nucl Med Biol. 2012;39(1):145–53.
34. Dabbagh Kakhki VR, et al. Effect of radiotracer injection volume on the success of sentinel node biopsy

in early-stage breast cancer patients. Nucl Med Commun. 2013;34(7):660–3.
35. Catarci M, et al. Preoperative lymphoscintigraphy and sentinel lymph node biopsy in papillary thyroid cancer. A pilot study. J Surg Oncol. 2001;77(1):21–4. discussion 25
36. Ogasawara Y, et al. Clinical significance of preoperative lymphoscintigraphy for sentinel lymph node biopsy in breast cancer. J Surg Res. 2008;148(2):191–6.
37. Marone U, et al. Lymphoscintigraphy defines new lymphatic pathways from cutaneous melanoma site: clinical implications and surgical management. Radiol Res Pract. 2011;2011:817043.
38. Liberman L. Lymphoscintigraphy for lymphatic mapping in breast carcinoma. Radiology. 2003;228(2):313–5.
39. Giudice G, et al. Unusual sentinel lymph nodes detected by lymphoscintigraphy in cutaneous melanoma patients. Recenti Prog Med. 2013;104(7–8):387–92.
40. Tsuchimochi M, Hayama K. Intraoperative gamma cameras for radioguided surgery: technical characteristics, performance parameters, and clinical applications. Phys Med. 2013;29(2):126–38.
41. Heller S, Zanzonico P. Nuclear probes and intraoperative gamma cameras. Semin Nucl Med. 2011;41(3):166–81.
42. Hellingman D, et al. Detecting near-the-injection-site sentinel nodes in head and neck melanomas with a high-resolution portable gamma camera. Clin Nucl Med. 2015;40(1):e11–6.
43. Duch J. Portable gamma cameras: the real value of an additional view in the operating theatre. Eur J Nucl Med Mol Imaging. 2011;38(4):633–5.
44. Goni Girones E, et al. Evaluation of the efficacy of sentinel node detection in breast cancer: chronological course and influence of the incorporation of an intra-operative portable gamma camera. Rev Esp Med Nucl Imagen Mol. 2013;32(6):343–9.
45. Sato K, et al. Clinically useful detection criteria for sentinel nodes in patients with breast cancer using a radioisotope technique. Jpn J Clin Oncol. 2002;32(10):403–6.
46. Carlson GW, et al. The definition of the sentinel lymph node in melanoma based on radioactive counts. Ann Surg Oncol. 2002;9(9):929–33.
47. Tanis PJ, et al. False negative sentinel node procedure established through palpation of the biopsy wound. Eur J Surg Oncol. 2000;26(7):714–5.
48. Kadkhodayan S, et al. Sentinel node biopsy for lymph nodal staging of uterine cervix cancer: a systematic review and meta-analysis of the pertinent literature. Eur J Surg Oncol. 2015;41(1):1–20.
49. Hassanzade M, et al. Lymphatic mapping and sentinel node biopsy in squamous cell carcinoma of the vulva: systematic review and meta-analysis of the literature. Gynecol Oncol. 2013;130(1):237–45.
50. Tehranian S, et al. Sentinel node mapping in anal canal cancer: systematic review and meta-analysis. J Gastrointestin Liver Dis. 2013;22(3):321–8.
51. Javan H, et al. The accuracy of sentinel node biopsy in breast cancer patients with the history of previous surgical biopsy of the primary lesion: systematic review and meta-analysis of the literature. Eur J Surg Oncol. 2012;38(2):95–109.
52. Manca G, et al. Sentinel lymph node biopsy in breast cancer: indications, contraindications, and controversies. Clin Nucl Med. 2016;41(2):126–33.
53. Tjalma WA. The contraindications for a sentinel node biopsy in breast cancer are actually indications. Surgeon. 2015;13(1):59.
54. Gradishar W, Salerno KE. NCCN guidelines update: breast cancer. J Natl Compr Cancer Netw. 2016;14(5S):641–4.
55. Stamatakos M, et al. Sentinel lymph node biopsy in breast cancer: a systematic review. Onkologie. 2010;33(3):121–6.
56. van der Ploeg IM, et al. Axillary recurrence after a tumour-negative sentinel node biopsy in breast cancer patients: a systematic review and meta-analysis of the literature. Eur J Surg Oncol. 2008;34(12):1277–84.
57. Sadeghi R, et al. Axillary concordance between superficial and deep sentinel node mapping material injections in breast cancer patients: systematic review and meta-analysis of the literature. Breast Cancer Res Treat. 2014;144(2):213–22.
58. Ferreres Garcia K, et al. Therapeutic attitude towards internal mammary chain drainage in patients with breast cancer. Breast. 2016;30:1–4.
59. Tan C, Caragata R, Bennett I. Is sentinel node biopsy of the internal mammary lymph nodes relevant in the management of breast cancer? Breast J. 2017;23(4):410–4.
60. Giuliano AE, et al. Axillary dissection vs no axillary dissection in women with invasive breast cancer and sentinel node metastasis: a randomized clinical trial. JAMA. 2011;305(6):569–75.
61. Morton DL, et al. Final trial report of sentinel-node biopsy versus nodal observation in melanoma. N Engl J Med. 2014;370(7):599–609.
62. Kim HL, et al. NCCN clinical practice guidelines in oncology™. Fort Washington, PA: NCCN; 2014.
63. Dunne JA, et al. Is sentinel lymph node biopsy warranted for desmoplastic melanoma? A systematic review. J Plast Reconstr Aesthet Surg. 2017;70(2):274–80.
64. de Rosa N, et al. Sentinel node biopsy for head and neck melanoma: a systematic review. Otolaryngol Head Neck Surg. 2011;145(3):375–82.
65. Manca G, et al. A critical reappraisal of false negative sentinel lymph node biopsy in melanoma. Q J Nucl Med Mol Imaging. 2014;58:105–13.
66. Tardelli E, et al. Sentinel lymph node biopsy in cutaneous melanoma: standard and new technical procedures and clinical advances. A systematic review of the literature. Clin Nucl Med. 2016;41(12):e498–507.
67. Valsecchi ME, et al. Lymphatic mapping and sentinel lymph node biopsy in patients with melanoma: a meta-analysis. J Clin Oncol. 2011;29(11):1479–87.

68. Rødgaard JC, Kramer S, Stolle LB. Sentinel node biopsy (SNB) in malignant melanoma as same day procedure vs delayed procedure: clinical and economic outcome. J Plast Surg Hand Surg. 2014;48(4):265–9.
69. Ribero S, et al. Multiple lymph node basin drainage in trunk melanoma is not associated with survival of sentinel lymph node-positive patients. Dermatology. 2017;233(2–3):205.
70. Tew K, Farlow D. SPECT/CT in melanoma lymphoscintigraphy. Clin Nucl Med. 2016;41(12):961–3.
71. Leiter U, et al. Complete lymph node dissection versus no dissection in patients with sentinel lymph node biopsy positive melanoma (DeCOG-SLT): a multicentre, randomised, phase 3 trial. Lancet Oncol. 2016;17(6):757–67.
72. Faries MB, et al. Completion dissection or observation for sentinel-node metastasis in melanoma. N Engl J Med. 2017;376(23):2211–22.
73. Salvo G, et al. Sensitivity and negative predictive value for sentinel lymph node biopsy in women with early-stage cervical cancer. Gynecol Oncol. 2017;145(1):96–101.
74. Dostálek L, et al. SLN biopsy in cervical cancer patients with tumors larger than 2 cm and 4 cm. Gynecol Oncol. 2018;148:456.
75. Bats A-S, et al. Feasibility and performance of lymphoscintigraphy in sentinel lymph node biopsy for early cervical cancer: results of the prospective multicenter SENTICOL study. Ann Nucl Med. 2015;29(1):63–70.
76. Kadkhodayan S, et al. Inappropriate intra-cervical injection of radiotracer for sentinel lymph node mapping in a uterine cervix cancer patient: importance of lymphoscintigraphy and blue dye injection. Asia Ocean J Nucl Med Biol. 2014;2(2):135.
77. Bats A-S, et al. Contribution of lymphoscintigraphy to intraoperative sentinel lymph node detection in early cervical cancer: analysis of the prospective multicenter SENTICOL cohort. Gynecol Oncol. 2015;137(2):264–9.
78. Hoogendam JP, et al. 99mTc SPECT/CT versus planar lymphoscintigraphy for preoperative sentinel lymph node detection in cervical cancer: a systematic review and metaanalysis. J Nucl Med. 2015;56(5):675–80.
79. Koh W-J, et al. Cervical cancer, version 2.2015. J Natl Compr Cancer Netw. 2015;13(4):395–404.
80. Amant F, Trum H. Sentinel-lymph-node mapping in endometrial cancer: routine practice? Lancet Oncol. 2017;18(3):281–2.
81. How JA, et al. Sentinel lymph node mapping in endometrial cancer: a systematic review and meta-analysis. Minerva Ginecol. 2018;70(2):194–214.
82. Geppert B, et al. Sentinel lymph node biopsy in endometrial cancer-feasibility, safety and lymphatic complications. Gynecol Oncol. 2018;148(3):491–8.
83. Kadkhodayan S, et al. Lymphatic mapping and sentinel node biopsy in endometrial cancer—a feasibility study using cervical injection of radiotracer and blue dye. Nucl Med Rev Cent East Eur. 2014;17(2):55–8.
84. Ansari M, et al. Sentinel node biopsy in endometrial cancer: systematic review and meta-analysis of the literature. Eur J Gynaecol Oncol. 2013;34(5):387–401.
85. Farazestanian M, et al. Concordance between intracervical and fundal injections for sentinel node mapping in patients with endometrial cancer?: A study using intracervical radiotracer and fundal blue dye injections. Clin Nucl Med. 2019;44(3):e123–e7.
86. Bogani G, et al. Sentinel lymph node detection in endometrial cancer: does injection site make a difference? J Gynecol Oncol. 2016;27(2):e23.
87. Buda A, Lissoni A, Milani R. Sentinel lymph node detection in endometrial cancer: hysteroscopic peritumoral versus cervical injection. J Gynecol Oncol. 2016;27(1):e11.
88. Naaman Y, et al. The added value of SPECT/CT in sentinel lymph nodes mapping for endometrial carcinoma. Ann Surg Oncol. 2016;23(2):450–5.
89. Levenback CF, et al. Lymphatic mapping and sentinel lymph node biopsy in women with squamous cell carcinoma of the vulva: a gynecologic oncology group study. J Clin Oncol. 2012;30(31):3786–91.
90. Van der Zee AG, et al. Sentinel node dissection is safe in the treatment of early-stage vulvar cancer. J Clin Oncol. 2008;26(6):884–9.
91. Oonk MH, et al. Size of sentinel-node metastasis and chances of non-sentinel-node involvement and survival in early stage vulvar cancer: results from GROINSS-V, a multicentre observational study. Lancet Oncol. 2010;11(7):646–52.
92. Covens A, et al. Sentinel lymph node biopsy in vulvar cancer: systematic review, meta-analysis and guideline recommendations. Gynecol Oncol. 2015;137(2):351–61.
93. Meads C, et al. Sentinel lymph node status in vulval cancer: systematic reviews of test accuracy and decision-analytic model-based economic evaluation. Health Technol Assess. 2013;17(60):1–216.
94. Ottenhof SR, et al. Advancements in staging and imaging for penile cancer. Curr Opin Urol. 2017;27(6):612–20.
95. Brouwer OR, et al. A hybrid radioactive and fluorescent tracer for sentinel node biopsy in penile carcinoma as a potential replacement for blue dye. Eur Urol. 2014;65(3):600–9.
96. Sadeghi R, et al. Accuracy of sentinel lymph node biopsy for inguinal lymph node staging of penile squamous cell carcinoma: systematic review and meta-analysis of the literature. J Urol. 2012;187(1):25–31.
97. Horenblas S. Sentinel lymph node biopsy in penile carcinoma. Semin Diagn Pathol. 2012;29(2):90–5.
98. Nicolai N. Has dynamic sentinel node biopsy achieved its top performance in penile cancer? What clinicians still need to manage lymph nodes in early stage penile cancer. Eur Urol. 2013;63(4):664–6.
99. Saad ZZ, et al. Investigating the role of SPECT/CT in dynamic sentinel lymph node biopsy for

penile cancers. Eur J Nucl Med Mol Imaging. 2017;44(7):1176–84.
100. Lutzen U, et al. A study on the value of computer-assisted assessment for SPECT/CT-scans in sentinel lymph node diagnostics of penile cancer as well as clinical reliability and morbidity of this procedure. Cancer Imaging. 2016;16(1):29.
101. Zou ZJ, et al. Radiocolloid-based dynamic sentinel lymph node biopsy in penile cancer with clinically negative inguinal lymph node: an updated systematic review and meta-analysis. Int Urol Nephrol. 2016;48(12):2001–13.
102. Bertelsen CA, et al. Pattern of colon cancer lymph node metastases in patients undergoing central Mesocolic lymph node excision: a systematic review. Dis Colon Rectum. 2016;59(12):1209–21.
103. van der Pas MH, et al. Sentinel-lymph-node procedure in colon and rectal cancer: a systematic review and meta-analysis. Lancet Oncol. 2011;12(6):540–50.
104. Oltedal S, et al. The prognostic relevance of sentinel lymph node metastases assessed by PHGR1 mRNA quantification in stage I to III colon cancer. Transl Oncol. 2018;11(2):436–43.
105. Weixler B, et al. Comparative analysis of tumor cell dissemination to the sentinel lymph nodes and to the bone marrow in patients with nonmetastasized colon cancer: a prospective multicenter study. JAMA Surg. 2017;152(10):912–20.
106. Sloothaak DAM, et al. Prognostic implications of occult nodal tumour cells in stage I and II colon cancer: the correlation between micrometastasis and disease recurrence. Eur J Surg Oncol. 2017;43(8):1456–62.
107. Lind GE, et al. Prognostic relevance of an epigenetic biomarker panel in sentinel lymph nodes from colon cancer patients. Clin Epigenetics. 2017;9:97.
108. Estrada O, et al. Sentinel lymph node biopsy as a prognostic factor in non-metastatic colon cancer: a prospective study. Clin Transl Oncol. 2017;19(4):432–9.
109. Andersen HS, et al. In vivo and ex vivo sentinel node mapping does not identify the same lymph nodes in colon cancer. Int J Color Dis. 2017;32(7):983–90.
110. Schaafsma BE, et al. Ex vivo sentinel node mapping in colon cancer combining blue dye staining and fluorescence imaging. J Surg Res. 2013;183(1):253–7.
111. Wong JH, et al. Validation of ex vivo lymphatic mapping in hematoxylin-eosin node-negative carcinoma of the colon and rectum. Ann Surg Oncol. 2004;11(8):772–7.
112. Saha S, et al. Sentinel lymph node mapping in colon and rectal cancer: its impact on staging, limitations, and pitfalls. Cancer Treat Res. 2005;127:105–22.
113. Braat AE, et al. Sentinel node detection after preoperative short-course radiotherapy in rectal carcinoma is not reliable. Br J Surg. 2005;92(12):1533–8.
114. Ahmed MM, Moore BA, Schmalbach CE. Utility of head and neck cutaneous squamous cell carcinoma sentinel node biopsy: a systematic review. Otolaryngol Head Neck Surg. 2014;150(2):180–7.
115. Miller MC, Goldenberg D. AHNS series: do you know your guidelines? Principles of surgery for head and neck cancer: a review of the National Comprehensive Cancer Network guidelines. Head Neck. 2017;39(4):791–6.
116. Garrel R, et al. Review of sentinel node procedure in cN0 head and neck squamous cell carcinomas. Guidelines from the French evaluation cooperative subgroup of GETTEC. Eur Ann Otorhinolaryngol Head Neck Dis. 2017;134(2):89–93.
117. Skubleny D, et al. Diagnostic evaluation of sentinel lymph node biopsy using indocyanine green and infrared or fluorescent imaging in gastric cancer: a systematic review and meta-analysis. Surg Endosc. 2018;32:2620.
118. Huang L, et al. Feasibility and diagnostic performance of dual-tracer-guided sentinel lymph node biopsy in cT1-2N0M0 gastric cancer: a systematic review and meta-analysis of diagnostic studies. World J Surg Oncol. 2017;15(1):103.
119. Bagheri R, et al. Sentinel node mapping in esophageal squamous cell carcinoma using intra-operative combined blue dye and radiotracer techniques. Esophagus. 2013;10(4):211–6.
120. Dabbagh Kakhki VR, et al. Accuracy of sentinel node biopsy in esophageal carcinoma: a systematic review and meta-analysis of the pertinent literature. Surg Today. 2014;44(4):607–19.
121. Khadivi E, et al. Intra-operative lymphatic mapping and sentinel node biopsy in laryngeal carcinoma: preliminary results. Iran J Otorhinolaryngol. 2015;27(81):285.
122. Sadeghi R, et al. Prognostic significance of sentinel lymph node mapping in Merkel cell carcinoma: systematic review and meta-analysis of prognostic studies. Biomed Res Int. 2014;2014:489536.
123. Taghizadeh Kermani A, et al. Lymphatic mapping and sentinel node biopsy in a patient with upper limb Merkel cell carcinoma: a case report and brief review of literature. Nucl Med Rev Cent East Eur. 2016;19(1):42–5.
124. Assadi M, et al. Sentinel node mapping in papillary thyroid carcinoma using combined radiotracer and blue dye methods. Endokrynol Pol. 2014;65(4):281–6.
125. Sadeghi R, et al. Sentinel node mapping in the prostate cancer. Meta-analysis. Nuklearmedizin. 2011;50(3):107–15.
126. Motamedolshariati M, et al. Sentinel node mapping in Marjolin's ulcers: is it feasible? Wounds. 2015;27(3):54–62.
127. Shafiei S, et al. Sentinel node mapping in non-small cell lung cancer using an intraoperative radiotracer technique. Asia Ocean J Nucl Med Biol. 2019;7(2):153–9.
128. Taghizadeh Kermani A, et al. Accuracy of sentinel node biopsy in the staging of non-small cell lung

carcinomas: systematic review and meta-analysis of the literature. Lung Cancer. 2013;80(1):5–14.
129. Hassanzadeh M, et al. Lymphatic mapping and sentinel node biopsy in ovarian tumors: a study using intra-operative Tc-99m-Phytate and lymphoscintigraphy imaging. J Ovarian Res. 2016;9(1):55.
130. Zarifmahmoudi L, Sadeghi R. Re: lymphatic path of the inguinal lymph node metastases in anorectal cancer: the Springbok pattern. Clin Nucl Med. 2016;41(9):747.
131. Zarifmahmoudi L, et al. Sentinel node biopsy in urothelial carcinoma of the bladder: systematic review and meta-analysis. Urol Intel. 2019;103(4):373–82.
132. Andreou D, et al. Sentinel node biopsy in soft tissue sarcoma subtypes with a high propensity for regional lymphatic spread—results of a large prospective trial. Ann Oncol. 2013;24(5):1400–5.
133. Maduekwe UN, et al. Role of sentinel lymph node biopsy in the staging of synovial, epithelioid, and clear cell sarcomas. Ann Surg Oncol. 2009;16(5):1356–63.

12 Lymphoscintigraphy in the Management of Lymphatic Disorders

Ramin Sadeghi and Hasan Ravari

12.1 Brief Introduction and Historical Perspective

Lymphedema is a chronic disorder of the lymphatic system that presents with limb swelling and can have a major impact on a person's quality of life [1, 2].

Lymphedema can be categorized according to the underlying cause in to two types: primary and secondary. Secondary lymphedema is very common and usually occurs following lymphadenectomy and radiation therapy of the regional lymphatic basins [3]. Primary lymphedema, on the other hand, is rare, and health care providers usually tend to ignore it because of its painless nature. Delayed diagnosis of lymphedema can be devastating for patients as early treatment of the disorder can prevent secondary fibrosis and its progression to irreversible swelling of the limbs [4].

In the past, radiological lymphography was used to evaluate the lymphatic system. However, this procedure is almost obsolete as it needs cannulation of the lymphatic vessels, which is technically difficult if not impossible [5, 6]. On the other hand, lymphoscintigraphy using radiolabeled particles is an easy, reproducible, and available method for lymphatic system evaluation [7]. Lymphoscintigraphy is one of the oldest procedures in nuclear medicine and has been used in medical practice since the 1960s [8]. It can play an important role in the early diagnosis of lymphedema, in the assessment of lymphedema's response to treatment, and in the evaluation of the integrity of the lymphatic system [9]. The application of lymphoscintigraphy in the management of lymphatic disorders will be featured in this chapter.

12.2 Radiopharmaceuticals

Various radiopharmaceuticals have been used for the evaluation of the lymphatic system. Almost all of these radiopharmaceuticals are radiolabeled particles that enter the lymphatic system upon administration. The single most important difference between these radiopharmaceuticals is particle size. Particles smaller than 0.005 nm in size penetrate into the capillary membranes and are not useful for lymphatic system imaging [10]. Particles larger than 500 nm in size mostly remain in the injection site and would not be available for lymphoscintigraphy either [11]. Different Tc-99m-labeled radiopharmaceuticals and their particle sizes are presented in Table 12.1 [11–13]. All of these radiopharmaceuticals have been used successfully in lymphoscintigraphy, and their use is dependent on their availability and cost in different countries.

R. Sadeghi (✉)
Nuclear Medicine Research Center, Mashhad University of Medical Sciences, Mashhad, Iran
e-mail: sadeghir@mums.ac.ir

H. Ravari
Vascular and Endovascular Surgery Research Center, Mashhad University of Medical Sciences, Mashhad, Iran

H. Ahmadzadehfar et al. (eds.), *Clinical Nuclear Medicine*,
https://doi.org/10.1007/978-3-030-39457-8_12

Table 12.1 The most frequently used Tc-99m-labeled radiopharmaceuticals for lymphoscintigraphy

Radiopharmaceutical	Particle size (nm)
Antimony sulfide colloid	<30
Nanocolloid	<80
Sulfur colloid	Mostly 100–600
Filtered sulfur colloid	10 nm
Phytate	150–1000

12.3 Methodology

Various aspects of lymphatic system evaluation by nuclear medicine techniques are controversial. In the following sections, the most important aspects of limb lymphoscintigraphy are discussed.

12.3.1 Prestudy Preparations

No preparation is needed. The patient is required to wash his/her feet or hands thoroughly before coming to the nuclear medicine department.

12.3.2 Injection Technique

12.3.2.1 Radiotracer Dose

The recommended dose of radiotracer is 0.25–1 mCi (9.25–37 MBq) in one or divided aliquots for each limb [9]. In departments with older generation gamma cameras that suffer from saturation upon imaging, lower dosage is recommended as quantification of the images could be affected (Fig. 12.1).

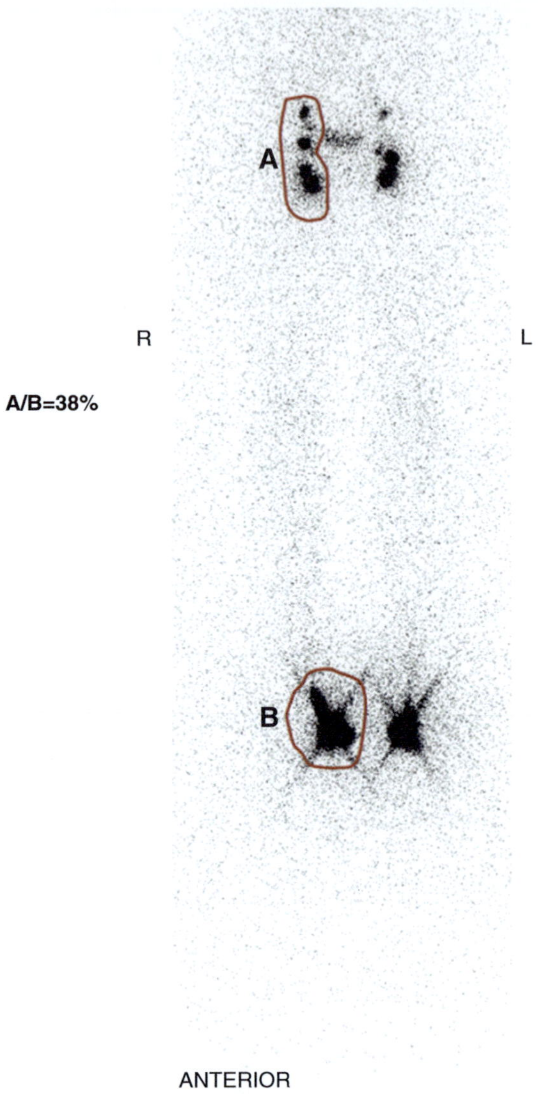

Fig. 12.1 Saturation effect: a 32-year-old patient with right leg swelling; 1.5 mCi (55.5 MBq) Tc-99m Antimony sulfide colloid was injected in each limb. Whole-body imaging in anterior view is shown. Note that saturation of counts in the injection site resulted in spuriously high inguinal to injection site area ratio

12.3.2.2 Injection Site and Numbers

Injection site is an important factor in the interpretation of limb lymphoscintigraphy. Two methods are used, namely, epifascial and subfascial injections. The scan patterns of epifascial and subfascial injections are strikingly different from each other (Fig. 12.2). Epifascial injection can be done by subcutaneous or intradermal injection of the tracer in the first interdigital webs (Fig. 12.3). Usually, one injection would be sufficient. Subfascial injection is done by deeply injecting into the calf or into the lateral aspect of the side of the foot at a depth of 1.5 cm.

Normally, intercalary nodes (epitrochlear and popliteal nodes) are not seen in epifascial injections, which is not the case in subfascial ones. In addition, dermal backflow (hallmark of lymphedema in epifascial injections) may not be visible in subfascial injections [14, 15]. Moreover, quantitative measurements can be affected considerably by the depth of the injection (Table 12.2).

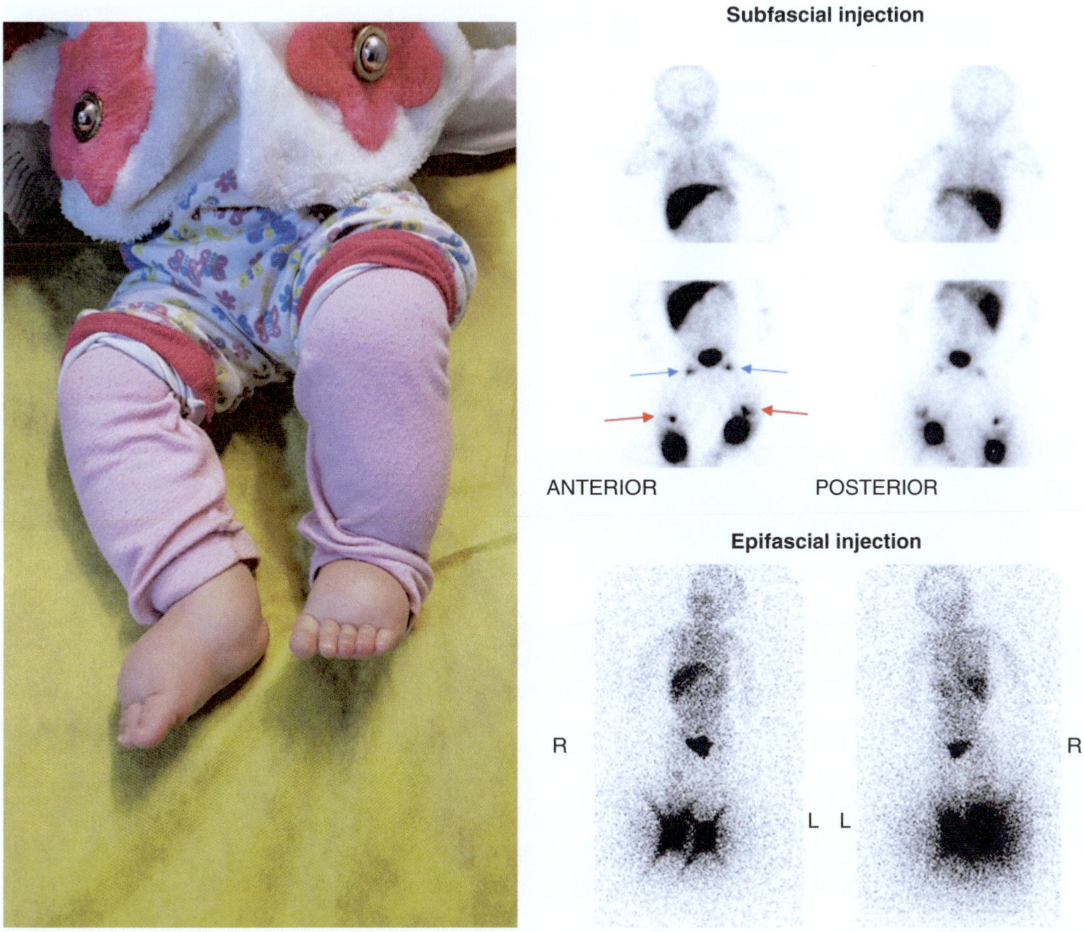

Fig. 12.2 Different patterns of subfascial and epifascial injections of the radiotracer: a 3-month-old female patient with bilateral congenital swelling of the legs (bottom images). Note the striking difference between subfascial injections in the calves and epifascial injections in the first interdigital webs. In the epifascial injections, no popliteal node was noted. Inguinal nodes were not visible either. This shows superficial lymphatic system agenesis as the cause of the patient's clinical presentations. Inguinal and popliteal nodes are shown with blue and red arrows in the subfascial injection, respectively

In our department, we use a single dose (0.5 mCi (18.5 MBq)) of Tc-99m phytate in the subcutaneous area of the first interdigital webs bilaterally using an insulin syringe.

12.3.3 Exercise Following Radiotracer Injections

Different departments have different protocols following injections. Some order the patient to walk around for a couple of minutes post injections. Others ask the patient to remain at rest before imaging. This can also have a striking effect on lymphoscintigraphy interpretation (Fig. 12.4). Dermal backflow and collateral vessels are more prominent on the postexercise images [15, 16], which can increase the sensitivity and specificity of the study [17].

In our department, we ask patients to walk around immediately for 15 min following injections.

For upper limb lymphoscintigraphy, exercise includes hand gripping or some other types of activity that can increase the lymph flow [18]. As we have normal uptake values for upper extremi-

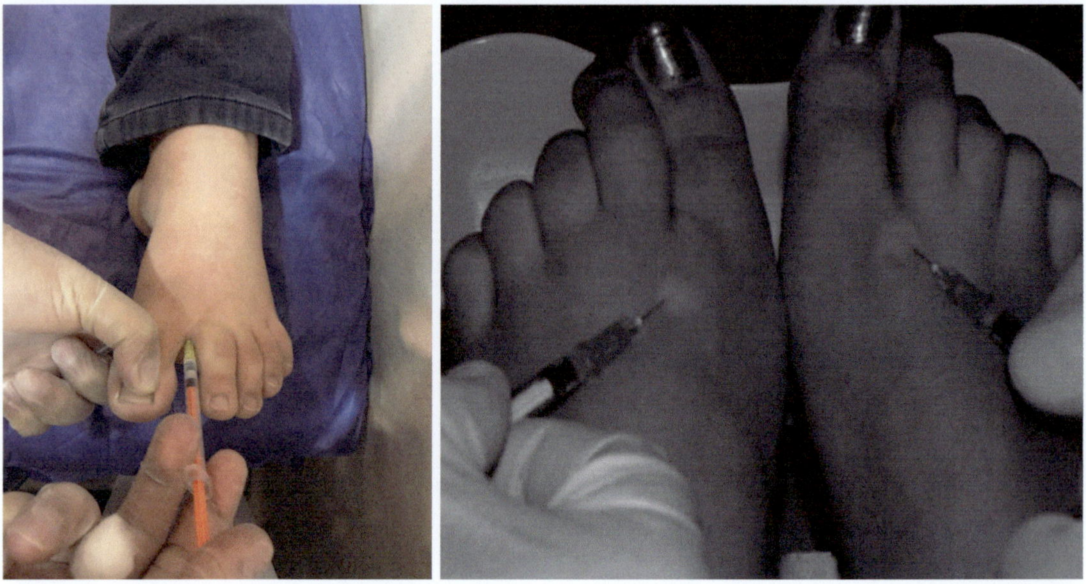

Fig. 12.3 Examples of intradermal (left) and subcutaneous (right) injections for lower limb lymphoscintigraphy. Note a wheal that was raised upon intradermal injections (The right side image was reproduced with permission from https://doi.org/10.1097/MNM.0b013e328338277d)

Table 12.2 Inguinal/axillary lymph nodes to injection site count ratio lower limits of normal at 1 h post injection

	With exercise			Without exercise		
	Epifascial			Epifascial		
	Subcutaneous, %	Intradermal, %	Subfascial, %	Subcutaneous, %	Intradermal, %	Subfascial
Upper limb	0.5	2	N/A	0.15	1	N/A
Lower limb	9	12	7	1.5	3	N/A

ties without exercise, in our department no exercise is used for upper extremity lymphoscintigraphy. Each department has to set up its own protocol based on the availability of normal values.

Some groups used both rest and exercise protocols in lymphoscintigraphy imaging. First, rest lymphoscintigraphy is done, and following exercise, another imaging is done with the same protocol [16].

12.3.4 Imaging

The time of imaging is highly dependent on whether the patient exercises following injections or not. If the patient exercises, a single set of image is sufficient at least 40 min post injection. No difference in the image pattern would be expected on the delayed images [19]. On the other hand, immediate dynamic imaging, as well as delayed lymphoscintigraphy, may be obligatory in patients who did not exercise following injections [20].

Imaging is performed in whole-body mode and should be continued from the injection site to at least the liver level. As the injection dose is not high, lower scan speed may be necessary; however, in gamma cameras with a saturation problem, the speed should not be less than 12 cm/min. If both upper and lower limbs are injected, injection sites of both upper and lower limbs should be included, and sometimes two sets of whole-body imaging may be necessary (Fig. 12.5).

In our department, patients undergo a single whole-body lymphoscintigraphy at least 1 h post injection. Imaging can be done from 1 to 6 h following tracer injection [21–23]. Delayed images do not yield any additional information in patients who stand up and walk following injections or do

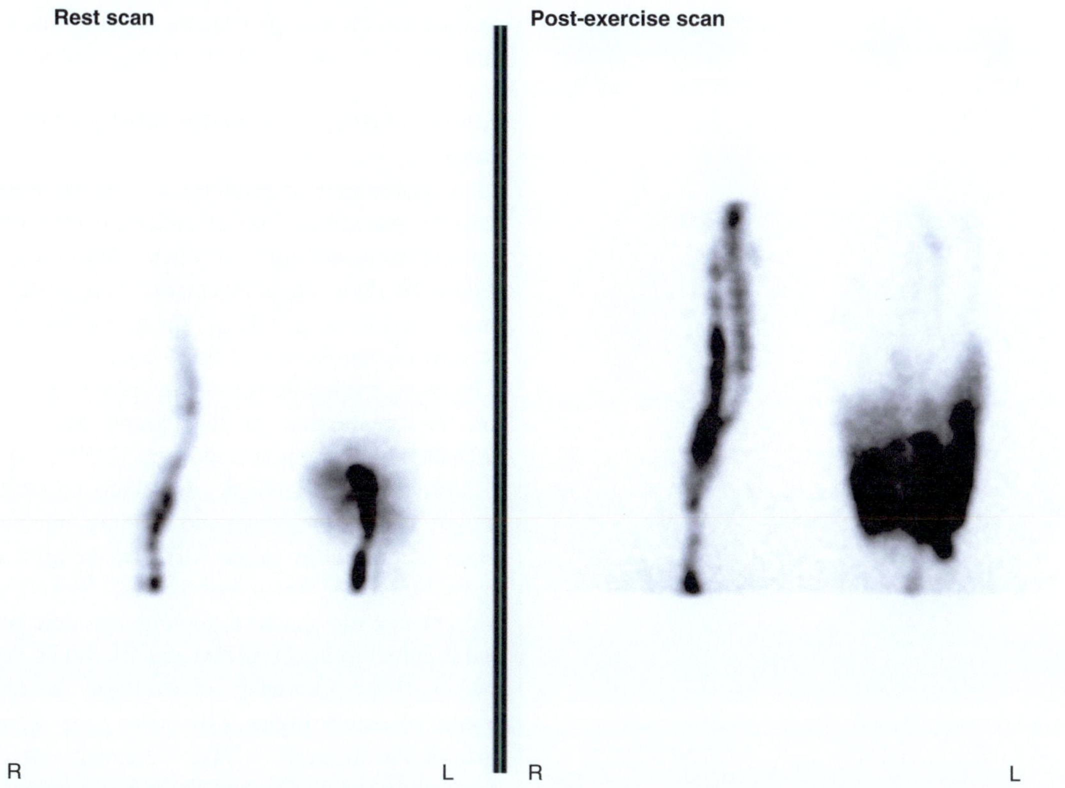

Fig. 12.4 Exercise lymphoscintigraphy of a patient with lower limb swelling. Note the difference between the rest and exercise scans, especially dermal backflow and collateral vessel visualization on the latter (Reproduced with permission from https://doi.org/10.1016/j.mvr.2010.09.003)

some other exercise for upper extremity lymphoscintigraphy (Fig. 12.6). Note that some radiotracers have renal excretion, and before imaging, patients should empty their bladders (this is especially important for Tc-99m phytate) [24].

12.4 Clinical Indications and Interpretation

12.4.1 Differentiation of Lymphedema From Other Causes of Limb Swelling

The main indication of lymphoscintigraphy is for the confirmation of lymphedema diagnosis in patients with extremity swelling. Table 12.3 shows the main differential diagnoses of limb swelling. For a correct interpretation of the lymphoscintigraphy images, qualitative and quantitative evaluations are both mandatory as they complement each other. The best accuracy is achieved by a combination of both quantitative and qualitative approaches [25].

12.4.1.1 Qualitative Criteria of Lymphedema

The normal pattern of lymphoscintigraphy is highly dependent on injection depth and patient activity following injection. Epifascial injection shows symmetrical activity in the inguinal/axillary lymph nodes with no abnormal finding such as dermal backflow or lymph lake, etc. Intercalary nodes (epitrochlear/popliteal nodes) are not visualized. Subfascial injection also shows symmetrical activity in the inguinal/axillary nodes with no other abnormal activity. However, intercalary nodes are usually visualized (Fig. 12.7).

Several findings are in favor of lymphedema diagnosis, any of which would suffice for diagno-

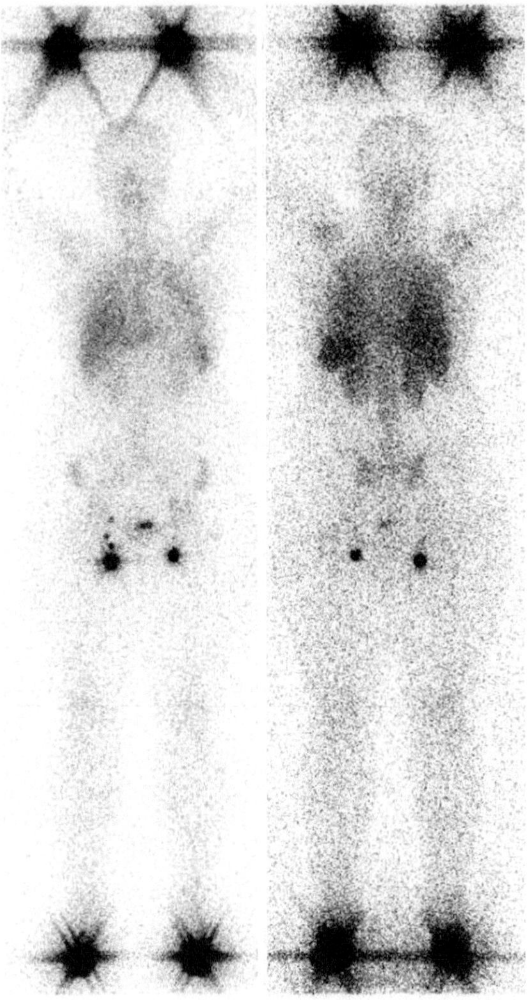

Fig. 12.5 Whole-body lymphoscintigraphy images of a patient with upper and lower limb swelling

sis confirmation. These findings are summarized in Table 12.4 [9, 26]. Some of these findings are only valid for intradermal injections of the tracer: visualization of ≥3 collateral vessels, as well as low number of inguinal lymph nodes. Figures 12.8, 12.9, 12.10, and 12.11 provide some examples of qualitative criteria of lymphedema diagnosis.

12.4.1.2 Semi-quantitative Approach of Image Interpretation

Semi-quantitative evaluation of the lymphoscintigraphy images is done by two basic methods: clearance of the activity from the injection site and ratio of lymph node uptake to the injection site.

Inguinal/Axillary to Injection Site Uptake Ratio

Semi-quantitative measurements can be easily done by placing regions of interest (ROIs) over inguinal areas and injection sites. Measurements should be done on both anterior and posterior images using a geometric mean method and background correction. A more accurate method is by using a standard activity in order to account for the attenuation of the lymph nodes, as described by Keramida et al. (Fig. 12.12) [27].

Normal values are highly dependent on patient activity between injection and imaging, injection depth (epifascial or subfascial), and the affected limbs (upper vs. lower extremities). In patients without free movement following injection, normal inguinal to injection site activity can be very low (1–10%); following leg exercise, the ratio would be much higher (10–30%) [28]. Semi-quantitative analysis is also dependent on the depth of injection. The lowest limit of inguinal to injection site ratio is usually 9–12% in the epifascial and 7% in the subfascial injections with exercise protocol [14, 29]. For upper limbs, data are very limited. For epifascial injection with and without exercise, the normal value of axillary to injection site ratio was 1.5–3% and 0.15–1%, respectively [30, 31].

In addition to the depth of the injection and activity of the patient following injection, the volume of the injected dose can affect the quantitative evaluation of the images [32]. Even subcutaneous and intradermal injections have been shown to be different quantitatively in the normal upper limbs (0.1% versus 1% in the subcutaneous and intradermal injections, respectively) [33]. Background and decay corrections should also be done for all quantitative evaluation.

Normal lymph node to injection site ratios are summarized in Table 12.2 based on injection depth and the activity of the patient. As many variables affect the quantitative evaluation of lymphoscintigraphy images, each department should stick to a strict method (injection depth,

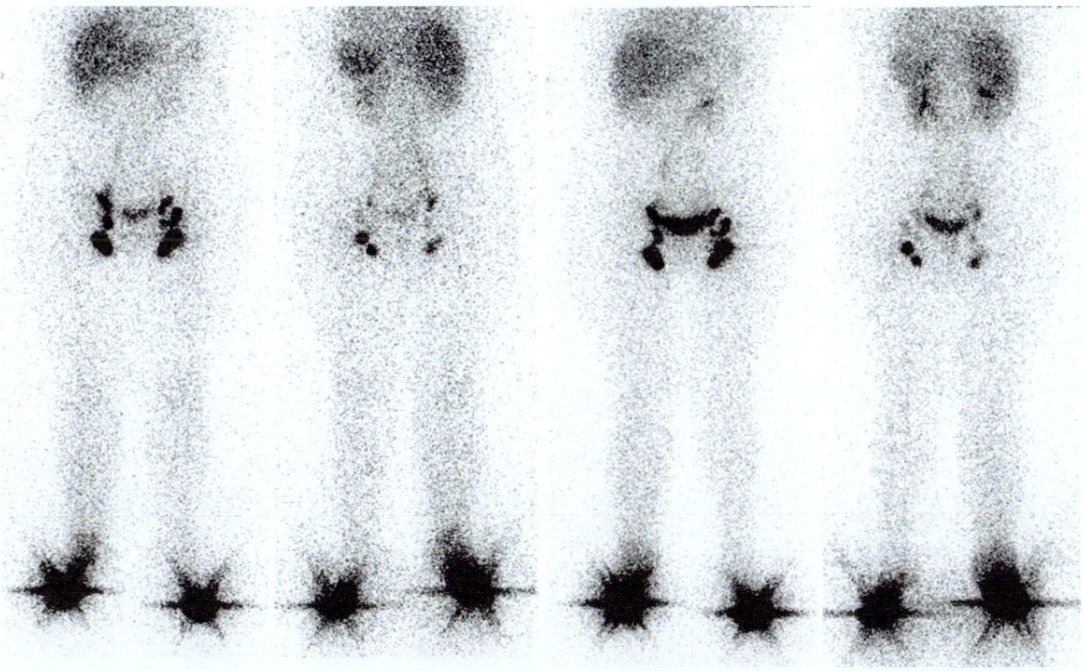

Fig. 12.6 Early and delayed lymphoscintigraphy images of a patient with bilateral lower limb swelling. Note that the scan patterns on the early and delayed images are exactly the same as the patient did some exercise following injection of the radiotracer

Table 12.3 Differential diagnoses of limb swelling

	Time frame	Findings	Uni- or bilateral	Location
Chronic venous insufficiency	Chronic onset	Soft pitting edema with more severe involvement of the calves, sometimes with venous ulcerations	Early stage unilateral, later stages bilateral	Lower limbs
Deep vein thrombosis	Acute onset	Painful pitting edema	Usually unilateral	Upper or lower limbs
Complex regional pain syndrome	Chronic onset	Early stage with warm painful skin, late in the course with atrophic changes of the skin	Unilateral	Upper or lower limbs
Lymphedema	Chronic slow progressing, in secondary cases following surgery or trauma	Pitting edema in early stage, skin thickening and nonpitting edema in the later stages	Predominantly unilateral or asymmetrical	Upper or lower limbs
Lipedema	Chronic onset	Puffy swelling involving calves and thighs sparing the feet	Bilateral	Lower limbs
Medical conditions (cardiac, hepatic, renal diseases, malabsorption)	Chronic progressive	Pitting edema without pain, accompanying signs or symptoms of the underlying cause	Bilateral	Upper and lower limbs

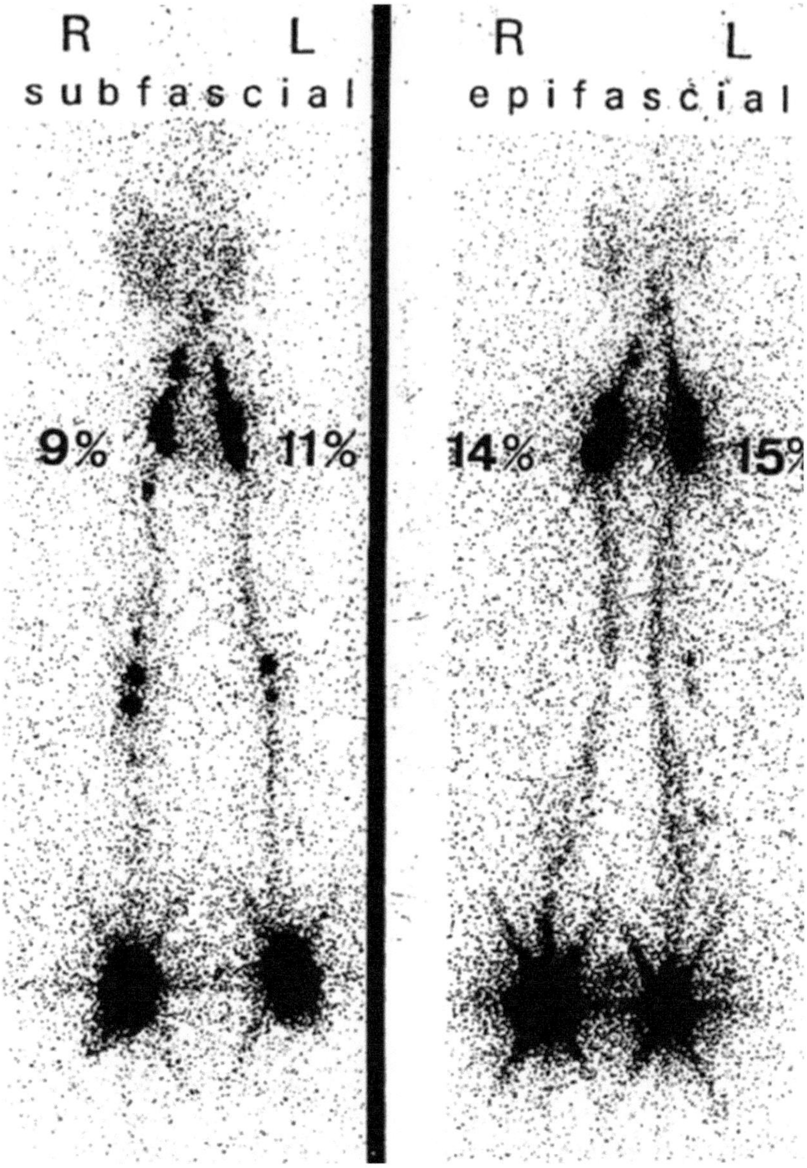

Fig. 12.7 Normal anterior view lymphoscintigraphies of a patient with epifascial and subfascial injections of the radiotracer. The tracer uptake values are also shown (% of injected dose). Note that intercalary node visualization is a normal finding in subfascial injection (Reproduced with permission from Analysis of lymphatic drainage in various forms of leg edema using two compartment lymphoscintigraphy: https://journals.uair.arizona.edu/index.php/lymph/article/view/17383)

Table 12.4 Criteria of abnormal lymphoscintigraphy

Collateral lymphatics in the dermis (dermal backflow Figs. 12.8 and 12.9) This finding is much more prominent in superficial injections
No visible inguinal or axillary lymph nodes (Fig. 12.10)
Asymmetry in the inguinal or axillary lymph node uptake
Visualization of the intercalary (popliteal or epitrochlear) nodes (Fig. 12.11) This finding is only reliable in superficial injections. Intercalary node visualization is normal in deep (subfascial) injections
Extravasation or pooling of the lymph in soft tissue (lymph lake)
Collateral vessels ≥ 3 This is a minor finding that is only visible using an intradermal injection
Reduced number of ilioinguinal nodes visualized (less than three) This is a minor finding that is only valid in the lower limb lymphoscintigraphy using intradermal injections For upper limb lymphoscintigraphy and for subcutaneous injections, this is not valid

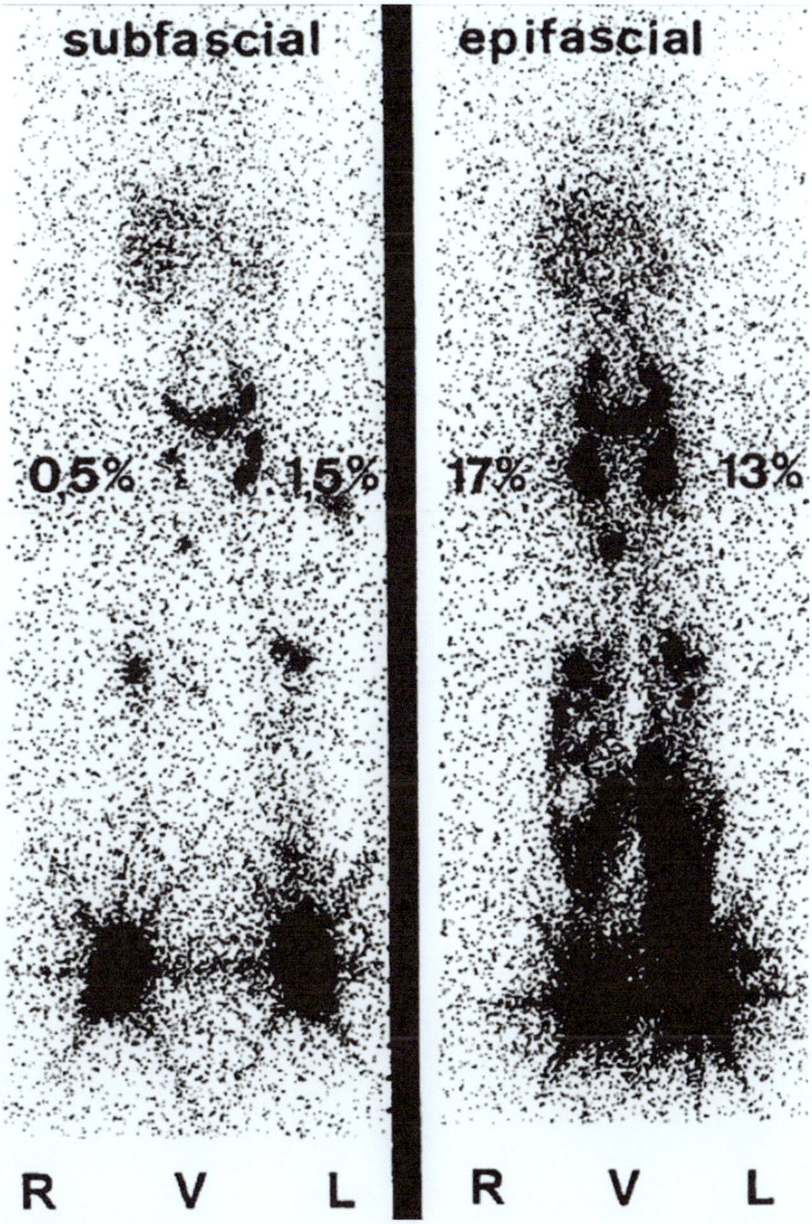

Fig. 12.8 Dermal backflow: abnormal anterior view lymphoscintigraphies of a patient with secondary lymphedema due to chronic venous insufficiency. Note that dermal backflow is prominent only on the epifascial injection image (Reproduced with permission from Analysis of lymphatic drainage in various forms of leg edema using two compartment lymphoscintigraphy: https://journals.uair.arizona.edu/index.php/lymph/article/view/17383)

patient activity, tracer dose and volume, time of imaging, and method of quantification).

Radiotracer Removal Constant Rates Based on Dynamic Imaging

Lymphoscintigraphy provides a unique opportunity to evaluate the clearance rate of the lymphatic system. Two different factors can be measured: clearance rate (κ) and volume of distribution (V_D). Usually, different ROIs are drawn proximal to the injection site (for example, in the forearm).

For clearance rate (κ), the count at each time point is divided by the count at the injection site. The natural logarithm of this ratio is plotted against time. Regression analysis of the plot gives a regression coefficient, or κ, for each site (unit of measurement is percentage per minute) [30] (see Fig. 12.13 for an example).

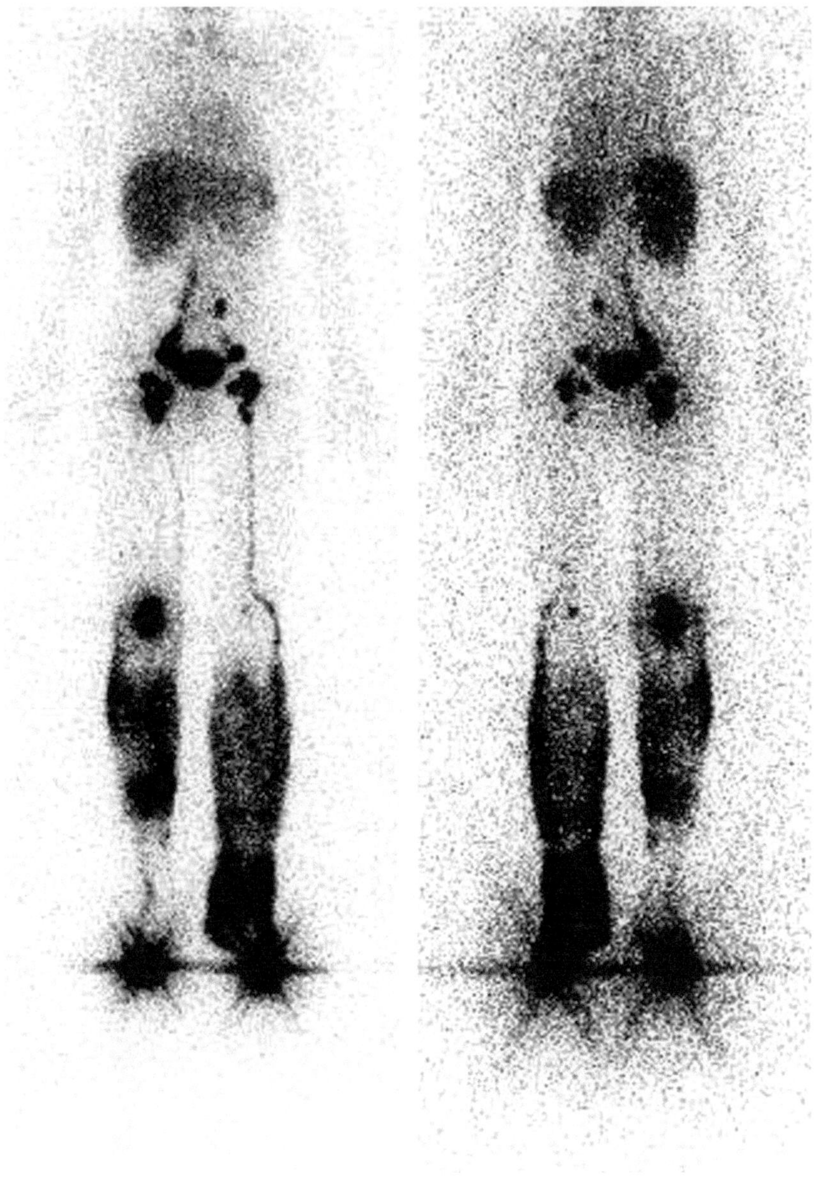

Fig. 12.9 Dermal backflow: 1 h post epifascial injection lymphoscintigraphy of a 15-year-old male with progressive swelling of the lower extremities (more on the left side). Note the prominent bilateral dermal backflow and right popliteal lymph node. These findings confirm the diagnosis of bilateral lymphedema despite good visualization of the inguinal lymph nodes

For the measurement of volume of distribution (V_D), usually the width of injection site through the time frame of dynamic imaging is used. The real V_D could not be measured but can be estimated from the images of the injection sites. Widths of each injection site are measured in cm at 10% of the peak and usually increase slightly with time (see Fig. 12.14 for an example).

Quantitative evaluation of the lymphoscintigraphy images should be an integral part of every lymphoscintigraphy study. Quantitative approach can increase the accuracy of lymphedema diagnosis considerably (Fig. 12.15).

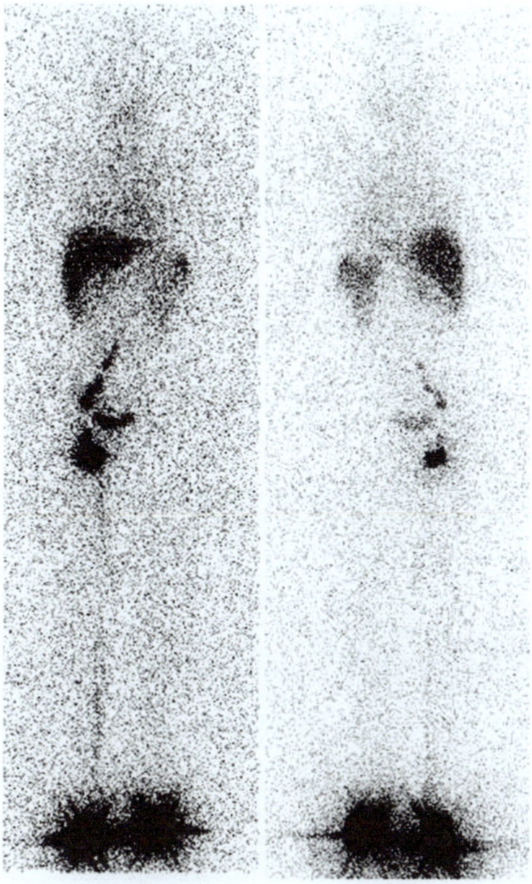

Fig. 12.10 Lymph node nonvisualization: 1 h post epifascial injection lymphoscintigraphy of a 31-year-old female with severe nonpitting edema of the left lower limb, which started since 10 years ago. Inguinal lymph node nonvisualization confirms the lymphedema diagnosis

12.4.1.3 Normal-Appearing Limbs and Lymphoscintigraphy Abnormalities

Despite unilateral presentation of lymphedema in a significant number of patients, primary lymphedema is a generalized disease and usually affects the limbs bilaterally. This is best shown in lymphoscintigraphy images. Many studies have shown that normal limbs of patients with primary lymphedema can have abnormal lymphoscintigraphy findings [26] (Fig. 12.16).

Overall, lymphoscintigraphy is very effective in the early diagnosis of lymphedema and the differentiation of lymphedema from other causes of limb swelling (Figs. 12.17 and 12.18).

12.4.2 Localization of Lymphatic System Defects

Lymphoscintigraphy, especially SPECT/CT, can be used for the localization of abnormalities in the lymphatic system. The application of lymphoscintigraphy has been proven in chylothorax, chylous ascites, etc. [21, 34] (Fig. 12.19).

12.4.3 Follow-Up of Patients With Lymphatic System Disorders

Lymphoscintigraphy has been proven to be an effective and objective method for the evaluation of treatment response [35–39]. Improvement of the lymphatic drainage has been confirmed after treatment by both qualitative evaluation and quantitative evaluation of the lymphoscintigraphy images (Fig. 12.20).

Lymphoscintigraphy can also be used for the prediction of treatment response before beginning treatment in lymphedematous limbs [40].

12.4.4 Prediction of the Development of Lymphedema

Lymphedema is a major health problem in patients with a history of oncology surgery, which is most commonly encountered in breast cancer patients. Lymphoscintigraphy studies showed that some breast cancer patients have an inherent predisposition to lymphedema development as their normal limbs showed impaired lymph drainage. In the future, lymphoscintigraphy may be used for determining patients who are more prone to lymphedema development before cancer surgery [41, 42].

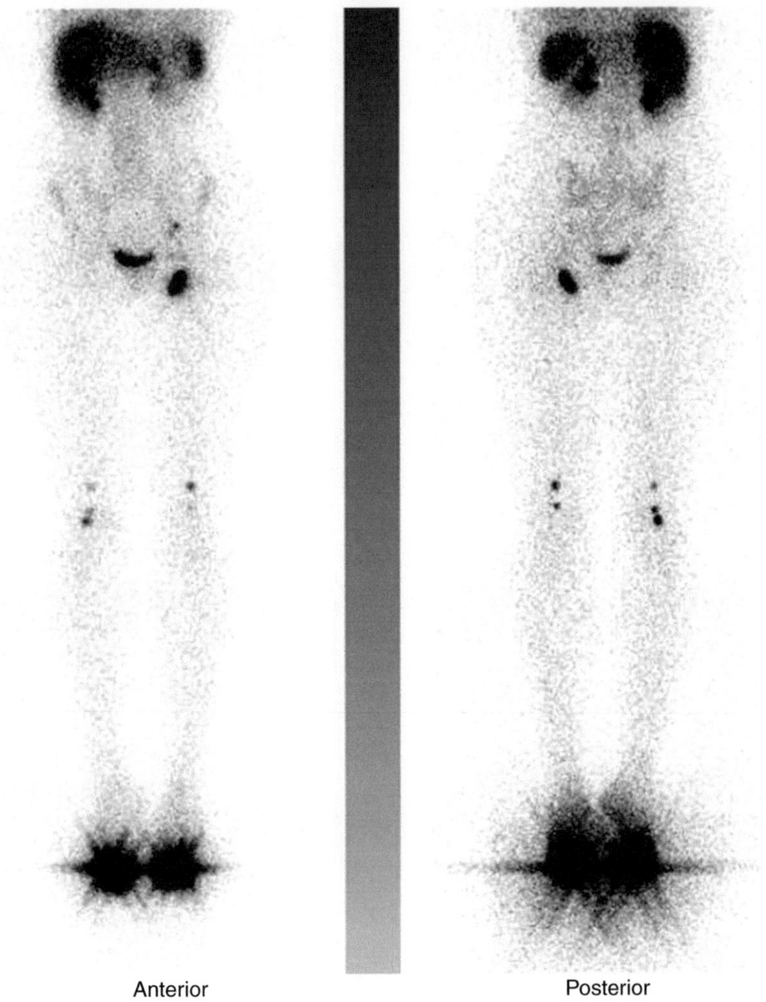

Fig. 12.11 Intercalary lymph node visualization: 1 h post epifascial injection lymphoscintigraphy of an 18-year-old female patient with a history of 2-year pitting edema of the right lower limb. Minimal intermittent swelling on the left side. Note bilateral popliteal node visualization, as well as the absence of inguinal lymph node on the right side. These findings confirm bilateral lower lymph lymphedema in this patient

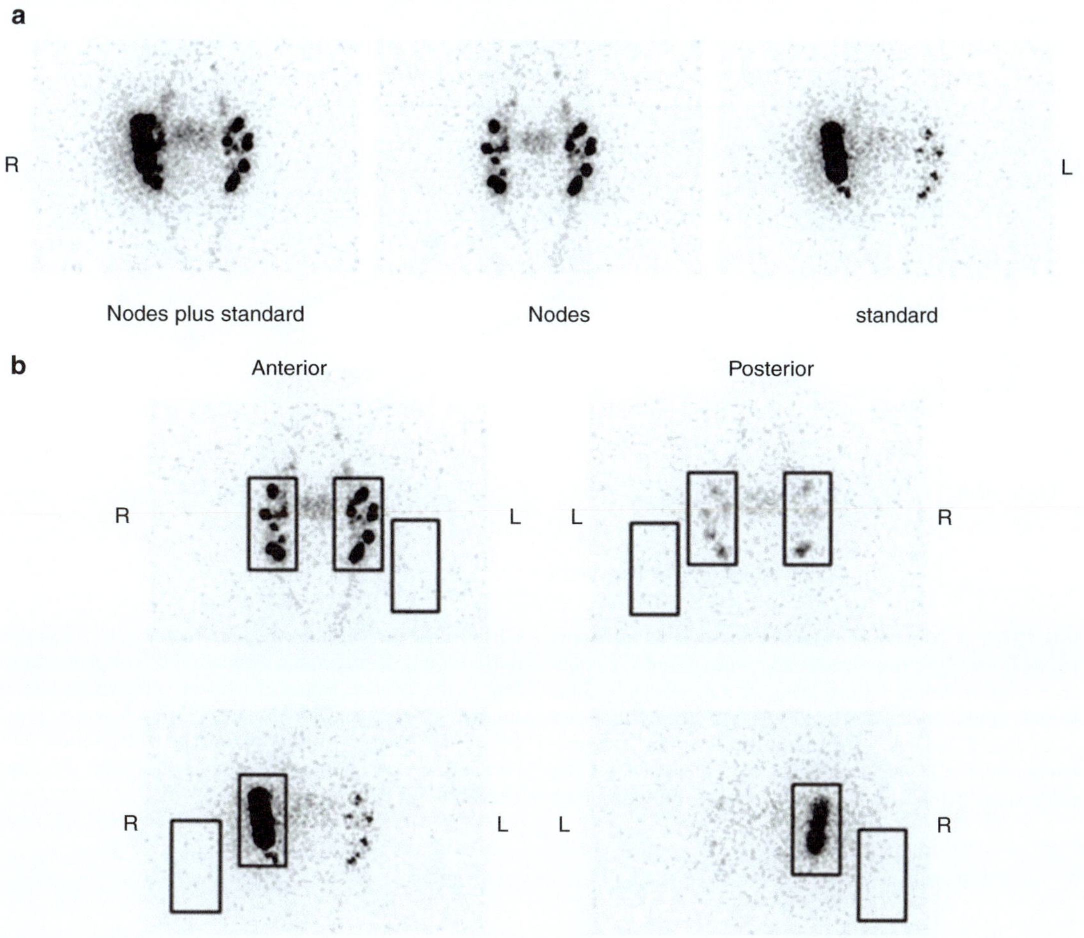

Fig. 12.12 Semi-quantitative evaluation of lymphoscintigraphy images using background-corrected geometric mean method. (**a**) Anterior images at 150 min post injection with (left) and without (middle) placement of the standard. The right panel is the subtraction image. (**b**) Regions of interest (ROI) were drawn over ilioinguinal nodes (upper) and standard (lower) on anterior and posterior images. The background ROI is also shown. The iIioinguinal node to injection site ratio after background correction and geometric mean calculation of the anterior and posterior counts would be 100 × (inguinal count/administered dose) × (standard activity/standard count on subtraction image)

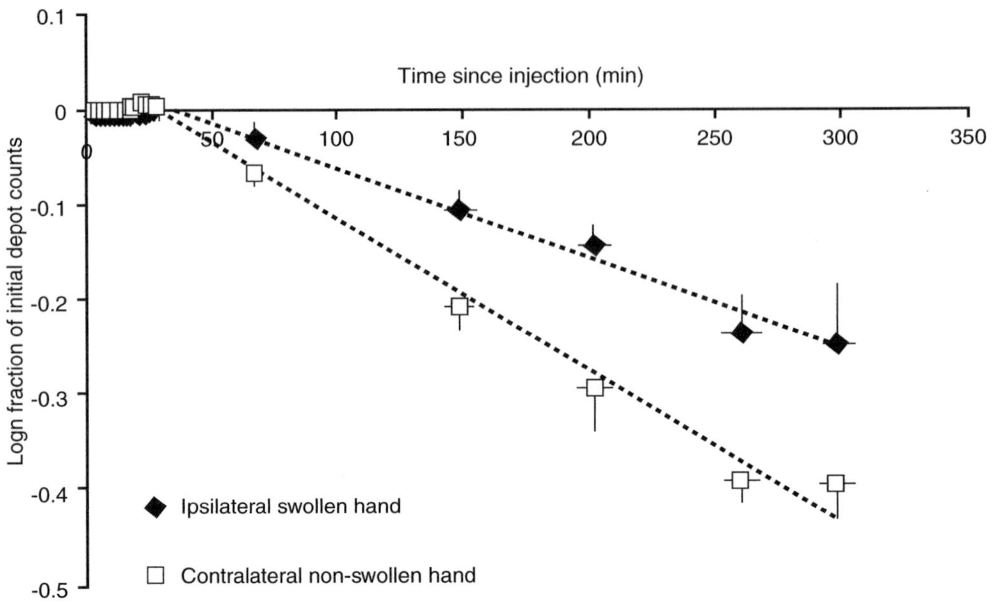

Fig. 12.13 Examples of clearance constant (κ) measurements in two lymphedematous and normal limbs. Counts rose slightly before falling from 30 min post injection. Counts in the edematous hand fell less steeply than the contralateral one, and κ ipsilateral was less than κ contralateral limb. Clearance rates (κ) are calculated by the regression method of the steep segment of the curves (Original figure was published in Stanton et al., A quantitative lymphoscintigraphic evaluation of lymphatic function in the swollen hands of women with lymphoedema following breast cancer treatment. Clinical Science (2006) 110, 553–561 https://doi.org/10.1042/CS20050277. Permission was granted by copyright holder Portland Press Ltd. for STM publishers)

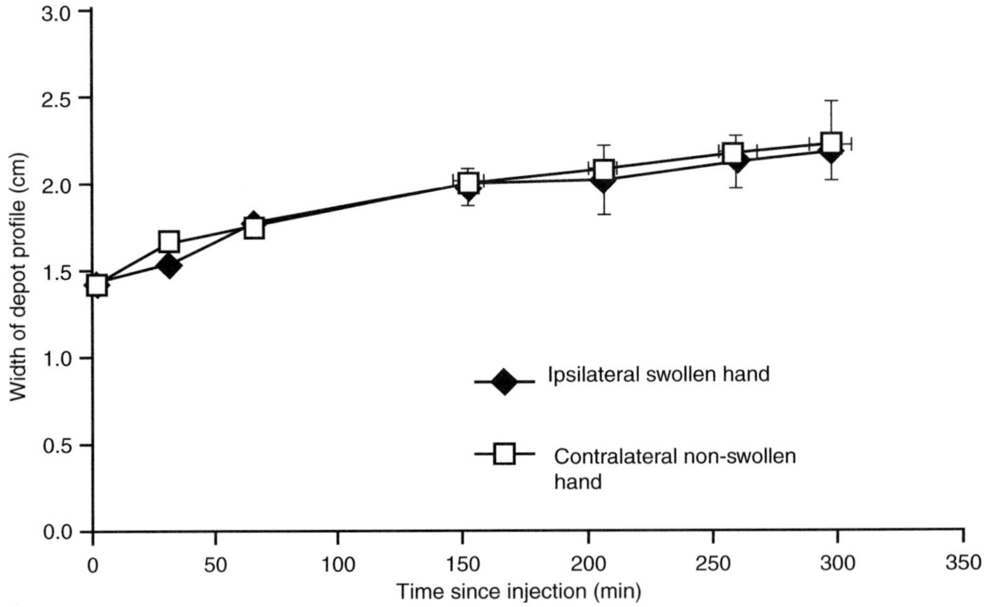

Fig. 12.14 Volume of distribution (V_D) measurements in two edematous and contralateral normal limbs, which use the width of injection site as a surrogate (Original figure was published in Stanton et al., A quantitative lymphoscintigraphic evaluation of lymphatic function in the swollen hands of women with lymphoedema following breast cancer treatment. Clinical Science (2006) 110, 553–561. https://doi.org/10.1042/CS20050277. Permission was granted by copyright holder Portland Press Ltd. for STM publishers)

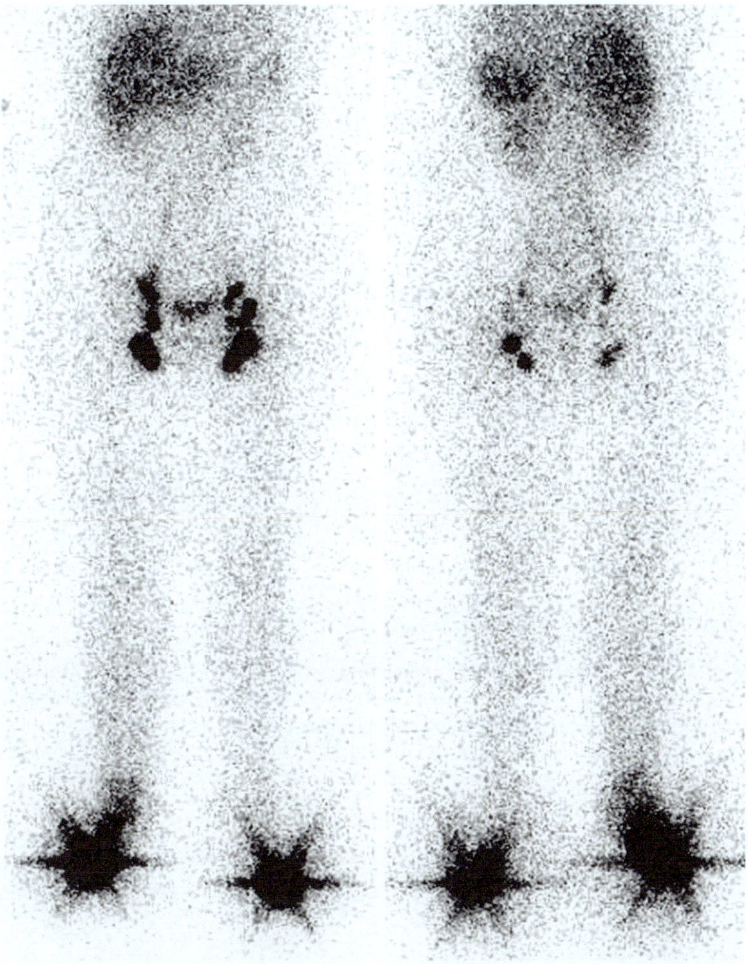

Fig. 12.15 One hour post epifascial injection of the tracer lymphoscintigraphy in a 38-year-old female patient with a history of right lower limb swelling for 2 months. Note a normal appearance of the scan except for a slight asymmetry in the inguinal nodes. Semi-quantitative evaluation showed 1% and 8% of the injection site activity in the inguinal nodes on the right and left sides, respectively. This finding confirmed the diagnosis of right lower limb lymphedema

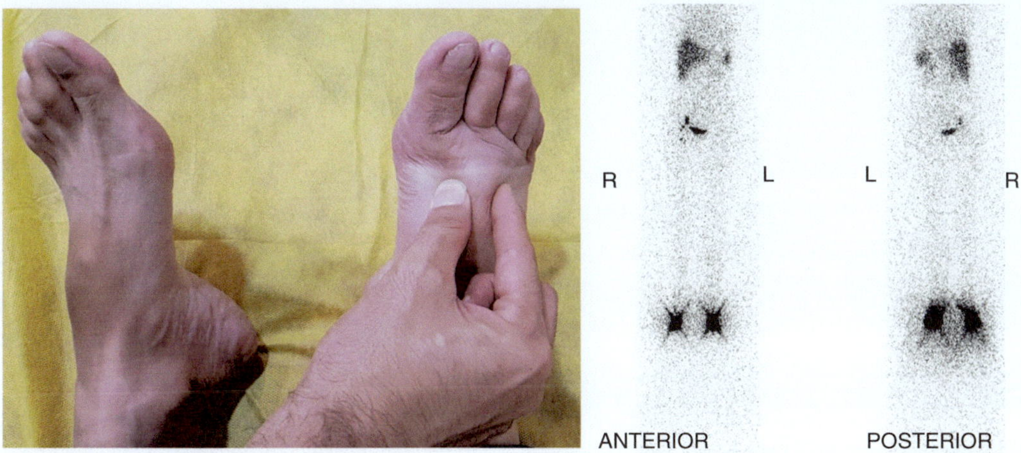

Fig. 12.16 Lymphoscintigraphy (1 h post epifascial injection of the tracer) of a patient with primary lymphedema of the right lower limb. Note inguinal lymph node nonvisualization on the right side. Quantitative analysis showed less than 1% of the injection site activity in the right inguinal nodes. The findings confirmed the diagnosis of right lower limb lymphedema, as well as lymphatic drainage compromise of the left side despite a normal-appearing left limb

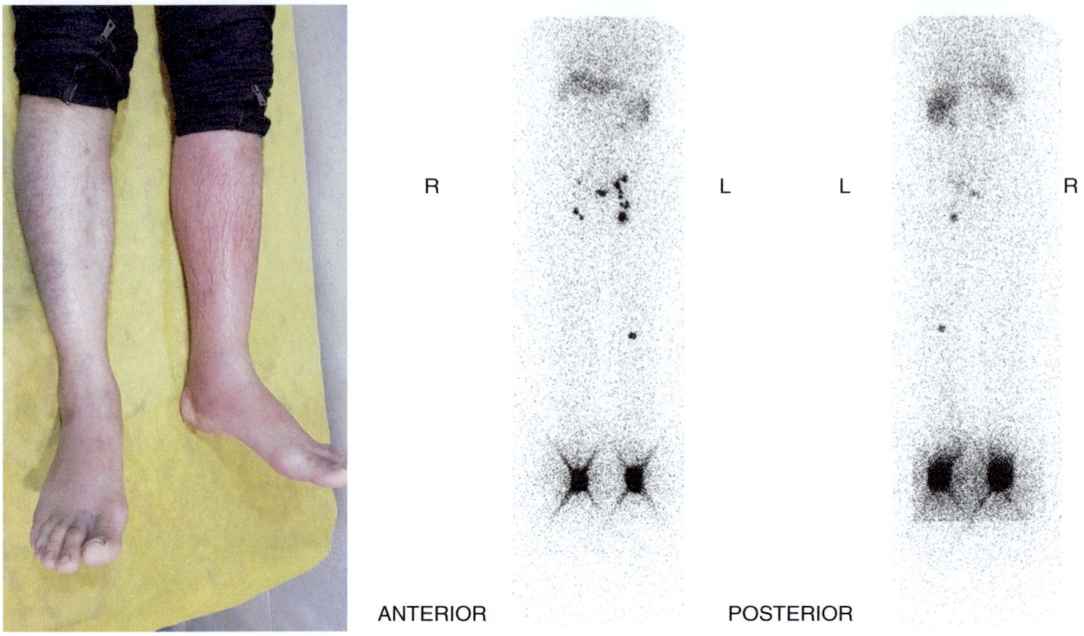

Fig. 12.17 A 17-year-old male patient with a history of recurrent cellulitis without apparent swelling of the limbs was referred for lymphoscintigraphy with the suspicion of early stages of primary lymphedema. Lymphoscintigraphy (1 h post epifascial injection of the tracer) showed asymmetrical uptake in the inguinal nodes, as well as a popliteal node on the left side. The findings confirmed lymphatic drainage compromise bilaterally

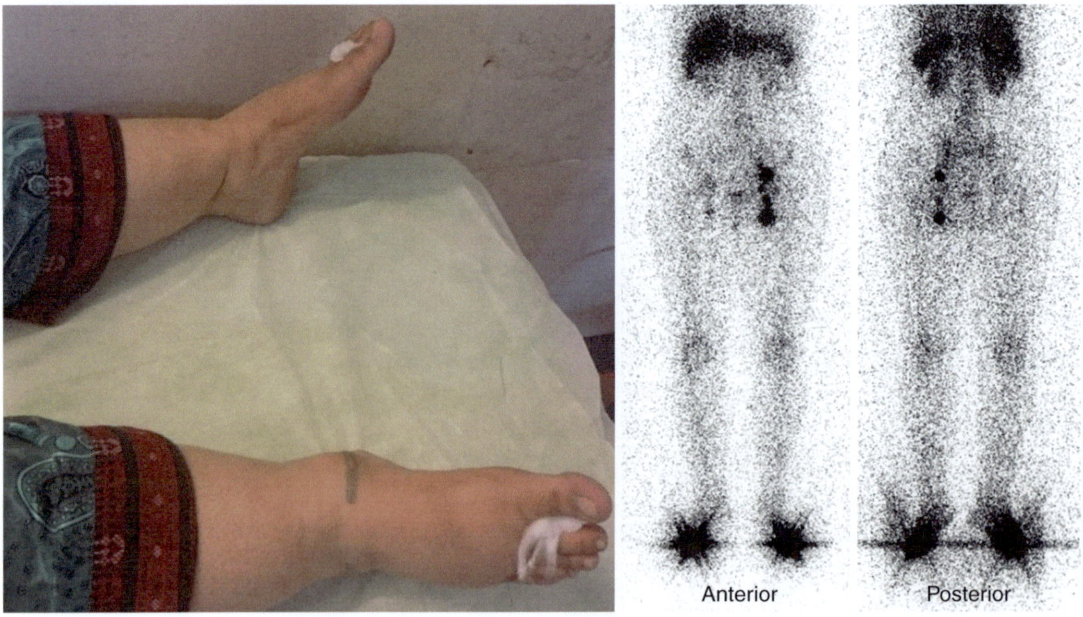

Fig. 12.18 A 33-year-old female patient with a history of leg swelling sparing the feet since childhood. Following a tattoo in the right ankle, the patient developed swelling of the right instep. With the suspicion of lipolymphedema, she was referred for lymphoscintigraphy. Lymphoscintigraphy (1 h post epifascial injection) showed almost no activity in the right inguinal lymph nodes, which confirmed the diagnosis of lipolymphedema on the right side

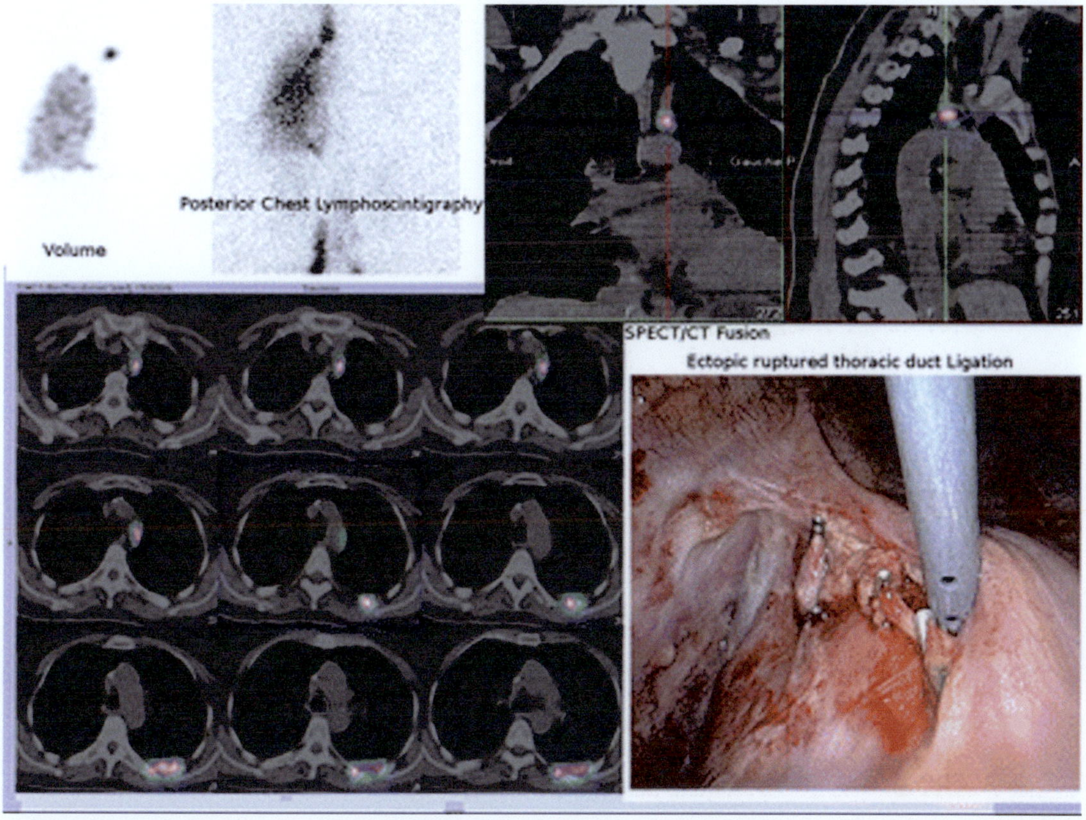

Fig. 12.19 A 60-year-old patient who developed chylothorax following thymectomy. SPECT/CT of the thorax showed abnormal tracer accumulation between the left common carotid artery and the left subclavian artery. This finding confirmed the rupture of a collateral thoracic lymph duct (Reproduced with permission from https://doi.org/10.1007/s00259-011-1793-1)

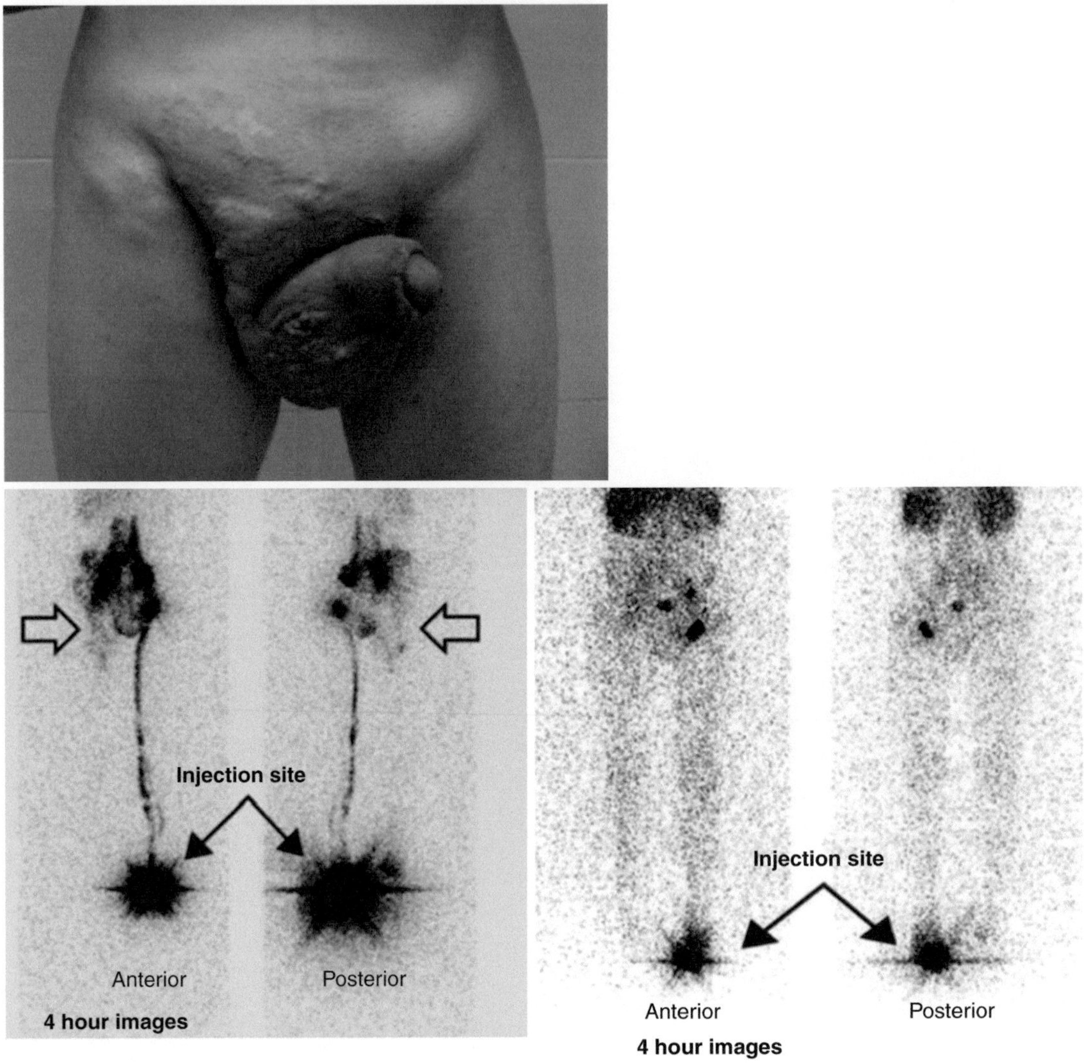

Fig. 12.20 A 23-year-old male patient with a history of lymphedema of the right groin and scrotal region (top image) was referred for lymphoscintigraphy of the lower limbs. Chylous reflux from normal limb to the affected limb was the suspicious cause of the lymphedema. The patient was only injected in the normal limb with the radiotracer, which showed a clear reflux to the affected limb (lower left). The patient underwent surgery for the removal of the defective lymph vessels connecting the lymphatic systems of the affected and normal limbs. Fifteen days following the surgery, another lymphoscintigraphy showed no reflux to the affected limb (lower right) (Reproduced with permission from https://doi.org/10.1097/RLU.0000000000000418)

References

1. Ahmed RL, Prizment A, Lazovich D, Schmitz KH, Folsom AR. Lymphedema and quality of life in breast cancer survivors: the Iowa Women's Health Study. J Clin Oncol. 2008;26:5689–96.
2. Herberger K, Blome C, Heyer K, Ellis F, Munter KC, Augustin M. Quality of life in patients with primary and secondary lymphedema in the community. Wound Repair Regen. 2017;25:466–73.
3. Jeffs E, Purushotham A. The prevalence of lymphoedema in women who attended an information and exercise class to reduce the risk of breast cancer-related upper limb lymphoedema. Springerplus. 2016;5:21.
4. Maclellan RA, Couto RA, Sullivan JE, Grant FD, Slavin SA, Greene AK. Management of primary and

secondary lymphedema: analysis of 225 referrals to a center. Ann Plast Surg. 2015;75:197–200.

5. de Roo T. The value of lymphography in lymphedema. Surg Gynecol Obstet. 1967;124:755–65.
6. Gan JL, Zhang DS, Fu KD, Luo JC, Chen H. Indirect lymphography with Isovist-300 in various forms of lymphedema. Chin Med J. 1991;104:49–53.
7. Sadeghi R, Kazemzadeh G, Keshtgar M. Diagnostic application of lymphoscintigraphy in the management of lymphoedema. Hell J Nucl Med. 2010;13:6–10.
8. Seitzman MD, Wright R, Halaby FA, Freeman JH. Radioactive lymphangiography as a therapeutic adjunct. Am J Roentgenol Radium Therapy, Nucl Med. 1963;89:140–9.
9. Szuba A, Shin WS, Strauss HW, Rockson S. The third circulation: radionuclide lymphoscintigraphy in the evaluation of lymphedema. J Nucl Med. 2003;44:43–57.
10. Henze E, Schelbert HR, Collins JD, Najafi A, Barrio JR, Bennett LR. Lymphoscintigraphy with Tc-99m-labeled dextran. J Nucl Med. 1982;23:923–9.
11. Eshima D, Fauconnier T, Eshima L, Thornback JR. Radiopharmaceuticals for lymphoscintigraphy: including dosimetry and radiation considerations. Semin Nucl Med. 2000;30:25–32.
12. Zarifmahmoudi L, Shabahang H, Shariati F, Dabbagh Kakhki VR, Mehrabibahar M, Sadat Alavifard R, et al. Dynamic lymphoscintigraphy in breast cancer patients: feasibility and added value. Iran J Nucl Med. 2016;24:130–5.
13. Sadri K, Ayati NK, Shabani G, Zakavi SR, Sadeghi R. Sentinel node detection failure due to defective labeling and large particle size of Tc-99m antimony sulfide colloid. Iran J Nucl Med. 2011;19:6–11.
14. Brautigam P, Foldi E, Schaiper I, Krause T, Vanscheidt W, Moser E. Analysis of lymphatic drainage in various forms of leg edema using two compartment lymphoscintigraphy. Lymphology. 1998;31:43–55.
15. Tartaglione G, Pagan M, Morese R, Cappellini GA, Zappala AR, Sebastiani C, et al. Intradermal lymphoscintigraphy at rest and after exercise: a new technique for the functional assessment of the lymphatic system in patients with lymphoedema. Nucl Med Commun. 2010;31:547–51.
16. Tartaglione G, Rubello D. The evolving methodology to perform limb lymphoscintigraphy: from rest to exercise acquisition protocol. Microvasc Res. 2010;80:540–4.
17. Ogawa Y, Hayashi K. 99mTc-DTPA-HSA lymphoscintigraphy in lymphedema of the lower extremities: diagnostic significance of dynamic study and muscular exercise. Kaku Igaku. 1999;36:31–6.
18. Lane KN, Dolan LB, Worsley D, McKenzie DC. Upper extremity lymphatic function at rest and during exercise in breast cancer survivors with and without lymphedema compared with healthy controls. J Appl Physiol. 2007;103:917–25.
19. Maclellan RA, Zurakowski D, Voss S, Greene AK. Correlation between lymphedema disease severity and lymphoscintigraphic findings: a clinical-radiologic study. J Am Coll Surg. 2017;225:366–70.
20. Nawaz K, Hamad MM, Sadek S, Awdeh M, Eklof B, Abdel-Dayem HM. Dynamic lymph flow imaging in lymphedema. Normal and abnormal patterns. Clin Nucl Med. 1986;11:653–8.
21. Ghahremani S, Shafiee S, Sabour M, Bazrafshan A, Sadeghi R. Tc-99m phytate lymphoscintigraphy: an excellent method for diagnosis of underlying cause of chylous ascites. Iran J Nucl Med. 2016;24:150–3.
22. Divband G, Ravari H, Kazemzadeh G, Shayegani H, Khosravi S, Sadeghi R. False positive lower limb lymphoscintigraphy due to inadvertent intra-vascular injection of the tracer: Importance of tracer re-injection. Iran J Nucl Med. 2017;25:136–8.
23. Gholami Malekshahi R, Dabbagh Kakhki VR, Zakavi SR, Aryana K, Sadeghi R. Visualization of a supraclavicular node on the lower extremity lymphoscintigraphy. Rev Esp Med Nucl. 2010;29:270.
24. Alivifard R, Yousefi Z, Kadkhodayan S, Hasanzadeh M, Sadeghi R. Pelvic kidney visualization on the lymphoscintigraphy images of a patient with uterine cervix cancer: importance of the delayed imaging. Clin Nucl Med. 2014;39:286–7.
25. Weissleder H, Weissleder R. Lymphedema: evaluation of qualitative and quantitative lymphoscintigraphy in 238 patients. Radiology. 1988;167:729–35.
26. Burnand KM, Glass DM, Mortimer PS, Peters AM. Lymphatic dysfunction in the apparently clinically normal contralateral limbs of patients with unilateral lower limb swelling. Clin Nucl Med. 2012;37:9–13.
27. Keramida G, Winterman N, Wroe E, Aplin M, Peters AM. Importance of accurate ilio-inguinal quantification in lower extremity lymphoscintigraphy. Nucl Med Commun. 2017;38:209–14.
28. Carena M, Campini R, Zelaschi G, Rossi G, Aprile C, Paroni G. Quantitative lymphoscintigraphy. Eur J Nucl Med. 1988;14:88–92.
29. Stewart G, Gaunt JI, Croft DN, Browse NL. Isotope lymphography: a new method of investigating the role of the lymphatics in chronic limb oedema. Br J Surg. 1985;72:906–9.
30. Stanton AW, Modi S, Mellor RH, Peters AM, Svensson WE, Levick JR, et al. A quantitative lymphoscintigraphic evaluation of lymphatic function in the swollen hands of women with lymphoedema following breast cancer treatment. Clin Sci (Lond). 2006;110:553–61.
31. Yoo JN, Cheong YS, Min YS, Lee SW, Park HY, Jung TD. Validity of quantitative lymphoscintigraphy as a lymphedema assessment tool for patients with breast cancer. Ann Rehabil Med. 2015;39:931–40.
32. Bourgeois P. Scintigraphic investigations of the lymphatic system: the influence of injected volume and quantity of labeled colloidal tracer. J Nucl Med. 2007;48:693.
33. Bourgeois P, Leduc O, Belgrado J, Leduc A. Scintigraphic investigations of the superficial lymphatic system: quantitative differences between intradermal and subcutaneous injections. Nucl Med Commun. 2009;30:270.
34. Prevot N, Tiffet O, Avet J, Quak E, Decousus M, Dubois F. Lymphoscintigraphy and SPECT/CT using

^{99m}Tc filtered sulphur colloid in chylothorax. Eur J Nucl Med Mol Imaging. 2011;38:1746.
35. Gloviczki P, Fisher J, Hollier LH, Pairolero PC, Schirger A, Wahner HW. Microsurgical lymphovenous anastomosis for treatment of lymphedema: a critical review. J Vasc Surg. 1988;7:647–52.
36. Kafejian-Haddad A, Perez J, Castiglioni M, Miranda JF, de Figueiredo L. Lymphscintigraphic evaluation of manual lymphatic drainage for lower extremity lymphedema. Lymphology. 2006;39:41.
37. de Godoy J, Batigalia F, Godoy MF. Preliminary evaluation of a new, more simplified physiotherapy technique for lymphatic drainage. Lymphology. 2002;35:91.
38. Pecking A, Février B, Wargon C, Pillion G. Efficacy of Daflon 500 mg in the treatment of lymphedema (secondary to conventional therapy of breast cancer). Angiology. 1997;48:93.
39. Hwang J, Kwon J, Lee K, Choi J, Kim B, Lee B, et al. Changes in lymphatic function after complex physical therapy for lymphedema. Lymphology. 1999;32:15.
40. Szuba A, Strauss W, Sirsikar S, Rockson S. Quantitative radionuclide lymphoscintigraphy predicts outcome of manual lymphatic therapy in breast cancer-related lymphedema of the upper extremity. Nucl Med Commun. 2002;23:1171.
41. Pain S, Purushotham A, Barber R, Ballinger J, Solanki C, Mortimer P, et al. Variation in lymphatic function may predispose to development of breast cancer-related lymphoedema. EJSO. 2004;30:508–14.
42. Stanton AW, Modi S, Mellor RH, Levick JR, Mortimer PS. Recent advances in breast cancer-related lymphedema of the arm: lymphatic pump failure and predisposing factors. Lymphat Res Biol. 2009;7:29–45.

13 Nuclear Medicine Imaging Techniques of the Neuroendocrine System

Alexander Haug

13.1 Neuroendocrine Tumors

Neuroendocrine tumors (NETs) are a challenge for diagnostics, and in particular imaging, for several reasons. NETs are a rare tumor entity but with a significant increase in incidence in recent years. Part of this increase, in addition to an increased awareness of NETs, can certainly be attributed to improved diagnostics in both imaging and pathology. Due to different secreted hormones, NETs can cause a large number of clinical symptoms, some of which are unspecific, such as diarrhea, and, in the absence of hormone secretion, can occur only very late in the course of the disease due to the size of the metastases. Therefore, the diagnosis of NET often takes place only after a long time of delay. Hence, the prognosis for NET is poor despite low growth dynamics due to the usually high degree of differentiation since there is often already a distant metastasis. In addition, the primary tumor is often small even after metastasis. NETs are derived from the neuroendocrine cell system, which is localized in almost all parts of the body. Accordingly, NET can in principle occur throughout the body. Nevertheless, there are predilection sites, such as the pancreas, lung, rectum, or ileum [1].

The localization of the primary tumor is of very great importance since the therapeutic algorithm and prognosis depend decisively on this. For example, NET of the ileum, unlike those of the pancreas, have no response to chemotherapy. Survival is longer, for example, with NET of the ileum than with NET of the pancreas. Thus, the choice of appropriate therapy is only possible with knowledge of the localization of the NET [1].

The most commonly used radiopharmaceutical in oncologic nuclear medicine imaging is ^{18}F-FDG (FDG). However, NETs in the vast majority of patients do not exhibit increased FDG uptake and are, therefore, not regularly positive in FDG PET, which hampers its use. On the other hand, several studies have shown a prognostic value of FDG PET: FDG positive NETs have a significantly shorter overall and progression-free survival as compared to FDG negative ones with high hazard ratios of 10.3 and 9.4, respectively [2]. A common feature of at least a NET with a high degree of differentiation (Ki67 < 20%, corresponding to NET grades 1 and 2) is the very high stocking of the cell membrane with somatostatin receptors (SSTR). There are five different SSTRs, with subtype 2 being expressed very frequently and being used for nuclear medicine imaging. This high receptor population has been used diagnostically for

A. Haug (✉)
Department of Biomedical Imaging and Image-guided Therapy, Medical University of Vienna, Vienna, Austria
e-mail: alexander.haug@meduniwien.ac.at

H. Ahmadzadehfar et al. (eds.), *Clinical Nuclear Medicine*,
https://doi.org/10.1007/978-3-030-39457-8_13

many years. Various agonist somatostatin analogs (SSA) with high affinity for SSTR type 2 were synthesized, provided with a chelator, and labeled with a radionuclide. [^{111}In] pentetreotide, or OctreoScan (Mallinckrodt), was the first approved radiopharmaceutical agent for NET imaging. Although high sensitivities and specificities were initially reported, [3] there are limitations in terms of local resolution and small NET detection due to the physical properties of Indium-111. The development of [^{68}Ga]-labeled SSA enabled significantly improved PET diagnostics. The three most common radiopharmaceuticals, [^{68}Ga]-DOTATATE, [^{68}Ga]-DOTATOC, and [^{68}Ga]-DOTANOC, each have different affinities for the different SSTR subtypes. In everyday clinical practice, however, they are to be regarded as equivalent without relevant differences. Although studies found significant differences in NET and organ storage between the three radiopharmaceuticals, these did not affect diagnostic accuracy [4, 5]. Several studies have shown the diagnostic gain of SSTR PET with significantly increased sensitivity (97% versus 52%) compared with OctreoScan and also with computed tomography (CT) (sensitivity 61%) [6]. In 87% of all patients with a negative or ambiguous OctreoScan, [^{68}Ga]-DOTATATE PET/CT was able to detect metastases [7]. In a prospective study of 131 patients, the highly significant diagnostic superiority of [^{68}Ga]-DOTATATE PET/CT (sensitivity of 95.1%), compared with OctreoScan SPECT/CT (30.9%) and also CT/MRI (45.3%), can be detected [8]. SSTR PET/CT is therefore to be regarded as the gold standard in the imaging of NETs. Also, due to significantly improved diagnostics, [^{68}Ga] DOTATATE has been approved by the Food and Drug Administration (FDA) in the US.

According to the guideline of the European Association of Nuclear Medicine (EANM), about 2 MBq/kg body weight is usually applied [9]. Typically, the acquisition of PET scan is started 45–60 min after application. The examination area usually covers the skull base to the thighs. There is no consensus on the need for a diagnostic CT with intravenous contrast, and many centers consider a native low-dose CT to be adequate.

SSA therapy such as octreotide or lanreotide is a standard therapy and is used in a majority of patients. Due to the fact that these SSA and radiopharmaceuticals bind to the same receptors and thus could theoretically be competitive and reduce the binding of radiopharmaceuticals, discontinuation of the medication before PET is often recommended [10]. However, this theoretical consideration could be refuted. In studies, chronic therapy with Sandostatin LAR has been shown to significantly reduce the uptake of organs, such as the liver and spleen, but does not affect the uptake of NETs [11]. There is thus no need to discontinue SSA before SSTR PET.

13.1.1 Primary Diagnosis

Primary diagnosis of patients suspected of having NET is challenging for several reasons. Either the diagnosis is due to the often nonspecific or missing clinical symptoms to a late, already metastatic stage, which often complicates the detection of small primary NETs, or in the case of a hormone-active NET, the primary tumor is still very small despite the sometimes pronounced symptoms and is thus difficult to represent in the imaging. One study examined [^{68}Ga] DOTATATE PET/CT for diagnostic ability in 104 patients suspected of having NET due to clinical complaints ($n = 70$), raised tumor markers ($n = 49$), or previous imaging ($n = 53$, multiple answers possible). Histologically, NET was confirmed in 36 patients, nonneuroendocrine malignancies in 12 patients, and benign tumors in seven patients. [^{68}Ga] DOTATATE PET/CT detected NET in 29/36 patients and excluded NET at 61/68, which corresponds to a sensitivity of 81% and a specificity of 90% [12]. Thus, SSTR PET/CT is considered to be a highly effective method for detecting or even excluding NET.

The so-called carcinoma unknown primary (CUP) syndrome, i.e., the presence of metastases without detection of the primary tumor, is comparatively common in NETs. In a study of 59 patients with NET and CUP syndrome, [^{68}Ga]-DOTANOC PET/CT was able to localize the primary tumor in 59% of these cases, most commonly in the pancreas (16 patients) and ileum/jejunum (14 patients) [13].

13.1.2 Therapy Management

The proven significantly better diagnostic accuracy of SSTR PET/CT should ideally also be reflected in improved therapy. Several studies have examined the influence of SSTR PET/CT on the therapeutic approach. In the prospective pivotal trial, [^{68}Ga] DOTATATE PETCT resulted in a change in therapy in 33% of patients [8]. In a recent meta-analysis of 14 trials involving 1561 patients, SSTR PET/CT changed the therapeutic approach in 40% of patients [14]. Some of these changes, such as the decision to perform a peptide receptor radionuclide therapy (PRRT) or SSA therapy, are certainly due to the nature of the study since prior to PRRT, storage in all tumor lesions is required, but serious changes are also noted, such as discarding a liver transplant when detecting extrahepatic metastases (Fig. 13.1).

[^{68}Ga] DOTATATE PET/CT also has a significant impact on the planning of surgical resection of well-differentiated NETs. In pancreatic NETs, the surgeon found SSTR PET/CT to be helpful in 100% of cases and changed the operative approach in 33% of cases [15]. SSTR PET/CT was also found to be helpful (in 96%) for NET of the ileum but had less impact on surgery (4% change), which is likely to be due to the standardized surgical procedure, a hemicolectomy.

Since SSA, a standard therapy for NET, have the same target structure as SSTR PET, SSTR PET may be useful for assessing therapeutic outcome. In fact, one study found that patients with a high expression of SSTR in SSTR PET had a significantly longer progression-free survival with a hazard ratio of 0.34 compared with patients with low uptake [16]. Even before a PRRT, the amount of SSTR expresion in the SSTR PET may predict the response to PRRT [17, 18].

13.1.3 Therapy Monitoring

The role of SSTR PET/CT for evaluating response to therapy is still the subject of debate, as a decrease in uptake may mean a reduction in tumor volume (and receptor number), but it does not rule out the development of undifferentiated cloning that may be SSTR negative, lead to this decrease in uptake. On the other hand, CT as a standard oncological imaging has limitations in NETs. While the response evaluation criteria in solid tumors (RECIST) are widely used in oncology, their applicability to gastroenteropancreatic neuroendocrine tumors (GEP-NETs) is questioned due to various issues. For example, slowly growing lesions are often erroneously interpreted as stable due to the small change in intervals. Despite proven effects on survival, therapies for NET rarely achieve size regression. The effect of targeted therapies is also more likely to be reflected by intralesional necrosis and diminished vascularization rather than size changes. In particular, intratumoral necrosis can visualize hepatic lesions for the first time, which could be misinterpreted as progress. In general, a disadvantage is the limited sensitivity of CT compared with SSTR PET, which affects liver metastases in particular [19]. In addition, liver metastases sometimes show cystic transformation under therapy, making size determination unreliable for therapy monitoring. Finally, morphological criteria for response to therapy are not always prognostic, at least in some PRRT studies in which patients who did not progress showed similar survival irrespective of remission status (size resistant versus unchanged) [20].

Due to the mentioned limitations, there is a need for better criteria for therapy response. An initial study has shown that [^{68}Ga]-DOTATOC PET can detect progression at an earlier stage than CT due to an earlier diagnosis of new metastases [20].

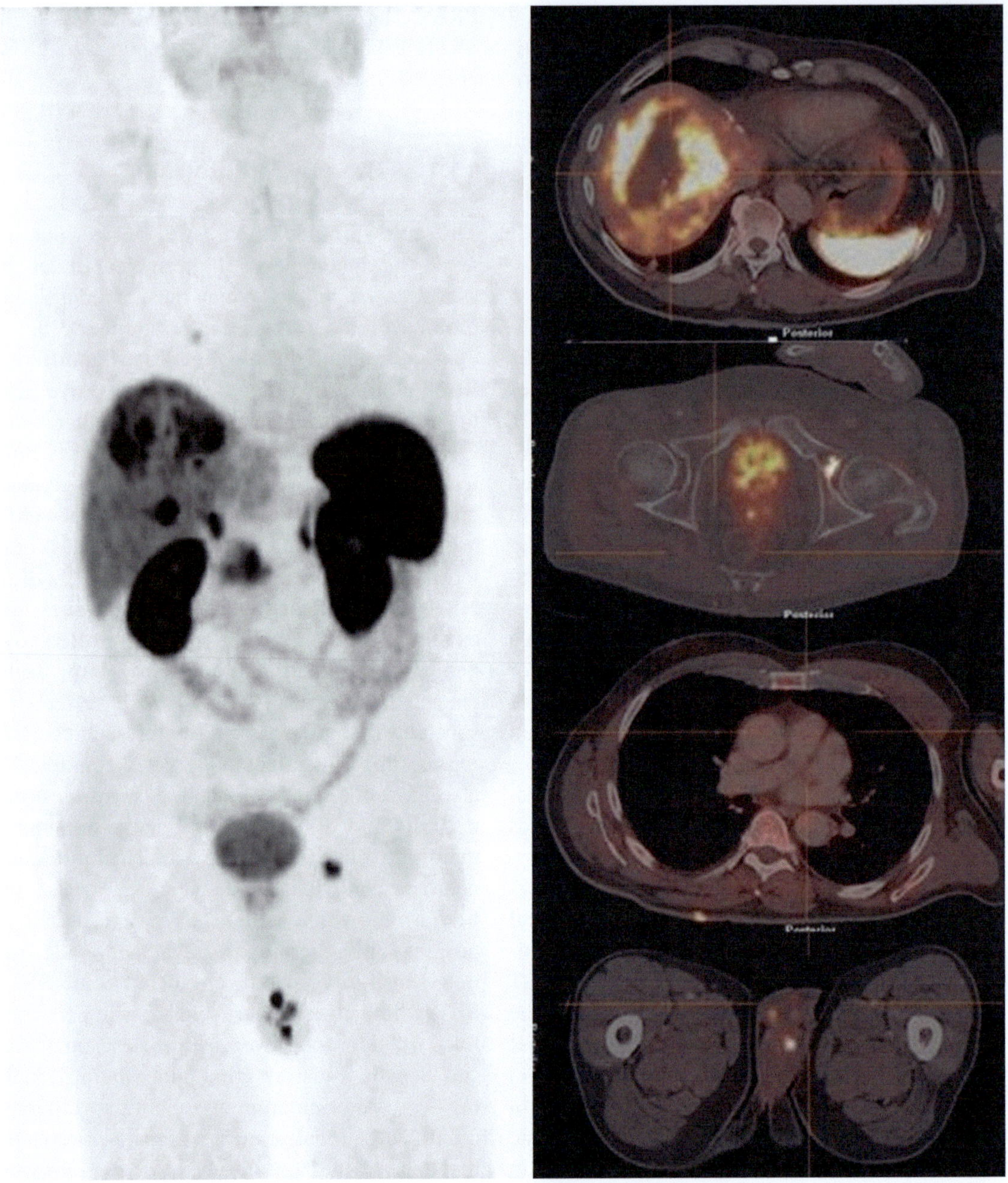

Fig. 13.1 Example of a patient with metastatic NET, which illustrates the high diagnostic accuracy of SSTR PET/CT and its influence on therapeutic management. In this patient, in whom only liver metastases were suspected, and therefore a local-liver-directed therapy was planned. In [^{68}Ga]-DOTANOC PET/CT, however, a single bone metastasis in the acetabulum, which was also recognizable in the CT, was also observed. In addition, it is not untypical for NET that metastases were also detectable at unusual sites, such as the skin and scrotum, which might otherwise have escaped detection. Thus, local therapy was no longer useful in systemic metastasis, and PRRT with [177Lu]-DOTATATE was performed

Furthermore, [^{68}Ga]-DOTATATE PET can be used for early therapy monitoring of PRRT. In a study of 33 patients, patients who had a decrease in tumor uptakes normalized to spleen SUV (tumor-spleen ratio) after the first cycle of PRRT had significantly longer progression-free survival [17].

13.1.4 Diagnosis of Recurrence

Even in patients with primary localized NET, there is potential for improvement in 5-year survival rates, which is around 80% [1], as relapse occurs in a relatively large number of patients. In a cohort of patients with pancreatic NET after curative resection, 42% developed recurrence, in most cases in the liver [21], whereas in a cohort of patients with small bowel, NET developed median relapse after 32 months in 59%. Given its proven diagnostic superiority, SSTR PET/CT is also applied in follow-ups after curative therapy. In fact, it was shown in 63 patients that [^{68}Ga]-DOTATATE PET/CT can be reliably used in follow-ups, with a sensitivity of 90% and a specificity of 82% [22]. In gastro-entero-pancreatic NETs, SSTR PET/CT gave even better results with a sensitivity of 94% and a specificity of 89%. This study also demonstrated the importance of accurate knowledge of clinical facts for diagnostic accuracy of SSTR PET/CT. A blinded evaluator had significantly lower diagnostic accuracy than an evaluator with access to clinical data.

13.1.5 SSTR PET/MRI

PET/MRI is becoming increasingly popular, and some studies are already working on SSTR PET/MRI. In a prospective study of 27 patients, [^{68}Ga]-DOTANOC PET/MRI demonstrated comparable sensitivity compared with PET/CT [23]. SSTR PET/MRI was superior in the detection of bone and liver metastases but showed weaknesses in lung and pleural metastases. Interobserver variability was comparable between PET/MRI and PET/CT. Another study with 30 patients shows a slightly higher sensitivity of [^{68}Ga]-DOTATOC PET/MRI compared with PET/CT (90.8% versus 86.7%) [24] (Fig. 13.2).

All in all, a comparable diagnostic accuracy of SSTR PET/MRI can thus be assumed, with advantages in the detection of liver and bone metastases. The drawback, however, must be the significantly higher logistical effort with a test duration of at least 30 min, but rather 60 min in the case of the use of liver-specific contrast agent or diffusion-weighted sequences, and the higher susceptibility of MRI to artifacts. Also, the problem of attenuation correction does not seem to have been finally resolved. Thus, although SSTR PET/MRI may be beneficial for selected patients, it is unlikely that it will be able to replace SSTR PET/CT as a standard procedure in the medium term.

13.1.6 SSR Antagonists

While radiolabeled SSA have been used for many years in the diagnosis of NET, antagonistic SSR have not been considered promising as they are not or hardly internalized into the tumor cell. However, these antagonists appear to recognize more binding sites on SSTR and have favorable pharmacokinetics [25]. Various antagonists have been evaluated, and [^{68}Ga] DOTA-JR11 (corresponding to [^{68}Ga] OPS202) has emerged as the most promising candidate. In a phase 1/2 study, [^{68}Ga]-OPS202 showed significantly lower background uptake, especially in the liver, intestine, and pancreas, compared to [^{68}Ga]-DOTATOC, resulting in significantly better tumor-background ratios (5.3 versus 1.9) and sensitivity (94% versus 88%) [26]. Currently, [^{68}Ga] OPS202 is being evaluated in a larger study. If promising results are confirmed, [^{68}Ga] OPS202 PET/CT certainly has the potential to become the new diagnostic standard.

13.1.7 Neuroendocrine Carcinoma

Neuroendocrine carcinomas (NECs) and grade 3 neuroendocrine tumors (NET G3) are defined as neuroendocrine neoplasm with a proliferation rate (Ki67) of more than 20%. NEC have a far

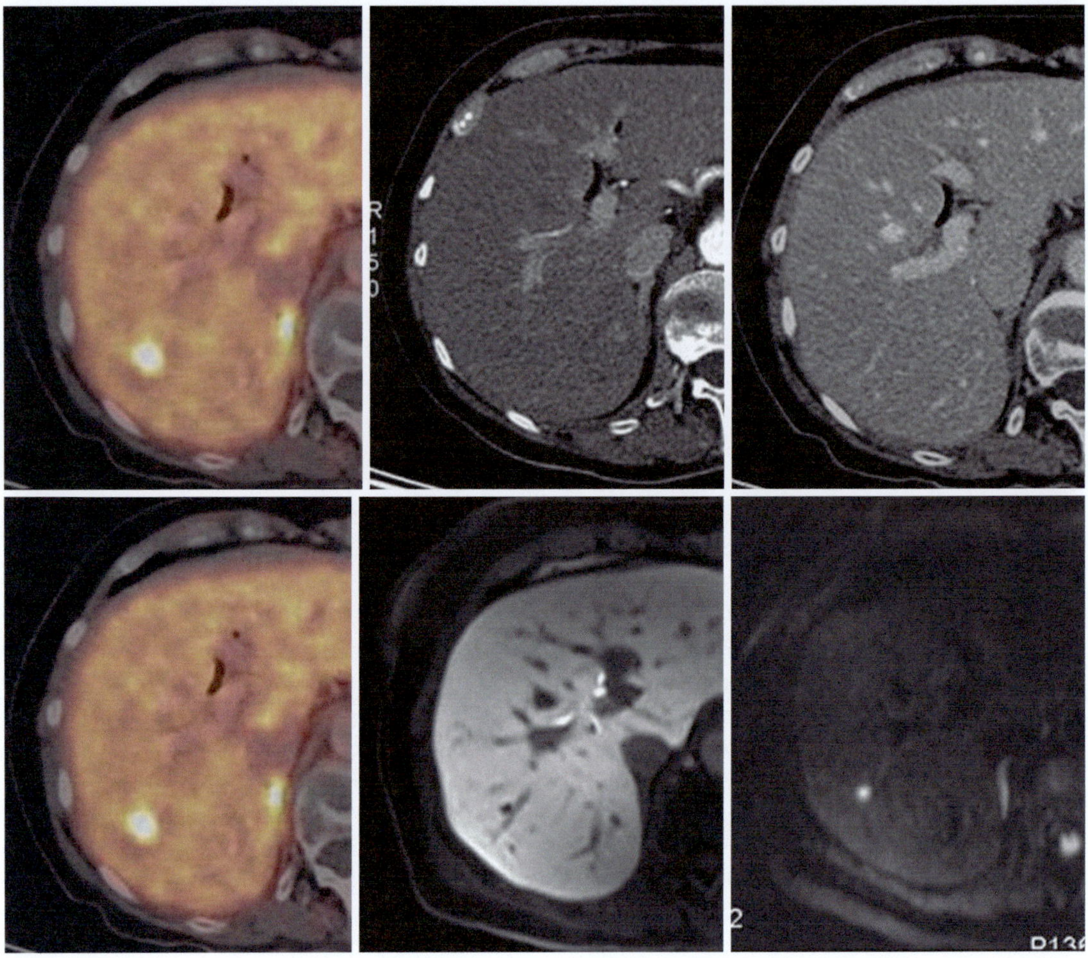

Fig. 13.2 Case of a young patient in follow-up after curative resection of pancreatic NET. In [68Ga]-DOTANOC PET/CT, a single suspicious focal storage can be detected, but there is no correlate in either arterial or venous CT. In PET/MRT with liver-specific contrast medium and diffusion-weighted sequences, liver metastasis can be clearly diagnosed. This case illustrates, on the one hand, the limited sensitivity of CT in liver metastases and, on the other hand, the high sensitivity of PET

worse prognosis than NET, and therapeutic as well as diagnostic approaches are differing. Although NEC partly express, SSTR PET/CT is not considered as standard imaging tool. In contrast to NETs, NECs present with increased FDG uptake in the majority of cases, which renders FDG PET/CT well suited for staging and restaging. NET G3 are considered as highly proliferating but well differentiated, and therefore SSTR PET/CT can be considered for imaging, especially as PRRT might be a treatment option in the course of the disease.

13.1.8 Pheochromocytoma and Paraganglioma

Pheochromocytoma is a disease of the chromaffin cells of the adrenal cord with an incidence of 1/100,000 persons/year. It is a tumor that produces catecholamines (noradrenaline, adrenaline, and metanephrine), which cause hypertension. Malignant pheochromocytoma, which accounts for approximately 10% of all pheochromocytomas, also forms dopamine. It is located 85% in the adrenal medulla. It is also found in the nerve tissues of the thoracic and abdominal border strand and is then named paraganglioma, where it produces almost exclusively noradrenaline. As these tumors are highly vascularized and can react with an excessive release of catecholamines in biopsies, this is often not feasible and the diagnosis must be made biochemically and by means of imaging. Since the early eighties, 123Iod-radiolabeled metaiodobenzylguanidine (MIBG), a functional analog of norepinephrine, has been used for the diagnosis and treatment of pheochromocytomas and paragangliomas. [^{123}I]-MIBG has to be injected slowly intravenously, and uptake by the thyroid must be blocked with sodium perchlorate. As some medications, such as antidepressants, influence MIBG uptake in tumors, these drugs have to be interrupted 48 h before administration [27]. Especially in pheochromocytoma, [^{123}I]-MIBG reported sensitivities show a wide variance, tend to be higher in older studies, and can be considered around 70% [28]. In contrast, PET imaging with [^{18}F]-DOPA has—in part due to the higher resolution of PET as compared to conventional scintigraphy—a substantially higher diagnostic accuracy with sensitivity around 90% and can be considered as superior [29]. Especially in non-catecholamine-secreting tumors, which tend to be MIBG- and [^{18}F]-DOPA-negative, FDG PET is a valuable imaging tool with a high sensitivity of 83% [30]. SSTR PET/CT offers similar diagnostic accuracy and can be considered as an equivalent alternative imaging modality [31]. A recent study showed that [^{123}I]-MIBG SPECT/CT was equally diagnostic accurate as SSTR PET/CT in the diagnosis of primary pheochromocytoma or paraganglioma [32]. However, [^{123}I]-MIBG SPECT/CT, as opposed to SSTR PET/CT, failed in detecting extraadrenal metastases.

13.2 Neuroblastoma

Neuroblastoma is the third most frequent malignoma in children. It arises from the adrenergic nervous system, secretes catecholamines in the majority of cases, and has already metastasized in half of the cases at the time of diagnosis, although its aggressiveness shows a wide variability. [^{123}I]-MIBG scintigraphy is well established in children suffering from neuroblastoma and has a high sensitivity of around 95%. [^{123}I]-MIBG scintigraphy is of special value in the diagnosis of bone marrow metastasis. Furthermore, it is very valuable in treatment monitoring and also for selecting patients suitable for treatment with [^{131}I]-MIBG [33] (Fig. 13.3). Preliminary studies report about the use of MIBG labeled with positron-emitting [^{124}I] and [^{18}F], which might improve diagnostic accuracy [34]. FDG PET also has a reported high sensitivity, which is significantly superior to whole-body MRI, which is frequently used in children due to its lack of ionizing radiation [35]. As neuroblastomas express SSTR in most cases, promising results, which even surpass [^{123}I]-MIBG scintigraphy in a small cohort of patients, have been reported by using [^{68}Ga]-DOTATATE PET/CT [36].

13.3 Medullary Thyroid Cancer

Recurrent and metastatic medullary cancer can be challenging for imaging. Especially in patients with elevated and rising levels of calcitonin, which serves as a tumor marker, imaging with CT/MRI fails to detect the site of recurrence quite often. Nuclear medicine offers several PET radiopharmaceuticals that perform with good efficacy. A recent meta-analysis has summarized the results of nine studies examining the accuracy of SSTR PET/CT in a recurrent medullary thyroid cancer [37]. The overall detection rate was 63.5% on a per-patient rate and increased with rising levels of calcitonin (83% for calcitonin >500 ng/ml). Similar detection rates (67%) were reported for FDG PET/CT. A study comparing the sensitivity of both radiopharmaceuticals in the same patients also found no significant differences (SSTR PET/CT 72%, FDG PET/CT 78%) [38]. [^{18}F]-DOPA PET/CT is likewise frequently used in medullary thyroid cancer. However, detection rates (63%) are within the same range as reported for FDG and SSTR PET [39]. In conclusion, there is no PET radiopharmaceutical that can be clearly recommended. The choice of the tracer depends

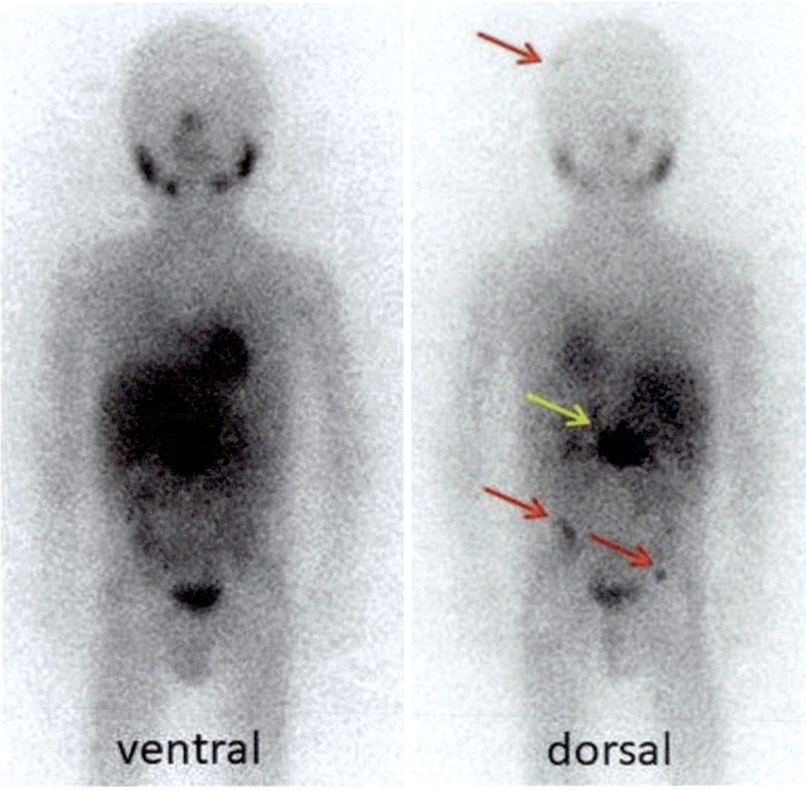

Fig. 13.3 Example of a child with metastasized neuroblastoma of the right adrenal gland (yellow arrow). Indicated are the bone metastases with clearly elevated MIBG uptake (red arrows). Note the high physiologic uptake of the salivary glands, the heart, the liver, and the bladder (renal excretion)

heavily on the expertise and availability of radiopharmaceuticals of the center as the diagnostic performance of theses tracers can be considered equivalent.

References

1. Yao JC, Hassan M, Phan A, et al. One hundred years after "carcinoid": epidemiology of and prognostic factors for neuroendocrine tumors in 35,825 cases in the United States. J Clin Oncol. 2008;26:3063–72.
2. Binderup T, Knigge U, Loft A, Federspiel B, Kjaer A. 18F-fluorodeoxyglucose positron emission tomography predicts survival of patients with neuroendocrine tumors. Clin Cancer Res. 2010;16:978–85.
3. Schillaci O. Somatostatin receptor imaging in patients with neuroendocrine tumors: not only SPECT? J Nucl Med. 2007;48:498–500.
4. Kabasakal L, Demirci E, Ocak M, et al. Comparison of (6)(8)Ga-DOTATATE and (6)(8)Ga-DOTANOC PET/CT imaging in the same patient group with neuroendocrine tumours. Eur J Nucl Med Mol Imaging. 2012;39:1271–7.
5. Poeppel TD, Binse I, Petersenn S, et al. 68Ga-DOTATOC versus 68Ga-DOTATATE PET/CT in functional imaging of neuroendocrine tumors. J Nucl Med. 2011;52:1864–70.
6. Gabriel M, Decristoforo C, Kendler D, et al. 68Ga-DOTA-Tyr3-octreotide PET in neuroendocrine tumors: comparison with somatostatin receptor scintigraphy and CT. J Nucl Med. 2007;48:508–18.
7. Srirajaskanthan R, Kayani I, Quigley AM, Soh J, Caplin ME, Bomanji J. The role of 68Ga-DOTATATE PET in patients with neuroendocrine tumors and negative or equivocal findings on 111In-DTPA-octreotide scintigraphy. J Nucl Med. 2010;51:875–82.
8. Sadowski SM, Neychev V, Millo C, et al. Prospective study of 68Ga-DOTATATE positron emission tomography/computed tomography for detecting gastro-entero-pancreatic neuroendocrine tumors and unknown primary sites. J Clin Oncol. 2016;34:588–96.
9. Bozkurt MF, Virgolini I, Balogova S, et al. Guideline for PET/CT imaging of neuroendocrine neoplasms with (68)Ga-DOTA-conjugated somatostatin receptor targeting peptides and (18)F-DOPA. Eur J Nucl Med Mol Imaging. 2017;44:1588–601.
10. Boy C, Poeppel T, Kotzerke J, et al. Somatostatin receptor PET/CT (SSTR-PET/CT). Nuklearmedizin. 2018;57:4–17.

11. Haug AR, Rominger A, Mustafa M, et al. Treatment with octreotide does not reduce tumor uptake of (68)Ga-DOTATATE as measured by PET/CT in patients with neuroendocrine tumors. J Nucl Med. 2011;52:1679–83.
12. Haug AR, Cindea-Drimus R, Auernhammer CJ, et al. The role of 68Ga-DOTATATE PET/CT in suspected neuroendocrine tumors. J Nucl Med. 2012;53:1686–92.
13. Prasad V, Ambrosini V, Hommann M, Hoersch D, Fanti S, Baum RP. Detection of unknown primary neuroendocrine tumours (CUP-NET) using (68) Ga-DOTA-NOC receptor PET/CT. Eur J Nucl Med Mol Imaging. 2010;37:67–77.
14. Barrio M, Czernin J, Fanti S, et al. The impact of somatostatin receptor-directed PET/CT on the management of patients with neuroendocrine tumor: a systematic review and meta-analysis. J Nucl Med. 2017;58:756–61.
15. Ilhan H, Fendler WP, Cyran CC, et al. Impact of (68) Ga-DOTATATE PET/CT on the surgical management of primary neuroendocrine tumors of the pancreas or ileum. Ann Surg Oncol. 2015;22:164–71.
16. Koch W, Auernhammer CJ, Geisler J, et al. Treatment with octreotide in patients with well-differentiated neuroendocrine tumors of the ileum: prognostic stratification with Ga-68-DOTA-TATE positron emission tomography. Mol Imaging. 2014;13:1–10.
17. Haug AR, Auernhammer CJ, Wangler B, et al. 68Ga-DOTATATE PET/CT for the early prediction of response to somatostatin receptor-mediated radionuclide therapy in patients with well-differentiated neuroendocrine tumors. J Nucl Med. 2010;51:1349–56.
18. Kratochwil C, Stefanova M, Mavriopoulou E, et al. SUV of [^{68}Ga]DOTATOC-PET/CT predicts response probability of PRRT in neuroendocrine tumors. Mol Imaging Biol. 2015;17(3):313–8.
19. Ruf J, Schiefer J, Furth C, et al. 68Ga-DOTATOC PET/CT of neuroendocrine tumors: spotlight on the CT phases of a triple-phase protocol. J Nucl Med. 2011;52:697–704.
20. Kwekkeboom DJ, de Herder WW, Kam BL, et al. Treatment with the radiolabeled somatostatin analog [177 Lu-DOTA 0,Tyr3]octreotate: toxicity, efficacy, and survival. J Clin Oncol. 2008;26:2124–30.
21. Boninsegna L, Panzuto F, Partelli S, et al. Malignant pancreatic neuroendocrine tumour: lymph node ratio and Ki67 are predictors of recurrence after curative resections. Eur J Cancer. 2012;48:1608–15.
22. Haug AR, Cindea-Drimus R, Auernhammer CJ, et al. Neuroendocrine tumor recurrence: diagnosis with 68Ga-DOTATATE PET/CT. Radiology. 2013;270(2):517–25.
23. Berzaczy D, Giraudo C, Haug AR, et al. Whole-body 68Ga-DOTANOC PET/MRI versus 68Ga-DOTANOC PET/CT in patients with neuroendocrine tumors: a prospective study in 28 patients. Clin Nucl Med. 2017;42:669–74.
24. Sawicki LM, Deuschl C, Beiderwellen K, et al. Evaluation of (68)Ga-DOTATOC PET/MRI for whole-body staging of neuroendocrine tumours in comparison with (68)Ga-DOTATOC PET/CT. Eur Radiol. 2017;27:4091–9.
25. Wang X, Fani M, Schulz S, Rivier J, Reubi JC, Maecke HR. Comprehensive evaluation of a somatostatin-based radiolabelled antagonist for diagnostic imaging and radionuclide therapy. Eur J Nucl Med Mol Imaging. 2012;39(12):1876–85.
26. Nicolas GP, Schreiter N, Kaul F, et al. Sensitivity comparison of (68)Ga-OPS202 and (68)Ga-DOTATOC PET/CT in patients with gastroenteropancreatic neuroendocrine tumors: a prospective phase II imaging study. J Nucl Med. 2018;59:915–21.
27. Bombardieri E, Aktolun C, Baum RP, et al. 131I/123I-metaiodobenzylguanidine (MIBG) scintigraphy: procedure guidelines for tumour imaging. Eur J Nucl Med Mol Imaging. 2003;30:BP132–9.
28. Rufini V, Treglia G, Castaldi P, Perotti G, Giordano A. Comparison of metaiodobenzylguanidine scintigraphy with positron emission tomography in the diagnostic work-up of pheochromocytoma and paraganglioma: a systematic review. Q J Nucl Med Mol Imaging. 2013;57:122–33.
29. Fiebrich HB, Brouwers AH, Kerstens MN, et al. 6-[F-18]Fluoro-L-dihydroxyphenylalanine positron emission tomography is superior to conventional imaging with (123)I-metaiodobenzylguanidine scintigraphy, computer tomography, and magnetic resonance imaging in localizing tumors causing catecholamine excess. J Clin Endocrinol Metab. 2009;94:3922–30.
30. Timmers HJ, Chen CC, Carrasquillo JA, et al. Comparison of 18F-fluoro-L-DOPA, 18F-fluoro-deoxyglucose, and 18F-fluorodopamine PET and 123I-MIBG scintigraphy in the localization of pheochromocytoma and paraganglioma. J Clin Endocrinol Metab. 2009;94:4757–67.
31. Chang CA, Pattison DA, Tothill RW, et al. (68) Ga-DOTATATE and (18)F-FDG PET/CT in paraganglioma and pheochromocytoma: utility, patterns and heterogeneity. Cancer Imaging. 2016;16:22.
32. Jing H, Li F, Wang L, et al. Comparison of the 68Ga-DOTATATA PET/CT, FDG PET/CT, and MIBG SPECT/CT in the evaluation of suspected primary pheochromocytomas and paragangliomas. Clin Nucl Med. 2017;42:525–9.
33. Howman-Giles R, Shaw PJ, Uren RF, Chung DK. Neuroblastoma and other neuroendocrine tumors. Semin Nucl Med. 2007;37:286–302.
34. Huang SY, Bolch WE, Lee C, et al. Patient-specific dosimetry using pretherapy [(1)(2)(4)I] m-iodobenzylguanidine ([(1)(2)(4)I]mIBG) dynamic PET/CT imaging before [(1)(3)(1)I]mIBG targeted radionuclide therapy for neuroblastoma. Mol Imaging Biol. 2015;17:284–94.
35. Ishiguchi H, Ito S, Kato K, et al. Diagnostic performance of (18)F-FDG PET/CT and whole-body diffusion-weighted imaging with background body suppression (DWIBS) in detection of lymph node and bone metastases from pediatric neuroblastoma. Ann Nucl Med. 2018;32:348–62.

36. Kong G, Hofman MS, Murray WK, et al. Initial experience with Gallium-68 DOTA-octreotate PET/CT and peptide receptor radionuclide therapy for pediatric patients with refractory metastatic neuroblastoma. J Pediatr Hematol Oncol. 2016;38:87–96.
37. Treglia G, Tamburello A, Giovanella L. Detection rate of somatostatin receptor PET in patients with recurrent medullary thyroid carcinoma: a systematic review and a meta-analysis. Hormones (Athens). 2017;16:362–72.
38. Conry BG, Papathanasiou ND, Prakash V, et al. Comparison of (68)Ga-DOTATATE and (18) F-fluorodeoxyglucose PET/CT in the detection of recurrent medullary thyroid carcinoma. Eur J Nucl Med Mol Imaging. 2009;37(1):49–57.
39. Hoegerle S, Altehoefer C, Ghanem N, Brink I, Moser E, Nitzsche E. 18F-DOPA positron emission tomography for tumour detection in patients with medullary thyroid carcinoma and elevated calcitonin levels. Eur J Nucl Med. 2001;28:64–71.

14 Thyroid and Parathyroid Imaging

Matthieu Pelletier-Galarneau, Frédéric Arsenault, and Lionel S. Zuckier

14.1 Thyroid

14.1.1 Thyroid Embryology, Anatomy and Physiology

The thyroid gland is an endocrine organ that produces and secretes thyroid hormones, thereby regulating a myriad aspects of energy expenditure and metabolism. Hormone release and production are governed by the hypothalamic-pituitary-thyroid axis by means of a negative feedback loop [1]. Thyrotropin-releasing hormone (TRH) is secreted by the hypothalamus in response to low serum thyroid hormone levels and stimulates the secretion of thyroid-stimulating hormone (TSH) by the pituitary gland, which in turn promotes the production and discharge of thyroid hormones by the thyroid. High levels of thyroid hormones inhibit the release of both TRH and TSH [2].

The thyroid gland normally lies anterior to the trachea at the level of the thyroid cartilage. It is comprised of two separate lobes, adjoined by the isthmus, which is situated at the level of the second or third tracheal ring (Fig. 14.1). Each lobe measures approximately 3 cm in height, 2 cm in width and a few millimetres in thickness. The weight of a normal thyroid gland is approximately 15–20 g [3, 4].

Embryologically, the thyroid derives from the second pharyngeal arch, between the first and second pharyngeal pouches, and is comprised of endoderm, mesoderm and ectoderm. During the fourth week of embryogenesis, a diverticulum arises from the midline floor of the primitive pharynx, from which develops the primitive thyroid (Fig. 14.2). During the ensuing 3 weeks, the thyroid migrates to its normal location, descending anterior to the hyoid bone and laryngeal cartilages, along the thyroglossal duct. Following migration, the thyroglossal duct atrophies to a variable degree; frequently, an extension of thyroid tissue can extend upwards from the main gland, forming the pyramidal lobe, a common benign anatomical variant [5, 6]. More infrequently, small remnants of thyroidal tissue are deposited along the duct, not in contiguity with the main thyroid gland, and present as thyroglossal duct cysts (Fig. 14.2).

Microscopically, a thyroid tissue is comprised of three main components: follicles, follicular

M. Pelletier-Galarneau (✉)
Department of Radiology and Nuclear Medicine, Institut de Cardiologie de Montréal, Montréal, QC, Canada
e-mail: matthieu.pelletier-galarneau@icm-mhi.org

F. Arsenault
Department of Medical Imaging–Nuclear Medicine, Centre Hospitalier de l'Université de Montréal (CHUM), Montréal, QC, Canada
e-mail: frederic.arsenault@umontreal.ca

L. S. Zuckier
Division of Nuclear Medicine, Department of Radiology, Montefiore Medical Center, Bronx, NY, USA

Albert Einstein College of Medicine, Bronx, NY, USA
e-mail: lzuckier@montefiore.org

H. Ahmadzadehfar et al. (eds.), *Clinical Nuclear Medicine*,
https://doi.org/10.1007/978-3-030-39457-8_14

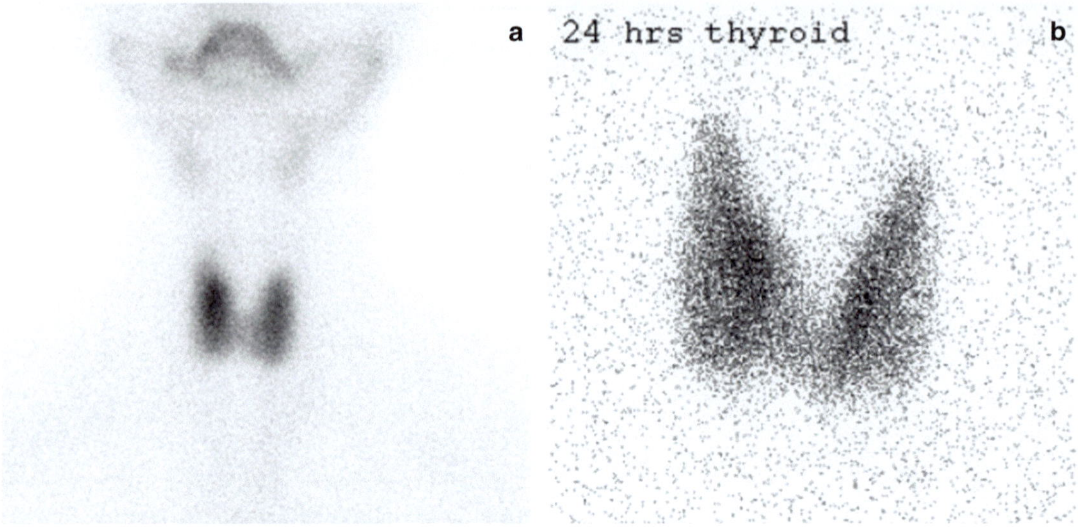

Fig. 14.1 Normal appearance of the thyroid on (**a**) $^{99m}TcO_4^-$ and (**b**) ^{123}I-NaI scintigraphy, performed in different patients. RAIU is 28% in the patient portrayed in (**b**)

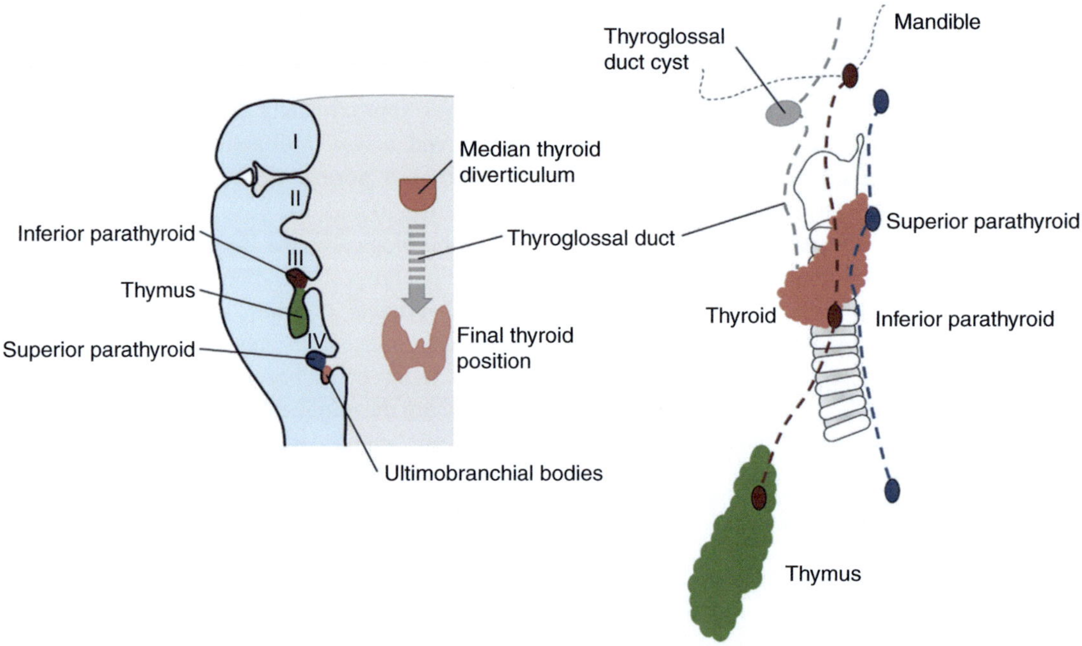

Fig. 14.2 Left panel. Embryological origins of the thyroid and parathyroid glands. Right panel. Illustration of possible orthotopic and ectopic locations of the parathyroid glands (blue and brown ovals) and thyroglossal duct cysts

cells and parafollicular cells. The follicles are highly vascularised spherical structures that are filled with viscous colloids, composed primarily of thyroglobulin, and are surrounded by a layer of follicular cells. Follicular cells and follicles are involved in the synthesis of the thyroid hormones triiodothyronine (T3) and thyroxine (T4). Parafollicular cells (also known as C cells) reside between the follicles, originate from the neural crest and are responsible for the secretion of calcitonin, a hormone involved in calcium regulation.

14.1.2 Thyroid Hormone Synthesis

Iodine is an essential component of thyroid hormones; T3 and T4 contain three and four atoms of iodine, respectively. Iodine is present in various forms in food, including inorganic salts (iodides and iodates), inorganic diatomic iodine and organic iodine [7]. Approximately 90% of ingested iodine is absorbed within an hour. Iodine-rich food includes vegetables, sea food, beans, dairy products and kelp. The daily dietary requirement of iodine is 150 μg, which increases to 200 μg during pregnancy and lactation. Iodine is added to table salt, making iodine deficiency virtually non-existent in developed countries. Nonetheless, iodine deficiency remains endemic in many regions of the world, leading to impaired thyroid hormone synthesis, hypothyroidism and the development of goitre [8, 9].

The synthesis of thyroid hormones follows well-defined steps (Fig. 14.3). Iodide (I^-), circulating in the bloodstream, is transported into the follicular cells by the sodium-iodide symporter (NIS), in conjunction with two sodium ions, which drives the gradient. Concentrations of iodide in the follicular cells are up to 50 times higher than in the plasma, a phenomenon classically known as iodide trapping. Other ion substrates of the NIS, of significance to nuclear medicine, include pertechnetate (TcO_4^-), perrhenate (ReO_4^-) and perchlorate (ClO_3^-) [10–12].

The protein thyroglobulin, synthesised in the rough endoplasmic reticulum within the cells, is released into the colloid, while iodide passively diffuses from the base of the follicular cell to the apex and is then transported into the colloid by pendrin, an anion exchange protein. Once in the colloid, inorganic iodide is oxidised to iodine (I_2), which in turn is organified on tyrosine residues within the thyroglobulin molecules, to create mono-iodo-tyrosine (MIT) and di-iodo-tyrosine (DIT). Subsequently, two DIT molecules can couple to form tetraiodothyronine (thyroxine or T4), while one MIT can couple with a single molecule of DIT to form triiodothyronine (T3).

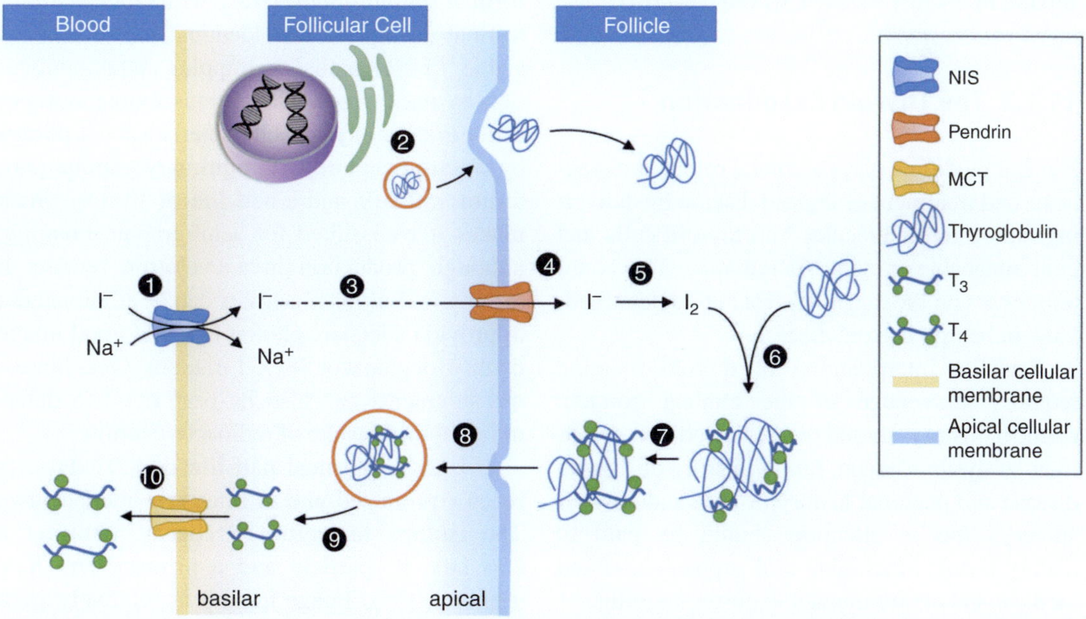

Fig. 14.3 Schematic representation of thyroid hormone production, including (1) iodide trapping (NIS), (2) thyroglobulin production, (3) passive diffusion of iodine through the follicular cell, (4) iodide transport into the follicle (pendrin), (5) oxidation, (6) organification, (7) coupling, (8) endocytosis, (9) proteolysis and (10) hormone release (MCT). Note that the basilar aspect of the follicular cell abuts the blood vessels, while the apical aspect borders the follicle and colloid matrix. *NIS* sodium iodide symporter, *MCT* monocarboxylate transporters

Following the production of thyroid hormone within the colloid, thyroglobulin is stored until needed, whereupon it is endocytosed from the colloid into the follicular cells. The endosome then fuses with a lysosome, leading to proteolysis and the release of T3, T4, MIT and DIT. MIT and DIT are rapidly deiodinated to yield tyrosine and free iodine, while T3 and T4 are released into the bloodstream at the base of the follicular cell via the monocarboxylate transporters (MCT).

Thyroid hormones circulate within the bloodstream primarily bound to circulating proteins, including thyroxine-binding globulin (70%), transthyretin (15%), albumin (10%) and lipoproteins. The unbound 'free' thyroid hormones are the metabolically active moieties. Serum concentrations of T4 are greater than those of T3, while T3 is the more metabolically active form of thyroid hormone. The thyroid secretes 15–20 times more T4 than T3, and the half-life of T4 is longer. Roughly 85% of T3 comes from peripheral conversion of T4 by iodothyronine deiodinases [13]. TSH stimulates all steps of production of thyroid hormones with the exception of peripheral conversion of T4 to T3 ([14, 15]; van der [16]).

14.1.3 The Thyroid Examination

Nuclear medicine plays a crucial role in the diagnosis and treatment of thyroid disease by delivering radioactive molecules into thyroid cells that emit imageable or cytotoxic radiation. This chapter focuses on the diagnostic role of nuclear medicine in benign thyroid disease.

Accurate interpretation of thyroid imaging requires knowledge of the clinical context. Clinical history should be reviewed for symptoms of dysthyroidism, family history of thyroid disease and personal history of neck radiation or surgery. Special attention should be paid to dietary history (including oral supplements) and medical and environmental exposure to iodine.

A focused physical examination is an important component of nuclear medicine evaluation to assess thyroid size, symmetry, nodules and tenderness, which will complement the findings on thyroid imaging [17]. Variable techniques can be employed to examine the thyroid gland; a common method is to stand behind the patient, using the tips of the second and third fingers of both hands for palpation. The thyroid is appreciated in the midline, just inferior to the larynx. Patients may be given a sip of water to swallow, which will cause the thyroid to move and facilitate examination. Any evidence of thyroid surgery or neck dissection, such as scars, should be noted, along with physical signs of hyperthyroidism, such as tachycardia, tremor, exophthalmos and hyperhidrosis. Basic biochemical thyroid indices, including the measurement of serum TSH and free serum T3 and T4, should be reviewed in all patients prior to imaging [18]. Chart review, history taking, physical examination and laboratory results are then combined with the scintigraphic findings and thyroid iodine uptake values to form an accurate comprehensive diagnosis.

14.1.3.1 Radiopharmaceuticals

Several radionuclides have been used in the imaging and therapy of the thyroid (Table 14.1). Iodine isotopes are administered orally in the form of sodium-iodide (NaI), with rapid gastrointestinal absorption and identical metabolism as stable ^{127}I-NaI, including trapping and organification by the thyroid. The various iodine isotopes differ in their physical characteristics. ^{123}I decays by electron capture with a primary gamma photon of 159 keV and a half-life of 13.2 h, which makes it well suited for scintigraphic imaging, although production in a cyclotron renders it expensive. Sufficient activity can be administered to provide adequate photon flux and good image quality for planar or SPECT imaging. Quantitative measurements can also be performed to determine thyroid uptake of radioactive iodine.

^{131}I has a physical half-life of 8.02 days, is reactor produced and is relatively inexpensive. The isotope undergoes β^- decay, emitting a 606 keV β^- particle and a primary 364 keV γ-photon [19]. Image quality is relatively poor due to the high energy of its γ-photon, which is subject to considerable septal penetration. As a general rule, only small amounts of ^{131}I activity (on the kBq or μCi scale) are administered, to minimise radiation exposure to thyroid and non-

Table 14.1 Properties of different isotopes used in thyroid imaging

Isotope	Half-life	Production	Decay	γ Energy, keV	Radiopharmaceutical	Application
^{123}I	13.2 h	Cyclotron	EC	159	NaI	Thyroid scintigraphy RAIU
^{124}I	4.2 days	Cyclotron	β+	511	NaI	PET thyroid imaging
^{125}I	59.4 days	Reactor	EC	<35	NaI	Biological assays Brachytherapy
^{131}I	8.02 days	Reactor	β-	364	NaI	RAIU Therapy
^{99m}Tc	6.02 h	Generator	IT	140	TcO_4^-	Thyroid scintigraphy
^{18}F	110 min	Cyclotron	β+	511	Fluorodeoxyglucose	PET oncologic imaging

EC electron capture, *IT* isomeric transition, *RAIU* radioactive iodide uptake

thyroid tissues. Today, this is typically done in order to perform 24-h radioactive iodine uptake (RAIU) measurements following thyroid scintigraphy with pertechnetate. In the therapy realm, ^{131}I-NaI is widely employed to treat benign and malignant conditions of the thyroid where the β^- emission is considered a desirable feature. Imaging is frequently performed following ^{131}I-NaI therapy for malignancy, as a means of verifying uptake, identifying metastases and allowing prognostication.

I-124, a positron-emitting isotope of iodine, has a half-life of 4.2 days and is imaged with a PET camera, which allows accurate quantification. This radionuclide still has only limited applicability in routine clinical settings [20], although it has potential to provide accurate dosimetry.

While not an isotope of iodine, ^{99m}Tc pertechnetate ($^{99m}TcO_4^-$) behaves in a physiologically similar manner to iodide and is therefore commonly used to image the thyroid gland. After intravenous injection, pertechnetate rapidly concentrates in the salivary glands, stomach and thyroid gland. It is trapped by the thyroid via the NIS symporter but does not undergo organification. Peak uptake within the thyroid is observed at 20–30 min post-injection [21]. ^{99m}Tc has a half-life of 6.02 h and emits a photon of 140 keV, with no particle emissions. It is readily available and inexpensive as it is directly eluted from a Mo-99/Tc-99m generator. As mentioned above, thyroid uptake can be achieved by administering a small amount of ^{131}I-NaI following the pertechnetate images.

Table 14.2 Indications for thyroid imaging in nuclear medicine. Adapted from [24]

Indications for thyroid imaging in nuclear medicine
Evaluation of the size and location of thyroid tissue
Evaluation of hyperthyroidism
Evaluation of suspected focal or diffuse thyroid disease
Evaluation of clinical laboratory tests suggestive of abnormal thyroid function
Evaluation of patients at risk of thyroid neoplasm
Assessment of the function of thyroid nodules identified on clinical examination or ultrasound or by other diagnostic imaging
Evaluation of congenital thyroid abnormalities

^{18}F-Fluorodeoxyglucose (FDG) is another positron-emitting radiopharmaceutical that is frequently used to image malignancies, such as lung cancer, colon cancer, and lymphoma. Not infrequently, a thyroid nodule can be incidentally seen to concentrate FDG in the course of oncologic imaging. Focal uptake implies a 25–50% risk of malignancy [22]; absence of uptake does not exclude malignancy [23].

14.1.3.2 Thyroid Scintigraphy

Scintigraphic imaging of the thyroid serves many purposes, generally related to the localisation and characterisation of thyroid tissues (Table 14.2) [25]. Thyroid scintigraphy is most commonly performed using iodine ^{123}I-NaI or $^{99m}TcO_4^-$ (pertechnetate). $^{99m}TcO_4^-$ is affordable, is readily available, and delivers a high photon flux at lower radiation exposure to the patient. Iodine isotopes have the added value of undergoing organification, which is not the case for pertechnetate. The use of ^{131}I-NaI is not recommended for routine thyroid scintigraphy due to its higher radiation exposure (6.6 mSv/MBq) when compared to ^{123}I-NaI (0.075 mSv/MBq) or pertechnetate (0.013 mSv/MBq). Thyroxine and iodine supplements should be discontinued 4–6 weeks, triiodothyronine 2 weeks and anti-thyroid medications 1 week prior to examination. Prior to thyroid scintigraphy, patients are fasted for 2 h [26]. Thyroid scintigraphy is performed 3–24 h following oral administration of 7–15 MBq ^{123}I-NaI or 5–30 min following intravenous injection of 75–370 MBq of $^{99m}TcO_4^-$. With either of these radiopharmaceuticals, pinhole or parallel-hole low-energy high-resolution (LEHR) collimators may be used, although a parallel-hole medium-energy general-purpose (MEGP) collimator has been recommended over LEHR when imaging ^{123}I-NaI to reduce septal penetration [27, 28]. Standard anterior and oblique views are obtained for 100,000–250,000 counts [17]. Additional images, such as lateral views, SPECT or SPECT-CT, may be indicated where anatomic variation is present, which requires more comprehensive elucidation.

Whole-body imaging with ^{123}I-NaI or ^{131}I-NaI may be performed in the staging and workup of thyroid cancer. This topic will be covered elsewhere in this volume.

14.1.3.3 Radioactive Iodine Uptake

Frequently, thyroid scintigraphy is combined with a radioactive iodine uptake (RAIU) measurement. RAIU represents the percentage of the total administered iodine that has been trapped and organified and is retained within the thyroid gland at the time of measurement, typically at 24 h. RAIU can be used to differentiate various etiologies of thyrotoxicosis and to estimate the optimal ^{131}I-NaI activity required for radioiodine therapy. Pertechnetate distribution and uptake can only be used as an approximate surrogate of radioiodine uptake [29].

RAIU measurement is most commonly performed using a γ-scintillation probe, though the γ-camera can be used for this purpose as well [30]. The typical γ-probe consists of a single small NaI-crystal detector coupled to a photomultiplier tube, collimated by a single-bore cylindrical collimator with an aperture of few centimetres in diameter. A linear ruler may be integrated in the device to standardise the distance from the neck to the probe detector surface. Accurate RAIU assessment requires measurement of the iodine capsule within an anthropomorphic neck phantom prior to administration, corrected for ambient room background. Approximately 24 h after administration of the iodine, the patient returns for counting of the neck and thigh, the latter used for in vivo neck background estimation. The percentage of radioiodine uptake can then be calculated using the following formula:

$$\mathrm{RAIU}(\%) = \frac{24\,\mathrm{h\ Neck\ CPM} - 24\,\mathrm{h\ Thigh\ CPM}}{\mathrm{Phantom\ CPM} - \mathrm{Background\ CPM}} \times 100 \times \mathrm{Decay\ Corrrection\ Factor}$$

The decay correction factor accounts for the degree of physical decay of the radionuclide occurring between measurement of the activity in the neck phantom and the patient measurements, which occur approximately 24 h thereafter. RAIU is a repeatable measurement with minimal detectable change of approximately 3% [31]. Current guidelines report normal 24-h RAIU as between 10% and 35% [32], though individual values vary depending on diet and medications, measurement techniques, among other factors. Population means have been noted to vary based on regional trends in diet [33]. Excess iodine intake from food, dietary supplements, iodine-containing drugs (such as amiodarone) and iodinated contrast competes with radioactive iodine and also down-regulates uptake, which can lead to the transient lowering of RAIU. A sudden excess of iodine intake, as seen in patients receiving intravenous iodinated contrast, causes a transient decrease in thyroid hormone production and release, a phenomenon called the Wolff-Chaikoff effect resulting in reduced RAIU values [34]. Conditions associated with abnormal RAIU are presented in Table 14.3.

Table 14.3 Conditions associated with abnormal RAIU

Increased RAIU
Graves' disease
Multinodular goitre
Autonomous toxic nodule
Type I amiodarone-induced thyrotoxicosis
Hydatidiform mole, choriocarcinoma, trophoblastic tumors
Hashitoxicosis
Decreased RAIU
Subacute thyroiditis
Thyrotoxicosis facticia
Jod-Basedow
Wolff-Chaikoff
Type II amiodarone-induced thyrotoxicosis
Struma ovarii

14.1.4 Normal Thyroid Scintigraphy

On scintigraphy, the left and right thyroid lobes appear relatively similar in size and are homogeneous in appearance, without areas of focal increased or decreased counts (Fig. 14.1). A pyramidal lobe may be present. The gland normally lies anterior to the trachea and in the midline of the neck. Anatomical variations may exist and should not be confused with thyroid nodules in the absence of palpable findings or correlative abnormalities on ultrasound.

14.1.5 Abnormal Thyroid

14.1.5.1 Congenital Abnormalities and Hypothyroidism

Congenital thyroid abnormalities include diseases associated with impaired or absent thyroid hormone production and anatomical variants. Anatomical variants occur during embryological development and range from subtle thyroid lobe asymmetry to complete agenesis of the gland. Abnormal thyroid gland migration during embryological development leads to ectopic thyroid tissue, which can present as cysts and be found anywhere from the foramen cecum at the base of the tongue to the anterior mediastinum, specifically along the course of the thyroglossal duct (Fig. 14.2) [35]. Ectopic thyroid tissue may coexist with an orthotopic thyroid gland or may comprise the entire inventory of functioning thyroid tissues. This is of relevance if surgical extirpation of the ectopic tissue is contemplated.

Absence or impairement of thyroid hormone production causes hypothyroidism, which is defined as the inability of the thyroid gland to produce sufficient thyroid hormones to meet the demands of normal bodily functions. The diagnostic role of nuclear medicine in hypothyroidism is primarily in the neonatal period. Untreated congenital hypothyroidism is one of the major causes of mental retardation (cretinism). Because physical signs may be subtle, this disease can go untreated for a prolonged period of time, leading to irreversible neurologic damage. The first systematic neonatal screening for congenital hypothyroidism began in 1973 in Quebec, Canada [36, 37]; currently, most developed countries perform newborn screening of TSH and/or T4 levels on a blood spot, leading to prompt investigation and treatment to prevent the dramatic consequences of this disease [38]. Congenital hypothyroidism can be caused by athyreosis, dyshormonogenesis or circulating maternal TSH receptor antibodies. Thyroid scintigraphy can differentiate these etiologies of congenital hypothyroidism, thereby providing useful information for counselling, genetic testing and prognosis. On thyroid scintigraphy, athyreosis and circulating maternal TSH receptor antibodies will manifest as absence of normal thyroid tissue, while dyshormonogenesis will present as a goitre that appears normal in position (Fig. 14.4) [39]. Thyroid ectopia is often associated with congenital hypothyroidism, presumably due to insufficient tissue to support the required hormone production.

14.1.5.2 Hyperthyroidism

Hyperthyroidism is defined by the presence of excessive amounts of thyroid hormone that can present with various signs and symptoms, including heat intolerance, tachycardia, irritability, paresis, diarrhea and insomnia. Its prevalence is estimated at 2.2% [40]. Hyperthyroidism is rarely central in origin, caused by TSH-secreting pituitary tumors or the pituitary resistance to thyroid hormone (PRTH) syndrome. More frequently, hyperthyroidism is associated with appropriately suppressed TSH, as seen in Graves' disease

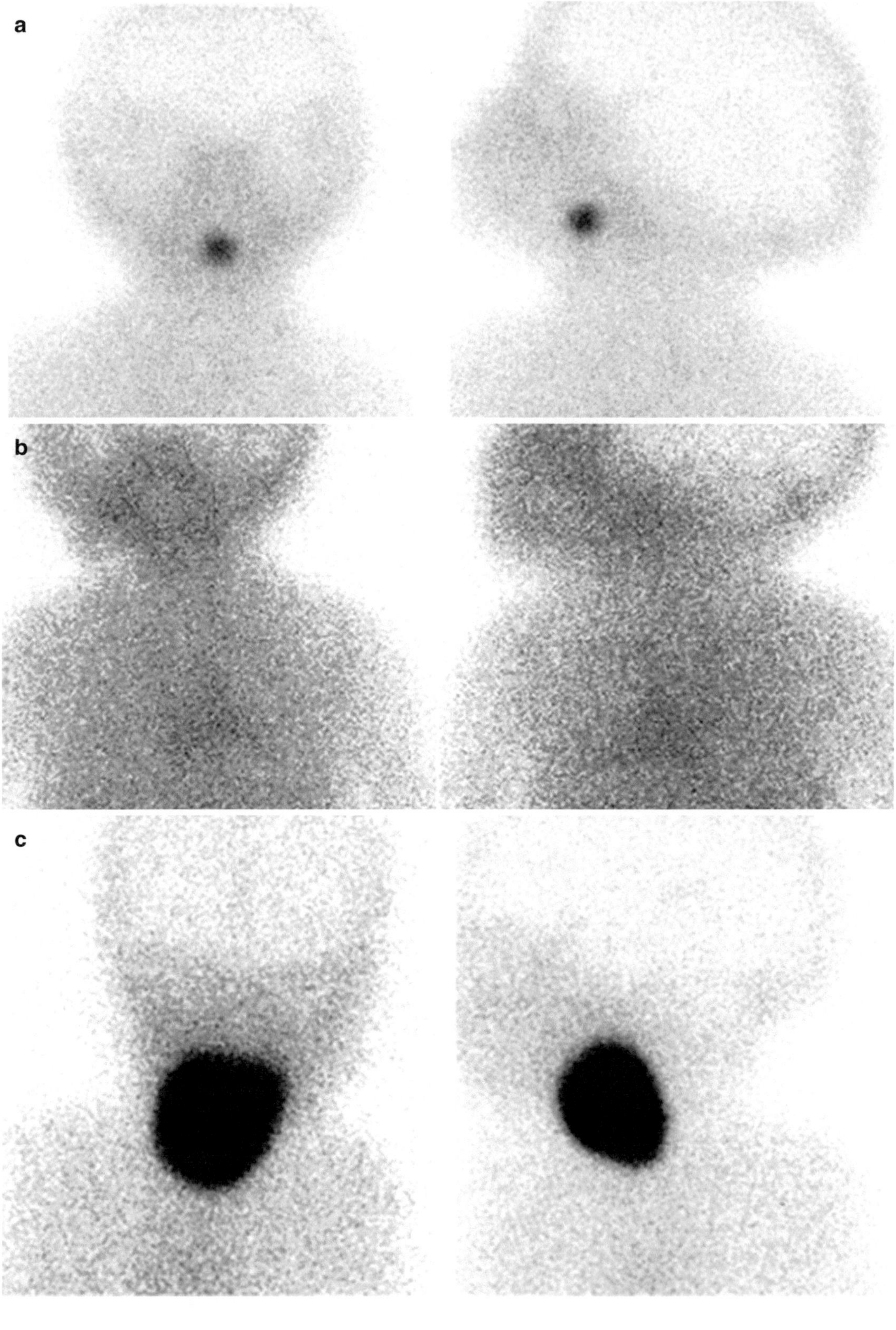
a
b
c

(GD), autonomous nodules and thyroiditis. Excessive iodine intake may lead to an increased production of thyroid hormones when the Wolff-Chaikoff mechanism fails, leading to the Jod-Basedow phenomenon [41, 42].

Graves' Disease

GD is the most frequent cause of hyperthyroidism, accounting for more than half of all cases, and is especially frequent in young women. This autoimmune disease is caused by TSH receptor antibodies stimulating the production of thyroid hormones and is characterised by very low or undetectable TSH and high levels of T4 and/or T3 blood levels. Clinically, GD can manifest with various signs and symptoms of hyperthyroidism, as well as some more specific findings, including thyromegaly, exophthalmos, lid lag and dry eyes. On scintigraphic imaging, the thyroid will demonstrate homogenous and increased uptake, with an associated increased 24-h RAIU (Figs. 14.5 and 14.6). There is an increased frequency of pyramidal lobe visualisation. In long-standing or recurrent GD, the thyroid can appear heterogeneous, mimicking a multinodular goitre (MNG) [43]. Not infrequently, a cold nodule can also be identified on thyroid scintigraphy in the context of GD, representing an appropriately hypofunctioning TSH-dependant thyroid nodule, which is referred to as Marine-Lenhart syndrome [44]. GD can be treated with anti-thyroid medications such as propylthiouracil (PTU) and methimazole (MMI), ^{131}I-NaI radioiodine ablation therapy or, less frequently, surgery [45]. Beta-blockers have a role in controlling adrenergic-mediated symptoms alone.

Thyroid Nodules

Thyroid nodules are very common, and most nodules are neither toxic nor malignant. More than 50% of patients without prior suspicion of harbouring thyroid nodules were found at autopsy to have at least one nodule [46]. Thyroid ultrasound (US), with or without fine needle aspiration (FNA), is usually the first imaging modality for the evaluation of suspected thyroid nodules [47]. The American Thyroid Association (ATA) guidelines recommend assessing nodules by FNA if they exceed 1.0 cm. Once a thyroid nodule is suspected, serum TSH should be measured. Nodules associated with normal or high TSH levels bear an increased risk of malignancy, and ultrasound remains the modality of choice for initial evaluation in these cases. A low TSH value is best evaluated with thyroid scintigraphy to assess the functional status of the nodule [47]. Thyrotoxicosis can result from autonomous thyroid tissue producing thyroid hormone despite reduced or suppressed TSH levels. Toxic nodules represent the second most frequent cause of hyperthyroidism, which is due to either solitary adenoma (historically known as Plummers disease) or multiple nodules (referred to as toxic multinodular goitre or MNG). The prevalence of toxic nodules increases with age, and females are more frequently affected. On scintigraphy, a single thyroid adenoma will present as a 'hot' nodule with relatively suppressed uptake in the remainder of the gland, while MNG will have a heterogeneous appearance, with several areas of focally increased uptake (Figs. 14.5 and 14.6). In both cases, RAIU can be inappropriately normal or mildly increased. The treatment of solitary adenoma and MNG includes radioiodine ablation therapy and surgery. The risk of malignancy associated with a solitary 'hot' nodule is less than 1%, compared with 15–20% for a non-functioning (cold) nodule or for a dominant (atypically prominent) non-functioning nodule in patients with

Fig. 14.4 Thyroid scintigraphy performed following intravenous administration of $^{99m}TcO_4^-$ in three babies presenting with congenital hypothyroidism. The first child (**a**) demonstrates a solitary focus of uptake along the posterior aspect of the oral cavity, compatible with ectopic thyroid tissue at the base of the tongue (foramen cecum). In the second child (**b**), there is complete absence of uptake in the head and neck region, compatible with thyroid agenesis or circulating maternal antibodies. Complete agenesis was confirmed by subsequent investigations. In the third child (**c**), a focus of intense uptake projects over the thyroid bed, compatible with dyshormonogenesis (Courtesy of Dr. Sophie Turpin, Centre Hospitalier Universitaire Sainte-Justine, Canada)

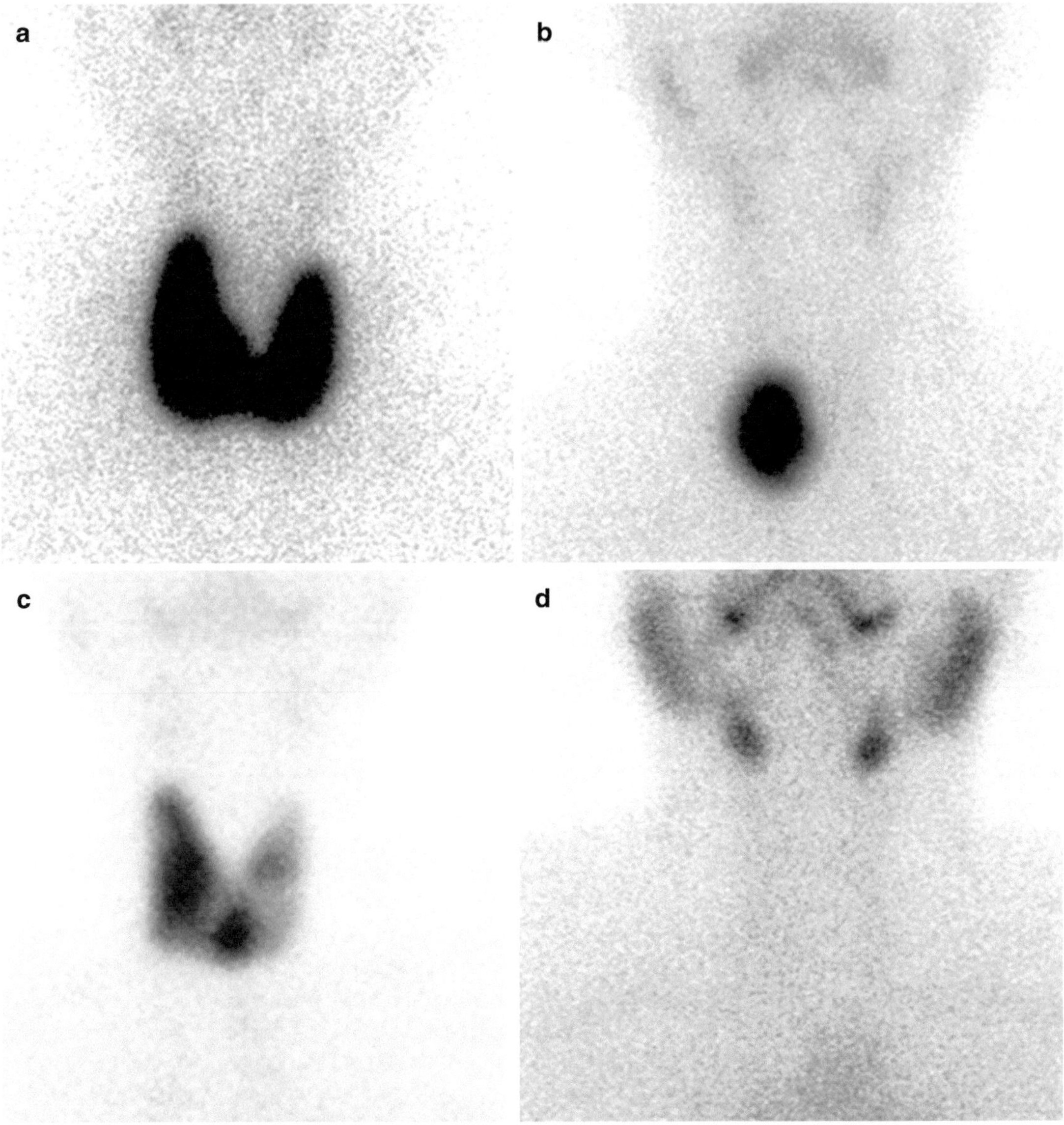

Fig. 14.5 Thyroid scintigraphy performed following intravenous administration of $^{99m}TcO_4^-$ in four adult patients with hyperthyroidism. (**a**) Homogeneous intense uptake in the thyroid compatible with Graves' disease. Non-visualisation of the salivary glands suggests that the thyroid uptake is increased. The 24-h RAIU in this patient was greater than 90%. (**b**) Intense uptake is noted in the right aspect of the thyroid, corresponding to a nodule on physical examination; uptake in the remainder of the thyroid gland is suppressed. These findings are compatible with a solitary toxic nodule. (**c**) Heterogeneous uptake in the thyroid gland, with several foci of increased uptake, compatible with a toxic multinodular goitre in the clinical context of suppressed TSH. (**d**) Absence of thyroid uptake in a patient with hyperthyroidism, compatible with thyroiditis. Note the relatively prominent appearance of the salivary glands

MNG [48, 49] (Fig. 14.6c). There is a rare occurrence where a thyroid nodule has the capacity to trap but not organify iodine, thereby appearing isointense on a pertechnetate image but 'cold' on the 24-h iodide scan. Because this feature would not be apparent on pertechnetate imaging, which relies on trapping alone, some favour imaging with sodium iodide to detect these 'discordant'

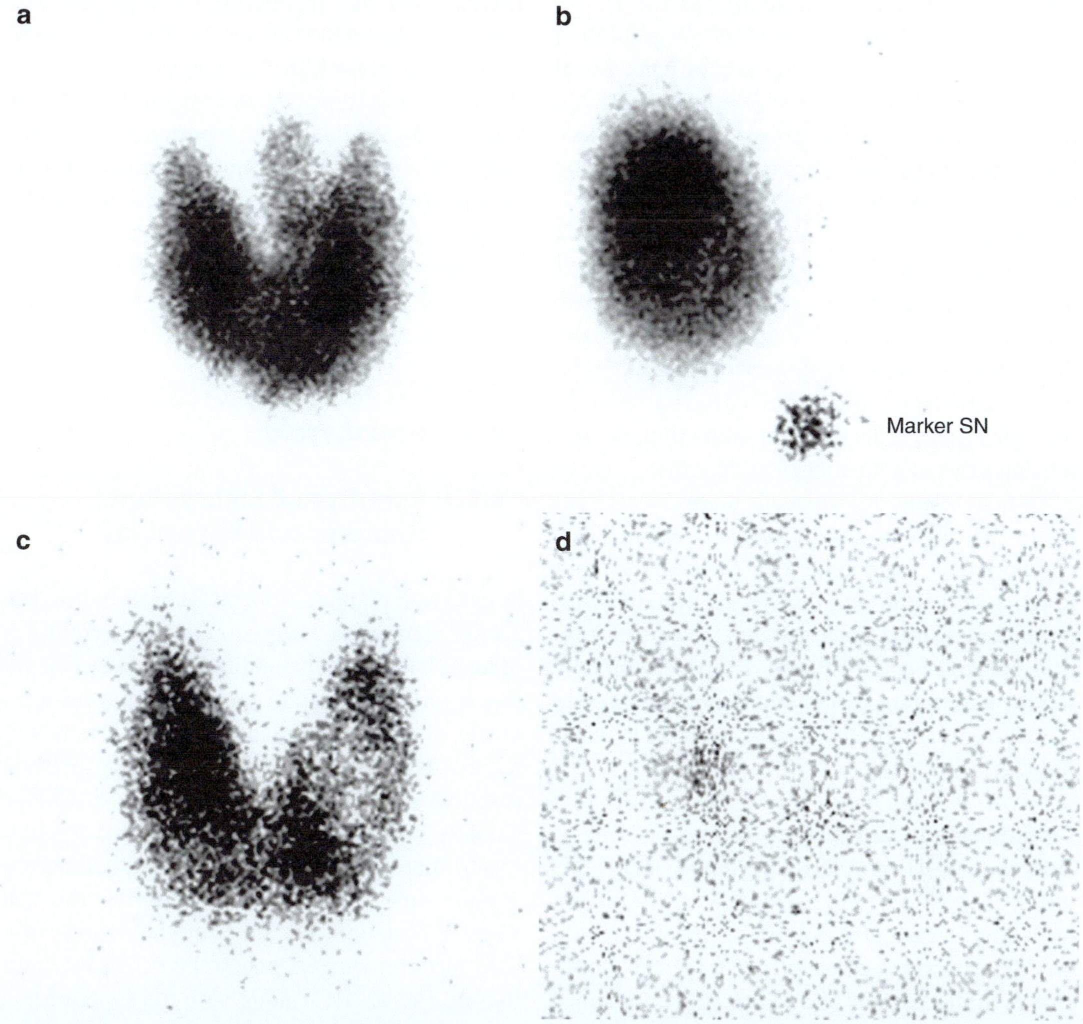

Fig. 14.6 Thyroid scintigraphy performed following oral administration of ^{123}I-NaI in four adult patients. (**a**) A 49-year-old female with Graves' disease. RAIU was 92%. Note the presence of a pyramidal lobe. (**b**) A 52-year-old female with palpable right-sided nodule and a diagnosis of hyperfunctioning nodule (Plummers disease). Twenty-four-hour RAIU is 45%. In this image, a hot marker has been placed over the sternal notch to provide anatomic reference. (**c**) A 66 year-old euthryoid woman with palpable left-sided thyroid nodule. RAIU was 23%. A large dominant cold nodule is noted in the mid-portion of the left lobe of the thyroid. Malignancy should be excluded by subsequent evaluations. (**d**) A 36-year-old male with fever, thyroid tenderness and suppressed TSH. RAIU is less than 1%. On physical examination, the pulse was 112 per minute and the thyroid was moderately enlarged and tender to palpation. Findings indicate subacute thyroiditis

nodules; however, this concern has been regarded as questionable [50].

Thyroiditis

Thyroiditis refers to inflammation of the thyroid gland, which can lead to thyrotoxicosis when cellular destruction causes leakage of thyroid hormone into the systemic circulation. As with GD and toxic nodules, women are more frequently affected than men and the patients are typically younger, between 20 and 50 years of age. Thyroiditis can be subcategorised according to the underlying causes. Silent thyroiditis, also called sporadic or painless thyroiditis, is characterised by an episode of thyrotoxicosis, followed by gradual improvement and a hypothyroid phase, without thyroid tenderness or pain. Silent thyroiditis is often seen post-partum and usually resolves on its own. Treatment consists of supportive care to prevent and treat symptoms related to thyrotoxicosis and to prevent complications.

Subacute thyroiditis, or de Quervain thyroiditis, is characterised by a transient phase of thyrotoxicosis associated with a painful thyroid gland, often preceded by viral infection and/or fever. Treatment includes administering non-steroidal anti-inflammatory drugs (NSAID) and steroids, with the aim to reduce the inflammation, as well as supportive care to control symptoms.

In both silent and subacute thyroiditis, circulating thyroid hormone is elevated and TSH is appropriately suppressed. Twenty-four-hour RAIU will be low, and thyroid scintigraphy will often demonstrate homogeneously reduced thyroid uptake (Figs. 14.5 and 14.6). Erythrocyte sedimentation rate (ESR) and C-reactive protein (CRP) levels can be elevated in subacute thyroiditis [51].

Amiodarone Induced Thyrotoxicosis

Amiodarone is an anti-arrhythmic drug frequently used for the treatment of recurrent arrhythmia. Each 200 mg tablet contains 75 mg of iodine, of which a portion can reach the bloodstream in the form of free iodide. Because amiodarone is lipophilic, it accumulates in adipose tissue, muscles and thyroid with a slow elimination half-life of 50–100 days. The effect of amiodarone on the thyroid can be seen as early as a few weeks after initiating treatment and can persist for up to several years thereafter. Amiodarone-induced thyrotoxicosis develops in 2–22% of North American patients and occurs more frequently in iodine-depleted regions [52].

Two types of amiodarone-induced thyrotoxicosis have been described. Type I is caused by excessive iodine leading to increased synthesis and the release of thyroid hormone (Jod-Basedow phenomenon) and is most often associated with concomitant thyroid pathology such as Graves' disease, autonomous toxic nodule or multinodular goitre. Type II is caused by direct amiodarone toxicity and the destruction of follicular cells, leading to the release of stored T3 and T4, as seen in subacute thyroiditis. Distinguishing between thyrotoxicosis types is crucial since treatment differs [53]. RAIU is often reported as elevated in Type I thyrotoxicosis, although it can be normal or mildly reduced, while RAIU is suppressed in Type II. Additionally, Type I amiodarone thyrotoxicosis will demonstrate diffuse ^{99m}Tc-sestamibi uptake, while ^{99m}Tc-sestamibi uptake in Type II disease is negligible [54].

14.2 Parathyroid

14.2.1 Parathyroid Embryology, Anatomy and Physiology

Parathyroid glands are involved in the homeostasis of calcium via a secretion of parathyroid hormones (PTH). Most commonly, two superior and two inferior glands are present on the posterior aspect of the thyroid gland (Fig. 14.2). In actuality, the total number of glands can vary, between two and six [6, 55]; approximately, 5–15% of patients have more than four glands and 5% have fewer than four glands [56]. The parathyroid glands undergo differentiation during the fifth week of gestation. The superior glands arise from the fourth pharyngeal pouch (hence called 'parathyroid IV' or 'P4') along with the superior pole of the thyroid gland and descend from the base of the tongue to the posterior borders of the upper thyroid lobes. The inferior parathyroid glands arise from the third brachial pouch (and are therefore referred to as 'parathyroid III' or 'P3'), as does the thymus, and they co-migrate to a variable degree caudally. The inferior glands are typically located more anteriorly than the superior glands and are situated lateral and inferior to the lower poles of the thyroid (Fig. 14.2). Ectopic inferior glands can be found as high as the angle of the mandible and as low as the anterior mediastinum (Table 14.4) [6].

A normal parathyroid gland is oblong in shape, measuring roughly 3 by 6 mm in diameter and weighing approximately 30–40 mg. Each gland is composed of equal parts parenchyma

Table 14.4 Possible location of ectopic parathyroid glands. Adapted from [57]

Possible location of ectopic parathyroid glands
Submandibular
Carotid sheath
Intrathyroidal
Prepharyngeal
Tracheoesophageal groove
Retroesophageal
Paraesophageal
Posterosuperior mediastinal
Anterosuperior mediastinal
Pericardium

and stroma, the latter consisting of adipose tissue and blood vessels, which support the parenchymal cells. The parenchyma is composed mainly of chief cells (or principal cells), which are responsible for the secretion of parathyroid hormone (PTH), in addition to the mitochondria-rich oxyphil cells that do not possess significant secretory function. PTH plays a central role in calcium homeostasis by acting directly and indirectly on multiple targets in order to increase serum calcium concentration. In the renal tubules, PTH promotes calcium reabsorption and phosphate excretion. PTH also stimulates the production of calcitriol, the active metabolite of vitamin D by the proximal tubules. In turn, calcitriol increases blood calcium by promoting calcium absorption by the small bowel, tubular resorption of calcium in the kidney and the release of calcium from the bones by indirect activation of osteoclasts.

14.2.2 Hyperparathyroidism

14.2.2.1 Primary Hyperparathyroidism

Primary hyperparathyroidism is relatively common with an incidence of 175 per 100,000 person years in women and 80 per 100,000 person years in men and a prevalence of one to four per 1000 persons [58]. Women are at higher risk of developing the disease, and the incidence increases with age, peaking between 50 and 70 years. Primary hyperparathyroidism is caused by parathyroid adenoma (85%), hyperplasia (10–15%) or, less frequently, parathyroid carcinoma (1–4%) (Table 14.5). Hereditary disorders, which account for up to 10% of cases of primary hyperparathyroidism, often involve multiple-gland hyperplasia, while spontaneous parathyroid adenomas are usually solitary; in only 2–10% of cases are two parathyroid adenomas present [59]. When multiple adenomas are detected, the possibility of four-gland hyperplasia of varying degrees should be raised [59].

Table 14.5 Causes of primary hyperparathyroidism

Causes of primary hyperparathyroidism
Sporadic (90%)
Familial hyperparathyroidism
MEN type 1
MEN type 2A
Hyperparathyroidism-jaw tumor syndrome
Familial hypocalciuric hypercalcemia

The diagnosis of primary hyperparathyroidism is characterised by persistent increased total serum calcium concentration associated with inappropriately elevated or normal serum PTH levels (Table 14.6). The total serum calcium concentration needs to be adjusted for albumin level, the principal binding protein of calcium in the blood. Other etiologies of increased calcium associated with elevated PTH include lithium use, thiazide use, tertiary hyperparathyroidism and familial hypocalciuric hypercalcemia [60]. In contrast, hypercalcemia of malignancy, the second most common cause of hypercalcemia, presents with an appropriately low or suppressed PTH level. Since the incorporation of serum calcium levels in the standard chemistry blood screening, primary hyperparathyroidism has often been detected incidentally in asymptomatic patients [60]. Approximately 20–25% of patients will present with non-specific symptoms or complications related to the disease at presentation, most commonly nephrolithiasis and reduced bone mineral density. Other non-specific symptoms include weakness, mild depression, fatigue, cognitive impairment and anorexia. Approximately a third of patients may demonstrate a progression of symptoms over the course of 15 years [61].

Table 14.6 Biochemical markers in different forms of hyperparathyroidism

	Hyperparathyroidism			
	Primary	Secondary	Tertiary	Paraneoplastic
PTH	↑	↑	↑	↓
Ca^{++}	↑	↔	↑	↑
PO_4	↓	↑	↓	–

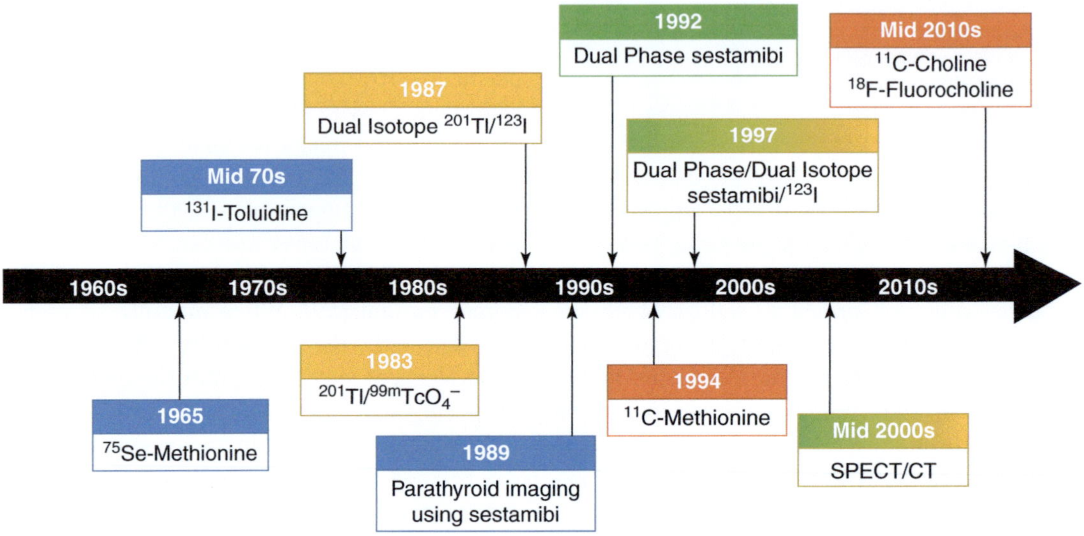

Fig. 14.7 Evolution of multiple scintigraphic imaging techniques used to localise abnormal parathyroid glands over the last five decades. Legend: blue banner—single time point, single-radiopharmaceutical method; yellow banner—'dual-isotope' single-photon method; green banner—'dual phase' method; orange banner—PET imaging method

The definitive treatment of primary hyperparathyroidism is surgery. Parathyroidectomy is recommended for all patients younger than 50 years old, as well as for symptomatic patients older than 50 years. For asymptomatic patients older than 50, parathyroidectomy is only recommended when serum calcium levels are elevated (>1.0 mg/dl or > 0.25 mmol/L above normal range), in the presence of osteoporosis, when glomerular filtration rate (GFR) is below 60 cc/min, or after the development of nephrolithiasis [62, 63]. For patients who do not undergo surgery, annual assessment of serum calcium level, GFR and bone mineral density (including the 1/3 distal radius) is therefore recommended. Minimally invasive parathyroidectomy is the surgical treatment of choice for patients without previous neck surgery or large thyroid goitre and is associated with shorter operative and recovery time, as well as lower complication rates, as compared with open surgery. For a successful minimally invasive surgery, preoperative localisation of parathyroid adenomas is necessary, thereby creating a niche for preoperative localisation.

14.2.2.2 Parathyroid Imaging

Historical Evolution

Parathyroid molecular imaging protocols have evolved over the past six decades (Fig. 14.7). Parathyroid imaging was first performed using ^{75}Se-methionine and ^{131}I-toluidine, but the technique was neither sensitive nor specific. In the 1980s, 'dual-isotope' methods were introduced using ^{201}Tl-thallous chloride in combination with $^{99m}TcO_4^-$ or $^{123}I^-$. The methods rely on the observation that the distribution of the two radiopharmaceuticals differs in the presence of parathyroid abnormalities. Pertechnetate and iodide are only taken up by functioning thyroid tissues, while thallous chloride is taken up by all cellular tissues, including the thyroid and parathyroid glands. A noticeable discrepancy will arise in the presence of prominent parathyroid tissues. After its introduction into cardiovascular nuclear medicine, ^{99m}Tc-sestamibi was then successfully substituted for thallous chloride in parathyroid imaging as well [64]. ^{99m}Tc-sestamibi is a lipophilic cation that diffuses across membranes and concentrates within the mitochondria due to their high membrane potential; accumulation in cells is proportional to the blood flow and mitochondrial density. Shortly after the introduction of ^{99m}Tc-sestamibi parathyroid imaging, 'dual-phase' imaging was described [65]. This method contrasts the early and delayed distribution of ^{99m}Tc-sestamibi relying on differences of washout between thyroid and parathyroid tissues. At present, ^{99m}Tc-sestamibi has largely replaced ^{201}Tl for parathyroid imaging due to its superior imaging quality, favourable dosimetry, improved accuracy and ability to be used with dual-phase imaging. Different radiopharmaceuticals, protocols, imaging methods and their interaction will be reviewed in more detail in the following sections.

Dual-Isotope Imaging

The method of dual-isotope, or dual-tracer, imaging relies on the principle that the distribution of a thyroid-specific and a cellularity-based radiopharmaceutical will differ in the presence of a significant non-thyroid tissue, such as a parathyroid adenoma. Dual-isotope imaging has been used with different combinations of isotopes and is currently performed with ^{99m}Tc-sestamibi and either ^{123}I-sodium iodide (^{123}I-NaI) or ^{99m}Tc-pertechnetate [24, 66].

Most parathyroid adenomas are enlarged and have increased oxyphil cell concentration and therefore have increased uptake and retention of ^{99m}Tc-sestamibi compared with normal glands. Abnormal parathyroid glands therefore demonstrate increased ^{99m}Tc-sestamibi uptake without corresponding uptake of ^{123}I-NaI or ^{99m}Tc-pertechnetate, while normal thyroid tissues and functioning thyroid adenomas demonstrate similar uptake with both radiopharmaceuticals (Fig. 14.8). Normal parathyroid glands are not visible on ^{99m}Tc-sestamibi imaging due to their small size. Malignant lesions such as thyroid carcinoma and lymph node metastases can mimic parathyroid lesions on dual-isotope imaging with increased ^{99m}Tc-sestamibi and absent ^{123}I-NaI/^{99m}Tc-pertechnetate uptake.

Parathyroid lesions are localised on dual-isotope imaging by performing visual comparison or digital subtraction of the paired images. When employing ^{123}I-NaI and ^{99m}Tc-sestamibi, simultaneous co-imaging of the two pharmaceuticals can be achieved based on the slightly different energy peaks of ^{123}I and ^{99m}Tc. Digital subtraction of the perfectly aligned images improves sensitivity while not affecting specificity compared with visual analysis alone [67]. If the images are acquired sequentially, caution should be exercised when applying digital subtraction as small misregistrations can lead to false positive findings.

Dual-Phase Imaging

Because ^{99m}Tc-sestamibi also accumulates in the normal thyroid glands, adenomas can be masked by physiological thyroid uptake. The method of dual-phase imaging was noted to circumvent this problem, making use of the observation that ^{99m}Tc-sestamibi washout from abnormal parathyroid tissues is slower than that of thyroid tissues [65]. Of note, ^{99m}Tc-tetrofosmin does not have the same washout properties as ^{99m}Tc-sestamibi, and therefore it should not be used for dual-phase imaging [68]. The dual-phase technique is simple and easy to perform and only requires a single injection of ^{99m}Tc-sestamibi, followed by imaging approximately 15 min and 90–150 min later. A persistent focus of activity on delayed images, relative to the thyroid gland activity, is indicative of a parathyroid lesion (Fig. 14.9). The technique is not specific, in that other non-thyroid abnormalities often also have relatively delayed washout characteristics.

If no clear-cut adenoma is apparent following the use of dual-phase imaging, pertechnetate or ^{123}I-NaI should be administered and a dual-isotope study performed, coupling the added thy-

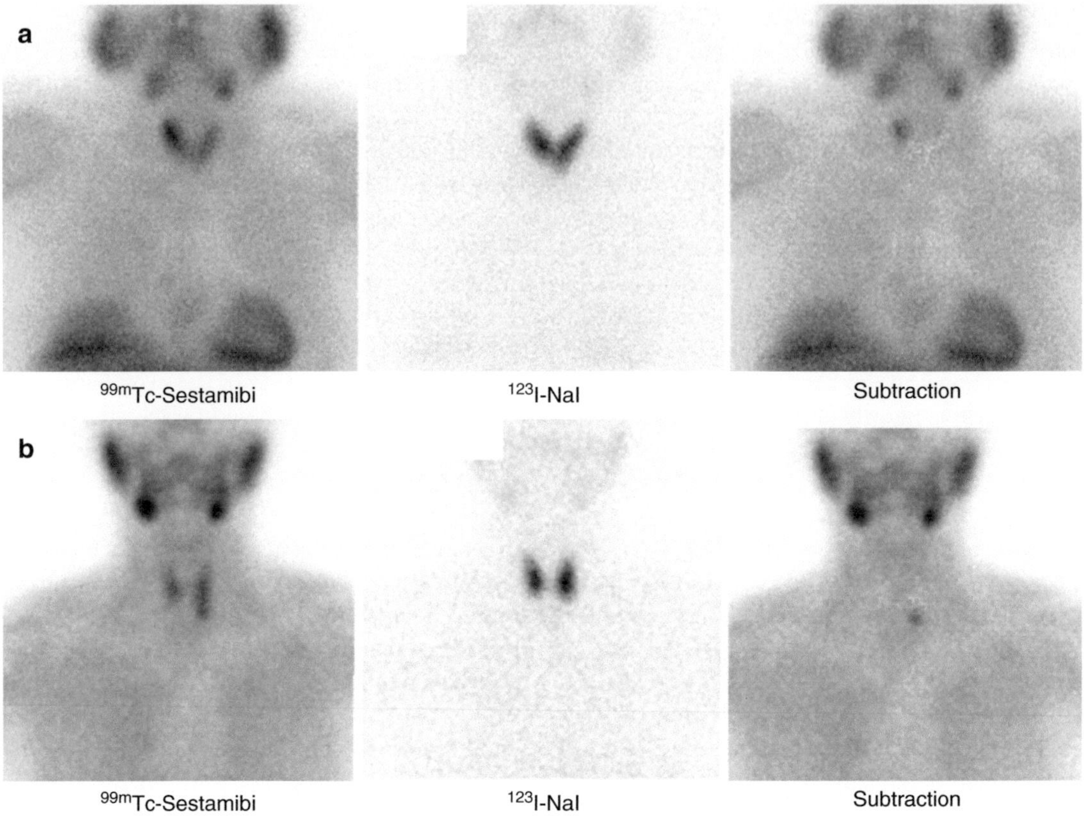

Fig. 14.8 Dual-isotope method. Two patients with primary hyperparathyroidism referred for parathyroid scintigraphy using a dual-isotope protocol. (**a**) ^{99m}Tc-sestamibi planar image demonstrates increased uptake in the right upper aspect of the thyroid, without concordant increased uptake on ^{123}I-NaI scintigraphy. Subtraction confirms the discrepancy. The patient was successfully treated with parathyroidectomy of the right upper parathyroid gland. (**b**) ^{99m}Tc-sestamibi, ^{123}I-NaI and subtraction images of a patient with primary hyperparathyroidism demonstrate a left lower parathyroid adenoma

roid image with the initial sestamibi image. The dual-isotope method has been shown to improve sensitivity as compared with dual-phase imaging alone, especially for hyperplastic glands [69, 70]. Furthermore, because many thyroid lesions concentrate both ^{99m}Tc-sestamibi and ^{123}I-NaI/^{99m}Tc-pertechnetate, no disparity of imaging will be present and the dual-isotope technique will improve the specificity of the test.

Pitfalls of Dual-Phase Imaging

Reported sensitivity of dual-phase imaging varies greatly, between 50% and 90% [65, 71–73]. This variability has been attributed to rapid ^{99m}Tc-sestamibi washout in a significant proportion of abnormal parathyroid glands, leading to no retention of activity on the delayed images [74]. Other causes of failure to locate parathyroid lesions are presented in Table 14.7. Because the diagnosis of hyperparathyroidism is established prior to imaging and imaging examinations are intended to *localize* the lesions, false positive results are seen when a study locates a lesion that is not involved in the autonomous secretion of PTH. Such ^{99m}Tc-sestamibi avid lesions include thyroid adenoma, thyroid carcinoma and, less frequently, malignant or benign lymphadenopathy [75] (Table 14.7). Evolution of imaging to include SPECT-CT has led to increased specificity of the technique.

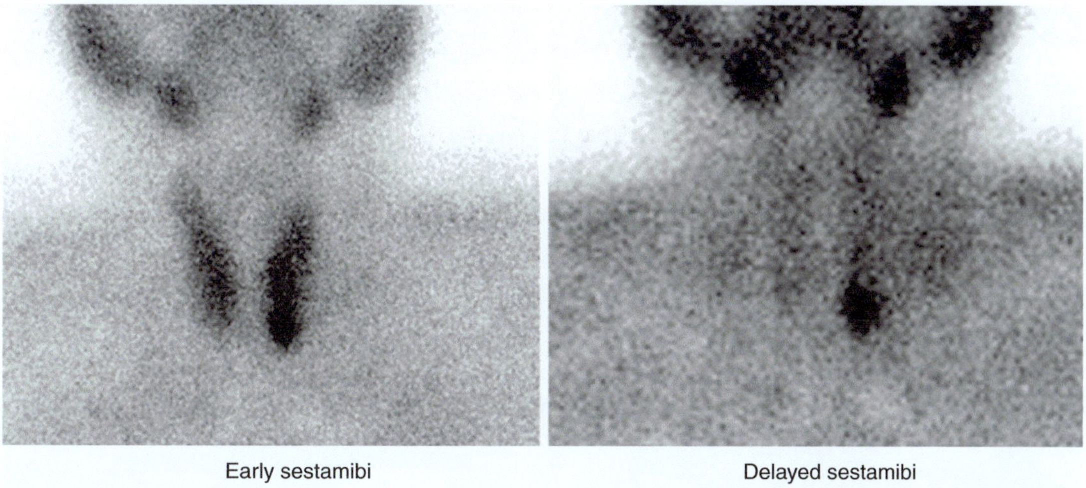

Fig. 14.9 Dual-phase method. Early ^{99m}Tc-sestamibi planar image obtained 15 min post injection of a patient with hyperparathyroidism demonstrates a focus of increased uptake projecting over the left lower thyroid pole. On delayed image obtained approximately 3 h post injection, the area of increased uptake shows a delayed washout compared with the rest of the gland, a suggestion of parathyroid adenoma (Courtesy of Dr. Raymonde Chartrand, Centre hospitalier universitaire de l'Université de Montréal, Canada)

Table 14.7 Causes of false positive and false negative dual-phase scan, adapted from [75]

False positive	False negative
Thyroid adenoma Thyroid carcinoma Lymphoma Lymphadenopathy Sarcoidosis	Small adenoma P-glycoprotein expression Multi-drug-resistance-related protein expression Hyperplasia Low oxyphil/mitochondrial concentration Multi-gland disease

SPECT/CT

SPECT/CT is useful in parathyroid scintigraphy as it provides precise information on localisation and is superior to SPECT or CT alone [76]. Given the small size of parathyroid lesions, near-simultaneous hybrid SPECT/CT imaging is preferred to avoid misregistration and to optimise imaging performance (Fig. 14.10). The CT component allows anatomic delineation of surrounding structures, which is especially useful for ectopic glands. SPECT/CT imaging with ^{99m}Tc-sestamibi has been shown to be superior to single- or dual-phase planar or SPECT [77–79]. The combination of early SPECT/CT images with any delayed imaging method (planar, SPECT or SPECT/CT) appears to be the most sensitive dual-phase protocol [72]. Early SPECT/CT is preferred over delayed SPECT/CT to improve the detection of lesions with rapid washout [24]. Therefore, when performing dual-phase imaging, early SPECT/CT should be acquired whenever possible.

Image Interpretation

The diagnosis of hyperparathyroidism is based on calcium and PTH plasma levels and not on imaging; the purpose of imaging is to localise the lesions and guide surgical approach rather than to establish the diagnosis. In that context, parathyroid scintigraphy should be interpreted with high sensitivity, and the report should include the size and location of abnormal parathyroid gland(s) (Figs. 14.8 and 14.9). Special care should be exercised to identify or explicitly exclude ectopic lesions and multiple-gland disease as these typically entail a different surgical approach and will not be identified at a standard surgical exploration. Furthermore, when available, detailed information regarding the location of the abnormal gland in relation to the surrounding structures, especially in the case of

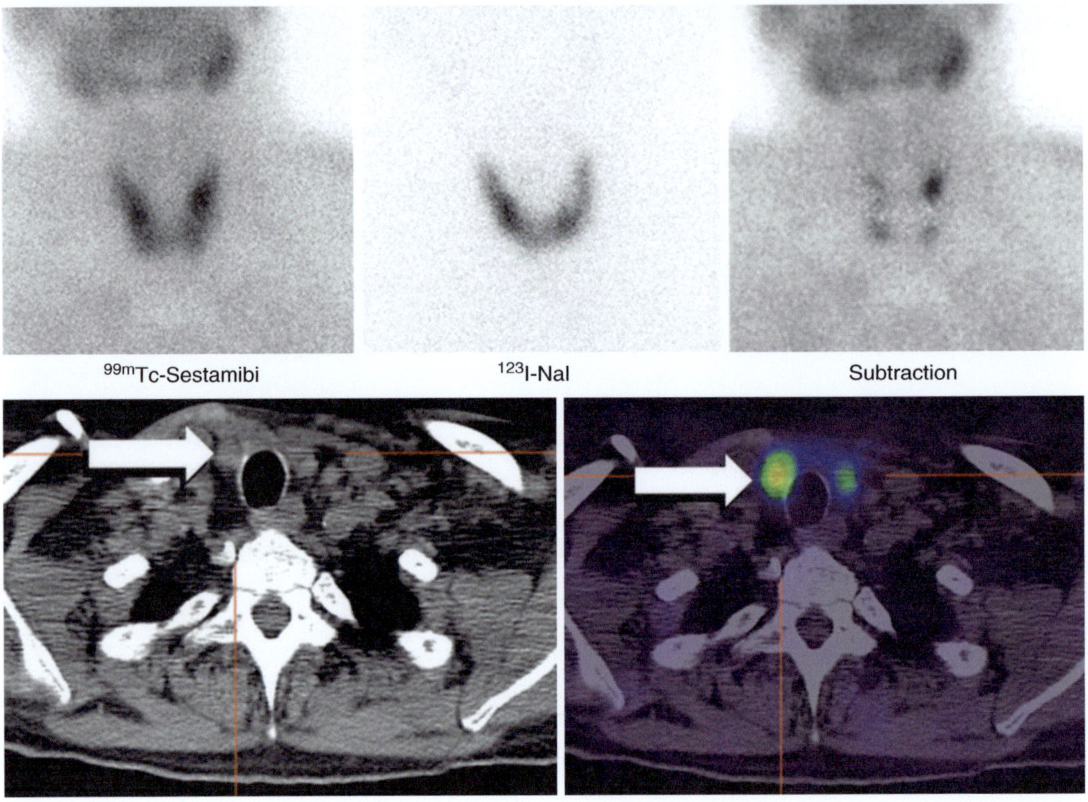

Fig. 14.10 ^{99m}Tc-sestamibi, ^{123}I-NaI and subtraction images of a patient with primary hyperparathyroidism demonstrate discordant uptake corresponding to all four parathyroid glands. SPECT-CT images localise the area of increased ^{99m}Tc-sestamibi uptake to enlarged parathyroid glands (example indicated by arrow). These findings suggest four-gland hyperplasia

ectopic glands, should be provided in the report, and SPECT/CT imaging is most helpful in this regard.

14.2.2.3 Secondary Hyperparathyroidism

In secondary hyperparathyroidism, there is physiological stimulation of the parathyroid glands to secrete PTH in order to maintain normal serum calcium. Multiple glands will be evident on imaging (Fig. 14.10). One of the most frequent causes of secondary hyperparathyroidism is chronic renal failure, which causes vitamin D deficiency, hyperphosphatemia and hypocalcemia. Secondary disease can also be associated with intestinal malabsorption. In chronic renal failure, vitamin D deficiency leads to impaired calcium homeostasis via a reduction of calcium absorption by the small bowel and impairment of the PTH effects on bone resorption. PTH secretion is then increased, leading to hyperplasia of all parathyroid glands and the normalisation of serum calcium [75, 80]. Parathyroid scintigraphy is indicated in cases of re-operation and can improve the success rate of parathyroidectomy in patients with secondary hyperparathyroidism by detecting ectopic or supernumerary glands. The parathyroid gland with the lowest ^{99m}Tc-sestamibi uptake is identified and can be autografted into the forearm or left in situ [81].

14.2.2.4 Tertiary Hyperparathyroidism

Tertiary hyperparathyroidism is caused by long-standing secondary hyperparathyroidism, which eventually leads to unregulated autonomous PTH secretion. Both tertiary hyperparathyroidism and secondary hyperparathyroidism are caused by prolonged increased PTH secretion. However, in tertiary disease, the unregulated secretion of PTH gives rise to hypercalcemia, while serum calcium is normal in secondary hyperparathyroidism. Because tertiary hyperparathyroidism is characterised by hyperplasia of all parathyroid glands, preoperative localisation is not routinely performed prior to initial neck exploration. However, in cases of persistent or recurrent hyperparathyroidism, imaging is recommended to locate a missed, supernumerary or ectopic parathyroid gland [82]. Because the prevalence of ectopic parathyroid glands is high in secondary/tertiary hyperparathyroidism, some authors argue that imaging should be performed routinely prior to surgical procedures [83].

14.2.3 PET/CT

Recently, attempts have been made to localise abnormal parathyroid glands using positron-emitting radiopharmaceuticals and PET/CT imaging. PET/CT presents the advantages of higher spatial resolution and shorter acquisition time and could potentially detect smaller lesions. Detection of parathyroid lesions has been attempted with several PET radiopharmaceuticals, including ^{18}F-FDG, ^{18}F-DOPA, ^{11}C-choline, ^{18}F-fluorocholine and ^{11}C-methionine. ^{18}F-FDG, which is by far the most widely available PET radiopharmaceutical, showed suboptimal results for the detection of parathyroid lesions [84]. ^{18}F-fluorocholine and ^{11}C-methionine have shown promising results, but only limited data are available [85]. Given the relatively low cost, widespread availability and high accuracy of MIBI SPECT/CT imaging, it remains the modality of choice to detect parathyroid lesions.

References

1. Chiamolera MI, Wondisford FE. Minireview: thyrotropin-releasing hormone and the thyroid hormone feedback mechanism. Endocrinology. 2009;150(3):1091–6. https://doi.org/10.1210/en.2008-1795.
2. Dietrich JW, Landgrafe G, Fotiadou EH. TSH and thyrotropic agonists: key actors in thyroid homeostasis. J Thyroid Res. 2012;2012:351864. https://doi.org/10.1155/2012/351864.
3. Ozgur Z, Celik S, Govsa F, Ozgur T. Anatomical and surgical aspects of the lobes of the thyroid glands. Eur Arch Otorhinolaryngol. 2011;268(9):1357–63. https://doi.org/10.1007/s00405-011-1502-5.
4. Pankow BG, Michalak J, McGee MK. Adult human thyroid weight. Health Phys. 1985;49(6):1097–103.
5. Braun EM, Windisch G, Wolf G, Hausleitner L, Anderhuber F. The pyramidal lobe: clinical anatomy and its importance in thyroid surgery. Surg Radiol Anat. 2007;29(1):21–7. https://doi.org/10.1007/s00276-006-0165-1.
6. Policeni BA, Smoker WR, Reede DL. Anatomy and embryology of the thyroid and parathyroid glands. Semin Ultrasound CT MR. 2012;33(2):104–14. https://doi.org/10.1053/j.sult.2011.12.005.
7. Rohner F, Zimmermann M, Jooste P, Pandav C, Caldwell K, Raghavan R, Raiten DJ. Biomarkers of nutrition for development—iodine review. J Nutr. 2014;144(8):1322S–42S. https://doi.org/10.3945/jn.113.181974.
8. Li JH, He ZH, Bansal V, Hennessey JV. Low iodine diet in differentiated thyroid cancer: a review. Clin Endocrinol. 2016;84(1):3–12. https://doi.org/10.1111/cen.12846.
9. Pretell, E. A., Pearce, E. N., Moreno, S. A., Dary, O., Kupka, R., Gizak, M., . . . Zimmermann, M. B. (2017). Elimination of iodine deficiency disorders from the Americas: a public health triumph. Lancet Diabetes Endocrinol, 5(6), 412–414. https://doi.org/10.1016/S2213-8587(17)30034-7.
10. Dohan O, Portulano C, Basquin C, Reyna-Neyra A, Amzel LM, Carrasco N. The Na+/I symporter (NIS) mediates electroneutral active transport of the environmental pollutant perchlorate. Proc Natl Acad Sci U S A. 2007;104(51):20250–5. https://doi.org/10.1073/pnas.0707207104.
11. Portulano C, Paroder-Belenitsky M, Carrasco N. The Na+/I-symporter (NIS): mechanism and medical impact. Endocr Rev. 2014;35(1):106–49. https://doi.org/10.1210/er.2012-1036.
12. Zuckier LS, Dohan O, Li Y, Chang CJ, Carrasco N, Dadachova E. Kinetics of perrhenate uptake and comparative biodistribution of perrhenate, pertechnetate, and iodide by NaI symporter-expressing tissues in vivo. J Nucl Med. 2004;45(3):500–7.
13. Pittman CS, Chambers JB Jr, Read VH. The extrathyroidal conversion rate of thyroxine to triiodothyronine in normal man. J Clin Invest. 1971;50(6):1187–96. https://doi.org/10.1172/JCI106596.
14. Maia AL, Kim BW, Huang SA, Harney JW, Larsen PR. Type 2 iodothyronine deiodinase is the major source of plasma T3 in euthyroid humans. J Clin Invest. 2005;115(9):2524–33. https://doi.org/10.1172/JCI25083.
15. Rousset B, Dupuy C, Miot F. Thyroid hormone synthesis and secretion. In: De Groot CG, Dungan

K, et al., editors. Endotext. South Dartmouth, MA: MDText.com, Inc; 2015.
16. van der Spek, A. H., Fliers, E., & Boelen, A. (2017). The classic pathways of thyroid hormone metabolism. Mol Cell Endocrinol 458 29. https://doi.org/10.1016/j.mce.2017.01.025
17. Balon, H. R., Silberstein, E. B., Meier, D. A., Charkes, D., Sarkar, S., Royal, H., & Donohoe, K. (2006). Society of nuclear medicine procedure guideline for thyroid scintigraphy, version 3.0. 2006. http://interactive.snm.org/index.cfm?PageID=772.
18. Parsa AA, Gharib H. History and examination for thyroid nodules. In: Gharib H, editor. Thyroid nodules. Contemporary endocrinology. Cham: Humana; 2018.
19. Mandel SJ, Shankar LK, Benard F, Yamamoto A, Alavi A. Superiority of iodine-123 compared with iodine-131 scanning for thyroid remnants in patients with differentiated thyroid cancer. Clin Nucl Med. 2001;26(1):6–9.
20. Pentlow, K. S., Graham, M. C., Lambrecht, R. M., Daghighian, F., Bacharach, S. L., Bendriem, B., . . . Larson, S. M. (1996). Quantitative imaging of iodine-124 with PET. J Nucl Med, 37(9), 1557–1562.
21. Meller J, Becker W. The continuing importance of thyroid scintigraphy in the era of high-resolution ultrasound. Eur J Nucl Med Mol Imaging. 2002;29(Suppl 2):S425–38. https://doi.org/10.1007/s00259-002-0811-8.
22. Liu Y. Clinical significance of thyroid uptake on F18-fluorodeoxyglucose positron emission tomography. Ann Nucl Med. 2009;23(1):17–23. https://doi.org/10.1007/s12149-008-0198-0.
23. Bae JS, Chae BJ, Park WC, Kim JS, Kim SH, Jung SS, Song BJ. Incidental thyroid lesions detected by FDG-PET/CT: prevalence and risk of thyroid cancer. World J Surg Oncol. 2009;7:63. https://doi.org/10.1186/1477-7819-7-63.
24. Greenspan, B. S., Dillehay, G., Intenzo, C., Lavely, W. C., O'Doherty, M., Palestro, C. J., . . . Tulchinsky, M. (2012). SNM practice guideline for parathyroid scintigraphy 4.0. J Nucl Med Technol, 40(2), 111–118. https://doi.org/10.2967/jnmt.112.105122.
25. Becker, D., Charles, N. D., Dworkin, H., Hurley, J., McDougall, I. R., Price, D., . . . Sarkar, S. (1996). Procedure guideline for thyroid scintigraphy: 1.0 Society of Nuclear MedicineJ Nucl Med, 37(7), 1264–1266.
26. National Institutes of Health. Patient education – procedures/diagnostic tests – thyroid scan/thyroid uptake study. Bethesda, MD: National Institutes of Health; 2000. https://www.cc.nih.gov/ccc/patient_education/procdiag/thyroidupt.pdf
27. Gregory, R. A., Murray, I., Gear, J., Aldridge, M. D., Levine, D., Fowkes, L., . . . Flux, G. (2017). Objective comparison of lesion detectability in low and medium-energy collimator iodine-123 mIBG images using a channelized Hotelling observer. Phys Med Biol, 62(1), 17–30. https://doi.org/10.1088/1361-6560/62/1/17.
28. Macey DJ, DeNardo GL, DeNardo SJ, Hines HH. Comparison of low- and medium-energy collimators for SPECT imaging with iodine-123-labeled antibodies. J Nucl Med. 1986;27(9):1467–74.
29. Pelletier-Galarneau M, Sogbein O, Zeng W, Zuckier L. Count rate of 99mTc-pertechnetate thyroid imaging can be used as a surrogate of 24 hour 131I radioactive iodide uptake (RAIU) in a clinically meaningful manner. Paper presented at the European Journal of Nuclear Medicine and Molecular Imaging. 2013.
30. Higgins HP, Ball D, Eastham S. 20-min 99mTc thyroid uptake: a simplified method using the gamma camera. J Nucl Med. 1973;14(12):907–11.
31. Pelletier-Galarneau M, Martineau P, Klein R, Henderson M, Zuckier LS. Reproducibility of radioactive iodine uptake (RAIU) measurements. J Appl Clin Med Phys. 2018;19(1):239–42. https://doi.org/10.1002/acm2.12217.
32. Balon HR, Silberstein EB, Meier DA, Charkes D, Royal H, Sarkar S, Donohoe K. Society of nuclear medicine procedure guideline for thyroid uptake measurement, version 3.0; 2006. http://interactive.snm.org/index.cfm?PageID=772.
33. Wong ET, Schultz AL. Changing values for the normal thyroid radioactive iodine uptake test. JAMA. 1977;238(16):1741–3.
34. Wolff J, Chaikoff IL, et al. The temporary nature of the inhibitory action of excess iodine on organic iodine synthesis in the normal thyroid. Endocrinology. 1949;45(5):504–13. https://doi.org/10.1210/endo-45-5-504.
35. Noussios G, Anagnostis P, Goulis DG, Lappas D, Natsis K. Ectopic thyroid tissue: anatomical, clinical, and surgical implications of a rare entity. Eur J Endocrinol. 2011;165(3):375–82. https://doi.org/10.1530/EJE-11-0461.
36. Dussault JH, Coulombe P, Laberge C, Letarte J, Guyda H, Khoury K. Preliminary report on a mass screening program for neonatal hypothyroidism. J Pediatr. 1975;86(5):670–4.
37. Dussault JH, Laberge C. Thyroxine (T4) determination by radioimmunological method in dried blood eluate: new diagnostic method of neonatal hypothyroidism? Union Med Can. 1973;102(10):2062–4.
38. Dussault JH. The anecdotal history of screening for congenital hypothyroidism. J Clin Endocrinol Metab. 1999;84(12):4332–4. https://doi.org/10.1210/jcem.84.12.6221.
39. Rastogi MV, LaFranchi SH. Congenital hypothyroidism. Orphanet J Rare Dis. 2010;5:17. https://doi.org/10.1186/1750-1172-5-17.
40. Canaris GJ, Manowitz NR, Mayor G, Ridgway EC. The Colorado thyroid disease prevalence study. Arch Intern Med. 2000;160(4):526–34.
41. Franklyn JA. The thyroid—too much and too little across the ages. The consequences of subclinical thyroid dysfunction. Clin Endocrinol. 2013;78(1):1–8. https://doi.org/10.1111/cen.12011.
42. Leung AM, Braverman LE. Consequences of excess iodine. Nat Rev Endocrinol. 2014;10(3):136–42. https://doi.org/10.1038/nrendo.2013.251.

43. Grammaticos P, Vasiliou O, Papanastasiou E, Gerasimou G, Balaris V, Alexandris R, et al. The clinical and laboratory findings in Graves' multinodular type disease. Hell J Nucl Med. 2006;9(1):53–9.
44. Charkes ND. Graves' disease with functioning nodules (Marine-Lenhart syndrome). J Nucl Med. 1972;13(12):885–92.
45. Torring O, Tallstedt L, Wallin G, Lundell G, Ljunggren JG, Taube A, et al. Graves' hyperthyroidism: treatment with antithyroid drugs, surgery, or radioiodine—a prospective, randomized study. Thyroid Study Group. J Clin Endocrinol Metab. 1996;81(8):2986–93. https://doi.org/10.1210/jcem.81.8.8768863.
46. Dean DS, Gharib H. Epidemiology of thyroid nodules. Best Pract Res Clin Endocrinol Metab. 2008;22(6):901–11. https://doi.org/10.1016/j.beem.2008.09.019.
47. Haugen, B. R., Alexander, E. K., Bible, K. C., Doherty, G. M., Mandel, S. J., Nikiforov, Y. E., . . . Wartofsky, L. (2016). 2015 American Thyroid Association management guidelines for adult patients with thyroid nodules and differentiated thyroid Cancer: the American Thyroid Association guidelines task force on thyroid nodules and differentiated thyroid Cancer. Thyroid, 26(1), 1–133. https://doi.org/10.1089/thy.2015.0020.
48. Giuffrida D, Gharib H. Controversies in the management of cold, hot, and occult thyroid nodules. Am J Med. 1995;99(6):642–50.
49. McCall A, Jarosz H, Lawrence AM, Paloyan E. The incidence of thyroid carcinoma in solitary cold nodules and in multinodular goiters. Surgery. 1986;100(6):1128–32.
50. Kusic Z, Becker DV, Saenger EL, Paras P, Gartside P, Wessler T, Spaventi S. Comparison of technetium-99m and iodine-123 imaging of thyroid nodules: correlation with pathologic findings. J Nucl Med. 1990;31(4):393–9.
51. Pearce EN, Farwell AP, Braverman LE. Thyroiditis. N Engl J Med. 2003;348(26):2646–55. https://doi.org/10.1056/NEJMra021194.
52. Epstein AE, Olshansky B, Naccarelli GV, Kennedy JI Jr, Murphy EJ, Goldschlager N. Practical management guide for clinicians who treat patients with amiodarone. Am J Med. 2016;129(5):468–75. https://doi.org/10.1016/j.amjmed.2015.08.039.
53. Tsang W, Houlden RL. Amiodarone-induced thyrotoxicosis: a review. Can J Cardiol. 2009;25(7):421–4.
54. Piga M, Cocco MC, Serra A, Boi F, Loy M, Mariotti S. The usefulness of 99mTc-sestaMIBI thyroid scan in the differential diagnosis and management of amiodarone-induced thyrotoxicosis. Eur J Endocrinol. 2008;159(4):423–9. https://doi.org/10.1530/EJE-08-0348.
55. Smith JR, Oates ME. Radionuclide imaging of the parathyroid glands: patterns, pearls, and pitfalls. Radiographics. 2004;24(4):1101–15. https://doi.org/10.1148/rg.244035718.
56. Johnson NA, Tublin ME, Ogilvie JB. Parathyroid imaging: technique and role in the preoperative evaluation of primary hyperparathyroidism. AJR Am J Roentgenol. 2007;188(6):1706–15. https://doi.org/10.2214/AJR.06.0938.
57. Eslamy HK, Ziessman HA. Parathyroid scintigraphy in patients with primary hyperparathyroidism: 99mTc sestamibi SPECT and SPECT/CT. Radiographics. 2008;28(5):1461–76. https://doi.org/10.1148/rg.285075055.
58. Clarke BL. Epidemiology of primary hyperparathyroidism. J Clin Densitom. 2013;16(1):8–13. https://doi.org/10.1016/j.jocd.2012.11.009.
59. Tezelman S, Shen W, Shaver JK, Siperstein AE, Duh QY, Klein H, Clark OH. Double parathyroid adenomas. Clinical and biochemical characteristics before and after parathyroidectomy. Ann Surg. 1993;218(3):300–7; discussion 307–309.
60. Marcocci C, Cetani F. Clinical practice. Primary hyperparathyroidism. N Engl J Med. 2011;365(25):2389–97. https://doi.org/10.1056/NEJMcp1106636.
61. Rubin, M. R., Bilezikian, J. P., McMahon, D. J., Jacobs, T., Shane, E., Siris, E., . . . Silverberg, S. J. (2008). The natural history of primary hyperparathyroidism with or without parathyroid surgery after 15 years. J Clin Endocrinol Metab, 93(9), 3462–3470. https://doi.org/10.1210/jc.2007-1215.
62. Bilezikian JP, Brandi ML, Eastell R, Silverberg SJ, Udelsman R, Marcocci C, Potts JT Jr. Guidelines for the management of asymptomatic primary hyperparathyroidism: summary statement from the fourth international workshop. J Clin Endocrinol Metab. 2014;99(10):3561–9. https://doi.org/10.1210/jc.2014-1413.
63. Wilhelm, S. M., Wang, T. S., Ruan, D. T., Lee, J. A., Asa, S. L., Duh, Q. Y., . . . Carty, S. E. (2016). The American Association of Endocrine Surgeons guidelines for definitive management of primary hyperparathyroidism. JAMA Surg, 151(10), 959–968. https://doi.org/10.1001/jamasurg.2016.2310.
64. Coakley A, Kettle A, Wells C, O'doherty M, Collins R. 99Tcm sestamibi-a new agent for parathyroid imaging. Nucl Med Commun. 1989;10(11):791–4.
65. Taillefer R, Boucher Y, Potvin C, Lambert R. Detection and localization of parathyroid adenomas in patients with hyperparathyroidism using a single radionuclide imaging procedure with technetium-99m-sestamibi (double-phase study). J Nucl Med. 1992;33(10):1801–7.
66. Hindie E, Ugur O, Fuster D, O'Doherty M, Grassetto G, Urena P, et al. 2009 EANM parathyroid guidelines. Eur J Nucl Med Mol Imaging. 2009;36(7):1201–16. https://doi.org/10.1007/s00259-009-1131-z.
67. Pelletier-Galarneau M, Sogbein OO, Dinh L, Zuckier LS. Superiority of digital subtraction for analysis of simultaneously-acquired dual-radiopharmaceutical parathyroid scintigraphy. Open J Med Imaging. 2015;5(2):7. https://doi.org/10.4236/ojmi.2015.52007.
68. Froberg AC, Valkema R, Bonjer HJ, Krenning EP. 99mTc-tetrofosmin or 99mTc-sestamibi for double-phase parathyroid scintigraphy? Eur J Nucl Med Mol

Imaging. 2003;30(2):193–6. https://doi.org/10.1007/s00259-002-1030-z.

69. Caveny SA, Klingensmith WC III, Martin WE, Sage-El A, McIntyre RC Jr, Raeburn C, Wolfe P. Parathyroid imaging: the importance of dual-radiopharmaceutical simultaneous acquisition with 99mTc-sestamibi and 123I. J Nucl Med Technol. 2012;40(2):104–10. https://doi.org/10.2967/jnmt.111.098400.
70. Hindie E, Melliere D, Jeanguillaume C, Perlemuter L, Chehade F, Galle P. Parathyroid imaging using simultaneous double-window recording of technetium-99m-sestamibi and iodine-123. J Nucl Med. 1998;39(6):1100–5.
71. Caixàs A, Bernà L, Piera J, Rigla M, Matías-Guiu X, Farrerons J, Puig-Domingo M. Utility of 99mTc-sestamibi scintigraphy as a first-line imaging procedure in the preoperative evaluation of hyperparathyroidism. Clin Endocrinol. 1995;43(5):525–30.
72. Lavely, W. C., Goetze, S., Friedman, K. P., Leal, J. P., Zhang, Z., Garret-Mayer, E., . . . Ziessman, H. A. (2007). Comparison of SPECT/CT, SPECT, and planar imaging with single- and dual-phase (99m)Tc-sestamibi parathyroid scintigraphy. J Nucl Med, 48(7), 1084–1089. https://doi.org/10.2967/jnumed.107.040428.
73. O'Doherty MJ, Kettle AG, Wells P, Collins R, Coakley AJ. Parathyroid imaging with technetium-99m-sestamibi: preoperative localization and tissue uptake studies. J Nucl Med. 1992;33(3):313–8.
74. Bénard F, Lefebvre B, Beuvon F, Langlois M-F, Bisson G. Rapid washout of technetium-99m-MIBI from a large parathyroid adenoma. J Nucl Med. 1995;36(2):241–3.
75. Palestro CJ, Tomas MB, Tronco GG. Radionuclide imaging of the parathyroid glands. Semin Nucl Med. 2005;35(4):266–76. https://doi.org/10.1053/j.semnuclmed.2005.06.001.
76. Wimmer, G., Profanter, C., Kovacs, P., Sieb, M., Gabriel, M., Putzer, D., . . . Prommegger, R. (2010). CT-MIBI-SPECT image fusion predicts multiglandular disease in hyperparathyroidism. Langenbeck's Arch Surg, 395(1), 73–80. https://doi.org/10.1007/s00423-009-0545-1.
77. Neumann DR, Obuchowski NA, Difilippo FP. Preoperative 123I/99mTc-sestamibi subtraction SPECT and SPECT/CT in primary hyperparathyroidism. J Nucl Med. 2008;49(12):2012–7. https://doi.org/10.2967/jnumed.108.054858.
78. Pelletier-Galarneau M, Sogbein B, Zuckier L. Coimaging of 123I-NaI can be eliminated from the scintigraphic evaluation of parathyroid adenoma with only minimal effect on final imaging diagnosis. J Nucl Med. 2013;54(Suppl 2):147.
79. Thomas DL, Bartel T, Menda Y, Howe J, Graham MM, Juweid ME. Single photon emission computed tomography (SPECT) should be routinely performed for the detection of parathyroid abnormalities utilizing technetium-99m sestamibi parathyroid scintigraphy. Clin Nucl Med. 2009;34(10):651–5. https://doi.org/10.1097/RLU.0b013e3181b591c9.
80. Jamal SA, Miller PD. Secondary and tertiary hyperparathyroidism. J Clin Densitom. 2013;16(1):64–8. https://doi.org/10.1016/j.jocd.2012.11.012.
81. Taïeb, D., Ureña-Torres, P., Zanotti-Fregonara, P., Rubello, D., Ferretti, A., Henter, I., . . . Blickman, J. G. (2013). Parathyroid scintigraphy in renal hyperparathyroidism: the added diagnostic value of SPECT and SPECT/CT. Clin Nucl Med, 38(8), 630.
82. Lai EC, Ching AS, Leong HT. Secondary and tertiary hyperparathyroidism: role of preoperative localization. ANZ J Surg. 2007;77(10):880–2. https://doi.org/10.1111/j.1445-2197.2007.04264.x.
83. Loftus KA, Anderson S, Mulloy AL, Terris DJ. Value of sestamibi scans in tertiary hyperparathyroidism. Laryngoscope. 2007;117(12):2135–8. https://doi.org/10.1097/MLG.0b013e31813e602a.
84. Liddy S, Worsley D, Torreggiani W, Feeney J. Preoperative imaging in primary hyperparathyroidism: literature review and recommendations. Can Assoc Radiol J. 2017;68(1):47–55. https://doi.org/10.1016/j.carj.2016.07.004.
85. Kluijfhout, W. P., Pasternak, J. D., Drake, F. T., Beninato, T., Gosnell, J. E., Shen, W. T., . . . Suh, I. (2016). Use of PET tracers for parathyroid localization: a systematic review and meta-analysis. Langenbeck's Arch Surg, 401(7), 925–935. https://doi.org/10.1007/s00423-016-1425-0.

15 Molecular Imaging of Inflammation and Infection

Christopher J. Palestro and Darlene Metter

15.1 Introduction

In spite of advances in its prevention and treatment, infection remains a major cause of morbidity and mortality throughout the world. While symptoms, signs, and abnormal laboratory tests may suggest infection, the diagnosis is not always obvious, and imaging tests often are used for confirmation and localization. Radiologic imaging such as X-rays, computed tomography, magnetic resonance imaging, and ultrasonography depicts structural alterations in tissues and organs that are caused by a combination of the infection itself and the host's response to the infection.

Molecular imaging procedures utilizing radiopharmaceuticals, such as labeled leukocytes, gallium-67, gallium-68, and fluorine-18 fluorodeoxyglucose, reflect the physiological changes that are part of the inflammatory process. This chapter reviews the role of these agents in the detection and localization of inflammation and infection.

C. J. Palestro (✉)
Donald and Barbara Zucker School of Medicine at Hofstra/Northwell, Hempstead, NY, USA

Nuclear Medicine and Molecular Imaging, Northwell Health, New Hyde Park, NY, USA
e-mail: palestro@northwell.edu

D. Metter
Department of Radiology, UT Health San Antonio, San Antonio, TX, USA

15.2 Single-Photon-Emitting Radiopharmaceuticals

15.2.1 Gallium-67 Citrate

The propensity of gallium-67 citrate (^{67}Ga) to concentrate in inflammation and infection was recognized more than 40 years ago. Uptake of this radiopharmaceutical is nonspecific, multifactorial, and related to the nature of the inflammatory response itself. Following intravenous injection, more than 90% of the ^{67}Ga in circulation is located in the plasma, and nearly all of this activity is bound to transferrin. Inflammation is characterized by increased blood flow and increased vascular membrane permeability. These factors result in increased delivery and increased accumulation of plasma proteins and hence increased ^{67}Ga uptake at inflammatory sites [1].

Bacteria are also involved in ^{67}Ga uptake in infection. Direct uptake mechanisms probably involve nonspecific binding and facilitated diffusion. Siderophores, which are small-molecule metal chelates produced by bacteria, have a high affinity for gallium. Presumably, the siderophore-gallium complex is transported into the bacterium where it cannot be released without destruction of the entire cell [1].

Plasma proteins also contribute to ^{67}Ga uptake in inflammation and infection. In addition to transferrin, ^{67}Ga binds to lactoferrin which is

H. Ahmadzadehfar et al. (eds.), *Clinical Nuclear Medicine*,
https://doi.org/10.1007/978-3-030-39457-8_15

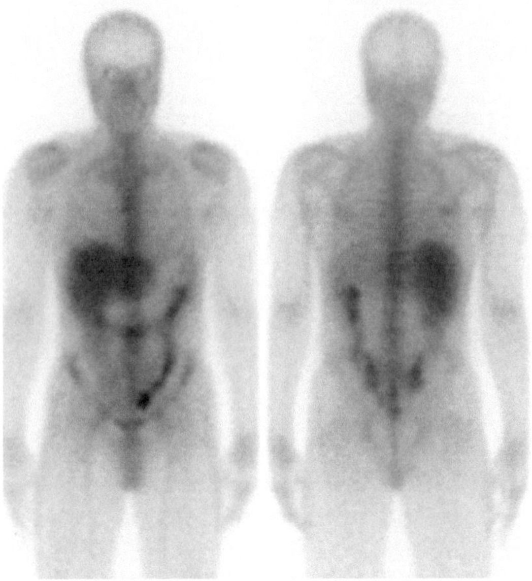

Anterior Posterior

Fig. 15.1 Normal gallium-67 scan. There is soft tissue, hepatic, colonic, and skeletal activity on these images, which were acquired approximately 48 h after radiopharmaceutical injection

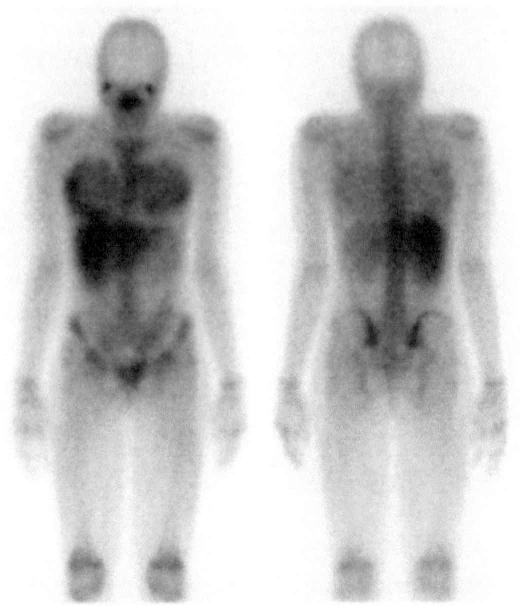

Anterior Posterior

Fig. 15.2 Normal gallium-67 scan. In this adolescent female, orbital, nasopharyngeal, and breast activity are prominent. The distal femoral and proximal tibial growth plates are also seen. Figures 15.1 and 15.2 illustrate the variable normal distribution of gallium-67

present in inflammatory exudates due to the secretion of lysosomal contents by stimulated neutrophils or as a result of cell death [1].

Although a small amount of ^{67}Ga is transported to inflammatory foci via leukocytes it is important to note that even in the absence of circulating leukocytes, ^{67}Ga will still accumulate at sites of inflammation and infection [1].

Imaging is usually performed 18–72 h after ^{67}Ga administration. The normal distribution of ^{67}Ga includes the skeleton, liver, gastrointestinal tract, urinary tract, and soft tissues (Fig. 15.1). Nasopharyngeal and lacrimal gland activity can be prominent. Breast uptake is increased in young women (Fig. 15.2) and also in hyperprolactinemic states related to pregnancy, lactation, certain drugs, and hypothalamic lesions. In patients who have undergone multiple transfusions, renal, bladder, and skeletal activity are increased, while hepatic and colonic activity are decreased. This altered pattern of uptake is presumably due to the saturation of iron receptors by exogenous iron from the transfused red blood cells. The MRI contrast agent gadolinium has also been reported to cause similar changes in the biodistribution of ^{67}Ga.

Disadvantages of this radiopharmaceutical include nonspecific uptake in tumors, trauma, aseptic inflammation, the long interval between injection and imaging (usually 48–72 h), and the wide range of emissions that adversely affects image quality [1].

Although labeled leukocytes and fluorine-18 fluorodeoxyglucose (^{18}F-FDG) have largely replaced ^{67}Ga, this radiopharmaceutical is still useful. It can provide information that is complementary to and under certain circumstances not available from other studies. ^{67}Ga is a sensitive indicator of pulmonary inflammation, accumulating in opportunistic infections, interstitial pneumonitis, drug reactions, and pneumoconioses [2] (Fig. 15.3). Sarcoidosis is a chronic inflammatory condition characterized by epithelioid noncaseating granulomas derived from bone marrow monocytes. These lesions are rich in lactoferrin which probably accounts for their gallium-avidity [3]. Pulmonary and extrapulmonary uptake of gallium in sarcoidosis is a well-known phenomenon, and when ^{18}F-FDG, the molecular imaging test of choice for sarcoid, is not available or cannot be performed, ^{67}Ga is an acceptable alternative (Fig. 15.4) [4, 5].

With reasonably good results, ^{67}Ga alone and in conjunction with bone scintigraphy has been used to diagnose spondylodiscitis [6]. Bone scintigraphy is often performed as a screening test, and if negative, ^{67}Ga imaging is not performed. There is, however, literature that indicates that ^{67}Ga is more sensitive than bone scintigraphy, especially in the elderly. ^{67}Ga is also more sensitive than bone scintigraphy for detecting soft tissue infections and abscesses that often accompany or mimic spondylodiscitis [7]. Thus in suspected spondylodiscitis, ^{67}Ga imaging should be performed regardless of the results of the bone scan. Recent investigations indicate that ^{67}Ga SPECT/CT is valuable in patients with suspected spondylodiscitis, by providing precise localization of radiopharmaceutical uptake and delineating the extent of infection (Fig. 15.5) [8–11].

Drug-induced acute interstitial nephritis is responsible for more than 10% of all cases of acute kidney injury. Pathologically this entity is characterized by interstitial edema and a mononuclear cellular infiltrate. Prompt diagnosis is important so that the offending agent can be removed and appropriate therapy instituted. Differentiating acute interstitial nephritis from acute tubular necrosis, the most common cause of acute kidney injury in hospitalized patients, can be difficult. Although definitive diagnosis is made by biopsy, ^{67}Ga imaging can be of value. Interstitial nephritis is characterized by renal uptake of ^{67}Ga, which is more intense than lumbar spine uptake (Fig. 15.6). In contrast, acute tubular necrosis is characterized by little or no renal uptake [12–14].

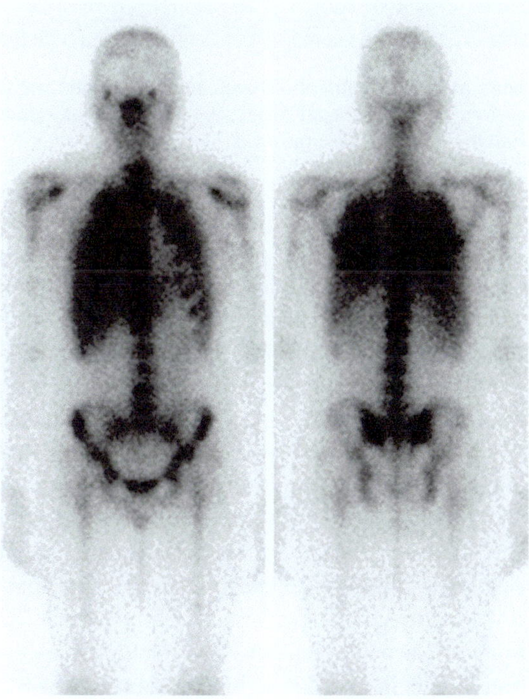

Anterior Posterior

Fig. 15.3 Pulmonary drug toxicity. There is diffusely increased activity in both lungs in a patient undergoing chemotherapy for lymphoma

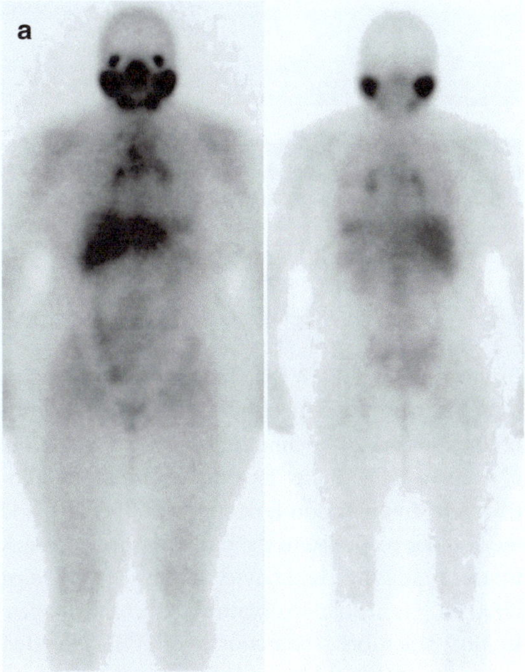

Anterior Posterior

Fig. 15.4 Sarcoidosis. On the whole body images, (**a**) there is increased activity in the orbits, nasopharynx, parotid, and submandibular glands and mediastinum. On the coronal SPECT/CT image, (**b**) the mediastinal abnormality involves hilar and subcarinal lymph nodes. The lungs are not involved

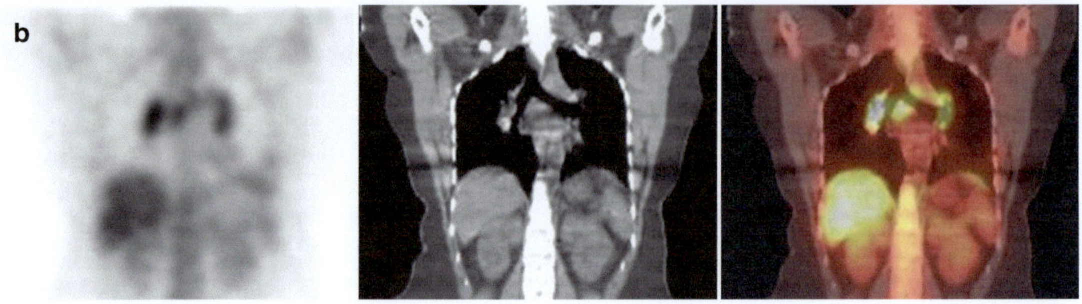

Fig. 15.4 (Continued)

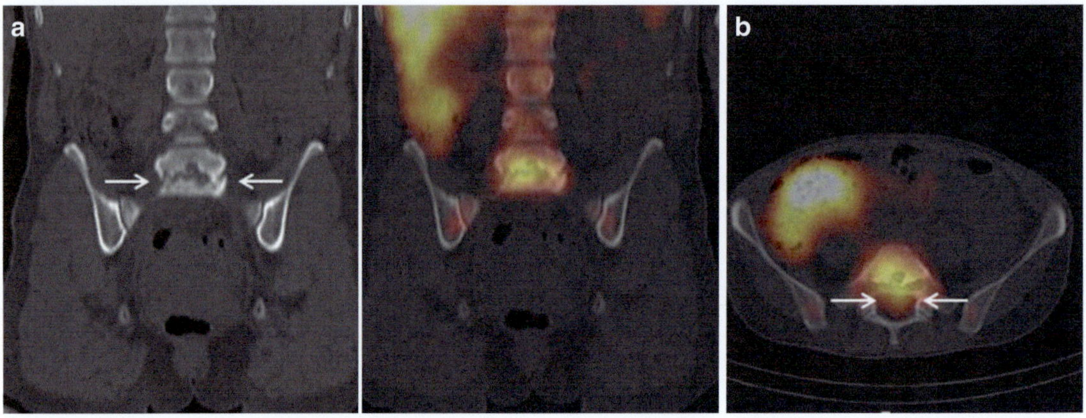

Fig. 15.5 (**a**) L4–L5 spondylodiscitis. Note the destructive changes involving the endplates of the L4 and L5 vertebrae (arrows) on the CT component of the SPECT/CT, with abnormal gallium-67 accumulation in the same region. (**b**) On the axial image, the abnormality extends into the epidural space (arrows)

15.3 Labeled Leukocytes

In vitro leukocyte (WBC) labeling is most commonly performed with either indium-111 oxyquinolone (^{111}In) or technetium-99m-exametazime (^{99m}Tc). WBC uptake depends on intact chemotaxis, the number and types of cells labeled, and the cellular response to the particular infection. A total circulating leukocyte count of at least 2000 μL^{-1} is needed to obtain satisfactory images. In most situations, the majority of WBCs labeled are neutrophils, and therefore the test is most sensitive for identifying neutrophil-mediated inflammatory/infectious processes, such as bacterial infections. WBC imaging is much less sensitive for inflammations and infections in which the predominant cellular response is not neutrophilic, such as sarcoid [15].

Advantages of using ^{111}In as the radiolabel include label stability; a normal 24-h post-reinfusion biodistribution limited to the liver, spleen, and bone marrow; and the ability to perform delayed imaging (Fig. 15.7). Disadvantages of ^{111}In-WBC imaging include limited resolution, the risk of handling blood products, and the 16–30-h interval between reinfusion of labeled leukocytes and imaging [16].

Complementary bone marrow imaging with ^{99m}Tc-sulfur colloid (SC) is frequently used in suspected musculoskeletal infection. Bone marrow imaging can be performed before ^{111}In-WBC imaging, as a simultaneous dual-isotope acquisition with ^{111}In-WBC imaging, or after ^{111}In-WBC imaging.

The normal distribution of ^{99m}Tc-WBCs is more variable than that of ^{111}In-WBCs. Normal physiologic ^{99m}Tc-WBC activity is seen in the

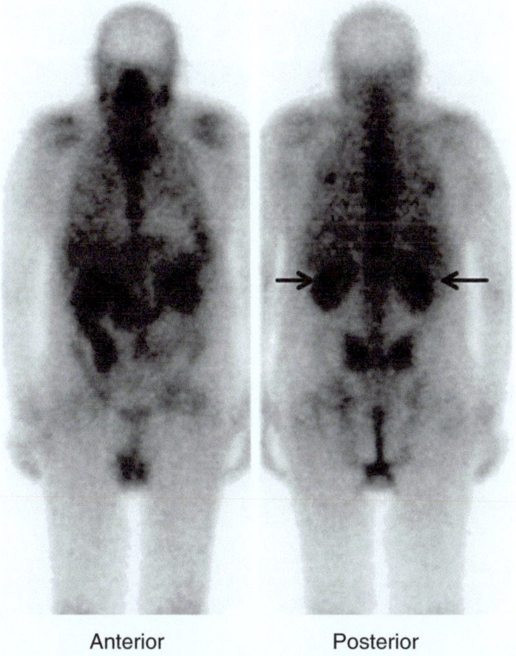

Fig. 15.6 Acute interstitial nephritis. Renal activity (arrows) is more intense than adjacent lumbar spine activity, which is the typical presentation of this entity on gallium-67 imaging

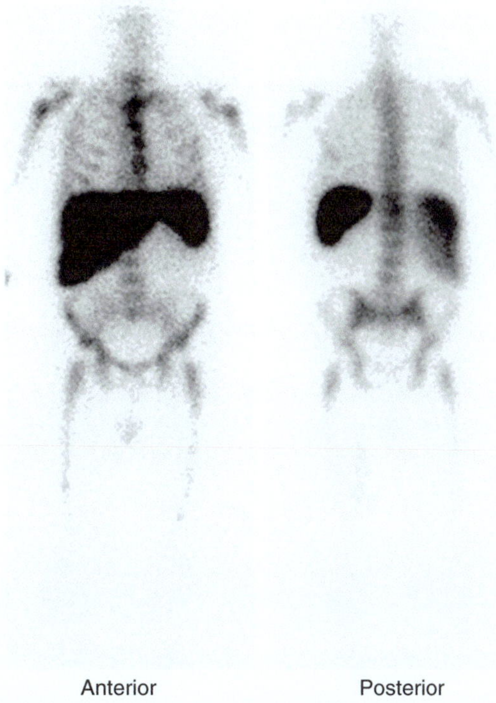

Fig. 15.7 Normal indium-111-labeled leukocyte scan. At 24 h after reinfusion of labeled cells, activity is confined to the liver, spleen, and bone marrow. Splenic activity usually is more intense than hepatic activity

reticuloendothelial system, urinary tract, large bowel (within 3–4 h after reinfusion of the labeled leukocytes), and occasionally the gall bladder (Fig. 15.8). ^{99m}Tc-WBC advantages include high-resolution images, which is especially useful when performing SPECT and SPECT/CT, and the ability to detect abnormalities within a few hours after reinfusion of labeled cells. Disadvantages include label instability, which accounts for the variable distribution of activity, and the 6-h half-life of ^{99m}Tc which limits delayed imaging. A 2- to 3-day interval between ^{99m}Tc-WBC and ^{99m}Tc-SC bone marrow imaging is also necessary [16].

During the first few hours after reinfusion, pulmonary uptake of labeled WBCs is a normal physiologic event. This phenomenon is likely due to leukocyte activation during labeling, hindering cellular movement through the pulmonary vascular bed and thereby prolonging WBC transit through the lungs (Fig. 15.9). At 24 h, pulmonary uptake is abnormal. Focal lobar or segmental pulmonary uptake is usually associated with bacterial pneumonia (Fig. 15.10). This pattern can also be seen in patients with cystic fibrosis due to WBC accumulation in pooled bronchiectasis secretions [17, 18].

Diffuse pulmonary activity on images obtained more than 4 h after reinfusion of labeled WBCs is associated with opportunistic infection, radiation pneumonitis, pulmonary drug toxicity, and adult respiratory distress syndrome (Fig. 15.11). This pattern is not associated with bacterial pneumonia. Diffuse pulmonary uptake also occurs in septic patients who have no clinical evidence of respiratory tract inflammation or infection. This diffuse uptake is presumably due to cytokine activation of circulating leukocytes, which makes it more difficult for the cells to undergo the cytoskeletal deformation required to maneuver through the pulmonary circulation. Cytokines also activate pulmonary vascular endothelial

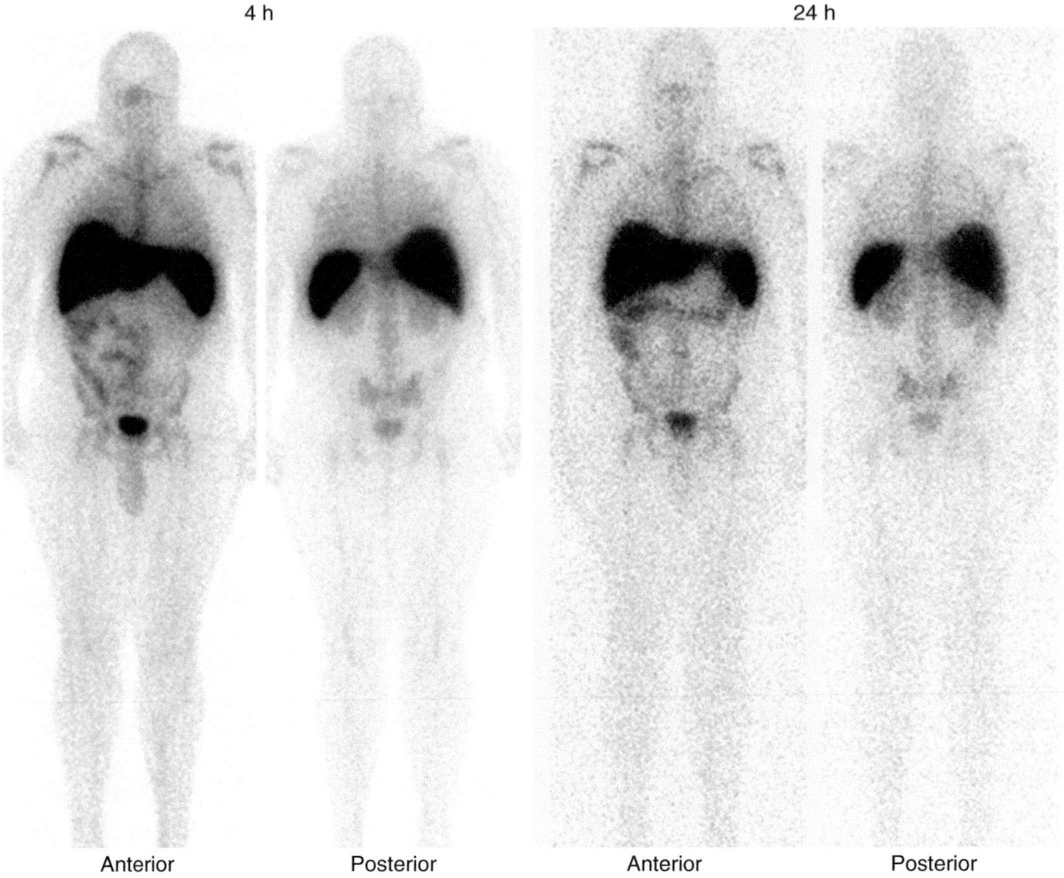

Fig. 15.8 Normal technetium-99m-labeled leukocyte scan. At 4 h after reinfusion of labeled cells (left), activity is present in the urinary tract and distal small bowel, in addition to the reticuloendothelial system. By 24 h, the intestinal activity has passed into the transverse colon

Fig. 15.9 Normal pulmonary transit of labeled leukocytes. Immediately after reinfusion of labeled leukocytes, intense activity is normally present in the lungs. This activity decreases rapidly as the leukocytes leave the lungs, until by 4 h, little pulmonary activity remains. Consequently pulmonary activity should be evaluated only on images acquired more than 4 h after labeled leukocyte administration

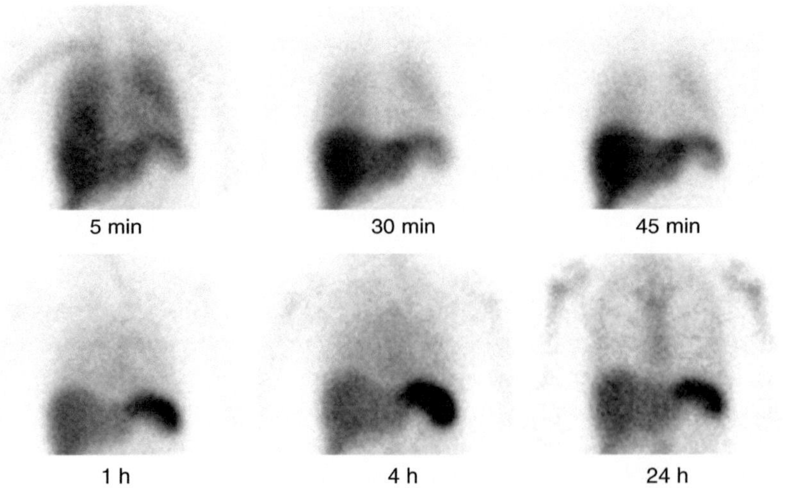

cells, causing increased adherence of leukocytes to the cell walls [17, 18].

^{111}In-WBCs do not accumulate in normal bowel. Such activity always is abnormal and is seen in infectious colitis, inflammatory bowel disease, ischemic colitis, and gastrointestinal bleeding [16, 18].

Radiolabeled WBCs do not accumulate in normally healing surgical wounds, and the presence of such activity usually indicates infection with some exceptions. Uninfected granulating wounds, such as tracheostomies, feeding gastrostomies, and colostomies, which heal by secondary intention, can appear as areas of focal increased activity that can be quite intense on WBC images [15, 19].

WBC imaging is the molecular imaging test of choice for most infections in the immunocompetent population. WBC imaging facilitates the differentiation of infection from other fluid collections, postoperative change, and tumor [15, 19] (Fig. 15.12). ^{99m}Tc-WBC is the molecular imaging test of choice for inflammatory bowel disease. It can be used as a screening test and as an alternative to radiography and endoscopy, when these procedures cannot be performed. ^{99m}Tc-WBC can also be used to monitor treatment response and to facilitate the differentiation between active infection and inflammation from scarring [15].

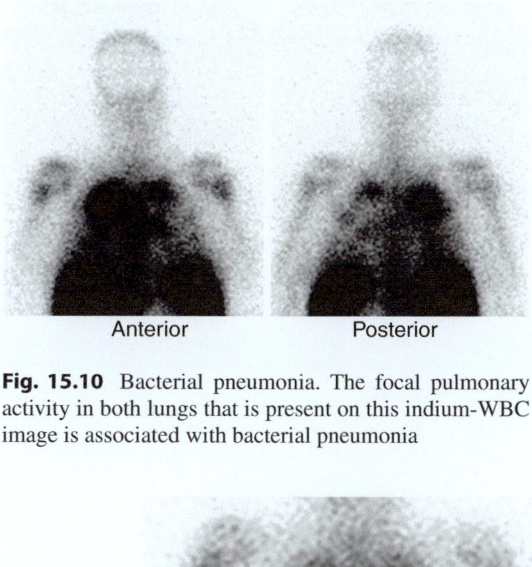

Fig. 15.10 Bacterial pneumonia. The focal pulmonary activity in both lungs that is present on this indium-WBC image is associated with bacterial pneumonia

In the brain, WBC imaging is a useful adjunct to computed tomography (CT) and magnetic resonance imaging (MRI) for differentiating tumor from abscess. Although WBC uptake has been observed in some tumors and following cerebrovascular accidents, the uptake usually is less intense than in abscesses. High- or medium-dose steroid treatment may decrease WBC sensitivity [16].

WBC imaging is useful for diagnosing prosthetic vascular graft infection. Sensitivity, which in most series exceeds 90%, is not affected by antibiotic therapy or duration of symptoms. Specificity is more variable, ranging from about 50% to 100%. False positive results can be caused by perigraft hematomas, lymphoceles, thrombosed grafts, bleeding, pseudoaneurysms, and uninfected grafts less than 1 month old [16]. SPECT/CT improves test accuracy [20–22]. In one series, SPECT/CT was more sensitive (100% vs. 81.5%) and more specific (100% vs. 62.5%) than SPECT alone and was especially useful for detecting, localizing, and defining the extent of infection [21] (Fig. 15.13).

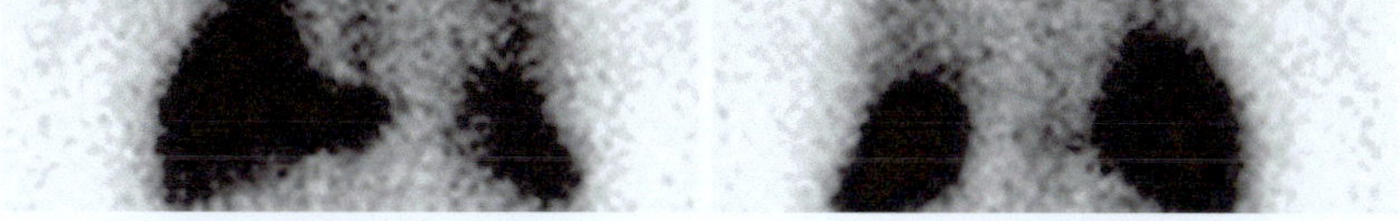

Fig. 15.11 Adult respiratory distress syndrome. There is diffuse bilateral pulmonary activity on this indium-WBC image acquired about 24 h after reinfusion of labeled cells. While this pattern is associated with many entities, it is not associated with bacterial pneumonia

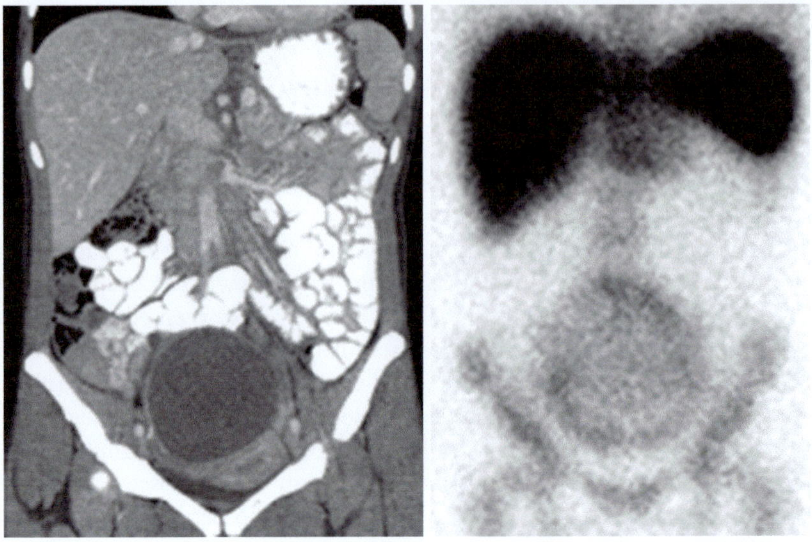

Fig. 15.12 Tubo-ovarian abscess. Although the CT scan (left) described a large right ovarian cyst, the indium-111-labeled leukocyte scan (right) shows a large area of circumferentially increased activity in this region. A tubo-ovarian abscess was found at surgery

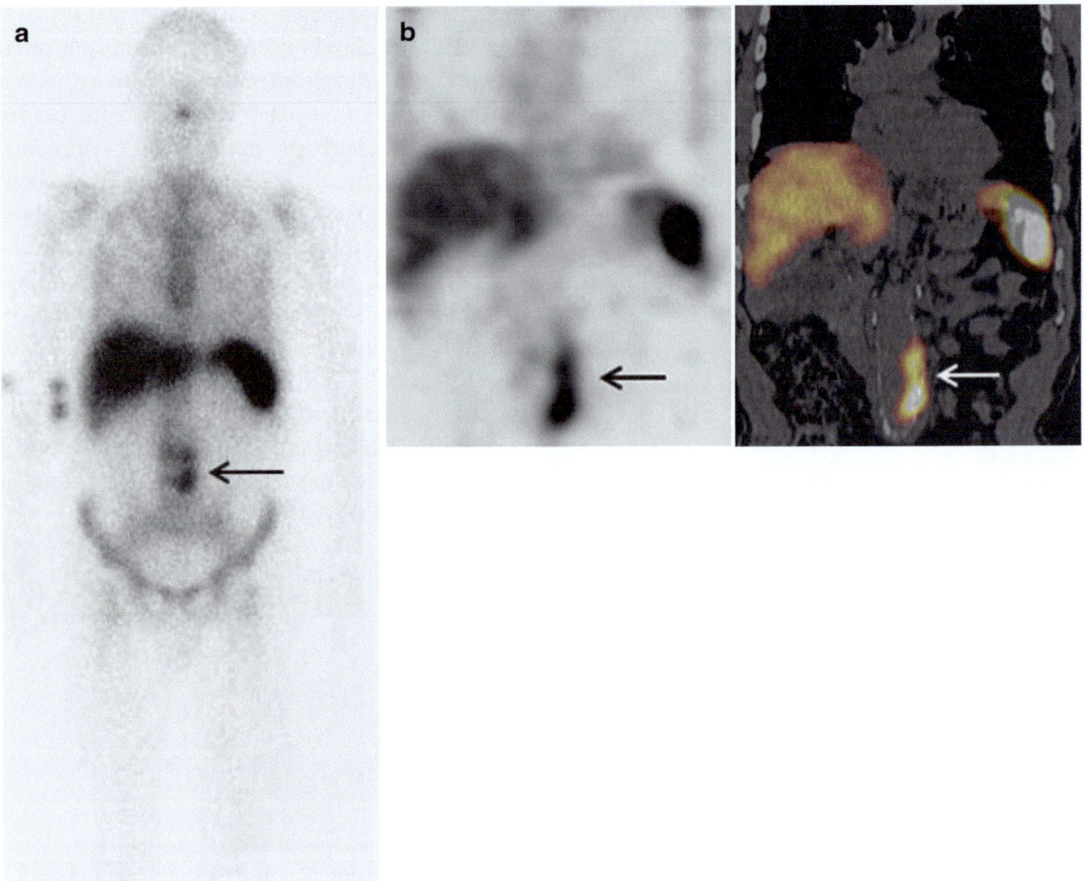

Fig. 15.13 (**a**) Infected abdominal aortic graft. There is an area of increased activity (arrow) overlying the mid-lumbar spine on the anterior indium-111-labeled leukocyte image, although it is hard to be sure of the exact location. (**b**) The SPECT/CT images confirm that this activity involves the prosthetic graft (arrows)

Cardiovascular implantable electronic device (CIED)-related infections are associated with significant morbidity and mortality. These infections, which usually originate in the surgical pocket, can extend through the pacemaker leads resulting in endocarditis and systemic infection. WBC SPECT/CT is useful for confirming the presence of CIED-associated infection, defining the location and extent of infection, and detecting associated complications [23, 24].

The development of SPECT/CT has led to a renaissance in molecular imaging for diagnosing infectious endocarditis (IE) and its complications. WBC SPECT/CT is useful for differentiating septic and marantic vegetations detected on echocardiography. When echocardiographic, laboratory, and clinical data are contradictory for infection and when valve involvement, especially in the setting of prosthetic valves, needs to be excluded during febrile episodes, sepsis, or postoperative infections, WBC SPECT/CT can be invaluable for diagnosing or excluding valvular infection (Fig. 15.14). Performing whole body imaging, in addition to SPECT/CT, may identify remote sites of infection and help to guide patient management [25, 26].

With the exception of the spine, WBC imaging is the molecular imaging test of choice for diagnosing complicating osteomyelitis. To maximize its accuracy and due to the fact that leukocytes accumulate in both the bone marrow and infection, the test frequently is performed in conjunction with ^{99m}Tc-sulfur colloid bone marrow imaging. Although the normal adult distribution of active bone marrow is assumed to be limited to the axial and proximal appendicular skeleton, the "normal" distribution of active bone marrow can be quite variable. Systemic processes such as tumors and sickle cell and Gaucher's diseases cause generalized alterations in marrow distribution, while heterotopic ossification, orthopedic hardware, fractures, and the neuropathic joint can produce more localized alterations in marrow distribution. The normal distribution of active marrow in children varies with age. Consequently, it may not be possible to determine if an area of activity on a WBC image represents infection or normal bone marrow. Performing complementary bone marrow imaging with ^{99m}Tc-sulfur colloid overcomes this problem. WBCs and sulfur colloid both accumulate in the bone marrow; WBCs also accumulate in infection, but sulfur colloid does not. The combined study is positive for infection when activity is present on the WBC image without concordant activity on the marrow image. Any other pattern is negative for infection (Figs. 15.15 and 15.16). Although WBC/marrow imaging has been most extensively investigated

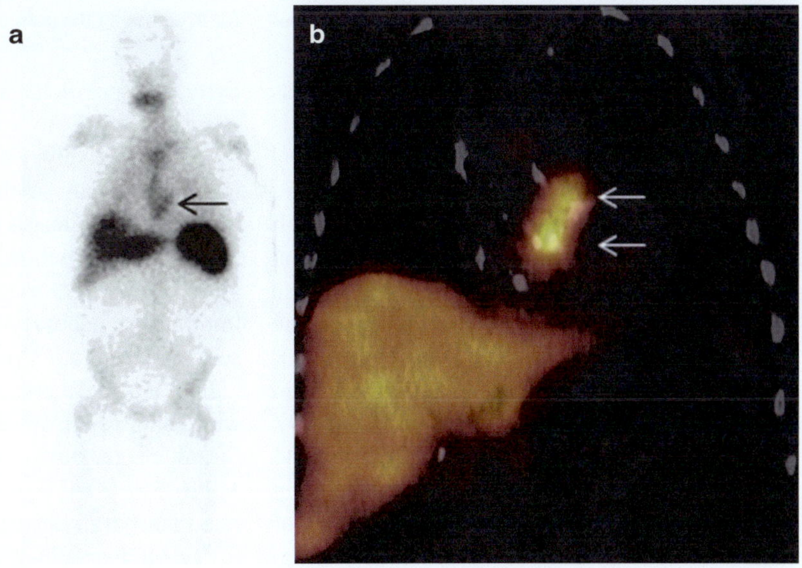

Fig. 15.14 (**a**) Infected prosthetic aortic valve. There is a poorly defined area of increased activity (arrow) along the left side of the sternum on the anterior indium-111-labeled leukocyte scan. (**b**) On the SPECT/CT images, the abnormal activity (arrows) involves the prosthetic valve and extends into the aorta. Transthoracic echocardiography (not shown) was negative. At surgery, an infected prosthetic valve and aortic root abscess were identified

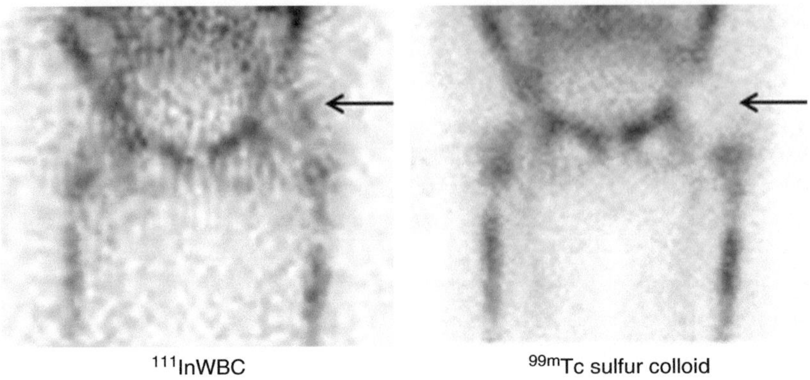

Fig. 15.15 Infected left hip arthroplasty. The indium-111-labeled leukocyte image (left), in isolation, could easily be interpreted as negative for infection. When viewed with the bone marrow image (right), however, the distribution of activity on the two images is discordant (arrows), and the combined study is positive for infection

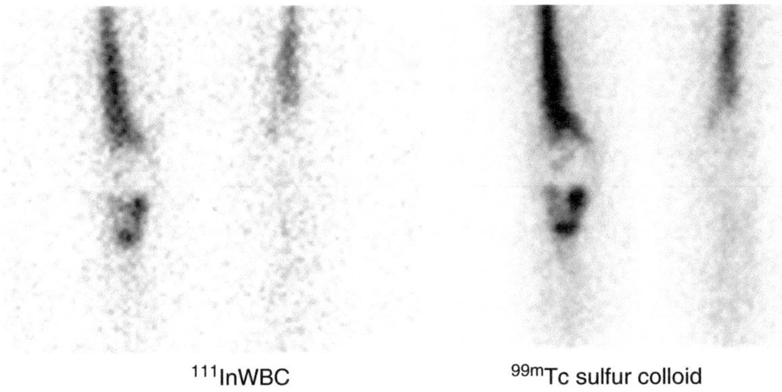

Fig. 15.16 Aseptically loosened right knee arthroplasty. The indium-111-labeled leukocyte image (left), in isolation, could easily be interpreted as positive for infection. When viewed with the bone marrow image (right), however, the distribution of activity on the two images is concordant, and the combined study is negative for infection. Compare the intensity of periprosthetic activity on the labeled leukocyte image in this illustration with that in Fig. 15.15. Intensity of uptake is not a reliable criterion for determining the presence or absence of infection

in prosthetic joint infection, this test, which has an overall accuracy of approximately 90%, is useful in any condition that potentially affects bone marrow biodistribution [27, 28].

Dual-time point imaging at 3–4 and 20–24 h after WBC infusion has been suggested as an alternative to WBC/marrow imaging. An increase in the size or intensity of WBC uptake over time is indicative of infection. Lack of WBC uptake or a decrease in size or intensity of uptake from early to late images is negative for infection [29].

WBC imaging is the molecular imaging "gold standard" for diagnosing pedal osteomyelitis in diabetics. The sensitivity and specificity of ^{111}In-WBC planar imaging range from 72% to 100% and 67% to 100%, respectively. The sensitivity and specificity of ^{99m}Tc-WBC planar imaging range from 86% to 93% and from 80% to 98%, respectively [30]. The majority of these infections occur in the distal forefoot, and the accuracy of the test is limited by low count rates, low spatial resolution, and low contrast. Several investigators have used SPECT/CT in an effort to improve the accuracy of the test [31–35]. In one series, investigators performed SPECT/CT using ^{111}In-WBC and bone scintigraphy, supplemented with bone marrow imaging when necessary. Simultaneous dual-isotope (^{111}In-WBC + ^{99m}Tc-MDP) SPECT/CT was significantly more accurate than both planar imaging and single-isotope (^{99m}Tc-MDP or ^{111}In-WBC) SPECT/CT. Performing bone SPECT/CT permitted more precise localiza-

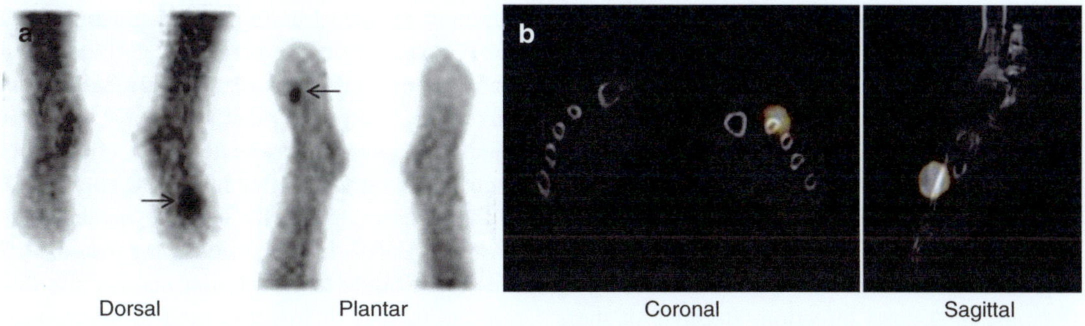

Fig. 15.17 (**a**) Diabetic pedal osteomyelitis. There is focally increased activity (arrows) in the left midfoot on the planar technetium-99m-labeled leukocyte images, which appears to involve the third or fourth metatarsal. (**b**) On the SPECT/CT images, however, it can be seen that the abnormality involves the second metatarsal of the left foot

tion of WBC accumulation, thereby improving both imaging accuracy and confidence of diagnosis [32]. In another investigation, dual-isotope SPECT/CT was more accurate than conventional imaging for diagnosing and localizing infection, providing guidance on treatment, and was associated with a shorter length of hospitalization compared to conventional imaging [33]. An alternative to dual-isotope SPECT/CT is to use ^{99m}Tc-WBC rather than ^{111}In-WBC. ^{99m}Tc-WBC image quality is superior, both labeling and imaging can be performed on the same day, and only one radiopharmaceutical is administered. Results are comparable to those obtained with dual-isotope SPECT/CT (Fig. 15.17) [34, 35].

In addition to its incremental value for diagnosis, WBC SPECT/CT may be useful for monitoring treatment response in diabetic pedal osteomyelitis. In one investigation, sensitivity, specificity, and positive and negative predictive values for predicting osteomyelitis relapse after completion of antibiotic treatment were 100%, 91.5%, 71.5%, and 100%, respectively. The authors concluded that a negative test reliably identifies diabetic pedal osteomyelitis remission and potentially could be useful for guiding antibiotic therapy [36]. In another investigation, the sensitivity, specificity, and positive and negative predictive values of WBC SPECT/CT for determining success of treatment were 90%, 56%, 69%, and 83%, respectively [37].

Molecular imaging is invaluable in the workup of the painful joint replacement. Differentiating aseptic loosening from infection is extremely important because their management is very different. A sensitive but nonspecific test can result in multiple unnecessary and costly operations when a single intervention would have sufficed. The specific but insensitive test will also result in additional surgical interventions, because undiagnosed infection will cause any revision implant to fail [28]. Currently, the best available imaging test for diagnosing prosthetic joint infection is WBC/marrow imaging with an accuracy of about 90%. Virtually all of the data published over the past 35 years confirm the high specificity of WBC/marrow imaging, and in most investigations, the test has proven to be sensitive as well [38–45]. SPECT/CT, using various radiopharmaceuticals, contributes useful information to the diagnostic workup of the painful joint replacement. SPECT/CT is helpful in differentiating periprosthetic and soft tissue infection, delineating the extent of infection, and identifying infectious and noninfectious conditions which may be responsible for the patient's symptoms (Fig. 15.18) [46–51].

It is important to note that, in contrast to other areas in the skeleton, WBC imaging is not useful for diagnosing spondylodiscitis. In adults with spondylodiscitis, 50% or more may present as areas of decreased or absent WBC activity (Fig. 15.19). Although the explanation for this phenomenon is uncertain, decreased uptake is not specific for infection and is associated with numerous other conditions including treated spondylodiscitis, tumor, and prior radiation treatment [7].

15.3.1 In Vivo Labeled Leukocytes

There are significant limitations to the in vitro leukocyte labeling procedure, which requires skilled personnel, is labor-intensive, is not always available, and involves direct contact with blood products. The procedure may be difficult to perform in leukopenic patients and children and usually needs to be combined with marrow imaging for musculoskeletal infection. Because of these issues, considerable effort has been devoted to develop methods for labeling leukocytes in vivo.

Besilesomab, a 150 kDa murine monoclonal antibody of the IgG1 kappa isotype, binds to nonspecific cross-reacting antigen-95 (NCA-95), an epitope expressed on the cell membrane of granulocytes and granulocyte precursors. Within 45 minutes after administration, about 10% of ^{99m}Tc-besilesomab is neutrophil bound, while 20% remains in the circulation, localizing in inflammatory sites through nonspecific mechanisms. This agent is reasonably accurate for diagnosing nonosseous infections and is comparable to WBC imaging for diagnosing diabetic pedal osteomyelitis. Results for diagnosing prosthetic joint infection have been variable [52].

A significant disadvantage of ^{99m}Tc-besilesomab is the incidence of human antimurine antibody (HAMA) response, which ranges from less than 5% in patients receiving a single administration to more than 30% in patients receiving repeated injections. Consequently, patients should be prescreened for HAMA, should receive no more than 50 μg of antibody, and should not undergo repeated administrations of this agent [52]. ^{99m}Tc-besilesomab is not available in the United States.

Antibody fragments do not induce a HAMA response and are a potential alternative to whole antibodies. ^{99m}Tc-sulesomab is a 50 kDa fragment antigen-binding (Fab') portion of an IgG1 class murine monoclonal antibody that binds to normal cross-reactive antigen-90 on leukocytes. Approximately 3–6% of the injected activity is associated with circulating neutrophils; at 24 h after injection, about 35% of the remaining activity localizes to the bone marrow. Early investigations suggested that this agent binds to circulating neutrophils that migrate to foci of infection and to neutrophils already present at the site of infection. Subsequent data, however, suggest that the accumulation in infection is nonspecific. ^{99m}Tc-sulesomab is reasonably accurate for diagnosing soft tissue infections, is useful in fever of unknown origin, and is sensitive for diagnosing musculoskeletal infection. Specificity is variable but can be improved by performing dual-time point imaging, time activity curve analysis, and bone marrow imaging [52]. ^{99m}Tc-sulesomab is no longer available.

Radiolabeled cytokines, which are low molecular weight proteins that interact with specific cell surface receptors on specific cell populations, have shown promise as in vivo leukocyte labeling agents, but no large-scale clinical trials have been conducted [52].

15.4 Positron-Emitting Radiopharmaceuticals

Positron-emitting radiopharmaceuticals have several advantages over single-photon-emitting radiopharmaceuticals. Positron emission tomography (PET) provides high-resolution three-dimensional images of the whole body especially when performed as PET/CT, which facilitates precise localization of the radiopharmaceutical uptake. Semiquantitative analysis is more feasible

Fig. 15.18 (**a**) Infected left hip arthroplasty (same patient illustrated in Fig. 15.15). Although the planar labeled leukocyte/bone marrow image is positive for infection, it provides only minimal information on the location and extent of the infection. (**b**) On the dual-isotope SPECT/CT, the abnormal labeled leukocyte accumulation extends from the hip jointly posteriorly into the adjacent soft tissues (arrows). Providing information on the extent of the infection is useful for surgical planning

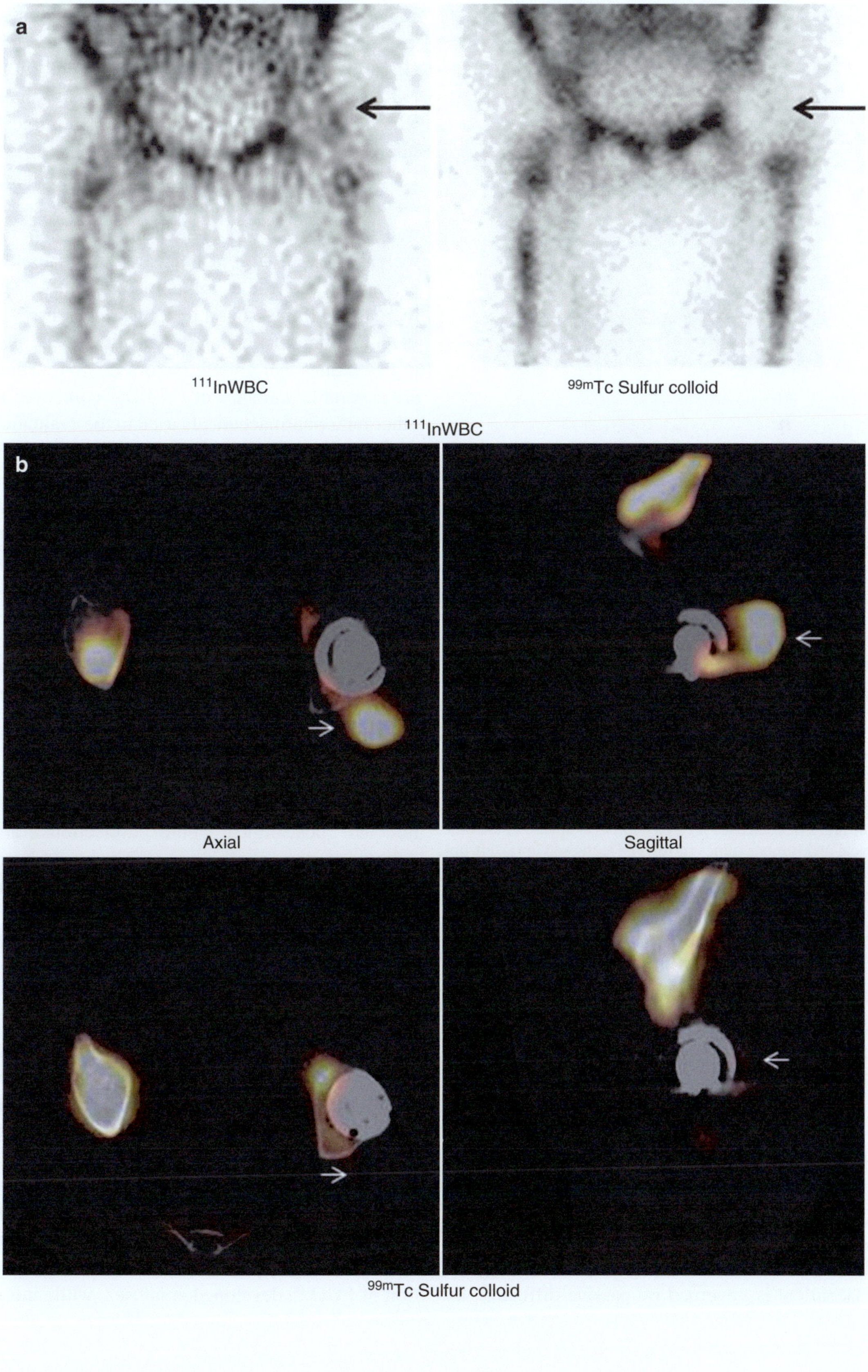
a
111InWBC
99mTc Sulfur colloid
111InWBC
b
Axial
Sagittal
99mTc Sulfur colloid

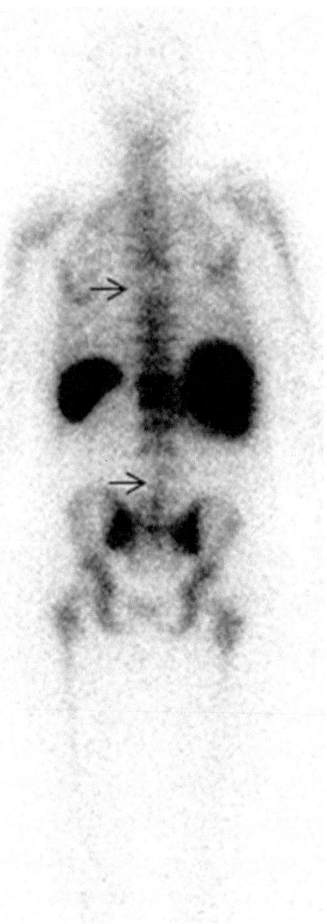

Fig. 15.19 Multifocal spondylodiscitis. There are multiple areas of decreased labeled leukocyte uptake in the thoracic and lumbar spines (arrows). Decreased uptake is not specific for infection and is associated with numerous other conditions, which is why labeled leukocyte imaging is not useful for this entity

with PET than with SPECT, may be useful for differentiating infectious from noninfectious conditions, and may be useful in monitoring response to therapy.

15.5 ^{18}F-Fluorodeoxyglucose

^{18}F-Fluorodeoxyglucose (^{18}F-FDG) is a structural analog of 2-deoxyglucose with a half-life of 110 minutes. Cellular uptake of this radiopharmaceutical is governed by passive diffusion, by active transport by a Na^+-dependent glucose transporter (GLUT), and via GLUT-1 through GLUT-13 transporters. Once inside the cell, ^{18}F-FDG is phosphorylated to ^{18}F-FDG-6-phosphate, which is not metabolized and is trapped intracellularly. ^{18}F-FDG accumulates in virtually all leukocytes, and its uptake in these cells is dependent on their metabolic rate and the number of glucose transporters. An increased number and an increased expression of glucose transporters are present in activated inflammatory cells. The increased affinity of these transporters for ^{18}F-FDG in inflammation is probably due to circulating cytokines and growth factors [53, 54]. There are several advantages of ^{18}F-FDG compared to other radiopharmaceuticals used in the evaluation of inflammation and infection. The small ^{18}F-FDG molecule rapidly enters poorly perfused regions, and the procedure is completed in 1–2 h. Uptake in normal bone marrow is usually low, which may facilitate the distinction of inflammatory cellular infiltrates from physiologic bone marrow activity. Following trauma or surgery, bone uptake generally normalizes relatively quickly, typically within 3–4 months. Degenerative bone disease is usually seen as faint increase in ^{18}F-FDG activity [54].

^{18}F-FDG is clinically helpful in approximately two-thirds of patients with suspected focal infection or inflammation. ^{18}F-FDG can identify infected postsurgical fluid collections and infected cysts in the kidney and liver and has a sensitivity of 90% for abdominal and pelvic abscesses, colitis, and diverticulitis [54, 55].

Fever of unknown origin (FUO) is a challenging clinical condition. There are no published guidelines, nor is there a recommended standard approach to its diagnostic workup. In up to 50% of cases, a definite diagnosis is not established. There are more than 200 causes of FUO, which usually are divided into four broad categories: infection (20–40%); malignancy (20–30%); noninfectious inflammatory diseases such as connective tissue diseases, vasculitis, and granulomatous diseases (10–30%); and miscellaneous (10–20%). Noninfectious inflammatory diseases and undiagnosed groups account for a higher proportion of FUO in developed countries, while infection and neoplasm are responsible for a higher proportion in underdeveloped countries [56].

The diagnostic workup of the patient with FUO begins with a comprehensive history, physical examination, and laboratory tests. ^{67}Ga and WBC imaging, typically used as second-line procedures, have met with only limited success. In contrast, ^{18}F-FDG has rapidly assumed an increasingly important role in the diagnostic workup of these patients (Figs. 15.20 and 15.21). Bleeker-Rovers et al. [54] reported that the positive and negative predictive values of ^{18}F-FDG PET were 87% and 95%, respectively. The positive and negative predictive values of chest and abdominal CT scans in a subgroup of these patients were 48% and 86%, respectively, compared to 65% and 90%, respectively, for ^{18}F-FDG-PET. Kubota et al. [57] found that ^{18}F-FDG PET sensitivity was highest (100%) in patients with tumors or granulomas and often provided additional information in patients with a final diagnosis of infection. A negative result reliably excluded malignancy and focal inflammatory disease. Bleeker-Rovers et al. [58] as part of a structured diagnostic protocol studied ^{18}F-FDG PET in 70 patients with FUO and reported that one third of these studies were clinically helpful. In a recent meta-analysis summary, sensitivity and specificity of ^{18}F-FDG-PET were 0.76 (0.66–0.83) and 0.50 (0.30–0.70), respectively [59].

Although initial investigations of FUO were conducted with ^{18}F-FDG-PET, ^{18}F-FDG-PET/CT has been used in more recent studies. The summary sensitivity and specificity of ^{18}F-FDG-PET/CT, as reported in a recent meta-analysis, were 0.86 (0.81–0.90) and 0.52 (0.36–0.67) vs. 0.76 (0.66–0.83) and 0.50 (0.30–0.70) for ^{18}F-FDG-PET [59]. The superiority of ^{18}F-FDG PET/CT is due to several factors, including improved anatomic localization of radiopharmaceutical uptake, better differentiation of physiologic and pathologic ^{18}F-FDG uptake, and additional information provided by the CT component [60].

^{18}F-FDG is more useful in patients with high fevers and in patients with continuous rather than intermittent fever. It is less useful in patients receiving empiric antibiotic therapy or steroids and in patients with normal erythrocyte sedimentation rate (ESR) and C-reactive protein (CRP). False-negative results have been reported in systemic lupus erythematosus, cytomegalovirus infection, toxoplasmosis, urinary infection, septicemia, pyelonephritis, and Crohn's disease [54, 57, 58, 61–64].

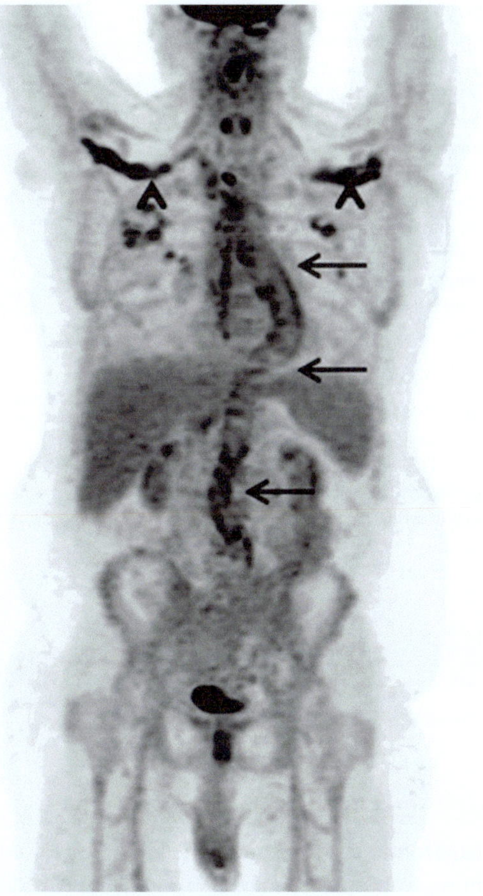

Fig. 15.20 Giant cell arteritis. There is diffusely increased ^{18}F-FDG uptake in the thoracic and abdominal aorta (arrows) and the subclavian arteries (arrowheads). Vasculitis is a well-recognized cause of fever of unknown origin in the elderly. ^{18}F-FDG is very sensitive for detecting large-vessel vasculitis and has shown promise for monitoring treatment response (Reproduced with permission from Palestro CJ. Imaging of Infection: The First Fifty Years. Sem Nucl Med. 2020;50:23–34)

Patients with occult bacteremia and no localizing signs can present a diagnostic dilemma similar to patients with classic FUO. ^{18}F-FDG provides useful information in this population by identifying the site of origin of the bacteremia, remote foci of infection, and complications such

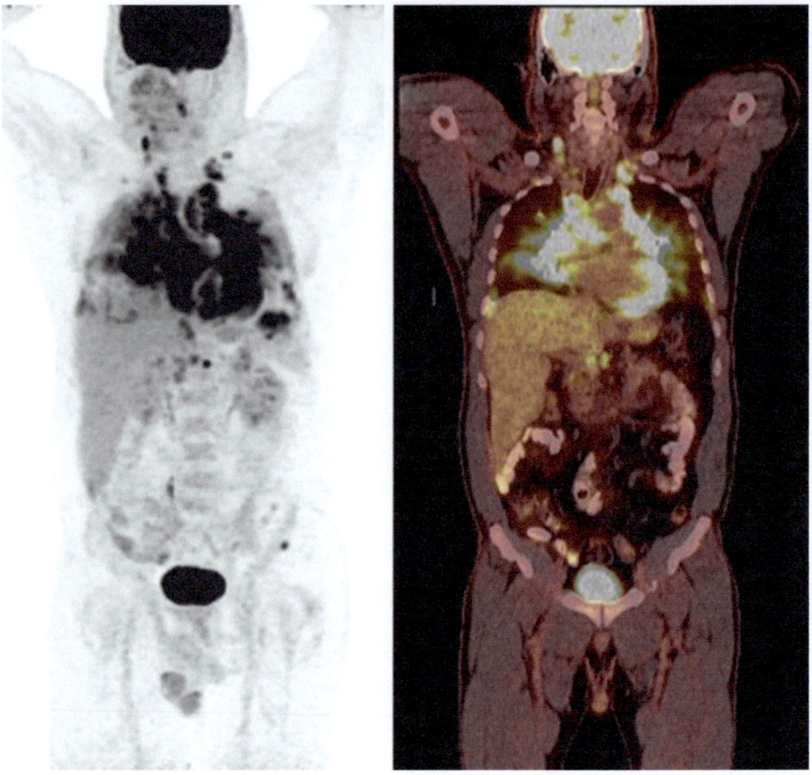

Fig. 15.21 Sarcoidosis. On the anterior maximum intensity projection (left) and coronal (right) images, there is extensive ^{18}F-FDG uptake in the supraclavicular regions, mediastinal and hilar lymph nodes, both lungs, upper abdominal lymph nodes, and left iliac crest. SUVmax ranged from 10.5 to 16.1. Sarcoid is another important cause of fever of unknown origin, and ^{18}F-FDG is very useful for determining the extent of disease and monitoring response to treatment

as thromboembolic phenomena, thereby contributing to patient management and improved outcomes. In patients with gram-positive bacteremia, ^{18}F-FDG PET facilitates earlier detection of clinically silent metastatic infectious foci and provides a cost-effective diagnostic tool by decreasing relapse rates, morbidity, and mortality [65, 66].

In children, FUO is defined as a persistent fever for at least 8 days, with no diagnosis after obtaining a thorough history, a complete physical examination, and laboratory data. In up to 20% of cases, a definitive diagnosis is not established [67]. The results of imaging studies have been disappointing, rarely identifying an unsuspected diagnosis [68]. ^{18}F-FDG, in contrast, contributes useful information in this population (Fig. 15.22). Jasper et al. [69] reviewed the results of ^{18}F-FDG-PET or PET/CT scans performed on children with FUO and reported that 19 of 44 scans (43%) were helpful in guiding focused evaluations in nine cases and eliminating additional workup in ten. Blokhuis et al. [70] retrospectively reviewed the results of ^{18}F-FDG PET/CT performed on 31 children with FUO and found that the test was helpful in about one third of the cases. Chang et al. [71] retrospectively reviewed the results of ^{18}F-FDG PET/CT performed on 19 critically ill children with FUO and reported that the test was helpful in 84% of the children.

The management of children with terminal chronic liver failure who are awaiting liver transplantation can be complicated by FUO. Extrahepatic infection may render the patient unsuitable for transplantation, while hepatic infection may necessitate liver resection for a cure. Sturm et al. [72] found that using ^{18}F-FDG PET to identify the source of fever can guide decisions on therapy and transplantation suitability.

In early investigations, ^{18}F-FDG was used as a second-line diagnostic tool in FUO. More recent data, however, suggest that this test should be performed earlier during the diagnostic evaluation. Using ^{18}F-FDG as a first-line diagnostic imaging procedure in FUO could reduce healthcare costs associated with this condition by decreasing the

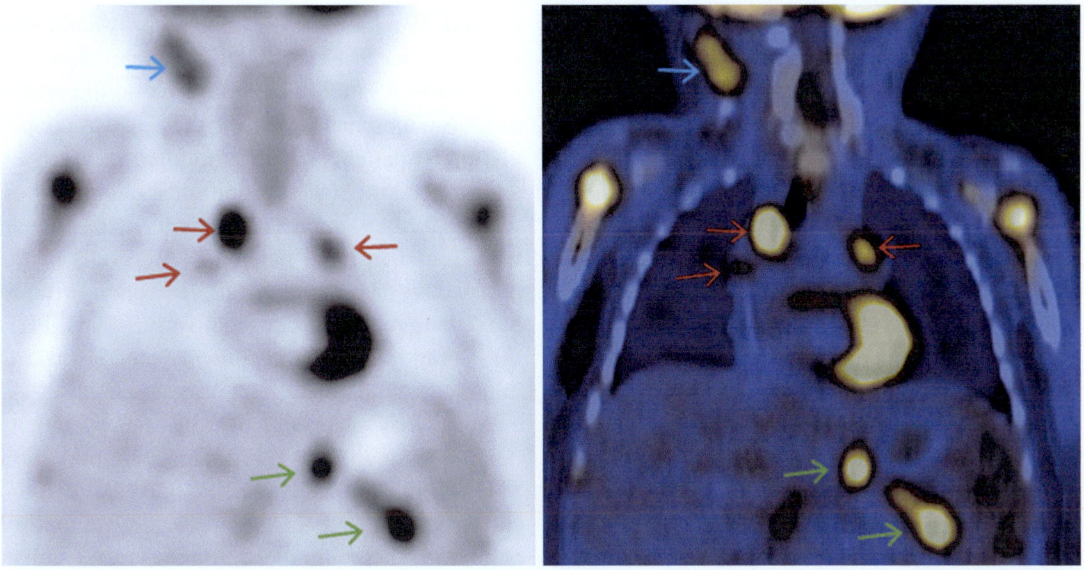

Fig. 15.22 X-Linked chronic granulomatous disease. On the coronal ^{18}F-FDG PET/CT, there are hypermetabolic lymph nodes in the right neck (blue arrow), mediastinum (red arrows), and abdomen (green arrows). Nodal biopsy revealed focal acute inflammation with non-necrotizing granulomas (Reproduced with permission, ref. (56))

number of diagnostic tests, obtaining a diagnosis and starting treatment earlier, decreasing morbidity and mortality, and shortening the length of hospitalization. Recent meta-analyses have supported these conclusions [73–75].

^{18}F-FDG is useful for diagnosing infections of the cardiovascular system, with a pooled sensitivity and specificity of 61% and 88%, respectively, for infectious endocarditis (IE). While overall sensitivity is low, ^{18}F-FDG is especially useful in patients with prosthetic heart valves [76]. ^{18}F-FDG is more sensitive but less specific than WBC imaging for diagnosing IE in this population. It has been suggested that WBC imaging should be utilized when ^{18}F-FDG results are inconclusive and during the first 2 months after cardiac surgery. ^{18}F-FDG, like WBC imaging, is also useful for detecting distant sites of infection [77, 78].

Results of ^{18}F-FDG for diagnosing infections of pacemakers and left ventricular assist devices also are encouraging [79–83]. ^{18}F-FDG PET/CT is useful for diagnosing pacemaker pocket infection, delineating the extent of infection, and facilitating the differentiation of device infection from postimplantation change. ^{18}F-FDG PET/CT improves the diagnostic accuracy of the modified Duke criteria for CIED infection and is potentially useful for making an early and accurate diagnosis of left ventricular assist device infection, determining the extent of infection, and monitoring response to therapy [82, 83]. In a recent meta-analysis, the pooled sensitivity of ^{18}F-FDG PET/CT for diagnosing CIED infection was 83% (95% CI 78–86%), and the pooled specificity was 89% (95% CI 84–94%). For diagnosing pocket infection, the sensitivity was 96% (95% CI 86–99%), and specificity was 97% (95% CI 86–99%). Accuracy for lead infections or CIED-IE was lower with pooled sensitivity of 76% (95% CI 65–85%) and specificity of 83% (95% CI 72–90%) [84].

False-negative results in IE and CIED infections are due to lesions that are below the limits of resolution for current PET/CT systems. Antibiotic treatment, especially for more than 1 week, also adversely affects sensitivity. False positive results are associated with postoperative inflammation and the presence of severe prosthetic valve thrombosis [79].

^{18}F-FDG is useful for diagnosing prosthetic vascular graft infection with high diagnostic accuracy and sensitivity, specificity, and positive predictive and negative predictive values ranging from 88% to 100% [85, 86]. Sah et al. [86] recently reported on a prospective investigation of ^{18}F-FDG PET/CT performed on 34 patients with suspected prosthetic vascular graft infection. Twenty-seven of the grafts were infected. Sensitivity, specificity, PPV, NPV, and accuracy of ^{18}F-FDG PET/CT for graft infection were 100%, 95%, 86%, 96%, and 97%, respectively.

Prosthetic vascular grafts can induce a foreign body inflammatory reaction, which can be associated with increased ^{18}F-FDG activity, even in the absence of infection. Knowledge of the typical uptake patterns associated with infection and foreign body reaction can improve the specificity of the test. Vascular graft infection typically presents as focal or heterogeneous uptake, while linear, diffuse, homogeneous uptake along the graft favors foreign body reaction (Fig. 15.23) [87, 88]. A "patched" pattern of ^{18}F-FDG uptake, which can be seen in patients in whom adhesives are used to secure the graft, is not indicative of infection [89].

^{18}F-FDG also may be useful for monitoring response to treatment in patients with prosthetic vascular graft infection. Husmann et al. [90] studied 25 patients with infected prosthetic vascular grafts. ^{18}F-FDG PET/CT had an impact on management in all patients. Based on the results of follow-up scans, antibiotic therapy was continued in 19 patients (76%), modified in 4 (16%), and stopped in 2 (8%). Additional abnormalities, which further impacted patient management, were found in eight patients. The results of the prospective Vascular Graft Infection Cohort Study suggest that consecutive ^{18}F-FDG PET/CTs could influence the clinical decision-making in patients with aortic graft infection [91].

Sensitivity in excess of 95% and specificity ranging from 75% to 99% have been reported for ^{18}F-FDG in acute and subacute bone and soft tissue infection. ^{18}F-FDG accurately diagnoses chronic and low-grade musculoskeletal infections, as well as non-arthroplasty orthopedic implant-associated infections [7, 92–94]. Published data strongly support the use of ^{18}F-FDG in suspected spondylodiscitis (Fig. 15.24). It is superior to bone, ^{67}Ga, and antigranulocyte antibody imaging and compares favorably to MRI for diagnosing these infections [10, 95–103]. It is especially useful for differentiating infection from severe degenerative changes involving the vertebral body endplates [97, 98]. There are data that

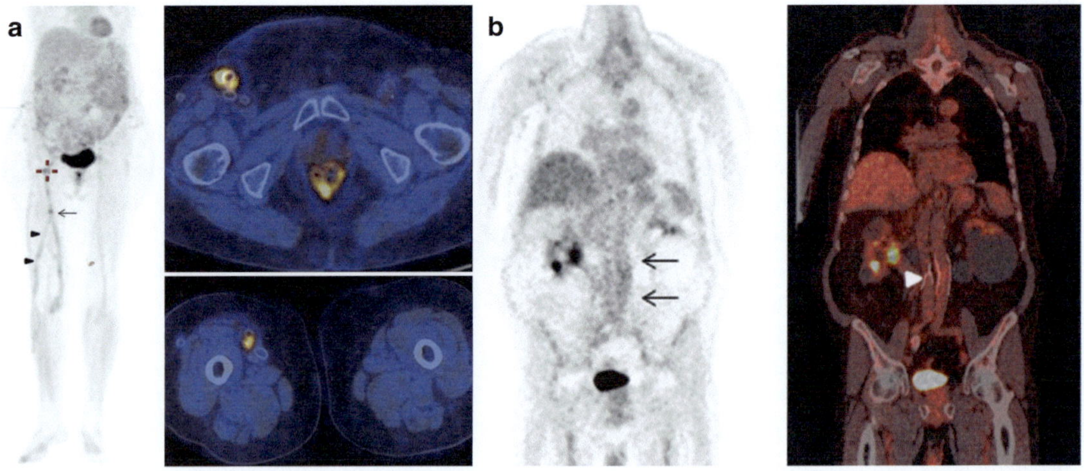

Fig. 15.23 (**a**) Infected prosthetic vascular graft. On the anterior MIP image (left), there is focally increased ^{18}F-FDG uptake in the upper (marker) and lower (arrow) parts of an infected right femoropopliteal graft. These abnormalities are better appreciated on the axial fused images (right). SUVmax ranged up to 6.3. There is homogeneous ^{18}F-FDG uptake in another, uninfected, graft (arrowheads), with an SUV max up to 3. This represents physiologic uptake in a foreign body reaction (courtesy Prof. Z. Keidar). (**b**) Uninfected prosthetic vascular graft. There is homogeneous ^{18}F-FDG uptake (SUV average: 2.8) in this 8-year-old uninfected abdominal aortic graft (arrows). Note the filter in the inferior vena cava (arrowhead)

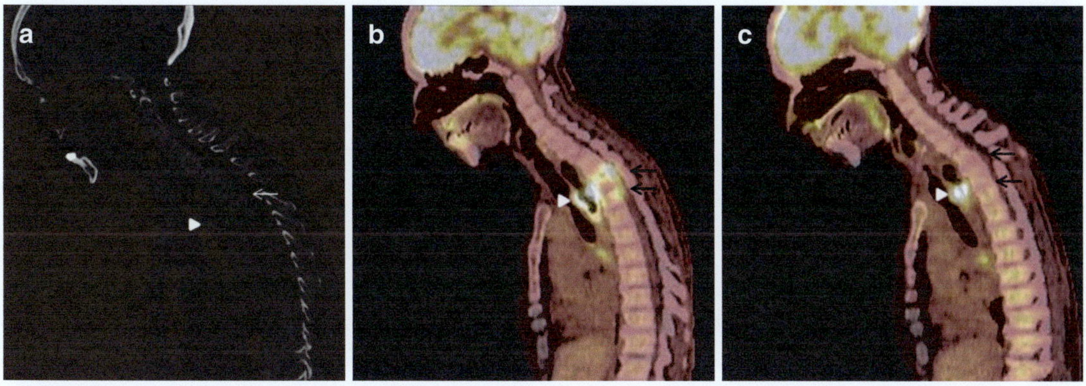

Fig. 15.24 (**a**) Spondylodiscitis. There is irregular fragmentation and destruction involving the T2 and T3 vertebral bodies (arrow) on the CT component of an ^{18}F-FDG PET/CT study performed on a 60-year-old woman with metastatic lung carcinoma. Note the esophageal stent (arrowhead). (**b**) On the fused image, there is increased ^{18}F-FDG uptake in the T2, T3, and T4 vertebrae (arrows) with SUVmax of 15.6. There is increased ^{18}F-FDG uptake around the esophageal stent (arrowhead) as well. (**c**) On the follow-up ^{18}F-FDG PET/CT performed approximately 3 months later, there is complete resolution of the vertebral body/disc space uptake (arrows). There is persistent activity around the esophageal stent (arrowhead) thought to represent foreign body reaction and/or metastatic disease. (Reproduced with permission from Palestro CJ. Imaging of Infection: The First Fifty Years. Sem Nucl Med. 2020;50:23–34)

suggest that ^{18}F-FDG may be useful for monitoring response to treatment in patients with spondylodiscitis, although the optimal criteria for assessing response have not yet been established (Fig. 15.24) [101, 102, 104–107].

There are some situations in which ^{18}F-FDG may be less useful. It is not clear that it is possible to differentiate pyogenic and tuberculous spondylodiscitis with this radiopharmaceutical. It is likely that it will be less reliable for differentiating infection from tumor and infection superimposed on tumor. Although uncommon, significant focal uptake in degenerative spine disease does occur. Increased uptake around uninfected spinal implants has been observed, which may adversely affect specificity [6].

Regardless of any limitations, ^{18}F-FDG accurately diagnoses spondylodiscitis, and published data support its role as the molecular imaging test of choice for this entity. Until more data are available, it should still be considered as an adjunct to MRI for the diagnosis of spondylodiscitis.

The results of ^{18}F-FDG for diagnosing diabetic foot osteomyelitis have been variable. Unfortunately, meaningful comparisons among investigations are not possible. In some studies only visual image interpretation was performed, and in others only semiquantitative analysis was used. Important details about the patients and their disease were also not consistently provided [7]. In one meta-analysis, the sensitivity and specificity of ^{18}F-FDG for diagnosing diabetic foot osteomyelitis were 74% and 91%, respectively, while in another, the sensitivity and specificity of ^{18}F-FDG were 89% and 92%, respectively [108, 109].

The role of ^{18}F-FDG for diagnosing prosthetic joint infection has been investigated extensively with conflicting, and often contradictory, results. Investigations comparing ^{18}F-FDG and bone or WBC imaging have also yielded contradictory results. In some investigations, ^{18}F-FDG was more accurate, while in others bone and/or WBC imaging were more accurate for diagnosing infection [7, 28, 42, 45, 110–115].

Molecular imaging is frequently used to differentiate prosthetic infection from aseptic loosening, the latter being the most common cause of prosthetic failure. ^{18}F-FDG cannot consistently differentiate between these two conditions because both infection and aseptic loosening can be accompanied by an inflammatory response characterized by intense leukocyte infiltration

[7]. The variability in published results may be related to the prevalence of infection and aseptic loosening in the populations studied; unfortunately, this information is often lacking. At the present time, ^{18}F-FDG does not have a role in the diagnosis of lower extremity prosthetic joint infection.

15.6 Other Positron-Emitting Radiopharmaceuticals

Investigators have studied both in vitro and in vivo leukocyte labeling with various PET agents. Although published results using leukocytes labeled in vitro with ^{18}F-FDG were encouraging, there are several drawbacks to this procedure. The 110-min half-life of fluorine-18 makes it impractical for labeling to be performed off-site, so the test would be limited to institutions capable of performing the labeling on-site. The short physical half-life of fluorine-18 also precludes delayed imaging. Labeling efficiency is significantly lower and more variable than with ^{111}In-oxine, and ^{18}F-FDG rapidly elutes from leukocytes [116–120].

The positron-emitting radionuclides, copper-64, and zirconium-89 have also been used to label leukocytes in vitro, but no clinical or even preclinical data are available for these agents [120, 121]. A copper-64-labeled peptide, cFLFLFK-PEG-64Cu, which targets the formyl peptide receptor (FPR) on leukocytes, has been studied in a murine model of *Klebsiella pneumoniae*. At 18 h postinjection, pulmonary uptake of this agent was five to six times higher than that of controls [122].

Recently the positron emitter gallium-68 (^{68}Ga) has become more widely available, and the potential of this agent for diagnosing infection is being investigated. ^{68}Ga-citrate reduces or eliminates some of the disadvantages of ^{67}Ga, such as poor image quality and the long interval between administration and imaging. The uptake mechanisms of both radiopharmaceuticals are the same however, and consequently, ^{68}Ga like ^{67}Ga lacks specificity [123, 124].

Numerous cells, including macrophages, express translocator protein (TSPO), which is upregulated in inflammation and downregulated by anti-inflammatory pharmacotherapies. TSPO is widely distributed throughout the body, and consequently its use has been limited to imaging in the central nervous system, where the background activity is low. Recently however, small-molecule TSPO-targeted ligands have been developed for imaging peripheral macrophage-expressing TSPO. One of the more promising of these ligands is DPA-713 which is retained by macrophages for up to 24 h postinjection. Due to its rapid clearance from most other TSPO-expressing tissues, imaging of the body outside the central nervous system can now be performed. Murine tuberculous granulomas have been successfully imaged with iodine-124 DPA-713 [125].

15.7 Infection-Specific Agents

15.7.1 Radiolabeled Antibiotics

Although useful, none of the clinically available radiopharmaceuticals is specific for infection, and the search continues for such an agent. Radiolabeled antibiotics have been investigated as infection-specific radiopharmaceuticals. The most extensively investigated of these compounds is ^{99m}Tc-ciprofloxacin, and early investigations reported high sensitivity and specificity. Unfortunately, subsequent studies have cast serious doubts about specificity, and much of the original enthusiasm for these compounds has faded [126].

15.7.2 ^{111}In-Biotin

Biotin, or vitamin B7, is used as a growth factor by certain bacteria. ^{111}In-biotin, alone and in combination with streptavidin, has been used for imaging musculoskeletal infection. Advantages of this radiopharmaceutical include same day imaging, minimal bone marrow uptake, and less patient radiation than WBC and ^{67}Ga studies.

Although the reported results have been encouraging, this radiopharmaceutical is available in only a very few centers [127, 128].

15.7.3 Radiolabeled Antimicrobial Peptides

Antimicrobial peptides (AMPs) are an important component of the natural defenses of most living organisms. Most are small, cationic, and amphipathic (hydrophilic and hydrophobic) and attack pathogens by multiple mechanisms. Their expression may be constant or induced on contact with microbes; they also may be transported by circulating leukocytes to sites of infection [52, 129].

Ubiquicidin (UBI) is a murine AMP present in the cytosolic fraction of macrophages [130]. ^{99m}Tc-UBI-29-41, a radiolabeled synthetic fragment of UBI, is sensitive and specific for a variety of infections and has shown potential for monitoring treatment response [131, 132]. While most investigations have used ^{99m}Tc as the radiolabel, ^{68}Ga-labeled antimicrobial peptides, including the UBI-29-41 fragment of ubiquicidin, are under investigation [133–135]. Over the past two decades and in spite of the favorable results that have been reported for these agents, no large-scale clinical trial of radiolabeled AMPS has ever been conducted.

Iodine-124-fialuridine. The radioiodinated thymidine analogue fialuridine (FIAU) was developed for reporter genes and for cells that were transfected with herpes simplex virus thymidine kinase (TK). This enzyme transfers a phosphate group from ATP to pyrimidine deoxynucleoside which then diffuses into the cell where the phosphorylated tracer is trapped with the TK activity [136]. In an initial clinical investigation, ^{124}I-FIAU showed promise as an infection-specific radiopharmaceutical [137]. Results of subsequent investigations involving diabetic foot and prosthetic joint infections were poor, and the future of this agent is doubtful [138, 139].

Bacteria-specific agents. Radiolabeled sugars, including fluorine-18-labeled maltose and maltohexose and fluorodeoxysorbitol (FDS), have demonstrated specificity for bacterial pathogens. ^{18}F-FDS rapidly and selectively accumulates in *E. coli* bacteria, but not in gram-positive bacteria, cancer, or normal mammalian cells. In an animal model, this agent differentiated infection from sterile inflammation and showed promise for monitoring response to treatment. In normal volunteers, it was safe, well tolerated, and rapidly cleared [140].

15.8 Summary

In spite of the fact that currently available molecular imaging tests reflect the host's response to inflammation and infection, these agents are nevertheless extremely useful. In the immunocompetent population, labeled leukocytes remain the molecular imaging test of choice for most infections. ^{67}Ga however is useful for the diagnosis of acute interstitial nephritis and is an alternative to ^{18}F-FDG, for indications such as spondylodiscitis and sarcoid, when ^{18}F-FDG cannot be performed. ^{18}F-FDG has emerged as the molecular imaging test of choice for FUO and spondylodiscitis and is useful for diagnosing cardiovascular infections. Moreover, data suggest that ^{18}F-FDG may have a role in monitoring response to therapy.

References

1. Palestro C. The current role of gallium imaging in infection. Semin Nucl Med. 1994;24:128–41.
2. Palestro CJ. Scintigraphic diagnosis of inflammation and infection. In: Brant WE, Helms CA, editors. Fundamentals of diagnostic radiology. 4th ed. Philadelphia, PA: Lippincott, Williams and Wilkins; 2012. p. 1339–52.
3. Palestro CJ, Schultz BG, Horowitz M, Swyer AJ. Indium-111-leukocyte and gallium-67 imaging in acute sarcoidosis: report of two cases. J Nucl Med. 1992;33:2027–9.
4. Sulavik SB, Spencer RP, Weed DA, Shapiro HR, Shiue ST, Castriotta RJ. Recognition of distinctive patterns of gallium-67 distribution in sarcoidosis. J Nucl Med. 1990;31:1909–14.
5. Rohatgi PK, Singh R, Vieras F. Extrapulmonary localization of gallium in sarcoidosis. Clin Nucl Med. 1987;12:9–16.

6. Raghavan M, Lazzeri E, Palestro CJ. Imaging of spondylodiscitis. Semin Nucl Med. 2018;48:131–47.
7. Palestro CJ. Radionuclide imaging of osteomyelitis. Semin Nucl Med. 2015;45:32–46.
8. Lievano P, De la Cueva L, Navarro P, et al. 67Ga SPECT/low-dose CT. A case report of spondylodiscitis and Schmorl's node. Rev Esp Med Nucl. 2009;28:288–90.
9. Domínguez ML, Lorente R, Rayo JI, et al. SPECT-CT with (67)Ga-citrate in the management of spondylodiscitis. Rev Esp Med Nucl Imaging Mol. 2012;31:34–9.
10. Fuster D, Solà O, Soriano A, et al. A prospective study comparing whole-body FDG PET/CT to combined planar bone scan with 67Ga SPECT/CT in the diagnosis of spondylodiskitis. Clin Nucl Med. 2012;37:827–32.
11. Tamm AS, Abele JT. Bone and gallium single-photon emission computed tomography-computed tomography is equivalent to magnetic resonance imaging in the diagnosis of infectious spondylodiscitis: a retrospective study. Can Assoc Radiol J. 2017;68:41–6.
12. Border WA, Holbrook JH, Peterson MC. Gallium citrate Ga 67 scanning in acute renal failure. West J Med. 1995;162:477–8.
13. Linton AL, Richmond JM, Clark WF, et al. Gallium67 scintigraphy in the diagnosis of acute renal disease. Clin Nephrol. 1985;24:84–7.
14. Joaquim AI, Mendes GEF, Patrícia FF, et al. Ga-67 scintigraphy in the differential diagnosis between acute interstitial nephritis and acute tubular necrosis: an experimental study. Nephrol Dial Transplant. 2010;25:3277–82.
15. Love C, Palestro CJ. Radionuclide imaging of inflammation and infection in the acute care setting. Semin Nucl Med. 2013;43:102–13.
16. Palestro CJ, Love C, Bhargava KK. Labeled leukocyte imaging: current status and future directions. Q J Nucl Med Mol Imaging. 2009;53:105–23.
17. Love C, Opoku-Agyemang P, Tomas MB, et al. Pulmonary activity on labeled leukocyte images: physiologic, pathologic, and imaging correlations. RadioGraphics. 2002;22:1385–93.
18. Love C, Palestro CJ. Radionuclide imaging of infection. J Nucl Med Technol. 2004;32:47–57.
19. Palestro CJ, Love C, Tronco GG, et al. Fever in the postoperative patient: role of radionuclide imaging in its diagnosis. Radiographics. 2000;20:1649–60.
20. Lou L, Alibhai KN, Winkelaar GB, et al. 99mTc-WBC scintigraphy with SPECT/CT in the evaluation of arterial graft infection. Nucl Med Commun. 2010;31:411–6.
21. Erba PA, Leo G, Sollini M, et al. Radiolabelled leucocyte scintigraphy versus conventional radiological imaging for the management of late, low-grade vascular prosthesis infections. Eur J Nucl Med Mol Imaging. 2014;41:357–68.
22. Bar-Shalom R, Yefremov N, Guralnik L, et al. SPECT/CT using 67Ga and 111 in-labeled leukocyte scintigraphy for diagnosis of infection. J Nucl Med. 2006;47:587–94.
23. Erba PA, Sollini M, Conti U, et al. Radiolabeled WBC scintigraphy in the diagnostic workup of patients with suspected device-related infections. JACC Cardiovasc Imaging. 2013;6:1075–86.
24. Litzler PY, Manrique A, Etienne M, et al. Leukocyte SPECT/CT for detecting infection of left-ventricular-assist devices: preliminary results. J Nucl Med. 2010;51:1044–8.
25. Erba PA, Conti U, Lazzeri E, et al. Added value of 99mTc-HMPAO-labeled leukocyte SPECT/CT in the characterization and management of patients with infectious endocarditis. J Nucl Med. 2012;53:1235–43.
26. Hyafil F, Rouzet F, Lepage L, et al. Role of radiolabelled leucocyte scintigraphy in patients with a suspicion of prosthetic valve endocarditis and inconclusive echocardiography. Eur Heart J Cardiovasc Imaging. 2013;14:586–94.
27. Palestro CJ, Love C, Tronco GG, et al. Combined labeled leukocyte and technetium-99m sulfur colloid marrow imaging for diagnosing musculoskeletal infection: principles, technique, interpretation, indications and limitations. RadioGraphics. 2006;26:859–70.
28. Palestro CJ. Radionuclide imaging of musculoskeletal infection: a review. J Nucl Med. 2016;57:1406–12.
29. Glaudemans AW, De Vries EF, Vermeulen LE, et al. A large retrospective single centre study to define best image acquisition protocols and interpretation criteria for white blood cell scintigraphy with 99mTc-HMPAO labelled leukocytes in musculoskeletal infections. Eur J Nucl Med Mol Imaging. 2013;40:1760–9.
30. Palestro CJ, Love C. Nuclear medicine and diabetic foot infections. Semin Nucl Med. 2009;39:52–65.
31. Przybylski MM, Holloway S, Vyce SD, Obando A. Diagnosing osteomyelitis in the diabetic foot: a pilot study to examine the sensitivity and specificity of Tc99mwhite blood cell-labelled single photon emission computed tomography/computed tomography. Int Wound J. 2016;13:382–9.
32. Heiba SI, Kolker D, Mocherla B, et al. The optimized evaluation of diabetic foot infection by dual isotope SPECT/CT imaging protocol. J Foot Ankle Surg. 2010;49:529–36.
33. Heiba S, Kolker D, Ong L, et al. Dual-isotope SPECT/CT impact on hospitalized patients with suspected diabetic foot infection: saving limbs, lives, and resources. Nucl Med Commun. 2013;34:877–84.
34. Filippi L, Uccioli L, Giurato L, et al. Diabetic foot infection: usefulness of SPECT/CT for 99mTc-HMPAO-labeled leukocyte imaging. J Nucl Med. 2009;50:1042–6.
35. Erdman WA, Buethe J, Bhore R, et al. Indexing severity of diabetic foot infection with 99mTc-WBC SPECT/CT hybrid imaging. Diabetes Care. 2012;35:1826–31.

36. Vouillarmet J, Morelec I, Thivolet C. Assessing diabetic foot osteomyelitis remission with white blood cell SPECT/CT imaging. Diabet Med. 2014;31:1093–9.
37. Lazaga F, Van Asten SA, Nichols A, et al. Hybrid imaging with 99mTc-WBC SPECT/CT to monitor the effect of therapy in diabetic foot osteomyelitis. Int Wound J. 2015;13:1158. https://doi.org/10.1111/iwj.12433.
38. Mulamba L'A H, Ferrant A, Leners N, et al. Indium-111 leucocyte scanning in the evaluation of painful hip arthroplasty. Acta Orthop Scand 1983;54:695–697.
39. Palestro CJ, Kim CK, Swyer AJ, et al. Total hip arthroplasty: periprosthetic indium-111-labeled leukocyte activity and complementary technetium-99m-sulfur colloid imaging in suspected infection. J Nucl Med. 1990;31:1950–5.
40. Palestro CJ, Swyer AJ, Kim CK, et al. Infected knee prostheses: diagnosis with in-111 leukocyte, Tc-99m sulfur colloid, and Tc-99m MDP imaging. Radiology. 1991;179:645–8.
41. Joseph TN, Mujitaba M, Chen AL, et al. Efficacy of combined technetium-99m sulfur colloid/indium-111 leukocyte scans to detect infected total hip and knee arthroplasties. J Arthroplast. 2001;16:753–8.
42. Love C, Marwin SE, Tomas MB, et al. Diagnosing infection in the failed joint replacement: a comparison of coincidence detection fluorine-18 FDG and indium-111-labeled leukocyte/technetium-99m-sulfur colloid marrow imaging. J Nucl Med. 2004;45:1864–71.
43. El Espera I, Blondet C, Moullart V, et al. The usefulness of 99mTc sulfur colloid bone marrow scintigraphy combined with 111In leucocyte scintigraphy in prosthetic joint infection. Nucl Med Commun. 2004;25:171–5.
44. Pill SG, Parvizi J, Tang PH, et al. Comparison of fluorodeoxyglucose positron emission tomography and (111)indium-white blood cell imaging in the diagnosis of periprosthetic infection of the hip. J Arthroplast. 2006;21:91–7.
45. Basu S, Kwee TC, Saboury B, et al. FDG-PET for diagnosing infection in hip and knee prostheses: prospective study in 221 prostheses and subgroup comparison with combined(111)in-labeled leukocyte/(99m)Tc-sulfur colloid bone marrow imaging in 88 prostheses. Clin Nucl Med. 2014;39:609–15.
46. Grate V, Feist M, Leaner S, et al. Detection of low-grade prosthetic joint infections using 99mTc-antigranulocyte SPECT/CT: initial clinical results. Eur J Nucl Med Mol Imaging. 2010;37:1751–9.
47. Tam HH, Balding B, Rahman F, et al. SPECT-CT in total hip arthroplasty. Clin Radiol. 2014;69:82–95.
48. Al-Nathan K, Michopoulou S, Allie R, et al. Painful knee prosthesis: can we help with bone SPECT/CT? Nucl Med Commun. 2014;35:182–8.
49. Kim HO, Na SJ, Oh SJ, et al. Usefulness of adding SPECT/CT to 99mTc-hexamethylpropylene amine oxime (HMPAO)-labeled leukocyte imaging for diagnosing prosthetic joint infections. J Comput Assist Tomogr. 2014;38(2):313–9.
50. Berber R, Henckel J, Khoo M, et al. Clinical usefulness of SPECT-CT in patients with an unexplained pain in metal on metal (MOM) total hip arthroplasty. J Arthroplast. 2015;30:687–94.
51. Mandegaran R, Agrawal K, Vijayanathan S. The value of 99mTc-MDP bone SPECT/CT in evaluation of patients with painful knee prosthesis. Nucl Med Commun. 2018;39:397–404.
52. Palestro CJ, Glaudemans AWJM, Dierckx RAJO. Multiagent imaging of inflammation and infection. Clin Transl Imaging. 2013;1:385–96.
53. Meller J, Sahlmann CO, Scheel AK. 18F-FDG PET and PET/CT in fever of unknown origin. J Nucl Med. 2007;48:35–45.
54. Bleeker-Rovers CP, de Kleijn EM, et al. Clinical value of FDG PET in patients with fever of unknown origin and patients suspected of focal infection or inflammation. Eur J Nucl Med Mol Imaging. 2004;31:29–37.
55. Petruzzi N, Shanthly N, Thakur M. Recent trends in soft-tissue infection imaging. Semin Nucl Med. 2009;39:115–23.
56. Palestro CJ, Love C. Nuclear medicine imaging in fever of unknown origin: the new paradigm. Curr Pharm Des. 2018;24:814–20.
57. Kubota K, Nakamoto Y, Tamaki N, et al. FDG-PET for the diagnosis of fever of unknown origin: a Japanese multi-center study. Ann Nucl Med. 2011;25:355–64.
58. Bleeker-Rovers CP, Vos FJ, Mudde AH, et al. A prospective multi-centre study of the value of FDG-PET as part of a structured diagnostic protocol in patients with fever of unknown origin. Eur J Nucl Med Mol Imaging. 2007;34:694–703.
59. Takeuchi M, Dahabreh IJ, Nihashi T, et al. Nuclear imaging for classic fever of unknown origin: meta-analysis. J Nucl Med. 2016;57:1913–9.
60. Kouijzer IJ, Bleeker-Rovers CP, Oyen WJ. FDG-PET in fever of unknown origin. Semin Nucl Med. 2013;43:333–9.
61. Gafter-Gvili A, Raibman S, Grossman A, et al. [18F] FDG-PET/CT for the diagnosis of patients with fever of unknown origin. QJM. 2015;108:289–98.
62. Crouzet J, Boudousq V, Lechiche C, et al. Place of (18)F-FDG-PET with computed tomography in the diagnostic algorithm of patients with fever of unknown origin. Eur J Clin Microbiol Infect Dis. 2012;31:1727–33.
63. Buysschaert I, Vanderschueren S. Blockmans et al. contribution of (18)fluoro-deoxyglucose positron emission tomography to the work-up of patients with fever of unknown origin. Eur J Intern Med. 2004;15:151–6.
64. Federici L, Blondet C, Imperiale A, Sibilia J, Pasquali JL, Pflumio F, et al. Value of (18)F-FDG-PET/CT in patients with fever of unknown origin and unexplained prolonged inflammatory syndrome:

a single centre analysis experience. Int J Clin Pract. 2010;64:55–60.
65. Vos FJ, Bleeker-Rovers CP, Kullberg BJ, et al. Cost-effectiveness of routine (18)F-FDG PET/CT in high-risk patients with gram-positive bacteremia. J Nucl Med. 2011;52:1673–8.
66. Berrevoets MAH, Kouijzer IJE, Aarntzen EHJG, et al. 18F-FDG PET/CT optimizes treatment in *Staphylococcus aureus* bacteremia and is associated with reduced mortality. J Nucl Med. 2017;58:1504–10.
67. Lorin MI, Feigin RD. Fever without localizing signs and fever of unknown origin. In: Feigin RD, Cherry JD, editors. Textbook of pediatric infectious diseases. 4th ed. Philadelphia, PA: WB Saunders; 1998. p. 820–30.
68. Steele RW, Jones SM, Lowe BA, Glasier CM. Usefulness of scanning procedures for diagnosis of fever of unknown origin in children. J Pediatr. 1991;119:526–30.
69. Jasper N, Däbritz J, Frosch M, et al. Diagnostic value of [18F]-FDG PET/CT in children with fever of unknown origin or unexplained signs of inflammation. Eur J Nucl Med Mol Imaging. 2010;37:136–45.
70. Blokhuis GJ, Bleeker-Rovers CP, Diender MG, et al. Diagnostic value of FDG-PET/(CT) in children with fever of unknown origin and unexplained fever during immune suppression. Eur J Nucl Med Mol Imaging. 2014;41:1916–23.
71. Chang L, Cheng MF, Jou ST, et al. Search of unknown fever focus using PET in critically ill children with complicated underlying diseases. Pediatr Crit Care Med. 2016;172:e58–65.
72. Sturm E, Rings EH, Scholvinck EH, et al. Fluordeoxyglucose positron emission tomography contributes to management of pediatric liver transplantation candidates with fever of unknown origin. Liver Transpl. 2006;12:1698–704.
73. Besson FL, Chaumet-Riffaud P, Playe M, Noel N, Lambotte O, Goujard C, et al. Contribution of (18) F-FDG PET in the diagnostic assessment of fever of unknown origin (FUO): a stratification-based meta-analysis. Eur J Nucl Med Mol Imaging. 2016;43:1887–95.
74. Sioka C, Assimakopoulos A, Fotopoulos A. The diagnostic role of (18)F fluorodeoxyglucose positron emission tomography in patients with fever of unknown origin. Eur J Clin Investig. 2015;45:601–8.
75. Dong MJ, Zhao K, Liu ZF, et al. A meta-analysis of the value of fluorodeoxyglucose-PET/PET-CT in the evaluation of fever of unknown origin. Eur J Radiol. 2011;80:834–44.
76. Yan J, Zhang C, Niu Y, et al. The role of 18F-FDG PET/CT in infectious endocarditis: a systematic review and meta- analysis. Int J Clin Pharmacol Ther. 2016;54:337–42.
77. Rouzet F, Chequer R, Benali K, et al. Respective performance of 18F-FDG PET and radiolabeled leukocyte scintigraphy for the diagnosis of prosthetic valve endocarditis. J Nucl Med. 2014;55:1980–5.
78. Kouijzer IJE, Berrevoets MAH, Aarntzen EHJG. 18F-fluorodeoxyglucose positron-emission tomography combined with computed tomography as a diagnostic tool in native valve endocarditis. Nucl Med Commun. 2018;39:747–52.
79. Pizzi MN, Roque A, Fernandez-Hidalgo N, et al. Improving the diagnosis of infective endocarditis in prosthetic valves and intracardiac devices with 18F-fluordeoxyglucose positron emission tomography computed tomography angiography initial results at an infective endocarditis referral center. Circulation. 2015;132:1113–26.
80. Bensimhon L, Lavergne T, Hugonnet F, et al. Whole body [(18) F]fluorodeoxyglucose positron emission tomography imaging for the diagnosis of pacemaker or implantable cardioverter defibrillator infection: a preliminary prospective study. Clin Microbiol Infect. 2011;17:836–44.
81. Sarrazin JF, Philippon F, Tessier M, et al. Usefulness of fluorine-18 positron emission tomography/computed tomography for identification of cardiovascular implantable electronic device infections. J Am Coll Cardiol. 2012;59:1616–25.
82. Graziosi M, Nanni C, Lorenzini M, et al. Role of ^{18}F-FDG PET/CT in the diagnosis of infective endocarditis in patients with an implanted cardiac device: a prospective study. Eur J Nucl Med Mol Imaging. 2014;41:1617–23.
83. Dell'Aquila AM, Mastrobuoni S, Alles S, et al. Contributory role of fluorine 18-fluorodeoxyglucose positron emission tomography/computed tomography in the diagnosis and clinical management of infections in patients supported with a continuous-flow left ventricular assist device. Ann Thorac Surg. 2016;101:87–94.
84. Mahmood M, Kendi AT, Farid S. Role of 18F-FDG PET/CT in the diagnosis of cardiovascular implantable electronic device infections: a meta-analysis. J Nucl Cardiol. 2017;26:958. https://doi.org/10.1007/s12350-017-1063-0.
85. Keidar Z, Engel A, Hoffman A, et al. Prosthetic vascular graft infection: the role of 18F-FDG PET/CT. J Nucl Med. 2007;48:1230–6.
86. Sah BR, Husmann L, Mayer D, et al. Diagnostic performance of 18F-FDG-PET/CT in vascular graft infections. Eur J Vasc Endovasc Surg. 2015;49:455–64.
87. Keidar Z, Pirmisashvili N, Leiderman M, et al. 18F-FDG uptake in noninfected prosthetic vascular grafts: incidence, patterns, and changes over time. J Nucl Med. 2014;55:392–5.
88. Saleem BR, Pol RA, Slart RH, et al. 18F-Fluorodeoxyglucose positron emission tomography/CT scanning in diagnosing vascular prosthetic graft infection. Biomed Res Int. 2014;1:471971.
89. Bowles H, Ambrosioni J, Mestres G, et al. Diagnostic yield of 18F-FDG PET/CT in suspected diagnosis of vascular graft infection: a prospective cohort

study. J Nucl Cardiol. 2018; https://doi.org/10.1007/s12350-018-1337-1.
90. Husmann L, Sah BR, Scherrer A, et al. ^{18}F-FDG PET/CT for therapy control in vascular graft infections: a first feasibility study. J Nucl Med. 2015;56:1024–9.
91. Husmann L, Ledergerber B, Anagnostopoulos A, et al. The role of FDG PET/CT in therapy control of aortic graft infection. Eur J Nucl Med Mol Imaging. 2018; https://doi.org/10.1007/s00259-018-4069-1.
92. Guhlmann A, Brecht-Krauss D, Suger G, et al. Chronic osteomyelitis: detection with FDG PET and correlation with histopathologic findings. Radiology. 1998;206:749–54.
93. de Winter F, van de Wiele C, Vogelaers D, et al. Fluorine-18 fluorodeoxyglucose positron emission tomography: a highly accurate imaging modality for the diagnosis of chronic musculoskeletal infections. J Bone Joint Surg. 2001;83-A:651–60.
94. Schiesser M, Stumpe KD, Trentz O, et al. Detection of metallic implant-associated infections with FDG PET in patients with trauma: correlation with microbiologic results. Radiology. 2003;226:391–8.
95. Guhlmann A, Brecht-Krauss D, Suger G, et al. Fluorine-18-FDG PET and technetium-99m antigranulocyte antibody scintigraphy in chronic osteomyelitis. J Nucl Med. 1998;39:2145–52.
96. Gratz S, Dorner J, Fischer U, Behr TM, et al. F-18-FDG hybrid PET in patients with suspected spondylitis. Eur J Nucl Med Mol Imaging. 2002;29:516–24.
97. Ohtori S, Suzuki M, Koshi T, et al. 18F-fluorodeoxyglucose-PET for patients with suspected spondylitis showing Modic change. Spine. 2010;35:E1599–603.
98. Stumpe KD, Zanetti M, Weishaupt D, et al. FDG positron emission tomography for differentiation of degenerative and infectious endplate abnormalities in the lumbar spine detected on MR imaging. AJR Am J Roentgenol. 2002;179:1151–7.
99. Seifen T, Rettenbacher L, Thaler C, et al. Prolonged back pain attributed to suspected spondylodiscitis. The value of 18F-FDG PET/CT imaging in the diagnostic work-up of patients. Nuklearmedizin. 2012;51:194–200.
100. Fuster D, Tomás X, Mayoral M, et al. Prospective comparison of whole-body 18F-FDG PET/CT and MRI of the spine in the diagnosis of haematogenous spondylodiscitis. Eur J Nucl Med Mol Imaging. 2015;42:264–71.
101. Skanjeti A, Penna D, Douroukas A, et al. PET in the clinical work-up of patients with spondylodiscitis: a new tool for the clinician? Q J Nucl Med Mol Imaging. 2012;56:569–76.
102. Ioannou S, Chatziioannou S, Pneumaticos SG, Zormpala A, Sipsas NV. Fluorine-18 fluoro-2-deoxy-D-glucose positron emission tomography/computed tomography scan contributes to the diagnosis and management of brucellar spondylodiskitis. BMC Infect Dis. 2013;13:73.
103. Nakahara M, Ito M, Hattori N, et al. 18F-FDG-PET/CT better localizes active spinal infection than MRI for successful minimally invasive surgery. Acta Radiol. 2015;56:829–36.
104. Nanni C, Boriani L, Salvadori C, et al. FDG PET/CT is useful for the interim evaluation of response to therapy in patients affected by haematogenous spondylodiscitis. Eur J Nucl Med Mol Imaging. 2012;39:1538–44.
105. Kim SJ, Kim IJ, Suh KT, et al. Prediction of residual disease of spine infection using F-18 FDG PET/CT. Spine. 2009;34:2424–30.
106. Riccio SA, Chu AK, Rabin HR, et al. Fluorodeoxyglucose positron emission tomography/computed tomography interpretation criteria for assessment of antibiotic treatment response in pyogenic spine infection. Can Assoc Radiol J. 2015;66:145–52.
107. Dauchy FA, Dutertre A, Lawson-Ayay S, et al. Interest of [18F]fluorodeoxyglucose positron emission tomography/computed tomography for the diagnosis of relapse in patients with spinal infection: a prospective study. Clin Microbiol Infect. 2016;22:438–43.
108. Treglia G, Sadeghib R, Annunziata S, et al. Diagnostic performance of Fluorine-18-Fluorodeoxyglucose positron emission tomography for the diagnosis of osteomyelitis related to diabetic foot: A systematic review and a meta-analysis. Foot. 2013;23:140–8.
109. Lauri C, Tamminga M, Glaudemans AWJM, et al. Detection of osteomyelitis in the diabetic foot by imaging techniques: a systematic review and meta-analysis comparing MRI, white blood cell scintigraphy, and FDG-PET. Diabetes Care. 2017;40:1111–20.
110. Zhuang H, Duarte PS, Pourdehnad M, et al. The promising role of 18F-FDG PET in detecting infected lower limb prosthesis implants. J Nucl Med. 2001;42:44–8.
111. Chacko TK, Zhuang H, Nakhoda KZ, et al. Applications of fluorodeoxyglucose positron emission tomography in the diagnosis of infection. Nucl Med Commun. 2003;24:615–24.
112. García-Barrecheguren E, Rodríguez Fraile M, et al. FDG-PET: a new diagnostic approach in hip prosthetic replacement. Rev Esp Med Nucl. 2007;26:208–20.
113. Delank KS, Schmidt M, Michael JW, et al. The implications of 18F-FDG PET for the diagnosis of endoprosthetic loosening and infection in hip and knee arthroplasty: results from a prospective, blinded study. BMC Musculoskelet Disord. 2006;7:20.
114. Reinartz P, Mumme T, Hermanns B, et al. Radionuclide imaging of the painful hip arthroplasty: positron-emission tomography versus triple-phase bone scanning. J Bone Joint Surg. 2005;87-B:465–70.
115. Stumpe KD, Notzli HP, Zanetti M, et al. FDG PET for differentiation of infection and aseptic loosening in total hip replacements: comparison with conventional radiography and three-phase bone scintigraphy. Radiology. 2004;231:333–41.

116. Dumarey N, Egrise D, Blocklet D, et al. Imaging infection with 18F-FDG-labeled leukocyte PET/CT: initial experience in 21 patients. J Nucl Med. 2006;47:625–32.
117. Rini JN, Bhargava KK, Tronco GG, et al. PET with FDG-labeled leukocytes versus scintigraphy with 111In-oxine-labeled leukocytes for detection of infection. Radiology. 2006;238:978–87.
118. Aksoy SY, Asa S, Ozhan M, et al. FDG and FDG-labelled leucocyte PET/CT in the imaging of prosthetic joint infection. Eur J Nucl Med Mol Imaging. 2014;41:556–64.
119. Bhattacharya A, Kochhar R, Sharma S, et al. PET/CT with 18F-FDG-labeled autologous leukocytes for the diagnosis of infected fluid collections in acute pancreatitis. J Nucl Med. 2014;55:1267–72.
120. Bhargava KK, Gupta RK, Nichols KJ, et al. In-vitro human leukocyte labeling with 64Cu: an intraindividual comparison with 111In-oxine and 18F-FDG. Nucl Med Biol. 2009;36:545–9.
121. Fairclough M, Prenant C, Ellis B, et al. A new technique for the radiolabelling of mixed leukocytes with zirconium-89 for inflammation imaging with positron emission tomography. J Label Comp Radiopharm. 2016;59:270–6.
122. Locke LW, Chordia MD, Zhang Y, et al. A novel neutrophil-specific PET imaging agent: cFLFLFK-PEG-64Cu. J Nucl Med. 2009;50:790–7.
123. Nanni C, Errani C, Boriani L, et al. 68Ga-citrate PET/CT for evaluating patients with infections of the bone: preliminary results. J Nucl Med. 2010;51:1932–6.
124. Vorster M, Maes A, Jacobs A, et al. Evaluating the possible role of 68Ga-citrate PET/CT in the characterization of indeterminate lung lesions. Ann Nucl Med. 2014;28:523–30.
125. Foss CA, Sanchez-Bautista J, Jain SK. Imaging macrophage-associated inflammation. Semin Nucl Med. 2018;48:242–5.
126. Chen DL, Scherer PM, Palestro CJ. Clinical imaging. In: Jain S, editor. Imaging infections: from bench to bedside. New York, NY: Springer; 2017. p. 17–41.
127. Lazzeri E, Pauwels EKJ, Erba P, et al. Clinical feasibility of two-step streptavidin/111In-biotin scintigraphy in patients with suspected vertebral osteomyelitis. Eur J Nucl Med Mol Imaging. 2004;31:1505–11.
128. Lazzeri E, Erba P, Perri M, et al. Clinical impact of SPECT/CT with in-111 biotin on the management of patients with suspected spine infection. Clin Nucl Med. 2010;35:12–7.
129. Wang G. Human antimicrobial peptides and proteins. Pharmaceuticals. 2014;7:545–94.
130. Hiemstra PS, van den Barselaar MT, Roest M, et al. Ubiquicidin, a novel murine microbicidal protein present in the cytosolic fraction of macrophages. J Leukoc Biol. 1999;66:423–8.
131. Lupetti A, Pauwels EK, Nibbering PH, et al. 99mTc-antimicrobial peptides: promising candidates for infection imaging. Q J Nucl Med. 2003;47:238–45.
132. Ostovar A, Assadi M, Vahdat K, et al. A pooled analysis of diagnostic value of 99mTc-ubiquicidin (UBI) scintigraphy in detection of an infectious process. Clin Nucl Med. 2013;38:413–6.
133. Ebenhan T, Chadwick N, Sathekge MM, et al. Peptide synthesis, characterization and ^{68}Ga-radiolabeling of NOTA-conjugated ubiquicidin fragments for prospective infection imaging with PET/CT. Nucl Med Biol. 2014;41:390–400.
134. Ebenhan T, Zeevaart JR, Venter JD, et al. Preclinical evaluation of 68Ga-labeled 1,4,7-triazacyclononane-1,4,7-triacetic acid-ubiquicidin as a radioligand for PET infection imaging. J Nucl Med. 2014;55:308–14.
135. Mokaleng BB, Ebenhan T, Ramesh S, et al. Synthesis, 68Ga-radiolabeling, and preliminary in vivo assessment of a depsipeptide-derived compound as a potential PET/CT infection imaging agent. Biomed Res Int. 2015;2015:284354.
136. Boerman OC, Laverman P, Oyen WJFIAU. From reporter gene imaging to imaging of bacterial proliferation. Am J Nucl Med Mol Imaging. 2012;2:271–2.
137. Diaz LA, Foss CA, Thornton K, et al. Imaging of musculoskeletal bacterial infections by [124I]FIAU-PET/CT. PLoS One. 2007;2(10):e1007.
138. Zhang XM, Zhang HH, McLeroth P, et al. [124I] FIAU: human dosimetry and infection imaging in patients with suspected prosthetic joint infection. Nucl Med Biol. 2016;43:273–9.
139. [124I]FIAU-PET/CT scanning in diagnosing osteomyelitis in patients with diabetic foot; 2016. infection.clinicaltrials.gov/ct2/show/NCT01764919. Accessed 15 Jul 2018.
140. Ordonez AA, Jain SK. Pathogen-specific bacterial imaging in nuclear medicine. Semin Nucl Med. 2018;48:182–94.

16 Imaging of Atherosclerosis with ^{18}F-FDG PET

Jan Bucerius

16.1 Introduction

Despite significant therapeutic advances, myocardial infarction and stroke, as the clinical consequences of atherosclerosis, are the two most common causes of death in Europe and worldwide [1, 2].

Atherosclerosis is a disease of the arterial wall with endothelial cell damage resulting in the accumulation of lipids and inflammatory cells within discrete areas of the intima, which also might affect the lumen of the artery. A sclerotic, collagen-rich fibrous cap protects the lipid core of an atherosclerotic plaque from the vessel lumen. However, by thinning and rupture of that protective cap through different mechanisms, embolic material can be released causing clinical events like stroke or myocardial infarction depending on the affected vessel (e.g., carotid or coronary arteries). Typically, atherosclerotic plaques slowly develop over many years and might only be detected once the clinical event occurred. At that time, an advanced stage of the disease already has been reached.

In clinical routine, evaluation of atherosclerosis still relies mainly on invasive of non-invasive assessment of the degree of intraluminal stenosis using invasive or CT angiography. However, angiography suffers from substantial limitations as it does not image the vessel wall nor does it provide information on the plaque vulnerability, i.e., the risk of plaque rupture. Therefore, there is a clear need for non-invasive, highly sensitive, measures to identify those high-risk plaques, which might be undetected by conventional imaging methods. Although some information on the plaque composition can be obtained using CT or MRI, *in vivo* molecular imaging of signature pathological mechanisms in atherosclerosis by using positron emission tomography (PET) gained more and more interest over the last two decades. Numerous studies were published regarding PET imaging in atherosclerosis providing insights into the biological processes within the atherosclerotic plaque, improving risk stratification, and enabling the evaluation of novel therapies and interventions (Fig. 16.1). Therefore, molecular imaging potentially facilitates further gains in cardiovascular care including a paradigm shift in diagnostic algorithm in atherosclerotic disease.

J. Bucerius (✉)
Department of Nuclear Medicine, University Medicine Göttingen, Göttingen, Germany

Georg-August-University Göttingen, Göttingen, Germany
e-mail: jan.bucerius@med.uni-goettingen.de

H. Ahmadzadehfar et al. (eds.), *Clinical Nuclear Medicine*,
https://doi.org/10.1007/978-3-030-39457-8_16

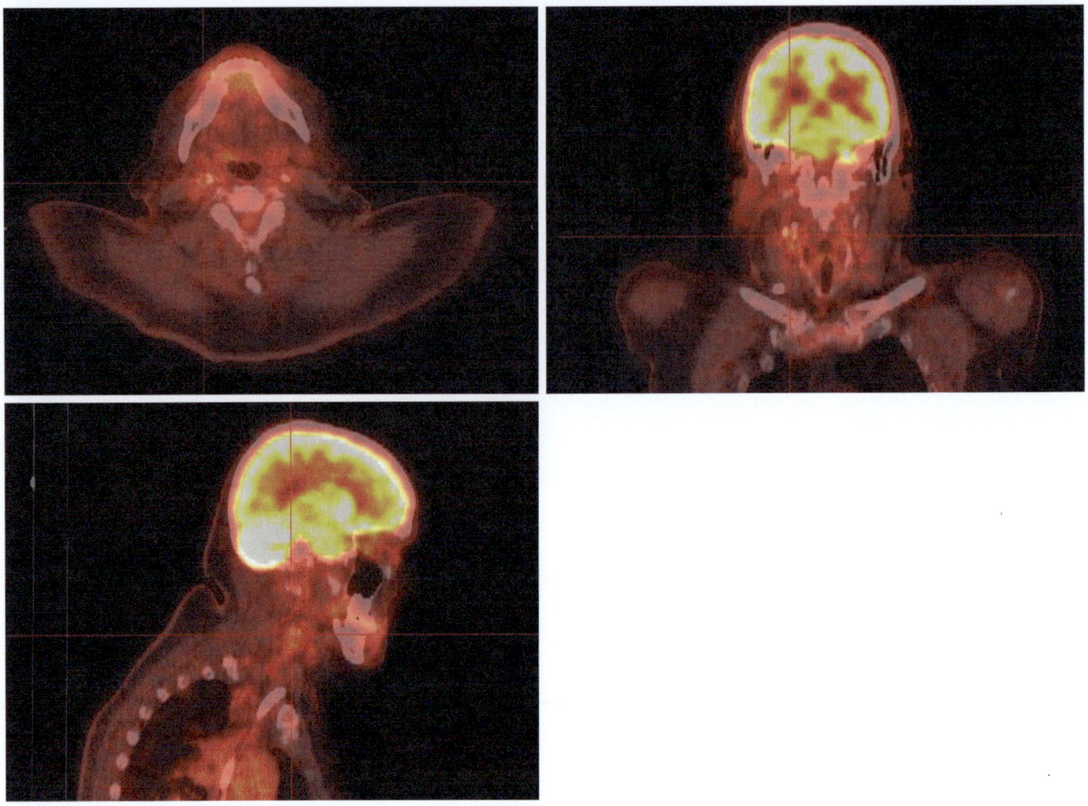

Fig. 16.1 Calcified lesion within the right common carotid artery showing an increased ^{18}F-FDG uptake in a patient known with systemic atherosclerosis. Transaxial (top), coronal (mid), and sagittal (bottom) view

16.2 Methodology

In 2016, the Cardiovascular Committee of the European Association of Nuclear Medicine (EANM) published a position paper on PET imaging of atherosclerosis [3]. This paper was intended to review the different parameters, which might influence the intensity of ^{18}F-fluorodeoxyglucose (FDG) measured in atherosclerotic plaques, and to propose optimal standardized scan protocols for imaging atherosclerosis with PET based on the existing literature in the field and the experience of the members of the EANM Cardiovascular Committee. By using more standardized protocols, interpretation and comparability of the results of different studies in atherosclerosis imaging with PET and steps toward implementation of that diagnostic approach into clinical routine are clearly facilitated.

The administered dose of FDG varies considerably among different clinical studies ranging from 185 to 925 MBq [4–7]. Factors, which need to be taken in consideration in order to define the dose of FDG administered to the patient, are the sensitivity of the PET scanner (in particular, 2D vs. 3D acquisitions), the duration of imaging steps, and the delay between tracer injection and image acquisition. Based on a circulation time (time period between injection of the tracer and start of the PET data acquisition) of 2 h for arterial imaging, injection of a FDG activity between 3 and 4 MBq/kg bodyweight is recommended to allow for a sufficient image quality.

Another crucial aspect in PET imaging of atherosclerosis is the delay between FDG injection and PET acquisitions (FDG circulation time, see above). For arterial imaging with PET, longer delays between FDG injection and PET imaging than the ones used for oncology are recommended in order to allow sufficient FDG accumulation in the arterial wall and to reduce the intensity of the FDG signal in the blood. This is critical as an optimal contrast between the target (plaque, arterial wall) and the background (blood) is essential to ensure accurate quantification of plaque or arterial wall FDG uptake, respectively [4, 5, 8–14]. At early time points (1 h) of data acquisition, the contrast between FDG uptake in the vessel wall and residual blood signal is likely suboptimal leading to the underestimation of FDG uptake in the vessel wall, whereas at later time points (2.5–3 h), the SUV signal measured with PET is approaching the true vascular (arterial) FDG uptake [14]. Therefore, acquisition of PET images 2 h p.i. for reliable quantification of the FDG uptake in the arterial vessel wall and/or plaques is recommended. This time delay is assumed to represent the best compromise between a low background signal in blood and an acceptable duration of the PET study for patients.

As diabetes is a major risk factor for atherosclerotic disease, the problem of elevated pre-scan glucose levels occurs frequently in patients scheduled for FDG PET imaging of arterial wall inflammation. It is known that in oncological studies, the intensity of FDG uptake in tumor tissues is indeed influenced by patient's pre-scan glucose levels [15–17]. One reason for the observed reduction of the FDG uptake is most likely the competition between stable glucose and FDG as facilitative transport via the glucose transporter protein (GLUT) system is the most important way for either types of glucose to enter human cells [18].

It has been recommended that arterial imaging should ideally be performed in patients with pre-scan glucose levels lower than 130 mg/dl (approximately 7.0–7.2 mmol/l) [4, 19, 20]. In patients in which these appropriate blood glucose levels cannot be achieved by other approaches, a correction of the vascular FDG uptake according to the EANM recommendations for oncological PET imaging can be considered but requires more extensive validation in the setting of vascular imaging with FDG PET. This approach was already applied in a previously published study on atherosclerotic PET imaging using a dedicated formula normalizing the measured glucose content for an overall population average of 90 mg/dl (5.0 mmol/l) [SUVgluc = SUV × patient's blood glucose (mg/dl or mmol/l, respectively)/90 mg/dl (5.0 mmol/l)] [3, 20].

Accurate quantification of radiotracer activity in the arterial wall or the atherosclerotic plaque on PET can be problematic. Whereas the determination of the SUV is the most commonly used parameter for measuring lesion activity among patients undergoing oncologic PET/CT, its applicability in atherosclerosis PET imaging might be limited to some degree and not the most optimal approach to quantify arterial tracer uptake. The SUV_{max} is, however, still a frequently used parameter to quantify FDG uptake in atherosclerotic plaque even though it may not accurately represent the lesion's overall activity. This is due to the fact that the tracer distribution is frequently not homogeneous within a lesion. Instead, SUV_{max} measurements in plaques rather reflect the part of the lesion with the highest FDG uptake. However, as most frequently regions of interest (ROI) in vascular imaging are placed around the entire lumen of the target vessel to avoid inaccuracies of the measurement due to partial volume effect (when just estimating the tracer uptake within a distinct plaque or small region of the vessel), determining the SUV within that ROI would also include the FDG uptake within the blood pool. In order to correct for the underlying blood activity and to give, as desired, a more reliable estimation of the tracer uptake within the arterial wall only, a target-to-background ratio (TBR) is frequently applied in vascular imaging. Over the last years, the TBR has been widely used in several studies after his first introduction in vascular imaging in 2006 [14]. Most frequently, the TBR is calculated as the ratio of the SUV (SUV_{mean} and/or SUV_{max}) measured in atherosclerotic plaques or the arterial vessel wall and the venous blood pool SUV_{mean} to correct for blood pool uptake (resulting in TBR_{mean} and/or TBR_{max} values). The TBR measured in atherosclerotic plaques on FDG PET/CT was shown to correlate well with plaque macrophage density on corresponding histological sections [7, 14, 21–23]. In addition, TBR values of different arterial territories demonstrated an excellent intra- and inter-reader agreement in patients imaged twice with FDG PET with a 2-week interval. Furthermore, TBR values were shown to be highly reproducible [24–26]. In order to compare different settings of data acquisition (e.g., in multicenter trial, etc.), it is important to know that the TBR is robust in different scanning settings of emission time and filter, while, in contrast, SUV has significant difference in each of these settings [21, 24].

Even though most clinical trials up to now used the TBR to estimate the arterial FDG uptake, its superiority compared to the use of the "uncorrected" SUV is still a matter of debate. In this context, a recent publication by Johnsrud et al. in 44 patients with a significant (≥70%) stenosis of the internal carotid artery showed a strong correlation between different quantification methods with and without background correction and also a significant correlation of the FDG uptake in the artery with the degree of inflammation as depicted by histology [27]. In this study, a superiority of TBR quantification compared to uncorrected estimation of the arterial FDG uptake could not be confirmed [27].

On the basis of the TBR calculation, three different approaches for the quantitative assessment of the arterial FDG uptake in a target (index) vessel were previously developed and tested in different study settings [4, 13, 14, 20, 25, 26, 28–30].

1. The average of the TBR (TBR_{mean} or TBR_{max}) values measured along all the axial segments that compose the target vessel (whole vessel mean TBR_{mean} or TBR_{max}) [4, 14, 20, 25, 26, 28, 30].
   - Well suited for the assessment of global vascular inflammation in patients as a marker of cardiovascular risk or for comparison with other surrogate markers of cardiovascular disease.
2. Measuring an average of the TBR_{max} activity in a small segment of the index vessel with the highest FDG uptake, the most diseased segment (MDS, e.g., defined as a 1.5 cm arterial segment centered on the slice of the target artery with the highest FDG uptake). The degree of the FDG uptake within the MDS is then calculated as a mean of the TBR_{max} values derived from three contiguous axial segments [30].
   - Particularly well suited when evaluating the degree of inflammation in an individual atherosclerotic plaque in a patient.
3. Active slice (AS) analysis. The idea of this approach is to analyze only arterial locations with a high, pre-defined, FDG uptake at baseline regarding the efficacy of therapeutic interventions on FDG uptake. All slices along the target vessels are first analyzed in each patient at baseline. Afterward, only slices with the pre-defined FDG uptake value (for instance, TBR ≥ 1.6) at baseline are then included for the evaluation of changes in FDG uptake under therapy [13, 29, 31].
   - This approach, which focuses only on parts of the artery with the highest inflammation, might improve the sensitivity of FDG PET imaging to identify changes in FDG uptake in atherosclerotic plaques in relation to the tested drug.

16.3 Arterial FDG PET Imaging in Clinical Studies

In order to evaluate the diagnostic performance of FDG PET in atherosclerosis and to estimate its clinical relevance, numerous studies in the human setting were performed over the last two decades. One of the very first studies in this field, still being a milestone publication, was published by Rudd et al. in 2002 [9]. In this prospective trial, patients with symptomatic carotid atherosclerosis were imaged with FDG PET/CT, and a 27% higher FDG uptake was observed in the symptomatic plaque compared to the asymptomatic contralateral lesions. Furthermore, no FDG uptake was seen in normal carotid arteries [9]. Four years later, Tawakol et al. published the second milestone publication in the field of atherosclerosis imaging with PET and provided histological evidence for the increased FDG uptake in carotid artery plaques when they reported a pretty high and highly significant correlation between the degree of arterial FDG uptake and the degree of inflammatory changes in the histological specimen [14].

From a more methodological point of view, several human studies indicated a specific arterial FDG uptake in different vascular territories like the carotid arteries; different aortic regions; the iliac, the femoral, and the popliteal arteries; and even the coronaries, even though imaging of the latter with PET still remains challenging due to the rather low spatial and temporal resolution and the high physiological uptake in the left ventricular myocardium, at least when FDG is used as tracer. However, PET imaging indeed offers not only the unique option to explore multiple vascular beds simultaneously but also an excellent intra- and inter-observer reproducibility, a fact which is crucial in order for PET/CT to be reliable for studying atherosclerotic plaques, especially when evaluating the efficacy of drug treatment for atherosclerosis and for tracking the changes that occur within the plaque over time.

16.4 Correlation with Clinical Cardiovascular Risk Factors

Arterial FDG uptake was increased in patients with an increased number of cardiovascular risk factors and with pre-existing disease such as diabetes mellitus and the metabolic syndrome [32, 33]. In a retrospective study in patients that underwent FDG PET imaging for cancer screening, Tahara et al. showed that carotid inflammation was associated with waist circumference, hypertension, glucose intolerance, and the metabolic syndrome [33]. In a case-control study of patients with type 2 diabetes, patients with impaired glucose tolerance, and controls, Kim et al. reported higher FDG uptake values in both study groups compared to controls [32]. They also observed increasing prevalence of diabetes with increments of maximum FDG uptake values as depicted by tertiles [32]. These findings were confirmed by two prospective trials published by Bucerius et al. showing a significant correlation between the carotid FDG uptake and hypertension, obesity, higher patient age, smoking, and male gender [34]. Interestingly, it was also observed that with an increasing number of components of the metabolic syndrome, the FDG uptake in the carotid arteries increased significantly [34]. Furthermore, a highly significant association between the FDG uptake in the carotid arteries and type 2 diabetes mellitus, being one of the most important cardiovascular risk factors, was reported by this group [20]. Most strikingly they also observed a significant relation between the arterial FDG uptake and increasing patient's fasting blood glucose values emphasizing the importance of an appropriate treatment regime in patients suffering from diabetes [20].

16.5 Prognostic Value of Arterial FDG PET Imaging on Cardiovascular-Related Outcome

Several efforts have been made over the last years to evaluate the predictive value of arterial FDG uptake and emerging cardiovascular events.

In 2009, Rominger et al. published one of the first studies on arterial FDG PET on identification of patients at risk for subsequent vascular events. They retrospectively included a cohort of 932 cancer patients who underwent a whole-body FDG PET/CT [35]. After a median follow-up time of 29 months, 279 died because of their oncological disease, and 15 out of the 932 patients (1.6%) suffered from a vascular event, which was defined as ischemic stroke, myocardial infarction, or revascularization. Increased arterial FDG uptake based on a TBR ≥ 1.7 was the strongest predictor of these vascular events and had a greater prognostic value than did the arterial calcified plaque burden in these patients [35]. In order to investigate the relation between inflammation-related FDG uptake in the carotid arteries and stroke recurrence, Marnane et al. included 60 patients (25 stroke, 29 TIA, 6 retinal embolism) of whom 13 (22%) suffered from stroke recurrence within the follow-up period of 90 days [36]. In patients with recurrent stroke during the follow-up period, the FDG uptake in the ipsilateral carotid plaque was significantly higher compared to asymptomatic patients. Furthermore, in a Cox regression model including age and degree of stenosis (50–69% or ≥70%), mean plaque FDG uptake was the only independent predictor of stroke recurrence [36]. In an interesting study published by the group of Ahmed Tawakol in Boston in 2013, the incremental value of arterial FDG PET imaging beyond traditional risk factors, as classified in the Framingham Risk Score (FRS), in predicting cardiovascular disease was evaluated [24]. Fifty-three individuals who underwent a FDG PET/CT were included in the study in case they met the inclusion criteria ≥30 years of age, no prior cardiovascular disease (CVD), and free of cancer. CVD events were defined as stroke, transient ischemic attack, acute coronary syndrome, revascularization, new-onset angina, peripheral arterial disease, heart failure, or CVD death. Forty-four patients out of the study population developed CVD during the follow-up period (median 4.2 years). The TBR, as measured in the ascending aorta, strongly predicted subsequent CVD independent of traditional risk factors (hazard ratio: 4.71; $p < 0.001$) and (hazard ratio: 4.13; $p = 0.004$) after further adjustment for coronary calcium score. Strikingly, TBR was also inversely associated with the timing of CVD (beta −0.096; $p < 0.0001$), meaning the higher the aortic TBR, the earlier the CVD event emerged [24]. Also to investigate the performance of arterial FDG uptake as an independent prognostic indicator of cardiovascular events (defined as myocardial infarction, any coronary intervention, angina requiring an emergency department visit, an ischemic stroke, or transient cerebral ischemic attack) and, in addition, to determine its incremental predictive value in addition to the FRS and carotid intima-media thickness (CIMT), Moon et al. analyzed 1089 asymptomatic adults who underwent FDG PET/CT [37]. The arterial FDG uptake was measured in the carotid arteries and quantified as TBR. During a mean follow-up period of 4.2 years, 19 individuals (1.74%) of the subjects included suffered from a cardiovascular event. High carotid FDG uptake (maximal TBR over the 75th percentile (right carotid ≥1.77 or left carotid ≥1.65)) and high CIMT (over the 75th percentile (right or left carotid artery ≥0.75 mm)) were identified as independent predictors of events (high FDG uptake (hazard ratio: 2.98; $p = 0.022$); high CIMT (hazard ratio: 2.82; $p = 0.026$)). By adding carotid FDG uptake, but not CIMT, to the FRS, the time-dependent area under the receiver-operating characteristic curve could be significantly increased from 0.60 to 0.73 ($p = 0.04$). Furthermore, adding carotid FDG uptake to the FRS plus CIMT increased the area under the receiver-operating characteristic curve from 0.65 to 0.75 reaching close to statistical significance ($p = 0.07$). Therefore, it can be concluded that high carotid FDG uptake not only predicts cardiovascular events independent of traditional risk factors and CIMT in asymptomatic adults but may also add to risk stratification beyond the FRS and CIMT [37].

Another interesting approach to evaluate the prognostic value of arterial FDG PET has just recently been published by Cho et al. in 2017 [38]. They investigated whether the FDG uptake in the large arteries (carotid arteries, ascending and abdominal aorta) is predictive of coronary artery calcium (CAC) progression in asymptomatic individuals ($n = 96$) undergoing FDG PET/CT and coronary calcium scoring (CAC) at baseline and follow-up CAC ≥1 after the baseline studies. FDG uptake in the carotid arteries as well as the ascending and abdominal aorta was quantified as TBR, and different scores were calculated to quantify the coronary calcium burden and the change over time. Afterwards, arterial FDG uptake and other clinical risk factors were compared between patients with CAC progression and those without. Thirty-one subjects (32.3%) were observed with CAC progression. Those patients indeed showed significantly higher TBR values in all of the three arteries analyzed compared to patients without CAC progression. Based on a multivariate regression analysis, peak TBR in the abdominal aorta and age ≥58 years and a positive baseline CAC were significantly associated with CAC progression. A higher TBR peak of the abdominal aorta (≥2.11), however, was only associated with CAC progression in patients with a negative baseline CAC. In contrast, in individuals with a positive baseline CAC, only the amount of baseline CAC showed a significant association with CAC progression [38].

16.6 FDG PET as a Surrogate Endpoint Marker in Clinical Interventional Trials

It was as early as in 2006 that arterial FDG PET was used as a surrogate endpoint marker to monitor changes in arterial inflammation in patients randomly assigned to a diet-only or a statin group. Low-dose simvastatin led to a significant decline of the arterial FDG uptake, whereas in the diet-only group, no significant change at all could be observed [13]. In a subsequent study, comparing the effect of 5 mg/day atorvastatin versus 20 mg/day using arterial FDG PET imaging, only treatment with 20 mg atorvastatin per day yielded to a significant reduction of the FDG uptake in the ascending aorta and the femoral artery after 6 months of treatment, whereas the respective changes in patients receiving 5 mg atorvastatin per day were not statistically significant [39]. In a well-designed prospective multicenter trial, this dose-dependent effect of atorvastatin on arterial inflammation was confirmed. Seventy-seven patients without high-dose statin treatment but with a cardiovascular risk profile or known atherosclerosis randomly received either 10 or 80 mg of atorvastatin per day. FDG PET/CT was performed on baseline and at 4 and 12 weeks, and the FDG uptake was measured in the carotid arteries and the ascending aorta [30]. A significant reduction in index vessel FDG uptake compared with baseline was observed at 4 weeks in both groups with an additional relative reduction at 12 weeks, which was only observed in the high-dose group receiving 80 mg of atorvastatin per day. Interestingly, changes in TBR did not correlate with lipid profile changes indicating an independent effect of statins on vascular inflammation [30].

Besides treatment with statins, the effects of several other drugs on arterial inflammation have been evaluated with FDG PET. In 2011, the results of a large double-blind multicenter trial on the effect of dalcetrapib, a modulator of the cholesteryl ester transfer protein (CETP), to raise high-density lipoprotein cholesterol (HDL-C) were published by Fayad et al. [40]. In this phase 2b trial, patients with, or with high risk of, coronary heart disease were randomly assigned to dalcetrapib 600 mg per day or placebo for 24 months. Co-primary endpoints of this trial were MRI-assessed indices after 24 months and assessment of arterial inflammation with FDG PET/CT within an index vessel (right carotid, left carotid, or ascending thoracic aorta) after 6 months. After 24 months, MRI revealed a reduction in total vessel enlargement in patients given dalcetrapib compared with those given placebo with an absolute change from baseline relative to placebo was −4.01 mm^2 (nominal $p = 0.04$). However, the index vessel most diseased segment TBR on PET was not different between groups. Furthermore, even though the carotid artery analysis showed a 7% reduction in most diseased segment TBR in the dalcetrapib group compared with the placebo group, this decline in arterial inflammation failed to be statistically significant ($p = 0.07$).

In 2012, the systemic anti-inflammatory properties of losmapimod (a p38 mitogen-activated protein kinase inhibitor) were demonstrated with FDG PET in patients with atherosclerosis as losmapimod reduced vascular inflammation in the most inflamed regions, concurrent with a reduction in inflammatory biomarkers and FDG uptake in visceral fat [29]. Further stressing the beneficial effect of statins on arterial inflammation, the results of a randomized, placebo-controlled, trial on a p38 mitogen-activated protein kinase (p38MAPK) inhibitor failed to show a significant reduction of atherosclerotic plaque inflammation as assessed by FDG PET imaging [31]. p38MAPK is an important element of inflammatory pathways in atherothrombosis. Whereas, as mentioned above, treatment with the p38MAPK inhibitor did not reduce arterial inflammation or hs-CRP relative to placebo, statin intensification was associated with significant reduction of hs-CRP and arterial inflammation in active slices as compared to placebo [31]. Just recently, a group from the Netherlands published the results on a randomized controlled trial on the anti-inflammatory effects of dipeptidyl peptidase (DPP)-4 inhibitors. DPP4-inhibitors are a class of oral anti-diabetic agents of which favorable cardiovascular effects are suggested. In experimental studies DPP-4 inhibitors reduce atherosclerotic plaque area and macrophage accumulation [41, 42]. After 26 weeks of treatment with the DPP-4 inhibitor linagliptin in 45 patients with early type 2 diabetes but without cardiovascular disease and naive to anti-diabetic treatment, the decrease in arterial FDG uptake under linagliptin exceeded that under placebo with 0.18 units ($p = 0.015$) [41].

FDG PET has also been used to assess the impact of rheumatoid arthritis on vascular inflammation. Rheumatoid arthritis is a systemic inflammatory condition associated with increased cardiovascular risk, and it is hypothesized that patients with this systemic inflammatory condition exhibit aortic inflammation. Indeed, in patients with rheumatoid arthritis, an increased aortic FDG uptake could be observed as compared to a control group of patients with stable cardiovascular disease. Furthermore, anti-tumor necrosis factor-α therapy reduced aortic inflammation in those patients, and this effect correlated with the decrease in aortic stiffness [43].

16.7 New Approaches in Imaging Atherosclerosis with PET

Although results on FDG PET imaging in atherosclerosis revealed promising results, several limitations still impede its application in clinical routine. Besides technical limitations of PET imaging like the rather low spatial and temporal resolution, mainly challenging direct imaging of atherosclerotic changes in the coronary arteries, FDG might not be the most optimal tracer for assessing arterial inflammation. Other PET tracers than FDG might not only be more specific in identifying inflammatory changes of the arterial wall and atherosclerotic plaques, they might also be more suitable for imaging of coronary artery disease as they are not physiologically taken up by the myocardium as is FDG. Therefore, much effort has been spent over the last years not only to develop new PET tracers for imaging of atherosclerosis but also to identify established PET tracer for different clinical indications like oncology which might be feasible to identify common pathways between those diseases and atherosclerosis. Two of the most intensively evaluated tracers in this context are ^{68}Ga-DOTATATE and ^{18}F-sodiumflouride (NaF). ^{68}Ga-labeled somatostatin receptor tracers like ^{68}Ga-DOTATATE gained entrance into clinical routine for imaging of neuroendocrine tumors, which typically express those types of receptors. Certain somatostatin receptors are also overexpressed in activated macrophages and damaged endothelial cells, where they have a role in modulating inflammation and angiogenesis [44–46]. Several studies have reported on vascular ^{68}Ga-DOTATATE imaging, of which one milestone paper was published by Tarkin et al. in 2017. In a first step, they confirmed ^{68}Ga-DOTATATE binding in macrophages and excised carotid plaques. Secondly, ^{68}Ga-DOTATATE PET imaging was compared to FDG PET imaging in 42 patients with atherosclerosis [46]. Here they found a specific ^{68}Ga-DOTATATE ligand binding to somatostatin receptors in CD68-positive macrophage-rich carotid plaque regions, and carotid somatostatin receptor mRNA was highly correlated with *in vivo* ^{68}Ga-DOTATATE PET signals ($r = 0.89$; $p = 0.02$). Most strikingly, the ^{68}Ga-DOTATATE uptake, expressed as maximum TBR, not only correctly identified culprit versus non-culprit arteries in patients with acute coronary syndrome (median difference: 0.69; $p = 0.008$) and transient ischemic attack/stroke (median difference: 0.13; $p = 0.003$) but also predicted high-risk coronary computed tomography features. Although FDG PET maximum TBR was also able to differentiate culprit from non-culprit carotid lesions and high-risk from low-risk coronary arteries, physiological myocardial FDG uptake led to uninterpretable coronary FDG uptake due to spillover from the myocardium in 27 patients (64%). In contrast, ^{68}Ga-DOTATATE rendered readable results in all patients [46].

The second "established" PET tracer, which gained great interest in imaging of atherosclerosis, is NaF. NaF is used in clinical routine for imaging of benign and malignant osseous lesions and has recently been reported being useful as a marker of valvular and vascular calcification activity in patients with aortic stenosis [47–50].

In 2014, a well-designed prospective clinical trial on NaF PET imaging of atherosclerosis was published by Joshi et al. [50]. Patients with myocardial infarction and stable angina (n = 40 in each group) underwent both, NaF and FDG PET/CT and invasive coronary angiography. Furthermore, NaF uptake was compared with histology in carotid endarterectomy specimens received from patients suffering from symptomatic carotid disease and with intravascular ultrasound in patients with stable angina. In the majority of patients with myocardial infarction (n = 37; 93%), the highest NaF uptake was observed in the culprit plaque (maximum TBR: culprit 1.66 versus highest non-culprit, 1.24; $p < 0.0001$). In contrast, FDG uptake in the coronary arteries was frequently obscured due to overspill from the myocardial FDG uptake. Furthermore, where discernible, no difference between culprit and non-culprit plaques (1.71 and 1.58; $p = 0.34$) was seen. In addition to these findings, a marked NaF uptake was identified at the site of all carotid plaques ruptures. Here, NaF uptake was associated with evidence of active calcification, macrophage infiltration, and apoptosis as well as necrosis in histology [50].

In addition to these two exemplary named PET tracers, several other promising PET tracers are currently evaluated for the assessment of atherosclerosis in both the pre-clinical and clinical setting, and it needs to be awaited whether those tracers further facilitate the introduction of arterial PET imaging into clinical routine.

References

1. Lozano R, Naghavi M, Foreman K, et al. Global and regional mortality from 235 causes of death for 20 age groups in 1990 and 2010: a systematic analysis for the Global Burden of Disease Study 2010. Lancet. 2012;380:2095.
2. Nichols M, Townsend N, Luengo-Fernandez R, et al. European cardiovascular disease statistics 2012 edition. Brussels: European Heart Network and European Society of Cardiology; 2012.
3. Bucerius J, Hyafil F, Verberne HJ, et al. Cardiovascular Committee of the European Association of nuclear medicine (EANM). Position paper of the cardiovascular Committee of the European Association of nuclear medicine (EANM) on PET imaging of atherosclerosis. Eur J Nucl Med Mol Imaging. 2016;43:780–92.
4. Bucerius J, Mani V, Moncrieff C, et al. Optimizing 18F-FDG PET/CT imaging of vessel wall inflammation: the impact of 18F-FDG circulation time, injected dose, uptake parameters, and fasting blood glucose levels. Eur J Nucl Med Mol Imaging. 2014a;41:369–83.
5. Davies JR, Rudd JH, Fryer TD, et al. Identification of culprit lesions after transient ischemic attack by combined 18F fluorodeoxyglucose positron-emission tomography and high-resolution magnetic resonance imaging. Stroke. 2005;36:2642–7.
6. Fifer KM, Qadir S, Subramanian S, et al. Positron emission tomography measurement of periodontal 18F-fluorodeoxyglucose uptake is associated with histologically determined carotid plaque inflammation. J Am Coll Cardiol. 2011;57:971–6.
7. Figueroa AL, Subramanian SS, Cury RC, et al. Distribution of inflammation within carotid atherosclerotic plaques with high-risk morphological features: a comparison between positron emission tomography activity, plaque morphology, and histopathology. Circ Cardiovasc Imaging. 2012;5:69–77.
8. Menezes LJ, Kotze CW, Hutton BF, et al. Vascular inflammation imaging with 18F-FDG PET/CT: when to image? J Nucl Med. 2009;50:854–7.
9. Rudd JH, Warburton EA, Fryer TD, et al. Imaging atherosclerotic plaque inflammation with [18F]-fluorodeoxyglucose positron emission tomography. Circulation. 2002;105:2708–11.
10. Rudd JH, Machac J, Fayad ZA. Simvastatin and plaque inflammation. J Am Coll Cardiol. 2007b;49:1991. Author reply 1991–1992.
11. Rudd JH, Fayad ZA, Machac J, et al. Imaging of vulnerable atherosclerotic plaques with FDG-microPET: no FDG accumulation. Atherosclerosis. 2007c;192:453–4. Author reply 451–452.
12. Rudd JH, Elkhawad M, Fayad ZA. Vascular imaging with 18F-FDG PET/CT: optimal 18F-FDG circulation time? J Nucl Med. 2009;50:1560.
13. Tahara N, Kai H, Ishibashi M, et al. Simvastatin attenuates plaque inflammation: evaluation by fluorodeoxyglucose positron emission tomography. J Am Coll Cardiol. 2006;48:1825–31.
14. Tawakol A, Migrino RQ, Bashian GG, et al. In vivo 18F-fluorodeoxyglucose positron emission tomography imaging provides a noninvasive measure of carotid plaque inflammation in patients. J Am Coll Cardiol. 2006;48:1818–24.
15. Lee WW, Chung JH, Jang SJ, et al. Consideration of serum glucose levels during malignant mediastinal

lymph node detection in non-small-cell lung cancer by FDG-PET. J Surg Oncol. 2006;94:607–13.
16. Rabkin Z, Israel O, Keidar Z. Do hyperglycemia and diabetes affect the incidence of false-negative 18F-FDG PET/CT studies in patients evaluated for infection or inflammation and cancer? A comparative analysis. J Nucl Med. 2010;51:1015–20.
17. Zhuang HM, Cortés-Blanco A, Pourdehnad M, et al. Do high glucose levels have differential effect on FDG uptake in inflammatory and malignant disorders? Nucl Med Commun. 2001;22:1123–8.
18. Shepherd PR, Kahn BB. Glucose transporters and insulin action – implications for insulin resistance and diabetes mellitus. N Engl J Med. 1999;341:248–57.
19. Boellaard R, Delgado-Bolton R, Oyen WJ, et al. FDG PET/CT: EANM procedure guidelines for tumour imaging: version 2.0. Eur J Nucl Med Mol Imaging. 2015;42:328–54.
20. Bucerius J, Mani V, Moncrieff C, et al. Impact of non insulin-dependent type 2 diabetes on carotid wall (18) F-fluorodeoxyglucose positron emission tomography uptake. J Am Coll Cardiol. 2012;59:2080–8.
21. Gholami S, Salavati A, Houshmand S, et al. Assessment of atherosclerosis in large vessel walls: a comprehensive review of FDG-PET/CT image acquisition protocols and methods for uptake quantification. J Nucl Cardiol. 2015;22:468–79.
22. Ogawa M, Ishino S, Mukai T, et al. (18)F-FDG accumulation in atherosclerotic plaques: immunohistochemical and PET imaging study. J Nucl Med. 2004;45:1245–50.
23. Zhao QM, Feng TT, Zhao X, et al. Imaging of atherosclerotic aorta of rabbit model by detection of plaque inflammation with fluorine-18 fluorodeoxyglucose positron emission tomography/computed tomography. Chin Med J. 2011;124:911–7.
24. Figueroa AL, Abdelbaky A, Truong QA, et al. Measurement of arterial activity on routine FDG PET/CT images improves prediction of risk of future CV events. JACC Cardiovasc Imaging. 2013;6:1250–9.
25. Rudd JH, Myers KS, Bansilal S, et al. (18) Fluorodeoxyglucose positron emission tomography imaging of atherosclerotic plaque inflammation is highly reproducible: implications for atherosclerosis therapy trials. J Am Coll Cardiol. 2007a;50:892–6.
26. Rudd JH, Myers KS, Bansilal S, et al. Atherosclerosis inflammation imaging with 18F-FDG PET: carotid, iliac, and femoral uptake reproducibility, quantification methods, and recommendations. J Nucl Med. 2008;49:871–8.
27. Johnsrud K, Skagen K, Seierstad T, et al. ^{18}F-FDG PET/CT for the quantification of inflammation in large carotid artery plaques. J Nucl Cardiol. 2019;26:883–93.
28. Bucerius J, Mani V, Wong S, et al. Arterial and fat tissue inflammation are highly correlated: a prospective 18F-FDG PET/CT study. Eur J Nucl Med Mol Imaging. 2014b;41:934–45.
29. Elkhawad M, Rudd JH, Sarov-Blat L, et al. Effects of p38 mitogen-activated protein kinase inhibition on vascular and systemic inflammation in patients with atherosclerosis. JACC Cardiovasc Imaging. 2012;5:911–22.
30. Tawakol A, Fayad ZA, Mogg R, et al. Intensification of statin therapy results in a rapid reduction in atherosclerotic inflammation: results of a multicenter fluorodeoxyglucose-positron emission tomography/computed tomography feasibility study. J Am Coll Cardiol. 2013;62:909–17.
31. Emami H, Vucic E, Subramanian S, et al. The effect of BMS-582949, a P38 mitogen-activated protein kinase (P38 MAPK) inhibitor on arterial inflammation: a multicenter FDG-PET trial. Atherosclerosis. 2015;240:490–6.
32. Kim TN, Kim S, Yang SJ, et al. Vascular inflammation in patients with impaired glucose tolerance and type 2 diabetes: analysis with 18F-fluorodeoxyglucose positron emission tomography. Circ Cardiovasc Imaging. 2010;3:142–8.
33. Tahara N, Kai H, Yamagishi S, et al. Vascular inflammation evaluated by [18F]-fluorodeoxyglucose positron emission tomography is associated with the metabolic syndrome. J Am Coll Cardiol. 2007;49:1533–9.
34. Bucerius J, Duivenvoorden R, Mani V, et al. Prevalence and risk factors of carotid vessel wall inflammation in coronary artery disease patients: FDG-PET and CT imaging study. JACC Cardiovasc Imaging. 2011;4:1195–205.
35. Rominger A, Saam T, Wolpers S, et al. 18F-FDG PET/CT identifies patients at risk for future vascular events in an otherwise asymptomatic cohort with neoplastic disease. J Nucl Med. 2009;50:1611–20.
36. Marnane M, Merwick A, Sheehan OC, et al. Carotid plaque inflammation on 18F-fluorodeoxyglucose positron emission tomography predicts early stroke recurrence. Ann Neurol. 2012;71:709–18.
37. Moon SH, Cho YS, Noh TS, et al. Carotid FDG uptake improves prediction of future cardiovascular events in asymptomatic individuals. JACC Cardiovasc Imaging. 2015;8:949–56.
38. Cho SG, Park KS, Kim J, et al. Prediction of coronary artery calcium progression by FDG uptake of large arteries in asymptomatic individuals. Eur J Nucl Med Mol Imaging. 2017;44:129–40.
39. Ishii H, Nishio M, Takahashi H, et al. Comparison of atorvastatin 5 and 20 mg/d for reducing F-18 fluorodeoxyglucose uptake in atherosclerotic plaques on positron emission tomography/computed tomography: a randomized, investigator-blinded, open-label, 6-month study in Japanese adults scheduled for percutaneous coronary intervention. Clin Ther. 2010;32:2337–47.
40. Fayad ZA, Mani V, Woodward M, et al. Dal-PLAQUE investigators. Safety and efficacy of dalcetrapib on atherosclerotic disease using novel non-invasive multimodality imaging (dal-PLAQUE): a randomised clinical trial. Lancet. 2011;378:1547–59.
41. de Boer SA, Heerspink HJ, Lefrandt JD, et al. Effect of Linagliptin on arterial 18F-Fluorodeoxyglucose

positron emission tomography uptake: a randomized controlled trial (RELEASE). J Am Coll Cardiol. 2017;69:1097–8.
42. Scheen AJ. Cardiovascular effects of gliptins. Nat Rev Cardiol. 2013;10:73–84.
43. Mäki-Petäjä KM, Elkhawad M, Cheriyan J, et al. Anti-tumor necrosis factor-α therapy reduces aortic inflammation and stiffness in patients with rheumatoid arthritis. Circulation. 2012;126:2473–80.
44. Adams RL, Adams IP, Lindow SW, et al. Somatostatin receptors 2 and 5 are preferentially expressed in proliferating endothelium. Br J Cancer. 2005;92:1493–8.
45. Armani C, Catalani E, Balbarini A, et al. Expression, pharmacology, and functional role of somatostatin receptor subtypes 1 and 2 in human macrophages. J Leukoc Biol. 2006;81:845–55.
46. Tarkin JM, Joshi FR, Evans NR, et al. Detection of atherosclerotic inflammation by 68Ga-DOTATATE PET compared to [18F]FDG PET imaging. J Am Coll Cardiol. 2017;69:1774–91.
47. Dweck MR, Chow MW, Joshi NV, et al. Coronary arterial 18F-sodium fluoride uptake: a novel marker of plaque biology. J Am Coll Cardiol. 2012a;59:1539–48.
48. Dweck MR, Jones C, Joshi NV, et al. Assessment of valvular calcification and inflammation by positron emission tomography in patients with aortic stenosis. Circulation. 2012b;125:76–86.
49. Dweck MR, Khaw HJ, Sng GK, et al. Aortic stenosis, atherosclerosis, and skeletal bone: is there a common link with calcification and inflammation? Eur Heart J. 2013;34:1567–74.
50. Joshi NV, Vesey AT, Williams MC, et al. 18F-fluoride positron emission tomography for identification of ruptured and high-risk coronary atherosclerotic plaques: a prospective clinical trial. Lancet. 2014;383:705–13.

17 PET/CT and PET/MRI, Normal Variations, and Artifacts

Mohsen Beheshti, Reyhaneh Manafi-Farid, Alireza Rezaee, and Werner Langsteger

17.1 Technical Artifacts

Technical artifacts are mainly due to the technical and physical limitations of the imaging system, systematic errors, and patient motion. They are independent of tracer and can cause apparent changing in the pattern of uptake and incorrect spatial registration between PET and CT in areas of potential clinical interest which may affect the interpretation.

M. Beheshti (✉)
Department of Nuclear Medicine, University Hospital, RWTH University, Aachen, Germany

Department of Nuclear Medicine & Endocrinology, Paracelsus Medical University, Salzburg, Austria
e-mail: mbeheshti@ukaachen.de

R. Manafi-Farid
Department of Nuclear Medicine, University Hospital, RWTH University, Aachen, Germany

Research Center for Nuclear Medicine, Shariati Hospital, Tehran University of Medical Sciences, Tehran, Iran

A. Rezaee
PET-CT Center Khatam, Khatamolanbia Hospital, Tehran, Iran

W. Langsteger
Department of Nuclear Medicine, University Hospital, RWTH University, Aachen, Germany

17.1.1 Partial Volume Effect

Partial volume effect is one of the common challenges in PET reading. The spatial resolution of PET scanner may reduce depiction of small, moderately active lesions, which may influence the interpretation particularly where a minimal change in apparent activity is important for correct assessment of disease. The current generation of PET scanners has a resolution of approximately 4–5 mm in small lesions [1, 2]. At this resolution, PET images of a 17-mm spherical phantom typically underrepresent activity by approximately 16%, increasing to 62% for a 10-mm lesion [3, 4].

The reconstruction parameters of the PET images regulate the adjustment between image noise and spatial resolution. Increasing PET acquisition time and injected activity to a certain extent leads to image noise reduction. The current generation of scanner systems further improves PET image resolution by using point spread function which can improve tumor detectability [5].

17.1.2 Motion Artifacts

Motion artifacts are typically presented as blurring in PET or as misalignment between PET and CT data sets, which can lead to both spatial localization errors and incorrect attenuation correction

H. Ahmadzadehfar et al. (eds.), *Clinical Nuclear Medicine*,
https://doi.org/10.1007/978-3-030-39457-8_17

[4]. The dimension of artifacts is mainly dependent on the number and spatial range of motion and the duration of acquisition. PET acquisition is usually performed by a series of consecutive bed positions of 15–20 cm with a duration of 2–3 min each. Therefore, motion particularly causes artifacts image in motion-affected regions. In contrast, the separately acquired helical CT scan acquires 15–20 cm in a few seconds, and motion-affected regions are usually obtained in a locally motion-free state [4].

Motion can be considered as either voluntary (e.g., head motion) or involuntary (e.g., cardiac contraction or respiratory motion). Artifacts can be developed by motion occurring during either the PET or the CT acquisition or from motion that occurs between the two acquisitions.

Patient movement may cause poor-quality and blurred PET images and regions of increased or decreased activity mainly due to incorrect attenuation correction. In addition, PET artifacts can result from erroneous scatter correction if the tracer distribution is not correctly adjusted with the CT due to regions of activity being incorrectly defined as scatter. Changing scatter correction parameters can often reduce this artifact. In addition, good communication with the patient, attention to careful positioning, physical supports, and occasionally, sedation may limit voluntary motion. However, careful inspection of PET/CT images to identify when motion has occurred is probably the most useful method to repeat local imaging when needed.

Involuntary motions causing artifact by respiratory-induced spatial misalignment between PET and CT data sets are potentially more difficult to control. It usually happened at the base part of the lung and the anterior wall of the heart and can lead to attenuation-correction errors and degrading of lesion detection and tumor quantitation (Fig. 17.1) [6–8].

Breath-hold methods, combining four-dimensional CT images, or obtaining motion-reduced images by either only retaining PET data from the quiescent phase of respiration or using respiratory gating to divide PET and CT acquisitions into matching states of respiration, are the most introduced available approaches to reduce respiratory motion artifacts [9–12]. Cardiac contractile motion can be diminished by PET acquisition corresponding to electrocardiogram gating using commercially available systems.

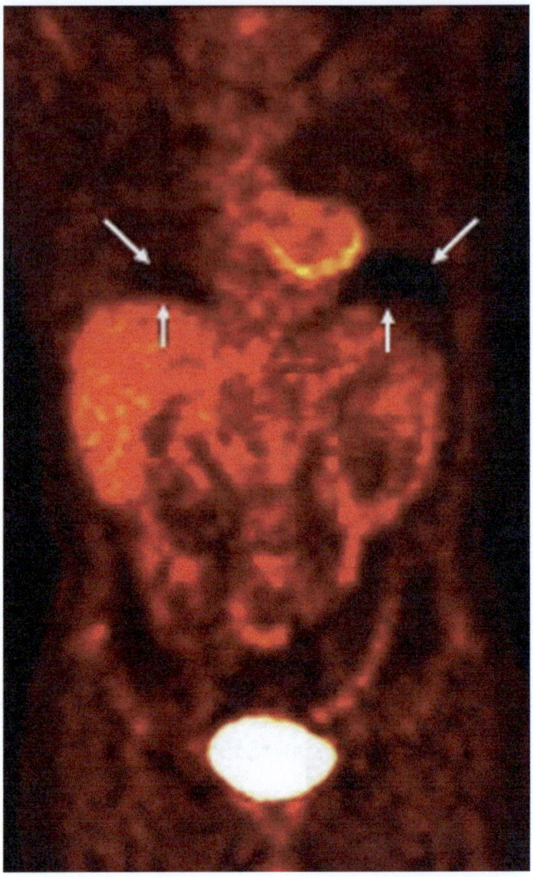

Fig. 17.1 ^{18}F-FDG PET (coronal view). Motion artifact. Involuntary motions causing artifact by respiratory-induced spatial misalignment between PET and CT data sets on the base of the lung, so-called mushroom sign, banana sign (arrows)

17.1.3 Artifacts Induced by High-Density Materials

CT contrast agents can cause artifacts in attenuation-corrected PET images. This is mainly due to failure of multilinear scaling used for converting CT data to PET attenuation-correction maps to correctly scale the contrast agents [4]. It leads to subsequent overestimation of attenuation and artificially elevated regions of PET activity

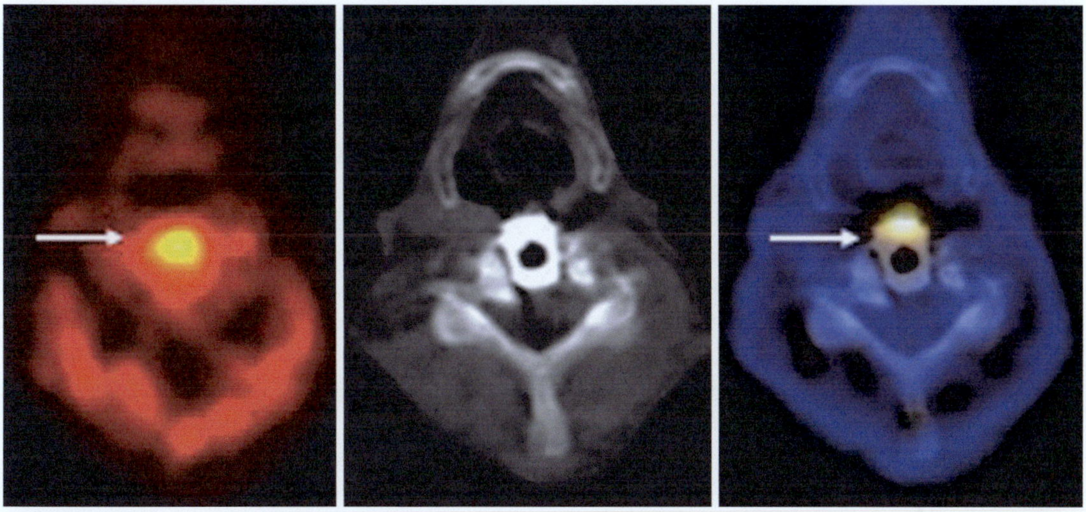

Fig. 17.2 ^{18}F-FDG PET/CT. *Trans-axial images*: *PET (left)*, *CT (middle)*, *fusion PET/CT (right)*. Metal artifact. There is an increasing band-shaped uptake on the anterior rim of a metal vertebral prosthesis which is caused by reconstruction artifacts due to metal prosthesis. Considering the non-attenuation-correction images helps to accurate interpretation of such uptakes

[13, 14]. Reducing the density of contrast agent by using of lower concentrations, negative oral contrast agents, or altering the time of intravenous administrations have been suggested to avoid or reduce artifacts [15]. Performing an additional ultralow-dose CT acquisition before the PET acquisition for attenuation correction is an alternative strategy.

A similar problem may occur at the sites of metal prostheses or implants (Fig. 17.2). However, such attenuation-correction artifacts are usually confined to the tissue immediately surrounding the metal substances.

17.1.4 Truncation Artifact

Truncation artifact occurs when body extends beyond the axial field of view of the scanner (e.g., 50 cm) and is usually seen in CT whole-body acquisition. PET acquisition is usually obtained over a larger axial field of view (e.g., 70 cm), and CT truncation can affect PET reconstruction data by causing regions of over- or under-correction of attenuation in the arms. However, such artifacts are mitigated in current modern devices that reconstruct attenuation-correction maps to 70 cm using data-extrapolation approach [16]. An alternative commonly used method to overcome with truncation artifact is positioning of patients with arms above their head and out of the field of view of the scanner.

17.1.5 Equipment Errors Causing Artifacts

Systematic errors and hardware failures can result in quantitative inaccuracy, PET/CT misalignment, and image artifacts, which may be difficult to identify in patient images. Accurate and regular quality control and preventative maintenance schedules can facilitate early detection of errors and minimize possible artifacts on images [17].

17.2 PET/MRI

Several studies have investigated techniques to improve the hybrid performance between molecular and anatomical information from PET and magnetic resonance imaging (MRI). The radiopharmaceutical-related physiologic uptakes and artifacts are mostly similar from PET/CT to PET/MRI; however, there are different technical artifacts which should be considered for accurate interpretation.

There are still several limitations in clinical imaging with PET/MRI. The long acquisition time and excessive imaging information of MRI, which are usually not used for the diagnosis, are the main components which may affect the work-flow of PET/MRI imaging [18].

Therefore, operating a PET/MRI center requires a comprehensive knowledge and expertise of molecular imaging using both magnetic resonance and nuclear medicine.

Lung imaging is considered as one of the main limitations of PET/MRI. Overall, detection of small lung nodules and destructive parenchymal lung disease is very time-consuming and challenging even when performing respiratory-triggered and motion-corrected sequences. [18].

In addition, there are several technical artifacts in clinical setting of PET/MRI. Fat-water swap is a common artifact in Dixon sequences which can cause a significant distortion on parts of the MRI image leading to nondiagnostic data. Changing the acquisition direction may help to overcome with such artifacts; however, it costs additional scanning time. Moreover, PET artifacts due to unexpected quantities of water in it can also result in distinctive situation. Such artifacts may happen when fluid-filled lesions (e.g., full urinary bladder) overlap two consequent bed positions.

Usual scatter correction artifacts around the lesions with intensive activity look generally similar to that on PET/CT. Another limitation of MRI-based attenuation correction is metal implant. This may lead to loss of MRI signals depending on the composition and size of the implant. Furthermore, hardware located in the field of view (e.g., specific MRI coil) is a potential source of PET bias [18]. Other artifacts relating to complex tissue classification have also been reported. For instance, "air leakage" into the lungs can happen when an MRI signal void (e.g., sternal metal suture) creates a connection between the background and the lungs leading to partial misclassification of lung tissue as air [18].

17.3 ^{18}F-FDG

^{18}F-fluorodeoxyglucose (FDG) is the most commonly used tracer for PET/CT imaging. Variable accumulation of FDG is reported in different tumors correlating with their characteristics and glycolysis. FDG uptake is also seen in nonmalignant tissue, notably in the brain, thyroid gland, digestive tract, myocardium, skeletal muscle, bone marrow, and genitourinary tract. Moreover, FDG is not a tumor-specific tracer, and its uptake can be seen in active inflammatory lesions including sarcoidosis, tuberculosis, fungal infection, inflammatory abscess, etc. Furthermore, different therapeutic procedures may affect the normal distribution of FDG and may cause various pattern of tracer uptake. Therefore, specific recognizing and proper categorizing of such physiologic variants and benign pathologic causes of FDG uptake are necessary for accurate interpretation.

17.3.1 Head and Neck

Due to complex anatomy and a lot of physiologic and FDG avid benign lesions, accurate interpretation of head and neck FDG PET/CT needs excellent knowledge and good experience to overcome possible pitfalls. Awareness of patient's past medical and surgical history or any prior radiation therapy which is a cornerstone of head and neck cancers management is crucial as well [19]. On the other hand, concomitant CT scan plays an important role for localization of any FDG avid lesion. It is also important to differentiate longitudinal versus focal FDG uptake, with the latter more concerning for a neoplastic process.

Parotids, sublingual, and submandibular salivary glands are of the most common organs with physiologic FDG uptake. However, the key point is their symmetricity and easy localization on CT.

The Waldeyer ring is composed of nasopharyngeal lymphoid tissue as well as lingual and palatine tonsils almost always shows mild-to-

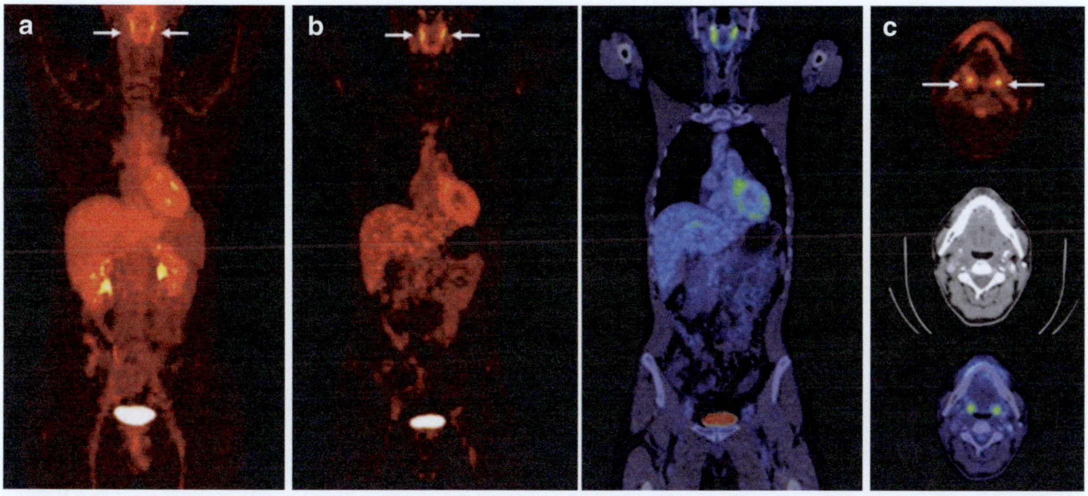

Fig. 17.3 ^{18}F-FDG PET/CT. Benign ^{18}F-FDG uptake in tonsils. A 37-year-old male with seminoma referred for restaging. (**a**) *MIP (maximum intensity projection) images*: mild symmetrical increased ^{18}F-FDG uptake is depicted in the tonsillar region. Otherwise, the study is unremarkable. (**b**) *Coronal PET (left) and fusion PET/CT (right)* and *C. trans-axial PET (upper), CT (middle), fusion (lower) images*: ^{18}F-FDG uptake is localized in the normal tonsillar tissue, bilaterally. The symmetrical uptake implies a benign finding, either a physiologic or inflammatory process

moderate physiologic FDG uptake [19, 20]. However, mild asymmetry in tonsillar metabolic activity is acceptable (Fig. 17.3) [19].

In addition, there are numerous tiny muscles in the neck which may demonstrate variable FDG uptake on PET based on their contraction (Fig. 17.4). Except after unilateral surgical removal, previous radiation therapy, or asymmetrical contractions, distribution of radiotracer should be symmetrical on the study [21].

Expectedly, teeth grinding and chewing cause increased metabolic activity of masticator muscles. This implies the importance of appropriate patient preparation after injection of FDG, particularly in the first 20 min.

As another example, speaking during uptake period may cause intense uptake of vocal cords in the larynx. Thus, vocal cord paralysis for any reason, including recurrent laryngeal nerve palsy, causes asymmetrically decreased FDG uptake on the paralyzed side [22].

The tongue as a powerful muscle may show uptake which is usually symmetrical.

The normal thyroid gland is non- or faintly FDG avid. However, diffuse tracer uptake could be either a normal variation or secondary to hyperthyroidism or chronic thyroiditis in appropriate clinical settings (Fig. 17.5). Nevertheless, focal FDG uptake may represent an adenoma. Other possibility which occurs in 30–50% of the cases is a primary thyroid cancer. In these cases, correlation with thyroid scintigraphy and/or ultrasound is warranted [23, 24].

Brown adipose tissues may show non-specific intensive tracer uptake (Fig. 17.6). Typical distribution of brown fat tissue in adults is suboccipital region, bilateral bases of the neck, and paraspinal areas with possible extension to perinephric fossa. Since it is a heat-producing tissue, the patient should be relaxed and rest in a warm room in uptake period. In addition, using medications such as β-blockers and benzodiazepines is of certain value [25, 26].

Dental implants and filling materials make both streak and attenuation-correction artifacts on CT and PET images, respectively [27].

The head and neck regions are prone to motion artifact and resultant misregistration, more than the other parts of the body. Furthermore, radiotherapy may affect the normal distribution of FDG and may cause various pattern of tracer uptake (Fig. 17.7).

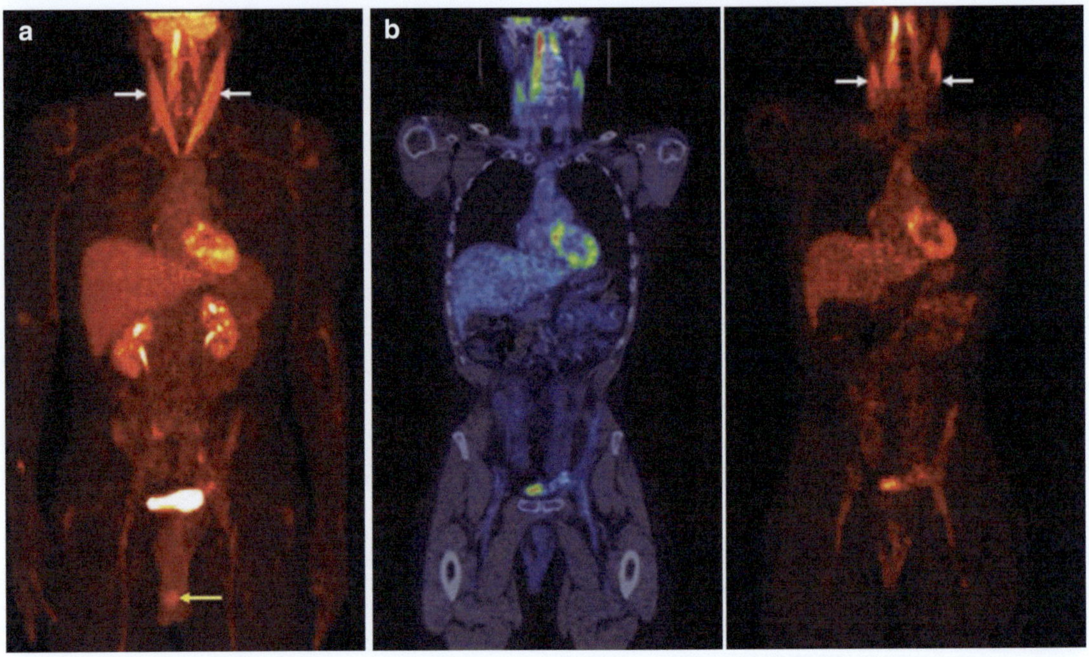

Fig. 17.4 ^{18}F-FDG PET/CT. Muscle uptake. A 50-year-old male with seminoma referred for evaluation of response to treatment. (**a**) *MIP (maximum intensity projection) image*: there is a linear ^{18}F-FDG uptake in bilateral cervical region (arrows). In addition, mild activity is seen in the scrotum (yellow arrow) which is due to inflammatory process secondary to surgical manipulation. (**b**) *Coronal fusion PET/CT (left) and PET (right) images*: the abnormal activity is localized in bilateral sternocleidomastoid muscles. Considering diffuse pattern, the uptake suggests a physiologic uptake or muscle strain

17.3.2 Chest

Knowledge of physiologic distribution of ^{18}F-FDG in the chest is very helpful to accurately interpret thoracic findings on FDG PET/CT. However, not only the malignant but also benign lesions such as inflammatory and infectious processes may take up FDG which are sometimes more avid than malignancies [28].

Physiologic FDG uptake in breasts reduces in advanced age and directly correlates with the volume of glandular tissue. It also depends on patient's menstrual cycle with the maximum activity after ovulation [29]. It is usually heterogeneously increased bilaterally in lactating mothers (Fig. 17.6). In general, nipples are also mildly FDG avid [28]. Due to enlargement of gland in men, increased FDG uptake may be noticed on PET in the case of gynecomastia [30].

As discussed before, this is expected that nonspecific uptake is seen in the brown adipose tissues in supraclavicular and paravertebral regions with quite high FDG uptake (Fig. 17.6). Providing a warm environment in PET clinics as well as pre-treatment with β-blockers and benzodiazepines is helpful to subside metabolic activity [25].

Similar to the other parts of the body, FDG uptake in bone marrow is variable but usually more prominent compared with blood pool activity [28]. Expectedly, traumatic changes and fractures of the rib cage normally represent with focal tracer uptake on FDG PET [31].

Muscle contraction causes increased FDG uptake. Therefore, chronic obstructive pulmonary disease may present with increased activity in respiratory accessory muscles such as intercostal muscles, diaphragm, and abdominal muscles, secondary to labored breathing (Fig. 17.8) [32].

Intact pleura usually shows symmetrical, mild FDG uptake with SUV less than 2. Pulmonary

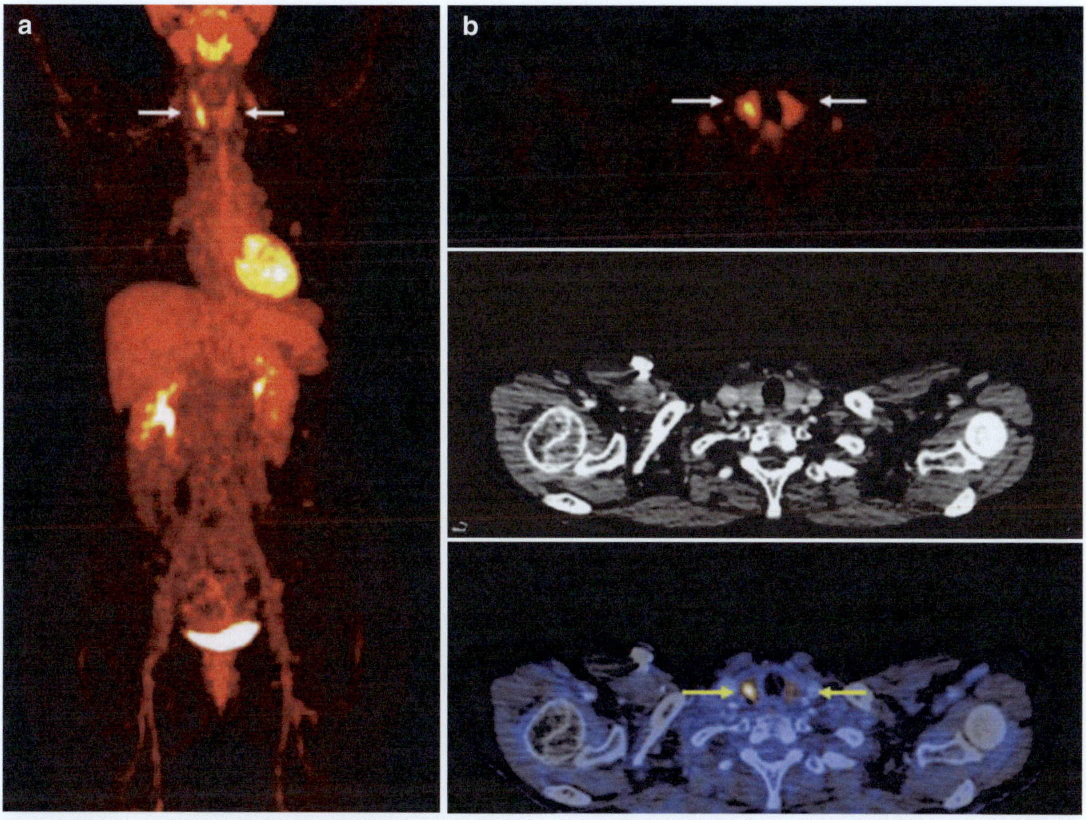

Fig. 17.5 ^{18}F-FDG PET/CT. Moderate diffuse ^{18}F-FDG uptake in the thyroid lobes. A 34-year-old female with right breast carcinoma referred for evaluation of residual disease. (**a**) *MIP (maximum intensity projection) image*: a moderate diffuse ^{18}F-FDG uptake is noted in the thyroid glands (arrows). (**b**) *Trans-axial PET (upper), CT (middle), and fusion PET/CT (lower) images*: the uptake is seen on both thyroid lobes suggesting a thyroid disease (arrows)

parenchyma demonstrates very low metabolic activity as well [28]. Diffuse and homogeneous FDG uptake is appreciated in atelectases which is directly correlated with the density of the collapsed lung [33]. The accurate differentiation of lung malignancy from corresponding atelectasis dramatically helps in radiation therapy planning to save the healthy lung parenchyma as much as possible [34]. In addition, a focal hot spot may be seen in the lung without morphologic correlation which is mainly due to non-specific retention of tracer in the pulmonary vessels and is known as FDG clot (Fig. 17.9). FDG clot may even show increasing pattern of tracer uptake on delayed images.

Thymic physiologic uptake is greatly dependent on the patient's age and is much higher under the age of 30. However, rebound thymic hyperplasia with moderately prominent FDG uptake in the enlarged gland may be observed after chemotherapy (Fig. 17.10) [35].

Adherent to minimum 6 h of fasting before FDG administration makes fatty acids as the dominant fuel for the myocytes, resulting in minimal FDG uptake in the heart. Nevertheless, myocardial tracer uptake is quite variable even in fasting state, in a spectrum from zero to complete avidity [36]. Inadequate patient preparation having meal shortly before PET examination may cause insulin secretion and diffuse muscle uptake (Fig. 17.11).

The activity in great vessels is based on the amount of FDG available in the blood pool. Considering the urinary system as the root of

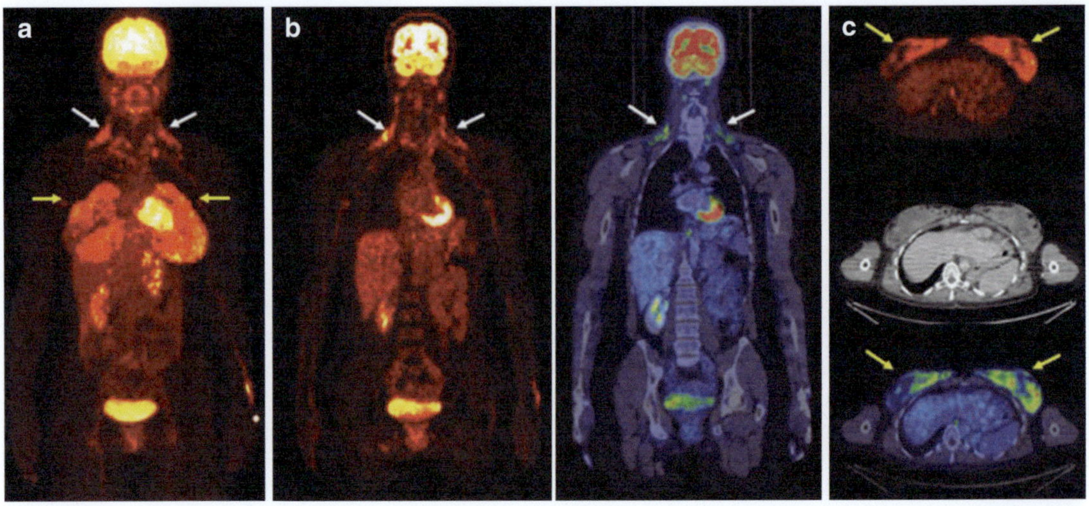

Fig. 17.6 ^{18}F-FDG PET/CT. Diffuse ^{18}F-FDG uptake in the cervical brown fat and breasts in breastfeeding. A 39-year-old female referred for evaluation of metabolic activity of a cervical cystic lesion. (**a**) *MIP (maximum intensity projection) image*: heterogeneous ^{18}F-FDG activity is visualized in the cervical region (white arrows), as well as a diffuse nonhomogeneous uptake in bilateral breasts (yellow arrows). (**b**) *Coronal PET (left) and fusion PET/CT (right) images*: the white arrows point the ^{18}F-FDG uptakes in the cervical brown fat. (**c**) *Trans-axial PET (upper), CT (middle), and fusion PET/CT (lower) images*: the diffuse heterogeneous ^{18}F-FDG activity is localized in the normal fibroglandular tissue of breasts indicative of physiologic uptake in breastfeeding

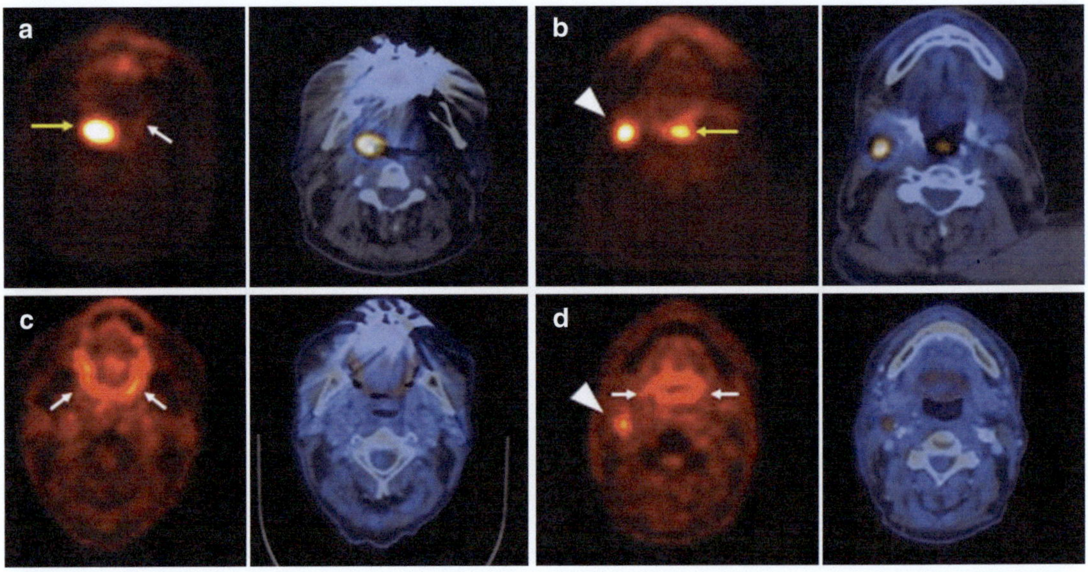

Fig. 17.7 ^{18}F-FDG PET/CT. Postradiation inflammation. A 59-year-old male with tonsil and epiglottis carcinoma referred for evaluation of response to treatment. (**a**, **b**) *Pre-treatment trans-axial PET (left) and fusion PET/CT (right) images:* hypermetabolic tumoral lesions are visualized in the right tonsil (**a**, yellow arrow), epiglottis (**b**, yellow arrow), and a right cervical lymph node (**b**, arrow head). (**c**, **d**) *Post-treatment trans-axial PET (left) and fusion PET/CT (right) images*: malignant lesions in the right tonsil and epiglottis are no longer seen. Also, the cervical lymph node shows a significant decrease in metabolic activity, indicating a remarkable response to treatment (**d**, arrow head). As a new finding, mild diffuse uptake (**c**, **d**, white arrows) is depicted in the oropharyngeal region which is correlated with the inflammatory process in the normal tissues after radiation therapy

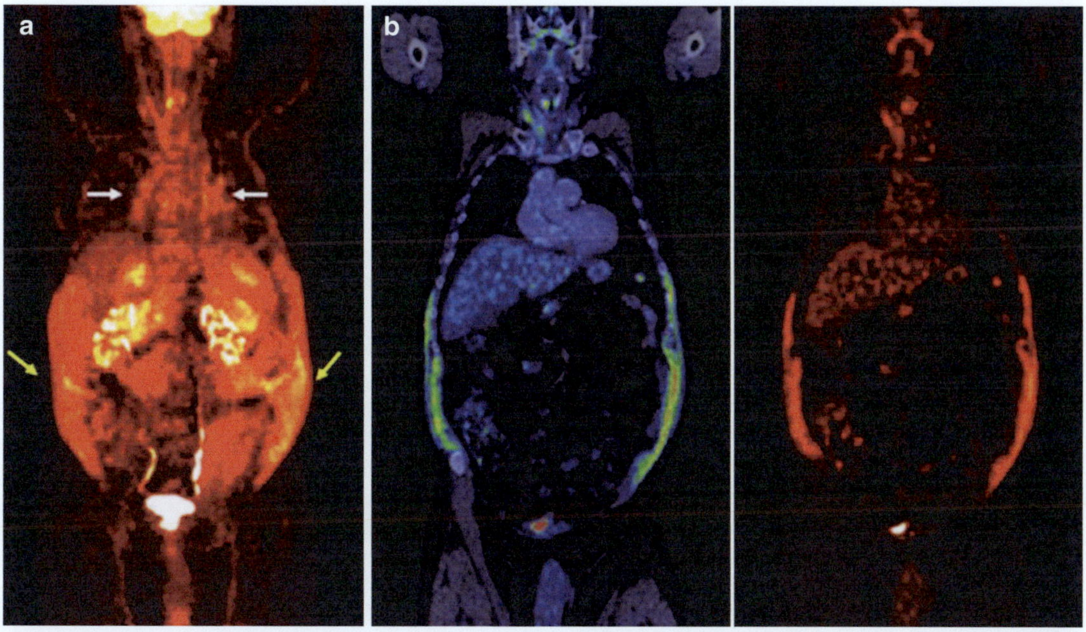

Fig. 17.8 ^{18}F-FDG PET/CT. Abdominal wall muscle uptake. A 73-year-old male with high-grade esophageal dysplasia. (**a**) *MIP (maximum intensity projection) image*: there is a diffuse abnormal ^{18}F-FDG uptake in the abdominal region (yellow arrows). Also, reactive mediastinal and hilar lymph nodes with mild metabolic activity are noted (white arrows). (**b**) *Coronal fusion PET/CT (left) and PET (right) images*: the abnormal activity is localized in the abdominal wall and intercostal muscles as well as diaphragm as a result of active abdominal breathing during the examination secondary to respiratory distress

tracer elimination from body, the blood pool activity is expectedly higher in patients with renal failure [37]. Due to subendothelial smooth muscle proliferation, mild-to-moderate increased FDG uptake is expected in major vessel walls in elderly patients [28].

Diffuse FDG uptake in the esophagus or mild focal FDG uptake in gastroesophageal junction is most likely benign in nature [38].

Mild-to-moderate normal FDG uptake may present in hilar regions which is usually symmetric. If it symmetrically persists on follow-up PET study of patients with non-pulmonary malignancies, it should be considered benign (Fig. 17.8) [28].

Metal objects such as chemotherapy ports make both streak and attenuation-correction artifacts on CT and PET images, respectively. Attenuation-correction artifact is also applied for calcified thoracic lymph nodes. Therefore, for a correct interpretation, it is necessary to check the same area on non-attenuation corrected PET/CT images [27, 39].

Diaphragmatic movement during respiration may make a mismatch between PET and CT images and cause a curvilinear cold region in upper abdomen (Fig. 17.1). This causes a part of the liver to be visualized in the chest, and using a breath-hold method is a solution. This causes a part of the liver to be visualized in the chest and using a breath-hold method is a solution. However, it may occurred less frequently using modern multi-slice CT scanners with fast scanning time or by applying the respiratory-gated method. This artifact is more important if the lesions are located in the base of the lungs or liver superior segments, causing a misdiagnosis [40, 41].

In order to reduce discomfort for patients and limit the chance of motion artifact, the imaging could be done with the patients arms down by the body. Nonetheless, this may lead to a beam hardening and streak artifact (truncation) on CT study.

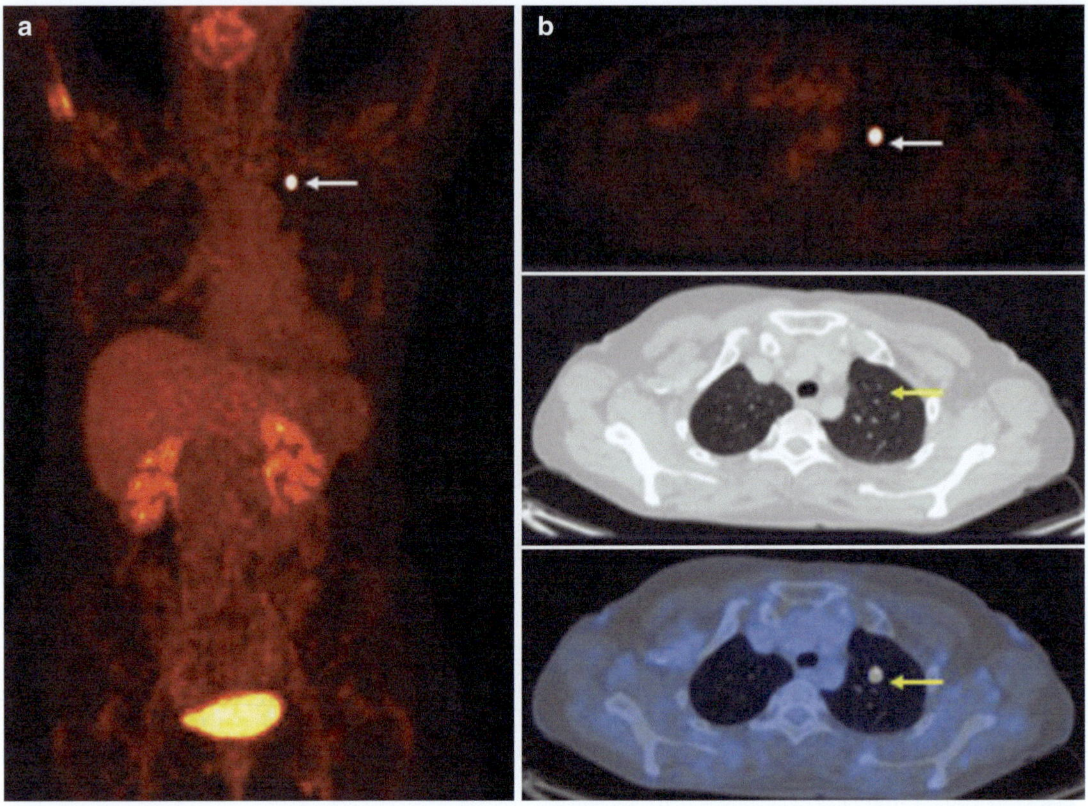

Fig. 17.9 ^{18}F-FDG PET/CT. FDG clot. A 59-year-old female with granulosa cell tumor referred for evaluation of recurrence. (**a**) *MIP (maximum intensity projection) image*: an intense focus of ^{18}F-FDG activity is depicted in the left upper thoracic region. (**b**) *Trans-axial PET (upper), CT (middle), and fusion PET/CT (lower) images*: the focus of ^{18}F-FDG activity is seen on the apicoposterior segment of the left lung without any morphological abnormality on CT suggesting of FDG clot

It would be resolved if all patients go to the scanner with their arms up, but in case of head and neck cancers, a dedicated head and neck PET/CT should be done with the arms down. The role of the technologist is very crucial in positioning the patients [39].

17.3.3 Abdomen

As the two major components of the abdomen, both alimentary tract and urinary system can show physiologic activity of ^{18}F-FDG on PET/CT. Thus, the hybrid imaging and correlation with CT scan for localization are very important for correct interpretation [42].

Although FDG uptake in alimentary tract is variable, however, a disseminated, mild-to-moderate activity is usually benign, causing from an inflammatory process, muscle contraction, uptake of lymphoid tissues, use of medications, and artifacts (Fig. 17.12). Among the different parts of the large intestine, the cecum and recto-sigmoid colon (more prominent in rectosigmoid junction) show the highest physiologic FDG uptake. Mild increased activity of gastroesophageal junction is acceptable [42].

In contrast, any focal and intense tracer uptake should be further evaluated to exclude malignancy. With an approximately 70% chance of malignancy, colonoscopic correlation is strongly warranted in these cases [43–45].

As the main root of FDG elimination from the body secondary to non-reabsorption of tracer from renal tubules, accumulation of radioactive urine is almost always seen in renal collecting

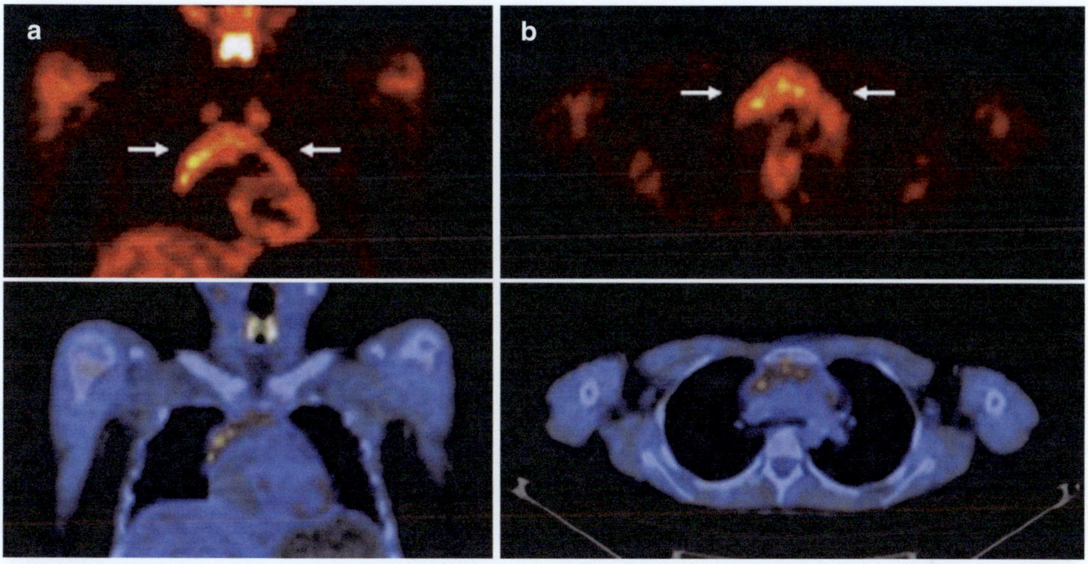

Fig. 17.10 ^{18}F-FDG PET/CT. (**a**) *Coronal PET (upper), fusion PET/CT (lower)* and (**b**) *trans-axial PET (upper), fusion PET/CT (lower) images*: physiologic reactive ^{18}F-FDG uptake is demonstrated in the normal thymus gland in a young patient

systems, ureters, and urinary bladder. This may obscure any underlying FDG malignant lesion. In addition, some GU tract neoplasms with cystic or necrotic features, mucinous histology, or low-grade pathology take up minimal radiotracer with resulting false-negative FDG PET/CT [46–48].

A mild, diffuse, homogenous FDG uptake is expected for the liver, spleen, adrenal glands, and pancreas, more prominent in the liver. But an intense, focal activity would be abnormal [42]. Adrenal nodule or masses are always compared with the liver. An intense tracer uptake which is markedly over the liver metabolic activity often represents a malignant process [49, 50].

With changing the cellular biology, some medications potentially alter distribution of FDG in the body [42].

One of them is metformin that increases FDG uptake in GI tract, more noticeable in the colon [51, 52]. This may result in missing an underlying FDG avid colon cancer and a false-negative interpretation [53]. Therefore, it is preferred that diabetic patients who are on metformin discontinue mediation at least 3 days before FDG PET imaging [54].

Another medication that can significantly change biodistribution of FDG in the body is granulocyte-colony stimulating factor (G-CSF). Normally, there is mild, diffuse tracer uptake in the spleen and bone marrow which is less than the liver. G-CSF consumption or recent courses of chemotherapy may cause diffuse intense increased FDG uptake in the spleen and bone marrow (Fig. 17.13) [55, 56].

Using oral contrast by the patient works as a metal object, causing streak beam artifact, and, due to increased CT numbers and elevated PET attenuation coefficient, causes a falsely increased FDG uptake in the bowels (attenuation-correction artifact). Review of non-attenuation corrected images plays a major role to avoid error in interpretation. However, intravenous contrast has minimal side effect on PET study [27, 57].

17.3.4 Pelvis

It has been shown that increased FDG uptake in the pelvis is not uncommon, and, in some investigations, it was reported that about 1% of people who underwent PET/CT had focal FDG uptake in the pelvis [58].

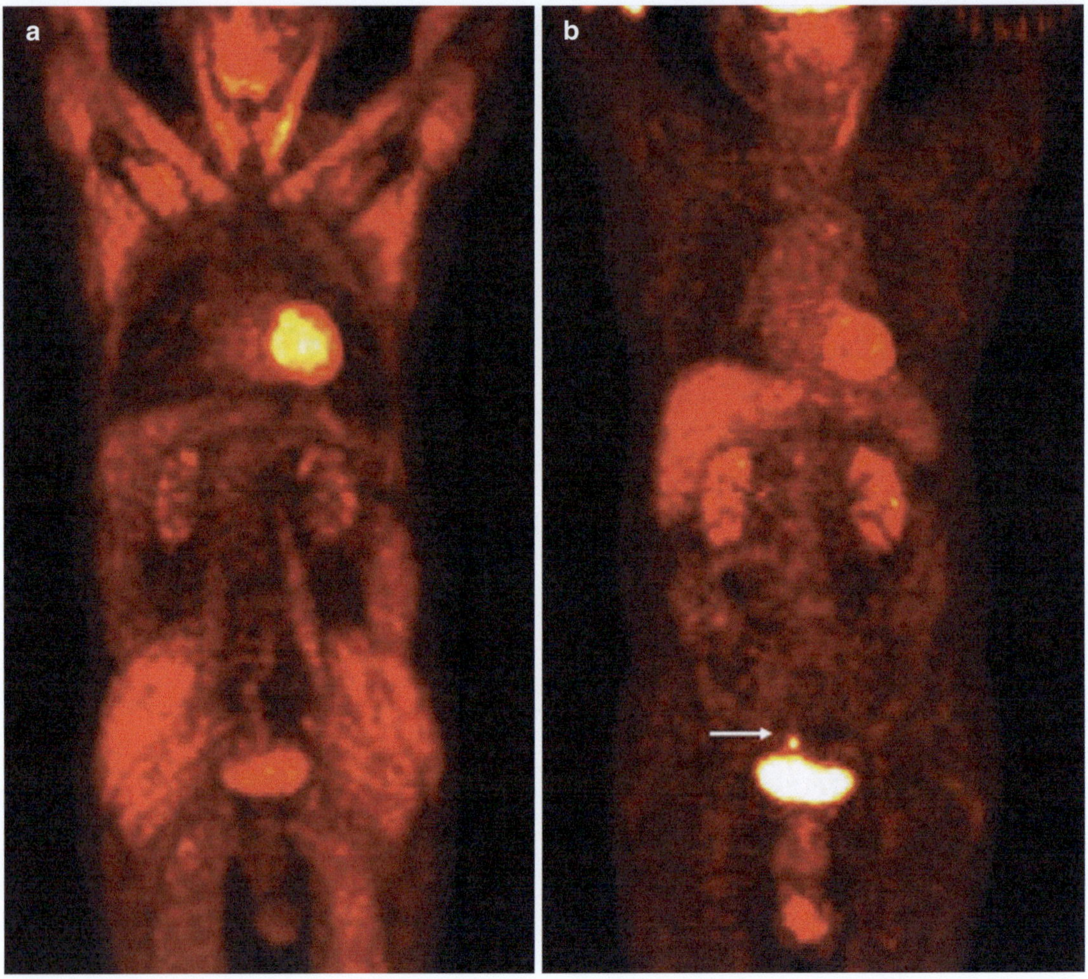

Fig. 17.11 ^{18}F-FDG PET/CT. A 73-year-old male with rectal adenocarcinoma referred for initial staging. (**a**) *MIP (maximum intensity projection) image*: diffuse ^{18}F-FDG uptake is visualized in almost all muscles due to inadequate preparation of patient having a meal shortly before examination which caused stimulation of insulin secretion and diffuse muscles uptakes. Owing to non-optimal quality, the ^{18}F-FDG PET/CT study was repeated on the next day. (**b**) *MIP image of the repeated examination*: no abnormal muscle activity is seen. Notably, a small focus of metabolically active tumoral lesion is depicted in the proximal part of the rectum (arrow), which was not detectable in the previous study as a result of compromised quality

As discussed before, in contrast to focal intense FDG uptake in the colon which usually warrants further evaluation, diffusely distributed tracer is often related to bowel wall smooth muscle activity or excretion of FDG in the lumen, most likely benign and a normal variation. It is sometimes related to metformin consumption in diabetic patients [58, 59].

Due to accumulation of radioactive urine in the bladder, FDG PET/CT is not quite sensitive to evaluate its malignancies. However, it is very important not to interpret bladder diverticula as a metastatic perivesical lymph node [58].

Faint FDG uptake in great vessels of pelvis, particularly in elderly patients, is physiologic. In some cases, apparent vessel wall calcification is also evident [60, 61].

The prostate gland normally shows mild, diffuse FDG uptake. However, focal activity warrants further evaluation to exclude a neoplastic process. Although FDG PET/CT is sub-optimal

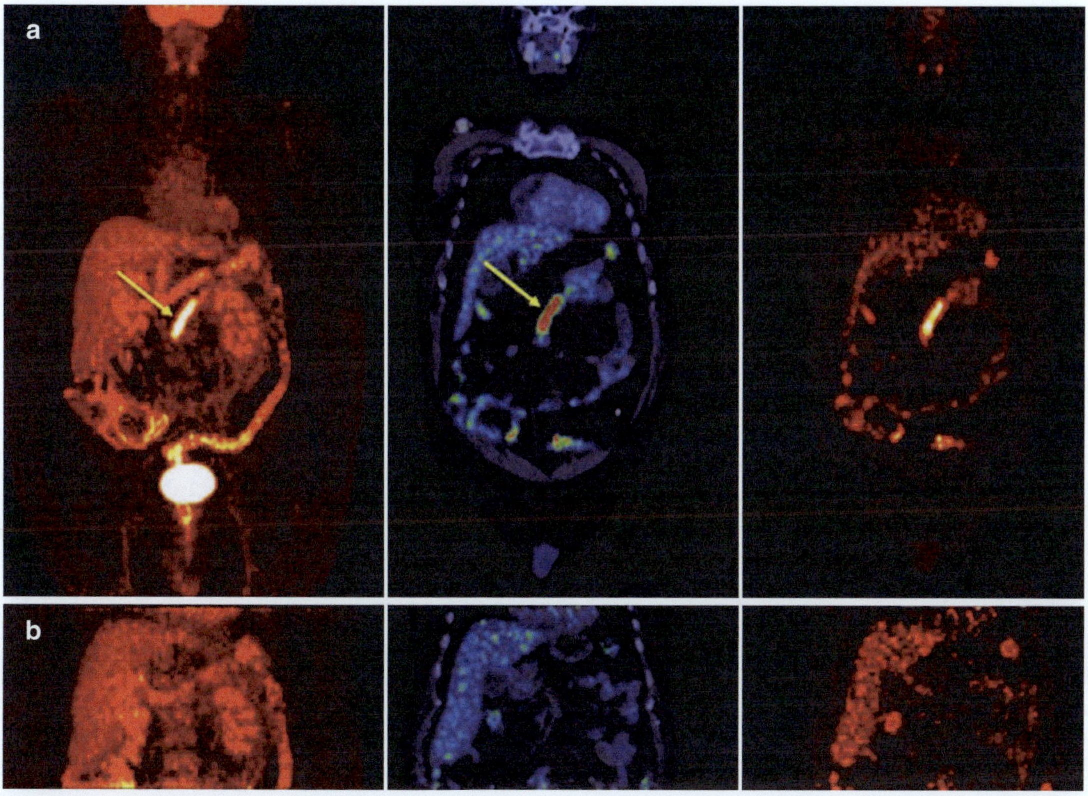

Fig. 17.12 ^{18}F-FDG PET/CT. Intense physiologic intestinal uptake. A 58-year-old male with esophageal cancer referred for surveillance. (**a**) *MIP (maximum intensity projection) (left), coronal fusion PET/CT (middle), and coronal PET (right) images*: there is an intense linear ^{18}F-FDG uptake (arrow) in the abdomen which is confined to the intestine on the fused images (arrows). At first glance, the intensity and pattern of the uptake imply an inflammatory process. (**b**) *Delayed examination. MIP (left), coronal fusion PET/CT (middle), and coronal PET (right) images*: the uptake disappeared after bowel movement on the delayed images, ruling out the inflammation, and indicating an advantage of the dual time imaging

for evaluation of prostate adenocarcinoma as a slow-growing malignancy, FDG avid prostate adenocarcinomas are almost always high grade that implies a prognostic role for this imaging modality [58, 62].

Mild-to-moderate homogenous FDG uptake in the testicles is well documented and could be due to metabolic activity in Leydig, Sertoli, or newborn spermatocytes [63]. The FDG uptake is inversely correlated with patient's age [64, 65]. It is important not to falsely interpret an undescended testis as an FDG avid lymphadenopathy [66].

Low FDG uptake is generally expected in uterus and ovaries in postmenopausal patients [58, 67]. FDG uptake is variable in premenopausal women. Increased FDG uptake may be seen in the uterus around mid-cycle, and if the patient is in her bleeding phase, radioactive blood could be visualized within the cavity. The metabolic activity is often unilateral in the ovaries and at its peak at mid-cycle but generally between the days 10 and 25 of the menstrual cycle. A luteal cyst may be FDG avid as well (Fig. 17.14) [58, 68–70].

17.3.5 Brain

Glucose is the only molecule that is used as the fuel by central nervous system neurons. Thus, and as a glucose analog, there is intense FDG uptake in the brain, much more prominent in

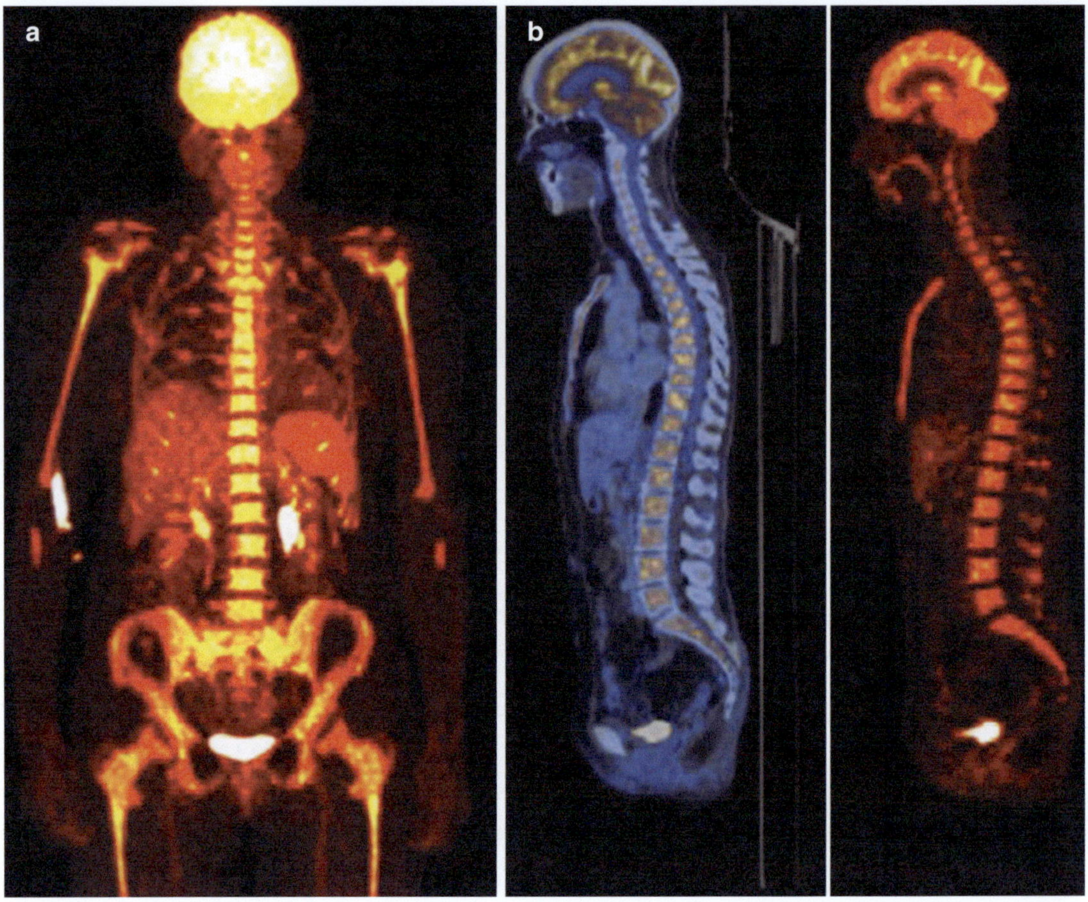

Fig. 17.13 18F-FDG PET/CT. Reactive bone marrow ^{18}F-FDG uptake. A 53-year-old female with breast carcinoma referred for evaluation of response to treatment. (**a**) *MIP (maximum intensity projection),* (**b**) *sagittal fusion PET/CT (left) sagittal PET (right) images*: diffuse homogeneous ^{18}F-FDG uptake is seen throughout the axial and proximal appendicular skeleton, which is compatible with reactive bone marrow hyperplasia secondary to G-CSF (granulocyte-colony stimulating factor) administration

cerebral cortex, basal ganglia, cerebellum, and thalamus compared with the white matter (with gray/white matter ratio ~2.5–4) [71–73].

Distribution of radiotracer is more prominent in the occipital, parietal, and frontal compared with temporal cortex [71].

It is approved that metabolic activity of brain reaches the level of adults at the age of 2 [74]. However, global brain metabolic rate shows a negative relationship with age [75]. In particular, advanced aging causes reduction in FDG uptake of frontal lobe [71]. However, in Alzheimer disease, hypometabolism of this lobe occurs only in advanced cases [76, 77].

On the other hand, review of literature to compare the brain metabolic rate in males and females is completely variable with no consensus [71].

The effect of medications also investigated and revealed that consumption of caffeine, ethanol, low-dose amphetamines, benzodiazepines, corticosteroids, and chemotherapeutic agents decreased cerebral metabolic activity and reduced FDG uptake. This also happened after radiation therapy of the brain [71, 78].

Elevated blood glucose level may cause global decreased of FDG uptake in the brain [71]. Also, patient motion artifact leads to attenuation-correction artifact and image blurring. Review of

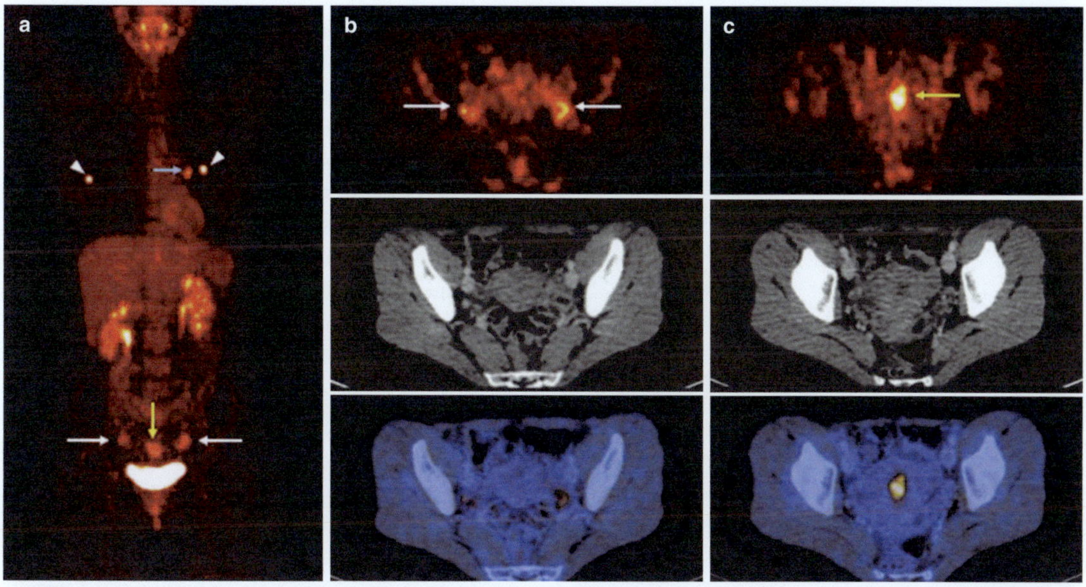

Fig. 17.14 ^{18}F-FDG PET/CT. Benign ^{18}F-FDG uptake in the uterus and ovaries. A 35-year-old female with breast carcinoma referred for initial staging. (**a**) *MIP (maximum intensity projection) images*: mild symmetrical ^{18}F-FDG activity is visualized in bilateral ovaries (**a**, **b**, white arrows) and uterus (**a**, **c**, yellow arrow). In addition, metabolically active tumoral lesions are noted in both breasts (arrow heads) and left hilum (blue arrow). (**b**) *Trans-axial PET (upper), CT (middle), fusion PET/CT (lower) images*: mild symmetrical ^{18}F-FDG uptake is depicted in both ovaries without morphologic abnormality. This finding is considered physiologic on the 17th day of the menstrual cycle which is due to metabolic activity in the corpus luteum after ovulation. (**c**) *Trans-axial PET (upper), CT (middle), and fusion PET/CT (lower) images:* a focus of ^{18}F-FDG uptake is localized in the uterus (yellow arrow), representing either a physiologic or inflammatory process

non-attenuation corrected study would be helpful [71]. Metal objects in the field of view cause false-positive PET images secondary to increased CT numbers. Again, review of non-attenuation corrected study is a clue for a correct interpretation [4, 71, 79].

17.4 ^{11}C- and ^{18}F-Choline

Three radiolabeled choline ligands have been commonly used in clinical routine practice: ^{11}C-choline, ^{18}F-methylcholine, and ^{18}F-ethylcholine. ^{11}C-choline has lower urinary excretion and a half-life of 20 min, whereas ^{18}F-methylcholine and ^{18}F-ethyl-choline have higher urinary excretion and longer half-life of 110 min (Fig. 17.15).

The phosphorylation pathway of ^{18}F-fluorocholine (FCH) is similar to that of ^{11}C-labeled choline and better than other choline analogs [80]. It has been reported that ^{18}F-labeled choline images show better sharpness comparing to ^{11}C-choline PET [81]. Furthermore, ^{11}C-choline examinations are limited to centers with an onsite cyclotron, while ^{18}F-labeled choline can be delivered commercially.

The uptake of the radiolabeled choline derivatives can be seen in physiologic or benign conditions that integrate cell membrane synthesis.

Therefore, knowledge of physiologic distribution, benign findings, and the potentially false-positive lesions is important for accurate interpretation.

17.4.1 Brain/Head and Neck

Brain shows usually low choline uptake compared to the extra-cerebral tissues. There are two kinds of energy-dependent transport systems for choline incorporation in the cell membrane, phosphorylcholine synthesis which is present on

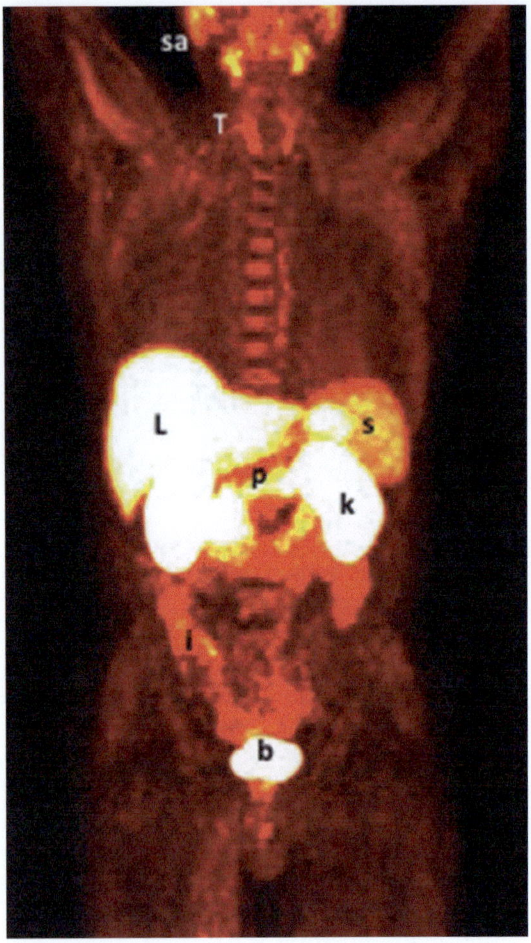

Fig. 17.15 Normal biodistribution of ^{118}F-fluorocholine PET. Physiologic uptake is presented in the salivary glands (sa), liver (L), spleen (s), pancreas (p), kidneys (k), intestine (i), and bladder (b)

all mammalian cells and acetyl-choline synthesis which is present in the synaptosomes, and the transport of choline is coupled to acetyl-choline synthesis [82, 83].

Choline based tracers have been applied in brain cancer imaging due to the fact that phosphorylcholine synthesis is increased in tumors. In a study evaluating the physiological distribution of ^{18}F-methylcholine [84], a range of uptake in different head and neck tissues have been reported, for instance, low-grade uptake in the normal brain parenchyma and moderate uptake in the choroid plexus, cavernous sinus, extraocular eye muscles, masticatory muscles, and bone marrow. Uptake in the pituitary gland was generally moderately intense, whereas uptake in the lacrimal glands and the mucosa of the nasal cavity was found to be variable. Parotid glands showed high-grade uptake. Tumors like glioblastomas and meningiomas were found to be moderately intense, whereas uptake in grade II and III gliomas was globally faint [83].

In another study, Calabria et al. reported a moderate abnormal tracer accumulation in mucosal thickening of the right maxillary sinus (SUVmax 4). The clinical and imaging follow-up studies were then suggestive of sinusitis [85].

In addition, asymmetrical FCH uptake may also be seen in the submandibular glands which are most likely functional caused by unilateral glandular hypo- and/or aplasia.

Thyroid gland may also show a mild uptake on FCH PET. However, the relationship between such choline uptakes and any thyroid disease is unclear (Fig. 17.15). Schillaci et al. [86] have presented a case of focal thyroid uptake on FCH PET which was found to be thyroiditis on clinical assessment.

Focal FCH uptake may also be related to parathyroid adenoma which should be further evaluated [87].

Inflammatory conditions such as sinusitis, thyroiditis, and otomastoiditis may also present increased ^{18}F-choline uptake which can be due to the proliferation of some cellular types involved in the genesis of phlogosis [85, 86, 88]. These findings should be correlated with clinical and laboratory findings. Recent trauma and bone fracture show also increased choline uptake.

17.4.2 Thorax

Lung parenchyma shows usually no radiolabeled choline uptake, apart from the lung bases where curvilinear uptake is seen along at the base of the lung mainly related to the supine position of the patients on PET/CT scanning [83].

However, diffuse increased uptake of choline in the lungs may reflect cardiac diseases (e.g., heart failure) with congestive changes in the lungs because of pulmonary venous imbalance.

Mediastinal, hilar, and axillary lymph nodes may also show mild increased tracer uptakes which are mostly reactive or related to an inflammatory process. The mean registered SUVmax of such lymph nodes is about 2.8 [83, 85].

Based on our experience, tracer intensity in the reactive lymph nodes is usually higher than blood pool activity and similar to the bone marrow uptake in the thoracic spine with ±20% difference [83]. Inflammatory lymph nodes resulting from granulomatous disease may show intensive tracer uptake. However, they mostly show the typical symmetrical pattern of tracer uptake in the mediastinum and hilum. Also, no significant myocardial uptake was seen in choline PET studies.

Brachial and/or cephalic vein may present a mild increased tracer uptake at the injection site which may be related to rapid and non-specific endothelial uptake.

An intensive choline uptake may be seen in thymoma with SUVmax of about 8 [85]. Pleuritis and esophagitis are other causes of increased choline uptake [86].

17.4.3 Abdomen

Angiotensin-converting enzyme converts acetylcholine into inactive choline metabolites and acetate in an intracellular and extracellular manner. Thus, the physiologic pattern of increased radiolabeled choline uptake is seen in liver parenchyma as the cholinergic components are also expressed in non-cancerous liver cells [89]. There is also a mild increased FCH uptake at the periphery of the liver as compared to the lobes toward the porta hepatis, similar to FDG. This may primarily be due to perfusion-related parameters rather than cell membrane-phospholipid proliferation.

Choline-labeled radiotracers can be detected in liver tumors like hepatoma [90, 91]. The gastrointestinal tract reveals a variable pattern of radiolabeled choline uptake. Once the choline is injected intravenously, there is hepatic and biliary uptake with subsequent excretion into the small bowel [83]. Physiological uptake of small intestine and colon is observed mainly due to the rapid turnover of the epithelial cells [92].

Pancreas is one of the most avid structures seen on choline PET as previously reported [86]. Pancreatic body and tail show variable moderate-to-intense uptake, while the pancreatic head is intensely avid [83]. Atrophic changes in the pancreas cause replacement of the pancreatic parenchyma with fat which may lead to inhomogeneous tracer distribution with a focal or diffuse reduction in choline uptake [93].

A moderate increased choline uptake is usually seen in the spleen. The adrenal glands show often no tracer uptake in all choline-labeled tracers; however, mild increased choline uptake can be seen uni- and/or bilaterally in the adrenal glands with mean SUVmax of ≤2.8 [85]. Adrenal adenoma may also show mild-to-moderate increased choline uptake corresponding with related findings on CT [83].

17.4.4 Pelvis/Genitourinary System

Generally, kidneys, ureters, and urinary bladder show intensive tracer accumulation, as the genitourinary organ is the main system of radiotracer excretion. Some centers use iv-hydration (500 ml of normal saline 0.9% intravenously) prior to scanning to overcome urinary pooling in the kidneys [86]. Physiologic tracer accumulation possesses a challenge for assessment of the pelvic region. Therefore, some centers perform an initial dynamic imaging of the pelvis before the excreted activity is seen in the bladder followed by delayed imaging of the whole body. Also, emptying the bladder prior to imaging minimizes the residual excreted activity in the urinary bladder. Bulbourethral gland may also show focal increased tracer uptake, especially in the early dynamic images [83].

Prostate cancer demonstrates an area of focal or diffuse increased tracer uptake, while normal prostate tissue may show only faint increased uptake [94–96]. Local inflammation of the prostate can also cause increased focal tracer accumulation and is the most common cause of false-positive choline uptake.

Inguinal lymph nodes showing mild-to-moderate increased choline uptake usually with rapid washout are usually considered as reactive [83].

17.4.5 Treatment Effect

A study reported a case of high blood pool activity on ^{18}F-methylcholine PET study in a patient receiving colchicine, whereas the activity was normalized on the repeated study after withdrawal of colchicine [97]. The authors suggested that colchicine and drugs with a possible similar effect like docetaxel and paclitaxel impair the normal choline pathway and must be stopped before ^{18}F-methylcholine PET/CT imaging [97]. However, no significant correlation between the duration of hormone therapy (HT) and FCH PET/CT positivity has been documented [95].

Moreover, patients with ongoing HT may show mildly increased and nonhomogenous bone marrow uptake in the axial skeleton which may cause false-positive results [83]. In our experience performing an additional delayed acquisition from undetermined lesions may help in differentiating malignant versus reactive/benign bony lesions [98].

17.5 ^{11}C-Acetate

The pathway of ^{11}C-acetate is related to the type of cells. In myocardial tissue, acetate is mainly metabolized to CO_2 via tricarboxylic acid cycle, while tumor cells stimulate fatty acid synthetase, thus converting acetate into fatty acids which will be incorporated into intracellular the cell membrane [99, 100].

^{11}C-acetate PET has been used to measure myocardial oxygen consumption, to study prostate cancer, hepatocellular carcinoma (HCC), renal cell carcinoma (RCC), bladder carcinoma, and brain tumors [101]. Previous studies reported incidentally depiction of thymoma [102], cerebellopontine angle schwannoma [103], angiomyolipoma of the kidney [104], encephalitis [105], and multiple myeloma by ^{11}C-acetate PET [106].

17.5.1 Brain/Head and Neck

Acetate metabolism in the normal rat brain is lower and more homogeneous than that of glucose and slightly increases during physiologic stimulation. This advantage of radiolabeled acetate provides a homogeneous low background activity and higher tumor to background ratio to delineate tumors. Increased uptake of ^{11}C-acetate was reported in meningeal tuberculoma probably due to increased macrophages activities [107].

Macroadenomas of pituitary gland and meningiomas showed high uptake of ^{11}C-acetate in previous studies [107, 108].

Benign thyroid nodes may reveal high tracer activity [109]. A moderate-to-high ^{11}C-acetate uptake may be observed in salivary glands and tonsils without remarkable activity in normal nasopharynx and other structures of the neck (Fig. 17.16) [110, 111].

17.5.2 Thorax

A very faint tracer uptake may be seen in the lung parenchyma, while the mediastinum presents a minor uptake. However, parenchymal lung disease may reveal a diffuse increased uptake [112]. Symmetrical pattern of lymph nodes ^{11}C-acetate uptake can be seen in mediastinum and hilum suggestive of reactive and/or inflammatory lymph nodes not related to the primary tumor. Myocardium shows usually no tracer uptake when performing routine oncologic protocol.

Minor uptake is presented in bone marrow, especially in dorsal vertebrae, while degenerative changes in the bones show an inhomogeneous moderate ^{11}C-acetate uptake.

17.5.3 Abdomen

Increasing pattern of ^{11}C-acetate uptake is often seen in the upper abdominal parenchymatous organs such as the liver, spleen, and pancreas. The highest uptake can be found in the pancreas followed by the spleen and then by the liver

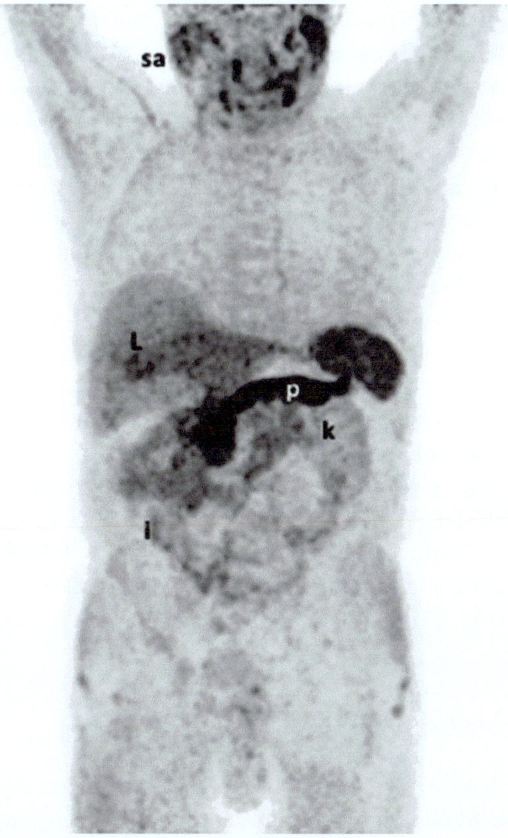

Fig. 17.16 Normal biodistribution of ^{11}C-acetate PET. Physiologic uptake is presented in the salivary glands (sa), liver (L), spleen (s), pancreas (p), intestine (i), and kidneys (k). *(Courtesy Georg Karanikas, Medical University of Vienna)*

(Fig. 17.16). Pancreatic tissue shows an early rapid uptake, visualized by 2-min post-injection and the most prominent organ in the imaging field in 10 min after tracer administration. By 30-min post-injection, the pancreas remains well-defined and is the only remaining conspicuous structure in the imaging field. Pancreas-to-liver ratio ranged from 2.1 to 4.5, with a mean of 3.1 in 20-min post-injection [113]. Chronic pancreatitis may lead to reduced ^{11}C-acetate uptake, while pancreatic endocrine insufficiency seems to have no remarkable influence of physiologic ^{11}C-acetate uptake in pancreas. The high ^{11}C-acetate tracer concentration within the pancreas is believed to be due to a high rate of lipid synthesis within pancreatic acinar cells [113, 114].

Focal nodular hyperplasia (FNH) and HCC reveal abnormal ^{11}C-acetate uptake. Nevertheless, using dual-time imaging may help to differentiate benign from malignant tissues. HCC presents an increasing pattern of tracer activity on delayed ^{11}C-acetate PET images, while rapid washout of the tracer activity is usually seen in FNH [115].

The previous studies reported that hemangioma; cholangiocarcinoma (pure primary adenocarcinoma of liver without HCC components); colon, breast, and lung cancers; as well as carcinoid tumors show no significant increased ^{11}C-acetate uptake. Increased tracer uptake may also be seen on the distal part of esophagus which is mainly due to inflammatory process when performing gastroscopy [113]. In addition, low tracer uptake is seen in muscles, intestines, and renal parenchyma [33].

In normal subjects, the renal cortex shows high tracer accumulation with rapid perfusion on early images (i.e., 60-s post-injection) and remains the most prominent organ in the imaging field through 10 min. However, no remarkable urinary activity appeared in the intrarenal collecting system. Interestingly, renal cortical tracer activity may readily identify even in patients with markedly reduced renal function due to chronic nephropathy with serum creatinine levels over 5 mg/dl [113].

17.5.4 Pelvis

The normal prostate tissue may reveal a minor tracer uptake. Dynamic ^{11}C-acetate PET acquisitions showed early perfusion of tracer in prostate with a maximum tracer uptake at about 5 min. No significant SUV changes were reported between 6- and 10-min and 15- and 20-min post-injection on individual time-activity curve analyses. Inflammatory processes in the prostate can cause increased ^{11}C-acetate accumulation [116]. Previous reports showed a range of SUVmax of 1.8–5.5 for primary prostate cancer, 1.5–2.6 for recurrent cancer, and 3.2–3.5 for BPH. SUV value was significantly different between BPH and recurrent cancer ($P = 0.02$), but primary cancer could not be differentiated from BPH [117].

Regularly, bowel shows a minor uptake, but rarely some patients present unusual high accumulation of ^{11}C-acetate. However, approximately half of the patients show remarkable increased tracer uptake in rectum. Additionally, in rare cases, marked tracer accumulation is seen in urinary bladder and urethra. False-positive ^{11}C-acetate uptake may be seen in urinary bladder in case of granulomatous cystitis [118].

Primary invasive transitional cell carcinoma (TCC) of the urinary bladder and its metastatic nodes showed increased ^{11}C-acetate uptake. However, false-positive findings may occur at sites of inflammation, in particular in patients pre-treated with Bacillus Calmette-Guérin (BCG) [118].

17.6 ^{18}F-DOPA

^{18}F-DOPA (L-6-[18F]fluoro-3,4-dihydroxyphenylalanine) is an amino acid-based radiopharmaceutical that was originally used in the assessment of the striatal dopaminergic system in patients with Parkinson disease.

L-DOPA (L-3,4-dihydroxyphenylalanine) is the precursor of the neurotransmitters dopamine, epinephrine (adrenaline), and norepinephrine (noradrenaline) which are known as catecholamines. ^{18}F-DOPA is a large amino acid with biochemical characteristics and kinetics similar to natural L-dopa. It interacts in the catecholamine metabolic pathway of endogenous L-DOPA both in the brain and peripherally [119]. By the emergence of hybrid PET/CT scanners, ^{18}F-DOPA is playing an important role in the management of neuroendocrine tumors (NET), brain tumors, and pancreatic cell hyperplasia [120–122].

The main clinical indications of ^{18}F-DOPA PET/CT are imaging of the striatum, brain tumors, medullary thyroid carcinoma, NETs, and hyperinsulinemic hypoglycemia [123].

17.6.1 CNS: Head and Neck

^{18}F-DOPA PET shows usually a symmetrical comma-shaped pattern of uptake in basal ganglia striatum (mean SUVmax 2.77, range 1.5–3.6), while the rest of the cerebral cortex reveals no remarkable activity. Thus, any tracer activity above the background level of the adjacent brain can be considered abnormal when assessing brain tumors. It provides sufficient tumor/background ratio for visual assessment of abnormal lesions. However, differentiation of postradiation necrosis from viable tumors seems to be challenging, as necrotic tissues may also show mild-to-moderate increased ^{18}F-DOPA uptake [121]. Therefore, different quantitative approaches have been introduced using tumor/background, tumor/striatum, or tumor/white matter ratios, which may significantly improve the specificity of ^{18}F-DOPA PET in brain tumors [121].

There is no appreciable physiologic ^{18}F-DOPA uptake in the oral cavity and pharyngeal regions (Fig. 17.17) [124].

17.6.2 Thorax

A mild ^{18}F-DOPA uptake can be seen in the myocardium, peripheral muscles, and esophagus and occasionally a very faint uptake in the mammary glands. Therefore, any abnormal tracer accumulation in the lungs corresponding to morphological changes may present tumoral involvement [123].

17.6.3 Abdomen

^{18}F-DOPA reveals physiologic uptake in various parts of abdomen mainly due to its excretion from abdominal organs. Intense and variable uptake can be seen in the gallbladder and biliary tract (mean SUVmax 8.5), kidneys (mean SUVmax 4.4), ureters, and urinary bladder (mean SUVmax 111) depending on individual elimination timing (Fig. 17.17) [124].

Mild diffuse uptake is usually visible in the liver (mean SUVmax 2.15, range 1.1–2.9). The pancreas shows variable and sometimes intensive ^{18}F-DOPA uptake mainly in the uncinate process (mean SUVmax 5.67, range 2.9–14.1) and less intense to the body–tail region (mean SUVmax 4.07, range 2.1–6.2). Similarly, the adrenal

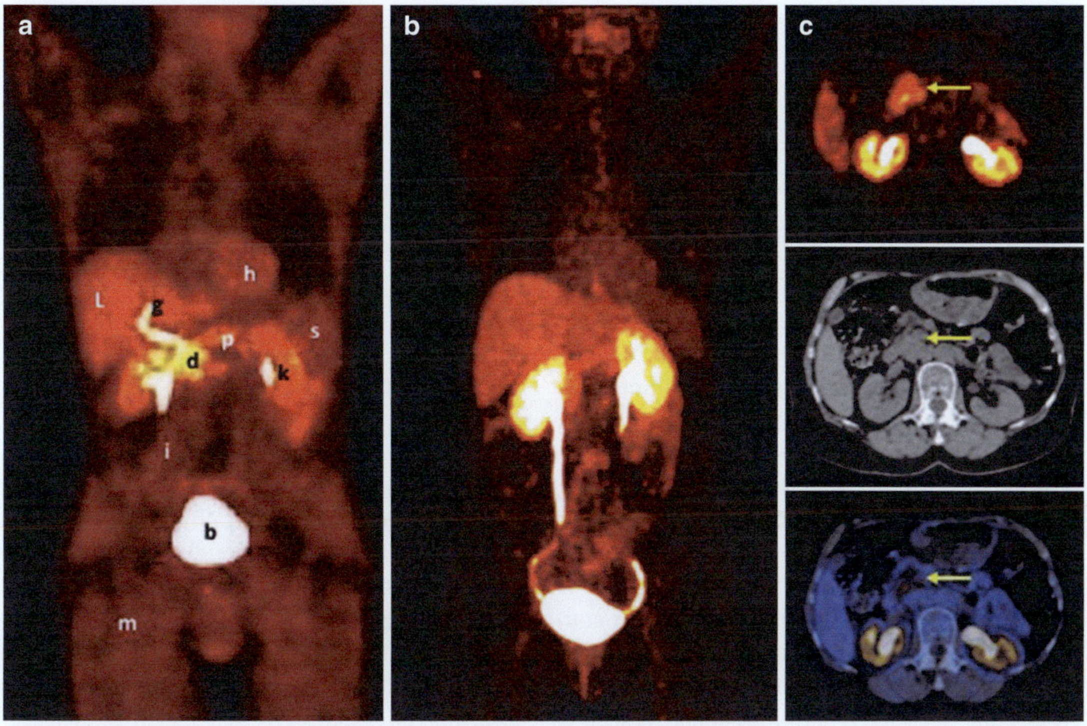

Fig. 17.17 Normal biodistribution of ^{18}F-DOPA PET in two different patients and different scanners (**a**, **b**). Physiologic uptake is presented in the liver (L), gallbladder and biliary tract (g), duodenum (d), spleen (s), pancreas (p), kidneys (k), and bladder (b), as well as, to a lesser extent, in the myocardium (h), muscles (m), and intestinal loops (i). However, by the administration of carbidopa (**b**), the uptake significantly decreases in the gallbladder and biliary tract. (**c**) *Trans-axial PET (upper), CT (middle), and fusion PET/CT (lower) images*: physiologic ^{18}F-DOPA uptake is visualized on uncinate process region without any abnormal morphological correlation on CT (arrows)

glands may also reveal variable tracer uptake (mean SUVmax 1.92, range 0.7–4.3) which should be taken into consideration to avoid any misinterpretation. Mild diffuse bowel activity (mean SUVmax 2.3) may also be seen in ^{18}F-DOPA PET images [123].

17.6.4 Effect of Carbidopa Premedication on the Biodistribution of ^{18}F-DOPA

Premedication with carbidopa may improve the diagnostic accuracy of ^{18}F-DOPA PET in the detection of paragangliomas and carcinoid tumors and can enhance striatum uptake [125, 126]. In fact, carbidopa administration leads to a higher ^{18}F-DOPA uptake in the basal ganglia, lungs, myocardium, and liver [126]. In contrast, it results in rapid tracer washout and markedly reduced tracer uptake in pancreas which is reported as the cause of false-negative results in patients with hyperinsulinemic hypoglycemia [126, 127]. It may also influence in physiologic excretion of ^{18}F-DOPA into the biliary ducts, the gallbladder, and the urinary system (Fig. 17.17) [123].

17.7 ^{68}Ga-DOTA-Peptides

Increased SSTR (somatostatin receptor) expression is a prominent characteristic of neuroendocrine tumors (NET). Novel radiotracers, targeting SSTR molecule, for PET/CT imaging have revolutionized the diagnosis of NET [128]. Several different compounds of radiotracers

[^{68}Ga-1,4,7,10-tetraazacyclododecane-1,4,7,10-tetraacetic acid (DOTA)-Peptides] have been developed and are increasingly used for imaging of NET [129]. ^{68}Ga-DOTA-Peptides PET/CT imaging is employed in staging/restaging, follow-up, detection of unknown primary tumor sites and selection of proper candidates for therapy with hot/cold somatostatin analogs in NET patients [129, 130]. ^{68}Ga-DOTA-Peptides uptake is highly associated with presence and density of SSTRs on NET cells; tumors with low, variable, or absent receptor expression may result in false-negative interpretation [129].

17.7.1 Brain / Head and Neck

Physiologic ^{68}Ga-DOTA-Peptides uptake is clearly visualized in the pituitary gland in contrary to the surrounding normal brain parenchyma with insignificant uptake [129, 131, 132]. Also, faint ^{68}Ga-DOTA-Peptides uptake is seen in the salivary and thyroid glands (Fig. 17.18) [129, 132]. There are several conditions that may cause false-positive interpretation of benign uptakes. SSTRs are expressed on activated lymphocytes, whether inflammatory or malignant. Hence, a special attention to areas that are the frequent site of inflammation such as thyroid, lymph nodes, or lymph nodes adjacent to areas of recent surgery/trauma is of great importance [129]. A thorough clinical history with particular attention to relevant inflammatory disorders such as sarcoidosis, chronic thyroiditis, thyroid nodules, recent invasive procedures, or trauma may often help precise image interpretation. Noteworthy, active osteoblastic activity secondary to any insult to the skeleton leads to increased ^{68}Ga-DOTA-Peptides uptake, such as osteoarthritis and fibrous dysplasia [133].

17.7.2 Thorax

According to the literature, any ^{68}Ga-SSTR uptake inside the rib cage is considered non-physiologic. However, low-grade uptake has been documented in the normal fibroglandular tissue of the breast [131]. In addition, a number of conditions, other than NET, have been reported to accumulate this tracer. Various inflammatory/infectious disorders, for instance, sarcoidosis, pneumonia, granulomatous disorders, and lung fibrosis, as well as inflammation/infection secondary to trauma or surgery, have been reported to pile up ^{68}Ga-DOTA-Peptides tracer [129].

17.7.3 Abdomen

Physiologic ^{68}Ga-DOTA-Peptides uptake is a challenging issue in the abdominal cavity since a number of organs reveal physiologic uptake. Significant ^{68}Ga-DOTA-Peptides uptake is demonstrated in the spleen, liver, adrenal glands, and intestine (Fig. 17.18) [129, 134]. More importantly, the presence of uptake in the head of the pancreas (exocrine) is a quite dilemma for the reporting physicians, in that pancreas is a frequent site of NET. On the other hand, considerable numbers of images show benign diffuse or focal ^{68}Ga-DOTA-Peptides uptake in the pancreas even with different compounds [134–136]. Particular attention to the uptake pattern and the comparison with other imaging techniques are mandatory to avoid misinterpretation [129]. Another benign condition that can be troublesome is the presence of accessory spleens associated with false-positive interpretation [131, 134]. Also, disparate amount of ^{68}Ga-DOTA-Peptides is excreted via the bile resulting in variable visualization of the gallbladder [134]. Finally, as is discussed before, any inflammatory/infectious process can exhibit ^{68}Ga-DOTA-Peptides activity.

17.7.4 Pelvis

Apart from physiologic uptake in the renal parenchyma, the main root of excretion from kidneys accounts for the significant ^{68}Ga-DOTA-Peptides activity in the urinary system [134]. The prostate gland also may reveal a low-grade ^{68}Ga-DOTA-Peptides uptake [134].

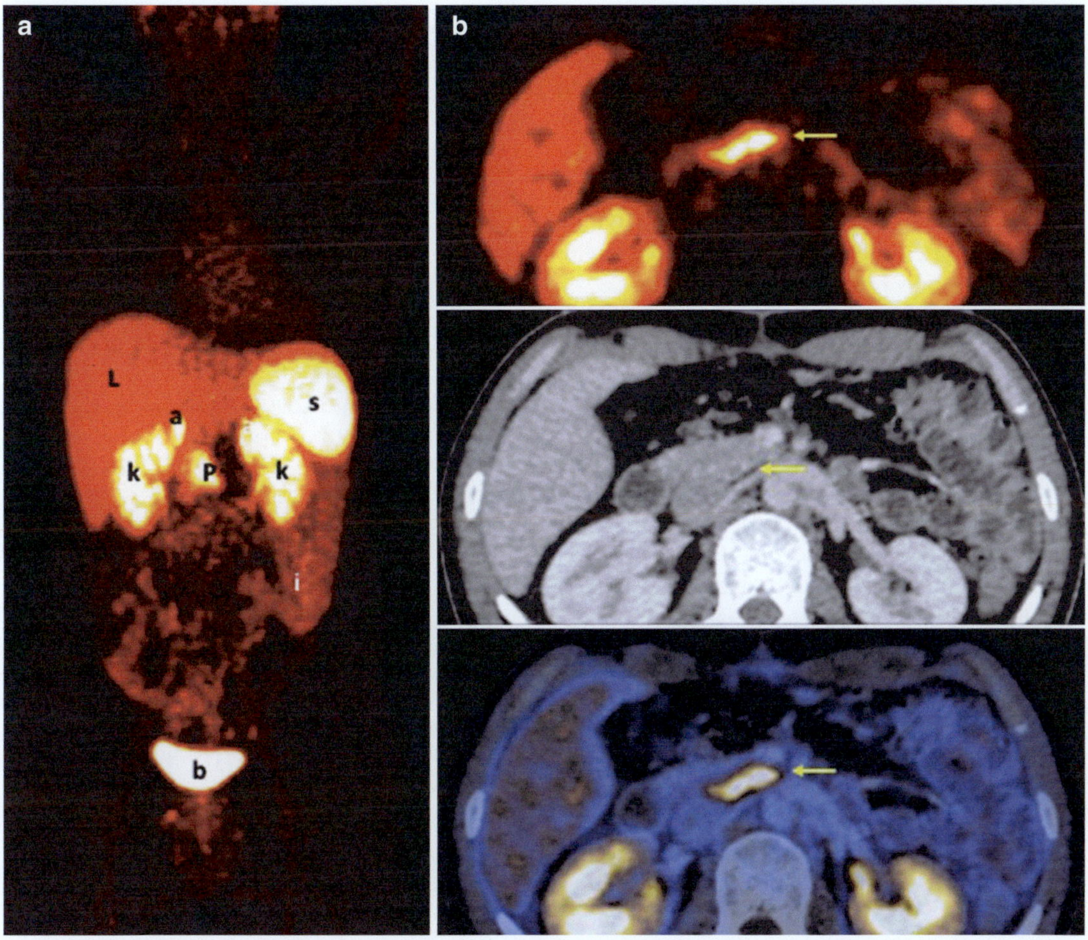

Fig. 17.18 Normal biodistribution of ^{68}Ga-DOTA-NOC PET/CT. (**a**) *MIP (maximum intensity projection)*: significant uptake is presented in the spleen (s), kidneys (k), adrenal glands (a), liver (L), and bladder (b). Faint uptake is also seen in the intestinal loops (i). (**b**) *Trans-axial PET (upper), CT (middle), and fusion PET/CT (lower) images:* physiologic ^{68}Ga-DOTA-NOC uptake is visualized on uncinate process region without any abnormal morphological correlation on CT (arrows)

17.7.5 Effects of Aging and Treatment

Although a potential effect of somatostatin analogs on tracer uptake has been assumed, current guidelines do not clearly recommend withdrawal before image acquisition [134, 137]. It has been demonstrated that liver and spleen background activity is reduced after treatment with cold somatostatin analogs; nevertheless, whether this phenomenon leads to better visualization of small-sized hepatic metastasis or conceals them is still a debated concept [134]. Epiphyseal growth plates in children also demonstrate a low-to-moderate increase in activity [138]. Otherwise, no particular difference in biodistribution of ^{68}Ga-DOTA-Peptides has been reported in children.

17.8 ^{68}Ga-PSMA

Prostate-specific membrane antigen (PSMA) is a transmembrane protein showing a considerable increased expression in prostate cancer cells [139, 140]. Advantages of performing ^{68}Ga-PSMA ligands PET/CT have been demonstrated in a multitude of studies, in primary prostate cancer [141, 142] and biochemical recurrence even with low PSA levels [143, 144]. PSMA expression is multiplied up to 1000 times in the prostate cancer cells making it an ideal tracer in seeking the tumoral cell deposits [145]. Even small lymph node metastases are frequently presented with excellent contrast [146].

17.8.1 Head and Neck

Intense physiologic ^{68}Ga-PSMA uptake is visualized in lacrimal glands and, to a lesser extent, in salivary glands (Fig. 17.19) [146, 147]. Tracer uptake in lacrimal and salivary glands also has been shown to demonstrate an increasing pattern which is of importance in the therapeutic application of PSMA ligands [146]. Radiotracer retention has been reported in nasal mucosa which could be due to either blood pool effect or PSMA expression in areas with tissue regeneration [146].

17.8.2 Thorax

Faint radiotracer uptake has been reported in the cervicothoracic (Stellate) ganglia in a limited number of patients (Fig. 17.20) [148]. Mild ^{68}Ga-PSMA uptake in the ribs without decisive morphologic correlation on CT should not be considered metastatic and seek for complementary data [147].

17.8.3 Abdomen

^{68}Ga-PSMA is accumulated in the liver, spleen, and pancreas (Fig. 17.19) [146, 147]. Furthermore, almost all studies show a high radiotracer uptake in the intestine which is more prominent in the proximal small intestine [146, 149]. Intense ^{68}Ga-PSMA activity in the liver potentially obscures metastatic lesions with small size or low avidity [147]. Another deceiving finding in ^{68}Ga-PSMA PET/CT study is the tracer uptake in the coeliac ganglia in a substantial number of patients that could be misinterpreted as metastatic lymph nodes (Fig. 17.20) [150]. Small amount of radiotracer is cleared through the biliary system; thus, visualization of the gallbladder seems to be a variable finding [146, 147].

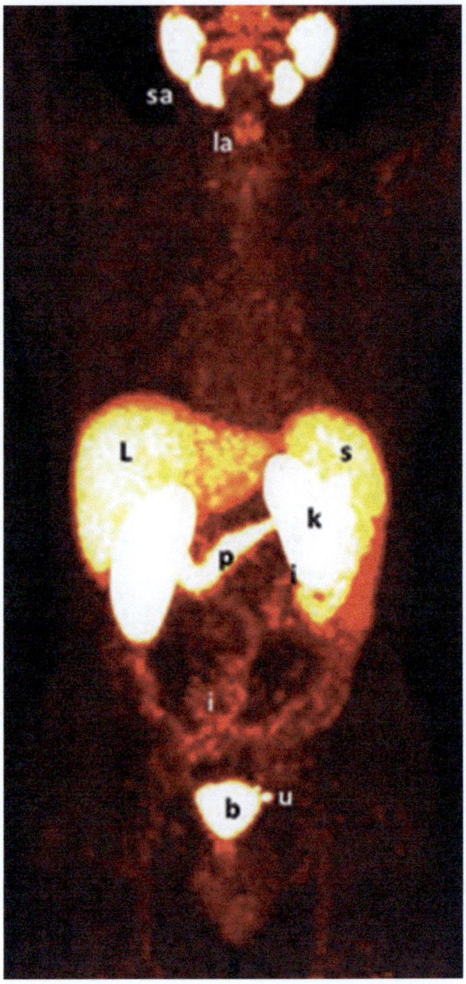

Fig. 17.19 Normal biodistribution of 68Ga-PSMA PET. Physiologic uptake is presented in the salivary glands (sa), larynx (la), liver (L), spleen (s), intestine (i), pancreas, kidneys (k), ureters (u), and bladder (b)

17.8.4 Pelvis

Importantly, moderate ^{68}Ga-PSMA uptake is presented in the normal prostate gland [151]. In addition, considerable ^{68}Ga-PSMA uptake is depicted in kidneys, the main pathway of tracer

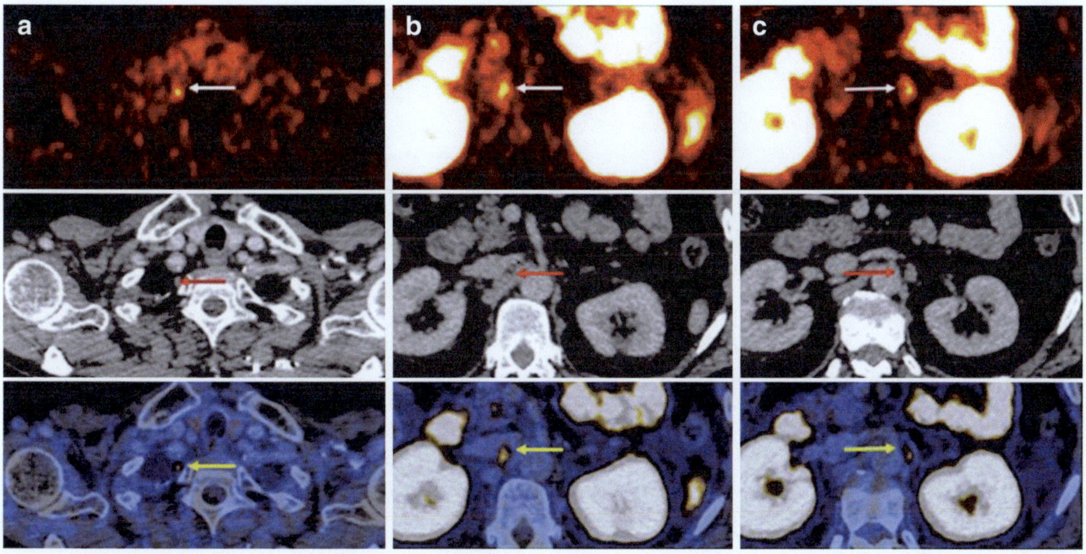

Fig. 17.20 ^{68}Ga-PSMA PET/CT. Physiologic uptake in cervicothoracic (Stellate) and coeliac ganglia. *Trans-axial PET (upper), CT (middle), and fusion (right) images*: physiologic ^{68}Ga-PSMA uptake is visualized in right cervicothoracic (Stellate) ganglion (**a**, arrows), and bilateral coeliac ganglia (**b**, **c**, arrows)

excretion (Fig. 17.19) [147]. Similar to most of the tracers, intensive urinary activity in the bladder can compromise the efficacy of ^{68}Ga-PSMA PET/CT in delineating malignant prostate tissue in surrounding areas [146]. Therefore, emptying bladder prior to the procedure is recommended. Furthermore, the impact of early dynamic imaging in the detection of local malignant tissue has been investigated and shown promising results [152].

17.8.5 Effects of Aging and Treatment

^{68}Ga-PSMA uptake is assumed to be upregulated after initiation of androgen deprivation therapy (ADT) and also may be after AR-targeted therapy (androgen receptor-targeted therapy); however, uptake alterations (increase or decrease) immediately after therapy could be misleading [147]. Moreover, the ^{68}Ga-PSMA uptake after proper treatment has shown to be a relevant finding regarding the evaluation of response to treatment [153, 154]. ^{68}Ga-PSMA scan is designed to detect prostate cancer which is performed in male patients, mostly in elderly, and its biodistribution is not investigated in children and young adults. No information is available regarding effects of aging on PSMA biodistribution.

17.9 ^{18}F-FLT

^{18}F-FLT (3′-deoxy-3′-[^{18}F]fluorothymidine) is a thymidine analog that reflects cell proliferation and has been mainly investigated for assessment of response to treatment in various malignancies [155].

17.9.1 Brain/Head and Neck

The physiologic ^{18}F-FLT uptake in the brain is low owing to its inability to cross the intact blood-brain barrier (BBB). However, significant ^{18}F-FLT retention is seen in a setting of damaged BBB [156, 157]. The physiologic ^{18}F-FLT uptake in the neck region is also unremarkable. ^{18}F-FLT PET was therefore believed to differentiate the inflammatory and neoplastic lymph nodes; however, false-positive ^{18}F-FLT uptake has been reported [158]. In addition, physiologic ^{18}F-FLT uptake is visualized in the proliferating bone

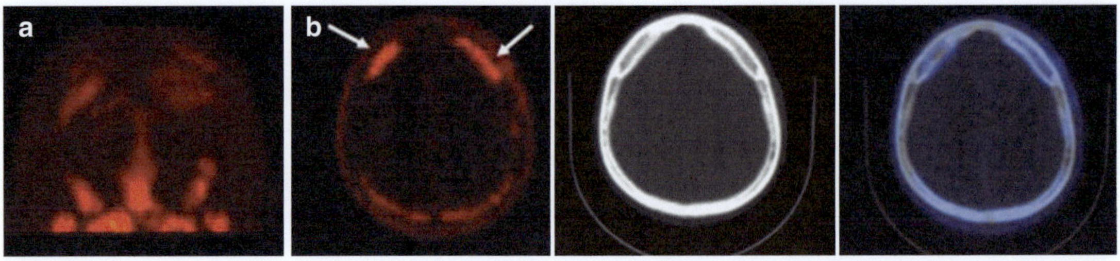

Fig. 17.21 ^{18}F-FLT PET/CT. Bone marrow uptake. A 48-year-old male with grade II astrocytoma. (**a**) *MIP (maximum intensity projection) of the skull: diffuse mild tracer uptake is noticed in the bone marrow of skull bones.* (**b**) *Trans-axial PET (left), CT (middle), and fusion PET/CT (right) images*: increased ^{18}F-FLT uptake is noticed in the skull bone marrow (arrows)

marrow of the cervical spine and, to a lesser extent, in the skull (Fig. 17.21). Unfortunately, this high physiologic ^{18}F-FLT uptake throughout the proliferating bone marrow can reduce the sensitivity regarding the malignant bone marrow infiltration [159, 160]. Noteworthy, the high physiologic ^{18}F-FLT uptake in proliferating bone marrow was successfully used to visualize the viable bone marrow in patients suffering from aplastic anemia and also to identify organs with ongoing extraosseous hematopoiesis [161].

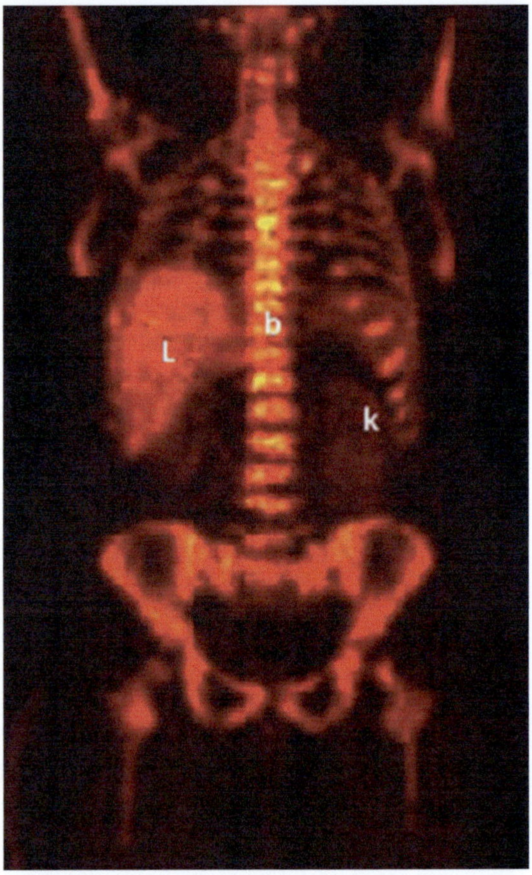

Fig. 17.22 Normal biodistribution of ^{18}F-FLT. Physiologic uptake is presented throughout the bone marrow (b), as well as in the liver (L) and kidneys (k)

17.9.2 Thorax

Lung parenchyma shows only a very low ^{18}F-FLT uptake allowing us to confidently interpret any focus of increased pulmonary ^{18}F-FLT uptake as highly suspicious for a malignant tumor. The accumulation of ^{18}F-FLT in the blood pool and muscle tissue of the left ventricular cavity results in increased heart uptake, potentially obscuring lung and breast lesions [162]. However, the blood pool activity in the heart showed a rapid washout leading to a good visualization of the thorax after around 45 min [162]. Presence of the proliferating bone marrow in the rib cage as well as in thoracic vertebrae accounts for the physiologic ^{18}F-FLT uptake in these areas [163].

17.9.3 Abdomen

A number of organs with increased physiologic ^{18}F-FLT uptake are located in the abdomen, including the liver and, to a lesser extent, the intestine, as well as the lower part of the ribs, lower thoracic and lumbar vertebrae (Fig. 17.22).

^{18}F-FLT undergoes extensive glucuronidation in the human liver resulting in approximately 25% of the plasma activity as ^{18}F-FLT-glucuronide at 60 min after injection [164–166]. Attempts to reduce the physiologic liver uptake of ^{18}F-FLT by use of probenecid have failed in a pilot evaluation [165].

Due to the rapid proliferation of gastrointestinal mucosa cells, the physiologic uptake is not unexpected. However, multiple groups have shown that physiologic gastrointestinal ^{18}F-FLT uptake does not significantly compromise the detection of gastric cancer [167, 168]. As previously discussed in the head and neck section, physiologic ^{18}F-FLT uptake is perceived throughout the proliferating bone marrow in the lower rib cage as well as in the lumbar spine.

17.9.4 Pelvis

Urinary uptake and contamination could be challenging, since the main root of excretion of ^{18}F-FLT is kidneys, mostly in its non-metabolized form and also as ^{18}F-FLT-glucuronide even after being metabolized in the liver [164]. At 60-min post-injection, there is only low-grade non-specific ^{18}F-FLT activity in the kidneys and the genitourinary system. Not surprising, high physiologic ^{18}F-FLT uptake is presented in the proliferating bone marrow of the pelvic bones and the lumbar vertebrae (Fig. 17.22). No remarkable physiologic ^{18}F-FLT uptake has been seen in other pelvic organs, such as uterus and ovaries, prostate, and seminal vesicles [163].

17.9.5 Effects of Aging and Treatment

17.9.5.1 Aging

The extent of proliferating bone marrow as a common region of physiologic ^{18}F-FLT uptake in humans is not constant in different ages. Otherwise, the physiologic ^{18}F-FLT uptake throughout the body is not affected by age alterations [163].

17.9.5.2 Treatment-Induced Effects

^{18}F-FLT PET has been employed in a multitude of studies and tumor entities for assessing response to treatment [155, 169]. Response to chemotherapy is expected to reduce the ^{18}F-FLT uptake, as previously reported in malignant lymphomas [170]. In contrast, increased ^{18}F-FLT uptake (i.e., flare phenomenon) was reported in aggressive non-Hodgkin lymphoma (NHL) after rituximab and 20 h after radiation therapy in a patient with a non-small cell lung cancer (NSCLC) [170, 171].

Radiation and chemoradiotherapy potentially alter the proliferating bone marrow, leading to a therapy-induced reduction of ^{18}F-FLT uptake, such as photogenic regions in the spine (Fig. 17.23). Decreased ^{18}F-FLT uptake in bone marrow has demonstrated to normalize again after 7 and 42 days in aggressive NHL patients with significantly decreased ^{18}F-FLT uptake 2 days after CHOP treatment [170]. In patients with renal cell carcinoma receiving sunitinib, an increase in ^{18}F-FLT uptake was visualized after withdrawal of sunitinib, a phenomenon which was called "withdrawal flare" by the authors [172].

17.10 ^{18}F-NaF

^{18}F-sodium fluoride (^{18}F-NaF) PET/CT is a praiseworthy method in the assessment of either benign or primary bone malignancies as well as bone metastases. Uptake mechanism of ^{18}F-NaF and ^{99m}Tc-MDP is similar. However, the former demonstrates significantly superior pharmacokinetic characteristics [173, 174]. ^{18}F-NaF ion exchanges with hydroxyl groups on hydroxyapatite forming fluorapatite and then incorporates into the bone matrix [175]. The high diagnostic efficiency of ^{18}F-NaF PET is justified to those bone lesions with high flow and bone turnover [175–177]. Since only a meager osteoblastic activity in the morphologically lytic or lucent lesions is spotted with ^{18}F-NaF, it offers a valuable sensitivity in detection of both sclerotic and lytic lesions [177, 178].

There is wide spectrum of patterns indicating a physiologic ^{18}F-NaF uptake in different parts

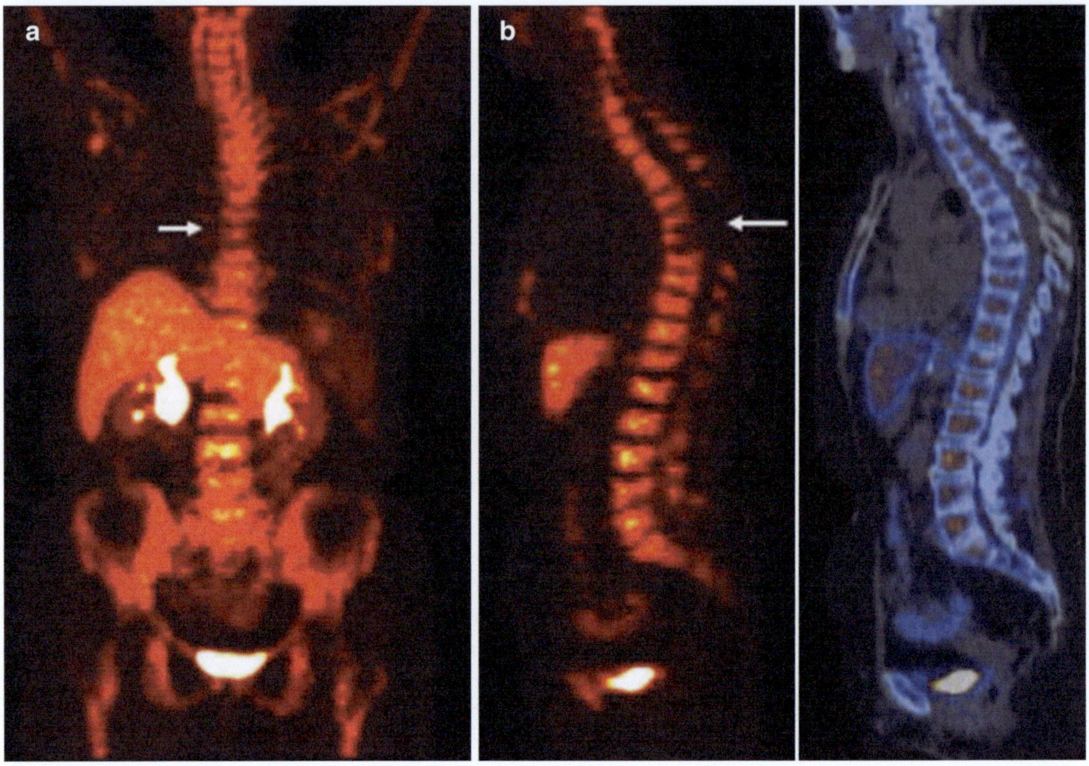

Fig. 17.23 ^{18}F-FLT PET/CT. Effect of therapy on biodistribution of ^{18}F-FLT. A 69-year-old female suffering from granulosa cell tumor with a history of lung metastasis referred for restaging. (**a**) *MIP (maximum intensity projection)*: diffuse physiologic bone marrow ^{18}F-FLT uptake is seen in the skeleton. However, an area of decreased ^{18}F-FLT uptake is noted in the mid-thoracic spine (arrow). (**b**) *Sagittal PET (left) and fusion PET/CT (right) images*: decreased metabolic activity in the mid-thoracic vertebrae is well demonstrated (arrow), which is secondary to previous radiation therapy aiming for lung metastasis

of the skeleton. While high-grade uptake is found in trabecular bones, characterized by greater bone turnover, cortical bones of the peripheral skeleton show modest activity [179, 180]. Nevertheless, a figure of rather uniform and symmetric ^{18}F-NaF uptake in the skeleton is mandatory for a negative interpretation (Fig. 17.24) [181]. Of note, owing to the substantially high sensitivity of ^{18}F-NaF, low-grade heterogeneity might be observed in the skeleton, demanding morphologic data to differentiate true bone abnormalities from normal variations [182]. Increased ^{18}F-NaF uptake is visualized in the metaphysis of both children and adults [182]. In the case of an intact renal function, there is a negligible soft tissue activity except for kidneys and the bladder [181].

^{18}F-NaF uptake is increased in a multitude of benign and malignant conditions. To catch a brief glimpse of an endless list, ^{18}F-NaF uptake can be seen in fibrosis dysplasia, Paget's disease, bone cyst, giant cell tumor, osteoid stoma and osteomyelitis as well as in osteosarcoma, Ewing's sarcoma, etc. [183].

Furthermore, ^{18}F-NaF PET/CT plays a role in the assessment of the condylar hyperplasia [184], jaw osteonecrosis [185, 186], low back pain [187–189], child abuse [190], vertebral abnormalities after fusion surgery [191], osteonecrosis of the femoral head [192], bone remodeling in patients with osteolytic acetabular defects after hip arthroplasty [193], unclear foot pain [194], metabolic bone conditions [195, 196], atherosclerotic plaques [197], and numerous other settings [198].

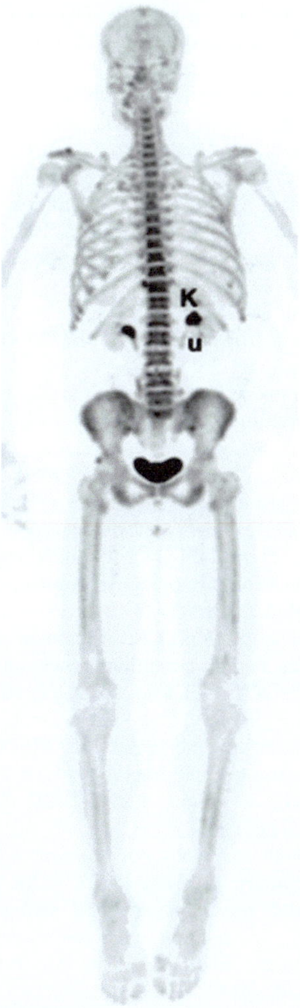

Fig. 17.24 ^{18}F-NaF PET. *MIP (maximum intensity projection)* image. Physiologic age-compatible ^{18}F-NaF distribution with symmetrical tracer uptake in the skeleton. Tracer accumulation is also seen in the pelvicalyceal system of the kidneys (k) and both ureters (u)

References

1. Soret M, Bacharach SL, Buvat I. Partial-volume effect in PET tumor imaging. J Nucl Med. 2007;48(6):932–45.
2. Moses WW. Fundamental limits of spatial resolution in PET. Nucl Instrum Methods Phys Res A. 2011;648(Suppl 1):S236–40.
3. Boellaard R, Oyen WJ, Hoekstra CJ, et al. The Netherlands protocol for standardisation and quantification of FDG whole body PET studies in multi-centre trials. Eur J Nucl Med Mol Imaging. 2008;35(12):2320–33.
4. Corrigan AJ, Schleyer PJ, Cook GJ. Pitfalls and artifacts in the use of PET/CT in oncology imaging. Semin Nucl Med. 2015;45(6):481–99.
5. Kadrmas DJ, Casey ME, Conti M, Jakoby BW, Lois C, Townsend DW. Impact of time-of-flight on PET tumor detection. J Nucl Med. 2009;50(8):1315–23.
6. Osman MM, Cohade C, Nakamoto Y, Wahl RL. Respiratory motion artifacts on PET emission images obtained using CT attenuation correction on PET-CT. Eur J Nucl Med Mol Imaging. 2003;30(4):603–6.
7. Erdi YE, Nehmeh SA, Pan T, et al. The CT motion quantitation of lung lesions and its impact on PET-measured SUVs. J Nucl Med. 2004;45(8):1287–92.
8. Liu C, Pierce LA 2nd, Alessio AM, Kinahan PE. The impact of respiratory motion on tumor quantification and delineation in static PET/CT imaging. Phys Med Biol. 2009;54(24):7345–62.
9. Pan T, Mawlawi O, Luo D, et al. Attenuation correction of PET cardiac data with low-dose average CT in PET/CT. Med Phys. 2006;33(10):3931–8.
10. Nehmeh SA, Haj-Ali AA, Qing C, et al. A novel respiratory tracking system for smart-gated PET acquisition. Med Phys. 2011;38(1):531–8.
11. Liu C, Alessio A, Pierce L, et al. Quiescent period respiratory gating for PET/CT. Med Phys. 2010;37(9):5037–43.
12. Nehmeh SA, Erdi YE, Pan T, et al. Four-dimensional (4D) PET/CT imaging of the thorax. Med Phys. 2004;31(12):3179–86.
13. Antoch G, Freudenberg LS, Beyer T, Bockisch A, Debatin JF. To enhance or not to enhance? 18F-FDG and CT contrast agents in dual-modality 18F-FDG PET/CT. J Nucl Med. 2004;45(Suppl 1):56S–65S.
14. Antoch G, Freudenberg LS, Egelhof T, et al. Focal tracer uptake: a potential artifact in contrast-enhanced dual-modality PET/CT scans. J Nucl Med. 2002;43(10):1339–42.
15. Beyer T, Antoch G, Muller S, et al. Acquisition protocol considerations for combined PET/CT imaging. J Nucl Med. 2004;45(Suppl 1):25S–35S.
16. Mawlawi O, Erasmus JJ, Pan T, et al. Truncation artifact on PET/CT: impact on measurements of activity concentration and assessment of a correction algorithm. AJR Am J Roentgenol. 2006;186(5):1458–67.
17. Pike L. Quality assurance of PET and PET/CT systems, vol. 108. York: Institute of Physics and Engineering in Medicine; 2013.
18. Delso G, ter Voert E, de Galiza Barbosa F, Veit-Haibach P. Pitfalls and limitations in simultaneous PET/MRI. Semin Nucl Med. 2015;45(6):552–9.
19. Bhargava P, Rahman S, Wendt J. Atlas of confounding factors in head and neck PET/CT imaging. Clin Nucl Med. 2011;36(5):e20–9.
20. Purohit BS, Ailianou A, Dulguerov N, Becker CD, Ratib O, Becker M. FDG-PET/CT pitfalls in oncological head and neck imaging. Insights Imaging. 2014;5(5):585–602.
21. Karunanithi S, Soundararajan R, Sharma P, Naswa N, Bal C, Kumar R. Spectrum of physiologic and patho-

logic skeletal muscle (18)F-FDG uptake on PET/CT. AJR Am J Roentgenol. 2015;205(2):W141–9.
22. Nakamura S, Okochi K, Murata Y, Shibuya H, Kurabayashi T. [18F]Fluorodeoxyglucose-PET/CT differentiation between physiological and pathological accumulations in head and neck. Nucl Med Commun. 2009;30(7):498–503.
23. Tsubaki F, Kurata S, Tani J, Sumi A, Fujimoto K, Abe T. Clinical significance of patterns of increased [(18)F]-FDG uptake in the thyroid gland: a pictorial review. Jpn J Radiol. 2018;36(3):181–93.
24. Makis W, Ciarallo A. Thyroid Incidentalomas on (18)F-FDG PET/CT: clinical significance and controversies. Mol Imaging Radionucl Ther. 2017;26(3):93–100.
25. Steinberg JD, Vogel W, Vegt E. Factors influencing brown fat activation in FDG PET/CT: a retrospective analysis of 15,000+ cases. Br J Radiol. 2017;90(1075):20170093.
26. Tatsumi M, Engles JM, Ishimori T, Nicely O, Cohade C, Wahl RL. Intense (18)F-FDG uptake in brown fat can be reduced pharmacologically. J Nucl Med. 2004;45(7):1189–93.
27. Sureshbabu W, Mawlawi O. PET/CT imaging artifacts. J Nucl Med Technol. 2005;33(3):156–61; quiz 163–154.
28. Wachsmann JW, Gerbaudo VH. Thorax: normal and benign pathologic patterns in FDG-PET/CT imaging. PET Clin. 2014;9(2):147–68.
29. An YS, Jung Y, Kim JY, et al. Metabolic activity of Normal glandular tissue on (18) F-Fluorodeoxyglucose positron emission tomography/computed tomography: correlation with menstrual cycles and parenchymal enhancements. J Breast Cancer. 2017;20(4):386–92.
30. Dong A, Wang Y, Lu J, Zuo C. Spectrum of the breast lesions with increased 18F-FDG uptake on PET/CT. Clin Nucl Med. 2016;41(7):543–57.
31. van Vliet KE, de Jong VM, Termaat MF, et al. FDG-PET/CT for differentiating between aseptic and septic delayed union in the lower extremity. Arch Orthop Trauma Surg. 2018;138(2):189–94.
32. Osman MM, Tran IT, Muzaffar R, Parkar N, Sachdeva A, Ruppel GL. Does (1)(8)F-FDG uptake by respiratory muscles on PET/CT correlate with chronic obstructive pulmonary disease? J Nucl Med Technol. 2011;39(4):252–7.
33. Gerbaudo VH, Julius B. Anatomo-metabolic characteristics of atelectasis in F-18 FDG-PET/CT imaging. Eur J Radiol. 2007;64(3):401–5.
34. Shusharina N, Liao Z, Mohan R, et al. Differences in lung injury after IMRT or proton therapy assessed by (18)FDG PET imaging. Radiother Oncol. 2018;128:147.
35. Chen CH, Hsiao CC, Chen YC, et al. Rebound thymic hyperplasia after chemotherapy in children with lymphoma. Pediatr Neonatol. 2017;58(2):151–7.
36. Maurer AH, Burshteyn M, Adler LP, Steiner RM. How to differentiate benign versus malignant cardiac and paracardiac 18F FDG uptake at oncologic PET/CT. Radiographics. 2011;31(5):1287–305.
37. Toriihara A, Kitazume Y, Nishida H, Kubota K, Nakadate M, Tateishi U. Comparison of FDG-PET/CT images between chronic renal failure patients on hemodialysis and controls. Am J Nucl Med Mol Imaging. 2015;5(2):204–11.
38. Jo K, Kim S, Cha J, et al. A comparison study of esophageal findings on (18)F-FDG PET/CT and esophagogastroduodenoscopy. Nucl Med Mol Imaging. 2016;50(2):123–9.
39. Blodgett TM, Mehta AS, Mehta AS, Laymon CM, Carney J, Townsend DW. PET/CT artifacts. Clin Imaging. 2011;35(1):49–63.
40. Lu Y, Fontaine K, Mulnix T, et al. Respiratory motion compensation for PET/CT with motion information derived from matched attenuation corrected gated PET data. J Nucl Med. 2018;59:1480.
41. Robin P, Bourhis D, Bernard B, et al. Feasibility of systematic respiratory-gated acquisition in unselected patients referred for (18)F-fluorodeoxyglucose positron emission tomography/computed tomography. Front Med. 2018;5:36.
42. Zukotynski K, Kim CK. Abdomen: normal variations and benign conditions resulting in uptake on FDG-PET/CT. PET Clin. 2014;9(2):169–83.
43. Shmidt E, Nehra V, Lowe V, Oxentenko AS. Clinical significance of incidental [18 F]FDG uptake in the gastrointestinal tract on PET/CT imaging: a retrospective cohort study. BMC Gastroenterol. 2016;16(1):125.
44. Kunawudhi A, Wong AK, Alkasab TK, Mahmood U. Accuracy of FDG-PET/CT for detection of incidental pre-malignant and malignant colonic lesions – correlation with colonoscopic and histopathologic findings. Asian Pac J Cancer Prev. 2016;17(8):4143–7.
45. Lee JC, Hartnett GF, Hughes BG, Ravi Kumar AS. The segmental distribution and clinical significance of colorectal fluorodeoxyglucose uptake incidentally detected on PET-CT. Nucl Med Commun. 2009;30(5):333–7.
46. Lakhani A, Khan SR, Bharwani N, et al. FDG PET/CT pitfalls in gynecologic and genitourinary oncologic imaging. Radiographics. 2017;37(2):577–94.
47. Zukotynski K, Lewis A, O'Regan K, et al. PET/CT and renal pathology: a blind spot for radiologists? Part 1, primary pathology. AJR Am J Roentgenol. 2012;199(2):W163–7.
48. Zukotynski K, Lewis A, O'Regan K, et al. PET/CT and renal pathology: a blind spot for radiologists? Part 2—lymphoma, leukemia, and metastatic disease. AJR Am J Roentgenol. 2012;199(2):W168–74.
49. Kim SJ, Lee SW, Pak K, Kim IJ, Kim K. Diagnostic accuracy of (18)F-FDG PET or PET/CT for the characterization of adrenal masses: a systematic review and meta-analysis. Br J Radiol. 2018;91(1086):20170520.

50. Yun M, Kim W, Alnafisi N, Lacorte L, Jang S, Alavi A. 18F-FDG PET in characterizing adrenal lesions detected on CT or MRI. J Nucl Med. 2001;42(12):1795–9.
51. Koffert JP, Mikkola K, Virtanen KA, et al. Metformin treatment significantly enhances intestinal glucose uptake in patients with type 2 diabetes: results from a randomized clinical trial. Diabetes Res Clin Pract. 2017;131:208–16.
52. Bahler L, Stroek K, Hoekstra JB, Verberne HJ, Holleman F. Metformin-related colonic glucose uptake; potential role for increasing glucose disposal? A retrospective analysis of (18)F-FDG uptake in the colon on PET-CT. Diabetes Res Clin Pract. 2016;114:55–63.
53. Steenkamp DW, McDonnell ME, Meibom S. Metformin may be associated with false-negative cancer detection in the gastrointestinal tract on PET/CT. Endocr Pract. 2014;20(10):1079–83.
54. Lee SH, Jin S, Lee HS, Ryu JS, Lee JJ. Metformin discontinuation less than 72 h is suboptimal for F-18 FDG PET/CT interpretation of the bowel. Ann Nucl Med. 2016;30(9):629–36.
55. Basu S, Baghel NS. Intense FDG uptake in the spleen due to recent granulocyte-macrophage colony-stimulating factor administration: follow-up scan clarifying the situation. J Cancer Res Ther. 2011;7(2):228–9.
56. Liu Y. Clinical significance of diffusely increased splenic uptake on FDG-PET. Nucl Med Commun. 2009;30(10):763–9.
57. Wang X, Koch S. Positron emission tomography/computed tomography potential pitfalls and artifacts. Curr Probl Diagn Radiol. 2009;38(4):156–69.
58. Kohan A, Avril NE. Pelvis: normal variants and benign findings in FDG-PET/CT imaging. PET Clin. 2014;9(2):185–93.
59. Ozulker T, Ozulker F, Mert M, Ozpacaci T. Clearance of the high intestinal (18)F-FDG uptake associated with metformin after stopping the drug. Eur J Nucl Med Mol Imaging. 2010;37(5):1011–7.
60. Buscombe JR. Exploring the nature of atheroma and cardiovascular inflammation in vivo using positron emission tomography (PET). Br J Radiol. 2015;88(1053):20140648.
61. Bucci M, Aparici CM, Hawkins R, et al. Validation of FDG uptake in the arterial wall as an imaging biomarker of atherosclerotic plaques with 18F-fluorodeoxyglucose positron emission tomography-computed tomography (FDG-PET/CT). J Neuroimaging. 2014;24(2):117–23.
62. Beauregard JM, Blouin AC, Fradet V, et al. FDG-PET/CT for pre-operative staging and prognostic stratification of patients with high-grade prostate cancer at biopsy. Cancer Imaging. 2015;15:2.
63. Dierickx LO, Huyghe E, Nogueira D, et al. Functional testicular evaluation using PET/CT with 18F-fluorodeoxyglucose. Eur J Nucl Med Mol Imaging. 2012;39(1):129–37.
64. Moon SH, Eo JS, Lee JJ, Chung JK, Lee DS, Lee MC. (18)F-FDG uptake of human testis on PET/CT: correlation with age, sex hormones, and vasectomy. Nucl Med Mol Imaging. 2011;45(4):291–8.
65. Well D, Yang H, Houseni M, et al. Age-related structural and metabolic changes in the pelvic reproductive end organs. Semin Nucl Med. 2007;37(3):173–84.
66. Groheux D, Teyton P, Vercellino L, Ferretti A, Rubello D, Hindie E. Cryptorchidism as a potential source of misinterpretation in (1)(8)FDG-PET imaging in restaging lymphoma patients. Biomed Pharmacother. 2013;67(6):533–8.
67. Liu Y. Benign ovarian and endometrial uptake on FDG PET-CT: patterns and pitfalls. Ann Nucl Med. 2009;23(2):107–12.
68. Park SA, Lee KM, Choi U, Kim HS, Kim HW, Song JH. Normal physiologic and benign foci with F-18 FDG avidity on PET/CT in patients with breast cancer. Nucl Med Mol Imaging. 2010;44(4):282–9.
69. Yun M, Cho A, Lee JH, Choi YJ, Lee JD, Kim CK. Physiologic 18F-FDG uptake in the fallopian tubes at mid cycle on PET/CT. J Nucl Med. 2010;51(5):682–5.
70. Schwarz EI, Ramach C, Mende KA, Strobel K. Physiologic FDG uptake in the ovary together with an abdominal wall leiomyoma mimicking metastasizing ovarian cancer on PET/CT imaging. Clin Nucl Med. 2009;34(4):249–50.
71. Berti V, Mosconi L, Pupi A. Brain: normal variations and benign findings in fluorodeoxyglucose-PET/computed tomography imaging. PET Clin. 2014;9(2):129–40.
72. Ahmad Sarji S. Physiological uptake in FDG PET simulating disease. Biomed Imaging Intervent J. 2006;2(4):e59.
73. Kostakoglu L, Hardoff R, Mirtcheva R, Goldsmith SJ. PET-CT fusion imaging in differentiating physiologic from pathologic FDG uptake. Radiographics. 2004;24(5):1411–31.
74. London K, Howman-Giles R. Normal cerebral FDG uptake during childhood. Eur J Nucl Med Mol Imaging. 2014;41(4):723–35.
75. Willis MW, Ketter TA, Kimbrell TA, et al. Age, sex and laterality effects on cerebral glucose metabolism in healthy adults. Psychiatry Res. 2002;114(1):23–37.
76. Chiaravalloti A, Barbagallo G, Ricci M, et al. Brain metabolic correlates of CSF tau protein in a large cohort of Alzheimer's disease patients: a CSF and FDG PET study. Brain Res. 2018;1678:116–22.
77. Croteau E, Castellano CA, Fortier M, et al. A cross-sectional comparison of brain glucose and ketone metabolism in cognitively healthy older adults, mild cognitive impairment and early Alzheimer's disease. Exp Gerontol. 2018;107:18–26.
78. Silva-Rodriguez J, Garcia-Varela L, Lopez-Arias E, et al. Impact of benzodiazepines on brain FDG-PET quantification after single-dose and chronic administration in rats. Nucl Med Biol. 2016;43(12):827–34.

79. Scholtens AM, Verberne HJ. Attenuation correction and metal artifact reduction in FDG PET/CT for prosthetic heart valve and cardiac implantable device endocarditis. J Nucl Cardiol. 2018;25:2172.
80. DeGrado TR, Baldwin SW, Wang S, et al. Synthesis and evaluation of (18)F-labeled choline analogs as oncologic PET tracers. J Nucl Med. 2001;42(12):1805–14.
81. Hara T, Kosaka N, Kishi H. Development of (18) F-fluoroethylcholine for cancer imaging with PET: synthesis, biochemistry, and prostate cancer imaging. J Nucl Med. 2002;43(2):187–99.
82. Friedland RP, Mathis CA, Budinger TF, Moyer BR, Rosen M. Labeled choline and phosphorylcholine: body distribution and brain autoradiography: concise communication. J Nucl Med. 1983;24(9):812–5.
83. Beheshti M, Haroon A, Bomanji JB, Langsteger W, Fluorocholine PET. Computed tomography: physiologic uptake, benign findings, and pitfalls. PET Clin. 2014;9(3):299–306.
84. Mertens K, Ham H, Deblaere K, et al. Distribution patterns of 18F-labelled fluoromethylcholine in normal structures and tumors of the head: a PET/MRI evaluation. Clin Nucl Med. 2012;37(8):e196–203.
85. Calabria F, Chiaravalloti A, Schillaci O. (18) F-choline PET/CT pitfalls in image interpretation: an update on 300 examined patients with prostate cancer. Clin Nucl Med. 2014;39(2):122–30.
86. Schillaci O, Calabria F, Tavolozza M, et al. 18F-choline PET/CT physiological distribution and pitfalls in image interpretation: experience in 80 patients with prostate cancer, Nucl Med Commun. 2019;31(1):39–45.
87. Beheshti M, Hehenwarter L, Paymani Z, et al. (18) F-fluorocholine PET/CT in the assessment of primary hyperparathyroidism compared with (99m) Tc-MIBI or (99m)Tc-tetrofosmin SPECT/CT: a prospective dual-centre study in 100 patients. Eur J Nucl Med Mol Imaging. 2018;45:1762.
88. Wyss MT, Weber B, Honer M, et al. 18F-choline in experimental soft tissue infection assessed with autoradiography and high-resolution PET. Eur J Nucl Med Mol Imaging. 2004;31(3):312–6.
89. Gu J. Primary liver cancer: challenges and perspectives. New York, NY: Springer; 2012.
90. de Certaines JD, Larsen VA, Podo F, Carpinelli G, Briot O, Henriksen O. In vivo 31P MRS of experimental tumours. NMR Biomed. 1993;6(6):345–65.
91. Sutinen E, Nurmi M, Roivainen A, et al. Kinetics of [(11)C]choline uptake in prostate cancer: a PET study. Eur J Nucl Med Mol Imaging. 2004;31(3):317–24.
92. Terauchi T, Tateishi U, Maeda T, et al. A case of colon cancer detected by carbon-11 choline positron emission tomography/computed tomography: an initial report. Jpn J Clin Oncol. 2007;37(10):797–800.
93. Katz DS, Hines J, Math KR, Nardi PM, Mindelzun RE, Lane MJ. Using CT to reveal fat-containing abnormalities of the pancreas. AJR Am J Roentgenol. 1999;172(2):393–6.
94. Beheshti M, Haim S, Zakavi R, et al. Impact of 18F-choline PET/CT in prostate cancer patients with biochemical recurrence: influence of androgen deprivation therapy and correlation with PSA kinetics. J Nucl Med. 2013;54(6):833–40.
95. Beheshti M, Imamovic L, Broinger G, et al. 18F choline PET/CT in the preoperative staging of prostate cancer in patients with intermediate or high risk of extracapsular disease: a prospective study of 130 patients. Radiology. 2010;254(3):925–33.
96. Ceci F, Castellucci P, Mamede M, et al. (11)C-choline PET/CT in patients with hormone-resistant prostate cancer showing biochemical relapse after radical prostatectomy. Eur J Nucl Med Mol Imaging. 2012;40(2):149–55.
97. Roef MJ, van der Poel H, van der Laken CJ, Vogel WV. Colchicine must be stopped before imaging with [18F]-methylcholine PET/CT, Nucl Med Commun. 2010;31(12):1075–7.
98. Haroon A, Zanoni L, Celli M, et al. Multicenter study evaluating extraprostatic uptake of 11C-choline, 18F-methylcholine, and 18F-ethylcholine in male patients: physiological distribution, statistical differences, imaging pearls, and normal variants. Nucl Med Commun. 2015;36(11):1065–75.
99. Swinnen JV, Heemers H, Deboel L, Foufelle F, Heyns W, Verhoeven G. Stimulation of tumor-associated fatty acid synthase expression by growth factor activation of the sterol regulatory element-binding protein pathway. Oncogene. 2000;19(45):5173–81.
100. Swinnen JV, Van Veldhoven PP, Timmermans L, et al. Fatty acid synthase drives the synthesis of phospholipids partitioning into detergent-resistant membrane microdomains. Biochem Biophys Res Commun. 2003;302(4):898–903.
101. Grassi I, Nanni C, Allegri V, et al. The clinical use of PET with (11)C-acetate. Am J Nucl Med Mol Imaging. 2012;2(1):33–47.
102. Ohtsuka T, Nomori H, Watanabe K, et al. Positive imaging of thymoma by 11C-acetate positron emission tomography. Ann Thorac Surg. 2006;81(3):1132–4.
103. Lee SM, Kim TS, Kim SK. Cerebellopontine angle schwannoma on C-11 acetate PET/CT. Clin Nucl Med. 2009;34(11):831–3.
104. Ho CL, Chen S, Ho KM, Ng WK, Leung YL, Cheng TK. 11C-acetate PET/CT in multicentric angiomyolipoma of the kidney. Clin Nucl Med. 2011;36(5):407–8.
105. Wang HC, Zhao J, Zuo CT, et al. Encephalitis depicted by a combination of C-11 acetate and F-18 FDG PET/CT. Clin Nucl Med. 2009;34(12):952–4.
106. Lee SM, Kim TS, Lee JW, et al. Incidental finding of an 11C-acetate PET-positive multiple myeloma. Ann Nucl Med. 2010;24(1):41–4.
107. Liu RS, Chang CP, Guo WY, et al. 1-11C-acetate versus 18F-FDG PET in detection of meningioma and monitoring the effect of gamma-knife radiosurgery. J Nucl Med. 2010;51(6):883–91.

108. Buchegger F, Garibotto V, Zilli T, et al. First imaging results of an intraindividual comparison of (11)C-acetate and (18)F-fluorocholine PET/CT in patients with prostate cancer at early biochemical first or second relapse after prostatectomy or radiotherapy. Eur J Nucl Med Mol Imaging. 2014;41(1):68–78.
109. Wachter S, Tomek S, Kurtaran A, et al. 11C-acetate positron emission tomography imaging and image fusion with computed tomography and magnetic resonance imaging in patients with recurrent prostate cancer. J Clin Oncol. 2006;24(16):2513–9.
110. Yeh SH, Liu RS, Wu LC, Yen SH, Chang CW, Chen KY. 11C-acetate clearance in nasopharyngeal carcinoma. Nucl Med Commun. 1999;20(2):131–4.
111. Sun A, Sorensen J, Karlsson M, et al. 1-[11C]-acetate PET imaging in head and neck cancer—a comparison with 18F-FDG-PET: implications for staging and radiotherapy planning. Eur J Nucl Med Mol Imaging. 2007;34(5):651–7.
112. Nomori H, Shibata H, Uno K, et al. 11C-acetate can be used in place of 18F-fluorodeoxyglucose for positron emission tomography imaging of non-small cell lung cancer with higher sensitivity for well-differentiated adenocarcinoma. J Thorac Oncol. 2008;3(12):1427–32.
113. Karanikas G, Beheshti M. (1)(1)C-acetate PET/CT imaging: physiologic uptake, variants, and pitfalls. PET Clin. 2014;9(3):339–44.
114. Shreve PD, Gross MD. Imaging of the pancreas and related diseases with PET carbon-11-acetate. J Nucl Med. 1997;38(8):1305–10.
115. Huo L, Wu Z, Zhuang H, Fu Z, Dang Y. Dual time point C-11 acetate PET imaging can potentially distinguish focal nodular hyperplasia from primary hepatocellular carcinoma. Clin Nucl Med. 2009;34(12):874–7.
116. Brogsitter C, Zöphel K, Kotzerke J. 18 F-choline, 11 C-choline and 11 C-acetate PET/CT: comparative analysis for imaging prostate cancer patients. Eur J Nucl Med Mol Imaging. 2013;40(1):18–27.
117. Karanikas G, Beheshti M. 11C-acetate PET/CT imaging: physiologic uptake, variants, and pitfalls. PET Clin. 2014;9(3):339–44.
118. Schöder H, Ong SC, Reuter VE, et al. Initial results with 11 C-acetate positron emission tomography/computed tomography (PET/CT) in the staging of urinary bladder cancer. Mol Imaging Biol. 2012;14(2):245–51.
119. Luxen A, Guillaume M, Melega W, Pike V, Solin O, Wagner R. Production of 6-[18F] fluoro-L-dopa and its metabolism in vivo—a critical review. Int J Radiat Appl Instrum B Nucl Med Biol. 1992;19(2):149–58.
120. Kauhanen S, Seppänen M, Ovaska J, et al. The clinical value of [18F] fluoro-dihydroxyphenylalanine positron emission tomography in primary diagnosis, staging, and restaging of neuroendocrine tumors. Endocr Relat Cancer. 2009;16(1):255–65.
121. Chen W. Clinical applications of PET in brain tumors. J Nucl Med. 2007;48(9):1468–81.
122. Kauhanen S, Seppanen M, Minn H, et al. Fluorine-18-L-dihydroxyphenylalanine (18F-DOPA) positron emission tomography as a tool to localize an insulinoma or β-cell hyperplasia in adult patients. J Clin Endocrinol Metabol. 2007;92(4):1237–44.
123. Chondrogiannis S, Marzola MC, Rubello D. 18F-DOPA PET/computed tomography imaging. PET Clin. 2014;9(3):307–21.
124. Chondrogiannis S, Grassetto G, Marzola MC, et al. 18F-DOPA PET/CT biodistribution consideration in 107 consecutive patients with neuroendocrine tumours. Nucl Med Commun. 2012;33(2):179–84.
125. Koopmans KP, de Vries EG, Kema IP, et al. Staging of carcinoid tumours with 18F-DOPA PET: a prospective, diagnostic accuracy study. Lancet Oncol. 2006;7(9):728–34.
126. Timmers H, Hadi M, Carrasquillo JA, et al. The effects of carbidopa on uptake of 6-18F-fluoro-L-DOPA in PET of pheochromocytoma and extraadrenal abdominal paraganglioma. J Nucl Med. 2007;48(10):1599–606.
127. Kauhanen SSM, Nuutila P. Premedication with carbidopa masks positive finding of insulinoma and beta-cell hyperplasia in [(18)F]-dihydroxy-phenyl-alanine positron emission tomography. J Clin Oncol. 2008;26(32):5307–8.
128. Krenning E, Kwekkeboom DJ, Wea B, et al. Somatostatin receptor scintigraphy with [111 in-DTPA-D-Phe 1]-and [123 I-Tyr 3]-octreotide: the Rotterdam experience with more than 1000 patients. Eur J Nucl Med. 1993;20(8):716–31.
129. Ambrosini V, Nanni C, Fanti S. The use of gallium-68 labeled somatostatin receptors in PET/CT imaging. PET Clin. 2014;9(3):323–9.
130. Prasad V, Ambrosini V, Hommann M, Hoersch D, Fanti S, Baum RP. Detection of unknown primary neuroendocrine tumours (CUP-NET) using 68 Ga-DOTA-NOC receptor PET/CT. Eur J Nucl Med Mol Imaging. 2010;37(1):67.
131. Virgolini I, Ambrosini V, Bomanji JB, et al. Procedure guidelines for PET/CT tumour imaging with 68 Ga-DOTA-conjugated peptides: 68 Ga-DOTA-TOC, 68 Ga-DOTA-NOC, 68 Ga-DOTA-TATE. Eur J Nucl Med Mol Imaging. 2010;37(10):2004–10.
132. Prasad V, Baum R. Biodistribution of the Ga-68 labeled somatostatin analogue DOTA-NOC in patients with neuroendocrine tumors: characterization of uptake in normal organs and tumor lesions. Q J Nucl Med Mol Imaging. 2010;54(1):61–7.
133. Hofman MS, Lau WE, Hicks RJ. Somatostatin receptor imaging with 68Ga DOTATATE PET/CT: clinical utility, normal patterns, pearls, and pitfalls in interpretation. Radiographics. 2015;35(2):500–16.
134. Agrawal K, Esmail AA, Gnanasegaran G, Navalkissoor S, Mittal BR, Fogelman I. Pitfalls and limitations of radionuclide imaging in endocrinology. Paper presented at seminars in nuclear medicine, 2015.
135. Gabriel M, Decristoforo C, Kendler D, et al. 68Ga-DOTA-Tyr3-octreotide PET in neuroendocrine

tumors: comparison with somatostatin receptor scintigraphy and CT. J Nucl Med. 2007;48(4):508–18.
136. Castellucci P, Pou Ucha J, Fuccio C, et al. Incidence of increased 68Ga-DOTANOC uptake in the pancreatic head in a large series of extrapancreatic NET patients studied with sequential PET/CT. J Nucl Med. 2011;52(6):886.
137. Poeppel TD, Binse I, Petersenn S, et al. ^{68}Ga-DOTATOC versus ^{68}Ga-DOTATATE PET/CT in Functional Imaging of Neuroendocrine Tumors. J Nucl Med. 2011;52(12):1864.
138. Hofman MS, Lau WF, Hicks RJ. Somatostatin receptor imaging with 68Ga DOTATATE PET/CT: clinical utility, normal patterns, pearls, and pitfalls in interpretation. Radiographics. 2015;35(2):500–16.
139. Sweat SD, Pacelli A, Murphy GP, Bostwick DG. Prostate-specific membrane antigen expression is greatest in prostate adenocarcinoma and lymph node metastases. Urology. 1998;52(4):637–40.
140. Mannweiler S, Amersdorfer P, Trajanoski S, Terrett JA, King D, Mehes G. Heterogeneity of prostate-specific membrane antigen (PSMA) expression in prostate carcinoma with distant metastasis. Pathol Oncol Res. 2009;15(2):167–72.
141. Uprimny C, Kroiss AS, Decristoforo C, et al. 68 Ga-PSMA-11 PET/CT in primary staging of prostate cancer: PSA and Gleason score predict the intensity of tracer accumulation in the primary tumour. Eur J Nucl Med Mol Imaging. 2017;44(6):941–9.
142. Maurer T, Gschwend JE, Rauscher I, et al. Diagnostic efficacy of 68gallium-PSMA positron emission tomography compared to conventional imaging for lymph node staging of 130 consecutive patients with intermediate to high risk prostate cancer. J Urol. 2016;195(5):1436–43.
143. Beheshti M, Paymani Z, Brilhante J, et al. Optimal time-point for 68 Ga-PSMA-11 PET/CT imaging in assessment of prostate cancer: feasibility of sterile cold-kit tracer preparation? Eur J Nucl Med Mol Imaging. 2018;45:1188–96.
144. Caroli P, Sandler I, Matteucci F, et al. 68 Ga-PSMA PET/CT in patients with recurrent prostate cancer after radical treatment: prospective results in 314 patients. Eur J Nucl Med Mol Imaging. 2018;45:2035–44.
145. Perera M, Papa N, Christidis D, et al. Sensitivity, specificity, and predictors of positive 68Ga-prostate-specific membrane antigen positron emission tomography in advanced prostate cancer: a systematic review and meta-analysis. Eur Urol. 2016;70(6):926–37.
146. Afshar-Oromieh A, Malcher A, Eder M, et al. PET imaging with a [68 Ga] gallium-labelled PSMA ligand for the diagnosis of prostate cancer: biodistribution in humans and first evaluation of tumour lesions. Eur J Nucl Med Mol Imaging. 2013;40(4):486–95.
147. Fendler WP, Eiber M, Beheshti M, et al. 68 Ga-PSMA PET/CT: joint EANM and SNMMI procedure guideline for prostate cancer imaging: version 1.0. Eur J Nucl Med Mol Imaging. 2017;44(6):1014–24.
148. Beheshti M, Rezaee A, Langsteger W. 68Ga-PSMA-HBED uptake on cervicothoracic (stellate) ganglia, a common pitfall on PET/CT. Clin Nucl Med. 2017;42(3):195–6.
149. Silver DA, Pellicer I, Fair WR, Heston W, Cordon-Cardo C. Prostate-specific membrane antigen expression in normal and malignant human tissues. Clin Cancer Res. 1997;3(1):81–5.
150. Krohn T, Verburg FA, Pufe T, et al. [68 Ga] PSMA-HBED uptake mimicking lymph node metastasis in coeliac ganglia: an important pitfall in clinical practice. Eur J Nucl Med Mol Imaging. 2015;42(2):210–4.
151. Wright Jr GL, Haley C, Beckett ML, Schellhammer PF. Expression of prostate-specific membrane antigen in normal, benign, and malignant prostate tissues. Paper presented at urologic oncology: seminars and original investigations, 1995.
152. Schmuck S, Mamach M, Wilke F, et al. Multiple time-point 68Ga-PSMA I&T PET/CT for characterization of primary prostate cancer: value of early dynamic and delayed imaging. Clin Nucl Med. 2017;42(6):e286–93.
153. Hillier SM, Kern AM, Maresca KP, et al. 123I-MIP-1072, a small-molecule inhibitor of prostate-specific membrane antigen, is effective at monitoring tumor response to taxane therapy. J Nucl Med. 2011;52(7):1087.
154. Schmidkonz C, Cordes M, Schmidt D, et al. 68 Ga-PSMA-11 PET/CT-derived metabolic parameters for determination of whole-body tumor burden and treatment response in prostate cancer. Eur J Nucl Med Mol Imaging. 2018;45:1862–72.
155. Tehrani OS, Shields AF. PET imaging of proliferation with pyrimidines. J Nucl Med. 2013;54(6):903–12.
156. Chen W, Cloughesy T, Kamdar N, et al. Imaging proliferation in brain tumors with 18F-FLT PET: comparison with 18F-FDG. J Nucl Med. 2005;46(6):945–52.
157. Choi SJ, Kim JS, Kim JH, et al. [18F]3′-deoxy-3′-fluorothymidine PET for the diagnosis and grading of brain tumors. Eur J Nucl Med Mol Imaging. 2005;32(6):653–9.
158. Troost EG, Vogel WV, Merkx MA, et al. 18F-FLT PET does not discriminate between reactive and metastatic lymph nodes in primary head and neck cancer patients. J Nucl Med. 2007;48(5):726–35.
159. Buck AK, Herrmann K, Shen C, Dechow T, Schwaiger M, Wester HJ. Molecular imaging of proliferation in vivo: positron emission tomography with [18F]fluorothymidine. Methods. 2009;48(2):205–15.
160. Buck AK, Bommer M, Stilgenbauer S, et al. Molecular imaging of proliferation in malignant lymphoma. Cancer Res. 2006;66(22):11055–61.
161. Agool A, Slart RH, Kluin PM, de Wolf JT, Dierckx RA, Vellenga E. F-18 FLT PET: a non-invasive diagnostic tool for visualization of the

bone marrow compartment in patients with aplastic anemia: a pilot study. Clin Nucl Med. 2011;36(4):286–9.
162. Gray KR, Contractor KB, Kenny LM, et al. Kinetic filtering of [(18)F]Fluorothymidine in positron emission tomography studies. Phys Med Biol. 2010;55(3):695–709.
163. Herrmann K, Buck AK. Proliferation imaging with 18F-fluorothymidine PET/computed tomography: physiologic uptake, variants, and pitfalls. PET Clin. 2014;9(3):331–8.
164. Muzi M, Mankoff DA, Grierson JR, Wells JM, Vesselle H, Krohn KA. Kinetic modeling of 3′-deoxy-3′-fluorothymidine in somatic tumors: mathematical studies. J Nucl Med. 2005;46(2):371–80.
165. Shields AF, Briston DA, Chandupatla S, et al. A simplified analysis of [18F]3′-deoxy-3′-fluorothymidine metabolism and retention. Eur J Nucl Med Mol Imaging. 2005;32(11):1269–75.
166. Visvikis D, Francis D, Mulligan R, et al. Comparison of methodologies for the in vivo assessment of 18FLT utilisation in colorectal cancer. Eur J Nucl Med Mol Imaging. 2004;31(2):169–78.
167. Kameyama R, Yamamoto Y, Izuishi K, et al. Detection of gastric cancer using 18F-FLT PET: comparison with 18F-FDG PET. Eur J Nucl Med Mol Imaging. 2009;36(3):382–8.
168. Herrmann K, Ott K, Buck AK, et al. Imaging gastric cancer with PET and the radiotracers 18F-FLT and 18F-FDG: a comparative analysis. J Nucl Med. 2007;48(12):1945–50.
169. Bading JR, Shields AF. Imaging of cell proliferation: status and prospects. J Nucl Med. 2008;49(Suppl 2):64S–80S.
170. Herrmann K, Wieder HA, Buck AK, et al. Early response assessment using 3′-deoxy-3′-[18F] fluorothymidine-positron emission tomography in high-grade non-Hodgkin's lymphoma. Clin Cancer Res. 2007;13(12):3552–8.
171. Everitt S, Hicks RJ, Ball D, et al. Imaging cellular proliferation during chemo-radiotherapy: a pilot study of serial 18F-FLT positron emission tomography/computed tomography imaging for non-small-cell lung cancer. Int J Radiat Oncol Biol Phys. 2009;75(4):1098–104.
172. Liu G, Jeraj R, Vanderhoek M, et al. Pharmacodynamic study using FLT PET/CT in patients with renal cell cancer and other solid malignancies treated with sunitinib malate. Clin Cancer Res. 2011;17(24):7634–44.
173. Blake GM, Park-Holohan S-J, Cook GJ, Fogelman I. Quantitative studies of bone with the use of 18F-fluoride and 99mTc-methylene diphosphonate. Paper presented at seminars in nuclear medicine, 2001.
174. Hoh CK, Hawkins RA, Dahlbom M, et al. Whole body skeletal imaging with [18F] fluoride ion and PET. J Comput Assist Tomogr. 1993;17(1):34–41.
175. Narita N, Kato K, Nakagaki H, Ohno N, Kameyama Y, Weatherell JA. Distribution of fluoride concentration in the rat's bone. Calcif Tissue Int. 1990;46(3):200–4.
176. Blau M, Ganatra R, Bender MA. 18F-fluoride for bone imaging. Paper presented at seminars in nuclear medicine, 1972.
177. Toegel S, Hoffmann O, Wadsak W, et al. Uptake of bone-seekers is solely associated with mineralisation! A study with 99m Tc-MDP, 153 Sm-EDTMP and 18 F-fluoride on osteoblasts. Eur J Nucl Med Mol Imaging. 2006;33(4):491–4.
178. Even-Sapir E, Metser U, Flusser G, et al. Assessment of malignant skeletal disease: initial experience with 18F-fluoride PET/CT and comparison between 18F-fluoride PET and 18F-fluoride PET/CT. J Nucl Med. 2004;45(2):272–8.
179. Schiepers C, Nuyts J, Bormans G, et al. Fluoride kinetics of the axial skeleton measured in vivo with fluorine-18-fluoride PET. J Nucl Med. 1997;38(12):1970–6.
180. Frost ML, Cook GJ, Blake GM, Marsden PK, Benatar NA, Fogelman I. A prospective study of Risedronate on regional bone metabolism and blood flow at the lumbar spine measured by18F-fluoride positron emission tomography. J Bone Miner Res. 2003;18(12):2215–22.
181. Segall G, Delbeke D, Stabin MG, et al. SNM practice guideline for sodium 18F-fluoride PET/CT bone scans 1.0. J Nucl Med. 2010;51(11):1813–20.
182. Even-Sapir E. 18F-fluoride PET/computed tomography imaging. PET Clin. 2014;9(3):277–85.
183. Beheshti M, Mottaghy F, Payche F, et al. 18 F-NaF PET/CT: EANM procedure guidelines for bone imaging. Eur J Nucl Med Mol Imaging. 2015;42(11):1767–77.
184. Laverick S, Bounds G, Wong WL. [18F]-fluoride positron emission tomography for imaging condylar hyperplasia. Br J Oral Maxillofac Surg. 2009;47(3):196–9.
185. Raje N, Woo S-B, Hande K, et al. Clinical, radiographic, and biochemical characterization of multiple myeloma patients with osteonecrosis of the jaw. Clin Cancer Res. 2008;14(8):2387–95.
186. Wilde F, Steinhoff K, Frerich B, et al. Positron-emission tomography imaging in the diagnosis of bisphosphonate-related osteonecrosis of the jaw. Oral Surg Oral Med Oral Pathol Oral Radiol Endodontol. 2009;107(3):412–9.
187. Lim R, Fahey FH, Drubach LA, Connolly LP, Treves ST. Early experience with fluorine-18 sodium fluoride bone PET in young patients with back pain. J Pediatr Orthop. 2007;27(3):277–82.
188. Ovadia D, Metser U, Lievshitz G, Yaniv M, Wientroub S, Even-Sapir E. Back pain in adolescents: assessment with integrated 18F-fluoride positron-emission tomography-computed tomography. J Pediatr Orthop. 2007;27(1):90–3.
189. Strobel K, Fischer DR, Tamborrini G, et al. 18 F-fluoride PET/CT for detection of sacroiliitis in ankylosing spondylitis. Eur J Nucl Med Mol Imaging. 2010;37(9):1760–5.

190. Drubach LA, Johnston PR, Newton AW, Perez-Rossello JM, Grant FD, Kleinman PK. Skeletal trauma in child abuse: detection with 18F-NaF PET. Radiology. 2010;255(1):173–81.
191. Gamie S, El-Maghraby T. The role of PET/CT in evaluation of facet and disc abnormalities in patients with low back pain using 18 F-fluoride. Nucl Med Rev. 2008;11(1):17–21.
192. Schiepers C, Broos P, Miserez M, Bormans G, De Roo M. Measurement of skeletal flow with positron emission tomography and 18 F-fluoride in femoral head osteonecrosis. Arch Orthop Trauma Surg. 1998;118(3):131–5.
193. Ullmark G, Sörensen J, Nilsson O. Bone healing of severe acetabular defects after revision arthroplasty: a clinical positron emission tomography study of 7 cases. Acta Orthop. 2009;80(2):179–83.
194. Fischer DR, Maquieira GJ, Espinosa N, et al. Therapeutic impact of [18 F] fluoride positron-emission tomography/computed tomography on patients with unclear foot pain. Skelet Radiol. 2010;39(10):987–97.
195. Frost ML, Fogelman I, Blake GM, Marsden PK, Cook GJ. Dissociation between global markers of bone formation and direct measurement of spinal bone formation in osteoporosis. J Bone Miner Res. 2004;19(11):1797–804.
196. Cook GJ, Lodge MA, Blake GM, Marsden PK, Fogelman I. Differences in skeletal kinetics between vertebral and humeral bone measured by 18F-fluoride positron emission tomography in postmenopausal women. J Bone Miner Res. 2000;15(4):763–9.
197. Derlin T, Richter U, Bannas P, et al. Feasibility of 18F-sodium fluoride PET/CT for imaging of atherosclerotic plaque. J Nucl Med. 2010;51(6):862.
198. Beheshti M, Mottaghy FM, Paycha F, et al. (18) F-NaF PET/CT: EANM procedure guidelines for bone imaging. Eur J Nucl Med Mol Imaging. 2015;42(11):1767–77.

18 PET in Head and Neck Cancer

Marcus Ruhlmann and Verena Ruhlmann

18.1 Introduction

Head and neck tumors (HNC) continue to be among the more common tumors. They include tumors in the oral cavity, pharynx, and larynx. About 90% of the tumors are squamous cell carcinomas, and adenocarcinomas, sarcomas, and adenoid cystic carcinomas are significantly rarer. According to the American Cancer Society, about 50,000 new cases of HNC in the USA are estimated to occur in 2017, with men being affected about 2.5 times more frequently than women. Some of the risk factors that have been known for some time and which promote the development of HNC include tobacco smoke, alcohol, and human papillomaviruses (HPV, predominantly type 16). Recent studies suggest that the Epstein-Barr virus (EBV) may also play an important role in the development of HNC [1, 2].

The therapy of HNC depends on the stage and the localization of the tumor. Smaller tumor stages can often be cured by surgery or laser surgery and have a good prognosis. Locally advanced or metastatic tumor diseases are often treated with a combination of chemotherapy, radiotherapy, and surgery. The 5-year survival rate is approximately 80% for the early and non-advanced HNCs and only 20% for the advanced diseases [3]. Early diagnosis of HNC is therefore important. In addition to endoscopic examination methods, which can also be used to obtain biopsies and ultrasound, computed tomography (CT) and magnetic resonance imaging (MRI) are also available. Compared to CT, the MRI shows a higher soft tissue contrast and lower artifacts due to dental prostheses, which enables better local staging [4, 5]. However, both methods miss out on small lymph node metastases [4, 6]. In recent decades, positron emission tomography (PET) with [^{18}F]FDG (FDG) becomes increasingly important in the diagnosis of HNC [7–9].

18.2 Initial Staging of Head and Neck Cancer

Correct initial staging is crucial for therapy planning and the further course of the disease. As a rule, the diagnosis of an HNC is made via biopsy as part of an endoscopic examination. In the next step, a staging must be carried out which includes both the evaluation of the primary tumor extension for the T-stage and a possible locoregional lymph node involvement for the N-stage. In addition, whole-body staging should be performed at least in the higher T-stages, since distant metastases are present in 10% of patients at the time of initial diagnosis [10].

PET can detect pathological metabolism as a functional procedure. This has made PET a very

M. Ruhlmann (✉) · V. Ruhlmann
Department of Nuclear Medicine, Medical Faculty, University Duisburg-Essen, Essen, Germany
e-mail: marcus.ruhlmann@uni-due.de

H. Ahmadzadehfar et al. (eds.), *Clinical Nuclear Medicine*,
https://doi.org/10.1007/978-3-030-39457-8_18

important tool in the assessment of lymph nodes. It has long been known that there are no hard morphological criteria in sonography, CT, or MRI that are able to distinguish between benign and malignant lymph nodes. The following criteria are often used to evaluate lymph nodes and categorize them as suspicious for malignancy: short axis diameter >10 mm, a spherical configuration, and contrast enhancement; in MRI additionally, a high signal on diffusion-weighted imaging (DWI) and a low signal on the corresponding apparent diffusion coefficient (ADC) map could be considered as a sign of malignancy. The frequently chosen size of more than 1 cm as a criterion for malignancy often includes reactive lymph nodes, and small lymph node metastases are often not diagnosed [4, 6, 11, 12]. PET, on the other hand, makes it possible to measure the glucose metabolism of lymph nodes independent of size criteria. In the combination of PET and CT as a hybrid examination method, a higher sensitivity and specificity can be achieved compared to the morphological methods alone [8, 13]. In meta-analyses, PET/CT achieved a sensitivity and specificity of over 80% in the staging of lymph nodes [14, 15]. PET/CT is also superior to MRI in local tumor staging, at least for T1–T2 tumors that are not yet advanced [16]. Another advantage of PET/CT is the whole-body examination in a single session to exclude distant metastases that would have major impact on the therapy concept [17–19]. In addition, the staging concept with a PET/CT examination detects more distant metastasis or synchronous cancer than the current concepts of the American and European guidelines, which recommend either an MRI of the head and neck with CT or a X-ray thorax, respectively [20] (Fig. 18.1).

18.3 Therapy Response and Residual Tumor Detection

In the case of locally advanced HNC, complete tumor resection is often no longer possible or would lead to a significant loss of quality of life. Therefore, in addition to neoadjuvant concepts with the aim of facilitating surgical resection, there is also the concept of definitive radiochemotherapy. Both concepts have in common that a therapy response assessment is necessary before continuing or changing the therapy. However, purely morphological criteria such as size reduction are only of limited use, especially after radiotherapy, as scarring post-therapeutic changes often occur. Furthermore, non-pathologically enlarged lymph node metastases can still be vital and escape the evidence with CT and MRI. On the other hand, necrotic lymph nodes can be enlarged post-therapeutically, although they are no longer vital.

In the scenario of therapy monitoring or restaging, FDG PET has already proven its particular significance in other tumor entities such as lymphoma [21]. If pathological glucose metabolism in the lymph nodes or the primary tumor is no longer detectable, a therapeutic success can be assumed. Various studies showed a very high sensitivity and specificity and high negative predictive value (NPV) of PET in the assessment of lymph nodes [22, 23].

Fig. 18.1 A 56-year-old male patient with CUP syndrome with swelling right cervical. Panendoscopy and tissue biopsy were inconspicuous. Whole-body ^{18}F-FDG PET/CT with dedicated head and neck protocol was performed for primary tumor search (**a–h**): PET/CT showed a focal increased FDG uptake at the right base of the tongue (**a**, **d**, **e**) without CT-morphological correlate (**c**, **e**) and a central necrotic pathologically enlarged lymph node right cervical (**f**, **h**) with increased tracer uptake at the edges (**a**, **g**, **h**), highly suspicious for a metastasis. In the rest of the whole-body was no metabolic evidence of malignant lesions in the PET images (**b**, maximum intensity projection (MIP)). MRI of the head and neck was performed to evaluate operability (**i–k**): In the contrast-enhanced T1-weighted MR images, an only weakly delimitable, marginally contrast-enhancing lesion on the base of the right tongue and the sulcus glossotonsillaris (**i**) with swelling all the way to the epiglottic vallecula (**j**) and a central necrotic enlarged lymph node right cervical (**k**) were found. A preoperative targeted tissue biopsy showed a squamous epithelial carcinoma of the right base of the tongue

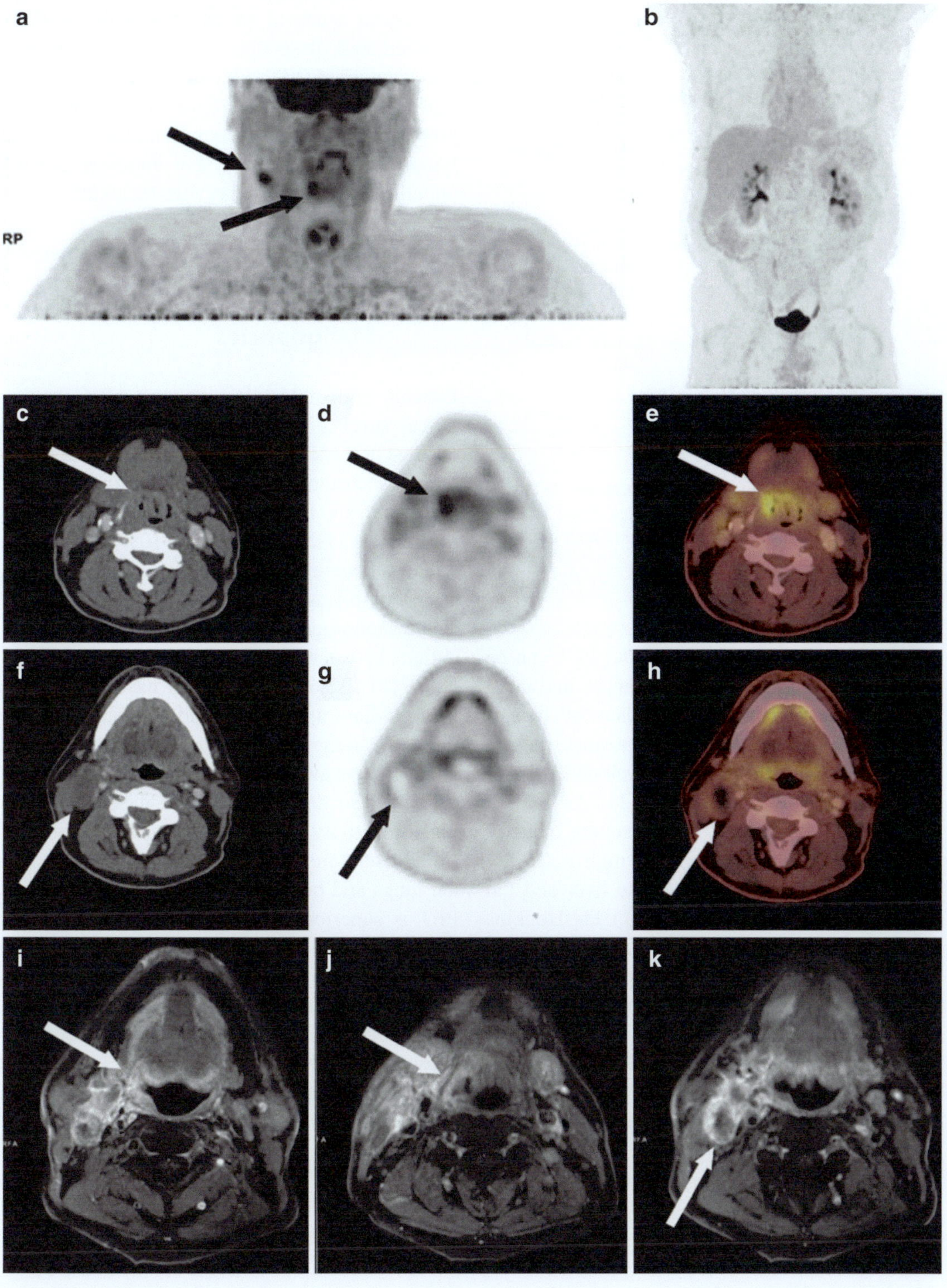
a
b
RP
c
d
e
f
g
h
i
j
k

Table 18.1 Hopkins criteria [24]

Score	^{18}F-FDG uptake pattern	Response category
1	^{18}F-FDG uptake at the primary site and nodes less than the IJV	Complete metabolic response
2	Focal ^{18}F-FDG uptake at the primary site and nodes greater than the IJV but less than the liver	Likely complete metabolic response
3	Diffuse ^{18}F-FDG uptake at the primary site or nodes is greater than the IJV or liver	Likely post-radiation inflammation
4	Focal ^{18}F-FDG uptake at the primary site or nodes greater than the liver	Likely residual tumor
5	Focal and intense ^{18}F-FDG uptake at the primary site or nodes	Residual tumor

Scores 1–3 correspond to a metabolic response and were considered as negative for tumor. Scores 4 and 5 correspond to residual, metabolic measureable tumor and were considered as positive for tumor
IJV internal jugular vein

However, the evaluation of FDG PET can be hampered by post-therapeutic changes and reactive increased glucose metabolism of benign lymph nodes that leads to false-positive results. Therefore, a working group developed the so-called Hopkins criteria for HNC [24]. An attempt is made to better classify the remaining metabolism in the primary tumor or lymph nodes by means of the FDG uptakes of the liver and the internal jugular vein (see Table 18.1). The Hopkins criteria can help to objectify PET findings [24–26]. These studies showed that overall survival and progression-free survival in patients with negative PET results according to Hopkins criteria are up to seven times higher [24–27]. In addition, the Hopkins criteria provide a high NPV of at least 92% [24, 25, 27], whereas the PET already achieved a high NPV of over 90% in a meta-analysis from 2011 without Hopkins criteria [28]. The inter-observer agreement was very high when the Hopkins criteria were applied [24, 25]. A good time interval between therapy and PET was determined in the studies of 12 weeks to minimize FDG uptake in post-therapeutic changes.

Finally, a study that prospectively examined 564 patients with advanced lymph node metastasis is worth mentioning. It could be shown that the 2-year survival in patients with regularly planned neck dissection after radiochemotherapy was comparable to those patients who underwent FDG PET/CT 12 weeks after radiochemotherapy, presented PET-negative lymph nodes (= no vital lymph node metastases), and therefore did not undergo neck dissection (Table 18.1) [29].

18.4 Restaging in Recurrent Disease and Second Malignancies

Patients with a locally advanced HNC have a 5-year survival rate of only 20% [3]. Fifty percentage of these patients experience a local recurrence or distant metastases [22]. In a current meta-analysis, the number of distant metastases in a relapse a HNC ranges from 10% to 32% [30].

Post-therapeutic changes after surgery or radiation complicate the diagnosis of a recurrence. The morphological methods often cannot differentiate between scarring changes and a recurrence [31, 32]. Meta-analyses have shown that PET/CT have a sensitivity and specificity of more than 90% in the detection of a recurrence [22, 33] and are superior to both CT and MRI [31]. PET/CT can also detect the distant metastases with high sensitivity and specificity during restaging [30]. Distant metastases occur most frequently in the lungs and bones [30]. In terms of specificity, PET is superior to CT in the detection of lung metastases [34]. Another problem that also affects mortality in HNC patients is the occurrence of secondary malignancies. Secondary tumors occur more frequently the longer patients survive the HNC [35]. About 20% of HNC patients develop a second malignancy with an incidence of 4% per year, predominantly in the aerodigestive tract [36, 37] (Fig. 18.2).

18.5 Thyroid Cancer

In most cases, thyroid carcinoma is papillary or follicular thyroid carcinoma, summarized as differentiated thyroid carcinoma (DTC). The vast majority of the DTC accumulates iodine in the tumor cells and can undergo radioiodine therapy

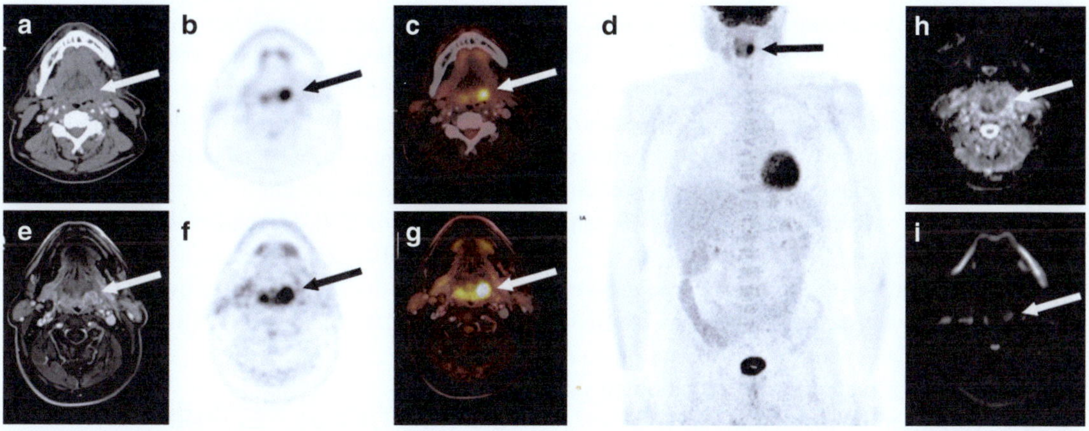

Fig. 18.2 A 65-year-old male patient with CUP syndrome after resection of the left glandula submandibularis and a lymph node left cervical with histological detection of squamous cell carcinoma. Whole-body ^{18}F-FDG PET/CT was performed for the initial staging and primary search to determine the further therapy concept (**a–c**): A conspicuous, side-asymmetric increased tracer uptake of the left base of the tongue (**b**, **c**) with questionable tissue asymmetry in CT (**a**) could be found. A whole-body ^{18}F-FDG PET/MRI followed immediately afterward (**d–i**): A pathologically focal increased tracer uptake of the left base of the tongue (**d**, **f**, **g**) with a clearly detectable marginal contrast-enhancing lesion in the contrast-enhanced T1-weighted MR images (**e**) and a corresponding diffusion restriction (**i**) with correlate in the ADC map (**h**) in the DWI sequences were detected. In the rest of the whole-body was no metabolic evidence of malignant lesions in the PET images (**d**, MIP). Later on, the carcinoma at the base of the tongue was histologically confirmed

(RIT). The overall prognosis for the most DTC patients is excellent [38]. However, there are two patient groups whose course of disease unfortunately differs from this. This includes high-risk patients with a high initial tumor stage or metastatic disease and patients with a persistent or recurrent disease. In these cases, additional diagnostic with PET can be helpful.

18.6 ^{124}I PET

While high-risk patients undergo at least one or several RIT with higher activities, the risk of side effects like bone marrow suppression or lung fibrosis is increased [39, 40]. A pretherapeutic risk stratification with ^{124}I PET can detect iodine avid metastases and offers the possibility of lesion dosimetry to decide which metastases can be treated successfully. Moreover, the activity of radioiodine can be adapted to the results of the lesion and blood dosimetry [41–43]. In cases of only low iodine uptake, other therapy like surgery might be the best choice for the patient. The same holds for patients with persistent or recurrent disease. Before undergoing additional RIT after initial treatment, the iodine uptake of the metastases or the recurrent/persistent tumor must be adequate for successful therapy.

Other iodine imaging uses ^{123}I or ^{131}I in combination with a gamma camera and single photon emission computed tomography (SPECT). Compared to ^{124}I PET, the gamma camera imaging needs higher activities of the iodine isotopes to achieve a comparable detection due to the lower spatial resolution and sensitivity of a gamma camera [41, 42, 44–46].

18.7 FDG PET

DTC patients with iodine-negative metastases or iodine-negative recurrent disease have a poorer prognosis [47, 48]. In addition to a surgery, which is not always possible, these patients usually only have a systemic therapy with, e.g., tyrosine kinase inhibitors or radiation therapy as a palliative therapy. In some cases, patients already have iodine-positive and iodine-negative metastases at the beginning of therapy.

FDG PET has been demonstrated to be a helpful diagnostic tool to detect iodine-negative metastases or recurrent tumor in case of advanced diseases. Moreover, FDG PET can unmask the initial iodine-negative metastases in the context of the first RIT and can improve the course of disease. Different studies showed high sensitivity and specificity of FDG PET(/CT) in detecting iodine-negative metastases of 95–98% and 81–94%, respectively [49–53].

Besides detecting iodine-negative metastases, FDG PET can evaluate the glucose metabolism of iodine-positive metastases. Iodine-positive metastases with a high glucose metabolism are positive correlated with shorter survival [54]. Moreover, the BRAF V600E mutations seem to be correlated with a higher glucose metabolism in DTC metastases, which requires further investigation [55] (Fig. 18.3).

18.8 Cancer of Unknown Primary (CUP)

In about 3–5% of patients with malignant epithelial tumors, the primary tumor is unknown [56]. Despite extensive diagnostics with panendoscopy and conventional imaging, the primary tumor is often not found [57]. The primary tumor is located in about 85% of patients with cervical lymph node metastases in the cervical region [58]. In order to optimize the therapy and minimize the necessity of, e.g., large-area radiotherapy, it is necessary to know the localization of the primary tumor [59]. CT and MRI can do this in only about 10–35% of cases [60–62]. PET or PET/CT, on the other hand, shows a recognition rate of 40–57% [62–64] (Fig. 18.4).

18.9 PET/CT vs. PET/MRI

The development from the PET scanner to the hybrid device PET/CT has yielded an enormous improvement. The metabolic and morphological findings were acquired in only one examination and could evaluated by fused images [65]. A further step in this development was the development of PET/MRI scanners.

MRI does not use any ionizing radiation and provides a high soft tissue contrast and a variety of additional functional parameters that go beyond the capabilities of the CT. This suggests that the combined PET/MRI is superior to PET/

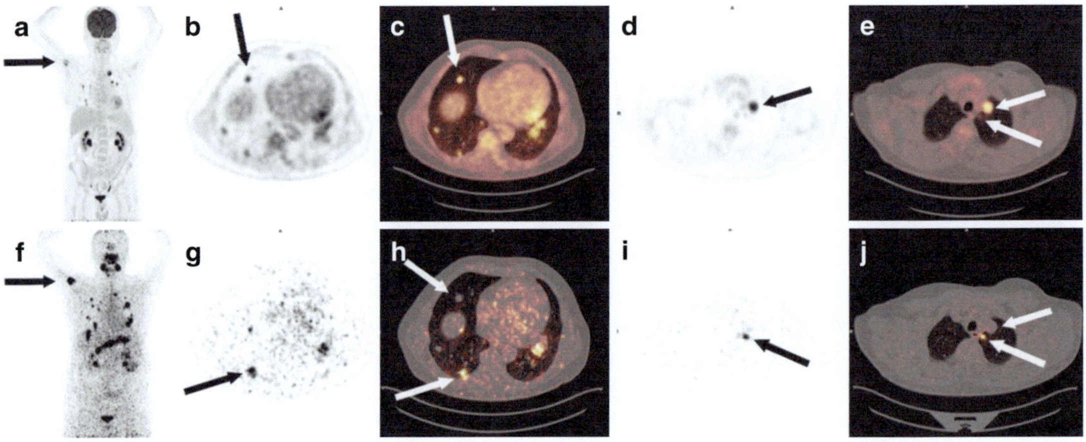

Fig. 18.3 A 72-year-old male patient with a differentiated follicular thyroid carcinoma after thyroidectomy and four radioiodine therapies with cumulative 29.8 GBq ^{131}I. Due to a pathologically increased and elevated tumor marker thyroglobulin (727 ng/ml), a whole-body ^{124}I PET/CT dosimetry (**f–j**) and FDG PET/CT (**a–e**, non-enhanced CT) imaging were performed. The iodine imaging shows multiple iodine-positive and iodine-negative bipulmonary metastases (**f–j**) as well as an iodine-positive osseous metastasis in the right proximal humerus (**f**, PET-MIP). FDG PET/CT showed the osseous metastasis in the right humerus as additionally FDG-positive (not only shine-through effect of existing iodine uptake) (**a**, PET-MIP) and multiple FDG-positive but iodine-negative bipulmonary metastases (**a**, **b**, **c**, **d**, **e**)

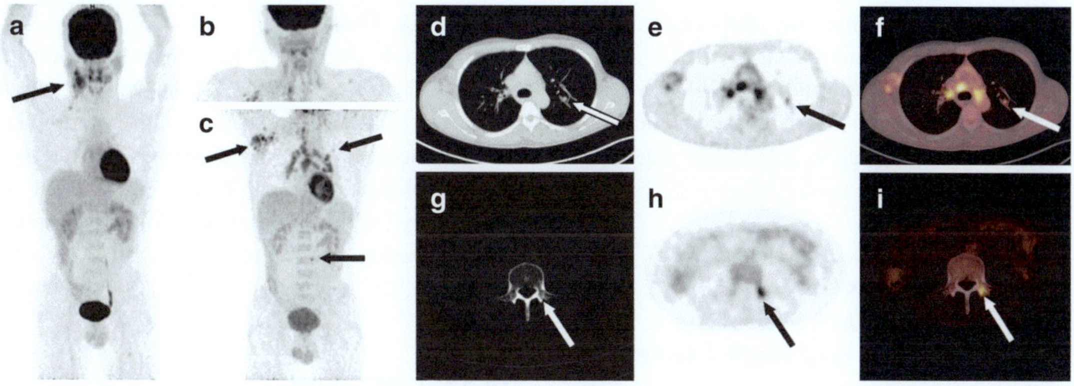

Fig. 18.4 A 35-year-old male patient with a metastatic nasopharyngeal carcinoma after neck dissection right cervical, chemotherapy, and radiation. Initially, cervical and periclavicular lymph node metastases were present in addition to the primary tumor (**a**, PET-MIP whole-body protocol). About 1.5 years later, whole-body ^{18}F-FDG PET/CT was performed for restaging while suspected for a recurrence (**b**–**i**): In the current PET/CT, multiple newly occurring, pathologically enlarged lymph node metastases right axillary, mediastinal, and hilar were detected (**b**, **c**, PET-MIP of dedicated head and neck and whole-body protocol). In the left upper lung lobe, a newly occurring, FDG-avid (**c**, **e**, **f**) and in the CT clearly distinguishable lesion (**d**, **f**) was found, highly suspicious for a metastasis. A newly occurring, moderately increased focal tracer uptake (**c**, **h**, **i**) in a questionable slight sclerosis (**g**, **i**) of the left processus transversus of LWK 3 was also detected, suspicious of a metastasis. Now a symmetrical, most likely physiological glucose metabolism of the nasopharynx was present (**b**, PET-MIP), therefore no evidence of a local relapse

CT in imaging of head and neck tumors. Numerous studies on different tumor entities such as tumors of the female and male pelvis, neuroendocrine primaries, and breast cancer showed comparable but not superior diagnostic competence of PET/CT and PET/MRI regarding whole-body staging as well as its superior diagnostic capacity regarding the assessment of parenchymatous and osseous metastases [66–68]. However, no significant advantage of using PET/MRI in the head and neck area could be found [9, 69–73]. PET/CT and PET/MRI are also equivalent in CUP imaging, with CT having advantages over MRI in the detection of lung metastases [74]. However, the inclusion of DWI can bring benefits in the reduction of false-positive findings in diagnosing HNC recurrence diagnostics and in lymph node staging [75, 76].

Due to the comparatively high acquisition costs of a PET/MRI device and the long examination duration of a whole-body PET/MRI protocol, first of all, the pre-dominant diagnostic procedure of the HNC will probably remain with performing a MRI of the head and neck in combination with a whole-body PET/CT.

18.10 Pitfalls

The most common problem is by far the artifacts of dental prostheses. These cause extinctions in the MRI and hardening artifacts in the CT. These CT artifacts influence the PET attenuation correction, and an increased focal FDG uptake can be simulated at this localization. In these cases, considering the non-attenuation-corrected PET images is necessary to exclude a false pathological FDG uptake.

The distinction between physiological, reactive, and malignant FDG uptake in the head and neck area is often a major challenge. Waldeyer's lymphatic ring (tonsilla pharyngealis, tubaria, palatina, et lingualis) often accumulates FDG, mostly physiologically and symmetrically. If the FDG uptake is significantly increased or very asymmetric, a biopsy is often necessary to exclude HNC or lymphoma.

Another problem can be brown adipose tissue. Especially children and slim, young women show an increased FDG uptake in the activated brown adipose tissue. A simple way to reduce the activity of the adipose tissue is to keep the patients warm before and after the FDG injection [77]. Also, the previous administration of, e.g., beta-blockers such as propranolol (in children, 1 mg propranolol per kilogram bodyweight with a maximum of 40 mg; in adults, 80 mg weight-independent) can be tried [78].

18.11 Examples for PET/CT and PET/MR Protocols for Head and Neck Cancer

The implementation of PET should follow the general guidelines. Patients should be fasting for at least 4 h and have only drunk water. Blood glucose levels should be below 150 mg/dl. After FDG injection (activity weight-adapted and depending on the PET scanner, e.g., time of flight), the examination should start about 60 min later.

18.11.1 PET/CT

In order to reduce the artifacts through the usually high positioned arms in the head and neck area, it is advisable to carry out the PET/CT examination in two stages:

18.11.1.1 Neck

A dedicated head and neck scan with one bed position from the skull base to the aortic arch. The patient's arms are placed beside the torso. The PET acquisition time is, for example, 4 min. The CT with intravenous application of contrast medium is performed according to the manufacturer's specifications with appropriate dose reduction programs and reconstruction in thin slices to improve the assessability of small structures in the head and neck area.

18.11.1.2 Whole Body

For the subsequent whole-body examination from the upper thorax to the mid-thighs, arms are placed over the patient's head. The PET measurements should be adapted to the usual hospital standard (e.g., 2 min per bed position). The CT should also be adapted to the otherwise valid clinical standard.

18.11.1.3 Thorax

As the whole-body PET data are acquired during shallow breathing and the CT in breath medium layer for better coregistration, the complementary thoracic examination in inspiration and low-dose technique for a better assessment of pulmonary lesions is a useful addition. A renewed administration of contrast medium is not necessary.

18.11.2 PET/MRI

Although the small size of the gantry allows the arms to be placed only beside the torso and not over the head, the division into the neck and whole body with appropriate protocol adaptation is also useful here. The attenuation correction should be performed according to the manufacturer's instructions. PET data acquisition is performed simultaneously to the extensive MR data acquisition, at least a duration of 2 min per bed position permits a sufficient image quality.

Before administration of the contrast agent, the following MRI sequences could be used:

1. Head and neck region
   (a) Non-enhanced T1 turbo spin echo (TSE) sequence in coronal orientation, slice thickness 5 mm
   (b) Non-enhanced T1 TSE sequence in transverse orientation, slice thickness 3 mm
   (c) T2 TSE sequence in transverse orientation, slice thickness 3 mm
   (d) Diffusion-weighted imaging (DWI) sequence with apparent diffusion coefficient (ADC) map in axial orientation
2. Whole body (from the upper thorax to the mid-thighs)
   (e) T2 TSE sequence in transverse orientation, slice thickness 5 mm
   (f) Non-enhanced T1 3D volume interpolated breath-hold examination (VIBE) sequence in transversal orientation, slice thickness of 3.5 mm
   (g) Diffusion-weighted echo-planar imaging (EPI) sequence in free breathing in transverse orientation, slice thickness of 5.0 mm

After administration of the contrast agent, the following MRI sequences could be used:

3. Head and neck region
   (h) Contrast-enhanced T1 TSE sequence with fat saturation in transverse orientation, slice thickness 3 mm
   (i) Contrast-enhanced T1 TSE sequence in coronal orientation, slice thickness 5 mm
4. Whole body
   (j) Contrast-enhanced T1 3D VIBE sequence in transversal orientation with fat saturation, slice thickness of 3.5 mm

References

1. She Y, Nong X, Zhang M, Wang M. Epstein-Barr virus infection and oral squamous cell carcinoma risk: a meta-analysis. PLoS One. 2017;12(10):e0186860.
2. He C, Huang X, Su X, Tang T, Zhang X, Ma J, et al. The association between circulating tumor cells and Epstein-Barr virus activation in patients with nasopharyngeal carcinoma. Cancer Biol Ther. 2017;18(11):888–94.
3. Sinevici N, O'sullivan J. Oral cancer: deregulated molecular events and their use as biomarkers. Oral Oncol. 2016;61:12–8.
4. Leslie A, Fyfe E, Guest P, Goddard P, Kabala JE. Staging of squamous cell carcinoma of the oral cavity and oropharynx: a comparison of MRI and CT in T- and N-staging. J Comput Assist Tomogr. 1999;23(1):43–9.
5. Hricak H, Gatsonis C, Coakley FV, Snyder B, Reinhold C, Schwartz LH, et al. Early invasive cervical cancer: CT and MR imaging in preoperative evaluation – ACRIN/GOG comparative study of diagnostic performance and interobser. Radiology. 2007;245(2):491–8.
6. Curtin HD, Ishwaran H, Mancuso AA, Dalley RW, Caudry DJ, McNeil BJ. Comparison of CT and MR imaging in staging of neck metastases. Radiology. 1998;207(1):123–30.
7. Minn H, Paul R, Ahonen A. Evaluation of treatment response to radiotherapy in head and neck cancer with fluorine-18 fluorodeoxyglucose. J Nucl Med. 1988;29(9):1521–5.
8. Czernin J, Allen-Auerbach M, Schelbert HR. Improvements in cancer staging with PET/CT: literature-based evidence as of September 2006. J Nucl Med. 2007;48(Suppl 1):78S–88S.
9. Schaarschmidt BM, Heusch P, Buchbender C, Ruhlmann M, Bergmann C, Ruhlmann V, et al. Locoregional tumour evaluation of squamous cell carcinoma in the head and neck area: a comparison between MRI, PET/CT and integrated PET/MRI. Eur J Nucl Med Mol Imaging. 2015;43(1):92–102.
10. de Bree R, Deurloo EE, Snow GB, Leemans CR. Screening for distant metastases in patients with head and neck cancer. Laryngoscope. 2000;110(3):397–401.
11. Leicher-Düber A, Bleier R, Düber C, Thelen M. Regional lymph node metastases in malignant tumors of the head and neck: value of diagnostic procedures. Laryngorhinootologie. 1991;70(1):27–31.
12. Lwin CT, Hanlon R, Lowe D, Brown JS, Woolgar JA, Triantafyllou A, et al. Accuracy of MRI in prediction of tumour thickness and nodal stage in oral squamous cell carcinoma. Oral Oncol. 2012;48(2):149–54.
13. Wax MK, Myers LL, Gona JM, Husain SS, Nabi HA. The role of positron emission tomography in the evaluation of the N-positive neck. Otolaryngol Head Neck Surg. 2016;129(3):163–7.
14. Yongkui L, Jian L, Wanghan JL. 18FDG-PET/CT for the detection of regional nodal metastasis in patients with primary head and neck cancer before treatment: a meta-analysis. Surg Oncol. 2013;22(2):e11–6.
15. Shen G, Zhang W, Jia Z, Li J, Wang Q, Deng H. Meta-analysis of diagnostic value of 18F-FDG PET or PET/CT for detecting lymph node and distant metastases in patients with nasopharyngeal carcinoma. Br Inst Radiol. 2014;87(1044):20140296.
16. Chaput A, Robin P, Podeur F, Ollivier M, Keromnes N, Tissot V, et al. Diagnostic performance of 18 fluorodeoxyglucose positron emission/computed tomography and magnetic resonance imaging in detecting T1-T2 head and neck squamous cell carcinoma. Laryngoscope. 2017;128(2):378–85.
17. de Bree R, Putten LVD, Brouwer J, Castelijns JA, Hoekstra OS, René Leemans C. Detection of locoregional recurrent head and neck cancer after (chemo) radiotherapy using modern imaging. Oral Oncol. 2009;45(4–5):386–93.
18. Argiris A, Karamouzis MV, Raben D, Ferris RL. Head and neck cancer. Lancet. 2008;371(9625):1695–709.
19. Goerres GW, Schmid DT, Grätz KW, Schulthess v GK, Eyrich GK. Impact of whole body positron emission tomography on initial staging and therapy in patients with squamous cell carcinoma of the oral cavity. Oral Oncol. 2003;39(6):547–51.
20. Rohde M, Nielsen AL, Johansen J, Sørensen JA, Nguyen N, Diaz A, et al. Head-to-head comparison of chest X-ray/head and neck MRI, chest CT/head and neck MRI, and 18F-FDG PET/CT for detection of distant metastases and synchronous cancer in oral, pharyngeal, and laryngeal cancer. J Nucl Med. 2017;58(12):1919–24.
21. Barrington SF, Mikhaeel NG, Kostakoglu L, Meignan M, Hutchings M, Müeller SP, et al. Role of imaging in the staging and response assessment of lymphoma: consensus of the international conference on malignant lymphomas imaging working group. J Clin Oncol. 2016;32(27):3048–58.

22. Kim S-A, Roh J-L, Kim JS, Lee JH, Lee SH, Choi S-H, et al. 18F-FDG PET/CT surveillance for the detection of recurrence in patients with head and neck cancer. Eur J Cancer. 2017;72:62–70.
23. Van den Wyngaert T, Helsen N, Carp L, Hakim S, Martens MJ, Hutsebaut I, et al. Fluorodeoxyglucose-positron emission tomography/computed tomography after concurrent chemoradiotherapy in locally advanced head-and-neck squamous C. J Clin Oncol. 2017;35(30):3458–64.
24. Marcus C, Ciarallo A, Tahari AK, Mena E, Koch W, Wahl RL, et al. Head and neck PET/CT: therapy response interpretation criteria (Hopkins criteria)-interreader reliability, accuracy, and survival outcomes. J Nucl Med. 2014;55(9):1411–6.
25. Kendi AT, Brandon D, Switchenko J, Wadsworth JT, El-Deiry MW, Saba NF, et al. Head and neck PET/CT therapy response interpretation criteria (Hopkins criteria) – external validation study. Am J Nucl Med Mol Imaging. 2017;7(4):174–80.
26. Wray R, Sheikhbahaei S, Marcus C, Zan E, Ferraro R, Rahmim A, et al. Therapy response assessment and patient outcomes in head and neck squamous cell carcinoma: FDG PET Hopkins criteria versus residual neck node size and morphologic features. AJR Am J Roentgenol. 2016;207(3):641–7.
27. Helsen N, Roothans D, Van Den Heuvel B, Van den Wyngaert T, Van den Weyngaert D, Carp L, et al. 18F-FDG-PET/CT for the detection of disease in patients with head and neck cancer treated with radiotherapy. Public Libr Sci. 2017;12(8):e0182350.
28. Gupta T, Master Z, Kannan S, Agarwal JP, Ghsoh-Laskar S, Rangarajan V, et al. Diagnostic performance of post-treatment FDG PET or FDG PET/CT imaging in head and neck cancer: a systematic review and meta-analysis. Eur J Nucl Med Mol Imaging. 2011;38(11):2083–95.
29. Mehanna H, Wong W-L, McConkey CC, Rahman JK, Robinson M, Hartley AGJ, et al. PET-CT surveillance versus neck dissection in advanced head and neck cancer. N Engl J Med. 2016;374(15):1444–54.
30. Gao S, Li S, Yang X, Tang Q. 18FDG PET-CT for distant metastases in patients with recurrent head and neck cancer after definitive treatment. A meta-analysis. Oral Oncol. 2014;50(3):163–7.
31. Evangelista L, Cervino AR, Chondrogiannis S, Marzola MC, Maffione AM, Colletti PM, et al. Comparison between anatomical cross-sectional imaging and 18F-FDG PET/CT in the staging, restaging, treatment response, and long-term surveillance of squamous cell head and neck cancer. Nucl Med Commun. 2014;35(2):123–34.
32. Kostakoglu L, Fardanesh R, Posner M, Som P, Rao S, Park E, et al. Early detection of recurrent disease by FDG-PET/CT leads to management changes in patients with squamous cell cancer of the head and neck. Oncologist. 2013;18(10):1108–17.
33. Sheikhbahaei S, Ahn SJ, Moriarty E, Kang H, Fakhry C, Subramaniam RM. Intratherapy or posttherapy FDG PET or FDG PET/CT for patients with head and neck cancer: a systematic review and meta-analysis of prognostic studies. Am J Roentgenol. 2015;205(5):1102–13.
34. Krabbe CA, Pruim J, van der Laan BFAM, Rödiger LA, Roodenburg JLN. FDG-PET and detection of distant metastases and simultaneous tumors in head and neck squamous cell carcinoma: a comparison with chest radiography and chest CT. Oral Oncol. 2009;45(3):234–40.
35. Spector JG, Sessions DG, Haughey BH, Chao KSC, Simpson J, Mofty El S, et al. Delayed regional metastases, distant metastases, and second primary malignancies in squamous cell carcinomas of the larynx and hypopharynx. Laryngoscope. 2001;111(6):1079–87.
36. León X, Quer M, Diez S, Orús C, López-Pousa A, Burgués J. Second neoplasm in patients with head and neck cancer. Head Neck. 1999;21(3):204–10.
37. León X, Prado Venegas M, Orús C, Kolañczak K, García J, Quer M. Metachronous second primary tumours in the aerodigestive tract in patients with early stage head and neck squamous cell carcinomas. Eur Arch Otorhinolaryngol. 2005;262(11):905–9.
38. Mazzaferri EL, Jhiang SM. Long-term impact of initial surgical and medical therapy on papillary and follicular thyroid cancer. Am J Med. 1994;97(5):418–28.
39. Dietlein M, Dressler J, Eschner W, Grünwald F, Lassmann M, Leisner B, et al. Procedure guidelines for radioiodine therapy of differentiated thyroid cancer (version 3). Nuklearmedizin. 2007;46:213–9.
40. Haugen BR, Alexander EK, Bible KC, Doherty GM, Mandel SJ, Nikiforov YE, et al. American Thyroid Association Management guidelines for adult patients with thyroid nodules and differentiated thyroid cancer: The American Thyroid Association Guidelines Task Force on thyroid nodules and differentiated thyroid cancer. Thyroid. 2016;26:1–133.
41. Pettinato C, Spezi E, Nanni C, Grassetto G, Monari F, Allegri V, et al. Pretherapeutic dosimetry in patients affected by metastatic thyroid cancer using 124I PET/CT sequential scans for 131I treatment planning. Clin Nucl Med. 2014;39(8):e367–74.
42. Pettinato C, Monari F, Nanni C, Allegri V, Marcatili S, Civollani S, et al. Usefulness of 124I PET/CT imaging to predict absorbed doses in patients affected by metastatic thyroid cancer and treated with 131I. Q J Nucl Med Mol Imaging. 2012;56(6):509–14.
43. Jentzen W, Bockisch A, Ruhlmann M. Assessment of simplified blood dose protocols for the estimation of the maximum tolerable activity in thyroid cancer patients undergoing radioiodine therapy using 124I. J Nucl Med. 2015;56(6):832–8.
44. Phan HTT, Jager PL, Paans AMJ, Plukker JTM, Sturkenboom MGG, Sluiter WJ, et al. The diagnostic value of 124I-PET in patients with differentiated thyroid cancer. Eur J Nucl Med Mol Imaging. 2008;35(5):958–65.
45. Beijst C, Kist JW, Elschot M, Viergever MA, Hoekstra OS, de Keizer B, et al. Quantitative comparison of 124I PET/CT and 131I SPECT/CT detectability. J Nucl Med. 2016;57(1):103–8.

46. Ruhlmann M, Jentzen W, Ruhlmann V, Pettinato C, Rossi G, Binse I, et al. High level of agreement between pretherapeutic 124I PET and intratherapeutic 131I imaging in detecting iodine-positive thyroid cancer metastases. J Nucl Med. 2016;57(9):1339–42.
47. Rouxel A, Hejblum G, Bernier M-O, Boëlle P-Y, Menegaux F, Mansour G, et al. Prognostic factors associated with the survival of patients developing loco-regional recurrences of differentiated thyroid carcinomas. J Clin Endocrinol Metab. 2004;89(11):5362–8.
48. Mirallié E, Guillan T, Bridji B, Resche I, Rousseau C, Ansquer C, et al. Therapeutic impact of 18FDG-PET/CT in the management of iodine-negative recurrence of differentiated thyroid carcinoma. Surgery. 2007;142(6):952–8.
49. Finkelstein SE, Grigsby PW, Siegel BA, Dehdashti F, Moley JF, Hall BL. Combined [18F]fluorodeoxyglucose positron emission tomography and computed tomography (FDG-PET/CT) for detection of recurrent, 131I-negative thyroid Cancer. Ann Surg Oncol. 2007;15(1):286–92.
50. Grünwald F, Kälicke T, Feine U, Lietzenmayer R, Scheidhauer K, Dietlein M, et al. Fluorine-18 fluorodeoxyglucose positron emission tomography in thyroid cancer: results of a multicentre study. Eur J Nucl Med Mol Imaging. 1999;26(12):1547–52.
51. Rosenbaum-Krumme SJ, Görges R, Bockisch A, Binse I. 18F-FDG PET/CT changes therapy management in high-risk DTC after first radioiodine therapy. Eur J Nucl Med Mol Imaging. 2012;39(9):1373–80.
52. Lee JW, Lee SM, Lee DH, Kim YJ. Clinical utility of 18F-FDG PET/CT concurrent with 131I therapy in intermediate-to-high-risk patients with differentiated thyroid cancer: dual-center experience with 286 patients. J Nucl Med. 2013;54(8):1230–6.
53. Palmedo H, Bucerius J, Joe A, Strunk H, Hortling N, Meyka S, et al. Integrated PET/CT in differentiated thyroid cancer: diagnostic accuracy and impact on patient management. J Nucl Med. 2006;47(4):616–24.
54. Robbins RJ, Wan Q, Grewal RK, Reibke R, Gonen M, Strauss HW, et al. Real-time prognosis for metastatic thyroid carcinoma based on 2-[18F]fluoro-2-deoxy-d-glucose-positron emission tomography scanning. J Clin Endocrinol Metab. 2006;91(2):498–505.
55. Nagarajah J, Ho AL, Tuttle RM, Weber WA, Grewal RK. Correlation of BRAFV600E mutation and glucose metabolism in thyroid cancer patients: an 18F-FDG PET study. J Nucl Med. 2015;56(5):662–7.
56. Pavlidis N, Pentheroudakis G. Cancer of unknown primary site. Lancet. 2012;379(9824):1428–35.
57. Cianchetti M, Mancuso AA, Amdur RJ, Werning JW, Kirwan J, Morris CG, et al. Diagnostic evaluation of squamous cell carcinoma metastatic to cervical lymph nodes from an unknown head and neck primary site. Laryngoscope. 2009;119(12):2348–54.
58. Nieder C, Gregoire V, Ang KK. Cervical lymph node metastases from occult squamous cell carcinoma: cut down a tree to get an apple? Int J Radiat Oncol Biol Phys. 2001;50(3):727–33.
59. Lell M, Mantsopoulos K, Uder M, Wuest W. Bildgebung der Kopf-Hals-Region. HNO. 2nd ed. Springer Berlin; 2016;64(3):189–210.
60. Nell S, Kist JW, Debray TPA, de Keizer B, van Oostenbrugge TJ, Rinkes IHMB, et al. Qualitative elastography can replace thyroid nodule fine-needle aspiration in patients with soft thyroid nodules. A systematic review and meta-analysis. Eur J Radiol. 2015;84(4):652–61.
61. Chorost MI, Lee MC, Yeoh CB, Molina M, Ghosh BC. Unknown primary. J Surg Oncol. 2004;87(4):191–203.
62. Freudenberg LS, Fischer M, Antoch G, Jentzen W, Gutzeit A, Rosenbaum SJ, et al. Dual modality of 18F-fluorodeoxyglucose-positron emission tomography/computed tomography in patients with cervical carcinoma of unknown primary. Med Princ Pract. 2005;14(3):155–60.
63. Rades D, Kühnel G, Wildfang I, Börner AR, Knapp W, Karstens JH. The value of positron emission tomography (PET) in the treatment of patients with cancer of unknown primary (CUP). Strahlenther Onkol. 2001;177(10):525–9.
64. Rades D, Kühnel G, Wildfang I, Börner AR, Schmoll HJ, Knapp W. Localised disease in cancer of unknown primary (CUP): the value of positron emission tomography (PET) for individual therapeutic management. Ann Oncol. 2001;12(11):1605–9.
65. Veit-Haibach P, Luczak C, Wanke I, Fischer M, Egelhof T, Beyer T, et al. TNM staging with FDG-PET/CT in patients with primary head and neck cancer. Eur J Nucl Med Mol Imaging. 2007;34(12):1953–62.
66. Beiderwellen K, Grueneisen J, Ruhlmann V, Buderath P, Aktas B, Heusch P, et al. [18F]FDG PET/MRI vs. PET/CT for whole-body staging in patients with recurrent malignancies of the female pelvis: initial results. Eur J Nucl Med Mol Imaging. 2014;42(1):56–65.
67. Beiderwellen K, Huebner M, Heusch P, Grueneisen J, Ruhlmann V, Nensa F, et al. Whole-body [^{18}F]FDG PET/MRI vs. PET/CT in the assessment of bone lesions in oncological patients: initial results. Eur Radiol. 2014;24(8):2023–30.
68. Beiderwellen K, Gomez B, Buchbender C, Hartung V, Poeppel TD, Nensa F, et al. Depiction and characterization of liver lesions in whole body [^{18}F]-FDG PET/MRI. Eur J Radiol. 2013;82(11):e669–75.
69. Schaarschmidt BM, Gomez B, Buchbender C, Grueneisen J, Nensa F, Sawicki LM, et al. Is integrated 18F-FDG PET/MRI superior to 18F-FDG PET/CT in the differentiation of incidental tracer uptake in the head and neck area? Diagn Interv Radiol. 2017;23(2):127–32.
70. Queiroz MA, Hüllner M, Kuhn F, Huber G, Meerwein C, Kollias S, et al. PET/MRI and PET/CT in follow-up of head and neck cancer patients. Eur J Nucl Med Mol Imaging. 2014;11(3):Doc08–1075.
71. Buchbender C, Heusner TA, Lauenstein TC, Bockisch A, Antoch G. Oncologic PET/MRI, part 1: tumors of the brain, head and neck, chest, abdomen, and pelvis. J Nucl Med. 2012;53(6):928–38.

72. Szyszko TA, Cook GJR. PET/CT and PET/MRI in head and neck malignancy. Clin Radiol. 2018;73(1):60–9.
73. Sekine T, de Galiza Barbosa F, Kuhn FP, Burger IA, Stolzmann P, Huber GF, et al. PET+MR versus PET/CT in the initial staging of head and neck cancer, using a trimodality PET/CT+MR system. Clin Imaging. 2017;42:232–9.
74. Ruhlmann V, Ruhlmann M, Bellendorf A, Grueneisen J, Sawicki LM, Grafe H, et al. Hybrid imaging for detection of carcinoma of unknown primary: a preliminary comparison trial of whole-body PET/MRI versus PET/CT. Eur J Radiol. 2016;85(11):1941–7.
75. Becker M, Zaidi H. Imaging in head and neck squamous cell carcinoma: the potential role of PET/MRI. BJR. 2014;87(1036):20130677–15.
76. Vandecaveye V, De Keyzer F, Vander Poorten V, Dirix P, Verbeken E, Nuyts S, et al. Head and neck squamous cell carcinoma: value of diffusion-weighted MR imaging for nodal staging. Radiology. 2009;251(1):134–46.
77. Parisi MT, Bermo MS, Alessio AM, Sharp SE, Gelfand MJ, Shulkin BL. Optimization of pediatric PET/CT. Semin Nucl Med. 2017;47(3):258–74.
78. Söderlund V, Larsson SA, Jacobsson H. Reduction of FDG uptake in brown adipose tissue in clinical patients by a single dose of propranolol. Eur J Nucl Med Mol Imaging. 2007;34(7):1018–22.

19 PET in Gastrointestinal, Pancreatic, and Liver Cancers

Majid Assadi

19.1 Esophageal Cancer

Esophageal cancer is one of the most prevalent malignancies, and its incidence is increasing rapidly. The two main histologic kinds of esophageal cancer are adenocarcinoma (AC) and squamous cell carcinoma (SCC), which are primarily distinguished in terms of risk factors and epidemiology [1, 2]. Most patients present with distant metastases or unresectable disease [3]. New therapy paradigms have tended to develop into multimodality approaches, including surgery and preoperative or definitive chemoradiation therapy [4, 5].

19.1.1 Diagnosis and Staging

The value of the use of ^{18}F-FDG PET (FDG PET) in the screening or initial diagnosis of esophageal cancer has not been proven. For initial tumor (T) staging of esophageal cancer, endoscopic ultrasound is the favored technique of choice because it measures the depth of invasion most precisely. In cases with negative endoscopic biopsy of an esophageal stricture, when doubt of an esophageal cancer is high, PET/CT may assist diagnostic and staging data [6]. However, PET/CT lacks the spatial resolution to delineate the depth of invasion. The sensitivity increases with increasing depth of invasion, the sensitivity being 83% for T2 tumors, 97% for T3 tumors, and 100% for T4 tumors [7], while early-stage tumors show minimal or no FDG uptake, probably resulting from a smaller degree of cellular proliferation in these smaller tumors [8]. Also, the sensitivity of FDG PET is diminished in non-FDG-avid esophageal malignancies, such as well-differentiated tumors (with low GLUT 1 expression) and mucus-secreting ones [9]. Gastroesophageal reflux or physiological smooth muscle esophageal uptake can cause false-positive findings [10]. In nodal staging, FDG PET/CT scanning has a low sensitivity of 55% but has a moderate specificity of 76% in identifying locoregional lymph node metastases [11]. It is noteworthy that FDG uptake in the primary tumor frequently obscures augmented uptake in more proximal locoregional nodes and causes lower sensitivity [11].

Given the lack of evidence of metastatic disease, locoregional staging with endoscopic ultrasound imaging is conducted, which helps provide a better evaluation of tumor invasion and the involvement of regional lymph node [12].

The principal value of FDG PET/CT scanning in the initial staging of esophageal cancer lies in its greater capability to reveal stage IV disease

M. Assadi (✉)
Nuclear Medicine and Molecular Imaging Research Center, Institute for Biomedical Sciences, Bushehr University of Medical Sciences School of Medicine, Bushehr, Iran
e-mail: asadi@bpums.ac.ir

H. Ahmadzadehfar et al. (eds.), *Clinical Nuclear Medicine*,
https://doi.org/10.1007/978-3-030-39457-8_19

[13] and to avoid futile intervention, and even in cases not suitable for surgery, the depiction of unsuspected metastases can guide palliative management [14, 15]. Distant metastases are seen in 20–30% of esophageal cancers at initial staging [16] and can be influenced by tumor histology; SCC tends to disseminate within the thorax, whereas AC inclines to spread within the abdomen and can comprise the liver and peritoneum [17].

The role of FDG PET/CT scanning has been promoted in some studies [18, 19] owing to its greater sensitivity and specificity over other imaging methods in the recognition of distant metastases. A systematic review presented pooled estimates for the sensitivity and specificity of FDG PET scanning for stage IV disease at 67% and 97%, respectively [20]. FDG PET/CT scanning has been revealed to provide improved staging in managing about one-third of patients, compared with EUS and CT techniques [21–24]. Researchers have also demonstrated the impact of tumor histology on the standardized uptake value (SUV) and found the median maximum SUV (SUV max) for AC to be considerably lower than that for SCC [25]. Recently, the percentage of alterations in the pretherapeutic stage by FDG PET/CT assessment has declined, presumably due to the advancement of other staging techniques [26–31].

PET/CT can also identify unsuspected synchronous tumors, which happen in 5.5% of patients with esophageal cancer [32]. These usually happen in the stomach, head and neck, and colon but have also been seen in the kidney, thyroid, and lung [14, 32].

Although FDG is the most frequently applied tracer, PET has also been conducted for esophageal cancer staging with other radiopharmaceuticals, such as [18F]-fluoro-3′-deoxy-3′-L-fluorothymidine ([18F]FLT), with promising results [33].

19.1.2 Recurrence/Restaging

Recurrent esophageal cancer is common and can happen near the surgical margins at anastomoses or in regional lymph nodes or distant organs [34]. PET/CT scanning is frequently ordered to monitor for recurrent or metastatic disease after esophagectomy [35, 36]. Even though recurrent disease after esophagostomy is considered incurable, they may be candidates for palliative chemotherapy or radiation therapy. In such patients, FDG PET/CT is valued for its diagnostic accuracy; for example, Flamen and colleagues [35] demonstrated a sensitivity of 94%, specificity of 82%, and accuracy of 87% for the depiction of recurrent esophageal tumors. They also found that FDG PET/CT scanning produces additional data to that acquired with conventional surveillance modalities in 27% of cases [35]. Moreover, FDG PET/CT scanning can depict interval distant metastatic disease, which is noted in 8–17% of cases upon restaging [37]. It is especially helpful in distinguishing new interval metastases that are either obscure or difficult to prospectively detect on conventional modalities and is, hence, valuable in the follow-up of esophageal cancer [38].

19.1.3 Prognosis/Response to Treatment

FDG PET/CT imaging parameters can deliver useful prognostic data before treatment. The principal concept is that the amount of FDG activity in the tumor associates with metabolism and the number of viable tumor cells and, therefore, with prognosis. The association between higher SUV and poorer overall survival has been reported in several studies [39–46]. Nevertheless, the cutoff of SUV is dissimilar in this issue.

However, measurement by SUV max does not include the significant heterogeneity of FDG uptake or account for the fact that most tumors have both malignant and nonmalignant components [47]. Novel PET metrics, such as texture analysis (as part of a radiomic technique; see Chap. 3), is an emerging tool to quantify the SUV heterogeneity in PET scans [48] and has been revealed to precisely prognosticate tumor response to treatment [49–51]. The next mathematical model parameter of FDG PET/CT is total lesion glycolysis (TLG), which is metabolic tumor volume (MTV) multiplied by the mean

SUV (SUV mean). It may be a helpful prognostic factor in esophageal cancer [52].

Overall, about 40–50% of patients have a remarkable response to neoadjuvant therapy [53]. Thus, to prevent treatment-related hazards without any significant advantage, personalizing management based on the use of PET parameters would be ideal [54–56]. Several imaging modalities applied to assess the response to treatment following neoadjuvant therapy include CT, EUS, and FDG PET/CT studies. One main benefit of clinical response assessment by EUS and CT imaging is the feasibility of application during and after therapy [57, 58]. Nonetheless, CT scanning has a relatively poor sensitivity (33–55%) and specificity (50–71%) in esophageal cancer response assessment [59]. Assessing the response to treatment can become more challenging after chemoradiotherapy (CRT) compared with after chemotherapy, since therapy-induced changes, such as inflammation, edema, and scarring, are considerably higher [37]. In addition, several novel cancer therapies are cytostatic instead of cytocidal, and a rational tumor response may take place without a significant decrease in tumor size [60]. Functional imaging by FDG PET scanning generates data on the metabolic activity of tumor cells and has become a valuable treatment response assessment tool. In total, the cutoffs range from 0% to 35% at assessment time points of 2–6 weeks after the beginning of therapy [41, 61–64].

In one large meta-analysis, FDG PET/CT scanning following CRT in cases with esophageal malignancy, sensitivities and specificities ranged from 71% to 100% and 55% to 100%, respectively [59]. A review of 26 studies entails 1544 patients with esophageal and gastroesophageal junction tumors who underwent neoadjuvant therapy depicted an evident association between post-therapeutic SUV and histopathologic response [65]. In another meta-analysis of 20 studies, the pooled sensitivity and specificity levels of FDG PET/CT scanning in the prediction of histopathologic tumor response were established to be 67% and 68%, respectively [66].

Rebollo Aguirre et al. analyzed the application of FDG PET in the assessment of neoadjuvant therapy response [67]. Ranges of sensitivity, specificity, positive predictive value, and negative predictive value for primary tumor response evaluation were 27.3–93.3%, 41.7–95.2%, 70.8–93.3%, and 71.4–93.5%, respectively, and for N restaging, they were 16.0–67.5%, 85.7–100%, 33–100%, and 91.7–93.3%, respectively [67].

An important issue is the timing of the post-treatment. Because radiation esophagitis regularly starts about 2 weeks following the initiation of therapy and is more common with higher radiation doses, the evaluation of response within the first 2 weeks of radiation treatment might prove to be more precise and less prone to false-positive results [14, 61].

Another source of potential error when looking at treatment response with PET/CT is respiratory motion artifacts, which are highest at the level of the diaphragm, and therefore, distal esophageal and gastroesophageal tumors are particularly susceptible to these artifacts, which can alter SUV max measurements by up to 30–50% [68].

Further, recent data have shown that ^{18}F-FLT PET (FLT PET) imaging may allow for better distinction between inflammation and a residual tumor during neoadjuvant treatment [69, 70].

Radiotherapy planning of primary esophageal tumors is mostly based on anatomical techniques that entail CT and EUS [71, 72]. Also, FDG PET/CT has been demonstrated to improve tumor volume outlining and to reduce geographic misses when compared with CT alone. In some patients, PET/CT also has a substantial effect on tumor staging. Generally, the addition of PET/CT seems to have an impact on radiation therapy planning for esophageal cancer, even if its long-term effect on treatment outcome remains uncertain [73–80].

19.2 Gastric Cancer

Gastric cancer is one of the most prevalent cancers worldwide and is among the leading causes of cancer mortality [81, 82]. The most frequent kind of gastric cancer is adenocarcinoma [83]. The behaviors of gastric cancers differ based on their histopathology; therefore, the treatment strategy is also tailored to the type of gastric cancer [84, 85].

19.2.1 Diagnosis and Staging

As with esophageal cancer, the most predominant diagnostic modality to use for patients with suspected gastric cancer is gastroscopy. Studies have shown a sensitivity of 93–94% of FDG PET for the diagnosis of gastric cancer, which is similar to the sensitivity of CT (93%). FDG PET has a greater specificity than CT (92% vs. 62%) [86, 87]. Overall, FDG PET has a higher sensitivity for more advanced malignancies (early gastric carcinoma, 63%; advanced gastric carcinoma, 98%) [87]. In contrast, FDG PET has a lower sensitivity in the diagnosis of primary gastric cancer in specific histologies, such as signet cell and mucinous adenocarcinomas, which have low FDG avidity [56, 88–91]. Likewise, a higher mean SUV is related to the intestinal type of gastric adenocarcinoma [87].

Pretreatment staging is crucial in defining potential curability and in designing optimal therapy [92]. Though FDG PET/CT may not have a role in the diagnosis of primary gastric tumors, it has an important role in the depiction of lymph node metastasis, particularly distant lymph node involvement and distant metastasis [93]. Furthermore, FDG PET/CT might have greater specificity and positive predictive value in the depiction of lymph node metastases than contrast-enhanced CT (CECT), which is widely applied. However, FDG PET/CT has had some contradictory results in that it may not be precise in the preoperative staging of gastric cancer due to its low sensitivity in predicting lymph node metastasis [94–101].

Also, FDG PET/CT is useful in cases with a probable synchronous second malignancy, since it not only assesses the stage of the primary gastric tumor but can also screen for synchronous tumors, as it permits an assessment of the whole body in one setting [91].

Choi and colleagues studied 256 patients and depicted that FDG PET/CT had high diagnostic accuracy (94.5%) in discerning synchronous colorectal cancer in 4.7% of their study population [102].

Furthermore, PET may be useful for the diagnosis of metastases in the liver, lungs, and distant lymph nodes but has a low sensitivity for the diagnosis of osseous metastases and peritoneal carcinomatosis due to the low spatial resolution [103].

In other studies, FLT PET has displayed a higher sensitivity than FDG PET and might apply as a valuable diagnostic tool for the quantitative evaluation of proliferation [104–106].

19.2.2 Recurrence/Restaging

In spite of complete resection, tumor recurrence represents more than half of cases with gastric adenocarcinomas [107, 108]. Systemic recurrence is more common than locoregional recurrence [109]. The most frequent sites of systemic recurrences are the liver and the peritoneal cavity, while for local recurrences, the most frequent sites are the luminal margin, the gastric bed, and locoregional lymph nodes [110].

In the diagnosis and assessment of gastric cancer recurrence, FDG PET/CT may have value as a moderately accurate predictor, particularly in FDG-avid primary tumors, leading to appropriate changes in management in these cases [100, 111–118]. A report by Kim and colleagues of 368 cases with advanced gastric cancer who underwent FDG PET/CT for initial staging and for recurrence surveillance following curative surgery revealed that of the 19.6% of cases who had recurrence, the sensitivity was greater in scans of patients with FDG-avid than non-avid tumors (81.0% vs. 52.4%) and nonanastomotic site recurrences (82.1% vs. 47.45%) [119]. A similar trend was also noted for detecting peritoneal recurrence. The sensitivity, specificity, and accuracy of FDG PET/CT's ability to diagnose recurrent gastric cancer disease range from 43% to 100%, 60% to 94%, and 57% to 89%, respectively [91].

19.2.3 Prognosis/Response to Treatment

Preoperative FDG PET/CT could be an effective tool in the prognosis after surgical resection in cases with gastric cancer. In this context, the

SUVmax cutoff values have measured from 5.74 to 8.2 in associating prognosis and outcome in the available studies [83, 120–123]. The FDG activity in metastatic lymph nodes can also offer prognostic data. Song and colleagues found that the preoperatively calculated nodal SUVmax is an independent risk factor for both recurrence-free survival ($P < 0.0001$, HR = 2.71) and overall survival ($P < 0.0001$, HR = 2.80) [124].

Overall, the metabolic changes in tumors in comparison to the baseline study can be assessed by FDG PET/CT, which is a useful indicator of response to systemic therapy [125, 126]. Ott and colleagues demonstrated a 35% decrease in uptake between prechemotherapy and a PET scan taken 2 weeks following the beginning of a prognosticated therapy response, with an accuracy of 85% [127]. Although using FDG PET/CT evidently has potential in the assessment response to treatment by tailoring the plan according to the tumor biology, well-designed studies are needed to establish both the clinical advantages and more standardized approaches to the quantification of metabolic response [128]. Recently data suggest that FLT PET/CT is considerably more sensitive than FDG in the diagnosis of gastric cancer and that it may be of use in the assessment of the response to treatment [104, 129].

19.3 Gastrointestinal Stroma Cell Tumors (GISTs)

Gastrointestinal stromal cell tumors (GISTs) are soft tissue tumors derived from the gastrointestinal tract that comprise only 0.1–3% of all gastrointestinal tumors [130]. More than 90% of GISTs are located in the stomach and small bowel, more frequently in the jejunum or ileum, but they can happen anywhere in the GI tract [131]. Mortality rates are very high, with only a 53% 2-year survival rate in advanced-stage disease [128, 132]. A unique characteristic of GISTs is that almost 95% of these tumors are immunoreactive with KIT (CD117), the c-kit receptor tyrosine kinase. Surgical resection and targeted therapy are the current standard treatments for GIST. Imatinib mesylate, a first-line medication that works as a tyrosine kinase inhibitor, was shown to have a remarkable response in the first single-patient trial presented in 2001 [133, 134]. The second drug countenance for the therapy of GIST is sunitinib, which also interacts with vascular endothelial growth factor receptors 1 through 3, fluorolevothymidine-3, and RET receptors, causing a potential antiangiogenic effect. Sunitinib is used for patients with unresectable disease who have shown primary or secondary resistance to imatinib and who are progressing in spite of higher doses of imatinib mesylate [135].

In terms of diagnosis and staging, PET/CT facilitates the detection of lesions in the majority of cases and assesses surgical resectability better [136]. The sensitivity and positive predictive values were 93% and 100%, respectively, for CT and 86% and 98%, respectively, for FDG PET/CT. No difference was noted in CT and FDG PET sensitivity or positive predictive values [137].

Deng and colleagues assessed the association between the tumor FDG uptake and the antigen Ki-67 (a tumor proliferation index) in a meta-analysis including 79 articles (n = 3242) and demonstrated a significant correlation between FDG uptake and Ki-67 expression in GIST in their subgroup analysis [138]. An association of the intensity of FDG uptake with the malignant potential and aggressiveness of a GIST [136, 139] has also been demonstrated. In malignant GISTs, recurrences and metastases are common, most often in the liver and peritoneum. Other metastatic sites entail the lungs, pleura, retroperitoneum, bone, and subcutaneous tissues [130].

The main role of PET in GIST is to assess the response to therapy and prognostication [140]. The CT-based Response Evaluation in Solid Tumors (RECIST) criteria are not very worthwhile in evaluation of the response to treatment since the size may not change in these tumors, while PET/CT responses based on changes in metabolic activity are in correlation with the clinical response [141, 142]. A positive response on FDG PET may be seen as early as 24 h after a single dose of imatinib [143].

FDG PET/CT is used before treatment in patients who are likely to need systemic therapy and also in the assessment of response to systemic therapy. A comparison of FDG PET and CT in the staging and assessment of treatment response to imatinib mesylate treatment in recurrent or metastatic GIST demonstrated that PET and CT were comparable in staging; nevertheless, FDG PET had better results than CT in predicting an early response to therapy [144]. Other studies have also demonstrated some evidence that serial PET study is more valuable for determining the response to treatment with imatinib mesylate in GIST cases (compared with only conventional CT monitoring) and that PET seems to be of potential value in initial disease assessment entailing the prediction of malignant potential in recently distinguished GISTs and in determining the optimal dose of imatinib for therapy [145].

Also, Demetri and colleagues evaluated the efficacy and safety of imatinib in advanced GISTs and used PET as a complement to CECT in 64 cases to evaluate metabolic changes in the tumors. In all responders, the evidence suggested that tumor-related glycolytic activity evaluated by PET diminished from baseline as early as 24 h after a single dose of imatinib. The PET findings were associated with subsequent evidence of response or progression on CECT or MR imaging [146]. In other studies, at baseline and day 8 of imatinib therapy, PET predicted CECT response at 8 weeks, and PET response was also correlated with longer progression-free survival [147, 148].

However, about 20% of GISTs do not reveal increased FDG uptake and cannot be monitored by PET [148]. Choi and colleagues demonstrated that monitoring tumor density on CECT is a good alternative and is superior over standard CT response criteria [148].

In spite of the success of imatinib, about 14% of cases present primary imatinib resistance, and half the cases with a good initial response show secondary resistance [132]. Prior and colleagues evaluated the response with PET after 4 weeks of therapy in 23 patients with GISTs who had aborted previous imatinib treatment due to recent tumor progression or undesirable imatinib toxicity [149]. A decrease in the SUVmax value of more than 25% between the baseline and after one therapeutic cycle of 4 weeks was highly predictive of progression-free survival. They concluded that even a single PET scan at 4 weeks was able to predict progression-free survival and to distinguish responders from nonresponders [149]. Also, in a multicenter study, Benjamin and colleagues assessed the efficacy and safety of motesanib in 138 patients with imatinib-resistant GISTs [150]. In conclusion, the early response assessment by CECT and PET demonstrated greater response rates than standard CT response criteria and better association with objective antitumor activity [150].

PET/CT has substantial value in the evaluation of response to treatment with imatinib or other drugs in GIST patients, enables an early assessment of response to therapy, and is a strong predictor of clinical outcome [144, 151–154] [132]. In addition, it is mentioned that for formerly treated patients, low FDG avidity in newly recurrent GISTs may be related to a poor response to tyrosine kinase inhibitor therapy [154].

Overall, the combination of PET and CECT seems to be the most valuable tool in the treatment of GIST patients, not only to make early assessments of the response to treatment but also to distinguish the development of resistance to imatinib [155].

19.4 Colorectal Cancer

Colorectal cancer (CRC) is the third most common cancer in both genders [156]. The most frequent type of primary tumor is adenocarcinoma. Mortality rates are decreasing due to the early diagnosis of precancerous lesions using screening programs and increasingly effective management. The average 5-year survival rate is about 64%. Surgery is curative without any further therapy in the early stage. Neoadjuvant or adjuvant chemotherapy is taken in patients with advanced colon cancer. In rectal cancer, chemoradiotherapy followed by surgery is highly useful.

19.4.1 Diagnosis and Staging

Due to its high accuracy, colonoscopy is the standard for the diagnosis of CRC. CT colonoscopy is a fair alternative, particularly if a complete colonoscopy is not possible or in patients where the exact tumor location cannot be distinguished. CT colonoscopy has a sensitivity of 96%, which is comparable to colonoscopy (95%) [157]. PET has no value in primary tumor diagnosis. Nonetheless, incidental focal bowel uptake on PET is frequently seen and warrants further evaluations. In a report with more than 10,000 PET scans, Peng and colleagues noted focal colonic uptake in 1.35% of the scans, and resulting cancerous and precancerous lesions in 20.5% and 23.5% of patients, respectively, are confirmed by colonoscopy and pathology [158].

For patients with CRC, it is imperative to ascertain the best treatment plan, which may be surgical intervention, chemotherapy, radiation therapy, or combinations thereof. When a patient is labeled with CRC and CT and in patients with rectum carcinoma, MR imaging are the main imaging methods for staging. Nevertheless, FDG PET/CT may have a complementary role in selected cases with higher disease stages.

Overall, in CRC, FDG PET/CT can affect patient management in 2–30% of patients [159, 160], and in rectal cancer, FDG PET/CT can influence patient management in 12–27% of patients [128, 161, 162].

Researchers agree that PET/CT gives slight added value for initial staging aims in cases with CRC without metastasis [163–166].

Niekel and colleagues conducted a meta-analysis including studies between 1990 and 2010 comparing CECT, MR imaging, and PET(/CECT) in the initial staging of CRC [167], and 39 eligible investigations were gathered, reporting on a total of 3391 cases. The pooled sensitivity levels of CECT, MR imaging, and PET on a per-lesion basis were 74.4%, 80.3%, and 81.4%, respectively (with no statistical differences among groups). On a per-patient basis, the sensitivities of CECT, MR imaging, and PET were 83.6%, 88.2%, and 94.1%, respectively (the sensitivity of CECT was meaningfully lower than that of PET). Per-patient specificity estimates were comparably high (>90%) for all techniques [167].

Overall, FDG PET/CT is not necessary unless CT results in a diagnosis of synchronous liver metastases, and the patient could be considered for curative liver surgery since FDG PET/CT is more sensitive than CT to rule out extrahepatic metastases. Also, FDG PET/CT should be done if staging a CT or MRI scan distinguishes nodal metastases in the common iliac region or equivocal results, such as uncertain pulmonary, liver, or bony lesions [168].

If other imaging methods have already depicted widespread metastatic disease and the patient would not be suitable for radical treatment, FDG PET/CT is not necessitated [169].

In terms of the evaluation of hepatic involvement, a meta-analysis of 3080 patients with CRC from 111 datasets was conducted by Kinkel et al. [103]. They demonstrated that the mean weighted sensitivity for the depiction of hepatic metastasis was 55% for ultrasound, 72% for CT, 76% for MRI, and 90% for FDG PET. Such points were presented in different studies [170–183].

Moreover, in a few small studies analyzing the ability of PET/CT and MRI to diagnose subcentimeter liver metastases, MRI outperformed PET/CT with a greater accuracy for detection, especially with the use of newer MR hepatobiliary-specific contrast agents [184–186]. Thus, MRI seems to be the modality of choice for detecting hepatic metastases smaller than 10 mm.

In cases with doubtful hepatic involvement on CECT or MRI imaging, PET could be applied as a second-line investigative tool for the assessment of hepatic involvement.

Considering the complementary benefits of PET and MRI imaging, the application of hybrid PET/MRI imaging could assist as a one-stop imaging plan that could potentially increase diagnostic accuracy in colorectal cancer. In colon cancer, substituting CT with MR imaging in hybrid FDG PET imaging has the benefit of being able to characterize liver lesions and to reveal small metastases, which has an effect on treatment strategy. The application of liver-specific contrast-enhanced MRI imaging has improved the diagnosis of small hepatic metastases [187]. PET/MRI can generate detailed data for the initial staging of colorectal cancer and particularly has the benefit of high-resolution MR imaging in determining the T stage of rectal cancer

[187–199]. PET/MRI has also been shown to have comparable diagnostic accuracy for N and M staging with PET/CT (true positive findings in 86% vs. 71%, respectively) [190]. A hybrid PET/MRI study demonstrated diagnostic accuracy of liver metastasis more than PET/CT (74% vs. 56%) and peritoneal seeding more than MRI (55% vs. 37%) [195]. In this report, the diagnostic accuracy of mucinous cancer diminished compared to non-mucinous cancer even with PET/MRI (52% vs. 76%).

19.4.2 Recurrence/Restaging

Recurrence develops in one-third of cases in the first 2 years after resection. Locoregional pelvic recurrence and liver metastases are the main places of relapse following the resection of colorectal cancer [196, 200–202]. The patterns of recurrence vary in colon cancer more than in rectal cancer. Local recurrence is more frequent with rectal cancers than colon cancer, ranging from 7% to 33% and 1% to 19%, respectively [203]. In addition, almost 30% of cases will develop synchronous liver metastases [204, 205]. Metachronous metastatic disease following locoregional treatment for colorectal cancer is more common. In spite of optimal primary therapy with proper management, approximately 30–50% of patients with colon cancer will relapse and die of their disease. The liver is the most frequent site of metastasis, and metastatic liver disease is the most common cause of death [206, 207].

Furthermore, an important issue in cases with prior CRC is the distinction of the sequelae of prior treatment that entail surgical scarring and radiation fibrosis from disease recurrence. This is most challenging with distal colon and rectal tumors, where presacral scarring and pelvic changes are common. The accuracy of FDG PET for the detection of local recurrent tumors was higher than 90% [208–212]. Ito et al. compared the results of FDG PET and MRI with histopathologic findings and showed that FDG PET could discriminate a scar from a local recurrent tumor [213].

Overall, the sensitivity of FDG PET imaging is in the range of 90%, and specificity is greater than 70%, which are both higher than CT in detecting recurrent or metastatic CRC. A meta-analysis of 11 clinical studies including 577 cases demonstrated that the sensitivity and specificity of FDG PET for detecting recurrent colorectal cancer were 97% and 76%, respectively [208].

In a meta-analysis including studies up to 2011, Maas and colleagues [211] depicted that the whole-body imaging modality had the greatest accuracy for the diagnosis of local and distant CRC recurrence in cases with clinically or biochemically suspected recurrence. They entailed 14 reports revealing that FDG PET and FDG PET/CT were more accurate than CT, with areas under the curves of 0.94 (0.90–0.97) for PET, 0.94 (0.87–0.98) for PET/CT, and 0.83 (0.72–0.90) for CT.

In general, the serial blood monitoring of carcinoembryonic antigen (CEA) levels is the most commonly used diagnostic test to detect asymptomatic recurrences [214]. It is estimated that tumors have recurred in 90% of cases with elevated CEA levels after surgery [215]. Nonetheless, serum CEA levels do not provide any data regarding the sites of recurrence, and it can be problematic when a patient has elevated CEA levels but no evident relapse can be localized. In 2013, Lu and colleagues [212] carried out a meta-analysis including 11 studies with 510 patients to assess the diagnostic accuracy of FDG PET or PET/CT in cases with elevated CEA levels and suspected recurrent disease. Diagnostic accuracy was acquired separately for FDG PET (seven studies) and FDG PET/CT (four studies). In the detection of the recurrence of cases with elevated CEA levels, pooled estimates of the sensitivity, specificity, and positive and negative likelihood ratios were respectively 90.3%, 80.0%, 2.88, and 0.12 for FDG PET. For FDG PET/CT, pooled estimates of the sensitivity, specificity, and positive and negative likelihood ratios were, respectively, 94.1%, 77.2%, 4.7, and 0.06. Such issue was reported in other studies [212, 216–218].

Some reports have indicated that PET/CT may be helpful in detecting recurrence in cases with normal CEA levels. Sanli and colleagues [219] compared the diagnostic value of FDG PET/CT in cases with normal and elevated CEA levels. In their retrospective investigation with 235 patients, 118 patients had normal CEA levels, and 117 patients had elevated CEA levels. Sensitivity and specificity for detecting recurrence were 100% and 84%, respectively, in the group with normal CEA; also, the sensitivity and specificity values for detecting recurrence were 97.1% and 84.6% for cases with elevated CEA levels. They demonstrated that, regardless of CEA levels, FDG PET/CT can detect recurrence. There have been several other supporting studies on this paramount point [220, 221].

Overall, the current evidence is convincing that PET/CT imaging should be the favored imaging modality in this setting, since it distinguishes and localizes the disease in one situation and can assist diagnostic or therapeutic interventions.

19.4.3 Prognosis/Response to Treatment

In manifold reports, PET has been applied to characterize CRC and to predict prognosis regarding therapy stratification and the early assessment of response to therapy [156, 200, 201, 222, 223]. PET may be used in the assessment of preoperative chemoradiotherapy in primary rectal cancer, in chemotherapy in advanced CRC, and in the assessment of impacts of local therapies for liver metastases [167, 224–230].

Follow-up of patients to acquire the effect of therapy in determining changes in the diameter of the lesions is usually based on RECIST. However, RECIST has restrictions, since a wane in tumor size does not always correspond with a better prognosis. Since FDG PET/CT focuses on metabolic alterations, it may be able to determine tumor response before anatomic changes happen.

Several studies have used the PET Response Criteria in Solid Tumors (PERCIST) to determine the FDG PET response to treatment [231]. A study by Skougaard and colleagues [232] involved 61 patients with metastatic CRC who were treated with cetuximab and irinotecan. Response assessment was carried out by CT using RECIST criteria and by FDG PET/CT using PERCIST criteria. A poor morphologic and metabolic agreement was found, mostly due to the fact that a large proportion of the patients who had stable disease on CT turned out to have partial metabolic response on FDG PET/CT. Janssen and colleagues [233] predicted response to therapy in the primary tumor in 30 cases with rectal cancer as early as 2 weeks following the start of a 3-month neoadjuvant chemoradiotherapy Scheme. A cutoff value of 48% SUVmax wane was acquired to discriminate responders from nonresponders (specificity of 100%, sensitivity of 64%).

This PET-based prediction may be applied to adjust the timing and extent of surgery.

Bystrom and colleagues [234] applied PET for the early assessment of response to palliative chemotherapy and to predict long-term outcomes following two cycles of chemotherapy entailing 51 cases with metastatic CRC. The response was evaluated by CECT after every four cycles of chemotherapy. The mean baseline SUV for all tumor lesions per patient was greater in nonresponders than in responders (mean 7.4 vs. 5.6). A robust association was observed between metabolic response (changes in SUV) and objective response ($r = 0.57$, $P = 0.0.00001$), with a sensitivity of 77% and a specificity of 76%. No substantial association between metabolic response and time to progression or overall survival was seen. Bystrom and colleagues demonstrated that although metabolic response evaluated by FDG PET reflects radiologic tumor volume changes, the accuracy is too low to encourage the routine application of PET in metastatic CRC. Likewise, PET failed to reflect long-term outcomes and should not be applied as a surrogate end point for a hard end point benefit. De Geus-Oei and colleagues demonstrated that FDG PET has a high predictive value in the therapeutic CRC strategy [235, 236]. Also, they carried out a systematic review of 15 studies evaluating PET for early preoperative therapy assessment and five studies assessing the predictive value of PET in early response monitoring in metastatic CRC [235].

They demonstrated that even if the studies included revealed large heterogeneity, PET was a noteworthy predictor of therapy outcome in both situations. The contradicting results may be due to the heterogeneity and small size of reports on these subjects. However, most studies have suggested that FDG PET/CT (or FDG PET) can be valuable in determining prognosis in cases involving the treatment of advanced or metastatic CRC.

Further, PET/CT is also appreciated for evaluating targeted therapies in cases with unresectable colorectal liver metastases. Treatment options for cases with unresectable liver metastases include selective internal radiation therapy (SIRT), radiofrequency ablation (RFA), and transcatheter arterial chemoembolization (TACE) [237]. In a review of 19 studies evaluating the impact of imaging on monitoring response to SIRT, the investigators showed that PET/CT and CEA results before and after radioembolization were most useful for assessing tumor response [238, 239]. Likewise, PET/CT has been revealed to be useful both in the evaluation of early response and in monitoring for relapse after RFA therapy [240, 241].

Since many newer localized therapy methods stabilize the disease rather than reduce tumor size, PET/CT can be especially useful in assessing the therapy response to novel therapies.

It should be mentioned that FDG PET/CT should be performed at least 4 weeks following surgery or the completion of chemoradiation to preclude the challenges from active postsurgical inflammatory changes and local inflammation after radiotherapy, which could mimic an active residual tumor [166, 230, 242].

Besides, the role of FDG PET/CT in radiation therapy planning in the demarcation of the target volume is evolving. FDG PET/CT increasingly contributes to determining the irradiation target volume, which is helpful when highly conformal radiation methods are to be deployed or when the dose is well adapted to local variations in tumor biology "dose painting." Substantial disparateness in tumor volumes can be visualized, depending on the modality for delineating the lesions [80, 243–247]. Hybrid PET/MR imaging may be of great value in staging of CRC, especially in rectal tumors. However, alterations in tumor volume demarcation may not always have a major effect on the total radiation field, so further well-designed studies are necessary to assess this issue.

19.5 Pancreatic Cancer

Pancreatic cancer is one of the most lethal of all solid tumors, despite diagnostic and therapeutic advances [248]. Invasive ductal adenocarcinoma is the most common pancreatic cancer, comprising more than 80% of pancreatic cancers [249, 250]. The head of the pancreas is the most common location (70%), with almost 20% of tumors originating from the body, 5% from the tail, and 15% involving more than one part [251]. Pancreatic adenocarcinoma is often locally advanced and/or metastatic at the time of diagnosis, so surgical resection is not done in most patients [252]. Analyzing the unique features of each tumor may assist in personalizing medical care and help to improve early detection, develop precise targeted therapies, and enhance prognostic prediction in these cases.

19.5.1 Diagnosis and Staging

Multidetector CT (MDCT) is the diagnostic modality of choice for the diagnosis and staging of pancreatic cancers [253]. MDCT has a high sensitivity for the detection of pancreatic cancers, ranging from 89% to 97% [254]. MRI and MRCP are now applied as problem-solving techniques for pancreatic cancer cases [7]. In small tumors, EUS is considered a precise tool for diagnosis of these focal lesions; in addition, histological information can also be acquired by EUS-FNA [255, 256].

No consensus has been reached to suggest that FDG PET/CT is greater than CT in this regard, although the debate is ongoing. In 2014, a meta-analysis of 35 investigations by Rijkers and colleagues measured pooled sensitivity, specificity, positive predictive value, and negative predictive value of 90%, 76%, 90%, and 76%, respectively, for FDG PET and 90%, 76%, 89%, and 78%, respectively, for FDG PET/CT in the diagnosis [257]. They compared their statistical parameters to the pooled sensitivity and specificity of 91% and 85% for CT and 84% and 82% for MR imaging from a prior meta-analysis; they demonstrated that FDG PET and FDG PET/CT delivered no additional advantages.

Though FDG PET/CT may not currently be the first diagnostic modality choice for the diagnosis of pancreatic cancer, it remains helpful in early work-up. Several studies have demonstrated the advantage of FDG PET/CT in the discrimination of carcinoma from inflammation, which is mostly based upon the distribution of uptake detected by FDG PET/CT: focal versus diffuse [258, 259].

Gambhir and colleagues presented a tabulated summary including 26 studies on pancreatic cancer and reported a weighted average sensitivity and specificity of 94% and 90%, respectively, compared with 82% and 75%, respectively, for CECT. Moreover, a change of management occurred in 50% of cases [260]. A meta-analysis comparing PET, PET/CT, and EUS presented overall pooled sensitivities of 88%, 90%, and 81%, respectively, and specificities of 83%, 80%, and 93%, respectively [261]. The role of FDG PET/CT for the discrimination of pancreatic adenocarcinoma from benign lesions, such as benign biliary strictures and focal pancreatitis, has been examined by various investigations, with the sensitivity ranging from 85% to 97% and the specificity from 64% to 94% for the primary tumor [262–269]. Also, an increased sensitivity for the diagnosis of pancreatic adenocarcinoma was noted when using a contrast-enhanced CT compared with an unenhanced CT on PET/CT reports [265]. The limitations of FDG PET/CT on the initial diagnosis of pancreatic adenocarcinoma include false-negative studies in cases with hyperglycemia [270] and small tumors (T1 or T2) [263, 271, 272] and false-positive findings associated with inflammatory changes (acute, chronic, and autoimmune pancreatitis), leading to decreased specificity [273–275].

Currently, most available PET/MR imaging data regarding pancreatic disease are based on retrospective fusion of PET and MR imaging information. Tatsumi and colleagues [276] evaluated the feasibility of retrospective PET and MR imaging fusion and demonstrated a benefit of fusing PET images with noncontrast T1-weighted MR images over PET/CT in the categorization of pancreatic tumors. Nagamachi and colleagues [277] noted substantially improved accuracy in the discrimination of pancreatic cancer from benign lesions using retrospectively fused PET and T2-weighted MR images compared with PET/CT (96.6% vs. 86.6%, respectively). Moreover, T2-weighted images result in better characterizations of pancreatic cystic lesions, helping to separate benign cysts from malignant cystic tumors.

Also, Herrmann and colleagues [278] studied the potential role of FLT PET in differentiating malignant pancreatic adenocarcinomas from benign pancreatic lesions in 31 patients with indeterminate lesions. They demonstrated a specificity of 100% and a sensitivity of 71.4%, and the missed malignancies were either well-differentiated or small tumors. More studies are necessary to assess the association of FLT uptake in pancreatic adenocarcinoma with histologic proliferation indices [279].

Furthermore, pancreatic cancer metastasizes most commonly in the liver, peritoneal cavity, lungs, pleura, and intrathoracic lymph nodes. At diagnosis, 50% of cases have liver metastases, 35% have peritoneal metastases, and 40% of cases will have locoregional lymph node metastases. FDG PET has been demonstrated to be superior to other imaging techniques for the diagnosis of metastatic disease [263, 280–283].

The advantages of contrast-enhanced FDG PET/CT, incorporating a three-phase CECT and FDG PET, have been demonstrated in the staging and treatment planning of pancreatic cancer [258].

PET/MR imaging has a potential value in the initial imaging of those cases with suspected carcinoma and with a pancreatic duct stricture in which no distinct mass is seen on contrast-enhanced CT. The combination of MR imaging with MRCP and FDG PET can detect small mass lesions at the stricture site and to direct endoscopic ultrasound-guided biopsy. The combination of MR imaging with DWI and FDG PET has a benefit over both contrast-enhanced CT and PET/CT in the diagnosis of early hepatic metastases and to preclude futile surgery. Both CT and FDG PET have a low sensitivity and accuracy for depiction of peritoneal implants, another main factor affecting surgical resectability. MR imaging with DWI as part of PET/MR imaging has a better sensitivity in revealing of peritoneal implants [284, 285].

19.5.2 Recurrence/Restaging

About 40% of pancreatic cancer subjects have recurrences within the first year after surgical resection [128]. The assessment of tumor recurrence in these subjects is challenging by conventional anatomic modalities, since postsurgical and fibrotic changes (mainly related to radiation therapy) are frequently difficult to discriminate from tumors. Likewise, tissue sampling of the suspicious areas for recurrence is problematic to attain, as pancreatic adenocarcinomas are related to marked desmoplastic reactions [286].

The value of FDG PET/CT for the depiction of suspected recurrence of pancreatic adenocarcinoma after surgery compared with CT/MR imaging was assessed in 31 subjects by Ruf and colleagues [286]. The FDG PET/CT and CT/MR imaging modalities depicted 96% (22 of 23) and 39% (9 of 23) of local recurrences and 42% (5 of 12) and 92% (11 of 12) of liver metastases, respectively. For subjects undergoing chemoradiation, residual disease was visualized by FDG PET/CT in 5 of 15 subjects, compared with none seen by CT in a study of Bang and colleagues [287]. Several other reports have concluded that FDG PET has greater accuracy in assessing pancreatic carcinoma local recurrence [288, 289].

Given that FDG is a nonspecific factor in glucose metabolism, other mechanisms, such as postsurgical inflammatory changes, the response to radiation therapy, and stent placement, can cause false-positive results, so it is recommended that FDG PET/CT should be carried out 6 weeks after surgery [286, 288]. Better anatomic outlining of the surgical bed by MR imaging and improved metabolic information from FDG activity via PET/MR hybrid imaging are encouraging because they have boosted depictions of local tumor recurrence.

19.5.3 Prognosis/Response to Treatment

By acquiring data on pretreatment studies, therapeutic strategies can be better tailored and personalized [290–294]. As such, FDG PET/CT may play a role in the prognosis of patients with pancreatic cancer [287, 295, 296].

Several investigations have demonstrated that the application of FDG PET/CT can assist in predicting patient outcomes in terms of both overall survival and progression-free survival [291, 292, 297] [298] [299, 300].

Furthermore, PET combined with CECT assists in monitoring the response to therapy in cases with unresectable pancreatic cancer [287, 301]. A noteworthy decline in FDG uptake may precede a volumetric CT decrease and may be proportionate to the change in tumor size at subsequent follow-up evaluations. Therefore, an earlier FDG PET assessment of tumor response to therapy could affect the continuation or withdrawal of therapy [288, 302].

Additionally, an incremental focus has been placed on the quantification of intratumoral heterogeneity, which, at a molecular level, can be associated with therapy failure and drug resistance [303]. Hyun and colleagues [304] studied the value of intratumoral heterogeneity texture analysis by FDG PET to predict outcomes in patients with pancreatic adenocarcinoma [252]. A novel metric for tumor quantification named generalized effective total uptake (gETU) was established by Rahmim and colleagues [305]. It involves various FDG PET metrics, such as SUVmax, TLG, and MTV, with different emphases on PET uptake versus volume.

An additional benefit of FLT PET/CT compared with FDG PET/CT is the lack of uptake interfering with hypoxia or inflammation, which can be visualized on FDG PET/CT. This is particularly imperative on the evaluation of response to therapy, in terms of increasing specificity and as a valuable method in the development of anticancer treatments.

Furthermore, subjects with locally advanced pancreatic cancer usually undergo radiation therapy, and CT-based radiation therapy planning continues to be the current standard technique of choice [306, 307]. Nonetheless, CT alone compared with FDG PET has low accuracy in describing the primary pancreatic tumor and in defining the adjacent lymphatic extension and distant metastasis disease [308–311]. Accordingly, it is rational that complementing CT with PET imaging may assist in delineating GTV and planning target volume and thereby reducing geographic misses and improving local disease control. Taken together, PET/CT-based target volume definition in subjects with locally advanced pancreatic cancer can be helpful.

19.6 Liver Cancer

Primary liver tumors are the sixth most commonly occurring cancer [312], and the most common type, comprising 90% of subjects, is hepatocellular carcinoma (HCC). The prognosis of primary liver tumors is very poor, with a 5-year survival rate ranging from 5% to 20% [128].

Secondary tumors of the liver are much more common than primary ones because the liver is a common organ for hematogenous metastatic spread. Tumors of the gastrointestinal system, especially colorectal cancers, are the main sources of liver metastases, though breast and lung cancers are also related to a high prevalence of liver spread.

Surgery is the main curative choice for most tumors, and earlier and more precise depiction may increase the likelihood of a timely intervention.

The outcomes of these cancers are related to the stage of the disease at diagnosis; larger cancers and metastatic disease have poorer outcomes. The staging of HCC is usually performed using a triple-phase contrast-enhanced CT scan or MRI of the abdominal region for local assessment, and metastatic work-up entails a bone scan and a chest CT scan.

HCC cells display different glucose receptor expressions, and thus, the uptake of FDG is variable [313, 314]. The sensitivity of FDG PET or PET/CT for the detection of primary HCC ranges from 50% to 65%, as observed in several studies [314–316]. Almost one-third of HCCs and most benign lesions do not show increased amounts of FDG and, therefore, cannot be reliably evaluated by PET/CT. Currently, PET/CT is not used in the screening of subjects who are at increased risk for HCC or in the assessment of focal liver lesions in the context of chronic hepatitis C, which can obscure trivial uptake in a malignant focus.

Gradually, FDG PET/CT has demonstrated that it can play a valuable role in the staging of liver cancers by identifying extrahepatic metastasis, thereby changing management planning.

Lin and colleagues [317] carried out a meta-analysis of eight investigations and demonstrated that FDG PET/CT assists in extrahepatic metastasis in patients with primary HCC, with a pooled sensitivity and specificity of 76.6% and 98%, respectively.

In addition, a few studies have assessed [318] its role as a biologic parameter and have noted that tumors with a higher density of glucose receptors tend to be aggressive; therefore, tumors which depict higher FDG uptake could demonstrate a disease with a bad biology [319–321].

Hybrid PET/MR imaging with hepatobiliary contrast agents and advanced MRI protocols that include dynamic contrast scans and diffusion weighted imaging could provide greater diagnostic value in terms of liver metastasis, as well as additive data for FDG non-avid lesions [322–328]. Sensitivity and negative predictive values of PET/MRI have been assessed to be 92.2% and 95.1%, respectively, which are greater than those of PET/CT (67.8% and 82.2%, respectively).

Non-FDG radiopharmaceuticals such as [11C]-acetate and [18F]-choline have been shown to have a high sensitivity for low-grade HCC, since uptake of these radiopharmaceuticals is associated with de novo lipid synthesis. As with FDG, these radiotracers also have a low sensitivity for small HCC, measuring less than 2 cm [329, 330].

Because primary liver tumors are described by an aggressive course, monitoring the disease is very important. A response assessment with FDG PET/CT is applied either by visual evaluation of the tumor site in the pre-therapy and post-therapy images in comparison with blood pool uptakes or by the measurement of the decrease of FDG uptake at the tumor site using different semiquantitative or quantitative techniques (e.g., the ratio of tumor SUV to the liver or mediastinum or SUV max). Several studies have reported better survival and event-free rates in subjects who reveal remarkable declines in uptakes at the tumor site [331, 332]. In comparison with conventional imaging modalities, such as CECT, FDG PET/CT demonstrated a greater sensitivity in identifying residual viable tissue, which is usually observed as a focal eccentric uptake on the periphery [333, 334].

The ideal time to evaluate response would be at 3 months post-therapy, allowing for posttreatment-related alterations, to avoid false-positive or equivocal results.

FDG PET/CT has been suggested for evaluating disease activity after nonoperative treatments such as transcatheter arterial chemoembolization or radiofrequency ablation [331, 335, 336]. FDG PET/CT for this issue should be done before the initiation of inflammatory changes, that is, within 6–12 h of the procedure, to preclude masking of the residual disease observed as a focal uptake on the periphery [337].

Besides, the early detection of local disease recurrence can suggest the need for salvage therapy, and thus, it is helpful to diagnose the extent of disease at restaging. FDG PET/CT has been revealed to be a useful mechanism to distinguish sites of local or distant recurrence when there is a clinical suspicion [338, 339]. A meta-analysis of eight reports demonstrated the pooled sensitivity and specificity of FDG PET (PET/CT) in the diagnosis of recurrent HCC to be 81.7% and 88.9%, respectively [317].

The FDG PET/CT modality plays a paramount role in the prognosis of subjects with HCC [299, 340–342]. Greater SUVs have been shown to be related to poor differentiations and worse prognoses [343, 344]. Also, PET is applied in pretransplant assessment in HCC, with high recurrence rates observed in cases with positive PET [345].

19.7 Conclusion

PET/CT is a valuable imaging modality that impacts the clinical management of patients with gastrointestinal, pancreas, and liver cancers and solves several challenges in this important field of oncology and facilitates the implementation of precision medicine, an emerging theme for future clinical practice.

Overall, PET/CT is most valuable in the evaluation of metastatic disease. It is most useful in patients suspected to have a metastatic disease and in patients with inconclusive findings on other imaging modalities. PET/CT generally does not outperform more conventional imaging modalities for the assessment of T status and the detection of lymph node involvement.

The role of PET/CT in the radiation treatment planning of gastrointestinal, pancreas, and liver cancers is evolving, but it could potentially improve tumor volume delineation, decrease geographic misses, and reduce treatment-related toxicities in some of the above tumors.

Likewise, there is good evidence supporting the ability of PET/CT in the areas of prognostication and response assessment in patients with gastrointestinal, pancreas, and liver cancers to assist in making precise therapy decisions and prognoses.

Furthermore, a growing body of evidence supports the use of hybrid PET/MRI imaging and alternative radiotracers in GI, pancreas, and liver cancers. Based on the initial clinical experience, PET/MR imaging has shown clinical utility in selected patients with GI, pancreas, and liver oncology for initial staging and for follow-up evaluations after treatment.

This overview provides insights into the usefulness of PET in gastrointestinal, pancreas, and liver oncology and how it can assist in providing optimal patient care.

References

1. Fitzmaurice C, Dicker D, Pain A, Hamavid H, Moradi-Lakeh M, MacIntyre MF, Allen C, Hansen G, Woodbrook R, Wolfe C, et al. The global burden of cancer. JAMA Oncol. 2013;1:505–27.
2. Rustgi AK, El-Serag HB. Esophageal carcinoma. N Engl J Med. 2014;371:2499–509.
3. Peery AF, Crockett SD, Barritt AS, Dellon ES, Eluri S, Gangarosa LM, Jensen ET, Lund JL, Pasricha S, Runge T, et al. Burden of gastrointestinal, liver, and pancreatic diseases in the United States. Gastroenterology. 2015;149:1731–41. e1733.
4. Korst RJ, Altorki NK. Imaging for esophageal tumors. Thorac Surg Clin. 2004;14:61–9.
5. Goel R, Subramaniam RM, Wachsmann JW. PET/computed tomography scanning and precision medicine: esophageal cancer. PET Clin. 2017;12:373–91.
6. Puli SR, Reddy JB, Bechtold ML, Antillon D, Ibdah JA, Antillon MR. Staging accuracy of esophageal cancer by endoscopic ultrasound: a meta-analysis and systematic review. World J Gastroenterol. 2008;14:1479–90.
7. Kato H, Miyazaki T, Nakajima M, Takita J, Kimura H, Faried A, Sohda M, Fukai Y, Masuda N, Fukuchi M, et al. The incremental effect of positron emission tomography on diagnostic accuracy in the initial staging of esophageal carcinoma. Cancer. 2005;103:148–56.
8. Muijs CT, Beukema JC, Pruim J, Mul VE, Groen H, Plukker JT, Langendijk JA. A systematic review on the role of FDG-PET/CT in tumour delineation and radiotherapy planning in patients with esophageal cancer. Radiother Oncol. 2010;97:165–71.
9. Flamen P. Positron emission tomography in gastric and esophageal cancer. Curr Opin Oncol. 2004;16:359–63.
10. Bruzzi JF, Truong MT, Marom EM, Mawlawi O, Podoloff DA, Macapinlac HA, Munden RF. Incidental findings on integrated PET/CT that do not accumulate 18F-FDG. AJR Am J Roentgenol. 2006;187:1116–23.
11. Shi W, Wang W, Wang J, Cheng H, Huo X. Meta-analysis of 18FDG PET-CT for nodal staging in patients with esophageal cancer. Surg Oncol. 2013;22:112–6.
12. Elsadek HM, Radwan MM. Diagnostic accuracy of mucosal biopsy versus endoscopic mucosal resection in Barrett's esophagus and related superficial lesions. Int Sch Res Notices. 2015;2015:735807.
13. Smyth EC, Shah MA. Role of (1)(8)F 2-fluoro-2-deoxyglucose positron emission tomography in upper gastrointestinal malignancies. World J Gastroenterol. 2011;17:5059–74.
14. Bruzzi JF, Munden RF, Truong MT, Marom EM, Sabloff BS, Gladish GW, Iyer RB, Pan TS, Macapinlac HA, Erasmus JJ. PET/CT of esophageal cancer: its role in clinical management. Radiographics. 2007;27:1635–52.
15. Heeren PA, Jager PL, Bongaerts F, van Dullemen H, Sluiter W, Plukker JT. Detection of distant metastases in esophageal cancer with (18)F-FDG PET. J Nucl Med. 2004;45:980–7.
16. Flanagan FL, Dehdashti F, Siegel BA, Trask DD, Sundaresan SR, Patterson GA, Cooper JD. Staging of esophageal cancer with 18F-fluorodeoxyglucose positron emission tomography. AJR Am J Roentgenol. 1997;168:417–24.
17. Alsop BR, Sharma P. Esophageal Cancer. Gastroenterol Clin N Am. 2016;45:399–412.
18. Varghese TK Jr, Hofstetter WL, Rizk NP, Low DE, Darling GE, Watson TJ, Mitchell JD, Krasna MJ. The society of thoracic surgeons guidelines on the diagnosis and staging of patients with esophageal cancer. Ann Thorac Surg. 2013;96:346–56.
19. Meyers BF, Downey RJ, Decker PA, Keenan RJ, Siegel BA, Cerfolio RJ, Landreneau RJ, Reed CE, Balfe DM, Dehdashti F, et al. The utility of positron emission tomography in staging of potentially operable carcinoma of the thoracic esophagus: results of the American College of Surgeons Oncology Group Z0060 trial. J Thorac Cardiovasc Surg. 2007;133:738–45.
20. van Westreenen HL, Westerterp M, Bossuyt PM, Pruim J, Sloof GW, van Lanschot JJ, Groen H, Plukker JT. Systematic review of the staging performance of 18F-fluorodeoxyglucose positron emission tomography in esophageal cancer. J Clin Oncol. 2004;22:3805–12.
21. Barber TW, Duong CP, Leong T, Bressel M, Drummond EG, Hicks RJ. 18F-FDG PET/CT has a high impact on patient management and provides powerful prognostic stratification in the primary staging of esophageal cancer: a prospective study with mature survival data. J Nucl Med. 2012;53:864–71.
22. Gillies RS, Middleton MR, Maynard ND, Bradley KM, Gleeson FV. Additional benefit of (1)(8) F-fluorodeoxyglucose integrated positron emission tomography/computed tomography in the staging of oesophageal cancer. Eur Radiol. 2011;21:274–80.
23. Duong CP, Demitriou H, Weih L, Thompson A, Williams D, Thomas RJ, Hicks RJ. Significant clinical impact and prognostic stratification provided by FDG-PET in the staging of oesophageal cancer. Eur J Nucl Med Mol Imaging. 2006;33:759–69.
24. Purandare NC, Pramesh CS, Karimundackal G, Jiwnani S, Agrawal A, Shah S, Kulkarni M, Laskar SG, Rangarajan V. Incremental value of 18F-FDG PET/CT in therapeutic decision-making of potentially curable esophageal adenocarcinoma. Nucl Med Commun. 2014;35:864–9.
25. Blencowe NS, Whistance RN, Strong S, Hotton EJ, Ganesh S, Roach H, Callaway M, Blazeby JM. Evaluating the role of fluorodeoxyglucose positron emission tomography-computed tomography in multi-disciplinary team recommendations for oesophago-gastric cancer. Br J Cancer. 2013;109:1445–50.

26. Foley KG, Lewis WG, Fielding P, Karran A, Chan D, Blake P, Roberts SA. N-staging of oesophageal and junctional carcinoma: is there still a role for EUS in patients staged N0 at PET/CT? Clin Radiol. 2014;69:959–64.
27. Pech O, May A, Manner H, Behrens A, Pohl J, Weferling M, Hartmann U, Manner N, Huijsmans J, Gossner L, et al. Long-term efficacy and safety of endoscopic resection for patients with mucosal adenocarcinoma of the esophagus. Gastroenterology. 2014;146:652–60. e651.
28. Moon SH, Kim HS, Hyun SH, Choi YS, Zo JI, Shim YM, Lee KH, Kim BT, Choi JY. Prediction of occult lymph node metastasis by metabolic parameters in patients with clinically N0 esophageal squamous cell carcinoma. J Nucl Med. 2014;55:743–8.
29. Blank S, Lordick F, Dobritz M, Grenacher L, Burian M, Langer R, Roth W, Schaible A, Becker K, Blaker H, et al. A reliable risk score for stage IV esophagogastric cancer. Eur J Surg Oncol. 2013;39:823–30.
30. Lordick F, Mariette C, Haustermans K, Obermannova R, Arnold D, Committee EG. Oesophageal cancer: ESMO clinical practice guidelines for diagnosis, treatment and follow-up. Ann Oncol. 2016;27:v50–7.
31. You JJ, Wong RK, Darling G, Gulenchyn K, Urbain JL, Evans WK. Clinical utility of 18F-fluorodeoxyglucose positron emission tomography/computed tomography in the staging of patients with potentially resectable esophageal cancer. J Thorac Oncol. 2013;8:1563–9.
32. van Westreenen HL, Westerterp M, Jager PL, van Dullemen HM, Sloof GW, Comans EF, van Lanschot JJ, Wiggers T, Plukker JT. Synchronous primary neoplasms detected on 18F-FDG PET in staging of patients with esophageal cancer. J Nucl Med. 2005;46:1321–5.
33. Han D, Yu J, Zhong X, Fu Z, Mu D, Zhang B, Xu G, Yang W, Zhao S. Comparison of the diagnostic value of 3-deoxy-3-18F-fluorothymidine and 18F-fluorodeoxyglucose positron emission tomography/computed tomography in the assessment of regional lymph node in thoracic esophageal squamous cell carcinoma: a pilot study. Dis Esophagus. 2012;25:416–26.
34. Mariette C, Balon JM, Piessen G, Fabre S, Van Seuningen I, Triboulet JP. Pattern of recurrence following complete resection of esophageal carcinoma and factors predictive of recurrent disease. Cancer. 2003;97:1616–23.
35. Flamen P, Lerut A, Van Cutsem E, Cambier JP, Maes A, De Wever W, Peeters M, De Leyn P, Van Raemdonck D, Mortelmans L. The utility of positron emission tomography for the diagnosis and staging of recurrent esophageal cancer. J Thorac Cardiovasc Surg. 2000;120:1085–92.
36. Cerfolio RJ, Bryant AS, Ohja B, Bartolucci AA, Eloubeidi MA. The accuracy of endoscopic ultrasonography with fine-needle aspiration, integrated positron emission tomography with computed tomography, and computed tomography in restaging patients with esophageal cancer after neoadjuvant chemoradiotherapy. J Thorac Cardiovasc Surg. 2005;129:1232–41.
37. Kim TJ, Kim HY, Lee KW, Kim MS. Multimodality assessment of esophageal cancer: preoperative staging and monitoring of response to therapy. Radiographics. 2009;29:403–21.
38. Bruzzi JF, Swisher SG, Truong MT, Munden RF, Hofstetter WL, Macapinlac HA, Correa AM, Mawlawi O, Ajani JA, Komaki RR, et al. Detection of interval distant metastases: clinical utility of integrated CT-PET imaging in patients with esophageal carcinoma after neoadjuvant therapy. Cancer. 2007;109:125–34.
39. Rizk N, Downey RJ, Akhurst T, Gonen M, Bains MS, Larson S, Rusch V. Preoperative 18[F]-fluorodeoxyglucose positron emission tomography standardized uptake values predict survival after esophageal adenocarcinoma resection. Ann Thorac Surg. 2006;81:1076–81.
40. Cerfolio RJ, Bryant AS. Maximum standardized uptake values on positron emission tomography of esophageal cancer predicts stage, tumor biology, and survival. Ann Thorac Surg. 2006;82:391–4; discussion 394–5.
41. Ott K, Weber WA, Lordick F, Becker K, Busch R, Herrmann K, Wieder H, Fink U, Schwaiger M, Siewert JR. Metabolic imaging predicts response, survival, and recurrence in adenocarcinomas of the esophagogastric junction. J Clin Oncol. 2006;24:4692–8.
42. Omloo JM, van Heijl M, Hoekstra OS, van Berge Henegouwen MI, van Lanschot JJ, Sloof GW. FDG-PET parameters as prognostic factor in esophageal cancer patients: a review. Ann Surg Oncol. 2011;18:3338–52.
43. Schreurs LM, Smit JK, Pavlov K, Pultrum BB, Pruim J, Groen H, Hollema H, Plukker JT. Prognostic impact of clinicopathological features and expression of biomarkers related to (18)F-FDG uptake in esophageal cancer. Ann Surg Oncol. 2014;21:3751–7.
44. Hsu PK, Lin KH, Wang SJ, Huang CS, Wu YC, Hsu WH. Preoperative positron emission tomography/computed tomography predicts advanced lymph node metastasis in esophageal squamous cell carcinoma patients. World J Surg. 2011;35:1321–6.
45. Choi JY, Jang HJ, Shim YM, Kim K, Lee KS, Lee KH, Choi Y, Choe YS, Kim BT. 18F-FDG PET in patients with esophageal squamous cell carcinoma undergoing curative surgery: prognostic implications. J Nucl Med. 2004;45:1843–50.
46. Atsumi K, Nakamura K, Abe K, Hirakawa M, Shioyama Y, Sasaki T, Baba S, Isoda T, Ohga S, Yoshitake T, et al. Prediction of outcome with FDG-PET in definitive chemoradiotherapy for esophageal cancer. J Radiat Res. 2013;54:890–8.
47. Zhao S, Kuge Y, Mochizuki T, Takahashi T, Nakada K, Sato M, Takei T, Tamaki N. Biologic correlates of intratumoral heterogeneity in 18F-FDG distribution with regional expression of glucose transporters and

hexokinase-II in experimental tumor. J Nucl Med. 2005;46:675–82.
48. Chicklore S, Goh V, Siddique M, Roy A, Marsden PK, Cook GJ. Quantifying tumour heterogeneity in 18F-FDG PET/CT imaging by texture analysis. Eur J Nucl Med Mol Imaging. 2013;40:133–40.
49. Tan S, Kligerman S, Chen W, Lu M, Kim G, Feigenberg S, D'Souza WD, Suntharalingam M, Lu W. Spatial-temporal [(1)(8)F]FDG-PET features for predicting pathologic response of esophageal cancer to neoadjuvant chemoradiation therapy. Int J Radiat Oncol Biol Phys. 2013;85:1375–82.
50. Zhang H, Tan S, Chen W, Kligerman S, Kim G, D'Souza WD, Suntharalingam M, Lu W. Modeling pathologic response of esophageal cancer to chemoradiation therapy using spatial-temporal 18F-FDG PET features, clinical parameters, and demographics. Int J Radiat Oncol Biol Phys. 2014;88:195–203.
51. Tixier F, Le Rest CC, Hatt M, Albarghach N, Pradier O, Metges JP, Corcos L, Visvikis D. Intratumor heterogeneity characterized by textural features on baseline 18F-FDG PET images predicts response to concomitant radiochemotherapy in esophageal cancer. J Nucl Med. 2011;52:369–78.
52. Li YM, Lin Q, Zhao L, Wang LC, Sun L, Dai MM, Luo ZM, Zheng H, Wu H. Pre-treatment metabolic tumor volume and total lesion glycolysis are useful prognostic factors for esophageal squamous cell cancer patients. Asian Pac J Cancer Prev. 2014;15:1369–73.
53. Krause BJ, Herrmann K, Wieder H, Zum Buschenfelde CM. 18F-FDG PET and 18F-FDG PET/CT for assessing response to therapy in esophageal cancer. J Nucl Med. 2009;50(Suppl 1):89S–96S.
54. Findlay JM, Bradley KM, Wang LM, Franklin JM, Teoh EJ, Gleeson FV, Maynard ND, Gillies RS, Middleton MR. Predicting pathologic response of esophageal cancer to neoadjuvant chemotherapy: the implications of metabolic nodal response for personalized therapy. J Nucl Med. 2017;58:266–75.
55. Choudhury PS, Gupta M. Personalized and precision medicine in cancer: a theragnostic approach. Curr Radiopharm. 2017;10(3):166–70.
56. Ghasemi M, Nabipour I, Omrani A, Alipour Z, Assadi M. Precision medicine and molecular imaging: new targeted approaches toward cancer therapeutic and diagnosis. Am J Nucl Med Mol Imaging. 2016;6:310–27.
57. Heger U, Bader F, Lordick F, Burian M, Langer R, Dobritz M, Blank S, Bruckner T, Becker K, Herrmann K, et al. Interim endoscopy results during neoadjuvant therapy for gastric cancer correlate with histopathological response and prognosis. Gastric Cancer. 2014;17:478–88.
58. Blank S, Lordick F, Bader F, Burian M, Dobritz M, Grenacher L, Becker K, Weichert W, Langer R, Sisic L, et al. Post-therapeutic response evaluation by a combination of endoscopy and CT scan in esophagogastric adenocarcinoma after chemotherapy: better than its reputation. Gastric Cancer. 2015;18:314–25.
59. Westerterp M, van Westreenen HL, Reitsma JB, Hoekstra OS, Stoker J, Fockens P, Jager PL, Van Eck-Smit BL, Plukker JT, van Lanschot JJ, Sloof GW. Esophageal cancer: CT, endoscopic US, and FDG PET for assessment of response to neoadjuvant therapy—systematic review. Radiology. 2005;236:841–51.
60. Tirkes T, Hollar MA, Tann M, Kohli MD, Akisik F, Sandrasegaran K. Response criteria in oncologic imaging: review of traditional and new criteria. Radiographics. 2013;33:1323–41.
61. Weber WA, Ott K, Becker K, Dittler HJ, Helmberger H, Avril NE, Meisetschlager G, Busch R, Siewert JR, Schwaiger M, Fink U. Prediction of response to preoperative chemotherapy in adenocarcinomas of the esophagogastric junction by metabolic imaging. J Clin Oncol. 2001;19:3058–65.
62. van Heijl M, Omloo JM, van Berge Henegouwen MI, Hoekstra OS, Boellaard R, Bossuyt PM, Busch OR, Tilanus HW, Hulshof MC, van der Gaast A, et al. Fluorodeoxyglucose positron emission tomography for evaluating early response during neoadjuvant chemoradiotherapy in patients with potentially curable esophageal cancer. Ann Surg. 2011;253:56–63.
63. Ilson DH, Minsky BD, Ku GY, Rusch V, Rizk N, Shah M, Kelsen DP, Capanu M, Tang L, Campbell J, Bains M. Phase 2 trial of induction and concurrent chemoradiotherapy with weekly irinotecan and cisplatin followed by surgery for esophageal cancer. Cancer. 2012;118:2820–7.
64. Wieder HA, Brucher BL, Zimmermann F, Becker K, Lordick F, Beer A, Schwaiger M, Fink U, Siewert JR, Stein HJ, Weber WA. Time course of tumor metabolic activity during chemoradiotherapy of esophageal squamous cell carcinoma and response to treatment. J Clin Oncol. 2004;22:900–8.
65. Schollaert P, Crott R, Bertrand C, D'Hondt L, Borght TV, Krug B. A systematic review of the predictive value of (18)FDG-PET in esophageal and esophagogastric junction cancer after neoadjuvant chemoradiation on the survival outcome stratification. J Gastrointest Surg. 2014;18:894–905.
66. Kwee RM. Prediction of tumor response to neoadjuvant therapy in patients with esophageal cancer with use of 18F FDG PET: a systematic review. Radiology. 2010;254:707–17.
67. Rebollo Aguirre AC, Ramos-Font C, Villegas Portero R, Cook GJ, Llamas Elvira JM, Tabares AR. 18F-fluorodeoxiglucose positron emission tomography for the evaluation of neoadjuvant therapy response in esophageal cancer: systematic review of the literature. Ann Surg. 2009;250:247–54.
68. Pan T, Mawlawi O, Nehmeh SA, Erdi YE, Luo D, Liu HH, Castillo R, Mohan R, Liao Z, Macapinlac HA. Attenuation correction of PET images with respiration-averaged CT images in PET/CT. J Nucl Med. 2005;46:1481–7.
69. Chao KS. Functional imaging for early prediction of response to chemoradiotherapy: 3′-deoxy-3′-18F-fluorothymidine positron emission tomography—a

clinical application model of esophageal cancer. Semin Oncol. 2006;33:S59–63.
70. Apisarnthanarax S, Alauddin MM, Mourtada F, Ariga H, Raju U, Mawlawi O, Han D, Bornmann WG, Ajani JA, Milas L, et al. Early detection of chemoradioresponse in esophageal carcinoma by 3′-deoxy-3′-3H-fluorothymidine using preclinical tumor models. Clin Cancer Res. 2006;12:4590–7.
71. Vrieze O, Haustermans K, De Wever W, Lerut T, Van Cutsem E, Ectors N, Hiele M, Flamen P. Is there a role for FGD-PET in radiotherapy planning in esophageal carcinoma? Radiother Oncol. 2004;73:269–75.
72. Leong T, Everitt C, Yuen K, Condron S, Hui A, Ngan SY, Pitman A, Lau EW, MacManus M, Binns D, et al. A prospective study to evaluate the impact of FDG-PET on CT-based radiotherapy treatment planning for oesophageal cancer. Radiother Oncol. 2006;78:254–61.
73. Konski A, Doss M, Milestone B, Haluszka O, Hanlon A, Freedman G, Adler L. The integration of 18-fluoro-deoxy-glucose positron emission tomography and endoscopic ultrasound in the treatment-planning process for esophageal carcinoma. Int J Radiat Oncol Biol Phys. 2005;61:1123–8.
74. Schreurs LM, Busz DM, Paardekooper GM, Beukema JC, Jager PL, Van der Jagt EJ, van Dam GM, Groen H, Plukker JT, Langendijk JA. Impact of 18-fluorodeoxyglucose positron emission tomography on computed tomography defined target volumes in radiation treatment planning of esophageal cancer: reduction in geographic misses with equal inter-observer variability: PET/CT improves esophageal target definition. Dis Esophagus. 2010;23:493–501.
75. Shimizu S, Hosokawa M, Itoh K, Fujita M, Takahashi H, Shirato H. Can hybrid FDG-PET/CT detect subclinical lymph node metastasis of esophageal cancer appropriately and contribute to radiation treatment planning? A comparison of image-based and pathological findings. Int J Clin Oncol. 2009;14:421–5.
76. MacManus M, Nestle U, Rosenzweig KE, Carrio I, Messa C, Belohlavek O, Danna M, Inoue T, Deniaud-Alexandre E, Schipani S, et al. Use of PET and PET/CT for radiation therapy planning: IAEA expert report 2006–2007. Radiother Oncol. 2009;91:85–94.
77. Schreurs LM, Pultrum BB, Koopmans KP, Verhoef CC, Jager PL, Van Dam GM, Groen H, Van Der Jagt EJ, Plukker JT. Better assessment of nodal metastases by PET/CT fusion compared to side-by-side PET/CT in oesophageal cancer. Anticancer Res. 2008;28:1867–73.
78. Vali FS, Nagda S, Hall W, Sinacore J, Gao M, Lee SH, Hong R, Shoup M, Emami B. Comparison of standardized uptake value-based positron emission tomography and computed tomography target volumes in esophageal cancer patients undergoing radiotherapy. Int J Radiat Oncol Biol Phys. 2010;78:1057–63.
79. Vesprini D, Ung Y, Dinniwell R, Breen S, Cheung F, Grabarz D, Kamra J, Mah K, Mansouri A, Pond G, et al. Improving observer variability in target delineation for gastro-oesophageal cancer—the role of (18F)fluoro-2-deoxy-D-glucose positron emission tomography/computed tomography. Clin Oncol (R Coll Radiol). 2008;20:631–8.
80. Tsai CJ, Das P. Impact of PET/CT-based radiation therapy planning in gastrointestinal malignancies. PET Clin. 2011;6:185–93.
81. Lozano R, Naghavi M, Foreman K, Lim S, Shibuya K, Aboyans V, Abraham J, Adair T, Aggarwal R, Ahn SY, et al. Global and regional mortality from 235 causes of death for 20 age groups in 1990 and 2010: a systematic analysis for the Global Burden of Disease Study 2010. Lancet. 2012;380:2095–128.
82. Chan AO, Wong BC, Lam SK. Gastric cancer: past, present and future. Can J Gastroenterol. 2001;15:469–74.
83. Malibari N, Hickeson M, Lisbona R. PET/computed tomography in the diagnosis and staging of gastric cancers. PET Clin. 2015;10:311–26.
84. Cheng XJ, Lin JC, Tu SP. Etiology and prevention of gastric cancer. Gastrointest Tumors. 2016;3:25–36.
85. Bordi C. Neuroendocrine pathology of the stomach: the parma contribution. Endocr Pathol. 2014;25:171–80.
86. Yeung HW, Macapinlac H, Karpeh M, Finn RD, Larson SM. Accuracy of FDG-PET in gastric cancer. Preliminary experience. Clin Positron Imaging. 1998;1:213–21.
87. Chen J, Cheong JH, Yun MJ, Kim J, Lim JS, Hyung WJ, Noh SH. Improvement in preoperative staging of gastric adenocarcinoma with positron emission tomography. Cancer. 2005;103:2383–90.
88. Mukai K, Ishida Y, Okajima K, Isozaki H, Morimoto T, Nishiyama S. Usefulness of preoperative FDG-PET for detection of gastric cancer. Gastric Cancer. 2006;9:192–6.
89. Kim EY, Lee WJ, Choi D, Lee SJ, Choi JY, Kim BT, Kim HS. The value of PET/CT for preoperative staging of advanced gastric cancer: comparison with contrast-enhanced CT. Eur J Radiol. 2011;79:183–8.
90. Yoshioka T, Yamaguchi K, Kubota K, Saginoya T, Yamazaki T, Ido T, Yamaura G, Takahashi H, Fukuda H, Kanamaru R. Evaluation of 18F-FDG PET in patients with advanced, metastatic, or recurrent gastric cancer. J Nucl Med. 2003;44:690–9.
91. Marcus C, Subramaniam RM. PET/computed tomography and precision medicine: gastric cancer. PET Clin. 2017;12:437–47.
92. Ajani JA, Bentrem DJ, Besh S, D'Amico TA, Das P, Denlinger C, Fakih MG, Fuchs CS, Gerdes H, Glasgow RE, et al. Gastric cancer, version 2.2013: featured updates to the NCCN guidelines. J Natl Compr Cancer Netw. 2013;11:531–46.
93. Dassen AE, Lips DJ, Hoekstra CJ, Pruijt JF, Bosscha K. FDG-PET has no definite role in preoperative imaging in gastric cancer. Eur J Surg Oncol. 2009;35:449–55.
94. Ha TK, Choi YY, Song SY, Kwon SJ. F18-fluorodeoxyglucose-positron emission tomography

and computed tomography is not accurate in preoperative staging of gastric cancer. J Korean Surg Soc. 2011;81:104–10.
95. Kawanaka Y, Kitajima K, Fukushima K, Mouri M, Doi H, Oshima T, Niwa H, Kaibe N, Sasako M, Tomita T, et al. Added value of pretreatment (18) F-FDG PET/CT for staging of advanced gastric cancer: comparison with contrast-enhanced MDCT. Eur J Radiol. 2016;85:989–95.
96. Altini C, Niccoli Asabella A, Di Palo A, Fanelli M, Ferrari C, Moschetta M, Rubini G. 18F-FDG PET/CT role in staging of gastric carcinomas: comparison with conventional contrast enhancement computed tomography. Medicine. 2015;94:e864.
97. Filik M, Kir KM, Aksel B, Soyda C, Ozkan E, Kucuk ON, Ibis E, Akgul H. The role of 18F-FDG PET/CT in the primary staging of gastric cancer. Mol Imaging Radionucl Ther. 2015;24:15–20.
98. Park K, Jang G, Baek S, Song H. Usefulness of combined PET/CT to assess regional lymph node involvement in gastric cancer. Tumori. 2014;100:201–6.
99. Namikawa T, Okabayshi T, Nogami M, Ogawa Y, Kobayashi M, Hanazaki K. Assessment of (18) F-fluorodeoxyglucose positron emission tomography combined with computed tomography in the preoperative management of patients with gastric cancer. Int J Clin Oncol. 2014;19:649–55.
100. Kim DW, Park SA, Kim CG. Detecting the recurrence of gastric cancer after curative resection: comparison of FDG PET/CT and contrast-enhanced abdominal CT. J Korean Med Sci. 2011;26:875–80.
101. Yang QM, Kawamura T, Itoh H, Bando E, Nemoto M, Akamoto S, Furukawa H, Yonemura Y. Is PET-CT suitable for predicting lymph node status for gastric cancer? Hepato-Gastroenterology. 2008;55:782–5.
102. Choi BW, Kim HW, Won KS, Song BI, Cho KB, Bae SU. Diagnostic accuracy of 18F-FDG PET/CT for detecting synchronous advanced colorectal neoplasia in patients with gastric cancer. Medicine. 2016;95:e4741.
103. Kinkel K, Lu Y, Both M, Warren RS, Thoeni RF. Detection of hepatic metastases from cancers of the gastrointestinal tract by using noninvasive imaging methods (US, CT, MR imaging, PET): a meta-analysis. Radiology. 2002;224:748–56.
104. Herrmann K, Ott K, Buck AK, Lordick F, Wilhelm D, Souvatzoglou M, Becker K, Schuster T, Wester HJ, Siewert JR, et al. Imaging gastric cancer with PET and the radiotracers 18F-FLT and 18F-FDG: a comparative analysis. J Nucl Med. 2007;48:1945–50.
105. Staniuk T, Malkowski B, Srutek E, Szlezak P, Zegarski W. Comparison of FLT-PET/CT and CECT in gastric cancer diagnosis. Abdom Radiol (NY). 2016;41:1349–56.
106. Staniuk T, Zegarski W, Malkowski B, Jankowski M, Klag M, Pietrzak T. Evaluation of FLT-PET/CT usefulness in diagnosis and qualification for surgical treatment of gastric cancer. Contemp Oncol (Pozn). 2013;17:165–70.
107. Roukos DH. Extended (D2) lymph node dissection for gastric cancer: do patients benefit? Ann Surg Oncol. 2000;7:253–5.
108. Lehnert T, Rudek B, Buhl K, Golling M. Surgical therapy for loco-regional recurrence and distant metastasis of gastric cancer. Eur J Surg Oncol. 2002;28:455–61.
109. Wanebo HJ, Kennedy BJ, Chmiel J, Steele G Jr, Winchester D, Osteen R. Cancer of the stomach. A patient care study by the American College of Surgeons. Ann Surg. 1993;218:583–92.
110. Shreve PD, Anzai Y, Wahl RL. Pitfalls in oncologic diagnosis with FDG PET imaging: physiologic and benign variants. Radiographics. 1999;19:61–77; quiz 150–1.
111. Li P, Liu Q, Wang C, Wang T, Liu J, Huang G, Song S. Fluorine-18-fluorodeoxyglucose positron emission tomography to evaluate recurrent gastric cancer after surgical resection: a systematic review and meta-analysis. Ann Nucl Med. 2016;30:179–87.
112. Lee JW, Lee SM, Son MW, Lee MS. Diagnostic performance of FDG PET/CT for surveillance in asymptomatic gastric cancer patients after curative surgical resection. Eur J Nucl Med Mol Imaging. 2016;43:881–8.
113. Cayvarli H, Bekis R, Akman T, Altun D. The role of 18F-FDG PET/CT in the evaluation of gastric cancer recurrence. Mol Imaging Radionucl Ther. 2014;23:76–83.
114. Zou H, Zhao Y. 18FDG PET-CT for detecting gastric cancer recurrence after surgical resection: a meta-analysis. Surg Oncol. 2013;22:162–6.
115. Lee JE, Hong SP, Ahn DH, Jeon TJ, Kang MK, Kwon CI, Ko KH, Hwang SG, Park PW, Rim KS. The role of 18F-FDG PET/CT in the evaluation of gastric cancer recurrence after curative gastrectomy. Yonsei Med J. 2011;52:81–8.
116. Sim SH, Kim YJ, Oh DY, Lee SH, Kim DW, Kang WJ, Im SA, Kim TY, Kim WH, Heo DS, Bang YJ. The role of PET/CT in detection of gastric cancer recurrence. BMC Cancer. 2009;9:73.
117. Nakamoto Y, Togashi K, Kaneta T, Fukuda H, Nakajima K, Kitajima K, Murakami K, Fujii H, Satake M, Tateishi U, et al. Clinical value of whole-body FDG-PET for recurrent gastric cancer: a multicenter study. Jpn J Clin Oncol. 2009;39:297–302.
118. Park MJ, Lee WJ, Lim HK, Park KW, Choi JY, Kim BT. Detecting recurrence of gastric cancer: the value of FDG PET/CT. Abdom Imaging. 2009;34:441–7.
119. Kim SJ, Cho YS, Moon SH, Bae JM, Kim S, Choe YS, Kim BT, Lee KH. Primary tumor (1)(8)F-FDG avidity affects the performance of (1)(8)F-FDG PET/CT for detecting gastric cancer recurrence. J Nucl Med. 2016;57:544–50.
120. Lee JW, Lee SM, Lee MS, Shin HC. Role of (1)(8) F-FDG PET/CT in the prediction of gastric cancer recurrence after curative surgical resection. Eur J Nucl Med Mol Imaging. 2012;39:1425–34.
121. Kim J, Lim ST, Na CJ, Han YH, Kim CY, Jeong HJ, Sohn MH. Pretreatment F-18 FDG PET/CT param-

eters to evaluate progression-free survival in gastric cancer. Nucl Med Mol Imaging. 2014;48:33–40.
122. Park JC, Lee JH, Cheoi K, Chung H, Yun MJ, Lee H, Shin SK, Lee SK, Lee YC. Predictive value of pretreatment metabolic activity measured by fluorodeoxyglucose positron emission tomography in patients with metastatic advanced gastric cancer: the maximal SUV of the stomach is a prognostic factor. Eur J Nucl Med Mol Imaging. 2012;39:1107–16.
123. Na SJ, O JH, Park JM, Lee HH, Lee SH, Song KY, Choi MG, Park CH. Prognostic value of metabolic parameters on preoperative 18F-fluorodeoxyglucose positron emission tomography/computed tomography in patients with stage III gastric cancer. Oncotarget. 2016;7:63968–80.
124. Song BI, Kim HW, Won KS, Ryu SW, Sohn SS, Kang YN. Preoperative standardized uptake value of metastatic lymph nodes measured by 18F-FDG PET/CT improves the prediction of prognosis in gastric cancer. Medicine. 2015;94:e1037.
125. Couper GW, McAteer D, Wallis F, Norton M, Welch A, Nicolson M, Park KG. Detection of response to chemotherapy using positron emission tomography in patients with oesophageal and gastric cancer. Br J Surg. 1998;85:1403–6.
126. Ferri LE, Ades S, Alcindor T, Chasen M, Marcus V, Hickeson M, Artho G, Thirlwell MP. Perioperative docetaxel, cisplatin, and 5-fluorouracil (DCF) for locally advanced esophageal and gastric adenocarcinoma: a multicenter phase II trial. Ann Oncol. 2012;23:1512–7.
127. Ott K, Herrmann K, Krause BJ, Lordick F. The value of PET imaging in patients with localized gastroesophageal cancer. Gastrointest Cancer Res. 2008;2:287–94.
128. Donswijk ML, Hess S, Mulders T. Lam MG: [18F]fluorodeoxyglucose PET/computed tomography in gastrointestinal malignancies. PET Clin. 2014;9:421–41, v–vi.
129. Kameyama R, Yamamoto Y, Izuishi K, Takebayashi R, Hagiike M, Murota M, Kaji M, Haba R, Nishiyama Y. Detection of gastric cancer using 18F-FLT PET: comparison with 18F-FDG PET. Eur J Nucl Med Mol Imaging. 2009;36:382–8.
130. Burkill GJ, Badran M, Al-Muderis O, Meirion Thomas J, Judson IR, Fisher C, Moskovic EC. Malignant gastrointestinal stromal tumor: distribution, imaging features, and pattern of metastatic spread. Radiology. 2003;226:527–32.
131. Ghanem N, Altehoefer C, Furtwangler A, Winterer J, Schafer O, Springer O, Kotter E, Langer M. Computed tomography in gastrointestinal stromal tumors. Eur Radiol. 2003;13:1669–78.
132. Treglia G, Mirk P, Stefanelli A, Rufini V, Giordano A, Bonomo L. 18F-Fluorodeoxyglucose positron emission tomography in evaluating treatment response to imatinib or other drugs in gastrointestinal stromal tumors: a systematic review. Clin Imaging. 2012;36:167–75.
133. Joensuu H, Roberts PJ, Sarlomo-Rikala M, Andersson LC, Tervahartiala P, Tuveson D, Silberman S, Capdeville R, Dimitrijevic S, Druker B, Demetri GD. Effect of the tyrosine kinase inhibitor STI571 in a patient with a metastatic gastrointestinal stromal tumor. N Engl J Med. 2001;344:1052–6.
134. Tuveson DA, Willis NA, Jacks T, Griffin JD, Singer S, Fletcher CD, Fletcher JA, Demetri GD. STI571 inactivation of the gastrointestinal stromal tumor c-KIT oncoprotein: biological and clinical implications. Oncogene. 2001;20:5054–8.
135. Demetri GD, van Oosterom AT, Garrett CR, Blackstein ME, Shah MH, Verweij J, McArthur G, Judson IR, Heinrich MC, Morgan JA, et al. Efficacy and safety of sunitinib in patients with advanced gastrointestinal stromal tumour after failure of imatinib: a randomised controlled trial. Lancet. 2006;368:1329–38.
136. Kamiyama Y, Aihara R, Nakabayashi T, Mochiki E, Asao T, Kuwano H, Oriuchi N, Endo K. 18F-fluorodeoxyglucose positron emission tomography: useful technique for predicting malignant potential of gastrointestinal stromal tumors. World J Surg. 2005;29:1429–35.
137. Goerres GW, Stupp R, Barghouth G, Hany TF, Pestalozzi B, Dizendorf E, Schnyder P, Luthi F, von Schulthess GK, Leyvraz S. The value of PET, CT and in-line PET/CT in patients with gastrointestinal stromal tumours: long-term outcome of treatment with imatinib mesylate. Eur J Nucl Med Mol Imaging. 2005;32:153–62.
138. Deng SM, Zhang W, Zhang B, Chen YY, Li JH, Wu YW. Correlation between the uptake of 18F-fluorodeoxyglucose (18F-FDG) and the expression of proliferation-associated antigen Ki-67 in cancer patients: a meta-analysis. PLoS One. 2015;10:e0129028.
139. Yamada M, Niwa Y, Matsuura T, Miyahara R, Ohashi A, Maeda O, Ando T, Ohmiya N, Itoh A, Hirooka Y, Goto H. Gastric GIST malignancy evaluated by 18FDG-PET as compared with EUS-FNA and endoscopic biopsy. Scand J Gastroenterol. 2007;42:633–41.
140. van Oosterom AT, Judson I, Verweij J, Stroobants S, Donato di Paola E, Dimitrijevic S, Martens M, Webb A, Sciot R, Van Glabbeke M, et al. Safety and efficacy of imatinib (STI571) in metastatic gastrointestinal stromal tumours: a phase I study. Lancet. 2001;358:1421–3.
141. Zukotynski K, Yap JT, Giobbie-Hurder A, Weber J, Gonzalez R, Gajewski TF, O'Day S, Kim K, Hodi FS, Van den Abbeele AD. Metabolic response by FDG-PET to imatinib correlates with exon 11 KIT mutation and predicts outcome in patients with mucosal melanoma. Cancer Imaging. 2014;14:30.
142. van Oosterom AT, Judson IR, Verweij J, Stroobants S, Dumez H, Donato di Paola E, Sciot R, Van Glabbeke M, Dimitrijevic S, Nielsen OS, et al. Update of phase I study of imatinib (STI571) in advanced soft tissue sarcomas and gastrointestinal stromal tumors: a

report of the EORTC Soft Tissue and Bone Sarcoma Group. Eur J Cancer. 2002;38(Suppl 5):S83–7.

143. Chen MY, Bechtold RE, Savage PD. Cystic changes in hepatic metastases from gastrointestinal stromal tumors (GISTs) treated with Gleevec (imatinib mesylate). AJR Am J Roentgenol. 2002;179:1059–62.
144. Gayed I, Vu T, Iyer R, Johnson M, Macapinlac H, Swanston N, Podoloff D. The role of 18F-FDG PET in staging and early prediction of response to therapy of recurrent gastrointestinal stromal tumors. J Nucl Med. 2004;45:17–21.
145. Basu S, Mohandas KM, Peshwe H, Asopa R, Vyawahare M. FDG-PET and PET/CT in the clinical management of gastrointestinal stromal tumor. Nucl Med Commun. 2008;29:1026–39.
146. Demetri GD, von Mehren M, Blanke CD, Van den Abbeele AD, Eisenberg B, Roberts PJ, Heinrich MC, Tuveson DA, Singer S, Janicek M, et al. Efficacy and safety of imatinib mesylate in advanced gastrointestinal stromal tumors. N Engl J Med. 2002;347:472–80.
147. Stroobants S, Goeminne J, Seegers M, Dimitrijevic S, Dupont P, Nuyts J, Martens M, van den Borne B, Cole P, Sciot R, et al. 18FDG-Positron emission tomography for the early prediction of response in advanced soft tissue sarcoma treated with imatinib mesylate (Glivec). Eur J Cancer. 2003;39:2012–20.
148. Choi H, Charnsangavej C, de Castro FS, Tamm EP, Benjamin RS, Johnson MM, Macapinlac HA, Podoloff DA. CT evaluation of the response of gastrointestinal stromal tumors after imatinib mesylate treatment: a quantitative analysis correlated with FDG PET findings. AJR Am J Roentgenol. 2004;183:1619–28.
149. Prior JO, Montemurro M, Orcurto MV, Michielin O, Luthi F, Benhattar J, Guillou L, Elsig V, Stupp R, Delaloye AB, Leyvraz S. Early prediction of response to sunitinib after imatinib failure by 18F-fluorodeoxyglucose positron emission tomography in patients with gastrointestinal stromal tumor. J Clin Oncol. 2009;27:439–45.
150. Benjamin RS, Schoffski P, Hartmann JT, Van Oosterom A, Bui BN, Duyster J, Schuetze S, Blay JY, Reichardt P, Rosen LS, et al. Efficacy and safety of motesanib, an oral inhibitor of VEGF, PDGF, and Kit receptors, in patients with imatinib-resistant gastrointestinal stromal tumors. Cancer Chemother Pharmacol. 2011;68:69–77.
151. Choi H, Charnsangavej C, Faria SC, Macapinlac HA, Burgess MA, Patel SR, Chen LL, Podoloff DA, Benjamin RS. Correlation of computed tomography and positron emission tomography in patients with metastatic gastrointestinal stromal tumor treated at a single institution with imatinib mesylate: proposal of new computed tomography response criteria. J Clin Oncol. 2007;25:1753–9.
152. Jager PL, Gietema JA, van der Graaf WT. Imatinib mesylate for the treatment of gastrointestinal stromal tumours: best monitored with FDG PET. Nucl Med Commun. 2004;25:433–8.
153. Heinicke T, Wardelmann E, Sauerbruch T, Tschampa HJ, Glasmacher A, Palmedo H. Very early detection of response to imatinib mesylate therapy of gastrointestinal stromal tumours using 18fluoro-deoxyglucose-positron emission tomography. Anticancer Res. 2005;25:4591–4.
154. Grimpen F, Yip D, McArthur G, Waring P, Goldstein D, Loughrey M, Beshay V, Chong G. Resistance to imatinib, low-grade FDG-avidity on PET, and acquired KIT exon 17 mutation in gastrointestinal stromal tumour. Lancet Oncol. 2005;6:724–7.
155. Van den Abbeele AD. The lessons of GIST—PET and PET/CT: a new paradigm for imaging. Oncologist. 2008;13(Suppl 2):8–13.
156. Maffione AM, Marzola MC, Capirci C, Colletti PM, Rubello D. Value of (18)F-FDG PET for predicting response to neoadjuvant therapy in rectal cancer: systematic review and meta-analysis. AJR Am J Roentgenol. 2015;204:1261–8.
157. Pickhardt PJ, Hassan C, Halligan S, Marmo R. Colorectal cancer: CT colonography and colonoscopy for detection—systematic review and meta-analysis. Radiology. 2011;259:393–405.
158. Peng J, He Y, Xu J, Sheng J, Cai S, Zhang Z. Detection of incidental colorectal tumours with 18F-labelled 2-fluoro-2-deoxyglucose positron emission tomography/computed tomography scans: results of a prospective study. Color Dis. 2011;13:e374–8.
159. Furukawa H, Ikuma H, Seki A, Yokoe K, Yuen S, Aramaki T, Yamagushi S. Positron emission tomography scanning is not superior to whole body multidetector helical computed tomography in the preoperative staging of colorectal cancer. Gut. 2006;55:1007–11.
160. Petersen RK, Hess S, Alavi A, Hoilund-Carlsen PF. Clinical impact of FDG-PET/CT on colorectal cancer staging and treatment strategy. Am J Nucl Med Mol Imaging. 2014;4:471–82.
161. Davey K, Heriot AG, Mackay J, Drummond E, Hogg A, Ngan S, Milner AD, Hicks RJ. The impact of 18-fluorodeoxyglucose positron emission tomography-computed tomography on the staging and management of primary rectal cancer. Dis Colon Rectum. 2008;51:997–1003.
162. Gearhart SL, Frassica D, Rosen R, Choti M, Schulick R, Wahl R. Improved staging with pretreatment positron emission tomography/computed tomography in low rectal cancer. Ann Surg Oncol. 2006;13:397–404.
163. Lee JE, Kim SW, Kim JS, Choi KY, Kang WK, Oh ST, Yoo Ie R, Kim SH. Prognostic value of 18-fluorodeoxyglucose positron emission tomography-computed tomography in resectable colorectal cancer. World J Gastroenterol. 2012;18:5072–7.
164. Brush J, Boyd K, Chappell F, Crawford F, Dozier M, Fenwick E, Glanville J, McIntosh H, Renehan A, Weller D, Dunlop M. The value of FDG positron

emission tomography/computerised tomography (PET/CT) in pre-operative staging of colorectal cancer: a systematic review and economic evaluation. Health Technol Assess. 2011;15:1–192, iii–iv.
165. Lu YY, Chen JH, Ding HJ, Chien CR, Lin WY, Kao CH. A systematic review and meta-analysis of pretherapeutic lymph node staging of colorectal cancer by 18F-FDG PET or PET/CT. Nucl Med Commun. 2012;33:1127–33.
166. Agarwal A, Marcus C, Xiao J, Nene P, Kachnic LA, Subramaniam RM. FDG PET/CT in the management of colorectal and anal cancers. AJR Am J Roentgenol. 2014;203:1109–19.
167. Niekel MC, Bipat S, Stoker J. Diagnostic imaging of colorectal liver metastases with CT, MR imaging, FDG PET, and/or FDG PET/CT: a meta-analysis of prospective studies including patients who have not previously undergone treatment. Radiology. 2010;257:674–84.
168. Laurens ST, Oyen WJ. Impact of fluorodeoxyglucose PET/computed tomography on the management of patients with colorectal cancer. PET Clin. 2015;10:345–60.
169. Schmoll HJ, Van Cutsem E, Stein A, Valentini V, Glimelius B, Haustermans K, Nordlinger B, van de Velde CJ, Balmana J, Regula J, et al. ESMO consensus guidelines for management of patients with colon and rectal cancer. a personalized approach to clinical decision making. Ann Oncol. 2012;23:2479–516.
170. Selzner M, Hany TF, Wildbrett P, McCormack L, Kadry Z, Clavien PA. Does the novel PET/CT imaging modality impact on the treatment of patients with metastatic colorectal cancer of the liver? Ann Surg. 2004;240:1027–34; discussion 1026–35.
171. Kochhar R, Liong S, Manoharan P. The role of FDG PET/CT in patients with colorectal cancer metastases. Cancer Biomark. 2010;7:235–48.
172. Lake ES, Wadhwani S, Subar D, Kauser A, Harris C, Chang D, Lapsia S. The influence of FDG PET-CT on the detection of extrahepatic disease in patients being considered for resection of colorectal liver metastasis. Ann R Coll Surg Engl. 2014;96:211–5.
173. Georgakopoulos A, Pianou N, Kelekis N, Chatziioannou S. Impact of 18F-FDG PET/CT on therapeutic decisions in patients with colorectal cancer and liver metastases. Clin Imaging. 2013;37:536–41.
174. Engledow AH, Skipworth JR, Pakzad F, Imber C, Ell PJ, Groves AM. The role of 18FDG PET/CT in the management of colorectal liver metastases. HPB (Oxford). 2012;14:20–5.
175. McLeish AR, Lee ST, Byrne AJ, Scott AM. Impact of (1)(8)F-FDG-PET in decision making for liver metastectomy of colorectal cancer. ANZ J Surg. 2012;82:30–5.
176. Ramos E, Valls C, Martinez L, Llado L, Torras J, Ruiz S, Gamez C, Serrano T, Fabregat J, Rafecas A. Preoperative staging of patients with liver metastases of colorectal carcinoma. Does PET/CT really add something to multidetector CT? Ann Surg Oncol. 2011;18:2654–61.
177. Briggs RH, Chowdhury FU, Lodge JP, Scarsbrook AF. Clinical impact of FDG PET-CT in patients with potentially operable metastatic colorectal cancer. Clin Radiol. 2011;66:1167–74.
178. Chua SC, Groves AM, Kayani I, Menezes L, Gacinovic S, Du Y, Bomanji JB, Ell PJ. The impact of 18F-FDG PET/CT in patients with liver metastases. Eur J Nucl Med Mol Imaging. 2007;34:1906–14.
179. Sorensen M, Mortensen FV, Hoyer M, Vilstrup H, Keiding S, Liver Tumour Board at Aarhus University H. FDG-PET improves management of patients with colorectal liver metastases allocated for local treatment: a consecutive prospective study. Scand J Surg. 2007;96:209–13.
180. Joyce DL, Wahl RL, Patel PV, Schulick RD, Gearhart SL, Choti MA. Preoperative positron emission tomography to evaluate potentially resectable hepatic colorectal metastases. Arch Surg. 2006;141:1220–6; discussion 1227.
181. Arulampalam TH, Francis DL, Visvikis D, Taylor I, Ell PJ. FDG-PET for the pre-operative evaluation of colorectal liver metastases. Eur J Surg Oncol. 2004;30:286–91.
182. Teague BD, Morrison CP, Court FG, Chin VT, Costello SP, Kirkwood ID, Maddern GJ. Role of FDG-PET in surgical management of patients with colorectal liver metastases. ANZ J Surg. 2004;74:646–52.
183. Ruers TJ, Langenhoff BS, Neeleman N, Jager GJ, Strijk S, Wobbes T, Corstens FH, Oyen WJ. Value of positron emission tomography with [F-18]fluorodeoxyglucose in patients with colorectal liver metastases: a prospective study. J Clin Oncol. 2002;20:388–95.
184. Frankel TL, Gian RK, Jarnagin WR. Preoperative imaging for hepatic resection of colorectal cancer metastasis. J Gastrointest Oncol. 2012;3:11–8.
185. Seo HJ, Kim MJ, Lee JD, Chung WS, Kim YE. Gadoxetate disodium-enhanced magnetic resonance imaging versus contrast-enhanced 18F-fluorodeoxyglucose positron emission tomography/computed tomography for the detection of colorectal liver metastases. Investig Radiol. 2011;46:548–55.
186. Donati OF, Reiner CS, Hany TF, Fornaro J, von Schulthess GK, Marincek B, Weishaupt D. 18F-FDG-PET and MRI in patients with malignancies of the liver and pancreas. Accuracy of retrospective multimodality image registration by using the CT-component of PET/CT. Nuklearmedizin. 2010;49:106–14.
187. Paspulati RM, Gupta A. PET/MR imaging in cancers of the gastrointestinal tract. PET Clin. 2016;11:403–23.
188. O'Neill BD, Brown G, Heald RJ, Cunningham D, Tait DM. Non-operative treatment after neoadjuvant chemoradiotherapy for rectal cancer. Lancet Oncol. 2007;8:625–33.

189. Dewhurst CE, Mortele KJ. Magnetic resonance imaging of rectal cancer. Radiol Clin N Am. 2013;51:121–31.
190. Paspulati RM, Partovi S, Herrmann KA, Krishnamurthi S, Delaney CP, Nguyen NC. Comparison of hybrid FDG PET/MRI compared with PET/CT in colorectal cancer staging and restaging: a pilot study. Abdom Imaging. 2015;40:1415–25.
191. Sassen S, de Booij M, Sosef M, Berendsen R, Lammering G, Clarijs R, Bakker M, Beets-Tan R, Warmerdam F, Vliegen R. Locally advanced rectal cancer: is diffusion weighted MRI helpful for the identification of complete responders (ypT0N0) after neoadjuvant chemoradiation therapy? Eur Radiol. 2013;23:3440–9.
192. Joye I, Deroose CM, Vandecaveye V, Haustermans K. The role of diffusion-weighted MRI and (18) F-FDG PET/CT in the prediction of pathologic complete response after radiochemotherapy for rectal cancer: a systematic review. Radiother Oncol. 2014;113:158–65.
193. Song I, Kim SH, Lee SJ, Choi JY, Kim MJ, Rhim H. Value of diffusion-weighted imaging in the detection of viable tumour after neoadjuvant chemoradiation therapy in patients with locally advanced rectal cancer: comparison with T2 weighted and PET/CT imaging. Br J Radiol. 2012;85:577–86.
194. Kwon HW, Becker AK, Goo JM, Cheon GJ. FDG whole-body PET/MRI in oncology: a systematic review. Nucl Med Mol Imaging. 2017;51:22–31.
195. Brendle C, Schwenzer NF, Rempp H, Schmidt H, Pfannenberg C, la Fougere C, Nikolaou K, Schraml C. Assessment of metastatic colorectal cancer with hybrid imaging: comparison of reading performance using different combinations of anatomical and functional imaging techniques in PET/MRI and PET/CT in a short case series. Eur J Nucl Med Mol Imaging. 2016;43:123–32.
196. de Jong EA, ten Berge JC, Dwarkasing RS, Rijkers AP, van Eijck CH. The accuracy of MRI, endorectal ultrasonography, and computed tomography in predicting the response of locally advanced rectal cancer after preoperative therapy: a metaanalysis. Surgery. 2016;159:688–99.
197. Wu LM, Zhu J, Hu J, Yin Y, Gu HY, Hua J, Chen J, Xu JR. Is there a benefit in using magnetic resonance imaging in the prediction of preoperative neoadjuvant therapy response in locally advanced rectal cancer? Int J Color Dis. 2013;28:1225–38.
198. Memon S, Lynch AC, Bressel M, Wise AG, Heriot AG. Systematic review and meta-analysis of the accuracy of MRI and endorectal ultrasound in the restaging and response assessment of rectal cancer following neoadjuvant therapy. Color Dis. 2015;17:748–61.
199. Li YL, Wu LM, Chen XX, Delproposto Z, Hu JN, Xu JR. Is diffusion-weighted MRI superior to FDG-PET or FDG-PET/CT in evaluating and predicting pathological response to preoperative neoadjuvant therapy in patients with rectal cancer? J Dig Dis. 2014;15:525–37.
200. Rymer B, Curtis NJ, Siddiqui MR, Chand M. FDG PET/CT can assess the response of locally advanced rectal cancer to neoadjuvant chemoradiotherapy: svidence From meta-analysis and systematic review. Clin Nucl Med. 2016;41:371–5.
201. Memon S, Lynch AC, Akhurst T, Ngan SY, Warrier SK, Michael M, Heriot AG. Systematic review of FDG-PET prediction of complete pathological response and survival in rectal cancer. Ann Surg Oncol. 2014;21:3598–607.
202. Jadvar H, Colletti P, Delgado-Bolton R, Esposito G, Krause B, Iagaru A, Nadel H, Quinn D, Rohren E, Subramaniam R, et al Appropriate use criteria for 18F-FDG PET/CT in restaging and treatment response assessment of malignant disease. J Nucl Med 2017 58(12):2026-2037.
203. Turk PS, Wanebo HJ. Results of surgical treatment of nonhepatic recurrence of colorectal carcinoma. Cancer. 1993;71:4267–77.
204. Hayashi M, Inoue Y, Komeda K, Shimizu T, Asakuma M, Hirokawa F, Miyamoto Y, Okuda J, Takeshita A, Shibayama Y, Tanigawa N. Clinicopathological analysis of recurrence patterns and prognostic factors for survival after hepatectomy for colorectal liver metastasis. BMC Surg. 2010;10:27.
205. Muratore A, Zorzi D, Bouzari H, Amisano M, Massucco P, Sperti E, Capussotti L. Asymptomatic colorectal cancer with un-resectable liver metastases: immediate colorectal resection or up-front systemic chemotherapy? Ann Surg Oncol. 2007;14:766–70.
206. Foster JH. Treatment of metastatic disease of the liver: a skeptic's view. Semin Liver Dis. 1984;4:170–9.
207. Tsai MS, Su YH, Ho MC, Liang JT, Chen TP, Lai HS, Lee PH. Clinicopathological features and prognosis in resectable synchronous and metachronous colorectal liver metastasis. Ann Surg Oncol. 2007;14:786–94.
208. Huebner RH, Park KC, Shepherd JE, Schwimmer J, Czernin J, Phelps ME, Gambhir SS. A meta-analysis of the literature for whole-body FDG PET detection of recurrent colorectal cancer. J Nucl Med. 2000;41:1177–89.
209. Zhang C, Chen Y, Xue H, Zheng P, Tong J, Liu J, Sun X, Huang G. Diagnostic value of FDG-PET in recurrent colorectal carcinoma: a meta-analysis. Int J Cancer. 2009;124:167–73.
210. Yu T, Meng N, Chi D, Zhao Y, Wang K, Luo Y. Diagnostic value of (18)F-FDG PET/CT in detecting local recurrent colorectal cancer: a pooled analysis of 26 individual studies. Cell Biochem Biophys. 2015;72:443–51.
211. Maas M, Rutten IJ, Nelemans PJ, Lambregts DM, Cappendijk VC, Beets GL, Beets-Tan RG. What is the most accurate whole-body imaging modality for assessment of local and distant recurrent disease in colorectal cancer? A meta-analysis : imaging for

recurrent colorectal cancer. Eur J Nucl Med Mol Imaging. 2011;38:1560–71.
212. Lu YY, Chen JH, Chien CR, Chen WT, Tsai SC, Lin WY, Kao CH. Use of FDG-PET or PET/CT to detect recurrent colorectal cancer in patients with elevated CEA: a systematic review and meta-analysis. Int J Color Dis. 2013;28:1039–47.
213. Ito K, Kato T, Tadokoro M, Ishiguchi T, Oshima M, Ishigaki T, Sakuma S. Recurrent rectal cancer and scar: differentiation with PET and MR imaging. Radiology. 1992;182:549–52.
214. Duffy MJ. Carcinoembryonic antigen as a marker for colorectal cancer: is it clinically useful? Clin Chem. 2001;47:624–30.
215. Moertel CG, Fleming TR, Macdonald JS, Haller DG, Laurie JA, Tangen C. An evaluation of the carcinoembryonic antigen (CEA) test for monitoring patients with resected colon cancer. JAMA. 1993;270:943–7.
216. Giacomobono S, Gallicchio R, Capacchione D, Nardelli A, Gattozzi D, Lettini G, Molinari L, Mainenti P, Cammarota A, Storto G. F-18 FDG PET/CT in the assessment of patients with unexplained CEA rise after surgical curative resection for colorectal cancer. Int J Color Dis. 2013;28:1699–705.
217. Ozkan E, Soydal C, Araz M, Kir KM, Ibis E. The role of 18F-FDG PET/CT in detecting colorectal cancer recurrence in patients with elevated CEA levels. Nucl Med Commun. 2012;33:395–402.
218. Panagiotidis E, Datseris IE, Rondogianni P, Vlontzou E, Skilakaki M, Exarhos D, Bamias A. Does CEA and CA 19-9 combined increase the likelihood of 18F-FDG in detecting recurrence in colorectal patients with negative CeCT? Nucl Med Commun. 2014;35:598–605.
219. Sanli Y, Kuyumcu S, Ozkan ZG, Kilic L, Balik E, Turkmen C, Has D, Isik G, Asoglu O, Kapran Y, Adalet I. The utility of FDG-PET/CT as an effective tool for detecting recurrent colorectal cancer regardless of serum CEA levels. Ann Nucl Med. 2012;26:551–8.
220. Bu W, Wei R, Li J, Wang L, Shi C, Song J, Ma S, Chen H, Cong N. Association between carcinoembryonic antigen levels and the applied value of 18F-fluorodeoxyglucose positron emission tomography/computed tomography in post-operative recurrent and metastatic colorectal cancer. Oncol Lett. 2014;8:2649–53.
221. Zhang Y, Feng B, Zhang GL, Hu M, Fu Z, Zhao F, Zhang XL, Kong L, Yu JM. Value of (1)(8)F-FDG PET-CT in surveillance of postoperative colorectal cancer patients with various carcinoembryonic antigen concentrations. World J Gastroenterol. 2014;20:6608–14.
222. Xia Q, Liu J, Wu C, Song S, Tong L, Huang G, Feng Y, Jiang Y, Liu Y, Yin T, Ni Y. Prognostic significance of (18)FDG PET/CT in colorectal cancer patients with liver metastases: a meta-analysis. Cancer Imaging. 2015;15:19.
223. Zhang C, Tong J, Sun X, Liu J, Wang Y, Huang G. 18F-FDG-PET evaluation of treatment response to neo-adjuvant therapy in patients with locally advanced rectal cancer: a meta-analysis. Int J Cancer. 2012;131:2604–11.
224. Bipat S, van Leeuwen MS, Comans EF, Pijl ME, Bossuyt PM, Zwinderman AH, Stoker J. Colorectal liver metastases: CT, MR imaging, and PET for diagnosis—meta-analysis. Radiology. 2005;237:123–31.
225. Ruers TJ, Wiering B, van der Sijp JR, Roumen RM, de Jong KP, Comans EF, Pruim J, Dekker HM, Krabbe PF, Oyen WJ. Improved selection of patients for hepatic surgery of colorectal liver metastases with (18)F-FDG PET: a randomized study. J Nucl Med. 2009;50:1036–41.
226. Moulton CA, Gu CS, Law CH, Tandan VR, Hart R, Quan D, Fairfull Smith RJ, Jalink DW, Husien M, Serrano PE, et al. Effect of PET before liver resection on surgical management for colorectal adenocarcinoma metastases: a randomized clinical trial. JAMA. 2014;311:1863–9.
227. Floriani I, Torri V, Rulli E, Garavaglia D, Compagnoni A, Salvolini L, Giovagnoni A. Performance of imaging modalities in diagnosis of liver metastases from colorectal cancer: a systematic review and meta-analysis. J Magn Reson Imaging. 2010;31:19–31.
228. Maffione AM, Lopci E, Bluemel C, Giammarile F, Herrmann K, Rubello D. Diagnostic accuracy and impact on management of (18)F-FDG PET and PET/CT in colorectal liver metastasis: a meta-analysis and systematic review. Eur J Nucl Med Mol Imaging. 2015;42:152–63.
229. Wiering B, Krabbe PF, Jager GJ, Oyen WJ, Ruers TJ. The impact of fluor-18-deoxyglucose-positron emission tomography in the management of colorectal liver metastases. Cancer. 2005;104:2658–70.
230. van Kessel CS, Buckens CF, van den Bosch MA, van Leeuwen MS, van Hillegersberg R, Verkooijen HM. Preoperative imaging of colorectal liver metastases after neoadjuvant chemotherapy: a meta-analysis. Ann Surg Oncol. 2012;19:2805–13.
231. Wahl RL, Jacene H, Kasamon Y, Lodge MA. From RECIST to PERCIST: evolving considerations for PET response criteria in solid tumors. J Nucl Med. 2009;50(Suppl 1):122S–50S.
232. Skougaard K, Johannesen HH, Nielsen D, Schou JV, Jensen BV, Hogdall EV, Hendel HW. CT versus FDG-PET/CT response evaluation in patients with metastatic colorectal cancer treated with irinotecan and cetuximab. Cancer Med. 2014;3:1294–301.
233. Janssen MH, Ollers MC, van Stiphout RG, Riedl RG, van den Bogaard J, Buijsen J, Lambin P, Lammering G. PET-based treatment response evaluation in rectal cancer: prediction and validation. Int J Radiat Oncol Biol Phys. 2012;82:871–6.
234. Bystrom P, Berglund A, Garske U, Jacobsson H, Sundin A, Nygren P, Frodin JE, Glimelius B. Early prediction of response to first-line chemotherapy by sequential [18F]-2-fluoro-2-deoxy-D-glucose posi-

tron emission tomography in patients with advanced colorectal cancer. Ann Oncol. 2009;20:1057–61.
235. de Geus-Oei LF, Vriens D, van Laarhoven HW, van der Graaf WT, Oyen WJ. Monitoring and predicting response to therapy with 18F-FDG PET in colorectal cancer: a systematic review. J Nucl Med. 2009;50(Suppl 1):43S–54S.
236. de Geus-Oei LF, van Laarhoven HW, Visser EP, Hermsen R, van Hoorn BA, Kamm YJ, Krabbe PF, Corstens FH, Punt CJ, Oyen WJ. Chemotherapy response evaluation with FDG-PET in patients with colorectal cancer. Ann Oncol. 2008;19:348–52.
237. Georgiades CS, Hong K, Geschwind JF. Radiofrequency ablation and chemoembolization for hepatocellular carcinoma. Cancer J. 2008;14:117–22.
238. Hipps D, Ausania F, Manas DM, Rose JD, French JJ. Selective interarterial radiation therapy (SIRT) in colorectal liver metastases: how do we monitor response? HPB Surg. 2013;2013:570808.
239. Wong CY, Salem R, Raman S, Gates VL, Dworkin HJ. Evaluating 90Y-glass microsphere treatment response of unresectable colorectal liver metastases by [18F]FDG PET: a comparison with CT or MRI. Eur J Nucl Med Mol Imaging. 2002;29:815–20.
240. Nielsen K, van Tilborg AA, Scheffer HJ, Meijerink MR, de Lange-de Klerk ES, Meijer S, Comans EF, van den Tol MP. PET-CT after radiofrequency ablation of colorectal liver metastases: suggestions for timing and image interpretation. Eur J Radiol. 2013;82:2169–75.
241. Poulou LS, Ziakas PD, Ziogas DC, Doxani C, Xyla V, Vakrinos G, Voulgarelis M, Thanos L. FDG-PET for detecting local tumor recurrence of ablated liver metastases: a diagnostic meta-analysis. Biomarkers. 2012;17:532–8.
242. Glazer ES, Beaty K, Abdalla EK, Vauthey JN, Curley SA. Effectiveness of positron emission tomography for predicting chemotherapy response in colorectal cancer liver metastases. Arch Surg. 2010;145:340–5; discussion 345.
243. Bassi MC, Turri L, Sacchetti G, Loi G, Cannillo B, La Mattina P, Brambilla M, Inglese E, Krengli M. FDG-PET/CT imaging for staging and target volume delineation in preoperative conformal radiotherapy of rectal cancer. Int J Radiat Oncol Biol Phys. 2008;70:1423–6.
244. Paskeviciute B, Bolling T, Brinkmann M, Rudykina G, Ernst I, Stegger L, Schober O, Willich N, Weckesser M, Konemann S. Impact of (18)F-FDG-PET/CT on staging and irradiation of patients with locally advanced rectal cancer. Strahlenther Onkol. 2009;185:260–5.
245. Ciernik IF, Huser M, Burger C, Davis JB, Szekely G. Automated functional image-guided radiation treatment planning for rectal cancer. Int J Radiat Oncol Biol Phys. 2005;62:893–900.
246. Patel DA, Chang ST, Goodman KA, Quon A, Thorndyke B, Gambhir SS, McMillan A, Loo BW Jr, Koong AC. Impact of integrated PET/CT on variability of target volume delineation in rectal cancer. Technol Cancer Res Treat. 2007;6:31–6.
247. Anderson C, Koshy M, Staley C, Esiashvili N, Ghavidel S, Fowler Z, Fox T, Esteves F, Landry J, Godette K. PET-CT fusion in radiation management of patients with anorectal tumors. Int J Radiat Oncol Biol Phys. 2007;69:155–62.
248. Siegel RL, Miller KD, Jemal A. Cancer statistics, 2017. CA Cancer J Clin. 2017;67:7–30.
249. Von Hoff DD, Ervin T, Arena FP, Chiorean EG, Infante J, Moore M, Seay T, Tjulandin SA, Ma WW, Saleh MN, et al. Increased survival in pancreatic cancer with nab-paclitaxel plus gemcitabine. N Engl J Med. 2013;369:1691–703.
250. Goldstein D, El-Maraghi RH, Hammel P, Heinemann V, Kunzmann V, Sastre J, Scheithauer W, Siena S, Tabernero J, Teixeira L, et al. nab-Paclitaxel plus gemcitabine for metastatic pancreatic cancer: long-term survival from a phase III trial. J Natl Cancer Inst. 2015;107:pii: dju413.
251. Rosewicz S, Wiedenmann B. Pancreatic carcinoma. Lancet. 1997;349:485–9.
252. Pinho DF, Subramaniam RM. PET-computed tomography and precision medicine in pancreatic adenocarcinoma and pancreatic neuroendocrine tumors. PET Clin. 2017;12:407–21.
253. Brennan DD, Zamboni GA, Raptopoulos VD, Kruskal JB. Comprehensive preoperative assessment of pancreatic adenocarcinoma with 64-section volumetric CT. Radiographics. 2007;27:1653–66.
254. Bronstein YL, Loyer EM, Kaur H, Choi H, David C, DuBrow RA, Broemeling LD, Cleary KR, Charnsangavej C. Detection of small pancreatic tumors with multiphasic helical CT. AJR Am J Roentgenol. 2004;182:619–23.
255. Cannon ME, Carpenter SL, Elta GH, Nostrant TT, Kochman ML, Ginsberg GG, Stotland B, Rosato EF, Morris JB, Eckhauser F, Scheiman JM. EUS compared with CT, magnetic resonance imaging, and angiography and the influence of biliary stenting on staging accuracy of ampullary neoplasms. Gastrointest Endosc. 1999;50:27–33.
256. Chen CH, Yang CC, Yeh YH, Chou DA, Nien CK. Reappraisal of endosonography of ampullary tumors: correlation with transabdominal sonography, CT, and MRI. J Clin Ultrasound. 2009;37:18–25.
257. Rijkers AP, Valkema R, Duivenvoorden HJ, van Eijck CH. Usefulness of F-18-fluorodeoxyglucose positron emission tomography to confirm suspected pancreatic cancer: a meta-analysis. Eur J Surg Oncol. 2014;40:794–804.
258. Dibble EH, Karantanis D, Mercier G, Peller PJ, Kachnic LA, Subramaniam RM. PET/CT of cancer patients: part 1, pancreatic neoplasms. AJR Am J Roentgenol. 2012;199:952–67.
259. Michl P, Pauls S, Gress TM. Evidence-based diagnosis and staging of pancreatic cancer. Best Pract Res Clin Gastroenterol. 2006;20:227–51.

260. Gambhir SS, Czernin J, Schwimmer J, Silverman DH, Coleman RE, Phelps ME. A tabulated summary of the FDG PET literature. J Nucl Med. 2001;42:1S–93S.
261. Tang S, Huang G, Liu J, Liu T, Treven L, Song S, Zhang C, Pan L, Zhang T. Usefulness of 18F-FDG PET, combined FDG-PET/CT and EUS in diagnosing primary pancreatic carcinoma: a meta-analysis. Eur J Radiol. 2011;78:142–50.
262. Kauhanen SP, Komar G, Seppanen MP, Dean KI, Minn HR, Kajander SA, Rinta-Kiikka I, Alanen K, Borra RJ, Puolakkainen PA, et al. A prospective diagnostic accuracy study of 18F-fluorodeoxyglucose positron emission tomography/computed tomography, multidetector row computed tomography, and magnetic resonance imaging in primary diagnosis and staging of pancreatic cancer. Ann Surg. 2009;250:957–63.
263. Heinrich S, Goerres GW, Schafer M, Sagmeister M, Bauerfeind P, Pestalozzi BC, Hany TF, von Schulthess GK, Clavien PA. Positron emission tomography/computed tomography influences on the management of resectable pancreatic cancer and its cost-effectiveness. Ann Surg. 2005;242:235–43.
264. Schick V, Franzius C, Beyna T, Oei ML, Schnekenburger J, Weckesser M, Domschke W, Schober O, Heindel W, Pohle T, Juergens KU. Diagnostic impact of 18F-FDG PET-CT evaluating solid pancreatic lesions versus endosonography, endoscopic retrograde cholangio-pancreatography with intraductal ultrasonography and abdominal ultrasound. Eur J Nucl Med Mol Imaging. 2008;35:1775–85.
265. Buchs NC, Buhler L, Bucher P, Willi JP, Frossard JL, Roth AD, Addeo P, Rosset A, Terraz S, Becker CD, et al. Value of contrast-enhanced 18F-fluorodeoxyglucose positron emission tomography/computed tomography in detection and presurgical assessment of pancreatic cancer: a prospective study. J Gastroenterol Hepatol. 2011;26:657–62.
266. Lemke AJ, Niehues SM, Hosten N, Amthauer H, Boehmig M, Stroszczynski C, Rohlfing T, Rosewicz S, Felix R. Retrospective digital image fusion of multidetector CT and 18F-FDG PET: clinical value in pancreatic lesions—a prospective study with 104 patients. J Nucl Med. 2004;45:1279–86.
267. Koyama K, Okamura T, Kawabe J, Nakata B, Chung KH, Ochi H, Yamada R. Diagnostic usefulness of FDG PET for pancreatic mass lesions. Ann Nucl Med. 2001;15:217–24.
268. Santhosh S, Mittal BR, Bhasin D, Srinivasan R, Rana S, Das A, Nada R, Bhattacharya A, Gupta R, Kapoor R. Role of (18)F-fluorodeoxyglucose positron emission tomography/computed tomography in the characterization of pancreatic masses: experience from tropics. J Gastroenterol Hepatol. 2013;28:255–61.
269. Rose DM, Delbeke D, Beauchamp RD, Chapman WC, Sandler MP, Sharp KW, Richards WO, Wright JK, Frexes ME, Pinson CW, Leach SD. 18Fluorodeoxyglucose-positron emission tomography in the management of patients with suspected pancreatic cancer. Ann Surg. 1999;229:729–37; discussion 737–28.
270. Diederichs CG, Staib L, Vogel J, Glasbrenner B, Glatting G, Brambs HJ, Beger HG, Reske SN. Values and limitations of 18F-fluorodeoxyglucose-positron-emission tomography with preoperative evaluation of patients with pancreatic masses. Pancreas. 2000;20:109–16.
271. Matsumoto I, Shirakawa S, Shinzeki M, Asari S, Goto T, Ajiki T, Fukumoto T, Kitajima K, Ku Y. 18-Fluorodeoxyglucose positron emission tomography does not aid in diagnosis of pancreatic ductal adenocarcinoma. Clin Gastroenterol Hepatol. 2013;11:712–8.
272. Strobel O, Buchler MW. Pancreatic cancer: FDG-PET is not useful in early pancreatic cancer diagnosis. Nat Rev Gastroenterol Hepatol. 2013;10:203–5.
273. Shreve PD. Focal fluorine-18 fluorodeoxyglucose accumulation in inflammatory pancreatic disease. Eur J Nucl Med. 1998;25:259–64.
274. Zimny M, Buell U, Diederichs CG, Reske SN. False-positive FDG PET in patients with pancreatic masses: an issue of proper patient selection? Eur J Nucl Med. 1998;25:1352.
275. Higashi T, Saga T, Nakamoto Y, Ishimori T, Fujimoto K, Doi R, Imamura M, Konishi J. Diagnosis of pancreatic cancer using fluorine-18 fluorodeoxyglucose positron emission tomography (FDG PET)—usefulness and limitations in "clinical reality". Ann Nucl Med. 2003;17:261–79.
276. Tatsumi M, Isohashi K, Onishi H, Hori M, Kim T, Higuchi I, Inoue A, Shimosegawa E, Takeda Y, Hatazawa J. 18F-FDG PET/MRI fusion in characterizing pancreatic tumors: comparison to PET/CT. Int J Clin Oncol. 2011;16:408–15.
277. Nagamachi S, Nishii R, Wakamatsu H, Mizutani Y, Kiyohara S, Fujita S, Futami S, Sakae T, Furukoji E, Tamura S, et al. The usefulness of (18)F-FDG PET/MRI fusion image in diagnosing pancreatic tumor: comparison with (18)F-FDG PET/CT. Ann Nucl Med. 2013;27:554–63.
278. Herrmann K, Eckel F, Schmidt S, Scheidhauer K, Krause BJ, Kleeff J, Schuster T, Wester HJ, Friess H, Schmid RM, et al. In vivo characterization of proliferation for discriminating cancer from pancreatic pseudotumors. J Nucl Med. 2008;49:1437–44.
279. Challapalli A, Barwick T, Pearson RA, Merchant S, Mauri F, Howell EC, Sumpter K, Maxwell RJ, Aboagye EO, Sharma R. 3′-Deoxy-3′-(1)(8)F-fluorothymidine positron emission tomography as an early predictor of disease progression in patients with advanced and metastatic pancreatic cancer. Eur J Nucl Med Mol Imaging. 2015;42:831–40.
280. Nishiyama Y, Yamamoto Y, Yokoe K, Monden T, Sasakawa Y, Tsutsui K, Satoh K, Ohkawa M. Contribution of whole body FDG-PET to the detection of distant metastasis in pancreatic cancer. Ann Nucl Med. 2005;19:491–7.

281. Franke C, Klapdor R, Meyerhoff K, Schauman M. 18-FDG positron emission tomography of the pancreas: diagnostic benefit in the follow-up of pancreatic carcinoma. Anticancer Res. 1999;19:2437–42.
282. Farma JM, Santillan AA, Melis M, Walters J, Belinc D, Chen DT, Eikman EA, Malafa M. PET/CT fusion scan enhances CT staging in patients with pancreatic neoplasms. Ann Surg Oncol. 2008;15:2465–71.
283. Strobel K, Heinrich S, Bhure U, Soyka J, Veit-Haibach P, Pestalozzi BC, Clavien PA, Hany TF. Contrast-enhanced 18F-FDG PET/CT: 1-stop-shop imaging for assessing the resectability of pancreatic cancer. J Nucl Med. 2008;49:1408–13.
284. Satoh Y, Ichikawa T, Motosugi U, Kimura K, Sou H, Sano K, Araki T. Diagnosis of peritoneal dissemination: comparison of 18F-FDG PET/CT, diffusion-weighted MRI, and contrast-enhanced MDCT. AJR Am J Roentgenol. 2011;196:447–53.
285. Soussan M, Des Guetz G, Barrau V, Aflalo-Hazan V, Pop G, Mehanna Z, Rust E, Aparicio T, Douard R, Benamouzig R, et al. Comparison of FDG-PET/CT and MR with diffusion-weighted imaging for assessing peritoneal carcinomatosis from gastrointestinal malignancy. Eur Radiol. 2012;22:1479–87.
286. Ruf J, Lopez Hanninen E, Oettle H, Plotkin M, Pelzer U, Stroszczynski C, Felix R, Amthauer H. Detection of recurrent pancreatic cancer: comparison of FDG-PET with CT/MRI. Pancreatology. 2005;5:266–72.
287. Bang S, Chung HW, Park SW, Chung JB, Yun M, Lee JD, Song SY. The clinical usefulness of 18-fluorodeoxyglucose positron emission tomography in the differential diagnosis, staging, and response evaluation after concurrent chemoradiotherapy for pancreatic cancer. J Clin Gastroenterol. 2006;40:923–9.
288. Yoshioka M, Sato T, Furuya T, Shibata S, Andoh H, Asanuma Y, Hatazawa J, Shimosegawa E, Koyama K, Yamamoto Y. Role of positron emission tomography with 2-deoxy-2-[18F]fluoro-D-glucose in evaluating the effects of arterial infusion chemotherapy and radiotherapy on pancreatic cancer. J Gastroenterol. 2004;39:50–5.
289. Asagi A, Ohta K, Nasu J, Tanada M, Nadano S, Nishimura R, Teramoto N, Yamamoto K, Inoue T, Iguchi H. Utility of contrast-enhanced FDG-PET/CT in the clinical management of pancreatic cancer: impact on diagnosis, staging, evaluation of treatment response, and detection of recurrence. Pancreas. 2013;42:11–9.
290. Sperti C, Pasquali C, Chierichetti F, Ferronato A, Decet G, Pedrazzoli S. 18-Fluorodeoxyglucose positron emission tomography in predicting survival of patients with pancreatic carcinoma. J Gastrointest Surg. 2003;7:953–9; discussion 959–60.
291. Schellenberg D, Quon A, Minn AY, Graves EE, Kunz P, Ford JM, Fisher GA, Goodman KA, Koong AC, Chang DT. 18Fluorodeoxyglucose PET is prognostic of progression-free and overall survival in locally advanced pancreas cancer treated with stereotactic radiotherapy. Int J Radiat Oncol Biol Phys. 2010;77:1420–5.
292. Xu HX, Chen T, Wang WQ, Wu CT, Liu C, Long J, Xu J, Zhang YJ, Chen RH, Liu L, Yu XJ. Metabolic tumour burden assessed by (1)(8)F-FDG PET/CT associated with serum CA19-9 predicts pancreatic cancer outcome after resection. Eur J Nucl Med Mol Imaging. 2014;41:1093–102.
293. Kang CM, Lee SH, Hwang HK, Yun M, Lee WJ. Preoperative volume-based pet parameter, MTV2.5, as a potential surrogate marker for tumor biology and recurrence in resected pancreatic cancer. Medicine. 2016;95:e2595.
294. Chirindel A, Alluri KC, Chaudhry MA, Wahl RL, Pawlik TM, Herman JM, Subramaniam RM. Prognostic value of FDG PET/CT-derived parameters in pancreatic adenocarcinoma at initial PET/CT staging. AJR Am J Roentgenol. 2015;204:1093–9.
295. Wakabayashi H, Nishiyama Y, Otani T, Sano T, Yachida S, Okano K, Izuishi K, Suzuki Y. Role of 18F-fluorodeoxyglucose positron emission tomography imaging in surgery for pancreatic cancer. World J Gastroenterol. 2008;14:64–9.
296. Maisey NR, Webb A, Flux GD, Padhani A, Cunningham DC, Ott RJ, Norman A. FDG-PET in the prediction of survival of patients with cancer of the pancreas: a pilot study. Br J Cancer. 2000;83:287–93.
297. Lee JW, Kang CM, Choi HJ, Lee WJ, Song SY, Lee JH, Lee JD. Prognostic value of metabolic tumor volume and total lesion glycolysis on preoperative (1)(8)F-FDG PET/CT in patients with pancreatic cancer. J Nucl Med. 2014;55:898–904.
298. Moon SY, Joo KR, So YR, Lim JU, Cha JM, Shin HP, Yang YJ. Predictive value of maximum standardized uptake value (SUVmax) on 18F-FDG PET/CT in patients with locally advanced or metastatic pancreatic cancer. Clin Nucl Med. 2013;38:778–83.
299. Parikh U, Marcus C, Sarangi R, Taghipour M, Subramaniam RM. FDG PET/CT in pancreatic and hepatobiliary carcinomas: value to patient management and patient outcomes. PET Clin. 2015;10:327–43.
300. Sheikhbahaei S, Wray R, Young B, Mena E, Taghipour M, Rahmim A, Subramaniam RM. 18F-FDG-PET/CT therapy assessment of locally advanced pancreatic adenocarcinoma: impact on management and utilization of quantitative parameters for patient survival prediction. Nucl Med Commun. 2016;37:231–8.
301. Kuwatani M, Kawakami H, Eto K, Haba S, Shiga T, Tamaki N, Asaka M. Modalities for evaluating chemotherapeutic efficacy and survival time in patients with advanced pancreatic cancer: comparison between FDG-PET, CT, and serum tumor markers. Intern Med. 2009;48:867–75.
302. Javery O, Shyn P, Mortele K. FDG PET or PET/CT in patients with pancreatic cancer: when does

it add to diagnostic CT or MRI? Clin Imaging. 2013;37:295–301.
303. Gerlinger M, Rowan AJ, Horswell S, Math M, Larkin J, Endesfelder D, Gronroos E, Martinez P, Matthews N, Stewart A, et al. Intratumor heterogeneity and branched evolution revealed by multiregion sequencing. N Engl J Med. 2012;366:883–92.
304. Hyun SH, Kim HS, Choi SH, Choi DW, Lee JK, Lee KH, Park JO, Lee KH, Kim BT, Choi JY. Intratumoral heterogeneity of (18)F-FDG uptake predicts survival in patients with pancreatic ductal adenocarcinoma. Eur J Nucl Med Mol Imaging. 2016;43:1461–8.
305. Rahmim A, Schmidtlein CR, Jackson A, Sheikhbahaei S, Marcus C, Ashrafinia S, Soltani M, Subramaniam RM. A novel metric for quantification of homogeneous and heterogeneous tumors in PET for enhanced clinical outcome prediction. Phys Med Biol. 2016;61:227–42.
306. Russo S, Butler J, Ove R, Blackstock AW. Locally advanced pancreatic cancer: a review. Semin Oncol. 2007;34:327–34.
307. Willett CG, Czito BG, Bendell JC, Ryan DP. Locally advanced pancreatic cancer. J Clin Oncol. 2005;23:4538–44.
308. Kitajima K, Murakami K, Yamasaki E, Kaji Y, Shimoda M, Kubota K, Suganuma N, Sugimura K. Performance of integrated FDG-PET/contrast-enhanced CT in the diagnosis of recurrent pancreatic cancer: comparison with integrated FDG-PET/non-contrast-enhanced CT and enhanced CT. Mol Imaging Biol. 2010;12:452–9.
309. Lachter J, Adler AC, Keidar Z, Haddad R. FDG-PET/CT identifies a curable pancreatic cancer surgical tract metastasis after failure by other imaging modalities. Isr Med Assoc J. 2008;10:243–4.
310. Antoch G, Saoudi N, Kuehl H, Dahmen G, Mueller SP, Beyer T, Bockisch A, Debatin JF, Freudenberg LS. Accuracy of whole-body dual-modality fluorine-18-2-fluoro-2-deoxy-D-glucose positron emission tomography and computed tomography (FDG-PET/CT) for tumor staging in solid tumors: comparison with CT and PET. J Clin Oncol. 2004;22:4357–68.
311. Kantorova I, Lipska L, Belohlavek O, Visokai V, Trubac M, Schneiderova M. Routine (18)F-FDG PET preoperative staging of colorectal cancer: comparison with conventional staging and its impact on treatment decision making. J Nucl Med. 2003;44:1784–8.
312. European Association For The Study Of The L, European Organisation For R, Treatment of C. EASL-EORTC clinical practice guidelines: management of hepatocellular carcinoma. J Hepatol. 2012;56:908–43.
313. Lee JD, Yang WI, Park YN, Kim KS, Choi JS, Yun M, Ko D, Kim TS, Cho AE, Kim HM, et al. Different glucose uptake and glycolytic mechanisms between hepatocellular carcinoma and intrahepatic mass-forming cholangiocarcinoma with increased (18) F-FDG uptake. J Nucl Med. 2005;46:1753–9.
314. Khan MA, Combs CS, Brunt EM, Lowe VJ, Wolverson MK, Solomon H, Collins BT, Di Bisceglie AM. Positron emission tomography scanning in the evaluation of hepatocellular carcinoma. J Hepatol. 2000;32:792–7.
315. Ho CL, Yu SC, Yeung DW. 11C-acetate PET imaging in hepatocellular carcinoma and other liver masses. J Nucl Med. 2003;44:213–21.
316. Wudel LJ Jr, Delbeke D, Morris D, Rice M, Washington MK, Shyr Y, Pinson CW, Chapman WC. The role of [18F]fluorodeoxyglucose positron emission tomography imaging in the evaluation of hepatocellular carcinoma. Am Surg. 2003;69:117–24; discussion 124–16.
317. Lin CY, Chen JH, Liang JA, Lin CC, Jeng LB, Kao CH. 18F-FDG PET or PET/CT for detecting extrahepatic metastases or recurrent hepatocellular carcinoma: a systematic review and meta-analysis. Eur J Radiol. 2012;81:2417–22.
318. Paudyal B, Paudyal P, Oriuchi N, Tsushima Y, Nakajima T, Endo K. Clinical implication of glucose transport and metabolism evaluated by 18F-FDG PET in hepatocellular carcinoma. Int J Oncol. 2008;33:1047–54.
319. Kwee TC, Basu S, Saboury B, Ambrosini V, Torigian DA, Alavi A. A new dimension of FDG-PET interpretation: assessment of tumor biology. Eur J Nucl Med Mol Imaging. 2011;38:1158–70.
320. Cho E, Jun CH, Kim BS, Son DJ, Choi WS, Choi SK. 18F-FDG PET CT as a prognostic factor in hepatocellular carcinoma. Turk J Gastroenterol. 2015;26:344–50.
321. Shiomi S, Nishiguchi S, Ishizu H, Iwata Y, Sasaki N, Tamori A, Habu D, Takeda T, Kubo S, Ochi H. Usefulness of positron emission tomography with fluorine-18-fluorodeoxyglucose for predicting outcome in patients with hepatocellular carcinoma. Am J Gastroenterol. 2001;96:1877–80.
322. Lee DH, Lee JM, Hur BY, Joo I, Yi NJ, Suh KS, Kang KW, Han JK. Colorectal cancer liver metastases: diagnostic performance and prognostic value of PET/MR imaging. Radiology. 2016;280:782–92.
323. Berger KL, Nicholson SA, Dehdashti F, Siegel BA. FDG PET evaluation of mucinous neoplasms: correlation of FDG uptake with histopathologic features. AJR Am J Roentgenol. 2000;174:1005–8.
324. Whiteford MH, Whiteford HM, Yee LF, Ogunbiyi OA, Dehdashti F, Siegel BA, Birnbaum EH, Fleshman JW, Kodner IJ, Read TE. Usefulness of FDG-PET scan in the assessment of suspected metastatic or recurrent adenocarcinoma of the colon and rectum. Dis Colon Rectum. 2000;43:759–67; discussion 767–70.
325. Donati OF, Hany TF, Reiner CS, von Schulthess GK, Marincek B, Seifert B, Weishaupt D. Value of retrospective fusion of PET and MR images in detection of hepatic metastases: comparison with 18F-FDG PET/CT and Gd-EOB-DTPA-enhanced MRI. J Nucl Med. 2010;51:692–9.

326. Beiderwellen K, Geraldo L, Ruhlmann V, Heusch P, Gomez B, Nensa F, Umutlu L, Lauenstein TC. Accuracy of [18F]FDG PET/MRI for the detection of liver metastases. PLoS One. 2015;10:e0137285.
327. Kuhn FP, Hullner M, Mader CE, Kastrinidis N, Huber GF, von Schulthess GK, Kollias S, Veit-Haibach P. Contrast-enhanced PET/MR imaging versus contrast-enhanced PET/CT in head and neck cancer: how much MR information is needed? J Nucl Med. 2014;55:551–8.
328. Beiderwellen K, Gomez B, Buchbender C, Hartung V, Poeppel TD, Nensa F, Kuehl H, Bockisch A, Lauenstein TC. Depiction and characterization of liver lesions in whole body [(1)(8)F]-FDG PET/MRI. Eur J Radiol. 2013;82:e669–75.
329. Park JW, Kim JH, Kim SK, Kang KW, Park KW, Choi JI, Lee WJ, Kim CM, Nam BH. A prospective evaluation of 18F-FDG and 11C-acetate PET/CT for detection of primary and metastatic hepatocellular carcinoma. J Nucl Med. 2008;49:1912–21.
330. Talbot JN, Fartoux L, Balogova S, Nataf V, Kerrou K, Gutman F, Huchet V, Ancel D, Grange JD, Rosmorduc O. Detection of hepatocellular carcinoma with PET/CT: a prospective comparison of 18F-fluorocholine and 18F-FDG in patients with cirrhosis or chronic liver disease. J Nucl Med. 2010;51:1699–706.
331. Song MJ, Bae SH, Lee SW, Song DS, Kim HY, Yoo Ie R, Choi JI, Lee YJ, Chun HJ, Lee HG, et al. 18F-fluorodeoxyglucose PET/CT predicts tumour progression after transarterial chemoembolization in hepatocellular carcinoma. Eur J Nucl Med Mol Imaging. 2013;40:865–73.
332. Ma W, Jia J, Wang S, Bai W, Yi J, Bai M, Quan Z, Yin Z, Fan D, Wang J, Han G. The prognostic value of 18F-FDG PET/CT for hepatocellular carcinoma treated with transarterial chemoembolization (TACE). Theranostics. 2014;4:736–44.
333. Kim HO, Kim JS, Shin YM, Ryu JS, Lee YS, Lee SG. Evaluation of metabolic characteristics and viability of lipiodolized hepatocellular carcinomas using 18F-FDG PET/CT. J Nucl Med. 2010;51:1849–56.
334. Song HJ, Cheng JY, Hu SL, Zhang GY, Fu Y, Zhang YJ. Value of 18F-FDG PET/CT in detecting viable tumour and predicting prognosis of hepatocellular carcinoma after TACE. Clin Radiol. 2015;70:128–37.
335. Higashi T, Hatano E, Ikai I, Nishii R, Nakamoto Y, Ishizu K, Suga T, Kawashima H, Togashi K, Seo S, et al. FDG PET as a prognostic predictor in the early post-therapeutic evaluation for unresectable hepatocellular carcinoma. Eur J Nucl Med Mol Imaging. 2010;37:468–82.
336. Huang WY, Kao CH, Huang WS, Chen CM, Chang LP, Lee MS, Chao HL, Chiu CH, Lo CH, Jen YM. 18F-FDG PET and combined 18F-FDG-contrast CT parameters as predictors of tumor control for hepatocellular carcinoma after stereotactic ablative radiotherapy. J Nucl Med. 2013;54:1710–6.
337. Purandare NC, Rangarajan V, Shah SA, Sharma AR, Kulkarni SS, Kulkarni AV, Dua SG. Therapeutic response to radiofrequency ablation of neoplastic lesions: FDG PET/CT findings. Radiographics. 2011;31:201–13.
338. Chen YK, Hsieh DS, Liao CS, Bai CH, Su CT, Shen YY, Hsieh JF, Liao AC, Kao CH. Utility of FDG-PET for investigating unexplained serum AFP elevation in patients with suspected hepatocellular carcinoma recurrence. Anticancer Res. 2005;25:4719–25.
339. Han AR, Gwak GY, Choi MS, Lee JH, Koh KC, Paik SW, Yoo BC. The clinical value of 18F-FDG PET/CT for investigating unexplained serum AFP elevation following interventional therapy for hepatocellular carcinoma. Hepato-Gastroenterology. 2009;56:1111–6.
340. Xia F, Wu L, Lau WY, Li G, Huan H, Qian C, Ma K, Bie P. Positive lymph node metastasis has a marked impact on the long-term survival of patients with hepatocellular carcinoma with extrahepatic metastasis. PLoS One. 2014;9:e95889.
341. Jo JE, Kim JY, Lee SH, Kim S, Kang T. Preoperative 18F-FDG PET/CT predicts disease-free survival in patients with primary invasive ductal breast cancer. Acta Radiol. 2015;56:1463–70.
342. Pant V, Sen IB, Soin AS. Role of (1)(8)F-FDG PET CT as an independent prognostic indicator in patients with hepatocellular carcinoma. Nucl Med Commun. 2013;34:749–57.
343. Hatano E, Ikai I, Higashi T, Teramukai S, Torizuka T, Saga T, Fujii H, Shimahara Y. Preoperative positron emission tomography with fluorine-18-fluorodeoxyglucose is predictive of prognosis in patients with hepatocellular carcinoma after resection. World J Surg. 2006;30:1736–41.
344. Seo S, Hatano E, Higashi T, Hara T, Tada M, Tamaki N, Iwaisako K, Ikai I, Uemoto S. Fluorine-18 fluorodeoxyglucose positron emission tomography predicts tumor differentiation, P-glycoprotein expression, and outcome after resection in hepatocellular carcinoma. Clin Cancer Res. 2007;13:427–33.
345. Kornberg A, Freesmeyer M, Barthel E, Jandt K, Katenkamp K, Steenbeck J, Sappler A, Habrecht O, Gottschild D, Settmacher U. 18F-FDG-uptake of hepatocellular carcinoma on PET predicts microvascular tumor invasion in liver transplant patients. Am J Transplant. 2009;9:592–600.

^{18}F-FDG-PET/CT in Breast and Gynecologic Cancer

20

Katrina E. Korhonen, Austin R. Pantel, and David A. Mankoff

20.1 Breast Cancer

20.1.1 Epidemiology

Breast cancer is the most common newly diagnosed cancer in women and the second leading cause of death from cancer among women, second only to lung cancer [1]. Commonly recognized risk factors for development of the disease include female sex, advanced age, family history, early menarche, late first pregnancy, obesity, genetic/inherited germline mutations (such as the BRCA-1 or BRCA-2 gene mutations), and history of mantle radiation for Hodgkin's disease [2]. Breast cancers may be classified based on histologic as well as phenotypic factors. Histologically, breast cancers arise from the epithelial cells in the breast ducts. The most important histologic feature in classifying breast cancer relates to the presence or absence of tumor invasion beyond the basement membrane of breast cancer ducts. Tumors which have not broken through the basement membrane are termed in situ and rarely metastasize; in contrast, tumors which have invaded through the basement membrane are termed *invasive*, for which there is an increased likelihood of either lymphatic or hematogenous metastases [3]. Additional important histologic features include type (ductal, lobular, or mixed architectural pattern), grade (low, intermediate, or high), and the presence or absence of lymphovascular invasion. In addition, several phenotypic features can be used to characterize breast cancers. These include hormone receptor status (such as estrogen receptor [ER] or progesterone receptor [PR]) as well as other receptors such as HER2/neu, a human epidermal growth factor receptor. Additional useful features of tumor evaluation include measuring levels of certain cellular biomarkers, which can also provide valuable information regarding tumor behavior. For example, Ki-67, a measure of cellular proliferation, can be assessed and provide information regarding tumor aggressivity. Together, evaluation of these phenotypic features can be used to predict tumor behavior and identify patients who might benefit from targeted therapies. For example, the assessment of tumoral ER/PR and HER2 expression is essential in helping identify which patients might benefit from endocrine and HER2-targeted treatments, respectively. These are the most commonly used targeted therapies in clinical practice [4]. Furthermore, the increased use of gene expression profiling has led to the recognition that breast cancer represents a heterogeneous spectrum of diseases with varying molecular patterns, resulting in several new subcategories of disease. As such, Perou et al. proposed four main breast cancer subtypes. In order of increasing aggressivity, these

K. E. Korhonen (✉) · A. R. Pantel · D. A. Mankoff
Department of Radiology, Division of Nuclear Medicine and Clinical Molecular Imaging, Hospital of the University of Pennsylvania, Philadelphia, PA, USA
e-mail: Katrina.Korhonen@pennmedicine.upenn.edu; mankoffd@pennmedicine.upenn.edu

H. Ahmadzadehfar et al. (eds.), *Clinical Nuclear Medicine*,
https://doi.org/10.1007/978-3-030-39457-8_20

are luminal A (generally ER/PR/HER2 positive and low grade), luminal B (ER/PR positive, HER2 negative, and generally intermediate to high grade), HER2 enriched (ER/PR negative, HER2 positive, usually intermediate to high grade), and basal-like (ER/PR/HER2 negative, usually high grade) [5].

20.1.2 Breast Cancer Detection, Diagnosis, and Staging

Mammography is the most common imaging modality used in breast cancer screening, detection, and diagnosis. Although full-field digital mammography has been commonly used in breast cancer screening, replacing the previously widespread screen-film mammography, digital breast tomosynthesis has demonstrated increased benefit over both modalities, with both an increase in cancer detection rate and a decrease in screening recalls compared to digital mammography [6–8]. Both ultrasound and MRI may serve as imaging adjuncts to mammography for the detection, characterization, and classification of extent of disease. Additionally, MRI is frequently utilized in breast cancer screening in women with greater than 20% lifetime risk of the disease, where it is typically used in an alternating fashion in combination with mammography [9].

Breast cancer staging is most commonly performed according to the AJCC system using a TNM approach. Groups of TNM categories form a staging classification ranging from early-stage disease (stage I) through late-stage, metastatic disease (stage IV) (SB [10]). Important factors in breast cancer staging include both regional lymph node status (which represents the *N* in TNM) and the presence of distant metastatic disease (which represents the *M* in TNM). Treatment options available to patients depend on tumor staging. Locoregional disease is typically treated with surgery (either lumpectomy or mastectomy) plus targeted radiotherapy in some patients. Distant metastatic disease is treated with systemic therapy, including chemotherapy, endocrine/hormonal therapy, or targeted biologic agents such as anti-HER2 therapies.

Regional lymph node staging is typically performed in all patients with invasive carcinoma, as axillary lymph node status is the most important prognostic factor in patients with breast cancer. Both disease-free and progression-free survival decreases as the number of positive axillary lymph nodes increases [3]. Metastatic axillary lymph nodes are also an important factor in determining further therapy following surgery [11]. Historically, axillary nodal staging involved a full axillary lymph node dissection in which the contents of the axilla were removed and examined; however, this procedure is associated with significant morbidity, with many patients suffering from lymphedema following the procedure. As a result, sentinel lymph node (SLN) sampling has largely replaced axillary lymph node dissection for axillary staging in patients with clinically negative axillae. In this procedure, the sentinel lymph node(s), the first lymphatic draining node(s) for a breast lesion, are sampled. If the sentinel lymph node(s) are negative, then the chance of further downstream nodal metastases is greatly reduced, and the patient is typically spared from a full axillary lymph node dissection. However, if the sentinel lymph node is positive, a full axillary lymph node dissection may be needed [11]. Radionuclide methods play a valuable role in SLN mapping, as a radiolabeled colloid pharmaceutical (most commonly, ^{99m}Tc-sulfur colloid) is injected, and SLN are identified via lymphoscintigraphy, gamma probes, or both [12]. Newer, more targeted agents have been used variably in clinical practice, such as ^{99m}Tc-tilmanocept (Lymphoseek), which binds to the mannose receptor, CD206, on activated macrophages [13]. Visible blue dye has also been used in SLN mapping (see also Chap. 11).

The most common sites of metastatic breast cancer include the bones, lymph nodes outside of the axillary and internal mammary chains, the liver, and the lungs. For patients with asymptomatic, early-stage breast cancer (stage I or stage IIA), no further imaging staging is suggested beyond diagnostic mammography (with ultrasound and MRI as needed) due to the low risk of metastatic disease and increased chance of false-positive findings [14]. Systemic staging is suggested only for patients with high-risk or advanced cancer, with recurrent breast cancer, with known metastatic disease, or with suspicious symptoms such as bone pain, for example. Systemic staging is most commonly performed with both anatomic imaging (CT of the chest, abdomen, and pelvis) and radionuclide methods including bone scan and ^{18}F-FDG-PET/CT. As previously mentioned, systemic staging is not currently recommended in asymptomatic patients with early-stage breast cancer. As such, the following discussion will focus on the role of ^{18}F-FDG-PET/CT in staging of patients with high-risk or locally advanced breast cancer (stage IIB and stage III). The role of ^{18}F-FDG-PET/CT in patients with advanced stage, metastatic breast cancer (stage IV) will then follow.

20.1.3 Role of ^{18}F-FDG-PET/CT in Staging Large or Locally Advanced Breast Cancer

^{18}F-FDG uptake and retention depends on the rate of cellular glycolysis, which is frequently elevated in malignant cells in comparison to most normal tissues. Among breast cancers, ^{18}F-FDG uptake varies depending upon tumor histology, histologic grade, and cellular proliferation indices. For example, invasive lobular carcinoma often demonstrates a lower ^{18}F-FDG uptake than invasive ductal carcinoma [15] and can be sometimes challenging to visualize by ^{18}F-FDG-PET/CT. Additionally, ^{18}F-FDG-PET/CT may be less sensitive for in situ or small, well-differentiated tumors, limiting the role of ^{18}F-FDG-PET/CT as a primary diagnostic modality for breast lesions. ^{18}F-FDG-PET has been reported to have a sensitivity of 64–96%, specificity of 73–100%, positive predictive value (PPV) of 81–100%, and negative predictive value (NPV) of 52–89% for the primary detection of breast cancer (reviewed in Scheidhauer et al. [16]).

For patients with stage IIB and stage III disease, ^{18}F-FDG-PET/CT plays a valuable role in the evaluation of both axillary and extra-axillary lymph node disease. While early studies of ^{18}F-FDG PET, preceding studies of sentinel lymph node methods, suggested that ^{18}F-FDG PET was both sensitive and specific for detecting axillary nodal metastases, later studies did not support such results. These later studies included breast cancers more representative of those seen clinically (including a larger number of smaller cancers) and demonstrated a sensitivity as low as 20–30% (reviewed in [17]). In one of the largest studies evaluating the role of ^{18}F-FDG-PET in detecting axillary nodal metastases by Wahl et al. of 360 women with newly diagnosed breast cancer, ^{18}F-FDG-PET demonstrated a sensitivity of 61%, specificity of 80%, PPV of 62%, and NPV of 79%. ^{18}F-FDG-PET demonstrated limited sensitivity for small or isolated lesions and is thus not a reasonable alternative to tissue sampling in axillary staging for patients with early-stage breast cancer [18]. Despite its limited sensitivity, the relatively higher specificity of ^{18}F-FDG-PET/CT for axillary nodal disease (ranging from 93% to 100% as reviewed in Rosen et al. [17]) could be of diagnostic value in patients who are at higher risk for axillary nodal spread, especially those with clinical evidence of nodal disease. In these patients, a positive ^{18}F-FDG-PET/CT could help direct axillary lymph node sampling and/or treatment by surgery or radiotherapy, while a negative study could direct the patient to SLN sampling for confirmation [17]. However, in current clinical practice, much of this evaluation is performed with ultrasound, which is cheaper, results in decreased radiation exposure to the patient, and may potentially direct targeted biopsy of a suspicious lesion [9].

In patients with stage IIB–stage III disease, ^{18}F-FDG-PET/CT may identify extra-axillary lymph node disease or additional sites of previously unknown disease. Such findings may change management or result in upstaging of disease. For example, in a study by Groheux et al. of 254 consecutive patients with stage II or III breast cancer, ^{18}F-FDG-PET/CT changed the clinical stage in 77/254 patients (30.3%) and found unsuspected N3 disease in 40 patients and unsuspected distant metastatic disease in 53 patients. Findings on ^{18}F-FDG-PET/CT also offered prognostic stratification for patients, where those with M1 disease on ^{18}F-FDG-PET/CT had a significantly reduced 3-year disease-specific survival than compared to those patients with M_0 disease on PET/CT (57% vs. 88%, respectively, $p < 0.001$) [19].

Regardless of initial staging, patients with primary tumors located in quadrants outside of the upper outer quadrant of the breast may drain to nodal basins outside the axilla [20] and may be more frequently understaged as compared to patients with a primary tumor in the outer quadrant of the breast. There is a higher propensity for inner-quadrant tumors to metastasize to extra-axillary nodal sites without metastasizing to the axillae. As such, these patients have been reported to have a higher mortality rate, and ^{18}F-FDG-PET/CT may be useful in detecting otherwise occult extra-axillary lymph node involvement. For example, in a study by Tran et al. of 141 patients with breast cancer, patients with inner-quadrant primary tumors had a sixfold increase in isolated extra-axillary lymph node metastases and a threefold risk for disease progression as compared to patients with outer-quadrant primary tumors [21].

Patients with locally advanced breast cancer (LABC) may benefit from staging with ^{18}F-FDG-PET/CT given its ability to detect regional nodal or distant metastatic disease. Such patients include those with a primary tumor larger than 5 cm, skin or chest wall involvement, fixed axillary lymph nodes, positive supraclavicular/infraclavicular/internal mammary lymph nodes, or inflammatory breast cancers. Patients with LABC have a greater chance for having or developing distant metastases during the course of their treatment, resulting in a poorer prognosis [22]. For untreated patients with apparent LABC discovered to have clinically occult distant metastatic disease, such findings could direct therapy options away from more aggressive, toxic, "curative" therapies that would ultimately prove futile. The benefit of ^{18}F-FDG-PET/CT is especially notable in inflammatory breast cancer, where its use may aid treatment decisions considerably [23] (Fig. 20.1).

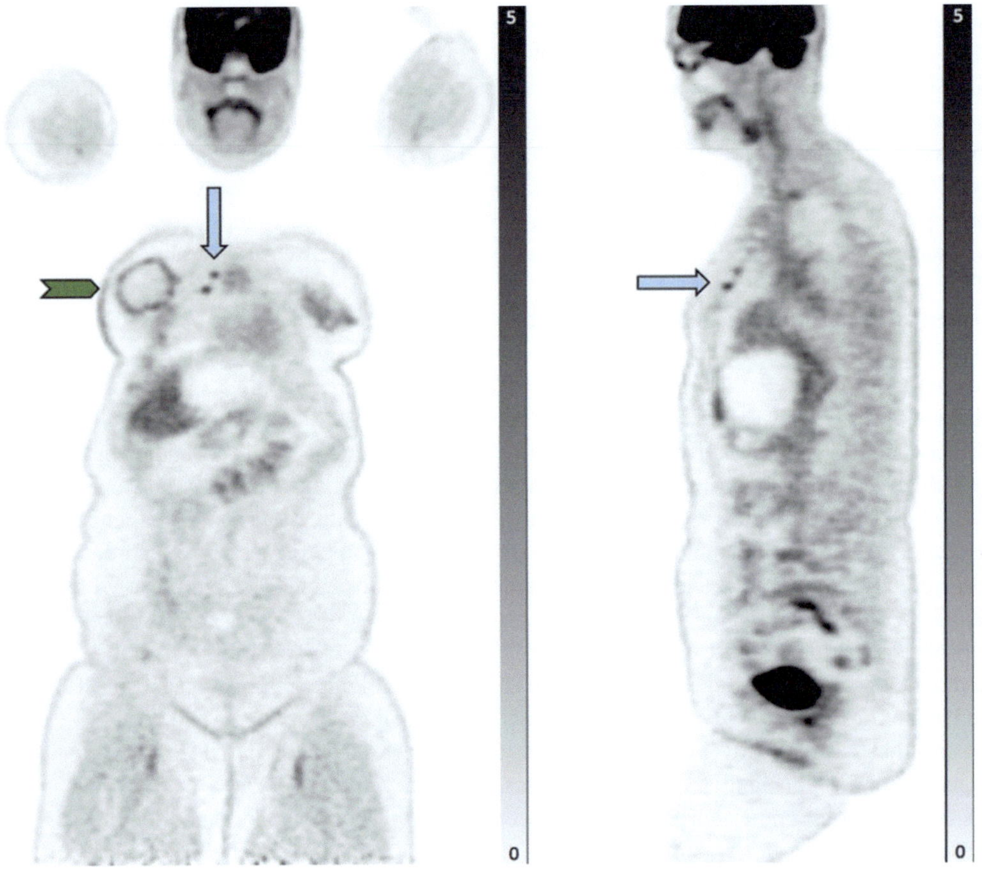

Fig. 20.1 Sixty-six-year-old female with well-differentiated, invasive ductal carcinoma of the right central breast status post lumpectomy. Coronal and sagittal FDG-PET images demonstrate two hypermetabolic right internal mammary lymph nodes (blue arrow) representing metastatic internal mammary lymphadenopathy. There is photopenia in the right breast with a rim of increased FDG uptake at the site of the patient's right seroma (green arrowhead) secondary to inflammatory change

20.1.4 Role of FDG-PET/CT in Staging of Distant Metastatic Breast Cancer

Approximately 5–6% of breast cancer patients have distant metastatic disease at diagnosis [24]. The bones are the most common site of metastatic involvement, representing the first site of metastatic disease in 26–50% of patients. Thirty to 85% of patients will experience osseous involvement during the course of the disease [25]. Anatomically, the spine and the pelvis are the most common locations for metastatic disease, followed by the ribs, the skull, and the femora. The liver, lungs, and distant nodal chains (including mediastinal lymph nodes) are other common sites of distant metastases.

Given the incidence of osseous metastatic disease in breast cancer patients, both bone scan with ^{99m}Tc-MDP (methylene diphosphonate) and ^{18}F-sodium fluoride (^{18}NaF) PET/CT have been used to detect and diagnose osseous metastatic disease. However, both modalities have limitations and potential pitfalls. The sensitivity and specificity for bone scintigraphy has been reported as 62–100% and 78–100%, respectively (reviewed in Hamaoka [25]). However, a variety of non-oncologic etiologies may demonstrate increased radiotracer uptake on bone scintigraphy, including trauma and degenerative change, and bone scan may be falsely negative in patients with lytic metastases. Some studies have suggested that ^{18}F-NaF-PET/CT offers additional advantage over bone scintigraphy. For example, in a study by Schirrmeister et al. of 34 patients with breast cancer, ^{18}F-NaF-PET/CT detected metastases in 17 patients, while bone scan detected metastases in only 11 patients; the clinical management of four patients was changed based on the findings on ^{18}F-NaF-PET/CT [26]. However, widespread clinical use of ^{18}F-NaF-PET/CT has been hindered by cost, lack of familiarity with the modality, and the dearth of data regarding its true clinical impact over bone scan.

^{18}F-FDG-PET/CT may play a valuable role in the evaluation of osseous metastatic disease in patients, especially those with more lytic-appearing metastases where bone scan may be limited. For example, in a study by Cook et al. of 23 patients with confirmed osseous metastatic disease from breast cancer, ^{18}F-FDG-PET, without correlative CT, detected an overall larger number of metastatic lesions than bone scan. ^{18}F-FDG-PET was superior to bone scan in patients with predominantly lytic or intramedullary metastases, and these patients had an overall poorer prognosis. However, in a subgroup of patients with predominantly osteoblastic disease, bone scan proved superior [27]. Further studies have indicated that the combination of ^{18}F-FDG PET and CT in PET/CT can detect lesions not seen by bone scan and misses few, if any, lesions identified by bone scan [28]. As such, bone scan and FDG-PET/CT may play a complementary, or even primary, role, in the evaluation of osseous metastatic disease.

Additionally, ^{18}F-FDG-PET/CT may have advantages over conventional contrast-enhanced CT of the chest, abdomen, and pelvis, which is commonly performed for patients requiring systemic disease staging. Although CT may identify suspicious osseous lesions, CT may not be able to distinguish a benign versus malignant etiology for an osseous lesion. Similarly, although CT may be used to detect visceral disease, ^{18}F-FDG-PET/CT may offer some advantages over CT, particularly with regard to identifying lymph node metastases that are not enlarged by anatomic size criteria. For example, in a study by Mahner et al. of 119 patients, ^{18}F-FDG-PET was superior to conventional imaging (chest radiograph, abdominal ultrasound, and bone scan) but had similar overall diagnostic accuracy as compared to CT. However, ^{18}F-FDG-PET demonstrated improved sensitivity as compared to CT with regard to the detection of metastases in the following locations: axillary, supraclavicular, or mediastinal lymph nodes (86%, 84%, and 96% for ^{18}F-FDG-PET as compared to 53%, 40%, and 31% for CT), bone (87% vs. 67%), lung (75% vs. 65%), and chest wall (86% vs. 67%) [29]. As such, ^{18}F-FDG-PET/CT may play a valuable role in the staging of both osseous and non-osseous metastatic disease (Fig. 20.2).

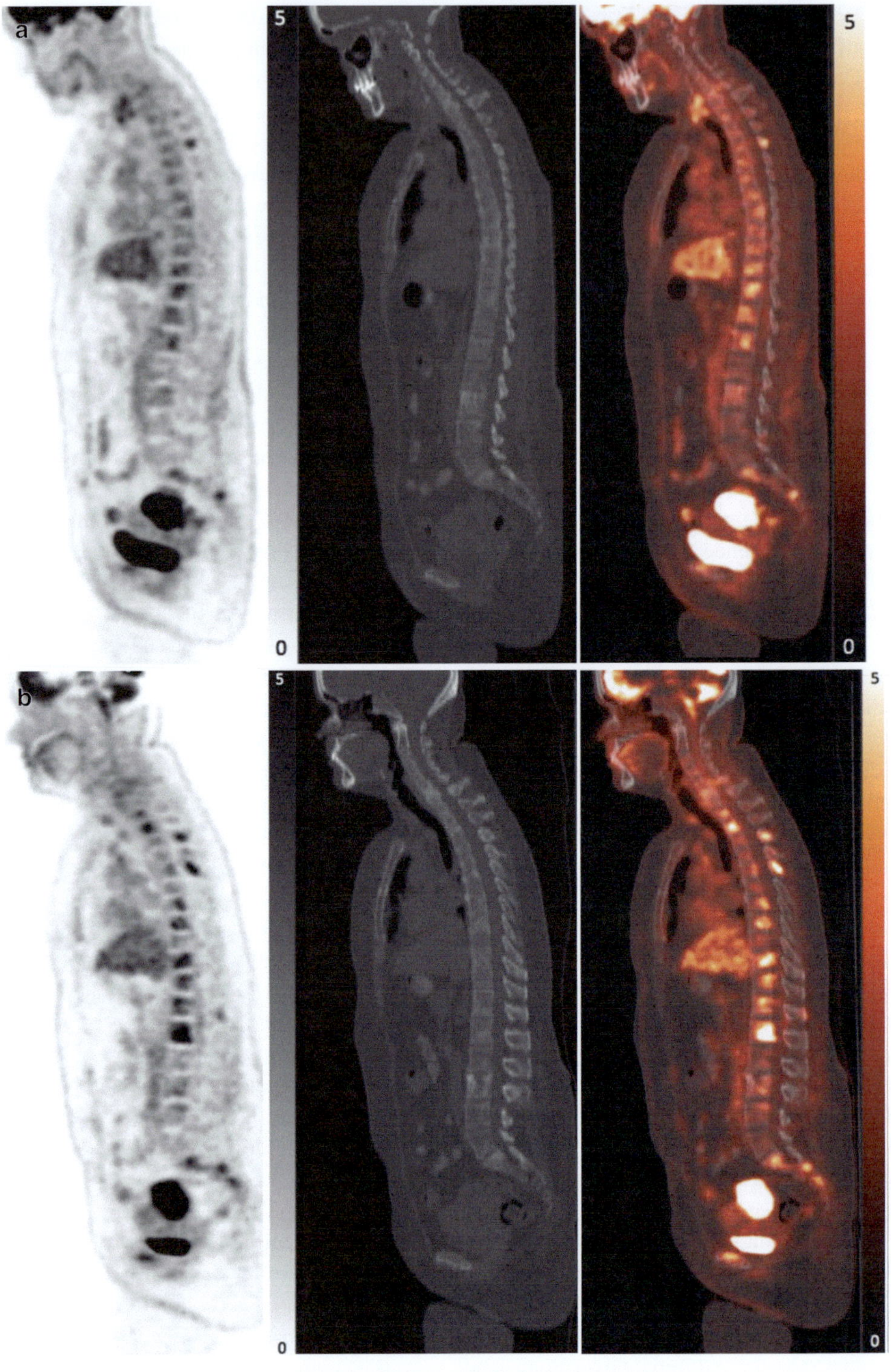

Fig. 20.2 Fifty-three-year-old female with a history of ER-positive, HER2-negative metastatic breast cancer. ^{18}F-FDG-PET, CT, and fused images (**a**, top row) demonstrate multiple mixed lytic and sclerotic osseous lesions. Images from a follow-up PET/CT performed 5 months later (**b**) demonstrate worsening of FDG avid osseous disease, with many new lesions seen and previously seen lesions demonstrating an increase in FDG uptake. Although some of the patient's previously seen lesions are unchanged anatomically on CT images, PET images add a component of functional imaging and confirm worsening osseous metastatic disease

20.1.5 Role of ^{18}F-FDG-PET/CT in Evaluating Response to Treatment in Breast Cancer

Patients may receive systemic therapy in either an adjuvant setting or a neoadjuvant setting. In the setting of adjuvant treatment where no macroscopic disease is expected, systemic therapy is given following surgery, and therapy is aimed at the treatment of residual microscopic disease. As such, there is no role for ^{18}F-FDG-PET/CT in evaluating treatment response in patients receiving adjuvant therapy, as PET/CT is not useful for identifying microscopic disease. In contrast, neoadjuvant therapy may be given prior to definitive surgery or as a primary treatment modality in patients with stage IV metastatic disease. Given the presence of macroscopic disease, ^{18}F-FDG-PET/CT may play a valuable role for evaluating the response to therapy in these clinical scenarios.

While various anatomic and functional imaging modalities have been used to evaluate treatment response, ^{18}F-FDG-PET/CT may offer additional benefits over the currently used modalities. For example, although contrast-enhanced CT may offer anatomic information regarding changes in size of index lesions, size-based approaches to evaluating treatment response may not be able to identify a pathologic complete response nor identify early treatment changes at a molecular level. ^{99m}Tc-sestamibi has also been used in both the primary diagnosis and the primary tumor response to treatment in the neoadjuvant setting, although it has not been widely utilized for either purpose. This radiopharmaceutical has been used in both scintimammography, where the breast is imaged using conventional nuclear medicine gamma cameras, and breast-specific gamma imaging, in which the breast is imaged using dedicated small field-of-view gamma cameras. Several studies have shown that serial imaging with ^{99m}Tc-sestamibi may predict pathologic response to treatment and that measures of response are similar to those of ^{18}F-FDG-PET [30, 31]. However, unlike ^{18}F-FDG-PET/CT, imaging with ^{99m}Tc-sestamibi is not as effective for evaluating disease outside of the breast—important in restaging patients receiving primary metastatic treatment—and as such, the modality has not gained widespread clinical use.

^{18}F-FDG-PET/CT may provide useful clinical information regarding treatment response, both prior to the completion of therapy and following the completion of therapy. For example, one of the earliest studies by Wahl et al. reported that there was a significant difference in SUV_{max} at baseline and SUV_{max} following 2 months of therapy (mid-cycle) between responders and non-responders, with non-responders demonstrating no significant change in SUV_{max} while responders generally experienced declines in SUV_{max} of 50% or more [32]. Similar findings have been reported in numerous subsequent studies (as reviewed in Mankoff et al. [33]). Several studies have evaluated the role of ^{18}F-FDG-PET/CT in treatment response as early as following one cycle of chemotherapy. For example, in a study by Rousseau et al., the authors found that a decline in SUV_{max} even after only one cycle of chemotherapy was suggestive of a good response to therapy and no change in SUV_{max} following one cycle of chemotherapy was suggestive of a poorer response to therapy [34]. Similarly, following the completion of treatment, ^{18}F-FDG-PET/CT may predict survival outcomes. In a study by Cachin et al. of patients with metastatic breast cancer who completed high-dose chemotherapy, patients with persistent ^{18}F-FDG uptake had a significantly poorer outcome than patients who achieved a complete metabolic response, suggesting that ^{18}F-FDG uptake could stratify survival outcomes [35].

It should be noted that, following chemotherapy, the absence of ^{18}F-FDG uptake may not necessarily indicate complete pathologic response – i.e., absence of disease at histopathologic analysis—as ^{18}F-FDG-PET/CT has reduced sensitivity for detecting small-volume disease, especially after treatment [36]. However, some recent studies have shown that the presence of FDG uptake following completion of therapy was highly predictive of disease relapse and/or disease progression [37]. As such, although ^{18}F-FDG-PET/CT may miss small volume residual disease following therapy, the qualitative presence or absence of FDG-avid disease may provide useful clinical prognostic information in patients.

In addition to chemotherapy, ^{18}F-FDG-PET/CT has also been utilized to follow the response to treatment of several targeted systemic therapies, most notably ER- and HER2-directed therapies. For example, Dehdashti et al. used ^{18}F-FDG-PET as an early indicator of the "flare" response to tamoxifen therapy, which was predictive of subsequent treatment response [38]. Later studies involving an estradiol challenge found that a rise in ^{18}F-FDG uptake of at least 12% (defined as a metabolic flare) was predictive of treatment response and time to progression [39]. Similarly, ^{18}F-FDG-PET/CT may be used to evaluate treatment response to other targeted molecular therapies. For example, early studies have shown promise in the use of serial ^{18}F-FDG-PET which has shown promise in evaluating the response to lapatinib, a HER2-targeted agent [40].

In patients with bone-only or bone-dominant metastatic breast cancer, ^{18}F-FDG-PET/CT provides a means of evaluating changes in osseous lesions. This is of particular value in the subset of patients in which anatomic imaging may be limited. Additionally, although bone scintigraphy may be helpful in the detection of osseous metastatic disease, changes in osseous metastases on bone scan may lag behind treatment response, and in some instances, bone scan may demonstrate a "flare" in response to successful therapy, providing a confusing clinical picture [41]. Stafford et al. found that changes in ^{18}F-FDG uptake in patients with bone-dominant metastatic breast cancer correlated with both the clinical assessment of treatment response and tumor markers [42]. A later study found that changes in ^{18}F-FDG uptake in osseous lesions predicted time to progression [43]. More recent studies utilizing the combined functional and anatomic information from ^{18}F-FDG-PET/CT have shown additional benefit. For example, in a study by Tateishi et al., changes in FDG uptake of index osseous lesions, along with structural changes of increased sclerosis on CT, were predictive of time to progression [44].

20.1.6 Novel Radiotracers

As precision medicine in breast cancer allows treatments to become increasingly personalized and individualized to patients, several new radiotracers—used in both the pre-clinical and the clinical setting—may provide potentially useful diagnostic information. Potential uses include staging of breast cancer, selection of patients for targeted therapies, and the evaluation of treatment response. Here we highlight a few of the most promising non-^{18}F-FDG PET radiotracers on the horizon, including tumor receptors and tumor proliferation markers. Several agents have targeted the imaging of tumor receptors, of which the estrogen receptor and, to a lesser extent, HER2 receptor have shown promise. The benefits of receptor imaging include its non-invasive nature as well as the ability to image expression in the tumor as a whole and avoid sampling error.

The most successful estrogen receptor imaging radiopharmaceutical to date has been 16 alpha-^{18}F-fluoro-17 beta-estradiol (^{18}F-FES). ^{18}F-FES uptake has been validated as a measure of estrogen receptor (ER) binding by both immunohistochemistry and radioligand binding. [45, 46] ^{18}F-FES PET can identify sites of heterogeneous ER expression, such as seen in the case of ER-negative metastatic disease arising from an ER-positive primary tumor [47, 48]. Additionally, multiple prior studies have shown that both qualitative and quantitative ^{18}F-FES uptake can identify patients that are most likely to benefit from estrogen receptor therapy with either selective estrogen receptor modulators or aromatase inhibitors. Greater ^{18}F-FES SUV_{max} on baseline studies correlated with a positive response to endocrine therapy [48–51]. Additional studies have reported that, following the initiation of endocrine therapy, the degree of ^{18}F-FES uptake corresponded to blockade of the ER and that decreases in SUV_{max} following treatment were predictive of treatment response. One of the earliest studies by Mortimer et al. of 40 patients with ER-positive breast cancer treated with tamoxifen demonstrated that, after 7–10 days of treatment, ^{18}F-FES uptake decreased compared to baseline representing an early blockade of the ER. The percent decrease in ^{18}F-FES uptake was greater in patients who ultimately had a clinical response as compared to those who did not [51]. Furthermore, ^{18}F-FES uptake may provide some information as to the dose of estrogen receptor antagonist required to block the estrogen receptor [49] (Fig. 20.3).

In addition to targeted imaging of the estrogen receptor, several potential agents aimed at imaging HER2 receptor expression have been

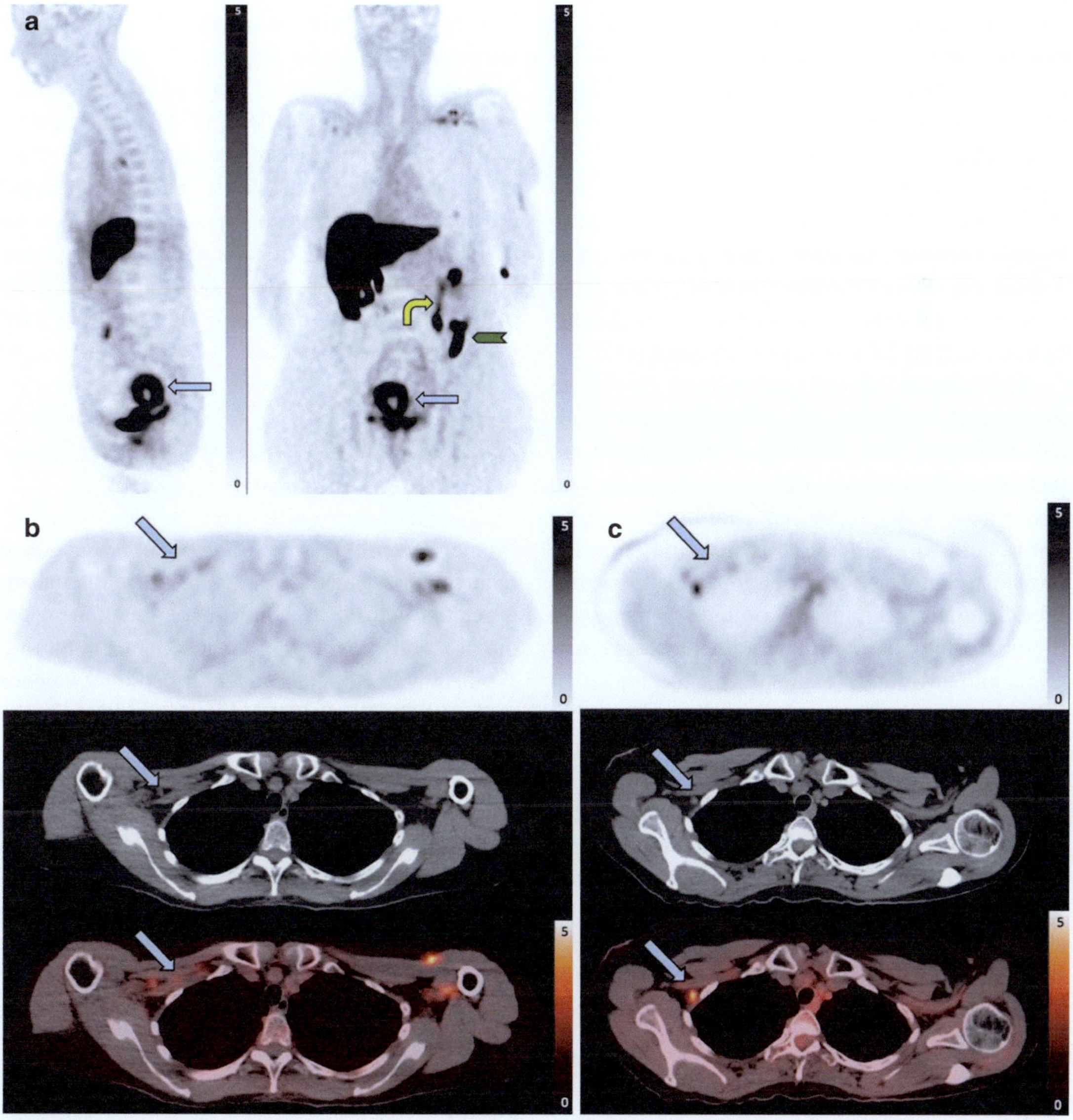

Fig. 20.3 Sixty-six-year-old female with ER/PR-positive, HER2-negative breast cancer status post bilateral mastectomy. ^{18}F-FES-PET (**a**) demonstrates physiologic distribution of ^{18}F-FES. In addition to gastrointestinal (green arrowhead) and renal excretion (curved yellow arrow), there is marked radiotracer uptake in the uterus (blue arrow), which can serve as an internal control during examinations. Axial ^{18}F-FES-PET/CT images (**b**) demonstrate mildly radiotracer avid right subpectoral lymph nodes. Radiotracer uptake in the left axilla is related to the injection of the tracer. Axial ^{18}F-FDG-PET/CT images (**c**) demonstrate that these right subpectoral lymph nodes are also mildly hypermetabolic. These lymph nodes are indeterminate in etiology but are suspicious for metastatic disease

developed. Radiolabeling of trastuzumab, a monoclonal antibody that binds to the extracellular domain of the HER2 receptor, has been studied with several radiopharmaceuticals, including ^{111}In- and ^{89}Zr-labeled radiotracers, which have shown the ability to image tumoral HER2 expression [52–56]. In a recent study of HER2 receptor imaging from Gebhart et al., 56 patients underwent pre-treatment HER2 PET/CT with ^{89}Zr-trastuzumab as well as ^{18}F-FDG-PET/CT at baseline and prior to a second cycle of treatment with trastuzumab emtansine. The authors found that combined HER2-PET/CT and ^{18}F-FDG-PET/CT accurately predicted morphological response and discriminated patients with a relatively short time-to-treatment-failure from those with a relatively longer time-to-treatment-failure (median 2.8 months vs. 15 months) [54].

Additionally, several radiotracers aimed at imaging of cellular proliferation have been studied. Increased rates of cellular proliferation are features of malignancy, and, in combination with tumor size, nodal status, and hormone receptor status, cellular proliferation indices may provide prognostic information for patients. Cellular proliferation has been most commonly measured by measuring Ki-67 using immunohistochemistry, a human protein expressed in the nuclei of cells during all phases of the cell cycle except G_0 [57]. Recently, several thymidine analogue radiotracers have been studied as a measure of cellular proliferation based on the activity of the enzyme thymidine-kinase 1, which is overexpressed during the S phase of the cell cycle and which has been shown to correlate with Ki-67 expression [58]. One of the earliest radiotracers, ^{11}C-thymidine, showed promise in tumoral proliferation imaging but is of limited clinical applicability due to its complex synthetic process as well as its short half-life (approximately 20 min) [59]. More recently, ^{18}F-fluorothymidine (FLT) has shown promise as a thymidine analogue for imaging cellular proliferation. Although larger-scale studies are needed, several studies have reported that ^{18}F-FLT-PET/CT has promise for imaging early treatment effects and potentially identifying early responders/non-responders to treatment [60–62].

20.2 Ovarian Cancer

20.2.1 Epidemiology

Ovarian cancer is the second most commonly diagnosed gynecologic cancer in the United States, with an estimated 21,290 new cases diagnosed in 2015. With an estimated 14,180 deaths attributable to the disease in 2015, ovarian cancer was the leading cause of death in women among gynecologic malignancies [1]. Ovarian cancers are most commonly surface epithelial tumors, of which serous, mucinous, and endometrioid are the most common subtypes [63]. Recognized risk factors for the disease include nulliparity, early menarche, late menopause, family history of ovarian cancer, increasing age, and personal history of breast cancer.

20.2.2 Ovarian Cancer Detection and Diagnosis

Women with ovarian cancer often present at a relatively advanced stage in the disease, which is related both to the clinical presentation of the disease and the lack of a good screening test. Women with certain cancer-susceptibility genes such as BRCA1, BRCA2, MLH1, and MSH2 are at an increased risk for developing the disease. Women with ovarian cancer may be asymptomatic or experience vague, non-specific symptoms such as abdominal fullness and bloating early in the disease. These symptoms may not be recognized by providers, leading to decreased detection of the disease at an early stage. Despite the highly lethal nature of the disease, screening of the general population with pelvic examination, pelvic ultrasound, or tumor markers such as serum cancer antigen-125 (CA-125) is not currently recommended by any national organization due to the overall low prevalence of the disease and lack of mortality benefit. However, for patients at a higher risk (such as those with BRCA1), screening with pelvic ultrasound may be of use [64].

Although serum CA-125 is the most commonly used tumor marker in the evaluation of ovarian cancer, its specificity for the disease is limited, particularly in pre-menopausal patients, as the marker may be elevated in a variety of benign conditions such as endometriosis, tubo-ovarian abscess, ovarian cystadenoma, and follicular cysts. Additionally, elevated levels of serum CA-125 may be seen in patients with non-ovarian malignancies including those with pancreatic, gastric, and colorectal cancer [65].

Ultrasound is the most commonly used modality to evaluate and characterize ovarian lesions, owing in part to its lack of ionizing radiation and relative cost. Although ultrasound may be used to identify suspicious imaging features such as mural nodularity or thick papillary projections, characterization with ultrasound alone may lead to unnecessary surgery for benign lesions [66]. As such, contrast-enhanced pelvic MRI may aid in characterization of sonographically indeterminate ovarian lesions and help in delineating benign versus malignant tumors [67]. Following suspicious findings on either ultrasound or MRI, consideration is usually given to surgery rather than biopsy due to the potential for peritoneal seeding and upstaging of the tumor [68].

20.2.3 Role of ^{18}F-FDG-PET/CT in the Primary Diagnosis of Ovarian Cancer

^{18}F-FDG-PET/CT is of limited use in the primary diagnosis of ovarian cancer due to its physiologic ovarian activity in pre-menopausal patients as well as both its false-negative and false-positive results. Increased ^{18}F-FDG uptake may be seen in the ovaries of pre-menopausal women both at ovulation and in the early luteal phase of the menstrual cycle [69]. As such, if practical, consideration can be given to scheduling ^{18}F-FDG-PET/CT for a few days after the menstrual flow phase of the menstrual cycle to diminish physiologic uptake, if desired [70]. However, any FDG uptake in the ovaries of a post-menopausal woman is considered abnormal.

Although patterns of ^{18}F-FDG uptake in ovarian lesions can suggest clues regarding their behavior, FDG uptake cannot reliably distinguish a benign versus a borderline or malignant ovarian lesion. For example, increased ^{18}F-FDG uptake may be seen in benign lesions such as endometriomas, fibromas, and dermoid cysts, and early-stage or low-grade ovarian tumors may not demonstrate increased ^{18}F-FDG uptake above that of background [63]. However, in general, malignant ovarian tumors demonstrate a higher SUV_{max} than benign ovarian lesions [71]. Additionally, several studies have found that ^{18}F-FDG uptake can be valuable in distinguishing benign versus malignant ovarian lesions. In a study by Nam et al. of 133 women with suspected ovarian cancer, ^{18}F-FDG-PET/CT had superior accuracy (92%) as compared to either pelvic ultrasound or CT/MRI (83% and 75%, respectively) in distinguishing benign versus borderline/malignant ovarian tumors [72]. However, the cystic nature of some ovarian lesions may limit the utility of ^{18}F-FDG-PET/CT, and a negative ^{18}F-FDG-PET/CT does not exclude early malignancy. As such, any suspicious ovarian lesion should be followed with pelvic ultrasound or MRI [67].

In patients with known ovarian malignancies, patterns of ^{18}F-FDG uptake cannot reliably predict the grade or histology of an ovarian tumor. In a study of 160 patients with suspected ovarian cancer (of which 67 patients were pathologically proven to have malignant tumors), Tanizaki et al. found that different subtypes of ovarian cancer trended toward varying patterns of ^{18}F-FDG uptake, with serous and endometrioid adenocarcinomas more often ^{18}F-FDG avid and with higher SUV_{max} values than patients with clear cell or mucinous adenocarcinoma or metastatic carcinoma, which were less frequently ^{18}F-FDG avid and with lower SUV_{max} values [73]. An additional study by Karantanis et al. found that ^{18}F-FDG uptake is not related to tumor grade or histology, as the authors found no statistically significant correlation between SUV_{max} and tumor grade, nor did they find a significant difference between SUV_{max} of serous versus endometrioid tumors [74].

20.2.4 Role of ^{18}F-FDG-PET/CT in Ovarian Cancer Staging

Ovarian cancer staging is based on the International Federation of Gynecology and

Obstetrics (FIGO) surgical-pathologic staging system as well as the Tumor Node Metastasis (TNM) classification system from the American Joint Committee on Cancer [10, 75]. ^{18}F-FDG-PET/CT may play a valuable role in the detection of locoregional lymph node and distant metastases in patients with ovarian cancer. The most common site of lymph node metastases in patients with ovarian cancer include the inguinal, pelvic, para-aortic and retroperitoneal, and mediastinal lymph node chains. Although contrast-enhanced CT and, less frequently, MRI have been the conventional modalities used for staging, ^{18}F-FDG-PET/CT has been increasingly utilized in primary ovarian cancer staging, and studies have suggested that the modality may be superior to CT. In a study by Nam et al., staging with ^{18}F-FDG-PET/CT was concordant with surgical staging in 78% of cases, and the authors found unexpected extra-abdominal metastases in 15.8% of patients. Unknown concomitant primary malignancies were found in 3.8% of patients, where ^{18}F-FDG-PET/CT detected five unknown primary malignancies: two thyroid cancers, two breast cancers, and one pancreatic neuroendocrine tumor [72]. Similarly, Castellucci et al. found that ^{18}F-FDG-PET/CT resulted in greater concordance with surgical staging than staging with contrast-enhanced CT (69% for ^{18}F-FDG-PET/CT vs. 53% for CT). Additionally, the authors found that CT incorrectly downstaged four out of six patients with stage IV cancer by missing distant metastases in the liver, pleura, mediastinum, and left supraclavicular lymph nodes [76]. Indeed, ^{18}F-FDG-PET/CT may be useful in identifying metastatic lymphadenopathy in otherwise normal-sized lymph nodes that do not meet CT size criteria for pathologic involvement. Despite its potential uses in ovarian cancer staging, it should be noted that ^{18}F-FDG-PET/CT may be of limited value in patients with peritoneal metastatic disease, where false-negative studies have been reported. A study by De Iaco et al. found that the percentage of false-negative cases was inversely related to the size of the lesion and noted that in patients with lesions smaller than 5 mm (such as seen in peritoneal carcinomatosis), there was a high rate of false-negative studies [77].

20.2.5 Role of ^{18}F-FDG-PET/CT in the Response to Treatment of Ovarian Cancer

Follow-up of patients with ovarian cancer most frequently consists of serial evaluation with tumor markers such as CA-125, which can suggest trends in treatment response, as well as imaging, most commonly with contrast-enhanced CT or, less commonly, MRI. These modalities can compare morphologic changes in index lesions as well as identify potential new sites of disease. However, there are inherent limitations of both CT and MRI in evaluating the response to treatment of the disease, as anatomic changes may require more time before they are evident and CT and MRI may have difficulty in identifying residual disease versus fibrosis [78].

During the course of treatment, ^{18}F-FDG-PET/CT may play a valuable role in identifying patients who fail to respond to therapy. In a study by Avril et al. of 33 patients with advanced ovarian cancer receiving neoadjuvant chemotherapy, the authors found a higher chance of overall survival in patients who achieved a >20% decrease in SUV_{max} after one cycle of chemotherapy and a >55% decrease in SUV_{max} after three cycles of chemotherapy [79]. In a study by Martoni et al. in 42 patients with advanced ovarian cancer who received ^{18}F-FDG-PET/CT at baseline and following both three and six cycles of neoadjuvant chemotherapy, patients who had a normalization of SUV_{max} values after three cycles of chemotherapy had a higher likelihood of achieving a complete pathologic response following an additional three cycles of chemotherapy than those who did not [80]. Similarly, ^{18}F-FDG-PET/CT may have a valuable role in evaluating response to treatment following treatment completion. In a study by Sironi et al. of 31 patients with ovarian cancer treated by primary cytoreductive surgery followed by chemotherapy, ^{18}F-FDG-PET/CT demonstrated an overall lesion-based sensitivity, specificity, accuracy, positive predictive value, and negative predictive value of 78% (90% for lesions greater than 1 cm), 75%, 77%, 89%, and 57%, respectively. No lesions larger than 0.5 cm were missed on ^{18}F-FDG-PET/CT [81]. In patients with advanced disease, ^{18}F-FDG-PET/CT could aid in preventing second look surgery. In a study by Lee et al. of 55 patients with advanced ovarian cancer who had undergone cytoreductive surgery and adjuvant chemotherapy, there was no significant difference in progression-free interval and disease-free interval in patients who had undergone ^{18}F-FDG-PET as compared to patients who underwent second look laparotomy [82].

20.2.6 Role of ^{18}F-FDG-PET/CT in Recurrent Ovarian Cancer

Patients with advanced ovarian cancer suffer a high rate of recurrence, estimated at 75–80% for patients with stage III disease and 90–95% for patients with stage IV disease [83]. Although rising CA-125 levels may suggest the presence of recurrent disease, imaging studies are needed for anatomic localization. CT and MRI are limited in that these modalities cannot identify metabolically active disease in normal-sized lymph nodes. As such, ^{18}F-FDG-PET/CT may have improved accuracy compared to either CT or CA-125 in detecting and localizing recurrent disease. In a study by Bristow et al. of 14 patients with asymptomatic rising serum CA-125 levels and negative or equivocal CT scans, ^{18}F-FDG-PET/CT detected recurrent ovarian cancer in retroperitoneal lymph nodes in 11/14 patients [84]. Similarly, in a prospective trial by Fulham et al. of 90 patients with recurrent ovarian cancer, pre-treatment evaluation with ^{18}F-FDG-PET/CT yielded additional, unknown sites of disease in 68% of patients resulting in a change in clinical management in 60% of patients [85]. This improved accuracy may be demonstrated in patients regardless of primary tumor grade. In a study by Antunovic et al. of 121 women with ovarian cancer, ^{18}F-FDG-PET/CT demonstrated superior accuracy compared to conventional CT for the detection of recurrent disease for patients with both low-grade and high-grade tumors [83].

20.2.7 Novel Radiotracers in Ovarian Cancer

Several non-^{18}F-FDG-labeled radiotracers have been studied both in the diagnosis and evaluation of treatment response in patients with ovarian cancer. These include ^{18}F-fluorothymidine (FLT), ^{11}C-methionine (MET), and ^{89}Zr-bevacizumab. As an essential amino acid, radiolabeling of methionine has been applied to evaluate both amino acid transport and tumor metabolism. In an early study of four patients with benign ovarian lesions, two patients with borderline ovarian tumors, and seven patients with malignant ovarian lesions, ^{11}C-MET accumulated in all ovarian carcinomas but did not accumulate in either the benign or borderline lesions [86]. With regard to treatment response, both ^{18}F-FLT and ^{89}Zr-bevacizumab have been studied with promising results. In a study by Munk Jensen et al. using a mouse model of human ovarian cancer treated with carboplatin and paclitaxel and evaluated both prior to and during treatment with ^{18}F-FDG and ^{18}F-FLT-PET, the authors found that both ^{18}F-FLT and ^{18}F-FDG-PET provided valuable information regarding treatment response. ^{18}F-FLT-PET showed an early, transient response to therapy, while ^{18}F-FDG-PET demonstrated a later, prolonged response [87]. Another radiotracer, ^{89}Zr-bevacizumab, has undergone early testing to monitor tumor VEGF-A expression as a biomarker of antiangiogenic effects in patients receiving everolimus, an mTOR inhibitor [88].

20.3 Endometrial Cancer

20.3.1 Epidemiology

Endometrial cancer is the most common gynecologic cancer in the United States and the fourth most common cancer in women, accounting for approximately 7% of all cancers diagnosed in women [1]. Commonly recognized risk factors for the disease include endometrial hyperplasia, tamoxifen use, and unopposed estrogen states such as obesity, anovulatory state, poly-cystic ovarian syndrome, and hyperinsulinemia [89, 90]. The two main subtypes of endometrial cancer are endometrioid (80–90% of cases) and non-endometrioid tumors, of which adenocarcinoma is the most common subtype. Additional less common histologies include adenosquamous, clear cell, and papillary serous carcinoma. Prognostic factors include tumor stage, histologic grade, lymph node status, and the presence and depth of myometrial invasion. Of note, clear cell and papillary serous carcinoma tend to carry an overall worse prognosis than other histologic subtypes, as these may spread in a pattern similar to that of ovarian cancer, with vascular invasion and peritoneal deposits [91].

20.3.2 Endometrial Cancer Detection, Diagnosis, and Staging

Patients with endometrial cancer most commonly present with abnormal uterine bleeding, typically in post-menopausal patients; however, due to early detection, over 70% of patients are stage I at diagnosis. Following clinical evaluation, transvaginal ultrasound is the most commonly used imaging modality in the evaluation of abnormal uterine bleeding, which may demonstrate a thickened endometrium (greater than 5 mm in post-menopausal patients) or a polypoid mass projecting into the endometrial cavity. Following biopsy and pathologic diagnosis, pelvic MRI is the most commonly utilized imaging modality in staging, as it aids in delineating local extent of tumor and potential myometrial or cervical invasion [92]. Several studies have demonstrated that contrast enhanced pelvic MRI was 84–93% accurate in assessing the depth of myometrial involvement and 90–92% accurate in assessing for cervical invasion (reviewed in Barwick et al. [92]). This is in contrast to CT, which is limited by poor soft tissue contrast and difficulty in delineating the primary tumor from the surrounding myometrium.

Endometrial cancer staging is surgical-pathological based on the FIGO staging system and includes exploratory laparotomy, total abdominal hysterectomy, bilateral salpingo-oophorectomy, and peritoneal lavage. Lymphadenectomy may be performed in patients with high-risk stage I disease and beyond or certain high-risk subtypes such as clear cell or papillary serous carcinoma [93]. When it spreads, endometrial cancer most commonly invades the myometrium first and then spreads distantly both lymphatically and hematogenously. Although the location of the primary tumor is usually known prior to staging, the location of the lymph node metastases can suggest the anatomic location of the primary tumor. Tumors in the middle and lower thirds of the uterus tend to drain laterally into the paracervical, parametrial, and obturator lymph nodes, while tumors in the upper third of the uterine corpus and the fundus tend to drain to the common iliac and obturator lymph nodes. Inguinal lymph nodes may also be involved, most commonly through tumor spread through the round ligament [94].

With regard to endometrial cancer, ^{18}F-FDG-PET/CT is most useful in the detection of distant metastatic disease. Several studies have demonstrated that it is highly specific, though only moderately sensitive, for the detection of locoregional lymph node metastases. For example, in a study by Picchio et al. of 32 patients with high-risk endometrial cancer, ^{18}F-FDG-PET/CT demonstrated a high sensitivity for both the detection of the primary tumor and distant metastatic disease (90.6% and 100%, respectively) but was markedly less sensitive in detecting nodal disease (57.1%) [95]. In a study by Kitajima et al. of 40 patients who underwent pre-operative ^{18}F-FDG-PET/CT prior to lymphadenectomy, ^{18}F-FDG-PET/CT was superior to conventional imaging in detecting nodal metastases but demonstrated only an overall 53% sensitivity (93% for lesions larger than 10 mm, 67% for lesions between 4 and 9 mm in diameter, and 16.7% for lesions less than 4 mm in diameter). As such, the authors concluded that even ^{18}F-FDG-PET/CT could not replace lymphadenectomy [96]. Despite its limitations in detecting locoregional lymph node metastases, ^{18}F-FDG-PET/CT plays a valuable role in identifying distant metastatic disease, with numerous studies suggesting that it is superior to either CT or MRI. For example, in a study by Suzuki et al. of 30 patients with endometrial cancer, ^{18}F-FDG-PET demonstrated superior sen-

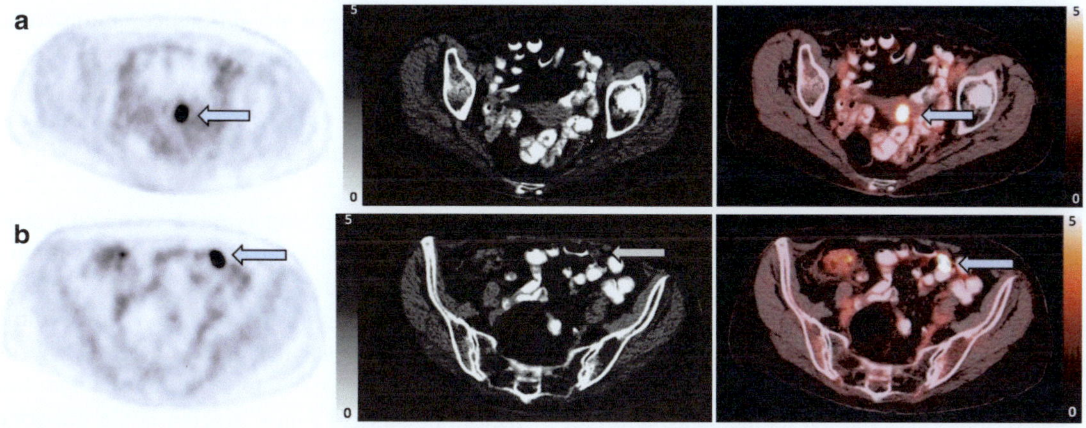

Fig. 20.4 Eighty-five-year-old female with a history of papillary adenocarcinoma of the endometrium. Staging ^{18}F-FDG-PET/CT demonstrates a hypermetabolic focus in the region of the endometrium (blue arrow, **a**) which represents the patient's primary tumor. An FDG avid omental implant is seen in the left lower quadrant (blue arrow, **b**) representing metastatic disease

sitivity as compared to either CT or MRI (83% as compared to 67%) in detecting extra-uterine, non-retroperitoneal lymph node metastases [97] (Fig. 20.4).

20.3.3 Role of ^{18}F-FDG-PET/CT in Evaluating Treatment Response in Endometrial Cancer

In patients in whom recurrent endometrial cancer is suspected, anatomic localization of sites of recurrent disease is critical. Patients with locally recurrent disease frequently are treated with surgery or radiation therapy, whereas patients with distant disease are treated with chemotherapy or endocrine therapy. In patients in whom recurrent disease is suspected, several studies have demonstrated that ^{18}F-FDG-PET/CT plays a valuable role in localizing tumor recurrence. In a study by Belhocine et al., ^{18}F-FDG-PET identified recurrent disease in 26 out of 41 studies, including on three studies in which recurrent disease was not suspected. The authors also reported that ^{18}F-FDG-PET impacted the clinical options in 9 out of 26 patients with confirmed recurrent disease [98]. Similarly, in a study by Chung et al. of 31 women with suspected recurrent endometrial cancer, the overall sensitivity, specificity, and accuracy of ^{18}F-FDG-PET/CT were 100%, 94.7%, and 92.3%, respectively. The authors reported that ^{18}F-FDG-PET/CT changed management in seven patients (22.6%), resulting in five patients undergoing previously unplanned procedures and preventing procedures in two patients [99].

20.3.4 Novel Radiotracers in Endometrial Cancer Imaging

Although there have been fewer studies in endometrial cancer as compared to breast cancer, a few studies have suggested a potential role of ^{18}F-FES in imaging endometrial cancer, which frequently expresses ER. The majority of published studies evaluated the role of ^{18}F-FES in primary tumor staging and evaluating tumor heterogeneity. For example, in a study by Tsujikawa et al. of 22 patients with endometrial adenocarcinoma and 9 patients with endometrial hyperplasia who underwent preoperative ^{18}F-FES-PET/CT and ^{18}F-FDG-PET/CT, the authors reported that there was a significant difference in SUV between high-risk and low-risk carcinoma for ^{18}F-FES but not ^{18}F-FDG. High-risk carcinomas had a significantly increased FDG-to-FES ratio compared to low-risk carcinomas. The authors concluded that, as endometrial carcinoma progresses to a higher grade, its glucose metabolism increases while its ER expression (and estrogen dependency) decreases. As such, the FDG-to-FES index could have a potential role in both noninvasive diagnosis and treatment planning [100].

20.4 Cervical Cancer

20.4.1 Epidemiology, Detection, and Diagnosis

Cervical cancer is the third most commonly diagnosed gynecologic malignancy in women in the United States [1]. Though its incidence and mortality have decreased over the past several decades thanks to population-based screening with pap smears, significant health disparities remain, with African-American and Hispanic women continuing to suffer a higher incidence and mortality from the disease as compared to Caucasian women [101]. Risk factors for the disease include high-risk HPV strains (16, 18, 31, 33), low socioeconomic status, chlamydia infection, HIV infection, cigarette smoking, and age at first pregnancy. Vaccines have been developed to help combat infection with HPV, and there are currently two FDA-approved vaccines available in the United States [102].

Early-stage cervical cancer is often asymptomatic, while more advanced tumors most commonly present with abnormal vaginal bleeding or post-coital bleeding. In some cases, advanced tumors may present with symptoms from urinary or bowel obstruction. Although many cases are detected with routine screening, symptomatic patients may undergo physical examination with pap smear as the first portion of their diagnostic workup. Patients with abnormal cells on pap smear usually undergo colposcopy or colposcopy-directed biopsy for further pathologic diagnosis. As such, imaging has little role in the primary detection of cervical cancer. When imaging is performed for the workup of abnormal vaginal bleeding, transvaginal ultrasound is the most commonly utilized modality [103]. Squamous cell carcinoma is the most common histologic subtype of cervical cancer, estimated to account for 80–90% of cases, with adenocarcinoma representing the second most common subtype. Some studies have suggested that adenocarcinomas may portend a slightly worse prognosis, while other studies have shown no difference in outcome based on histologic subtype [104].

20.4.2 Cervical Cancer Staging

Cervical cancer staging is most commonly performed clinically with the International Federation of Gynecology and Obstetrics (FIGO) staging system ('FIGO staging classifications and clinical practice guidelines in the management of gynecologic cancers', [75]). One of the most important factors in cervical cancer staging is the presence or absence of parametrial invasion. While patients with tumors confined to the uterus and upper two-thirds of the vagina (FIGO stage IIA and below) may be treated with surgery, those with parametrial involvement (FIGO stage IIB and above) or tumors larger than 4 cm are typically treated with chemotherapy and radiation therapy [103].

As the disease spreads, local and regional structures are typically first affected, followed by hematogenous spread of the disease to distant sites. Pelvic and para-aortic lymph nodes are commonly affected when there is nodal spread of disease. The liver, lungs, bones, and brain are the most common sites of distant metastatic disease. Although the FIGO classification system is clinical and does not factor lymph node status into staging subcategories, lymph node status is important for treatment planning purposes and disease prognosis [105].

MRI is the most common modality used for evaluating local extent of disease and is preferred over both CT and US due to its superior soft tissue resolution. Although ^{18}F-FDG-PET/CT is most commonly performed during staging to detect nodal or extra-pelvic sites of disease, ^{18}F-FDG uptake may be identified in the primary cervical tumor on staging studies, and the degree of ^{18}F-FDG uptake by the tumor has been shown to vary both with tumor histology and grade. In a study by Kidd et al. of 240 patients with cervical cancer undergoing pre-treatment PET/CT, the authors reported that SUV_{max} was significantly different for squamous compared to non-squamous tumors, as well as well-differentiated versus poorly differentiated tumors [104]. As such, although not performed for the purposes of evaluation of local tumor, findings on ^{18}F-FDG-PET/CT may be suggestive of certain primary tumor characteristics.

Contrast-enhanced CT is commonly performed as part of cervical cancer staging, as it may detect nodal or other extra-pelvic sites of disease not imaged with pelvic MRI. Metastatic lymph nodes may also be identified on MRI imaging. However, both CT and MRI are limited by their ability to detect disease in normal-sized lymph nodes that do not meet size criteria for pathologic involvement. Several studies have reported that ^{18}F-FDG-PET/CT offers improved sensitivity and specificity for lymph node metastases compared to these anatomic modalities. For example, a study by Reinhardt et al. compared the diagnostic accuracy of ^{18}F-FDG-PET to MRI and found that ^{18}F-FDG-PET had improved sensitivity and specificity compared to MRI (91% and 100% for PET as compared to 73% and 83% for MRI) [106]. A study by Grigsby et al. compared ^{18}F-FDG-PET to CT and found that PET identified abnormal lymph nodes more often than did CT and that PET-positive para-aortic lymphadenopathy was a significant prognostic factor for progression-free survival [107]. These studies have supported the use of ^{18}F-FDG PET/CT as a tool for cervical cancer staging.

Despite the utility of PET/CT for lymph node evaluation, ^{18}F-FDG-PET/CT may be falsely negative in cases of microscopic disease or when involved lymph nodes are relatively small in size. For example, in a study by Sironi et al. of 47 patients with cervical cancer who underwent PET/CT prior to surgery, PET/CT correctly identified nodal metastatic disease in 13/18 patients; lymph nodes that were not correctly identified on PET/CT all had a short axis diameter of 0.5 cm or less [108]. Additional studies have questioned the value of PET/CT in patients with early-stage cervical cancer. In a study by Wright et al. of 59 patients with early-stage cervical cancer (stage IIA or below) who underwent ^{18}F-FDG-PET prior to pelvic lymphadenectomy, PET had relatively poor sensitivity (53%) for lymph node metastases, while the specificity was considerably higher (90%) [109]. As such, PET/CT may be of more limited value in patients with early-stage cervical cancer.

In addition to providing clinical information regarding the extent of disease, ^{18}F-FDG-PET/CT may also provide prognostic information and may be a predictor of disease-free survival. For example, in a study by Lee et al. of 44 patients with FIGO stage IB to IIA cervical cancer, the SUV_{max} of the primary cervical tumor was compared to pathologic prognostic factors. Patients with a high primary tumor SUV_{max} prior to treatment (>13.4) had significantly reduced disease-free survival compared to those who did not, and an SUV_{max} of greater than 13.4 was an independent predictor of cervical cancer recurrence following treatment [110]. Additionally, the presence of nodal disease on ^{18}F-FDG-PET/CT can predict cause-specific survival. A study by Singh et al. of 47 patients with FIGO stage IIIB cervical cancer who underwent ^{18}F-FDG-PET prior to therapy found that 3-year cause-specific survival was highly dependent on extent of lymph node disease; for those patients with no lymph node metastases, 3-year cause-specific survival was 73% compared to 58% for those with only pelvic lymph node metastases, 29% for those with pelvic and para-aortic lymph node metastases, and 0% for those with pelvic, para-aortic, and supraclavicular lymph node metastases [111] (Fig. 20.5).

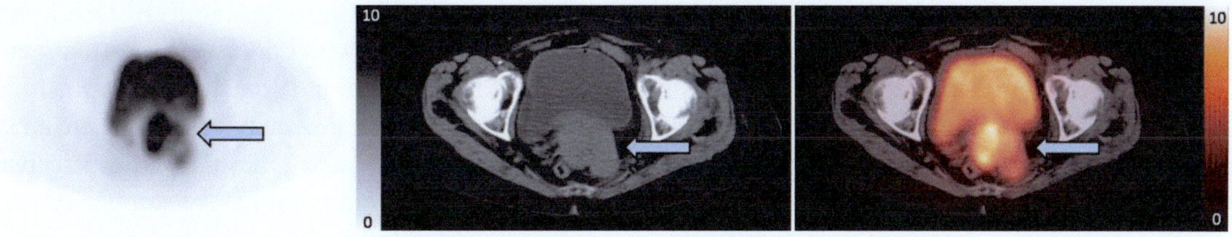

Fig. 20.5 Sixty-nine-year-old female with newly diagnosed cervical cancer. Axial PET, CT, and fused images from the patient's staging ^{18}F-FDG-PET/CT demonstrate a markedly FDG avid, friable cervical mass (blue arrows) representing her primary cervical cancer

20.4.3 PET/CT in the Evaluation of the Response to Treatment of Cervical Cancer

^{18}F-FDG-PET/CT has a valuable role in evaluating both the response to treatment in patients receiving neoadjuvant chemotherapy as well as detecting recurrent disease. Several studies have demonstrated that persistent ^{18}F-FDG uptake in patients following the completion of therapy may predict cause-specific survival. For example, Schwarz et al. studied 92 women who underwent ^{18}F-FDG-PET at 3 months following completion of external irradiation, brachytherapy, and concurrent chemotherapy. Post-therapy PET demonstrated a complete metabolic response in 70% of patients, a partial metabolic response in 16% of patients, and progressive disease in 13% of patients. The 3-year progression-free survival rates differed significantly between groups, with 78% for those achieving a complete metabolic response, 33% for those achieving only a partial metabolic response, and 0% for those with disease progression on the 3-month ^{18}F-FDG-PET [112]. Similarly, in a study by Grigsby et al. of 152 patients with cervical carcinoma who underwent pre- and post-treatment ^{18}F-FDG-PET, new or persistent ^{18}F-FDG uptake following completion of therapy was the most significant prognostic factor for developing metastatic disease and death from cervical cancer when compared to both pre-treatment factors such as lymph node status as well as treatment-related prognostic factors [113].

^{18}F-FDG-PET/CT is useful for detecting recurrent disease in patients both in whom recurrent disease is clinically expected and asymptomatic patients. For example, in a study by Havrilesky et al. of patients with suspected recurrent cervical cancer undergoing post-treatment FDG-PET, the authors reported the sensitivity and specificity of ^{18}F-FDG-PET for detecting recurrent cervical cancer as 86% and 87%, respectively. A positive predictive value was calculated at 86% with a negative predictive value of 87% [114]. Several studies have found that ^{18}F-FDG-PET detected recurrent disease in asymptomatic patients or patients in whom recurrent disease was not clinically suspected [115–117]. For example, in a study by Brooks et al. of 103 patients treated with definitive chemoradiation for advanced cervical cancer, ^{18}F-FDG-PET found recurrent disease in nine asymptomatic patients (eight patients with locoregional recurrent disease and one patient with distant metastatic disease) [115]. Similarly, a retrospective study by Mittra et al. of 30 symptomatic and asymptomatic women who underwent ^{18}F-FDG-PET/CT following therapy reported true-positive recurrent disease in 44% of asymptomatic women. For symptomatic patients, 71% of patients had true-positive findings on PET/CT [116]. As such, ^{18}F-FDG-PET/CT may play a valuable role in surveillance for recurrent disease both in a symptomatic and asymptomatic population.

20.4.4 Novel Radiotracers

Although several new radiotracers have been studied for both the diagnosis and treatment of cervical cancer, the most promising early work involves new radiotracers aimed at imaging tumor hypoxia. Hypoxia is a component of malignancy, and tumoral hypoxia contributes to the progression of malignant disease by several potential mechanisms including the elimination of p53 tumor suppressor activity as well as angiogenesis. Several studies have explored the role of radiocopper-labeled diacetyl-bis(N_4-methylthiosemicarbazone) (Cu-ATSM) in imaging tumoral hypoxia. For example, Grigsby et al. imaged 15 patients with cervical cancer prior to treatment with ^{60}CU-ATSM-PET and found that patients with hypoxic tumors ($n = 6$) had a significantly worse 4-year overall survival than those patients with non-hypoxic tumors ($n = 9$), with 4-year survival estimates of 33% versus 75%, respectively [118]. Similarly, a study by Dehdashti et al. of 38 women who underwent pre-treatment ^{60}CU-ATSM-PET found that tumoral uptake of the radiotracer was inversely related to progression-free survival and cause-specific survival [119]. Although most studies of copper-ATSM have utilized radiolabeling to ^{60}CU, ^{64}CU-ATSM-PET may be superior to ^{60}CU-ATSM-PET for hypoxia imaging. ^{64}CU-ATSM has a longer half-life (12.7 h vs. 0.4 h for ^{60}CU-ATSM) and results in images with less noise compared to ^{60}CU-ATSM-PET [120]. However, further larger-scale studies are needed to continue to explore the potential role of tumoral hypoxia imaging in the treatment of patients with cervical cancer.

20.4.5 PET/MRI

Although this chapter has focused on the use of PET/CT, the role of PET/MRI is being further explored in patients with pelvic gynecologic malignancies. Compared to CT, MRI has improved soft tissue resolution, which may lead to better delineation of local extent of tumor, and is less affected by streak artifact from bone or metal in the pelvis. MRI further benefits from the lack of ionizing radiation, which is a clinical consideration in patients who might be undergoing numerous follow-up studies. In a study of 19 patients with suspected recurrent pelvic malignancies, Beiderwellen et al. found that, although PET/MRI and PET/CT offered equivalently high diagnostic value, PET/MRI offered improved diagnostic confidence in discriminating benign versus malignant lesions [121]. However, there are still many hurdles limiting the broad application of PET/MRI, including long scan times and addressing a means to correct for photon attenuation, as MR data cannot be directly extrapolated in the same way as CT data for attenuation correction [122]. Although preliminary studies are promising, more research is needed to delineate the future value of PET/MRI.

References

1. Siegel RL, Miller KD, Jemal A. Cancer statistics, 2015. CA Cancer J Clin. 2015;65(1):5–29.
2. Howell A, Anderson AS, Clarke RB, Duffy SW, Evans DG, Garcia-Closas M, Gescher AJ, Key TJ, Saxton JM, Harvie MN. Risk determination and prevention of breast cancer. Breast Cancer Res. 2014;16(5):1–19.
3. Schnitt SJ. Traditional and newer pathologic factors. JNCI Monogr. 2001;2001(30):22–6.
4. Walker RA. Immunohistochemical markers as predictive tools for breast cancer. J Clin Pathol. 2008;61(6):689–96.
5. Perou CM, Sorlie T, Eisen MB, van de Rijn M, Jeffrey SS, Rees CA, Pollack JR, Ross DT, Johnsen H, Akslen LA, Fluge O, Pergamenschikov A, Williams C, Zhu SX, Lonning PE, Borresen-Dale A-L, Brown PO, Botstein D. Molecular portraits of human breast tumours. Nature. 2000;533:747–52.
6. Friedewald SM, Rafferty EA, Rose SL, Durand MA, Plecha DM, Greenberg JS, Hayes MK, Copit DS, Carlson KL, Cink TM, Barke LD, Greer LN, Miller DP, Conant EF. Breast Cancer screening using tomosynthesis in combination with digital mammography. JAMA. 2014;311(24):2499–507.
7. McDonald ES, McCarthy AM, Akhtar A, Synnestvedt MB, Schnall M, Conant EF. Baseline screening mammography: performance of full-field digital mammography versus digital breast Tomosynthesis. AJR. 2015;205:1143–8.
8. Skaane P, Bandos AI, Gullien R, Eben EB, Ekseth U, Haakenaasen U, Izadi M, Jebsen IN, Krager M, Niklason L, Hofvind S, Gur D. Comparison of digital mammography alone and digital mammography plus tomosynthesis in a population-based screening program. Radiology. 2013;267(1):47–56.
9. Mainiero MB, Lourenco A, Mahoney MC, Newell MS, Bailey L, Barke LD, D'Orsi C, Harvey JA, Hayes MK, Huynh PT, Jokich PM, Lee S-J, Lehman CD, Mankoff DA, Nepute JA, Patel SB, Reynolds HE, Sutherland ML, Haffty BG. ACR appropriateness criteria breast cancer screening. J Am Coll Radiol. 2013;10(1):11–4.
10. Edge S, Byrd D, Compton C, Green F, Trotti A. AJCC cancer staging manual. 7th ed. New York, NY: Springer; 2010.
11. Newman EA, Newman LA. Lymphatic mapping techniques and sentinel lymph node biopsy in breast cancer. Surg Clin N Am. 2007;87(2):353–64.
12. Aarsvold JN, Alazraki NP. Update on detection of sentinel lymph nodes in patients with breast cancer. Seminars in Nuclear Medicine. 2005;35(2):116–28.
13. Azad AK, Rajaram MVS, Metz WL, Cope FO, Blue MS, Vera DR, Schlesinger LS. γ-Tilmanocept, a new radiopharmaceutical tracer for Cancer sentinel lymph nodes, binds to the mannose receptor (CD206). J Immunol. 2015;195(5):2019–29.
14. Gradishar WJ, Anderson BO, Balassanian R, Blair SL, Burstein HJ, Cyr A, Elias AD, Farrar WB, Forero A, Giordano SH, Goetz M, Goldstein LJ, Hudis CA, Isakoff SJ, Marcom PK, Mayer IA, McCormick B, Moran M, Patel SA, Pierce LJ, Reed EC, Salerno KE, Schwartzberg LS, Smith KL, Smith Lou M, Soliman H, Somlo G, Telli M, Ward JH, Shead DA, Kumar R. Invasive breast cancer version 1.2016, NCCN clinical practice guidelines in oncology. J Natl Compr Canc Netw. 2016;14(3):324–54.
15. Bos R, van Der Hoeven JJM, van Der Wall E, van Der Groep P, van Diest PJ, Comans EFI, Joshi U, Semenza GL, Hoekstra OS, Lammertsma AA, Molthoff CFM. Biologic correlates of (18)fluorodeoxyglucose uptake in human breast cancer measured

by positron emission tomography. J Clin Oncol. 2002;20(2):379–87.
16. Scheidhauer K, Walter C, Seemann MD. FDG PET and other imaging modalities in the primary diagnosis of suspicious breast lesions. Eur J Nucl Med Mol Imaging. 2004;31(0):S70–9.
17. Rosen EL, Eubank WB, Mankoff DA. FDG PET, PET/CT, and breast cancer imaging. Radiographics. 2007;27(Suppl 1):S215–29.
18. Wahl RL, Siegel BA, Coleman RE, Gatsonis CG, Group PETS. Prospective multicenter study of axillary nodal staging by positron emission tomography in breast Cancer: a report of the staging breast cancer with PET study group. J Clin Oncol. 2003;22(2):277–85.
19. Groheux D, Hindié E, Delord M, Giacchetti S, Hamy A, de Bazelaire C, de Roquancourt A, Vercellino L, Toubert M-E, Merlet P, Espié M. Prognostic impact of (18)FDG-PET-CT findings in clinical stage III and IIB breast cancer. J Natl Cancer Inst. 2012;104(24):1879–87.
20. Byrd DR, Dunnwald LK, Mankoff DA, Anderson BO, Moe RE, Yeung RS, Schubert EK, Eary JF. Internal mammary lymph node drainage patterns in patients with breast cancer documented by breast lymphoscintigraphy. Ann Surg Oncol. 2001;8(3):234–40.
21. Tran A, Pio BS, Khatibi B, Czernin J, Phelps ME, Silverman DHS. ^{18}F-FDG PET for staging breast cancer in patients with inner-quadrant versus outer-quadrant tumors: comparison with long-term clinical outcome. J Nucl Med. 2005;46(9):1455–9.
22. Chia S, Swain SM, Byrd DR, Mankoff DA. Locally advanced and inflammatory breast cancer. J Clin Oncol. 2008;26(5):786–90.
23. Walker GV, Niikura N, Yang W, Rohren E, Valero V, Woodward WA, Alvarez RH, Lucci A, Ueno NT, Buchholz TA. Pretreatment staging positron emission tomography/computed tomography in patients with inflammatory breast cancer influences radiation treatment field designs. Int J Rad Oncol Biol Phys. 2012;83(5):1381–6.
24. Jensen AØ, Jacobsen JB, Nørgaard M, Yong M, Fryzek JP, Sørensen HT. Incidence of bone metastases and skeletal-related events in breast cancer patients: a population-based cohort study in Denmark. BMC Cancer. 2011;11(1):29.
25. Hamaoka T, Madewell JE, Podoloff DA, Hortobagyi GN, Ueno NT. Bone imaging in metastatic breast cancer. J Clin Oncol. 2004;22(14):2942–53.
26. Schirrmeister H, Guhlmann A, Santjohanser C, Ku T, Kreienberg R, Messer P, Nu K, Elsner K, Glatting G, Tra H, Neumaier B, Diederichs C, Reske SN. Early detection and accurate description of extent of metastatic bone disease in breast cancer with fluoride ion and positron emission tomography. J Clin Oncol. 2017;17(8):2381–9.
27. Cook GJ, Houston S, Rubens R, Maisey MN, Fogelman I. Detection of bone metastases in breast cancer by ^{18}FDG PET: differing metabolic activity in osteoblastic and osteolytic lesions. J Clin Oncol. 1998;16(10):3375–9.
28. Morris PG, Lynch C, Feeney JN, Patil S, Howard J, Larson SM, Dickler M, Hudis CA, Jochelson M, McArthur HL. Integrated positron emission tomography/computed tomography may render bone scintigraphy unnecessary to investigate suspected metastatic breast cancer. J Clin Oncol. 2010;28(19):3154–9.
29. Mahner S, Schirrmacher S, Brenner W, Jenicke L, Habermann CR, Avril N, Dose-Schwarz J. Comparison between positron emission tomography using 2-[fluorine-18]fluoro-2-deoxy-D-glucose, conventional imaging and computed tomography for staging of breast cancer. Ann Oncol. 2008;19(7):1249–54.
30. Mankoff D, Dunnwald L, Gralow J, Ellis G, Drucker M, Livingston R. Monitoring the response of patients with locally advanced breast carcinoma to neoadjuvant chemotherapy using technetium 99m-sestamibi scintimammography. Cancer. 1999;85:2410–23.
31. Tiling R, Linke R, Untch M. ^{18}F-FDG PET and ^{99m}Tc-sestamibi scintimammography for monitoring breast cancer response to neoadjuvant chemotherapy: a comparative study. Eur J Nucl Med Mol Imaging. 2001;28:711–20.
32. Wahl RL, Zasadny K, Helvie M, Hutchins GD, Weber B, Cody R. Metabolic monitoring of breast cancer chemohormonotherapy using positron emission tomography: initial evaluation. J Clin Oncol. 1993;11(11):2101–11.
33. Mankoff DA, Dunnwald LK. Changes in glucose metabolism and blood flow following chemotherapy for breast cancer. PET Clin. 2006;1(1):71–81.
34. Rousseau C, Devillers A, Sagan C, Ferrer L, Bridji B, Campion L, Ricaud M, Bourbouloux E, Doutriaux I, Clouet M, Berton-Rigaud D, Bouriel C, Delecroix V, Garin E, Rouquette S, Resche I, Kerbrat P, Chatal JF, Campone M. Monitoring of early response to neoadjuvant chemotherapy in stage II and III breast cancer by [^{18}F]fluorodeoxyglucose positron emission tomography. J Clin Oncol. 2006;24(34):5366–72.
35. Cachin F, Prince HM, Hogg A, Ware RE, Hicks RJ. Powerful prognostic stratification by [^{18}F]fluorodeoxyglucose positron emission tomography in patients with metastatic breast Cancer treated with high-Dose chemotherapy. J Clin Oncol. 2006;24(19):3026–31.
36. Burcombe RJ, Makris A, Pittam M, Lowe J, Emmott J, Wong WL. Evaluation of good clinical response to neoadjuvant chemotherapy in primary breast cancer using [^{18}F]-fluorodeoxyglucose positron emission tomography. Eur J Cancer. 2002;38(3):375–9.
37. Emmering J, Krak NC, Van der Hoeven JJM, Spreeuwenberg MD, Twisk JWR, Meijer S, Pinedo HM, Hoekstra OS. Preoperative [^{18}F] FDG–PET after chemotherapy in locally advanced breast cancer: prognostic value as compared with histopathology. Ann Oncol. 2008;19(9):1573–7.
38. Dehdashti F, Mortimer JE, Trinkaus K, Naughton MJ, Ellis M, Katzenellenbogen JA, Welch MJ, Siegel BA. PET-based estradiol challenge as a predictive biomarker of response to endocrine therapy in women

with estrogen-receptor-positive breast cancer. Breast Cancer Res Treat. 2009;113(3):509–17.
39. Ellis MJ, Gao F, Dehdashti F, Jeffe DB, Marcom PK, Carey LA, Dickler MN, Silverman P, Crowder R, Siegel BA. Lower-dose vs high-dose oral estradiol therapy of hormone receptor–positive, aromatase inhibitor–resistant advanced breast cancer: a phase 2 randomized study. JAMA. 2009;302(7):774–80.
40. Kawada K, Murakami K, Sato T, Kojima Y, Ebi H, Mukai H, Tahara M, Shimokata K, Minami H. Prospective study of positron emission tomography for evaluation of the activity of lapatinib, a dual inhibitor of the ErbB1 and ErbB2 tyrosine kinases, in patients with advanced tumors. Jpn J Clin Oncol. 2007;37(1):44–8.
41. Coleman RE, Mashiter G, Whitaker KB, Moss DW, Rubens RD, Fogelman I. Bone scan flare predicts successful systemic therapy for bone metastases. J Nucl Med. 1988;29(8):1354–9.
42. Stafford SE, Gralow JR, Schubert EK, Rinn KJ, Dunnwald LK, Livingston RB, Mankoff DA. Use of serial FDG PET to measure the response of bone-dominant breast cancer to therapy. Acad Radiol. 2002;9(8):913–21.
43. Specht JM, Tam SL, Kurland BF, Gralow JR, Livingston RB, Linden HM, Ellis GK, Schubert EK, Dunnwald LK, Mankoff DA. Serial 2-[^{18}F] fluoro-2-deoxy-d-glucose positron emission tomography (FDG-PET) to monitor treatment of bone-dominant metastatic breast cancer predicts time to progression (TTP). Breast Cancer Res Treat. 2007;105(1):87–94.
44. Emmering J, Krak NC, Van der Hoeven JJM, Spreeuwenberg MD, Twisk JWR, Meijer S, Pinedo HM, Hoekstra OS. Preoperative [^{18}F] FDG–PET after chemotherapy in locally advanced breast cancer: prognostic value as compared with histopathology. Ann Oncol. 2008;19(9):1573–7.
45. Mintun MA, Welch MJ, Siegel BA, Mathias CJ, Brodack JW, McGuire AH, Katzenellenbogen JA. Breast cancer: PET imaging of estrogen receptors. Radiology. 1988;169(1):45–8.
46. Peterson LM, Mankoff DA, Lawton T, Yagle K, Schubert EK, Stekhova S, Gown A, Link JM, Tewson T, Krohn KA. Quantitative imaging of estrogen receptor expression in breast Cancer with PET and ^{18}F-Fluoroestradiol. J Nucl Med. 2008;49(3):367–74.
47. Dehdashti F, Mortimer JE, Siegel BA, Griffeth LK, Bonasera TJ, Fusselman MJ, Detert DD, Cutler PD, Katzenellenbogen JA, Welch MJ. Positron tomographic assessment of estrogen receptors in breast cancer: comparison with FDG-PET and in vitro receptor assays. J Nucl Med. 1995;36(10):1766–74.
48. Linden HM, Stekhova SA, Link JM, Gralow JR, Livingston RB, Ellis GK, Petra PH, Peterson LM, Schubert EK, Dunnwald LK, Krohn KA, Mankoff DA. Quantitative fluoroestradiol positron emission tomography imaging predicts response to endocrine treatment in breast cancer. J Clin Oncol. 2006;24(18):2793–9.
49. van Kruchten M, de Vries EG, Glaudemans AW, van Lanschot MC, van Faassen M, Kema IP, Brown M, Schröder CP, de Vries EF, Hospers GA. Measuring residual estrogen receptor availability during fulvestrant therapy in patients with metastatic breast cancer. Cancer Discov. 2015;5(1):72–81.
50. Linden HM, Kurland BF, Peterson LM, Schubert EK, Gralow JR, Specht JM, Ellis GK, Lawton TJ, Livingston RB, Petra PH, Link JM, Krohn KA, Mankoff DA. Fluoroestradiol positron emission tomography reveals differences in pharmacodynamics of aromatase inhibitors, tamoxifen, and Fulvestrant in patients with metastatic breast cancer. Clin Cancer Res. 2011;17(14):4799–805.
51. Mortimer JE, Dehdashti F, Siegel BA, Trinkaus K, Katzenellenbogen JA, Welch MJ. Metabolic flare: Indicator of hormone responsiveness in advanced breast cancer. J Clin Oncol. 2001;19(11):2797–803.
52. Clark AS, DeMichele A, Mankoff D. HER2 imaging in the ZEPHIR study. Ann Oncol. 2016;27(4):555–7.
53. Dijkers ECF, Kosterink JGW, Rademaker AP, Perk LR, van Dongen GAMS, Bart J, de Jong JR, de Vries EGE, Hooge MNL. Development and characterization of clinical-grade ^{89}Zr-Trastuzumab for HER2/neu ImmunoPET imaging. J Nucl Med. 2009;50(6):974–81.
54. Gebhart G, Lamberts LE, Wimana Z, Garcia C, Emonts P, Ameye L, Stroobants S, Huizing M, Aftimos P, Tol J, Oyen WJG, Vugts DJ, Hoekstra OS, Schröder CP, Menke-van der Houven van Oordt CW, Guiot T, Brouwers AH, Awada A, de Vries EGE, Flamen P. Molecular imaging as a tool to investigate heterogeneity of advanced HER2-positive breast cancer and to predict patient outcome under trastuzumab emtansine (T-DM1): the ZEPHIR trial. Ann Oncol. 2016;27(4):619–24.
55. de Korte MA, de Vries EGE, Lub-de Hooge MN, Jager PL, Gietema JA, van der Graaf WTA, Sluiter WJ, van Veldhuisen DJ, Suter TM, Sleijfer DT, Perik PJ. ^{111}Indium-trastuzumab visualises myocardial human epidermal growth factor receptor 2 expression shortly after anthracycline treatment but not during heart failure: a clue to uncover the mechanisms of trastuzumab-related cardiotoxicity. Eur J Cancer. 2007;43(14):2046–51.
56. Perik PJ, Lub-De Hooge MN, Gietema JA, Van Der Graaf WTA, De Korte MA, Jonkman S, Kosterink JGW, Van Veldhuisen DJ, Sleijfer DT, Jager PL, De Vries EGE. Indium-111-labeled trastuzumab scintigraphy in patients with human epidermal growth factor receptor 2-positive metastatic breast cancer. J Clin Oncol. 2006;24(15):2276–82.
57. Edmonds CE, Mankoff DA. Molecular pathology of breast cancer. In: Badve S, Gökmen-Polar Y, editors. Molecular pathology of breast cancer. Cham: Springer; 2016. p. 187–206.
58. Chudgar AV, Mankoff DA. Molecular imaging and precision medicine in breast cancer. PET Clin. 2017;12(1):39–51.

59. Mankoff DA, Shields AF, Krohn KA. PET imaging of cellular proliferation. Radiol Clin N Am. 2005;43(1):153–67.
60. Kenny L. The use of novel PET tracers to image breast cancer biologic processes such as proliferation, DNA damage and repair, and angiogenesis. J Nucl Med. 2016;57(Suppl 1):89S–95S.
61. Kenny L, Coombes RC, Vigushin DM, Al-Nahhas A, Shousha S, Aboagye EO. Imaging early changes in proliferation at 1 week post chemotherapy: a pilot study in breast cancer patients with 3′-deoxy-3′-[^{18}F] fluorothymidine positron emission tomography. Eur J Nucl Med Mol Imaging. 2007;34(9):1339–47.
62. Kostakoglu L, Duan F, Idowu MO, Jolles PR, Bear HD, Muzi M, Cormack J, Muzi JP, Pryma DA, Specht JM, Hovanessian-Larsen L, Miliziano J, Mallett S, Shields AF, Mankoff DA. A phase II study of 3'-deoxy-3′-^{18}F-fluorothymidine PET in the assessment of early response of breast cancer to neoadjuvant chemotherapy: results from ACRIN 6688. J Nucl Med. 2015;56(11):1681–9.
63. Khiewvan B, Torigian DA, Emamzadehfard S, Paydary K, Salavati A, Houshmand S, Werner TJ, Alavi A. An update on the role of PET/CT and PET/MRI in ovarian cancer. Eur J Nucl Med Mol Imaging. 2017;44(6):1079–91.
64. Schorge JO, Modesitt SC, Coleman RL, Cohn DE, Kauff ND, Duska LR, Herzog TJ. SGO white paper on ovarian cancer: etiology, screening and surveillance. Gynecol Oncol. 2010;119(1):7–17.
65. Holcomb K, Vucetic Z, Miller MC, Knapp RC. Human epididymis protein 4 offers superior specificity in the differentiation of benign and malignant adnexal masses in premenopausal women. Am J Obstet Gynecol. 2011;205(4):358.e1–6.
66. Outwater EK, Dunton CJ. Imaging of the ovary and adnexa: clinical issues and applications of MR imaging. Radiology. 1995;194(1):1–18.
67. Grab D, Flock F, Stöhr I, Nüssle K, Rieber A, Fenchel S, Brambs H-J, Reske SN, Kreienberg R. Classification of asymptomatic adnexal masses by ultrasound, magnetic resonance imaging, and positron emission tomography. Gynecol Oncol. 2000;77(3):454–9.
68. Mohaghegh P, Rockall AG. Imaging strategy for early ovarian cancer: characterization of adnexal masses with conventional and advanced imaging techniques. Radiographics. 2012;32(6):1751–73.
69. Kim S-K, Kang KW, Roh JW, Sim JS, Lee ES, Park S-Y. Incidental ovarian ^{18}F-FDG accumulation on PET: correlation with the menstrual cycle. Eur J Nucl Med Mol Imaging. 2005;32(7):757–63.
70. Nishizawa S, Inubushi M, Ozawa F, Kido A, Okada H. Physiological FDG uptake in the ovaries after hysterectomy. Ann Nucl Med. 2007;21(6):345–8.
71. Yamamoto Y, Oguri H, Yamada R, Maeda N, Kohsaki S, Fukaya T. Preoperative evaluation of pelvic masses with combined ^{18}F-fluorodeoxyglucose positron emission tomography and computed tomography. Int J Gynecol Obstet. 2008;102(2):124–7.
72. Nam EJ, Yun MJ, Oh YT, Kim JW, Kim JH, Kim S, Jung YW, Kim SW, Kim YT. Diagnosis and staging of primary ovarian cancer: correlation between PET/CT, Doppler US, and CT or MRI. Gynecol Oncol. 2010;116(3):389–94.
73. Tanizaki Y, Kobayashi A, Shiro M, Ota N, Takano R, Mabuchi Y, Yagi S, Minami S, Terada M, Ino K. Diagnostic value of preoperative SUVmax on FDG-PET/CT for the detection of ovarian cancer. Int J Gynecol Cancer. 2014;24(3):454–60.
74. Karantanis D, Allen-Auerbach M, Czernin J. Relationship among glycolytic phenotype, grade, and histological subtype in ovarian carcinoma. Clin Nucl Med. 2012;37(1):49–53.
75. Benedet JL, Bender H, Jones H, Ngan HY, Pecorelli S. FIGO staging classifications and clinical practice guidelines in the management of gynecologic cancers. Int J Gynecol Obstet. 2000;70(2):209–62.
76. Castellucci P, Perrone AM, Picchio M, Ghi T, Farsad M, Nanni C, Messa C, Meriggiola MC, Pelusi G, Al-Nahhas A, Rubello D, Fazio F, Fanti S. Diagnostic accuracy of ^{18}F-FDG PET/CT in characterizing ovarian lesions and staging ovarian cancer: correlation with transvaginal ultrasonography, computed tomography, and histology. Nucl Med Commun. 2007;28(8):589–95.
77. De Iaco P, Musto A, Orazi L, Zamagni C, Rosati M, Allegri V, Cacciari N, Al-Nahhas A, Rubello D, Venturoli S, Fanti S. FDG-PET/CT in advanced ovarian cancer staging: value and pitfalls in detecting lesions in different abdominal and pelvic quadrants compared with laparoscopy. Eur J Radiol. 2011;80(2):e98–e103.
78. Schwarz JK, Grigsby PW, Dehdashti F, Delbeke D. The role of ^{18}F-FDG PET in assessing therapy response in cancer of the cervix and ovaries. J Nucl Med. 2009;50(Suppl 1):64S–73S.
79. Avril N, Sassen S, Schmalfeldt B, Naehrig J, Rutke S, Weber WA, Werner M, Graeff H, Schwaiger M, Kuhn W. Prediction of response to neoadjuvant chemotherapy by sequential F-18-Fluorodeoxyglucose positron emission tomography in patients with advanced-stage ovarian cancer. J Clin Oncol. 2005;23(30):7445–53.
80. Martoni A, Fanti S, Zamagni C, Rosati M, De Iaco P, D'Errico Grigioni A, et al. [^{18}F]FDG-PET/CT monitoring early identifies advanced ovarian cancer patients who will benefit from prolonged neoadjuvant chemotherapy. Nucl Med Mol Imaging. 2011;55:81–90.
81. Sironi S, Messa C, Mangili G, Zangheri B, Aletti G, Garavaglia E, Vigano R, Picchio M, Taccagni G, Del Maschio A, Fazio F. Integrated FDG PET/CT in patients with persistent ovarian cancer: correlation with histologic findings. Radiology. 2004;233(2):433–40.
82. Lee MC, Kim S, Chung J-K, Kang S-B, Kim M-H, Jeong JM, Lee DS. [^{18}F]FDG PET as a substitute for second-look laparotomy in patients with advanced ovarian carcinoma. Eur J Nucl Med Mol Imaging. 2004;31(2):196–201.

83. Antunovic L, Cimitan M, Borsatti E, Baresic T, Sorio R, Giorda G, Steffan A, Balestreri L, Tatta R, Pepe G, Rubello D, Cecchin D, Canzonieri V. Revisiting the clinical value of ^{18}F-FDG PET/CT in detection of recurrent epithelial ovarian carcinomas: correlation with histology, serum CA-125 assay, and conventional radiological modalities. Clin Nucl Med. 2012;37(8):184–8.
84. Bristow RE, Giuntoli RL, Pannu HK, Schulick RD, Fishman EK, Wahl RL. Combined PET/CT for detecting recurrent ovarian cancer limited to retroperitoneal lymph nodes. Gynecol Oncol. 2005;99(2):294–300.
85. Fulham MJ, Carter J, Baldey A, Hicks RJ, Ramshaw JE, Gibson M. The impact of PET-CT in suspected recurrent ovarian cancer: a prospective multi-centre study as part of the Australian PET data collection project. Gynecol Oncol. 2009;112(3):462–8.
86. Lapela M, Leskinen-Kallio S, Varpula M, Grénman S, Salmi T, Alanen K, Någren K, Lehikoinen P, Ruotsalainen U, Teräs M. Metabolic imaging of ovarian tumors with carbon-11-methionine: a PET study. J Nucl Med. 1995;36(12):2196–200.
87. Munk Jensen M, Erichsen K, Bjorkling F, Madsen J, Buhl Jensen P, Sehested M, Hojgaard L, Kjær A. Imaging of treatment response to the combination of carboplatin and paclitaxel in human ovarian cancer xenograft tumors in mice using FDG and FLT PET. PLoS One. 2013;8(12):e85126.
88. van der Bilt ARM, van Scheltinga AGTT, Timmer-Bosscha H, Schröder CP, Pot L, Kosterink JGW, van der Zee AGJ, Hooge MNL, de Jong S, de Vries EGE, Reyners AKL. Measurement of tumor VEGF-A levels with ^{89}Zr-bevacizumab PET as an early biomarker for the antiangiogenic effect of Everolimus treatment in an ovarian cancer xenograft model. Clin Cancer Res. 2012;18(22):6306–14.
89. Nead KT, Sharp SJ, Thompson DJ, Painter JN, Savage DB, Semple RK, Barker A, Australian National Endometrial Cancer Study Group, Perry JRB, Attia J, Dunning AM, Easton DF, Holliday E, Lotta LA, O'Mara T, McEvoy M, Pharoah PDP, Scott RJ, Spurdle AB, Langenberg C, Wareham NJ, Scott RA. Evidence of a causal association between insulinemia and endometrial cancer: a mendelian randomization analysis. J Natl Cancer Inst. 2015;107(9):djv178.
90. Ziel HK, Finkle WD. Increased risk of endometrial carcinoma among users of conjugated estrogens. N Engl J Med. 1975;293(23):1167–70.
91. Peungjesada S, Bhosale PR, Balachandran A, Iyer RB. Magnetic resonance imaging of endometrial carcinoma. J Comp Assist Tomogr. 2009;33(4):601.
92. Barwick TD, Rockall AG, Barton DP, Sohaib SA. Imaging of endometrial adenocarcinoma. Clin Radiol. 2006;61(7):545–55.
93. Petru E, Lück H-J, Stuart G, Gaffney D, Millan D, Vergote I. Gynecologic cancer intergroup (GCIG) proposals for changes of the current FIGO staging system. Eur J Obstet Gynecol Reprod Biol. 2009;143(2):69–74.
94. Mariani A, Webb MJ, Keeney GL, Podratz KC. Routes of lymphatic spread: a study of 112 consecutive patients with endometrial cancer. Gynecol Oncol. 2001;81(1):100–4.
95. Picchio M, Mangili G, Gajate AMS, De Marzi P, Spinapolice EG, Mapelli P, Giovacchini G, Sigismondi C, Viganò R, Sironi S, Messa C. High-grade endometrial cancer: value of [^{18}F]FDG PET/CT in preoperative staging. Nucl Med Commun. 2010;31(6):506–12.
96. Kitajima K, Murakami K, Yamasaki E, Fukasawa I, Inaba N, Kaji Y, Sugimura K. Accuracy of ^{18}F-FDG PET/CT in detecting pelvic and paraaortic lymph node metastasis in patients with endometrial cancer. Am J Roentgenol. 2008;190(6):1652–8.
97. Suzuki R, Miyagi E, Takahashi N, Sukegawa A, Suzuki A, Koike I, Sugiura K, Okamoto N, Inoe T, Hirahara F. Validity of positron emission tomography using fluoro-2-deoxyglucose for the preoperative evaluation of endometrial cancer. Int J Gynecol Cancer. 2007;17(4):890–6.
98. Belhocine T, De Barsy C, Hustinx R, Willems-Foidart J. Usefulness of ^{18}F-FDG PET in the post-therapy surveillance of endometrial carcinoma. Eur J Nucl Med Mol Imaging. 2002;29(9):1132–9.
99. Chung HH, Kang WJ, Kim JW, Park N-H, Song Y-S, Chung J-K, Kang S-B. The clinical impact of [^{18}F]FDG PET/CT for the management of recurrent endometrial cancer: correlation with clinical and histological findings. Eur J Nucl Med Mol Imaging. 2008;35(6):1081–8.
100. Tsujikawa T, Yoshida Y, Kudo T, Kiyono Y, Kurokawa T, Kobayashi M, Tsuchida T, Fujibayashi Y, Kotsuji F, Okazawa H. Functional images reflect aggressiveness of endometrial carcinoma: estrogen receptor expression combined with ^{18}F-FDG PET. J Nucl Med. 2009;50(10):1598–604.
101. Sawaya GF, Huchko MJ. Cervical Cancer screening. Med Clin N Am. 2017;101(4):743–53.
102. American Cancer Society. Cancer facts and figures 2016. Atlanta, GA: American Cancer Society; 2016.
103. Wildenberg JC, Yam BL, Langer JE, Jones LP. US of the nongravid cervix with multimodality imaging correlation: normal appearance, pathologic conditions, and diagnostic pitfalls. Radiographics. 2016;36(2):596–617.
104. Kidd EA, Spencer CR, Huettner PC, Siegel BA, Dehdashti F, Rader JS, Grigsby PW. Cervical cancer histology and tumor differentiation affect ^{18}F-fluorodeoxyglucose uptake. Cancer. 2009;115(15):3548–54.
105. Rauch GM, Kaur H, Choi H, Ernst RD, Klopp AH, Boonsirikamchai P, Westin SN, Marcal LP. Optimization of MR imaging for pretreatment evaluation of patients with endometrial and cervical cancer. Radiographics. 2014;34(4):1082–98.
106. Reinhardt MJ, Ehritt-Braun C, Vogelgesang D, Ihling C, Högerle S, Mix M, Moser E, Krause TM. Metastatic lymph nodes in patients with cer-

vical cancer: detection with MR imaging and FDG PET. Radiology. 2001;218(3):776–82.
107. Grigsby PW, Siegel BA, Dehdashti F. Lymph node staging by positron emission tomography in patients with carcinoma of the cervix. J Clin Oncol. 2001;19(17):3745–9.
108. Sironi S, Buda A, Picchio M, Perego P, Moreni R, Pellegrino A, Colombo M, Mangioni C, Messa C, Fazio F. Lymph node metastasis in patients with clinical early-stage cervical Cancer: detection with integrated FDG PET/CT. Radiology. 2006;238(1):272–9.
109. Wright JD, Dehdashti F, Herzog TJ, Mutch DG, Huettner PC, Rader JS, Gibb RK, Powell MA, Gao F, Siegel BA, Grigsby PW. Preoperative lymph node staging of early-stage cervical carcinoma by [^{18}F]-fluoro-2-deoxy-D-glucose-positron emission tomography. Cancer. 2005;104(11):2484–91.
110. Lee Y-Y, Choi CH, Kim CJ, Kang H, Kim T-J, Lee J-W, Lee J-H, Bae D-S, Kim B-G. The prognostic significance of the SUV_{max} (maximum standardized uptake value) for F-18 fluorodeoxyglucose of the cervical tumor in PET imaging for early cervical cancer: preliminary results. Gynecol Oncol. 2009;115(1):65–8.
111. Singh AK, Grigsby PW, Dehdashti F, Herzog TJ, Siegel BA. FDG-PET lymph node staging and survival of patients with FIGO stage IIIb cervical carcinoma. Int J Rad Oncol Biol Phys. 2003;56(2):489–93.
112. Schwarz JK, Siegel BA, Dehdashti F, Grigsby PW. Association of posttherapy positron emission tomography with tumor response and survival in cervical carcinoma. JAMA. 2007;298(19):2289–95.
113. Grigsby PW, Siegel BA, Dehdashti F, Rader J, Zoberi I. Posttherapy [^{18}F]fluorodeoxyglucose positron emission tomography in carcinoma of the cervix: response and outcome. J Clin Oncol. 2004;22(11):2167–71.
114. Havrilesky LJ, Wong TZ, Secord AA, Berchuck A, Clarke-Pearson DL, Jones EL. The role of PET scanning in the detection of recurrent cervical cancer. Gynecol Oncol. 2003;90(1):186–90.
115. Brooks RA, Rader JS, Dehdashti F, Mutch DG, Powell MA, Thaker PH, Siegel BA, Grigsby PW. Surveillance FDG-PET detection of asymptomatic recurrences in patients with cervical cancer. Gynecol Oncol. 2009;112(1):104–9.
116. Mittra E, El-Maghraby T, Rodriguez CA, Quon A, McDougall IR, Gambhir SS, Iagaru A. Efficacy of ^{18}F-FDG PET/CT in the evaluation of patients with recurrent cervical carcinoma. Eur J Nucl Med Mol Imaging. 2009;36(12):1952–9.
117. Ryu S-Y, Kim M-H, Choi S-C, Choi C-W, Lee K-H. Detection of early recurrence with ^{18}F-FDG PET in patients with cervical cancer. J Nucl Med. 2003;44(3):347–52.
118. Grigsby PW, Malyapa RS, Higashikubo R, Schwarz JK, Welch MJ, Huettner PC, Dehdashti F. Comparison of molecular markers of hypoxia and imaging with ^{60}Cu-ATSM in cancer of the uterine cervix. Mol Imaging Biol. 2007;9(5):278–83.
119. Dehdashti F, Grigsby PW, Lewis JS, Laforest R, Siegel BA, Welch MJ. Assessing tumor hypoxia in cervical cancer by PET with ^{60}Cu-labeled diacetyl-Bis(N_4-methylthiosemicarbazone). J Nucl Med. 2008;49(2):201–5.
120. Lewis JS, Laforest R, Dehdashti F, Grigsby PW, Welch MJ, Siegel BA. An imaging comparison of ^{64}Cu-ATSM and ^{60}Cu-ATSM in cancer of the uterine cervix. J Nucl Med. 2008;49(7):1177–82.
121. Beiderwellen K, Grueneisen J, Ruhlmann V, Buderath P, Aktas B, Heusch P, Kraff O, Forsting M, Lauenstein TC, Umutlu L. [^{18}F]FDG PET/MRI vs. PET/CT for whole-body staging in patients with recurrent malignancies of the female pelvis: initial results. Eur J Nucl Med Mol Imaging. 2015;42(1):56–65.
122. Lee SI, Catalano OA, Dehdashti F. Evaluation of gynecologic cancer with MR imaging, ^{18}F-FDG PET/CT, and PET/MR imaging. J Nucl Med. 2015;56(3):436–43.

21 PET in Lung Cancer and Mediastinal Malignancies

Florian C. Gaertner

21.1 Lung Cancer

Lung cancer is the main cause of cancer death in the United States, in male and in female patients. It accounts for about one quarter of all cancer-related deaths [1].

Though lung cancer is characterized by a variety of different histologic subtypes [2], traditionally the differentiation between non-small cell lung cancer (NSCLC) and small cell lung cancer (SCLC) is most important for clinical therapy decisions, next to less frequent tumors such as well-differentiated neuroendocrine tumors of the lung (carcinoids) and mesenchymal tumors. NSCLC is a very heterogeneous group of carcinomas, encompassing many different histological subtypes such as adenocarcinoma, squamous cell carcinoma, and large cell carcinoma. NSCLC is diagnosed most frequently, accounting for about 85% of lung cancer cases. SCLC is a neuroendocrine tumor entity with a high proliferation rate. It is typically characterized by a quite aggressive clinical phenotype and makes up for about 15% of lung cancer cases. NSCLC and SCLC show large differences regarding tumor growth dynamics, clinical aggressiveness, and pattern of metastasis and they differ in the employed methods of staging, clinical therapy regimen, and overall prognosis.

^{18}F-Fluorodeoxyglucose (FDG) positron emission tomography/computed tomography (PET/CT) plays an important role in the clinical management of lung cancer. Before a definite diagnosis of lung cancer is established, FDG PET/CT may be helpful in the clinical work-up of solitary pulmonary nodules. In patients with non-metastatic NSCLC, guidelines propose the use of FDG PET/CT in the algorithm for preoperative locoregional staging [3]. Also, in patients with SCLC, FDG PET/CT can be helpful to guide the initial therapy approach. Furthermore, FDG PET/CT can help in the detection of recurrences.

21.1.1 Solitary Pulmonary Nodules

Pulmonary nodules are defined by the Fleischner Society as rounded opacities, well or poorly defined, measuring up to 3 cm in diameter on CT or chest x-ray studies [4]. They are a common incidental finding on whole-body CT scans, with an incidence of about 15% in asymptomatic patients [5].

The etiology of solitary pulmonary nodules can be subsumed under five categories: infectious causes, inflammatory diseases, vascular lesions, benign neoplasms, and malignancies. The size, growth, and margins of a lesion are important predictors of malignancy. Lesions less than 5 mm

F. C. Gaertner (✉)
Department of Nuclear Medicine, University Hospital Bonn, Bonn, Germany
e-mail: florian.gaertner@ukbonn.de

H. Ahmadzadehfar et al. (eds.), *Clinical Nuclear Medicine*,
https://doi.org/10.1007/978-3-030-39457-8_21

in diameter are malignant in less than 1% of cases, whereas the rate of malignancy rises to 6–28% for nodules of 5–10 mm in diameter and reaches 64–82% for lesions larger than 20 mm in diameter. The doubling time of a malignant lesion (regarding volume, not diameter) is typically in the rage between 1 month and 1 year. A lesion that does not show any growth in a 2-year interval is most likely of a benign etiology. Irregularly shaped lesions with spiculae or a lobulated appearance have a high risk of malignancy. However, a well-defined lesion with smooth margins does not exclude malignancy, as 21% of malignant nodules exhibit well-defined margins. Lesion calcifications (central, laminated, diffuse solid, and "popcorn" patterns) are associated with benign etiologies (granulomatous-infectious and hamartomas), as well as evidence of intralesional fat on CT imaging (hamartomas) [6].

Still, in a number of cases, the etiology of solitary pulmonary nodules remains unclear on CT imaging. These nodules require further work-up, e.g., by follow-up imaging or by histopathologic sampling. Especially in cases where histologic sampling is problematic, FDG PET/CT can help to further characterize lesion dignity (Fig. 21.1). Though FDG PET/CT cannot deliver a definite diagnosis, a negative FDG PET/CT result can help to justify an initial conservative approach and may help reduce the number of unnecessary biopsies and thoracotomies due to benign pulmonary nodules [6].

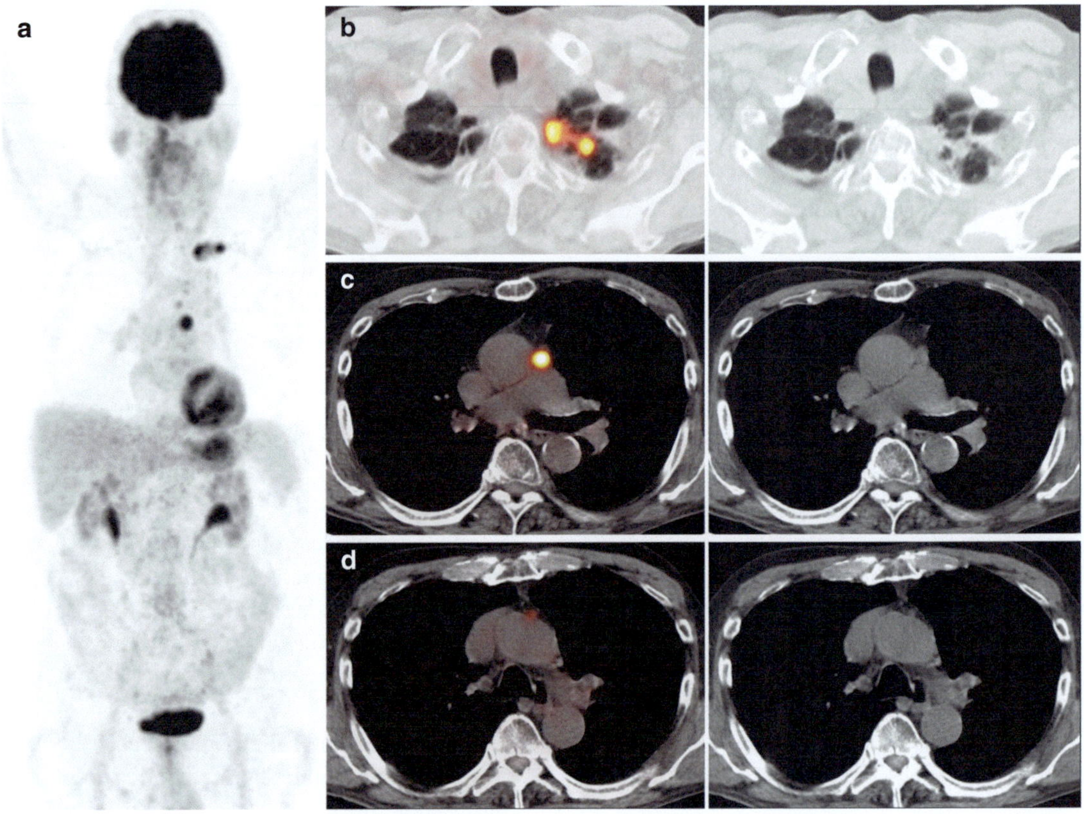

Fig. 21.1 (**a**) FDG PET/CT in an 81-year-old male patient with unclear pulmonary nodules in the left upper lobe next to thickening of the apical pleura. The patient had a history of pulmonary tuberculosis 53 years ago and suffers from bronchial asthma, coronary artery disease, and kidney failure grade III. (**b**) Bifocal hypermetabolism in the region of the mass in the left upper lobe, suspicious of malignancy. (**c, d**) Hypermetabolic ipsilateral mediastinal lymph nodes, suspicious for lymph node metastases. The patient subsequently underwent surgery with evidence of NSCLC (squamous cell carcinoma)

Meta-analyses have shown a sensitivity of 97% and a specificity of 78% for FDG PET in the detection of malignant pulmonary nodules [7], and with the use of combined PET/CT, the specificity further increases to 85% in the differentiation of malignant from benign solitary pulmonary nodules [8].

Regarding sensitivity and specificity, false-positive results are typically encountered more frequently than false negatives. False-positive results can be caused by infectious diseases (e.g., tuberculosis, aspergillosis, histoplasmosis) and inflammatory/granulomatous processes (e.g., sarcoidosis). Especially in geographical regions with high incidence of infectious lung disease, such as histoplasmosis in the South Central United States, specificity can be impaired significantly.

False-negative results may occur due to partial volume effects in small lesions showing less than 8–10 mm in diameter. Also, low- or non-glucose avid malignant processes, such as adenocarcinoma in situ (bronchioloalveolar carcinoma, lepidic growth adenocarcinoma), well-differentiated neuroendocrine tumors (pulmonary carcinoids), or metastases of low-glucose avid malignancies such as renal cell carcinoma or prostate cancer can lead to false-negative results. Furthermore, insufficient patient preparation such as non-fasting state, insulin injection, or hyperglycemia may result in impaired lesional FDG uptake.

Several studies evaluated threshold values for SUV_{max} with the intent to differentiate benign from malignant nodules, with reported cutoff values varying between 2.0 and 3.5. However, there is growing evidence that the use of SUV_{max} as a threshold for differentiation between benign and malignant pulmonary nodules is unrealistic, as it only represents a semi-quantitative measurement which is furthermore influenced by a number of factors, such as scanner type, reconstruction algorithm, partial volume effects, as well as patient parameters such as incubation time, body size, and blood glucose level [6].

Studies evaluating the role of dual-time-point FDG PET/CT imaging to increase accuracy in distinguishing benign from malignant nodules delivered mixed results. Overall, a meta-analysis of ten studies evaluating dual-time-point FDG PET in this indication resulted in a pooled sensitivity of 85% and specificity of 77%, which did not show an improvement over single time-point studies, questioning the added value of dual-time-point FDG PET [9].

21.1.2 NSCLC Primary Staging

For patients with NSCLC, primary staging is pivotal for the decision between curative resection and palliative (radio-)chemotherapy. The UICC TNM classification of NSCLC and SCLC in the 8th edition of 2016 is shown in Table 21.1, and the clinical staging system is shown in Table 21.2 [10]. Complete resection of the tumor in curative intent is the main goal in

Table 21.1 The UICC TNM classification of NSCLC and SCLC (8th edition, 2016) [10]

T: Primary tumor	
TX	Primary tumor cannot be assessed or tumor proven by the presence of malignant cells in sputum or bronchial washings but not visualized by imaging or bronchoscopy
T0	No evidence of primary tumor
Tis	Carcinoma in situ[a]
T1	Tumor 3 cm or less in greatest dimension, surrounded by lung or visceral pleura, without bronchoscopic evidence of invasion more proximal than the lobar bronchus (i.e., not in the main bronchus)[b] • T1mi: Minimally invasive adenocarcinoma[c] • T1a: Tumor 1 cm or less in greatest dimension[b] • T1b: Tumor more than 1 cm but not more than 2 cm in greatest dimension[b] • T1c: Tumor more than 2 cm but not more than 3 cm in greatest dimension[b]
T2	Tumor more than 3 cm but not more than 5 cm or tumor with any of the following features[d]: • Involves the main bronchus regardless of distance to the carina, but without involvement of the carina • Invades visceral pleura • Associated with atelectasis or obstructive pneumonitis that extends to the hilar region involving either part of or the entire lung T2a: Tumor more than 3 cm but not more than 4 cm in greatest dimension T2b: Tumor more than 4 cm but not more than 5 cm in greatest dimension

(continued)

Table 21.1 (continued)

T3	Tumor more than 5 cm but not more than 7 cm in greatest dimension or one that directly invades any of the following, parietal pleura, chest wall (including superior sulcus tumors), phrenic nerve, and parietal pericardium, or separate tumor nodule(s) in the same lobe as the primary
T4	Tumor more than 7 cm or of any size that invades any of the following, diaphragm, mediastinum, heart, great vessels, trachea, recurrent laryngeal nerve, esophagus, vertebral body, and carina, or separate tumor nodule(s) in a different ipsilateral lobe to that of primary
N: Regional lymph nodes	
NX	Regional lymph nodes cannot be assessed
N0	No regional lymph node metastasis
N1	Metastasis in ipsilateral peribronchial and/or ipsilateral hilar lymph nodes and intrapulmonary nodes, including involvement by direct extension
N2	Metastasis in ipsilateral mediastinal and/or subcarinal lymph node(s)
N3	Metastasis in contralateral mediastinal, contralateral hilar, ipsilateral or contralateral scalene, or supraclavicular lymph node(s)
M: Distant metastasis	
M0	No distant metastasis
M1	Distant metastasis M1a: Separate tumor nodule(s) in a contralateral lobe; tumor with pleural or pericardial nodules or malignant pleural or pericardial effusion[e] M1b: Single extrathoracic metastasis in a single organ[f] M1c: Multiple extrathoracic metastasis in a single or multiple organs

[a]This includes adenocarcinoma in situ and squamous carcinoma in situ
[b]The uncommon superficial spreading of tumor of any size with its invasive component limited to the bronchial wall, which may extend proximal to the main bronchus, is also classified as T1a
[c]Solitary adenocarcinoma (not more than 3 cm in greatest dimension), with a predominantly lepidic pattern and not more than 5 mm invasion in greatest dimension in any one focus
[d]T2 tumors with these features are classified as T2a if 4 cm or less or if size cannot be determined and T2b if greater than 4 cm but not larger than 5 cm
[e]Most pleural (pericardial) effusions with lung cancer are due to tumor. In a few patients, however, multiple microscopic examinations of pleural (pericardial) fluid are negative for tumor, and the fluid is non-bloody and is not an exudate. Where these elements and clinical judgment dictate that the effusion is not related to the tumor, the effusion should be excluded as a staging descriptor
[f]This includes involvement of a single non-regional node

Table 21.2 The UICC clinical staging system of NSCLC and SCLC (8th edition, 2016) [10]

Occult carcinoma	TX	N0	M0
Stage 0	Tis	N0	M0
Stage IA	T1	N0	M0
Stage IA1	T1mi, T1a	N0	M0
Stage IA2	T1b	N0	M0
Stage IA3	T1c	N0	M0
Stage IB	T2a	N0	M0
Stage IIA	T2b	N0	M0
Stage IIB	T1a–c, T2a,b T3	N1 N0	M0 M0
Stage IIIA	T1a–c, T2a,b T3 T4	N2 N1 N0,N1	M0 M0 M0
Stage IIIB	T1a–c, T2a,b T3, T4	N3 N2	M0 M0
Stage IIIC	T3, T4	N3	M0
Stage IV	Any T	Any N	M1
Stage IVA	Any T	Any N	M1a, M1b
Stage IVB	Any T	Any N	M1c

clinical stages up to IIIA. Stages IIIB and upward (thus any N3 and any M1) are usually categorized as inoperable—though this threshold becomes increasingly diffuse with the development of new surgical techniques and diagnostic possibilities.

FDG PET/CT plays an important role in primary staging of NSCLC as it has been shown to improve staging accuracy. Examples are shown in Figs. 21.2 and 21.3. The use of FDG PET/CT for primary staging of NSCLC is guideline-recommended and deemed mandatory if the patient is potentially eligible for a curative resection [3].

Assessment of the stage of the primary tumor (T-staging) is mostly dependent on morphological imaging methods, mostly CT (exceptionally also MRI), as T-stage is defined by tumor size, invasion of surrounding structures (pleura, bronchi, chest wall, mediastinum, etc.), and presence of separate tumor nodules in the lung, which is best achieved by high-resolution morphological imaging.

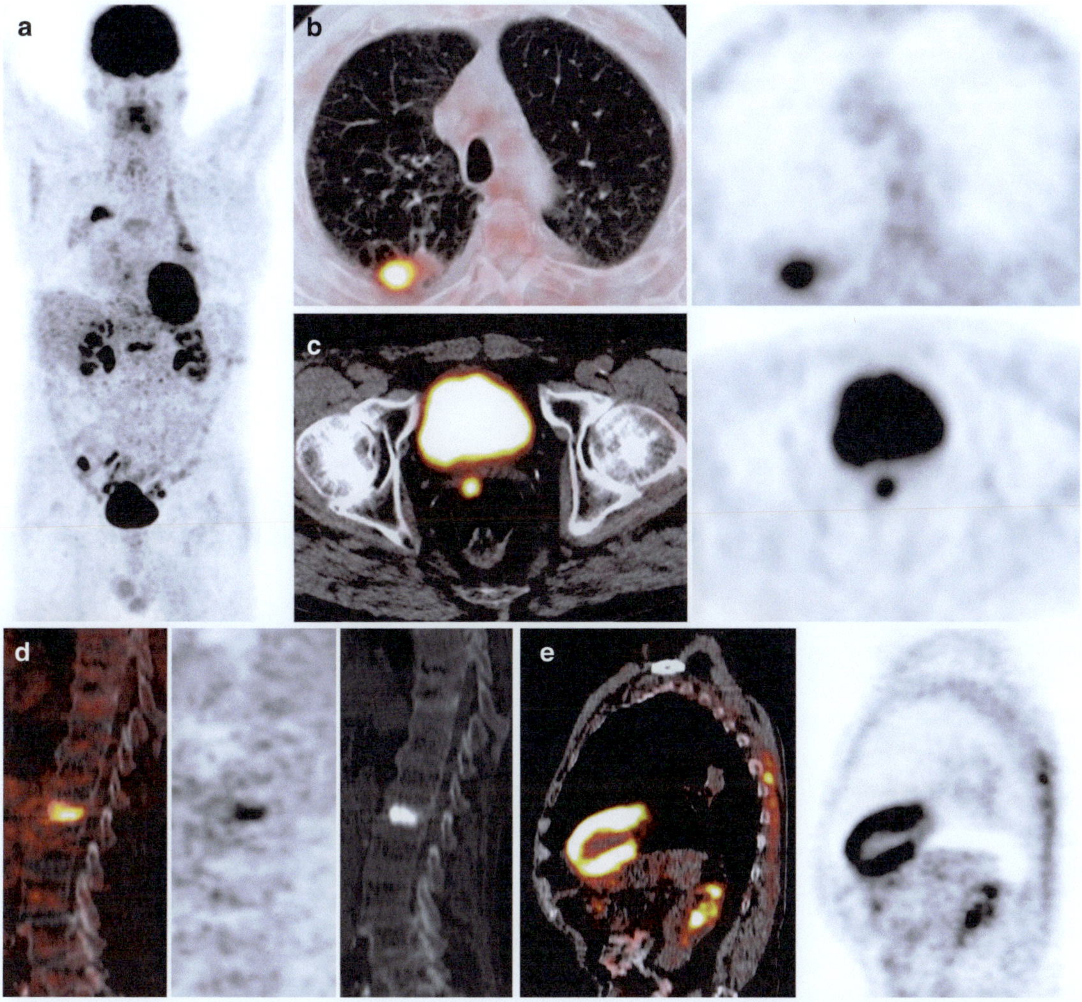

Fig. 21.2 (**a**) Primary staging in a 76-year-old male patient with histologically proven NSCLC (SCC) in the right upper lobe of the lung. (**b**) Intense uptake of FDG was observed in the primary tumor. (**c**) As an incidental finding, intense focal uptake was observed in the rectum, suspicious of a dysplastic adenoma/carcinoma of the rectum. (**d**, **e**) Non-specific uptake in the lumbar vertebrae 1 after vertebroplasty due to an osteoporotic fracture and in the back musculature on the left side

FDG PET/CT is most beneficial regarding N- and M-staging. While N0 and N1 stages are candidates for curative surgery, surgical multimodality treatment is recommended for N2, and N3 is usually deemed non-resectable [3]. Sensitivity and specificity are 83% and 89% for FDG PET/CT for the differentiation between N0/1 and N2/3 stages (i.e., detection of mediastinal lymph node involvement), which is superior compared to CT-staging which shows a sensitivity and specificity of 56% and 81%, respectively [11]. FDG-positive (and also morphologically enlarged) lymph nodes should be confirmed by endosonographic biopsy or subsequent surgical staging (mediastinoscopy) to exclude false-positive results caused by non-specific FDG uptake in inflammatory lymph nodes [3].

For the detection of distant metastases (M-staging), FDG PET/CT has a very high

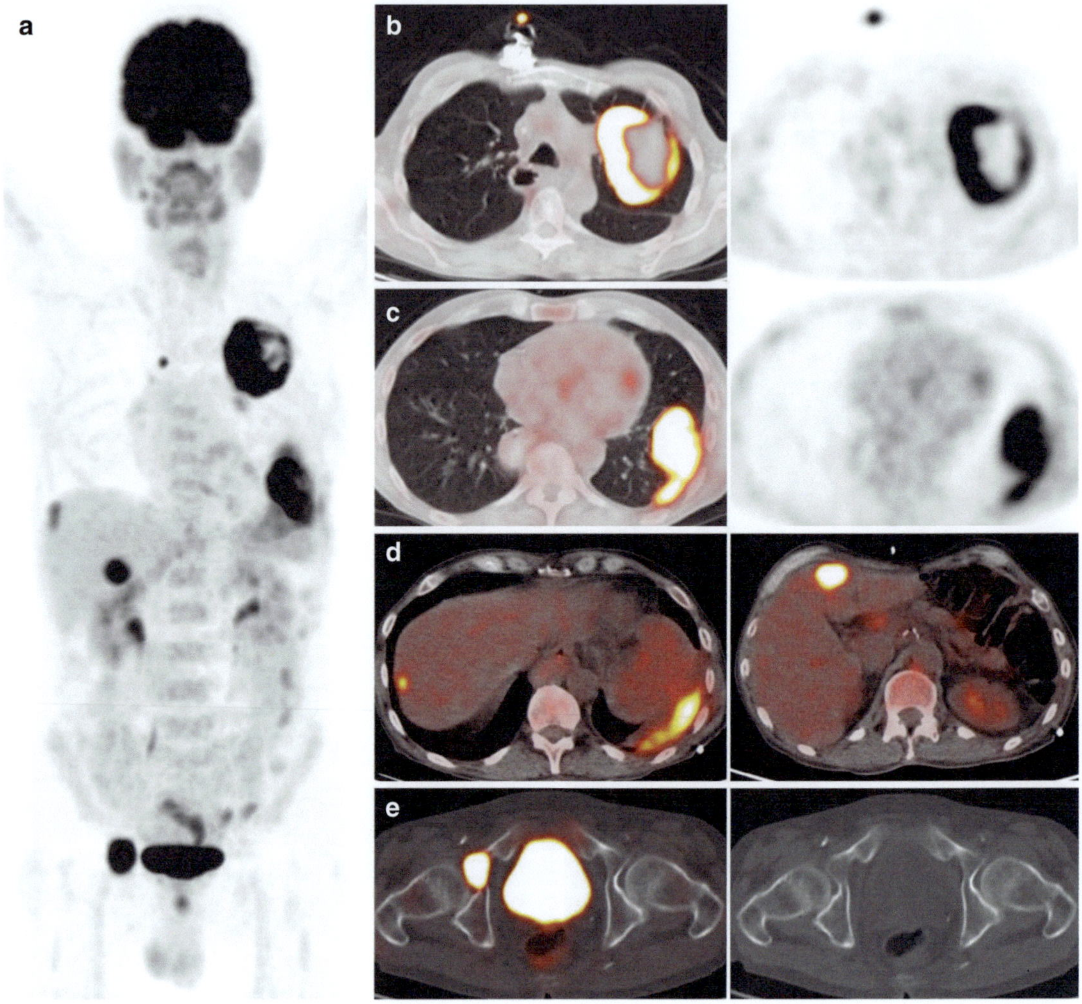

Fig. 21.3 (**a**) Primary staging in a 58-year-old male patient with histologically proven NSCLC (large cell lung cancer). The patient had a history of recurrent esophageal cancer 9 and 7 years ago and colorectal cancer 5 years ago. (**b**) Intense uptake of FDG was observed in the NSCLC of the right upper lobe with a central zone of necrosis. Activity in the region of the injection site (central port). (**c**) Another region of uptake suspicious for malignancy with extension into the pleural space was observed in the left lower lobe; however, this was later shown to correspond to a pleural empyema. (**d**, **e**) Two hypermetabolic lesions were observed in the liver, and another one was observed in the bone (right acetabulum), corresponding to distant metastases

accuracy of 97%, which is superior to CT-staging alone (accuracy for M-staging: 88%) [12]. FDG PET/CT also has a higher sensitivity (91%) and specificity (98%) for the detection of bone metastases compared to bone scintigraphy (sensitivity 82%, specificity 62%); thus, bone scintigraphy may be waived after staging with FDG PET/CT [13, 14]. However, the sensitivity of FDG PET/CT for the detection of brain metastases is very low (less than 30%); thus, an additional cranial MRI is necessary for a complete staging of NSCLC patients [13]. M1 stages of NSCLC are usually considered inoperable and undergo palliative chemotherapy. It should be noted that pathological confirmation is recommended for single PET-positive distant lesions [3].

Overall, FDG PET/CT has been reported to lead to changes in staging in 51% of patients with NSCLC (41% upstaging, 10% downstaging), impacting therapeutic decisions (change in treatment modality or curative intent) in 42% [15].

21.1.3 SCLC Primary Staging

For patients with SCLC, the differentiation between limited disease (LD) and extensive disease (ED) based on the VALG (Veterans Administration Lung Cancer Study Group) and IASLC (International Association for the Study of Lung Cancer) criteria is highly important regarding the choice of therapy [16]. LD is characterized by the disease being limited to one hemithorax with lymph node metastases limited to the pulmonary hilum (ipsilateral and contralateral), mediastinum (ipsilateral and contralateral), ipsilateral supraclavicular region, and ipsilateral pleural effusion (independent of cytology results), if all tumor sites can be included in a radiotherapy field. Tumor spread outside these limits is staged as ED. Most clinical therapy decisions are based on the differentiation between LD and ED, as most clinical trials have utilized this system. The UICC TNM classification and clinical staging system for SCLC (which are the same as those for NSCLC shown in Tables 21.1 and 21.2 [10]) are featured less prominently in current clinical SCLC therapy algorithms.

SCLC in the limited stage is potentially curable, and the standard therapy regimen consists of concomitant chemotherapy and thoracic radiotherapy and potentially prophylactic cranial irradiation in responders, achieving long-term survival in about 20% of patients. Surgical procedures followed by chemotherapy might be considered in T1–2, N0–1 stages. Patients with extended-stage SCLC usually are treated with palliative chemotherapy, potentially with prophylactic cranial irradiation in responders to chemotherapy; however, prognosis is poor in extended-stage SCLC with a 2-year survival of only 5% [14, 16].

SCLC is highly glucose avid, with a reported sensitivity of 100% for FDG PET in the detection of the primary tumor [16]. Regarding SCLC staging, a prospective study showed a sensitivity of 93% and a specificity of 100% of FDG PET for the detection of ED versus LD in SCLC patients, compared to standard staging (CT, bone scan, and bone marrow biopsy) with a sensitivity of 79% and a specificity of 100% [17]. In patients initially staged as LD by conventional methods, FDG PET lead to upstaging to ED in 19% of cases, and conversely, 11% of patients initially staged as ED were downstaged to LD by FDG PET. Analogous to NSCLC staging, FDG PET was inferior to MRI in the detection of brain metastases in SCLC patients. Overall, FDG PET lead to a change in patient management in 27% of cases [16].

These results show that FDG PET/CT does have an impact on staging of patients with SCLC, more frequently leading to upstaging than downstaging; however, the impact of FDG PET/CT on clinical management is less pronounced in patients with SCLC compared to NSCLC. This might be explained by the more aggressive nature of SCLC compared to NSCLC, leading to more pronounced metastases which are more apparent on conventional staging.

Bone scan and bone marrow biopsy are standard procedures in conventional staging of SCLC; however when FDG PET/CT (including diagnostic CT scans of the chest and abdomen) and MRI of the brain are performed, these procedures may be skipped. Overall, the use of FDG PET/CT in SCLC staging proved to be beneficial, though further prospective trials are needed to confirm the clinical value of PET in this indication [16].

21.1.4 Recurrence of NSCLC

The risk of recurrence of NSCLC is highest in the first 2 years after initial surgery [10]. One study in 55 patients with the suspicion of NSCLC recurrence showed inconclusive results of CT imaging in 51% of patients, while all patients could be classified as positive or negative for recurrence by FDG PET/CT. This resulted in an overall sensitivity of 100% and a specificity of 83% of FDG PET/CT for recurrence detection. In the subgroup of patients with inconclusive CT results, FDG PET/CT showed a sensitivity of 100% and a specificity of 78%. The authors reported an impact of FDG PET/CT on therapeutic decisions in 79% of patients in whom both CT and FDG PET/CT were performed, which were changes from local to systemic treatment, changes in radiotherapy field size, initiation of treatment, and avoidance of unnecessary treatment [18].

Though FDG PET/CT is more accurate for NSCLC recurrence detection compared to CT imaging, FDG PET/CT is currently not recommended for routine follow-up of patients with NSCLC. However, if tumor recurrence is suspected or confirmed, FDG PET/CT can be helpful to distinguish local from distant recurrence and thus have an impact on therapy decisions, i.e., local therapy vs. systemic treatment (Fig. 21.4) [19].

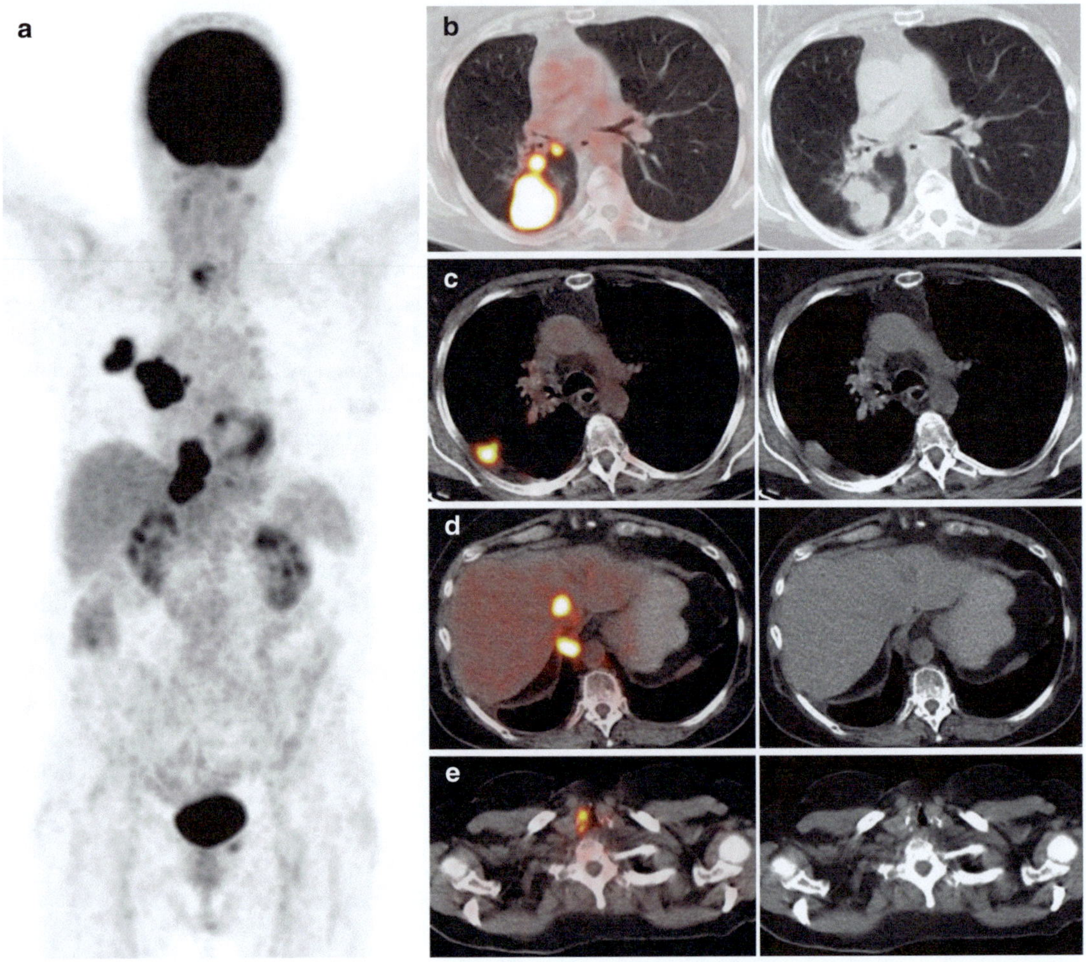

Fig. 21.4 (**a**) FDG PET/CT in a 72-year-old female patient with suspicion of NSCLC recurrence. The patient underwent radiotherapy due to NSCLC of the right upper lobe 7 years ago. (**b**) Intense focal uptake of FDG in the mass of the right upper lobe, suspicious of recurrence, and hypermetabolic lymph node metastases in the ipsilateral hilar region. (**c**, **d**) Pleural thickening on the right side with focal FDG uptake, suspicious of pleural metastases. (**d**) Intense focal uptake in the liver, suspicious of metastasis. (**e**) Asymmetric uptake of the vocal cords (right side) due to vocal cord paresis on the left side

21.2 Malignant Pleural Effusion

The accumulation of fluid in the pleural space caused by a neoplastic process is called a "malignant pleural effusion" (MPE), which adversely affects patient prognosis and may alter the therapeutic approach [20]. Not all pleural effusions are caused by malignancy—in fact most pleural effusions are of benign origin, and most of them are caused by congestive heart failure (46% of cases). However, malignancy is the second leading cause of pleural effusions (22% of cases), followed by parapneumonic effusions (17%) and pulmonary emboli (6%) [21]. The definite diagnosis of an MPE is based on the detection of malignant cells in a pleural fluid aspirate, and non-invasive imaging cannot replace aspiration cytology to establish a definite diagnosis.

Regarding CT imaging, the most accurate parameter for the detection of an MPE is the density of the effusion, with a cutoff at 3.2 Hounsfield units. This parameter reaches an accuracy of 69% with a specificity of 95%; however, the sensitivity is low, reaching only 29%. The size of the pleural effusion and visual pleural abnormalities on CT imaging are less accurate, with accuracy values of only 64% and 56%, respectively [20].

FDG PET/CT seems to perform better in the detection of an MPE compared to CT. A study with 36 patients showed that visual pleural uptake was the most accurate PET parameter for MPE detection, with an accuracy of 78% (sensitivity 57%, specificity 91%). The best semi-quantitative parameter was the uptake ratio pleura to the 12th thoracic vertebrae (cutoff value 0.95), with an accuracy of 75% (sensitivity 93%, specificity 68%) and a negative predictive value of 88%. The use of SUV_{max} was not as efficient for the detection of MPE (accuracy 69%). Due to the high negative predictive value, this modality may provide valuable information for evaluating pleural disease when a pleural effusion analysis is not possible, when the results are questionable, or when it is difficult to obtain enough pleural fluid [20].

These results are in line with a meta-analysis of 14 studies, overall including 639 patients. Visual analysis was best suited for the detection of MPE, with a sensitivity of 91%. In comparison, semi-quantitative analysis reached a sensitivity of 82%. Though FDG PET/CT was more accurate than CT in the detection of MPE, the accuracy of FDG PET/CT still was only in the moderate range. Thus, FDG PET/CT is not generally recommended for the routine evaluation to discriminate malignant from benign effusions [22]; however, it might be helpful in selected individual cases. Examples are shown in Figs. 21.5 and 21.6.

21.3 Pleural Mesothelioma

Mesothelioma is the most common primary tumor of the pleura. Other pleural tumors, such as solitary fibrous tumors and pleural liposarcomas, are infrequent. Pleural mesothelioma mostly affects men (80% of patients with pleural mesothelioma are male), and it has a strong association with previous exposure to asbestos, with a long latency period of 30–40 years. Symptoms are usually unspecific (dyspnea, chest wall pain) which may delay diagnosis. The disease easily spreads along the tissue planes in the pleural cavity, and often patients are diagnosed with advanced-stage disease with a median survival of less than 12 months [23].

In patients with asbestos exposure, benign abnormalities of the pleura such as pleural plaques and benign asbestos-related effusion may complicate the differential diagnosis to malignant pleural mesothelioma by CT imaging, which is the primary imaging method in this indication [23]. One study showed that FDG PET/CT may help to differentiate malignant mesothelioma from benign asbestos-related disease, with a reported sensitivity of 94% and a specificity of 100% (positive predictive value, 100%; negative predictive value, 93%) when a SUV cutoff of 2.2 was used; however, the study population was small (31 patients) [24]. These results are in line with an earlier study using FDG PET, resulting in similar values regarding sensitivity and specificity, using an SUV cutoff of 2.0 (28 patients) [25].

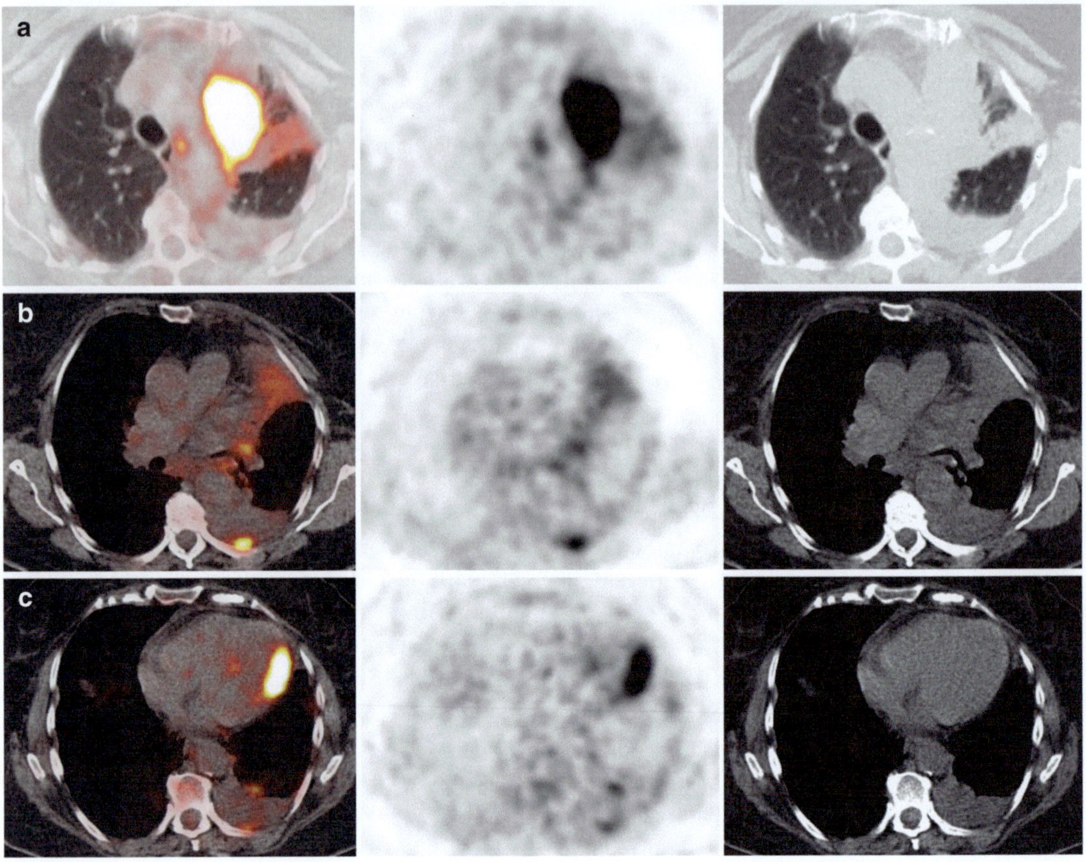

Fig. 21.5 Staging with FDG PET/CT in a 79-year-old female patient with histologically proven adenocarcinoma of the lung (left upper lobe). (**a**) Intense uptake of FDG in the primary tumor of the lung, as well as hypermetabolic mediastinal lymph nodes, suspicious of metastases. (**b**, **c**) Multiple foci of increased uptake in the region of the left pleural effusion, consistent with pleural metastatic spread

Routine staging of patients with pleural mesothelioma is mainly performed with CT, though it tends to underestimate lymph node metastases. However, correct staging of lymph node metastases and distant metastases is important due to poor outcome of patients with extrapleural tumor involvement who undergo radical resection. Patients with T4 (locally advanced tumor with infiltration of surrounding structures), N3 (presence supraclavicular or contralateral intrathoracic lymph nodes), or M1 status are usually deemed unresectable.

In a retrospective analysis of 60 patients who underwent surgery with histopathologic analysis of nodal involvement, PET/CT correctly staged lymph node involvement in 63% of cases, compared to 45% for CT. Regarding the detection of distant metastases, FDG PET/CT showed a very good sensitivity of 92% in comparison to CT (33% sensitivity) [26]. Erasmus et al. found that FDG PET/CT precluded surgery in 41% of patients initially deemed candidates for extrapleural pneumonectomy, with the detection of extrathoracic metastases being the main advantage of FDG PET [27].

Overall, the strength of FDG PET in assessment of pleural mesothelioma lies in the detection of extrathoracic metastases. However, PET/CT does not seem to be superior to CT or MRI to identify the locoregional disease stage or to evaluate the mediastinal lymph node status [23].

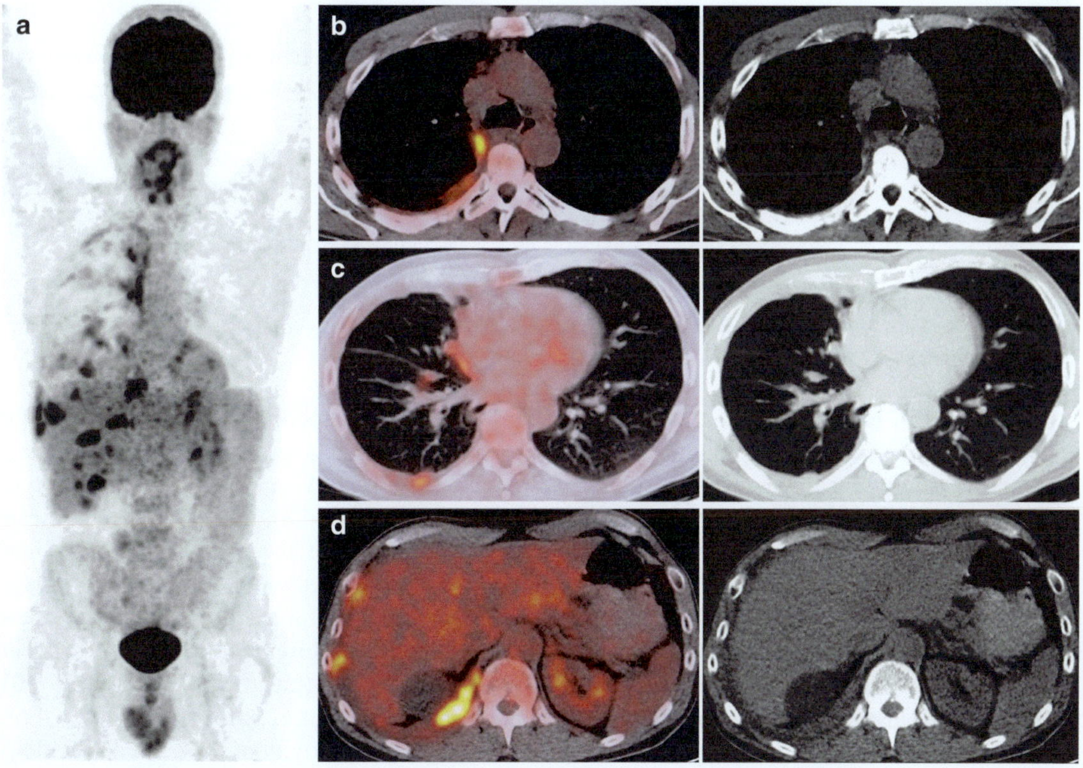

Fig. 21.6 (**a**) FDG PET/CT in a 47-year-old male patient with pleural effusion and pleural thickening on the right side. (**b–d**) Multifocal intense uptake in the right pleura, suspicious of malignancy. Pleural biopsy revealed an adenocarcinoma of unknown primary

21.4 Thymic Epithelial Tumors (TETs): Thymoma and Thymic Carcinoma

Thymoma and thymic carcinoma are rare thoracic cancers with an incidence of 1.3–3.2 per million per year, with a mean diagnosis at around 50–60 years of age. Despite the low incidence, these tumors are the most frequent cause of anterior mediastinal masses (accounting for ~35%), followed by lymphoma (~25%) and germ cell tumors (~20%). TETs are frequently associated with autoimmune disorders, mostly myasthenia gravis (occurring in up to 45% of patients) [28], and red cell aplasia and hypogammaglobulinemia may occur, among others. Thymomas lacking histological features of cell atypia may also exhibit a local invasive growth; thus, all thymomas should be considered as potentially malignant, and the term "benign thymoma" should be avoided [29, 30].

The WHO classification differentiates several types of thymic neoplasias based on their histologic appearance, as listed in Table 21.3. Survival is excellent in type A and still good in types AB–B2, while types B3 and C (thymic carcinoma, TC) have a significantly worse prognosis.

All TETs without metastases should undergo surgery (usually complete thymectomy) if the tumor is resectable, and depending on histologic type and stage, followed by postoperative radiotherapy and—less frequently—also postoperative chemotherapy. Tumor resection is a major prognostic factor, with a 5-year overall survival of 81% in resected tumors vs. 28% in non-resected tumors [29]. TETs with lymph node metastases or distant metastases are deemed unresectable and should undergo definitive chemotherapy [30].

Table 21.3 WHO histological subtypes of TET, data from [29, 30]

Type	Relative frequency (%)	Association with myasthenia gravis (%)	Overall 5-year survival (%)	Relative survival[a] (%)
A	12	15	88	100
AB	28	20	83	93
B1	18	40	82	87
B2	26	50	82	86
B3	16	50	53	57
C (thymic carcinoma, TC)	18	<5	38	42

[a]Relative survival: the ratio of the observed to the expected survival, as an estimator of the excess risk of death compared to the standard population

TETs need to be differentiated from benign causes of thymic enlargement: thymic rebound hyperplasia (caused by chemotherapy, radiotherapy, anti-hormonal treatment, corticosteroids, stress, injuries) and non-involuted thymus. The standard imaging procedure for diagnosis and staging is contrast-enhanced CT and possibly also MRI. Signs on CT imaging for a benign cause are preservation of the physiologic pyramidal shape of the thymus and patterns of fatty infiltration. MRI (chemical shift imaging) may be helpful to detect these fatty infiltrations on the microscopic level in unclear cases. Though there is no general recommendation to use FDG PET in the evaluation of thymic masses, it can be helpful to detect higher-grade thymomas and thymic carcinomas for staging of advanced-stage disease and tumors with histological signs of aggressiveness and to detect recurrences [30].

Preoperative biopsy usually is not performed if a mediastinal mass is highly suspicious of TET and the lesion is deemed resectable. Nevertheless, preoperative information regarding the grade of malignancy of the lesion might be helpful in some cases to select the best therapeutic strategy. For example, patients with a high suspicion of thymic carcinoma could be excluded from a minimally invasive surgical approach, and patients with locally advanced disease or biologically aggressive tumors might undergo neoadjuvant treatment. The morphological imaging methods CT and MRI are not useful to distinguish between the histological subtypes of TET [31]. Only a few studies exist on the role of FDG PET/CT in this indication, attributable to the low incidence of TETs. One of the largest studies included 112 patients who underwent FDG PET/CT before the resection of a TET. Though the authors observed a gradual increase of tracer uptake from type A (mean SUV_{max} 3.5) to type B3 (mean SUV_{max} 4.8), there was no significant difference between low-risk (A, AB, B1) and high-risk (B2, B3) thymomas, caused by a high variability of SUV in each type. However, there was a significant difference in SUV_{max} between thymoma and TC (mean SUV_{max} for TC: 8.0), and the optimal cutoff value was SUV_{max} 4.58, resulting in a sensitivity of 80% and a specificity of 78% for the detection of TC vs. thymoma. In small lesions less than 3 cm, a cutoff value of SUV_{max} 4.57 resulted in a sensitivity of 75% and a specificity of 94%. Previous studies including smaller numbers of patients reported cutoff values between 5.0 and 6.3 [32]. In a meta-analysis of 11 studies, significant differences of SUV_{max} were found between TC and low-risk thymoma, TC and high-risk thymoma, and even low-risk and high-risk thymoma, though in the meta-analysis no cutoff values could be defined due to large overlaps of SUV_{max} among the different subgroups [31].

TET in the advanced stage may spread locally in the thoracic cavity resulting in mediastinal, pleural, and pericardial metastases. Hematogenous distant metastases of TET are rare and usually associated with TC [33]. Data regarding the detection of TET metastases with FDG PET/CT is limited; however, it seems that TET metastases usually are FDG-positive. Thus, FDG PET/CT might be helpful in patients with advanced-stage and high-risk TET/TC for identification of distant metastases, which are sometimes difficult to detect using other imaging modalities [34].

Lifetime follow-up of TET is recommended and is mainly based on thoracic CT. Recurrences occur in 10–15% of all TET after complete resection, at an average time of 5 years after surgery (range 3–7 years). Patients with recurrences undergo the same therapeutic strategy as patients with newly diagnosed tumors, and complete resection of recurrences is a major prognostic factor for a favorable outcome [30]. FDG PET/CT seems favorable over thoracic CT to detect thymoma recurrence. A study in 37 patients after thymoma resection showed a sensitivity of 82% and a specificity of 95% for FDG PET/CT for recurrence detection, whereas sensitivity and specificity for CT were 71% and 85%, respectively. In the anterior mediastinum, a sensitivity of FDG PET/CT of 100% was observed, compared to 55% sensitivity of CT, while sensitivity of FDG PET/CT for detection of pleural recurrence was worse compared to CT imaging [35]. Overall, data regarding thymoma recurrence detection with FDG PET/CT is limited; thus, there is no general recommendation for its use in follow-up after thymoma resection; however, the data available indicates that FDG PET/CT might be beneficial in select cases, especially when CT results are inconclusive.

References

1. Siegel RL, Miller KD, Jemal A. Cancer statistics, 2017. CA Cancer J Clin. 2017;67:7–30.
2. Travis WD, Brambilla E, Nicholson AG, et al. The 2015 World Health Organization classification of lung tumors. J Thorac Oncol. 2015;10:1243–60.
3. Postmus PE, Kerr KM, Oudkerk M, et al. Early and locally advanced non-small-cell lung cancer (NSCLC): ESMO Clinical Practice Guidelines for diagnosis, treatment and follow-up. Ann Oncol. 2017;28:iv1–iv21.
4. Hansell DM, Bankier AA, MacMahon H, et al. Fleischner Society: glossary of terms for thoracic imaging. Radiology. 2008;246:697–722.
5. Furtado CD, Aguirre DA, Sirlin CB, et al. Whole-body CT screening: spectrum of findings and recommendations in 1192 patients. Radiology. 2005;237:385–94.
6. Sim YT, Poon FW. Imaging of solitary pulmonary nodule-a clinical review. Quant Imaging Med Surg. 2013;3:316–26.
7. Gould M, Maclean C, Kuschner W. Accuracy of positron emission tomography for diagnosis of pulmonary nodules and mass lesions: a meta-analysis. JAMA. 2001;285:914.
8. Kim SK, Allen-Auerbach M, Goldin J, et al. Accuracy of PET/CT in characterization of solitary pulmonary lesions. J Nucl Med. 2007;48:214–20.
9. Barger RL, Nandalur KR. Diagnostic performance of dual-time 18F-FDG PET in the diagnosis of pulmonary nodules: a meta-analysis. Acad Radiol. 2012;19:153–8.
10. Brierley JD, Gospodarowicz MK, Wittekind C. TNM classification of malignant tumours. 8th ed. Chichester: Wiley Blackwell; 2016.
11. Hellwig D, Baum RP, Kirsch CM. FDG-PET, PET/CT and conventional nuclear medicine procedures in the evaluation of lung cancer: a systematic review. Nuklearmedizin. 2009;48:59–69.
12. De Wever W, Vankan Y, Stroobants S, et al. Detection of extrapulmonary lesions with integrated PET/CT in the staging of lung cancer. Eur Respir J. 2007;29:995–1002.
13. Wu Y, Li P, Zhang H, et al. Diagnostic value of fluorine 18 fluorodeoxyglucose positron emission tomography/computed tomography for the detection of metastases in non-small-cell lung cancer patients. Int J Cancer. 2013;132:E37–47.
14. Goeckenjan G, Sitter H, Thomas M, et al. [Prevention, diagnosis, therapy, and follow-up of lung cancer]. Pneumologie. 2010;64(Suppl 2):e1–164.
15. Gregory DL, Hicks RJ, Hogg A, et al. Effect of PET/CT on management of patients with non-small cell lung cancer: results of a prospective study with 5-year survival data. J Nucl Med. 2012;53:1007–15.
16. Kalemkerian GP. Staging and imaging of small cell lung cancer. Cancer Imaging. 2011;11:253–8.
17. Fischer BM, Mortensen J, Langer SW, et al. A prospective study of PET/CT in initial staging of small-cell lung cancer: comparison with CT, bone scintigraphy and bone marrow analysis. Ann Oncol. 2007;18:338–45.
18. Jiménez-Bonilla JF, Quirce R, Martínez-Rodríguez I, et al. Diagnosis of recurrence and assessment of post-recurrence survival in patients with extracranial non-small cell lung cancer evaluated by 18F-FDG PET/CT. Lung Cancer. 2013;81:71–6.
19. Jimenez Bonilla JF, Quirce Pisano MR, Martínez Rodríguez MI, et al. The role of PET/CT molecular imaging in the diagnosis of recurrence and surveillance of patients treated for non-small cell lung cancer. Diagnostics. 2016;2016(6):36.
20. Nakajima R, Abe K, Sakai S. Diagnostic ability of FDG-PET/CT in the detection of malignant pleural effusion. Medicine (Baltimore). 2015;94:e1010.
21. Marel M, Zrustova M, Stasny B, et al. The incidence of pleural effusion in a well-defined region: epidemiologic study in Central Bohemia. Chest. 1993;104:1486–9.
22. Porcel JM, Hernández P, Martínez-Alonso M, et al. Accuracy of fluorodeoxyglucose-PET imaging for differentiating benign from malignant pleural effusions: a meta-analysis. Chest. 2015;147:502–12.

23. Kruse M, Sherry SJ, Paidpally V, et al. FDG PET/CT in the management of primary pleural tumors and pleural metastases. Am J Roentgenol. 2013;201:W215.
24. Yildirim H, Metintas M, Entok E, et al. Clinical value of fluorodeoxyglucose-positron emission tomography/computed tomography in differentiation of malignant mesothelioma from asbestos-related benign pleural disease: an observational pilot study. J Thorac Oncol. 2009;4:1480–4.
25. Benard F, Sterman D, Smith RJ, et al. Metabolic imaging of malignant pleural mesothelioma with fluorodeoxyglucose positron emission tomography. Chest. 1998;114:713–22.
26. Elliott HS, Metser U, de Perrot M, et al. 18 F-FDG PET/CT in the management of patients with malignant pleural mesothelioma being considered for multimodality therapy: experience of a tertiary referral center. Br J Radiol. 2018;91:20170814.
27. Erasmus JJ, Truong MT, Smythe WR, et al. Integrated computed tomography-positron emission tomography in patients with potentially resectable malignant pleural mesothelioma: staging implications. J Thorac Cardiovasc Surg. 2005;129:1364–70.
28. Detterbeck FC, Parsons AM. Thymic tumors. Ann Thorac Surg. 2004;77:1860–9.
29. de Jong WK, Blaauwgeers JLG, Schaapveld M, et al. Thymic epithelial tumours: a population-based study of the incidence, diagnostic procedures and therapy. Eur J Cancer. 2008;44:123–30.
30. Girard N, Ruffini E, Marx A, et al. Thymic epithelial tumours: ESMO clinical practice guidelines for diagnosis, treatment and follow-up. Ann Oncol. 2015;26:v40–55.
31. Treglia G, Sadeghi R, Giovanella L, et al. Is 18F-FDG PET useful in predicting the WHO grade of malignancy in thymic epithelial tumors? A meta-analysis. Lung Cancer. 2014;86:5–13.
32. Nakagawa K, Takahashi S, Endo M, et al. Can 18F-FDG PET predict the grade of malignancy in thymic epithelial tumors? An evaluation of only resected tumors. Cancer Manag Res. 2017;9:761–8.
33. Passuello N, Pozza G, Blandamura S, et al. Thymoma metastatic to liver and pancreas: case report and review of the literature. J Int Med Res. 2017;45:868–74.
34. Otsuka H. The utility of FDG-PET in the diagnosis of thymic epithelial tumors. J Med Investig. 2012;59:225–34.
35. El-Bawab HY, Abouzied MM, Rafay MA, et al. Clinical use of combined positron emission tomography and computed tomography in thymoma recurrence. Interact Cardiovasc Thorac Surg. 2010;11:395–9.

22 Nuclear Medicine Imaging Techniques in Melanoma

Ismaheel O. Lawal and Mike M. Sathekge

22.1 Introduction

Melanoma is the least common type of skin cancer but the deadliest of all [1]. It arises from the melanocytes of the dermo-epidermal junction of the skin. The skin is the commonest site of melanoma occurrence. In addition to the skin, melanoma also arises from the mucosal membranes of the respiratory tract, gastrointestinal tract, and urogenital system, meninges, and the uveal tract of the eye [2]. The exact etiology of melanoma is unknown. Certain predisposing factors have been identified. Intermittent sun exposure rather than high continuous pattern of sun exposure is a strong risk factor for the development of cutaneous melanoma [3]. Other risk factors include high number of common and atypical naevi, family history of melanoma, fair skin color, high density of freckles, phenotypic factors such as blue eye color and red hair color, actinic skin damage, and the presence of other skin tumors [4–6].

I. O. Lawal · M. M. Sathekge (✉)
Department of Nuclear Medicine, University of Pretoria and Steve Biko Academic Hospital, Pretoria, South Africa
e-mail: mike.sathekge@up.ac.za

H. Ahmadzadehfar et al. (eds.), *Clinical Nuclear Medicine*,
https://doi.org/10.1007/978-3-030-39457-8_22

22.2 Morphology

Morphologically, melanoma appears as a flat or slightly raised naevus with irregular or notched borders. Malignant melanoma may arise de novo or from a preexisting benign naevus. Features suggestive of malignant melanoma are described by the acronym ABCDE: Asymmetry, Border irregularity, Color change, Diameter increasing, and Evolution of time. Melanomas exhibit two growth patterns, radial and vertical growth phases [2]. In the radial growth phase, the lesion spreads horizontally within the epidermis and superficial dermis. Melanomas in the radial growth phase probably lack the capacity for metastasis, and they fall in the following clinicopathologic classes:

- Superficial spreading—it is the commonest type of melanoma and may occur anywhere on the skin except the palms and soles. It has a relatively long radial growth phase before vertical growth begins. It usually measures 10–20 mm in diameter at the time of diagnosis.
- Lentigo maligna—it is seen mostly in older individuals with sun-damaged skin. It appears as flat, deeply pigmented lesion with irregular borders. It is slow growing and has the best prognosis among the different types of melanoma.

- Acral lentiginous—it occurs on the palms and soles as well as in the subungual areas. It is more common among dark-skinned individuals. The diagnosis is often delayed giving it a poor prognostic outcome.

After a variable and often unpredictable length of time, melanoma changes the pattern of growth from radial to a vertical growth pattern where the deeper dermal and subdermal tissues are invaded. It is during this latter phase of growth that metastatic potential is acquired. Melanomas in the vertical phase of growth often clinically appear as a nodule.

- Nodular melanoma—vertical growth pattern starts early in the history of this subtype of melanoma. Nodular melanoma carries the worse prognosis among all melanoma subtypes.

22.3 Prognostic Factors

The thickness and presence of ulceration in the melanoma lesion are the most important prognostic factors which influence management. The thickness of the lesion correlates with the probability of distant metastasis [7]. The thickness of the melanoma is measured by the distance from the superficial epidermal granular cell layer to the deepest depth point of tumor invasion. This measurement is known as the Breslow thickness.

Due to high level of awareness, melanomas are now diagnosed at an early tumor stage. Surgical excision is commonly offered for these thin lesions. A number of clinical and pathologic characteristics of the excised lesions are used to predict the likelihood of distant metastasis and for prognostication. These characteristics indicative of favorable prognosis are as follows [8–10]:

Pathologic

1. Thin Breslow thickness
2. No or one mitoses per mm^2 of lesion
3. The presence of lymphocyte infiltration of the tumor
4. The absence of ulceration on the lesion

Clinical

5. Female gender
6. Location in the limbs

Biochemical

7. Normal levels of lactate dehydrogenase

There is no significant difference in prognosis according to melanoma subtype. When matched for Breslow thickness, gender, and other prognostic indicators, nodular melanoma has the same prognostic as superficial spreading melanoma [11]. The poor prognosis ascribed to nodular melanoma lies in its early vertical growth making it relatively thicker than other melanoma subtypes at the time of diagnosis. Tumor regression is a marker of immune activation against the melanoma lesion. Its presence may impair correct assessment of the Breslow thickness. There is no consensus on how its impact on prognosis in patients with melanoma. While some studies have found it predictive of a poor outcome, others have reported a good outcome in its presence [12]. The eighth edition of the American Joint Committee on Cancer (AJCC) staging of melanoma provides a risk stratification of patients into prognostic stage groups and is shown in Tables 22.1, 22.2, 22.3, and 22.4 [13].

22.4 Sentinel Lymph Node Scintigraphy

Wide local excision is the mainstay treatment for localized melanoma. Metastatic spread of melanoma is common. Early spread is via the lymphatic to the regional lymph nodes [14]. Lymph node metastasis is the strongest prognostic factor in patients with melanoma, and its determination is necessary for appropriate staging of disease [7, 8]. The risk of nodal metastasis varies with Breslow thickness. Less than 5% of melanoma with Breslow thickness ≤1 mm (thin melanoma) have nodal metastases [15]. In patients with intermediate thickness melanoma, Breslow 1.01–4 mm, nodal metastasis is present in only about 20% [16]. The highest prevalence of nodal metastasis

Table 22.1 Eighth edition AJCC staging for melanoma. Description of primary tumor (T)

T Category	Thickness	Ulceration status
TX: Primary tumor cannot be assessed	Not applicable	Not applicable
T0: No evidence of primary tumor	Not applicable	Not applicable
Tis: Melanoma in situ	Not applicable	Not applicable
T1	≤1.0 mm	Unknown or unspecified
T1a	<0.8 mm	Without ulceration
T1b	<0.8 mm	With ulceration
	0.8–1.0 mm	With or without ulceration
T2	>1.0–2.0 mm	Unknown or unspecified
T2a	>1.0–2.0 mm	Without ulceration
T2b	>1.0–2.0 mm	With ulceration
T3	>2.0–4.0 mm	Unknown or unspecified
T3a	>2.0–4.0 mm	Without ulceration
T3b	>2.0–4.0 mm	With ulceration
T4	>4.0 mm	Unknown or unspecified
T4a	>4.0 mm	Without ulceration
T4b	>4.0 mm	With ulceration

Table 22.2 Eighth edition AJCC staging for melanoma. Description of regional lymph node metastasis (N)

N category	No. of tumor-involved regional lymph nodes	Presence of in-transit, satellite, and/or microsatellite metastases
NX	Regional nodes not assessed	No
N0	No regional metastasis	No
N1	One tumor-involved node or any number of in-transit, satellite, and/or microsatellite metastases with no tumor-involved nodes	
N1a	One clinically occult node	No
N1b	One clinically detected node	No
N1c	No regional lymph node involvement	Yes
N2	Two or three tumor-involved nodes or any number of in-transit, satellite, and/or microsatellite metastases with one tumor-involved node	
N2a	Two or three clinically occult	No
N2b	Two or three nodes, at least one of which was clinically detectable	No
N2c	One clinically occult or clinically detected	Yes
N3	Four or more tumor-involved nodes or any number of in-transit, satellite, and/or microsatellite metastases with two or more tumor-involved nodes, or any number of matted nodes without or with in-transit, satellite, and/or microsatellite metastases	
N3a	Four or more clinically occult	No
N3b	Four or more nodes, at least one of which was clinically detected, or presence of any number of matted nodes	No
N3c	Two or more clinically occult or clinically detected and/or presence of any number of matted nodes	Yes

Clinically occult (previously described as microscopic nodal metastases): Detectable by sentinel lymph node biopsy
Clinically detected (previously described as macroscopic nodal metastases): Detectable clinically by palpation
Satellite metastases: Clinically evident cutaneous and/or subcutaneous metastases occurring within 2 cm of the primary melanoma
Microsatellites: Microscopic cutaneous and/or subcutaneous metastases found adjacent or deep to a primary melanoma lesion on histological examination
In-transit metastases: Clinically evident cutaneous and/or subcutaneous metastases occurring at a distance more than 2 cm from the primary melanoma in the region between the primary and the first echelon of regional lymph nodes

Table 22.3 Eighth edition AJCC staging for melanoma. Description of distant metastases

M category	Anatomic site	Lactate dehydrogenase level
M0	No evidence of distant metastasis	Not applicable
M1	Evidence of distant metastasis	
M1a	Distant metastasis to skin, soft tissue, and/or non-regional lymph node	Not recorded or unspecified
M1a(0)		Not elevated
M1a(1)		Elevated
M1b	Distant metastasis to lung with or without M1a sites of disease	Not recorded or unspecified
M1b(0)		Not elevated
M1b(1)		Elevated
M1c	Distant metastasis to non-central nervous system visceral sites with or without M1a or M1b sites of metastasis	Not recorded or unspecified
M1c(0)		Not elevated
M1c(1)		Elevated
M1d	Distant metastasis to the central nervous system with or without M1a, M1b, or M1c sites of metastasis	Not recorded or unspecified
M1d(0)		Not elevated
M1d(1)		Elevated

Table 22.4 Eighth edition AJCC staging for melanoma. Description of AJCC pathological prognostic stage groups

Pathological stage group	T	N	M
0	Tis	N0	M0
IA	T1a	N0	M0
IB	T1b	N0	M0
IB	T2a	N0	M0
IIA	T2b	N0	M0
IIA	T3a	N0	M0
IIB	T3b	N0	M0
IIB	T4a	N0	M0
IIC	T4b	N0	M0
IIIB	T0	N1b, N1c	M0
IIIC	T0	N2b, N2c, N3b or N3c	M0
IIIA	T1a/b–T2a	N1a or N2a	M0
IIIB	T1a/b–T2a	N1b/c or N2b	M0
IIIB	T2b/T3a	N1a–N2b	M0
IIIC	T1a–T3a	N2c or N3a/b/c	M0
IIIC	T3b/T4a	Any N ≥ N1	M0
IIIC	T4b	N1a–N2c	M0
IIID	T4b	N3a/b/c	M0
IV	Any T, Tis	Any N	M1

is seen in patients with thick melanoma, Breslow >4 mm in which nodal spread is seen in more than 30% of patients [7, 17, 18]. Complete lymph node dissection (CLND) is associated with severe morbidities including severe bleeding, neurological damage, lymphedema, lymphatic fistula, and wound infection. Therefore, CLND is not justifiable in patients with thin melanoma due to the low prevalence of nodal metastases.

Sentinel lymph node biopsy (SLNB) has emerged as a preferred method for evaluating the draining lymph node basin for nodal metastasis in patients with intermediate thickness melanoma. The technique, first described by Morton and colleagues, is based on the paradigm that lymphatic drainage from a melanoma lesion follows an orderly manner in which drainage occurs first to a single or a few nodes—the sentinel node(s)—and then to the other lymph nodes in the draining basin [19]. If the sentinel lymph node (SLN) is identified, histologically examined, and tumor free, the other lymph nodes in the draining basin are unlikely to contain metastatic deposit, and the patient can be spared CLND and the potential complications therefrom. Fewer lymph nodes are removed and examined during a SLNB biopsy procedure compared with the number of nodes resected during CLND. This allows the pathologist to analyze these fewer nodes more intensively for microscopic metastasis and tumor isolates [20].

22.4.1 Radiopharmaceuticals

The ideal radiopharmaceutical for lymphoscintigraphy should have a rapid and predictable transport within the lymphatics to the sentinel node and a persistent retention within it. Persistent retention within sentinel node will ensure visualization of the sentinel nodes and reduce the number of resected numbers that may occur with tracer transit into second and third echelon of nodes. Resection of fewer nodes allows for more extensive examination of these nodes for metastases as well as reduces procedure-related morbidities. The size of the particles of the radiopharmaceutical is a strong determinant of its kinetics within the lymphatics. Small particle size <100 nm is required for the radiopharmaceutical to transit from the injection site to the lymphatic channels and the lymph nodes [21]. Particles larger than 500 nm remained trapped at the injection site, while particles smaller than 5 nm may penetrate the capillaries and therefore transit via the venous circulation. This is seen clinically as an early liver visualization on scintigraphy.

Three radiopharmaceuticals are in common use in clinical application.

1. Tc-99m sulfur colloid (Tc-99m SC) is prepared by the addition of Tc-99m eluate to a sulfur colloid (SC) kit. The reaction vial is heated at 100 °C for 5–10 min. The radiopharmaceutical so prepared has a low pH and causes burning sensation when injected into the skin. This may be prevented by neutralizing the tracer prior to injection using a phosphate buffer. The typical size of the particles ranges from 100 to 1000 nm [21]. This is filtered through a filter with pore size of less 220 nm to obtain smaller particle size suitable for lymphoscintigraphy.
2. Tc-99m nanocolloid is licensed in Europe for lymphoscintigraphy. It has typical particle size of 5–100 nm [20]. It is available in kit form with Stannous II chloride as a reducing agent. Its smaller particle size compared with Tc-99m SC may cause to transit faster from the injected site.
3. Tc-99m antimony trisulfide is available for clinical use in Australia. With a typical particle size of 3–30 nm, it has the smallest particle size among the three agents in common use in the clinics presently [20, 21].

Tc-99m tilmanocept (Tc-99m diethylenetriamine penta-acetic-acid-mannosyl-dextran) is a newer agent that recently received the United States Food and Drug Administration's approval for use in lymphatic mapping studies in breast cancer, melanoma, and other solid cancers. Tc-99m tilmanocept consists of dextran backbone surrounded by many mannose moieties. It binds to the mannose receptors (CD206) expressed on reticuloendothelial cells in the lymph nodes. It has an effective particle size of 7 nm. Consequent to its receptor binding property and its small size, Tc-99m tilmanocept has a more rapid clearance from the injection site and sustained sentinel lymph node uptake without distal transit to second and third echelon nodes [22, 23].

Lymphatic drainage mapping can be done with nonradioactive dyes alone or in combination with radioactive tracers. In the initial technique described by Morton et al., isosulfan blue dye alone was injected for sentinel node detection in patients with melanoma [19]. The blue dye was injected at the site of the melanoma lesion, and the drainage via the lymphatic was followed intraoperatively until it reached the sentinel node. Isosulfan blue dye is associated with about 1% risk of anaphylactic reaction [24]. Methylene blue dye is now used as a cheaper substitute for isosulfan blue dye with similar effectiveness at detecting sentinel nodes [25]. In melanoma patients, SLN is identified in about 84% of patients using blue dye alone, while with the use of radiopharmaceutical, SLN is detected in about 99% of cases [26]. The combination of both techniques yields a higher SLN detection rate.

A major limitation of the use of blue dyes is in their limited visibility through the skin or overlying tissue. Indocyanine green (ICG) is an alternative agent for optical imaging of the SLN. Following intradermal injections, ICG transits quickly through the lymphatics and accumulates within the SLN. ICG fluoresces at near-infrared region and is not visible to the unaided eyes. Dedicated near-infrared florescent camera is necessary for visualization of its tissue distribution [27]. The better tissue penetration and spatial resolution of ICG compared with blue dyes is responsible for its higher rate of SLN detection [27, 28].

A clinical trial of 80 patients comparing the SLN detection rates of Tc-99m nanocolloid versus ICG reported 21% detection rate for ICG before skin incision. This detection rate improved to 96% after skin incision. Tc-99m nanocolloid detected all SLN (100%) [29]. ICG has a small molecular weight of 774 Da and binds to albumin with a combined diameter of about 2.6 nm [30, 31]. On the basis of the studies reporting lower SLN detection rate for ICG, it is not recommended that this florescent technique be used alone. Florescence signal of ICG is limited to about 1–1.5 cm, and hence deeper lying nodes may not be seen. This will present a specific challenge especially in the obese patients.

Hybrid tracers in the form ICG-Tc-99m—nanocolloid for lymphatic mapping and SLN detection—have been described taking advantage of the merits of the two individual methods (radionuclide lymphoscintigraphy and florescent imaging). Stoffels et al. randomized 40 patients mostly with malignant melanoma of the head and neck into two groups—group A received ICG-Tc-99m nanocolloid hybrid tracer for SLN detection, while group B received standard Tc-99m nanocolloid. The end points were number of excised SLN and the duration of surgical procedure. The time to SLN excision was slightly shorter in group A compared with group B, but this difference did not reach statistical significance. SLN basins were identified preoperatively in all patients in group A but identified in 18/20 of patients in group B. The intraoperative SLN identification rate was higher in group A than in group B but again without statistical significance [32].

22.4.2 Methodology

22.4.2.1 Patient Preparation

No special patient preparation is necessary. Local anesthetic cream or spray may be applied for local pain control especially in mucosal melanoma or in children. Tight fitting clothing and jewelry must be removed before injection to prevent impaired lymphatic flow.

22.4.2.2 Injection Technique

Tuberculin syringes mounted with a narrow bore needle (25G or 27G) are preferred for tracer injection. Intradermal injection is the recommended method of injection because of the rich network of dermal lymphatics and the fact that cutaneous melanomas arise from melanocyte located in the dermoepidermal junction. The intradermal injection should be done 1 cm from the edge of the lesion or excisional biopsy scar. A distance more than 1 cm may be maintained between the injection site and the lesion/scar in a case of hypertrophic scar or scared skin [20]. The needle should be inserted tangential to the skin surface and about 0.1–0.2 ml of the tracer deposited a few millimeters within the skin [33]. A small volume of tracer should be deposited enough to raise a wheal as a larger volume may collapse the lymphatics. Care must be taken to prevent skin contamination, a potential false-positive interpretation.

The total injected activity depends on the time interval between lymphoscintigraphy and the proposed time of surgery and its range from 5 and 120 MBq with higher activity administered if lymphoscintigraphy is planned for the day before surgery [33]. The number of aliquots of tracer injected around the lesion/scar depends on the site of melanoma. Two injections on either side of the lesion/scar are generally adequate for melanoma of the extremities because of the predictable nature of the lymphatic drainage from these lesions. Head and neck lesions and, to a lesser extent, truncal melanoma have variable lymphatic drainage, and drainage may be cranial and caudal and across the midline of the body plane [34]. For this reason, tracer must be injected in four equal aliquots around the lesion/scar (at 3, 6, 9, and 12 O'clock positions) [33].

22.4.3 Preoperative Imaging

22.4.3.1 Dynamic Imaging

Following tracer injection, a dynamic lymphoscintigraphy is done using a large field of view gamma camera to cover all draining lymph node basins that may receive metastasis from the tumor. The European Association of Nuclear Medicine (EANM) recommends that the initial dynamic imaging be done using these imaging parameters: 1 min per frame for 10–20 min in a 128 × 128 matrix in word mode [33]. The use of a double-headed gamma camera reduces imaging time. Sentinel lymph node(s) is/are the node(s) that receive direct drainage from the tumor. Therefore, the dynamic imaging allows for the determination of the SLN. On a delayed image with visualization of multiple nodes, it may not be possible to distinguish between sentinel node(s) from second and third echelon nodes. Other merits of the dynamic imaging are the ability to detect lymph nodes lying close to the injection site, detection of in-transit node which may be the only site of metastasis, and detection of drainage to unusual lymph node basins [20, 33–35].

22.4.3.2 Static Images

After the dynamic image, an early static planar image is acquired for 5 min with a 256 × 256 matrix over the draining lymph node basin. Both anterior-posterior and lateral static images are acquired. For melanoma of the trunk, both axillae and groins must be images as direct drainage may be to any of these lymph node basins.

A second set of static planar images are acquired 1–3 h post tracer injection (delayed static images). The purpose of this delayed imaging is for skin marking which may facilitate intraoperative identification and resection. It is important to do skin marking at the same position the patient will be operated upon. Only node which meets criteria for SLNs must be marked to prevent unnecessary removal of non-sentinel nodes (second and third echelon nodes).

Imaging with body contouring adds topographic information to the acquired image and facilitates SLN localization. Co-57 flood source can be used to produce body silhouette. The source is placed below the bed during imaging of the trunk. Imaging may be repeated without the flood source to prevent the source from masking the visualization of a faint activity within a SLN.

22.4.3.3 SPECT and SPECT/CT Imaging

SPECT imaging provides superior contrast resolution above planar imaging and provides additional benefit in the form of more lymph node detection [36]. The addition of anatomic data in the form of CT provides better localization. CT data is also useful for attenuation correction of SPECT data and hence better image quality. The EANM has recommended the following parameters for SPECT acquisition: matrix size of 128 × 128, 180° in the anterior L-mode rotation, and a 3° angle step with 20–25 s per frame [33]. 3D volume rendering of CT images is now done in some departments, and this facilitates intraoperative localization and may shorten surgical time.

22.4.4 Intraoperative Procedure

A number of imaging and non-imaging techniques are now available to aid intraoperative identification of SLNs and their removal. The gamma probe is a handheld device that is useful to guide SLN identification intraoperatively. The gamma probe is used to localize the preoperatively localized SLN. After the removal of SLN, the gamma probe is applied to it so that it is indeed the radioactive node identified on imaging. The probe is also applied to the lymph node basin where a low count is recorded after successful excision of the hot SLN.

The blue dye technique improves SLN detection and may be used in combination with the gamma probe as a non-imaging intraoperative technique.

Portable gamma cameras are now available for intraoperative imaging of radioactive SLNs. They provide real-time visualization of the SLNs, and their successful resection can also be confirmed on imaging. Combined intraoperative florescent and SPECT imaging with hybrid tracers are now being reported [37]. This technique may be useful in SLNB of melanoma in the neck and neck region due to the complex anatomy of this region.

22.4.5 Indications and Contraindications

The SLNB is indicated in patients with intermediate thickness melanoma (Breslow thickness 1.01–4 mm). There is <5% risk of nodal metastasis in patients with thin melanoma (Breslow thickness

≤1 mm), and routine SLNB is not recommended. The National Comprehensive Cancer Network (NCCN) recommends SLNB in thin melanomas in the following scenarios [38]:

- Breslow thickness <0.8 mm with any of these adverse features alone or in combination—ulceration, mitotic index ≥2/mm^2 (especially in young patients), lymphovascular invasion
- Breslow thickness 0.8–1 mm with or without ulceration
- Significant uncertainty on the adequacy of Breslow thickness measurement

SLNB is not routinely done in patients with thick melanoma (Breslow >4 mm). This high rate of nodal metastasis in this category of patients justifies a CLND.

SLNB is not indicated in the following settings:

- Clinically detectable metastatic melanoma including patients with satellitosis and in-transit metastasis
- Extensive surgical dissection including reconstructive surgery at the site of the primary tumor or the lymph node basin that causes distortion of the lymphatics [39]
- Extreme old age (>80 years) due to atrophic lymphatics [39]
- Poor general health status, severe concurrent illness

22.5 ^{18}F-FDG PET/CT Imaging of Melanoma

^{18}F-FDG PET/CT (FDG PET/CT) has a widespread utility in the imaging of various human solid tumors. Thick melanomas are a highly metastatic tumor. FDG PET/CT is becoming an increasingly useful imaging modality in melanoma patients.

22.5.1 Staging

FDG PET/CT is not indicated in all stages of melanoma for initial staging. Melanoma is staged using the AJCC staging system (Tables 22.1, 22.2, 22.3, and 22.4). The staging of the primary tumor (T staging) is based on the thickness of the tumor which is obtained at histology. Metastasis occurs early to lymph nodes [14]. Visceral metastasis occurs in more advanced disease. FDG PET/CT is useful in evaluating for nodal (N staging) and distant metastasis (M staging). F-18 FDG PET/CT has low yield in patients with stage I and II disease [40–42]. This is because the PET camera has poor sensitivity for the detection of micrometastasis or tumor isolates owing to its limited spatial resolution. SLNB techniques are more sensitive for the evaluation of micrometastasis [43]. FDG PET/CT is therefore not recommended in this category of patients.

Conversely, in patients with palpable nodal disease (macrometastases), FDG PET/CT is useful in N and M staging. For this indication, FDG PET/CT outperforms conventional radiological techniques in detecting distant metastases with a sensitivity and specificity of 80% and 87%, respectively, compared with 51% and 69%, respectively, for CT [44]. FDG PET/CT obtained for initial staging in AJCC stage III melanoma may upstage disease to stage IV by detecting previously unknown sites of metastases [45]. It helps to detect sites of deep tissue, lymph node, and visceral metastases [46]. In a meta-analysis, FDG PET led to a change in planned patient management in 33% of cases (range = 15–64%) [47]. FDG PET/CT scan performed for initial staging in stage III and IV disease has prognostic utility. Limited or no disease on such scans confers survival benefit on the patients, while patients with extensive disease have a lower 5-year melanoma-specific survival rates [48].

22.5.2 Therapy Response Assessment

Previously, FDG PET/CT played limited role in therapy response assessment. This was largely due to the fact that only few effective therapeutic options were available for the treatment of widely metastatic melanoma. Then, response assessment was based on changes in standardized uptake values and other PET metabolic parameters such as total lesion glycolysis (TLG) between the baseline and posttreatment scans [49]. These FDG PET parameters outperform soluble biomarkers such as S-100B in response to therapy assessment [49, 50] (Fig. 22.1).

The management of metastatic malignant melanomas received a boost with the introduction of immune modulation therapy and mutation-targeted therapy [46]. Immune modulation therapy uses monoclonal antibodies to turn on the host immune system to attack the cancer cells. Two broad categories of immune modulating therapy are currently approved for treatment of metastatic malignant melanoma. One group acts by targeting the cytotoxic T-lymphocyte antigen-4 (CTLA-4), while the other group targets the programmed cell death 1 protein (PD-1) and its ligands (PD-L1 and PD-L2) [51]. Mutation-targeted therapy is directed against the common mutations in malignant melanoma. BRAF is a serine/threonine kinase that is downstream of RAS, and its activating mutations are seen in 40–50% of melanomas [2]. MEK1 and MEK2 are effector proteins downstream of BRAF and have also been targeted in the treatment of metastatic melanoma. All of these immune modulation and mutation-targeted therapies have been shown to prolong survival in advanced melanoma patients [52, 53] (Fig. 22.2).

The utility of FDG PET/CT in therapy response assessment to immune checkpoint modulators is emerging. In a group of melanoma patients with BRAF mutations, McArthur and colleagues showed a reduction of 80% in SUVmax following therapy with vemurafenib including three patients with complete metabolic response [54]. The changes in SUVmax in response to therapy occur early (15 days) after

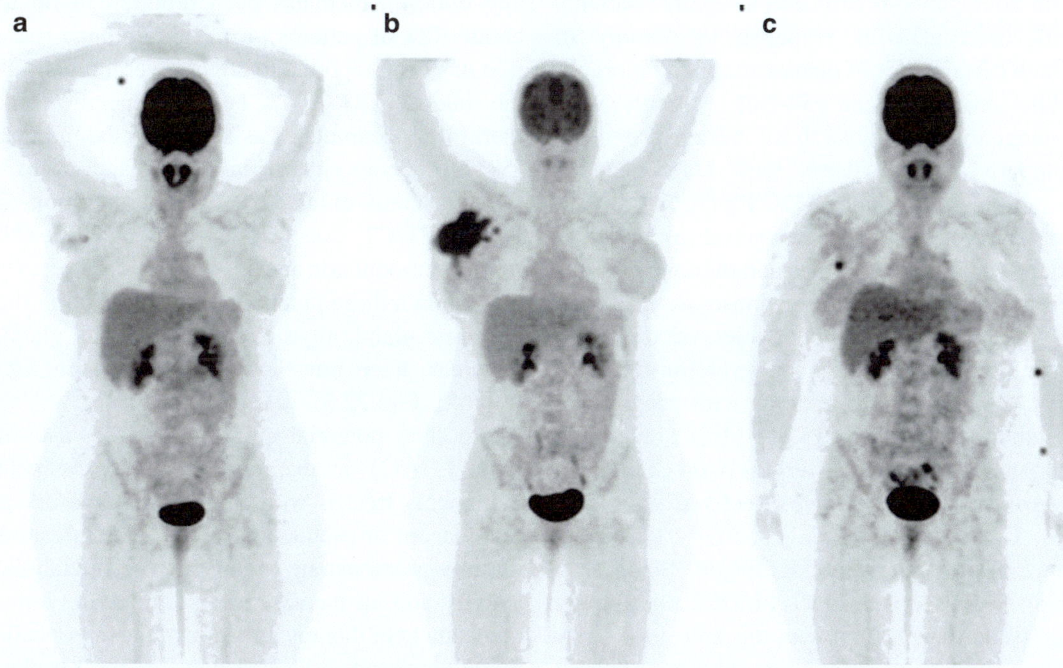

Fig. 22.1 F18 FDG PET/CT for recurrence and monitoring of response to therapy. A 41-year-old female Caucasian status post excision of a superficial spreading malignant melanoma from the tip of her right shoulder and right axillary lymphadenectomy. Three sets of F-18 FDG PET/CT were acquired in 2015, 2016, and 2017. (**a**) F-18 FDG PET/CT of October 2015 post-surgery showed low grade soft tissue FDG uptake at surgical site in the right axilla consistent with postoperative changes. (**b**) F-18 FDG PET/CT acquired in May 2016 showed metabolically active conglomerate of right axillary lymph nodes consistent with melanoma recurrence. (**c**) A repeat F-18 FDG PET/CT of August 2017 postchemotherapy showed significant reduction in right axillary mass as well as its metabolic activity consistent with response to chemotherapy

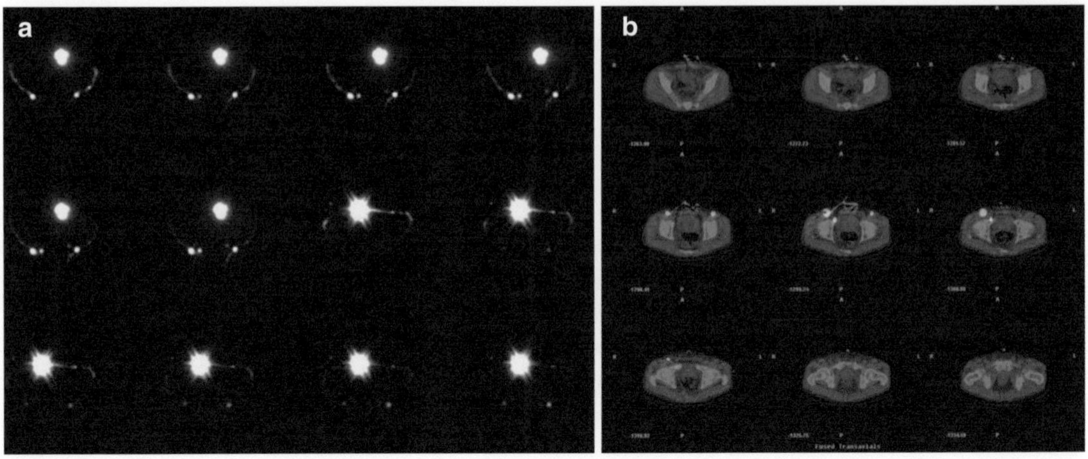

Fig. 22.2 Sentinel lymph node for melanoma. A 72-year-old male Caucasian with an intermediate thickness malignant melanoma excised from his back in the midline. Sentinel lymph node study was done. (**a**) Dynamic imaging showed drainage to bilateral inguinal regions. (**b**) Fused SPECT/CT images showed sentinel nodes in the groins bilaterally

treatment. FDG PET may also show patients with homogeneous response as against patients with heterogeneous response to therapy in which certain sites of disease respond favorably while other do not [54–56]. Patients with homogenous response have better prognosis compared with patients with heterogeneous response. Additionally, FDG PET/CT is able to predict progression-free survival as early as after two cycles of ipilimumab therapy. Patients with stable metabolic response assessed on FDG PET/CT after two cycles of treatment have significantly longer progression-free survival compared with patients with progressive metabolic response [57]. Most oncologic response assessment criteria rely on changes in size of tumor to determine effectiveness of therapy. Changes in metabolic activity of tumor, however, precede any significant changes in size. The use of F-FDG PET/CT in therapy assessment may, therefore, be able to stratify patient into good responders who may benefit from continuation of therapy and nonresponders in whom it may be more appropriate to interrupt therapy.

Immune modulation therapy potentiates the activity of T lymphocytes. This causes a high rate of immune-related side effects of this therapy option which has been reported in up to about 70% of patients [46]. This immune reaction has been reported to affect several organs of the body. FDG PET/CT is nonspecific and, therefore, accumulates as sites of inflammation [58, 59]. These sites of immune reaction are a potential cause of false-positive interpretation on FDG PET/CT done in patients treated with immune modulator agents. Several case reports have shown these potential pitfalls involving the pituitary gland, thyroid gland, adrenal gland, pancreas, liver, bowel, lymph nodes, skin, etc. [60–62] (Fig. 22.3).

Another potential pitfall with the use of FDG PET/CT in therapy response assessment in patients treated with immune modulators is the concept of pseudoprogression where lesions initially demonstrate more intense metabolic activity and an increase in size following commencement of therapy. Invasion of the tumor cells by inflammatory cells is responsible for this phenomenon. The disease initially progresses before showing documented response [63]. This may be erroneously interpreted as therapy failure leading to discontinuation of a beneficial treatment. This peculiarity of response to immune modulation

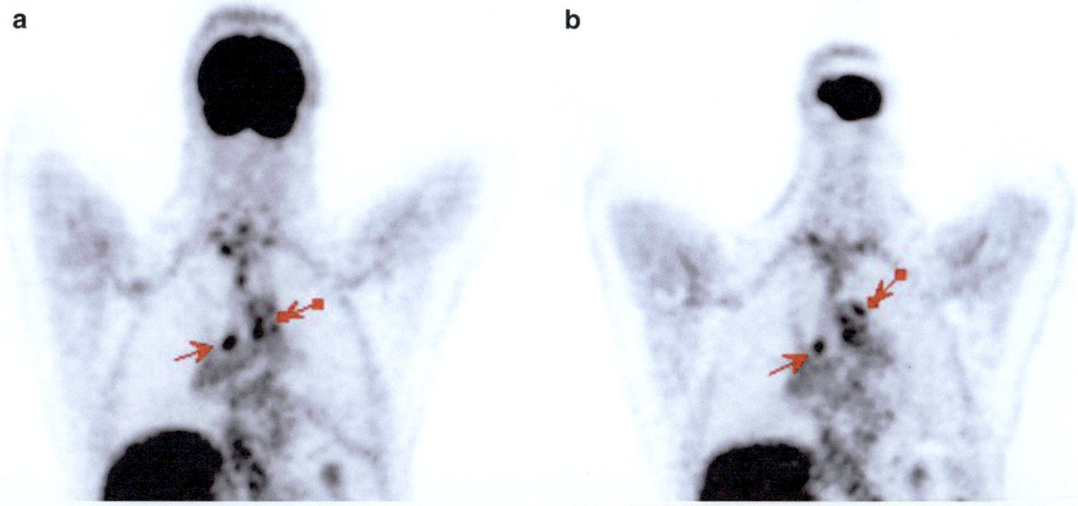

Fig. 22.3 False-positive on F-18 FDG PET/CT. A 79-year-old female Caucasian had malignant melanoma excised from her right shoulder. One of four right supraclavicular nodes resected was positive for micrometastasis. (**a**) Baseline F-18 FDG PET/CT acquired in April 2016 showed metabolic activity in multiple meditational lymph nodes (red arrows). (**b**) A follow-up F-18 FDG PET/CT done in July 2017 with no treatment in the interval showed that mediastinal nodes have remained the same size and in the level of metabolic activity. This was interpreted as benign lymphadenopathy

therapy has led to the development of a dedicated response assessment criteria by the response evaluation criteria in solid tumors (RECIST) working group called immune Response Criteria in Solid Tumor (iRECIST) [64] (Fig. 22.4).

22.5.3 Surveillance

Melanoma frequently recurs following initial treatment. Rate of recurrence is higher in more advanced disease (stage III) compared with early-staged disease (stage I and II). The 5-year relapse-free survival at any site is 63% for stage IIIA, 32% for stage IIIB, and 11% for stage III [65]. The commonest sites of disease relapse are local/in-transit, lymph nodes, liver, and lungs [66]. It is important to detect recurrence early when salvage therapy (metastectomy) may be offered with curative intent. Diagnosis of advanced recurrent disease is now important due to the availability of effective therapies including immune modulators and mutation-targeted therapy [46]. Surveillance for melanoma can be done using clinical examination and tumor markers, e.g., S-100B, or with imaging. Addition of imaging to patients' follow-up detects more cases of recurrence [67]. Imaging may also be able to detect disease recurrence before it becomes clinically apparent [66]. The NCCN guidelines do not recommend routine imaging in the follow-up of asymptomatic patients with stage IA–IIA disease. For stage IIB–IV, imaging every 3–12 months is recommended but not beyond 3–5 years in asymptomatic patients [38] (Figs. 22.5, 22.6, 22.7, 22.8, and 22.9).

FDG PET outperforms standard diagnostic procedures (including clinical examination, ultrasound, CT, and MRI) in the evaluation of patients with symptomatic recurrent melanoma. In a per-patient analysis, FDG PET has sensitivity and specificity of 74% and 86%, respectively, compared with 58% and 45% for standard diagnostic procedures. PET was more accurate in detecting local regional recurrence and distant metastases than standard diagnostic procedures. PET and CT performed equally for the detection

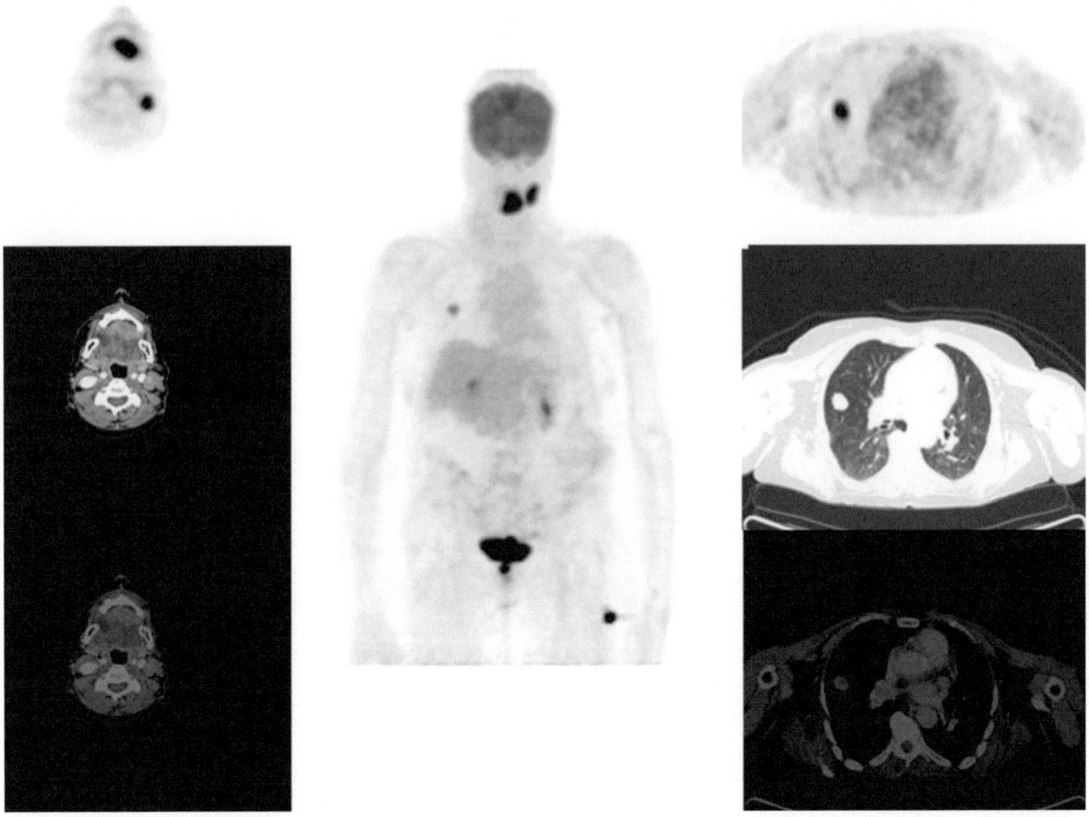

Fig. 22.4 F-18 FDG PET/CT upstages disease and led to change in management plan. A 64-year-old Black female with malignant melanoma of the tongue and a palpable level Va cervical lymph node. F-18 FDG PET/C was acquired for staging. Images show primary lesion on the dorsum of the tongue, metastatic left cervical lymph node, and a previously unknown right middle lobe lung metastasis

of pulmonary recurrence. However, PET was less sensitive for brain metastases compared with MRI [68]. Compared with S-100B, FDG PET/CT has better diagnostic performance with a sensitivity, specificity, positive predictive value, and negative predictive value 98.5%, 90.9%, 98.5%, and 90.9%, respectively, in the detection of disease recurrence among melanoma patients with symptomatic recurrence versus 33.8%, 90.9%, 96.0%, and 17.5% for S-100B [69].

In view of the need to detect recurrence early, FDG PET/CT has been evaluated for the detection of asymptomatic recurrence. In a retrospective review of 144 patients with stage I–III malignant melanoma asymptomatic for recurrence who had FDG PET/CT for surveillance, recurrence was detected in 25.7% of the patients after a median follow-up of 50.5 months with a median time to recurrence of 20 months (range = 5.6–37 months). FDG PET/CT had a sensitivity of 94.5%, specificity of 87.6%, and accuracy of 89.6% for the detection of recurrence in the study [66]. In a more selective study including patients with stage IIIB and IIIC disease who were followed up with FDG PET/CT every 6 months, PET was 91% sensitive and 95% specific for the detection of asymptomatic recurrence. All recurrences detected had S-100B in the normal range emphasizing the superiority of imaging above tumor markers for surveillance [70]. Imaging can detect the site of recurrence and extent of recurrence, two important pieces of information needed to decide on therapy option.

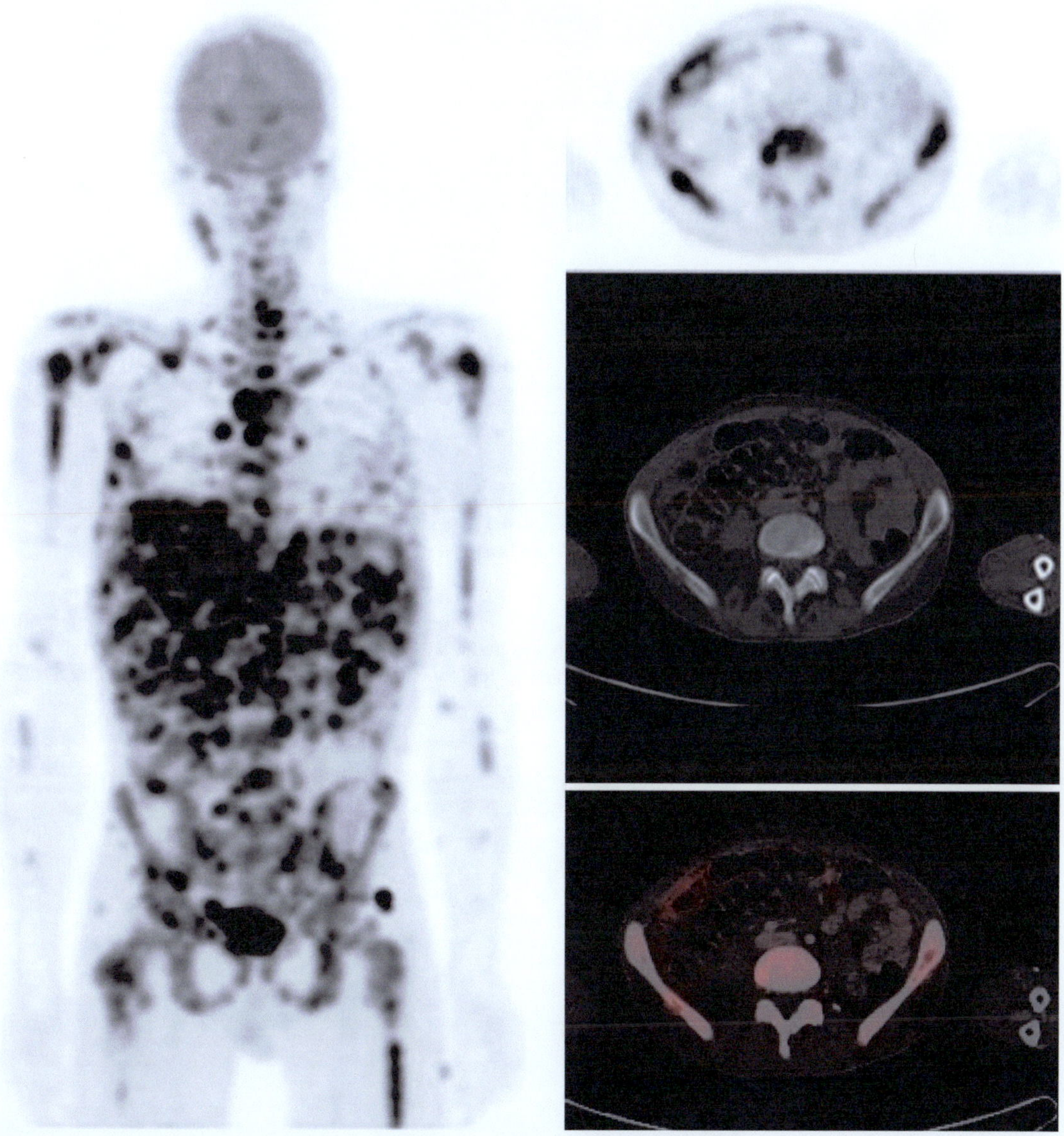

Fig. 22.5 F-18 FDG PET for surveillance. A 33-year-old Caucasian male with melanoma of the back. Baseline F-18 FDG PET/CT showed a solitary metastatic right inguinal node and a metastatic right gluteal cutaneous nodule. Metastectomy was performed and patient was followed up with a repeat F-18 FDG PET/CT 8 months later. Repeat imaging showed widespread metastases to the nodes, bones, liver, and lung

The scan reader must be aware of the potential pitfalls associated with FDG PET/CT obtained for surveillance. Due to the limited resolution of the PET system, micrometastases are not detected. This is a potential cause of false-negative interpretation. Intense physiologic uptake in the brain may obscure visualization of brain metastases. Conversely, F-18 FDG uptake in non-malignant inflammatory or infectious focus may be wrongly interpreted as disease recurrence. These potential causes of false-positive interpretation may constitute a big challenge in regions where granulomatous inflammatory conditions such as tuberculous infection and fungal infections are endemic [66].

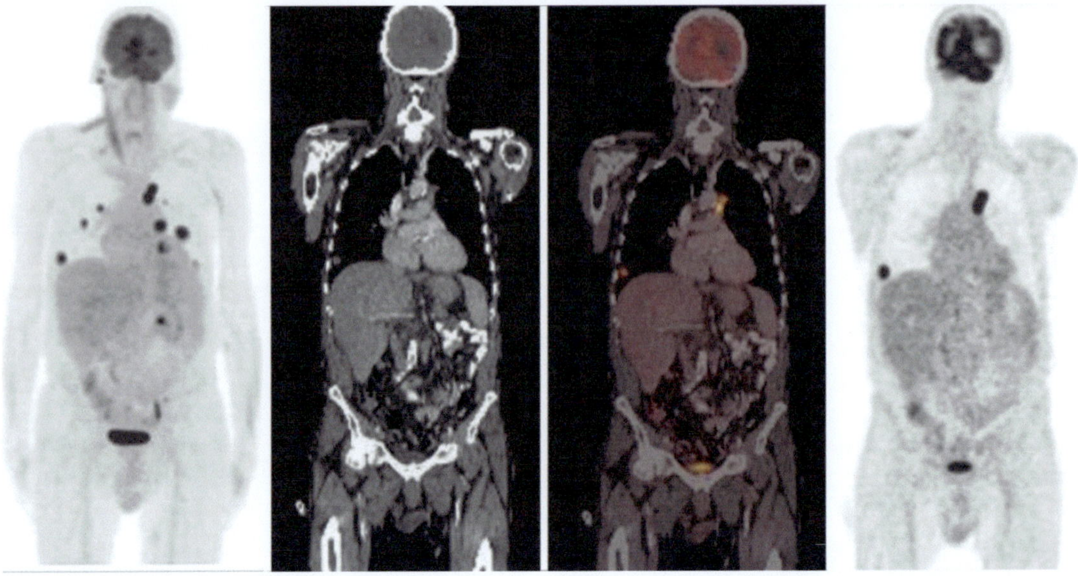

Fig. 22.6 F-18 FDG PET/CT for initial staging. In a 77-year-old Caucasian male, an ulcerated nodular malignant melanoma was excised from the right ear lobe, Breslow thickness = 18.6 mm. One of right cervical nodes resected on supraomohyoid neck dissection was positive for metastasis. F-18 FDG obtained for restaging postsurgery showed metastases to the right multiple mediastinal node, both lungs and left iliac bone. Benign right sternocleidomastoid and trapezius muscles' metabolic activity were seen

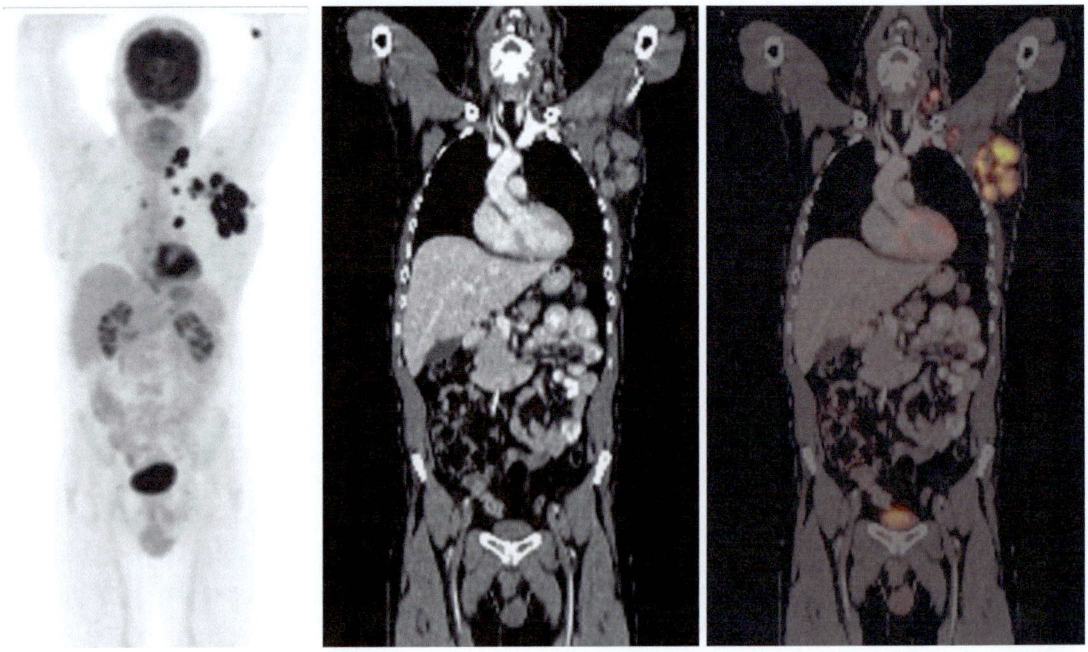

Fig. 22.7 F-18 FDG PET/CT for initial staging. A 51-year-old Caucasian male with malignant melanoma diagnosed from biopsy of left axillary node. F-18 FDG PET/CT was acquired for staging. Images showed multiple nodal metastases. Site of primary melanoma remained unknown

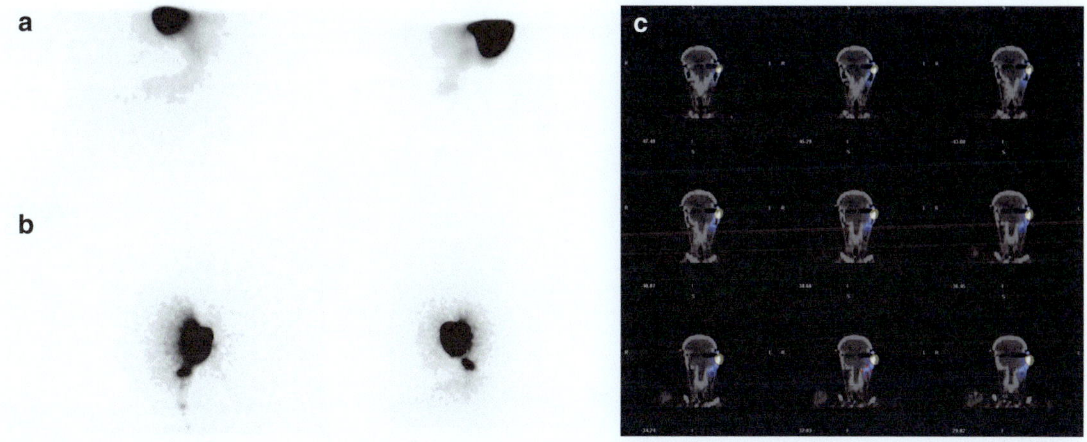

Fig. 22.8 F-18 FDG PET negative but positive SLNB for micrometastasis. An 85-year-old Caucasian female with a 2.5 mm malignant melanoma excised from the helix of the left ear. F-18 FDG PET/CT obtained was negative for residual malignant disease postsurgery. A sentinel lymph node biopsy procedure was done. (**a**, **b**) No sentinel node was visualized on static images obtained at 60 min but seen on the static images obtained at 120 min. (**c**) This was confirmed on SPECT/CT images. Histological examination showed micrometastasis in the resected sentinel node. Failure to visualize sentinel node on 60 min images was probably related to atrophic lymphatic seen in older patients. Negative F-18 FDG PET is related to poor sensitivity of this imaging technique for micrometastasis

22.6 Tracers for Specific Targeting of Melanoma

Despite the good performance reported for FDG PET in the imaging of patients with melanoma, significant challenges still exist in its clinical application. Following the introduction of immune modulator agents for the treatment of advanced melanoma, by far, the greatest challenge with FDG PET use lies in its lack for specificity to differentiate between malignancies from inflammatory conditions [71]. Immune-related side effects may be seen in up to 70% of these patients [46]. The development of a molecular probe that targets the cancer cells and capable of differentiating melanoma from other malignant tissues or inflammatory condition is, therefore, necessary. Wei and co-authors have recently presented the various efforts undertaken to achieving this goal [72]. The details of the agents with potential for specific targeting of melanoma is, however, beyond the scope of this chapter.

High level of melanin is synthesized in melanoma. This has made its targeting for melanoma imaging attractive. Radiolabeled benzamide and its derivatives are currently being explored for targeting melanin for melanoma imaging. ^{123}I-BZA2 is a benzamide analogue that targets melanin of melanin-positive melanomas. In a study of 87 patients with melanoma, in a per lesion analysis, ^{123}I-BZA2 demonstrated better specificity for detecting metastases compared with FDG PET (86% versus 54%, $p < 0.05$). In the study, ^{123}I-BZA2 had a lower sensitivity compared with F-18 FDG PET probably due to the small number of lesions with high melanin expression as confirmed on histological examination [73]. ^{18}F-5-FPN is another benzamide derivative for PET imaging. It was shown in a mice model of melanoma to have better sensitivity for the detection of lung metastases as well as subcentimeter metastatic lymph nodes [74].

α-Melanocyte-stimulating hormone (α-MSH) is a ligand for the melanocortin 1 receptor (MC1R) overexpressed in melanoma. Several analogues of (α-MSH) have been explored for specific melanoma imaging. MC1R receptor is expressed by both melanotic and amelanotic melanoma [72]; hence, its targeting may have broader application compared with benzamide analogues which are only useful for imaging of melanoma with high melanin production.

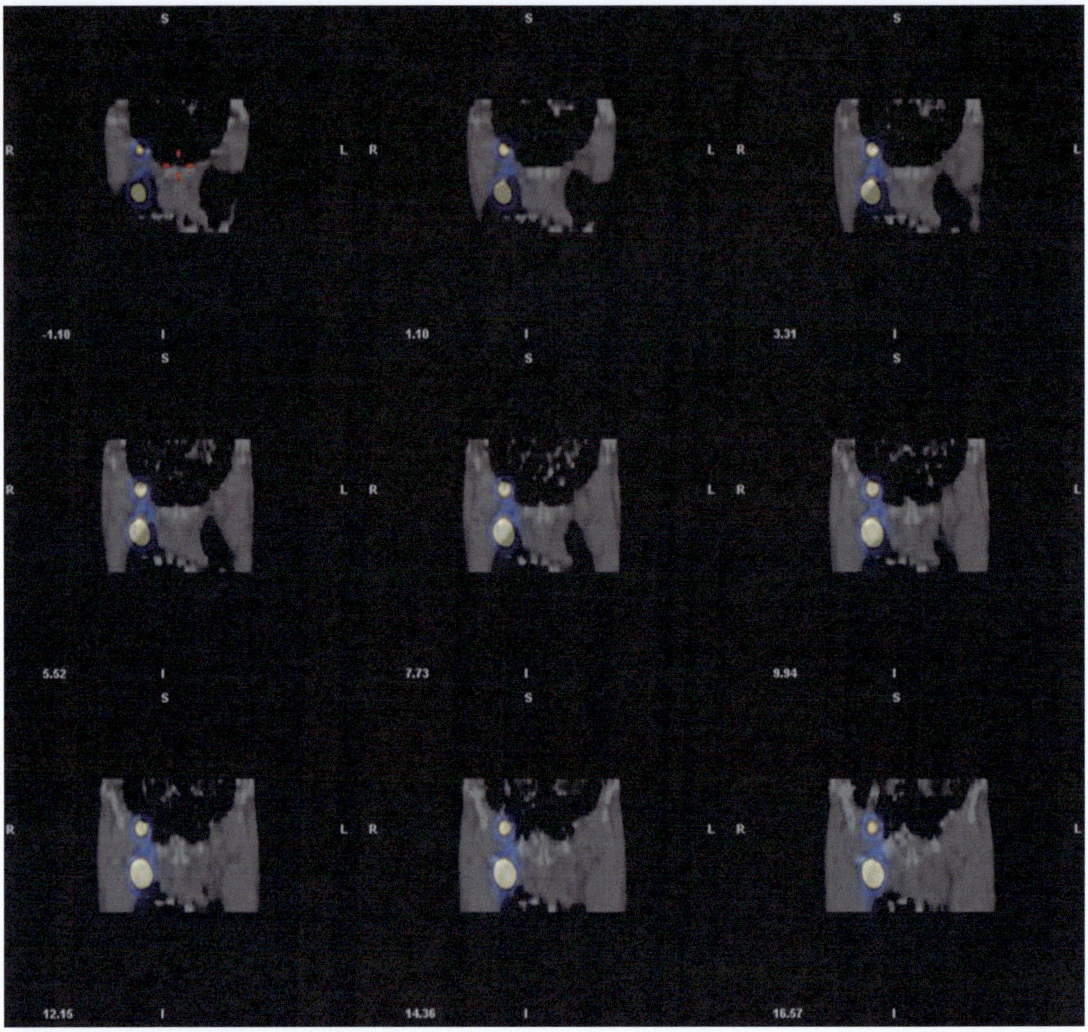

Fig. 22.9 SLNB. A 77-year-old Black male with acral lentiginous malignant melanoma of the right heel scheduled for wide local excision. Sentinel lymph node study was done which showed a sentinel node in the right inguinal region and a second echelon node in the right external iliac region. Frozen section of the resected right inguinal node was positive for metastasis necessitating right groin dissection and complete lymphadenectomy

I-111 diethylenetriaminepentacetic acid (DTPA)-anti-PD-L1 is a novel tracer that has been shown to be capable to identify tumor that overexpresses PD-L1 and consequently patients who may benefit from immunomodulation therapy targeting this ligand [75].

References

1. American Cancer Society. Cancer facts & figures 2017. http://www.cancer.org/research/cancer-facts-statistics/all-cancer-facts-figures/cancer-facts-figures-2017.html. Accessed 3 Dec 2017.
2. Lazar AJF, Murphy GF. The skin. In: Kumar V, Abbas AK, Aster JC, editors. Robbins and Cotran pathologic basis of disease. 9th ed. Philadelphia: Elsevier Saunders; 2015. p. 1141–78.
3. Gandini S, Sera F, Cattaruzza MS, Pasquini P, Picconi O, Boyle P, et al. Meta-analysis of risk factors for cutaneous melanoma: II. Sun exposure. Eur J Cancer. 2005;41:45–60.
4. Gandini S, Sera F, Cattruzza MS, Pasquini P, Abeni D, Boyle P, et al. Meta-analysis of risk factors for cutaneous melanoma: I. Common and atypical naevi. Eur J Cancer. 2005;41:28–44.
5. Gandini S, Sera F, Cattaruzza MS, Pasquini P, Zanetti R, Masini C, et al. Meta-analysis of risk factors for cutaneous melanoma: III. Family history, actinic damage and phenotypic factors. Eur J Cancer. 2005;41:2040–59.

6. Markovic SN, Erickson L, Rao RD, McWilliams RR, Kottschade LA, Creagan ET, et al. Malignant melanoma in the 21st century, Part 1: Epidemiology, risk factors, screening, prevention, and diagnosis. Mayo Clin Proc. 2007;82:364–80.
7. Balch CM, Soong SJ, Gershenwald JE, Thompson JF, Reintgen DS, Cascinelli N, et al. Prognostic factors analysis of 17,600 melanoma patients: validation of the American Joint Committee on Cancer Melanoma Staging System. J Clin Oncol. 2001;16:3622–34.
8. Mandalà M, Imberti GL, Piazzalunga D, Belfiglio M, Labianca R, Barberis M, et al. Clinical and histopathological risk factors to predict sentinel lymph node positivity, disease-free and overall survival in clinical stages I–II AJCC skin melanoma: outcome analysis from a single-institution prospectively collected database. Eur J Cancer. 2009;45:2537–45.
9. Mandalà M, Galli F, Cattaneo L, Merelli B, Rulli E, Ribero S, et al. Mitotic rate correlates with sentinel lymph node status and outcome in cutaneous greater than 1 millimeter in thickness: a multi-institutional study of 1524 cases. J Am Acad Dermatol. 2017;76:264–73.
10. Ettl T, Irga S, Müller S, Rohrmeier C, Reichert TE, Schreml S, et al. Value of anatomic site, histology and clinicopathological parameters for prediction of lymph node metastasis and overall survival in head and neck melanomas. J Craniomaxillofac Surg. 2014;42:e252–8.
11. Pizzichetta MA, Massi D, Mandalà M, Queirolo P, Stanganelli I, De Giogi V, et al. Clinicopathologic predictors of recurrence in nodular and superficial spreading cutaneous melanoma: a multivariate analysis of 214 cases. J Transl Med. 2017;15:227. https://doi.org/10.1186/s12967-017-1332-3.
12. Zugna D, Senetta R, Osella-Abate S, Fierro MT, Pisacane A, Zaccagna A, et al. Favourable prognostic role of histological regression in stage III positive sentinel lymph node melanoma patients. Br J Cancer. 2017;118:398. https://doi.org/10.1038/bjc.2017.397.
13. Gershenwald JE, Scolyer RA, Hess KR, Sondak VK, Long GV, Ross MI, et al. Melanoma of the skin. In: Amin MB, Edge SB, Greene FL, et al., editors. AJCC cancer staging manual. 8th ed. New York: Springer International Publishing; 2017. p. 563–85.
14. Reintgen D, Cruse CW, Wells K, Berman C, Fenske N, Glass F, et al. The orderly progression of melanoma nodal metastases. Ann Surg. 1994;220:759–67.
15. Gershenwald JE, Thompson W, Mansfield PF, Lee JE, Colome MI, Tseng C, et al. Multi-institutional melanoma lymphatic mapping experience: the prognostic value of sentinel lymph node status in 612 stage I or II melanoma patients. J Clin Oncol. 1999;17:976–83.
16. Morton DL, Thompson JF, Cochran AJ, Mozzillo N, Elashoff R, Essner R, et al. Sentinel-node biopsy or nodal observation in melanoma. N Engl J Med. 2006;355:1307–17.
17. Slingluff CL, Stidham KR, Ricci WM, Stanley WE, Seigler HF. Surgical management of regional lymph nodes in patients with melanoma. Experience in 4682 patients. Ann Surg. 1994;219:120–30.
18. Gershenwald JE, Mansfield PF, Lee JE, Ross MI. Role for lymphatic mapping and sentinel lymph node biopsy in patients with thick (≥4 mm) primary melanoma. Ann Surg Oncol. 2000;7:160–5.
19. Morton DL, Wen DR, Wong JH, Economou JS, Cagle LA, Storm FK, et al. Technical details of intraoperative lymphatic mapping for early stage melanoma. Arch Surg. 1992;127:392–9.
20. Tardelli E, Mazzarri S, Rubello D, Gennaro M, Fantechi L, Duce V, et al. Sentinel lymph node biopsy in cutaneous melanoma: standard and new technical procedures and clinical advances. A systematic review of the literature. Clin Nucl Med. 2016;41:e498–507.
21. Wilhelm AJ, Mijnhout GS, Franssen EJF. Radiopharmaceuticals in sentinel lymph-node dissection—an overview. Eur J Nucl Med. 1999;26(Suppl 1):S36–42.
22. Surasi DS, O'Malley J, Bhambhvani P. ^{99m}Tc-tilmanocept: a novel molecular agent for lymphatic mapping and sentinel lymph node localization. J Nucl Med Technol. 2015;43:87–91.
23. Baker JL, Pu M, Tokin CA, Hoh CK, Vera DR, Messer K, et al. Comparison of [^{99m}Tc]Tilmanocept and filtered [^{99m}Tc]sulfur colloid for identification of SLNs in breast cancer patients. Ann Surg Oncol. 2015;22:40–5.
24. Leong SP, Donegan E, Heffernon W, Dean S, Katz JA. Adverse reactions to isosulfan blue during selective sentinel lymph node dissection in melanoma. Ann Surg Oncol. 2000;7:361–6.
25. Simmons R, Thevarajah S, Brennan MB, Christos P, Osborne M. Methylene blue dye as an alternative to isosulfan blue dye for sentinel lymph node localization. Ann Surg Oncol. 2003;10:242–7.
26. Niebling MG, Pleijhuis RG, Bastiaannet E, Brouwers AH, van Dam GM, Hoekstra HJ. A systematic review and meta-analyses of sentinel lymph node identification in breast cancer and melanoma, a plea for tracer mapping. Eur J Surg Oncol. 2016;42:466–73.
27. Burnier P, Niddam J, Bosc R, Hersant B, Meninguad JP. Indocyanine green applications in plastic surgery: a review of the literature. J Plast Reconstr Aesthet Surg. 2017;70:814–27.
28. Sugie T, Sawada T, Tagaya N, Kinoshita T, Yamagami K, Suwa H, et al. Comparison of the indocyanine green florescence and blue dye methods in detection of sentinel lymph nodes in early-stage breast cancer. Ann Surg Oncol. 2013;20:2213–8.
29. Stoffels I, Dissemond J, Pöppel T, Schadendorf D, Klode J. Intraoperative fluorescence imaging for sentinel lymph node detection. Prospective clinical trial to compare the usefulness of indocyanine green vs technetium Tc 99m for identification of sentinel lymph nodes. JAMA Surg. 2015;150:617–23.
30. Furukawa N, Oi H, Shigetomi H, Kanyama S, Kobayashi H. The usefulness of Photodynamic Eye for sentinel lymph node identification in patients with cervical cancer. Tumori. 2010;96:936–40.
31. Takayama S, Furuhama K, Ohura K, Onodera T, Akimoto T. Experimental studies on the usefulness

of Indocyanine green (ICG) as a lymphatic vital dye. Oyo Yakuri Pharmacometrics. 1980;19:603–14.
32. Stoffels I, Leyh J, Pöppel T, Schadendorf D, Klode J. Evaluation of a radioactive and fluorescent hybrid tracer for sentinel lymph node biopsy in head and neck malignancies: prospective randomized clinical to compare ICG-^{99m}Tc-nanocolloid hybrid tracer versus ^{99m}Tc-nanocolloid. Eur J Nucl Med Mol Imaging. 2015;42:1631–8.
33. Bluemel C, Herrmann K, Giammarile F, Nieweg OE, Dubreuil J, Testori A, et al. EANM practice guidelines for lymphoscintigraphy and sentinel lymph node biopsy in melanoma. Eur J Nucl Med Mol Imaging. 2015;42:1750–66.
34. Voinea S, Sandru A, Gherghe M, Blidaru A. Peculiarities of lymphatic drainage in cutaneous malignant melanoma: clinical experience in 75 cases. Chirurgia. 2014;109:26–33.
35. Voinea S, Sandru A, Gherghe M. Pitfalls in cutaneous melanoma lymphatic drainage. Chirurgia. 2016;III:87–9.
36. Doepker MP, Yamamoto M, Applebaum MA, Patel NU, Montilla-Soler MJ, Sarnaik AA, et al. Comparison of single-photon emission computed tomography-computed tomography (SPECT/CT) and conventional planar lymphoscintigraphy for sentinel node localization in patients with cutaneous malignancies. Ann Surg Oncol. 2017;24:355–61.
37. KleinJan GH, Karakullukçu B, Klop MC, Engelen T, van den Berg N, van Leeuwen FWB. Introducing navigation during melanoma-related sentinel lymph node procedures in the head-and-neck region. EJNMMI Res. 2017;7:65. https://doi.org/10.1186/s13550-017-0312-1.
38. Coit DG, Thompson JA, Albertini MR, Algazi A, Andtbacka R, Bichakjian CK, et al. NCCN clinical practice guidelines in oncology. Melanoma. Version I. 2018.
39. Schuitevoerder D, Grinlington L, Stevens J, Nance R, Fortino J, Vetto JT. Nonvisualised sentinel lymph nodes on lymphoscintigraphy in melanoma: predictive factors and surgical outcomes. Nucl Med Commun. 2017;38:383–7.
40. Holtkamp LHJ, Read RL, Emmett L, Thompson JF, Nieweg OE. Futility of imaging to stage melanoma patients with a positive sentinel lymph node. Melanoma Res. 2017;27:457–62.
41. Wagner T, Meyer N, Zerdoud S, Julian A, Payoux P, Courbon F. Fluorodeoxyglucose positron emission tomography fails to detect distant metastases at initial staging of melanoma patients with metastatic involvement of sentinel lymph node. Br J Dermatol. 2011;164:1235–40.
42. Clark PB, Soo V, Kraas J, Shen P, Levine EA. Futility of fluorodeoxyglucose F 18 positron emission tomography in initial evaluation of patients with T2 to T4 melanoma. Arch Surg. 2006;141:284–8.
43. Singh B, Ezziddin S, Palmedo H, Reinhardt M, Strunk H, Tüting T, et al. Preoperative 18F-FDG-PET/CT imaging and sentinel node biopsy in the detection of regional lymph node metastases in malignant melanoma. Melanoma Res. 2008;18:346–52.
44. Xing Y, Bronstein Y, Ross MI, Askew RL, Lee JE, Gershenwald JE, et al. Contemporary diagnostic imaging modalities for the staging and surveillance of melanoma patients: a meta-analysis. J Natl Cancer Inst. 2011;103:129–42.
45. Singnurkar A, Wang J, Joshua AM, Langer DL, Metser U. ^{18}F-FDG-PET/CT in the staging and management of melanoma. A prospective Multicenter Ontario PET Registry Study. Clin Nucl Med. 2016;41:189–93.
46. Perng P, Marcus C, Subramaniam RM. ^{18}F-FDG PET/CT and melanoma: staging, immune modulation and mutation-targeted therapy assessment, and prognosis. AJR. 2015;205:259–70.
47. Krug B, Crott R, Lonneux M, Baurain JF, Pirson AS, Borght TV. Role of PET in the initial staging of cutaneous malignant melanoma: systematic review. Radiology. 2008;249:836–44.
48. Niebling MG, Bastiaannet E, Hoekstra OS, Bonen-Kamp JJ, Koelemij R, Hoekstra HJ. Outcome of clinical stage III melanoma patients with FDG-PET and whole-body CT added to the diagnostic work-up. Ann Surg Oncol. 2013;20:3098–105.
49. Strobel K, Skalsky J, Steinert HC, Dummer R, Hany TF, Bhure U, et al. S-100B and FDG-PET/CT in therapy response assessment of melanoma patients. Dermatology. 2007;215:192–201.
50. Strobel K, Dummer R, Steinert HC, Conzett KB, Schad K, Lago MP, et al. Chemotherapy response assessment in stage IV melanoma patients—comparison of 18F-FDG-PET/CT, CT, brain MRI, and tumor marker S-100B. Eur J Nucl Med Mol Imaging. 2008;35:1786–95.
51. Ott PA, Hodi FS, Robert C. CTLA-4 and PD-1/PD-L1 blockage: new immunotherapeutic modalities with durable clinical benefit in melanoma. Clin Cancer Res. 2013;19:5300–9.
52. Li X, Wang J, Yao Y, Yang L, Li Z, Yu C, et al. Comparative efficacy and safety of immune checkpoint inhibitor-related therapies for advanced melanoma: a Bayesian network analysis. Oncotarget. 2017;8:83637–49.
53. Flaherty KT, Infante JR, Daud A, Gonzalez R, Kefford RF, Sosman J, et al. Combined BRAF and MEK inhibition in melanoma with BRAF V600 mutations. N Engl J Med. 2012;367:1694–703.
54. McArthur GA, Puzanov I, Amaravadi R, Ribas A, Chapman P, Kim KB, et al. Marked, homogeneous, and early [18F]fluorodeoxyglucose-positron emission tomography responses to vemurafenib in BRAF-mutant advanced melanoma. J Clin Oncol. 2012;30:1628–34.
55. Yordanova A, Schlenkhoff C, Palmedo H, Essler M, Ahmadzadehfar H. [^{18}F]Fluorodeoxyglucose positron emission tomography reveals a complete remission of refractory metastatic melanoma after therapy with ipilimumab. Indian J Nucl Med. 2017;32:66–7.
56. Carlino MS, Saunders CA, Haydu LE, Menzies AM, Martin C Jr, Lebowitz PF, et al. (18)F-labelled

fluorodeoxyglucose-positron emission tomography (FDG-PET) heterogeneity of response is prognostic in dabrafenib treated BRAF mutant metastatic melanoma. Eur J Cancer. 2013;49:395–402.
57. Sachpekidis C, Larribere L, Pan L, Haberkorn U, Dimitrakopoulou-Strauss A, Hassel JC. Predictive value of early ^{18}F-FDG PET/CT studies for treatment response evaluation to ipilimumab in metastatic melanoma: preliminary results of an ongoing study. Eur J Nucl Med Mol Imaging. 2015;42:386–96.
58. Lawal I, Zeevaart JR, Ebenhan T, Ankrah A, Vorster M, Kruger H, et al. Metabolic imaging of infection. J Nucl Med. 2017;58:1727–32.
59. Lawal I, Sathekge M. F-18 FDG PET/CT imaging of cardiac and vascular inflammation and infection. Br Med Bull. 2016;120:55–74.
60. Wachsmann JW, Ganti R, Peng F. Immune-mediated disease in ipilimumab immunotherapy of melanoma with FDG PET-CT. Acad Radiol. 2017;24:111–5.
61. Lyall A, Vargas HA, Carvajal RD, Ulaner G. Ipilimumab-induced colitis on FDG PET/CT. Clin Nucl Med. 2012;37:629–30.
62. Bacanovic S, Burger IA, Stolzmann P, Hafner J, Heullner MW. Ipilimumab-induced adrenalitis: a possible pitfall in 18F-FDG-PET/CT. Clin Nucl Med. 2015;40:e518–9.
63. Queirolo P, Spangnolo F. Atypical responses in patients with advanced melanoma, lung cancer, renal-cell carcinoma and other solid tumors treated with anti-PD-1 drugs. A systematic review. Cancer Treat Rev. 2017;59:71–8.
64. Seymour L, Bogaerts J, Perrone A, Ford R, Schwartz LH, Mandrekar S, et al. iRECIST: guideline for response criteria for use in trials testing immunotherapeutics. Lancet Oncol. 2017;18:e143–52.
65. Romano E, Scordo M, Dusza SW, Coit DG, Chapman PB. Site and timing of first relapse in stage III melanoma patients: implications for follow-up guidelines. J Clin Oncol. 2010;20:3042–7.
66. Lawal I, Lengana T, Ololade K, Boshomane T, Reyneke F, Modiselle M, et al. ^{18}F-FDG PET/CT in the detection of asymptomatic malignant melanoma recurrence. Nukleamedizin. 2017;56:83–9.
67. Kurtz J, Beasley GM, Agnese D, Kendra K, Olencki TE, Terando A, et al. Surveillance strategies in the follow-up of melanoma patients: too much or not enough? J Surg Res. 2017;214:32–7.
68. Fuster D, Chiang S, Johnson G, Schuchter LM, Zhuang H, Alavi A. Is ^{18}F-FDG PET accurate than standard diagnostic procedures in the detection of suspected recurrent melanoma? J Nucl Med. 2004;45:1323–7.
69. Peric B, Zagar I, Novakovic S, Zgajnar J, Hocevar M. Role of serum S100B and PET-CT in follow-up of patients with cutaneous melanoma. BMC Cancer. 2011;11:328. https://doi.org/10.1186/1471-2407-11-328.
70. Madu MF, Timmerman P, Eouters MWJM, van der Hiel B, van der Hage JA, van Akkooi ACJ. PET/CT surveillance detects asymptomatic recurrences in stage IIIB and IIIc melanoma patients: a prospective cohort study. Melanoma Res. 2017;27:251–7.
71. Wong ANM, McArthur GA, Hofman MS, Hicks RJ. The advantages and challenges of using FDG PET/CT for response assessment in melanoma in the era of targeted agents and immunotherapy. Eur J Nucl Med Mol Imaging. 2017;44(Suppl 1):67–77.
72. Wei W, Ehlerding EB, Lan X, Luo Q, Cai W. PET and SPECT imaging of melanoma: the state of the art. Eur J Nucl Med Mol Imaging. 2018;45:132–50.
73. Cachin F, Miot-Noirault E, Gillet B, Isnardi V, Labeille B, Payoux P, et al. (123)I-BZA2 as a melanin-targeted radiotracer for the identification of melanoma metastases: results and perspectives of a multicenter phase III clinical trial. J Nucl Med. 2014;55:15–22.
74. Wang Y, Li M, Zhang Y, Zhang F, Liu C, Song Y, et al. Detection of melanoma with PET-comparison of 18F-5-FPN with 18F-FDG. Nucl Med Biol. 2017;50:33–8.
75. Nedrow JR, Josefsson A, Park S, Ranka S, Roy S, Sgouros G. Imaging of programmed cell death ligand 1: impact of protein concentration on distribution of anti-PD-L1 SPECT agents in an immunocompetent murine model of melanoma. J Nucl Med. 2017;58:1560–6.

PET in Lymphoma

23

Nasrin Ghesani, Somali Gavane, Anthony Hafez, and Lale Kostakoglu

23.1 Introduction

Lymphoma is a cancer that begins in cells of the lymph system. The lymph system is part of the immune system, which helps the body fight infection and disease. Because lymph tissue is found all throughout the body, lymphoma can begin almost anywhere [1].

The two main types of lymphoma are Hodgkin lymphoma and non-Hodgkin lymphoma (NHL). These can occur in both children and adults. Non-Hodgkin lymphoma differ from HL with respect to their biologic and clinical characteristics. Whereas ~80–85% of patients with HL will be cured of their lymphoma by chemotherapy with or without radiotherapy, the prognosis and natural history of NHL tend to be more variable. There are many different types of NHL that derive from different types of white blood cells (B-cells, T-cells, NK cells). Within each category are lymphomas that grow quickly and behave aggressively, as well as lymphomas that are more indolent or slow growing in nature. The most common types of NHL in adults originate from B-cells, and the most common entity is diffuse large B-cell lymphoma, which is usually aggressive, and follicular lymphoma, which is usually indolent.

In 2017, over 72,000 new cases of NHL were diagnosed in the United States, about 4% of all new cancers in both males and females making it the eighth and ninth most common cause of cancer-related death in women and men, respectively. Approximately 2.1% of men and women will be diagnosed with non-Hodgkin lymphoma at some point during their lifetime, based on 2013–2015 data. The incidence is nearly ten times the incidence of Hodgkin lymphoma. The incidence of NHL has nearly doubled over the last 20–40 years and continues to rise by 1.5–2% each year. Patients with both primary and secondary immunodeficiency states are predisposed to developing NHL. These include patients with HIV infection, patients who have undergone organ transplantation, and patients with inherited immune deficiencies and autoimmune conditions. The 5-year survival rates for NHL is 72% for Caucasians and 63% for African Americans [2].

A functional or metabolic diagnostic imaging modality can contribute to the assessment of a patient in various ways. Functional imaging can complement anatomic imaging modalities, mainly

N. Ghesani (✉) · S. Gavane · A. Hafez
Nuclear Medicine, Radiology, Icahn School of Medicine at Mount Sinai,
New York, NY, USA
e-mail: Nasrin.Ghesani@mountsinai.org; somali.gavane@mssm.edu

L. Kostakoglu
Mount Sinai School of Medicine, New York, NY, USA

Radiology, Nuclear Medicine and Molecular Imaging, Department of Radiology and Medical Imaging, University of Virginia Health System,
Charlottesville, VA, USA
e-mail: lale.kostakoglu@mountsinai.org, lk3qf@virginia.edu

H. Ahmadzadehfar et al. (eds.), *Clinical Nuclear Medicine*,
https://doi.org/10.1007/978-3-030-39457-8_23

CT, and thereby enhances the accuracy of defining the extent of disease prior to therapy. In the post-therapy setting, the ability to differentiate residual viable disease from benign post-therapy changes could impact patient management and outcome, particularly if it helps to select patients who would require additional therapy or a change in treatment regimen. The limitations associated with anatomic imaging modalities, mainly with computed tomography (CT), to identify disease in the lymph nodes as well as in the extranodal sites have long been recognized. Historically, functional imaging techniques such as Ga-67 citrate, Thallium-201, and Tc-99m-sestamibi single-photon emission tomography (SPECT) have complemented CT, particularly in the post-therapy setting, although the sensitivity of this imaging technique is suboptimal in infradiaphragmatic disease and low-grade lymphomas. Since the advent of ^{18}F-fluorodeoxyglucose positron emission tomography (FDG-PET) and later combined modality PET/CT fusion technology, sufficient evidence has accumulated to demonstrate that FDG-PET/CT is a more accurate imaging modality compared to conventional imaging studies in the staging and restaging as well as in the evaluation of treatment response in lymphomas (Fig. 23.1).

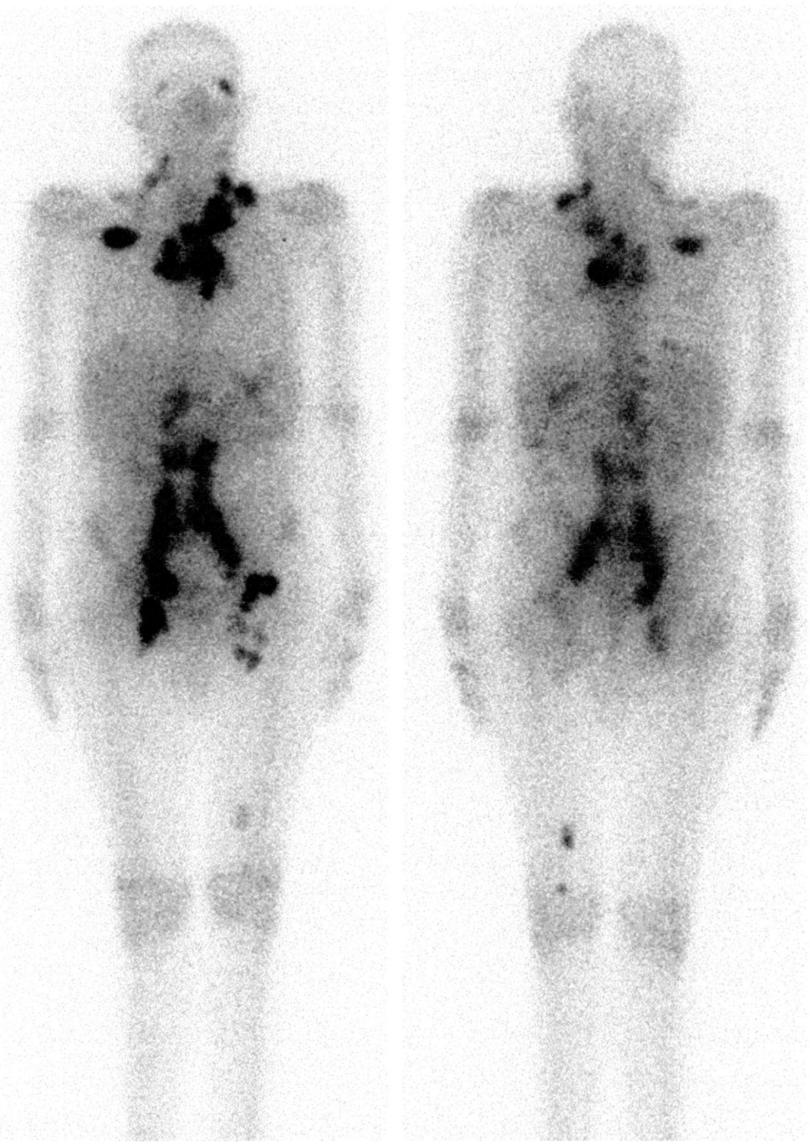

Fig. 23.1 Anterior (left) and posterior (right) whole-body images of Gallium-67 showing tracer avid lymph nodes in the neck, chest, abdomen, pelvis and left popliteal region

23.2 Classification and Staging

The proper staging and management of lymphomas depend on an accurate pathological diagnosis, classification, and determination of the extent of disease (Table 23.1). Most malignancies arise as localized disease within the tissue of origin; in contrast, lymphoma is regarded as a systemic disease due to the widespread distribution of the lymphoid tissues and tendency of lymphoid cells to migrate. Thus, the TNM staging system, which requires the knowledge of the exact origin of the malignancy, cannot be used in lymphomas. The established classification system, the Revised European-American Classification of Lymphoid Neoplasms (REAL) (National Cancer Institute 1982) [8], and first introduced in 2001 [9], and subsequently updated in 2008 [3] and 2016 (Table 23.2) [10], World Health

Table 23.1 Recommendations for the diagnostic evaluation of patients with lymphoma

A. Mandatory procedures
1. Biopsy (preferably excisional), with interpretation by a qualified pathologist. Diagnosis from a core biopsy should be based on multiple core biopsies. Appropriate IHC and ancillary studies should be performed to establish a diagnosis [3]
2. History, with special attention to the presence and duration of fever, night sweats, and unexplained loss of 10% or more of body weight in the previous 6 months (B symptoms should be recorded in the medical record; in HL, they are part of staging)
3. Physical examination
4. Laboratory evaluation
(a) Complete blood cell count and platelet count with differential and slide review
(b) ESR (HL patients)
(c) Comprehensive metabolic panel (electrolytes, blood urea nitrogen, creatinine, calcium, aspartate transaminase (AST; serum glutamic oxaloacetic transaminase (SGOT))), alanine transaminase (ALT; serum glutamic-pyruvic transaminase (SGPT)), bilirubin, total protein, albumin, alkaline phosphatase
(d) LDH, phosphorus, uric acid
(e) HIV testing
(f) Hepatitis B core antibody and hepatitis B surface antigen, especially in patients being considered for anti-CD20 therapy
5. Radiographic examination
(a) CT of the neck, chest, abdomen, and pelvis with intravenous (IV) contrast (if safe)
(b) Functional (metabolic) imaging with FDG-PET
6. Bone marrow aspiration and biopsy in selected cases
B. Examples of ancillary procedures
1. Plain bone radiographs and/or MR imaging in patients with bone disease on functional imaging to evaluate for fracture
2. Esophagogastroduodenoscopy (EGD), colonoscopy, and/or GI series in patients with GI presentations
3. MR imaging of the spine in patients with suspected leptomeningeal disease
4. MR imaging of the brain in patients with cranial nerve palsy or suspicion of leptomeningeal or parenchymal brain disease
5. CSF cytology with flow cytometry in patients with:
(a) DLBCL
(i) CNS risk score[a] [4] 4–6
(ii) CNS risk score 2–3 and double expressor (BCL2 and MYC by IHC) [4]
(iii) HIV infection
(iv) Testicular involvement [5]
(v) Breast involvement [6]
(vi) Children
(b) Burkitt's lymphoma

[a]CNS risk score: 1 point for each of the following risk factors: age >60 years; performance status (PS) ≤2; LDH greater than upper limit of normal; two or more extralymphatic sites; Stage III/IV; adrenal or renal involvement

Adapted from AJCC Cancer Staging Manual. Springer International Publishing. ISBN-10: 3-319-40617-5, ISBN-13: 978-3-319-40617-6 [7]

Table 23.2 Adapted from the 2016 revision of the World Health Organization classification of lymphoid neoplasms

B-cell
Mature (peripheral) B-cell neoplasms
Lymphoplasmacytic lymphoma (Waldenstrom's macroglobulinemia)
Hairy cell leukemia
Splenic marginal zone B-cell lymphoma
Extranodal marginal zone B-cell lymphoma of MALT type
Nodal marginal zone B-cell lymphoma
Follicular lymphoma
Mantle cell lymphoma
Diffuse large B-cell lymphoma (including subtypes)
High grade B-cell lymphoma with MYC and BCL2 and/or BCL6 rearrangements
High grade B-cell lymphoma NOS
Burkitt's lymphoma/Burkitt's cell leukemia
Primary mediastinal large B-cell lymphoma
Plasmablastic lymphoma
Primary effusion lymphoma
HHV8+ DLBCL NOS
Intravascular large B-cell lymphoma
ALK+ large B-cell lymphoma
T-cell
Mature (peripheral) T-cell neoplasms
T-cell granular lymphocytic leukemia
Adult T-cell leukemia/lymphoma (HTLV-1+)
Extranodal NK/T-cell lymphoma, nasal type
Enteropathy-associated T-cell lymphoma
Hepatosplenic T-cell lymphoma
Subcutaneous panniculitis-like T-cell lymphoma
Mycosis fungoides
Sezary syndrome
Peripheral T-cell lymphoma, NOS
Angioimmunoblastic T-cell lymphoma
Anaplastic large cell lymphoma, ALK+
Anaplastic large cell lymphoma, ALK−
Hodgkin lymphoma
Nodular lymphocyte-predominant Hodgkin lymphoma
Classical Hodgkin lymphoma
Nodular sclerosis classical Hodgkin lymphoma
Lymphocyte-rich classical Hodgkin lymphoma
Mixed cellularity classical Hodgkin lymphoma
Lymphocyte-depleted classical Hodgkin lymphoma
Posttransplant lymphoproliferative disorders (PTLD)
Plasmacytic hyperplasia PTLD
Infectious mononucleosis PTLD
Florid follicular hyperplasia PTLD
Polymorphic PTLD
Monomorphic PTLD (B- and T-/NK-cell types)
Classical Hodgkin lymphoma PTLD

Swerdlow SH, Campo E, Pileri SA, Harris NL, Stein H, Siebert R, et al. Blood. 2016;127(20):2375–90 [10]

Organization classification integrate the cytogenetic, molecular, and immunologic information in lymphoma staging.

Staging defines disease location and extent, suggests prognostic information, allows comparisons among studies, and provides a baseline against which response or disease progression can be compared. Initial staging criteria were designed primarily for Hodgkin lymphoma (HL) [11–13] and were superseded by the Ann Arbor classification [14]. With the aim to develop improved staging and response criteria for HL and NHL, a workshop was held at the 11th International Conference on Malignant Lymphoma in Lugano (Table 23.3), Switzerland, in June 2011, that included leading hematologists, oncologists, radiation oncologists, pathologists, radiologists, and nuclear medicine physicians, representing major international lymphoma clinical trial groups and cancer centers. Clinical and imaging subcommittees presented their conclusions at a subsequent workshop at the 12th International Conference on Malignant Lymphoma, leading to revised criteria for staging—Lugano classification [15].

Table 23.3 Lugano classification for Hodgkin and non-Hodgkin lymphoma

Stage	Stage description
Limited stage	
I	Involvement of a single lymphatic site (i.e., nodal region, Waldeyer's ring, thymus, or spleen)
IE	Single extralymphatic site in the absence of nodal involvement (rare in Hodgkin lymphoma)
II	Involvement of two or more lymph node regions on the same side of the diaphragm
IIE	Contiguous extralymphatic extension from a nodal site with or without involvement of other lymph node regions on the same side of the diaphragm
II bulky[a]	*Stage II with disease bulk*[b]
Advanced stage	
III	Involvement of lymph node regions on both sides of the diaphragm; nodes above the diaphragm with spleen involvement

Table 23.3 (continued)

Stage	Stage description
IV	Diffuse or disseminated involvement of one or more extralymphatic organs, with or without associated lymph node involvement, or *noncontiguous* extralymphatic organ involvement in conjunction with nodal stage II disease or *any* extralymphatic organ involvement in nodal stage III disease Stage IV includes *any* involvement of the CSF, bone marrow, liver, or multiple lung lesions (other than by direct extension in stage IIE disease)

Note: Hodgkin lymphoma uses A or B designation with stage group. A/B is no longer used in NHL

Note: Extent of disease is determined by positron emission tomography–computed tomography for avid lymphomas and computed tomography for non-avid histologies. Tonsils, Waldeyer's ring, and spleen are considered nodal tissue

Adapted from AJCC CANCER STAGING MANUAL—8th Ed. (2017). American College of Surgeons 2017, Corrected at 3rd printing 2017 [7, 15]

[a]Stage II bulky may be considered either early or advanced stage based on lymphoma histology and prognostic factors (see discussion of Hodgkin lymphoma prognostic factors)

[b]The definition of disease bulk varies according to lymphoma histology. In the Lugano classification [15], bulk in Hodgkin lymphoma is defined as a mass greater than one third of the thoracic diameter on CT of the chest or a mass >10 cm. For NHL, the recommended definitions of bulk vary by lymphoma histology. In follicular lymphoma, 6 cm has been suggested based on the Follicular Lymphoma International Prognostic Index-2 (FLIPI-2) and its validation [16, 17]. In DLBCL, cutoffs ranging from 5 to 10 cm have been used, although 10 cm is recommended [18]

23.3 Imaging for Staging in Lymphoma

Lymphoma may be unifocal, multifocal, or diffuse, affecting isolated lymph nodes or any organ system. Normal lymph nodes often have an elongated shape and a fatty hilum. Lymph nodes infiltrated with lymphoma are often visualized incidentally or during a targeted assessment at ultrasonography (US), demonstrating homogeneous echotexture and enlargement. They are often rounded, with a hypoechoic, "pseudocystic" appearance caused by replacement of the node with lymphomatous tissue. The traditional imaging modality of choice for the diagnosis of lymphoma has been computed tomography (CT), which may be accompanied by sonography or endoscopy in some selected cases. MRI images are comparable diagnostic quality using faster acquisition sequences. Additionally, MRI offers advantages including better tissue discrimination, lack of ionizing radiation, and use of contrast agents with less risk of systemic effects [19–21]. On computed tomographic (CT) images, involved lymph nodes are generally enlarged and of homogeneous density. Some lymphoma subtypes, namely, small cell lymphocytic lymphoma/chronic lymphocytic leukemia, may manifest as an increased number of small nodes [22]. Nevertheless, the accuracy of CT and MRI is limited in staging of lymphoma as diagnosis depends on lymph node enlargement and multiplicity; thus, false-negative results are obtained in normal-sized lymph nodes that harbor lymphoma. Alternatively, in lymph nodes that are enlarged due to reactive changes they can give rise to false positive findings. CT lacks functional information, which impedes identification of disease in normal-sized organs [23].

As per Lugano classification (Fig. 23.2), for patients staged with CT, up to six of the largest target nodes, nodal masses, or other lymphomatous lesions that are measurable in two diameters (longest diameter (LDi) and shortest diameter) should be identified from different body regions representative of the patient's overall disease burden and include mediastinal and retroperitoneal disease, if involved. A measurable node must have an LDi greater than 1.5 cm. Measurable extranodal disease (e.g., hepatic nodules) may be included in the six representative, measured lesions. A measurable extranodal lesion should have an LDi greater than 1.0 cm. All other lesions (including nodal, extranodal, and assessable disease) should be followed as non-measured disease (e.g., cutaneous, GI, bone, spleen, liver, kidneys, pleural or pericardial effusions, ascites) [15].

^{18}F-Fluorodeoxyglucose (FDG) positron emission tomography/computed tomography(PET/CT) is a widely used critical tool in lymphomas as a baseline measurement before therapy to increase

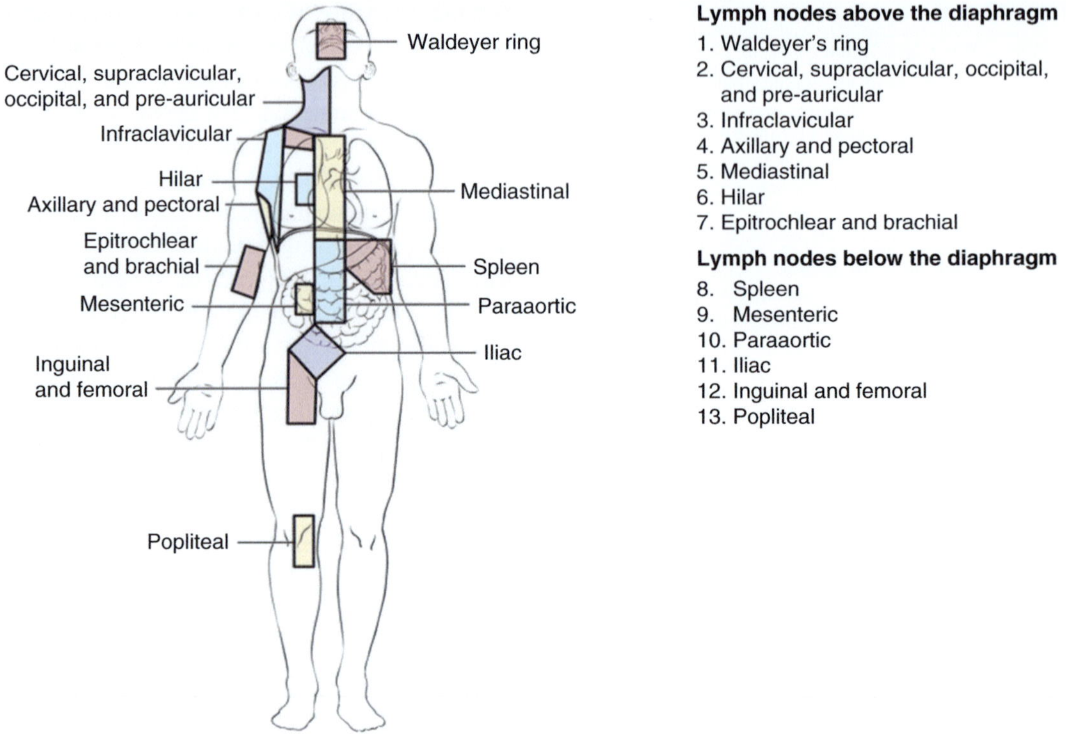

Fig. 23.2 Lymph nodes above and below the diaphragm (Ann Arbor/Lugano classification). Adapted from © AJCC CANCER STAGING MANUAL—8th Ed. (2017). American College of Surgeons 2017, Corrected at 3rd printing 2017 [7]

the accuracy of subsequent response assessment [24, 25]. The Lugano classification formally incorporated PET/CT into standard staging for FDG-avid lymphomas (essentially all histologies except chronic lymphocytic leukemia/small lymphocytic lymphoma, lymphoplasmacytic lymphoma/Waldenstrom's macroglobulinemia, mycosis fungoides, and marginal zone NHLs, unless there is a suspicion of aggressive transformation) [15]. Combined FDG PET/CT has been found to be more accurate than CT alone for staging and response assessment. For example, in a retrospective analysis, Schaefer et al. demonstrated that in identifying lymph node involvement, FDG PET/CT was 94% sensitive and 100% specific, while contrast-enhanced CT alone was 88% sensitive and 86% specific. For organ involvement, FDG PET/CT showed sensitivity of 88% and specificity of 100%, whereas contrast-enhanced CT alone had sensitivity of 50% and specificity of 90% [26]. With FDG PET/CT, non-Hodgkin lymphoma will be upstaged in 31% and downstaged in 1% of patients relative to CT (usually patients with stage I or II disease), thereby potentially changing treatment in 25%. Hodgkin lymphoma will be upstaged in 32% and downstaged in 15% of patients with FDG PET/CT, thus possibly leading to treatment change in up to 33% [27].

23.3.1 International Prognostic Index (IPI) and Score (IPS)

The Ann Arbor staging system is not highly accurate in identifying prognostic subgroups which usually determines the therapy strategy (The Non-Hodgkin's Lymphoma Classification Project 1997) [28]. Consequently, a pretreatment predictive model, International Prognostic Index

(IPI) was developed for patients with aggressive NHL (The International Non-Hodgkin's Lymphoma Prognostic Factors Project 1993) [29] to provide useful information for determination of proper therapy for subgroups based on risk profile. The International Prognostic Score (IPS) is designed to predict outcome in advanced Hodgkin disease to avoid overtreating some patients and to identify others in whom standard treatment is likely to fail and is described based on the number of adverse prognostic factors present at diagnosis [30]. In the IPS, seven factors are considered for adverse prognostic effects: a serum albumin level <4 g/dl, a hemoglobin level <10.5 g/dl, male sex, age ≥45 years, stage IV disease by Ann Arbor classification, leukocytosis (a white cell count ≥15,000/mm^3), and lymphocytopenia (a lymphocyte count <600/mm^3, a count <8% of the white cell count, or both).

The International Prognostic Index (IPI) has been the basis for determining prognosis in patients with aggressive non-Hodgkin lymphoma (NHL) for the past 20 years. Using raw clinical data from the National Comprehensive Cancer Network (NCCN) database collected during the rituximab era, an enhanced NCCN-IPI was built with the goal of improving risk stratification. Compared with the IPI, the NCCN-IPI better discriminated low- and high-risk subgroups (5-year overall survival: 96% vs. 33%) than the IPI (5-year OS: 90% vs. 54%), respectively (Table 23.4). The NCCN-IPI is easy to apply and more powerful than the IPI for predicting survival in the rituximab era [31].

Table 23.4 The NCCN-IPI

NCCN-IPI	Score
Age (years)	
>40 to ≤60	1
>60 to ≤75	2
>75	3
LDH, normalized	
> 1 to ≤3	1
>3	2
Ann Arbor stages III–IV	1
Extranodal disease[a]	1
Performance status (ECOG) ≥2	1

[a]Disease in the bone marrow, CNS, liver/GI tract, or lung

23.4 Clinically Relevant Issues About Lymphomas

The lymphomas are traditionally divided into two broad categories, HD and NHLs, based on the therapeutic and management implications [1]. An estimated 82,310 new cases of lymphoma will be diagnosed in the United States in 2019, with Hodgkin lymphoma (8110 cases) or non-Hodgkin lymphoma (NHL, 74,200 cases), and an estimated 1000 deaths from Hodgkin lymphoma and 19,970 deaths from NHL [32].

NHL accounts for more than 85% of the lymphomas. The non-Hodgkin lymphomas (NHLs) are a heterogeneous group of lymphoproliferative malignancies with differing patterns of behavior and responses to treatment [33]. NHL has a predilection to disseminate to extranodal sites, and the prognosis depends on the histologic type, stage, and treatment. NHL can be divided into two prognostic groups: indolent lymphomas and aggressive lymphomas [34]. Aggressive lymphomas constitute approximately 60% of NHL series, while indolent lymphomas account for approximately 40% of new diagnoses.

Indolent NHL types are nodular (or follicular) in morphology and have a relatively good prognosis with a median survival as long as 20 years, but they usually are not curable in advanced clinical stages [35]. While indolent NHL is responsive to immunotherapy, radiation therapy, and chemotherapy, a continuous rate of relapse is usually seen in advanced stages. Patients, however, can often be re-treated with considerable success as long as the disease histology remains low grade. Patients who present with or convert to aggressive forms of NHL may have sustained complete remissions with combination chemotherapy regimens or aggressive consolidation with marrow or stem cell support [36, 37].

The aggressive type of NHL has a shorter natural history, but a significant number of these patients can be cured with intensive combination chemotherapy regimens. In general, with modern treatment of patients with NHL, overall survival at 5 years is over 60%. Of patients with aggressive NHL, more than 50% can be cured. The vast majority of relapses occur in the first 2 years after therapy. The risk of late relapse is higher in patients who manifest both indolent and aggressive histologies [38].

HD accounts for 10–15% of lymphomas and is composed of two different entities, classical HD representing 95% of cases and nodular lymphocyte-predominant HD making up 5% of cases. Classical HD is further subdivided into nodular sclerosis (most common), mixed cellularity, and lymphocyte-rich and lymphocyte depletion types. Patients with nodular lymphocyte-predominant HD usually present with isolated peripheral lymph node involvement. These patients have a clinical course resembling NHL with an indolent growth pattern, which thus is considered to have a different biology than classical HD.

Unlike HD, NHL is much less predictable and has a far greater predilection to have a disseminated pattern. Only 10% of patients with low-grade follicular NHL have localized disease at diagnosis [39], and the majority of patients with aggressive lymphomas have advanced-stage disease.

In both HD and NHL, prognosis and treatment depend on histological type and grade as well as disease stage. For patients with non-bulky early-stage classical HD (favorable prognosis), radiation therapy alone has been the primary treatment. However, the late effects of radiation therapy consisting of occurrence of solid tumors and cardiovascular disease render this therapy modality a less attractive option for patients with favorable prognosis. The use of combination therapy with non-alkylating agents and involved field radiotherapy (IF RT) has proven more effective to reduce the relapse rate compared to the use of radiotherapy alone [40]. For patients with bulky stage I–II disease, treatment usually consists of a full course of chemotherapy followed by IF RT. Patients with advanced-stage disease are treated with full-course chemotherapy, with the consideration of delivering IF RT to bulky disease sites.

Accurate staging is particularly important in initial staging to determine extent of disease to modify therapy protocols. With polychemotherapy the cure rate for HD is greater than 80% of patients with first-line therapy. The detection of additional disease sites would have a significant impact on management of both aggressive NHL and classical HD patients in whom a stage migration occurs from apparently early stage to advanced stage. In these patients, a number of chemotherapy cycles can be modified, and/or combined modality therapy can be initiated in addition to or in lieu of radiotherapy alone. Furthermore, detection of unknown disease sites and better definition of metabolically active tumor volume could alter radiotherapy fields and gross tumor volume alike. Nonetheless, this is an evolving area and FDG-PET based changes in therapy planning require further evaluation. The lymphocyte-predominant HD has a relatively indolent course, and radiation therapy alone can be an option for these patients [41]; thus, imaging findings are less conducive to a dramatic change in management in this subtype of HD. It is generally accepted that there is little therapeutic benefit in distinguishing between stage III and stage IV disease, since the treatment options are nearly identical.

Evaluation of therapy response is equally important in both HD and NHL to determine whether fewer cycles of chemotherapy can be administered in rapidly responding patients to avoid unnecessary therapy and morbidity. Moreover, imaging can determine whether or not radiation therapy is indicated for an individual lymphoma patient. This is essential as unnecessary use of radiation may lead to development of untoward effects such as cardiac disease, pulmonary fibrosis, and secondary malignancies, while appropriate use could potentially decrease the risk of recurrence and allow for administration of fewer chemotherapy cycles than the conventional six cycles [42].

23.5 ^{18}F-FDG PET/CT in Initial Staging of Lymphoma

As per recommendations of the workshop at the 12th International Conference on Malignant Lymphoma, FDG PET/CT is formally incorporated into standard staging for FDG-avid lymphomas. Almost all lymphomas are FDG avid (Table 23.5), but most published data are related to the use of PET in HL, diffuse large B-cell lymphoma (DLBCL), and follicular lymphoma (FL). PET scans are usually reported using visual assessment [51], noting the location of increased focal uptake in nodal and extranodal sites, which is distinguished from physiologic uptake and other patterns of disease with increased FDG uptake including infection and inflammation, according to distribution and/or CT characteristics [52, 53]. On PET-CT scan, focal uptake in nodal and extranodal sites, according to the distribution and/or CT characteristics, is considered involvement with lymphoma, including the spleen, liver, bone, thyroid, and so on. In patients in whom a discordant histology or malignant transformation is suspected, a PET-CT may identify the optimal site to biopsy for confirmation.

Table 23.5 FDG avidity according to the WHO classification

Histology	No. of patients	FDG avid (%)
HL	489	97–100
DLBCL	446	97–100
FL	622	91–100
Mantle cell lymphoma	83	100
Burkitt's lymphoma	24	100
Marginal zone lymphoma, nodal	14	100
Lymphoblastic lymphoma	6	100
Anaplastic large T-cell lymphoma	37	94–100[a]
NK-/T-cell lymphoma	80	83–100
Angioimmunoblastic T-cell lymphoma	31	78–100
Peripheral T-cell lymphoma	93	86–98
MALT marginal zone lymphoma	27	54–81
Small lymphocytic lymphoma	49	47–83
Enteropathy-type T-cell lymphoma	20	67–100
Marginal zone lymphoma, splenic	13	53–67
Marginal zone lymphoma, unspecified	12	67
Mycosis fungoides	24	83–100
Sezary syndrome	8	100[b]
Primary cutaneous anaplastic large T-cell lymphoma	14	40–60
Lymphomatoid papulosis	2	50
Subcutaneous panniculitis-like T-cell lymphoma	7	71
Cutaneous B-cell lymphoma	2	0

Note: Data adapted from Weiler-Sagie M, Bushelev O, Epelbaum R, Dann EJ, Haim N, Avivi I, et al. (18)F-FDG avidity in lymphoma readdressed: a study of 766 patients. Journal of nuclear medicine: official publication, Society of Nuclear Medicine. 2010;51(1):25–30 [43, 44] with additional updates [45–50]

Abbreviations: *DLBCL* diffuse large B-cell lymphoma, *FDG-(^{18}F)* fluorodeoxyglucose, *FL* follicular lymphoma, *HL* Hodgkin lymphoma, *MALT* mucosa-associated lymphoid tissue, *NK* natural killer

[a]Only 27% of cutaneous sites

[b]Only 62% of cutaneous sites

FDG PET imaging results better correlate with increased metabolic activity at sites with lymphoma involvement than CT-based size measurements. In 2005, Isasi et al. published a meta-analysis of early studies of FDG PET or PET/CT which included 854 subjects, and 7 studies and lesion-based data, of 3658 lesions. Among those studies with patient-based data, the median sensitivity was 90.3% and the median specificity was 91.1%. The pooled sensitivity was 90.9% (95% confidence interval (95% CI), 88.0–93.4), and the pooled false-positive rate was 10.3% (95% CI, 7.4–13.8). The maximum joint sensitivity and specificity was 87.8% (95% CI, 85.0–90.7). The pooled sensitivity and false-positive rate appeared to be higher in patients with Hodgkin disease compared with those with non-Hodgkin lymphoma [54].

At initial staging, FDG PET leads to upstaging in as many as 30% of patients [55–61]. Schaefer et al. reported that the sensitivity of PET/CT and CECT for both nodal diseases in HL and aggressive NHL was higher than that of CT (94% vs. 88%), while the specificity was 100% vs. 86% [26, 62]. For extranodal involvement, the sensitivity of PET/CT was almost twofold better than that of CECT (88% vs. 50%), while the specificities were similar (100% vs. 90%). In a systematic review, Kwee et al. reported that the sensitivity and specificity of CT and FDG PET were 87.5% and 85.6% vs. 87.5% and 100%, respectively, in initial staging of lymphomas [23]. The sensitivity of PET was somewhat lower in NHL at 83% with no change in specificity; this was probably because of the inclusion of lower-grade lymphomas (Fig. 23.3).

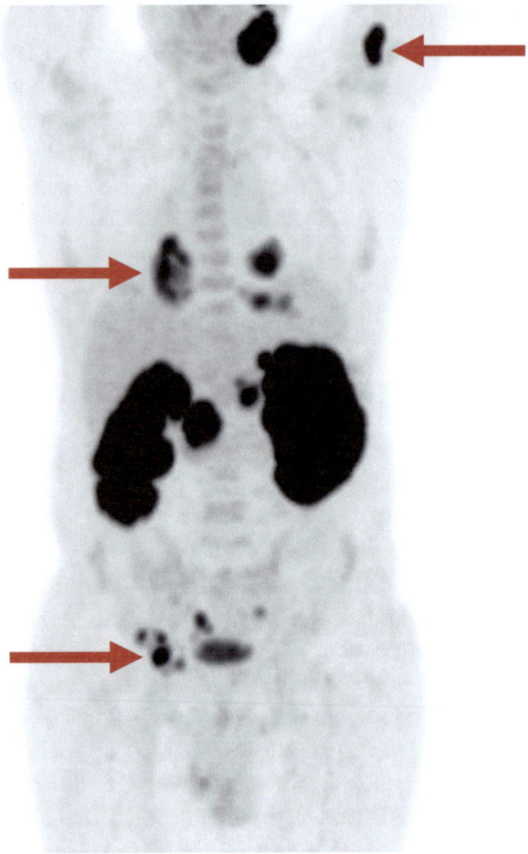

Fig. 23.3 A 54-year-old man newly diagnosed with diffuse large B-cell lymphoma of the kidneys and left neck. ^{18}F-FDG MIP demonstrating occult involvement of the left humerus, myocardium, and the right acetabulum (red arrows)

It is important, however, to realize that treatment is changed in only 10–15% of patients and also there is no evidence that superior PET results improve survival [55–58, 62–70]. It is equally important to recognize that CECT is a valuable diagnostic test for distinguishing lymph nodes from vessels and unopacified bowel loops in the abdomen and pelvis (Table 23.6).

23.5.1 Bone Marrow Involvement

The detection of bone marrow (BM) involvement identifies a group of high-risk patients and changes disease management. Hence, this is particularly important in early-stage patients given

Table 23.6 Summary of recommendations

Recommendations
Section 1: Interpretation of PET-CT scans
1. Staging of FDG-avid lymphomas is recommended using visual assessment, with PET-CT images scaled to fixed SUV display and color table; focal uptake in HL and aggressive NHL is sensitive for bone marrow involvement and may obviate need for biopsy; MRI is modality of choice for suspected CNS lymphoma (type 1)
2. Five-point scale is recommended for reporting PET-CT; results should be interpreted in the context of anticipated prognosis, clinical findings, and other markers of response; scores 1 and 2 represent CMR; score 3 also probably represents CMR in patients receiving standard treatment (type 1)
3. Score 4 or 5 with reduced uptake from baseline likely represents partial metabolic response but at end of treatment represents residual metabolic disease; increase in FDG uptake to score 5, score 5 with no decrease in uptake, and new FDG-avid foci consistent with lymphoma represent treatment failure and/or progression (type 2)
Section 2: Role of PET-CT for staging
1. PET-CT should be used for staging in clinical practice and clinical trials but is not routinely recommended in lymphomas with low FDG avidity; PET-CT may be used to select best site to biopsy (type 1)
2. Contrast-enhanced CT when used at staging or restaging should ideally occur during single visit combined with PET-CT, if not already performed; baseline findings will determine whether contrast-enhanced PET-CT or lower-dose unenhanced PET-CT will suffice for additional imaging examinations (type 2)
3. Bulk remains an important prognostic factor in some lymphomas; volumetric measurement of tumor bulk and total tumor burden, including methods combining metabolic activity and anatomical size or volume, should be explored as potential prognosticators (type 3)
Section 3: Role of interim PET
1. If midtherapy imaging is performed, PET-CT is superior to CT alone to assess early response; trials are evaluating role of PET response-adapted therapy; currently, it is not recommended to change treatment solely on the basis of interim PET-CT unless there is clear evidence of progression (type 1)
2. Standardization of PET methods is mandatory for use of quantitative approaches and desirable for routine clinical practice (type 1)
3. Data suggest that quantitative measures (e.g., δSUVmax) could be used to improve on visual analysis for response assessment in DLBCL, but this requires further validation in clinical trials (type 2)

Table 23.6 (continued)

Recommendations
Section 4: Role of PET at end of treatment
1. PET-CT is standard of care for remission assessment in FDG-avid lymphoma; in the presence of residual metabolically active tissue, where salvage treatment is being considered, biopsy is recommended (type 1)
2. Investigation of significance of PET-negative residual masses should be collected prospectively in clinical trials; residual mass size and location should be recorded on end-of-treatment PET-CT reports where possible (type 3)
3. Emerging data support use of PET-CT after rituximab-containing chemotherapy in high-tumor-burden FL; studies are warranted to confirm this finding in patients receiving maintenance therapy (type 2)
4. Assessment with PET-CT could be used to guide decisions before high-dose chemotherapy and ASCT, but additional studies are warranted (type 3)

Summary of the Recommendation of Fourth International Workshop on PET in Lymphoma in Menton, France, and the 12th ICML in Lugano, Switzerland, and the International Harmonization Project guidance regarding PET [43]

the trend toward less intensive treatment in this group of patients. The incidence of BM involvement at diagnosis varies according to the subtype of lymphoma with occurrence of 39% of low-grade, 36% of intermediate-grade, and 18% of high-grade lymphomas. Bone marrow involvement (BMI) was associated with significantly shorter survivals in patients with intermediate- or high-grade lymphomas. In general, the incidence is rather low in patients with HD (1–2%), while it is common in low-grade lymphoma (mainly follicular cell subtype, 60–70%), chronic lymphocytic leukemia, and mantle cell lymphoma (90–100%) [71]. In aggressive NHL (mainly diffuse large cell lymphoma), BM infiltration is observed in 25–40% of patients [72]. In the NCCN Guidelines, bone marrow biopsy with or without aspirate is included as part of essential workup for all lymphomas [73]. Several studies in HL and DLBCL showed improved sensitivity of FDG/PET scans over trephine bone marrow biopsies [74, 75]. Thus, this procedure was no longer considered essential in the routine staging of HL, and in most patients with DLBCL, unless in the latter, the FDG/PET was negative, and it was important to determine if a discordant histology was present in the bone marrow. In patients with low-bulk indolent disease with radiographic clinical stage III disease, an initial staging bone marrow evaluation can be deferred if observation is recommended as it will not change the clinical recommendations. However, in the evaluation of potential early-stage indolent lymphoma (stage I or II), bone marrow biopsy is essential [76–78]. It is well recognized that BMB has several limitations, including the possibility of missing a patchy pattern of marrow involvement, as reflected in studies comparing bilateral versus unilateral BMB [79]. MRI is especially useful in detecting BMI; however, benign entities such as hemangiomas, inflammatory processes, and post-therapy changes diminish its specificity by mimicking lymphoma features. BM is a metabolically active organ, and depending on the marrow turnover, the degree of FDG uptake varies between faintly noticeable and prominent. Overall, focal FDG uptake suggests pathological BM activity, a pattern more commonly seen in HD patients. In aggressive NHL, the degree of BM involvement may range from a few cells to complete marrow replacement. In cases with the latter condition, FDG uptake is usually diffuse and somewhat heterogeneous but never specific. Diffusely increased FDG uptake is also seen in patients with BM hyperplasia, particularly following administration of colony-stimulating factors (e.g., G-CSF) [80, 81] (Fig. 23.4).

Numerous recent studies have suggested that PET-CT is a highly sensitive and specific method for determining BMI in HL and DLBCL [74, 82–87]. A retrospective study of 454 patients with newly diagnosed HL, identified through the Danish Lymphoma Registry, determined the sensitivity and specificity of PET-CT to be 85% and 86%, respectively [74]. The negative predictive value was 99%, further supporting the irrelevance of a bone marrow biopsy in patients with negative PET-CT skeletal results. In a study involving the 530 patients with DLBCL, Alzahrani et al. demonstrated that PET/CT accurately assessed BM involvement in the majority of patients with DLBCL. The authors also demonstrated that BMB was negative in 94/146 (64%) patients with

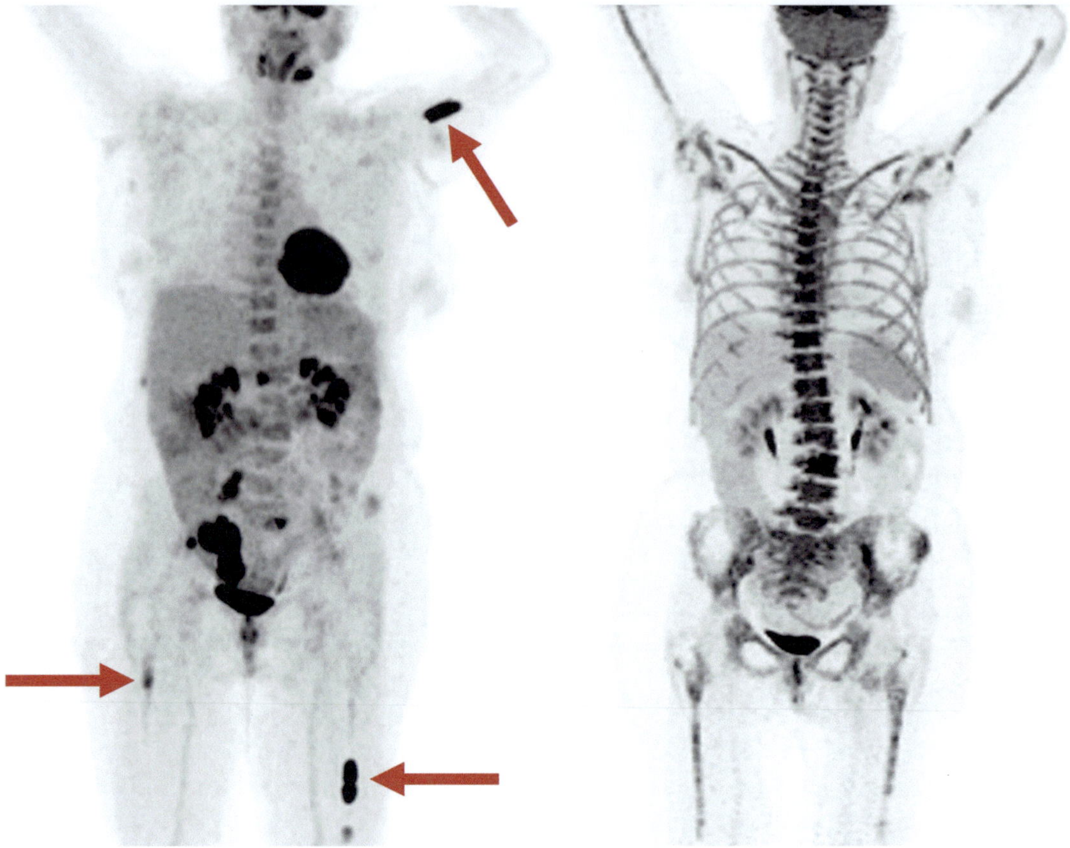

Fig. 23.4 A 48-year-old patient with ileocecal and bone involvement of DLBCL on pretherapy FDG PET/CT scan (left). Post-therapy PET/CT scan (right) shows diffuse increased uptake in the bone marrow related to GCSF administration

positive PET/CT and, thus, missed disease that altered staging assessment and management, suggesting that routine BMB is not a critical element of disease staging in all patients with newly diagnosed DLBCL undergoing upfront PET/CT staging [88]. Retrospective study by Ujjani et al. aimed to evaluate the role of PET-CT in detecting BMI in DLBCL and HL and to explore its usefulness in other subtypes demonstrated that PET-CT was highly accurate for detecting BMI at diagnosis in DLBCL and HL and highly specific in FL at diagnosis and relapse [89]. Overall, the negative predictive value for FDG-PET in the detection of BM involvement is higher than the positive predictive value. Nevertheless, a minimal degree of BM involvement can result in false-negative findings due to the inherent resolution limits of FDG-PET imaging (Fig. 23.5).

23.5.2 Spleen Involvement

A wide range of normal spleen sizes has been reported [18, 90, 91], related to race, body size, and height. A spleen may be of normal size and still contain lymphoma or may be enlarged as a result of variations in blood volume, use of hematopoietic growth factors, or lymphoma-unrelated causes. Splenic involvement is best determined by PET-CT and may be characterized by homogeneous splenomegaly, diffuse infiltration with miliary lesions, focal nodular lesions, or a large solitary mass [92]. There is no agreement on whether single, multiple, or volumetric measurements should be used to measure spleen size or what cutoff to use for splenomegaly. For simplicity, a single measurement that correlates well with volume [93, 94] is preferable to a volumetric

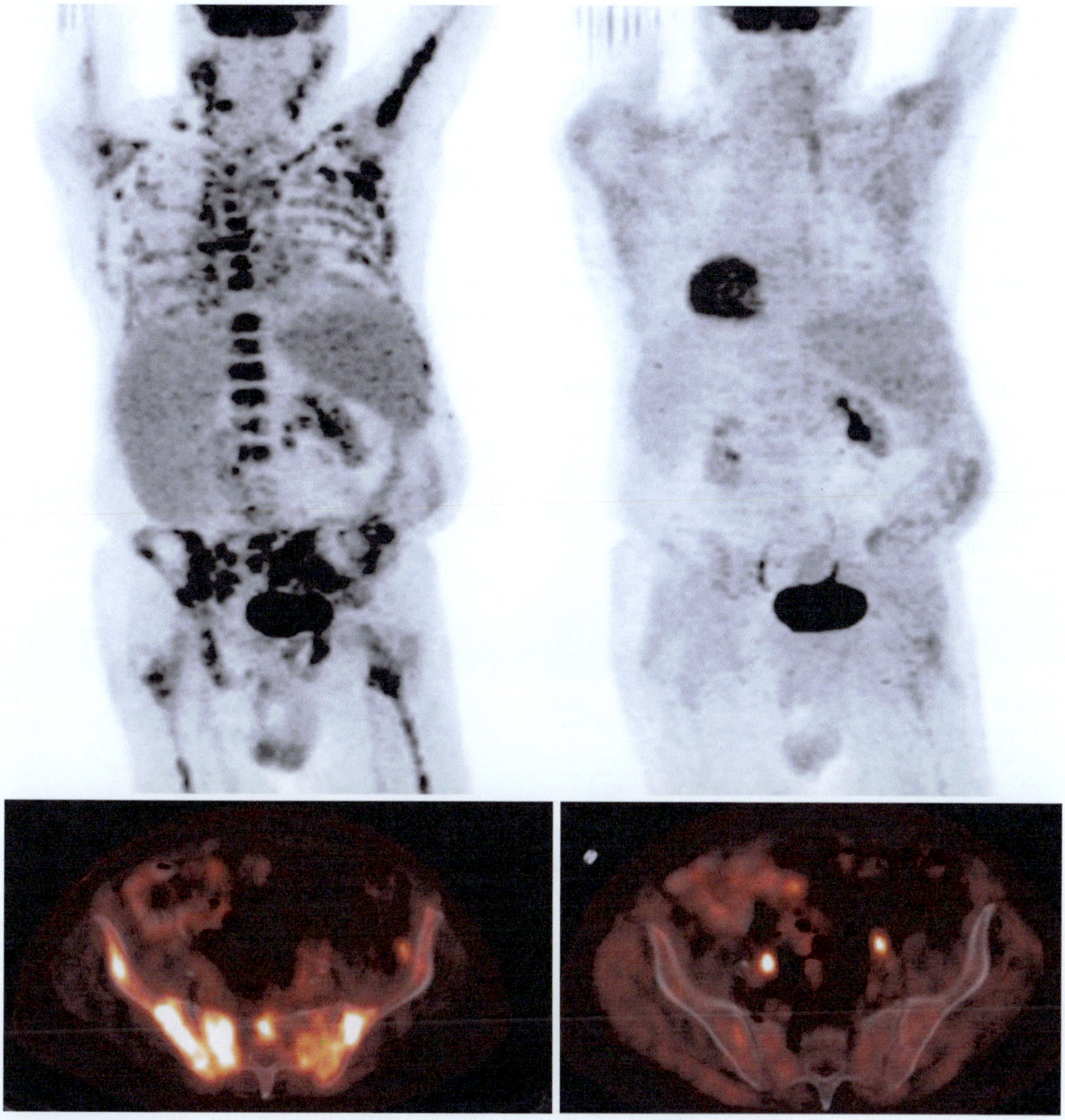

Fig. 23.5 Patient with DLBCL. Pretherapy PET/CT MIP (upper left image) and axial fused PET/CT (left lower) shows patchy increased uptake throughout the osseous structures consistent with bone marrow involvement. Post-therapy PET/CT MIP (upper right image) and axial fused PET/CT (lower right image) shows interval resolution of osseous uptake

measurement or estimation by equations, with special software, which are unlikely to be used routinely. Most studies use 10–12 cm for vertical length. Our recommendation is to use a cutoff for splenomegaly of more than 13 cm [15].

Splenic involvement is observed as an element of systemic involvement in 40% of DLBCL [95–97]. The diagnostic efficiency of FDG-PET is superior to that of CT. FDG-PET localizes approximately 25% more lesions than does CT in the liver and spleen [96, 98]. For initial staging of splenic involvement in malignant lymphoma, De Jong et al. showed the sensitivity and specificity of PET/CT can reach 100% and 95% [99]. In a recent retrospective review of 93 patients with FDG-avid lymphomas, defined by the presence of at least a single nodal or extranodal site, using the 13-cm splenic craniocaudal diameter cutoff, Berzaczy et al. found a sensitivity of 74.1% and a specificity of 47% for splenic involvement by lymphoma. The study revealed that currently recommended vertical length cut-off value of 13 cm for detection of splenic involvement offers a reasonable sensitivity but cannot rule out the presence of lymphomatous organ infiltration, whereas specificity is clearly lacking; and thus, detection of splenic involvement by means of organ diameter measurements is not reliable [100] (Fig. 23.6).

23.5.3 Liver Involvement

Given the variability in body habitus and the impact of numerous medical conditions, liver size by physical examination or CT scan is not a

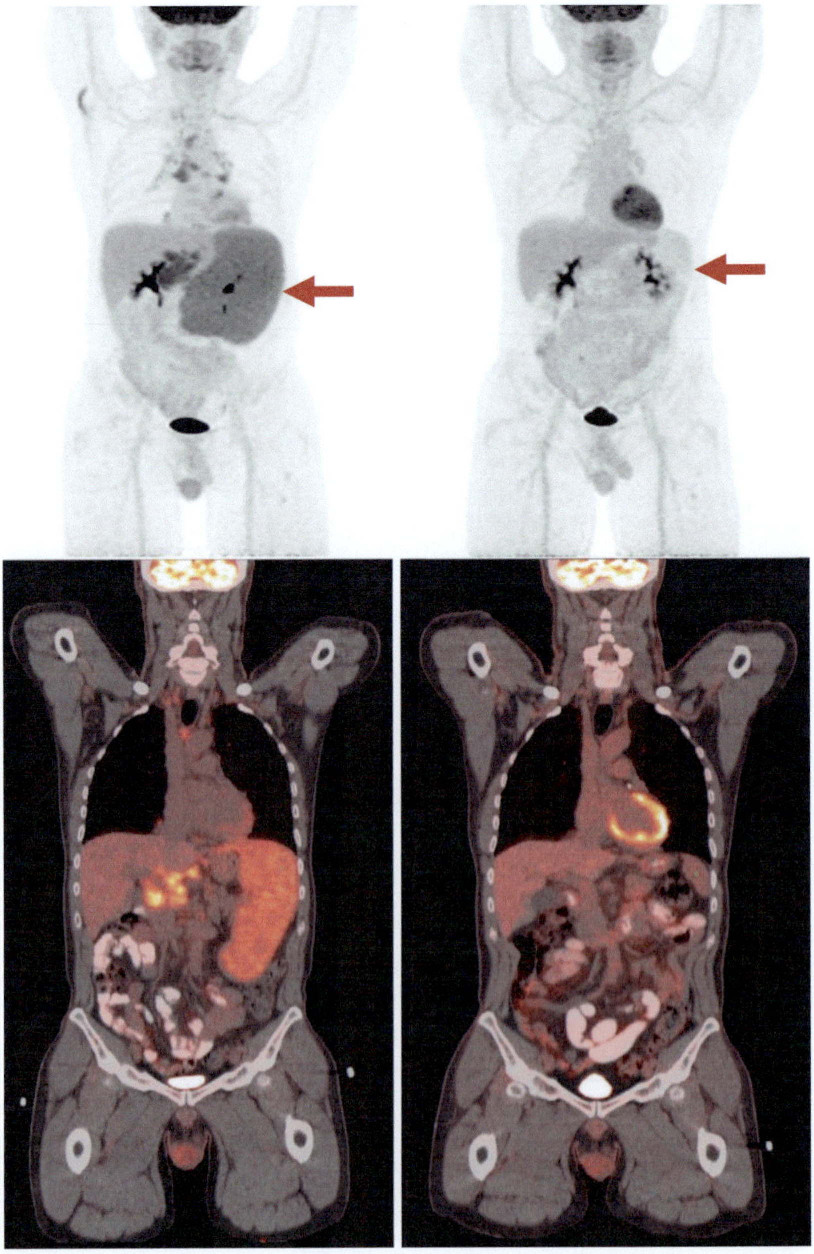

Fig. 23.6 A 52-year-old male with marginal zone lymphoma. Pretherapy PET/CT MIP (upper left) and coronal fused images (lower left) shows diffuse increased uptake in enlarged spleen (arrow) along with hypermetabolic adenopathy in the chest and abdomen. Post-therapy scan PET/CT MIP (upper right) and coronal fused (lower right) show interval resolution of hypermetabolic adenopathy as well as interval decrease in size of enlarged spleen and uptake

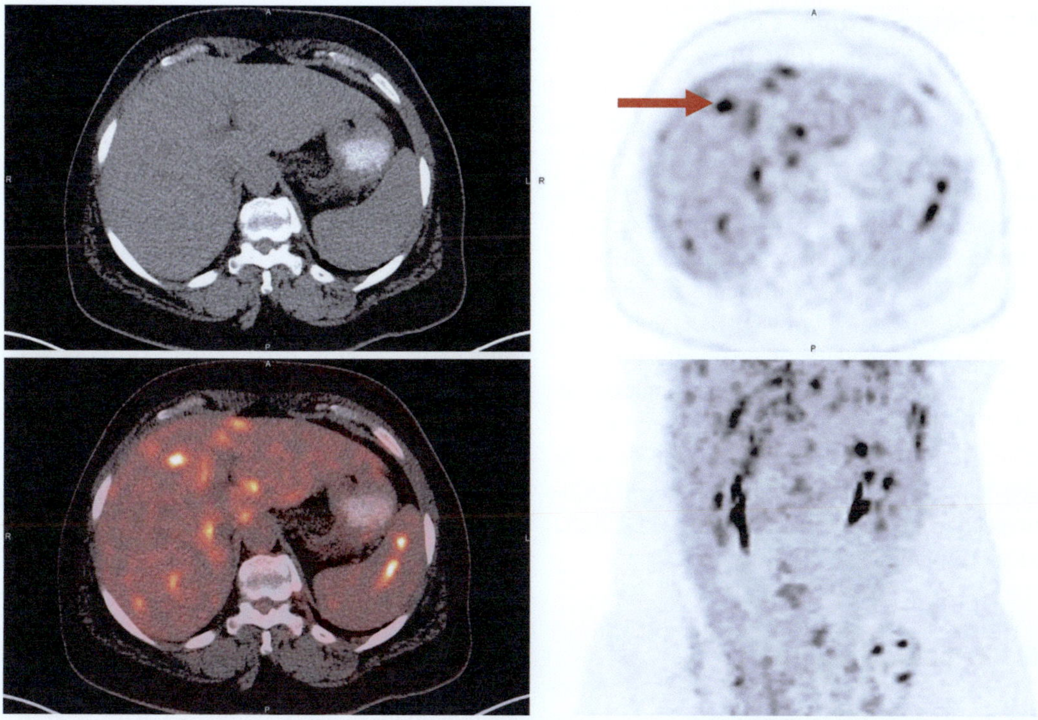

Fig. 23.7 Patient with newly diagnosed lymphoma. FDG PET/CT images (axial PET upper left) shows scattered foci of increased uptake in the liver (arrow). Axial fused PET/CT (lower right) shows foci of uptake in the spleen

reliable measure of hepatic involvement by lymphoma. Similar to splenic involvement, diffusely increased or focal uptake, with or without focal or disseminated nodules, supports liver involvement [15] (Fig. 23.7).

23.6 PET/CT Response Assessment

23.6.1 Hodgkin Disease

A multitude of FDG-PET studies have been conducted in HL. More recent data have further proven the superior sensitivity of FDG-PET, which is achieved without diminished specificity. *FDG-PET/CT as a potential replacement for* contrast-enhanced CT (CECT) detects a higher number of lesions than conventional CECT in 25–30% of patients [55, 56, 68]. The meta-analysis by Isasi et al. showed that the median sensitivity and specificity of FDG-PET in various lymphomas were 90% and 91%, respectively, and 93% and 88%, respectively, in Hodgkin lymphoma [54]. PET-CT upstaged the disease in 9–41% of patients and downstaged in 0–12% of patients, which translated into a change of treatment in 3–25% of cases [55, 57, 62, 64, 65, 98]. The most common reason for the downstaging was due to the absence of abnormal uptake in the lymph nodes with a longitudinal dimension greater than 15 mm; in CT, this is often considered to be associated with the lymphoproliferative process. The most common cause of disease upstaging is the identification of bone marrow or bone involvement, which confers stage IV disease affecting both treatment and prognosis. The introduction of PET-CT has led to a significant improvement, with a twofold increase in diagnosed cases of bone marrow involvement in Hodgkin lymphoma, when compared to diagnosis by histopathology alone. The sensitivity of FDG-PET/CT in the detection of bone marrow involvement is very high close to 97%, and the proportion of FDG-PET/CT-negative patients with a positive bone marrow biopsy among all cases is only 1.1% [83, 101, 102].

23.6.2 Diffuse Large B-Cell Lymphoma (DLBCL)

DLBCLs are the largest subgroup of aggressive non-Hodgkin lymphomas (NHLs) and exhibit FDG avidity in about 97% of the cases [44]. The combination of rituximab, cyclophosphamide, doxorubicin, vincristine, and prednisone (R-CHOP) achieves long-term cure in approximately 70% of patients with DLBCL and is the current first-line standard of care. Interim PET has been evaluated as a possible biomarker of early R-CHOP success or failure in several retrospective and prospective studies. About 39–87% patients achieve a negative interim FDG-PET/CT in prospective studies of advanced-stage DLBCL initially receiving R-CHOP (Fig. 23.8).

23.6.3 Other Lymphomas

23.6.3.1 Follicular Lymphoma

FL is the second most common subtype of NHL in the United States. The treatment goal for indolent FL is non-curative; however, overall survival (OS) can be significantly prolonged with therapy. The superiority of PET/CT is seen in a metanalysis of three multicenter prospective studies [103]: the PRIMA, PET-FL, and FOLL05. All three studies used both PET-CT and conventional CT to follow PFS and OS in patients receiving first-line or induction immunochemotherapy for advanced follicular lymphoma. The study pooled available information from 246 patients whose scans reviewed centrally rather than at each center. Three blinded nuclear medicine physicians read baseline and postinduction scans of these patients. The postinduction scans were undertaken within 3 months following induction therapy.

The results show that a positive PET-CT scan after induction therapy was associated with worse clinical outcomes. The 4-year PFS rate for patients with a positive PET-CT scan was 23% vs. 63% for patients with a negative PET-CT. Similarly, OS after 4 years was 87% for patients with a positive postinduction PET-CT compared with 97% for patients with a negative PET-CT. In contrast, responses on conventional CT scans were weakly predictive of PFS (hazard ratio, 1.7; $P = 0.017$).

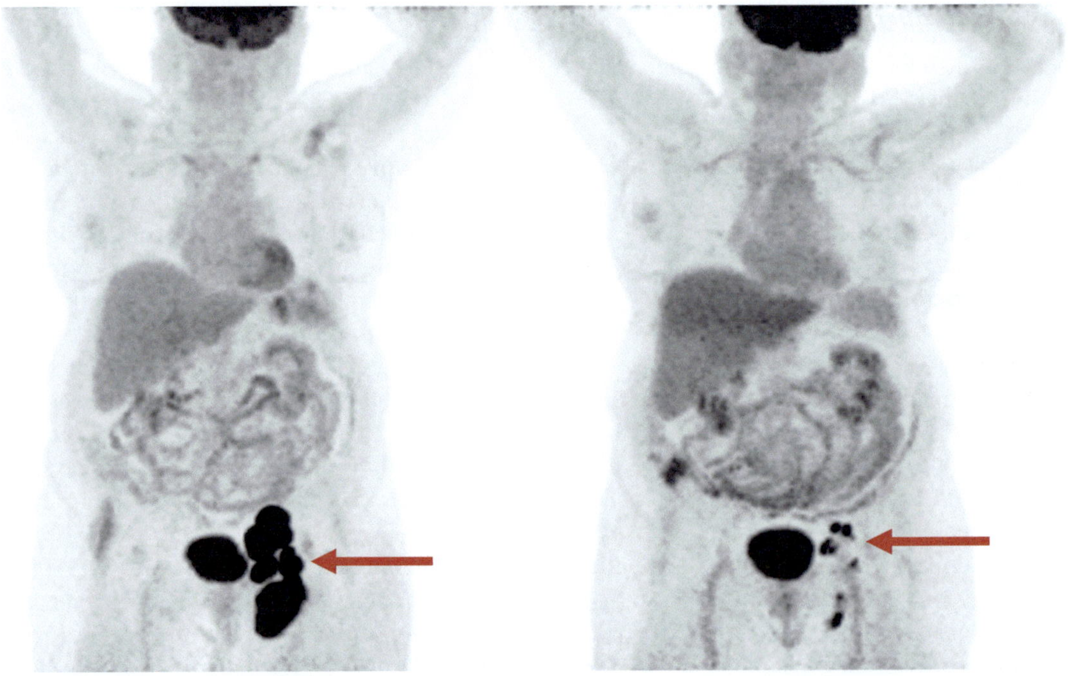

Fig. 23.8 A 84-year-old female with DLBCL. Pretherapy PET/CT (left panel) showed hypermetabolic left inguinal adenopathy. Post-therapy PET/CT scan (right panel) showed interval decrease in size and FDG uptake in the left inguinal nodes consistent with Deauville score of 4

In the setting of incurable disease, the impact of FDG-PET/CT on changes in patient management has been less compared with the impact in curable diseases. Current guidelines recommend that all patients with FL have a pretherapy staging FDG-PET/CT [15, 73]. The baseline PET study could serve as a tool to select the best modality for posttreatment response assessment in FL. For indolent FL without FDG avidity or in cases in which FDG-avid lesions do not have significantly high uptake to be able to adequately assess for change post therapy, continued use of CT response criteria for follow-up is warranted [1].

Although indolent FL is an incurable disease, proper posttreatment response assessments have prognostic implications and highlight patients who may require further therapy. Similar to aggressive lymphomas, patients with even minimal residual disease on post-therapy assessment have a worse prognosis [104], and patients with an excellent response to conventional therapy have a significantly better prognosis and prolonged OS. Several individual studies have shown that results on post-therapy FDG-PET correlate with progression-free survival (PFS), providing prognostic information, with a negative PET associated with longer PFS and a positive PET associated with shorter PFS [28, 34, 37]. In a meta-analysis of eight studies, FDG-PET was found to be an independent predictor of progression (HR = 5.1; 95% confidence interval 3.7–7.2), whereas CT fared worse than PET (HR = 2.6; 95% confidence interval 1.2–5.8). PET-based response criteria yielded better results than did CT-based criteria at differentiating complete response from non-complete response [105, 106] (Fig. 23.9).

23.6.4 T-Cell Lymphoma

A disease in which lymphoid cells called T-cell (or T-lymphocytes) becomes malignant. The two NHL subtypes were described by Alibert as early as 1806 and Sezary in 1938 [107, 108], but B- and T-cell diseases were not differentiated until the 1970s [109]. The incidence of T-cell lymphomas (TCL) is lower than B-cell lymphomas, accounting for a minority (about 15%) of non-Hodgkin lymphomas in the Western countries, with a higher incidence in Asia, and accounting for about half of pediatric lymphomas [28, 110]. TCLs, originating from mature T-cells, are a broad group of heterogeneous diseases, further categorized into peripheral T-cell lymphomas (PTCL) and cutaneous T-cell lymphomas (CTCL). Most subtypes are considered PTCL, where CTCL is relatively rare, only comprising for 2–3% of all NHL cases [111]. CTCLs tend to appear on the skin due to the expression of the cutaneous lymphocyte antigen [112].

T-cell lymphomas are highly diverse and include the following:

1. Anaplastic large cell lymphoma (ALCL), which can be primary cutaneous, systemic, or breast implant-associated
2. Lymphoblastic lymphoma (mainly in children and adolescents)
3. Mycosis fungoides (called Sezary syndrome if the malignant T-cells circulate in blood)
4. Peripheral T-cell lymphoma (a heterogenous group of generally aggressive diseases)

T-cell lymphomas (Table 23.7) show a spectrum of clinical behavior, from chronic indolent to aggressive variants; extranodal involvement is frequently seen. A description of the radiologic features associated with specific disease subtypes has been made [114]. The utility of ^{18}F-FDG PET/CT in T-cell lymphoma has been extensively studied [115–123]. Feeney et al. in their study that included 135 patients demonstrated clear role of FDG PET/CT in evaluation of T-cell lymphoma. FDG avidity was detected throughout the range of T-cell histologies, and it ranged from 78% in angioimmunoblastic T-cell lymphoma to 90–100% in anaplastic large cell lymphoma, subcutaneous panniculitis-like T-cell lymphoma, and adult T-cell leukemia lymphoma [49]. In contrast, a phase II pivotal study of romidepsin for relapsed and refractory PTCL, Horwitz et al. [124] found an avidity of 95%. Regarding the predictive value of interim and end-of-treatment PET/CT for PTCL, the data are based on retrospective studies and are even less conclusive. Some retrospective studies have shown that positive end-of-treatment PET/CT findings are associated with a poor prognosis [124–126]. In a retrospective review that included 99 patients

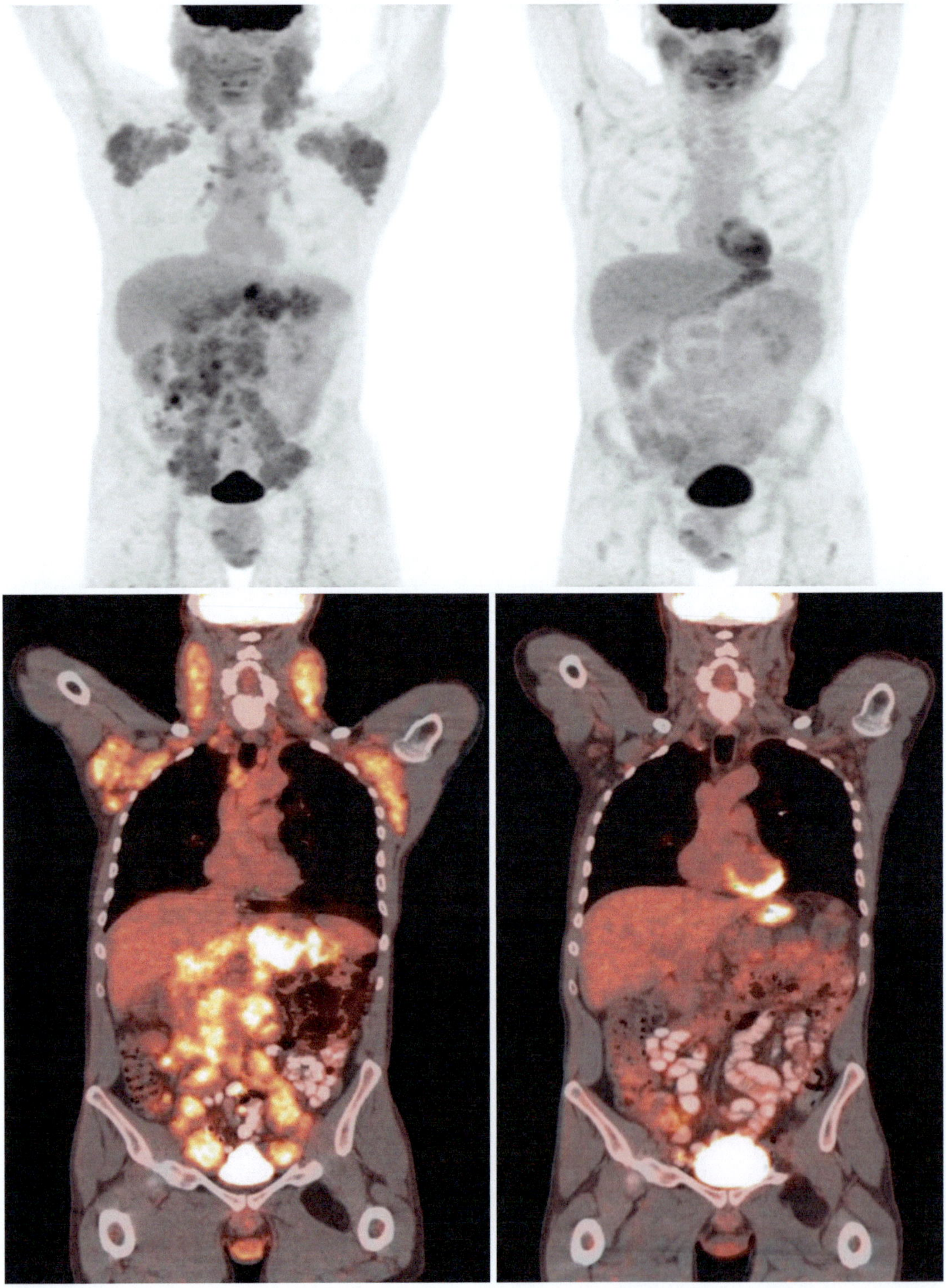

Fig. 23.9 A 61-year-old patient with CLL. Pretherapy FDG PET MIP (upper left) and coronal fused (lower left) showing hypermetabolic adenopathy in the neck, chest abdomen, and pelvis. Post-therapy FDG PET/CT MIP (upper right) and coronal fused (lower right) showing resolution of hypermetabolic adenopathy

Table 23.7 World Health Organization–European Organization for Research and Treatment of Cancer classification of primary cutaneous T-cell and natural killer cell lymphomas [10, 113]

T-cell lymphoma
I. Mycosis fungoides (MF)
A. MF variants and subtypes
1. Folliculotropic MF
2. Pagetoid reticulosis
3. Granulomatous slack skin
II. Sézary syndrome
III. Adult T-cell leukemia/lymphoma
IV. Primary cutaneous CD30+ lymphoproliferative disorders
A. Primary cutaneous anaplastic large cell lymphoma
B. Lymphomatoid papulosis
V. Subcutaneous panniculitis-like T-cell lymphoma
VI. Extranodal natural killer/T-cell lymphoma, nasal type
VII. Primary cutaneous peripheral T-cell lymphoma, unspecified
A. Primary cutaneous aggressive epidermotropic CD8+ T-cell lymphoma (provisional)
B. Cutaneous γ/δ T-cell lymphoma (provisional)
C. Primary cutaneous CD4+ small-/medium-sized pleomorphic T-cell lymphoma (provisional)
VIII. Precursor hematologic neoplasm
A. CD4+/CD56+ hematodermic neoplasm (blastic NK-cell lymphoma)

with peripheral T-cell lymphoma, Mehta-Shah et al. demonstrated that baseline total metabolic tumor volume (TMTV) and interim 5-point scores (5PS) are both independent prognostic factors in patients with PTCL. In this series, the use of interim 5PS in PTCL was independently predictive of outcome. Interim PET evaluation also identified a particularly high-risk group that may benefit from alternative treatment strategies earlier in the treatment course [127].

Another inconclusive question for lymphoma in general and PTCL in particular is the additional value of conducting a bone marrow biopsy (BMB). According to the Lugano classification, with HL, if a PET/CT scan is performed, a BMB is no longer required for routine evaluation. For DLBCL, if the PET/CT findings are negative, a BMB is indicated only if relevant for a clinical trial or for patient treatment [15]. However, this remains an open question for PTCL.

23.6.5 Mantle Cell Lymphoma

MCL is a relatively rare lymphoma subtype, accounting for approximately 2–7% of all cases of NHL. MCL presents with a broad histological spectrum, and the prognostic value of various morphological subtypes is still under debate [128]. Most authors agree that the blastoid variant of MCL has an even more aggressive clinical behavior with a very poor prognosis [129–131].

The current NCCN guidelines do not recommend the use of FDG-PET/CT for response assessment of MCL [73]. The data favoring the use of FDG-PET/CT for response assessment are mixed and less robust than the data available for other FDG-avid lymphomas including HL, DLBCL, and FL. Many studies have not shown a significant advantage of FDG-PET/CT over conventional evaluation with CT for MCL [132–134].

23.6.6 Chronic Lymphocytic Leukemia/Small Lymphocytic Lymphoma

CLL/SLL is a mature B-cell lymphoproliferative disorder characterized by accumulation of large numbers of incompetent lymphocytes in the blood or lymph nodes. On FDG-PET/CT, lymphadenopathy with low levels of FDG uptake (SUVs < 5) may be seen. The spleen may also be enlarged with FDG uptake mildly greater than the liver. Changes in size of lymph nodes and the spleen on CT is best for monitoring tumor response when treatment is initiated because of the low level of FDG uptake in this lymphoma subtype. CLL/SLL can behave indolently for many years, but histologically aggressive CLL has been described, and CLL/SLL can also transform to a high-grade lymphoma (or Richter transformation) in about 8% of patients. SUVmax is rather low for histologically indolent CLL/SLL, intermediate for histologically aggressive CLL, and highest for Richter transformation. SUVmax >10 in patients with CLL/SLL, regardless of subtype, is a poor prognostic factor [135, 136]. Transformation to an aggressive lymphoma phenotype can be suggested on FDG-PET/CT imaging either with the evidence of disproportionately high uptake in one or more nodes vs. others or with much higher uptake on a follow-up vs. previous scans. In a study of patients with NHL, SUV > 10 has an 81% specificity for excluding low-grade lymphoma [137]. Diagnostic performance of FDG-PET/CT for detecting transformation is better for CLL/SLL, which typically has homogeneous low-level FDG uptake, compared with the wide baseline range of uptake that can be seen in FL (Fig. 23.10).

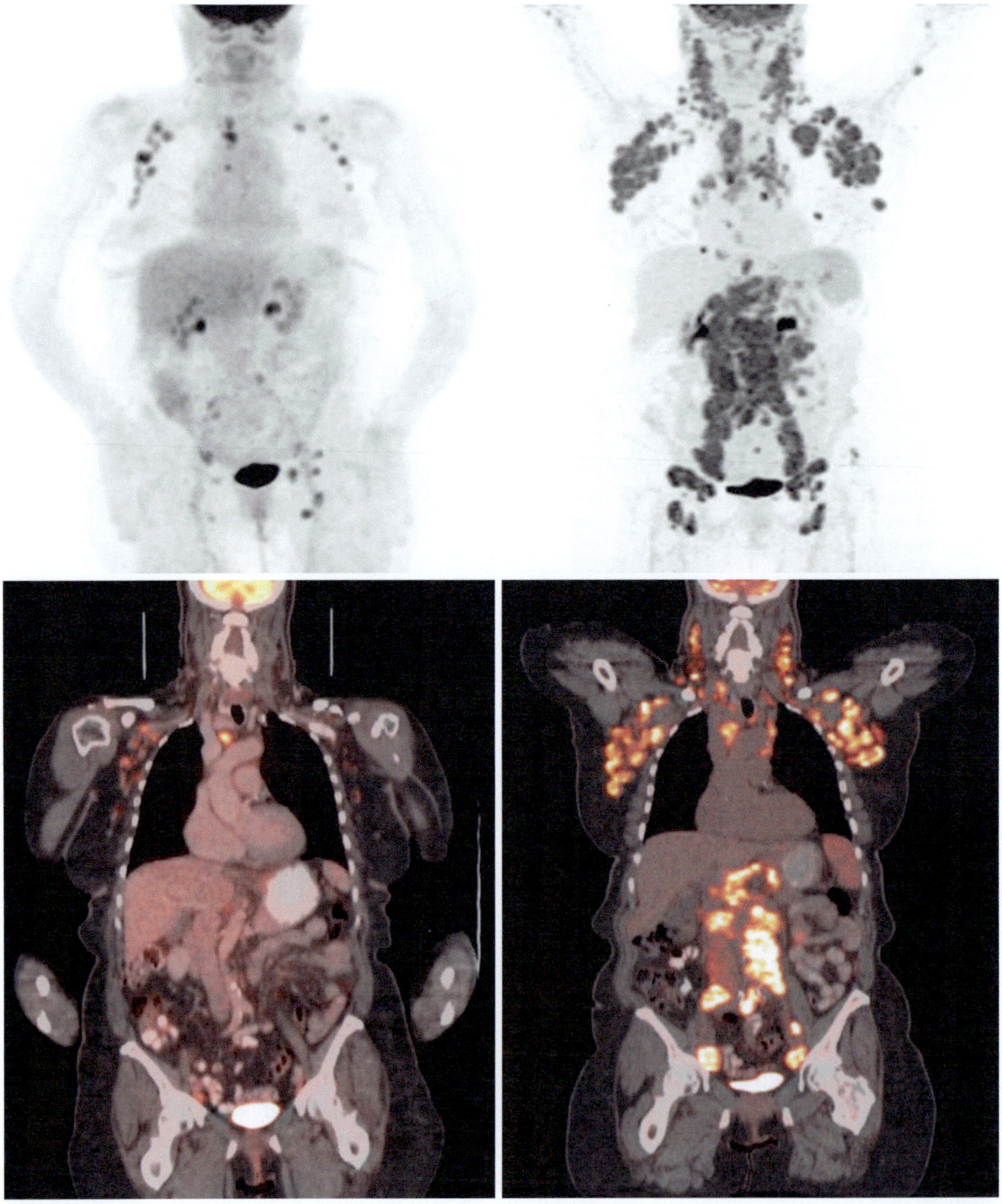

Fig. 23.10 A 74-year-old female with history of small cell lymphoma with transformation into DLBCL non-Hodgkin lymphoma. Baseline whole-body MIP (top left) and coronal PET/CT fused image (bottom left) and whole-body MIP (top right) and coronal PET/CT fused image (bottom right) demonstrating increase in number and intensity of FDG uptake in the involved lymph nodes

The NPV of FDG-PET/CT for excluding transformation is quite high at ≥95% [138]. Tissue confirmation is still necessary, and FDG-PET/CT can help guide biopsy.

23.6.7 Marginal Zone Lymphomas

There are several types of marginal zone lymphomas, including extranodal marginal zone lymphoma of mucosa-associated lymphoid tissue lymphoma, nodal marginal zone lymphoma, and splenic marginal zone lymphoma. The benefit of using PET/CT in MZL has scarcely been explored because of the supposed variable avidity for ^{18}F-FDG in this tumor. FDG-PET/CT is suggested as an alternative to diagnostic CT by NCCN guidelines at baseline in these lymphomas [23, 73], particularly if disease is limited and smaller radiation fields with involved site radiation are being considered. Like CLL/SLL, FDG-PET/CT is also useful for excluding transformation to a higher-grade lymphoma and guiding biopsy in this scenario when suspected. Several groups have reported an absence of ^{18}F-FDG avidity in MZL, mostly in cases with gastric involvement [139]. In Hoffman's series, 6 patients diagnosed with NMZL were shown to be avid in contrast to the 14 patients with MALT lymphomas in which PET gave completely negative results. Similarly, Jerusalem and Beguin failed to prove avidity in the 4 patients with MALT lymphoma in a series of 42 low-grade NHLs [140].

23.6.8 Posttransplant Lymphoproliferative Disorders

Posttransplant lymphoproliferative disorder (PTLD) is a rare but serious complication of both solid organ and bone marrow transplantation. PTLD represents a diverse and heterogenous group of lymphoproliferative disorders, ranging from abnormal lymphoid hyperplasia to frank malignant neoplasms [141]. Most cases of PTLD are of B-cell origin, and the pathogenesis in most patients appears to be related to Epstein–Barr virus infection, occurring primarily in the context of immunosuppression [142]. T-cell PTLD occurs in 10% of cases and tends to be more aggressive and less responsive to conventional treatment [143, 144]. FDG-PET/CT is useful in the evaluation and staging of select cases of PTLD as per the NCCN guidelines [73]. Depending on the type of PTLD, treatment generally involves reducing the immunosuppressive medication as well as immunotherapy and chemotherapy with a potential curative intention while being able to preserve the transplanted graft. The NCCN guidelines currently do not give recommendations on posttreatment response evaluation of PTLD; however, there are several small series that have shown promising results regarding the use of FDG-PET/CT in assessing response to therapy [145–148] (Fig. 23.11).

23.6.9 FDG-PET in Extranodal Lymphoma

Extranodal disease is defined as lymphomatous infiltration of anatomical sites other than the lymph nodes or lymphatic tissue. Approximately 50% of patients will develop extranodal disease (secondary extranodal disease), while between 10% and 35% of patients will have primary extranodal lymphoma at initial diagnosis [39]. The most commonly involved extranodal sites in lymphoma include BM, spleen, liver, primary central nervous system (PCNS), and gastrointestinal tract (GIT) [149]. Other sites involved with aggressive NHLs at presentation include the testis, bone, and kidney. Rare sites include the prostate, bladder, ovary, orbit, heart, breast, salivary glands, thyroid, and adrenal glands (Figs. 23.12 and 23.13).

Symptoms due to extralymphatic disease are usually associated with aggressive NHL and are uncommon in the indolent lymphomas. Extranodal involvement in primary nodal lymphomas is generally classified as stage IV lymphoma and affects prognosis. Given the high sensitivity of FDG-PET/CT in staging, treatment evaluation, and recurrence detection, we are detecting an increasing number of

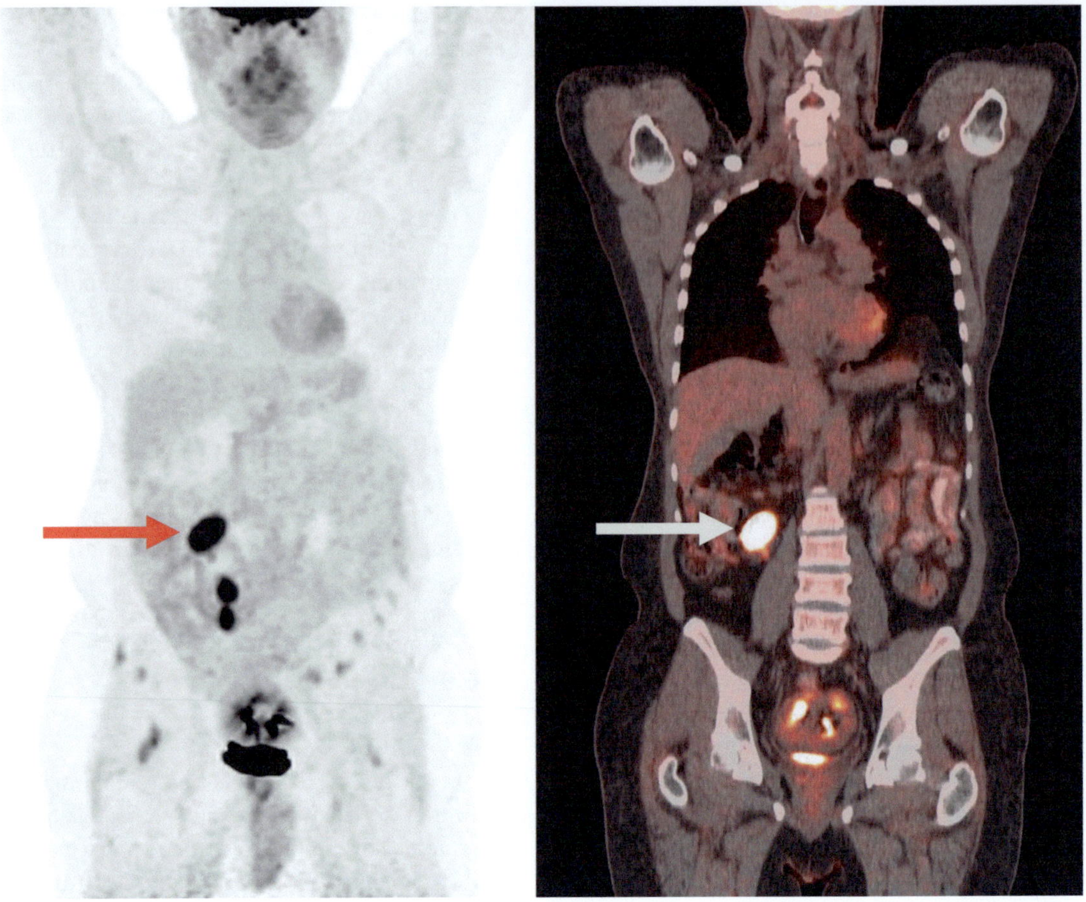

Fig. 23.11 A 54-year-old male with renal transplant. FDG PET/CT MIP image (left) and fused coronal image (right) showing transplanted kidney in the pelvis with hypermetabolic adenopathy in the right abdomen (arrow) consistent with PTLD

extranodal sites, be it primary or secondary involvement [150]. The FDG avidity of extranodal site is dependent on the histological subtype, with the indolent subtypes showing less FDG avidity or sometimes non-avidity [44]. A multitude of studies have reported that FDG-PET may provide more information about the extent of disease in cases with extranodal lymphoma compared to CT [82, 151, 152]. Schaefer et al. reported that for extranodal involvement, the sensitivity of PET/CT was almost twofold better than that of contrast-enhanced CT (88% vs. 50%), while the specificities were similar (100% vs. 90%) [26].

Primary extranodal lymphoma can involve any organs or systems, sometimes at unexpected sites with nonspecific presentations, mimicking carcinoma or infection [153] (Fig. 23.14).

The therapeutic strategy in patients with primary extranodal lymphomas is, in general, analogous. The results obtained, thus far, in extranodal lymphoma are similar to those with nodal lymphoma.

Primary CNS lymphoma (PCNSL) is a highly aggressive non-Hodgkin lymphoma confined to the CNS, including the brain, spine, cerebrospinal fluid (CSF), and eyes. PCNSL can develop in immunosuppressed (HIV/AIDS, organ transplant,

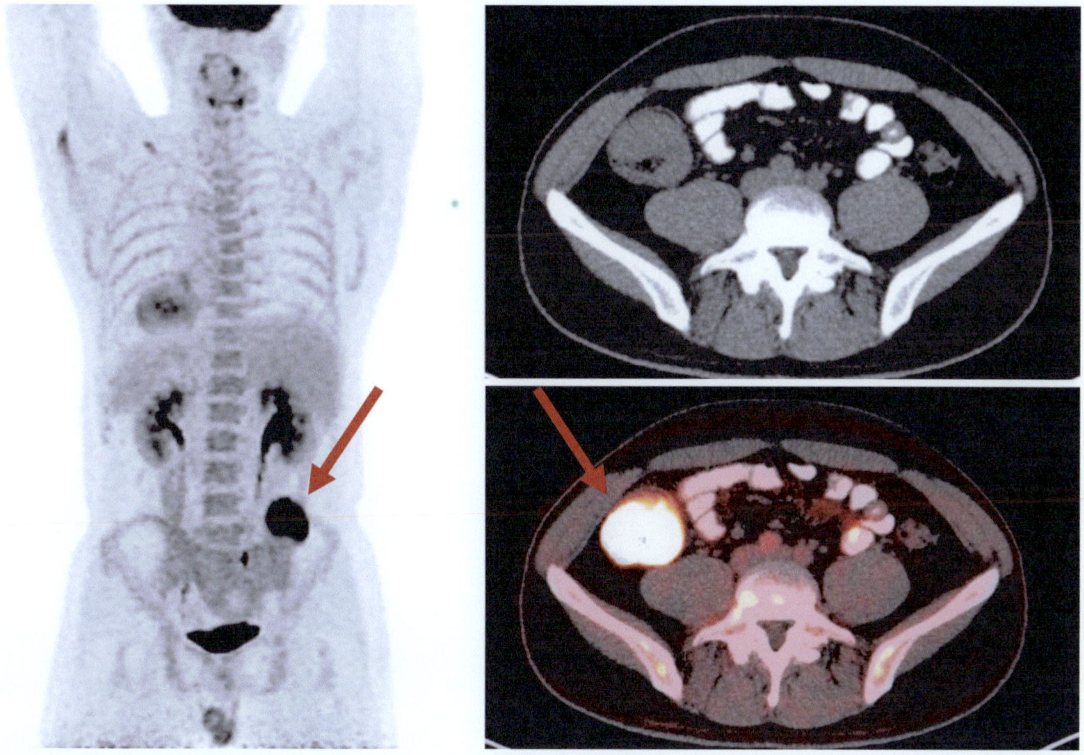

Fig. 23.12 A 50-year-old man with newly diagnosed primary lymphoma of the cecum (red arrow)

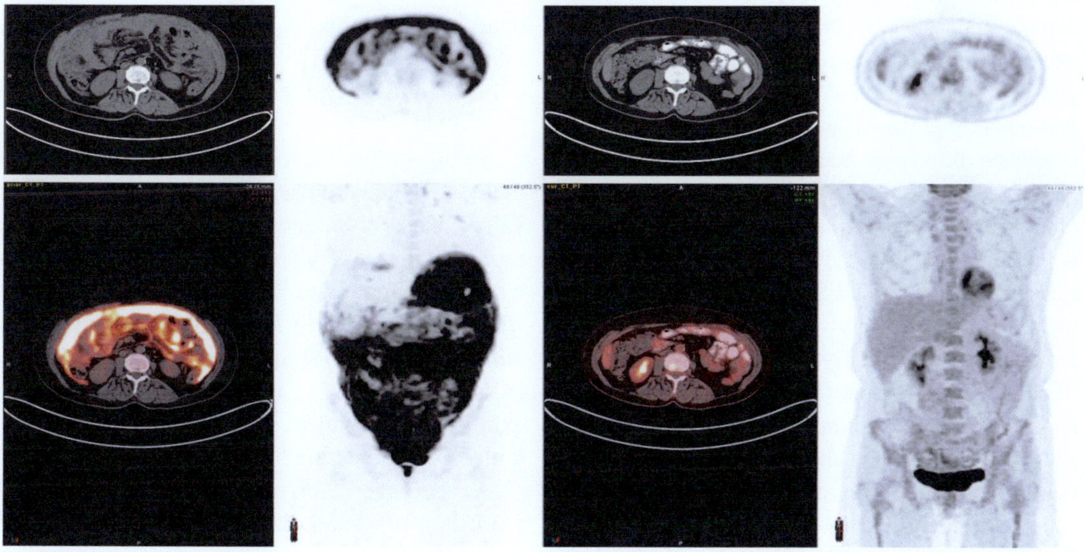

Fig. 23.13 A 61-year-old woman with DLBCL. ^{18}F-FDG PET/CT scan demonstrating extensive peritoneal involvement

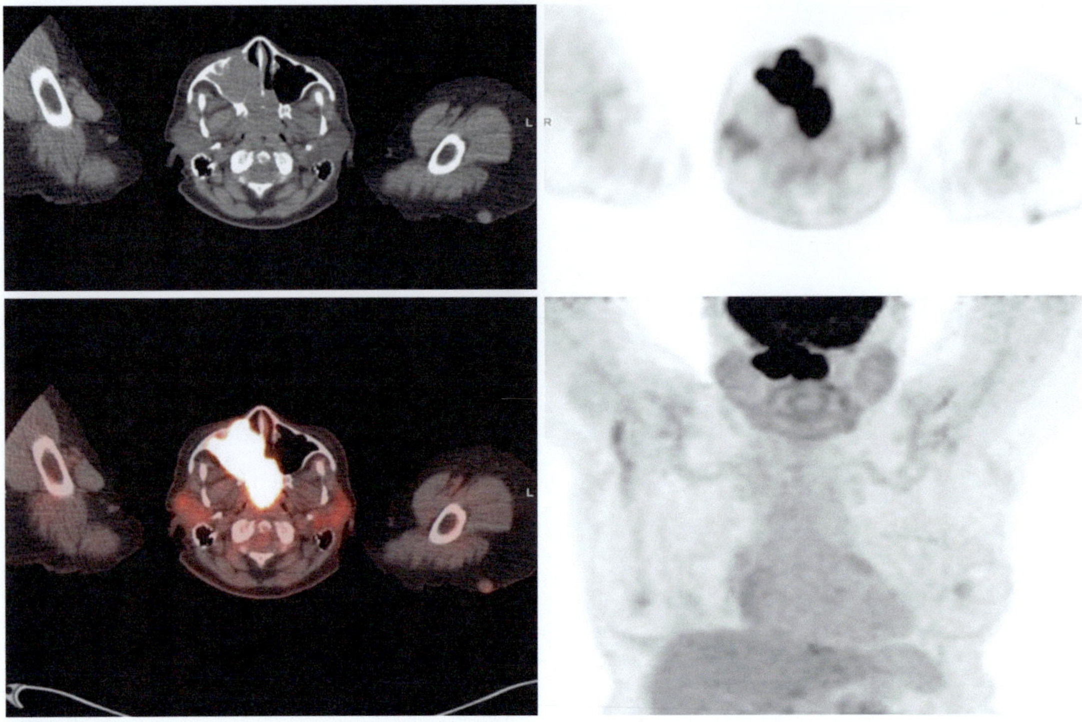

Fig. 23.14 An 84-year-old woman presenting with symptoms of sinus infection was ultimately diagnosed with DLBCL of the sinus

immunosuppressive agents) or immunocompetent patients [154]. PCNSL in immunocompetent patients is rare and represents 4% of all intracranial neoplasms and 4–6% of all extranodal lymphomas [155]. However, in recent years, a rising incidence has been recognized, particularly in patients older than 60 years, with an incidence rate of 0.5 per 100,000 per year [156]. Approximately 1500 new patients are diagnosed each year in the United States. PCNSL has a very high cellular density and increased glucose metabolism and usually shows strong uptake of ^{18}F-FDG in the tumor [157, 158]. In a literature review, Kawai et al. demonstrated ^{18}F-FDG uptake value in PCNSL to be about 2.5 times higher than that in the normal gray matter, and the tumor can usually be identified in the brain visually [159]. Total body ^{18}F-FDG-PET has an important role in PCNSL staging at diagnosis or in the follow-up, as it can diagnose a systemic disease with higher sensitivity than conventional imaging. Mohile et al. showed that 7% of patients with suspected PCNSL were found to have systemic NHL by total body FDG-PET, while body CT scans and bone marrow biopsies were negative. Moreover, total body FDG-PET was positive in 27% of patients during restaging for recurrent disease [160, 161].

Some studies have suggested that pretreatment ^{18}F-FDG uptake may have a prognostic value in newly diagnosed PCNSL. Kawai et al. reported that overall survival time of patients with low to moderate ^{18}F-FDG uptake (SUV max <12) was significantly longer than that of patients with high ^{18}F-FDG uptake (SUV max ≥12). PCNSL with high ^{18}F-FDG uptake tended to exhibit poor treatment response compared to that with low to moderate ^{18}F-FDG uptake [162].

As per the 2005 report of an international workshop to standardize baseline evaluation and response criteria for primary CNS lymphoma, gadolinium-enhanced MRI scans are the standard for treatment response evaluation of the bulky parenchymal brain disease [163]. Subsequent studies have supported that FDG-PET is suitable for early therapeutic monitoring after chemotherapy [164]. Birsen et al. reported that early PET evaluation after two cycles of methotrexate-based treatment strongly correlated to end-of-treatment MRI-assessed response and to progression-free survival. The study also supported that early PET may better identify early responders than MRI, suggesting that future risk-stratified therapeutic strategies might take advantage of PET evaluation to identify patients requiring frontline intensification or de-escalation, aiming for optimal, personalized medicine strategies in this frequently fatal disease [165] (Fig. 23.15).

Infection with human immunodeficiency virus (HIV) predisposes individuals to the development of neoplasm, including primary central nervous system lymphoma (PCL). Incidence of CNS lymphoma among persons with AIDS is several thousand-fold higher than that in the general population [166]. Distinguishing infectious etiology such as toxoplasmosis can be a challenge for morphological imaging studies including CT and MRI. Historically, Tl-201 is also known as a valuable imaging tool in the differentiation of

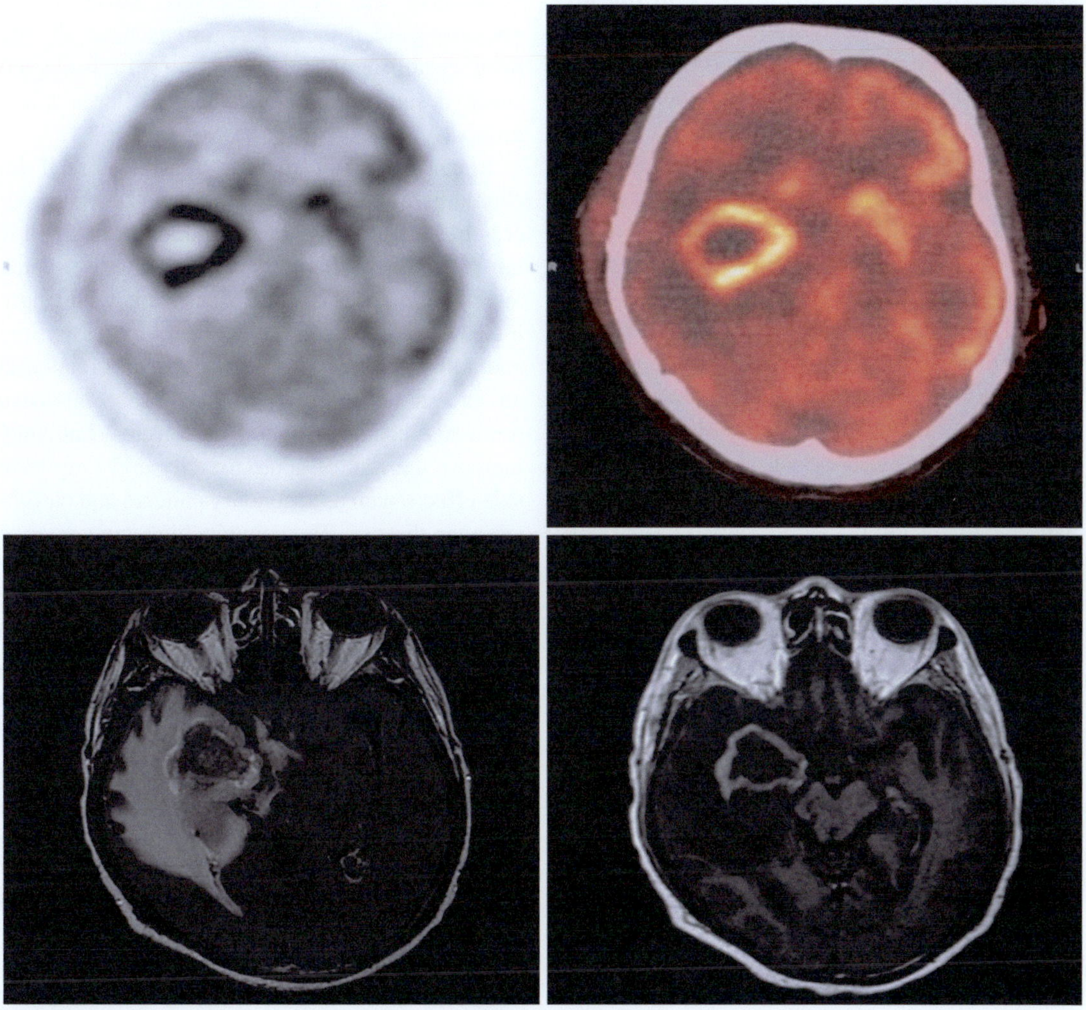

Fig. 23.15 Patient with CNS lymphoma. FDG PET/CT images show a centrally necrotic lesion in the right parietal lobe with peripheral increased uptake on axial PET (upper right), axial fused (upper left). (Lower right) Axial FLAIR and T1 post-contrast images (lower left) showing edema in surrounding brain parenchyma and rim-enhancing lesion

CNS lymphoma from infectious causes [167, 168]. Another possible method to increase the specificity is to combine imaging with measurement of EBV DNA in a cerebrospinal fluid sample. One study considered the value of combined thallium SPECT and measurement of EBV DNA in 13 patients with PCL and 18 patients with non-tumor disorders. The presence of increased uptake and/or positive EBV DNA had 100% sensitivity and almost 100% negative predictive value, suggesting that brain biopsy could be avoided in these patients [169]. In a recent study, FDG-PET proved superior to Tl-201 SPECT in the differentiation of CNS lymphomas from toxoplasmosis with an accuracy of 100% vs. 44% [170]. On FDG-PET imaging, a lesion with an FDG uptake higher than the adjacent gray matter is highly suggestive of a malignant process. FDG-PET can differentiate primary lymphomas of the CNS from infectious processes with a reported accuracy of 89% [171, 172]. Difficulty arises, however, when CNS lymphoma undergoes necrosis or is below the resolution limits of PET systems.

Primary bone lymphoma (PBL) is an extranodal lymphoma that arises from the medullary cavity and manifests as a localized, solitary lesion, which represents ~3% of all primary malignant bone tumors, 4–5% of extranodal lymphoma and less than 1% of all non-Hodgkin lymphoma [173, 174].

In a small series involving 19 patients, Wang et al. demonstrated that ^{18}F-FDG PET/CT was a sensitive imaging modality for diagnosis and treatment response evaluation for primary bone lymphoma [175].

Primary splenic DLBCL is considered extremely rare, with a prevalence of less than 1% [176, 177]. In a small study of 17 patients with primary splenic lymphoma, Karunanithi et al. demonstrated that PET/CT was true positive during initial staging with an accuracy of 100% and in those studies performed for restaging (35/50), sensitivity was 90.9%, specificity was 91.7%, and accuracy was 91.4% [178].

23.7 Response Assessment Criteria on FDG PET/CT

Over the course of many decades, combined chemotherapy and radiotherapy adapted to the stage of disease have become the optimal and standard treatment for Hodgkin lymphoma (HL) and diffuse large B-cell lymphoma. Besides achieving optimized cure rates of the underlying disease, reduction of toxicity has become a major goal. Since the introduction of FDG-PET for the staging and restaging of patients with lymphoma, a high predictive value of ^{18}F-FDG PET in response assessment has been observed. Several PET response-guided therapy regimens have already been established, and even more PET-adapted study designs are being tested in large study groups.

Stage-dependent therapy regimes based on chemotherapy or radiotherapy have become successful [179]. A PET-based reduction of therapy has proven helpful and is being further evaluated after commencement of treatment with more intensive regimens [180]. Both radiotherapy and chemotherapy carry high risks, directly related to an excess long-term mortality. More intensive regimens achieve higher cure rates but may increase the risk of acute toxicity and long-term side effects such as secondary cancers and cardiovascular disease. To maintain high cure rates, a strong and reliable indicator is needed to identify those patients in which therapy can be reduced. The metabolic therapy response can be seen in early interim PET after a few cycles of chemotherapy and in end-of-treatment (EOT) PET. The uptake of the tracer ^{18}F-fluorodeoxyglucose markedly decreases or is lower or no longer visible as soon as the tumor responds to therapy, and the majority of patients do respond to the treatments available today. Several prospective, risk-adapted trials have demonstrated that the use of PET can improve outcome in high-risk (interim PET-positive) patients and can limit the amount of treatment in lower-risk (interim PET-negative) patients [181–188]. Combining a PET-based response with biomarkers may improve the predictive value of PET, not only during interim assessment but also prior to treatment.

Although some authors suggested that EOT PET might not be necessary when interim PET results are negative, Hindie et al. pointed out that interim PET has a lower sensitivity than EOT PET so that EOT PET should not be omitted even in cases of a negative interim PET [189, 190]. Metabolic imaging using FDG-PET is superior to all other prognostic markers in HL [191], not only early in the course of treatment but also after first-line chemotherapy [70, 192]. The negative predictive value of PET after first-line treatment was consistently high in several studies and reached values of >95%, even in advanced-stage patients with residual tissue. A negative PET scan was found to be the strongest indicator for successful treatment [70, 193–195]. Unlike PET-negative patients, PET-positive patients after chemotherapy are at an increased risk of progression or relapse. However, the rate of such events is strongly dependent on initial risk factors and on the intensity of chemotherapy given and of subsequent radiotherapy. At the end of treatment, PET has proved to be highly predictive of disease remission, which is the goal of treatment. Negative predictive values of 90–100% have been reported for HL [194, 196–200] and aggressive NHL. The positive predictive value is lower, because while FDG accumulates in residual tumor, it may also be taken up in inflammation induced by treatment. Published positive predictive values range from 50% to 100% [194, 197–200] with variability again related to the initial disease prognosis. To minimize inflammatory uptake, imaging should be delayed for a minimum of 3 weeks, and preferably for 6–8 weeks, after chemotherapy at the end of treatment, 2 weeks after granulocyte colony-stimulating factor (GCSF) treatment, and 3 months after radiotherapy (RT).

23.7.1 Response Evaluation Methods

The introduction of radiation therapy and clinical introduction of CT and later FDG PET/CT imaging contributed significantly to the evolution of staging and response assessment systems in lymphoma. In 1971, The Ann Arbor staging classification was published, with anatomic stages related to radiation therapy fields [201]. Cotswolds modifications were added to create the modified Ann Arbor system after the introduction of CT for staging assessment in 1989 [202]. In 1999, the International Working Group criteria defined five categories of clinical response based on CT imaging of lesion size [202]. The category "complete remission—unconfirmed" applied to residual adenopathy after treatment and caused confusion. The International Harmonization Project criteria for response assessment defined clinical response based on PET/CT imaging of metabolic activity in 2007 [203, 204]. The FDG avidity was defined relative to the mediastinal blood pool. The Deauville criteria were subsequently proposed in 2009 [51] for grading FDG avidity on PET. In 2014, The Lugano classification was published [15].

The 5-point scale incorporates the Deauville criteria initially proposed for assessment on interim FDG PET/CT images. The 5-point scale includes the following categories:

1. No FDG uptake > background
2. FDG uptake ≤ mediastinum
3. FDG uptake > mediastinum but ≤ liver
4. FDG uptake moderately > liver
5. FDG uptake markedly > liver and/or new lesions

X. New areas of FDG uptake unlikely to be related to lymphoma

In interpreting the 5-point scale, a score of 1 or 2 is interpreted as negative for lymphoma, while a score of 4 or 5 is considered positive. A score of 3 likely also represents complete metabolic response at interim with resulting good prognosis and is therefore usually also considered as negative. However, in some trials pursuing a de-escalation of therapy strategy, a score of 3 may be considered as inadequate response to avoid undertreatment [205]. The Lugano classification represents a major change from the Ann

Arbor staging system and the International Working Group criteria for response assessment. The classification was developed following meetings in 2011 and 2013. The goal of the Lugano classification is the simplification and standardization of response assessment and reporting. The new classification also addresses the role of FDG PET/CT for staging and interim treatment response assessment. Given the expected rapid clinical application of the new staging criteria, it is important for radiologists and nuclear medicine specialists to be aware of the associated implications for lymphoma imaging.

23.7.1.1 Eligible Lesions

- Lymph nodes: the longest diameter in axial plane should be >1.5 cm.
- Extranodal lesions: the longest diameter in the axial plane should be >1.0 cm.

23.7.1.2 Selection of Lesions

Lesions chosen should be measurable in two dimensions.

CT (or ^{18}F-FDG PET-CT): tumor burden is to be calculated at baseline staging:

- Choose up to six of the largest nodes, nodal complexes, or other lymphoma deposits.
- Measure the longest diameter and shortest diameter of each lesion in the axial plane.
- Multiply the longest diameter and shortest diameter for each lesion to give the "product of the diameters."
- Add these to give the "sum of the product of the diameters" (SPD)—the SPD calculated at the time of staging will serve as the baseline for sequential quantification of tumor burden at interim and end-of-therapy FDG PET-CT.

Spleen measurement includes the largest transverse diameter and the perpendicular diameter in the axial plane, besides the craniocaudal diameter in the coronal plane. Splenomegaly is defined as vertical splenic length >13.0 cm. Four categories for CT have been outlined: (a) complete radiologic response, all nodes less than or equal to 1.5 cm in longest diameter, disappearance of all CT findings of lymphoma; (b) partial remission, 50% or greater decrease in disease burden; (c) stable disease, less than 50% decrease in disease burden; and (d) progressive disease, new or increased adenopathy or new extranodal lymphoma.

New response evaluation criteria: RECIL 2017 New criteria for evaluating response in lymphoma clinical trials—RECIL 2017—have been developed by an International Working Group with the aim of harmonizing criteria with the RECIST criteria used for solid tumors [206]. The standard response criteria currently in use for lymphoma are the Lugano Criteria which are based on (^{18}F)2-fluoro-2-deoxy-D-glucose positron emission tomography or bidimensional tumor measurements on computed tomography scans. These differ from the RECIST criteria used in solid tumors, which use unidimensional measurements. The RECIL group hypothesized that single-dimension measurement could be used to assess response to therapy in lymphoma patients, producing results similar to the standard criteria. They tested this hypothesis by analyzing 47,828 imaging measurements from 2983 individual adult and pediatric lymphoma patients enrolled in ten multicenter clinical trials and developed new lymphoma response criteria. A new provisional category of MR is included in the response assessment.

23.7.2 Response Categories Based on Assessment of Target Lesions

Complete Response

- Complete disappearance of all target lesions and all nodes with long axis <10 mm.
- ≥30% decrease in the sum of longest diameters of target lesions (partial response) plus normalization of FDG-PET.
- Normalization of FDG-PET (Deauville score 1–3).
- No bone marrow involvement.
- No new lesions.
- Reduction in the sum of diameters by ≤30% with normalization of FDG-PET uptake should not be considered a complete response unless documented by negative tissue biopsy.

Partial Response

- ≥30% decrease in the sum of longest diameters of target lesions but not a complete response.
- Positive FDG-PET (Deauville score 4–5).
- Any bone marrow involvement.
- No new lesions.

Minor Response

- ≥10% decrease in the sum of longest diameters of target lesions but not a partial response.
- Any FDG-PET finding.
- Any bone marrow involvement.
- No new lesions.

Stable Disease

- <10% decrease or ≤20% increase in the sum of longest diameters of target lesions.
- Any FDG-PET finding.
- Any bone marrow involvement.
- No new lesions.

Progressive Disease

- >20% increase in the sum of longest diameter of target lesions.
- For small lymph nodes of <15 mm post-therapy, minimum absolute increase of 5 mm and long diameter >15 mm.
- Appearance of new lesion.
- Any FDG-PET finding.
- Any bone marrow involvement.
- New or no new lesions.

23.7.3 Disease Progression After Initial Response

After initial response, and in the absence of appearance of new lesions, progressive disease is defined as an increase of the nadir sum of diameters by >20%.

23.7.3.1 Response Assessment to Immune-Modulating Agents, Including Checkpoint Inhibitors

To account for potential "pseudo-progression," immune-related response criteria should be used, requiring confirmation of progressive disease in two consecutive scans at least 4 weeks apart and inclusion of new lesion measurements in the total tumor burden.

23.7.4 Appearance of New Extranodal Lesion

A minimum of 1 cm in largest diameter of new extranodal lesions is required to confirm progressive disease. New smaller but suspicious lesions should be designated as equivocal; if later they are confirmed (by CT or biopsy) as due to lymphoma, the documented date of disease progression should be the date of identification as equivocal.

23.7.5 Quantification of Treatment Response with FDG PET/CT

Quantification of treatment response has become an interesting research area and is the subject of ongoing investigations in lymphoma imaging [207–209]. Several retrospective studies have shown a potential benefit for PET quantitative metrics to predict survival. In 127 early-stage HL patients (20% bulky) treated with six cycles of Adriamycin (doxorubicin), bleomycin, vinblastine, and dacarbazine (ABVD), Song et al. showed that only older age, B symptoms, and high MTV status were independently associated with PFS ($P = 0.008$) and OS ($P = 0.007$) [210, 211]. In this study, a fixed threshold method of $SUV_{max} \geq 2.5$ was used to determine the disease volume. Similarly, in a cohort of 59 HL patients (stages II–IV), Kanoun et al. [212] showed that patients with a low baseline MTV had a significantly better 4-year PFS than those with a high MTV (85% vs. 42%, $P = 0.001$, 88% vs. 45%, $P = 0.0015$, respectively). The MTVs were measured with a semiautomatic method using a 41% SUV_{max} threshold. In a multivariate analysis, only baseline MTV ($P < 0.006$, relative risk (RR) 4.4) and ΔSUV_{max} at PET2 (71%, $P = 0.0005$, RR 6.3) remained independent predictors of PFS when tumor bulk (>10 cm) did not reach statistical significance. In contrast, Tseng et al. reported that baseline PET metrics including SUV_{max}, SUV_{mean}, and MTV did not predict survival in 30 HL patients (stages IIB–IV, 63%) treated with varying chemotherapy regimens with or without IFRT, whereas ΔMTV ($P < 0.01$), ΔSUV_{max} ($P = 0.01$), and ΔSUV_{mean} ($P < 0.05$) at interim PET were associated with PFS and OS [84]. The International Prognostic Score (IPS) was also associated with PFS ($P < 0.05$) and OS ($P < 0.01$) [211–213].

The quantitative PET assessment appears to be a highly promising method to use for adaptive studies if externally proven valid. However, this methodology is still in an evolutionary phase and the published data are not always consistent. This may be on the basis of retrospective designs, small sample sizes translating to insufficient representation of risk and stage groups, differences in treatments, as well as the varying methodologies used to measure MTVs. Currently, there is no consensus regarding the most optimal segmentation algorithm or the quantitative index to assess the actual metabolic disease burden. Further trials investigating the prognostic and predictive value of MTV are warranted in large, standardized, homogeneous data sets for both internal and external validation of this exciting method to prove or refute a role to improve on the prognostic value of conventional risk-stratifying systems.

23.8 Pitfalls in Lymphoma Imaging

23.8.1 Sarcoid-Like Granulomas

Sarcoid-like reactions in enlarged hilar and mediastinal lymph nodes as well as in lung nodules can be identified in lymphoma patients after therapy, particularly in the HD population [214–217]. In the case of HD, these noncaseating epithelioid-cell granulomata may occur synchronous to the disease or many years later. This inflammatory manifestation may arise directly in direct relation with the tumor or distant to the lesion. It is deemed that the granulomatous formations represent a secondary reaction to the chronic stimulation of tumoral antigens disseminated through the body or as a particular side effect of certain drugs including bleomycin and more rarely vinblastine and doxorubicin [216, 218–221]. Recently, development of pulmonary sarcoidosis has been described in patients receiving immunotherapy from blockade of the cytotoxic T-lymphocyte-associated antigen-4 [222–224] (Fig. 23.16).

23.8.2 Benign Lymphoproliferative Disorders

The benign lymphoproliferative disorders (LPD) most frequently manifest in the thorax either in the lymph nodes or in the bronchus-associated lymphoid tissue of the lung [225]. Entities such as plasma cell granuloma, posttransplant lymphoproliferative disorders, lymphoid interstitial pneumonia, and lymphomatoid granulomatosis involve the pulmonary parenchyma, while Castleman's disease, infectious mononucleosis, and angioimmunoblastic lymphadenopathy involve intrathoracic lymph nodes. It is important to differentiate the benign forms of LPD from the aggressive lymphomas. There is a considerable overlap between benign LPD and NHL, especially in the immunocompromised patients. One might assume that the FDG uptake would be lower in this benign form of LPD than that seen in aggressive NHL and HD [226, 227]. It is expected that in the indolent forms of NHL, the differentiation between benign LPD and lymphoma may not be possible (Fig. 23.17).

23.8.3 Other Nonspecific Lymphadenopathies

As ^{18}F-FDG PET/CT has become an essential tool in lymphoma for monitoring treatment response and surveillance, nonspecific FDG uptake is often seen in lymph node follow-up scans. Cervical lymph nodes are often visualized at the end of treatment on ^{18}F-FDG-PET/CT imaging, often being reactive from the upper respiratory tract infections. In a retrospective review by Young-Sil An et al., only 9% positive

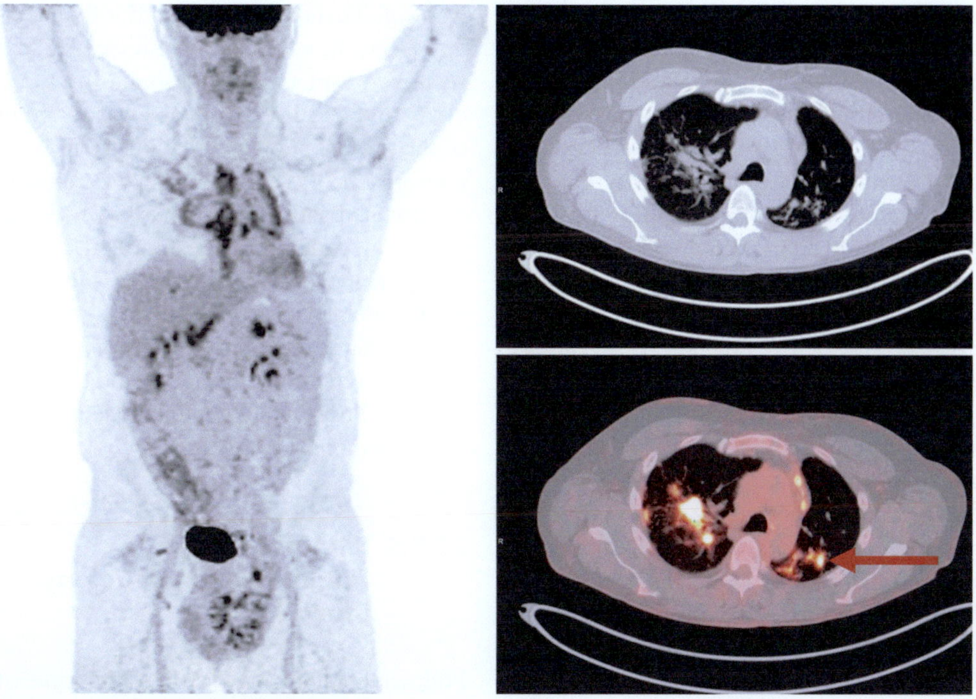

Fig. 23.16 A 48-year-old male with history of Hodgkin disease. Post-therapy FDG PET/CT demonstrating foci of FDG uptake in the lung parenchyma (red arrow). Subsequent CT-guided biopsy revealed sarcoidosis

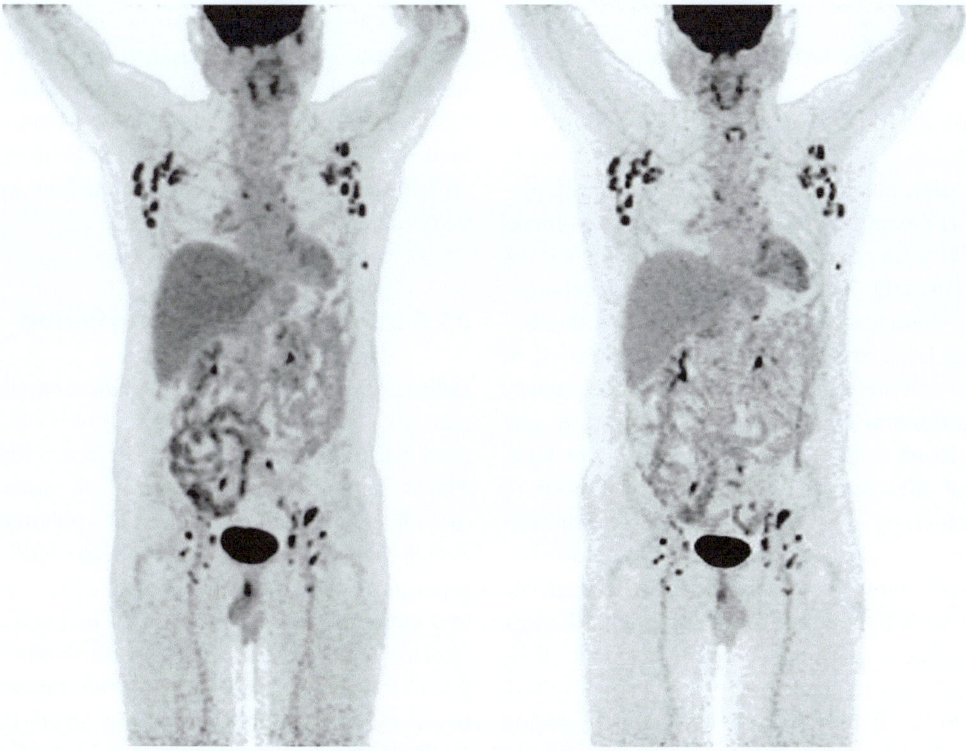

Fig. 23.17 FDG PET/CT MIP image (left) and follow-up FDG PET/CT (right) showing stable mildly FDG avid lesions in the axilla and inguinal region consistent with biopsy-proven lymphoid hyperplasia

cervical lymph nodes in the follow-up scans were positive for lymphoma [228]. Isolated FDG uptake in the axillary lymph nodes is often seen from the radiotracer extravasation at the injection site [229, 230]. These lymph nodes are morphologically normal and demonstrate fatty hila. The axillary lymph node uptake after treatment should be considered as pathologic only if there are additional abnormal findings, increasing the rate of true positivity from 20.8% to 79.6% [231]. In case of symmetric bilateral FDG uptake, benign lymphoid hyperplasia should also be considered [232]. Increased FDG uptake is observed in the inguinal lymph nodes with similar frequency and is often from the distal extremity infections. Patient with single and morphologically normal-appearing inguinal lymph node should not be subjected to biopsy, especially if the lymph node was not involved at initial diagnosis.

Generalized nodal FDG uptake is seen in a variety of infectious condition such as syphilis, tuberculosis, and cat scratch disease and in autoimmune conditions such as lupus [233–235].

23.8.4 Thymic Uptake

Physiologic ^{18}F-FDG uptake in the thymus has been reported in children and in sporadic cases in adults after chemotherapy [236]. Thymic hyperplasia is a common phenomenon after treatment, especially in children with an incidence of approximately 20% [237–239]. This phenomenon is characterized by lymph follicles demonstrating large nuclear centers and infiltration of plasma cells following thymic aplasia secondary to inhibition of lymphocyte proliferation. In one study, Brink et al. found increased FDG uptake in 73% of the children with malignancy prior to chemotherapy and in 75% of the children with malignancy following chemotherapy. However, they also found increased uptake in 5% of the adults with lymphoma following chemotherapy [240]. These findings support the idea that, although thymic uptake may be a normal finding in children, it may also be expected in young adults after therapy [238]. In a study of pediatric patients, thymic FDG uptake after chemotherapy was significantly higher than during chemotherapy [239]. In a retrospective review of 559 consecutive ^{18}F-FDG PET/CT studies by Jerushalmi et al., thymic ^{18}F-FDG uptake was found in 28% of the present study population, more frequently after treatment. Thymic uptake was found in 73% of untreated patients up to the age of 13 years and in 8% of patients in the fourth decade of life [241]. Knowledge of this age- and treatment-related incidence of physiologic thymic ^{18}F-FDG avidity can reduce the number of potential pitfalls in reporting PET/CT studies in cancer patients. Post-therapy thymic uptake may persist for 6–18 months (Fig. 23.18).

23.8.5 BM Uptake After Administration of Colony Stimulators

Following administration of granulocyte colony-stimulating factor or granulocyte-macrophage colony-stimulating factor, the BM demonstrates diffuse, increased FDG accumulation [80, 81]. However, diffuse bone marrow FDG uptake can also be caused by bone marrow involvement by lymphoma, which may be indistinguishable from hematopoietic cytokine-mediated FDG bone marrow uptake [242]. Of note, colony-stimulating factors can also cause increased splenic uptake, which should not be misinterpreted as splenic involvement by lymphoma.

23.8.6 Posttransplantation Period

Following bone marrow transplantation (BMT), patients can develop cellular immunodeficiency until the full engraftment of transplanted marrow. These patients are susceptible to infections including idiopathic interstitial pneumonitis, *Pneumocystis carinii*, cytomegalovirus, and aspergillus [243]. About 35–50% of hematopoietic stem cell transplant (HSCT) recipients will develop acute GVHD [244]. Additionally, acute graft vs. host disease (GVHD) often occurs during the first 3 months following an allogeneic BMT [245]. To minimize the risk of graft rejection and GVHD, allogeneic BMT patients are

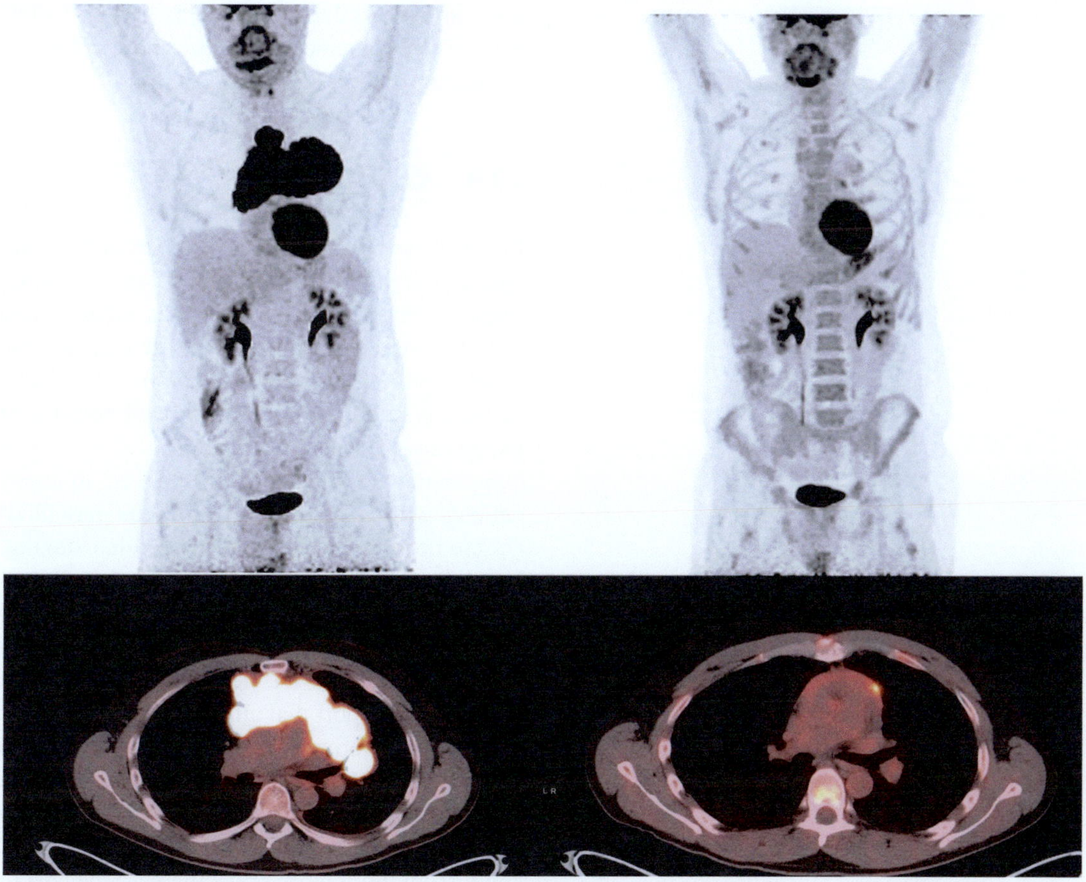

Fig. 23.18 A 36-year-old man with mediastinal B-cell lymphoma. Treated with R-EPOCH. Pretreatment PET/CT scan on the left showing large mediastinal mass. Posttreatment scan on the right demonstrating resolution of lymphoma with residual FDG uptake in the anterior mediastinum, compatible with thymic rebound

given immunosuppressants to prevent GVHD before and after transplant. Use of these drugs, however, increases the risk of infection. Therefore, caution should be exercised when interpreting FDG-PET images in immunocompromised patients.

23.8.7 AIDS-Related Lymphoma

There has been a rising incidence of AIDS-related cancers, possibly because antiretroviral therapy (ART) prolongs patient survival and causes dysfunctional cell-mediated immunity [246]. AIDS-related lymphomas are characterized by the presence of B-symptoms (weight loss, night sweats, and fevers) in approximately 90% of patients, advanced clinical stage in greater than 60%, and clinical aggressiveness with poor therapeutic outcomes. Extranodal involvement is a particularly distinctive feature, with the gastrointestinal tract being the most common location. Other sites of involvement include the central nervous system, the bone marrow, the oral cavity, the lungs, and the skin. Recently, a primary effusion lymphoma has been described in association with HIV [247].

^{18}F-FDG PET/CT can demonstrate abnormal foci of increased FDG accumulation in HIV-infected individuals with suspected malignancy or fever of unknown origin (FUO) by localizing to malignant or inflammatory cells such as neutrophils and macrophages [248, 249]. Activated lymphocytes exhibit increased glucose utilization, and HIV-infected individuals have a greater accumulation of FDG in their lymph nodes than

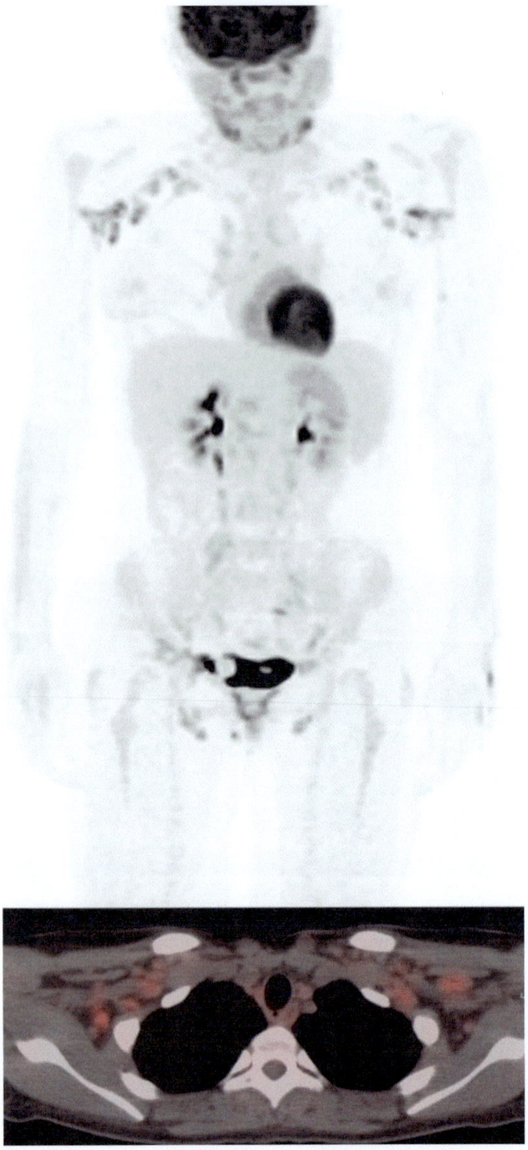

Fig. 23.19 A 38-year-old male with past history of Hodgkin lymphoma PET/CT MIP (top) and axial fused (bottom) shows mildly hypermetabolic lymph nodes in bilateral axillae which are related to HIV infection

patients without HIV infection [250, 251]. FDG PET/CT scan can be used to differentiate HIV-associated lymphoma from HIV-associated reactive adenopathy using quantitative FDG PET and symmetry. Quantitative PET metabolic metrics as well as the qualitative assessment of symmetry of nodal uptake appear to be valuable tools for differentiating lymphoma from reactive adenopathy in HIV-infected patients using FDG PET. These parameters appear more robust in aviremic patients [252] (Fig. 23.19).

23.9 Conclusions

PET/CT has become an integral part of the management of patients with DLBCL. In the revised response criteria of 2007, it was incorporated into the restaging evaluation. More recently, the ICML Working Group has recommended that it be incorporated into staging as well because of its increased sensitivity and specificity when compared with CT alone. Moreover, in many patients with HL and DLBCL, a scan may obviate the need for a BMB during routine staging. However, this practice will make historical comparisons with older studies difficult because of stage migration. Nevertheless, the role of interim and surveillance PET remains controversial. Data fail to support that altering treatment on the basis of an interim study improves outcome in DLBCL; however, suggestive retrospective data in advanced HL have led to a number of prospective studies attempting to validate this potential application. Follow-up scans increase the cost of patient care in a time when cost containment should be considered, with no evidence that these studies detect relapse prior to clinical signs or symptoms, yet are associated with anxiety, expense, a risk of radiation, and a false-positive rate that leads to additional scans or unnecessary invasive studies. CECT is desirable if the measurement of lymph node size is important or to better delineate intra-abdominal disease. The quantitative PET assessment appears to be a highly promising method to use for adaptive studies if externally proven valid. However, this methodology is still in an evolutionary phase and the published data are not always consistent. This may be on the basis of retrospective designs, small sample sizes translating to insufficient representation of risk and stage groups, differences in treatments, as well as the varying methodologies used to measure MTVs. Currently, there is no consensus regarding the most optimal segmentation algorithm or the quantitative index to assess the actual metabolic disease burden. Further trials investigating the prognostic and predictive value of MTV are warranted in large, standardized, homogeneous data sets for both internal and external validation of this exciting method to prove or refute a role to improve on the prognostic value of conventional risk-stratifying systems. More uniform standardization of scan conduct and interpretation with the 5PS will enhance the ability to compare results amongst trials.

References

1. Howlader N, Noone AM, Krapcho M, Miller D, Brest A, Yu M, Ruhl J, Tatalovich Z, Mariotto A, Lewis DR, Chen HS, Feuer EJ, Cronin KA, editors. SEER cancer stat facts: non-Hodgkin lymphoma. Bethesda, MD: National Cancer Institute; 2018. https://seer.cancer.gov/statfacts/html/nhl.html
2. Jacobson CA, Longo DL. Non-Hodgkin's lymphoma. New York, NY: McGraw-Hill Education; 2018.
3. Swerdlow SH, Campo E Harris NL, Bosman FT, Jaffe ES, Lakhani SR, Ohgaki H, eds. , WHO classification of tumours of haematopoietic and lymphoid tissues. The International Agency for Research on Cancer (IARC) 2008; 2008; Lyon, France: World Health Organization classification of tumours.
4. Savage KJ, Zeynalova S, Kansara RR. Validation of a prognostic model to assess the risk of CNS disease in patients with aggressive B-cell lymphoma. Blood. 2014;124(21):394.
5. Vitolo U, Chiappella A, Ferreri AJ, Martelli M, Baldi I, Balzarotti M, et al. First-line treatment for primary testicular diffuse large B-cell lymphoma with rituximab-CHOP, CNS prophylaxis, and contralateral testis irradiation: final results of an international phase II trial. J Clin Oncol. 2011;29(20):2766–72.
6. Hosein PJ, Maragulia JC, Salzberg MP, Press OW, Habermann TM, Vose JM, et al. A multicentre study of primary breast diffuse large B-cell lymphoma in the rituximab era. Br J Haematol. 2014;165(3):358–63.
7. Mahul B, Amin MF, editors. AJCC cancer staging manual. New York: Springer International Publishing; 2017.
8. National Cancer Institute sponsored study of classifications of non-Hodgkin's lymphomas: summary and description of a working formulation for clinical usage. The Non-Hodgkin's Lymphoma Pathologic Classification Project. Cancer. 1982;49(10):2112–35.
9. Harris NL, Jaffe ES, Diebold J, Flandrin G, Muller-Hermelink HK, Vardiman J, et al. The World Health Organization classification of neoplasms of the hematopoietic and lymphoid tissues: report of the Clinical Advisory Committee meeting—Airlie House, Virginia, November, 1997. Hematol J. 2000;1(1):53–66.
10. Swerdlow SH, Campo E, Pileri SA, Harris NL, Stein H, Siebert R, et al. The 2016 revision of the World Health Organization classification of lymphoid neoplasms. Blood. 2016;127(20):2375–90.
11. Peters M. A study of survival in Hodgkin's disease treated radiologically. Am J Roentgenol. 1950;62:299–311.
12. Rosenberg SA, Boiron M, DeVita VT Jr, Johnson RE, Lee BJ, Ultmann JE, Viamonte M Jr. Report of the committee on Hodgkin's disease staging procedures. Cancer Res. 1971;31(11):1862–3.
13. Carbone PP, Kaplan H, Musshoff K, et al. Report of the committee on Hodgkin's disease. Cancer Res. 1971;31(11):1860–1.
14. Rosenberg SA. Validity of the Ann Arbor staging classification for the non-Hodgkin's lymphomas. Cancer Treat Rep. 1977;61(6):1023–7.
15. Cheson BD, Fisher RI, Barrington SF, Cavalli F, Schwartz LH, Zucca E, et al. Recommendations for initial evaluation, staging, and response assessment of Hodgkin and non-Hodgkin lymphoma: the Lugano classification. J Clin Oncol. 2014;32(27):3059–67.
16. Arcaini L, Rattotti S, Gotti M, Luminari S. Prognostic assessment in patients with indolent B-cell lymphomas. TheScientificWorldJournal. 2012;2012:107892.
17. Federico M, Bellei M, Marcheselli L, Luminari S, Lopez-Guillermo A, Vitolo U, et al. Follicular lymphoma international prognostic index 2: a new prognostic index for follicular lymphoma developed by the international follicular lymphoma prognostic factor project. J Clin Oncol. 2009;27(27):4555–62.
18. Pfreundschuh M, Ho AD, Cavallin-Stahl E, Wolf M, Pettengell R, Vasova I, et al. Prognostic significance of maximum tumour (bulk) diameter in young patients with good-prognosis diffuse large-B-cell lymphoma treated with CHOP-like chemotherapy with or without rituximab: an exploratory analysis of the MabThera International Trial Group (MInT) study. Lancet Oncol. 2008;9(5):435–44.
19. Hoane BR, Shields AF, Porter BA, Borrow JW. Comparison of initial lymphoma staging using computed tomography (CT) and magnetic resonance (MR) imaging. Am J Hematol. 1994;47(2):100–5.
20. Jung G, Heindel W, von Bergwelt-Baildon M, Bredenfeld H, Gossmann A, Zahringer M, et al. Abdominal lymphoma staging: is MR imaging with T2-weighted turbo-spin-echo sequence a diagnostic alternative to contrast-enhanced spiral CT? J Comput Assist Tomogr. 2000;24(5):783–7.
21. Ferrucci JT. Advances in abdominal MR imaging. Radiographics. 1998;18(6):1569–86.
22. Johnson SA, Kumar A, Matasar MJ, Schoder H, Rademaker J. Imaging for staging and response assessment in lymphoma. Radiology. 2015;276(2):323–38.

23. Kwee TC, Kwee RM, Nievelstein RA. Imaging in staging of malignant lymphoma: a systematic review. Blood. 2008;111(2):504–16.
24. Barrington SF, Mackewn JE, Schleyer P, Marsden PK, Mikhaeel NG, Qian W, et al. Establishment of a UK-wide network to facilitate the acquisition of quality assured FDG-PET data for clinical trials in lymphoma. Ann Oncol. 2011;22(3):739–45.
25. Quarles van Ufford H, Hoekstra O, de Haas M, Fijnheer R, Wittebol S, Tieks B, et al. On the added value of baseline FDG-PET in malignant lymphoma. Mol Imaging Biol. 2010;12(2):225–32.
26. Schaefer NG, Hany TF, Taverna C, Seifert B, Stumpe KDM, von Schulthess GK, et al. Non-Hodgkin lymphoma and Hodgkin disease: coregistered FDG PET and CT at staging and restaging—do we need contrast-enhanced CT? Radiology. 2004;232(3):823–9.
27. Johnson SA, Kumar A, Matasar MJ, Schöder H, Rademaker J. Imaging for staging and response assessment in lymphoma. Radiology. 2015;276(2):323–38.
28. A clinical evaluation of the International Lymphoma Study Group classification of non-Hodgkin's lymphoma. The Non-Hodgkin's Lymphoma Classification Project. Blood. 1997;89(11):3909–18.
29. A predictive model for aggressive non-Hodgkin's lymphoma. N Engl J Med. 1993;329(14):987–94.
30. Hasenclever D, Diehl V. A prognostic score for advanced Hodgkin's disease. International Prognostic Factors Project on Advanced Hodgkin's Disease. N Engl J Med. 1998;339(21):1506–14.
31. Zhou Z, Sehn LH, Rademaker AW, Gordon LI, Lacasce AS, Crosby-Thompson A, et al. An enhanced International Prognostic Index (NCCN-IPI) for patients with diffuse large B-cell lymphoma treated in the rituximab era. Blood. 2014;123(6):837–42.
32. American Cancer Society. American Cancer Society: Cancer facts and figures 2019. 2019. https://www.cancer.org/content/dam/cancer-org/research/cancer-facts-and-statistics/annual-cancer-facts-and-figures/2019/cancer-facts-and-figures-2019.pdf.
33. Shankland KR, Armitage JO, Hancock BW. Non-Hodgkin lymphoma. Lancet. 2012;380(9844):848–57.
34. Armitage JO, Weisenburger DD. New approach to classifying non-Hodgkin's lymphomas: clinical features of the major histologic subtypes. Non-Hodgkin's Lymphoma Classification Project. J Clin Oncol. 1998;16(8):2780–95.
35. Tan D, Horning SJ, Hoppe RT, Levy R, Rosenberg SA, Sigal BM, et al. Improvements in observed and relative survival in follicular grade 1–2 lymphoma during 4 decades: the Stanford University experience. Blood. 2013;122(6):981–7.
36. Bastion Y, Sebban C, Berger F, Felman P, Salles G, Dumontet C, et al. Incidence, predictive factors, and outcome of lymphoma transformation in follicular lymphoma patients. J Clin Oncol. 1997;15(4):1587–94.
37. Yuen AR, Kamel OW, Halpern J, Horning SJ. Long-term survival after histologic transformation of low-grade follicular lymphoma. J Clin Oncol. 1995;13(7):1726–33.
38. Cabanillas F, Velasquez WS, Hagemeister FB, McLaughlin P, Redman JR. Clinical, biologic, and histologic features of late relapses in diffuse large cell lymphoma. Blood. 1992;79(4):1024–8.
39. Anderson T, Chabner BA, Young RC, Berard CW, Garvin AJ, Simon RM, et al. Malignant lymphoma. 1. The histology and staging of 473 patients at the National Cancer Institute. Cancer. 1982;50(12):2699–707.
40. Tubiana M, Henry-Amar M, Carde P, Burgers JM, Hayat M, Van der Schueren E, et al. Toward comprehensive management tailored to prognostic factors of patients with clinical stages I and II in Hodgkin's disease. The EORTC Lymphoma Group controlled clinical trials: 1964–1987. Blood. 1989;73(1):47–56.
41. Diehl V, Sextro M, Franklin J, Hansmann ML, Harris N, Jaffe E, et al. Clinical presentation, course, and prognostic factors in lymphocyte-predominant Hodgkin's disease and lymphocyte-rich classical Hodgkin's disease: report from the European Task Force on Lymphoma Project on Lymphocyte-Predominant Hodgkin's Disease. J Clin Oncol. 1999;17(3):776–83.
42. Ng AK, Bernardo MV, Weller E, Backstrand K, Silver B, Marcus KC, et al. Second malignancy after Hodgkin disease treated with radiation therapy with or without chemotherapy: long-term risks and risk factors. Blood. 2002;100(6):1989–96.
43. Barrington SF, Mikhaeel NG, Kostakoglu L, Meignan M, Hutchings M, Mueller SP, et al. Role of imaging in the staging and response assessment of lymphoma: consensus of the International Conference on Malignant Lymphomas Imaging Working Group. J Clin Oncol. 2014;32(27):3048–58.
44. Weiler-Sagie M, Bushelev O, Epelbaum R, Dann EJ, Haim N, Avivi I, et al. (18)F-FDG avidity in lymphoma readdressed: a study of 766 patients. J Nucl Med. 2010;51(1):25–30.
45. Luminari S, Biasoli I, Arcaini L, Versari A, Rusconi C, Merli F, et al. The use of FDG-PET in the initial staging of 142 patients with follicular lymphoma: a retrospective study from the FOLL05 randomized trial of the Fondazione Italiana Linfomi. Ann Oncol. 2013;24(8):2108–12.
46. Trotman J, Fournier M, Lamy T, Seymour JF, Sonet A, Janikova A, et al. Positron emission tomography-computed tomography (PET-CT) after induction therapy is highly predictive of patient outcome in follicular lymphoma: analysis of PET-CT in a subset of PRIMA trial participants. J Clin Oncol. 2011;29(23):3194–200.
47. Dupuis J, Berriolo-Riedinger A, Julian A, Brice P, Tychyj-Pinel C, Tilly H, et al. Impact of [(18)F] fluorodeoxyglucose positron emission tomography response evaluation in patients with high-tumor

burden follicular lymphoma treated with immunochemotherapy: a prospective study from the Groupe d'Etudes des Lymphomes de l'Adulte and GOELAMS. J Clin Oncol. 2012;30(35):4317–22.
48. Bodet-Milin C, Touzeau C, Leux C, Sahin M, Moreau A, Maisonneuve H, et al. Prognostic impact of 18F-fluoro-deoxyglucose positron emission tomography in untreated mantle cell lymphoma: a retrospective study from the GOELAMS group. Eur J Nucl Med Mol Imaging. 2010;37(9):1633–42.
49. Feeney J, Horwitz S, Gonen M, Schoder H. Characterization of T-cell lymphomas by FDG PET/CT. AJR Am J Roentgenol. 2010;195(2):333–40.
50. Cahu X, Bodet-Milin C, Brissot E, Maisonneuve H, Houot R, Morineau N, et al. 18F-fluorodeoxyglucose-positron emission tomography before, during and after treatment in mature T/NK lymphomas: a study from the GOELAMS group. Ann Oncol. 2011;22(3):705–11.
51. Meignan M, Gallamini A, Meignan M, Gallamini A, Haioun C. Report on the First International Workshop on Interim-PET-Scan in Lymphoma. Leuk Lymphoma. 2009;50(8):1257–60.
52. Cook GJ, Wegner EA, Fogelman I. Pitfalls and artifacts in 18FDG PET and PET/CT oncologic imaging. Semin Nucl Med. 2004;34(2):122–33.
53. Barrington SF, O'Doherty MJ. Limitations of PET for imaging lymphoma. Eur J Nucl Med Mol Imaging. 2003;30(Suppl 1):S117–27.
54. Isasi CR, Lu P, Blaufox MD. A metaanalysis of 18F-2-deoxy-2-fluoro-D-glucose positron emission tomography in the staging and restaging of patients with lymphoma. Cancer. 2005;104(5):1066–74.
55. Naumann R, Beuthien-Baumann B, Reiss A, Schulze J, Hanel A, Bredow J, et al. Substantial impact of FDG PET imaging on the therapy decision in patients with early-stage Hodgkin's lymphoma. Br J Cancer. 2004;90(3):620–5.
56. Hutchings M, Loft A, Hansen M, Pedersen LM, Berthelsen AK, Keiding S, et al. Position emission tomography with or without computed tomography in the primary staging of Hodgkin's lymphoma. Haematologica. 2006;91(4):482–9.
57. Jerusalem G, Beguin Y, Fassotte MF, Najjar F, Paulus P, Rigo P, et al. Whole-body positron emission tomography using 18F-fluorodeoxyglucose compared to standard procedures for staging patients with Hodgkin's disease. Haematologica. 2001;86(3):266–73.
58. Weihrauch MR, Re D, Bischoff S, Dietlein M, Scheidhauer K, Krug B, et al. Whole-body positron emission tomography using 18F-fluorodeoxyglucose for initial staging of patients with Hodgkin's disease. Ann Hematol. 2002;81(1):20–5.
59. Picardi M, Soricelli A, Grimaldi F, Nicolai E, Gallamini A, Pane F. Fused FDG-PET/contrast-enhanced CT detects occult subdiaphragmatic involvement of Hodgkin's lymphoma thereby identifying patients requiring six cycles of anthracycline-containing chemotherapy and consolidation radiation of spleen. Ann Oncol. 2011;22(3):671–80.
60. Carr R, Barrington SF, Madan B, O'Doherty MJ, Saunders CA, van der Walt J, et al. Detection of lymphoma in bone marrow by whole-body positron emission tomography. Blood. 1998;91(9):3340–6.
61. Tatsumi M, Cohade C, Nakamoto Y, Fishman EK, Wahl RL. Direct comparison of FDG PET and CT findings in patients with lymphoma: initial experience. Radiology. 2005;237(3):1038–45.
62. Bangerter M, Moog F, Buchmann I, Kotzerke J, Griesshammer M, Hafner M, et al. Whole-body 2-[18F]-fluoro-2-deoxy-D-glucose positron emission tomography (FDG-PET) for accurate staging of Hodgkin's disease. Ann Oncol. 1998;9(10):1117–22.
63. Buchmann I, Reinhardt M, Elsner K, Bunjes D, Altehoefer C, Finke J, et al. 2-(fluorine-18)fluoro-2-deoxy-D-glucose positron emission tomography in the detection and staging of malignant lymphoma. A bicenter trial. Cancer. 2001;91(5):889–99.
64. Munker R, Glass J, Griffeth LK, Sattar T, Zamani R, Heldmann M, et al. Contribution of PET imaging to the initial staging and prognosis of patients with Hodgkin's disease. Ann Oncol. 2004;15(11):1699–704.
65. Partridge S, Timothy A, O'Doherty MJ, Hain SF, Rankin S, Mikhaeel G. 2-Fluorine-18-fluoro-2-deoxy-D glucose positron emission tomography in the pretreatment staging of Hodgkin's disease: influence on patient management in a single institution. Ann Oncol. 2000;11(10):1273–9.
66. Pelosi E, Pregno P, Penna D, Deandreis D, Chiappella A, Limerutti G, et al. Role of whole-body [18F] fluorodeoxyglucose positron emission tomography/computed tomography (FDG-PET/CT) and conventional techniques in the staging of patients with Hodgkin and aggressive non Hodgkin lymphoma. Radiol Med. 2008;113(4):578–90.
67. Raanani P, Shasha Y, Perry C, Metser U, Naparstek E, Apter S, et al. Is CT scan still necessary for staging in Hodgkin and non-Hodgkin lymphoma patients in the PET/CT era? Ann Oncol. 2006;17(1):117–22.
68. Rigacci L, Vitolo U, Nassi L, Merli F, Gallamini A, Pregno P, et al. Positron emission tomography in the staging of patients with Hodgkin's lymphoma. A prospective multicentric study by the Intergruppo Italiano Linfomi. Ann Hematol. 2007;86(12):897–903.
69. Rodriguez-Vigil B, Gomez-Leon N, Pinilla I, Hernandez-Maraver D, Coya J, Martin-Curto L, et al. PET/CT in lymphoma: prospective study of enhanced full-dose PET/CT versus unenhanced low-dose PET/CT. J Nucl Med. 2006;47(10):1643–8.
70. Schaefer NG, Taverna C, Strobel K, Wastl C, Kurrer M, Hany TF. Hodgkin disease: diagnostic value of FDG PET/CT after first-line therapy—is biopsy of FDG-avid lesions still needed? Radiology. 2007;244(1):257–62.

71. DeVita VT Jr, Canellos GP. The lymphomas. Semin Hematol. 1999;36(4 Suppl 7):84–94.
72. Shipp MA. Prognostic factors in aggressive non-Hodgkin's lymphoma: who has "high-risk" disease? Blood. 1994;83(5):1165–73.
73. Zelenetz AD, Gordon LI, Abramson JS, et al. NCCN clinical practice guidelines in oncology: B-cell lymphomas. Version 2.2019. 2019. https://www.nccn.org/professionals/physician_gls/pdf/b-cell.pdf.
74. El-Galaly TC, d'Amore F, Mylam KJ, de Nully Brown P, Bogsted M, Bukh A, et al. Routine bone marrow biopsy has little or no therapeutic consequence for positron emission tomography/computed tomography-staged treatment-naive patients with Hodgkin lymphoma. J Clin Oncol. 2012;30(36):4508–14.
75. Khan AB, Barrington SF, Mikhaeel NG, Hunt AA, Cameron L, Morris T, et al. PET-CT staging of DLBCL accurately identifies and provides new insight into the clinical significance of bone marrow involvement. Blood. 2013;122(1):61–7.
76. Conlan MG, Bast M, Armitage JO, Weisenburger DD. Bone marrow involvement by non-Hodgkin's lymphoma: the clinical significance of morphologic discordance between the lymph node and bone marrow. Nebraska Lymphoma Study Group. J Clin Oncol. 1990;8(7):1163–72.
77. Senff NJ, Kluin-Nelemans HC, Willemze R. Results of bone marrow examination in 275 patients with histological features that suggest an indolent type of cutaneous B-cell lymphoma. Br J Haematol. 2008;142(1):52–6.
78. Juneja SK, Wolf MM, Cooper IA. Value of bilateral bone marrow biopsy specimens in non-Hodgkin's lymphoma. J Clin Pathol. 1990;43(8):630–2.
79. Brunning RD, Bloomfield CD, McKenna RW, Peterson LA. Bilateral trephine bone marrow biopsies in lymphoma and other neoplastic diseases. Ann Intern Med. 1975;82(3):365–6.
80. Abdel-Dayem HM, Rosen G, El-Zeftawy H, Naddaf S, Kumar M, Atay S, et al. Fluorine-18 fluorodeoxyglucose splenic uptake from extramedullary hematopoiesis after granulocyte colony-stimulating factor stimulation. Clin Nucl Med. 1999;24(5):319–22.
81. Gundlapalli S, Ojha B, Mountz JM. Granulocyte colony-stimulating factor: confounding F-18 FDG uptake in outpatient positron emission tomographic facilities for patients receiving ongoing treatment of lymphoma. Clin Nucl Med. 2002;27(2):140–1.
82. Moog F, Bangerter M, Diederichs CG, Guhlmann A, Merkle E, Frickhofen N, et al. Extranodal malignant lymphoma: detection with FDG PET versus CT. Radiology. 1998;206(2):475–81.
83. Pakos EE, Fotopoulos AD, Ioannidis JP. 18F-FDG PET for evaluation of bone marrow infiltration in staging of lymphoma: a meta-analysis. J Nucl Med. 2005;46(6):958–63.
84. Pelosi E, Penna D, Douroukas A, Bello M, Amati A, Arena V, et al. Bone marrow disease detection with FDG-PET/CT and bone marrow biopsy during the staging of malignant lymphoma: results from a large multicentre study. Q J Nucl Med Mol Imaging. 2011;55(4):469–75.
85. Cortes-Romera M, Sabate-Llobera A, Mercadal-Vilchez S, Climent-Esteller F, Serrano-Maestro A, Gamez-Cenzano C, et al. Bone marrow evaluation in initial staging of lymphoma: 18F-FDG PET/CT versus bone marrow biopsy. Clin Nucl Med. 2014;39(1):e46–52.
86. Muzahir S, Mian M, Munir I, Nawaz MK, Faruqui ZS, Mufti KA, et al. Clinical utility of (1)(8)F FDG-PET/CT in the detection of bone marrow disease in Hodgkin's lymphoma. Br J Radiol. 2012;85(1016):e490–6.
87. Weiler-Sagie M, Kagna O, Dann EJ, Ben-Barak A, Israel O. Characterizing bone marrow involvement in Hodgkin's lymphoma by FDG-PET/CT. Eur J Nucl Med Mol Imaging. 2014;41(6):1133–40.
88. Alzahrani M, El-Galaly TC, Hutchings M, Hansen JW, Loft A, Johnsen HE, et al. The value of routine bone marrow biopsy in patients with diffuse large B-cell lymphoma staged with PET/CT: a Danish-Canadian study. Ann Oncol. 2016;27(6):1095–9.
89. Ujjani CS, Hill EM, Wang H, Nassif S, Esposito G, Ozdemirli M, et al. (18)F-FDG PET-CT and trephine biopsy assessment of bone marrow involvement in lymphoma. Br J Haematol. 2016;174(3):410–6.
90. Prassopoulos P, Daskalogiannaki M, Raissaki M, Hatjidakis A, Gourtsoyiannis N. Determination of normal splenic volume on computed tomography in relation to age, gender and body habitus. Eur Radiol. 1997;7(2):246–8.
91. Loftus WK, Chow LT, Metreweli C. Sonographic measurement of splenic length: correlation with measurement at autopsy. J Clin Ultrasound. 1999;27(2):71–4.
92. Saboo SS, Krajewski KM, O'Regan KN, Giardino A, Brown JR, Ramaiya N, et al. Spleen in haematological malignancies: spectrum of imaging findings. Br J Radiol. 2012;85(1009):81–92.
93. Lamb PM, Lund A, Kanagasabay RR, Martin A, Webb JA, Reznek RH. Spleen size: how well do linear ultrasound measurements correlate with three-dimensional CT volume assessments? Br J Radiol. 2002;75(895):573–7.
94. Bezerra AS, D'Ippolito G, Faintuch S, Szejnfeld J, Ahmed M. Determination of splenomegaly by CT: is there a place for a single measurement? AJR Am J Roentgenol. 2005;184(5):1510–3.
95. Kashimura M, Noro M, Akikusa B, Okuhara A, Momose S, Miura I, et al. Primary splenic diffuse large B-cell lymphoma manifesting in red pulp. Virchows Arch. 2008;453(5):501–9.
96. Shimono J, Miyoshi H, Kamimura T, Eto T, Miyagishima T, Sasaki Y, et al. Clinicopathological features of primary splenic follicular lymphoma. Ann Hematol. 2017;96(12):2063–70.
97. Shimono J, Miyoshi H, Kiyasu J, Sato K, Kamimura T, Eto T, et al. Clinicopathological analysis of

primary splenic diffuse large B-cell lymphoma. Br J Haematol. 2017;178(5):719–27.
98. Bednaruk-Mlynski E, Pienkowska J, Skorzak A, Malkowski B, Kulikowski W, Subocz E, et al. Comparison of positron emission tomography/computed tomography with classical contrast-enhanced computed tomography in the initial staging of Hodgkin lymphoma. Leuk Lymphoma. 2015;56(2):377–82.
99. de Jong PA, van Ufford HM, Baarslag HJ, de Haas MJ, Wittebol SH, Quekel LG, et al. CT and 18F-FDG PET for noninvasive detection of splenic involvement in patients with malignant lymphoma. AJR Am J Roentgenol. 2009;192(3):745–53.
100. Berzaczy D, Haug AR, Raderer M, Kiesewetter B, Berzaczy G, Weber M, et al. Is there a reliable size cut-off for splenic involvement in lymphoma? A [18F]FDG-PET controlled study. PLoS One. 2019;14(3):e0213551.
101. Wu LM, Chen FY, Jiang XX, Gu HY, Yin Y, Xu JR. 18F-FDG PET, combined FDG-PET/CT and MRI for evaluation of bone marrow infiltration in staging of lymphoma: a systematic review and meta-analysis. Eur J Radiol. 2012;81(2):303–11.
102. Adams HJ, Kwee TC, de Keizer B, Fijnheer R, de Klerk JM, Littooij AS, et al. Systematic review and meta-analysis on the diagnostic performance of FDG-PET/CT in detecting bone marrow involvement in newly diagnosed Hodgkin lymphoma: is bone marrow biopsy still necessary? Ann Oncol. 2014;25(5):921–7.
103. Trotman J, Luminari S, Boussetta S, Versari A, Dupuis J, Tychyj C, et al. Prognostic value of PET-CT after first-line therapy in patients with follicular lymphoma: a pooled analysis of central scan review in three multicentre studies. Lancet Haematol. 2014;1(1):e17–27.
104. Galimberti S, Luminari S, Ciabatti E, Grassi S, Guerrini F, Dondi A, et al. Minimal residual disease after conventional treatment significantly impacts on progression-free survival of patients with follicular lymphoma: the FIL FOLL05 trial. Clin Cancer Res. 2014;20(24):6398–405.
105. Pyo J, Won Kim K, Jacene HA, Sakellis CG, Brown JR, Van den Abbeele AD. End-therapy positron emission tomography for treatment response assessment in follicular lymphoma: a systematic review and meta-analysis. Clin Cancer Res. 2013;19(23):6566–77.
106. Dreyling M, Ghielmini M, Rule S, Salles G, Vitolo U, Ladetto M. Newly diagnosed and relapsed follicular lymphoma: ESMO Clinical Practice Guidelines for diagnosis, treatment and follow-up. Ann Oncol. 2016;27(Suppl 5):v83–90.
107. Whang-Peng J, Bunn PA Jr, Knutsen T, Matthews MJ, Schechter G, Minna JD. Clinical implications of cytogenetic studies in cutaneous T-cell lymphoma (CTCL). Cancer. 1982;50(8):1539–53.
108. Sezary A, Bouvrain Y. Erythrodermie avec présence de cellules monstrueses dans le derme et dans lang circulant. Bull Soc Fr Dermatol Syphiligr. 1938;45:254–60.
109. Pinkus GS, Said JW, Hargreaves H. Malignant lymphoma, T-cell type. A distinct morphologic variant with large multilobated nuclei, with a report of four cases. Am J Clin Pathol. 1979;72(4):540–50.
110. Wang SS, Vose JM. Epidemiology and prognosis of T-cell lymphoma. In: Foss F, editor. T-cell lymphomas. Totowa, NJ: Humana; 2013.
111. Daly PA, O'Briain DS, Robinson I, Guckian M, Prichard JS. Hodgkin's disease with a granulomatous pulmonary presentation mimicking sarcoidosis. Thorax. 1988;43(5):407–9.
112. Geskin LJ. Cutaneous T-cell lymphoma (mycosis fungoides and SéZary syndrome). In: Kaushansky K, Lichtman MA, Prchal JT, Levi MM, Press OW, Burns LJ, et al., editors. Williams hematology. 9th ed. New York, NY: McGraw-Hill Education; 2015.
113. Olsen E, Vonderheid E, Pimpinelli N, Willemze R, Kim Y, Knobler R, et al. Revisions to the staging and classification of mycosis fungoides and Sezary syndrome: a proposal of the International Society for Cutaneous Lymphomas (ISCL) and the cutaneous lymphoma task force of the European Organization of Research and Treatment of Cancer (EORTC). Blood. 2007;110(6):1713–22.
114. Lee HJ, Im JG, Goo JM, Kim KW, Choi BI, Chang KH, et al. Peripheral T-cell lymphoma: spectrum of imaging findings with clinical and pathologic features. Radiographics. 2003;23(1):7–26; discussion 26-8.
115. Casulo C, Schoder H, Feeney J, Lim R, Maragulia J, Zelenetz AD, et al. 18F-fluorodeoxyglucose positron emission tomography in the staging and prognosis of T cell lymphoma. Leuk Lymphoma. 2013;54(10):2163–7.
116. Kim CY, Hong CM, Kim DH, Son SH, Jeong SY, Lee SW, et al. Prognostic value of whole-body metabolic tumour volume and total lesion glycolysis measured on (1)(8)F-FDG PET/CT in patients with extranodal NK/T-cell lymphoma. Eur J Nucl Med Mol Imaging. 2013;40(9):1321–9.
117. Zhou X, Lu K, Geng L, Li X, Jiang Y, Wang X. Utility of PET/CT in the diagnosis and staging of extranodal natural killer/T-cell lymphoma: a systematic review and meta-analysis. Medicine. 2014;93(28):e258.
118. Jiang C, Su M, Kosik RO, Zou L, Jiang M, Tian R. The Deauville 5-point scale improves the prognostic value of interim FDG PET/CT in extranodal natural killer/T-cell lymphoma. Clin Nucl Med. 2015;40(10):767–73.
119. Jiang C, Zhang X, Jiang M, Zou L, Su M, Kosik RO, et al. Assessment of the prognostic capacity of pretreatment, interim, and post-therapy (18)F-FDG PET/CT in extranodal natural killer/T-cell lymphoma, nasal type. Ann Nucl Med. 2015;29(5):442–51.
120. Zhou Z, Chen C, Li X, Li Z, Zhang X, Chang Y, et al. Evaluation of bone marrow involvement in extranodal NK/T cell lymphoma by FDG-PET/CT. Ann Hematol. 2015;94(6):963–7.

121. Chang Y, Fu X, Sun Z, Xie X, Wang R, Li Z, et al. Utility of baseline, interim and end-of-treatment (18)F-FDG PET/CT in extranodal natural killer/T--cell lymphoma patients treated with L-asparaginase/pegaspargase. Sci Rep. 2017;7:41057.
122. Shao D, Gao Q, Liang CH, Wang SX. Discussion of 18F-FDG PET/CT imaging characteristics and diagnostic values of angioimmunoblastic T-cell lymphoma. Leuk Lymphoma. 2017;58(7):1581–8.
123. Wang H, Shen G, Jiang C, Li L, Cui F, Tian R. Prognostic value of baseline, interim and end-of-treatment 18F-FDG PET/CT parameters in extranodal natural killer/T-cell lymphoma: a meta-analysis. PLoS One. 2018;13(3):e0194435.
124. Horwitz S, Coiffier B, Foss F, Prince HM, Sokol L, Greenwood M, et al. Utility of (1)(8)fluorodeoxyglucose positron emission tomography for prognosis and response assessments in a phase 2 study of romidepsin in patients with relapsed or refractory peripheral T-cell lymphoma. Ann Oncol. 2015;26(4):774–9.
125. El-Galaly TC, Pedersen MB, Hutchings M, Mylam KJ, Madsen J, Gang AO, et al. Utility of interim and end-of-treatment PET/CT in peripheral T-cell lymphomas: a review of 124 patients. Am J Hematol. 2015;90(11):975–80.
126. Tomita N, Hattori Y, Fujisawa S, Hashimoto C, Taguchi J, Takasaki H, et al. Post-therapy (18) F-fluorodeoxyglucose positron emission tomography for predicting outcome in patients with peripheral T cell lymphoma. Ann Hematol. 2015;94(3):431–6.
127. Mehta-Shah N, Ito K, Bantilan K, Moskowitz AJ, Sauter C, Horwitz SM, et al. Baseline and interim functional imaging with PET effectively risk stratifies patients with peripheral T-cell lymphoma. Blood Adv. 2019;3(2):187–97.
128. Tiemann M, Schrader C, Klapper W, Dreyling MH, Campo E, Norton A, et al. Histopathology, cell proliferation indices and clinical outcome in 304 patients with mantle cell lymphoma (MCL): a clinicopathological study from the European MCL Network. Br J Haematol. 2005;131(1):29–38.
129. Weigert O, Unterhalt M, Hiddemann W, Dreyling M. Current management of mantle cell lymphoma. Drugs. 2007;67(12):1689–702.
130. Bosch F, Lopez-Guillermo A, Campo E, Ribera JM, Conde E, Piris MA, et al. Mantle cell lymphoma: presenting features, response to therapy, and prognostic factors. Cancer. 1998;82(3):567–75.
131. Argatoff LH, Connors JM, Klasa RJ, Horsman DE, Gascoyne RD. Mantle cell lymphoma: a clinicopathologic study of 80 cases. Blood. 1997;89(6):2067–78.
132. Gill S, Wolf M, Prince HM, Januszewicz H, Ritchie D, Hicks RJ, et al. [18F]fluorodeoxyglucose positron emission tomography scanning for staging, response assessment, and disease surveillance in patients with mantle cell lymphoma. Clin Lymphoma Myeloma. 2008;8(3):159–65.
133. Hosein PJ, Pastorini VH, Paes FM, Eber D, Chapman JR, Serafini AN, et al. Utility of positron emission tomography scans in mantle cell lymphoma. Am J Hematol. 2011;86(10):841–5.
134. Kedmi M, Avivi I, Ribakovsky E, Benyamini N, Davidson T, Goshen E, et al. Is there a role for therapy response assessment with 2-[fluorine-18]fluoro-2-deoxy-D-glucose-positron emission tomography/computed tomography in mantle cell lymphoma? Leuk Lymphoma. 2014;55(11):2484–9.
135. Bruzzi JF, Macapinlac H, Tsimberidou AM, Truong MT, Keating MJ, Marom EM, et al. Detection of Richter's transformation of chronic lymphocytic leukemia by PET/CT. J Nucl Med. 2006;47(8):1267–73.
136. Falchi L, Keating MJ, Marom EM, Truong MT, Schlette EJ, Sargent RL, et al. Correlation between FDG/PET, histology, characteristics, and survival in 332 patients with chronic lymphoid leukemia. Blood. 2014;123(18):2783–90.
137. Schoder H, Noy A, Gonen M, Weng L, Green D, Erdi YE, et al. Intensity of 18fluorodeoxyglucose uptake in positron emission tomography distinguishes between indolent and aggressive non-Hodgkin's lymphoma. J Clin Oncol. 2005;23(21):4643–51.
138. Bodet-Milin C, Kraeber-Bodere F, Moreau P, Campion L, Dupas B, Le Gouill S. Investigation of FDG-PET/CT imaging to guide biopsies in the detection of histological transformation of indolent lymphoma. Haematologica. 2008;93(3):471–2.
139. Hoffmann M, Kletter K, Becherer A, Jager U, Chott A, Raderer M. 18F-fluorodeoxyglucose positron emission tomography (18F-FDG-PET) for staging and follow-up of marginal zone B-cell lymphoma. Oncology. 2003;64(4):336–40.
140. Jerusalem GH, Beguin YP. Positron emission tomography in non-Hodgkin's lymphoma (NHL): relationship between tracer uptake and pathological findings, including preliminary experience in the staging of low-grade NHL. Clin Lymphoma. 2002;3(1):56–61.
141. Borhani AA, Hosseinzadeh K, Almusa O, Furlan A, Nalesnik M. Imaging of posttransplantation lymphoproliferative disorder after solid organ transplantation. Radiographics. 2009;29(4):981–1000; discussion 1000–2.
142. Loren AW, Porter DL, Stadtmauer EA, Tsai DE. Post-transplant lymphoproliferative disorder: a review. Bone Marrow Transplant. 2003;31(3):145–55.
143. Tsai DE, Aqui NA, Vogl DT, Bloom RD, Schuster SJ, Nasta SD, et al. Successful treatment of T-cell post-transplant lymphoproliferative disorder with the retinoid analog bexarotene. Am J Transplant. 2005;5(8):2070–3.
144. Birsen R, Blanc E, Burroni B, Broudin C, Willems L, Legoff M, Leray E, Pilorge S, Salah S, Quentin A, Deau-Fisher B, Franchi P, Vignon M, Mabille L, Nguyen C, Kirova Y, Varlet P, Tauziede-Espariat A, Edjlali M, Edouard D, Hoang-Xuan K, Houillier C, Soussain C, Pallud J, Damotte D, Bouscary D, Tamburini Bonnefoy J. Prognostic value of early 18F-FDG PET/CT scanner evaluation in immuno-

competent primary CNS lymphoma patients. Blood. 2017;130:4169. http://www.bloodjournal.org/content/130/Suppl_1/4169
145. McCormack L, Hany TI, Hubner M, Petrowsky H, Mullhaupt B, Knuth A, et al. How useful is PET/CT imaging in the management of post-transplant lymphoproliferative disease after liver transplantation? Am J Transplant. 2006;6(7):1731–6.
146. Bianchi E, Pascual M, Nicod M, Delaloye AB, Duchosal MA. Clinical usefulness of FDG-PET/CT scan imaging in the management of posttransplant lymphoproliferative disease. Transplantation. 2008;85(5):707–12.
147. Takehana CS, Twist CJ, Mosci C, Quon A, Mittra E, Iagaru A. (18)F-FDG PET/CT in the management of patients with post-transplant lymphoproliferative disorder. Nucl Med Commun. 2014;35(3):276–81.
148. Metser U, Lo G. FDG-PET/CT in abdominal post-transplant lymphoproliferative disease. Br J Radiol. 2016;89(1057):20150844.
149. Friedberg JW, Mauch PM, Rimsza LM, Fisher RI. Non-Hodgkin's lymphomas. In: DeVita VT, Lawrence TS, Rosenberg SA, editors. DeVita, Hellman, and Rosenberg's cancer: principles and practice of oncology. 8th ed. Philadelphia, PA: Lippincott Williams & Wilkins; 2008.
150. Kostakoglu L, Cheson BD. Current role of FDG PET/CT in lymphoma. Eur J Nucl Med Mol Imaging. 2014;41(5):1004–27.
151. Thill R, Neuerburg J, Fabry U, Cremerius U, Wagenknecht G, Hellwig D, et al. [Comparison of findings with 18-FDG PET and CT in pretherapeutic staging of malignant lymphoma]. Nuklearmedizin. 1997;36(7):234–239.
152. Rodriguez M, Ahlstrom H, Sundin A, Rehn S, Sundstrom C, Hagberg H, et al. [18F] FDG PET in gastric non-Hodgkin's lymphoma. Acta Oncol. 1997;36(6):577–84.
153. Paes FM, Kalkanis DG, Sideras PA, Serafini AN. FDG PET/CT of extranodal involvement in non-Hodgkin lymphoma and Hodgkin disease. Radiographics. 2010;30(1):269–91.
154. Grommes C, DeAngelis LM. Primary CNS lymphoma. J Clin Oncol. 2017;35(21):2410–8.
155. Villano JL, Koshy M, Shaikh H, Dolecek TA, McCarthy BJ. Age, gender, and racial differences in incidence and survival in primary CNS lymphoma. Br J Cancer. 2011;105(9):1414–8.
156. O'Neill BP, Decker PA, Tieu C, Cerhan JR. The changing incidence of primary central nervous system lymphoma is driven primarily by the changing incidence in young and middle-aged men and differs from time trends in systemic diffuse large B-cell non-Hodgkin's lymphoma. Am J Hematol. 2013;88(12):997–1000.
157. Rosenfeld SS, Hoffman JM, Coleman RE, Glantz MJ, Hanson MW, Schold SC. Studies of primary central nervous system lymphoma with fluorine-18-fluorodeoxyglucose positron emission tomography. J Nucl Med. 1992;33(4):532–6.
158. Kosaka N, Tsuchida T, Uematsu H, Kimura H, Okazawa H, Itoh H. 18F-FDG PET of common enhancing malignant brain tumors. Am J Roentgenol. 2008;190(6):W365–W9.
159. Kawai N, Miyake K, Yamamoto Y, Nishiyama Y, Tamiya T. 18F-FDG PET in the diagnosis and treatment of primary central nervous system lymphoma. J Biomed Res Int. 2013;2013:8.
160. Mohile NA, Deangelis LM, Abrey LE. Utility of brain FDG-PET in primary CNS lymphoma. Clin Adv Hematol Oncol. 2008;6(11):818–20, 40.
161. Chiavazza C, Pellerino A, Ferrio F, Cistaro A, Soffietti R, Rudà R, et al. Primary CNS lymphomas: challenges in diagnosis and monitoring. J Biomed Res Int. 2018;2018:16.
162. Kawai N, Zhen H-N, Miyake K, Yamamaoto Y, Nishiyama Y, Tamiya T. Prognostic value of pretreatment 18F-FDG PET in patients with primary central nervous system lymphoma: SUV-based assessment. J Neurooncol. 2010;100(2):225–32.
163. Abrey LE, Batchelor TT, Ferreri AJM, Gospodarowicz M, Pulczynski EJ, Zucca E, et al. Report of an International Workshop to standardize baseline evaluation and response criteria for primary CNS lymphoma. J Clin Oncol. 2005;23(22):5034–43.
164. Palmedo H, Urbach H, Bender H, Schlegel U, Schmidt-Wolf IGH, Matthies A, et al. FDG-PET in immunocompetent patients with primary central nervous system lymphoma: correlation with MRI and clinical follow-up. Eur J Nucl Med Mol Imaging. 2006;33(2):164–8.
165. Birsen R, Blanc E, Willems L, Burroni B, Legoff M, Le Ray E, et al. Prognostic value of early 18F-FDG PET scanning evaluation in immunocompetent primary CNS lymphoma patients. Oncotarget. 2018;9(24):16822–31.
166. Cote TR, Manns A, Hardy CR, Yellin FJ, Hartge P. Epidemiology of brain lymphoma among people with or without acquired immunodeficiency syndrome. AIDS/Cancer Study Group. J Natl Cancer Inst. 1996;88(10):675–9.
167. Skiest DJ, Erdman W, Chang WE, Oz OK, Ware A, Fleckenstein J. SPECT thallium-201 combined with Toxoplasma serology for the presumptive diagnosis of focal central nervous system mass lesions in patients with AIDS. J Infect. 2000;40(3):274–81.
168. D'Amico A, Messa C, Castagna A, Zito F, Galli L, Pepe G, et al. Diagnostic accuracy and predictive value of 201T1 SPET for the differential diagnosis of cerebral lesions in AIDS patients. Nucl Med Commun. 1997;18(8):741–50.
169. Antinori A, De Rossi G, Ammassari A, Cingolani A, Murri R, Di Giuda D, et al. Value of combined approach with thallium-201 single-photon emission computed tomography and Epstein-Barr virus DNA polymerase chain reaction in CSF for the diagnosis of AIDS-related primary CNS lymphoma. J Clin Oncol. 1999;17(2):554–60.

170. Vidan E, Kostakoglu L, Goldsmith S. Superiority of F-18 FDG PET over Tl-201 SPECT in the evaluation of AIDS-associated brain lesions. J Nucl Med. 2006;47(suppl 1):238P.
171. Heald AE, Hoffman JM, Bartlett JA, Waskin HA. Differentiation of central nervous system lesions in AIDS patients using positron emission tomography (PET). Int J STD AIDS. 1996;7(5):337–46.
172. Westwood TD, Hogan C, Julyan PJ, Coutts G, Bonington S, Carrington B, et al. Utility of FDG-PETCT and magnetic resonance spectroscopy in differentiating between cerebral lymphoma and non-malignant CNS lesions in HIV-infected patients. Eur J Radiol. 2013;82(8):e374–9.
173. Singh T, Satheesh CT, Lakshmaiah KC, Suresh TM, Babu GK, Lokanatha D, et al. Primary bone lymphoma: a report of two cases and review of the literature. J Cancer Res Ther. 2010;6(3):296–8.
174. Mulligan ME, McRae GA, Murphey MD. Imaging features of primary lymphoma of bone. Am J Roentgenol. 1999;173(6):1691–7.
175. Wang LJ, Wu HB, Wang M, Han YJ, Li HS, Zhou WL, et al. Utility of F-18 FDG PET/CT on the evaluation of primary bone lymphoma. Eur J Radiol. 2015;84(11):2275–9.
176. Ahmann DL, Kiely JM, Harrison EG Jr, Payne WS. Malignant lymphoma of the spleen. A review of 49 cases in which the diagnosis was made at splenectomy. Cancer. 1966;19(4):461–9.
177. Grosskreutz C, Troy K, Cuttner J. Primary splenic lymphoma: report of 10 cases using the REAL classification. Cancer Investig. 2002;20(5–6):749–53.
178. Karunanithi S, Sharma P, Roy SG, Vettiyil B, Sharma A, Thulkar S, et al. Use of 18F-FDG PET/CT imaging for evaluation of patients with primary splenic lymphoma. Clin Nucl Med. 2014;39(9):772–6.
179. Diehl V, Franklin J, Pfreundschuh M, Lathan B, Paulus U, Hasenclever D, et al. Standard and increased-dose BEACOPP chemotherapy compared with COPP-ABVD for advanced Hodgkin's disease. N Engl J Med. 2003;348(24):2386–95.
180. Kobe C, Dietlein M, Franklin J, Markova J, Lohri A, Amthauer H, et al. Positron emission tomography has a high negative predictive value for progression or early relapse for patients with residual disease after first-line chemotherapy in advanced-stage Hodgkin lymphoma. Blood. 2008;112(10):3989–94.
181. Andre MPE, Girinsky T, Federico M, Reman O, Fortpied C, Gotti M, et al. Early positron emission tomography response-adapted treatment in stage I and II Hodgkin lymphoma: final results of the randomized EORTC/LYSA/FIL H10 trial. J Clin Oncol. 2017;35(16):1786–94.
182. Gallamini A, Patti C, Viviani S, Rossi A, Fiore F, Di Raimondo F, et al. Early chemotherapy intensification with BEACOPP in advanced-stage Hodgkin lymphoma patients with a interim-PET positive after two ABVD courses. Br J Haematol. 2011;152(5):551–60.
183. Johnson P, Federico M, Kirkwood A, Fossa A, Berkahn L, Carella A, et al. Adapted treatment guided by interim PET-CT scan in advanced Hodgkin's lymphoma. N Engl J Med. 2016;374(25):2419–29.
184. Meyer RM, Gospodarowicz MK, Connors JM, Pearcey RG, Bezjak A, Wells WA, et al. Randomized comparison of ABVD chemotherapy with a strategy that includes radiation therapy in patients with limited-stage Hodgkin's lymphoma: National Cancer Institute of Canada Clinical Trials Group and the Eastern Cooperative Oncology Group. J Clin Oncol. 2005;23(21):4634–42.
185. Press OW, Li H, Schoder H, Straus DJ, Moskowitz CH, LeBlanc M, et al. US intergroup trial of response-adapted therapy for stage III to IV Hodgkin lymphoma using early interim fluorodeoxyglucose-positron emission tomography imaging: Southwest Oncology Group S0816. J Clin Oncol. 2016;34(17):2020–7.
186. Radford J, Illidge T, Counsell N, Hancock B, Pettengell R, Johnson P, et al. Results of a trial of PET-directed therapy for early-stage Hodgkin's lymphoma. N Engl J Med. 2015;372(17):1598–607.
187. Raemaekers JM, Andre MP, Federico M, Girinsky T, Oumedaly R, Brusamolino E, et al. Omitting radiotherapy in early positron emission tomography-negative stage I/II Hodgkin lymphoma is associated with an increased risk of early relapse: clinical results of the preplanned interim analysis of the randomized EORTC/LYSA/FIL H10 trial. J Clin Oncol. 2014;32(12):1188–94.
188. Straus DJ, Jung SH, Pitcher B, Kostakoglu L, Grecula JC, Hsi ED, et al. CALGB 50604: risk-adapted treatment of nonbulky early-stage Hodgkin lymphoma based on interim PET. Blood. 2018;132(10):1013–21.
189. Hindie E, Mesguich C, Bouabdallah K, Milpied N. Advanced Hodgkin's lymphoma: end-of-treatment FDG-PET should be maintained. Eur J Nucl Med Mol Imaging. 2017;44(8):1254–7.
190. Mesguich C, Cazeau AL, Bouabdallah K, Soubeyran P, Guyot M, Milpied N, et al. Hodgkin lymphoma: a negative interim-PET cannot circumvent the need for end-of-treatment-PET evaluation. Br J Haematol. 2016;175(4):652–60.
191. Gallamini A, Hutchings M, Rigacci L, Specht L, Merli F, Hansen M, et al. Early interim 2-[18F] fluoro-2-deoxy-D-glucose positron emission tomography is prognostically superior to international prognostic score in advanced-stage Hodgkin's lymphoma: a report from a joint Italian-Danish study. J Clin Oncol. 2007;25(24):3746–52.
192. Markova J, Kahraman D, Kobe C, Skopalova M, Mocikova H, Klaskova K, et al. Role of [18F]-fluoro-2-deoxy-D-glucose positron emission tomography in early and late therapy assessment of patients with advanced Hodgkin lymphoma treated with bleomycin, etoposide, adriamycin, cyclophosphamide, vincristine, procarbazine and prednisone. Leuk Lymphoma. 2012;53(1):64–70.

193. de Wit M, Bohuslavizki KH, Buchert R, Bumann D, Clausen M, Hossfeld DK. 18FDG-PET following treatment as valid predictor for disease-free survival in Hodgkin's lymphoma. Ann Oncol. 2001;12(1):29–37.
194. Spaepen K, Stroobants S, Dupont P, Thomas J, Vandenberghe P, Balzarini J, et al. Can positron emission tomography with [(18)F]-fluorodeoxyglucose after first-line treatment distinguish Hodgkin's disease patients who need additional therapy from others in whom additional therapy would mean avoidable toxicity? Br J Haematol. 2001;115(2):272–8.
195. Weihrauch MR, Re D, Scheidhauer K, Ansen S, Dietlein M, Bischoff S, et al. Thoracic positron emission tomography using 18F-fluorodeoxyglucose for the evaluation of residual mediastinal Hodgkin disease. Blood. 2001;98(10):2930–4.
196. Cerci JJ, Pracchia LF, Linardi CC, Pitella FA, Delbeke D, Izaki M, et al. 18F-FDG PET after 2 cycles of ABVD predicts event-free survival in early and advanced Hodgkin lymphoma. J Nucl Med. 2010;51(9):1337–43.
197. Engert A, Haverkamp H, Kobe C, Markova J, Renner C, Ho A, et al. Reduced-intensity chemotherapy and PET-guided radiotherapy in patients with advanced stage Hodgkin's lymphoma (HD15 trial): a randomised, open-label, phase 3 non-inferiority trial. Lancet. 2012;379(9828):1791–9.
198. Micallef IN, Maurer MJ, Wiseman GA, Nikcevich DA, Kurtin PJ, Cannon MW, et al. Epratuzumab with rituximab, cyclophosphamide, doxorubicin, vincristine, and prednisone chemotherapy in patients with previously untreated diffuse large B-cell lymphoma. Blood. 2011;118(15):4053–61.
199. Spaepen K, Stroobants S, Dupont P, Van Steenweghen S, Thomas J, Vandenberghe P, et al. Prognostic value of positron emission tomography (PET) with fluorine-18 fluorodeoxyglucose ([18F] FDG) after first-line chemotherapy in non-Hodgkin's lymphoma: is [18F]FDG-PET a valid alternative to conventional diagnostic methods? J Clin Oncol. 2001;19(2):414–9.
200. Zinzani PL, Rigacci L, Stefoni V, Broccoli A, Puccini B, Castagnoli A, et al. Early interim 18F-FDG PET in Hodgkin's lymphoma: evaluation on 304 patients. Eur J Nucl Med Mol Imaging. 2012;39(1):4–12.
201. Carbone PP, Kaplan HS, Musshoff K, Smithers DW, Tubiana M. Report of the committee on Hodgkin's disease staging classification. Cancer Res. 1971;31(11):1860–1.
202. Cheson BD, Horning SJ, Coiffier B, Shipp MA, Fisher RI, Connors JM, et al. Report of an international workshop to standardize response criteria for non-Hodgkin's lymphomas. NCI Sponsored International Working Group. J Clin Oncol. 1999;17(4):1244.
203. Cheson BD, Pfistner B, Juweid ME, Gascoyne RD, Specht L, Horning SJ, et al. Revised response criteria for malignant lymphoma. J Clin Oncol. 2007;25(5):579–86.
204. Cheson BD. The International Harmonization Project for response criteria in lymphoma clinical trials. Hematol Oncol Clin North Am. 2007;21(5): 841–54.
205. Barrington SF, Qian W, Somer EJ, Franceschetto A, Bagni B, Brun E, et al. Concordance between four European centres of PET reporting criteria designed for use in multicentre trials in Hodgkin lymphoma. Eur J Nucl Med Mol Imaging. 2010;37(10):1824–33.
206. Younes A, Hilden P, Coiffier B, Hagenbeek A, Salles G, Wilson W, et al. International Working Group consensus response evaluation criteria in lymphoma (RECIL 2017). Ann Oncol. 2017;28(7):1436–47.
207. Hasenclever D, Kurch L, Mauz-Korholz C, Elsner A, Georgi T, Wallace H, et al. qPET—a quantitative extension of the Deauville scale to assess response in interim FDG-PET scans in lymphoma. Eur J Nucl Med Mol Imaging. 2014;41(7):1301–8.
208. Rossi C, Kanoun S, Berriolo-Riedinger A, Dygai-Cochet I, Humbert O, Legouge C, et al. Interim 18F-FDG PET SUVmax reduction is superior to visual analysis in predicting outcome early in Hodgkin lymphoma patients. J Nucl Med. 2014;55(4):569–73.
209. Sattarivand M, Caldwell C, Poon I, Soliman H, Mah K. Effects of ROI placement on PET-based assessment of tumor response to therapy. Int J Mol Imaging. 2013;2013:132804.
210. Kostakoglu L, Chauvie S. Metabolic tumor volume metrics in lymphoma. Semin Nucl Med. 2018;48(1):50–66.
211. Song M-K, Chung J-S, Lee J-J, Jeong SY, Lee S-M, Hong J-S, et al. Metabolic tumor volume by positron emission tomography/computed tomography as a clinical parameter to determine therapeutic modality for early stage Hodgkin's lymphoma. Cancer Sci. 2013;104(12):1656–61.
212. Kanoun S, Rossi C, Berriolo-Riedinger A, Dygai-Cochet I, Cochet A, Humbert O, et al. Baseline metabolic tumour volume is an independent prognostic factor in Hodgkin lymphoma. Eur J Nucl Med Mol Imaging. 2014;41(9):1735–43.
213. Tseng D, Rachakonda LP, Su Z, Advani R, Horning S, Hoppe RT, et al. Interim-treatment quantitative PET parameters predict progression and death among patients with Hodgkin's disease. Radiat Oncol. 2012;7(1):5.
214. Cherk MH, Pham A, Haydon A. 18F-fluorodeoxyglucose positron emission tomography-positive sarcoidosis after chemoradiotherapy for Hodgkin's disease: a case report. J Med Case Rep. 2011;5:247.
215. Subbiah V, Ly UK, Khiyami A, O'Brien T. Tissue is the issue-sarcoidosis following ABVD chemotherapy for Hodgkin's lymphoma: a case report. J Med Case Rep. 2007;1:148.
216. London J, Grados A, Ferme C, Charmillon A, Maurier F, Deau B, et al. Sarcoidosis occurring after lymphoma: report of 14 patients and review of the literature. Medicine. 2014;93(21):e121.

217. de Hemricourt E, De Boeck K, Hilte F, Abib A, Kockx M, Vandevivere J, et al. Sarcoidosis and sarcoid-like reaction following Hodgkin's disease. Report of two cases. Mol Imaging Biol. 2003;5(1):15–9.
218. Koo HJ, Kim MY, Shin SY, Shin S, Kim SS, Lee SW, et al. Evaluation of mediastinal lymph nodes in sarcoidosis, sarcoid reaction, and malignant lymph nodes using CT and FDG-PET/CT. Medicine. 2015;94(27):e1095.
219. Mustafa M, Patel D, Shen L, Shetty A, Mansberg R. Granulomatous lymphangitis masquerading as relapsed Hodgkin disease on FDG PET/CT. Tomography. 2018;4(1):1–3.
220. Talcott JA, Garnick MB, Stomper PC, Godleski JJ, Richie JP. Cavitary lung nodules associated with combination chemotherapy containing bleomycin. J Urol. 1987;138(3):619–20.
221. Brincker H. The sarcoidosis-lymphoma syndrome. Br J Cancer. 1986;54(3):467–73.
222. Wilgenhof S, Morlion V, Seghers AC, Du Four S, Vanderlinden E, Hanon S, et al. Sarcoidosis in a patient with metastatic melanoma sequentially treated with anti-CTLA-4 monoclonal antibody and selective BRAF inhibitor. Anticancer Res. 2012;32(4):1355–9.
223. Montaudie H, Pradelli J, Passeron T, Lacour JP, Leroy S. Pulmonary sarcoid-like granulomatosis induced by nivolumab. Br J Dermatol. 2017;176(4):1060–3.
224. Cousin S, Toulmonde M, Kind M, Cazeau AL, Bechade D, Coindre JM, et al. Pulmonary sarcoidosis induced by the anti-PD1 monoclonal antibody pembrolizumab. Ann Oncol. 2016;27(6):1178–9.
225. Koss MN. Pulmonary lymphoid disorders. Semin Diagn Pathol. 1995;12(2):158–71.
226. Murphy SP, Nathan MA, Karwal MW. FDG-PET appearance of pelvic Castleman's disease. J Nucl Med. 1997;38(8):1211–2.
227. Reddy MP, Graham MM. FDG positron emission tomographic imaging of thoracic Castleman's disease. Clin Nucl Med. 2003;28(4):325–6.
228. An YS, Yoon JK, Lee SJ, Jeong SH, Lee HW. Clinical significance of post-treatment (18) F-fluorodeoxyglucose uptake in cervical lymph nodes in patients with diffuse large B-cell lymphoma. Eur Radiol. 2016;26(12):4632–9.
229. Chiang SB, Rebenstock A, Guan L, Burns J, Alavi A, Zhuang H. Potential false-positive FDG PET imaging caused by subcutaneous radiotracer infiltration. Clin Nucl Med. 2003;28(9):786–8.
230. Wagner T, Brucher N, Julian A, Hitzel A. A false-positive finding in therapeutic evaluation: hypermetabolic axillary lymph node in a lymphoma patient following FDG extravasation. Nucl Med Rev Cent East Eur. 2011;14(2):109–11.
231. Tsamita CS, Golemi A, Egesta L, Castellucci P, Nanni C, Stefoni V, et al. Clinical significance of axillary findings in patients with lymphoma during follow-up with 18F-fluorodeoxyglucose-PET. Nucl Med Commun. 2008;29(8):705–10.
232. Muthukrishnan A, Joyce JM, Islam M. Follicular hyperplasia: a potential false-positive finding on PET/CT imaging in the evaluation of lymphoma. Clin Nucl Med. 2006;31(7):401–2.
233. Ranganath P, Kapila R, Vadehra V, Wang Q, Capitle E, Ghesani N. Generalized lymphadenopathy and 18-fluorine fluorodeoxyglucose positron emission tomography/computed tomography targeting diagnostic intervention, characterizing disease extent, and assessing treatment efficacy in syphilis. Sex Transm Dis. 2015;42(2):68–70.
234. Shrestha D, Dhakal AK, Raj KCS, Shakya A, Shah SC, Shakya H. Systemic lupus erythematosus and granulomatous lymphadenopathy. BMC Pediatr. 2013;13:179.
235. Haroon A, Zumla A, Bomanji J. Role of fluorine 18 fluorodeoxyglucose positron emission tomography-computed tomography in focal and generalized infectious and inflammatory disorders. Clin Infect Dis. 2012;54(9):1333–41.
236. Patel PM, Alibazoglu H, Ali A, Fordham E, LaMonica G. Normal thymic uptake of FDG on PET imaging. Clin Nucl Med. 1996;21(10):772–5.
237. Weinblatt ME, Zanzi I, Belakhlef A, Babchyck B, Kochen J. False-positive FDG-PET imaging of the thymus of a child with Hodgkin's disease. J Nucl Med. 1997;38(6):888–90.
238. Ferdinand B, Gupta P, Kramer EL. Spectrum of thymic uptake at 18F-FDG PET. Radiographics. 2004;24(6):1611–6.
239. Kawano T, Suzuki A, Ishida A, Takahashi N, Lee J, Tayama Y, et al. The clinical relevance of thymic fluorodeoxyglucose uptake in pediatric patients after chemotherapy. Eur J Nucl Med Mol Imaging. 2004;31(6):831–6.
240. Brink I, Reinhardt MJ, Hoegerle S, Altehoefer C, Moser E, Nitzsche EU. Increased metabolic activity in the thymus gland studied with 18F-FDG PET: age dependency and frequency after chemotherapy. J Nucl Med. 2001;42(4):591–5.
241. Jerushalmi J, Frenkel A, Bar-Shalom R, Khoury J, Israel O. Physiologic thymic uptake of 18F-FDG in children and young adults: a PET/CT evaluation of incidence, patterns, and relationship to treatment. J Nucl Med. 2009;50(6):849–53.
242. Mayer D, Bednarczyk EM. Interaction of colony-stimulating factors and fluorodeoxyglucose F(18) positron emission tomography. Ann Pharmacother. 2002;36(11):1796–9.
243. Gea-Banacloche J, Komanduri KV, Carpenter P, Paczesny S, Sarantopoulos S, Young JA, et al. National Institutes of Health Hematopoietic Cell Transplantation Late Effects Initiative: The Immune dysregulation and Pathobiology Working Group Report. Biol Blood Marrow Transplant. 2017;23(6):870–81.
244. Jacobsohn DA, Vogelsang GB. Acute graft versus host disease. Orphanet J Rare Dis. 2007;2:35.
245. Ichiki Y, Bowlus CL, Shimoda S, Ishibashi H, Vierling JM, Gershwin ME. T cell immunity and

graft-versus-host disease (GVHD). Autoimmun Rev. 2006;5(1):1–9.
246. Bower M, Palmieri C, Dhillon T. AIDS-related malignancies: changing epidemiology and the impact of highly active antiretroviral therapy. Curr Opin Infect Dis. 2006;19(1):14–9.
247. O'Doherty MJ, Barrington SF, Campbell M, Lowe J, Bradbeer CS. PET scanning and the human immunodeficiency virus-positive patient. J Nucl Med. 1997;38(10):1575–83.
248. Love C, Tomas MB, Tronco GG, Palestro CJ. FDG PET of infection and inflammation. Radiographics. 2005;25(5):1357–68.
249. Scharko AM, Perlman SB, Pyzalski RW, Graziano FM, Sosman J, Pauza CD. Whole-body positron emission tomography in patients with HIV-1 infection. Lancet. 2003;362(9388):959–61.
250. Bental M, Deutsch C. Metabolic changes in activated T cells: an NMR study of human peripheral blood lymphocytes. Magn Reson Med. 1993;29(3):317–26.
251. Liu YY. Demonstrations of AIDS-associated malignancies and infections at FDG PET-CT. Ann Nucl Med. 2011;25(8):536–46.
252. Mhlanga JC, Durand D, Tsai HL, Durand CM, Leal JP, Wang H, et al. Differentiation of HIV-associated lymphoma from HIV-associated reactive adenopathy using quantitative FDG PET and symmetry. Eur J Nucl Med Mol Imaging. 2014;41(4):596–604.

24 PET/CT in Renal, Bladder, and Testicular Cancer

Kirsten Bouchelouche and Peter L. Choyke

Abbreviations

AFP	Alpha-fetoprotein
BC	Bladder cancer
CAIX	Carbonic anhydrase 9
CSD	Cancer-specific death
CT	Computed tomography
DOTATATE	1,4,7,10-Tetraazacyclododecane-1,4,7,10-tetraacetic acid-octreotate
DSS	Disease-specific survival
FDG	Fluorodeoxyglucose
FLT	Fluorothymidine
GCT	Germ cell tumor
hCG	Human chorionic gonadotropin
LDH	Lactate dehydrogenase
LN	Lymph node
MRI	Magnetic resonance imaging
MTV	Metabolic tumor volume
NPV	Negative predictive value
NSGCT	Non-seminomatous germ cell tumor
OS	Overall survival
PFS	Progression-free survival
PLND	Pelvic lymph node dissection
PPV	Positive predictive value
PSMA	Prostate-specific membrane antigen
RCC	Renal cell carcinoma
RECIST	Response evaluation criteria in solid tumors
SUV	Standardized uptake value
TLG	Total lesion glycolysis

K. Bouchelouche (✉)
Department of Nuclear Medicine & PET Centre, Aarhus University Hospital, Skejby, Aarhus, Denmark
e-mail: kirsbouc@rm.dk

P. L. Choyke
Molecular Imaging Program, Center for Cancer Research, National Cancer Institute (NCI), Bethesda, MD, USA

Keypoints

- PET/CT with ^{18}F-FDG is not widely used in most primary renal cancers. However, ^{18}F-FDG PET/CT may be used in selected high-risk patients and when conventional imaging is negative or if there is a potential tumor thrombus. In metastatic renal cancer, ^{18}F-FDG PET/CT is increasingly used to monitor targeted molecular therapies. Metabolic tumor volume (MTV) and SUVmax are prognostic for survival and response to targeted therapies. Several other PET agents targeting carbonic anhydrase IX, PSMA, DOTATATE, hypoxia, and fatty acid synthesis have been proposed and tested but none are in widespread use.
- In bladder cancer, ^{18}F-FDG PET/CT is not very useful for the detection of primary tumors due to urinary excretion of ^{18}F-FDG. However, several methods have been suggested to overcome interference with radioactivity in the

H. Ahmadzadehfar et al. (eds.), *Clinical Nuclear Medicine*,
https://doi.org/10.1007/978-3-030-39457-8_24

urine. ^{18}F-FDG PET/CT is increasingly used for staging and restaging in muscle-invasive bladder cancer, and the scan may add important prognostic information. Other PET agents with no urinary excretion, like ^{11}C-choline, have been tested in clinical studies.
- In testicular cancer, ^{18}F-FDG PET/CT is clinically useful for initial staging and determining the viability of residual masses after treatment, especially in patients with seminoma.

24.1 Introduction

Hybrid imaging with positron emission tomography (PET)/computed tomography (CT) has become one of the most important imaging modalities in oncology, and PET/CT with F-18 fluorodeoxyglucose (FDG) has become ubiquitous as a tool for staging and follow-up of many cancer patients. In urology, FDG is the most common PET radiotracer used in renal, bladder, and testicular cancer, but its role is hampered by physiological urinary excretion of FDG through the urinary system masking FDG uptake in primary renal and bladder carcinomas. Thus, new PET radiotracers have been introduced and tested in both malignancies. In this review, we focus on the role of PET/CT in the clinical management of patients with renal, bladder, and testicular cancer.

24.2 Use of PET in Renal Cell Carcinoma

24.2.1 Overview of RCC

Renal cell carcinoma (RCC) represents approximately 3% of human cancers. With the advent of widespread cross-sectional imaging, the detection of small renal cancers has increased, and the majority of these are well-differentiated and are cured by surgical resection [1]. Nonetheless, renal cancer remains a significant cause of cancer death due to the variable aggressiveness of some tumors. Renal cancers are categorized as clear cell (60–80%), papillary (10%), chromophobe-oncocytic (5%), and other tumors such as sarcomatoid, squamous cell, and leiomyosarcoma. Accompanying the increase in small RCCs, there has been an increase in the diagnosis of small benign tumors such as oncocytomas and angiomyolipomas that can mimic RCC [1]. Since RCCs can be highly lethal it is important to identify them, characterize and stage them, and then monitor them during treatment. A decade ago PET played almost no role in RCC. In recent years, a fuller understanding of the role of PET in the management of RCC has been realized.

Renal cancers can be stratified as localized, locally advanced, and metastatic. Here, we consider the role of FDG PET in each of these settings. In the final section, we will consider other PET agents that have been proposed to evaluate RCC.

24.2.2 Primary RCC

Traditionally, FDG PET has played a minor role in the diagnosis of RCC. Contrast-enhanced CT and MRI have proven very effective at detecting solid renal masses suspicious for RCC. However, both modalities are non-specific and cannot distinguish benign and malignant lesions. For many small lesions that are indeterminant, a biopsy is recommended to rule out benign disease prior to intervention, although this recommendation is often not followed [1]. It would be tempting to use FDG PET in this setting however, PET/CT has a sensitivity of only approximately 60% for RCC although it is 90% specific for malignancy [2]. Recent data confirm that CT and MRI are superior to FDG PET/CT for primary diagnosis [3]. Thus, a negative FDG PET is not often clinically helpful. This is in part due to the lower metabolic status of many RCCs but also because FDG PET is primarily excreted through the kidneys making RCCs isointense with renal parenchyma [4]. If they were located elsewhere in the body, where the background was lower, they might be considered positive, but in the kidney they are often difficult to detect. The uptake of FDG in renal tumors is size dependent [4]. FDG is exquisitely sensitive for type II papillary renal cancers (Figs. 24.1 and 24.2) especially when found in conjunction with the hereditary leiomyoma renal cell carcinoma (HLRCC) syndrome and are useful not only in

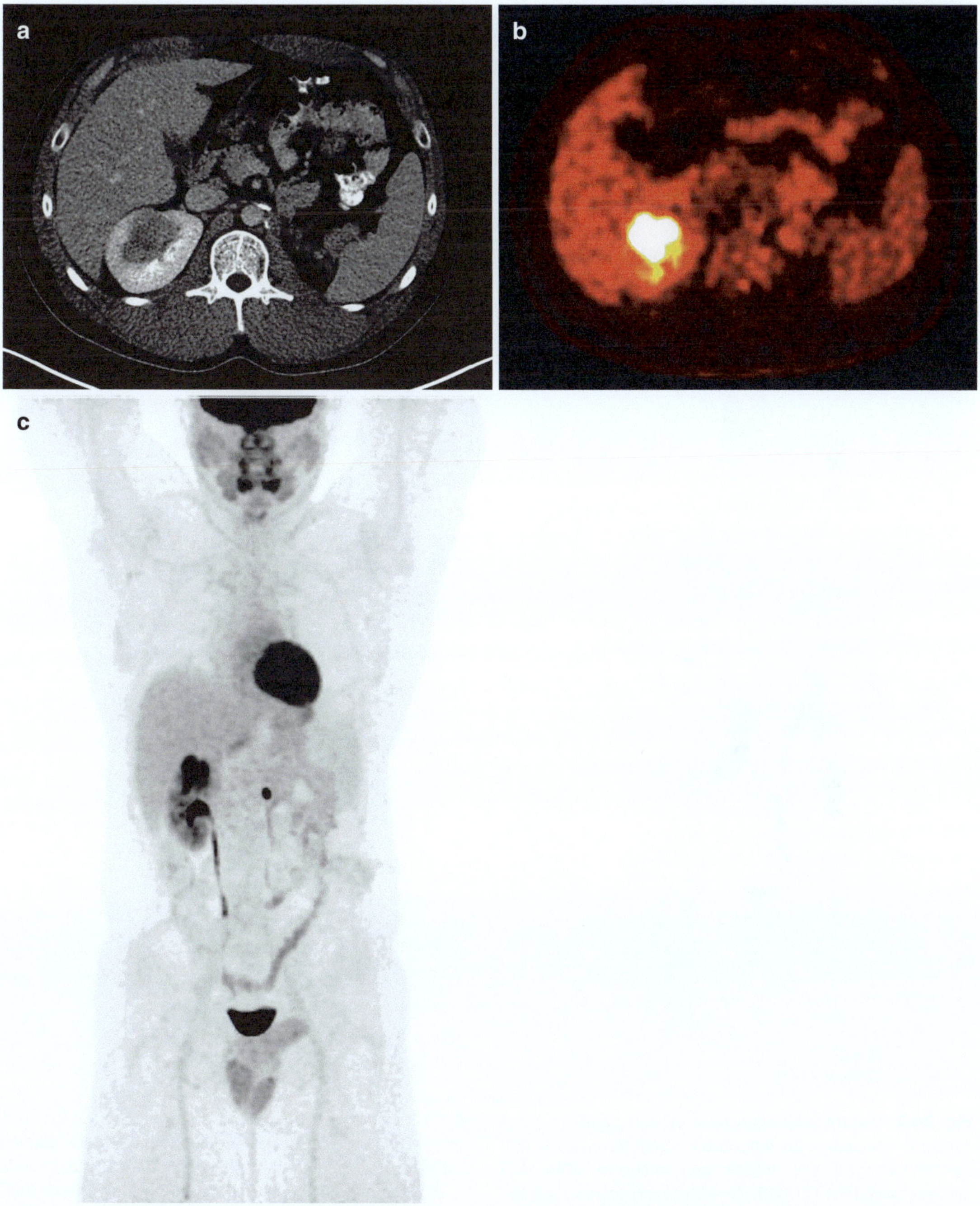

Fig. 24.1 Solitary renal cancer in the right upper pole. This patient had a type II papillary renal cancer in the right kidney (**a**) and was considered high risk for metastatic disease. The FDG PET/CT demonstrates increased activity in the upper pole of the kidney corresponding the mass on CT (**b**) and no evidence of metastatic disease elsewhere (**c**) [61]

diagnosis but also in restaging [4]. Sarcomatoid tumors are also reliably FDG avid [4]. However, in general, FDG has modest uptake and can also be taken up in benign renal tumors [4]. Thus, FDG PET has played a minor role in primary RCC evaluation. Moreover, FDG has proven insensitive in cystic renal masses due to the low burden of solid tissue in such lesions [5].

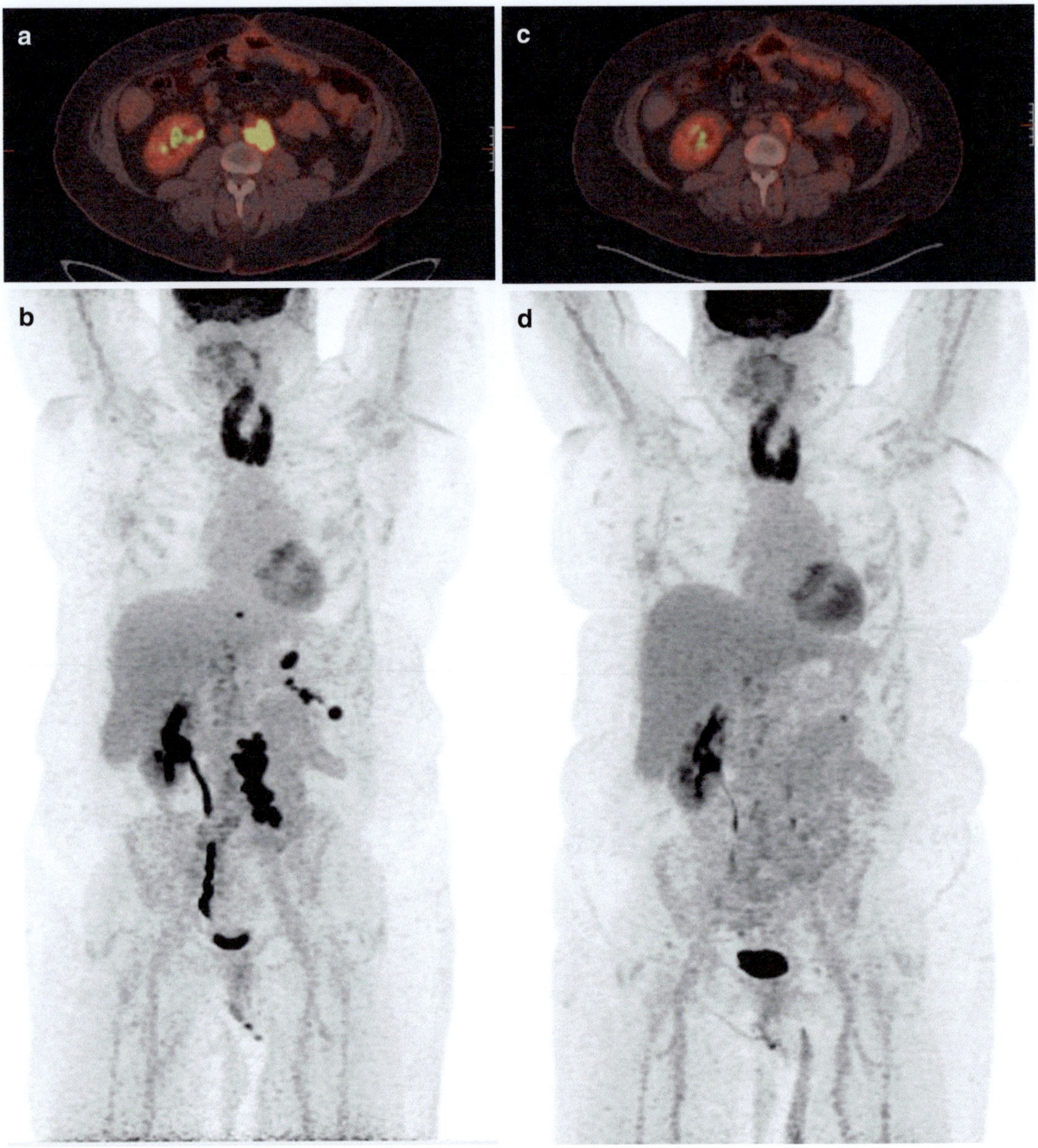

Fig. 24.2 Patient with aggressive type II papillary renal cancer associated with hereditary leiomyoma renal cell carcinoma syndrome which has recurred after left nephrectomy. PET CT with ^{18}F-FDG demonstrates intense uptake in the left para-aortic adenopathy on transverse PET/CT (**a**) and coronal projection image (**b**). After therapy with a combination of targeted therapies, the activity and size of the adenopathy have dramatically decreased (**c**, **d**). The patient has maintained a good response for 2 years [61]

Interestingly, ^{11}C-acetate has been reported to be useful in this setting, having a 100% positive predictive value (PPV), although a sensitivity of only 50%. ^{11}C-acetate is excreted via the pancreas and therefore avoids the confusion of renal parenchymal enhancement found with FDG. However, ^{11}C-acetate is limited to masses >1.5 cm in diameter [5] and has the unavoidable disadvantage of a short half-life ($t½$ = 20 min), limiting the study to sites with cyclotrons and radiochemistry facilities. Occasionally, an FDG PET scan performed for another malignancy will reveal a lesion within the kidney. It is uncertain whether this lesion represents a metastasis or another primary tumor [6]. Unfortunately, uptake in the lesion is not specific in this regard, and a biopsy is usually performed to clarify this dilemma. Diagnosis is generally made on CT and/or MRI and if questions arise, a biopsy is usually recommended. FDG plays an important role in particular subtypes of renal cancer such as aggressive type II papillary and sarcomatoid.

24.2.3 Staging of RCC

FDG PET is playing an increasing role in the initial staging of RCC. The majority of cancers discovered on CT or MRI are small and localized with a low risk of metastases, therefore additional studies are unwarranted. However, higher risk, larger tumors are more FDG PET avid. Initial SUVmax values of metastatic lesions are highly prognostic for survival [7]. For local staging FDG PET has been found useful in determining whether thrombus in the renal vein and inferior vena cava is malignant or "bland" [8], a distinction that is considered important by some surgeons [9]. In general, CT, MRI, and bone scan in symptomatic patients are considered sufficient staging studies to clear a patient for surgery. Occasionally, when an isolated potential metastasis is detected, FDG PET can be used to confirm metabolic activity thereby confirming the diagnosis of metastatic disease (Fig. 24.3). However, in general FDG PET is not widely used for RCC staging. This may change with the results of a new exploratory study (REMAP) combining FDG PET and MRI launched recently [10]. Surveillance imaging after surgery is also discouraged as there is no level 1 evidence that early intervention improves survival [11]. American Urologic Association guidelines suggest that more advanced initial tumors may warrant increased surveillance and FDG PET could play a role here, although this has not been studied [11].

24.2.4 Metastatic RCC

FDG PET in RCC is most often used in patients with metastatic disease who are on novel targeted therapies. Renal cancer is not responsive to conventional chemotherapy and thus, this therapy is rarely, if ever, employed. However, a variety of targeted therapies, which include tyrosine kinase inhibitors, such as sorafenib and sunitinib, that have antiangiogenic mechanisms and mTOR inhibitors such as everolimus, have demonstrated efficacy and small but important improvements in overall survival [7]. These targeted agents do not generally behave in the same manner as conventional cytotoxic agents. Although tumor size measurements, embodied in the RECIST criteria, have proven adequate for monitoring chemotherapy, for other cancers with modern targeted therapies, there is often little change in the size of the lesions and some metastases even increase even while the drug is prolonging survival [12]. Thus, FDG PET activity could play a role in monitoring the effectiveness of targeted therapies with tyrosine kinase inhibitors.

Ferda et al. demonstrated that initial uptake of lesions correlated with prognosis, with patients whose renal tumors exhibit SUVmax >10 having significantly worse survival than those with SUV max <10 [13]. Decreases in FDG uptake also correlated with outcome [12–14] and were independent of where the lesion was located (e.g., bone, lung, node, etc.). More dramatic decreases in SUV max correlated with better progression-free survival (PFS) and overall survival (OS) [2]. The advantage of FDG PET over conventional modalities is most apparent in bone and musculoskeletal metastases, which are difficult to assess on CT and MRI because the bone damage continues to be seen even when the lesion is responding. There is a trend toward using a metabolic tumor volume (MTV) or total lesion glycolysis (TLG) as an overall measure of disease burden [15, 16] rather than individual SUVmax scores. This is calculated by multiplying the SUVmax and the number of lesions. Both MTV and TLG have been shown to be predictive of response and outcome [17]. Thus, FDG PET is increasingly used to monitor the efficacy of treatment of patients with metastatic disease who are receiving tyrosine kinase inhibitors and other targeted therapies.

24.2.5 Other Agents for RCC

A number of other PET agents have been used for renal cancer. Sodium fluoride PET has not been commonly reported in RCC but recent reports suggest it will be more sensitive than conventional

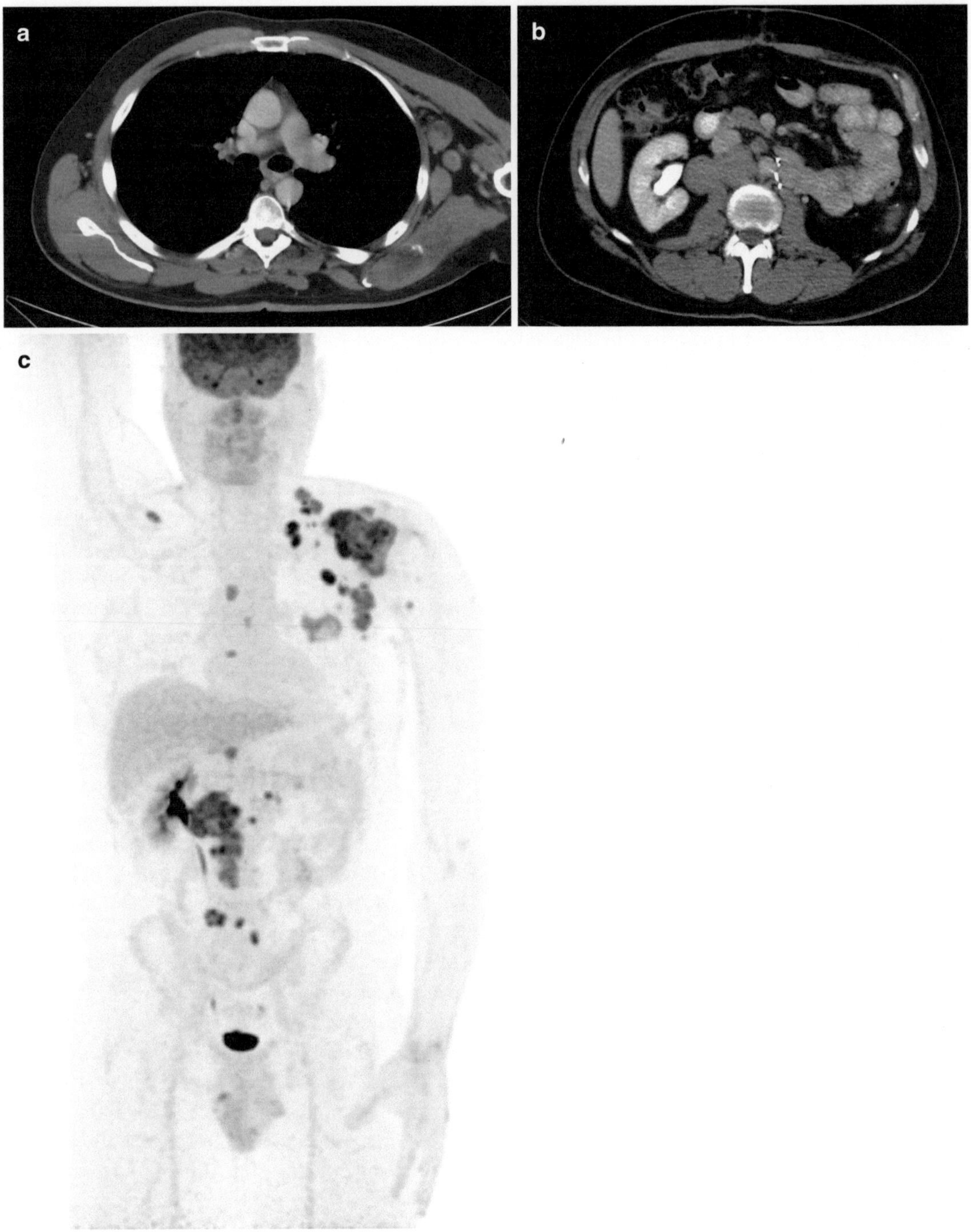

Fig. 24.3 Patient with a history of clear cell renal cancer with recurrent disease in the axilla and retroperitoneum. Transverse CT scan shows several abnormal nodes in the left axilla (**a**). Retroperitoneal adenopathy is also seen (**b**). Coronal PET demonstrates extensive uptake in the Axilla and shoulder muscles as well as retroperitoneal adenopathy (**c**) [61]

bone scans, much as it in other malignancies. This is true even for predominantly lytic renal cancer bone metastases [18].

Over 95% of clear cell renal cancers express carbonic anhydrase IX on their cell membrane. An antibody, cG250, was developed as a potential therapeutic agent, but results of early trials showed modest or no benefit [19]. However, it was thought that labeling the antibody with ^{124}I could produce an effective imaging agent for clear cell carcinoma [19]. The REDECT trial of ^{124}I Girentuximab (cG250) showed an 86% sensitivity and 86% specificity for clear cell carcinoma [19]. The agent was not as useful for lesions <2 cm in diameter or in non-clear-cell renal cancers. The advantages of this agent are that it is specific for clear cell carcinoma and has a sensitivity comparable to biopsy [19] but the disadvantage is that less common, but nevertheless aggressive cancers may be negative. It may play a role in patients too ill to undergo biopsy or in those patients for whom adequate conventional studies cannot be obtained. However, the study requires 3–7 days because of the long clearance time of the antibody and this may make it impractical [8]. Moreover, it is unclear whether the niche applications of this agent would make it economically sustainable. Suggestions have been made to exchange the ^{124}I with ^{89}Zr, which may result in better imaging, but this does not clarify the actual clinical role of this agent [8, 20]. A small molecule affinity agent for CAIX, named VM-4, was tested in patients undergoing resection for renal cancer. While the uptake in the primary tumor was confounded by normal uptake in the kidney, metastases showed much higher uptake suggesting this agent may play a role in detecting metastases and assessing treatment response to metastases [21].

^{18}F-MISO has also been suggested as an imaging agent for RCC based on the level of hypoxia in many renal tumors; however, this agent has not been extensively studied and early reports show only modest uptake in RCCs and it was not predictive of response to therapy [22]. Interestingly, initial studies show a decrease in hypoxia after initiating TKI therapy likely due to "vascular normalization", followed by an increase in hypoxia as antiangiogenic effects begin to predominate [22].

As mentioned earlier ^{11}C-acetate has been proposed as an alternative agent for imaging RCC as it is not excreted through the kidney. However, the technical limitations of this agent are likely to inhibit its widespread use.

There are several more recent entries into the category of PET agents that might be useful for renal cancer metastases, those targeting prostate-specific membrane antigen (PSMA) and those targeting somatostatin receptor (DOTATATE). In both cases, the reports are largely anecdotal. In the case of PSMA PET affinity agents, it is thought that the neovascularity associated with renal cancer harbors sufficient expression of PSMA to take up on PET scans. It has been observed with both ^{18}F and ^{68}Ga labeled compounds [23–27]. In the case of DOTATATE imaging, several similar reports have appeared [28, 29]. The number and diversity of reports supporting a role for PSMA currently outweigh the data for DOTATATE but more studies are needed to define their role.

Finally, ^{89}Zr-bevacizumab (anti-VEGF) has been proposed as an imaging agent to monitor tyrosine kinase inhibitor therapy. Renal cancer is driven by VEGF and thus, is a promising antibody-based imaging agent for monitoring treatment response [30].

24.2.6 Summary

FDG PET/CT is not widely used in most primary RCCs although particular RCC subtypes are quite avid for the agent. In high risk, larger patients' FDG PET may be useful in pre-operative staging and is particularly useful when conventional imaging is negative or there is a potential tumor thrombus. In metastatic RCC, FDG PET/CT is increasingly used to monitor targeted molecular therapies such as tyrosine kinase inhibitors. Clinically meaningful relationships between FDG uptake as measured by SUVmax and MTV and patient outcome are now established. Sodium fluoride PET appears to be a useful method in detecting subtle bone metastases but it has not yet replaced conventional bone scan. Several other PET agents targeting carbonic anhydrase IX, hypoxia and fatty acid synthesis, PSMA and DOTATATE have been reported but none are in widespread use. The role of PSMA PET is particularly promising given the rapid rise of this agent in prostate cancer imaging.

24.3 Use of PET in Bladder Cancer

24.3.1 Overview of Bladder Cancer

Bladder cancer (BC) is the most common cancer in the urinary system and is the fifth most common malignancy in men worldwide, following prostate, lung, colon/rectum, and liver cancer [31]. In the last 30 years, BC has not changed substantially, indicating gaps between diagnosis and management of BC. Little or no change in BC control outcomes has been achieved [32]. Incidence of BC peaks in the sixth and seventh decades of life [33], and rates in males are three to four times those in females [34]. Smoking is the most common risk factor in BC and accounts for approximately half of all BCs [35]. While urothelial carcinoma of the bladder and upper tract urothelial carcinoma are two distinct diseases [36], cigarette smoking is the most established risk factor for both [37]. Current smoking increases the risk of developing urothelial carcinoma by as much as fourfold and sixfold, respectively [37], and 30–50% of all BC is caused by cigarette smoking [38]. A meta-analysis demonstrated a significant association of BC for both current and former cigarette smokers [39]. The latency period is approximately 20–30 years. The second most important risk factor for BC is occupational exposure to chemicals, and work-related cases account for 20–25% of all BCs [35]. Other possible factors include genetic predisposition, external-beam radiotherapy for gynecology cancer resulting in secondary BC, Schistosoma hematobium bladder infections, exposure to arsenic in drinking water, while other dietary factors have been discussed [40]. Painless hematuria or gross hematuria is the most common presenting complaint in patients with BC [33]. The standard method of diagnosing BC is based on direct visualization of the bladder with cystoscopy and subsequent biopsy/resection [41, 42]. CIS is diagnosed by a combination of cystoscopy, urine cytology, and histological evaluation of multiple bladder biopsies [43], and urinary cytology continues to play an important role in the diagnosis and surveillance of BC [44]. In an effort to improve the sensitivity of BC diagnosis, fluorescence cystoscopy continues to evolve [45–47]. In the following, we present an overview of PET/CT in BC.

24.3.2 Primary Bladder Cancer

Proper and accurate staging of the BC is essential for optimal treatment of the patients [48]. After diagnosing BC, the first aspect that has to be assessed is whether the patient has a superficial or a muscle-invasive tumor (T1 vs. T2) since infiltration beyond the lamina propria will require more aggressive treatment than transurethral resection. Histology of the biopsy at the time of initial cystoscopic examination reveals the tumor's cell type, grade, and depth of invasion. More than 90% of BCs are urothelial (transitional cell) carcinomas, 5% are squamous cell carcinomas, and less than 2% are adenocarcinomas [33]. The primary tumor in the urinary bladder may present a thickening of the bladder wall or as an intraluminal tumor mass. Currently, the most accurate method for differentiating T1 from T2 tumors is with a biopsy obtained from the muscularis propria of the tumor base [32, 48]. Both conventional CT and MRI may be used for assessment of local invasion, but both modalities are unable to accurately detect microscopic invasion of perivesical fat (T2 versus T3a) [49–52]. Therefore, the role of CT and MRI is to detect T3b disease or higher. CT has sensitivities in the range of 79–89.7% and specificities ranging from 91% to 94.7% in detecting BC [53–55]. MRI is superior to CT for determining the depth of bladder wall infiltration [56, 57], while CT and MRI yield similar results in demonstrating invasion of perivesical structures [56, 58, 59]. For local tumor assessment, MRI is reported to be more accurate than CT [60], and MRI imaging is considered by some to be the modality of choice for primary T staging of urinary BC [59]. Excretory-phase CT urography is used for upper urinary tract urothelial tumors and has replaced conventional i.v. urography and ultrasound in high-risk patients.

The role of FDG PET/CT in the detection of localized BC is limited because of the difficulty in differentiating ^{18}F-FDG activity excreted into the urine from tumor activity in the bladder wall. Several methods have been proposed to overcome radioactivity interference in the urine, i.e., FDG wash out, early images, late images after voiding, dual-phase imaging, catheterization, bladder irrigation, and forced diuresis [40, 56, 61–69]. In a recent study, it was demonstrated that on early dynamic PET, SUVmax was significantly correlated with muscle invasiveness, histological grade, and pathological tumor size [69]. A meta-analysis including six studies evaluated the diagnostic accuracy of FDG PET/CT for detecting BC lesions [70]. The pooled sensitivity and specificity of PET or PET/CT for the detection of BC was 80.0% and 84.0%, respectively [70].

Recently, two small studies have used simultaneous PET/MRI systems in the evaluation of BC [71, 72], since PET/MRI combine the unique benefits of both modalities (high contrast resolution and multiparametric nature of MRI; metabolic information on PET). Hybrid PET/MRI scanners perform spatially and temporally simultaneous acquisitions, thereby improving the alignment of structures between the two modalities. The two studies indicate a possible role of FDG PET/MRI in the evaluation of BC patients [71, 72]. However, larger prospective studies are needed to clarify the possible role of PET/MRI in the clinical management of BC patients.

24.3.3 Staging

At clinical presentation, approximately 30% of patients have muscle-invasive BC [60]. Muscle-invasive BC is an aggressive epithelial tumor with a high rate of early systemic metastases. The common sites of metastatic disease include LNs, liver, lung, bone, and adrenal glands. The optimal management of BC patients is dependent on accurate staging and detection of metastatic disease. The sensitivity of conventional CT and MRI for detection of LN metastases is low since LN metastases rely on size criteria. Thus, both modalities may not detect metastases in normal-sized LNs. Furthermore, the specificity is low since enlarged LN may be due to benign disease. Since FDG PET may detect metabolic activity in not enlarged LNs, FDG PET/CT has been used in clinical studies for primary NM staging (Figs. 24.4 and 24.5) [73–83]. Studies have demonstrated that FDG PET/CT detects more malignant disease than conventional CT/MRI in 20–40% of patients [78, 79], and important is that FDG PET/CT may change the clinical management in up to 68% of the patients [79]. Upstaging is more frequent than downstaging [78]. A recent meta-analysis evaluated the diagnostic accuracy of FDG PET in detecting LN metastases [84]. Eight studies fulfilled the criteria in the analysis [73, 77, 80, 84–88]. The pooled sensitivity of FDG PET/CT for detecting LN metastases was 0.565 (95% CI 0.473–0.653); specificity, 0.954 (95% CI 0.922–0.976); positive LR, 9.02 (95% CI 4.48–18.16); and negative LR, 0.50 (95% CI 0.39–0.64). The pooled measures for CT alone in five of the included studies were: sensitivity 0.35, specificity 0.95, positive LR 4.91, and negative LR 0.7. The authors concluded that FDG PET/CT is better to detect LN metastases as compared to CT alone. With a pooled sensitivity of 35%, CT alone correctly identified 22% fewer patients with LN metastasis, as compared to FDG PET/CT. Thus, FDG PET/CT offered additional metabolic information, as compared to CT alone, and therefore is more accurate for staging BC [84]. In another meta-analysis of FDG PET/CT for the staging

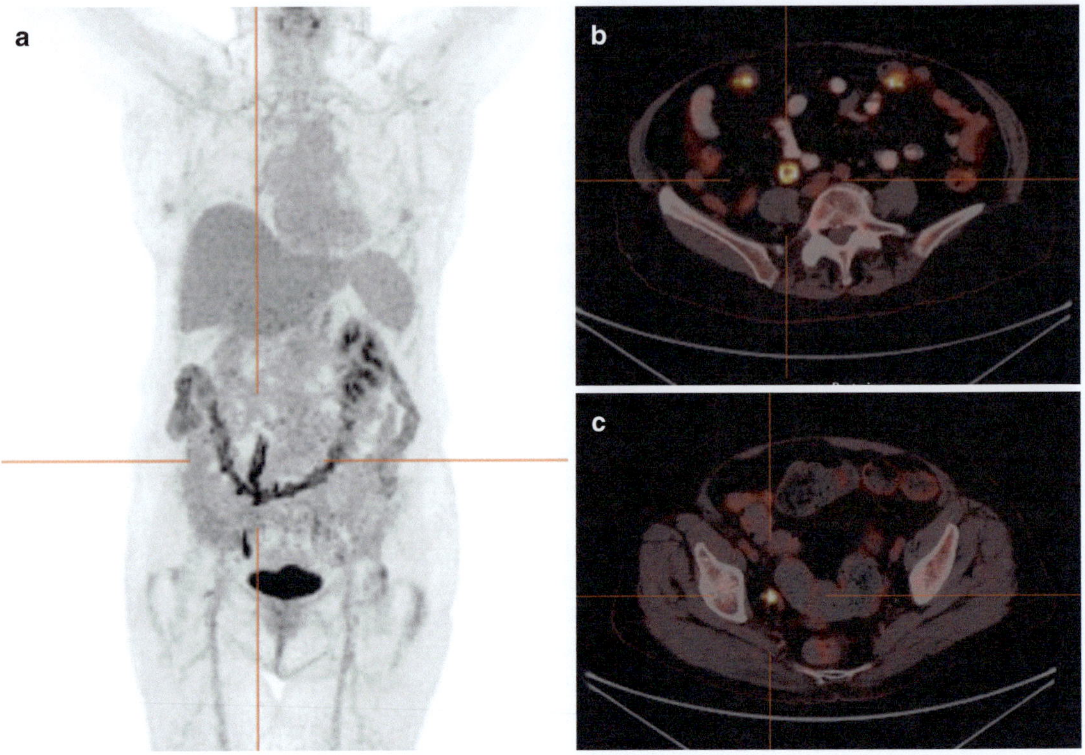

Fig. 24.4 Patient with newly diagnosed muscle-invasive bladder cancer. Tumor in the bladder wall could not be visualized with FDG PET due to FDG activity in the urine. However, unexpected focal increased FDG activity in the right ureter was seen (**a**, **b**), which was due to malignancy. A lymph node metastasis was also seen in the right side of pelvis (**c**) [61]

and restaging of BC, the pooled sensitivity was 82%, the pooled specificity was 89%, and the global accuracy was 92% [89]. Six studies met the inclusion criteria [65, 67, 74, 79, 80, 90]. The pooled sensitivity and specificity of PET/CT for primary lesion detection of BC were 0.90 (95% CI: 0.70–0.99) and 1.00 (95% CI: 0.74–1.00), respectively. The pooled sensitivity and specificity of FDG PET or PET/CT for staging or restaging (metastatic lesions) of BC were 0.82 (95% CI: 0.72–0.89) and 0.89 (95% CI: 0.81–0.95), respectively. It was concluded that the diagnostic accuracy of FDG PET/CT is good in metastatic lesions of BC [89]. Recently, a study evaluated the value of SUVmax of LNs on FDG PET/CT in patients with BC before cystectomy with PLND, and compared with histology [83]. It was demonstrated that on SUVmax >2 analysis the sensitivity was 79.4% and specificity 66.5%, and on SUVmax >4 analysis the sensitivity was 61.8% and specificity was 84.5%. Two years of follow-up implied that higher SUVmax is correlated with higher recurrence risk, independent of conventional pathological findings [83]. Thus, FDG PET/CT using SUVmax of LNs may be a useful tool for preoperative evaluation of pelvic LN metastases from muscle-invasive BC and may contribute to the selection of patients for personalized treatment.

FDG PET/CT has been compared to MRI for LN staging in patients with BC [82]. The study demonstrated specificities for the detection of LN metastases for MRI and FDG PET/CT to be 80% and 93.33%, respectively. The negative predictive values (NPV) were 80% and 87.5% for MRI and FDG PET/CT, respectively. However, the differences in specificity and NPV were not statistically significant but the trend of the data indicates an advantage of FDG PET/CT over MRI [82].

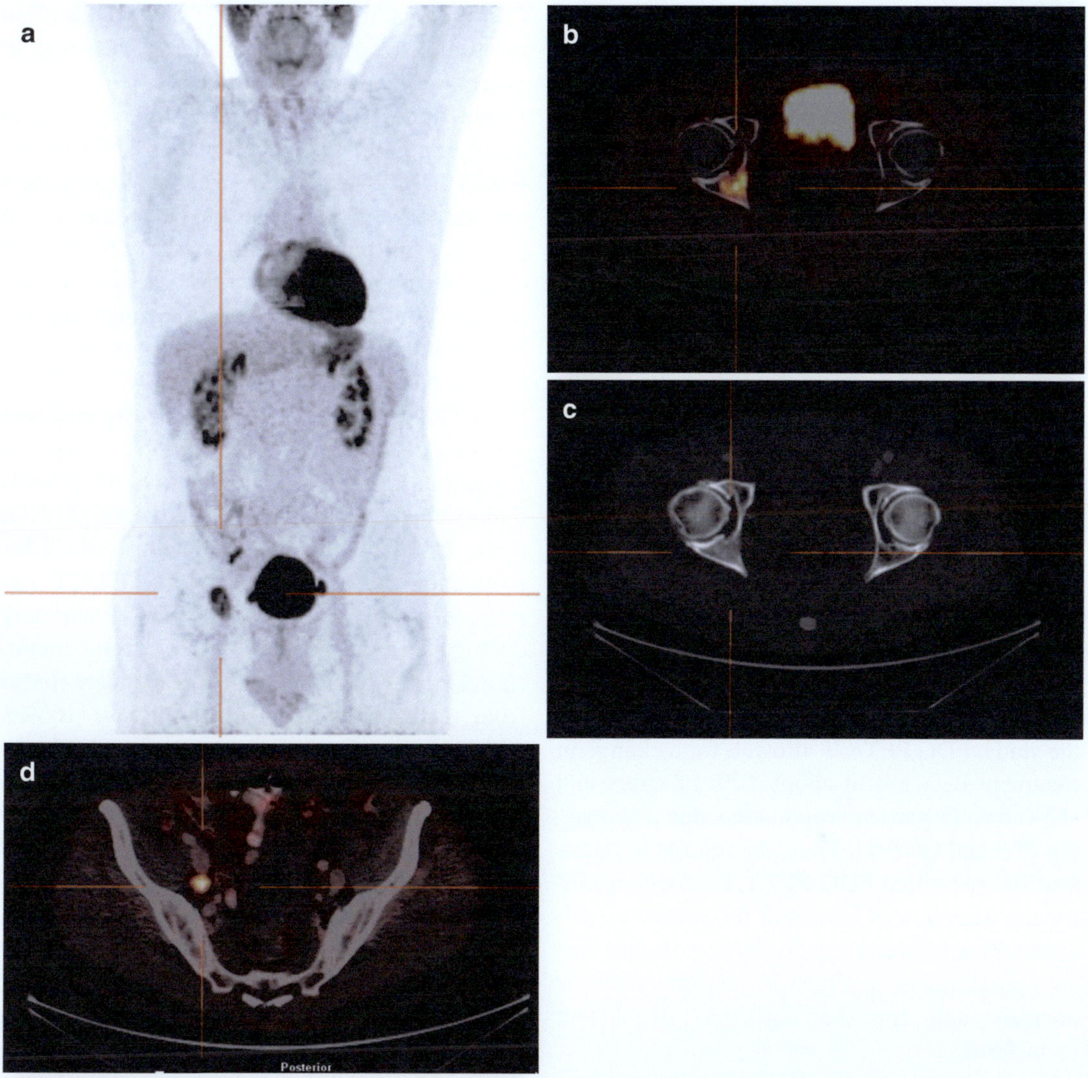

Fig. 24.5 Patient with newly diagnosed muscle-invasive bladder cancer. A bone metastasis in right acetabulum can be seen on FDG PET/CT (**a**, **b**) but with only minimal changes on CT (**c**). A lymph node metastasis is seen in the right side of the pelvis (**d**) [61]

24.3.4 Restaging

In recurrent BC, the overall prognosis is poor. Muscle-invasive BC is a disease with a known pattern of predominantly distant and early recurrences, and approximately 50% of these patients will have relapse after radical cystectomy. Local occurrence accounts for 30% of relapses, whereas distant metastases are more common. Salvage and/or palliative therapies are prompted when recurrent disease is discovered. Accurate restaging is therefore important before additional costly and toxic therapies are considered [61]. Only a few data are available on the utility of FDG PET/CT in assessing for recurrence and metastatic disease in patients who have previously undergone treatment for their primary BC [65, 67, 90, 91]. In a study, FDG PET/CT was used to evaluate the diagnostic ability of FDG PET or PET/CT in recurrent and metastatic BC [90]. In the study, all the BC patients were previously treated for their primary disease. The metastatic sites detected in the study included mediastinum, lung, and bone. FDG PET/CT affected the clinical management in 17% of patients, by prompting either additional therapy or a wait-and-watch strategy. A recent study evaluated the accuracy, the effect upon treatment decision, and the prognostic value of FDG PET/CT in patients with suspected recurrent BC [91]. Sensitivity, specificity, positive predictive value, negative predictive value, and accuracy of FDG PET/CT were 87%, 94%, 95%, 85%, and 90%. PFS was significantly longer in patients with negative scan vs. those with pathological findings (85% vs. 24%). Moreover, a normal scan was associated with a longer OS (88% vs. 47% after 2 years and 87% vs. 25% after 3 years, respectively, $p < 0.05$). SUVmax > 6 and TLG > 8.5 were recognized as the most accurate thresholds to predict PFS (2-year PFS 62% for SUVmax < 6 vs. 15% for SUVmax > 6, $p = 0.018$; 2-year PFS 66% for TLG < 8.5 vs. 18% for TLG > 8.5, $p = 0.09$). In the study, FDG PET/CT allowed for a change in treatment decision in about 40% of cases and showed an important prognostic value in assessing PFS and OS [91]. Thus, the reports in recurrent BC show that FDG PET/CT may be useful for the detection of recurrent local lesions, differentiation between local recurrent disease versus postsurgical or post-irradiation fibrosis/necrosis and for the detection of distant metastases.

24.3.5 Response to Therapy

Patients with BC and regional LN metastases could be treated with neoadjuvant chemotherapy, and patients with distant metastases should be spared the unnecessary morbidity of radical cystectomy. It has been shown that neoadjuvant cisplatin-based combination chemotherapy improves outcomes for muscle-invasive BC [92]. Since nonresponse rate to neoadjuvant chemotherapy is relatively high, monitoring the LN response to neoadjuvant chemotherapy may guide the selection of patients for further surgery. Conventional imaging with CT and MRI is often not useful for evaluation of therapy response in metastases because of difficulty in identifying viable tumor in residual necrotic masses and small tumors in LNs of normal size. Therefore, FDG PET/CT has been used for evaluating therapy response to neoadjuvant chemotherapy in patients with muscle-invasive BC [93–95]. In a study, metabolic response was assessed according to EORTC (European Organization for Research and Treatment of Cancer) recommendations based on the change in FDG uptake on FDG PET/CT [93]. Radiological response was assessed on CT according to RECIST (Response Evaluation Criteria in Solid Tumors). All patients underwent pelvic lymph node dissection (PLND) with histopathological evaluation of LNs. Evaluating the LN response with PET/CT was feasible in all patients. FDG PET/CT correctly distinguished responders (95%) from nonresponders (79%) and complete responders (68%) from patients with residual disease (63%). Although no definitive conclusions can be drawn from this small study, FDG PET/CT may be feasible for evaluating the LN response to neoadjuvant chemotherapy and distinguishing responders from nonresponders [93]. Recently, a study evaluated the role of FDG PET/CT for response evaluation of neoadjuvant or induction chemotherapy for muscle-invasive BC [95]. The results were compared with response on pathological analysis of radical prostatectomy specimens (golden standard). FDG PET/CT bladder tumor downstaging was identified with 83% sensitivity and 80% specificity, and the authors concluded that response monitoring might be used to adjust neoadjuvant treatment. In a study, it was demonstrated that, in comparison with CT, the response after two cycles of first-line chemotherapy detected by FDG PET/CT was associated with longer PFS and OS in patients with advanced BC [96]. Another recent study also suggests a role of FDG PET/CT for response evaluation of induction chemotherapy for oligometastatic BC [94]. The role of FDG PET/CT for assessment of therapy response has to be confirmed in larger prospective studies.

24.3.6 Prognostic Value

The prognosis and treatment of BC depends on tumor grade and stage [58]. The overall 5-year survival rate is 82%. It is 94% for localized and superficial BCs, but it is only 6% for metastatic BCs [40, 53]. Only a few studies have focused on the prognostic value of FDG PET/CT. A study reported sensitivity, specificity, PPV, and NPV of 70%, 94%, 78%, and 91%, respectively, for FDG PET/CT in 42 BC patients [80]. The median follow-up was 14.9 months. It was shown that FDG PET/CT detected occult metastatic disease in 17% of the BC patients with negative conventional preoperative evaluations. Recurrence-free survival, OS, and disease-specific survival (DSS) were all significantly poorer in the patients with positive FDG PET/CT than in those with negative FDG-PET/CT. In the study, FDG PET/CT was strongly correlated with survival. In a large bi-institutional study including 211 patients with muscle-invasive BC underwent FDG PET/CT and CT for primary staging [97]. In the study, the patients were divided into two groups, a PET/CT positive and a PET/CT negative group data on staging, and mortality were retrospectively analyzed from prospective databases. Median follow-up was 18 months. Patients with a positive PET/CT had a significantly shorter OS and DSS (median OS: 14 vs. 50 months, $p = 0.001$; DSS: 16 vs. 50 months, $p < 0.001$). In multivariable analysis, the presence of extravesical lesions on PET/CT was an independent prognostic indicator of mortality (OS: hazard ratio = 3.0, confidence interval 95% 1.7–5.1). This association was not statistically significant for conventional CT (hazard ratio = 1.6, 95% confidence interval 0.9–2.7). The study demonstrated that the presence of extravesical metastatic lesions on PET/CT might be an independent indicator of mortality [97].

24.3.7 Other Agents for Bladder Cancer

In order to improve the sensitivity of PET by using tracers that are not excreted in the urine like FDG, other PET agents like ^{11}C-choline, ^{11}C-acetate, and ^{11}C-methionine have been used in BC [40, 61]. Furthermore, sodium fluoride has been used for the detection of bone metastasis [40, 61]. PSMA PET/CT is widely used in prostate cancer [98], but may not be useful in BC due to scant expression of PSMA in urothelial cancer [99].

Choline: Studies have evaluated the role of ^{11}C-choline PET/CT in BC [100–106]. The sensitivity for the detection of LN metastasis is relatively low [100, 102, 103]. A study reported the diagnostic accuracy of ^{11}C-choline PET/CT in preoperative LN staging of BC suitable for radical cystectomy and extended PLND [102]. On a patient-based analysis, choline PET/CT showed a sensitivity of 42% and specificity of 84%, whereas CT showed a sensitivity of 14% and specificity of 89%. On an LN-based analysis, choline PET/CT showed a sensitivity of 10% and specificity of 64%, whereas CT showed a sensitivity of 2% and specificity of 63%. In contrast, in another study, choline PET/CT was not able to improve the diagnostic efficacy in preoperative LN staging compared with CT [106]. However, ^{11}C-choline PET/CT may be more useful for restaging of BC suspected of relapse, especially for LN evaluation and distant metastases [105].

The prognostic value of ^{11}C-choline PET/CT in preoperative staging of muscle-invasive BC has been investigated in a prospective study [104]. In the study, 44 patients with localized BC were staged with choline PET/CT before radical cystectomy with PLND. The results of imaging were correlated to OS and cancer-specific death (CSD). There was no statistically significant difference in OS and CSD between the patient groups when stratified for organ-confined versus non-organ-confined disease or LN involvement defined by either choline PET/CT or CT. The authors concluded that neither CT nor ^{11}C-choline PET/CT was able to sufficiently predict OS or CSD in BC patients treated with radical cystectomy. However, a major limitation of the study is the relatively small number of patients included.

Methionine. ^{11}C-methionine uptake in tissue is an indication of amino acid transport and metabolism, which is often increased in malignant tumors. In a small study, methionine was superior to FDG; however, tumor was identified with a sensitivity of 78% only with methionine PET [107]. Methionine uptake was correlated to tumor grade, but methionine did not improve the staging of BC. In another study, methionine PET was used for the evaluation of therapy response in patients with varying stages of BC treated with chemotherapy [108]. The diagnostic accuracy of PET was poor and the technique could not monitor the therapeutic effect of neoadjuvant chemotherapy, producing results that correlated with therapy outcome.

Acetate. A small study prospectively evaluated MRI, ^{11}C-acetate PET/CT, and CT for the staging of BC [109]. MRI, acetate PET/CT, and CT demonstrated similar levels of accuracy. For all modalities, a history of intravesical and/or systemic chemotherapy affected staging accuracy. In another small study, acetate PET/CT was compared with choline PET/CT in BC [110]. Acetate and choline PET/CT scans were performed within 1 week. The two tracers demonstrated equivalent results in the preoperative evaluation.

Sodium fluoride. Lytic bone metastases of BC may be better detected using sodium fluoride PET/CT, as compared with a conventional ^{99m}Tc-MDP bone scan. Sodium fluoride PET has been compared with MDP bone scan in the detection of skeletal metastases in BC [111]. In this prospective study, patients with BC underwent PET and bone scan within 48 h. Skeletal metastases diagnosed on each of these techniques was compared against a final diagnosis based on CT, MRI, skeletal survey, clinical follow-up, and histological correlation [111]. The sensitivity, specificity, positive PPV, NPV, and accuracy of MDP planar bone scan were 82.35%, 64.51%, 56%, 86.95%, and 70.83%; of MDP SPECT/CT were 88.23%, 74.19%, 65.21%, 92%, and 79.16%; and of fluoride PET/CT were 100%, 87.09%, 80.95%, 100%, and 91.66%, respectively [111]. In the study, fluoride PET/CT was superior to both MDP planar bone scan and MDP SPECT/CT. Fluoride PET/CT identified bony metastases and changed the management in 35% of the patients [111].

24.3.8 Pelvic and Ureter Cancer

Local evaluation of the primary pelvic or ureter tumor on ^{18}F-FDG PET/CT is often limited due to urinary excretion of ^{18}F-FDG which may mask the tumors, particular if the tumor is small and is confined to the mucosa or wall, but in some cases assessment of metabolic activity may still be possible through close correlation with CT images [112]. However, FDG PET/CT may be useful for the detection of primary tumor [113], LN or distant metastases [114], site of recurrence [115], and the assessment of early treatment response [96]. FDG PET/CT may change the clinical management in 20% of the patients [114].

24.3.9 Summary

^{18}F-FDG PET/CT is not useful for the evaluation of primary tumor in the urinary bladder because of urinary excretion of ^{18}F-FDG. Several methods have been proposed to overcome interference from radioactivity in the urine. However, ^{18}F-FDG PET/CT is increasingly used for staging and restaging in muscle-invasive BC, and FDG PET/CT may add important prognostic information. Recently, ^{18}F-FDG PET/CT has been used for assessment of treatment response, but further studies are needed. Tracers with no or little urinary excretion have been proposed and tested in BC, but are not recommended in international guidelines.

24.4 Use of PET in Testicular Cancer

24.4.1 Overview of Testicular Cancer

Testicular cancer represents between 1% and 1.5% of male cancers and 5% of urological tumors, with 3–10 new cases occurring per 100,000 males/year [116]. Over the last 30 years, the incidence of testicular cancer has increased [117]. Only 1–2% is bilateral at diagnosis. The histological type varies; although there is a clear predominance (90–95%) of germ cell tumors

(GCT) [116]. Testicular cancers are classified as seminomas, which account for approximately 40% of GCT or non-seminomatous germ cell tumors (NSGCT), which account for approximately 60% [118]. The clinical management of testicular GCT depends on the pathology, staging, and prognostic stratification [119]. Testicular tumors show excellent cure rates [118]. This is mainly due to careful staging at the time of diagnosis, adequate early treatment based on chemotherapeutic combinations, with or without radiotherapy and surgery; and very strict follow-up and salvage therapies [61]. Testicular cancer typically spreads by the lymphatic route through channels along testicular vessels to the retroperitoneum [120]. Hematogenous spread is predominantly to the lungs. Testicular cancer normally appears as a painless, unilateral scrotal mass [118]. In approximately 20% of cases, the first symptom is scrotal pain. Orchidectomy and pathological examination of the testis are necessary to confirm the diagnosis and to define the local extension [116]. Serum tumor markers (AFP, hCG, LDH) are prognostic factors and contribute to diagnosis and staging [116]. Imaging plays an important role in the clinical management of testicular cancer. In the following, we give an overview of PET/CT in testicular cancer.

24.4.2 Primary Testicular Cancer

Currently, diagnostic ultrasound (US) serves to confirm the presence of a testicular mass and to explore the contralateral testis [121]. The sensitivity of US to detect testicular tumor is almost 100%, and it has an important role in determining whether a mass is intra- or extratesticular [121]. MRI offers higher sensitivity and specificity than US for diagnosing tumors [121, 122]. MRI of the scrotum has a sensitivity of 100% and a specificity of 95–100% [123], but its high cost does not justify its clinical use. Recently, a study evaluated the differential diagnostic value of FDG PET/CT for benign and malign testicular lesions [124]. An SUVmax of 3.75 was the optimal cut-off value to differentiate between benign and malignant testicular lesions [124]. The diagnostic sensitivity, specificity, accuracy, positive predictive value, and negative predictive value of this PET/CT modality in the differential diagnosis of benign versus malignant testicular lesions were 90.6%, 80.9%, 86.8%, 87.9%, and 85.0%, respectively [124]. However, the role of FDG PET/CT in the primary investigation of scrotal masses needs further evaluation in prospective studies.

24.4.3 Staging

In order to determine the presence of metastatic disease, the LN pathway must be screened and the presence of visceral metastases must be determined [116]. Retroperitoneal and mediastinal LNs are most often assessed by CT. The supraclavicular nodes can be assessed by physical examination. CT has a sensitivity of 70–80% in determining the state of the retroperitoneal LN, and MRI produces similar results to CT [116]. However, MRI is not recommended for routine imaging in staging of testicular cancer because of the high cost and limited access to MRI, but MRI may be useful when CT and US are inconclusive, when the patients have an allergy to CT contrast media or in cases where the radiation dose should be reduced. FDG PET is a potentially useful diagnostic tool for initial staging in patients with GCT. Studies have suggested improved diagnostic accuracy of FDG PET compared with CT imaging in a range of settings [125–128]. In one study, 70% of patients with normal-sized nodes who subsequently developed relapse could be identified at presentation by the use of PET [127]. Recently, Ambrosini et al. performed a retrospective study in 51 seminoma and 70 NSGCT [129]. FDG demonstrated good sensitivity and specificity for seminoma lesions (92% and 84%, respectively), but its sensitivity was lower for NSGCT (sensitivity and specificity were 77% and 95%, respectively). The FDG scan influenced the clinical management of 92% (47/51) seminomas, and 84% (59/70) NSGCT [129]. Sharma et al. demonstrated high diagnostic accuracy of FDG PET/CT for restaging both seminomatous and non-seminomatous malignant GCTs in a large patient population ($n = 96$) [130]. FDG PET/CT showed sensitivity, specificity, PPV, NPV, and accuracy of 94.2%, 75.0%, 83.0%, 90.9%, and 85.8% overall; 90.0%, 74.0%, 72.0%, 90.9%, and 80.8% in seminomatous GCT; and 96.8%, 76.9%, 91.1%, 90.9%, and 91.1% in non-seminomatous GCT, respectively [130]. The difference in PET/CT accuracy for seminomatous and non-seminomatous GCTs was not significant. A meta-analysis including 16 studies focusing on the diagnostic accuracy of ^{18}F-FDG PET/CT in testicular cancer reported a pooled sensitivity and specificity of 75% and 87%, respectively [131]. The results support the potential usefulness of FDG PET/CT for the assessment of patients with GCT.

24.4.4 Residual Disease

In patients with metastatic seminoma, post-chemotherapy residual masses are present in 55–80% [61]. In lesions >3 cm, viable tumor is expected in 11–37% of cases. Surgery is technically demanding due to fibrosis and it is often incomplete and associated with increased morbidity. Thus, it is important to discriminate between residual tumor and fibrosis/necrosis. CT and MRI cannot adequately predict the histology of residual masses [132]. For many years, FDG PET has been considered as the gold standard for discriminating between residual tumors and necrosis/fibrosis (Fig. 24.6). Several prospective and retrospective studies evaluated the diagnostic

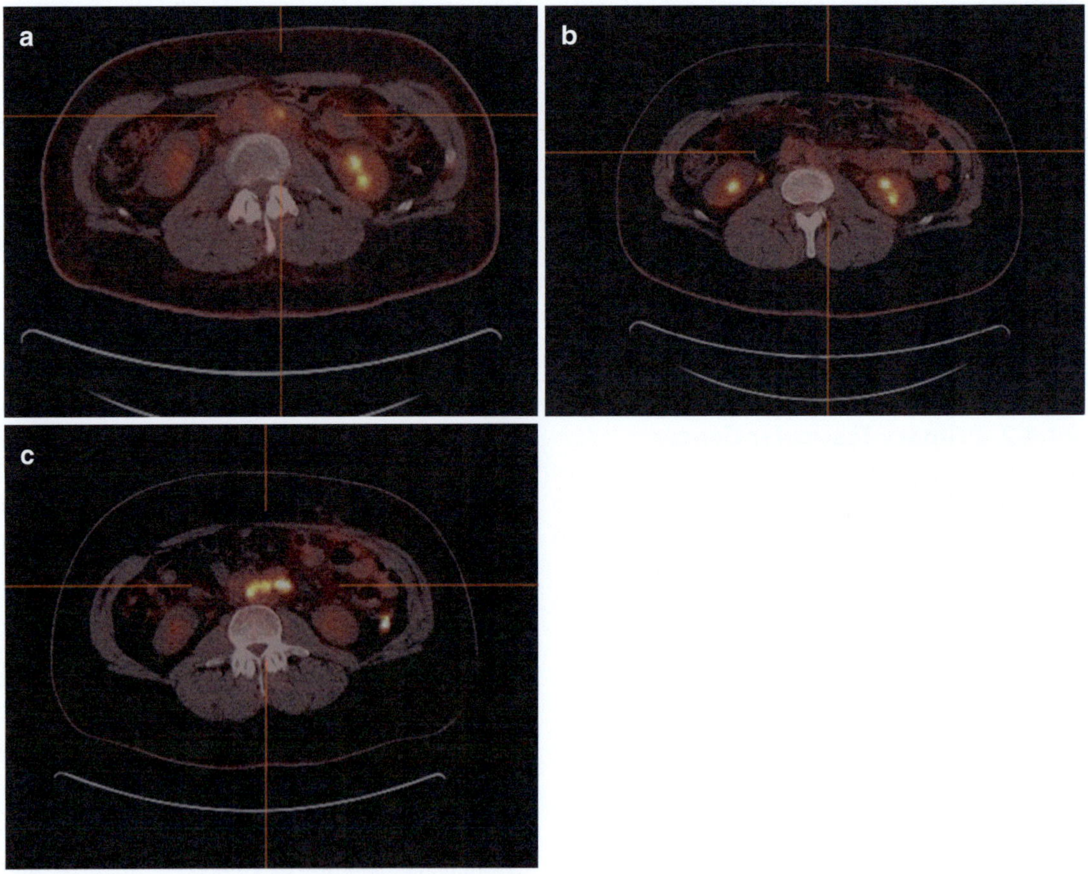

Fig. 24.6 Patient with seminoma treated with chemotherapy, where a retroperitoneal residual mass was seen on CT. FDG PET/CT demonstrated moderate activity in a small area of the known residual mass (**a**). After a new cycle of chemotherapy FDG PET/CT showed complete regression of FDG activity in the residual mass (**b**). However, control FDG PET/CT 3 months later demonstrated relapse in the retroperitoneal mass (**c**) and multiples peritoneal metastases (**d**). After one more cycle of chemotherapy FDG PET/CT demonstrated complete regression (**e**). Only few benign inflammatory elements in cutis were seen [61]

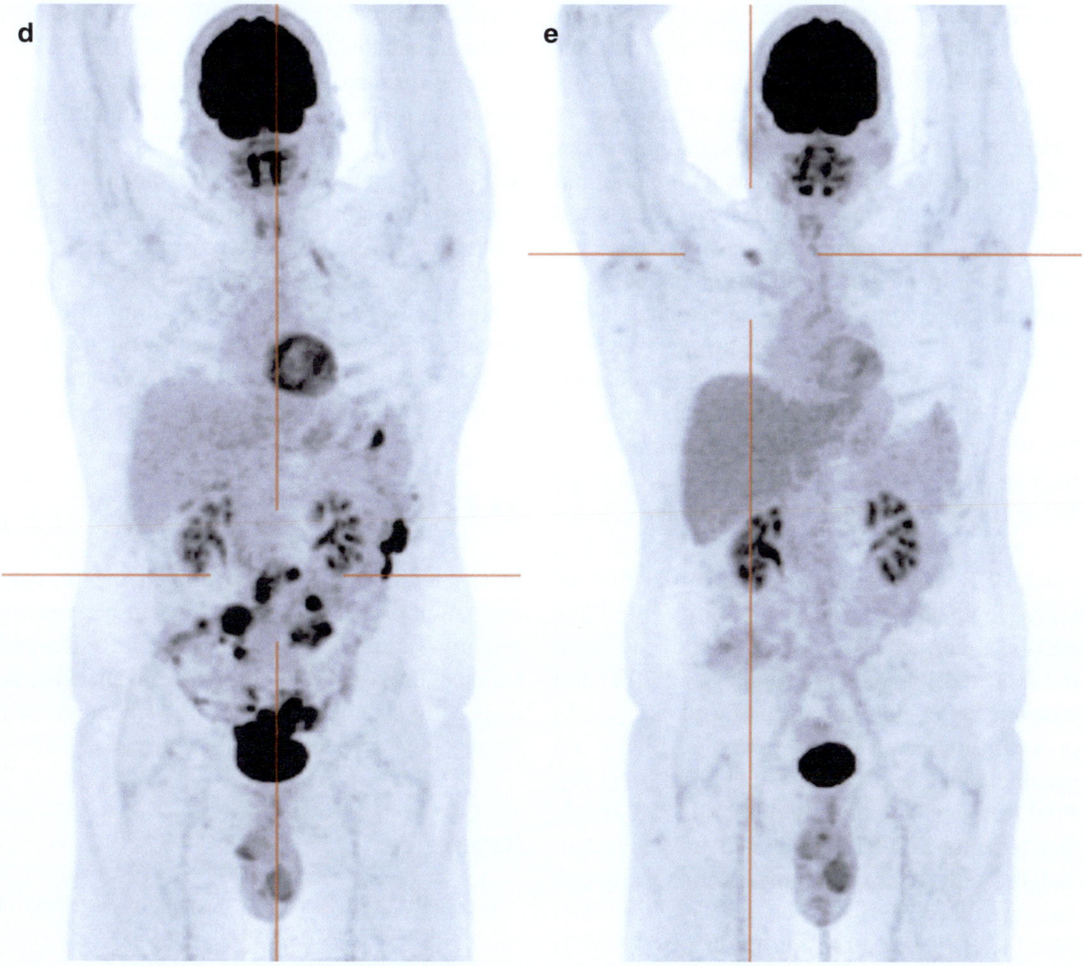

Fig. 24.6 (continued)

performance of FDG PET or PET/CT in the post-chemotherapy management of patients with GCT [125, 129, 133–143]. Recently, Treglia et al. published a meta-analysis about the diagnostic performance of FDG PET and PET/CT in the post-chemotherapy management of patients with seminoma [144]. Nine studies including 375 scans were included. The pooled analysis demonstrated sensitivity 78%, specificity 86%, PPV 58%, NPV 94%, and accuracy 84%. A better diagnostic accuracy of FDG PET or PET/CT in evaluating residual/recurrent lesions >3 cm compared to those <3 cm was found. However, possible sources of false-negative and false-positive results for post-chemotherapy residual/recurrent seminoma at FDG PET or PET/CT should be kept in mind. False-negative findings may be due to small lesions (with size below the resolution of the method) or with low proliferative activity (and consequently low FDG uptake). False-positive results may be due to inflammatory lesions. The results of the meta-analysis support the role of FDG PET or PET/CT in the post-chemotherapy management of patients with seminoma [144]. Bachner et al. [133] performed a retrospective validation of the large SEMPET trial published in 2004 [136]. A total of 11 centers participated and a total of 127 FDG PET studies were evaluated. The authors compared PET scans carried out before and after a cut-off level of 6 weeks after the end of the last chemotherapy cycle. PET sensitivity, specificity, NPV, and PPV were 50%, 77%, 91%, and 25%, respectively, before the cut-off and 82%, 90%, 95%, and 69% after the cut-off. PET accuracy significantly improved from 73% before to 88% after the cut-off ($p = 0.032$).

The presence of vital carcinoma and mature teratoma is common (55%) in residual masses in patients with NSGCT. In patients with metastatic NSGCT, residual masses after cisplatin-based combination chemotherapy consist of necrosis in 40%, persisting vital carcinoma in 20%, and mature teratoma in 40% of patients [145]. Oechsle et al. conducted a large prospective multicenter study in order to evaluate the accuracy of FDG PET in NSGCT for the prediction of histology compared with CT and serum tumor markers [139]. A total of 121 patients with stage IIC or III NSGCT scheduled for secondary resection after cisplatin-based CTX were included. FDG PET was performed after completion of CTX. Prediction of tumor viability with FDG PET was correct in 56%, which did not reach the expected clinically relevant level of 70%, and was not better than the accuracy of CT (55%) or serum tumor markers (56%). Sensitivity and specificity of FDG PET were 70% and 48% [139]. PPV were not significantly different (55%, 61%, and 59% for CT, STM, and PET, respectively). Judging only vital carcinoma as true malignant finding, the NPV increased to 83% for FDG PET [139]. The results indicate that in NSGCT, FDG-PET is less helpful in predicting histology in residual masses after chemotherapy than in patients with pure seminomatous GCT. Whether NSGCT has lower FDG uptake than seminoma remains to be evaluated further in the future in prospective large-scale studies.

24.4.4.1 Other Agents for Testicular Cancer

Until recently, FDG has been the only radiotracer used for PET imaging of GCT. Increased uptake of FDG is regarded as an indicator of viable tumor. However, FDG uptake is not specific for tumor; inflammatory and granulomatous tissues also show FDG accumulation. The role of FDG PET in staging non-seminomatous GCT residues is limited because FDG PET cannot differentiate mature teratoma from necrosis and fibrosis. The thymidine analog F-18-fluorothymidine (FLT) is a cell proliferation marker. Recently, A small study investigated the addition of FLT PET to FDG PET for early response monitoring and prediction of the histology of residual tumor masses in patients with metastatic GCT [87, 146]. The authors concluded that despite the lower incidence of false-positive results with FLT PET than with FDG PET, PET-negative residual masses after chemotherapy of metastatic non-seminomatous GCT still require resection, because the low negative predictive value of FDG PET cannot be improved by the application of the proliferation marker FLT [146].

24.4.5 Summary

FDG PET/CT has still no role in the primary evaluation of a scrotal mass, but can be used for primary staging in GCT. For the detection of residual disease, FDG PET/CT is an accurate diagnostic method in the post-chemotherapy management of patients with seminoma.

References

1. Sahni VA, Silverman SG. Imaging management of incidentally detected small renal masses. Semin Intervent Radiol. 2014;31:9–19.
2. Caldarella C, Muoio B, Isgro MA, Porfiri E, Treglia G, Giovanella L. The role of fluorine-18-fluorodeoxyglucose positron emission tomography in evaluating the response to tyrosine-kinase inhibitors in patients with metastatic primary renal cell carcinoma. Radiol Oncol. 2014;48:219–27.
3. Gofrit ON, Orevi M. Diagnostic challenges of kidney cancer: a systematic review of the role of positron emission tomography-computerized tomography. J Urol. 2016;196:648–57.
4. Makis W, Ciarallo A, Rakheja R, Probst S, Hickeson M, Rush C, Novales-Diaz JA, Derbekyan V, Stern J, Lisbona R. Spectrum of malignant renal and urinary bladder tumors on 18F-FDG PET/CT: a pictorial essay. Clin Imaging. 2012;36:660–73.
5. Oyama N, Ito H, Takahara N, Miwa Y, Akino H, Kudo T, Okazawa H, Fujibayashi Y, Komatsu K, Tsukahara K, et al. Diagnosis of complex renal cystic masses and solid renal lesions using PET imaging: comparison of 11C-acetate and 18F-FDG PET imaging. Clin Nucl Med. 2014;39:e208–14.
6. Aras M, Dede F, Ones T, Inanir S, Erdil TY, Turoglu HT. Is the value of FDG PET/CT in evaluating renal

metastasis underestimated? A case report and review of the literature. Mol Imaging Radionucl Ther. 2013;22:109–12.
7. Nakaigawa N, Kondo K, Tateishi U, Minamimoto R, Kaneta T, Namura K, Ueno D, Kobayashi K, Kishida T, Ikeda I, et al. FDG PET/CT as a prognostic biomarker in the era of molecular-targeting therapies: max SUVmax predicts survival of patients with advanced renal cell carcinoma. BMC Cancer. 2015;16:67.
8. Czarnecka AM, Kornakiewicz A, Kukwa W, Szczylik C. Frontiers in clinical and molecular diagnostics and staging of metastatic clear cell renal cell carcinoma. Future Oncol. 2014;10:1095–111.
9. Ravina M, Hess S, Chauhan MS, Jacob MJ, Alavi A. Tumor thrombus: ancillary findings on FDG PET/CT in an oncologic population. Clin Nucl Med. 2014;39:767–71.
10. Kelly-Morland C, Rudman S, Nathan P, Mallett S, Montana G, Cook G, Goh V. Evaluation of treatment response and resistance in metastatic renal cell cancer (mRCC) using integrated (18)F-Fluorodeoxyglucose ((18)F-FDG) positron emission tomography/magnetic resonance imaging (PET/MRI); The REMAP study. BMC Cancer. 2017;17:392.
11. Smaldone MC, Uzzo RG. Balancing process and risk: standardizing posttreatment surveillance for renal cell carcinoma. J Urol. 2013;190:417–8.
12. Chen JL, Appelbaum DE, Kocherginsky M, Cowey CL, Rathmell WK, McDermott DF, Stadler WM. FDG-PET as a predictive biomarker for therapy with everolimus in metastatic renal cell cancer. Cancer Med. 2013;2:545–52.
13. Ferda J, Ferdova E, Hora M, Hes O, Finek J, Topolcan O, Kreuzberg B. 18F-FDG-PET/CT in potentially advanced renal cell carcinoma: a role in treatment decisions and prognosis estimation. Anticancer Res. 2013;33:2665–72.
14. Kakizoe M, Yao M, Tateishi U, Minamimoto R, Ueno D, Namura K, Makiyama K, Hayashi N, Sano F, Kishida T, et al. The early response of renal cell carcinoma to tyrosine kinase inhibitors evaluated by FDG PET/CT was not influenced by metastatic organ. BMC Cancer. 2014;14:390.
15. Farnebo J, Gryback P, Harmenberg U, Laurell A, Wersall P, Blomqvist LK, Ullen A, Sandstrom P. Volumetric FDG-PET predicts overall and progression-free survival after 14 days of targeted therapy in metastatic renal cell carcinoma. BMC Cancer. 2014;14:408.
16. Yoon HJ, Paeng JC, Kwak C, Park YH, Kim TM, Lee SH, Chung JK, Edmund Kim E, Lee DS. Prognostic implication of extrarenal metabolic tumor burden in advanced renal cell carcinoma treated with targeted therapy after nephrectomy. Ann Nucl Med. 2013;27:748–55.
17. Nakajima R, Matsuo Y, Kondo T, Abe K, Sakai S. Prognostic value of metabolic tumor volume and total lesion glycolysis on preoperative 18F-FDG PET/CT in patients with renal cell carcinoma. Clin Nucl Med. 2017;42:e177–82.
18. Fuccio C, Spinapolice EG, Cavalli C, Palumbo R, D'Ambrosio D, Trifiro G. 18F-Fluoride PET/CT in the detection of bone metastases in clear cell renal cell carcinoma: discordance with bone scintigraphy. Eur J Nucl Med Mol Imaging. 2013;40:1930–1.
19. Divgi CR, Uzzo RG, Gatsonis C, Bartz R, Treutner S, Yu JQ, Chen D, Carrasquillo JA, Larson S, Bevan P, et al. Positron emission tomography/computed tomography identification of clear cell renal cell carcinoma: results from the REDECT trial. J Clin Oncol. 2013;31:187–94.
20. Cheal SM, Punzalan B, Doran MG, Evans MJ, Osborne JR, Lewis JS, Zanzonico P, Larson SM. Pairwise comparison of 89Zr- and 124I-labeled cG250 based on positron emission tomography imaging and nonlinear immunokinetic modeling: in vivo carbonic anhydrase IX receptor binding and internalization in mouse xenografts of clear-cell renal cell carcinoma. Eur J Nucl Med Mol Imaging. 2014;41:985–94.
21. Turkbey B, Lindenberg ML, Adler S, Kurdziel KA, McKinney YL, Weaver J, Vocke CD, Anver M, Bratslavsky G, Eclarinal P, et al. PET/CT imaging of renal cell carcinoma with (18)F-VM4-037: a phase II pilot study. Abdom Radiol (NY). 2016;41:109–18.
22. Ammari S, Thiam R, Cuenod CA, Oudard S, Hernigou A, Grataloup C, Siauve N, Medioni J, Fournier LS. Radiological evaluation of response to treatment: application to metastatic renal cancers receiving anti-angiogenic treatment. Diagn Interv Imaging. 2014;95:527–39.
23. Einspieler I, Tauber R, Maurer T, Schwaiger M, Eiber M. 68Ga prostate-specific membrane antigen uptake in renal cell cancer lymph node metastases. Clin Nucl Med. 2016;41:e261–2.
24. Sawicki LM, Buchbender C, Boos J, Giessing M, Ermert J, Antke C, Antoch G, Hautzel H. Diagnostic potential of PET/CT using a (68)Ga-labelled prostate-specific membrane antigen ligand in whole-body staging of renal cell carcinoma: initial experience. Eur J Nucl Med Mol Imaging. 2017;44:102–7.
25. Rhee H, Ng KL, Tse BW, Yeh MC, Russell PJ, Nelson C, Thomas P, Samaratunga H, Vela I, Gobe G, et al. Using prostate specific membrane antigen (PSMA) expression in clear cell renal cell carcinoma for imaging advanced disease. Pathology. 2016;48:613–6.
26. Rowe SP, Gorin MA, Hammers HJ, Pomper MG, Allaf ME, Javadi MS. Detection of 18F-FDG PET/CT occult lesions with 18F-DCFPyL PET/CT in a patient with metastatic renal cell carcinoma. Clin Nucl Med. 2016;41:83–5.
27. Rowe SP, Gorin MA, Hammers HJ, Som Javadi M, Hawasli H, Szabo Z, Cho SY, Pomper MG, Allaf ME. Imaging of metastatic clear cell renal cell carcinoma with PSMA-targeted (18)F-DCFPyL PET/CT. Ann Nucl Med. 2015;29:877–82.

28. Vamadevan S, Le K, Shen L, Loh H, Mansberg R. 68Ga-DOTATATE uptake in solitary pancreatic metastasis from clear cell renal cancer. Clin Nucl Med. 2017;42:700–1.
29. Vamadevan S, Le K, Shen L, Stevanovic A, Loh H, Mansberg R. 68Ga-DOTATATE uptake in a soft tissue metastasis from clear cell renal cell cancer. Clin Nucl Med. 2018;43:44–5.
30. van Es SC, Brouwers AH, Mahesh SVK, Leliveld-Kors AM, de Jong IJ, Lub-de Hooge MN, de Vries EGE, Gietema JA, Oosting SF. (89)Zr-Bevacizumab PET: potential early indicator of everolimus efficacy in patients with metastatic renal cell carcinoma. J Nucl Med. 2017;58:905–10.
31. Siegel RL, Miller KD, Jemal A. Cancer statistics, 2016. CA Cancer J Clin. 2016;66:7–30.
32. Abdollah F, Gandaglia G, Thuret R, Schmitges J, Tian Z, Jeldres C, Passoni NM, Briganti A, Shariat SF, Perrotte P, et al. Incidence, survival and mortality rates of stage-specific bladder cancer in United States: a trend analysis. Cancer Epidemiol. 2013;37:219–25.
33. Kaufman DS, Shipley WU, Feldman AS. Bladder cancer. Lancet. 2009;374:239–49.
34. Parkin DM. The global burden of urinary bladder cancer. Scand J Urol Nephrol Suppl. 2008:12–20.
35. Burger M, Catto JW, Dalbagni G, Grossman HB, Herr H, Karakiewicz P, Kassouf W, Kiemeney LA, La Vecchia C, Shariat S, et al. Epidemiology and risk factors of urothelial bladder cancer. Eur Urol. 2013;63:234–41.
36. Green DA, Rink M, Xylinas E, Matin SF, Stenzl A, Roupret M, Karakiewicz PI, Scherr DS, Shariat SF. Urothelial carcinoma of the bladder and the upper tract: disparate twins. J Urol. 2013;189:1214–21.
37. Crivelli JJ, Xylinas E, Kluth LA, Rieken M, Rink M, Shariat SF. Effect of smoking on outcomes of urothelial carcinoma: a systematic review of the literature. Eur Urol. 2014;65:742–54.
38. Kirkali Z, Chan T, Manoharan M, Algaba F, Busch C, Cheng L, Kiemeney L, Kriegmair M, Montironi R, Murphy WM, et al. Bladder cancer: epidemiology, staging and grading, and diagnosis. Urology. 2005;66:4–34.
39. Gandini S, Botteri E, Iodice S, Boniol M, Lowenfels AB, Maisonneuve P, Boyle P. Tobacco smoking and cancer: a meta-analysis. Int J Cancer. 2008;122:155–64.
40. Bouchelouche K. Diagnostic applications of nuclear medicine: kidney and bladder cancer. In: Strauss HW, Mariani G, Volterrani D, Larson SM, editors. Nuclear oncology. From pathophysiology to clinical applications. 2nd ed. New York: Springer; 2017. p. 839–81.
41. Barocas DA, Clark PE. Bladder cancer. Curr Opin Oncol. 2008;20:307–14.
42. Bischoff CJ, Clark PE. Bladder cancer. Curr Opin Oncol. 2009;21:272–7.
43. Kurth KH, Schellhammer PF, Okajima E, Akdas A, Jakse G, Herr HW, Calais da Silva F, Fukushima S, Nagayama T. Current methods of assessing and treating carcinoma in situ of the bladder with or without involvement of the prostatic urethra. Int J Urol. 1995;2(Suppl 2):8–22.
44. van Rhijn BW, van der Poel HG, van der Kwast TH. Urine markers for bladder cancer surveillance: a systematic review. Eur Urol. 2005;47:736–48.
45. Burger M, Grossman HB, Droller M, Schmidbauer J, Hermann G, Dragoescu O, Ray E, Fradet Y, Karl A, Burgues JP, et al. Photodynamic diagnosis of non-muscle-invasive bladder cancer with hexaminolevulinate cystoscopy: a meta-analysis of detection and recurrence based on raw data. Eur Urol. 2013;64:846–54.
46. Rink M, Babjuk M, Catto JW, Jichlinski P, Shariat SF, Stenzl A, Stepp H, Zaak D, Witjes JA. Hexyl aminolevulinate-guided fluorescence cystoscopy in the diagnosis and follow-up of patients with non-muscle-invasive bladder cancer: a critical review of the current literature. Eur Urol. 2013;64:624–38.
47. Malmstrom PU, Grabe M, Haug ES, Hellstrom P, Hermann GG, Mogensen K, Raitanen M, Wahlqvist R. Role of hexaminolevulinate-guided fluorescence cystoscopy in bladder cancer: critical analysis of the latest data and European guidance. Scand J Urol Nephrol. 2012;46:108–16.
48. Tsakiris P, de la Rosette J. Imaging in genitourinary cancer from the urologists' perspective. Cancer Imaging. 2007;7:84–92.
49. Lawrentschuk N, Lee ST, Scott AM. Current role of PET, CT, MR for invasive bladder cancer. Curr Urol Rep. 2013;14:84–9.
50. Takeuchi M, Sasaki S, Naiki T, Kawai N, Kohri K, Hara M, Shibamoto Y. MR imaging of urinary bladder cancer for T-staging: a review and a pictorial essay of diffusion-weighted imaging. J Magn Reson Imaging. 2013;38:1299–309.
51. Paik ML, Scolieri MJ, Brown SL, Spirnak JP, Resnick MI. Limitations of computerized tomography in staging invasive bladder cancer before radical cystectomy. J Urol. 2000;163:1693–6.
52. Hafeez S, Huddart R. Advances in bladder cancer imaging. BMC Med. 2013;11:104.
53. Vikram R, Sandler CM, Ng CS. Imaging and staging of transitional cell carcinoma: Part 1, Lower urinary tract. AJR Am J Roentgenol. 2009;192:1481–7.
54. Knox MK, Cowan NC, Rivers-Bowerman MD, Turney BW. Evaluation of multidetector computed tomography urography and ultrasonography for diagnosing bladder cancer. Clin Radiol. 2008;63:1317–25.
55. Sadow CA, Silverman SG, O'Leary MP, Signorovitch JE. Bladder cancer detection with CT urography in an Academic Medical Center. Radiology. 2008;249:195–202.
56. Bouchelouche K, Turkbey B, Choyke PL. PET/CT and MRI in bladder cancer. J Cancer Sci Ther. 2012;S14:7692.
57. Verma S, Rajesh A, Prasad SR, Gaitonde K, Lall CG, Mouraviev V, Aeron G, Bracken RB, Sandrasegaran

K. Urinary bladder cancer: role of MR imaging. Radiographics. 2012;32:371–87.
58. Beyersdorff D, Zhang J, Schoder H, Bochner B, Hricak H. Bladder cancer: can imaging change patient management? Curr Opin Urol. 2008;18:98–104.
59. Zhang J, Gerst S, Lefkowitz RA, Bach A. Imaging of bladder cancer. Radiol Clin N Am. 2007;45:183–205.
60. Witjes JA, Comperat E, Cowan NC, De Santis M, Gakis G, Lebret T, Ribal MJ, Van der Heijden AG, Sherif A, European Association of Urology. EAU guidelines on muscle-invasive and metastatic bladder cancer: summary of the 2013 guidelines. Eur Urol. 2014;65:778–92.
61. Bouchelouche K, Choyke PL. PET/computed tomography in renal, bladder, and testicular cancer. PET Clin. 2015;10:361–74.
62. Mertens LS, Bruin NM, Vegt E, de Blok WM, Fioole-Bruining A, van Rhijn BW, Horenblas S, Vogel WV. Catheter-assisted 18F-FDG-PET/CT imaging of primary bladder cancer: a prospective study. Nucl Med Commun. 2012;33:1195–201.
63. Mertens LS, Fioole-Bruining A, Vegt E, Vogel WV, van Rhijn BW, Horenblas S. Detecting primary bladder cancer using delayed (18)F-2-fluoro-2-deoxy-D-glucose-positron emission tomography/computed tomography imaging after forced diuresis. Indian J Nucl Med. 2012;27:145–50.
64. Chondrogiannis S, Marzola MC, Colletti PM, Rubello D. Proposal of a new acquisition protocol for bladder cancer visualization with 18F-FDG PET/CT. Clin Nucl Med. 2015;40:e78–80.
65. Anjos DA, Etchebehere EC, Ramos CD, Santos AO, Albertotti C, Camargo EE. 18F-FDG PET/CT delayed images after diuretic for restaging invasive bladder cancer. J Nucl Med. 2007;48:764–70.
66. Yang Z, Cheng J, Pan L, Hu S, Xu J, Zhang Y, Wang M, Zhang J, Ye D, Zhang Y. Is whole-body fluorine-18 fluorodeoxyglucose PET/CT plus additional pelvic images (oral hydration-voiding-refilling) useful for detecting recurrent bladder cancer? Ann Nucl Med. 2012;26:571–7.
67. Harkirat S, Anand S, Jacob M. Forced diuresis and dual-phase F-fluorodeoxyglucose-PET/CT scan for restaging of urinary bladder cancers. Indian J Radiol Imaging. 2010;20:13–9.
68. Yildirim-Poyraz N, Ozdemir E, Uzun B, Turkolmez S. Dual phase 18F-fluorodeoxyglucose positron emission tomography/computed tomography with forced diuresis in diagnostic imaging evaluation of bladder cancer. Rev Esp Med Nucl Imagen Mol. 2013;32:214–21.
69. Yoon HJ, Yoo J, Kim Y, Lee DH, Kim BS. Enhanced application of 18F-FDG PET/CT in bladder cancer by adding early dynamic acquisition to a standard delayed PET protocol. Clin Nucl Med. 2017;42:749–55.
70. Wang N, Jiang P, Lu Y. Is fluorine-18 fluorodeoxyglucose positron emission tomography useful for detecting bladder lesions? A meta-analysis of the literature. Urol Int. 2014;92:143–9.
71. Rosenkrantz AB, Balar AV, Huang WC, Jackson K, Friedman KP. Comparison of coregistration accuracy of pelvic structures between sequential and simultaneous imaging during hybrid PET/MRI in patients with bladder cancer. Clin Nucl Med. 2015;40:637–41.
72. Rosenkrantz AB, Friedman KP, Ponzo F, Raad RA, Jackson K, Huang WC, Balar AV. Prospective pilot study to evaluate the incremental value of PET information in patients with bladder cancer undergoing 18F-FDG simultaneous PET/MRI. Clin Nucl Med. 2017;42:e8–e15.
73. Swinnen G, Maes A, Pottel H, Vanneste A, Billiet I, Lesage K, Werbrouck P. FDG-PET/CT for the preoperative lymph node staging of invasive bladder cancer. Eur Urol. 2010;57:641–7.
74. Drieskens O, Oyen R, Van Poppel H, Vankan Y, Flamen P, Mortelmans L. FDG-PET for preoperative staging of bladder cancer. Eur J Nucl Med Mol Imaging. 2005;32:1412–7.
75. Bachor R, Kotzerke J, Reske SN, Hautmann R. [Lymph node staging of bladder neck carcinoma with positron emission tomography]. Urologe A. 1999;38:46–50.
76. Kosuda S, Kison PV, Greenough R, Grossman HB, Wahl RL. Preliminary assessment of fluorine-18 fluorodeoxyglucose positron emission tomography in patients with bladder cancer. Eur J Nucl Med. 1997;24:615–20.
77. Jensen JB, Ulhoi BP, Jensen KM. Lymph node mapping in patients with bladder cancer undergoing radical cystectomy and lymph node dissection to the level of the inferior mesenteric artery. BJU Int. 2010;106:199–205.
78. Mertens LS, Fioole-Bruining A, Vegt E, Vogel WV, van Rhijn BW, Horenblas S. Impact of (18) F-fluorodeoxyglucose (FDG)-positron-emission tomography/computed tomography (PET/CT) on management of patients with carcinoma invading bladder muscle. BJU Int. 2013;112:729–34.
79. Apolo AB, Riches J, Schoder H, Akin O, Trout A, Milowsky MI, Bajorin DF. Clinical value of fluorine-18 2-fluoro-2-deoxy-D-glucose positron emission tomography/computed tomography in bladder cancer. J Clin Oncol. 2010;28:3973–8.
80. Kibel AS, Dehdashti F, Katz MD, Klim AP, Grubb RL, Humphrey PA, Siegel C, Cao D, Gao F, Siegel BA. Prospective study of [18F]fluorodeoxyglucose positron emission tomography/computed tomography for staging of muscle-invasive bladder carcinoma. J Clin Oncol. 2009;27:4314–20.
81. Liu IJ, Lai YH, Espiritu JI, Segall GM, Srinivas S, Nino-Murcia M, Terris MK. Evaluation of fluorodeoxyglucose positron emission tomography imaging in metastatic transitional cell carcinoma with and without prior chemotherapy. Urol Int. 2006;77:69–75.
82. Jensen TK, Holt P, Gerke O, Riehmann M, Svolgaard B, Marcussen N, Bouchelouche K. Preoperative lymph-node staging of invasive urothelial bladder

cancer with 18F-fluorodeoxyglucose positron emission tomography/computed axial tomography and magnetic resonance imaging: correlation with histopathology. Scand J Urol Nephrol. 2011;45:122–8.
83. Vind-Kezunovic S, Bouchelouche K, Ipsen P, Hoyer S, Bell C, Bjerggaard Jensen J. Detection of lymph node metastasis in patients with bladder cancer using maximum standardised uptake value and (18) F-fluorodeoxyglucose positron emission tomography/computed tomography: results from a high-volume centre including long-term follow-up. Eur Urol Focus. 2019;5(1):90–6.
84. Soubra A, Hayward D, Dahm P, Goldfarb R, Froehlich J, Jha G, Konety BR. The diagnostic accuracy of 18F-fluorodeoxyglucose positron emission tomography and computed tomography in staging bladder cancer: a single-institution study and a systematic review with meta-analysis. World J Urol. 2016;34(9):1229–37.
85. Lodde M, Lacombe L, Friede J, Morin F, Saourine A, Fradet Y. Evaluation of fluorodeoxyglucose positron-emission tomography with computed tomography for staging of urothelial carcinoma. BJU Int. 2010;106:658–63.
86. Nayak B, Dogra PN, Naswa N, Kumar R. Diuretic 18F-FDG PET/CT imaging for detection and locoregional staging of urinary bladder cancer: prospective evaluation of a novel technique. Eur J Nucl Med Mol Imaging. 2013;40:386–93.
87. Goodfellow H, Viney Z, Hughes P, Rankin S, Rottenberg G, Hughes S, Evison F, Dasgupta P, O'Brien T, Khan MS. Role of fluorodeoxyglucose positron emission tomography (FDG PET)-computed tomography (CT) in the staging of bladder cancer. BJU Int. 2014;114:389–95.
88. Hitier-Berthault M, Ansquer C, Branchereau J, Renaudin K, Bodere F, Bouchot O, Rigaud J. 18 F-fluorodeoxyglucose positron emission tomography-computed tomography for preoperative lymph node staging in patients undergoing radical cystectomy for bladder cancer: a prospective study. Int J Urol. 2013;20:788–96.
89. Lu YY, Chen JH, Liang JA, Wang HY, Lin CC, Lin WY, Kao CH. Clinical value of FDG PET or PET/CT in urinary bladder cancer: a systemic review and meta-analysis. Eur J Radiol. 2012;81:2411–6.
90. Jadvar H, Quan V, Henderson RW, Conti PS. [F-18]-Fluorodeoxyglucose PET and PET-CT in diagnostic imaging evaluation of locally recurrent and metastatic bladder transitional cell carcinoma. Int J Clin Oncol. 2008;13:42–7.
91. Alongi P, Caobelli F, Gentile R, Stefano A, Russo G, Albano D, Baldari S, Gilardi MC, Midiri M. Recurrent bladder carcinoma: clinical and prognostic role of 18 F-FDG PET/CT. Eur J Nucl Med Mol Imaging. 2017;44:224–33.
92. Meeks JJ, Bellmunt J, Bochner BH, Clarke NW, Daneshmand S, Galsky MD, Hahn NM, Lerner SP, Mason M, Powles T, et al. A systematic review of neoadjuvant and adjuvant chemotherapy for muscle-invasive bladder cancer. Eur Urol. 2012;62:523–33.
93. Mertens LS, Fioole-Bruining A, van Rhijn BW, Kerst JM, Bergman AM, Vogel WV, Vegt E, Horenblas S. FDG-positron emission tomography/computerized tomography for monitoring the response of pelvic lymph node metastasis to neoadjuvant chemotherapy for bladder cancer. J Urol. 2013;189:1687–91.
94. Kollberg P, Almquist H, Blackberg M, Cwikiel M, Gudjonsson S, Lyttkens K, Patschan O, Liedberg F. [(18)F]Fluorodeoxyglucose-positron emission tomography/computed tomography response evaluation can predict histological response at surgery after induction chemotherapy for oligometastatic bladder cancer. Scand J Urol. 2017;51:308–13.
95. van de Putte EEF, Vegt E, Mertens LS, Bruining A, Hendricksen K, van der Heijden MS, Horenblas S, van Rhijn BWG. FDG-PET/CT for response evaluation of invasive bladder cancer following neoadjuvant chemotherapy. Int Urol Nephrol. 2017;49:1585–91.
96. Giannatempo P, Alessi A, Miceli R, Raggi D, Fare E, Nicolai N, Serafini G, Padovano B, Piva L, Biasoni D, et al. Interim fluorine-18 fluorodeoxyglucose positron emission tomography for early metabolic assessment of therapeutic response to chemotherapy for metastatic transitional cell carcinoma. Clin Genitourin Cancer. 2014;12:433–9.
97. Mertens LS, Mir MC, Scott AM, Lee ST, Fioole-Bruining A, Vegt E, Vogel WV, Manecksha R, Bolton D, Davis ID, et al. 18F-fluorodeoxyglucose—positron emission tomography/computed tomography aids staging and predicts mortality in patients with muscle-invasive bladder cancer. Urology. 2014;83:393–8.
98. Bouchelouche K, Turkbey B, Choyke PL. PSMA PET and radionuclide therapy in prostate cancer. Semin Nucl Med. 2016;46:522–35.
99. Campbell SP, Baras AS, Ball MW, Kates M, Hahn NM, Bivalacqua TJ, Johnson MH, Pomper MG, Allaf ME, Rowe SP, et al. Low levels of PSMA expression limit the utility of (18)F-DCFPyL PET/CT for imaging urothelial carcinoma. Ann Nucl Med. 2018;32:69–74.
100. Picchio M, Treiber U, Beer AJ, Metz S, Bossner P, van Randenborgh H, Paul R, Weirich G, Souvatzoglou M, Hartung R, et al. Value of 11C-choline PET and contrast-enhanced CT for staging of bladder cancer: correlation with histopathologic findings. J Nucl Med. 2006;47:938–44.
101. Gofrit ON, Mishani E, Orevi M, Klein M, Freedman N, Pode D, Shapiro A, Katz R, Libson E, Chisin R. Contribution of 11C-choline positron emission tomography/computerized tomography to preoperative staging of advanced transitional cell carcinoma. J Urol. 2006;176:940–4; discussion 944.
102. Brunocilla E, Ceci F, Schiavina R, Castellucci P, Maffione AM, Cevenini M, Bianchi L, Borghesi M, Giunchi F, Fiorentino M, et al. Diagnostic accuracy of (11)C-choline PET/CT in preoperative lymph

node staging of bladder cancer: a systematic comparison with contrast-enhanced CT and histologic findings. Clin Nucl Med. 2014;39:e308–12.
103. de Jong IJ, Pruim J, Elsinga PH, Jongen MM, Mensink HJ, Vaalburg W. Visualisation of bladder cancer using (11)C-choline PET: first clinical experience. Eur J Nucl Med Mol Imaging. 2002;29:1283–8.
104. Maurer T, Horn T, Souvatzoglou M, Eiber M, Beer AJ, Heck MM, Haller B, Gschwend JE, Schwaiger M, Treiber U, et al. Prognostic value of 11C-choline PET/CT and CT for predicting survival of bladder cancer patients treated with radical cystectomy. Urol Int. 2014;93:207–13.
105. Graziani T, Ceci F, Lopes FL, Chichero J, Castellucci P, Schiavina R, Bianchi L, Chondrogiannis S, Colletti PM, Costa S, et al. 11C-choline PET/CT for restaging of bladder cancer. Clin Nucl Med. 2015;40:e1–5.
106. Maurer T, Souvatzoglou M, Kubler H, Opercan K, Schmidt S, Herrmann K, Stollfuss J, Weirich G, Haller B, Gschwend JE, et al. Diagnostic efficacy of [11C]choline positron emission tomography/computed tomography compared with conventional computed tomography in lymph node staging of patients with bladder cancer prior to radical cystectomy. Eur Urol. 2012;61:1031–8.
107. Ahlstrom H, Malmstrom PU, Letocha H, Andersson J, Langstrom B, Nilsson S. Positron emission tomography in the diagnosis and staging of urinary bladder cancer. Acta Radiol. 1996;37:180–5.
108. Letocha H, Ahlstrom H, Malmstrom PU, Westlin JE, Fasth KJ, Nilsson S. Positron emission tomography with L-methyl-11C-methionine in the monitoring of therapy response in muscle-invasive transitional cell carcinoma of the urinary bladder. Br J Urol. 1994;74:767–74.
109. Vargas HA, Akin O, Schoder H, Olgac S, Dalbagni G, Hricak H, Bochner BH. Prospective evaluation of MRI, (1)(1)C-acetate PET/CT and contrast-enhanced CT for staging of bladder cancer. Eur J Radiol. 2012;81:4131–7.
110. Orevi M, Klein M, Mishani E, Chisin R, Freedman N, Gofrit ON. 11C-acetate PET/CT in bladder urothelial carcinoma: intraindividual comparison with 11C-choline. Clin Nucl Med. 2012;37:e67–72.
111. Chakraborty D, Bhattacharya A, Mete UK, Mittal BR. Comparison of 18F fluoride PET/CT and 99mTc-MDP bone scan in the detection of skeletal metastases in urinary bladder carcinoma. Clin Nucl Med. 2013;38:616–21.
112. Patil VV, Wang ZJ, Sollitto RA, Chuang KW, Konety BR, Hawkins RA, Coakley FV. 18F-FDG PET/CT of transitional cell carcinoma. AJR Am J Roentgenol. 2009;193:W497–504.
113. Asai S, Fukumoto T, Tanji N, Miura N, Miyagawa M, Nishimura K, Yanagihara Y, Shirato A, Miyauchi Y, Kikugawa T, et al. Fluorodeoxyglucose positron emission tomography/computed tomography for diagnosis of upper urinary tract urothelial carcinoma. Int J Clin Oncol. 2015;20:1042–7.
114. Tanaka H, Yoshida S, Komai Y, Sakai Y, Urakami S, Yuasa T, Yamamoto S, Masuda H, Koizumi M, Kohno A, et al. Clinical value of 18F-fluorodeoxyglucose positron emission tomography/computed tomography in upper tract urothelial carcinoma: impact on detection of metastases and patient management. Urol Int. 2016;96:65–72.
115. Kitajima K, Yamamoto S, Fukushima K, Yamakado K, Katsuura T, Igarashi Y, Kawanaka Y, Mouri M, Hirota S. FDG-PET/CT as a post-treatment restaging tool in urothelial carcinoma: comparison with contrast-enhanced CT. Eur J Radiol. 2016;85:593–8.
116. Albers P, Albrecht W, Algaba F, Bokemeyer C, Cohn-Cedermark G, Fizazi K, Horwich A, Laguna MP, European Association of Urology. EAU guidelines on testicular cancer: 2011 update. Eur Urol. 2011;60:304–19.
117. Manecksha RP, Fitzpatrick JM. Epidemiology of testicular cancer. BJU Int. 2009;104:1329–33.
118. Horwich A, Shipley J, Huddart R. Testicular germ-cell cancer. Lancet. 2006;367:754–65.
119. Flechon A, Rivoire M, Droz JP. Management of advanced germ-cell tumors of the testis. Nat Clin Pract Urol. 2008;5:262–76.
120. Jana S, Blaufox MD. Nuclear medicine studies of the prostate, testes, and bladder. Semin Nucl Med. 2006;36:51–72.
121. Kim W, Rosen MA, Langer JE, Banner MP, Siegelman ES, Ramchandani P. US MR imaging correlation in pathologic conditions of the scrotum. Radiographics. 2007;27:1239–53.
122. Cassidy FH, Ishioka KM, McMahon CJ, Chu P, Sakamoto K, Lee KS, Aganovic L. MR imaging of scrotal tumors and pseudotumors. Radiographics. 2010;30:665–83.
123. Johnson JO, Mattrey RF, Phillipson J. Differentiation of seminomatous from nonseminomatous testicular tumors with MR imaging. AJR Am J Roentgenol. 1990;154:539–43.
124. Shao D, Gao Q, Tian XW, Wang SY, Liang CH, Wang SX. Differentiation and diagnosis of benign and malignant testicular lesions using 18F-FDG PET/CT. Eur J Radiol. 2017;93:114–20.
125. Hain SF, O'Doherty MJ, Timothy AR, Leslie MD, Harper PG, Huddart RA. Fluorodeoxyglucose positron emission tomography in the evaluation of germ cell tumours at relapse. Br J Cancer. 2000;83:863–9.
126. Hain SF, O'Doherty MJ, Timothy AR, Leslie MD, Partridge SE, Huddart RA. Fluorodeoxyglucose PET in the initial staging of germ cell tumours. Eur J Nucl Med. 2000;27:590–4.
127. Lassen U, Daugaard G, Eigtved A, Hojgaard L, Damgaard K, Rorth M. Whole-body FDG-PET in patients with stage I non-seminomatous germ cell tumours. Eur J Nucl Med Mol Imaging. 2003;30:396–402.
128. Cremerius U, Wildberger JE, Borchers H, Zimny M, Jakse G, Gunther RW, Buell U. Does positron emission tomography using 18-fluoro-2-deoxyglucose improve clinical staging of testicular

cancer?—Results of a study in 50 patients. Urology. 1999;54:900–4.
129. Ambrosini V, Zucchini G, Nicolini S, Berselli A, Nanni C, Allegri V, Martoni A, Rubello D, Cricca A, Fanti S. 18F-FDG PET/CT impact on testicular tumours clinical management. Eur J Nucl Med Mol Imaging. 2014;41:668–73.
130. Sharma P, Jain TK, Parida GK, Karunanithi S, Patel C, Sharma A, Thulkar S, Julka PK, Bal C, Kumar R. Diagnostic accuracy of integrated (18)F-FDG PET/CT for restaging patients with malignant germ cell tumours. Br J Radiol. 2014;87:20140263.
131. Zhao JY, Ma XL, Li YY, Zhang BL, Li MM, Ma XL, Liu L. Diagnostic accuracy of 18F-FDG-PET in patients with testicular cancer: a meta-analysis. Asian Pac J Cancer Prev. 2014;15:3525–31.
132. Stomper PC, Kalish LA, Garnick MB, Richie JP, Kantoff PW. CT and pathologic predictive features of residual mass histologic findings after chemotherapy for nonseminomatous germ cell tumors: can residual malignancy or teratoma be excluded? Radiology. 1991;180:711–4.
133. Bachner M, Loriot Y, Gross-Goupil M, Zucali PA, Horwich A, Germa-Lluch JR, Kollmannsberger C, Stoiber F, Flechon A, Oechsle K, et al. 2-(1)(8) fluoro-deoxy-D-glucose positron emission tomography (FDG-PET) for postchemotherapy seminoma residual lesions: a retrospective validation of the SEMPET trial. Ann Oncol. 2012;23:59–64.
134. Hinz S, Schrader M, Kempkensteffen C, Bares R, Brenner W, Krege S, Franzius C, Kliesch S, Heicappel R, Miller K, et al. The role of positron emission tomography in the evaluation of residual masses after chemotherapy for advanced stage seminoma. J Urol. 2008;179:936–940; discussion 940.
135. Lewis DA, Tann M, Kesler K, McCool A, Foster RS, Einhorn LH. Positron emission tomography scans in postchemotherapy seminoma patients with residual masses: a retrospective review from Indiana University Hospital. J Clin Oncol. 2006;24:e54–5.
136. De Santis M, Becherer A, Bokemeyer C, Stoiber F, Oechsle K, Sellner F, Lang A, Kletter K, Dohmen BM, Dittrich C, et al. 2-18fluoro-deoxy-D-glucose positron emission tomography is a reliable predictor for viable tumor in postchemotherapy seminoma: an update of the prospective multicentric SEMPET trial. J Clin Oncol. 2004;22:1034–9.
137. Spermon JR, De Geus-Oei LF, Kiemeney LA, Witjes JA, Oyen WJ. The role of (18)fluoro-2-deoxyglucose positron emission tomography in initial staging and re-staging after chemotherapy for testicular germ cell tumours. BJU Int. 2002;89:549–56.
138. Ganjoo KN, Chan RJ, Sharma M, Einhorn LH. Positron emission tomography scans in the evaluation of postchemotherapy residual masses in patients with seminoma. J Clin Oncol. 1999;17:3457–60.
139. Oechsle K, Hartmann M, Brenner W, Venz S, Weissbach L, Franzius C, Kliesch S, Mueller S, Krege S, Heicappell R, et al. [18F]Fluorodeoxyglucose positron emission tomography in nonseminomatous germ cell tumors after chemotherapy: the German multicenter positron emission tomography study group. J Clin Oncol. 2008;26:5930–5.
140. Becherer A, De Santis M, Karanikas G, Szabo M, Bokemeyer C, Dohmen BM, Pont J, Dudczak R, Dittrich C, Kletter K. FDG PET is superior to CT in the prediction of viable tumour in post-chemotherapy seminoma residuals. Eur J Radiol. 2005;54:284–8.
141. De Santis M, Bokemeyer C, Becherer A, Stoiber F, Oechsle K, Kletter K, Dohmen BM, Dittrich C, Pont J. Predictive impact of 2-18fluoro-2-deoxy-D-glucose positron emission tomography for residual postchemotherapy masses in patients with bulky seminoma. J Clin Oncol. 2001;19:3740–4.
142. Siekiera J, Malkowski B, Jozwicki W, Jasinski M, Wronczewski A, Pietrzak T, Chmielowska E, Petrus A, Kamecki K, Mikolajczak W, et al. Can we rely on PET in the follow-up of advanced seminoma patients? Urol Int. 2012;88:405–9.
143. Cook GJ, Sohaib A, Huddart RA, Dearnaley DP, Horwich A, Chua S. The role of 18F-FDG PET/CT in the management of testicular cancers. Nucl Med Commun. 2015;36:702–8.
144. Treglia G, Sadeghi R, Annunziata S, Caldarella C, Bertagna F, Giovanella L. Diagnostic performance of fluorine-18-fluorodeoxyglucose positron emission tomography in the postchemotherapy management of patients with seminoma: systematic review and meta-analysis. Biomed Res Int. 2014;2014:852681.
145. Hartmann JT, Schmoll HJ, Kuczyk MA, Candelaria M, Bokemeyer C. Postchemotherapy resections of residual masses from metastatic non-seminomatous testicular germ cell tumors. Ann Oncol. 1997;8:531–8.
146. Pfannenberg C, Aschoff P, Dittmann H, Mayer F, Reischl G, von Weyhern C, Kanz L, Claussen CD, Bares R, Hartmann JT. PET/CT with 18F-FLT: does it improve the therapeutic management of metastatic germ cell tumors? J Nucl Med. 2010;51:845–53.

25 PSMA-Ligand Imaging in the Diagnosis of Prostate Cancer

Ali Afshar-Oromieh

During the past years, the prostate-specific membrane antigen (PSMA) has received increased attention as an excellent target for prostate carcinoma (PC) imaging and therapy. PSMA, also known as glutamate carboxypeptidase II, *N*-acetyl-α-linked acidic dipeptidase I, or folate hydrolase, is an enzyme which is significantly overexpressed in prostate cancer cells. Another advantages of PSMA are its transmembraneous location with a large extracellular domain and its enzyme activity which allows the development of specific inhibitors and their internalization after ligand binding.

Following many years of preclinical research in order to create PSMA-ligands, the broad clinical breakthrough was achieved in 2011 with the introduction of ^{68}Ga-PSMA-11 for imaging with positron emission tomography (PET) [1]. Technetium-labeled PSMA-ligands for SPECT-imaging are currently being established. This chapter, therefore, focuses on results obtained with PSMA-ligands for PET-imaging.

Currently, several PSMA-ligands are available for PET-imaging such as ^{68}Ga-PSMA-11 [2], ^{68}Ga-PSMA-I&T [3], ^{68}Ga-PSMA-617 [4], ^{18}F-DCFBC [5], ^{18}F-DCFPyL [6], and ^{18}F-PSMA-1007 [7]. However, ^{68}Ga-labelled PSMA-11 was the first tracer used for clinical routine and has also become the most frequently used ligand due to its favorable characteristics such as high tumor uptake and fast pharmacokinetics which allow favorable tumor contrast as early as 1 h post-injection. Consequently, the significant majority of publications and experiences including data about sensitivities and specificities derive from the utilization of ^{68}Ga-PSMA-11.

25.1 Physiologic Distribution of PSMA-Ligands

Despite its name, PSMA is not specific to the prostate gland. The majority of PSMA-ligands show physiological uptake in the lacrimal glands, nasal mucosa, salivary glands, glottis, spleen, liver, kidneys, and proximal parts of the small intestines and in some parts of the colon (Fig. 25.1). PSMA-ligands for imaging are mainly excreted via the urinary tract as also shown by Fig. 25.1. A physiological uptake is also seen in healthy prostate tissue. In addition, ganglions of the vegetative nervous system as well as inflammatory lymph nodes can show a slight uptake of PSMA-ligands as well (Figs. 25.2 and 25.3) [8, 9]. Ganglia can be differentiated from lymph nodes by their typical elongated extensions. Inflammatory lymph nodes present with decreasing tracer uptake intensities by time

A. Afshar-Oromieh (✉)
Department of Nuclear Medicine, Bern University Hospital, Bern, Switzerland
e-mail: ali.afshar@insel.ch

H. Ahmadzadehfar et al. (eds.), *Clinical Nuclear Medicine*,
https://doi.org/10.1007/978-3-030-39457-8_25

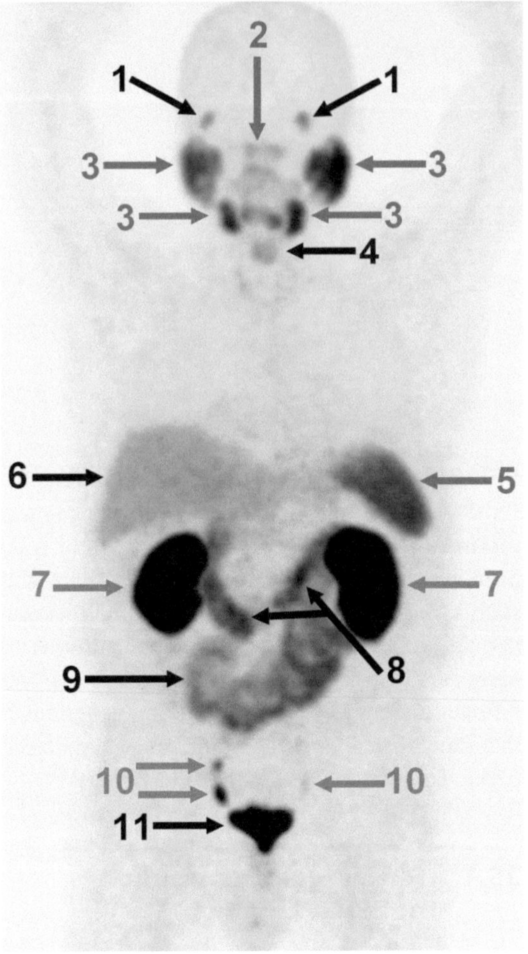

Fig. 25.1 This figure presents the maximum intensity projection of a PET scan showing the physiological distribution of the PSMA-ligand ^{68}Ga-PSMA-11. Despite its name, PSMA is not specific to the prostate gland. The majority of PSMA-ligands show physiological uptake in the lacrimal glands (1), nasal mucosa (2), salivary glands (3), glottis (4), spleen (5), liver (6), kidneys (7), and proximal parts of the small intestines (8) and in some parts of the colon (9). The tracer is excreted via the urinary tract (10: ureters and 11: urinary bladder). In addition, ganglions of the vegetative nervous system showed an uptake of the PSMA-ligand as well (not visible in the image)

in the majority of cases. In case of unclear lymph nodes (inflammatory vs. metastatic), it is recommended to conduct late scans, e.g., at 3 h p.i.: while the majority of inflammatory lymph nodes present with a decreasing uptake, the majority of lymph node metastases of prostate cancer show the opposite.

25.2 Lesion Characteristics for Prostate Cancer

Lesions of PC often present with intense uptake and contrast in PSMA-ligand PET/CT (Fig. 25.4). There is a strong variation of tracer uptake which is dependent on the PSMA expression of the lesions, though (Fig. 25.4). So far, ^{68}Ga-PSMA-11 has demonstrated a very high positive predictive value of >95% for PC in several studies [10–15]. Therefore, any uptake of ^{68}Ga-PSMA-11 above local background in lesions which are morphologically visible is highly specific for PC. However, this statement is currently valid in patients with recurrent or high-risk primary PC since uptake of PSMA-ligands in various nonprostatic tissues of benign and malignant origin has been reported in multiple publications [16]. Among the malignant tissues were the neovasculature of various solid tumors such as lymphoma, thyroid cancer, multiple myeloma, gastrointestinal stromal tumor, pancreatic cancer, hepatocellular carcinoma, colon/rectal cancer, oropharynx cancer, non-small cell lung cancer, urothelial and renal cell carcinoma, or high grade astrocytoma. Among the benign tissues were hemangiomas, desmoid tumors, thyroid adenomas, Paget disease, inflammatory processes (including sarcoidosis and activated lymph nodes), neuronal ganglia or myxomas, fibromas, or fasciitis. Probably, more PSMA-positive tissues of nonprostatic origin will be reported in the future. However, compared to most PC lesions, all of the abovementioned entities usually present with an often significantly lower PSMA-ligand uptake. Therefore, PSMA-ligand PET/CT has not yet been established for the diagnosis of any other entity than PC.

25.3 Imaging Recurrent Prostate Cancer

The detection of recurrent PC is often challenging for conventional imaging modalities such as CT or MRI. Currently, PSMA-ligand PET/CT is regarded as the most sensitive and specific

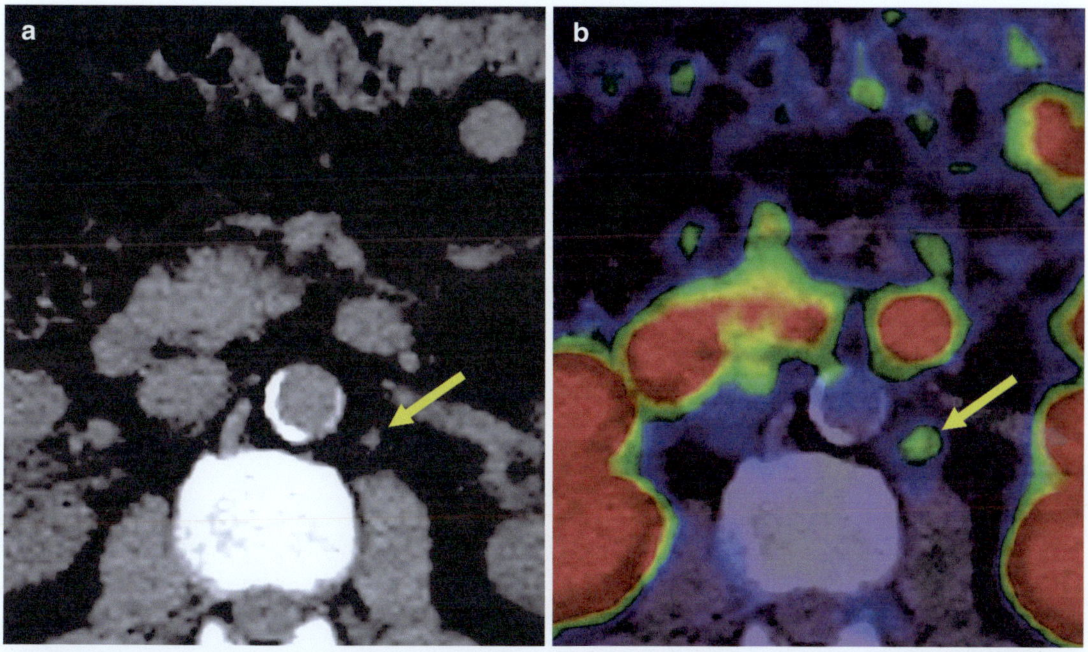

Fig. 25.2 Ganglions of the vegetative nervous system can present with a slight uptake of PSMA-ligands as well (yellow arrows point on such a ganglion). However, by analyzing several slices of the CT scan, ganglia can be differentiated from lymph nodes by their typical elongated extensions. (**a**) Low dose CT. (**b**) Fusion of PET and CT

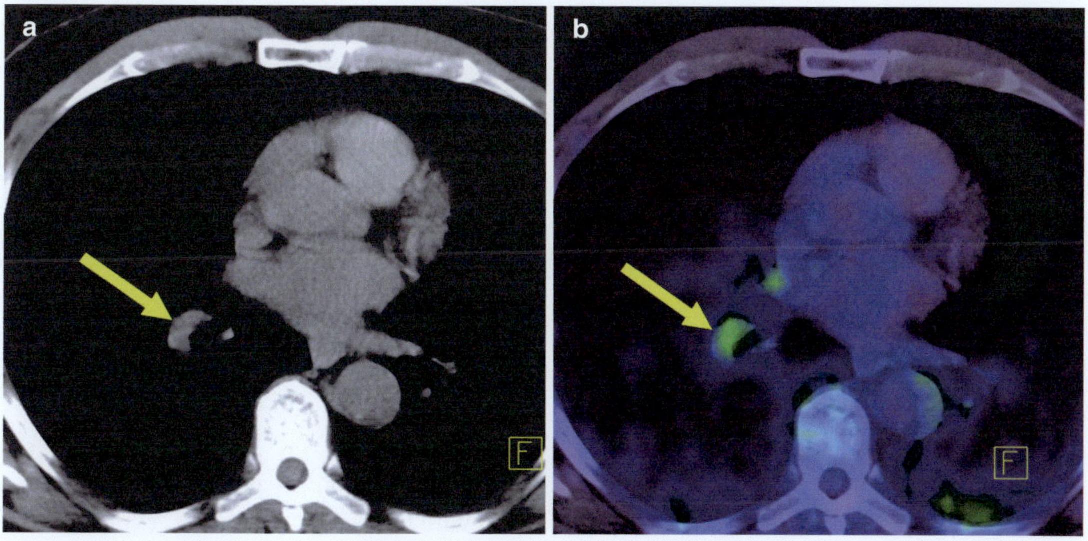

Fig. 25.3 Inflammatory mediastinal and para-aortal lymph nodes also show a slight uptake of PSMA-ligands (yellow arrows point on such a lymph node). However, the uptake intensity decreases by time in the majority of cases. (**a**) Low dose CT. (**b**) Fusion of PET and CT

modality for detecting recurrent PC. As a consequence, recurrent prostate cancer is the most frequent indication for PSMA-ligand imaging. Figures 25.4 and 25.5 present different examples of recurrent PC. As mentioned above, all available relevant statistical data concern ^{68}Ga-PSMA-11: among all patients referred to PET/CT, 80–90% present with at least one lesion

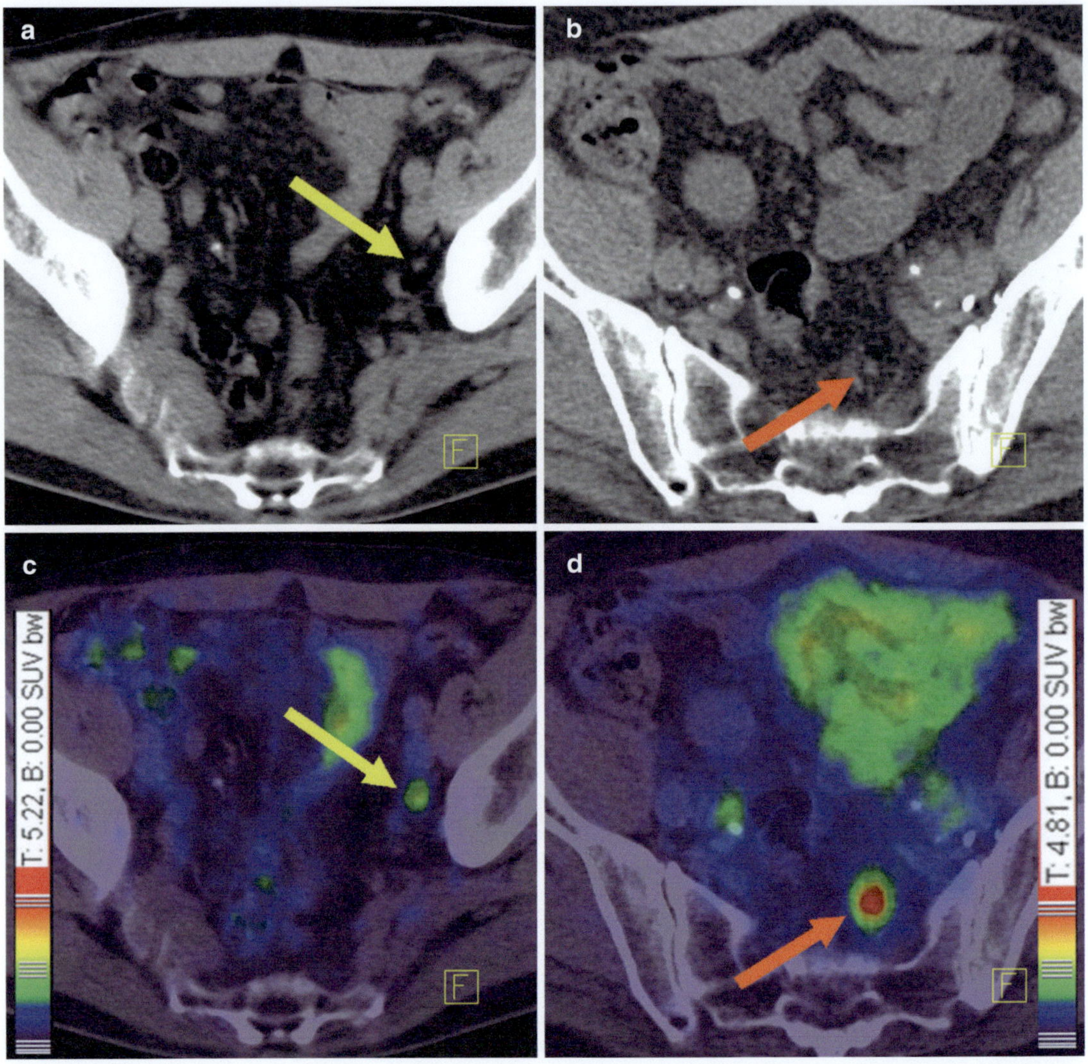

Fig. 25.4 Two different patients (patient 1: **a** + **c**; patient 2: **b** + **d**) presenting with lymph node metastases of PC (yellow and orange arrows). Although of similar size, the two lesions show different intensities of tracer uptake, typically according to the grade of their PSMA expression. (**a**, **b**) CT without contrast medium. (**c**, **d**) Fusion of PET and CT. (Image reprinted from Ref. [10] (an open access publication))

characteristic for PC [10, 17, 18]. These rates comply with the patient-based sensitivities. However, the sensitivity of ^{68}Ga-PSMA-11 PET/CT significantly correlates with PSA values at scanning time [10, 17, 18]. At PSA less than 0.5 ng/ml, the probability of a pathologic scan is estimated to be around 50% (Fig. 25.6). This value must not be confused with the tumor detection rate which includes the rate of detected tumor lesions existent in a patient. At PSA between 0.5 and 1.0 ng/ml, the probability of a pathologic scan rises to 70–80%. From PSA values of >2.0 ng/ml, the probability remains around 90–95%. This result is concordant with the fact that not all PC expresses sufficiently PSMA. For those tumors, alternative proved tracers such as choline or FDG PET/CT (latter used at dedifferentiated states) should be recommended. However, the time point of such alternative PET scans can be challenging. Considering Fig. 25.6, one option could be to conduct PSMA-ligand PET/CT for PSA values of up to 5.0 ng/ml (about 90% probability of a pathologic scan). At PSA >5.0 ng/ml, higher

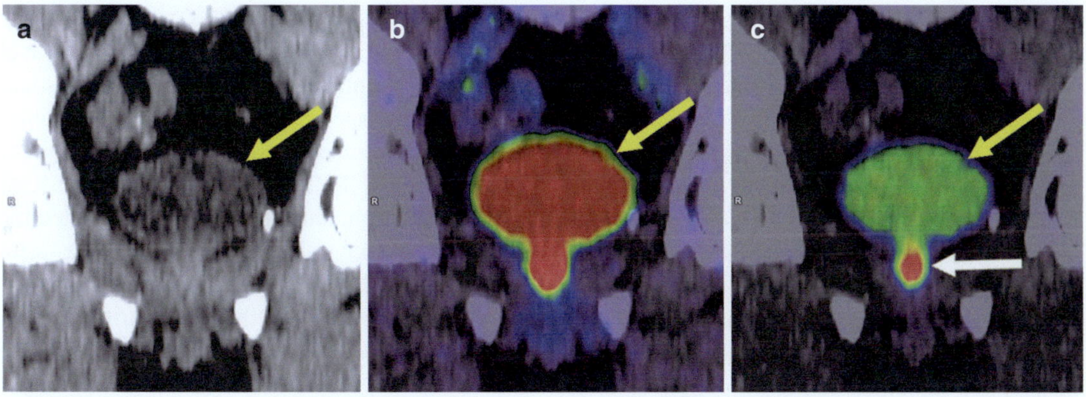

Fig. 25.5 Local relapse of PC (white arrow) which cannot be distinguished from the urinary bladder (yellow arrow) in the normal windowing of the scan. By adjusting manually the PET-windowing (in this case, the PET signal was reduced), the local relapse presents with significantly more intense tracer uptake compared to the urinary bladder. (**a**) CT without contrast medium; (**b**) fusion of PET and CT provided automatically by the scanner; (**c**) fusion of PET and CT with manually reduced PET signal

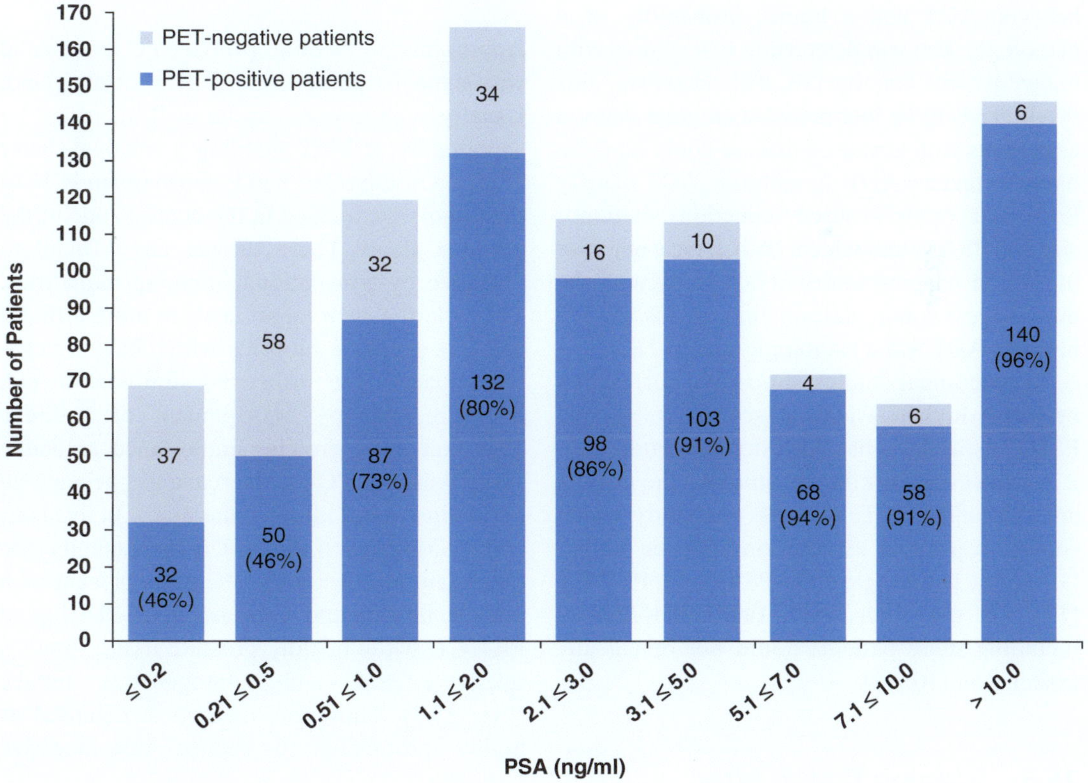

Fig. 25.6 Probabilities of a pathological ^{68}Ga-PSMA-11 PET/CT scan in relation to PSA values in a cohort of 971 patients. (Image reprinted from Ref. [10] (an open access publication))

PSA values do not lead to a significantly higher probability of a pathologic scan. Therefore, patients who do not present with a pathologic PSMA-ligand PET/CT at PSA higher than 5.0 ng/ml might rather be referred to PET/CT with alternative ligands instead of waiting until higher PSA values have been reached and then conduct a second PSMA-ligand PET/CT.

25.4 Impact of Different Factors on PSMA-Ligand PET/CT in Recurrent Prostate Cancer

Several studies have analyzed the impact of different factors on the probability of PC detection in PSMA-ligand PET/CT. For age, amount of injected tracer, and PSA doubling time, no impact was detected in studies with patient cohorts including more than 100 patients [10, 17, 18]. The results regarding an association between faster PSA velocities and a pathologic scan are contradictory [17, 18].

A significant association was detected between a positive PET and the PSA level as demonstrated by Fig. 25.6. With regard to an ongoing androgen deprivation therapy (ADT), the results are ambivalent: an association between ADT and a higher probability of a pathologic scan was detected in two studies with bigger patient cohorts [10, 18]. However, this result needs to be interpreted with great caution as patients with advanced disease could be more likely to receive ADT. In addition, ADT usually leads to apoptosis-caused reductions in tumor size and PSA values which, both, have a negative impact on imaging sensitivity. A study with the third largest cohort did not find an association between ADT and a pathologic scan [17].

In preclinical studies, a positive correlation between higher Gleason scores (GS) and PSMA expression has been demonstrated [19–21]. However, in clinical studies, the results are contradictory. There exist one study which showed a positive association between higher GS and a pathologic ^{68}Ga-PSMA-11 PET/CT [17]. On the other hand, two other studies including more patients could not reveal any association [10, 18].

25.5 Imaging Timing After Application

^{68}Ga-PSMA-11 PET/CT is routinely conducted 1 h after the injection (p.i.) according to its first described clinical set-up [1]. However, several studies have shown that the majority of PC lesions present with higher uptake and contrast at later time points [1, 22–26]. In a very small patient group ($n = 4$) and therefore of significantly reduced value, the optimal imaging timing for ^{68}Ga-PSMA-11 PET/CT seemed to be at 3 h p.i [22]. In addition, one study has demonstrated the positive impact of additional imaging with ^{68}Ga-PSMA-11 PET/CT at 3 h p.i. which can be used as a powerful method to clarify unclear findings at 1 h p.i. [26]. For alternative PSMA-ligands, the optimal imaging timing has not yet been analyzed.

25.6 Imaging Primary Prostate Cancer and Primary Staging of Prostate Cancer

Approximately ¾ of all primary PC are located within the peripheral zone of the prostate gland. Usually such tumors can be well identified by sonography or MRI enabling a relatively easy biopsy. On the other hand, approximately ¼ of the tumors are located in the central zone of the prostate gland. These tumors are difficult to visualize by conventional imaging modalities. The lack of a clear target leads to more difficult and less sensitive biopsies which have a negative impact on the further risk stratification and, therefore, therapy management of patients. This fact is of growing importance as active surveillance of PC has increasingly become an option instead of invasive therapies. In this context, PSMA-ligand PET/CT is increasingly getting attention. Lesions of PC often present with intense uptake and contrast in PSMA-ligand PET/CT, while healthy prostate tissue shows a relatively low and homogeneous uptake (Fig. 25.7). Thus, this method is regarded as highly promising to reduce false-negative biopsies.

Primary staging in high-risk prostate cancer with PSMA-ligand PET/CT has also shown to be superior when compared to conventional imaging modalities such as computed tomography or MRI [15, 27, 28]. The detection of radiologically

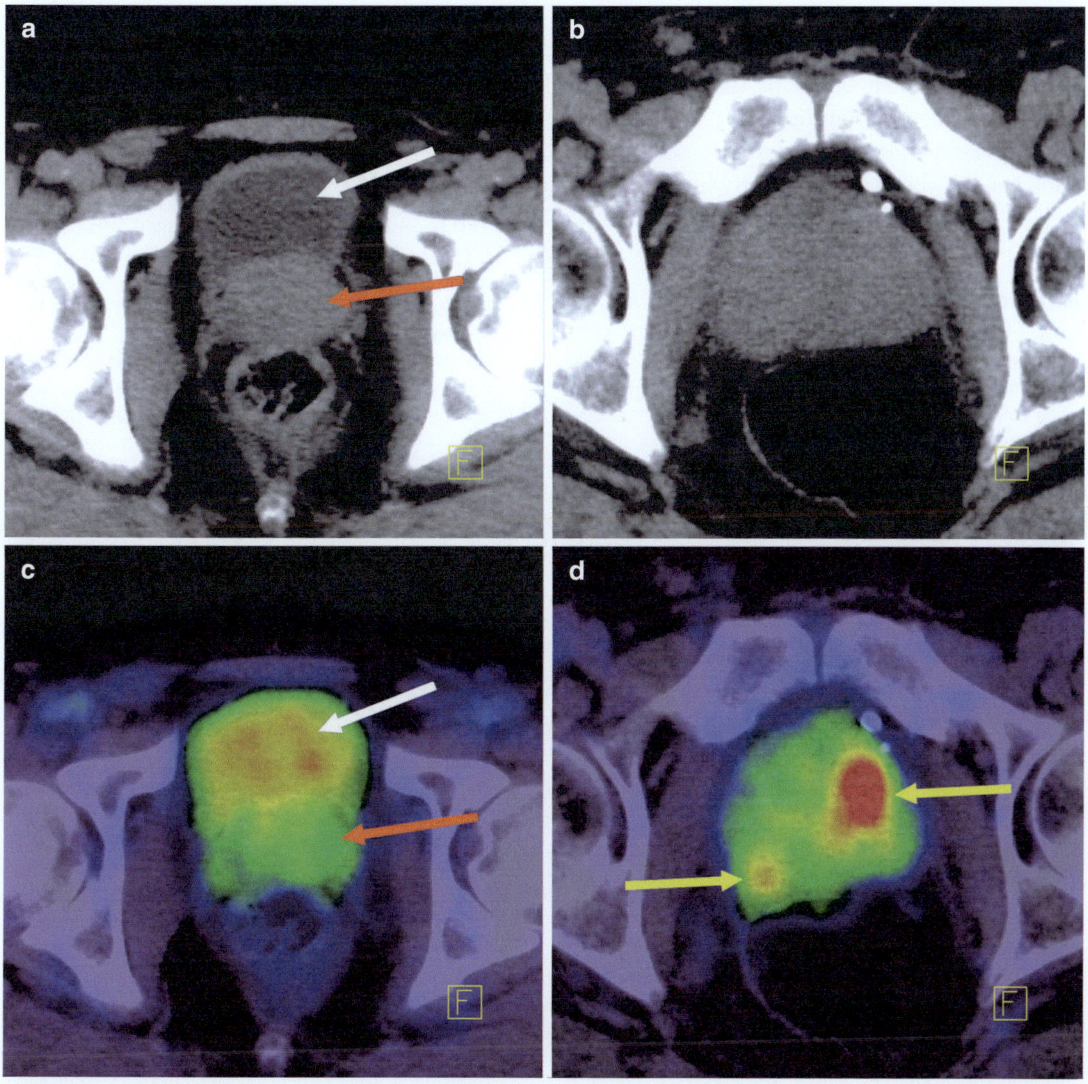

Fig. 25.7 The normal prostate tissue presents with a diffuse and moderate PSMA expression (orange arrows). On the other hand, and depending on the tumor size, the majority of prostate cancers show focal increase of PSMA expression: yellow arrows point to a bifocal prostate cancer (one small and one of bigger size). White arrows point to the urinary bladder which excretes the surplus tracer. (**a**) Low-dose CT and (**c**) fusion of PET with ^{68}Ga-PSMA-11 and CT of a patient with normal prostate tissue. (**b**) Low-dose CT and (**d**) fusion of PET with ^{68}Ga-PSMA-11 and CT of a patient with bifocal prostate cancer

occult metastases by PSMA-ligand PET/CT has an impact on the further therapy management [29, 30]. While the impact of PSMA-ligand PET/CT on the management of low-risk PC is expected to be very low due to the minimal probability of expansive disease, the impact on intermediate risk PC has not yet been sufficiently investigated.

25.7 Other Indications of PSMA-Ligand Imaging

PSMA-ligand imaging (PET or SPECT) is currently mandatory to evaluate a possible PSMA-based radioligand therapy of metastatic prostate cancer. Only a PSMA-positive tumor phenotype can be treated by an appropriate radioligand therapy. However, the still unsolved question is how intense the tracer uptake needs to be in order to achieve a sufficient effect of the PSMA-based radioligand therapy. Furthermore, the impact of PSMA-ligand imaging in therapy response evaluation has not yet been sufficiently investigated.

References

1. Afshar-Oromieh A, Malcher A, Eder M, Eisenhut M, Linhart HG, Hadaschik BA, et al. PET imaging with a [68Ga]gallium-labelled PSMA ligand for the diagnosis of prostate cancer: biodistribution in humans and first evaluation of tumour lesions. Eur J Nucl Med Mol Imaging. 2013;40:486–95.
2. Eder M, Schäfer M, Bauder-Wüst U, Hull W-E, Wängler C, Mier W, et al. 68Ga-complex lipophilicity and the targeting property of a urea-based PSMA inhibitor for PET imaging. Bioconjug Chem. 2012;23:688–97.
3. Weineisen M, Schottelius M, Simecek J, Baum RP, Yildiz A, Beykan S, et al. 68Ga- and 177Lu-labeled PSMA I&T: optimization of a PSMA-targeted theranostic concept and first proof-of-concept human studies. J Nucl Med. 2015;56:1169–76.
4. Benešová M, Schäfer M, Bauder-Wüst U, Afshar-Oromieh A, Kratochwil C, Mier W, et al. Preclinical evaluation of a tailor-made DOTA-conjugated PSMA inhibitor with optimized linker moiety for imaging and endoradiotherapy of prostate cancer. J Nucl Med. 2015;56:914–20.
5. Mease RC, Dusich CL, Foss CA, Ravert HT, Dannals RF, Seidel J, et al. N-[N-[(S)-1,3-Dicarboxypropyl] carbamoyl]-4-[18F]fluorobenzyl-L-cysteine, [18F] DCFBC: a new imaging probe for prostate cancer. Clin Cancer Res. 2008;14:3036–43.
6. Szabo Z, Mena E, Rowe SP, Plyku D, Nidal R, Eisenberger MA, et al. Initial evaluation of [(18)F] DCFPyL for prostate-specific membrane antigen (PSMA)-targeted PET imaging of prostate cancer. Mol Imaging Biol. 2015;17:565–74.
7. Cardinale J, Schäfer M, Benešová M, Bauder-Wüst U, Leotta K, Eder M, et al. Preclinical evaluation of [18F]PSMA-1007: a new PSMA-ligand for prostate cancer imaging. J Nucl Med. 2017;58(3):425–31.
8. Rischpler C, Beck TI, Okamoto S, Schlitter AM, Knorr K, Schwaiger M, et al. 68Ga-PSMA-HBED-CC uptake in cervical, coeliac and sacral ganglia as an important pitfall in prostate cancer PET imaging. J Nucl Med. 2018;59(9):1406–11.
9. Afshar-Oromieh A, Sattler LP, Steiger K, Holland-Letz T, da Cunha ML, Mier W, et al. Tracer uptake in mediastinal and paraaortal thoracic lymph nodes as a potential pitfall in image interpretation of PSMA ligand PET/CT. Eur J Nucl Med Mol Imaging. 2018;45(7):1179–87.
10. Afshar-Oromieh A, Avtzi E, Giesel FL, Holland-Letz T, Linhart HG, Eder M, et al. The diagnostic value of PET/CT imaging with the (68)Ga-labelled PSMA ligand HBED-CC in the diagnosis of recurrent prostate cancer. Eur J Nucl Med Mol Imaging. 2015;42:197–209.
11. Morigi JJ, Stricker PD, van Leeuwen PJ, Tang R, Ho B, Nguyen Q, et al. Prospective comparison of 18F-fluoromethylcholine versus 68Ga-PSMA PET/CT in prostate cancer patients who have rising PSA after curative treatment and are being considered for targeted therapy. J Nucl Med. 2015;56:1185–90.
12. Sahlmann C-O, Meller B, Bouter C, Ritter CO, Ströbel P, Lotz J, et al. Biphasic ^{68}Ga-PSMA-HBED-CC-PET/CT in patients with recurrent and high-risk prostate carcinoma. Eur J Nucl Med Mol Imaging. 2016;43:898–905.
13. Herlemann A, Wenter V, Kretschmer A, Thierfelder KM, Bartenstein P, Faber C, et al. 68Ga-PSMA positron emission tomography/computed tomography provides accurate staging of lymph node regions prior to lymph node dissection in patients with prostate cancer. Eur Urol. 2016;70:553–7.
14. Maurer T, Weirich G, Schottelius M, Weineisen M, Frisch B, Okur A, et al. Prostate-specific membrane antigen-radioguided surgery for metastatic lymph nodes in prostate cancer. Eur Urol. 2015;68:530–4.
15. Hijazi S, Meller B, Leitsmann C, Strauss A, Meller J, Ritter CO, et al. Pelvic lymph node dissection for nodal oligometastatic prostate cancer detected by 68Ga-PSMA-positron emission tomography/computerized tomography. Prostate. 2015;75:1934–40.
16. Sheikhbahaei S, Afshar-Oromieh A, Eiber M, Solnes LB, Javadi MS, Ross AE, et al. Pearls and pitfalls in clinical interpretation of prostate-specific membrane antigen (PSMA)-targeted PET imaging. Eur J Nucl Med Mol Imaging. 2017;44:2117–36.
17. Eiber M, Maurer T, Souvatzoglou M, Beer AJ, Ruffani A, Haller B, et al. Evaluation of hybrid ^{68}Ga-PSMA ligand PET/CT in 248 patients with biochemical recurrence after radical prostatectomy. J Nucl Med. 2015;56:668–74.
18. Afshar-Oromieh A, Holland-Letz T, Giesel FL, Kratochwil C, Mier W, Haufe S, et al. Diagnostic performance of 68Ga-PSMA-11 (HBED-CC) PET/CT in patients with recurrent prostate cancer: evaluation in 1007 patients. Eur J Nucl Med Mol Imaging. 2017;44:1258–68.
19. Marchal C, Redondo M, Padilla M, Caballero J, Rodrigo I, García J, et al. Expression of prostate specific membrane antigen (PSMA) in prostatic adenocarcinoma and prostatic intraepithelial neoplasia. Histol Histopathol. 2004;19:715–8.
20. Kasperzyk JL, Finn SP, Flavin R, Fiorentino M, Lis R, Hendrickson WK, et al. Prostate-specific membrane antigen protein expression in tumor tissue and risk of lethal prostate cancer. Cancer Epidemiol Biomarkers Prev. 2013;22:2354–63.
21. Minner S, Wittmer C, Graefen M, Salomon G, Steuber T, Haese A, et al. High level PSMA expression is

associated with early PSA recurrence in surgically treated prostate cancer. Prostate. 2011;71:281–8.
22. Afshar-Oromieh A, Hetzheim H, Kübler W, Kratochwil C, Giesel FL, Hope TA, et al. Radiation dosimetry of (68)Ga-PSMA-11 (HBED-CC) and preliminary evaluation of optimal imaging timing. Eur J Nucl Med Mol Imaging. 2016;43:1611–20.
23. Afshar-Oromieh A, Hetzheim H, Kratochwil C, Benesova M, Eder M, Neels OC, et al. The theranostic PSMA ligand PSMA-617 in the diagnosis of prostate cancer by PET/CT: biodistribution in humans, radiation dosimetry, and first evaluation of tumor lesions. J Nucl Med. 2015;56:1697–705.
24. Herrmann K, Bluemel C, Weineisen M, Schottelius M, Wester H-J, Czernin J, et al. Biodistribution and radiation dosimetry for a probe targeting prostate-specific membrane antigen for imaging and therapy. J Nucl Med. 2015;56:855–61.
25. Wondergem M, van der Zant F, Knol R, Lazarenko S, Pruim J, de Jong IJ. (18)F-DCFPyL PET/CT in the detection of prostate cancer at 60 and 120 minutes; detection rate, image quality, activity kinetics and biodistribution. J Nucl Med. 2017;58(11):1797–804.
26. Afshar-Oromieh A, Sattler LP, Mier W, Hadaschik B, Debus J, Holland-Letz T, et al. The clinical impact of additional late PET/CT imaging with 68Ga-PSMA-11 (HBED-CC) in the diagnosis of prostate cancer. J Nucl Med. 2017;58(5):750–5.
27. Maurer T, Gschwend JE, Rauscher I, Souvatzoglou M, Haller B, Weirich G, et al. Diagnostic efficacy of (68) gallium-PSMA positron emission tomography compared to conventional imaging for lymph node staging of 130 consecutive patients with intermediate to high risk prostate cancer. J Urol. 2016;195:1436–43.
28. Herlemann A, Wenter V, Kretschmer A, Thierfelder KM, Bartenstein P, Faber C, et al. (68)Ga-PSMA positron emission tomography/computed tomography provides accurate staging of lymph node regions prior to lymph node dissection in patients with prostate cancer. Eur Urol. 2016;70:553–7.
29. Sterzing F, Kratochwil C, Fiedler H, Katayama S, Habl G, Kopka K, et al. (68)Ga-PSMA-11 PET/CT: a new technique with high potential for the radiotherapeutic management of prostate cancer patients. Eur J Nucl Med Mol Imaging. 2016;43:34–41.
30. Roach PJ, Francis R, Emmett L, Hsiao E, Kneebone A, Hruby G, et al. The impact of (68)Ga-PSMA PET/CT on management intent in prostate cancer: results of an Australian prospective multicenter study. J Nucl Med. 2018;59(1):82–8.

Lacrimal Dacryoscintigraphy, Radionuclide Hysterosalpingography, and Scrotal Scintigraphy

26

László Pavics

26.1 Lacrimal Dacryoscintigraphy

Several methods are available to examine the function and morphology of the lacrimal drainage system under physiological conditions. Radionuclide scintigraphy is a sensitive method that is not cumbersome for the patient. Dacryoscintigraphy was first introduced by Rossomondo et al. in 1972 [1]. Since then the method has been modified by several groups and its significance supported by numerous studies. Indications of dacryoscintigraphy are obstructive disorders of the lacrimal drainage system. The method is helpful in the diagnosis of tear flow disturbances and in the follow-up for the detection of therapy response [2, 3].

The lacrimal drainage system begins with the puncta. One punctum is present at the medial end of both the superior and inferior eyelids. The puncta are situated on slight elevations called the lacrimal papillae. Malposition or stenosis of the puncta may cause epiphora. Through the puncta the lacrima flows into the superior and inferior vertical canaliculus, which is about 2 mm long and joins in the 8-mm-long horizontal canaliculus at a right angle called the ampulla. These usually join and form the common canaliculus, which immediately enters the (naso)lacrimal sac through the valve of Rosenmüller (a flap of mucosa to prevent reflux). The (naso)lacrimal sac is about 10 mm long and funnels into the 12-mm-long nasolacrimal duct. It opens into the inferior nasal meatus. The valve of Rasner closes the opening. Within the nasolacrimal duct other valves are also present. The number of these valves differs between individuals.

Capillarity ensures that 70% of the tears enter the inferior canaliculus and 30% through the superior canaliculus. On blinking, the attachment of the preseptal orbicular muscle helps create positive and negative pressure in the lacrimal sac, which sucks the tears into it (the tear pump). Gravity then helps to keep the sac empty.

Obstruction or stenosis of the lacrimal drainage system is related predominantly to inflammation or trauma. ^{99m}Tc-pertechnetate in physiologic saline solution has been established as the most useful tracer for dacryoscintigraphy. The dose should be 2–4 MBq in about 10 μl volume. The investigation can be performed with the patient in the lying or sitting position, and the patient's head should be held firmly during the investigation so that the use of a headholder or slit-lamp headrest is recommended. The drop of radiopharmaceutical should be carefully applied to the conjunctiva preferably simultaneously on both sides in front of the gamma camera. The overflowing tracer is wiped away. The camera is equipped with a low energy high-resolution (LEHR) collimator,

L. Pavics (✉)
Department of Nuclear Medicine, Albert Szent-Gyorgyi Medical University, Szeged, Hungary
e-mail: pavicsl@ss10.numed.szote.u-szeged.hu

H. Ahmadzadehfar et al. (eds.), *Clinical Nuclear Medicine*,
https://doi.org/10.1007/978-3-030-39457-8_26

zoom ×1.6, matrix, e.g. 64 × 64 or even higher. The dynamic data acquisition is started immediately with a 10-s/image frequency up to 2 min, followed by static images after 5, 10, 15, and 20 min. If available the use of a pinhole collimator (aperture 1–2 mm) is of advantage for static imaging. After finishing the acquisition, the eye is flashed with physiologic saline to reduce the absorbed dose in the eye. The dynamic study is evaluated by the ROI technique. The generation of time-activity curves from the different regions (conjunctival sac, nasolacrimal sac, nasolacrimal duct, and nose) is recommended.

The normal dynamics of tear flow vary over a wide range (comparison to the contralateral symptom-free side is helpful). As a rule, the tracer flows through the canaliculi in a few seconds (~10 s), and the tracer should appear within 10 min in the cavity of the nose.

Several investigations have shown that dacryoscintigraphy is a highly sensitive method. A normal finding excludes with a high probability disturbance of the tear flow. With abnormal results further morphological investigations are needed for the exact definition of the abnormality. In the follow-up because of its high sensitivity and lower radiation exposure, radionuclide dacryoscintigraphy is recommended.

The advantage of the method is its high sensitivity; the limitation of the technique is related to its spatial resolution.

The radiation exposure of the lens in normal lacrimal drainage is 0.14–0.21 mGy, and under pathological conditions it is about four times higher, but these values are well below the absorbed dose of a skull X-ray (30 mGy) [4, 5].

26.2 Radionuclide Hysterosalpingography

Radionuclide hysterosalpingography, or hysterosalpingo-radionuclide scintigraphy, was designed to evaluate the migration of a particulate radiopharmaceutical from the vagina to the peritoneal cavity and ovaries as well as to image and functionally outline the pathways between these two extremities of the female reproductive system.

The female reproductive system comprises the ovaries, fallopian tubes, uterus, vagina accessory glands, and external genital organs. The two fallopian tubes extend outwards from the uterus to embrace the ovaries. The end of the tube near the ovary expands to form a funnel-shaped infundibulum, which is surrounded by fingerlike extensions called fimbriae. The oocyte enters the peritoneal cavity before it enters the fallopian tube. At the time of ovulation the fimbriae increase their activity and create currents in the peritoneal fluid in the direction of the tube. Inside the fallopian tube, the oocyte is moved along by the rhythmic beating of cilia and by peristaltic action of the muscle of the tube. Successful fertilization requires coordinated migration of sperm from the vagina (deposited near the external os of the cervix) and an ovum from the ovarium. The fertilization usually occurs in the ampullary portion (next to the infundibulum) of the fallopian tube.

Obstruction of the fallopian tubes is a common cause of infertility.

Radionuclide hysterosalpingography is used as a method to investigate fallopian tube patency under physiological conditions, and was first described by Iturralde and Venter in 1981 [6]. The original method was modified and the activity used has been decreased to 18 MBq of ^{99m}Tc-human serum albumin macroaggregate (HSA MAA), which should be placed in less than 1 ml in the posterior cervical fornix. Data acquisition starts promptly using a gamma camera equipped with a predominantly parallel collimator and continues for 2 h or until bilateral spillage in the peritoneum. When necessary, oblique images can help to separate the anatomic structures [7]. Other groups recommend the use of ^{99m}Tc-hexamethylene-propyleneamine-oxime (HMPAO) labeled spermatozoa as a radiopharmaceutical (an intrauterine device, IUD, inhibits the migration of sperm only), but in other conditions ^{99m}Tc-pertechnetate has also been used successfully.

Under physiological conditions patency is indicated by the prompt flow of activity through the uterus and fallopian tubes with hot spots at the sites of the ovaries or spillage into the peritoneum. On the dominant side radiopharmaceutical transport is accelerated.

In the case of obstructed transport, the failure of visualization from the cornu of the uterine cavity to the fallopian tube ("cornu cut off sign") is diagnostic. Misinterpretation of the images is possible by the overlap of vaginal or uterine activity with intraperitoneal accumulation or by confusing the activity remaining in the vagina with the uterus.

Radionuclide hysterosalpingography is helpful in patients with unexplained infertility also when X-ray contrast salpingography is normal, in the follow-up after reanastomosis surgery or when there is suspected tubal ligation, and beneficial in aiding the selection of the method of artificial insemination.

The advantage of the method is that it makes possible to investigate tubal patency under physiological conditions in quite a sensitive way. But we should take into account that spermatic transport is menstrual cycle dependent; therefore, the timing of the investigation plays a role in the correct interpretation. Radionuclide hysterosalpingography purports the spermatic transport function, but does not demonstrate the capability of the oviduct to transport ova or embryos in the reverse direction.

The radiation exposure of the ovaria during radionuclide hysterosalpingography is 0.6–1.5 mGy/MBq [8].

26.3 Scrotal Scintigraphy

Scrotal scintigraphy was introduced for the differentiation from other conditions of acute torsion of the testicle, which needs urgent surgical intervention and inflammation or appendicular torsion, for which treatments are conservative. The method was first described by Nadel et al. in 1973 [9].

The scrotum comprises a thin layer of dartos muscle continuous with the superficial fascia of the groin and peritoneum covered by skin. The medial extension of the dartos muscle separates the scrotum into left and right compartments. Each hemiscrotum contains a testicle (size range 14–35 cm^3) covered by a dense capsule, the tunica albuginea. The testicle descends down the retroperitoneum, bringing with it the spermatic cord, and its vascular lymphatic and neural lifeline. On top of the testis is the epididymis, the distal tail of which leads to the vas deferens, ascends the spermatic cord and ends in the ejaculatory duct. The testis and epididymis are covered by a double layer of the tunica vaginalis, which is a contiguous extension of the peritoneum. The lower pole of the testis is loosely attached to the floor of the scrotum by the gubernaculum.

Four other vestigial structures are also of importance because these structures can twist themselves, mimicking testicular torsion. These are: the appendix testis (remnant of the müllerian tube), the appendix epididymis, the paradidymis, and the vas aberrans (these are mesonephric remnants). The testicular artery (the principal arterial supply of the testicle) originates from the abdominal aorta, inferior to the renal artery. Branches of the deferential artery originating from the internal iliac artery and cremasteric branches of the inferior epigastric artery also run within the spermatic cord and anastomose with the testicular artery. The scrotum is supplied by the internal superficial and deep pudendal vessels, which have no anastomoses with the testicle supplying vessels. Testicular veins drain into the plexus pampiniformis, which as an anastomosing venous complex surrounds the spermatic cord and leads to the testicular and cremasteric veins. Valves within the testicular veins prevent the retrograde reflux of the blood.

Two types of testicular torsion have been described, intravaginal torsion in children and adults and extravaginal torsion in neonates. The exact cause of intravaginal torsion is unknown. Patients generally complain of acute onset of testicular pain. Nausea and vomiting might also be present. Within 6–12 h perfusion should be restored otherwise irreversible damage of spermatogenetic function develops. Extravaginal torsion usually occurs during the testicular descent. The scrotum is generally swollen at birth, blue red discoloration is present and testicular necrosis is almost uniform.

Nowadays scrotal scintigraphy is performed with ^{99m}Tc-pertechnetate or for lowering the radiation exposure with ^{99m}Tc-DTPA. In adults the dose is 550–750 MBq, and the minimal dose in children is 100 MBq. The patient is positioned supine under the gamma camera or stands in front of it. The penis is taped upwards to the abdominal wall and a thin layer of lead plate is placed under the scrotum to diminish soft tissue activity. At the time of injection a dynamic study is started with an image frequency of 1–3 s/frame with a duration of 1 min. Two and 10 min after injection static images are obtained from the anterior view with about 0.5–1 million counts. Markers can help to clear the correct anatomical positions of the testicles. For better visualization of the structures, zoomed images are helpful [10].

In normal cases the flow in the testicular artery is poorly visualized and significant intrascrotal activity is not present because of the low perfusion normally present. On static images the scrotum appears with symmetrical and homogeneous distribution of activity.

Extravaginal torsion in neonates is clinically obvious; therefore, scintigraphy is not needed. In the early phase (5–7 h after symptoms onset) of intravaginal testicular torsion the perfusion is decreased but it is not always discernible on the dynamic images of the investigation because of the low baseline flow. On static blood pool images, a unilateral decrease of activity is observed on the affected side. In the case of spontaneous detorsion, a normal distribution or diffuse hyperemia of the involved side may be present. Later (until 24 h after onset) perfusion is absent and due to the increasing inflammation a hyperemic rim with progressively increasing activity surrounds the photopenic testicle ("bull's-eye"; "halo" or "rim" sign). As time elapses after the symptom onset, the rim becomes pronounced but it is difficult to completely exclude testicular viability according to the result of the scintigraphy. In epididymo-orchitis, static images demonstrate diffusely increased activity and increased blood flow. The radionuclide appearance is normal or mild hyperemia with focal or diffuse photopenic defects is visible in torsion of the testicular appendices. Other conditions such as abscess, hydrocele, hematoma, or hernia can simulate acute or missed torsion on scintigraphy; therefore, a comprehensive examination of the patient and clinical data is necessary for the correct image interpretation.

The sensitivity of the examination is high (96%). The positive predictive value of cold lesion is about 63%, but most of the "false–positive" cases require surgery as well. The procedure is also highly acceptable in the evaluation of the effects of surgical interventions during the follow-up [10, 11].

Scrotal scintigraphy frequently contributes to patient management and minimizes unnecessary interventions.

References

1. Rossomondo RM, Carlton WH, Trueblood JH, Thomas RP. A new method of evaluating lacrimal drainage. Arch Ophthalmol. 1972;88(5):523–5.
2. Brockmann H, Wilhelm K, Joe A, Palmedo H, Biersack HJ. Nasolacrimal drainage obstruction after radioiodine therapy: case report and a review of the literature. Clin Nucl Med. 2005;30(8):543–5.
3. von Denffer H, Dressler J, Pabst HW. Lacrimal dacryoscintigraphy. Semin Nucl Med. 1984;14(1):8–15.
4. Brizel HE, Sheils WC, Brown M. The effects of radiotherapy on the nasolacrimal system as evaluated by dacryoscintigraphy. Radiology. 1975;116(2):373–81.
5. Robertson JS, Brown ML, Colvard DM. Radiation absorbed dose to the lens in dacryoscintigraphy with $^{99m}TcO_4^-$. Radiology. 1979;133(3):747–50.
6. Iturralde M, Venter PF. Hysterosalpingo-radionuclide scintigraphy (HERS). Semin Nucl Med. 1981;11(4):301–14.
7. Becker W, Steck T, Albert P, Borner W. Hysterosalpingoscintigraphy: a simple and accurate method of evaluating fallopian tube patency. Nuklearmedizin. 1988;27(6):252–7.

8. Yang KT, Chiang JH, Chen BS, Liang CH, Lee SF, Liao SC. Radionuclide hysterosalpingography with technetium-99m-pertechnetate: application and radiation dose to the ovaries. J Nucl Med. 1992;33(2):282–6.
9. Nadel NS, Gitter MH, Hahn LC, Vernon AR. Preoperative diagnosis of testicular torsion. Urology. 1973;1(5):478–9.
10. Bockisch A, van Ahlen H, Makarewitsch J, Ruhlmann J, Hotze A, Biersack HJ. The significance of testicular scintigraphy for the differential diagnosis of the acute scrotum. Nuklearmedizin. 1989;28(3):84–7.
11. Lutzker LG, Zuckier LS. Testicular scanning and other applications of radionuclide imaging of the genital tract. Semin Nucl Med. 1990;20(2):159–88.

Radionuclide Imaging of Children

27

Reza Vali, Susan McQuattie, and Amer Shammas

27.1 Introduction

Although many types of radionuclide studies are similar in adults and children, there are specific consideration to be aware of in the pediatric population. Nuclear medicine physicians and technologists are often faced with frightened children and anxious parents, and as such careful planning and good communication is essential. Having the appropriate tools, environment, and enough time is of pivotal importance to acquire an optimum study. In addition, it is important to be aware of the normal variances and appropriate thresholds in order to interpret an activity as abnormal in children as compared with adults. In this chapter we review the common nuclear medicine procedures in children, focusing on the indication of the study, patient preparation, dose of the radioactivity, and the interpretation of the studies. Similar to the previous edition, the effective radiation doses listed are for a 20-kg 5-year-old child except where indicated.

It should be noted that the protocols suggested in the following pages are institutional specific and may vary to some degree from those currently in practice in other pediatric facilities. As with any nuclear medicine procedure, it is beneficial to consult local regulations and guidelines such as the EANM, SNMMI, and Image Gently Alliance when establishing pediatric specific protocols.

R. Vali (✉) · S. McQuattie · A. Shammas
Nuclear Medicine, The Hospital for Sick Children, University of Toronto, Toronto, ON, Canada
e-mail: reza.vali@sickkids.ca

27.2 Genitourinary System

Radionuclide studies of the genitourinary system are perhaps one of the most common procedures in children. There are various clinical indications in pediatric nephro-urology imaging including:

- Cortical imaging of acute pyelonephritis, scars, and infarction
- Evaluation of congenital anomalies (duplication and ectopia)
- Assessment of the renal function in hydronephrosis (suspected ureteropelvic junction or ureterovesical junction obstruction) or after renal trauma
- Evaluation of renal transplant
- GFR studies
- Evaluation of vesicoureteral reflux

Most nuclear medicine studies in genitourinary system disorders can be categorized into three main groups:

1. Evaluation of renal function (including both glomerular and tubular studies)

H. Ahmadzadehfar et al. (eds.), *Clinical Nuclear Medicine*,
https://doi.org/10.1007/978-3-030-39457-8_27

2. Evaluation of renal cortex
3. Evaluation of the bladder

Other radionuclide studies such as scintigraphy of the testis, evaluation of tumors (e.g., MIBG scan for neuroblastoma), etc. can also be seen in pediatric population. This section will focus on the most common radionuclide studies in pediatric nephro-urological disorders.

27.3 Dynamic Renography

Similar to the adults, dynamic renal imaging is generally acquired after intravenous injection of a glomerular radiotracer [e.g., ^{99m}Tc-diethylene triamine pentaacetic acid (DTPA)] or a tubular agent [e.g., ^{99m}Tc-mercaptoacetyltriglycine (MAG3) and ^{99m}Tc-ethylenedicysteine (^{99m}Tc-EC)]. In children 2 years of age and younger (because of immature nephrons and low GFR), ^{99m}Tc-MAG3 is the preferred radiotracer due to its better quality and higher target-to-background activity. However, when GFR measurement is of interest, ^{99m}Tc-DTPA should be used. Similar protocols can be used for both ^{99m}Tc-DTPA and ^{99m}Tc-MAG3 renal scans (Box 27.1).

Box 27.1 Protocol Summary for Dynamic Renography

Indications

To evaluate renal function and to distinguish between retention in the calyceal system due to obstruction and a dilated system without mechanical obstruction.

Contraindication

None. However, it is better to postpone the study or interpret with caution in the first 2 weeks of age.

Patients sensitive to sulfonamides may also be sensitive to furosemide.

Patient Preparation

Make sure the patient doesn't have any contraindication to furosemide administration.

If the patient has a cardiac disease, prophylactic antibiotic may be needed prior to urethral catheterization (consult with the cardiologists). Hydration fluid volume may need to be modified to guard against fluid overload.

Hydration: Via IV, hydrate the child with normal saline. Give 10 cc per kg if the child is under 6 months and 15 cc per kg if over 6 months. Allow half of the total volume to infuse 15 min prior to the MAG3 injection—the other half can infuse during the image acquisition. Older, compliant children can be given oral hydration. Record the total amount of hydration on the requisition.

Have the child void just prior to the scan if he/she is not catheterized.

Radiopharmaceutical

^{99m}Tc-DTPA, 3.7 MBq (100 μCi)/kg; minimum, 20–37 MBq (1 mCi)*.

^{99m}Tc-MAG3, 1.9 MBq (50 μCi)/kg; minimum, 15–37 MBq (1 mCi)*.

Effective dose (mSv/MBq): 0.015 for ^{99m}Tc-MAG3 and 0.012 for ^{99m}Tc-DTPA [1].

Image Acquisition

Position the patient supine with the bladder at the bottom of the field of view.

Acquire serial 30–60 s images (64 × 64 or 128 × 128 matrix) for 30–60 min, depending on the technique chosen.

Acquire 1–3 min dynamic images after upright positioning (child sit up or have the parent hold a baby upright for about 5–15 min). Late PM images acquired after 60 min are also useful in certain cases.

Processing and Analysis

Please refer to the text for more detailed processing in different methods of Lasix injection. Renogram, DRF, T max, T½ of the furosemide curve, PM images after the upright positioning or at 60 min, and NORA are useful parameters for interpretation.

*EANM (2) suggests a minimum activity of 15 MBq for ^{99m}Tc-MAG3 and 20 MBq for ^{99m}Tc-DTPA. The minimum activity is 37 MBq for both radiotracers according to the SNM guideline (3).

PM, post-micturition; DRF, differential renal function; T max, time of maximum activity; NORA, normalized residual activity.

The child should be hydrated before the study (Box 27.1). Urinary catheterization is suggested in younger children to allow for free flow of urine from the bladder during the study. Catheterization may not be necessary for older and compliant children. However, it is especially useful when there is history of vesicoureteral reflux, severely dilated pelvicalyceal system, and suspected UVJ obstruction or in patients with a pelvic kidney. Children undergoing renal scintigraphy in conjunction with GFR measurement are not routinely catheterized; however, a post-void image is taken where possible.

Patient preparation and the technique of scanning are summarized in Box 27.1. Similar to adults, a few seconds after the administration of the radiotracer, both kidneys are visualized symmetrically (flow or perfusion phase). Evaluation of perfusion phase is important in patients with hypertension or after renal transplantation. Within 1–3 min the activity accumulates in both kidneys' parenchyma (extraction, uptake or cortical phase). The uptake phase is perhaps one of the most important phases of a renal scan. The cortical uptake in the first 1–3 min is used to evaluate the differential renal function (DRF). It is important to pay attention to the region of interest (ROI) over the kidneys and background activity particularly on follow-up scans (to be consistent). In the case of a poor renal function, or when the kidney is not located in the normal position, evaluation of the DRF is more accurate with a renal cortical radiotracer such as ^{99m}Tc-DMSA. Excretion of the radiotracer starts very early but will be more prominent within a few minutes after injection (excretory phase). The tracer then clears from the kidneys into the ureters and bladder gradually (drainage or clearance phase).

Furosemide (1 mg/kg IV; maximum 40 mg) is commonly used to distinguish between retention in the calyceal system due to obstruction and a dilated system without mechanical obstruction. The pelvicalyceal system may be dilated due to congenital malformation, vesicoureteral reflux, previous obstruction, and bladder abnormalities, such as neurogenic bladder or posterior urethral valve (PUV), rather than a current mechanical obstruction. A number of different protocols exist in terms of the timing of furosemide injection; however the results of all protocols are similar. Some centers inject furosemide when the dilated renal pelvis is maximally distended with radiotracer. Injection of furosemide 20 min after the radiotracer administration (F+20) is more common in adult centers. The F+20 method has the advantage in that the diuretic will be injected only if there is retention in one of the kidneys. In our institution furosemide is injected immediately after the radiotracer administration (F-0). The F-0 method has the advantage of a shorter acquisition time, and no need for a separate injection. Furosemide can also be injected 15 min before the radiotracer administration [2].

A renogram (time–activity curve that represents the cortical uptake, excretion, and drainage of the kidneys over time) is drawn by placing a ROI over the kidneys and background. Some descriptive parameters are useful to interpret a renogram. The time to reach the peak of activity in the parenchyma is called T max which is normally about 2–5 min after radiotracer administration. Typically, an ROI over the collecting system that excludes the renal parenchyma is used in adults to evaluate the diuresis phase. However, in the pediatric population, especially in small children, it is difficult and perhaps not very accurate to exclude the parenchyma. Thus, in practice, a similar ROI to that which is drawn for the evaluation of cortical uptake is used for the assessment of diuresis. If there is evidence of hydroureter, another ROI can be drawn to include the ureters. T½ which is the time that the activity in the collecting system reaches 50% of the maximum activity is commonly used to assess the drainage or clearance of the collecting systems. Normalized residual activity (NORA) which is the ratio of the residual activity in the kidney at time *t* (over a period of 1 min) to time 1–2 min is also a useful parameter to evaluate the drainage of the kidney [2]. In many cases, post-upright positioning images, post-micturition (PM) image, and delayed images (e.g., at 60 min) are of pivotal importance to assess the obstruction and the prognosis (Fig. 27.1).

T½ is normally used with furosemide. In case of a mechanical obstruction, the drainage of the calyceal system may be delayed by the narrowed area, and the T½ is prolonged. Therefore, the time–activity curve may show minimal or no evidence of downsloping. On the other hand, in a nonobstructive system, the drainage is improved

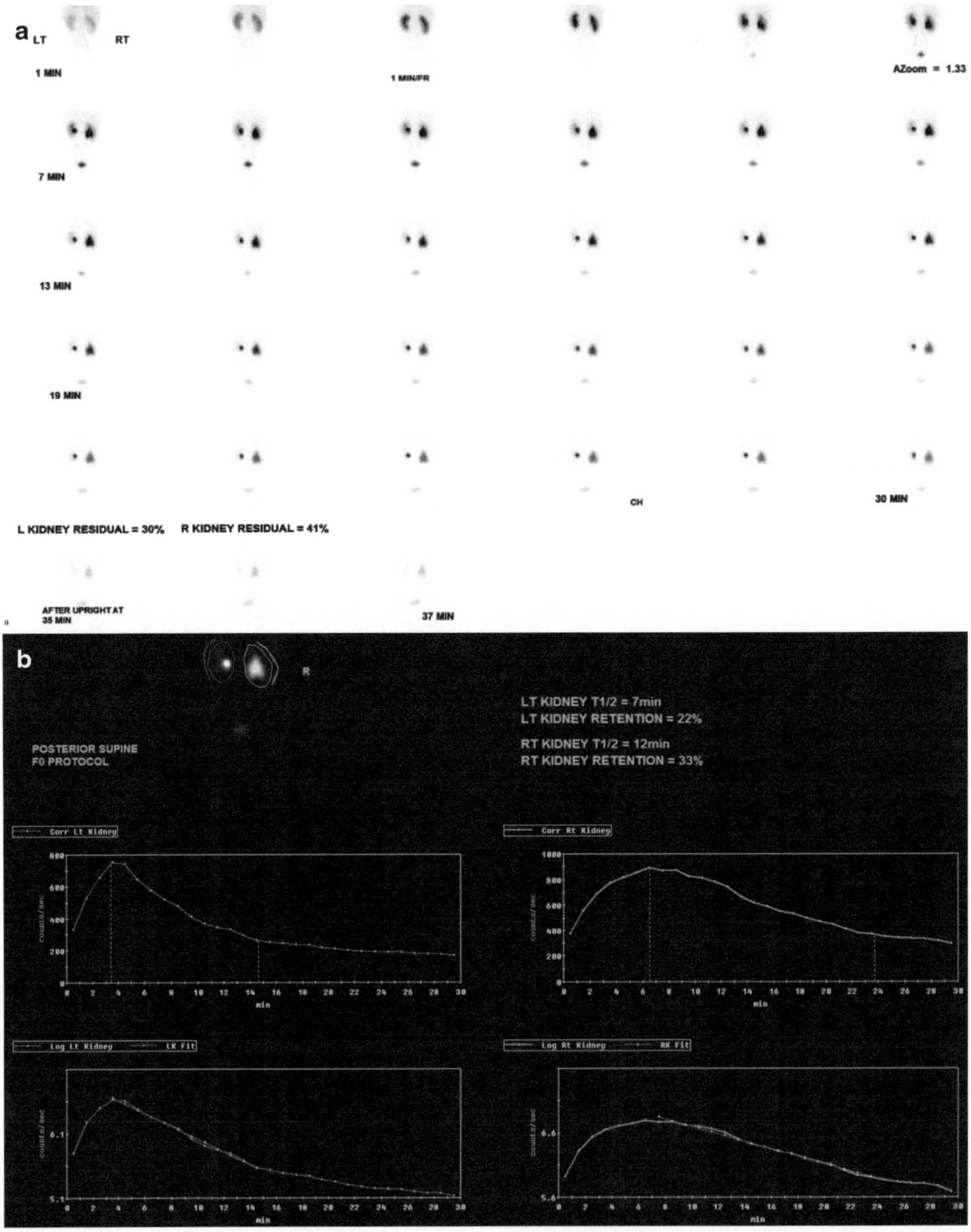

Fig. 27.1 Renal scan with ^{99m}Tc-MAG3 in a 2-year-old child with prominent left renal pelvis and dilated right pelvicalyceal system on ultrasound. There is mild retention of activity in the right pelvicalyceal system (**a**) with a T½ of 12 min (**b**). There is further drainage of the activity on both sides after the upright positioning (**a**) with no evidence of mechanical obstruction

after administration of furosemide. In general, if the T½ values are less than 10 min, the study is accurate to exclude obstruction. Alternatively, if the T½ is markedly prolonged, the study is suggestive of high-grade obstruction. For values in between, the T½ is relatively equivocal, and other clinical parameters or follow-up is needed to confirm or exclude a mechanical obstruction. In uncomplicated cases (e.g., preserved cortical function), if there is no evidence of a high-grade obstruction, a close follow-up may be the best approach for equivocal T½ [4]. This is particularly true in neonatal hydronephrosis as the natural behavior of hydronephrosis is variable and may change over time [3].

There are other conditions in which the interpretation of drainage values should be done cautiously. For example, if furosemide is injected at 20 min and the radiotracer has already cleared from the kidney, the T½ after the injection of furosemide is invalid as the collecting system has been already emptied. In large hydronephrotic kidneys (pelvic volume greater than 75 mL), there will be a delay in clearance of the activity due to a dilution effect, even with no significant mechanical obstruction. Finally, in cases of poor renal function, the drainage of the kidneys cannot be accurately evaluated due to delayed accumulation of the activity within the kidneys. In other words, with incomplete input, evaluation of kidney output is not so reliable. Moreover, in severely decreased renal function response to the furosemide, stimulation is not optimum.

27.4 Renal Cortical Imaging

^{99m}Tc-DMSA (dimercaptosuccinic acid) is the radiotracer of choice for the assessment of renal cortex. ^{99m}Tc-DMSA is bound to proximal tubular cells with 40–65% of the injected dose present in the cortex 2 h after injection. Image acquisitions are usually obtained 2–3 h after the injection of 1.85 MBq/kg (0.05 mCi/kg) of ^{99m}Tc-DMSA (minimum dose 18.5 MBq) (Box 27.2). This study consists of two sets of acquisitions—one set, using the LEHR collimator, provides images for calculation of the differential function, and the other set, using the pinhole collimator or SPECT, provides multi-projection images for high-resolution assessment of the renal cortex. In our institute we acquire SPECT for patient older than 5 years. In some institutes SPECT images are obtained for the patients older than 1–3 years. Pinhole images are obtained in posterior and posterior oblique views. For the renal transplant patients, imaging should be acquired in anterior and oblique views. For pelvic kidney the anterior and anterior oblique views should be added to the acquired images of the normally positioned posterior kidney.

Box 27.2 Protocol Summary for DMSA

Indications

To evaluate for renal scarring, acute pyelonephritis, differential renal function, solitary or ectopic renal tissue, horseshoe kidney, space-occupying lesions, renal trauma, and hydronephrosis.

Contraindication

None. If there is any nuclear medicine scan performed in the last 24–48 h, it is better to postpone the study if possible.

Patient Preparation

No special requirements. Patients should have normal hydration—oral hydration is encouraged. Prior to imaging, patient should void or diaper is changed.

Radiopharmaceutical

^{99m}Tc-DMSA, 1.85 MBq/kg or 0.05 mCi/kg; minimum dose 18.5 MBq or 0.5 mCi.

Effective dose (mSv/MBq): 0.039 [12].

Image Acquisition

Image the patient 2–4 h following injection. If there is poor renal function, delayed imaging (up to 24 h) is useful.

Image the patient in anterior and posterior projection with a low-energy high-resolution collimator for 500k or 2 min for calculation of the differential function.

Continue with planar pinhole imaging (for younger children) or SPECT acquisition (for older children) for high-resolution assessment of the renal cortex.

Pinhole imaging: For 8 min or 100k counts per view in posterior and posterior oblique projections for each kidney separately. The pinhole collimator should be within the same distance from patient for both kidneys.

SPECT acquisition: 128 matrix, 64 images, 180°; step and shoot 20 s/frame; zoom as required.

Processing and Analysis

Depending on the camera and the available software: for ordered subset expectation maximization (OSEM), use Butterworth filter with 0.52 critical frequency or Hanning filter with high cutoff smoothing kernel. Motion correction or attenuation correction can be done if needed.

The normal finding is the homogeneous uptake of the radiotracer in both kidneys with no definite focal cortical defect. The shape of the kidneys may be variable. There is usually mild decreased activity over the area of the pelvicalyceal system. Upper lateral region of the left kidney may be flattened due to splenic impression (Fig. 27.2). Indentations in the border of the kidneys may be seen due to fetal lobulation. The normal differential function is in the range of 43–57% for each kidney.

In addition to the usual indication of ^{99m}Tc-DMSA renal scan in acute pyelonephritis and detection of renal scars, it can also be helpful in the assessment of functioning cortical tissue in a dysplastic or small kidney, to evaluate the differential renal function, to evaluate ectopic kidney and horseshoe kidney, and to differentiate the hypertrophic columns of Bertin versus a tumor.

^{99m}Tc-DMSA can be helpful in evaluating a child with febrile UTI to evaluate for acute pyelonephritis. Recently, some authors have suggested to start with a DMSA scan when approaching a patient with acute pyelonephritis (the so-called top-down approach) instead of a radionuclide cystography due to the relative importance of renal damage rather than reflux in these patients [6]. Acute pyelonephritis shows as a single or multifocal area of decreased DMSA activity without volume loss or may present as a diffuse decrease in radiotracer activity (Fig. 27.3a). Reduced cortical activity after an episode of acute pyelonephritis may completely resolve within several months or may lead to a permanent scar formation (Fig. 27.3b). A follow-up ^{99m}Tc-DMSA study (at least 6 months after the acute pyelonephritis) is useful to detect scarring [7].

^{99m}Tc-DMSA scans are also useful to evaluate kidneys in other conditions. In ectopic kidneys, unlike intravenous pyelogram (IVP) and ultrasound, bowel gas or bony structures cannot obscure the ectopic kidney. ^{99m}Tc-DMSA can be helpful to distinguish renal ectopia from hypoplasia or agenesis. A DMSA scan is useful to evaluate function of the horseshoe kidney and also function of each moiety in a duplex kidney.

27.5 Radionuclide Cystography

Vesicoureteral reflux (VUR) is seen in approximately 1–2% of the pediatric population and up to 40% in children with acute pyelonephritis. Almost half of the patients with VUR diagnosed before birth or at neonate show spontaneous resolution by the age of 2–3 years. Thus, frequent imaging may be needed in some patients. In general, radionuclide VUR studies are indicated for evaluation at diagnosis (for females), for siblings of patients with reflux, and for follow-up studies in both females and males. For males or those patients with a suspicion of anatomic abnormalities, it is suggested to start with radiographic voiding cystography (VCUG) due to anatomical resolution [8]. In contrast to VCUG, continuous recordings during radionuclide cystography (RNC) with no extra patient radiation can increase the sensitivity and higher detection rate for the intermittent reflux. Quantification of the bladder volume at initiation of reflux and measurement of the residual bladder volume after voiding are other parameters that are useful for follow-up studies.

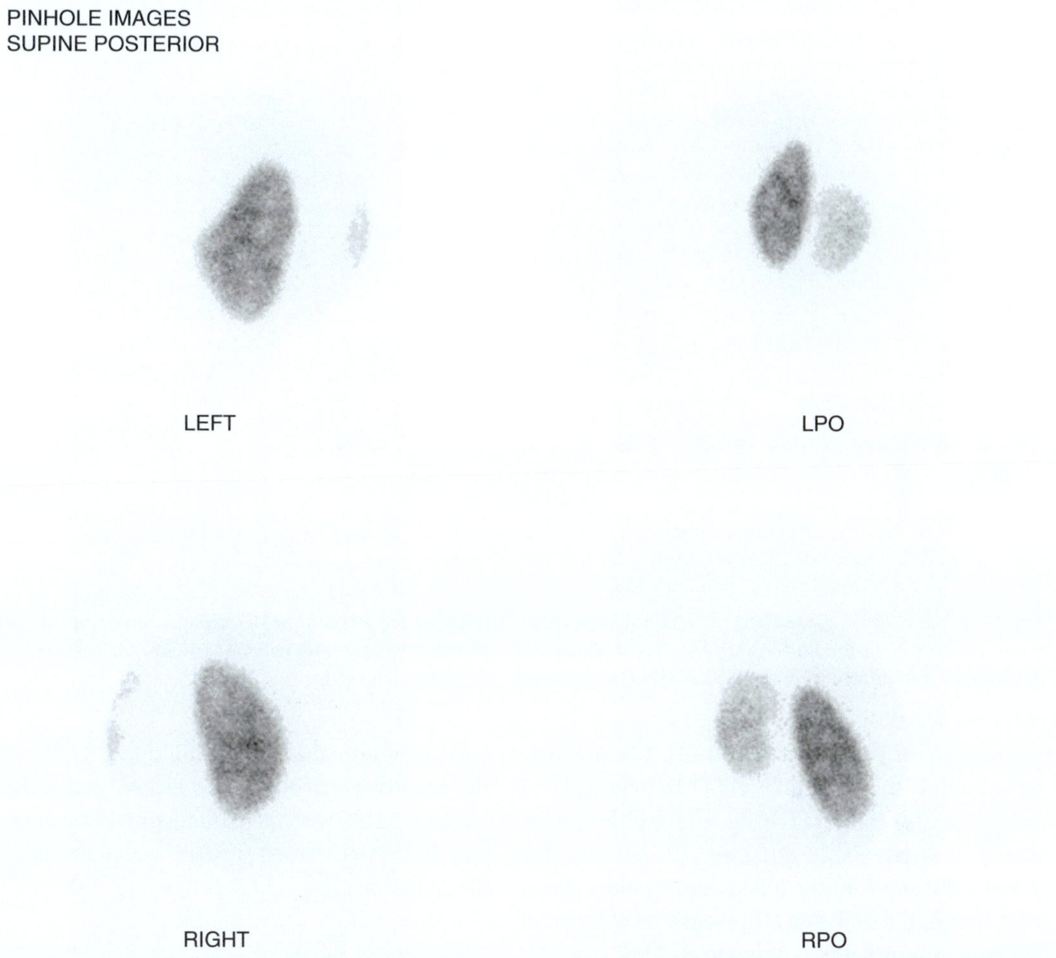

Fig. 27.2 Splenic impression: ^{99m}Tc-DMSA scan in a 4-year-old child with history of urinary tract infection. No definite focal cortical defect or loss of volume is visualized to suggest scarring. There is a flattening in the upper lateral region of the left kidney due to splenic impression

In direct radionuclide cystography (DRC), ^{99m}Tc-pertechnetate or ^{99m}Tc-sulfur colloid (total maximum dose is 37 MBq; 1 mCi) is infused into the bladder with saline via a urinary catheter. The filling phase can be completed when the optimum pre-estimated volume is achieved, when the patient has spontaneously voided, or when the flow from the bottle of solution is stopped in a non-voiding patient (back-pressure effect), and finally when bilateral severe reflux is visualized (the last one is controversial) [5]. Pre-estimated volume is calculated based on this formula: (age in years + 2) × 30 cc = bladder volume. For patients less than 1 year, the same formula is used (if the patient is 6 months old, the age will be 0.5) or is calculated based on this formula: weight in kg × 7 cc = bladder volume. Second or third attempts at filling the bladder may be considered if the target volume is not achieved.

The acquisition starts with filling of the bladder, and when reflux is noted, the bladder volume should be recorded. A single-head camera with a large FOV all-purpose collimator is used for imaging (for newborn less than 1 year, a converg-

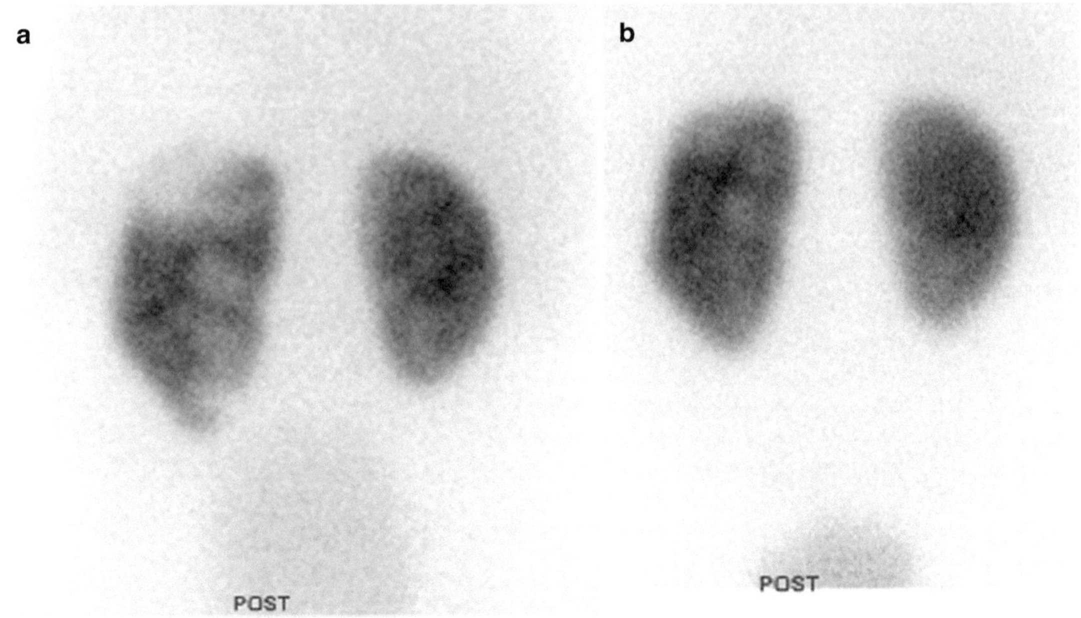

Fig. 27.3 Acute pyelonephritis: ^{99m}Tc-DMSA scan (posterior view) in a 12-month-old girl with fever showed a geographic photopenic defects in the upper and lower poles of the left kidney (**a**). Complete interval resolution of the photopenic defects was noted on follow-up scan 8 months later (**b**)

ing collimator is usually preferred). The acquisitions include dynamic imaging (128 matrix, 10 s/frame for 200 frames) during filling phase, continued with dynamic imaging (2 s/frame for 2 min) during voiding phase and a static post-void imaging (for 1 min). Presence of activity in the ureters or renal pelvis suggests VUR.

The grading system of RNC is different from VCUG. Grade 1 (or mild) reflux in RNC is the visualization of the activity in the ureter (equal to grade 1 in VCUG), a grade 2 (or moderate) is the visualization of activity in the collecting system (equal to grades 2 and 3 in VCUG), and grade 3 (or severe) is the visualization of activity in the collecting system with a dilatation of the collecting system and ureter (equal to grades 4 and 5 in VCUG) (Fig. 27.4).

Another method to detect vesicoureteric reflux is indirect radionuclide cystography (IRC). After a ^{99m}Tc-DTPA or MAG3 renal scan, when the radioisotope has completely cleared from the upper urinary tract and accumulated in the bladder, the child is asked to void and the reflux is assessed. This method has the advantages of additional information about the renal function, there is no need for catheterization, and it is more physiological (avoiding bladder overfilling) [9]. However, the sensitivity of the study is less than DRC or VCUG. Moreover, the patient should be cooperative and toilet trained (usually >3 years old), and the radiation dose is higher than DRC (Box 27.3).

Box 27.3 Protocol Summary for DRC

Indications

To evaluate for vesicoureteral reflux (evaluation of girls at diagnosis, siblings of patients with reflux, and for follow-up studies).

Contraindication

If the child has an active UTI, catheterization may be deferred until after treatment. Please follow your institutional policy for catheter instillation.

Patient Preparation

No special requirements. However if the patient has history of cardiac disease, then prophylactic antibiotics may be necessary. The referring physician is responsible for prescribing the antibiotics and must be informed at the time of booking.

Radiopharmaceutical

^{99m}Tc-SC administered via catheter: 18.5–37 MBq (0.5–1 mCi).

Effective dose (mSv/MBq): 0.0024 [5].

Image Acquisition

Dynamic imaging (128 matrix, 10 s/frame for 200 frames) during filling phase, continued with dynamic imaging (2 s/frame for 2 min) during voiding phase and a static post-void image (for 1 min).

Single-head, large FOV all-purpose collimator (for newborn less than 1 year, a converging collimator) is usually preferred.

Processing and Analysis

Typical evaluation of DRC is visual, reviewing the dynamic imaging for detection of reflux and measuring the bladder volume at the time of reflux. Measurement of the post-residual bladder volume is also helpful.

27.6 Gastric Emptying

A gastric emptying scan is a noninvasive and physiologic imaging technique to measure gastric emptying and to assess response to medication or surgery on the upper GI tract. A barium study is useful for evaluation of anatomic abnormalities. However, barium studies do not provide quantitative measurements and are not completely physiologic. Patients with delayed gastric emptying may present with nausea, vomiting, early satiety, epigastric fullness, or failure to thrive. Patients with diabetes, pyloric stenosis, duodenal stenosis, duodenal web, SLE, dermatomyositis, polymyositis, myotonic dystrophy, hypokalemia, acidosis, hypothyroidism, vagotomy, and gastric inflammation/infection and neurologically impaired children may have delayed gastric emptying. Certain clinical conditions such as partial gastric resection, damage to the vagus nerve, Zollinger–Ellison syndrome, carcinoid syndrome, and duodenal ulcer may

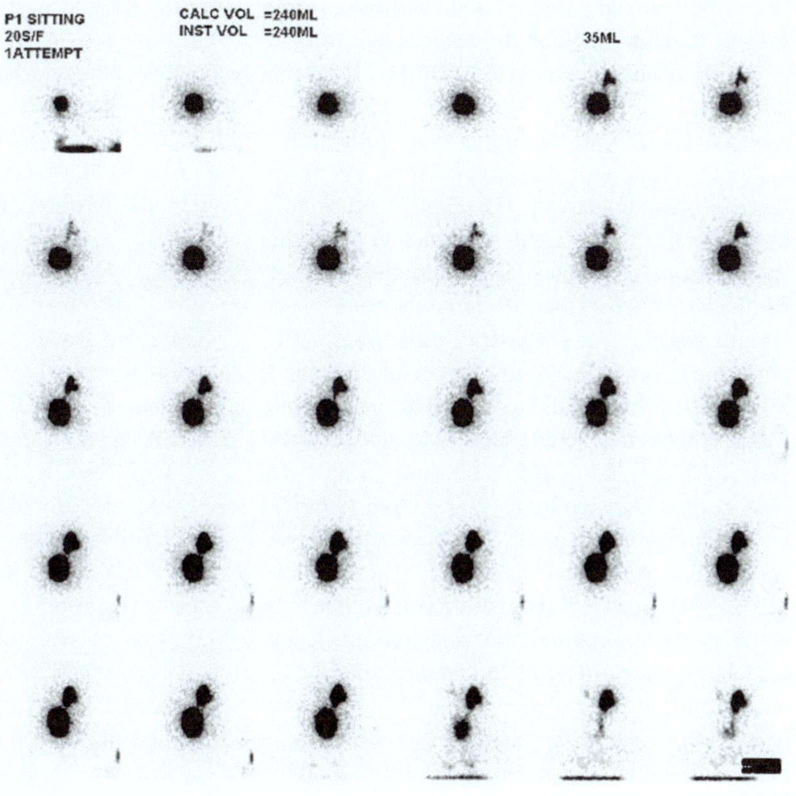

Fig. 27.4 Vesicoureteral reflux: direct radionuclide cystography in a 6-year-old child with history of pyelonephritis. Reflux of the tracer into the right dilated pelvicalyceal system (grade: severe) is noted during filling phase (at 35 cc filling). There is also reflux of the tracer into the left renal pelvis (grade: moderate) visualized during voiding

accelerate the gastric emptying. Medications may also affect the gastric emptying. Opioid or anticholinergic medications may delay gastric emptying, while cisapride, metoclopramide, erythromycin, and ondansetron may accelerate it.

Many factors affect the rate of gastric emptying. Liquid meals usually empty faster than solid meals with an exponential clearance of activity. Solid meals usually empty after a lag phase period followed by a relatively linear pattern. Higher fat content and calorie, increased osmolality, and larger particles may slow gastric emptying. A standardized meal (content, volume, and calories) is necessary to obtain a reliable study but can sometimes be challenging in children.

Milk or formula is usually used to measure gastric emptying in infants (the so-called milk scan). In a milk scan, gastroesophageal reflux and pulmonary aspiration can also be evaluated. The patient should be fasting for 2–4 h before the study. The volume of feed to be given to the child is determined in consultation with the child's physician, dietitian, or parent. The aim is to fill the stomach as much as the patient can tolerate. The milk is mixed with ^{99m}Tc-SC (sulfur colloid) since it remains stable in the acidic environment of the stomach and cannot be absorbed from the GI mucosa. ^{99m} Tc-SC (9.0 MBq; 0.25 mCi) is mixed in 50–75% of the liquid meal (radioactive or "hot" milk) with the remainder to be given "cold" (nonradioactive). The "hot" feed is followed by the "cold" liquid in order to clear the activity from the esophagus. The liquid should be administered in less than 10 min either orally, via NG (nasogastric) or G (gastric) tube. Imaging is performed immediately after the "feeding" phase is finished. The patient is imaged for 60 min using a dynamic acquisition (two consecutive sets of 30 min), 64 matrix, 5 s/frame. Infants are held upright between images, and older children are encouraged to sit up or walk between images. As the milk study is usually done in younger children, a posterior view acquisition is adequate (for solid gastric emptying, anterior and posterior acquisitions for a dual-head camera; anterior or left anterior oblique view for a single-head camera). Static posterior view acquisitions for 1 min (128 matrix) are suggested at 60 and 120 min. Although there is a range of normative values for a milk study in children, in our practice the study is considered to be normal if the half time of emptying is more than 50% at 1 h for children over the age of 2 and more than 50% at 2 h for children less than 2.

An egg sandwich (120 cc white egg) containing ^{99m}Tc-sulfur colloid (9.0 MBq; 0.25 mCi) with two pieces of white bread toasted, two packets of strawberry jam, and 120 mL of water is usually used for the solid gastric emptying study. The geometric mean activity (by simultaneously obtaining anterior and posterior images) is used to overcome the variability of counts with the posteroanterior migration of gastric contents during the acquisition. This is particularly important in older and obese children. If a single-head camera is used, left anterior oblique acquisition is the preferred projection. Static images (with an LEHR collimator and 128 matrix) for 1 min are acquired immediately after feeding (time 0) and at 30, 60, 120, and 240 min. There is limited information available for the normative values of different solid meals among different age groups of children. In young children the normal gastric emptying is 24–48% at 60 min and 48–70% at 120 min [11]. The normal values for adults, where the upper limits of normal range for gastric retention are 90%, 60%, 30%, and 10%, 1 h, 2 h, 3 h, and 4 h after ingestion of a meal, respectively [12], may be useful as a guide for older children (Box 27.4).

Box 27.4 Protocol Summary for Gastric Emptying Study

Indications

Nausea, vomiting, early satiety, epigastric fullness, or failure to thrive.

Contraindication

Food allergy to peanut butter or egg.

Patient Preparation

NPO for 4–6 h. Medications that delay gastric emptying, such as opiates or antispasmodic agents and prokinetic agents such as metoclopramide, tegaserod, domperidone, and erythromycin, are generally stopped 2 days before the test unless the test is done to assess the efficacy of these drugs. Other medications that may have an effect on the rate of gastric emptying include anticholinergic agents atropine, calcium channel blockers, antacids, somatostatin progesterone, octreotide, theophylline, benzodiazepine, and phentolamine. Barium swallow study should not be performed within 72 h prior to this procedure.

Radiopharmaceutical

For solid study, ^{99m}Tc-SC egg white sandwich (120 cc) with water: 9 MBq (0.25 mCi).

For liquid study, ^{99m}Tc-SC (9 MBq; 0.25 mCi) is mixed in 50–75% of the liquid meal (radioactive or "hot" milk) with the remainder to be given "cold" (nonradioactive).

Effective dose (mSv/MBq): 0.024 [5].

Critical organ: proximal colon [12].

Image Acquisition

For liquid study, the patient is imaged for 60 min dynamic acquisition (two sets of 30 min) (with a low-energy high-resolution collimator and 64 matrix), 5 s/frame followed by static posterior view acquisitions for 1 min (128 matrix) at 60 and 120 min. Posterior view is adequate.

For solid study, static images (with a low-energy high-resolution collimator and 128 × 128 matrix) for 1 min are acquired immediately after feeding (time 0) and at 30, 60, 120, and 240 min. Obtain a simultaneous anterior and posterior views with a dual head camera and left anterior oblique view with a single-head camera.

Processing and Analysis

A region of interest is drawn over the stomach in different times. Background subtraction and radioactive decay correction should be performed.

27.7 Pulmonary Aspiration

Pulmonary aspiration can be seen in patients with congenital malformations of the head and neck (e.g., cleft palate) or after upper aerodigestive tract surgery or in neurologically impaired children. The patient may present with recurrent pneumonia. A liquid gastric emptying study (milk scan) and salivagram may be used for the assessment of the pulmonary aspiration in children.

Reviewing the images in a milk scan is helpful to detect gastroesophageal reflux (GER) as well as pulmonary aspiration. The technique is similar to the milk scan with the addition of a delayed static view (with a low-energy high-resolution collimator and 128 matrix for at least 5 min) of the chest added to the typical protocol. A milk scan can detect the aspiration related to GER (retrograde events). The detection rate of aspiration varies in different studies and is relatively low (up to 25%) [13]. The low detection rate of aspiration by a milk study is perhaps due to the low concentration of radiotracer and faster clearance of the radiotracer from the esophagus and stomach in some patients. Protective mechanisms such as cough reflex and mucociliary action can also reduce the sensitivity of the milk scan to detect pulmonary aspiration. Moreover, if the mechanism of pulmonary aspiration is an antegrade aspiration, it can be missed by a milk scan which is based on a retrograde aspiration detection. However, a milk scan has the advantage of evaluating the gastric emptying, GER, and pulmonary aspiration in one study.

A salivagram is a simple, noninvasive study used to evaluate pulmonary aspiration due to antegrade aspiration. The radiation dose is minimal (0.05 mSv) [14], and there is no specific preparation required for the study. The detection rate for this study is higher than a milk study. Since the frequency of antegrade reflux events as a cause of aspiration may be higher than that of retrograde reflux, particularly in neurologically impaired children, the sensitivity of a salivagram is higher than the milk scan. The higher concentration of radiotracer in a salivagram comparing with a milk scan is probably another reason for the higher sensitivity. In a study by Baikie et al. on 63 children with severe spastic quadriplegic cerebral palsy, the salivagram was most frequently positive (56%). Barium video-fluoroscopy was positive in 39%, and milk scan was positive in 6% of the cases [15].

In a salivagram, a drop of liquid containing a small amount of radioactivity (11 MBq; 0.3 mCi of ^{99m}Tc-SC) in 0.1 mL of saline is placed in the oral cavity usually under the tongue. Dynamic images (128 matrix, 30 s for 30 frames) followed by static images of the chest (one in posterior and one lateral projections for 5 min each with 256 matrix) are acquired immediately after administration of the radiotracer. After 5–10 min, 1 cc of water can be placed under the patient's tongue to promote mixing of the saliva in the mouth (this is controversial as it may change a salivagram into a swallow study). The pulmonary aspiration (antegrade aspiration) is diagnosed if there is evidence of tracheobronchial visualization or pulmonary aspiration. In general, the acquisition time is completed by 60 min. However, in the majority of cases, evidence of aspiration is seen in the first 15 min. The acquisition can be continued until the oral radioactivity is no longer present.

27.8 Gastroesophageal Reflux Study

Gastroesophageal reflux (GER) can be detected by pH probe. Reduced pH level over longer than standardized references values for age is often suggestive of an acid reflux event. The PH probe has the benefit of detecting late prandial reflux of nocturnal episodes of reflux. However, it is an invasive procedure and may have false negative results (due to elevation of pH by milk during the test). A milk scan is a physiologic, noninvasive, and simple study to detect GER especially in infants. In infants, the symptoms of GER are usually nonspecific and cannot reliably be used to diagnose GERD or predict the response to treatment. These symptoms include recurrent regurgitation with/without vomiting, symptoms related to pulmonary aspiration, and weight loss or inadequate weight gain. In older children and adolescents, a history and physical examination may be enough to make a diagnosis. Detection of non-acid reflux is another advantage of a milk scan which is reported in approximately 16% of children with GER [16]. The technique of a milk scan is described before. Visual dynamic review of computer-enhanced images is used to assess reflux. The number of episodes of reflux, the duration of each episode, the level reached within the esophagus, and the timing (early versus late) are the parameters that should be reported (Fig. 27.5).

27.9 Meckel's Diverticulum Scan

Meckel's diverticulum is the most common congenital abnormality of the small intestine (1–3% of the population). It is a true diverticulum caused by an incomplete closure of the omphalomesenteric duct. Meckel's diverticulum contains heterotopic gastric mucosa in as many as 50–60% of the cases; these patients usually present with bleeding and/or abdominal pain. Intermittent and painless bleeding per rectum is usually seen in patients less than 2 years old but may occur at any age. In certain cases, the ulceration of the diverticulum or adjacent small bowel mucosa may cause pain with or without bleeding. Other complications include perforation of the small bowel, partial or complete small bowel obstruction, and Meckel's diverticulitis.

Ultrasound is the first investigation to exclude other causes of abdominal pain or bleeding. However, Meckel's diverticulum may be missed in ultrasound or small bowel contrast radiography. ^{99m}Tc scintigraphy is a noninvasive common procedure for the diagnosis of Meckel's diverticulum containing heterotopic gastric mucosa. Approximately 25% of the administered activity accumulates in gastric mucosa. A focal uptake in the abdomen, commonly in the right lower abdomen, increasing over time at a rate similar to the gastric uptake is suggestive of a Meckel's diverticulum containing heterotopic gastric mucosa (Fig. 27.6). The sensitivity and specificity of a Meckel's scan to detect a Meckel's diverticulum are about 85% and 95%, respectively [17].

The patient should be fasted for 2–4 h as the lesion may be obscured by a full stomach or bladder. If possible, the study should be postponed for a few days after a barium study, or a radionuclide scan (Box 27.5). Certain procedures on GI (such as colonoscopy) or some medications (e.g., ethosuximide) may cause nonspecific uptake of the radioisotope due to bowel irritation and inflammation. Potassium perchlorate should not be used as it can reduce the uptake in the heterotopic gastric mucosa.

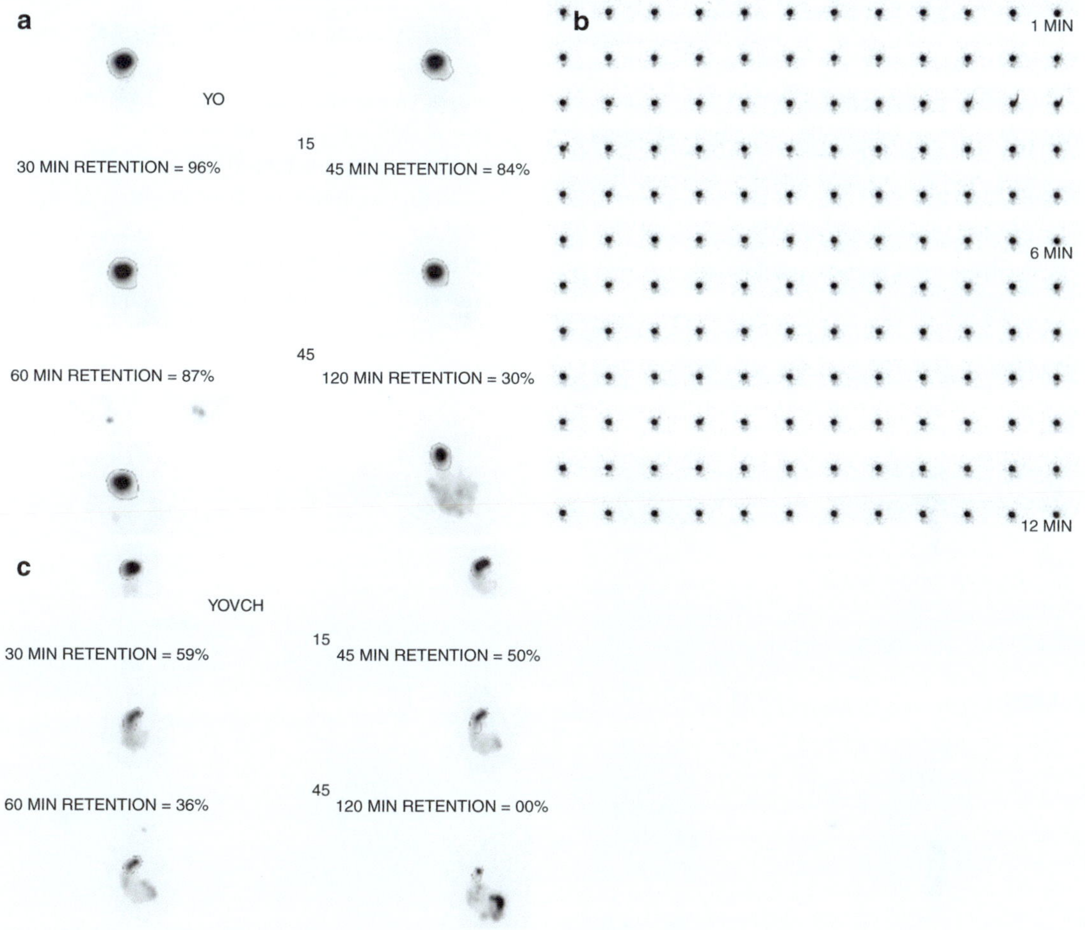

Fig. 27.5 Delayed gastric emptying with gastroesophageal reflux: gastric emptying study in a 7-year-old boy with nausea and vomiting showed delayed gastric emptying (**a**). Dynamic images revealed multiple episodes of gastroesophageal reflux (**b**), some of them reached to the upper esophagus, and it lasts for 20 s (only the first 12 min of dynamic images are shown here). Follow-up study after treatment with domperidone showed interval resolution of the gastric emptying (**c**)

Box 27.5 Protocol Summary for Meckel's Scan

Indications

Bleeding per rectum (painless or with pain) in a child, abdominal pain (in particular if there is questionable finding in other modalities such as ultrasound).

Contraindication

No pre-treatment with sodium perchlorate should be done. The study should be postponed at least 3–4 days after a barium study. The study should be postponed for at least 24–48 h for in vitro RBC scan. It is preferred to postpone the study longer (if possible) if DTPA, MDP, or a stannous agent was used (the stannous from these radiopharmaceuticals remains in the body for approximately 1–2 weeks, and when pertechnetate is administered, it binds to the stannous resulting in a label to RBCs).

Patient Preparation

NPO for 2–4 h.

Premedication with cimetidine (20 mg/kg p.o. for 2 days) or ranitidine (1 mg/kg, IV, 1 h before the study infused over 20 min) or glucagon (50 mg/kg IV over 10 min after the Tc99m pertechnetate administration) with or without pentagastrin (6 mg/kg IV).

Radiopharmaceutical

^{99m}Tc-Pertechnetate: 1.85 MBq/kg (0.05 mCi/kg). Minimum dose of 9 MBq (0.25 mCi).

Effective dose (mSv/MBq): 0.013 [18].

Critical organ: proximal colon.

Image Acquisition

Dynamic imaging (with 128 word matrix, 60 s/frame) for 15 frames followed by static images (256 word matrix, 60 s per image, to include the following views: anterior, right lateral, and posterior abdomen) up to 60 min.

Processing and Analysis

Visual assessment. Pay attention to the other causes of a focal activity in the abdomen rather than heterotopic gastric mucosa and also causes of a false negative study (see text).

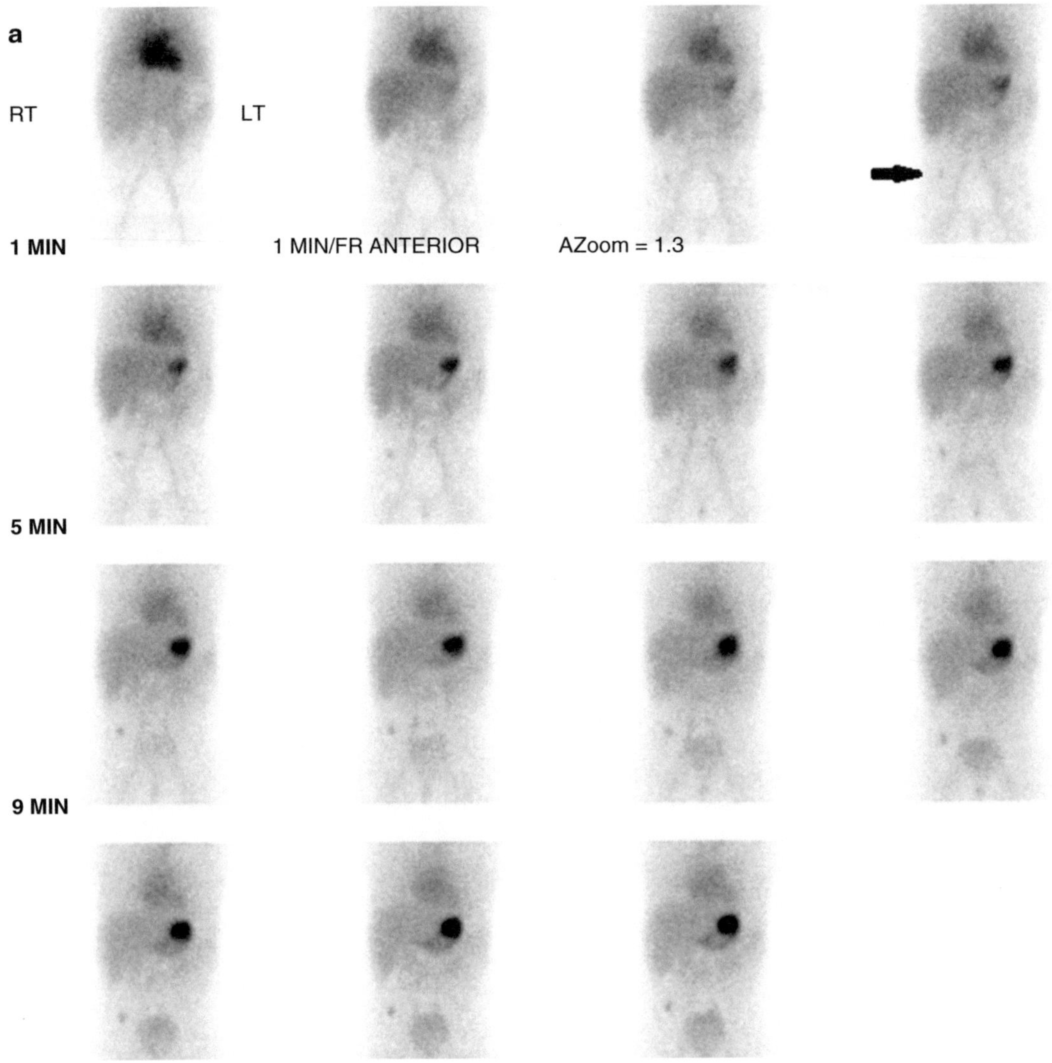

Fig. 27.6 Meckel's diverticulum containing heterotopic gastric mucosa: a small focal activity (arrow) was seen in the right lower quadrant at a rate similar to the gastric uptake (**a**). The activity was seen more lateral at 16 min (**b**) and moved close to the bladder at 30 min (**c**) image. The activity was clearly separated from the adjacent bladder on post-void image at 60 min (**d**)

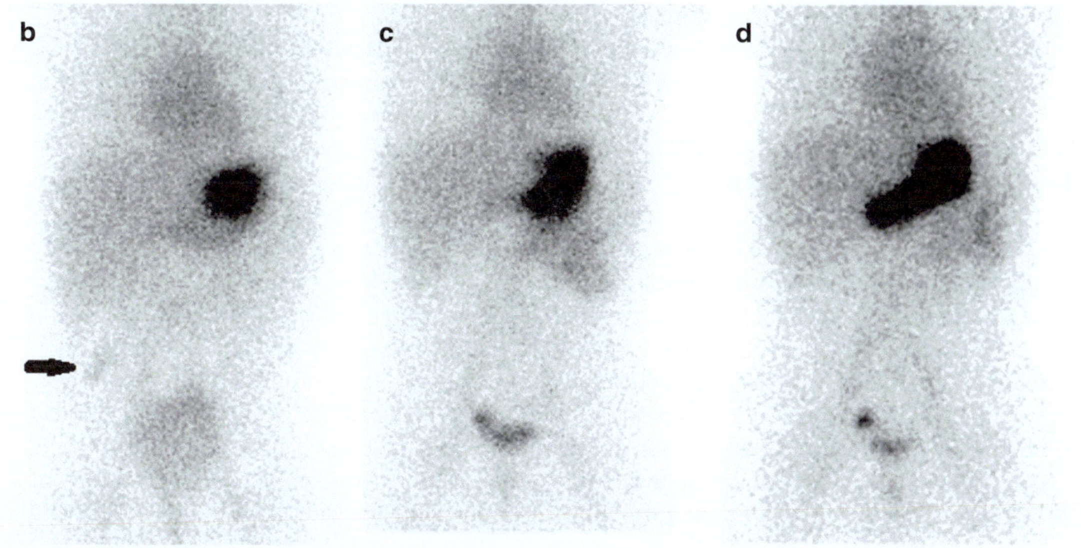

Fig. 27.6 (continued)

The sensitivity of the test can be increased by premedication options:

1. Histamine H2 blockers (cimetidine, ranitidine, famotidine) can increase the uptake of ^{99m}Tc-pertechnetate by inhibiting the release of the activity from the gastric mucosa. The dose is 20 mg/kg p.o. for 2 days for cimetidine or 1 mg/kg, IV, 1 h before the study infused over 20 min for ranitidine.
2. Pentagastrin, with a dose of 6 mg/kg IV, increases the duration and intensity of the ^{99m}Tc-pertechnetate uptake in the gastric mucosa. However, pentagastrin may increase intestinal motility and increase the activity washout.
3. Glucagon, with a dose of 50 mg/kg IV 10 min after the ^{99m}Tc-pertechnetate administration, can be used with pentagastrin or alone to reduce bowel motility.

If the patient is in emergency situation, there is no need for premedication. After the IV injection of 1.85 MBq/kg (0.05 mCi/kg) of ^{99m}Tc-pertechnetate (minimum dose of 9 MBq or 0.25 mCi), dynamic imaging (with 128 matrix, 60 s/frame) is obtained for 15 frames followed by static images (256 matrix, 60 s per image), to include the following views: anterior, right lateral, and posterior abdomen up to 60 min (Box 27.5).

A focal activity in the right lower quadrant, increasing over the time at a rate similar to the gastric uptake, is suggestive of a Meckel's diverticulum containing heterotopic gastric mucosa. However, other possibilities may mimic this pattern including vascular malformations, contamination, ulcers, hypervascular tumors, ectopic gastric mucosa other than Meckel's diverticulum (duplication cysts, Barrett's esophagus), ectopic kidney, accessory spleen, inflammation due to intestinal obstruction, intussusception, irritation due to consumption of certain drugs (ethosuximide or laxatives), and various urinary tract abnormalities such as dilated pelvis or ureters, extrarenal pelvis, hydronephrosis, bladder diverticulum, vesicoureteral reflux, obstruction, or vesicoureteral reflux.

In certain cases, the study may not show the heterotopic gastric mucosa in a Meckel's scan. These include insufficient gastric mucosa, washout of the secreted ^{99m}Tc-pertechnetate, dilution of radioactivity in small bowel due to hemorrhage, fast washout due to increased bowel movement, and impaired vascular supply due to intussusception, obstruction, or pressure from the adjacent organs (dilated ureter, bladder, or bowel). Poor techniques (inadequate preparation, no fasting, no premedication prior administration of potassium perchlorate, previous barium study, inadequate timing of imaging, and lack of appropriate lateral and post-void images) are other important considerations for a false negative study [19].

27.10 Hepatobiliary Scan

Various indications are available for hepatobiliary scintigraphy including suspected cases of biliary atresia, choledochal cyst, cholecystitis, and biliary leakage. ^{99m}Tc-disofenin (2,6-diisopropylacetanilido iminodiacetic acid) and ^{99m}Tc-mebrofenin (bromo-2,4,6-trimethylacetanilido iminodiacetic acid) are usually used for hepatobiliary scintigraphy. ^{99m}Tc-mebrofenin (0.05 mCi/kg or 1.85 MBq/kg) is the preferred radiotracer to differentiate obstructive biliary tract diseases, such as biliary atresia from hepatocellular disorders (Box 27.6). The patient doesn't need to be NPO. Pre-treatment with phenobarbital (5 mg/kg/day divided bid for 3–5 days) or ursodeoxycholic acid (20 mg/kg/day in two divided doses for 2–3 days) prior to scintigraphy increases the test accuracy. The sensitivity and specificity of the test for biliary atresia are about 97% and 82%, respectively [10].

Box 27.6 Protocol Summary for Hepatobiliary Scan in Biliary Atresia

Indications

In suspected cases of biliary atresia (conjugated hyperbilirubinemia in early infancy).

Contraindication

Hypersensitivity to a hepatobiliary compound.

Patient Preparation

The patient doesn't need to be NPO (for non-biliary atresia scan, the patient should fast for 2–4 h).

Pre-treatment with phenobarbital (5 mg/kg/day divided bid for 3–5 days) or ursodeoxycholic acid (20 mg/kg/day in two divided doses for 2–3 days) prior to scintigraphy.

Radiopharmaceutical

^{99m}Tc-disofenin or ^{99m}Tc-mebrofenin 1.8 MBq/kg (0.05 mCi/kg), with a minimum administered activity of 18.5 MBq (0.5 mCi).

Effective dose: 1–2 mSv.

Critical organ: colon.

Image Acquisition

Dynamic anterior images (128 matrix, 60 s per frame using appropriate zoom setting) for 30 min followed by static images (256 matrix for 2 min each) in anterior and right lateral views at 1 h.

If no bowel activity is seen after 1 h of imaging, delayed static images (2, 4, 6, and 24 h) up to 24 h are acquired to detect any radiotracer excretion into the bowel.

Processing and Analysis

Visual assessment. Visualization of bowel activity excludes biliary atresia.

Immediately following injection of the radiotracer, dynamic abdominal images (128 matrix, 60 s per frame for 30 min using appropriate zoom setting) are acquired in anterior projection. At 1 h after injection, static (256 matrix for 2 min each, anterior and right lateral views) images are obtained. If no bowel activity is seen after 1 h of imaging, delayed static images (2, 4, 6, and 24 h) up to 24 h are acquired to detect any radiotracer excretion into the bowel. Excretion into the bowel excludes the presence of biliary atresia (Fig. 27.7). If there is no bowel activity, the study is suggestive of biliary atresia (Fig. 27.8). However, this pattern may be seen in severe cases of hepatocellular disease, sepsis, dehydration, TPN cholestasis, and bile plug syndrome in cystic fibrosis [11]. Thus, in practice, the value of hepatobiliary scan is to exclude biliary atresia (in case of visualization of bowel activity), not to diagnose it.

In children, acute cholecystitis may be due to gallbladder obstruction, or may be acalculous, secondary to sepsis, prolonged illness, vasculitis, or infections. Similar to the adults, non-visualization of the gallbladder is suggestive of acute cholecystitis. However, there is still

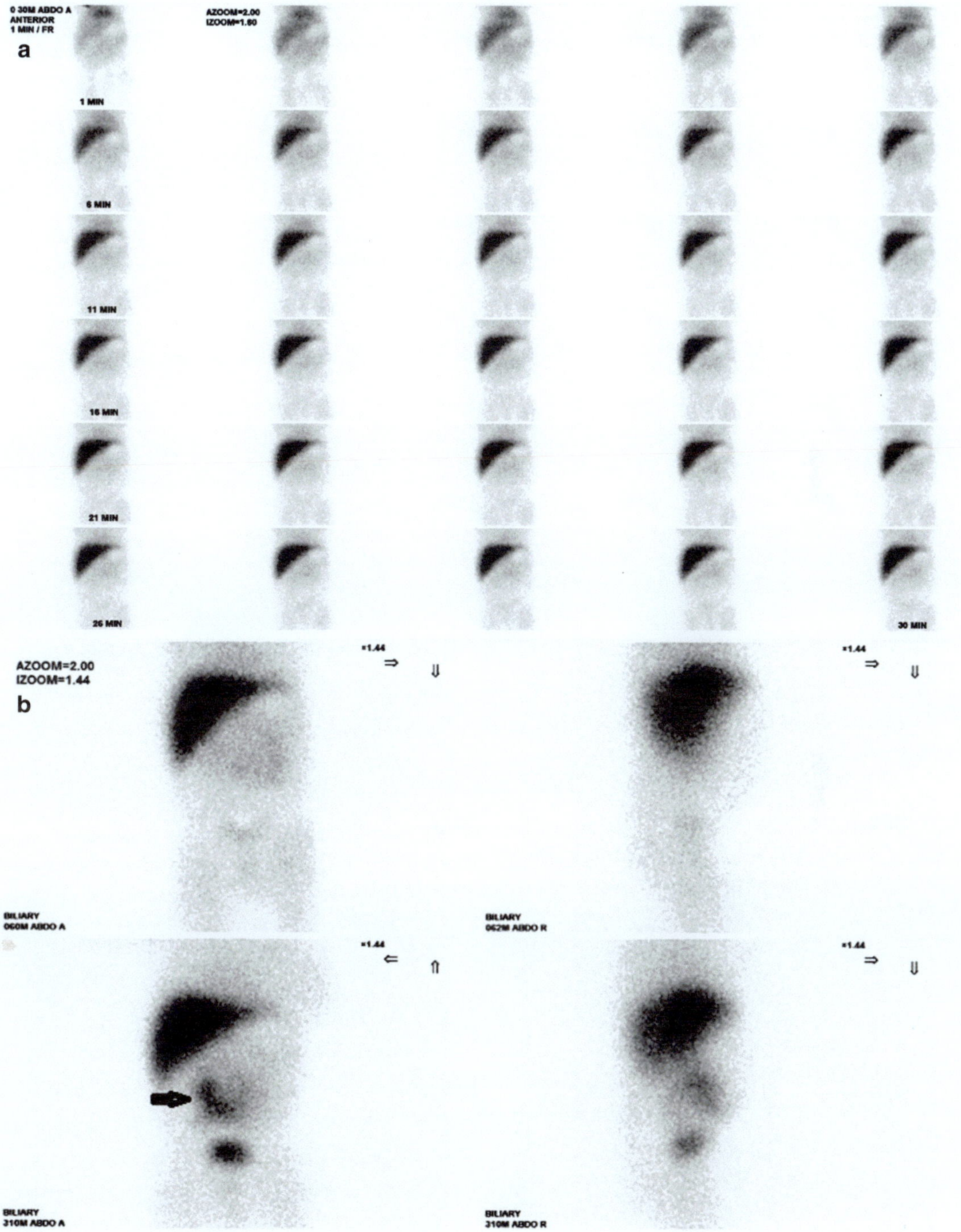

Fig. 27.7 No evidence of biliary atresia: hepatobiliary scan in a 4-week-old boy with conjugated hyperbilirubinemia showed good hepatic uptake with no drainage of activity into the bowel in the first 30 min (**a**). Bowel activity (arrow) was visualized on delayed images (4–6 h) which excluded the diagnosis of biliary atresia (**b**)

possibility of acalculous cholecystitis. If the gallbladder is visualized, response to a fatty meal or infusion of sincalide (0.02 mg/kg) is helpful to assess the contraction of the gallbladder. Hepatobiliary scintigraphy is also helpful to evaluate a biliary leak secondary to trauma or surgery.

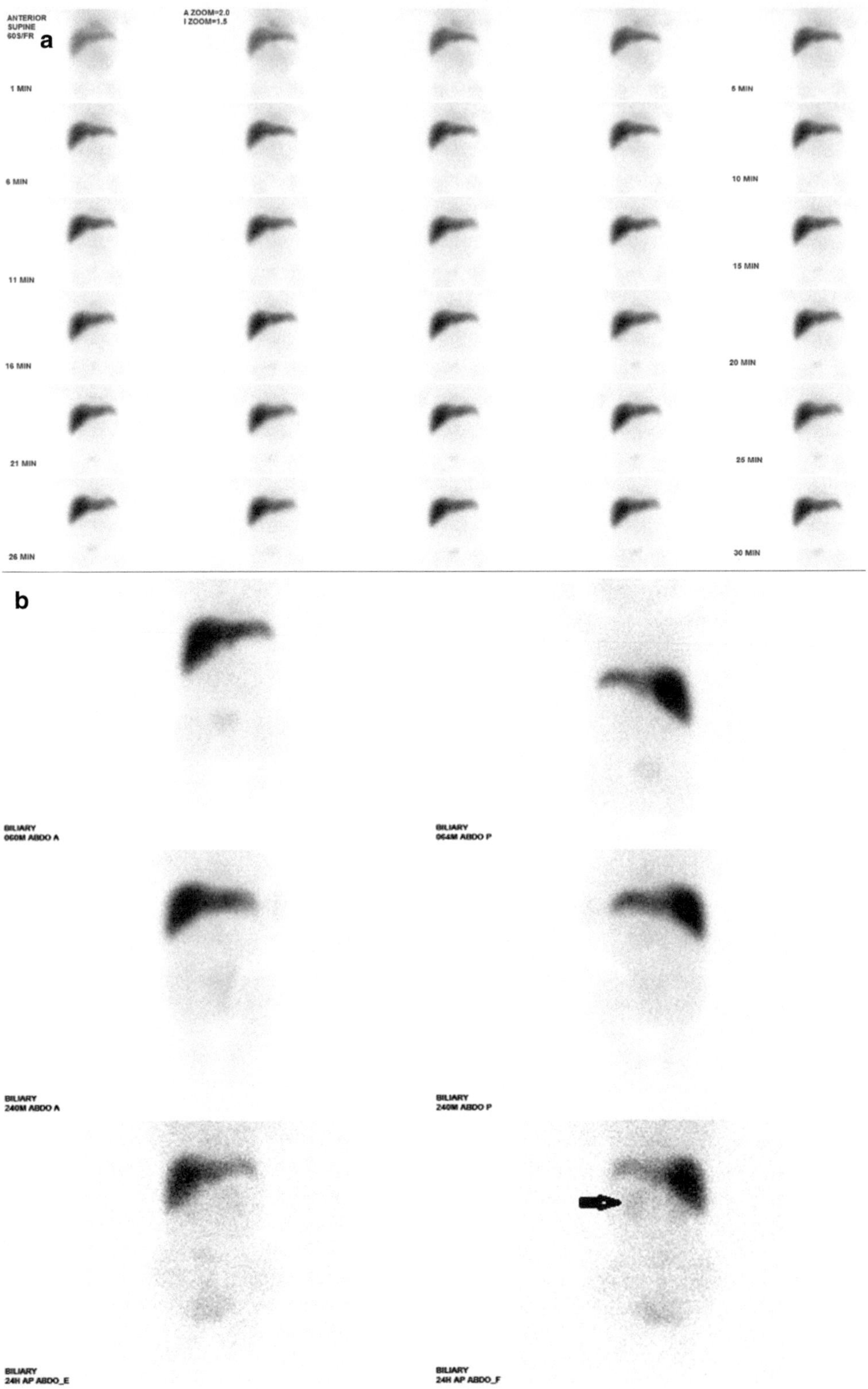

Fig. 27.8 Biliary atresia: hepatobiliary scan in a 5-week-old boy with conjugated hyperbilirubinemia showed good hepatic uptake with no drainage of activity into the bowel on early images (**a**) and delayed views (**b**) up to 24 h. Note the renal activity (arrow) seen in the abdomen on delayed images which is more prominent on posterior view

A biliary leak may be suspected by visualization of a fluid collection on US or CT scan. A hepatobiliary scan is a sensitive and noninvasive method that is able to establish an active hepatobiliary component associated with the fluid collection.

27.11 Bone Scintigraphy

Bone scintigraphy is a very sensitive modality to evaluate benign and neoplastic bone diseases in both adults and children. ^{99m}Tc-Methylene diphosphonate (^{99m}Tc-MDP) is the most commonly used radiopharmaceutical for bone scintigraphy. This tracer concentrates in the amorphous calcium phosphate and crystalline hydroxyapatite reflecting both blood flow and osteoblastic reaction of bone. In accordance with the North American Consensus Guidelines, the recommended dose is 9.3 MBq/kg (0.25 mCi/kg) for children with a minimum dose of 37 MBq (1.0 mCi) [20]. The most recent version of EANM Paediatric Dose Card can also be used for optimal administered activities [21].

PET imaging using ^{18}F-NaF is being explored as an alternative method to bone scintigraphy with ^{99m}Tc-MDP. PET scanners have a greater ability than gamma cameras to image the high-energy photons of ^{18}F-NaF with similar radiation dosimetry and offer better sensitivity by improving spatial resolution [22, 23]. In addition, scanning can be acquired as early as 30 min after injection comparing with bone scintigraphy (using ^{99m}Tc-MDP), which requires imaging to be done 2–4 h after injection. This reduced time allows for faster and increased patient scheduling which can be beneficial for a busy nuclear medicine department.

Bone scintigraphy may include blood flow, blood pool, and delayed imaging and is known as three-phase imaging. Osteomyelitis is one of the most common indications for acquiring a three-phase bone scan in children. A blood flow study is obtained immediately after intravenous radiotracer injection for 1 min followed by blood pool images. Skeletal phase or delayed images are performed 2–4 h later (Box 27.7). Whole-body images are highly recommended in children regardless of the location of symptoms. For younger or small children, multiple static images can be acquired to avoid longer immobilization periods and thus minimize motion artifacts. In addition, this technique allows for better positioning of extremities [24].

Box 27.7 Protocol Summary for Bone Scintigraphy

Indications

Evaluate benign and neoplastic bone diseases.

Contraindication

Previously administered radiopharmaceutical (within 24–48 h).

Patient Preparation

No special requirements.

A topical anesthetic such as Maxilene can be applied prior to intravenous injection if needed.

Have patient void prior to imaging the pelvis or check if a diaper change is needed.

Radiopharmaceutical

^{99m}Tc-MDP: 9.3 MBq/kg (0.25 mCi/kg). Minimum 37 MBq (1 mCi) [44].

Effective dose: 2.7 mSv [1].

Critical organ: urinary bladder.

Image Acquisition

- **Flow Phase**: Dynamic images (1–3 s per frame) for 60 s.
- **Blood Pool Phase**: Immediate static images. 128 × 128 or greater matrix.
- 3–5 min/image or approximately 300,000 counts/image.
- **Skeletal Phase**: 2–3 h after tracer injection.
- Low-energy, high-resolution collimator is commonly used.
- Whole-body scan with speed 8–12 cm/min. 256 × 1024 matrix or greater.
- Spot views with 5 min/view or 300–500k counts/view. 128 or 256 matrix.
- **SPECT**: 60–64 images (20 s/view), 128 matrix or greater; zoom as required.
- **SPECT/CT**: CT acquisition should be strictly limited to the body segment of interest.

- CT settings should be individually adjusted according to the age and BMI.
- **Pinhole Collimator**: With 2 or 5 mm insert. Approximately 75k–100k counts/view.
- Dynamic acquisition could be used for motion correction to create a composite image.

Magnification technique with pinhole collimation improves resolution and can be particularly helpful in imaging small bony structures such as the femoral capital epiphysis. SPECT (single-photon emission computed tomography) can improve the sensitivity and specificity of planar images while providing better anatomic localization. Generally, SPECT studies are superior to planar images and are particularly useful in the evaluation of back pain [23, 25]. Combining the functional imaging of SPECT with the anatomic imaging of CT can further improve diagnostic accuracy and localization. SPECT/CT imaging systems are readily available and rapidly emerging as an important diagnostic tool in pediatric musculoskeletal imaging. In adult patients, SPECT/CT may be used for localization of osteomyelitis, inflammation, and both benign and malignant bone disease. Potential applications in children may include back pain and evaluation for suspected spondylolysis or enthesitis in the spinous processes [26, 27].

In order to appropriately interpret pediatric bone scintigraphy images, it is essential to know the unique normal physiologic distribution as well as pathologic findings in children. The normal distribution in pediatric bone scans may differ from adults. In children, high physeal and apophyseal uptake due to rich blood supply and active enchondral ossification is often noted. Absence of uptake in nonossified cartilaginous structures should not be mistaken for avascular necrosis. Regions where this may be of concern in younger children include the femoral capital epiphysis, patella, and navicular bone. Before ossification, the ischiopubic synchondrosis appears as a discontinuity of the inferior pubic ramus. During ossification, increased uptake in ischiopubic synchondroses is a common normal variant and should not be misinterpreted as a pathologic lesion [28].

Acute osteomyelitis is a common pediatric disease that can occur at any age, most often affecting children less than 5 years. Usually, it is the result of hematogenous spread of infection due to the rich vascular supply of the growing skeleton. It can be seen following direct puncture or spread of infection from contiguous structure [29]. Circulating organisms tend to infect the metaphyseal ends of the long bones (i.e., femur, tibia, and humerus), especially in the lower extremities, because of the high vascularity of the metaphyseal capillaries. In children less than 18 months, the presence of transphyseal vessels extending between the metaphysis and the epiphysis makes them particularly prone to septic arthritis of the adjacent joint. In older children, the growth plate is a relative barrier to the spread of infection into the epiphysis. Osteomyelitis in flat bones such as ilium and vertebrae is less frequent than in long bones [30]. Limping or refusal to bear weight is often the only symptom in older children. Radiography may be normal or only show deep soft tissue swelling within 48 h of infection. Three-phase bone scintigraphy is highly sensitive for the detection of osteomyelitis. Typically, a bone scan becomes positive 24–72 h after the onset of infection. The sensitivity of three-phase bone scan has been estimated as 94% with a specificity of 95% [31]. Ideally, the bone scan should be obtained before joint aspiration. However, diagnostic aspiration and antibiotic therapy should not be delayed until the bone scan is completed, as fine needle aspiration does not alter bone scan findings, nor does antibiotic therapy lead to a rapid change in bone scan [30]. A delayed whole-body scan on skeletal phase should be routinely obtained as osteomyelitis in children can be multifocal or present with referred pain. In addition, malignant disease such as leukemia and sarcoma may mimic acute osteomyelitis [25]. Blood flow, blood pool, and delayed images show focally high uptake in the affected bone. Occasionally, the affected bone in children shows low uptake [32]. This is most likely due to reduced tracer delivery by increased intraosseous pressure from inflammation, edema, and joint effusion. Cellulitis can be differentiated from osteomyelitis as it typically demonstrates diffuse increased activity in the soft tissues on the dynamic and blood pool images, without focal osseous abnormality on delayed images.

Septic arthritis is more common in children younger than 3 years old with the hip and knee joints being the most commonly involved areas. Clinical findings include fever, pain, swelling, and erythema of the involved joint. Pain with passive motion is the most consistent finding in septic arthritis. Transient synovitis is the most common condition that mimics septic arthritis and is commonly seen in children less than 10 years old. It is typically preceded by a viral upper respiratory infection. Transient synovitis is a self-limited condition that most commonly involves the juvenile hip. It may be clinically indistinguishable from septic arthritis, and joint aspiration is often required. Early radiography may demonstrate the presence of a joint effusion with joint space widening and subluxation. Ultrasound can help in the detection of joint effusion. Echogenic material within the effusion suggests septic arthritis. In transient synovitis, the three-phase bone scan may be normal or can demonstrate diffuse increased flow and blood pool activity. Delayed images may demonstrate periarticular increased activity in the affected joint. If a bone scan is performed before joint aspiration, decreased tracer uptake on delayed images may be seen as a result of vascular compression by the joint effusion. The proper course of action is to aspirate the joint promptly. Generally, a bone scan is obtained after aspiration to detect any associated osteomyelitis [25].

Chronic recurrent multifocal osteomyelitis (CRMO) occurs most frequently in the latter half of the first decade and the first half of the second decade of life. Girls are more affected than boys. The clinical spectrum is often nonspecific with an insidious onset of localized warmth, tenderness, pain, and swelling. New sites of involvement can present as old sites resolve or are in various phases of healing. The disorder typically has a benign, self-limited clinical course with periodic exacerbations and remissions. Bone biopsy demonstrates fibrosis and inflammatory cells, but bone and blood cultures are negative. The metaphysis is the most common location of CRMO (Fig. 27.9). The most common anatomical sites are the long bones, spine, pelvis, and clavicles. Bone scintigraphy is helpful in identifying the multifocal bone lesions and typically demonstrates high uptake in both symptomatic and asymptomatic lesions [30, 33].

Legg–Calvé–Perthes disease is idiopathic ischemic necrosis of the femoral head in children. This disorder is most commonly seen in children between the ages of 5 and 8 years. Patients typically present with limping and pain in the affected hip. Bone scintigraphy is more sensitive than radiography for early diagnosis and is comparable to MRI [25]. In children, pinhole images can be obtained to improve the resolution. Generally, studies performed early after the onset of clinical symptoms show the absence of activity in the capital femoral epiphysis (Fig. 27.10) and can precede radiographic manifestations [34]. Later scans may demonstrate increased activity due to revascularization and remodeling.

Skeletal trauma can be evaluated by radiography. However, some injuries may be occult, and bone scintigraphy can help localize the abnormality and assist in diagnosis. Bone scintigraphy is highly sensitive and becomes abnormal as early as a few hours after injury. A toddler's fracture is a spiral or oblique fracture that most commonly involves the tibiae. Radiographic findings are often subtle and fractures may not be apparent. As such bone scintigraphy is a valuable tool for detecting this injury early before radiographic changes are present. Typically, the bone scan shows diffuse increased uptake in the tibial diaphysis (Fig. 27.11). A linear or spiral pattern of high uptake may be seen in some children [30].

Stress injury occurs due to repetitive stress on normal bone causing internal remodeling involving osteoclastic resorption and osteoblastic repair. Stress fractures can occur when resorption exceeds bone replacement which temporarily weakens the cortex [35]. Bone scintigraphy is

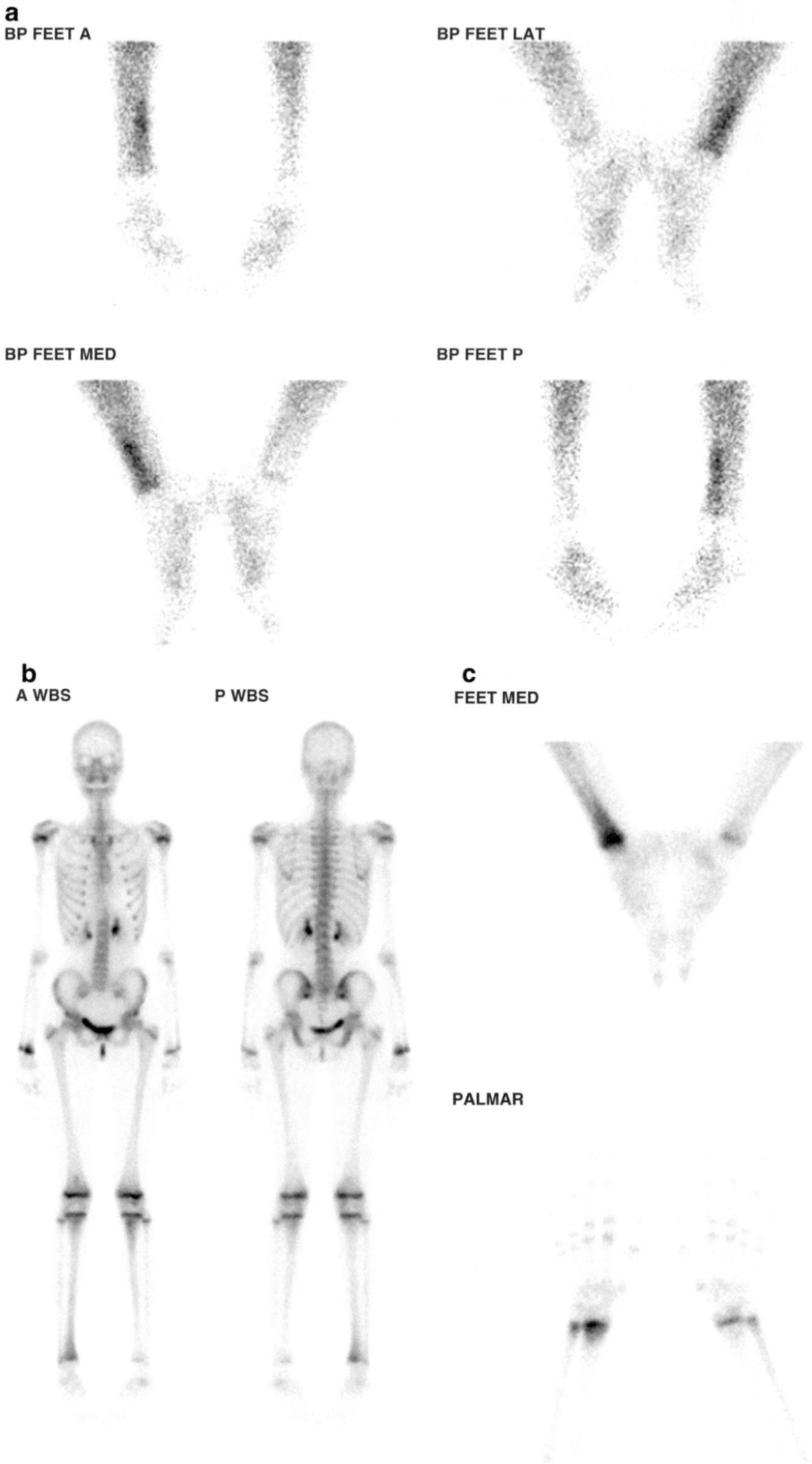

Fig. 27.9 CRMO: bone scan in a 15-year-old girl with CRMO presenting with right ankle swelling and redness. Blood pool images (**a**) showed asymmetric increased activity in the distal right tibia suggestive of hyperemia. On delayed whole-body scan (**b**) and spot views (**c**), there are multiple foci of increased activity in the distal right tibia, bilateral distal femurs, proximal left tibia, and distal right radius

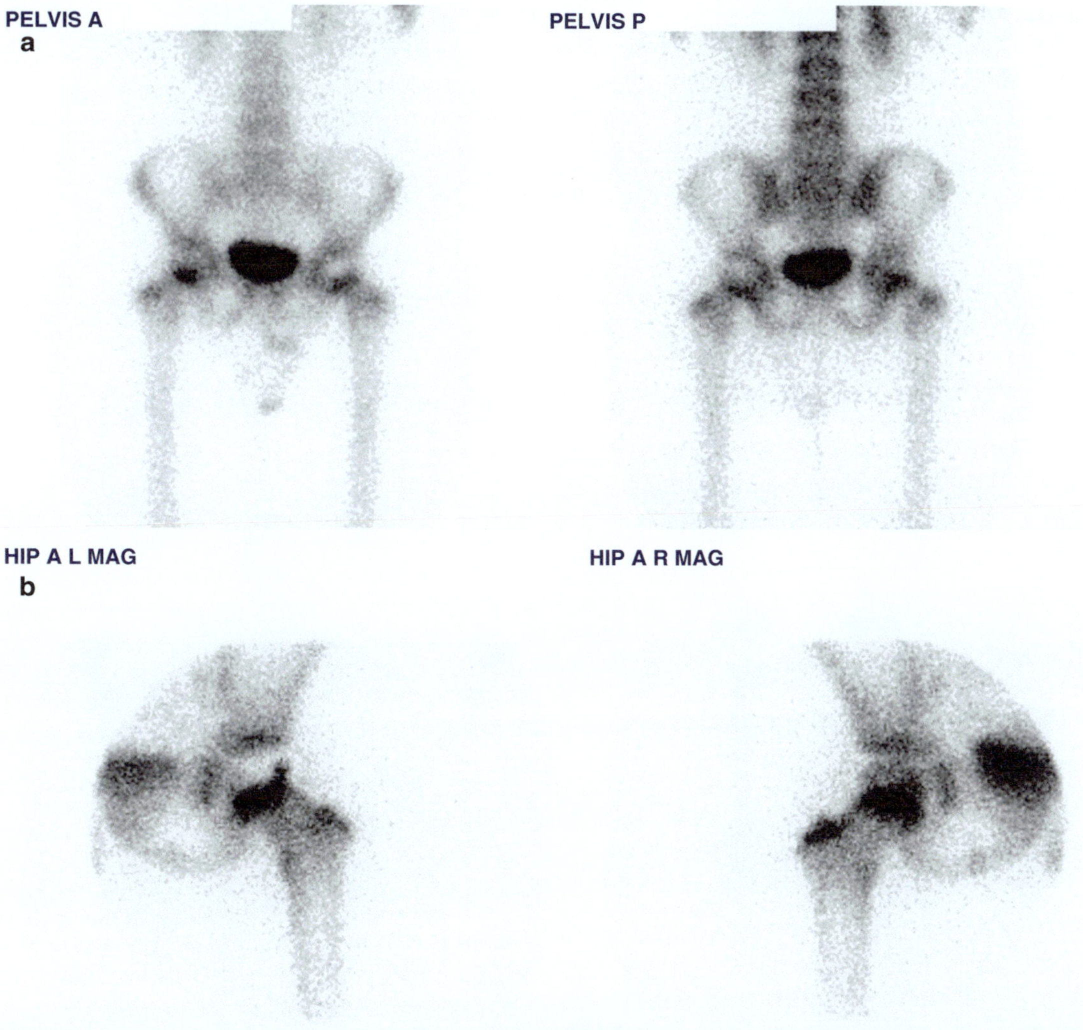

Fig. 27.10 Legg–Calvé–Perthes disease: planar (**a**) and pinhole (**b**) bone scan in a 6-year-old boy with limping shows decreased activity in the left femoral head suggestive of avascular necrosis

more sensitive than radiographs in detecting stress fractures. The bone scan is usually abnormal at the time of presentation and can precede plain film changes. MRI can be used in stress injury; however, unlike bone scintigraphy the entire skeleton cannot be easily screened on MRI.

Spondylolysis represents a stress fracture of the pars interarticularis of the vertebrae that occurs most commonly in the lower lumbar spine secondary to repetitive minor trauma such as hyperextension. However, congenital weakness of the pars as a result of hereditary factors also plays a role in its pathogenesis. Most patients present with either acute or chronic back pain. Sports such as gymnastics, diving, ballet, and contact sports such as football, hockey, and lacrosse are most commonly associated with spondylolysis. Bilateral spondylolysis may cause spondylolisthesis. Pars defects can be imaged with plain radiography, bone scintigraphy, computed tomography (CT), and magnetic resonance imaging (MRI). In bone scintigraphy, spondylolysis produces little or no abnormality on blood pool images. Delayed images typically show focally high uptake in the region of the pars interarticularis. SPECT imaging (or SPECT/CT) is more sensitive than planar studies and is recommended in evaluation of low back pain in young athletes [36]. Low back pain may arise from a lumbosacral transitional vertebral articulation

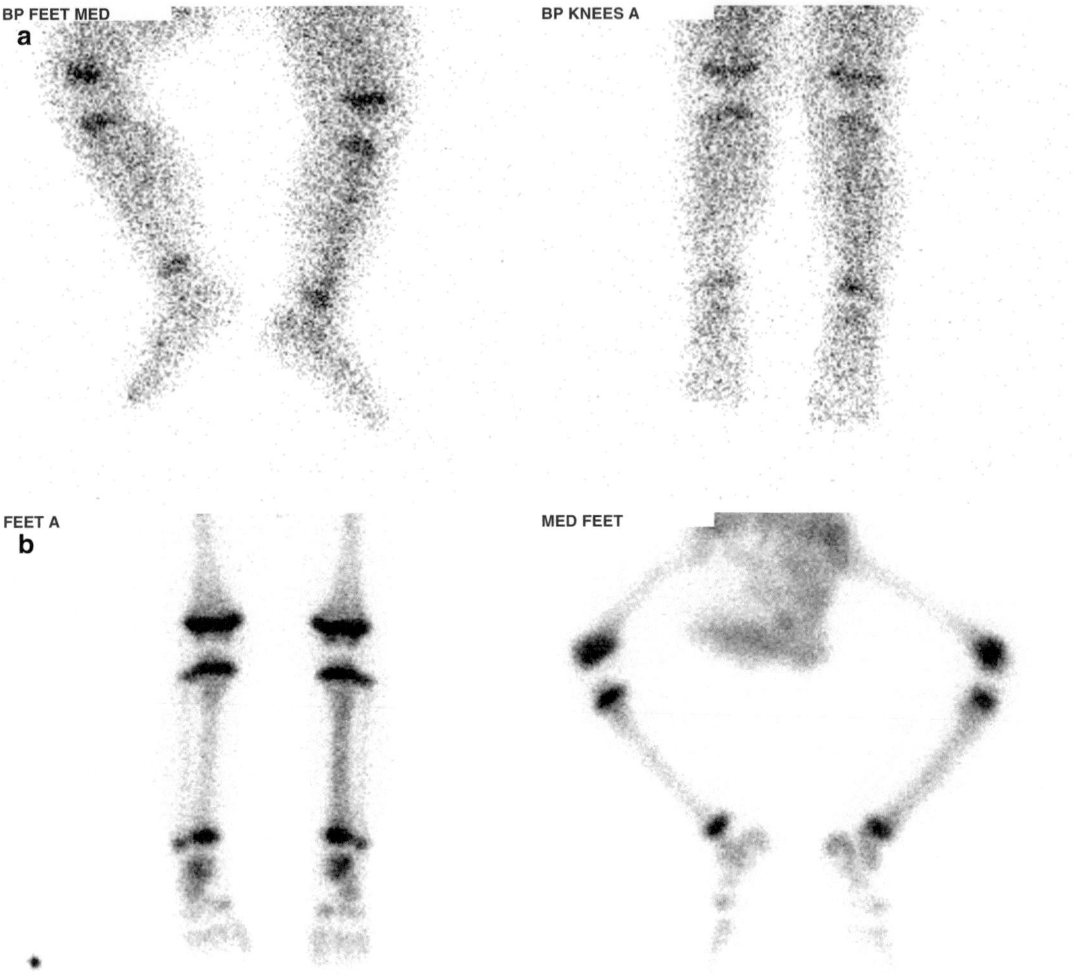

Fig. 27.11 Toddler's fracture: bone scan in an 18-month-old infant who fell down at daycare and was unable to bear his weight on the left side. Blood pool images (**a**) and delayed spot views (**b**) showed diffuse increased uptake in the left tibial diaphysis suggestive of toddler's fracture

which is a common congenital anomaly. Skeletal scintigraphy can show focally increased uptake along the transverse-sacral articulation of the transitional vertebra which supports the diagnosis of stress-associated injury with lumbosacral transitional vertebrae. As for spondylolysis, a SPECT study is superior to planar images (Fig. 27.12) and is recommended [23, 37].

In child abuse, bone scintigraphy is a complementary imaging modality to skeletal survey in diagnosis and management. Both modalities can be performed when child abuse is suspected [38]. Bone scintigraphy is useful when radiographs are normal, or detection of additional fractures would be helpful in confirming the diagnosis. It can provide a quick assessment to characterize the extent and severity of trauma and is more sensitive than radiographs for detection of rib fractures and nondisplaced diaphyses fractures of the extremities but is less sensitive for skull or symmetric metaphyseal fractures. Typically, rib fractures occur laterally, anteriorly, and posteriorly close to the costovertebral junction where the ribs are compressed against

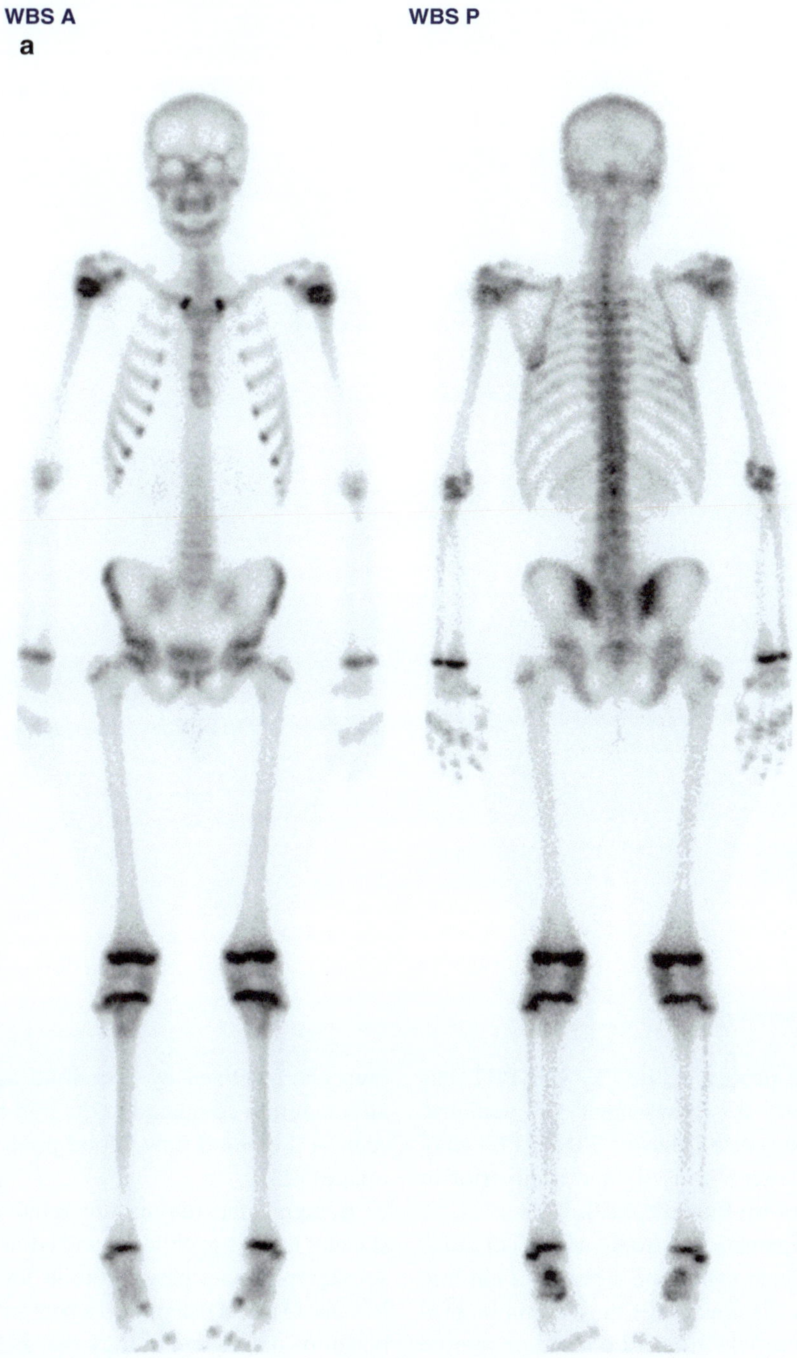

Fig. 27.12 Spondylolysis: bone scan in a 14-year-old by with low back pain. Whole-body scan (**a**) didn't show any significant abnormality. SPECT study showed a focal increased activity in the left pars interarticularis visualized on coronal (**b**), axial (**c**), and sagittal (**d**) views

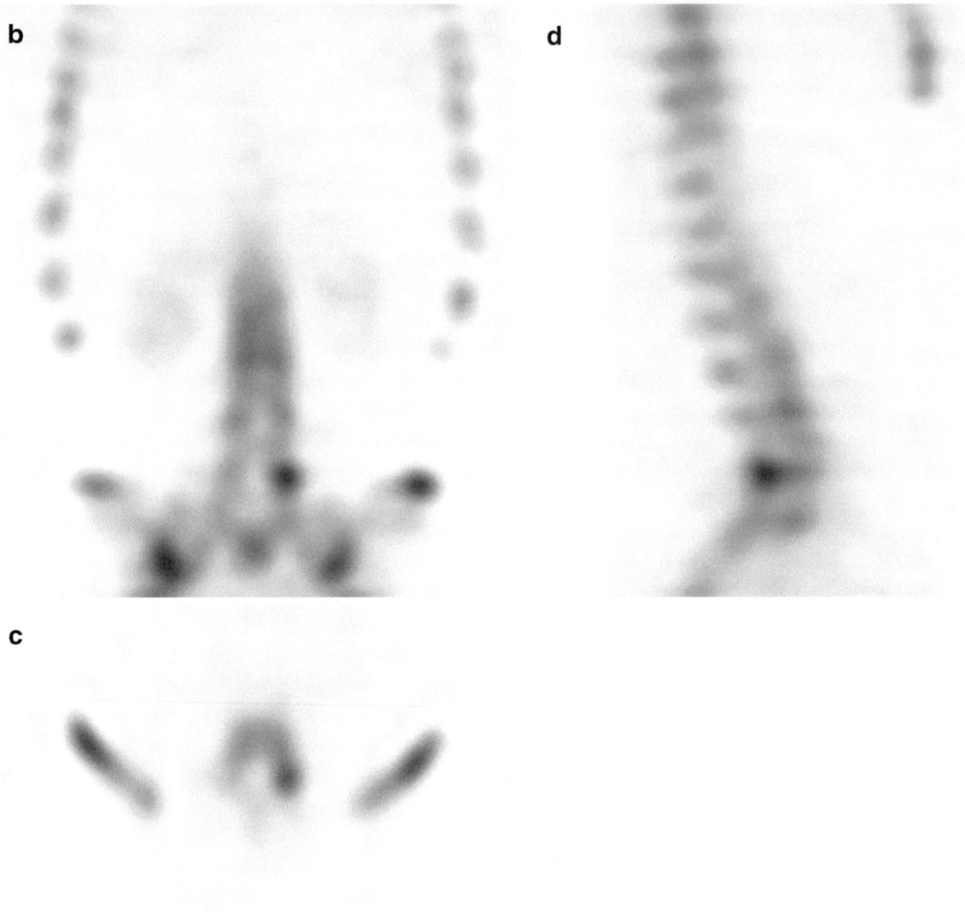

Fig. 27.12 (continued)

the transverse process [39]. ^{18}F-NaF PET has been evaluated for assessment of pediatric patients with suspected abuse. ^{18}F-NaF PET may have overall better sensitivity and is superior in the detection of rib fractures [40].

Reflex sympathetic dystrophy (RSD) or complex regional pain syndrome type I is a chronic pain syndrome. Trauma is the most common precipitating factor, which may be acute or remote by several months. RSD should be considered in a child who presents with persistent pain in the absence of laboratory and clinical findings. The typical findings on bone scan are hyperemia on blood flow and blood pool images with intense periarticular activity in the affected extremity. A cold variant of RSD has been reported in children characterized by decreased activity in the affected limb compared to the non-affected limb seen in the blood flow, blood pool, and delayed images [23].

Benign bone tumors are relatively common skeletal lesions in children and adolescents. Bone scintigraphy may play a role in localizing these lesions. Osteoid osteoma is a benign skeletal neoplasm of unknown etiology that is composed of highly vascular central nidus surrounded by reactive trabecular bone. The central nidus is usually smaller than 1.5 cm in diameter. The lesion can be cortical (most common), medullary, or periosteal. It can occur in any bone commonly in femur, tibia, and spine, but appendicular lesions are more common than vertebral lesions. Vertebral lesions occur most often in the posterior elements and are frequently associated with a painful scoliosis. The most common location for a spinal lesion is the lumbar spine [36]. Osteoid osteomas occur most commonly in adolescents and young adults. The classic presentation is that of focal bone pain at the site of the tumor. The pain worsens at night and increases with activity. Bone scintigraphy is highly sensitive and usually shows increased activity in the flow and blood pool images. Delayed images demonstrate a focus of intense uptake in the nidus surrounded by diffuse and less intense uptake in the reactive bone [41]. Fibrous dysplasia is a development anomaly in which the normal medullary bone is replaced by fibrous tissue and can affect any bone. The monostotic form is more common and most frequently affects the ribs, femur, tibia, and craniofacial bones. The polyostotic form tends to occur in a unilateral distribution. However, bilateral involvement may occur with asymmetric involvement. The most common affected sites are the femur, tibia, and pelvis. Bone scintigraphy typically shows markedly increased uptake in both early blood pool and delayed images. At the initial presentation, bone scintigraphy is useful to demonstrate the extent of the disease [42].

Osteochondroma is the most common benign bone tumor and is defined as a cartilage-covered bony projection on the external surface of a bone. Most osteochondromas arise from tubular bones and are metaphyseal in location. It is found most commonly around the knee and the proximal humerus; however, it can occur in any bone. Bone scintigraphy shows varied accumulation of activity. Non-ossifying fibromas are well-circumscribed fibrous proliferations that occur most commonly in the juxta-epiphyseal regions of long bones. The most common site is the femur, followed by the tibia. The lesion is usually asymptomatic and discovered incidentally. The lesion usually regresses spontaneously. On bone scan, the lesion typically shows normal or mildly increased uptake. However, lesions that are ossifying may become quite active on bone scan during adolescence [43].

Osteosarcoma is the most common primary malignant bone tumor in children. The peak incidence is in adolescence and young adulthood. Children younger than 7 years are rarely affected. Osteosarcoma predominantly affects the metaphyseal regions of long bones. The most common locations for primary osteosarcoma are distal femur, proximal tibia, and proximal humerus. Flat bones are less frequently involved. Common sites for metastases are the lungs and bones. After radiography, initial imaging work up for osteosarcoma typically includes CT, MRI, and bone scintigraphy. CT of the chest is necessary to detect lung metastases. MRI of the primary lesion is used to assess the extent of intramedullary disease and surrounding soft tissue and to later distinguish postoperative changes from residual or recurrent disease. Bone scintigraphy typically is used to detect distant metastases or skip lesions and later to evaluate therapy response and recurrent disease. Primary tumors and skeletal metastases typically show marked uptake. Occasionally bone scintigraphy demonstrates pulmonary metastases due to osteoid production by the metastatic deposits. However, it is much less sensitive than CT in the detection of pulmonary metastases [25].

Ewing sarcoma is the second most common primary bone malignancy in children arising from mesenchymal origin. It often occurs in the second decade of life with peak age range from 4 to 15 years. Males are affected more than females. The most common presenting symptoms are pain and swelling. Although any bone can be affected typically, the bones of the pelvis, femur, tibia, spine, ribs, and humerus are involved with lungs and skeleton being the most common sites of metastases [30]. The diagnosis of Ewing sarcoma is usually made by radiographs which typically show an aggressive lytic lesion in the metaphysis or diaphysis of the bone, with a soft tissue mass extending from the bone. CT scanning helps to define the bone destruction that is associated with Ewing sarcoma. MRI can also be used to assess the extent of Ewing sarcoma. Whole-body bone scans can provide information about the primary lesion, presence of any skip lesions, or distant metastases during tumor staging. It is also recommended for end of treatment evaluation [23].

27.12 MIBG Scan

MIBG scans (labeled with I-131 or I-123 and recently I-124) have been used in neuroectodermal tumors including pheochromocytoma (Pheo) and neuroblastoma (NBL) for about 40 years. ^{123}I-MIBG is the preferred radiotracer in children due to lower radiation dose and better image characteristics (shorter half-life, 13 h; ideal energy of γ-ray: 159 keV). Moreover, the study can be completed in a shorter period of time. Patient preparation is important for MIBG scan. The pre-treatment with sodium or potassium perchlorate (300–600 mg/m^2 BSA) daily (5 days before scanning for ^{131}I-MIBG or 1 day for ^{123}I-MIBG) or Lugol's iodine solution (0.3 mL) three times a day (3 days before for ^{131}I-MIBG or 1 day for ^{123}I-MIBG) to block the thyroid uptake is necessary (Box 27.8). These medications should be continued for 1–2 days for ^{123}I-MIBG, or 2–3 days for ^{131}I-MIBG after scanning [56]. A number of drugs may interfere with MIBG uptake and should be discontinued before the exam (please refer to EANM procedure guidelines for ^{131}I-MIBG therapy. Eur J Nucl Med Mol Imaging. 2008). Foods containing vanillin and catecholamine-like compounds (e.g., chocolate and blue-veined cheeses) may also interfere with MIBG uptake [56].

Box 27.8 Protocol Summary for MIBG Scan

Indications

For confirmation, staging, response to therapy, and evaluation of relapse in neuroectodermal tumors.

Contraindication

Contraindicated in patients medicated with certain agents; please refer to the EANM 2010 guideline for MIBG therapy [60].

Patient Preparation

Pre-treatment with sodium or potassium perchlorate (300–600 mg/m^2 BSA) daily (5 days before scanning for ^{131}I-MIBG or 1 day for ^{123}I-MIBG) or Lugol's iodine solution (0.3 mL) three times a day (3 days before for ^{131}I-MIBG or 1 day for ^{123}-MIBG) to block the thyroid uptake.

These medications should be continued for 1–2 days for ^{123}I-MIBG or 2–3 days for ^{131}I-MIBG after scanning. Patient should be encouraged to drink water and void frequently.

Radiopharmaceutical

^{123}I-MIBG, 7.4 MBq/kg; minimum, 37 MBq, maximum, 400 MBq.

Effective dose (mSv): 3.7 [1].

Critical organ: urinary bladder [58] and liver [56].

Image Acquisition

Whole-body scan (scan speed 5 cm/s, matrix of 256 × 1024, in supine position) or spot views (5–10 min/view, 256 matrix, and zoom as required) with either a low-energy high-resolution (LEHR) or a medium-energy high-resolution (MEHR) collimator (20% energy window centered at 159 keV).

SPECT consists of 120 projections, in steps of 3° (in continuous or step and shoot mode), 25–35 s per step (matrix 128). In noncooperative patients, the acquisition time can be reduced using steps of 6° or a 64 × 64 matrix [60].

Processing and Analysis

The processing parameters depend on the camera. Iterative reconstruction with a low-pass post-filter often provides better images than filtered back projection [60].

Visual interpretation. Any focal activity other than physiologic MIBG uptake is considered suspicious. Semiquantitative evaluation (e.g., Curie score) can also be recorded.

The radiotracer should be infused slowly (over 5 min) with a dose of 0.52 MBq/kg (3.7–18.5 MBq) for ^{131}I-MIBG and 7.4 MBq/kg (37–400 MBq) for ^{123}I-MIBG. The recommended minimum and maximum doses are 37 MBq and

400 MBq for ^{123}I-MIBG and 3.7 MBq and 18.5 MBq for ^{131}I-MIBG, respectively [57]. Imaging is acquired at 24, 48, and 72–96 h (for ^{131}I-MIBG), or at 24 and 48 h (for ^{123}I-MIBG) after radiotracer administration (please see Box 27.8 for the technique of acquisition). SPECT views from the chest, abdomen, and pelvis are usually obtained with ^{123}I-MIBG scan.

The uptake of MIBG is varied in different types of neuroectodermal tumors; it is not possible to differentiate different types of neuroectodermal tumors based on the positivity and intensity of MIBG uptake [59]. However, neuroblastoma (NBL) usually shows a good uptake of MIBG. NBL is the most common extracranial solid tumor in children frequently seen during infancy. The clinical behavior and prognosis of NBL are variable in different patients and different age groups; some may regress spontaneously even without treatment, and some may progress and metastasize rapidly with poor prognosis despite aggressive therapy. One of the tools to evaluate patient prognosis is staging based on the International Neuroblastoma Staging System (INSS). The classification evaluates the disease distribution using radiographic and scintigraphic studies, surgical operability, and lymph node and bone marrow involvement. As metastases are relatively common at presentation, accurate staging depends on multimodality imaging. An MIBG scan is a sensitive (approximately 90%) and very specific (approximately 95–100%) modality for the detection of NBL (Fig. 27.13) [57, 59]. However, in up to 10% of NBL, the tumor is not MIBG avid. MIBG-negative NBL tumors are a clinical challenge and are usually seen in stage I and II tumors [61]. As NBL cell lines may have somatostatin receptors, new radiotracers with DOTA-conjugated peptides (e.g., ^{68}Ga-DOTATATE, ^{68}Ga-DOTATOC) may have a role in NBL, in particular when a radionuclide therapy (e.g., ^{177}Lu-DOTATATE) is an option [62, 63]. If the tumor is MIBG avid at diagnosis, MIBG scan can be used for evaluation of response to treatment, prognosis, and follow-up surveillance and when the treatment regimen changes.

27.13 ^{18}F-FDG PET/CT

The clinical application of PET/CT in the management of pediatric malignancies has been shown in several studies during the last decade. In general, the clinical application and the technique are similar to adults including staging, response to therapy and evaluation of relapse in a variety of tumors, as well as selection of the best site for biopsy and for the evaluation of fever of unknown origin (FUO) [67, 74, 75]. There are, however, physiologic variations in FDG biodistribution and potential pitfalls in the pediatric population which merit special attention.

The palatine and lingual tonsils are very active during childhood. Moreover, clinical or subclinical upper respiratory infection is relatively common in children. Thus, it is not uncommon to see increased ^{18}F-FDG activity in these structures, even without apparent inflammation (Fig. 27.14a). The intensity of the activity and the symmetric/asymmetric pattern of activity and correlative CT findings may be helpful to differentiate a normal variant versus pathology. In a physiologic uptake, the activity is usually symmetric, and the intensity of the uptake is mild to moderate with no correlative CT findings.

The activity in the thymus is more prominent in pediatric population. The thymus often shows mild to moderate homogeneous increased activity with a quadrilateral shape during early childhood and a more triangular shape during adolescence (Fig. 27.14b). Thymus activity may also increase in thymus hyperplasia after chemotherapy, particularly in young patients with lymphoma or testicular cancer. An abnormality is suspected if the thymus activity is heterogeneous or focal, or the intensity is high, or there are any abnormal findings on the correlated CT. In a study by Sasaki et al., the average SUV for thymic carcinoma was much higher (7.2 ± 2.9) than invasive thymoma (3.8 ± 1.3) and noninvasive thymoma (3 ± 1) [77]. Ferdinand et al. suggested an SUV cutoff of 5 to differentiate thymic carcinoma from thymoma with a sensitivity of 84.6%, specificity of 92.3%, and accuracy of 88.5% [76].

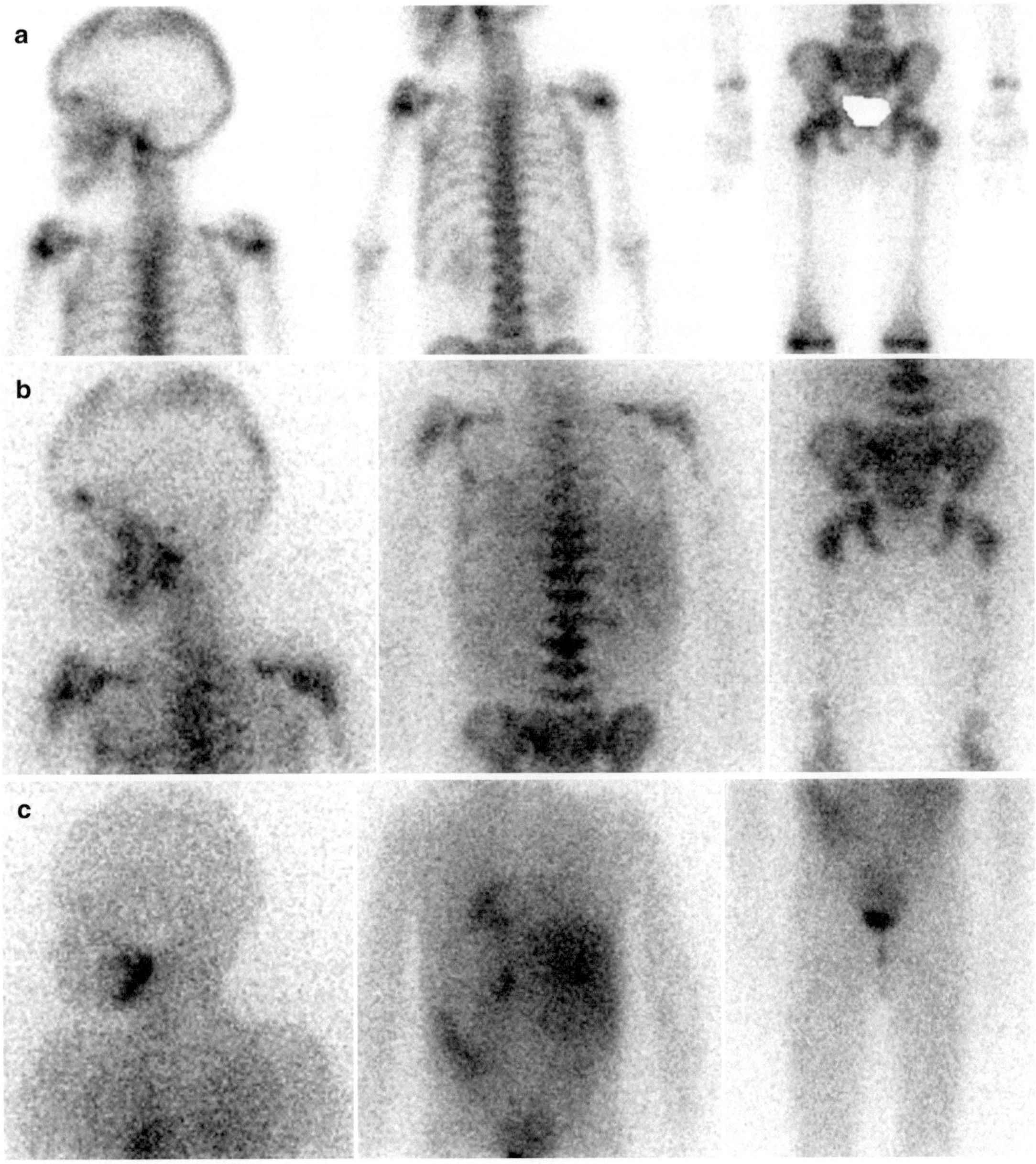

Fig. 27.13 Bone/bone marrow metastases on MIBG scan: bone scan in a 4-year-old boy with NBL showed an abnormal activity in the skull with no significant abnormal uptake in the vertebrae, pelvis, and femurs (**a**). ^{123}I-MIBG scan revealed multiple bone/bone marrow metastases (**b**). Complete resolution of the lesions was noted on a follow-up ^{123}I-MIBG scans 5 months after treatment (**c**)

Increased activity in the brown fat is more common in children than in adults. The brown fat uptake is usually seen in the neck region extending inferiorly in the upper shoulders, superior and posterior mediastinum, diaphragmatic hiatus, and suprarenal area (Fig. 27.14c). Brown fat uptake corresponds to hypodense regions on CT and should be differentiated from lymph nodes activity. Some medication such as propranolol and diazepam may reduce brown fat uptake. As there is an association between brown fat uptake and cold temperature, we control the room tem-

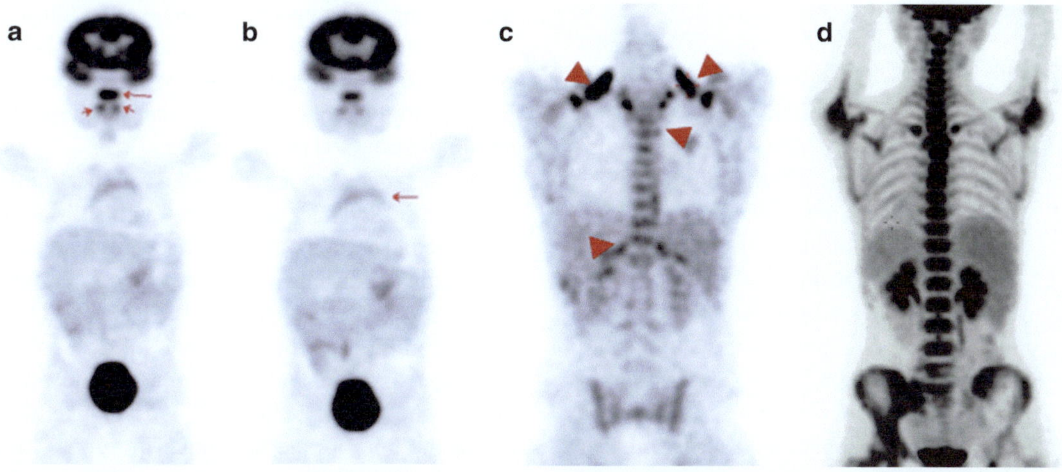

Fig. 27.14 FDG PET in children: physiologic increased activity in the tonsils (arrow) (**a**), thymic activity (arrow) (**b**), brown fat uptake (arrow head) (**c**), and increased bone marrow activity after G-CSF administration (**d**)

perature of the injection room in our hospital and often place a warm blanket over the patient during the uptake phase.

There are other special considerations that are useful for interpretation of PET/CT findings in children. Bone marrow activity is often more active in children than adults, likely due to greater red marrow component. Bone marrow uptake may be more prominent following a hematopoietic drug stimulators injection such as granulocyte colony-stimulating factor (G-CSF) (Fig. 27.14d). It is suggested to perform the PET study 2–3 weeks postinjection of G-CSF, if possible. Children may move a lot during the uptake phase. Therefore, it is not infrequent to see increased activity in a group of muscles. Patient movement during scanning may cause misregistration of PET and CT images and can create artifacts. Reviewing the non-attenuation corrected images is helpful for interpretation of these cases. Increased activity in the vocal cords or accessory respiratory muscles may be also seen due to the child's screaming or crying. The vocal cords uptake in these scenarios is usually symmetrical. In case of asymmetric vocal cord activity, correlation with CT scan is helpful to diagnose any possible pathology.

Finally, the standardized uptake value (SUV) of the lesions cannot be simply extrapolated from the adults' numbers. Additionally, the consistency of SUVs is more challenging in children as the body composition is changing over time. Fat has lower FDG uptake than other tissues. The percentage of fat to body weight is about 11% in newborn, rises to about 26% at 5 months, and then decreases gradually until 12 months of age [78]. This may affect the SUV consistency during infancy. The technique of PET/CT in children is varied in different centers depending on the camera information and institutional policy (Box 27.9).

Box 27.9 Protocol Summary for PET/CT Scan

Indications

For staging, response to therapy, and evaluation of relapse in different tumors; for selection of the best site for biopsy in malignancies; for evaluation of fever of unknown origin (FUO).

Contraindication

Nothing.

Patient Preparation

No heavy exercise for at least 48 h. NPO for 4 h (except for water).

Check the glucose level (should be <11 mmol/L or 200 mg/dL). For diabetic patients follow specific guidelines.

The patient should be relaxed and in a warm room during the uptake phase.

G-CSF should be stopped 2–3 weeks before the exam if possible.

Radiopharmaceutical

^{18}F-FDG: 5.2 MBq/kg; minimum, 37 MBq, maximum, 370 MBq.

Effective dose (mSv/MBq): 0.056 [79].

Critical organ: urinary bladder [79].

Image Acquisition

Imaging starts 60 min after radiotracer injection. Acquisition parameters and patient positioning will vary depending on the indication provided on the requisition and the PET/CT camera. In general, for lymphoma patients, with no evidence of bone involvement, imaging from basal skull to mid-thigh is adequate. For certain conditions such as sarcoma, Langerhans cell histiocytosis, neuroblastoma, and thyroid, whole-body acquisition (to include skull and extremities) is required.

PET acquisition time: 2–3 min/bed position.

CT can be done as a low-dose CT for attenuation correction or a diagnostic CT scan when it is needed.

Processing and Analysis

Filtered back projection or iterative reconstruction depending on the camera parameters.

Other PET tracers have also been used in children. The use of ^{18}F-fluoro-L-DOPA (^{18}F-DOPA) PET/CT in congenital hyperinsulinism (CHI) is a good example. The result of surgery in CHI has been improved recently, mainly because of the better delineation of the lesion using ^{18}F-DOPA PET/CT [64]. Congenital hyperinsulinism may be due to a focal area of secreting insulin cells, a diffuse form of lesions, and atypical forms of scattered segmental mosaic lesions. In focal CHI, or a segmental mosaic form, surgical resection is the main treatment. However, it is important to resect enough tissues to minimize relapse and to avoid too much resection in order not to induce diabetes. This is especially important in the segmental mosaic form. In diffuse CHI, however, there is a recent tendency toward medical therapy due to high frequency of relapse or surgical induced diabetes [66]. There is also a possibility of spontaneous improvement of hyperinsulinemic hypoglycemia (perhaps because of apoptosis) in diffuse CHI [64].

As the focal lesions are mainly an accumulation of diseased islet cells secreting insulin without control (but not a tumor), it is very hard to be distinguished during surgery even with magnifying lenses [65]. ^{18}F-DOPA PET/CT is very useful to guide the surgeon for appropriate surgical resection of focal and segmental mosaic forms during the surgery. PET/CT is also useful to select the appropriate technique of surgery. For example, if PET-CT shows a lesion in the pancreatic tail, primary laparoscopic resection is probably a better approach.

27.14 PET/MR

Combined PET/MRI has been recently used as important clinical and research tools. There are many clinical indications for PET/MR in children including staging, response to therapy (e.g., lymphoma, sarcoma, neuroblastoma, and neurofibromatosis type 1), and surveillance of cancers and in neurology [68–71]. The main advantages of PET/MR to PET/CT are the low radiation and better delineation of soft tissue. Using MR instead of CT will reduce the radiation dose by about 50–80% [72, 73]. Attenuation correction is technically difficult with MR. However, there are some improvements in terms of measurement of SUV using a specific technique called segmentation-based attenuation correction [73].

27.15 Brain Scintigraphy for Brain Death

Brain death in neonates, infants, and children relies on a clinical diagnosis that is based on the absence of neurologic function with a known irreversible cause of coma. Coma and apnea must coexist to diagnose brain death. This diagnosis should be made by physicians who have evaluated the history and completed the neurologic examinations [80, 81]. The diagnosis of brain death should not be made based on neurologic examination alone if high therapeutic levels of sedative agents have been administered. If uncertainty remains, an additional study such as brain scintigraphy should be performed, although this study is not a substitute for the neurologic examination.

Additional studies can be used to help in making the diagnosis of brain death to reduce the observation period, or when components of the examination or apnea testing cannot be completed safely, or if there is uncertainty about the results of the neurologic examination, or if a medication effect may interfere with evaluation of the patient. If the ancillary study supports the diagnosis, the second examination and apnea testing can then be performed [80]. In some countries other than the United States, a confirmatory test is required by law [82].

Conventional cerebral radionuclide angiography followed by planar scintigraphy with ^{99m}Tc-pertechnetate or ^{99m}Tc-diethylenetriaminepentaacetic acid (DTPA) can be used in children with an equivocal clinical diagnosis of brain death which is based on flow images followed by static planar images in anterior and lateral projections [83]. However, imaging with brain-specific tracers such as ^{99m}Tc-ECD or ^{99m}Tc-HMPAO has currently been used more frequently, allowing for better visualization of posterior fossa and brain stem perfusion [84]. Brain-specific radiotracers are preferred as interpretation is less dependent on the quality of the bolus and early dynamic images. These radiotracers provide an assessment of cerebral flow on the first pass flow images as well as on delayed planar and SPECT views [83]. The typical dose for children is 11.1 MBq/kg (0.3 mCi/kg) with a minimum dose of 185 MBq (5 mCi). Flow images are acquired at the time of tracer injection at 1 s per frame for 60 s. If better spatial resolution is required, images can be combined into 2 s per frame for display purposes. If nonspecific radiotracers are used, static planar images are acquired in anterior and lateral views and posterior if possible. Planar images should be acquired approximately 20 min after injection in addition to the flow images [83]. Single-photon emission computed tomography (SPECT) can be performed to provide a better visualization as it can be helpful for differentiating overlying scalp from intracranial activity and for evaluating the posterior fossa [85].

When nonspecific radiotracers are used, the lack of flow in dynamic flow study on anterior view, in combination with the absence of activity in the venous sinus on static images, suggests the diagnosis of brain death. However, faint activity of venous sinuses may be seen in children with nonspecific brain tracers, which makes it difficult to interpret. Coker et al. reported sinus activity in 14 of 55 children who had confirmed brain death [86].

Using specific agents such as ^{99m}TC-HMPAO, the planar or SPECT images should demonstrate no cerebral or cerebellar activity in addition to absent of brain flow (Fig. 27.15) [87]. Usually, this brain imaging study is not affected by drug intoxication or hypothermia (as the EEG may be) and is more specific for brain death. The sensitivity of planar imaging using ^{99m}Tc-HMPAO is very high, and the specificity is virtually 100%. To evaluate the reliability of SPECT imaging in the diagnosis of brain death, Facoo et al. evaluated 50 comatose patients with SPECT imaging using ^{99m}Tc-HMPAO. SPECT imaging confirmed the diagnosis of brain death in 45 out of 47 patients (95.7%). Activity in the basal ganglia, thalamus, or brain stem was noted in two clinically brain-dead infants [88]. In certain cases, the intracranial pressure may not increase significantly (due to open fontanels) in infants. Therefore, brain uptake may be present despite the clinical diagnosis of brain death. Ashwal et al. reported a brain uptake in 6 of 17 infants with clinical brain death; three of them were preterm infants [89]. The remaining 11 infants had no cerebral blood flow. Okuyaz et al. also reported two newborns needed a second image to confirm the diagnosis. In this study, eight patients who fulfilled the clinical criteria of brain death were evaluated using ^{99m}Tc-HMPAO SPECT, and six patients demonstrated lack of perfusion activity in the cerebrum in their first SPECT study [84]. Thus, a brain death study should be interpreted with caution especially in infants.

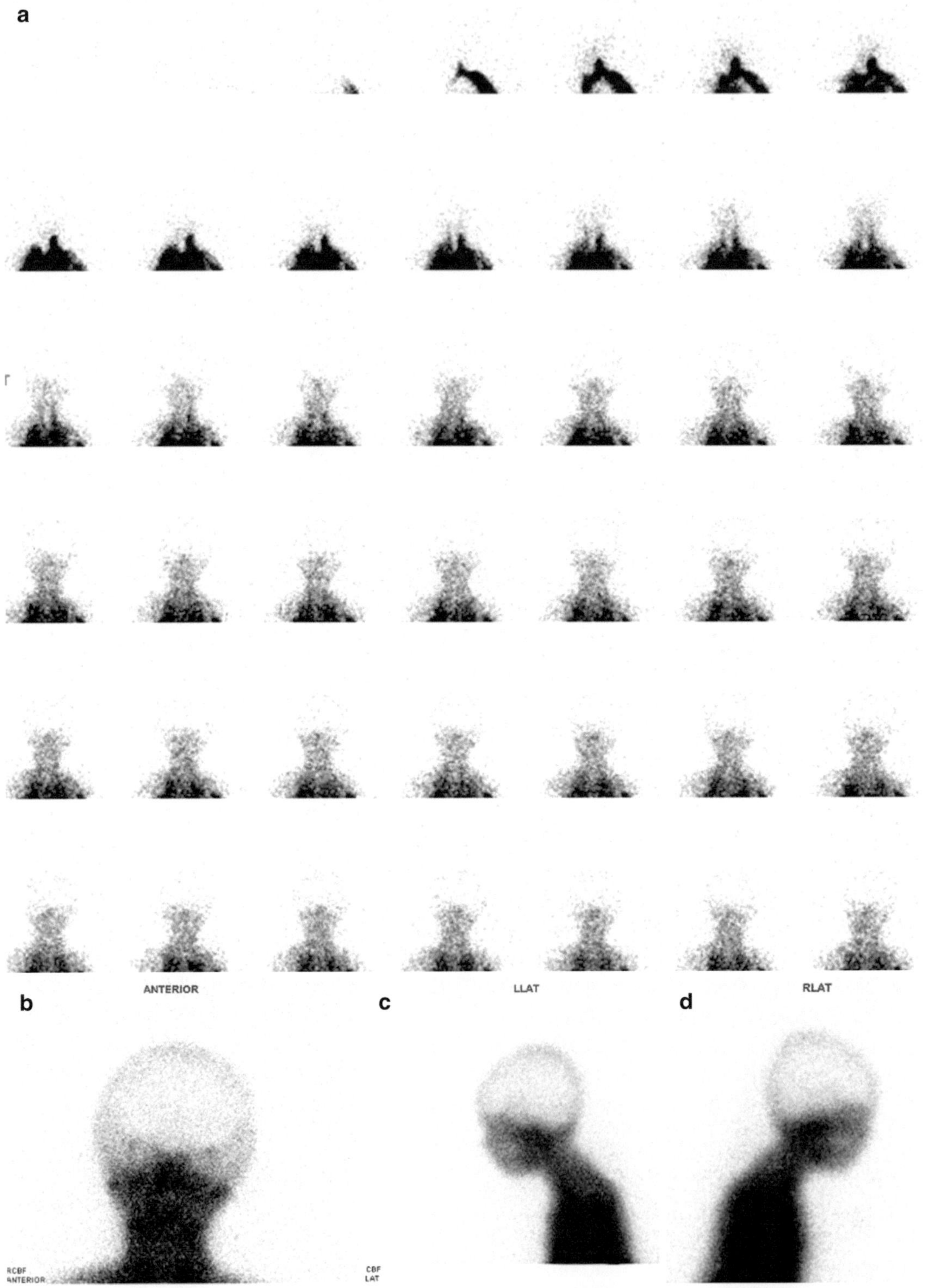

Fig. 27.15 Brain death: a 4-year-old boy with brain death after drowning. Early dynamic images (**a**) as well as delayed static views after 20 min in anterior (**b**) and lateral projections (**c**, **d**) didn't show any activity in the brain

27.16 Ventilation/Perfusion Scans for Pulmonary Embolism

Pulmonary embolism (PE) in the pediatric population is relatively less common than in adults. However, improvements in pediatric care have led to an increase in the survival of chronic or critically ill children and, thus, an increase in the risk and incidence of common complications encountered by such patients, including PE [45]. Buck et al. reviewed autopsies performed in children and found a PE incidence of 4%. They concluded that PE in children is underdiagnosed and using lung perfusion scintigraphy should be encouraged [46].

Cancer, immobility, central venous lines, vascular malformations, nephrotic syndrome, long-term total parenteral nutrition administration, systemic lupus erythematosus, ventriculoatrial shunts, congenital and/or acquired thrombotic tendencies, and acute DVT are all recognizable risk factors associated with PE in children [47].

The clinical findings of PE in children are similar to those encountered in adults. However, none of these signs and symptoms is specific to establish the diagnosis of PE and could be associated with underlying comorbid disease, reducing the level of suspicion by clinicians. The symptoms of PE in children may include shortness of breath, pleuritic chest pain, and hemoptysis. However, the clinical presentation may vary and may be subtle and mimic other diseases [45]. In adolescents, pleuritic chest pain is the most common presenting complaint, followed by dyspnea, cough, and hemoptysis [47]. Other signs and symptoms may include wheezing, rales, sweating, tachycardia, nausea, vomiting, syncope, murmur, and cyanosis. Pleurisy with friction rub may also be present. Arterial blood oxygen is frequently reduced. However, normal blood gases do not exclude PE. The erythrocyte sedimentation rate (ESR) is elevated in approximately 40% of patients, and electrocardiogram (ECG) may show right ventricle strain [47].

Chest X-ray is often normal in patients with pediatric PE. The signs such as atelectasis, pleural effusion, elevated hemidiaphragm, and infiltrate or consolidation are variable and not specific for PE. Oligemia distal to PE (Westermark sign) or a shallow, wedge-shaped opacity with its base against the pleura (Hampton hump) is not frequently seen [47]. CT pulmonary angiography (CTPA) can be performed quickly in critically ill patients. With the availability of CTA and its high sensitivity and specificity, pulmonary CTA is now more common procedure for the diagnosis of PE [48]. Pulmonary embolism appears as filling defects in the pulmonary arteries. A normal helical CT scan reduces the probability of pulmonary embolism; however, the use of iodinated contrast and the presence of radiation exposure are disadvantages of CTPA. If the patient has an allergy to iodinated contrast material or renal insufficiency or CTA is not available, a V/Q scan may be considered. Stein et al. suggest performing a V/Q if the chest radiograph is normal and acquiring CTA if there is an abnormality on the chest X-ray [49].

The radiopharmaceutical used for lung perfusion imaging is ^{99m}Tc-macroaggregated albumin (^{99m}Tc-MAA). After slow intravenous injection with the patient in a supine position, ^{99m}Tc-MAA particles lodge in pre-capillary arterioles, causing a temporary occlusion in a distribution proportional to regional arterial blood flow in lungs. The number of occluded arterioles by ^{99m}Tc-MAA particles is approximately 0.1% of their total number which is relatively small [50]. The particles clear by enzymatic hydrolysis and are eventually phagocytized by reticuloendothelial system and eliminated in the bile, with a biologic half-life in the lungs of between 6 and 8 h. The particle size is generally between 10 and 90 μm (90% of particles), with an average number of 500,000 particles in adult dose. In children, the number of particles should be adjusted to the age or weight to keep the number as low as possible in order to embolize no more than 0.1% of the total lung capillary vessels. It is estimated that neonates have about 10% of the eventual number of adult pulmonary capillaries. The number of capillaries increases to half of the adult value by age 3 years and reaches an adult level by age 8–12 years. The number of injected particles should not exceed 50,000 in the newborn and 165,000 for children at 1 year old. The recommended number of particles for 5–10 years old with average weight of 20–35 kg is from 200,000 to 300,000 [50]. In infants and children with right-to-left shunt or pulmonary hypertension, the number of particles should be reduced (10,000–30,000 particles) depending on the age of the patient and the severity of involvement. The recommended dose by North American Consensus Guidelines is 2.59 MBq/kg (0.07 mCi/kg) if ^{99m}Tc is used for ventilation study and 1.11 MBq/kg (0.03 mCi/kg) if no concomitant ^{99m}Tc ventilation study is performed, with a minimum dose of 14.8 MBq (0.4 mCi) [20]. When administering ^{99m}Tc-MAA, withdrawing blood into the syringe should be avoided as small clots may occur with hot spots appearing on the images. If ^{99m}Tc-labeled radioaerosols or Technegas is used for the ventilation scan, this should be performed before the perfusion scan. If ^{81m}Kr gas is used for the ventilation scan, this can be acquired before or after the perfusion scan, or both examinations may be performed simultaneously as a dual-isotope scan [50].

Images can be acquired after radiotracer administration using a high-resolution, low-energy collimator. Planar images are obtained in a 128 × 128 or 256 × 256 matrix format, with a zoom large enough to include both lungs in the field of view with good margins. Multiple projections should be obtained including anterior, posterior, anterior and posterior oblique, and both lateral projections. SPECT or SPECT/CT study can also be performed. The CT portion is acquired with a low-dose CT for attenuation and anatomic correlation [50, 51].

^{99m}Tc-DTPA Aerosol: ^{99m}Tc-DTPA aerosol is the most commonly used radiopharmaceutical. Many different aerosols have been used, but DTPA is preferred in children because of the fast renal clearance, which lowers the radiation burden. ^{99m}Tc-DTPA aerosol can be inhaled through a mask connected to a nebulizer containing a saline solution of the radiopharmaceutical or preferably using a mouthpiece and nose clips in older children [50]. Swallowing of saliva may cause high gastric signal with possible difficult visualization of the left lower lung field. Cooperative children can be asked to rinse their mouth with water before beginning image acquisition. Aerosolized ^{99m}Tc-DTPA crosses the alveolar-capillary membrane and enters the bloodstream where it is then filtered by the kidneys. Increased permeability of alveolar-capillary membrane and thus lung clearance can be seen after exercise or certain lung disease such as cystic fibrosis.

Ventilation imaging is usually performed before perfusion imaging. Since both agents are labeled with ^{99m}Tc, it is extremely important that the count rate of the second study be at least three times the count rate of the first study. One advantage of ^{99m}Tc-DTPA aerosol is the persistence of activity in the lungs which allows for the acquisition of multiple projections or SPECT to match the perfusion images. Also, collection systems (required when using radioactive gases) are not necessary with the use of radioactive aerosols [50].

Xenon-133: Xenon is an inert gas with low solubility in body fluids and higher solubility in fat. After ^{133}Xe inhalation in single breath, the pattern of distribution reflects the regional ventilation. It has a physical half-life of 5.24 days and a low-energy gamma emission (81 keV). However, it rapidly washes out from the lungs with a half time of 5–30 s. The usual dose for children is 10–12 MBq/kg (0.3 mCi/kg) with a minimum dose of 100–120 MBq. The Xe-133 ventilation scan is generally performed prior to the Tc-99m MAA perfusion exam, as down-scatter from the Tc-99m would severely degrade image quality. A posterior projection is generally used, while a bolus of ^{133}Xe is injected into the mouthpiece of the spirometer system at a time when the patient begins maximal inspiration. The imaging room should provide appropriate exhaust for radioactive gas. The advantage of a xenon exam is the ability to obtain single breath, equilibrium, and washout images providing better sensitivity and evaluation of ventilation in patients with obstructive lung disease [50].

Krypton-81m: ^{81m}Kr gas is produced by a rubidium generator (^{81}Rb/^{81m}Kr) with a half-life of 13 s and emission of a 190 keV gamma ray. The gas is administered by continuous inhalation mixed with atmospheric air during the acquisition of the images. Because it has a short half-life, Krypton-81m is not considered an environmental hazard, and storage or exhaust systems are not necessary. The radiation dose to the lungs is lower than with other agents. However, the generator is expensive and can be used only for one working day which makes it impractical for most clinical situations. In addition, it is currently not available in the United States [51].

Several diagnostic schemes have been suggested for interpretation of V/Q scans, such as the modified PIOPED II with the proposed criteria for a very low probability interpretation to improve the accuracy and minimize the number of nonconclusive results [52]. However, in the daily practice of nuclear medicine, experienced physicians may not follow a strict single interpretive criteria but rather use integrated knowledge of different published criteria and their own experience ("Gestalt" interpretation) [53]. Several studies were performed to evaluate the performance of different readers with different experience using different widespread algorithms such as PIOPED criteria, earlier schemes developed by McNeil and Biello. In general, the ideal scheme would minimize the frequency of intermediate or indeterminate results. Glaser et al. suggested a trinary interpretation for V/Q scanning considering normal, very low probability, and low probability read as no evidence of PE, high probability as PE present, and intermediate probability as nondiagnostic [54]. Single segmental mismatches were considered positive for PE. The trinary interpretation group included 664 examinations, with 8.4% being PE present, 3.5% nondiagnostic, and 88.1% PE negative. Pediatric subgroup analysis in 20 children showed positive in 10%, nondiagnostic in 5%, and negative in 85%, with no false negatives using either scheme. They concluded that the trinary interpretation can safely be used. In children, Gelfand et al. evaluated the frequency of indeterminate findings in children without known lung disease or previous extensive PE and reported a low rate of indeterminate studies using criteria of Biello et al. with minimal modification. It was concluded that V/Q scans are still appropriate for imaging children with suspected PE [55].

27.17 Thyroid Scan for Congenital Hypothyroidism

Thyroid hormone deficiency at birth is most commonly caused by a problem with thyroid gland development (dysgenesis), including ectopic thyroid tissue, no thyroid tissue (athyreosis), and less frequently hypoplasia, or a disorder of thyroid hormone biosynthesis (dyshormonogenesis). These disorders result in primary hypothyroidism [90]. Thyroid dysgenesis is generally sporadic, but thyroid dyshormonogenesis is associated with hormone synthesis protein gene mutations [91].

Congenital hypothyroidism (CH) is classified into two main types: transient and permanent. Permanent CH is mainly due to primary hypothyroidism presented with elevated thyroid-stimulating hormone (TSH) levels. Transient hypothyroidism can be due to maternal antithyroid medications, transplacental thyrotropin receptor blocking antibodies, and iodine imbalance (deficiency or excess) as well as genetic defects such as mutations in the genes encoding for DUOX and DUOXA2 [90].

The incidence of CH initially increased after the introduction of newborn screening with a range of 1:3000 to 1:4000. However, recent reports showed that the incidence is increased with rates ranging from 1:1400 to 1:2800 in many countries. The rise in incidence could be attributed to the change in demographics, change in newborn screening strategies such as lowering cutoff values, and increase in preterm birth [92]. A higher incidence was reported in the Asian, Native American, and Hispanic populations and lower in the African American population. It is more common in females with approximately a 2:1 female to male ratio [90]. Early treatment with thyroid hormone replacement is essential for normal neurodevelopment. The treatment should be started once the diagnosis is confirmed based on serum thyroid function test results [90].

Diagnostic studies may be performed to determine an underlying etiology. These include thyroid scintigraphy, thyroid ultrasonography, serum thyroglobulin (Tg) measurement, antithyroid antibody determinations, and measurement of urinary iodine. Thyroid imaging can be helpful in differentiating underlying etiology (either thyroid dysgenesis or dyshormonogenesis).

Iodine-123 (^{123}I) or sodium pertechnetate-99m (^{99m}Tc) can be used for thyroid imaging. Iodine-131 (^{131}I) is not recommended due to higher radiation dose to the thyroid. ^{99m}Tc is taken up by the thyroid through sodium–iodine symporter (NIS) but unlike iodine is not organified. More prominent physiologic activity in salivary glands is seen in ^{99m}Tc compared to iodine scans. ^{99m}Tc is commonly used due to its availability, lower cost, and faster exam times. The intravenous administered dose for children is 1.1 MBq/kg with a minimum dose of 7 MBq [93]. Imaging is started 20 min after injection. Static images with the neck extended can be obtained for 5 min. Anterior views of the neck and thorax are acquired using a low-energy high-resolution collimator and a 128 × 128 matrix. Lateral views can be acquired with a chin marker for better anatomic localization [94].

Unlike ^{99m}Tc, ^{123}I is organified and then incorporated into thyroid hormones. The administered dose is 0.28 MBq/kg with a minimum dose of 1 MBq [93]. Imagining can be acquired 2–4 h after administration. ^{123}I is the preferred agent particularly if a perchlorate discharge test is required for dyshormonogeneses in children with eutopic thyroid. If there is defective organification of iodide, the uptake in the thyroid gland will be decreased by more than 10% when perchlorate is given [94]. However, ^{123}I is more expensive and less readily available and requires a longer time to complete.

Absent thyroid activity is likely to represent athyreosis (Fig. 27.16). Ultrasound can be performed to confirm the diagnosis as absence of uptake can also be seen with TSHβ gene mutations, TSH receptor-inactivating mutations, iodide trapping defects, and maternal thyrotropin receptor blocking antibodies [90].

Ectopic activity in a thyroid scan can be found along the embryological migration pathway from the foramen cecum at the base of the tongue to the mediastinum. Lingual thyroid is typically presented with small focus of uptake in the midline at the base of the tongue

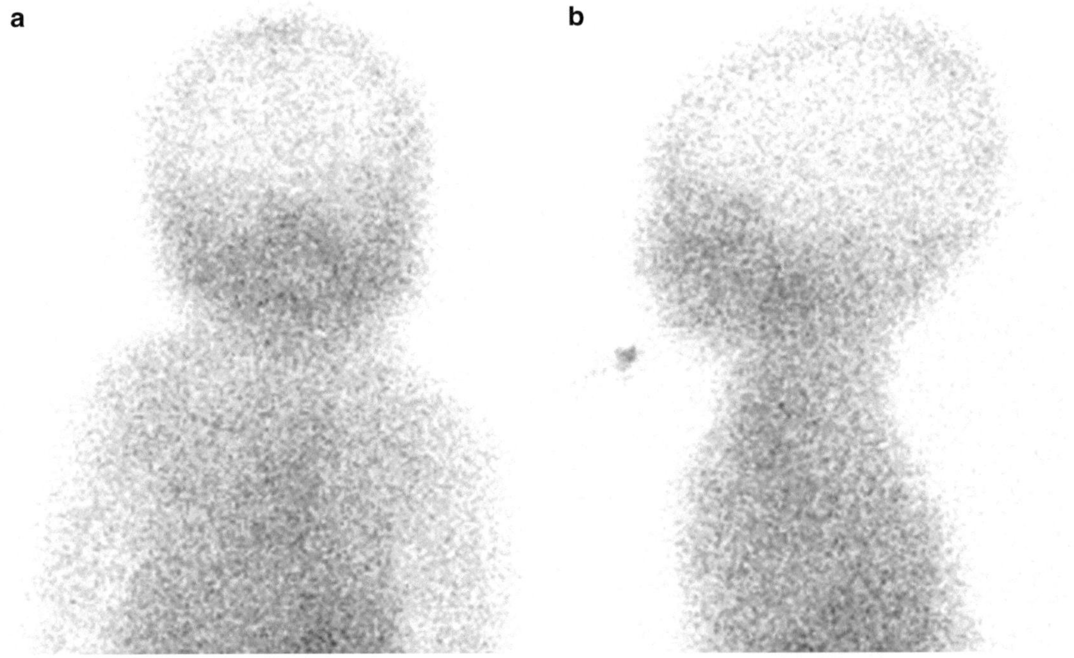

Fig. 27.16 Thyroid agenesis congenital hypothyroidism: thyroid scan (**a**, anterior; **b**, lateral) in a 4-day-old boy with congenital hypothyroidism shows no activity in the thyroid bed suggestive of agenesis or a suppressed thyroid

(Fig. 27.17). In hypoplasia, the uptake is usually low in the thyroid gland and could be unilateral causing asymmetric uptake [94].

In dyshormonogenesis, a patient may present with a palpable goiter. The thyroid scan may demonstrate an enlarged gland in eutopic location with increased uptake, suggesting dyshormonogeneses beyond trapping (Fig. 27.18). I-123 uptake can be followed by a perchlorate discharge test [95].

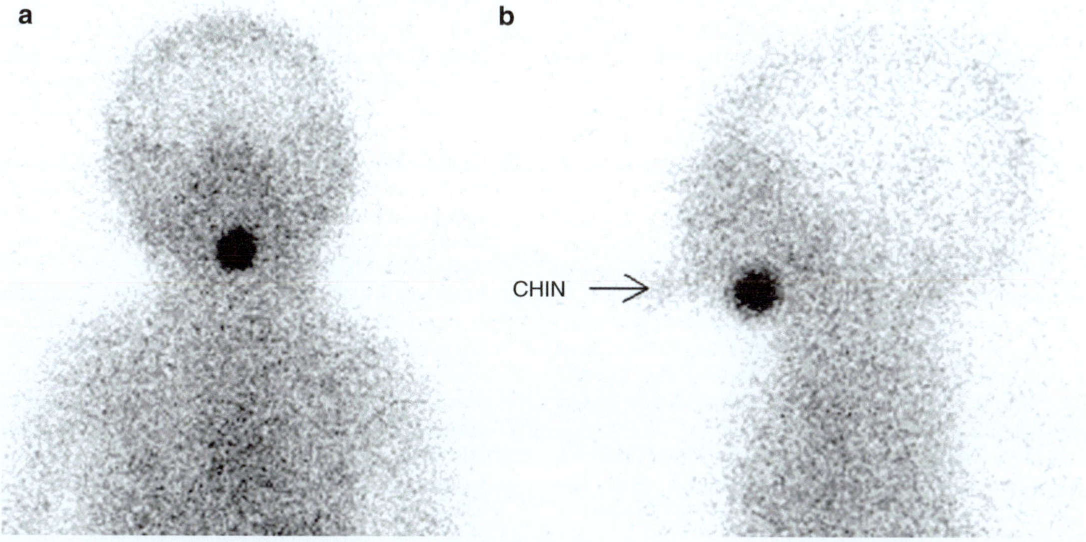

Fig. 27.17 Lingual thyroid; thyroid scan (**a**, anterior; **b**, lateral) in a 7-day-old infant with congenital hypothyroidism shows a focal activity at the base of the tongue

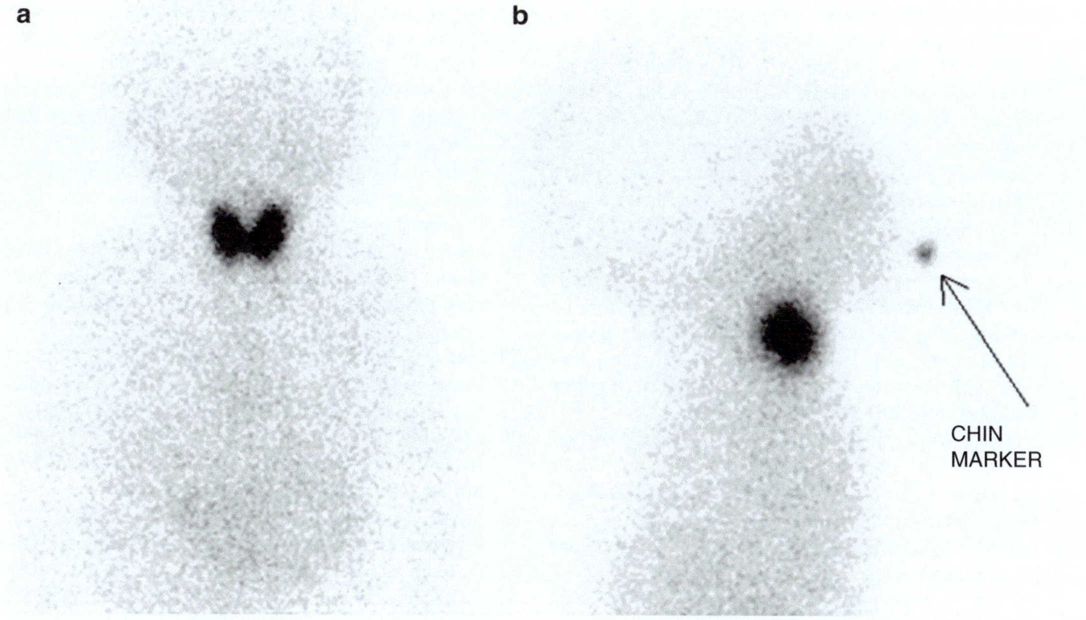

Fig. 27.18 Dyshormonogenesis: thyroid scan (**a**, anterior; **b**, lateral) in a 6-day-old infant with congenital hypothyroidism shows marked increased activity in both thyroid lobes suggestive of organification enzyme defect (dyshormonogenesis)

References

1. Stabin MG, Gelfand MJ. Dosimetry of pediatric nuclear medicine procedures. Q J Nucl Med. 1998;42(2):93–112.
2. Gordon I, Piepsz A, Sixt R. Guidelines for standard and diuretic renogram in children; guideline. Eur J Nucl Med Mol Imaging. 2011;38:1175.
3. Shulkin BL, Mandell GA, Cooper JA, et al. Procedure guideline for diuretic renography in children 3.0. J Nucl Med Technol. 2008;36(3):162–8.
4. Chotipanich C, Rubin J, Lin J, Charron M. Clinical follow-up of children with low differential function on diuretic renogram. J Med Assoc Thai. 2007;90(4):754–61.
5. Mandell G, Eggli D, Gilday D, et al. Society of nuclear medicine procedure guideline for renal cortical scintigraphy in children version 3.0. Approved June 20, 2003.
6. Ajdinovic B, Jaukovic L, Krstic Z, Dopuda M. Impact of micturating cystourethrography and DMSA renal scintigraphy on the investigation scheme in children with urinary tract infection. Ann Nucl Med. 2008;22(8):661–5.
7. Hoberman A, Charron M, Hickey RW, Baskin M, Kearney DH, Wald ER. Imaging studies after a first febrile urinary tract infection in young children. N Engl J Med. 2003;348(3):195–202.
8. Lim R. Vesicoureteral reflux and urinary tract infection: evolving practices and current controversies in pediatric imaging. AJR Am J Roentgenol. 2009;192(5):1197–208.
9. Pollet JE, Sharp PF, Smith FW. Radionuclide imaging for vesico-renal reflux using intravenous 99mTc--D.T.P.A. Pediatr Radiol. 1979;8(3):165–7.
10. Gerhold JP, Klingensmith WC III, Kuni CC, et al. Diagnosis of biliary atresia with radionuclide hepatobiliary imaging. Radiology. 1983;146(2):499–504.
11. Warrington JC, Charron M. Pediatric gastrointestinal nuclear medicine. Semin Nucl Med. 2007;37(4):269–85.
12. Donohoe KJ, Maurer AH, Ziessman HA, et al. Procedure guideline for adult solid-meal gastric-emptying study 3.0. J Nucl Med Technol. 2009;37(3):196–200.
13. Fawcett HD, Hayden CK, Adams JC, Swischuk LE. How useful is gastroesophageal reflux scintigraphy in suspected childhood aspiration? Pediatr Radiol. 1988;18(4):311–3.
14. Siegel J, Wu R, Knight L, Zelac R, Stern H, Malmud L. Radiation dose estimates for oral agents used in upper gastrointestinal disease. J Nucl Med. 1983;24:835–37.
15. Baikie G, South MJ, Reddihough DS, et al. Agreement of aspiration tests using barium videofluoroscopy, salivagram, and milk scan in children with cerebral palsy. Dev Med Child Neurol. 2005;47(2):86–93.
16. Sonneville A, Ait-Tahar H, Baulieu F, et al. [Value of esophageal scintigraphy in exploration of a gastroesophageal reflux in a respiratory patient]. Allerg Immunol 2000;32(5):207–208.
17. Sfakianakis GN, Conway JJ. Detection of ectopic gastric mucosa in Meckel's diverticulum and in other aberrations by scintigraphy: II. Indications and methods–a 10-year experience. J Nucl Med. 1981;22(8):732–8.
18. Spottswood SE, Pfluger T, Bartold S, et al. SNMMI and EANM Practice Guideline for meckel diverticulum scintigraphy. J Nucl Med Technol. 2014;42(3):163–9.
19. Vali R, Daneman A, McQuattie S, Shammas A. The value of repeat scintigraphy in patients with a high clinical suspicion for Meckel diverticulum after a negative or equivocal first Meckel scan. Pediatr Radiol. 2015;45:1506–14.
20. Gelfand MJ, Parisi MT, Treves ST, Pediatric Nuclear Medicine Dose Reduction Workgroup. Pediatric radiopharmaceutical administered doses: 2010 North American consensus guidelines. J Nucl Med. 2011;52(2):318–22.
21. Lassmann M, Treves ST, EANM/SNMMI Paediatric Dosage Harmonization Working Group. Paediatric radiopharmaceutical administration: harmonization of the 2007 EANM paediatric dosage card (version 1.5.2008) and the 2010 North American consensus guidelines. Eur J Nucl Med Mol Imaging. 2014;41(5):1036–41.
22. Grant FD. 18F-Fluoride PET and PET/CT in children and young adults. PET Clin. 2014;9(3):287–97.
23. Nadel HR. Pediatric bone scintigraphy update. Semin Nucl Med. 2010;40(1):31–40.
24. De Palma D. Radionuclide studies with bone-seeking radiophamaceuticals in pediatric benign diseases. In: Mansi L, et al., editors. Clinical nuclear medicine in pediatrics. New York, NY: Springer; 2016.
25. Ma JJ, Kang BK, Treves ST. Pediatric musculoskeletal nuclear medicine. Semin Musculoskelet Radiol. 2007;11(4):322–34.
26. De Palma D, Nadel HR, Bar-Sever Z. Skeletal scintigraphy with SPECT/CT in benign pediatric bone conditions. Clin Transl Imag. 2016;4:191.
27. Bybel B, Brunken RC, DiFilippo FP, et al. SPECT/CT imaging: clinical utility of an emerging technology. Radiographics. 2008;28(4):1097–113.
28. Treves ST. Skeletal scintigraphy: general considerations. In: Treves ST, editor. Pediatric nuclear medicine and molecular imaging. 4th ed. New York, NY: Springer; 2014.
29. Faden H, Grossi M. Acute osteomyelitis in children. Reassessment of etiologic agents and their clinical characteristics. Am J Dis Child. 1991;145(1):65–9.
30. Connolly LP, Drubach SA, Connolly SA, et al. Bone. In: Treves ST, editor. Pediatric nuclear medicine/PET. 3rd ed. New York, NY: Springer; 2007.
31. Schauwecker DS. The scintigraphic diagnosis of osteomyelitis. AJR Am J Roentgenol. 1992;158(1):9–18.
32. Pennington WT, Mott MP, Thometz JG, et al. Photopenic bone scan osteomyelitis: a clinical perspective. J Pediatr Orthop. 1999;19(6):695–8.
33. Acikgoz G, Averill L. Chronic recurrent multifocal osteomyelitis: typical patterns of bone involvement in whole-body bone scintigraphy. Nucl Med Commun. 2014;35(10):1097.

34. Connolly LP, Treves ST. Assessing the limping child with skeletal scintigraphy. J Nucl Med. 1998;39(6):1056–61.
35. Drubach LA, Connolly LP, D'Hemecourt PA, et al. Assessment of the clinical significance of asymptomatic lower extremity uptake in young athletes. J Nucl Med. 2001;42(2):209–12.
36. Sty JR, Wells RG, Conway JJ. Spine pain in children. Semin Nucl Med. 1993;23(4):296–320.
37. Pekindil G, Sarikaya A, Pekindil Y, et al. Lumbosacral transitional vertebral articulation: evaluation by planar and SPECT bone scintigraphy. Nucl Med Commun. 2004;25(1):29–37.
38. Mandelstam SA, Cook D, Fitzgerald M, et al. Complementary use of radiological skeletal survey and bone scintigraphy in detection of bony injuries in suspected child abuse. Arch Dis Child. 2003;88(5):387–90.
39. Conway JJ, Collins M, Tanz RR, et al. The role of bone scintigraphy in detecting child abuse. Semin Nucl Med. 1993;23(4):321–33.
40. Drubach LA, Johnston PR, Newton AW, et al. Skeletal trauma in child abuse: detection with 18F-NaF PET. Radiology. 2010;255(1):173–81.
41. Villani MF, Falappa P, Pizzoferro M, Toniolo RM, Lembo A, Chiapparelli S, Garganese MC. Role of three-phase bone scintigraphy in paediatric osteoid osteoma eligible for radiofrequency ablation. Nucl Med Commun. 2013;34(7):638–44.
42. Zhibin Y, Quanyong L, Libo C, et al. The role of radionuclide bone scintigraphy in fibrous dysplasia of bone. Clin Nucl Med. 2004;29:177–80.
43. Connolly LP, Drubach LA, Treves ST. Pediatric skeletal scintigraphy. In: Henkin RE, Bova D, Dillehay GL, Karesh SM, Halama JR, Wagner RH, editors. Nuclear medicine. 2nd ed. Philadelphia, PA: Mosby-Elsevier; 2006. p. 1721–44.
44. Stauss J, Hahn K, Mann M, De Palma D. Guidelines for paediatric bone scanning with 99mTc-labelled radiopharmaceuticals and 18F-fluoride. Eur J Nucl Med Mol Imaging. 2010;37(8):1621–8.
45. Patocka C, Nemeth J. Pulmonary embolism in pediatrics. J Emerg Med. 2012;42(1):105–16.
46. Buck JR, Connors RH, Coon WW, et al. Pulmonary embolism in children. J Pediatr Surg. 1981;16(3):385–91.
47. Brandão LR, Labarque V, Diab Y, et al. Pulmonary embolism in children. Semin Thromb Hemost. 2011;37(7):772–85.
48. Hunt JM, Bull TM. Clinical review of pulmonary embolism: diagnosis, prognosis, and treatment. Med Clin North Am. 2011;95(6):1203–22.
49. Stein EG, Haramati LB, Chamarthy M, Sprayregen S, Davitt MM, Freeman LM. Success of a safe and simple algorithm to reduce use of CT pulmonary angiography in the emergency department. AJR Am J Roentgenol. 2010;194(2):392–7.
50. Ciofetta G, Piepsz A, Roca I, et al. Guidelines for lung scintigraphy in children. Eur J Nucl Med Mol Imaging. 2007;34(9):1518–26.
51. Parker JA, Coleman RE, Grady E, et al. SNM practice guideline for lung scintigraphy 4.0. J Nucl Med Technol. 2012;40(1):57–65.
52. Gottschalk A, Stein PD, Sostman HD, et al. Very low probability interpretation of V/Q lung scans in combination with low probability objective clinical assessment reliably excludes pulmonary embolism: data from PIOPED II. J Nucl Med. 2007;48(9):1411–5.
53. Shammas A, Vali R, Charron M. Pediatric Nuclear Medicine in Acute Care. Semin Nucl Med. 2013;43(2):139–56.
54. Glaser JE, Chamarthy M, Haramati LB, et al. Successful and safe implementation of a trinary interpretation and reporting strategy for V/Q lung scintigraphy. J Nucl Med. 2011;52(10):1508–12.
55. Gelfand MJ, Gruppo RA, Nasser MP. Ventilation-perfusion scintigraphy in children and adolescents is associated with a low rate of indeterminate studies. Clin Nucl Med. 2008;33(9):606–9.
56. Bodei L, Lam M, Chiesa C, et al. EANM procedure guideline for treatment of refractory metastatic bone pain. Eur J Nucl Med Mol Imaging. 2008;35(10):934–1940.
57. Olivier P, Colarinha P, Fettich J, et al. Guidelines for radioiodinated MIBG scintigraphy in children. Eur J Nucl Med Mol Imaging. 2003;30(5):B45–50.
58. Kowalsky RJ, Falen SW. Radiopharmaceuticals in nuclear pharmacy and nuclear medicine. 2nd ed. Washington DC: American Pharmacists Association; 2004.
59. Lonergan GJ, Schwab CM, Suarez ES, et al. Neuroblastoma, ganglioneuroblastoma, and ganglioneuroma: radiologic-pathologic correlation. Radiographics. 2002;22(4):911–34.
60. Bombardieri E, Giammarile F, Aktolun C, et al. 131I/123I-Metaiodobenzylguanidine (mIBG) scintigraphy: procedure guidelines for tumour imaging. Eur J Nucl Med Mol Imaging. 2010;37:2436–46.
61. Boubaker A, Bischof Delaloye A. Nuclear medicine procedures and neuroblastoma in childhood. Their value in the diagnosis, staging and assessment of response to therapy. Q J Nucl Med. 2003;47(1):31–40.
62. Alexander N, Vali R, Ahmadzadehfar H, Shammas A, Baruchel S. Review: the role of radiolabeled DOTA-conjugated peptides for imaging and treatment of childhood neuroblastoma. Curr Radiopharm. 2018;11(1):14–21.
63. Zhang L, Vines D, Scollard D, et al. Correlation of somatostatin receptor-2 expression with gallium-68-DOTA-TATE uptake in neuroblastoma xenograft models. Contrast Media Mol Imaging. 2017;2017:9481276.
64. Barthlen W, Mohnike W, Mohnike K. Techniques in pediatric surgery: congenital hyperinsulinism. Horm Res Paediatr. 2010;74:438–43.
65. Arnoux JB, de Lonlay P, et al. Congenital hyperinsulinism. Early Hum Dev. 2010;86:287–94.
66. McAndrew HF, Smith V, et al. Surgical complications of pancreatectomy for persistent hyperinsulinaemic hypoglycaemia of infancy. J Pediatr Surg. 2003;38:13–6. discussion 13–16.

67. McCarville M. PET-CT imaging in pediatric oncology. Cancer Imaging. 2009;9(1):35–43.
68. Krohmer S, Sorge I, Krausse A, Kluge R, Bierbach U, Marwede D, et al. Whole-body MRI for primary evaluation of malignant disease in children. Eur J Radiol. 2010;74(1):256–261.6.
69. Volker T, Denecke T, Steffen I, Misch D, Schonberger S, Plotkin M, et al. Positron emission tomography for staging of pediatric sarcoma patients: results of a prospective multicenter trial. J Clin Oncol. 2007;25(34):5435–41.
70. Bisdas S, Ritz R, Bender B, Braun C, Pfannenberg C, Reimold M, et al. Metabolic mapping of gliomas using hybrid MR-PET imaging: feasibility of the method and spatial distribution of metabolic changes. Invest Radiol. 2013;48(5):295–301.
71. Warbey VS, Ferner RE, Dunn JT, Calonje E, O'Doherty MJ. [^{18}F] FDG PET/CT in the diagnosis of malignant peripheral nerve sheath tumours in neurofibromatosis type-1. Eur J Nucl Med Mol Imaging. 2009;36(5):751–7.
72. Gatidis S, Schmidt H, Gucke B, Bezrukov I, Seitz G, Ebinger M, et al. Comprehensive oncologic imaging in infants and preschool children with substantially reduced radiation exposure using combined simultaneous ^{18}F-fluorodeoxyglucose positron emission tomography/magnetic resonance imaging: a direct comparison to ^{18}F fluorodeoxyglucose positron emission tomography/computed tomography. Invest Radiol. 2016;51(1):7–14.
73. Schafer JF, Gatidis S, Schmidt H, Guckel B, Bezrukov I, Pfannenberg CA, et al. Simultaneous whole-body PET/MR imaging in comparison to PET/CT in pediatric oncology: initial results. Radiology. 2014;273(1):220–31.
74. Nihayah S, Shammas A, Vali R, Parra D, Alexander S, Amaral J, Connolly B. Correlation of PET/CT and image-guided biopsies of pediatric malignancies. AJR Am J Roentgenol. 2017;208(3):656–62.
75. Blokhuis GJ, Bleeker-Rovers CP, Diender MG, Oyen WJ, Draaisma JM, de Geus-Oei LF. Diagnostic value of FDG-PET/(CT) in children with fever of unknown origin and unexplained fever during immune suppression. Eur J Nucl Med Mol Imaging. 2014;41(10):1916–23.
76. Ferdinand B, Gupta P, Kramer EL. Spectrum of thymic uptake at 18F-FDG PET. Radiographics. 2004;24(6):1611–6.
77. Sasaki M, Kuwabara Y, Ichiya Y, et al. Differential diagnosis of thymic tumors using a combination of 11C-methionine PET and FDG PET. J Nucl Med. 1999;40(10):1595–601.
78. Bemben MG, Massey BH, Bemben DA, et al. Age-related variability in body composition methods for assessment of percent fat and fat-free mass in men aged 20–74 years. Age Ageing. 1998;27(2):147–53.
79. Delbeke D, Coleman R, Milton J, et al. Procedure guideline for tumor imaging with 18F-FDG PET/CT 1.0. In: SNM guideline. Reston, VA: SNM; 2006.
80. Nakagawa TA, Ashwal S, Mathur M, et al. Guidelines for the determination of brain death in infants and children: an update of the 1987 Task Force recommendations. Crit Care Med. 2011;39(9):2139–55.
81. Banasiak KJ, Lister G. Brain death in children. Curr Opin Pediatr. 2003;15(3):288–93.
82. Friedman NC, Burt RW. Cerebral perfusion imaging. In: Henkin RE, Bova D, Dillehay GL, et al., editors. Nuclear medicine. 2nd ed. Philadelphia, PA: Mosby-Elsevier; 2006.
83. Donohoe KJ, Agrawal G, Frey KA, et al. SNM practice guideline for brain death scintigraphy 2.0. J Nucl Med Technol. 2012;40(3):198–203.
84. Okuyaz C, Gücüyener K, Karabacak NI, et al. Tc-99m-HMPAO SPECT in the diagnosis of brain death in children. Pediatr Int. 2004;46(6):711–4.
85. Sinha P, Conrad GR. Scintigraphic confirmation of brain death. Semin Nucl Med. 2012;42(1):27–32.
86. Coker SB, Dillehay GL. Radionuclide cerebral imaging for confirmation of brain death in children: the significance of dural sinus activity. Pediatr Neurol. 1986;2(1):43–6.
87. Wieler H, Marohl K, Kaiser KP, et al. Tc-99m HMPAO cerebral scintigraphy. A reliable, noninvasive method for determination of brain death. Clin Nucl Med. 1993;18:104–9.
88. Facco E, Zucchetta P, Munari M, Baratto F, et al. 99mTc-HMPAO SPECT in the diagnosis of brain death. Intensive Care Med. 1998;24(9):911–7.
89. Ashwal S, Schneider S. Brain death in the newborn. Pediatrics. 1989;84(3):429–37.
90. Rastogi MV, LaFranchi SH. Congenital hypothyroidism. Orphanet J Rare Dis. 2010;5:17. https://doi.org/10.1186/1750-1172-5-17.
91. Léger J, Olivieri A, Donaldson M, Torresani T, Krude H, van Vliet G, et al. European Society for Paediatric Endocrinology consensus guidelines on screening, diagnosis, and management of congenital hypothyroidism. J Clin Endocrinol Metab. 2014;99:363 84.
92. Wassner AJ, Brown RS. Congenital hypothyroidism: recent advances. Curr Opin Endocrinol Diabetes Obes. 2015;22(5):407–12.
93. Treves ST, Gelfand MJ, Fahey FH, Parisi MT. 2016 Update of the North American Consensus Guidelines for pediatric administered radiopharmaceutical activities. J Nucl Med. 2016;57(12):15N–8N.
94. Keller-Petrot I, Leger J, Sergent-Alaoui A, de Labriolle-Vaylet C. Congenital hypothyroidism: role of nuclear medicine. Semin Nucl Med. 2017;47(2):135–42.
95. Volkan-Salancı B, Özgen Kıratlı P. Nuclear medicine in thyroid diseases in pediatric and adolescent patients. Mol Imaging Radionucl Ther. 2015;24(2):47–59. https://doi.org/10.4274/mirt.76476.

Part III

Nuclear Medicine Therapy

28 Radioiodine Therapy for Benign Thyroid Disease

Markus Dietlein

Abbreviations

Ab	Antibody
ATD	Antithyroid drug
FNAB	Fine needle aspiration biopsy
fT4	Free levothyroxine in serum
fT3	Free triiodothyronine in serum
I-131	Iodine-131 (radioiodine)
LT4	Levothyroxine medication
mrhTSH	Modified recombinant human TSH
PTU	Propylthiouracil
rhTSH	Recombinant human TSH
SD	Standard deviation
Tg	Thyroglobulin
TPO	Thyroidal peroxidase
Xe-131	Xenon-131

28.1 Introduction

Oral administration of I-131 has been used to treat benign conditions of the thyroid gland since the 1940s. For practical purposes, it is helpful to define three subpopulations [1]:

(a) Patients with *hyperthyroidism* as the consequence of solitary hyperfunctioning thyroid nodule or toxic multinodular goiter (Plummer's disease). Recently, there is an emerging role for I-131 in the treatment for so-called subclinical hyperthyroidism [2–4]. Even a TSH level in the lower normal range may increase the risk of atrial fibrillation in elderly patients, predominately in males [5, 6]. In patients with hyperthyroidism, the aim of treatment with I-131 is to achieve a non-hyperthyroid status, which can be euthyroid or hypothyroid, recompensated by levothyroxine medication.

(b) Patients with large *nontoxic goiter (NTG)* or goiter recurrence who are euthyroid but may benefit of diminishment of thyroid volume. In these patients, the aim of treatment with I-131 is to diminish the size of the goiter and, consequently, to reduce the symptoms related to gland enlargement and nodule formation. With more effective strategies for goiter shrinkage, more patients will require levothyroxine medication.

(c) Patients with *Graves' disease (GD)* are sent to radioiodine therapy in two different constellations: relapse of thyrotoxicosis after the withdrawal of antithyroid drugs or persistence of Graves' thyrotoxicosis after 12–24 months of antithyroid drugs. Radioiodine therapy should be considered as first-line treatment in patients with an initially high risk of recurrent thyrotoxicosis when they stop taking antithyroid drugs after 12–24 months. This high-risk

M. Dietlein (✉)
Department of Nuclear Medicine, University Hospital of Cologne, Cologne, Germany
e-mail: markus.dietlein@uk-koeln.de

H. Ahmadzadehfar et al. (eds.), *Clinical Nuclear Medicine*,
https://doi.org/10.1007/978-3-030-39457-8_28

group consists of patients with young age at the time of the first manifestation of Graves' disease, with larger goiter of >40 mL, or with persistent high TSH-receptor antibodies of >10 IU/L after 6 months of antithyroid drugs. In all constellations, the risk of relapse is increased in smokers.

28.2 Treatment Options for Hyperthyroidism and Nontoxic Goiter

Antithyroid drugs (ATD), surgery, and radioiodine therapy are useful options for treatment of hyperthyroidism (Table 28.1). Although antithyroid drugs—propylthiouracil, and methimazole, or its derivative carbimazole—can all normalize serum-free T4 (fT4), serum-free T3 (fT3), and thyroid-stimulating hormone (TSH) concentrations, thyrotoxicosis recurrence after cessation of therapy is greater than 90% for multinodular goiter [8] and about 50% for Graves' disease. In nonimmune hyperthyroidism, there is no chance for permanent inhibition of the thyroid hormone production, activated by somatic mutations. Apart from that, ATD treatment is not without the risk of adverse reactions, including minor rashes and, in rare instances, agranulocytosis and hepatitis.

Surgery is preferably performed in selected cases of nodular goiter, when there is additionally a suspicion of malignancy, when there is a severe compression of neighboring structures, or when an immediate effectiveness of therapy is necessary due to severe adverse effects of ATDs.

Radioiodine therapy is in most cases the first-line treatment for solitary hyperfunctioning thyroid nodules and toxic multinodular goiter without hypofunctioning nodules or large cystic degenerations. The main indications for radioiodine treatment of NTG are to reduce the size of a goiter that is causing cosmetic difficulties for the patient and to relieve compressive signs or symptoms. The available treatment options in NTG patients in whom the risk of malignancy is considered low are "wait and see" policy, surgery, iodine supplementation, levothyroxine (LT4, in a non-TSH-suppressive dosage), and radioiodine administration (Table 28.2). In patients with postoperative goiter recurrence, radioiodine therapy is often considered first-line therapy, and the physician should not wait until the patient becomes symptomatic. The recommendation to

Table 28.1 Main features of the three available treatments for hyperthyroidism due to toxic goiters or Graves' disease (Modified from [7])

	Antithyroid drug	Surgery	Radioiodine
Time to initial improvement	2–4 weeks	Needs antithyroid drug pretreatment (toxic goiters) Success immediately	Needs antithyroid drug pretreatment; 4–8 weeks after RIT
Recurrence	90–100% (toxic goiters)	1–4%	5–10%
Use in pregnancy/ breast feeding	Yes (first trimester: PTU preferred)	Second trimester	No
Adverse effect on eye disease in toxic goiter	No	No	0.1% (1% risk of immune hyperthyroidism; rarely eye symptoms)
Adverse effect on eye disease in Graves' disease	Spontaneous course	Spontaneous course	Glucocorticoids in patients with Graves' ophthalmopathy
Interference with daily activities	No	Requires hospital admission	Need for radiation precautions and in some countries requires hospital admission
Key adverse effects	Rash; arthralgia; hepatitis; agranulocytosis	Surgical; vocal cord paralysis; hypoparathyroidism; hypothyroidism	Hypothyroidism

Table 28.2 Main features of the three available treatments for nontoxic goiter (Modified from [7])

	Levothyroxine	Surgery	Radioiodine
Efficacy	Poor	Excellent	50% reduction in the 1st year, 70% reduction after 4 years
Relief of symptoms	Slow	Immediate	Medium term
Recurrence	If treatment stopped	1–40% (depend on size of thyroid remnant)	Unlikely; repeat treatment feasible
Special indications	Small goiter; patient wish	Suspicion of malignancy; severe compression of neighboring structures	Patient wish; elderly with surgical risk factors; postoperative goiter recurrence
Exclusions	Suppressed TSH	Surgical contraindications	Radiation protection issues
Key adverse effects	Depending on TSH-level: cardiac arrhythmia, osteopenia	Surgical; vocal cord paralysis; hypoparathyroidism; hypothyroidism	Hypothyroidism

radioiodine therapy should be given early in an asymptomatic status with a goiter volume of about 30–40 mL for patients with preexisting paralysis of the N. recurrens (with or without previous thyroid surgery), especially if paralysis is contralateral to a unilateral recurrent goiter, and for patients with temporary postoperative hypoparathyroidism after the first operation. With levothyroxine medication, some patients may achieve clinically relevant (more than 50%) nodule or goiter shrinkage; however, it occurs only in 10–20% of patients [9]. The only available controlled long-term investigation [10] showed no significant nodule size reduction after 5 years of continuous LT4 therapy. Additionally, a comparative study showed the superiority of I-131 treatment over LT4 therapy [11]. Radioiodine treatment is indicated in patients with medical contraindications to thyroid surgery, patients with slight or moderate compressive symptoms, patients with large goiter, or patients who wish to avoid operation. The interdisciplinary approach to patients followed by well-balanced decision-making and informed consent allows for an individualized selection between alternative treatment options. Special consideration should be given to the patient's profession as I-131 is without risk for paralysis of the recurrent laryngeal nerve. There are well-known regional differences in the choice of treatment for initial or recurrent hyperthyroidism, but radioiodine is increasingly used as first-line treatment as ever more data accumulate proving its safety.

In patients with Graves' disease, radioiodine therapy can be offered as first-line treatment or in case of a relapse of the thyrotoxicosis. Smokers with an active Graves' ophthalmopathy are not suitable candidates for radioiodine therapy. To avoid hyperthyroidism or the need for antithyroid drugs during pregnancy in the future, young women are suitable candidates for radioiodine therapy. Because the TSH receptor antibodies remain high for about 1 or 2 years after the radioiodine therapy, it is better to treat young women during their early lifetime when conception is not intended. If conception becomes an urgent matter, the family planning had to be postponed for about 4 months after radioiodine therapy. The contraception after the radioiodine therapy is necessary until a stable euthyroidism is reached taking levothyroxine medication.

28.3 Physical and Radiobiological Properties of Radioiodine

Iodine is an indispensable component of thyroid hormones levothyroxine (T4) and triiodothyronine (T3). Thyroid cells extract and concentrate iodide from plasma. Shortly after administration, radioiodine is taken up from the blood via the sodium-iodine symporter and accumulates within thyroid follicular cells (Fig. 28.1). About 20% of the iodide perfusing the thyroid is removed at each passage through the gland. Ingested iodine is absorbed through the small intestine and trans-

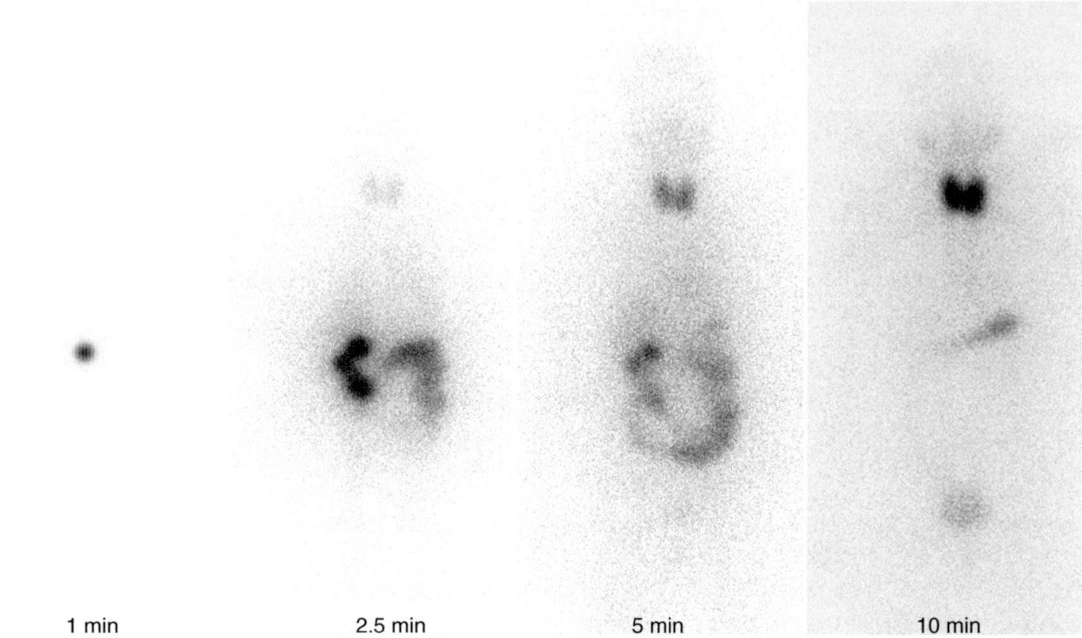

Fig. 28.1 Example for the rapid I-131 thyroidal uptake demonstrated by dynamic whole-body images: *1 min* after the application of an I-131 therapy capsule, the activity is visible in the stomach, after *2.5 min* activity in the gut, after *5 min* increasing thyroidal accumulation, and after *10 min* the thyroidal accumulation dominating

ported in the plasma to the thyroid, where it is concentrated, oxidized, and then incorporated into thyroglobulin (Tg) and later T4 and T3. After storage in thyroid follicles, Tg is subjected to proteolysis, and the released hormones are secreted into the circulation. In subjects with normal thyroid function, up to 20–30% of orally administered iodine is taken up by the thyroid. In hyperthyroid patients, this fraction is increased—in individual cases up to more than 80% (rationale for pretherapeutic radioiodine testing). The fraction of radioiodine which is not taken up by the thyroid gland is mainly excreted via the urine (Fig. 28.2).

I-131 is a beta- and gamma-emitting radionuclide (principle $\beta^- = 0.807$ MeV; gamma rays ranging from 80 to 637 keV, most abundant γ: 364 keV) with a physical half-life of 8.02 days. The average range of the 0.807 MeV beta particles in soft tissue approximates 1 mm which allows high intrathyroidal doses. Radiobiological effects of radioiodine on tissues are direct (radiation deposit within DNA) or indirect. Indirect effects produce free radicals that in turn react with the critical macromolecules. I-131 used for treatment of thyroid disorders decays to stable Xe-131 by beta emission.

The radiopharmaceutical I-131 sodium iodine is administered orally in capsules, but in patients with severe swallowing difficulties, it can be administered in liquid or intravenously in patients in whom vomiting is a problem.

28.4 Contraindication for Radioiodine Therapy and Precautions

28.4.1 Pregnancy and Breast Feeding

Pregnancy and breast feeding are all absolute contraindications to radioiodine treatment. Most recommendations stipulate that pregnancy should be avoided for 4 months after radioiodine treatment in women and in men [12, 13]. Arguments for this waiting period are radiation protection and stability of thyroid function in women, the cycle of spermatogenesis in men. This in turn

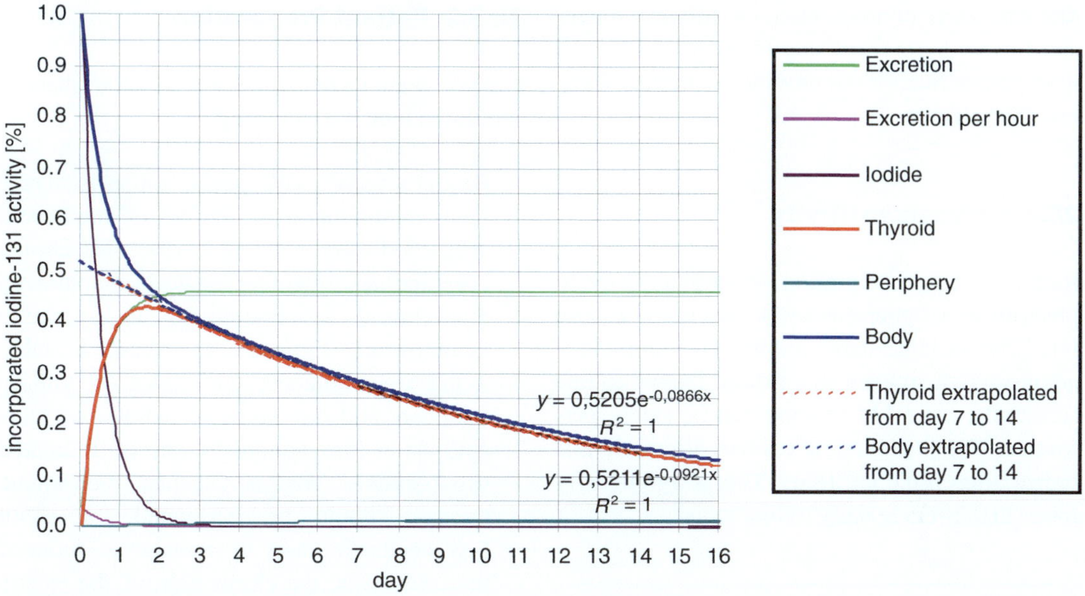

Fig. 28.2 Modeling of iodine kinetics

implies that the clinician must have a careful discussion with each patient for whom there may be plans for conception, and treatment must be planned with this in mind. More generally, each patient requires a careful explanation of all treatment options provided by a specialist accredited in the treatment of thyroid disease. To keep the organ dose of the breast low, the interval between cessation of breast feeding and start of radioiodine therapy should be at least 8 weeks.

28.4.2 Uncontrolled Hyperthyroidism

Since radioiodine administration may cause a transient elevation in fT4 and fT3 levels approximately 7 days following administration, uncontrolled symptoms of hyperthyroidism or high level of fT3 constitutes relative contraindications for therapy (further elevation of thyroid hormone may trigger atrial fibrillation or heart failure or, rarely, lead to thyroid storm). In that case, pretreatment with antithyroid drugs combined, if necessary, with β-blockers should be administered first. In the symptomatically well-controlled patient, radioiodine therapy will have little effect on patient clinical symptoms. In highly selected cases where antithyroid drug is contraindicated (e.g., due to agranulocytosis or posttherapy liver failure) and surgery cannot be performed due to symptoms of hyperthyroidism, I-131 may be administered under the cover of β-blockers, preferably propranolol, which blocks T4 to T3 conversion. The American Thyroid Association Guidelines recommend for management of thyroid storm additionally steroids, usually hydrocortisone hemisuccinate 300 mg as intravenous load, then 100 mg i.v. every 8 h, or dexamethasone as an alternative drug [14].

28.4.3 Tracheal Stenosis

Patients with large goiter with tracheal narrowing <1 cm may be treated under the cover of steroids though in the authors experience clinically harmful thyroid swelling was never observed with tracheal diameters ≥5–6 mm. If tracheal diameter is <5–6 mm, due to risk of severe dyspnea, surgery rather than radioiodine therapy should be performed. Patients with high risk of severe posttreatment complications (elderly with a risk of heart failure, patients with narrow tracheal diameter, large thyroid goiter, or with uncompensated hyperthyroidism) should always be treated in in-patient facilities to provide continuous medical surveillance.

28.4.4 Hypersensitivity

Radioiodine administration is very unlikely to precipitate a hypersensitivity reaction because I-131 free of large stable iodine contamination is administered, so even in cases of known iodine sensitivity, the I-131 therapy can be safely performed. The stable iodine content of radioiodine preparations is 0.05–0.18 μg. This is significantly lower than average daily iodine intake.

28.5 Procedure

28.5.1 Facility and Legislation

The facilities required to perform radioiodine therapy will depend on the national legislation for the emission of pure beta- or beta–gamma-emitting therapy agents. The requirement to admit patients due to administered I-131 activity varies considerably across the different countries. If in-patient therapy is required by national legislation, this should take place in an approved environment with appropriately shielded rooms. The facility in which treatment is performed must have appropriate personnel, radiation safety equipment, and procedures available for waste handling and disposal and handling of incidental contamination, monitoring personnel for accidental contamination, and controlling/limiting its spread.

The restrictions on work and contact with small children depend on national dose limits. Generally in Europe, the exposition from radioiodine radiation should not exceed 1 mSv for other individuals in the general population. Usually, the patient is advised to keep as much distance as possible between themselves and others, including children, and of keeping contact times as short as possible [15–18].

28.5.2 Patient Preparation

Patient evaluation before radioiodine therapy should include the following:

1. Patient's history with special emphasis on previous treatments (e.g., the use of antithyroid drugs, iodinated contrast media, amiodarone, other iodine-containing medication, iodinated multivitamin combinations) and urinary incontinence. Exposure to excessive stable iodine may influence the choice of primary treatment and the timing of radioiodine therapy. After the administration of iodinated water-soluble contrast agents, radioiodine therapy should be postponed for about 6–8 weeks. In cases of *amiodarone*-induced thyrotoxicosis, the elimination of the excess iodine load can take up to 1–2 years (on average 6 months) in amiodarone-induced thyrotoxicosis [19]. In doubtful cases, measurement of iodine excretion in the urine is possible. If amiodarone cannot be stopped because of the underlying heart problem, then radioiodine treatment will not be feasible.

   In patients presenting with unmanageable urinary incontinence, a lifelong medication with ATDs may be justified in case of overt hyperthyroidism, if surgery is too risky due to comorbidity. TSH level should be kept in the lower range to avoid increase of the thyroid volume. Consequently, information on this is important and should be part of the patients' evaluation before therapy.
2. Laboratory testing, including fT4, fT3, TSH, TSHR-Ab, TPO-Ab, and Tg-Ab.
3. Thyroid scintigraphy and radioiodine testing with radioiodine 24 h uptake: The 24 h uptake should be >20%, if lower other treatment modalities should be considered. Uptake measurements are not absolutely required when fixed activities are used in the countries where Graves' disease is the predominant cause of hyperthyroidism and the thyroid volume is uniformly low.
4. Assessment of thyroid target volume (ultrasonography) [20] and intrathoracic extension in

case of large goiters (magnetic resonance imaging/computed tomography) [21].

5. Fine needle aspiration biopsy (FNAB) in nodules larger than 1–1.5 cm with a suspicious sonographic appearance or scintigraphically hypofunctioning. In elderly patients with large goiters, the combination of hyperfunctioning nodules (indication for radioiodine therapy) and hypofunctioning nodules (surgery as preferred option) is a common constellation. An individual risk stratification is necessary. In autonomous nodules, as the risk of malignancy is very low, FNAB should only be considered in case of suspicious sonographic features [13]. Alternatively, I-123 scintigraphy with late imaging 24 h p.i. is a strategy to confirm autonomously functioning nodules and to exclude Tc-99m-pertechnetate "trapping-only" nodules.
6. Female patients with child-bearing potential should be routinely tested for pregnancy within 72 h or less before the administration of I-131. When patient history clearly indicates that pregnancy is excluded, a pregnancy test may be omitted at the discretion of the treating physician. Consequently, posttherapeutic contraception for 4 months after I-131 therapy is also a prerequisite.

28.5.3 Special Considerations for Medication

Antithyroid drugs are often used in the initial treatment of patients with hyperthyroidism. As pretreatment with ATDs depletes thyroid hormone stores, it constitutes a safe patient preparation for radioiodine treatment, especially beneficial in patients with overt hyperthyroidism or distinctly elevated fT3. However, since thyrostatic drugs may lower the uptake of radioiodine as well as the effective half-life, they can decrease effectiveness of radioiodine treatment. Another side effect of ATDs is the possible radioprotective effect which seems to depend on chemical compounds contained in the thyrostatic medication. Radioresistance, which may be associated with thiourea-based medication, may result from the presence of a sulfhydryl group. Methimazole and carbimazole, which do not possess sulfhydryl groups, will probably do not offer radioprotective effects, and this may explain the difference to propylthiouracil [22]. The potentially negative impact of thyrostatic drugs can be compensated for by discontinuing medication shortly before treatment; carbimazole and methimazole should be withdrawn respectively for at least 2 days before planned radioiodine administration [23–25] if tolerated by the patient. Propylthiouracil (PTU) which has a more distinct radioprotective action that may further reduce the effectiveness of radioiodine should be stopped at least 2–3 weeks before radioiodine treatment. When data from an individual pretherapeutic dosimetry (radioiodine testing with measurement of the effective half-life) are available, a withdrawal of PTU 2 days before "radioiodine testing" and radioiodine therapy may be sufficient [26, 27]. Beta-adrenergic antagonists (usually propranolol in dose adjusted to clinical symptoms) may be helpful for interim hyperthyroidism symptom relief during ATD withdrawal, provided that there are no contraindications.

Levothyroxine medication decreases radioiodine uptake, but may be used to optimize the distribution of radioiodine within the nodular thyroid. In patients with autonomously functioning nodules and a pretherapeutic TSH level of more than 0.3 mU L^{-1}, the levothyroxine medication leads to an exogenous suppression of the thyrotropin secretion and may be favorable to achieve posttherapeutic euthyroidism without levothyroxine substitution in the long-term perspective. If reduction of goiter size is given priority, TSH suppression is not necessary.

Lithium can block radioiodine release from the thyroid but does not interfere with radioiodine uptake. It may enhance the effectiveness of radioiodine when given for a few days immediately after treatment, but the available data are controversial, and side effects may be experienced by 10% of patients. In one prospective, randomized, controlled trial from Italy, lithium treatment (900 mg/day for 6 days from the time of radioiodine treatment) increased the cure rate by 11% and induced a more rapid control of hyperthyroidism [28]. However, another randomized, controlled trial from India has found no evidence of an effect of lithium on outcome after radioiodine treatment [29]. Therefore, the off-label use of lithium (e.g., 2 × 250 mg) is not routinely recommended.

Modified recombinant human TSH (mrhTSH) may be used to maximize I-131 uptake in the thyroid gland and to minimize the radiation dose to the remainder of the body in patients with nontoxic multinodular goiter [30–33]. However, mrhTSH is not yet approved for this indication, and administration in a patient with nontoxic goiter represents an off-label use.

28.6 Patient Information and Instruction

Patients should receive both written and verbal information about the procedure before receiving therapy. Written informed consent must be obtained from the patient. The following items should be discussed:

- Therapeutic options and alternatives including watchful waiting
- More than one I-131 treatment course may be necessary. Pretherapeutic dosimetry before I-131 therapy and intended absorbed doses of about 100–150 Gy for toxic goiters and nontoxic goiters, of about 300–400 Gy for toxic nodules, and of about 300 Gy for Graves' disease offer high rates of success of a single I-131 therapy.
- Recommendations for radiation protection after discharge from hospital or as outpatient
- Early and late side effects
- Need for contraception for 4 months for female and male patients
- Need for lifelong follow-up

28.7 Radiation Dosimetry and I-131 Activity

The aim for radioiodine treatment in toxic nodules or toxic goiters is often to restore euthyroidism [12]. There have been many studies attempting to identify an optimal regimen for radioiodine treatment that minimizes the risks of developing hypothyroidism while maximizing the cure rate of hyperthyroidism. However, this is a challenging issue: first because a maximum cure rate inevitably results in the highest rate of hypothyroidism and second because any single dosage method cannot practically encompass all of the variables affecting outcome. These variables include age, sex, thyroid size, severity of hyperthyroidism, innate differences in radiation sensitivity, iodine intake, and preceding use of antithyroid drugs. Nevertheless, there is an ongoing discussion on the establishment of the optimal method to determine the activity that can be recommended for clinical practice: estimation (the so-called fixed dose) versus calculation (based on radioiodine uptake measurements). Council directive Euratom 97/43 requires that for all medical exposure of individuals for radiotherapeutic purposes, exposures of target volumes will be individually planned. In principle, formulas which calculate the therapeutic I-131 activity for an individual patient differ in the time points when radioiodine uptake is measured during the radioiodine test. The Marinelli formula takes the 24 h radioiodine uptake and a late uptake for the calculation of the effective half-life of I-131, while Hänscheid-Bockisch formula focuses on a late uptake about 5 days after ingestion of a test capsule [34, 35].

In either toxic or nontoxic multinodular goiter, radioiodine doses have been empirically established. The optimal radioiodine therapy should be a single-dose cure. Currently, an absorbed radiation dose of 100–150 Gy is recommended (Table 28.3), requiring about 3.7–5.5 MBq per gram of thyroid tissue corrected for the 24 h

Table 28.3 Recommendations for intended target dose

	Target volume	Dose (Gy) per g tissue
Toxic goiter	Thyroid	120
Hyperfunctioning nodule	Nodule	300–400
Nontoxic goiter	Thyroid	120
Graves' disease	Thyroid	300
Retreatment >6 months after first dose of radioiodine		Original dose

I-131 uptake [36]. To increase radioiodine uptake and retention in nontoxic goiter, mrhTSH was used in some studies [23, 24]. mrhTSH can increase the absorbed radiation dose and permits a more equal distribution in the gland [31–33, 37]. Its future role, however, still has to be established. In patients with autonomous nodules, the recommended dose is 300–400 Gy.

Hyperthyroidism due to Graves' disease is usually treated by an ablative dosage concept of about 300 Gy. The substitution with levothyroxine becomes necessary within 3 months after the radioiodine therapy. The ablative dosage concept of radioiodine therapy is comparable with the surgical strategy of a near-total thyroidectomy in the surgically treated patients with Graves' disease.

The recommended formula to calculate the activity which is required to achieve the dose in the thyroid is as follows:

$$A[\mathrm{MBq}] = \frac{F}{\ln 2} \cdot \frac{M[\mathrm{g}] \cdot D[\mathrm{Gy}]}{\int_0^\infty \mathrm{RIU}(t)\,\mathrm{d}t}$$

A = activity; F = correction factor; M = mass of target volume; D = required dose

In this respect, the radioiodine uptake (RI)U can be calculated as follows:

$$\mathrm{RIU} = \frac{\text{Activity in thyroid gland}}{\text{Administered activity}} \times 100\%$$

The range of activities currently prescribed, irrespective of the method used, varies between 200 and 800 MBq depending on gland size or nodule size, with the majority of patients receiving 400–600 MBq. To get more insight into the procedure guidelines for pretherapeutic "radioiodine testing," some papers are recommended in which comprehensive updates are provided for clinical practice [7, 26, 27, 38–45].

Kobe et al. [41] analyzed the radioiodine half-life and uptake in a region with a mean alimentary iodine supply of 130–150 μg daily. Inclusion criteria were the control of hyperthyroidism and withdrawal of ATDs 2 days before preliminary radioiodine testing and therapy. Patients were treated for toxic goiter (n = 639), toxic solitary nodule (n = 365), or nontoxic goiter (n = 50). The effective half-life and uptake of I-131 were estimated by uptake measurements after 24 h and 5 days during the preliminary radioiodine test and serial measurements over 5 days during therapy. The mean effective half-life of I-131 measured during radioiodine therapy was 6.6 days in toxic goiter, 5.7 days in toxic solitary nodule, 6.4 days in nontoxic goiter, and 5.4 days in Graves' disease. The mean maximal uptake of I-131 measured during radioiodine therapy was 38% in toxic goiter, 31% in toxic nodule, 42% in nontoxic goiter, and 64% in Graves' disease (Table 28.4).

Another advantage of an individual pre- and posttherapeutical dosimetry is the early detection of an unexpected low thyroid dose. If the post-therapeutically achieved dose is much lower than the intended dose, a second I-131 capsule can be administered, while patient is still hospitalized (2–3 days after the first I-131 administration). Monitoring of radioiodine kinetics during therapy in an individual patient allows to intervene in case of impending therapy failure which lowers the rate of patients requiring a second therapy and represents a highly personalized approach to radioiodine therapy (Fig. 28.3) [12, 26].

Patients with end-stage renal failure cannot excrete radioiodine normally, reducing the dose

Table 28.4 Effective thyroidal half-life and thyroidal I-131 uptake measured in 639 patients with toxic goiter, in 365 patients with solitary hyperfunctioning nodules, in 50 patients with nontoxic goiter, and in 363 patients with Graves' disease [41]

	Toxic goiter	Toxic solitary nodule	Nontoxic goiter	Graves' disease
Half-life of I-131 (test) [days ± SD]	7.3 ± 1.0	6.5 ± 1.4	7.4 ± 0.9	5.5 ± 1.5
Half-life of I-131 (therapy) [days ± SD]	6.6 ± 1.2	5.7 ± 1.5	6.4 ± 1.1	5.4 ± 1.6
Maximal uptake of I-131 (test) [% ± SD]	37 ± 15	31 ± 12	38 ± 15	63 ± 17
Maximal uptake of I-131 (therapy) [% ± SD]	38 ± 15	31 ± 23	42 ± 13	64 ± 18

Inclusion criteria were the control of hyperthyroidism and withdrawal of antithyroid drugs 2 days before preliminary radioiodine testing and therapy. *SD* standard deviation

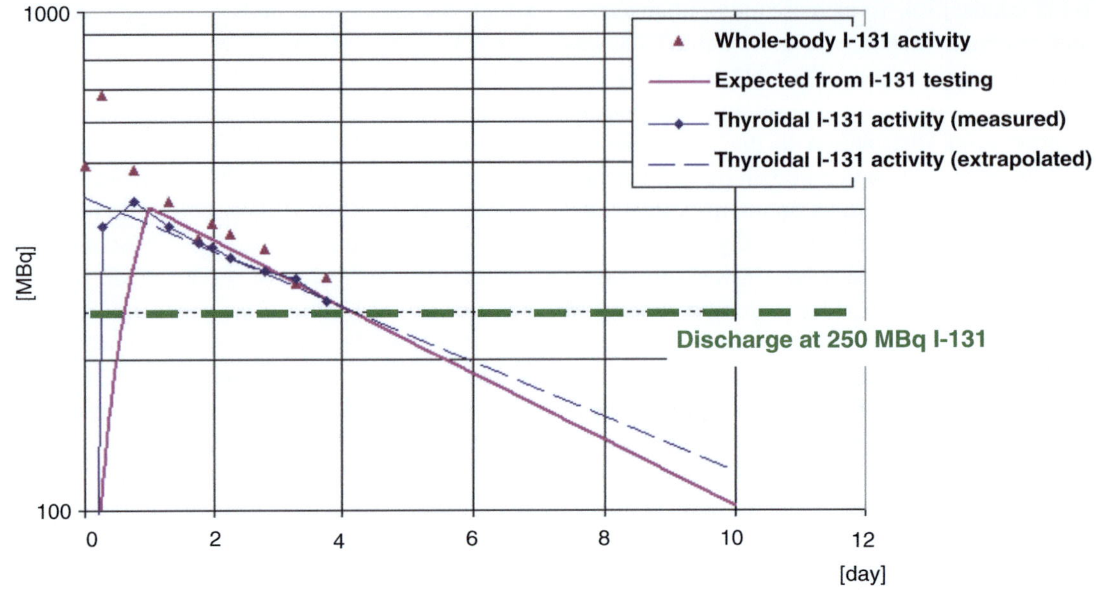

Fig. 28.3 Time activity curves during I-131 therapy of a toxic goiter. Whole-body activity (*triangle*) and thyroidal activity after the application of an I-131 therapy capsule (*rhombus, thin line*) were measured twice a day. Extrapolated values of the posttherapeutic thyroidal activity are represented by the *dashed line*. The time activity curve from the pretherapeutic I-131 testing is also visible (*broader line*) and allows a comparison between the expected and the achieved thyroidal dose. The national laws in Germany allow discharge from hospital at 250 MBq I-131 residual activity

required for treatment, and the effects of hemodialysis or peritoneal dialysis add further complications to calculating the activity required [46].

28.8 Side Effects of I-131 Therapy

28.8.1 Acute Side Effects

Patients with large goiters may notice transient swelling of the goiter. Thyroid swelling lasts until approximately 1 week following therapy, and some discomfort may be associated with it. Treatment strategy is the sequence cooling with ice, antiphlogistic drugs, and glucocorticoids. Slight discomfort of the salivary glands may be present, but sialadenitis is transient and permanent injury uncommon. There may be a transient rise in fT4 and fT3 levels 7–10 days following radioiodine treatment, and patients who have been poorly controlled before radioiodine therapy may experience an exacerbation of heart arrhythmias and heart failure. In some patients, a thyroid storm may develop. This rare condition must be treated with intravenous infusion of antithyroid drugs, corticosteroids, and β-blockers.

28.8.2 Hypothyroidism

The main side effect of radioiodine treatment is hypothyroidism [38, 47]. Its rates vary, and incidence continues to increase over time, so that life-long follow-up is essential. Pretreatment prediction is not possible using current variables; however, the incidence is higher in small gland size than in large toxic goiter. In solitary hyperfunctioning nodules, the volume of the surrounding thyroid tissue is the decisive factor. The ablative dosage concept due to Graves' thyrotoxicosis leads to the consequence of levothyroxine substitution in nearly all successfully treated patients. Using a thyroid function preserving dose concept in toxic goiter, levothyroxine medication is needed in patients under 65 years with elevated TSH > 4 mU L^{-1} after I-131 therapy, also in older patients over 65 years with subclinical hypothyroidism and TSH > 7 mU L^{-1} after I-131 therapy.

28.8.3 Autoimmune Thyroiditis

This phenomenon is observed in 1% of the patients following radioiodine therapy of goiter/autonomy. The risk is increased up to 10% in patients with preexisting thyroid peroxidase or thyroglobulin antibodies [48]. In case of autoimmune thyroiditis after radioiodine therapy, about 10% of patients will develop ophthalmopathy. Thus, the risk of ophthalmopathy is in the range of 0.1% for patients without a preexisting elevation of thyroid antibodies.

28.8.4 Radiation-Induced Cancers

A small excess of mortality from malignancy (standardized mortality ratio 1.09; confidence intervals 1.03–1.16) was reported [49], but the study was biased by the increased surveillance, changes in reporting, and a higher proportion of smokers in the hyperthyroid patients. A small increase in relative risk of diagnosis or death from thyroid cancer after radioiodine treatment has been reported in large epidemiological studies carried out in different countries. The reported absolute risk, however, is still very small in these studies, and in addition, it seems to be more associated with the underlying disease than treatment with radioiodine [50–54].

28.9 Success Rate

The success rate of radioiodine therapy depends on thyroid volume, compensation of hyperthyroidism, time of the withdrawal of antithyroid drugs, alimentary iodine intake, and the dose concepts in the different thyroid diseases. The superiority of dosimetric approaches over the use of fixed activities or of volume-adapted activities remains controversial. The dosimetric approach is mandatory in some European countries; it allows early therapeutic intervention, should the posttherapeutically achieved thyroid dose fall unexpectedly below the intended dose. In this constellation, the application of a second I-131 capsule may be appropriate.

28.9.1 Toxic Multinodular Goiter

Two studies with an intended absorbed dose of 150 Gy to the thyroid and higher doses in selected patients with a high Tc-99m pertechnetate uptake under suppression reported a success rate of more than 90% [55, 56]. In a comparative study from Switzerland, 3 days of carbimazole withdrawal was sufficient for a high success rate of radioiodine therapy [57].

28.9.2 Solitary Hyperfunctioning Nodule

Studies in which the radiation-absorbed dose to the hyperfunctioning nodule has been measured posttherapeutically or, at least, a target-absorbed dose has been determined pretherapeutically have shown a success rate of 85–100% and an incidence of hypothyroidism of 10–20% [58]. In a comparative study, successful elimination of functional thyroid autonomy occurred at 12 months after radioiodine therapy in 90% of patients receiving 300 Gy to the nodule volume and in 94% of patients receiving 400 Gy to the nodule volume [59].

28.9.3 Nontoxic Multinodular Goiter

The success of radioiodine treatment in reducing the size of a NTG depends on many factors. Cystic and fibrotic areas will be resistant to shrinkage, and their extent varies between patients. The volume reduction in radioiodine-accumulating goiter areas increases with higher I-131 activities per gram thyroid tissue, higher achieved thyroid doses, and a homogeneous distribution of I-131 within the goiter. In most previous reports, the administered amount of radioiodine has been approximately 3.7 MBq per gram thyroid tissue, corrected for 100% uptake in the thyroid after 24 h, leading to an absorbed dose of about 100 Gy in the thyroid. The decrease in thyroid volume ranged between 30% and 60% [60]. Most of the shrinkage occurred within the first year, and goiter volumes continued to decrease for several years. Symptomatic swelling of the goiter is uncommon as severe stenosis of the trachea can be excluded by adequate imaging procedures. Calculations based on pretherapeutic uptake measurements over 5 days and an intended thyroid dose of 150 Gy—resulting in mean activities of 1721 ± 440 MBq I-131, equivalent to 14 ± 4.19 MBq I-131 per gram of thyroid tissue—led to a mean volume reduction of 42% after 3 months, 66% after 1 year, 70% after 2 years, and nearly 75% after 3 years in a patient group with goiters of at least 80 mL residing in an area of longstanding iodine deficiency [61].

Volume measurements of large goiters can be optimized by magnetic resonance imaging (MRI) or CT without contrast agent, which provides more objective results and less intra-/interobserver variability than ultrasound as precise volume measurements become more difficult with increasing thyroid size [62]. Additionally, MRI or CT evaluates the size of an accompanying retrosternal goiters and the diameter of the trachea. SPECT/CT with Tc-99m pertechnetate or I-123 offers the advantage to combine anatomical and functional imaging.

A more homogeneous radioiodine uptake and an improvement of goiter volume reduction results from radioiodine therapy after stimulation with a low dose of recombinant human thyrotropin, especially prepared for a delayed release in randomized trials [63].

Radioiodine therapy for reducing the size of a NTG can be recommended as effective therapy especially for elderly people, for those with comorbidity and for patients who want to avoid surgery.

28.9.4 Graves' Disease

Graves' hyperthyroidism is eliminated in >90% of patients following radioiodine testing and the ablative dosage concept with an intended dose of 300 Gy.

First manifestation or worsening of ophthalmopathy is possible in the spontaneous course of Graves' disease. The risk after the radioiodine therapy is not increased compared to the operative or conservative treatment under the following precautions: Radioiodine therapy starts when euthyroidism is achieved by antithyroid drugs. The radioiodine therapy eliminates successfully the thyrotoxicosis by a single-dose cure. Patients with Graves' ophthalmopathy receive glucocorticoids. Levothyroxine medication should start early after the radioiodine therapy to prevent hypothyroidism. Smokers with a Graves' ophthalmopathy undergo radioiodine therapy only if the ophthalmopathy has become inactive.

28.10 Follow-Up After Radioiodine Treatment

Regular review of thyroid function tests in patients who have undergone radioiodine treatment for thyroid disease is essential to assess the efficacy of the treatment and for timely detection of developing hypothyroidism or post-radioiodine immunogenic hyperthyroidism. First TSH and fT4 examination should be performed not longer than 4–6 weeks after radioiodine therapy. Shorter intervals of about 2–3 weeks are recommended for patients who received ATDs. If the treatment was performed for (overt) hyperthyroidism, about 3–5 days after the radioiodine administration restart of antithyroid drugs should be recommended. In case of persistent hyperthyroidism, radioiodine treatment can be repeated after 6–12 months. In case of post-radioiodine immunogenic hyperthyroidism, ATDs for some months appear to be adequate, and a second radioiodine therapy is not necessary in most patients. Laboratory tests (at least including TSH) in annual intervals are necessary lifelong, even in patients with euthyroidism after I-131 therapy.

The material was originally published by Dietlein M, Schmidt M. Radioiodine Therapy of Hyperthyroidism (Toxic Goiter, Hyperfunctioning Nodule) and Non-Toxic Goiter: Procedures and Guidelines (Pages 335–346). In: Baum RP (Ed).

Therapeutic Nuclear Medicine. Springer-Verlag Berlin Heidelberg 2014. ISBN 978-3-540-36718-5. DOI 10.1007/978-3-540-36719-2. "With permission of Springer Nature"

References

1. Stokkel M, Handkiewicz J, Lassmann M, Dietlein M, Luster M. EANM procedure guidelines for therapy of benign thyroid disease. Eur J Nucl Med Mol Imaging. 2010;37:2218.
2. Col NF, Surks MI, Daniels GH. Subclinical thyroid disease. Clinical applications. JAMA. 2004;291:239–43.
3. McDermott MT, Woodmansee WW, Haugen BR, Smart A, Ridgway EC. The management of subclinical hyperthyroidism by thyroid specialists. Thyroid. 2003;13:1133–9.
4. Surks MI, Ortiz E, Daniels GH, et al. Subclinical thyroid disease. Scientific review and guidelines for diagnosis and management. JAMA. 2004;291:229–38.
5. Gammage MD, Parle JV, Holder RL, Roberts LM, Hobbs FDR, Wilson S, Sheppard MC, Franklyn JA. Association between serum free thyroxine concentration and atrial fibrillation. Arch Intern Med. 2007;167:928–34.
6. Heeringa J, Hoogendoorn EH, van der Deure WM, Hofman A, Peeters RP, Hop CJ, den Heijer M, Visser TJ, Witteman JCM. High-normal thyroid function and risk of atrial fibrillation - The Rotterdam Study. Arch Intern Med. 2008;168:2219–24.
7. Weetman AP. Radioiodine treatment for benign thyroid diseases. Clin Endocrinol (Oxf). 2007;66:757–64.
8. Freitas JE. Therapeutic options in the management of toxic and nontoxic nodular goiter. Semin Nucl Med. 2000;30:88–97.
9. Fast S, Nielsen V, Bonnema S, Hegedus L. Time to reconsider nonsurgical therapy of benign nontoxic multinodular goiter. Focus on recombinant human TSH (rhTSH) augmented radioiodine therapy. Eur J Endocrinol. 2008;160:517–28.
10. Papini E, Petrucci L, Guglielmi R, Panunzi C, Rinaldi R, Bacci V, Crescenzi A, Nardi F, Fabbrini R, Pacella CM. Long-term changes in nodular goiter: a 5-year prospective randomized trial of levothyroxine suppressive therapy for benign cold thyroid nodules. J Clin Endocrinol Metab. 1998;83:780–3.
11. Wesche MF, Tiel-V Buul MM, Lips P, Smits NJ, Wiersinga WM. A randomized trial comparing levothyroxine with radioactive iodine in the treatment of sporadic nontoxic goiter. J Clin Endocrinol Metab. 2001;86:998–1005.
12. Dietlein M, Grünwald F, Schmidt M, Schneider P, Verburg FA, Luster M. Guideline for radioiodine therapy for benign thyroid diseases (version 5). [German]. Nuklearmedizin. 2016;55:213–20.
13. Haugen BR, Alexander EK, Bible KC, Doherty GM, Mandel SJ, Nikiforov YE, Pacini F, Randolph GW, Sawka AM, Schlumberger M, Schuff KG, Sherman SI, Sosa JA, Steward DL, Tuttle RM, Wartowsky L. 2015 American Thyroid Association management guidelines for adult patients with thyroid nodules and differentiated thyroid cancer. Thyroid. 2016;26:1–133.
14. Ross DS, Burch HB, Cooper DS, Greenlee MC, Laurberg P, Maria AL, Rivkees SA, Samuels M, Sosa JA, Stan MN, Malter MA. 2016 American Thyroid Association guidelines for diagnosis and management of hyperthyroidism and other causes of thyrotoxicosis. Thyroid. 2015;26:1343–421.
15. Cappelen T, Unhjem JF, Amundsen AL, Kravdal G, Følling I. Radiation exposure to family members of patients with thyrotoxicosis treated with iodine-131. Eur J Nucl Med Mol Imaging. 2006;33:81–6.
16. Dillehay GL, Ellerbroek NA, Balon H, Brill DR, Grigsby PW, Macklis RM, Mauch PM, Mian TA, Potters L, Silberstein EB, Williams TR, Wong JC, Gaspar LE. American Society for Therapeutic Radiology and Oncology. Practice guideline for the performance of therapy with unsealed radiopharmaceutical sources. Int J Radiat Oncol Biol Phys. 2006;64:1299–307.
17. International Commission on Radiological Protection. Release of patients after therapy with unsealed radionuclides. Ann ICRP. 2004;34:1–79. Erratum in: Ann ICRP 34(3–4): 281.
18. Koch W, Rosa F, Knesewitsch P, Hahn K. Guideline on radiation protection in medicine requires documentation of radioiodine therapy and follow-up: what are the benefits of an electronic database? Nuklearmedizin. 2005;44:49–55.
19. Eskes SA, Wiersinga WM. Amiodarone and thyroid. Best Pract Res Clin Endocrinol Metab. 2009;23:735–51.
20. Brunn J, Block U, Ruf G, Bos I, Kunze WP, Schriba PC. Volumetric analysis of thyroid lobes by real-time ultrasound. Dtsch Med Wschr. 1981;106:1338–40.
21. Moschetta M, Ianora AA, Testini M, Vacca M, Scardapane A, Angelelli G. Multidetector computed tomography in the preoperative evaluation of retrosternal goiters: a useful procedure for patients for whom magnetic resonance imaging is contraindicated. Thyroid. 2010;20:181–7.
22. Moka D, Dietlein M, Schicha H. Radioiodine therapy and thyrostatic drugs and iodine. Eur J Nucl Med Mol Imaging. 2002;29(Suppl 2):S486–91.
23. Bonnema SJ, Bennedbaek FN, Veje A, Marving J, Hegedus L. Propylthiouracil before I-131 therapy of hyperthyroid diseases; effect on cure rate evaluated by a randomized clinical trial. J Clin Endocrinol Metab. 2004;89:4439–44.
24. Braga M, Walpert N, Burch HB, Solomon BL, Cooper DS. The effect of methimazole on cure rates after radioiodine treatment for Graves' hyperthyroidism: a randomized clinical trial. Thyroid. 2002;12:135–9.
25. Santos RB, Romaldini JH, Ward LS. Propylthiouracil reduces the effectiveness of radioiodine treatment in hyperthyroid patients with Graves' disease. Thyroid. 2004;14:525–30.

26. Kobe C, Eschner W, Sudbrock F, Weber I, Marx K, Dietlein M, Schicha H. Graves' disease and radioiodine therapy: is success of ablation dependent on the achieved dose above 200 Gy? Nuklearmedizin. 2008a;47:13–7.
27. Kobe C, Weber I, Eschner W, Sudbrock F, Schmidt M, Dietlein M, Schicha H. Graves' disease and radioiodine therapy: is success of ablation dependent on the choice of thyreostatic medication? Nuklearmedizin. 2008b;47:153–66.
28. Bogazzi F, Bartalena L, Brogioni S, Scarcello G, Burelli A, Compomori A, Manetti L, Rossi G, Pinchera A, Martino E. Comparison of radioiodine with radioiodine plus lithium in the treatment of Graves' hyperthyroidism. J Clin Endocrinol Metab. 1999;84:499–530.
29. Bal CS, Kumar A, Pandey RM. A randomized controlled trial to evaluate the adjuvant effect of lithium on radioiodine treatment of hyperthyroidism. Thyroid. 2002;12:399–405.
30. Fast S, Nielsen VE, Grupe P, Bonnema SJ, Hegedus L. Optimizing 131I uptake after rhTSH stimulation in patients with nontoxic multinodular goiter: evidence from a prospective, randomized, double-blind study. J Nucl Med. 2009;50:732–7.
31. Nielsen VE, Bonnema SJ, Hegedus L. Transient goiter enlargement after administration of 0.3 mg of recombinant human thyrotropin in patients with benign non-toxic nodular goiter: a randomized, double-blind, cross-over trial. J Clin Endocrinol Metab. 2006a;91:1317–22.
32. Nielsen VE, Bonnema SJ, Boel-Jorgensen H, Grupe P, Hegedus L. Stimulation with 0.3 mg recombinant human thyrotropin prior to iodine 131 therapy to improve the size reduction of benign non-toxic nodular goiter: a prospective randomized double-blind trial. Arch Intern Med. 2006b;166:1476–82.
33. Silva MN, Rubió IG, Romão R, Gebrin EM, Buchpiguel C, Tomimori E, Camargo R, Cardia MS, Medeiros-Neto G. Administration of a single dose of recombinant human thyrotropin enhances the efficacy of radioiodine treatment of large compressive multinodular goiters. Clin Endocrinol (Oxf). 2004;60:300–8.
34. Bockisch A, Jamitzky T, Derwanz R, Biersack HJ. Optimized dose planning of radioiodine therapy of benign thyroidal diseases. J Nucl Med. 1993;34:1632–8.
35. Marinelli LD, Quimby EH, Hine G. [Dosimetry of radioactive isotopes; biological observations and practical applications]. Strahlentherapie 1950;81:587–594
36. Hegedus L, Bonnema SJ, Bennedbaek FN. Management of simple nodular goiter: current status and future perspectives. Endocr Rev. 2003;24:102–32.
37. Nieuwlaat WA, Huysmans DA, van den Bosch HC, Sweep CG, Ross HA, Corstens FH, Hermus AR. Pretreatment with a single, low dose of recombinant human thyrotropin allows dose reduction of radioiodine therapy in patients with nodular goiter. J Clin Endocrinol Metab. 2003;88:3121–9.
38. Boeleart K, Syed AA, Manji N, Sheppard MC, Holder RL, Gough SC, Franklyn JA. Prediction of cure and risk of hypothyroidism in patients receiving I-131 for hyperthyroidism. Clin Endocrinol (Oxf). 2009;70:129–38.
39. de Rooy A, Vandenbroucke JP, Smit JW, Stokkel MP, Dekkers OM. Clinical outcomes after estimated versus calculated activity of radioiodine for the treatment of hyperthyroidism: systematic review and meta-analysis. Eur J Endocrinol. 2009;161:771–7.
40. Dietlein M, Dressler J, Eschner W, Lassman M, Leisner B, Reiners C, Schicla H. Procedure guideline for radioiodine test (version 3). [German]. Nuklearmedizin. 2007;46:198–202.
41. Kobe C, Eschner W, Wild M, Rahlff I, Sudbrock F, Schmidt M, Dietlein M, Schicha H. Radioiodine therapy of benign thyroid disorders: what are the effective thyroidal half-life and uptake of I-131. Nucl Med Commun. 2010;31:201–5.
42. Leslie WD, Ward L, Salamon EA, Ludwig S, Rowe RC, Cowden EA. A randomized comparison of radioiodine in Graves' hyperthyroidism. J Clin Endocrinol Metab. 2003;88:978–83.
43. Salvatori M, Luster M. Radioiodine therapy dosimetry in benign thyroid disease and differentiated thyroid carcinoma. Eur J Nucl Med Mol Imaging. 2010;37:821–8.
44. Sisson JC, Avram AM, Rubello D, Gross MD. Radioiodine treatment of hyperthyroidism: fixed or calculated doses; intelligent design of science? Eur J Nucl Med Mol Imaging. 2007;34:1129–30.
45. Stabin MG, Brill AB. State of the art in nuclear medicine dose assessment. Semin Nucl Med. 2008;38:308–20.
46. Kaptein EM, Levenson H, Siege ME, Gadallah M, Akmal M. Radioiodine dosimetry in patients with end-stage renal disease receiving continuous ambulatory peritoneal dialysis therapy. J Clin Endocrinol Metabol. 2000;85:3058–64.
47. Hall P, Holm LE. Late consequences of radioiodine for diagnosis and therapy in Sweden. Thyroid. 1997;7:205–8.
48. Schmidt M, Gorbauch E, Dietlein M, Faust M, Stützer H, Eschner W, Theissen P, Schicha H. Incidence of postradioiodine immunogenic hyperthyroidism/Graves' disease in relation to a temporary increase in thyrotropin receptor antibodies after radioiodine therapy for autonomous thyroid disease. Thyroid. 2006;16:281–8.
49. Hall P, Lundell G, Holm LE. Mortality in patients treated for hyperthyroidism with iodine-131. Acta Endocrinol. 1993;128:230–4.
50. Boice JD Jr. Radiation induced thyroid cancer – what's new? J Natl Cancer Inst. 2005;97:703–5.
51. Dickman PW, Holm LE, Lundell G, Boice JD Jr, Hall P. Thyroid cancer risk after thyroid examination with I-131: a population-based cohort study in Sweden. Int J Cancer. 2003;106:580–7.
52. Dobyns BM, Sheline GE, Workman JB, Tompkins EA, McConahey WM, Becker DV. Malignant and benign neoplasms of the thyroid in patients treated

for hyperthyroidism: a report of the cooperative thyrotoxicosis therapy follow-up study. J Clin Endocrinol Metab. 1974;38:976–98.
53. Franklyn JA, Maisonneuve P, Sheppard M, Betteridge J, Boyle P. Cancer incidence and mortality after radioiodine treatment for hyperthyroidism: a population based cohort study. Lancet. 1999;353:2111–5.
54. Lucignani G. Long-term risks in hyperthyroid patients treated with radioiodine: is there anything new? Eur J Nucl Med Mol Imaging. 2007;34:1504–9.
55. Dunkelmann S, Endlicher D, Prillwitz A, Rudolph F, Groth P, Schuemichen C. Results of a TcTUs-optimized radioiodine therapy of multifocal and disseminated functional thyroid autonomy. Nuklearmedizin. 1999;38:131–9.
56. Reinhardt MJ, Joe A, von Mallek D, Zimmerlin M, Manka-Waluch A, Palmedo H, Krause TM. Dose selection for radioiodine therapy of borderline hyperthyroid patients with multifocal and disseminated autonomy on the basis of ^{99m}Tc-pertechnetate thyroid uptake. Eur J Nucl Med Mol Imaging. 2002;29:480–5.
57. Walter MA, Crist-Crain M, Schindler C, Mueller-Brand J, Mueller B. Outcome of radioiodine therapy without, on or 3 days off carbimazole: a prospective interventional three-group comparison. Eur J Nucl Med Mol Imaging. 2006;33:730–7.
58. Reiners C, Schneider P. Radioiodine therapy of thyroid autonomy. Eur J Nucl Med. 2002;29(Suppl 2):S471–8.
59. Reinhardt MJ, Kim B, Wissmeyer M, Juengling F, Brockmann H, von Mallek D, Ezziddin S, Joe AY, Krause T. Dose selection for radioiodine therapy of borderline hyperthyroid patients according to thyroid uptake of ^{99m}Tc-pertechnetate: applicability to unifocal thyroid autonomy? Eur J Nucl Med Mol Imaging. 2006;33:608–12.
60. Manders JMB, Corstens FHM. Radioiodine therapy of euthyroid multinodular goiters. Eur J Nucl Med. 2002;29(Suppl 2):S466–70.
61. Bachmann J, Kobe C, Bor S, Rahlff I, Dietlein M, Schicha H, Schmidt M. Radioiodine therapy for thyroid volume reduction of large goiters. Nucl Med Commun. 2009;30:466–71.
62. Bonnema SJ, Andersen PB, Knudsen DU, Hegedus L. MR Imaging of large multinodular goiters: observer agreement on volume versus observer disagreement on dimension of the involved trachea. Am J Roentgenol. 2002;179:259–66.
63. Bonnema SJ, Nielsen VE, Boel-Jørgensen H, Grupe P, Andersen PB, Bastholt L, Hegedus L. Improvement of goiter volume reduction after 0.3mg recombinant human thyrotropin-stimulated radioiodine therapy in patients with a very large goiter: a double-blinded, randomized trial. J Clin Endocrinol Metab. 2007;92:3424–34.

29 Differentiated Thyroid Cancer: Radioiodine Therapy

Frederik A. Verburg

29.1 Introduction

29.1.1 Historical Perspective

In 1942, Dr. Samuel M. Seidlin of the Memorial Hospital in New York was faced with a 51-year-old patient in poor condition: overtly hyperthyroid, dramatically underweight, and in severe pain. The patient had undergone a thyroidectomy for what had been histologically diagnosed as a 'malignant adenoma' of the thyroid in 1923. A decade and a half later, he returned with overt signs of hyperthyroidism and lower back pain. A metastasis was found in the lower spine and was surgically removed. Nonetheless, the patient progressed in the years after, developing additional bone metastases. The patient was given radioiodine, which in 1942 had just become available. The patient responded favourably to the I-131 treatment and received several more courses. As a result the hyperthyroidism subsided, the body weight increased from 38 to 53 kg, and the pain diminished. In addition to the therapeutic effect, the diagnostic capabilities of radioiodine were demonstrated after Geiger counter examinations of the patient revealed two previously unknown metastases.

The report of a potential cure for a terminally ill patient caused I-131 availability to become a political issue. As a result, on August 1, 1946, the American Atomic Energy Act made radioisotopes available for 'atomic medicine', later renamed nuclear medicine.

29.1.2 Differentiated Thyroid Cancer

Although it concerns fewer than 1% of all cancer cases, and its incidence varies throughout the world [1], thyroid carcinoma is the most common endocrine malignancy [2]. Thyroid carcinoma spans a considerable oncological width with respect to natural history and prognosis. About 10% of cases concern an anaplastic thyroid carcinoma (ATC), which originates from thyroid cells and is one of the most lethal human cancers. It has a cause-specific mortality of nearly 100% within a year of diagnosis. A further 10% of cases involve patients with a thyroidal c-cell-derived medullary thyroid carcinoma (MTC). The 5-year cause-specific mortality of this entity is about 50%.

The remaining about 80% of thyroid carcinoma cases comprise the so-called differentiated thyroid carcinoma (DTC): papillary thyroid carcinoma (PTC) or follicular thyroid carcinoma (FTC). These tumours derive from the follicular thyrocytes and are referred to as 'differentiated' thyroid cancer because the tumour cells retain

F. A. Verburg (✉)
Department of Nuclear Medicine, University Hospital Marburg, Marburg, Germany
e-mail: Verburg@med.uni-marburg.de

H. Ahmadzadehfar et al. (eds.), *Clinical Nuclear Medicine*,
https://doi.org/10.1007/978-3-030-39457-8_29

some of normal thyrocytes' properties. Most importantly the ability to take up and store iodine and to respond to thyrotropin (thyroid-stimulating hormone, TSH) stimulation is retained, which allows for treatment and imaging using radioactive iodine analogues. The relative frequency of FTC and PTC in part depends on the iodine sufficiency and therefore varies by geographic area, but generally, PTC is more common [3]. DTC cases typically have a good prognosis, with long-term survival ranging from about 70% to more than 95%, depending on the extent of disease at the time of diagnosis [4]. Consequently, in >85% of DTC patients, life expectancy is unimpaired [5, 6].

29.1.2.1 Incidence

The incidence of DTC has steadily increased over the past few years [7], although this rise now seems to be abating [8]. The rise in incidence for the largest part appears to be due to an increasing use and quality of ultrasound diagnostics. DTC is more frequent in females than in males, with reported incidences of 2.0–3.8 per 100,000 in females vs. 1.2–2.6 per 100,000 in males [1, 8–11]. DTC-specific mortality varies from 0.4 to 2.8 per 100,000 in females and from 0.2 to 1.2 per 100,000 in males [12]. The gender differences are most prominent in the reproductive period. The mean age at diagnosis is about 45 years, with younger patients almost exclusively having papillary thyroid cancers and older patients showing an increased frequency of follicular carcinomas [4].

29.1.2.2 Histology and Clinical Behaviour

PTC

The classical form of PTC is an unencapsulated tumour with papillary and follicular structures. It is characterized by overlapping cell nuclei that have a ground-glass appearance and longitudinal grooves, with invaginations of cytoplasm into the nuclei [13, 14]. PTC histologic variants among others include the encapsulated, follicular, tall cell, columnar cell, clear cell, diffuse sclerosing, solid or trabecular, and oxyphilic forms [2, 15]. PTCs are often multifocal, with many of the lesions of different clonal origin, i.e., arising independently [16]. PTC metastasis tends to be lymphogenic, before spreading to the lungs and bones.

FTC

FTC is characterized by follicular differentiation, without the nuclear changes seen in PTC [13, 14]. FTCs are encapsulated tumours, distinguishable from follicular adenomas by the presence of invasion of the capsule and/or vessels. According to the pattern of invasion, FTCs can be divided into two categories: minimally invasive and widely invasive. FTCs are less often multifocal than are PTCs. FTC tends to metastasize to the lungs, bone, and liver; regional lymph node metastases are much less common than in PTC.

Hürthle cell carcinoma is a variety of FTC that consists of at least 75% oxyphilic cells [15]. An important characteristic of Hürthle cell carcinomas is their reputedly poor or even absent iodine uptake, which renders this entity more difficult to treat.

The TNM staging system for differentiated thyroid cancer is demonstrated in Table 29.1.

29.1.2.3 DTC Treatment

In the treatment of DTC, multiple modalities are involved, each of which will be discussed separately.

Surgery

Surgery is the first and most important component of the primary treatment of DTC. In Europe, the Americas and much of Australasia (near), total thyroidectomy is usually performed in almost all patients. Only for papillary microcarcinoma hemithyroidectomy is deemed to suffice by most patients [16, 19–26]. More recently, a discussion has erupted on the need for total thyroidectomy in non-metastatic, not locally invasive DTC with a diameter up to 4 cm [27]; this strategy however has yet to prove itself.

For DTC in general, the vast majority of authors have found the therapeutic effect to be related to the extent of surgery [19]. Relapse-free survival and thyroid cancer-specific survival are better after (near) total thyroidectomy than after unilateral thyroid lobectomy.

Table 29.1 The staging criteria for the seventh [17] and eighth [18] edition of the UICC/AJCC TNM staging system for differentiated thyroid cancer

TNM, version 7: for differentiated thyroid carcinoma		
T0: no evidence for primary tumour		
T1a: primary tumour ≤1 cm, confined to the thyroid gland		
T1b: primary tumour >1 and ≤2 cm, confined to the thyroid gland		
T2: primary tumour >2 cm and ≤4 cm, confined to the thyroid gland		
T3: primary tumour >4 cm, confined to the thyroid gland *or* any tumour with minimal extrathyroid extension		
T4a: primary tumour with invasion of subcutaneous soft tissues, larynx, trachea, oesophagus, recurrent laryngeal nerve		
T4b: primary tumour with invasion of prevertebral fascia, mediastinal vessels, encasing of carotid artery		
N0: no lymph node metastases		
N1a: metastasis in level VI (pre- and paratracheal)		
N1b: metastasis in lymph nodes outside of level VI, including mediastinal lymph nodes		
M0: no distant metastases		
M1: distant metastases present		
STAGE	Age <45 years	Age ≥45 years
I	M0	T1a, T1b
II	M1	T2
III	T3 or N1a	
IVa	T1-3N1bM0, T4aN0-1M0	
IVb	T4bN0-1M0	
IVc	M1	
TNM, version 8: for differentiated thyroid carcinoma		
T0: no evidence for primary tumour		
T1a: primary tumour ≤1 cm, confined to the thyroid gland		
T1b: primary tumour >1 and ≤2 cm, confined to the thyroid gland		
T2: primary tumour >2 cm and ≤4 cm, confined to the thyroid gland		
T3a: primary tumour >4 cm, confined to the thyroid gland		
T3b: primary tumour of any size with gross extrathyroidal extension involving only the sternothyroid, sternohyoid, or omohyoid muscles		
T4a: primary tumour with invasion of subcutaneous soft tissues, larynx, trachea, oesophagus, recurrent laryngeal nerve, regardless of diameters		
T4b: primary tumour with invasion of prevertebral fascia, mediastinal vessels, encasing of carotid artery, regardless of diameter		
N0: no lymph node metastases		
N1a: metastasis in level VI (pre- and paratracheal)		
N1b: metastasis in lymph nodes outside of level VI, including mediastinal lymph nodes		
M0: no distant metastases		
M1: distant metastases present		
STAGE	Age <55 years	Age ≥55 years
I	M0	T1a, T1b, T2
II	M1	T3 or T0-3N1
III	T4aN0-1M0	
IVa	T4bN0-1M0	
IVb	M1 T4bNxM0	

Moreover, in >50% of patients undergoing a completion thyroidectomy after initial unilateral lobectomy, malignant tissue is found in the thyroid remnant [26]. This observation is unsurprising in light of the frequently multifocal, multiclonal nature of PTC [16].

Arguments against total thyroidectomy in early-stage PTC are also available. PTC often is found in post-mortem studies without a single clinical symptom during life [28, 29], raising questions regarding the clinical relevance of papillary microcarcinomas.

The prognosis of DTC and the effectiveness of adjuvant treatment with I-131 (also called ablation; see below) are so good [30–32] that without at least cytologic proof of the necessity of a radical neck dissection, this procedure, which is associated with significant morbidity, appears to be unjustifiable in any case. A modified radical lateral neck dissection should be performed only after a diagnosis of lymph node metastases [2]. The less invasive central or pretracheal compartment lymph node dissection is however advocated as a standard procedure in thyroidectomy for any DTC by many authors, as it both facilitates the accurate staging with regard to lymph node status and may prevent locoregional DTC recurrence [33].

The most serious potential complications of thyroid surgery are hypoparathyroidism and recurrent laryngeal nerve damage [34, 35]. Identification and electronic monitoring of the recurrent laryngeal nerve can significantly reduce the rate of nerve damage [36]. The incidence and impact of complications can be reduced by performing the procedure in expert centres [35] as well as intensive post-operative monitoring; especially serum calcium levels should be monitored frequently in the immediate post-operative phase.

Thyroid Hormone Replacement Therapy

As by definition the production of endogenous thyroxine is discontinued by thyroidectomy procedure, DTC patients require thyroid hormone (levothyroxine, LT4) replacement therapy [27].

Differentiated thyroid cancer cells still react to TSH stimulation; for this reason LT4 is usually administered in such doses that TSH levels fall to very low levels of <0.1 mU/l [37]. Especially for low-risk patients TSH suppression is not generally advocated [27]. The exact dose of LT4 required to achieve TSH suppression varies from patient to patient and depends in part on body weight.

Radioiodine (I-131) Therapy

The Effectivity of Radioiodine Therapy

A landmark study by Mazzaferri and Jhiang published in 1994 on a population of over 1500 patients followed for four decades or more clearly showed that both recurrence rates and death rates related to DTC were much lower in patients who received radioiodine treatment (RIT) after surgery than in those who did not receive I-131 [22]. In fact, now that I-131 therapy belongs to the standard treatment of DTC, life expectancy in patients without extensive neck or distant metastases is unimpaired [5].

A primary cause of the good prognosis of DTC is the use of I-131 both in an ablative and therapeutic setting. I-131-NaI closely approaches the ideal oncologic drug: due to thyroid cells' role as the body's main iodine reservoir and primary locus of expression of the sodium-iodide symporter (NIS) [38], I-131 is largely specific for the target cancer cell and generally has relatively limited side effects. Additionally, this isotope emits therapeutically useful beta radiation as well as gamma rays suitable for imaging the drug distribution.

Practical Considerations

The majority of current guidelines recommend post-surgical application of a high ('ablative') I-131 activity as a second component of the primary treatment of DTC in some or most (near) totally thyroidectomized patients [39–42]. The radioiodine is administered as sodium iodide, either orally or by intravenous injection.

In clinical practice, I-131 therapy after surgery has four possible goals [2]:

- To destroy occult microscopic DTC foci, thereby decreasing the long-term risk of recurrent disease [19, 22, 31, 43, 44] (adjuvant therapy).
- To eliminate any remaining healthy thyroid tissue, thereby increasing the specificity of detectable serum thyroglobulin (Tg) and positive WBS as markers for persistent or recurrent DTC cells [2, 43, 45]. Additionally, by destroying healthy thyroid cells, ablation may remove a locus for new neoplastic transformation [46], given the multiclonal nature of many DTC cases [16] (Remnant ablation).
- Through use of a large I-131 activity, to permit sensitive post-ablation WBS to detect previously unknown persistent locoregional dis-

ease or, because the abundance of tracer overwhelms any ‘monopolization’ of uptake by the thyroid bed, to detect previously unknown metastases [47, 48]. Post-ablation scintigraphy also allows precise probe-guided removal of the newly detected disease foci in selected cases [49].
- To treat known remaining tumour tissue (treatment of advanced disease).

Although the medical use of the second goal can be debated in the current day and age of highly sensitive and stable Tg assays, the first (and in a sense also the third) objective solidly positions I-131 treatment as an adjuvant oncological therapy. Achieving these goals should lead to decreased rates and to more timely detection of persistent or recurrent disease and, more importantly, to improved tumour-specific survival in (near) totally thyroidectomized patients with DTC [19, 22, 50]. The preferred I-131 activity for initial post-operative I-131 treatment has been a matter of debate [51–57]. Although good results may be obtained with 1.1 GBq [52, 53], some literature has suggested that remnant eradication rates seem to improve with increasing activities [57]. A plateauing of the I-131 activity-response curve has been noted for ablation activities over 1.85 GBq [51]. On the other hand, in low- as well as in high-risk DTC patients higher activities in long-term follow-up were associated with lower DTC-related death and recurrence rates. Nonetheless, published papers have contained no clear answer from randomized controlled trials regarding the optimal activity for I-131 ablation. Those trials that have been published [58–60] unfortunately only targeted successful ablation and no long-term follow-up in patients is as yet available from these trials.

Although as noted above, I-131 is highly specific for thyroid cells, physiological uptake occurs in other tissues expressing NIS, including the salivary glands and the breasts. Relatively high radiation exposure also occurs in the gastrointestinal and urinary tracts, since the body excretes from iodine via the faeces and, especially, the urine. Measures to minimize extra-thyroidal radiation exposure include abundant hydration to encourage frequent micturation, lemon juice or lemon candy ingestion to stimulate salivary secretion (but started only with at least 24-h distance to I-131 administration as otherwise the radiation dose to the salivary glands will paradoxically be increased), and laxative administration to decrease faecal transit time.

Iodine also is secreted in milk [61], so breastfeeding must be discontinued at least 6–8 weeks before I-131 administration. This discontinuation serves two objectives: (1) preventing I-131 ingestion by the infant and (2) avoiding unduly high radiation doses to the mother’s breasts. Discontinuation of breastfeeding stops milk production and consequently decreases the mammary gland’s uptake of circulating iodine. However, as the mammary glands require some time to reduce their mass and activity once lactation stops, a waiting period between discontinuation of lactation and I-131 is in order.

Relative contraindications for radioiodine therapy in patients with thyroid cancer include:

- High-grade bone marrow depression in cases of treatment with high activities of radioiodine
- Considerable reduction of pulmonary function in patients with lung metastases and high radioiodine uptake
- Considerable xerostomia due to proven impairment of salivary gland function

Side effects and complications from I-131 therapy potentially include acute or chronic salivary gland problems ranging from mild sialoadenitis to complete xerostomia, the latter occurring only in a small minority of patients. Other potential complications include temporary loss of taste or smell and transient haematologic abnormalities. The incidence of such complications depends on the administered activities as well as on the cumulative life time activity [62, 63]. Evidence of earlier onset of menopause was found in women treated with I-131 for DTC [64]. Additionally, an excess of second primary malignancies can be observed after I-131 treatment of DTC [65–67]. The risk of second primary malignancies also may relate to administered radioiodine activities; that risk presumably is smaller when only a single activity, especially a lower one, is given for ablation versus when multiple radioiodine therapy courses are applied for metastatic disease, as was the case in many patients in epidemiological studies examining second primary malignancy incidence in the radioiodine-treated DTC setting. Also, whether the I-131 therapy is the sole cause of excess second primary malignancies, or whether a genetic predisposition to cancers among DTC patients also is involved, is open to debate [68].

29.1.2.4 A Short How-to

Low-Iodine Diet

Before I-131 treatment, the patient should be prepared adequately. A low-iodine diet for 2–3 weeks before iodine administration is strongly recommended, even more important is the avoidance of iodine-containing drugs (e.g. X-ray contrast media, reagents for disinfection, ophthalmologic agents, amiodarone, iodide medication) or food or food additives with high iodine content (e.g. seaweed, kelp, dietary supplements) [69–73].

Pre-ablation Uptake Measurement/ Scanning

The application of a diagnostic activity of I-131 immediately before radioiodine treatment may induce 'stunning', i.e. reduced I-131 uptake or changed I-131 kinetics during consecutive radioiodine therapy that may be the cause for significant impairment of the efficacy of radioiodine therapy [74]. Therefore it is recommended not to use diagnostic activities of I-131 necessary for scintigraphy, i.e. more than 10–20 MBq [75]. With smaller activities of I-131 (<10 MBq), 24-h uptake measurements may be performed to estimate roughly the mass of thyroid remnant after surgery [76]. As an alternative for I-131, short-lived I-123 (half-life 13.2 h, gamma emitter) may be used. The advantage of I-123 is that no stunning is involved. However, this radionuclide does not allow late scans with low background activity after more than 24 h leading to a lower sensitivity of I-123 scintigraphy as compared to I-131 scanning. I-124 is an interesting positron and gamma-emitting radionuclide suitable for high sensitive and specific PET-CT imaging with half-life 4.2 days, but so far high costs and limited availability have limited its use.

rhTSH Stimulation

High thyrotropin levels (above 30 mU/l) are generally considered to be necessary for I-131 ablation and therapy of both benign post-surgical thyroid remnants and DTC metastases in order to induce sufficient I-131 uptake [39–41]. Such high TSH levels can be achieved either by thyroid hormone withdrawal (THW) for 3–4 weeks or by intramuscular injections of recombinant human TSH. Through avoidance of hypothyroidism, the use of rhTSH results in an unimpaired quality of life [77–79]. A further advantage of rhTSH is that it results in a lower radiation exposure to the remainder of the body, including the bone marrow [80], the reproductive system, and the salivary glands [81, 82].

Over time, many studies have shown the equivalence of rhTSH to THW for both TSH-stimulated Tg testing with or without concurrent dxWBS [83] and for initial I-131 ablation of patients without distant metastases. Furthermore, rhTSH is likely cost-effective from several points of view [84, 85].

Considering all the above-mentioned advantages the American Thyroid Association [40], the European Society for Medical Oncology [42], and the European Association for Nuclear Medicine [39] currently recommend patient preparation for radioiodine ablation with rhTSH as method of choice.

Although an increasing number of smaller studies indicate that rhTSH administration is able to stimulate I-131 uptake in distant DTC metastases to such a degree that a response to therapy is seen in a significant fraction of the patients [86–88], there are no prospective studies in literature in which THW was compared with rhTSH for the treatment of DTC metastases. Therefore the use of rhTSH in I-131 therapy of patients with persistent local or metastatic DTC remains a form of off-label use, which should only be opted for with all the due caution that is required in such situations.

I-131 Activities

Usually standard I-131 activities of between 1 and 3.7 GBq are recommended for treatment; a standard activity of 3.7 GBq is prescribed in the registration studies of rhTSH. Between 1 and 3.7 GBq I-131, higher activities seem to coincide with higher success rates [89] and better recurrence-free and overall survival [90] most likely due to a higher bioavailability of I-131 [91].

In the case of microscopically non-radical resections, aggressive subtypes of differentiated thyroid cancer or other high-risk constellations, higher standard activities of up to 7.4 GBq I-131 can be administered in a single course without special precautions. If higher activities of radioiodine are considered for ablative treatment, dosimetric approaches should be used to estimate the radiation dose to the bone marrow [46, 92].

I-131 Therapy of Advanced DTC and Dosimetry

For I-131 therapy, patients usually are given a standard fixed activity. This activity reflects the physician's or institution's estimation of the amount of radioiodine needed to deliver the highest safe radiation dose to neoplastic foci, given the patient's tumour burden or histology, age group, etc. However, because there is great inter- and even intra-patient (i.e. between different lesions in the same individual) variation in radioiodine kinetics, such fixed activities frequently pose a risk of either under-dosing the patient or—much more worrying—of exceeding commonly accepted safety limits [93, 94]. To avoid both risks, it is possible to perform a pre-therapeutic dosimetry using a small test activity of I-131.

The rationale for basing treatment activities on such dosimetry is to allow the administered activity, and with it, the absorbed dose to iodine-avid thyroid tissue, to be maximized for each individual while avoiding bone marrow toxicity, pulmonary fibrosis, or (presumably) other severe or serious side effects.

Multiple administrations of lower activities in a 'fractionated' therapy could lead to changes in tumour/lesion biokinetics as has been shown by Samuel et al. [95] and Chiesa et al. [96]. Their findings suggest that the repetition of treatment of a lesion drastically reduces its uptake, with a loss of therapeutic efficacy along the sequence of fixed activity administrations. This is also corroborated by clinical evidence showing that prognosis progressively worsens with increasing number of therapy courses, but not with increasing cumulative activities given [30].

One well-accepted concept for treating advanced DTC uses the activity that is as high as safely administrable (AHASA) and based on calculation of the individualized activity to be administered to deliver a 2 Gy absorbed dose to the blood. Blood, as a surrogate for the red bone marrow, was considered the critical organ at risk in the approach originally reported by Benua et al. [97, 98] and Benua and Leeper [98]. This 'safety dosimetry' concept also specifies that the whole-body retention be <4.4 GBq at 48 h after radioiodine administration. Additionally, in the presence of diffuse pulmonary metastases, lung uptake should be <3 GBq at 24 h post-therapy to avoid pulmonary fibrosis [98].

In radioiodine therapy of differentiated thyroid carcinoma, several parameters are equally or even more important than the administered activity for the radiation-absorbed dose to the target tissue, namely, its iodine avidity depending on stimulation and differentiation, the residence time of the radioiodine per volume of blood plasma representing the bioavailability of the I-131, the effective half-life in the target volume, and the mean energy deposited per decay being mainly determined by size and shape of the accumulating mass [99]. The high individual variation of all mentioned parameters [99] fundamentally questions value and feasibility of the quest for the 'best' fixed therapeutic activity, not unlikely dooming any study disregarding these dependencies to fail.

To overcome the uncertainty of individual biokinetics, two dosimetry-based approaches have been introduced by Benua and Maxon. As early as in 1962, Benua et al. [97] used the easily measureable absorbed dose to the blood as conservative estimate of the absorbed dose to the organ at risk, the red marrow, and settled a limit of 2 Gy to be used to determine the highest activity that is safely administrable to the individual without severe damage to the haematopoietic system. The limit of 2 Gy absorbed dose to the blood is however based on only a few cases of severe bone marrow suppression [97]. A study targeting at 3 Gy red marrow dose [100] and the observation that patients treated with fixed activities of 7.4 or 11.1 GBq frequently exceed Benua's safety limit [93, 101] while no studies report on correspondent rates of severe haematotoxic reactions indicate that the limit of 2 Gy might be regarded as conservative. The blood dose closely reflects the true amount of I-131 available to the target tissue [102] and, in thyroid remnant ablation, seems to correlate better with therapeutic success than the administered activity alone [91, 103]. For further details on dosimetry-based activity selection we refer to papers by Van Nostrand [94] or Lassmann [104].

Later, Maxon et al. [105, 106] first aimed at a specified radiation-absorbed dose to the target tissue, namely, 300 Gy to thyroid remnants and 80 Gy for the treatment of cervical lymph node metastases. Although these values fixed by Maxon have been quoted often and used widely, they have not been verified by independent prospective trials. In Maxon's approach of lesion dosimetry, the recommended values mainly suffer from uncertainties in the determination of the target mass and how much of the energy is imparted to surrounding tissue, a question which is always a challenge to answer for small and irregular shaped tissues. More recent studies based on measurements with improved equipment support the hypothesis that therapeutic outcome correlates with the absorbed dose administered to the target tissue [96, 100, 107] but do not generally confirm the values settled by Maxon.

The main argument against Maxon's approach arises from the fact that absorbed doses may vary considerably between different lesions within the same patient and that the distribution of the absorbed dose in a tumour may be inhomogeneous [96, 108]. This may lead to undertreatment of lesions not included in the dosimetric evaluation or with supposedly sufficient absorbed dose but inhomogeneous activity distribution. It remains to prospective studies to clarify whether or not improved techniques for dosimetry and the introduction of formalisms to weigh the measurements like the calculation of the biologically effective dose BED or the equivalent uniform dose UED [109, 110] will result unique and reliable recommendations for lesion dosimetry in DTC.

Recently, the EANM published a standard operational procedure (SOP) for determining the AHASA I-131 activity for DTC therapy using the 2 Gy absorbed blood radiation dose threshold [92]. In brief, patients should be given 5–10 MBq I-131, followed by whole-body scanning together with a standard 1, 4, 24, 48, 72, 96, and 168 h after I-131 administration; at the same time blood samples should be drawn. Based on the results of these measurements the AHASA activity can then be calculated. Initial clinical experience with this methodology indicates that it is safe and effective [111]. Iodine-124 PET-CT has been advocated because it can also be used for tumour dosimetry [108, 112–114]. Using three-dimensional voxel-based dosimetry highly variable dose estimates were found for individual metastases in individual patients. Although large-scale data correlating these estimates with response are lacking, the prospect of calculating the minimally effective activity/dose while at the same time being able to calculate the activity that is as high as safely administrable (AHASA) using whole-body retention, organ and blood/bone marrow dose to individualize treatment seems very appealing and of high oncologic relevance.

29.2 Side Effects and Complications

The risk of malignancy due to I-131 therapy in DTC patients has not been clarified definitively. Also further side effects of I-131 therapy like xerostomia (prevalence range, 16–54%), lacrimal gland dysfunction (prevalence, 11%), transient male gonadal dysfunction, or transient female gonadal dysfunction may occur [115]. The prevalence and severity of adverse effects seem to be correlated to the cumulative I-131 activity. These late effects can severely impact quality of life [115].

It is furthermore well known that high I-131 activities may induce acute myeloid leukaemia. This was already observed in some of the first DTC patients treated with I-131 therapy [116] and has been confirmed in multiple subsequent case reports. These reports included patients treated with low activities or multiple times within a short time frame. However, it could also be established that a more frequent radiation exposure or an exposure to higher cumulative doses will lead to a higher risk of complications. It is however unclear to what degree and at what point. Furthermore, it was reported that the risk of second primary solid tumours could be elevated after I-131 therapy [117], but also before [68]—the latter finding pointing to constitutively elevated risks rather than an effect of I-131. Hay et al. report a statistically significant excess mortality due to non-thyroid malignancies in survivors of paediatric PTC first occurring 30–50 years after diagnosis [118]. However, as in the latter study only a minority of patients received I-131 therapy, the excess mortality may also be due to other, e.g. genetic, causes.

In contrast with such negative reports, Reiners et al. reported on the results of treatment from a large cohort of children and adolescents with high-risk radiation-induced PTC after the Chernobyl reactor meltdown. These children mostly received multiple courses of high body weight-adapted activities (100 MBq/kg). The authors did however not observe secondary malignancies during a median 11.3-year follow-up after the last RAI [119].

As paediatric PTC patients have a long remaining life expectancy, the risk of developing secondary tumours over the course of a lifetime is non-negligible. This risk is related to the cumulative lifetime I-131 activity as well as to other, potentially predisposing, factors such as genetic ones. Furthermore, especially in patients with extensive lung metastases, the risk of pulmonary fibrosis which is also related to the cumulative radiation exposure needs to be considered as a rare but potentially lethal complication. When one then considers recent evidence [120] that long-term prognosis in patients who do eventually become disease-free does not markedly improve after more than four courses of I-131 therapy or a cumulative lifetime activity of 22 GBq compared to those who never become disease-free, the harms in the long term may outweigh the benefits. Therefore for the future it may be advisable in paediatric PTC patients to consider cessation of further I-131 therapy courses if a complete remission of disease is not achieved with 3–4 courses of I-131 therapy.

29.3 Conclusion

The diagnosis, treatment, and follow-up of DTC are a complex matter with which entire books can be filled. Although some principles of I-131 therapy have been employed with little change for over 70 years, many aspects of DTC care are rapidly evolving and will continue to change in the future.

References

1. Parkin DM, Muir CS, Whelan SL, Gao YT, Ferlay J, Powell J. Cancer incidence in five continents. Vol 6. IARC scientific publications ed. Lyon: International Agency for Research on Cancer; 1992.
2. Schlumberger MJ. Papillary and follicular thyroid carcinoma. N Engl J Med. 1998;338:297–306.
3. Busnardo B, De Vido D. The epidemiology and etiology of differentiated thyroid carcinoma. Biomed Pharmacother. 2000;54:322–6.
4. Verburg FA, Mader U, Luster M, Reiners C. Histology does not influence prognosis in differentiated thyroid carcinoma when accounting for age,

tumour diameter, invasive growth and metastases. Eur J Endocrinol. 2009;160:619–24.

5. Verburg FA, Mader U, Tanase K, Thies ED, Diessl S, Buck AK, et al. Life expectancy is reduced in differentiated thyroid cancer patients >= 45 years old with extensive local tumor invasion, lateral lymph node, or distant metastases at diagnosis and normal in all other DTC patients. J Clin Endocrinol Metab. 2013;98:172–80.
6. Tanase K, Thies ED, Mader U, Reiners C, Verburg FA. The TNM system (version 7) is the most accurate staging system for the prediction of loss of life expectancy in differentiated thyroid cancer. Clin Endocrinol (Oxf). 2015;84:284.
7. Leenhardt L, Grosclaude P, Cherie-Challine L. Increased incidence of thyroid carcinoma in France: a true epidemic or thyroid nodule management effects? Report from the French Thyroid Cancer Committee. Thyroid. 2004;14:1056–60.
8. Sassolas G, Hafdi-Nejjari Z, Remontet L, Bossard N, Belot A, Berger-Dutrieux N, et al. Thyroid cancer: is the incidence rise abating? Eur J Endocrinol. 2009;160:71–9.
9. Burgess JR, Dwyer T, McArdle K, Tucker P, Shugg D. The changing incidence and spectrum of thyroid carcinoma in Tasmania (1978-1998) during a transition from iodine sufficiency to iodine deficiency. J Clin Endocrinol Metab. 2000;85:1513–7.
10. Davies L, Welch HG. Increasing incidence of thyroid cancer in the United States, 1973-2002. JAMA. 2006;295:2164–7.
11. Farahati J, Geling M, Mader U, Mortl M, Luster M, Muller JG, et al. Changing trends of incidence and prognosis of thyroid carcinoma in lower Franconia, Germany, from 1981-1995. Thyroid. 2004;14:141–7.
12. Schlumberger MJ, Pacini F. Thyroid tumors. Paris: Editions Nucleon; 2003.
13. Hedinger C, Williams ED, Sobin LH. Histological typing of thyroid tumours. No. 11 of international histologic classification of tumours. Berlin: Springer; 1988.
14. Rosai J, Carcangiu ML, Delellis RA. Tumors of the thyroid gland. Atlas of tumor pathology, 3rd series. Fascicle 5. Washington, DC: Armed Forces Institute of Pathology; 1992.
15. Kloos RT, Mazzaferri E. Thyroid carcinoma. In: Cooper DS, editor. Medical management of thyroid disease. New York, NY: Marcel Dekker Inc.; 2001.
16. Shattuck TM, Westra WH, Ladenson PW, Arnold A. Independent clonal origins of distinct tumor foci in multifocal papillary thyroid carcinoma. N Engl J Med. 2005;352:2406–12.
17. Sobin LH, Gospodarowicz MK, Wittekind C. TNM classification of malignant tumours. 7th ed. New York, NY: Wiley-Blackwell; 2009.
18. Brierley J, Gospodarowicz MK, Wittekind C. TNM classification of malignant tumours. 8th ed. Hoboken, NJ: Wiley-Blackwell; 2017.
19. Simpson WJ, Panzarella T, Carruthers JS, Gospodarowicz MK, Sutcliffe SB. Papillary and follicular thyroid cancer: impact of treatment in 1578 patients. Int J Radiat Oncol Biol Phys. 1988;14:1063–75.
20. Hay ID, Bergstralh EJ, Grant CS, McIver B, Thompson GB, van Heerden JA, et al. Impact of primary surgery on outcome in 300 patients with pathologic tumor-node-metastasis stage III papillary thyroid carcinoma treated at one institution from 1940 through 1989. Surgery. 1999;126:1173–81.
21. Hay ID, Grant CS, Bergstralh EJ, Thompson GB, van Heerden JA, Goellner JR. Unilateral total lobectomy: is it sufficient surgical treatment for patients with AMES low-risk papillary thyroid carcinoma? Surgery. 1998;124:958–64.
22. Mazzaferri EL, Jhiang SM. Long-term impact of initial surgical and medical therapy on papillary and follicular thyroid cancer. Am J Med. 1994;97:418–28.
23. Tsang RW, Brierley JD, Simpson WJ, Panzarella T, Gospodarowicz MK, Sutcliffe SB. The effects of surgery, radioiodine, and external radiation therapy on the clinical outcome of patients with differentiated thyroid carcinoma. Cancer. 1998;82:375–88.
24. Hay ID, Grant CS, Taylor WF, McConahey WM. Ipsilateral lobectomy versus bilateral lobar resection in papillary thyroid carcinoma: a retrospective analysis of surgical outcome using a novel prognostic scoring system. Surgery. 1987;102:1088–95.
25. Duren M, Yavuz N, Bukey Y, Ozyegin MA, Gundogdu S, Acbay O, et al. Impact of initial surgical treatment on survival of patients with differentiated thyroid cancer: experience of an endocrine surgery center in an iodine-deficient region. World J Surg. 2000;24:1290–4.
26. Pasieka JL, Thompson NW, McLeod MK, Burney RE, Macha M. The incidence of bilateral well-differentiated thyroid cancer found at completion thyroidectomy. World J Surg. 1992;16:711–6.
27. Haugen BR, Alexander EK, Bible KC, Doherty GM, Mandel SJ, Nikiforov YE, et al. 2015 American Thyroid Association Management Guidelines for adult patients with thyroid nodules and differentiated thyroid cancer: The American Thyroid Association Guidelines Task Force on thyroid nodules and differentiated thyroid cancer. Thyroid. 2016;26:1–133.
28. Franssila KO, Harach HR. Occult papillary carcinoma of the thyroid in children and young adults. A systemic autopsy study in Finland. Cancer. 1986;58:715–9.
29. Solares CA, Penalonzo MA, Xu M, Orellana E. Occult papillary thyroid carcinoma in postmortem species: prevalence at autopsy. Am J Otolaryngol. 2005;26:87–90.
30. Thies ED, Tanase K, Maeder U, Luster M, Buck AK, Hanscheid H, et al. The number of 131I therapy courses needed to achieve complete remission is an indicator of prognosis in patients with differentiated thyroid carcinoma. Eur J Nucl Med Mol Imaging. 2014;41:2281–90.

31. Verburg FA, de Keizer B, Lips CJ, Zelissen PM, de Klerk JM. Prognostic significance of successful ablation with radioiodine of differentiated thyroid cancer patients. Eur J Endocrinol. 2005;152:33–7.
32. Verburg FA, Stokkel MP, Duren C, Verkooijen RB, Mader U, van Isselt JW, et al. No survival difference after successful (131)I ablation between patients with initially low-risk and high-risk differentiated thyroid cancer. Eur J Nucl Med Mol Imaging. 2010;37:276–83.
33. Pereira JA, Jimeno J, Miquel J, Iglesias M, Munne A, Sancho JJ, et al. Nodal yield, morbidity, and recurrence after central neck dissection for papillary thyroid carcinoma. Surgery. 2005;138:1095–100. discussion.
34. Cheah WK, Arici C, Ituarte PH, Siperstein AE, Duh QY, Clark OH. Complications of neck dissection for thyroid cancer. World J Surg. 2002;26:1013–6.
35. Thomusch O, Machens A, Sekulla C, Ukkat J, Lippert H, Gastinger I, et al. Multivariate analysis of risk factors for postoperative complications in benign goiter surgery: prospective multicenter study in Germany. World J Surg. 2000;24:1335–41.
36. Dralle H, Sekulla C, Lorenz K, Brauckhoff M, Machens A. Intraoperative monitoring of the recurrent laryngeal nerve in thyroid surgery. World J Surg. 2008;32:1358–66.
37. Diessl S, Holzberger B, Mader U, Grelle I, Smit JW, Buck AK, et al. Impact of moderate vs stringent TSH suppression on survival in advanced differentiated thyroid carcinoma. Clin Endocrinol (Oxf). 2012;76:586–92.
38. Eskandari S, Loo DD, Dai G, Levy O, Wright EM, Carrasco N. Thyroid Na+/I- symporter. Mechanism, stoichiometry, and specificity. J Biol Chem. 1997;272:27230–8.
39. Luster M, Clarke SE, Dietlein M, Lassmann M, Lind P, Oyen WJ, et al. Guidelines for radioiodine therapy of differentiated thyroid cancer. Eur J Nucl Med Mol Imaging. 2008;35:1941–59.
40. Cooper DS, Doherty GM, Haugen BR, Kloos RT, Lee SL, Mandel SJ, et al. Revised American Thyroid Association management guidelines for patients with thyroid nodules and differentiated thyroid cancer. Thyroid. 2009;19:1167–214.
41. Pacini F, Schlumberger M, Dralle H, Elisei R, Smit JW, Wiersinga W. European consensus for the management of patients with differentiated thyroid carcinoma of the follicular epithelium. Eur J Endocrinol. 2006;154:787–803.
42. Pacini F, Castagna MG, Brilli L, Pentheroudakis G. Thyroid cancer: ESMO Clinical Practice Guidelines for diagnosis, treatment and follow-up. Ann Oncol. 2010;21(Suppl 5):v214–9.
43. Mazzaferri EL, Kloos RT. Clinical review 128: current approaches to primary therapy for papillary and follicular thyroid cancer. J Clin Endocrinol Metab. 2001;86:1447–63.
44. Tubiana M, Schlumberger M, Rougier P, Laplanche A, Benhamou E, Gardet P, et al. Long-term results and prognostic factors in patients with differentiated thyroid carcinoma. Cancer. 1985;55:794–804.
45. Utiger RD. Follow-up of patients with thyroid carcinoma. N Engl J Med. 1997;337:928–30.
46. Verburg FA, Dietlein M, Lassmann M, Luster M, Reiners C. Why radioiodine remnant ablation is right for most patients with differentiated thyroid carcinoma. Eur J Nucl Med Mol Imaging. 2009;36:343–6.
47. Sherman SI, Tielens ET, Sostre S, Wharam MDJ, Ladenson PW. Clinical utility of posttreatment radioiodine scans in the management of patients with thyroid carcinoma. J Clin Endocrinol Metab. 1994;78:629–34.
48. Tenenbaum F, Corone C, Schlumberger M, Parmentier C. Thyroglobulin measurement and postablative iodine-131 total body scan after total thyroidectomy for differentiated thyroid carcinoma in patients with no evidence of disease. Eur J Cancer. 1996;32A:1262.
49. Travagli JP, Cailleux AF, Ricard M, Baudin E, Caillou B, Parmentier C, et al. Combination of radioiodine (131I) and probe-guided surgery for persistent or recurrent thyroid carcinoma. J Clin Endocrinol Metab. 1998;83:2675–80.
50. Taylor T, Specker B, Robbins J, Sperling M, Ho M, Ain K, et al. Outcome after treatment of high-risk papillary and non-Hurthle-cell follicular thyroid carcinoma. Ann Intern Med. 1998;129:622–7.
51. Bal C, Padhy AK, Jana S, Pant GS, Basu AK. Prospective randomized clinical trial to evaluate the optimal dose of 131 I for remnant ablation in patients with differentiated thyroid carcinoma. Cancer. 1996;77:2574–80.
52. Vermiglio F, Violi MA, Finocchiaro MD, Baldari S, Castagna MG, Moleti M, et al. Short-term effectiveness of low-dose radioiodune ablative treatment of thyroid remnants after thyroidectomy for differentiated thyroid cancer. Thyroid. 1999;9:387–91.
53. Johansen K, Woodhouse NJ, Odugbesan O. Comparison of 1073 MBq and 3700 MBq iodine-131 in postoperative ablation of residual thyroid tissue in patients with differentiated thyroid cancer. J Nucl Med. 1991;32:252–4.
54. Leung SF, Law MW, Ho SK. Efficacy of low-dose iodine-131 ablation of post-operative thyroid remnants: a study of 69 cases. Br J Radiol. 1992;65:905–9.
55. Kuni CC, Klingensmith WC III. Failure of low doses of 131I to ablate residual thyroid tissue following surgery for thyroid cancer. Radiology. 1980;137:773–4.
56. DeGroot LJ, Reilly M. Comparison of 30- and 50-mCi doses of iodine-131 for thyroid ablation. Ann Intern Med. 1982;96:51–3.
57. de Klerk JM, de Keizer B, Zelissen PM, Lips CM, Koppeschaar HP. Fixed dosage of 131I for remnant ablation in patients with differentiated thyroid carcinoma without pre-ablative diagnostic 131I scintigraphy. Nucl Med Commun. 2000;21:529–32.

58. Bal CS, Kumar A, Pant GS. Radioiodine dose for remnant ablation in differentiated thyroid carcinoma: a randomized clinical trial in 509 patients. J Clin Endocrinol Metab. 2004;89:1666–73.
59. Schlumberger M, Catargi B, Borget I, Deandreis D, Zerdoud S, Bridji B, et al. Strategies of radioiodine ablation in patients with low-risk thyroid cancer. N Engl J Med. 2012;366:1663–73.
60. Mallick U, Harmer C, Yap B, Wadsley J, Clarke S, Moss L, et al. Ablation with low-dose radioiodine and thyrotropin alfa in thyroid cancer. N Engl J Med. 2012;366:1674–85.
61. Mountford PJ, Coakley AJ. A review of the secretion of radioactivity in human breast milk: data, quantitative analysis and recommendations. Nucl Med Commun. 1989;10:15–27.
62. Alexander C, Bader JB, Schaefer A, Finke C, Kirsch CM. Intermediate and long-term side effects of high-dose radioiodine therapy for thyroid carcinoma. J Nucl Med. 1998;39:1551–4.
63. DiRusso G, Kern KA. Comparative analysis of complications from I-131 radioablation for well-differentiated thyroid cancer. Surgery. 1994;116:1024–30.
64. Ceccarelli C, Bencivelli W, Morciano D, Pinchera A, Pacini F. 131I therapy for differentiated thyroid cancer leads to an earlier onset of menopause: results of a retrospective study. J Clin Endocrinol Metab. 2001;86:3512–5.
65. Subramanian S, Goldstein DP, Parlea L, Thabane L, Ezzat S, Ibrahim-Zada I, et al. Second primary malignancy risk in thyroid cancer survivors: a systematic review and meta-analysis. Thyroid. 2007;17:1277–88.
66. Brown AP, Chen J, Hitchcock YJ, Szabo A, Shrieve DC, Tward JD. The risk of second primary malignancies up to three decades after the treatment of differentiated thyroid cancer. J Clin Endocrinol Metab. 2008;93:504–15.
67. Rubino C, De Vathaire F, Dottorini ME, Hall P, Schvartz C, Couette JE, et al. Second primary malignancies in thyroid cancer patients. Br J Cancer. 2003;89:1638–44.
68. Verkooijen RB, Smit JW, Romijn JA, Stokkel MP. The incidence of second primary tumors in thyroid cancer patients is increased, but not related to treatment of thyroid cancer. Eur J Endocrinol. 2006;155:801–6.
69. Pluijmen MJ, Eustatia-Rutten C, Goslings BM, Stokkel MP, Arias AM, Diamant M, et al. Effects of low-iodide diet on postsurgical radioiodide ablation therapy in patients with differentiated thyroid carcinoma. Clin Endocrinol (Oxf). 2003;58:428–35.
70. Sonenberg M. Low-iodine diet in the treatment of differentiated thyroid cancer with radioactive iodine. Endocrine. 2002;17:141–3.
71. Morris LF, Wilder MS, Waxman AD, Braunstein GD. Reevaluation of the impact of a stringent low-iodine diet on ablation rates in radioiodine treatment of thyroid carcinoma. Thyroid. 2001;11:749–55.
72. Maxon HR, Thomas SR, Boehringer A, Drilling J, Sperling MI, Sparks JC, et al. Low iodine diet in I-131 ablation of thyroid remnants. Clin Nucl Med. 1983;8:123–6.
73. Goslings BM. Proceedings: effect of a low iodine diet on 131-I therapy in follicular thyroid carcinomata. J Endocrinol. 1975;64:30P.
74. Lassmann M, Luster M, Hanscheid H, Reiners C. Impact of (131)i diagnostic activities on the biokinetics of thyroid remnants. J Nucl Med. 2004;45:619–25.
75. Medvedec M. Thyroid stunning in vivo and in vitro. Nucl Med Commun. 2005;26:731–5.
76. Verburg FA, Mader U, Luster M, Reiners C. Primary tumor diameter as a risk factor for advanced disease features of differentiated thyroid carcinoma. Clin Endocrinol (Oxf). 2008;71:291–7.
77. Luster M, Felbinger R, Dietlein M, Reiners C. Thyroid hormone withdrawal in patients with differentiated thyroid carcinoma: a one hundred thirty-patient pilot survey on consequences of hypothyroidism and a pharmacoeconomic comparison to recombinant thyrotropin administration. Thyroid. 2005;15:1147–55.
78. Dow KH, Ferrell BR, Anello C. Quality-of-life changes in patients with thyroid cancer after withdrawal of thyroid hormone therapy. Thyroid. 1997;7:613–9.
79. Schroeder PR, Haugen BR, Pacini F, Reiners C, Schlumberger M, Sherman SI, et al. A comparison of short-term changes in health-related quality of life in thyroid carcinoma patients undergoing diagnostic evaluation with recombinant human thyrotropin compared with thyroid hormone withdrawal. J Clin Endocrinol Metab. 2006;91:878–84.
80. Hanscheid H, Lassmann M, Luster M, Thomas SR, Pacini F, Ceccarelli C, et al. Iodine biokinetics and dosimetry in radioiodine therapy of thyroid cancer: procedures and results of a prospective international controlled study of ablation after rhTSH or hormone withdrawal. J Nucl Med. 2006;47:654.
81. Rosario PW, Borges MA, Purisch S. Preparation with recombinant human thyroid-stimulating hormone for thyroid remnant ablation with 131I is associated with lowered radiotoxicity. J Nucl Med. 2008;49:1776–82.
82. Frigo A, Dardano A, Danese E, Davi MV, Moghetti P, Colato C, et al. Chromosome translocation frequency after radioiodine thyroid remnant ablation: a comparison between recombinant human thyrotropin stimulation and prolonged levothyroxine withdrawal. J Clin Endocrinol Metab. 2009;94:3472–6.
83. Haugen BR, Pacini F, Reiners C, Schlumberger M, Ladenson PW, Sherman SI, et al. A comparison of recombinant human thyrotropin and thyroid hormone withdrawal for the detection of thyroid remnant or cancer. J Clin Endocrinol Metab. 1999;84:3877–85.
84. Borget I, Remy H, Chevalier J, Ricard M, Allyn M, Schlumberger M, et al. Length and cost of hospital

stay of radioiodine ablation in thyroid cancer patients: comparison between preparation with thyroid hormone withdrawal and thyrogen. Eur J Nucl Med Mol Imaging. 2008;35:1457–63.
85. Borget I, Corone C, Nocaudie M, Allyn M, Iacobelli S, Schlumberger M, et al. Sick leave for follow-up control in thyroid cancer patients: comparison between stimulation with Thyrogen and thyroid hormone withdrawal. Eur J Endocrinol. 2007;156:531–8.
86. Luster M, Lassmann M, Haenscheid H, Michalowski U, Incerti C, Reiners C. Use of recombinant human thyrotropin before radioiodine therapy in patients with advanced differentiated thyroid carcinoma. J Clin Endocrinol Metab. 2000;85:3640–5.
87. de Keizer B, Brans B, Hoekstra A, Zelissen PM, Koppeschaar HP, Lips CJ, et al. Tumour dosimetry and response in patients with metastatic differentiated thyroid cancer using recombinant human thyrotropin before radioiodine therapy. Eur J Nucl Med Mol Imaging. 2003;30:367–73.
88. Robbins RJ, Driedger A, Magner J. Recombinant human thyrotropin-assisted radioiodine therapy for patients with metastatic thyroid cancer who could not elevate endogenous thyrotropin or be withdrawn from thyroxine. Thyroid. 2006;16:1121–30.
89. Sawka AM, Thephamongkhol K, Brouwers M, Thabane L, Browman G, Gerstein HC. Clinical review 170: a systematic review and metaanalysis of the effectiveness of radioactive iodine remnant ablation for well-differentiated thyroid cancer. J Clin Endocrinol Metab. 2004;89:3668–76.
90. Verburg FA, Mader U, Reiners C, Hanscheid H. Long-term survival in differentiated thyroid cancer is worse after low-activity initial post-surgical (131)i therapy in both high- and low-risk patients. J Clin Endocrinol Metab. 2014;99:4487–96.
91. Verburg FA, Lassmann M, Mader U, Luster M, Reiners C, Hanscheid H. The absorbed dose to the blood is a better predictor of ablation success than the administered (131)I activity in thyroid cancer patients. Eur J Nucl Med Mol Imaging. 2011;38:673–80.
92. Lassmann M, Haenscheid H, Chiesa C, Hindorf C, Flux G, Luster M. EANM dosimetry committee series on standard operational procedures for pretherapeutic dosimetry I: blood and bone marrow dosimetry in differentiated thyroid cancer therapy. Eur J Nucl Med Mol Imaging. 2008;35:1405–12.
93. Tuttle RM, Leboeuf R, Robbins RJ, Qualey R, Pentlow K, Larson SM, et al. Empiric radioactive iodine dosing regimens frequently exceed maximum tolerated activity levels in elderly patients with thyroid cancer. J Nucl Med. 2006;47:1587–91.
94. Van Nostrand D, Atkins F, Yeganeh F, Acio E, Bursaw R, Wartofsky L. Dosimetrically determined doses of radioiodine for the treatment of metastatic thyroid carcinoma. Thyroid. 2002;12:121–34.
95. Samuel AM, Rajashekharrao B, Shah DH. Pulmonary metastases in children and adolescents with well-differentiated thyroid cancer. J Nucl Med. 1998;39:1531–6.
96. Chiesa C, Castellani MR, Vellani C, Orunesu E, Negri A, Azzeroni R, et al. Individualized dosimetry in the management of metastatic differentiated thyroid cancer. Q J Nucl Med Mol Imaging. 2009;53:546–61.
97. Benua RS, Cicale NR, Sonenberg M, Rawson RW. The relation of radioiodine dosimetry to results and complications in the treatment of metastatic thyroid cancer. Am J Roentgenol Radium Ther Nucl Med. 1962;87:171–82.
98. Benua RS, Leeper RD. A method and rationale for treating metastatic thyroid carcinoma with the largest safe dose of I-131. In: Medeiros-Neto G, Gaitan G, editors. Frontiers in thyroidology. New York, NY: Plenum Medical Book Co; 1986. p. 1317–21.
99. Hanscheid H, Lassmann M, Luster M, Thomas SR, Pacini F, Ceccarelli C, et al. Iodine biokinetics and dosimetry in radioiodine therapy of thyroid cancer: procedures and results of a prospective international controlled study of ablation after rhTSH or hormone withdrawal. J Nucl Med. 2006;47:648–54.
100. Dorn R, Kopp J, Vogt H, Heidenreich P, Carroll RG, Gulec SA. Dosimetry-guided radioactive iodine treatment in patients with metastatic differentiated thyroid cancer: largest safe dose using a risk-adapted approach. J Nucl Med. 2003;44:451–6.
101. Kulkarni K, Van Nostrand D, Atkins F, Aiken M, Burman K, Wartofsky L. The relative frequency in which empiric dosages of radioiodine would potentially overtreat or undertreat patients who have metastatic well-differentiated thyroid cancer. Thyroid. 2006;16:1019–23.
102. Hanscheid H, Lassmann M, Luster M, Kloos R, Reiners C. Blood dosimetry from a single measurement of the whole body radioiodine retention in patients with differentiated thyroid carcinoma. Endocr Relat Cancer. 2009;16:1283.
103. Hanscheid H, Verburg FA, Biko J, Diessl S, Demidchik YE, Drozd V, et al. Success of the postoperative (131)I therapy in young Belarusian patients with differentiated thyroid cancer after Chernobyl depends on the radiation absorbed dose to the blood and the thyroglobulin level. Eur J Nucl Med Mol Imaging. 2011;38:1296–302.
104. Lassmann M, Reiners C, Luster M. Dosimetry and thyroid cancer: the individual dosage of radioiodine. Endocr Relat Cancer. 2010;17:R161–72.
105. Maxon HR, Thomas SR, Hertzberg VS, Kereiakes JG, Chen IW, Sperling MI, et al. Relation between effective radiation dose and outcome of radioiodine therapy for thyroid cancer. N Engl J Med. 1983;309:937–41.
106. Maxon HR III, Englaro EE, Thomas SR, Hertzberg VS, Hinnefeld JD, Chen LS, et al. Radioiodine-131 therapy for well-differentiated thyroid cancer--a quantitative radiation dosimetric approach: outcome and validation in 85 patients. J Nucl Med. 1992;33:1132–6.

107. Flux GD, Haq M, Chittenden SJ, Buckley S, Hindorf C, Newbold K, et al. A dose-effect correlation for radioiodine ablation in differentiated thyroid cancer. Eur J Nucl Med Mol Imaging. 2010;37:270–5.
108. Sgouros G, Kolbert KS, Sheikh A, Pentlow KS, Mun EF, Barth A, et al. Patient-specific dosimetry for 131I thyroid cancer therapy using 124I PET and 3-dimensional-internal dosimetry (3D-ID) software. J Nucl Med. 2004;45:1366–72.
109. Bolch WE, Eckerman KF, Sgouros G, Thomas SR. MIRD pamphlet No. 21: a generalized schema for radiopharmaceutical dosimetry--standardization of nomenclature. J Nucl Med. 2009;50:477–84.
110. Prideaux AR, Song H, Hobbs RF, He B, Frey EC, Ladenson PW, et al. Three-dimensional radiobiologic dosimetry: application of radiobiologic modeling to patient-specific 3-dimensional imaging-based internal dosimetry. J Nucl Med. 2007;48:1008–16.
111. Verburg FA, Hanscheid H, Biko J, Hategan MC, Lassmann M, Kreissl MC, et al. Dosimetry-guided high-activity (131)I therapy in patients with advanced differentiated thyroid carcinoma: initial experience. Eur J Nucl Med Mol Imaging. 2010;37:896–903.
112. Freudenberg LS, Jentzen W, Görges R, Petrich T, Marlowe RJ, Knust J, et al. 124I-PET dosimetry in advanced differentiated thyroid cancer: therapeutic impact. Nuklearmedizin. 2007;46:121–8.
113. Jentzen W, Freudenberg L, Eising E, Sonnenschein WJ, Knust J, Bockisch A. Optimized 124I PET dosimetry protocol for radioiodine therapy of differentiated thyroid cancer. J Nucl Med. 2008;49:1017–23.
114. Jentzen W, Weise R, Kupferschlager J, Freudenberg L, Brandau W, Bares R, et al. Iodine-124 PET dosimetry in differentiated thyroid cancer: recovery coefficient in 2D and 3D modes for PET(/CT) systems. Eur J Nucl Med Mol Imaging. 2008;35:623.
115. Clement SC, Peeters RP, Ronckers CM, Links TP, van den Heuvel-Eibrink MM, Nieveen van Dijkum EJ, et al. Intermediate and long-term adverse effects of radioiodine therapy for differentiated thyroid carcinoma--a systematic review. Cancer Treat Rev. 2015;41:925–34.
116. Seidlin SM, Siegal E, Yalow AA, Melamed S. Acute myeloid leukemia following prolonged iodine-131 therapy for metastatic thyroid carcinoma. Science. 1956;123:800–1.
117. Iyer NG, Morris LG, Tuttle RM, Shaha AR, Ganly I. Rising incidence of second cancers in patients with low-risk (T1N0) thyroid cancer who receive radioactive iodine therapy. Cancer. 2011;117:4439.
118. Hay ID, Gonzalez-Losada T, Reinalda MS, Honetschlager JA, Richards ML, Thompson GB. Long-term outcome in 215 children and adolescents with papillary thyroid cancer treated during 1940 through 2008. World J Surg. 2010;34:1192–202.
119. Reiners C, Biko J, Haenscheid H, Hebestreit H, Kirinjuk S, Baranowski O, et al. Twenty-five years after Chernobyl: outcome of radioiodine treatment in children and adolescents with very-high-risk radiation-induced differentiated thyroid carcinoma. J Clin Endocrinol Metab. 2013;98:3039–48.
120. Biko J, Reiners C, Kreissl MC, Verburg FA, Demidchik Y, Drozd V. Favourable course of disease after incomplete remission on (131)I therapy in children with pulmonary metastases of papillary thyroid carcinoma: 10 years follow-up. Eur J Nucl Med Mol Imaging. 2011;38:651–5.

Palliation of Metastatic Bone Pain with Radiolabeled Phosphonates

30

Jiaqiong Wang and Aldo N. Serafini

30.1 Introduction

Bone metastases occur most commonly in the advanced stages of cancer and may induce intractable bone pain and not be amenable to conventional treatment plans as advocated by the World Health Organization guidelines for the management of pain in the cancer patient [1]. This results in a significant decrease in the patient's quality of life. The majority of skeletal metastases originate from prostate cancer and breast cancer [2], with up to 90% of prostate cancer patients and about 65–75% of breast cancer patients developing bone metastases [3, 4].

The treatment of bone pain secondary to metastatic bone disease requires a multidisciplinary approach, with multiple services providing support in the appropriate use of various therapeutic agents including analgesics, steroids, bisphosphonates, hormone or antiandrogen agents, and chemotherapeutic agents given alone or in combination. In certain circumstances, the added value of pain palliation from using local treatments such as nerve blocking agents, surgery, radiofrequency, external beam, and systemic radioisotope radiotherapy may be indicated.

Several radioisotopes used alone or as conjugates have been investigated and utilized for treating painful bone metastases, including Phosphorus-32 (32P), Strontium-89 (89Sr), Yttrium-90 (90Y), Tin-117m (117mSn), Samarium-153 (153Sm), Holmium-166 (166Ho), Thulium-170 (170Tm), Lutetium-177 (177Lu), Rhenium-186 (186Re), Rhenium-188 (188Re), and Radium-223 [5–16]. These are characterized as being either beta minus (β−) emitting particles, alpha (α) emitting particles, or Auger electrons [5–11, 13, 16]. The most commonly utilized agents for tumor-targeted systemic radioisotope therapy have been β− emitting radioisotopes, such as sodium phosphate P-32, Strontium-89, Samarium-153m, Rhenium-186, and Lutetium 177 [6, 7, 10, 17–20].

In addition, an increasing role for alpha emitting radioisotopes such as Radium-223 (Chap. 33) which is administered monthly over 6 months as a course of treatment has also been utilized and shown to be effective in bone palliation as well as improving overall survival [11, 21–24].

J. Wang
Nuclear Medicine, Department of Radiology, Jackson Memorial Hospital, Sylvester Comprehensive Cancer Center Miller School of Medicine, University of Miami, Miami, FL, USA
e-mail: jiaqiong.wang@jhsmiami.org

A. N. Serafini (✉)
Nuclear Medicine, Department of Radiology, Sylvester Comprehensive Cancer Center, Miller School of Medicine, University of Miami, Miami, FL, USA
e-mail: aserafini@miami.edu

H. Ahmadzadehfar et al. (eds.), *Clinical Nuclear Medicine*,
https://doi.org/10.1007/978-3-030-39457-8_30

30.2 Radiolabeled Phosphonates in the Treatment of Bone Pain

More recently, different radionuclides attached to a variety of phosphonates have been shown to be useful for the palliation of pain from bone metastases [25]. They have a high affinity for localizing at reactive osteoblastic metastatic sites for effective pain relief. Further, they can be used alone or in combination with cold bisphosphonates, chemotherapy, and external beam radiation therapy to treat pain from osteoblastic metastases. These radiopharmaceuticals include Samarium-153 ethylenediaminetetramethylenephosphonate (Samarium-153 EDTMP) [13], Rhenium-186 hydroxyethylidenediphosphonate (Rhenium-186 HEDP) [26–30], Rhenium-188-HEDP [31–33], and Lutetium-177 ethylenediaminetetramethylene phosphonic acid (Lutetium-177 EDTMP) [5].

30.2.1 Samarium-153 EDTMP

Samarium (153Sm) lexidronam (chemical name Samarium-153 ethylenediaminetetramethylenephosphonate, abbreviated Samarium-153 EDTMP) is a chelated complex of a radioisotope of the element Samarium with EDTMP.

A significant body of literature has been developed over the years showing the utility of Samarium-153 EDTMP in reducing bone pain in many centers worldwide. Samarium-153 is generated by neutron irradiation of Samarium-152 oxide which can then be chelated with the calcium salt of ethylenediaminetetramethylene phosphonic acid (EDTMP) to form Samarium-153 EDTMP. It has a purity of 100%. Samariumm-153 emits beta particles (640, 710, and 810 keV, with maximum energy of 810 keV) and gamma particles (103 keV), with a physical half-life of 46.3 hours and an average penetration distance of 0.83 mm in water [34]. Additionally, the gamma rays emitted by Samarium-153 can be utilized for imaging the biodistribution of therapeutic Samarium-153 EDTMP with a gamma camera for dosimetry purposes and to correlate its efficacy in targeting lesions previously seen on the Technetium99m diphosphonate bone scan obtained prior to the treatment.

30.2.1.1 Samarium-153 EDTMP Binding Mechanism and Biodistribution

Samarium-153 EDTMP binds to the hydroxyapatite crystals by chemi-absorption similar to Technetium99m radiolabeled diphosphonates specifically in locations with a high bone turnover rate. Bone metastases accumulate Samarium-153 EDTMP about five times more than normal bone tissue, resulting in higher doses of radiation to the metastatic sites than to normal adjacent bone. Samarium-153 EDTMP once injected is removed rapidly from the circulation bi-exponentially with estimated half-lives of 5.5 and 65 minutes [35]. There is less than 1% left in the blood at 5 hours after injection [35]. Urinary excretion is the major route of elimination and is completed within 6 hours [34, 36, 37].

Dose-escalation trials to determine the maximally tolerated dose were conducted with Samarium-153 EDTMP dosage ranging from 37 to 111 MBq/kg (1.0–3.0 mCi/kg) by Collins and colleagues in the early 1990s, and the dose of 92.5 MBq/kg (2.5 mCi/kg) was found to be the maximum tolerated dose [38]. Patients who received 92.5 MBq/kg (2.5 mCi/kg) showed more improvement in self-reported pain scores, greater reduction in opioid pain medication, more significant decrease in serum prostate-specific antigen (PSA) and serum prostatic acid phosphatase (PAP) levels, as well as longer survival than those who received 37 MBq/kg (1.0 mCi/kg) (median survival of 9 months versus 6 months; [38]). The only toxicity was the marrow suppression which increased with dose escalation [38].

An early dosimetry study by Eary et al. [36] showed that the skeletal doses (ranging from 20,000 to 32,000 mrad/mCi (5300–8800 Gy/MBq)) were several folds greater than the marrow doses (ranging from 4600 to 7500 mrad/mCi (1200–2000 Gy/MBq)) and the urinary bladder doses (ranging from 1300 to 4700 mrad/mCi (360–1300 Gy/MBq)). The total absorbed marrow doses were estimated between 1277 and

2250 rad (12.8–22.5 Gy) in patients that received the 111 MBq/kg (3.0 mCi/kg) dose, indicating that higher doses of Samarium-153 EDTMP were tolerable for palliation of bone pain from metastases [36]. The present standard utilized dose of Samarium-153 EDTMP is 37 MBq/kg (1 mCi/kg) administered intravenously, which has proven safe and effective, inducing only mild reversible bone marrow suppression in patients with preexisting normal hematological levels [13].

30.2.1.2 Samarium-153 EDTMP Single-Dose Treatment

Following several open-label studies in animals and humans [39], prospective controlled clinical trials were performed investigating the treatment efficacy of Samarium-153 EDTMP for the palliation of bone pain from metastases in a large population of patients in North America, Europe, South America, Asia, and Mexico [12, 13, 40–45]. Cost-effective studies have demonstrated that the cost of pain control for Samarium-153 EDTMP therapy was cheaper than the conventional pain therapy in Spain [46] and Portugal [47].

In the first reported prospective double-blind placebo-controlled clinical trial by Serafini et al. [13], 118 patients diagnosed with painful bone metastases originating from various types of primary tumors were randomly treated with either placebo ($n = 39$), or 18.5 MBq/kg (0.5 mCi/kg, $n = 40$), or 37 MBq/kg (1.0 mCi/kg, $n = 39$) of Samarium-153 EDTMP. Patient and physician evaluations were used to assess pain relief, as well as associated changes in opioid use. Both the low and high dose groups showed reduced pain scores from baseline at each of 4 weeks after treatment for 16 weeks, with the higher-dose group showing greater reduction, while the placebo group did not show any change from the baseline. Pain relief occurred in 62–75% of those patients who were treated with the higher 1 mCi/kg dose during the first 4 weeks with marked to complete responses seen in 31% of the patients by week 4. Pain relief was seen to persist beyond 16 weeks in 43 patients treated with the 1 mCi/kg dose. There was a significant correlation observed in the reductions in opioid analgesic use. Furthermore, the authors demonstrated that the higher dose of 1.0 mCi/kg of Samarium-153 EDTMP produces a relatively rapid onset of pain control in comparison with the placebo during the first week after drug injection. This early response is beneficial to the patient in terms of immediate relief of pain and allowing for an early decrease in the utilization of opioid analgesics and other supportive care. Additionally, the analgesic effects of 1.0 mCi/kg of Samarium-153 EDTMP were enduring at 16 weeks after drug administration for more than half of the patients who were given this dose. The only significant adverse pharmacologic effect observed in this study was a mild, transient, dose-related myelosuppression [13].

Resche et al. [42] demonstrated the efficacy and safety of Samarium-153 EDTMP in a single-blind, dose-controlled study involving 114 patients with painful bone metastases from a variety of primary tumors. Samarium-153 EDTMP was administered at a single dose of either 18.5 MBq/kg (0.5 mCi/kg) ($n = 55$) or 37 MBq/kg (1.0 mCi/kg) ($n = 59$). Significant difference in pain scores was observed between different doses at week 4. Both dose levels relieved the patient's pain, with the higher-dose group achieving greater magnitude of improvement at each week after dose administration, with substantial pain decreases from baseline at week 3 and week 4 ($p < 0.005$; [42]). Female breast cancer patients who received a higher dose of 37 MBq/kg (1.0 mCi/kg) showed the most significant pain relief. A patient global assessment (PGA) of the pain response also revealed some degree of pain relief in each dose group, with 55% of patients in the 18.5 MBq/kg (0.5 mCi/kg) dose group and 70% of patients in the 37 MBq/kg (1.0 mCi/kg) dose group experiencing pain relief at week 4 [42]. Additionally, a long-term follow-up study demonstrated that breast cancer patients who had received the higher dose (37 MBq/kg (1.0 mCi/kg)) had longer survival than those patients who had received the lower dose (18.5 MBq/kg (0.5 mCi/kg)) [42].

Similarly, a multicenter trial in China involving 105 patients with painful bone metastases from various tumors was evaluated for the efficacy and toxicity of single-dose Samarium-153 EDTMP as a palliative treatment for painful skeletal metastases. The patients were treated with Samarium-153 EDTMP at a dose of 37 MBq/kg (1 mCi/kg, group I) or 18.5 MBq/kg (0.5 mCi/kg, group II), and 83.8% of patients showed effective palliation response to a dose of 37 MBq/kg (1 mCi/kg) of Samarium-153 EDTMP [45].

Another study by Tripathi et al. [48] evaluated 86 patients with metastatic bone pain from various primary cancers who received treatment with Samarium-153 EDTMP at a dose of 37 MBq/kg (1 mCi/kg). The overall palliation response rate reached 73%, with 80.3% breast cancer patients and 80.5% prostate cancer patients responding. All responders reduced analgesic consumption and demonstrated better Karnofsky and mobility scores [48].

Dolezal [49] evaluated 43 women with breast cancer associated with painful bone metastases who underwent therapy with Samarium-153 EDTMP. At 1 month after administration, significant pain relief was obtained in 51% of the patients, while mild relief was obtained in 30% of the patients. At 3 months after administration, significant pain relief was obtained in 42% of the patients, and mild relief was obtained in 30% of the patients [49].

Similarly, Petersen et al. [50] reported clinical pain reduction in 22 patients with metastatic, hormone-refractory prostate cancer after single-dose administration of 37 MBq/kg (1.0 mCi/kg) of Samarium-153 EDTMP at weeks 4, 16, and 28 after treatment. Particularly, analgesic scores according to WHO declined by 50% or more in 50% of patients at 4 weeks, in 70% of patients at 16 weeks, and in 71% of patients at 28 weeks after treatment.

Most recently, a study performed by Correa-Gonzalez and colleagues [40] evaluated 277 patients with severe and painful bone metastases from prostate and breast cancer and other malignancies, who received Samarium-153 EDTMP at a dose of 37 MBq/kg (1.0 mCi/kg). The pain intensity was reduced 54% at 3 weeks and 74% at 12 weeks in the pain relief score scales [40].

30.2.1.3 Samarium-153 EDTMP Repeated Sequential Treatment

Several studies have demonstrated the safety and effectiveness of repeated doses of Samarium-153 EDTMP for the treatment of painful multifocal skeletal metastases. As early as 1991, Turner and Claringbold conducted a phase II study of Samarium-153 EDTMP and reported that the patients in the retreated group had longer median duration of pain control (24 weeks) and survival (9 months) as compared to patients who received only single dose. The latter had shorter median duration of pain control (8 weeks) and survival (4 months) [51].

Menda et al. [52] reported repeated treatment response in a patient with prostate cancer complicated with metastatic bone pain. This patient was given 11 doses of Samarium-153 EDTMP, 37 MBq/kg (1 mCi/kg) per dose, over a period of 28 months. With the first five doses, pain assessment scores and the impact of pain on daily living showed the patient's bone pain decreased appreciatively, and his quality of life improved. With doses 6–11, the beneficial effects were apparent but not as obvious; the pain score declined; however the patient also began to increase his use of opioid analgesics. During the 28-month treatment period, Samarium-153 EDTMP induced transient reductions in white blood cell (WBC) and platelet counts which were not of clinical significance or concern.

Sartor et al. [53] investigated the safety and efficacy of repeated treatments of Samarium-153 EDTMP in patients with metastatic bone pain. They prospectively evaluated 55 patients who were given ≥2 doses 37 MBq/kg (1.0 mCi/kg) of Samarium-153 EDTMP. Samarium-153 EDTMP retreatment was given to patients who had pain improvement by week 4 after the first treatment, but whose pain subsequently recurred by week 8 or later. They documented significantly reduced pain scores ($p < 0.001$) at week 4 after each of the first three doses and maintained at week 8 after the first 2 doses ($p < 0.003$) but not after the third dose. Pain scores reduced in 70%, 63%, and 80% of patients, after doses 1, 2, and 3, respectively. The most common adverse events after treatment were mild, transient suppression of platelets and

WBC counts. Nadirs reached approximately half of baseline at 4 weeks after dosing, with recovery in 90% of patients by week 8. Transient grade 3 thrombocytopenia happened in 11%, 12%, and 17% of patients after the first, second, and third dose administration, respectively. The data demonstrated that repeated administration with Samarium-153 EDTMP is both safe and effective to treat patients with metastatic bone pain, provided that platelet and WBC counts are adequate prior to retreatment.

Higano et al. [54] evaluated the safety of repeated high doses of Samarium-153 EDTMP in 18 male patients with hormone-naive prostate cancer metastatic to bone. They found that the safe dose and schedule for repeated high-dose treatment of Samarium-153 EDTMP was three doses of 74 MBq/kg (2 mCi/kg) per dose every 12 weeks [54].

These studies suggest that whenever a patient demonstrates a good response to a single treatment dose of Samarium-153 EDTMP, repeated doses may be considered.

30.2.1.4 Samarium-153 EDTMP Combined with Chemotherapy

Radiopharmaceuticals have been used in combination with chemotherapy. Chemosensitization is a method to improve efficacy of radiation-based therapy. Chemotherapy can induce the tumor cells to become more sensitive to radiation damage and improve the efficacy of the bone-seeking agents. Combining a radiopharmaceutical such as Samarium-153 EDTMP and first-line chemotherapy with docetaxel may improve the clinical outcome by offering independent effects that in combination provide additive tumoricidal benefit to the patient.

A phase II clinical trial conducted by Fizazi et al. [55] evaluated the combined therapy of docetaxel and Samarium-153 EDTMP for 43 patients with bone metastases from castration-resistant prostate cancer (CRPC). Initially, four cycles of docetaxel and estramustine were administered to patients to obtain a response or stabilization. Then a consolidation regimen was performed by utilizing docetaxel at a dose of 20 mg/m^2/week for 6 weeks and Samarium-153 EDTMP at a dose of 37 MBq/kg (1.0 mCi/kg) during week 1. A favorable PSA response was achieved in 77%. The positive pain response rate was 69% and long-term pain control was attained. The median PSA-PFS was 6.4 months, median survival was 29 months, the 1-year survival rate was 77%, and the 2-year survival rate was 56% [55]. These positive results indicate that the combination of docetaxel and Samarium-153 EDTMP is well tolerated in patients with bone metastases from CRPC and that it results in major long-term pain relief [55].

Similarly, a phase I clinical trial study evaluated the toxicity and efficacy of the combination of docetaxel and Samarium-153 EDTMP for patients with metastatic CRPC. This study showed that concurrent 6-month treatment of four doses (75 mg/m^2) of docetaxel every 3 weeks with two infusions every 3 months of 37 MBq/kg (1 mCi/kg) Samarium-153 EDTMP is feasible with reversible bone marrow suppression [56].

Autio et al. [57] evaluated the efficacy and toxicity of the combination of repetitive Samarium-153 EDTMP and docetaxel for patients with metastatic CRPC and more than three bone lesions. Thirty patients were involved in this study and treated with Samarium-153 EDTMP at 37 MBq/kg (1 mCi/kg) per dose every 9 weeks and docetaxel at 75 mg/m^2 per dose every 3 weeks. Patients completed approximately 2.5 cycles of treatment (6.5 doses of docetaxel and 2.5 doses of Samarium-153 EDTMP). The PSA level decreased over 50% in 12 patients (40%). Median progression-free survival was 7.0 months. Overall survival was 14.3 months. The authors concluded that it can be safe to combine Samarium-153 EDTMP with docetaxel at full doses as an antitumor strategy for metastatic CRPC [57].

These studies suggest that the combined therapy of docetaxel and Samarium-153 EDTMP is safe and efficacious for patients with bone metastases from CRPC.

30.2.1.5 Samarium-153 EDTMP Combined with External Beam Radiotherapy

Another type of combined therapy is the combination of external beam radiotherapy (EBRT) with Samarium-153 EDTMP. In a prospective randomized clinical trial by Baczyk et al. [58], 177 patients with metastatic CRPC were divided into two groups, with 89 patients receiving the Samarium-153 EDTMP monotherapy at 37 MBq/kg (1 mCi/kg) and the other 88 patients receiving the combined therapy including Samarium-153 EDTMP 37 MBq/kg (1 mCi/kg) and local EBRT; the EBRT was performed from 3 to 14 days after the radiopharmaceutical administration with the irradiation field limited to the area of the highest pain intensity. It was found that the combination of Samarium-153 EDTMP therapy with local EBRT provided more analgesic effect than solo Samarium-153 EDTMP therapy ($p < 0.001$). The biggest pain relief was obtained in the first weeks following treatment termination. In the whole population, 154 patients (87%) showed a total or partial analgesic effect [58]. No statistically significant differences were observed between the Samarium-153 EDTMP monotherapy group and the combined therapy group in the decline of hemoglobin concentration, the number of erythrocytes, thrombocytes, blood platelets, and neutrophils [58]. These results suggest that the combination of the Samarium-153 EDTMP therapy with local EBRT has greater analgesic effect than monotherapy with Samarium-153 EDTMP and is safe for patients with metastatic CRPC [58].

30.2.1.6 Samarium-153 EDTMP Combined with Bisphosphonates

Some preliminary studies have demonstrated that the therapeutic effect of the combination of radiolabeled phosphonates such as Samarium-153 EDTMP and cold (nonradioactive) bisphosphonates is better than that of mono-treatment with cold bisphosphonates or radiolabeled phosphonates to relieve bone pain [59, 60].

As early as 2003, Baczyk and colleagues evaluated the effectiveness of combined application of Strontium-89 chloride or Samarium-153 EDTMP and nonradioactive "cold" bisphosphonate therapy in 16 breast cancer patients with multiple painful osteoblastic-osteolytic (mixed) bone metastases. Each patient was given a standard dose of Strontium-89 chloride or Samarium-153 EDTMP combined with pamidronate or zoledronate intravenously repeated every month [59]. This contrasted with the control group who received only bisphosphonate. They found that the combined palliative approach employing radioisotope and bisphosphonates was more beneficial than treatment with bisphosphonates or Samarium-153 EDTM only. The combined therapy was effective for pain reduction with a 66–75% "good" and "moderate" response rate, the analgesic requirements reduced to 30% of dose on average, and there was significant improvement in motor activity [59].

Later, Lam et al. [61] from the Netherlands reported a case of a patient with hormone-refractory prostate cancer with multiple painful osseous metastases, who received the combination therapy of Samarium-153 EDTMP with zoledronic acid. Zoledronic acid was administered at 4 mg intravenously every 4 weeks for 6 months, and Samarium-153 EDTMP was given at a dose of 37 MBq/kg (1 mCi/kg) every 3 months. The first dose of zoledronic acid began 2 days prior to the first dose of Samarium-153 EDTMP. In total, the patient received seven doses of zoledronic acid and three doses of Samarium-153 EDTMP (37 MBq/kg) with a cumulative dosage of 13,173 MBq. The patient had total pain relief at 2 weeks after the initial treatment with zoledronic acid in combination with Samarium-153 EDTMP. The patient's PSA decreased 71% in comparison to baseline value. After the third dose of Samarium-153 EDTMP, bone scintigraphy revealed a substantial resolution of skeletal lesions over the treatment period. There was no negative interaction and the toxicity was low [61].

Rasulova et al. [60] evaluated the timing of bisphosphonate administration in combinational therapy with Samarium-153 oxabifore in order to obtain optimal palliation of bone pain. They found that the combination therapy of zoledronic acid administered 48–72 hours prior to Samarium-153 oxabifore induces greater and faster pain relief following the initiation of the combination therapy than other alternative dosing schedules [60].

30.2.2 Rhenium-188 HEDP

In addition to Samarium-153 EDTMP, there are other radiolabeled phosphonates under investigation, such as Lutetium-177 EDTMP and Rhenium-188 HEDP [28, 29, 31, 62]. Rhenium-188 is of special interest in clinical applications due to its availability and cost-effectiveness as it is the product of an 188tungsten/188Re generator [31–33, 62–64].

Rhenium-188 (188Re) is well suited for effective treatment: it has a short physical half-life of 16.8 hours; it is mainly a beta emitter with the energy of 2.1 MeV, and it has a 15% gamma component with the energy of 155 keV, allowing for imaging, biodistribution, and absorbed radiation dose studies. The penetration depth in tissue for 188Re is approximately 10 mm.

Rhenium-188 HEDP is a specific bone-targeting therapeutic radiopharmaceutical that accumulates in the skeletal system and bone lesions. Liepe et al. [65] performed a dosimetry study of Rhenium-188 HEDP in prostate cancer patients with skeletal metastases by injecting 2700–3459 MBq Rhenium-188 HEDP. The radiation absorbed dose was 3.83 ± 2.01 mGy/MBq for bone metastases, higher than the radiation absorbed dose by the bone marrow (0.61 ± 0.21 mGy/MBq), the whole body (0.07 ± 0.02 mGy/MBq), and the kidney (0.71 ± 0.22 mGy/MBq). Rhenium-188 HEDP was rapidly excreted in the urine, with 41% of the administered dose excreted within the first 8 h after therapy.

In a dose-escalation study in prostate cancer patients with painful bone metastases, Palmedo showed that the maximum tolerated dose of Rhenium-188 HEDP is 3.3 GBq if the baseline thrombocyte count is below 200 × 10^9/l and that 4.4 GBq might be tolerable if thrombocyte counts over 200 × 10^9/l. The most important side effects were thrombopenia and leukopenia, with the overall nadir of thrombopenia at week 4 [32].

An early study utilizing single-dose Rhenium-188 HEDP treatment in prostate cancer patients with osseous metastases showed that a single dose of 2.6 GBq or more of Rhenium-188 HEDP resulted in pain palliation in 60–75% of patients [32]. Later studies demonstrated that repeated Rhenium-188 HEDP treatment can enhance pain palliation effect and prolong the progression-free and overall survival [33]. In a phase II clinical trial, Palmedo et al. [33] randomly assigned 64 patients with hormone-refractory prostate carcinoma and bone pain into two different groups for radionuclide bone-targeted therapy with Rhenium-188 HEDP; the Group A patients received a single injection, and the Group B patients received two injections with an 8-week interval. Both groups showed low toxicity with moderate thrombopenia and leukopenia. Repeated Rhenium-188 HEDP therapies (Group B) achieved better pain palliation effectiveness with a response rate of 92% and time of response of 5.66 months, respectively (p = 0.006 and p = 0.001). The PSA level decreased more than 50% for at least 8 weeks in 11/28 patients (39%) in Group B, compared with 2/30 patients (7%) in the Group A. Repeated Rhenium-188 HEDP therapies also demonstrated longer median times to progression, which was 7.0 months (0–24.1 months) in Group B compared to 2.3 months (0–12.2 months) in Group A (p = 0.0013). Repeated Rhenium-188 HEDP therapies also had longer median overall survival time, which was 12.7 months (range, 4.1–32.2 months) in Group B, compared to 7.0 months (range, 1.3–36.7 months) in Group A (p = 0.043; [33]).

Recently in a retrospective study, Biersack et al. [31] also showed the positive effect of repeated Rhenium-188 HEDP therapy on overall survival in patients with hormone-refractory prostate cancer and bone metastases. In this study, 60 patients were divided into three different groups according to the number of Rhenium-188 HEDP injections. Group A patients received only one injection (n = 19), Group B patients received two injections (n = 19), and Group C patients received three or more injections (n = 22). Pain palliation effect was gained in 89.5% of Group A, 94.7% of Group B, and 90.9% of Group C; no significant pain palliation differences were observed between the three groups. Mean survival after the first Rhenium-188 HEDP therapy was 4.5 months in Group A, prolonged to 9.98 months in Group B, and improved to 15.7 months in Group C [31].

Recently, Lange and colleagues from the Netherlands showed that treatment with Rhenium-188 HEDP resulted in significant pain palliation effect and better overall quality of life in both prostate and breast cancer patients with painful bone metastases [66].

30.2.3 Lutetium-177 EDTMP

Lutetium-177 (177Lu) has a half-life of 6.73 days, emits both beta particles and gamma particles, and has been utilized for therapy and imaging [67]. In early studies, 177Lu was successfully labeled with ethylene diphosphonate (MDP) with a very high radiochemical purity of greater than 99%. An animal study in rats showed its high skeletal uptake and relative low biodistribution in soft tissue [68]. Another radiopharmaceutical 177Lu-ethylenediaminetetramethylene propionate (Lutetium-177 EDTMP) has been successfully formulated with a radiochemical purity greater than 99%. Biodistribution studies using mice and rabbits showed that it almost exclusively accumulated in the skeletal system, specifically in regions of remodeling bone [69].

Recent human studies have demonstrated that Lutetium-177 EDTMP is safe and effective for metastatic bone pain palliation. In a clinical trial in Iran, 30 patients with metastatic bone pain received Lutetium-177 EDTMP IV injections at a dose of 29.6 MBq/kg [5]. Significant pain relief was achieved in 25 patients (83%) as early as 2 weeks after the administration and lasted up to 12 weeks [5]. Similarly, another phase II study from India demonstrated the efficacy and safety of Lutetium-177 EDTMP for palliation of pain from bone metastases in 44 patients with documented breast cancer ($n = 12$) or CRPC ($n = 32$) [70]. The patients were randomly divided into high-dose (2590 MBq) and low-dose (1295 MBq) groups. The overall response rate was 86%, with 92% of the breast cancer patients and 84% of the prostate cancer patients showing a favorable response [70]. The low-dose group showed an overall response rate of 77%, and the high-dose group showed an overall response rate of 95% [70]. Both groups showed an obvious reduction in visual analogue scores (VAS) and analgesic scores (AS), together with improvement in quality of life [70]. No significant differences in efficacy or hematological toxicity existed between the low-dose group and the high-dose group [70]. Therefore, Lutetium-177 EDTMP is a novel and promising radiopharmaceutical for palliation therapy in patients with disseminated bone metastases from various types of cancer [67].

Additionally, several prospective studies reported similar therapeutic efficacy of Lutetium-177 EDTMP and Samarium-153 EDTMP in pain relief and improvement in patients' quality of life, without significant differences in blood parameters [16, 71].

30.3 Conclusion

A variety of therapeutic radiopharmaceuticals are available and continue to be developed for the palliative treatment of bone pain from metastatic bone disease. Radiolabeled phosphonates may be administered as single treatments (monotherapy) at high doses or as multiple fractionated treatments at lower doses (as is done with external beam radiation). For recurrent bone pain retreatment, repeated multidose regimens have been shown to be safe and efficacious as well.

In addition, any adjuvant chemotherapy regimens which are needed to treat residual solid cancers in non-osseous sites can be restarted as early as 6 weeks post Samarium-153 EDTMP withdrawal once hematological status has normalized. Hematological status may normalize spontaneously or can be advanced by the introduction of supportive colony stimulating agents.

More recently the combination of beta-emitting radiopharmaceuticals such as Samarium-153 EDTMP, with chemotherapy, external beam therapy, and cold bisphosphonates has been shown to be promising in both palliating bone pain and enhancing the tumoricidal effects.

In addition to Samarium-153 EDTMP, Renium-188 HEDP and Lutetium-177 EDTMP are effective and safe for palliation of bone pain from metastatic bone disease.

References

1. World Health Organization. Cancer pain relief: with a guide to opioid availability. 2nd ed. Geneva: World Health Organization; 1996.
2. Cecchini M, Wetterwald A, Pluijm G, Thalmann G. Molecular and biological mechanisms of bone metastasis. EAU Upd Ser. 2005;3:214–26.
3. Bubendorf L, Schöpfer A, Wagner U, Sauter G, Moch H, Willi N, Gasser TC, Mihatsch MJ. Metastatic patterns of prostate cancer: an autopsy study of 1,589 patients. Hum Pathol. 2000;31(5):578–83.
4. Macedo F, Ladeira K, Pinho F, Saraiva N, Bonito N, Pinto L, Goncalves F. Bone metastases: an overview. Oncol Rev. 2017;11(1):321.
5. Alavi M, Omidvari S, Mehdizadeh A, Jalilian AR, Bahrami-Samani A. Metastatic bone pain palliation using (177) Lu-ethylenediaminetetramethylene phosphonic acid. World J Nucl Med. 2015;14(2):109–15.
6. Blake GM, Wood JF, Wood PJ, Zivanovic MA, Lewington VJ. 89Sr therapy: strontium plasma clearance in disseminated prostatic carcinoma. Eur J Nucl Med. 1989a;15(1):49–54.
7. Blake GM, Zivanovic MA, Lewington VJ. Measurements of the strontium plasma clearance rate in patients receiving Sr89 radionuclide therapy. Eur J Nucl Med. 1989b;15(12):780–3.
8. Guerra Liberal FDC, Tavares AAS, Tavares JMRS. Palliative treatment of metastatic bone pain with radiopharmaceuticals: a perspective beyond Strontium-89 and Samarium-153. Appl Radiat Isot. 2016;110:87–99.
9. Guerra Liberal FD, Tavares AA, Tavares JM. Comparative analysis of 11 different radioisotopes for palliative treatment of bone metastases by computational methods. Med Phys. 2014;41(11):114101. https://doi.org/10.1118/1.4897240.
10. Nair N. Relative efficacy of 32P and 89Sr in palliation in skeletal metastases. J Nucl Med. 1999;40(2):256–61.
11. Parker C, Nilsson S, Heinrich D, Helle SI, O'Sullivan JM, Fosså SD, Chodacki A, Wiechno P, Logue J, Seke M, Widmark A, Johannessen DC, Hoskin P, Bottomley D, James ND, Solberg A, Syndikus I, Kliment J, Wedel S, Boehmer S, Dall'Oglio M, Franzén L, Coleman R, Vogelzang NJ, O'Bryan-Tear CG, Staudacher K, Garcia-Vargas J, Shan M, Bruland ØS, Sartor O, Investigators ALSYMPACA. Alpha emitter radium-223 and survival in metastatic prostate cancer. N Engl J Med. 2013;369(3):213–23.
12. Serafini AN. Samarium Sm-153 lexidronam for the palliation of bone pain associated with metastases. Cancer. 2000;88(12 Suppl):2934–9.
13. Serafini AN, Houston SJ, Resche I, Quick DP, Grund FM, Ell PJ, Bertrand A, Ahmann FR, Orihuela E, Reid RH, Lerski RA, Collier BD, McKillop JH, Purnell GL, Pecking AP, Thomas FD, Harrison KA. Palliation of pain associated with metastatic bone cancer using samarium-153 lexidronam: a double-blind placebo-controlled clinical trial. J Clin Oncol. 1998;16(4):1574–81.
14. Srivastava SC, Aktins HL, Krishnamurthy GT, Zanzi I, Silberstein EB, Meinken G, Mausner LF, Swailem F, D'Alessandro T, Cabahug CJ, Lau Y, Park T, Madajewicz S. Treatment of metastatic bone pain with tin-177m Stannic diethylenetriaminepentaacetic acid: a phase I/II clinical study. Clin Cancer Res. 1998;4(1):61–8.
15. Srivastava SC, Meinken GE, Richards P, et al. The development and in-vivo behavior of tin containing radiopharmaceuticals I. Chemistry, preparation and biodistribution in small animals. Int J Nucl Med Biol. 1985;12:167–74.
16. Thapa P, Nikam D, Das T, Sonawane G, Agarwal JP, Basu S. Clinical efficacy and safety comparison of 177Lu-EDTMP with 153Sm-EDTMP on an equidose basis in patients with painful skeletal metastases. J Nucl Med. 2015;56(10):1513–9.
17. Blake GM, Zivanovic MA, McEwan AJ, Ackery DM. Sr-89 therapy: strontium kinetics in disseminated carcinoma of the prostate. Eur J Nucl Med. 1986;12(9):447–54.
18. Kaplan E, Fels IG, Kotlowski BR. Therapy of carcinoma of the prostate metastatic to bone with P-32 labeled condensed phosphate. J Nucl Med. 1960;1:1–13.
19. Karasawa K. Cancer therapy using unsealed radioisotopes-the present and future. Gan To Kagaku Ryoho. 2014;41(13):2555–8.
20. Kutzner J, Dähnert W, Schreyer T, Grimm W, Bord KH, Becker M. Yttrium-90 zur Strahlentherapie von Knochenmetastasen. Nucl Med. 1981;20:229–35.
21. Bertolaso P, Leroy L, Gross-Goupil M, Aupee O, Ravaud A, Roubaud G, Cazeau AL, Le Moulec S. Principles, modalities and indications of the administration of Radium in cancers, focus on metastatic prostate cancer: state of arts. Bull Cancer. 2017;104(9):762–70.
22. Hoskin P, Sartor O, O'Sullivan JM, Johannessen DC, Helle SI, Logue J, Bottomley D, Nilsson S, Vogelzang NJ, Fang F, Wahba M, Aksnes AK, Parker C. Efficacy and safety of radium-223 dichloride in patients with castration-resistant prostate cancer and symptomatic bone metastases, with or without previous docetaxel use: a prespecified subgroup analysis from the randomised, double-blind, phase 3 ALSYMPCA trial. Lancet Oncol. 2014;15(12):1397–406.
23. Saad F, Carles J, Gillessen S, Heidenreich A, Heinrich D, Gratt J, Lévy J, Miller K, Nilsson S, Petrenciuc O, Tucci M, Wirth M, Federhofer J, O'Sullivan JM, Radium-223 International Early Access Program Investigators. Radium-223 and concomitant therapies in patients with metastatic castration-resistant prostate cancer: an international, early access, open-label, single-arm phase 3b trial. Lancet Oncol. 2016;17(9):1306–16.
24. Sartor O, Coleman R, Nilsson S, Heinrich D, Helle SI, O'Sullivan JM, Fosså SD, Chodacki A, Wiechno P, Logue J, Widmark A, Johannessen DC, Hoskin

P, James ND, Solberg A, Syndikus I, Vogelzang NJ, O'Bryan-Tear CG, Shan M, Bruland ØS, Parker C. Effect of radium-223 dichloride on symptomatic skeletal events in patients with castration-resistant prostate cancer and bone metastases: results from a phase 3, double-blind, randomised trial. Lancet Oncol. 2014;15(7):738–46.
25. Ando A, Ando I, Tonami N, Kinuya S, Kazuma K, Kataiwa A, Nakagawa M, Fujita N. 177Lu-EDTMP: a potential therapeutic bone agent. Nucl Med Commun. 1998;19(6):587–91.
26. De Klerk JM, van Dijk A, van het Schip AD, Zonnenberg BA, van Rijk PP. Pharmacokinetics of rhenium-186 after administration of rhenium-186-HEDP to patients with bone metastases. J Nucl Med. 1992;33(5):646–51.
27. Ketring AR. 153 Sm-EDTMP and 186 Re-HEDP as bone therapeutic radiopharmaceuticals. Int J Rad Appl Instrum B. 1987;14(3):223–32.
28. Palmedo H, Bender H, Dierke-Dzierzon C, Carl UM, Risse J, Krebs D, Biersack HJ. Pain palliation with rhenium-186 HEDP in breast cancer patients with disseminated bone metastases. Clin Nucl Med. 1999;24(9):643–8.
29. Palmedo H, Bender H, Schomburg A, Grünwald F, Schöneich G, Zamorra P, Reichmann K, Dierke-Dzierzon C, Mallmann P, Biersack HJ. Pain therapy with rhenium-186 HEDP in multiple bone metastases. Nuklearmedizin. 1996;35(2):63–7. German.
30. Palmedo H, Grünwald F, Wagner U, Köhler S, Krebs D, Biersack HJ. Remission of bone metastases after combined chemotherapy and radionuclide therapy with Re-186 HEDP. Clin Nucl Med. 1998;23(8):501–4.
31. Biersack HJ, Palmedo H, Andris A, Rogenhofer S, Knapp FF, Guhlke S, Ezziddin S, Bucerius J, von Mallek D. Palliation and survival after repeated (188) Re-HEDP therapy of hormone-refractory bone metastases of prostate cancer: a retrospective analysis. J Nucl Med. 2011;52(11):1721–6.
32. Palmedo H, Guhlke S, Bender H, Sartor J, Schoeneich G, Risse J, Grünwald F, Knapp FF Jr, Biersack HJ. Dose escalation study with rhenium-188 hydroxyethylidene diphosphonate in prostate cancer patients with osseous metastases. Eur J Nucl Med. 2000;27(2):123–30.
33. Palmedo H, Manka-Waluch A, Albers P, Schmidt-Wolf IG, Reinhardt M, Ezziddin S, Joe A, Roedel R, Fimmers R, Knapp FF Jr, Guhlke S, Biersack HJ. Repeated bone-targeted therapy for hormone-refractory prostate carcinoma: tandomized phase II trial with the new, high-energy radiopharmaceutical rhenium-188 hydroxyethylidenediphosphonate. J Clin Oncol. 2003;21(15):2869–75.
34. Farhanghi M, Holmes RA, Volkert WA, Logan KW, Singh A. Samarium-153-EDTMP: pharmacokinetic, toxicity and pain response using an escalating dose schedule in treatment of metastatic bone cancer. J Nucl Med. 1992;33(8):1451–8.
35. Bayouth JE, Macey DJ, Kasi LP, Fossella FV. Dosimetry and toxicity of samarium-153-EDTMP administered for bone pain due to skeletal metastases. J Nucl Med. 1994;35(1):63–9.
36. Eary JF, Collins C, Stabin M, Vernon C, Petersdorf S, Baker M, Hartnett S, Ferency S, Addison SJ, Appelbaum F, et al. Samarium-153-EDTMP biodistribution and dosimetry estimation. J Nucl Med. 1993;34(7):1031–6.
37. Singh A, Holmes RA, Farhangi M, Volkert WA, Williams A, Stringham LM, Ketring AR. Human pharmacokinetics of samarium-153 EDTMP in metastatic cancer. J Nucl Med. 1989;30(11):1814–8.
38. Collins C, Eary JF, Donaldson G, Vernon C, Bush NE, Petersdorf S, Livingston RB, Gordon EE, Chapman CR, Appelbaum FR. Samarium-153-EDTMP in bone metastases of hormone refractory prostate carcinoma: a phase I/II trial. J Nucl Med. 1993;34(11):1839–44.
39. Alberts AS, Smit BJ, Louw WK, van Rensburg AJ, van Beek A, Kritzinger V, Nel JS. Dose response relationship and multiple dose efficacy and toxicity of samarium-153-EDTMP in metastatic cancer to bone. Radiother Oncol. 1997;43(2):175–9.
40. Correa-González L, Arteaga de Murphy C, Pichardo-Romero P, Pedraza-López M, Moreno-García C, Correa-Hernández L. (153)Sm-EDTMP for pain relief of bone metastases from prostate and breast cancer and other malignancies. Arch Med Res. 2014;45(4):301–8.
41. Paes FM, Serafini AN. Systemic metabolic radiopharmaceutical therapy in the treatment of metastatic bone pain. Semin Nucl Med. 2010;40(2):89–104.
42. Resche I, Chatal JF, Pecking A, Ell P, Duchesne G, Rubens R, Fogelman I, Houston S, Fauser A, Fischer M, Wilkins D. A dose-controlled study of 153Sm-ethylenediaminetetramethylenephosphonate (EDTMP) in the treatment of patients with painful bone metastases. Eur J Cancer. 1997;33(10):1583–91.
43. Sapienza MT, Ono CR, Guimarães MI, Watanabe T, Costa PA, Buchpiguel CA. Retrospective evaluation of bone pain palliation after samarium-153-EDTMP therapy. Rev Hosp Clin Fac Med Sao Paulo. 2004;59(6):321–8.
44. Sartor O, Reid RH, Hoskin PJ, Quick DP, Ell PJ, Coleman RE, Kotler JA, Freeman LM, Olivier P, Quadramet 424Sm10/11 Study Group. Samarium-153-Lexidronam complex for treatment of painful bone metastases in hormone-refractory prostate cancer. Urology. 2004;63(5):940–5.
45. Tian JH, Zhang JM, Hou QT, Oyang QH, Wang JM, Luan ZS, Chuan L, He YJ. Multicentre trial on the efficacy and toxicity of single-dose samarium-153-ethylene diamine tetramethylene phosphonate as a palliative treatment for painful skeletal metastases in China. Eur J Nucl Med. 1999;26(1):2–7.
46. Velasco Latrás M, Carreras Coderch L, Antoñanzas Villar F, Coya Viña J, Martín Comín J, Martínez Carderón F, Nieto Martín-Bejarano J, Sáenz Cusí

A, Serrano Bermúdez G, Echevarría IA. Cost-effectiveness analysis of samarium153 (Quadramet) for the treatment of patients with prostate cancer and bone metastases. Clin Transl Oncol. 2005;7(5):198–204.
47. Macedo A, Araújo A, Melo FC, Nunes G, Cantinho G, Amorin I. Cost-effectiveness of samarium-153-EDTMP for the treatment of pain due to multiple bone metastases in hormone-refractory prostate cancer versus conventional pain therapy, in Portugal. Acta Med Port. 2006;19(5):421–6.
48. Tripathi M, Singhal T, Chandrasekhar N, Kumar P, Bal C, Jhulka PK, Bandopadhyaya G, Malhotra A. Samarium-153 ethylenediamine tetramethylene phosphonate therapy for bone pain palliation in skeletal metastases. Indian J Cancer. 2006;43(2):86–92.
49. Dolezal J. Efficacy and toxicity of 153samarium-EDTMP in painful breast cancer bone metastases. Onkologie. 2009;32(1-2):35–9.
50. Petersen LJ, Lund L, Jønler M, Jakobsen M, Abrahamsen J. Samarium-153 treatment of bone pain in patients with metastatic prostate cancer. Dan Med Bull. 2010;57(6):A4154.
51. Turner JH, Claringbold PG. A phase II study of treatment of painful multifocal skeletal metastases with single and repeated dose samarium-153 ethylenediaminetetramethylene phosphonate. Eur J Cancer. 1991;27(9):1084–6.
52. Menda Y, Bushnell DL, Williams RD, et al. Efficacy and safety of repeated samarium-153 lexidronam treatment in a patient with prostate cancer and metastatic bone pain. Clin Nucl Med. 2000;25:698–700.
53. Sartor O, Reid RH, Bushnell DL, et al. Safety and efficacy of repeat administration of samarium Sm-153 lexidronam to patients with metastatic bone pain. Cancer. 2007;109:637–43.
54. Higano CS, Quick DP, Bushnell D, Sartor O. Safety analysis of repeated high doses of samarium-153 lexidronam in men with hormone-naive prostate cancer metastatic to bone. Clin Genitourin Cancer. 2008;6(1):40–5.
55. Fizazi K, Beuzeboc P, Lumbroso J, et al. Phase II trial of consolidation docetaxel and samarium-153 in patients with bone metastases from castration-resistant prostate cancer. J Clin Oncol. 2009;27:2429.
56. Lin J, Sinibaldi VJ, Carducci MA, Denmeade S, Song D, DeWeese T, Eisenberger MA. Phase I trial with a combination of docetaxel and 153Sm-lexidronam in patients with castration-resistant metastatic prostate cancer. Urol Oncol. 2011;29:670–5.
57. Autio KA, Pandit-Taskar N, Carrasquillo JA, Stephenson RD, Slovin SF, Rathkopf DE, Hong C, Heller G, Scher HI, Larson SM, Morris MJ. Repetitively dosed docetaxel and 153-samarium-EDTMP as an antitumor strategy for metastatic castration-resistant prostate cancer. Cancer. 2013;119:3186–94.
58. Baczyk M, Milecki P, Pisarek M, Gut P, Antczak A, Hrab M. A prospective randomized trial: a comparison of the analgesic effect and toxicity of 153Sm radioisotope treatment in monotherapy and combined therapy including local external beam radiotherapy (EBRT) among metastatic castrate resistance prostate cancer (mCRPC) patients with painful bone metastases. Neoplasma. 2013;60(3):328–33.
59. Baczyk M, Baczyk E, Sowiński J. Preliminary results of combined application of radioisotopes and biphosphonates in the management of pain associated with osteoblastic-osteolytic bone metastases of breast cancer. Ortop Traumatol Rehabil. 2003;5(2):234–7.
60. Rasulova N, Lyubshin V, Arybzhanov D, Sagdullaev S, Krylov V, Khodjibekov M. Optimal timing of bisphosphonate administration in combination with samarium-153 oxabifore in the treatment of painful metastatic bone disease. World J Nucl Med. 2013;12(1):14–8.
61. Lam MG, de Klerk JM, Zonnenberg BA. Treatment of painful bone metastases in hormone-refractory prostate cancer with zoledronic acid and samarium-153-ethylenediaminetetramethylphosphonic acid combined. J Palliat Med. 2009;12(7):649–51.
62. Ahmadzadehfar H. Targeted therapy for metastatic prostate cancer with radionuclides. In: Mohan R, editor. Prostate cancer. Rijeka: IntechOpen; 2016. https://doi.org/10.5772/64016. Available from https://www.intechopen.com/books/prostate-cancer-leading-edge-diagnostic-procedures-and-treatments/targeted-therapy-for-metastatic-prostate-cancer-with-radionuclides.
63. Chhabra A, Rathore Y, Bhusari P, Vatsa R, Mittal BR, Shukla J. Concentration protocol of rhenium-188 perrhenate eluted from tungsten-188/rhenium-188 generator for the preparation of high-yield rhenium-188-labelled radiopharmaceuticals. Nucl Med Commun. 2018;39:957. https://doi.org/10.1097/MNM.0000000000000893.
64. Knapp FF Jr, Beets AL, Guhlke S, Zamora PO, Bender H, Palmedo H, Biersack HJ. Availability of rhenium-188 from the alumina-based tungsten-188/rhenium-188 generator for preparation of rhenium-188-labeled radiopharmaceuticals for cancer treatment. Anticancer Res. 1997;17(3B):1783–95.
65. Liepe K, Hliscs R, Kropp J, Runge R, Knapp FF Jr, Franke WG. Dosimetry of 188Re-hydroxyethylidene diphosphonate in human prostate cancer skeletal metastases. J Nucl Med. 2003;44(6):953–60.
66. Lange R, Overbeek F, de Klerk JM, Pasker-de Jong PC, van den Berk AM, Ter Heine R, Rodenburg CJ, Kooistra A, Hendrikse NH, Bloemendal HJ. Treatment of painful bone metastases in prostate and breast cancer patients with the therapeutic radiopharmaceutical rhenium-188-HEDP. Clinical benefit in a real-world study. Nuklearmedizin. 2016;55(5):188–95.
67. Mazzarri S, Guidoccio F, Mariani G. The emerging potential of 177Lu-EDTMP: an attractive novel option for radio metabolic therapy of skeletal metastases. Clin Transl Imag. 2015;3(2):167–8.
68. Abbasi IA. Studies on 177Lu-labeled methylene diphosphonate as potential bone-seeking radiopharmaceutical for bone pain palliation. Nucl Med Biol. 2011;38(3):417–25.

69. Máthé D, Balogh L, Polyák A, Király R, Márián T, Pawlak D, Zaknun JJ, Pillai MR, Jánoki GA. Multispecies animal investigation on biodistribution, pharmacokinetics and toxicity of 177Lu-EDTMP, a potential bone pain palliation agent. Nucl Med Biol. 2010;37(2):215–26.
70. Agarwal KK, Singla S, Arora G, Bal C. (177) Lu-EDTMP for palliation of pain from bone metastases in patients with prostate and breast cancer: a phase II study. Eur J Nucl Med Mol Imaging. 2015;42(1):79–88.
71. Sharma S, Singh B, Koul A, Mittal BR. Comparative therapeutic efficacy of 153Sm-EDTMP and 177Lu-EDTMP for bone pain palliation in patients with skeletal metastases: patients' pain score analysis and personalized dosimetry. Front Med (Lausanne). 2017;4:46. https://doi.org/10.3389/fmed.2017.00046.

31 Radionuclide Therapy of Bone Metastases with Radium-223 Chloride in Prostate Cancer Patients

Holger Palmedo

31.1 Introduction

Radionuclide therapy of bone metastases represents a systemic antitumour therapy administering open radioactive agents intravenously. It is the aim of each radiation therapy to apply a maximal dose to the target – in this case bone metastases – and a minimal dose to the rest of the whole body. The dose to the rest of the body determines the frequency and intensity of side effects and limits treatment efficacy [1].

Bone metastases are frequent and will occur to every physician treating oncologic patients. Many solid tumours generate bone metastases. Mainly, patients with breast, prostate and lung cancer are concerned. Over 60% of all breast cancer patients develop osseous metastases of the osteolytic or combined osteolytic/osteoblastic type during the course of disease [2]. Half of prostate cancer and a third of lung cancer patients will come up with metastatic bone disease. In prostate cancer, bone metastases are predominantly osteoblastic [3].

Once bone metastases are diagnosed, the disease must be classified as incurable. At this stage, quality of life and prolongation of survival are the important parameters that build the basis of further medical decision-making.

Bone metastases can lead to serious complications and, finally, often induce lethal disease progression. Thirty to sixty percent of patients develop pain symptoms of diverse intensity. Predominantly, the osteolytic type has the tendency to develop fractures resulting in severe morbidity. But also osteoblastic metastases might cause bone fracture. Furthermore, a hypercalcaemic syndrome due to increased bone resorption of osteolytic metastases can occur; this can also appear as a paraneoplastic syndrome. If there is extensive metastatic disease, the bone marrow can be destroyed and clinically relevant alterations of the blood counts can be observed.

With the introduction of the new radiopharmaceutical radium-223 chloride (Ra-223), significance of radionuclide therapy has rapidly increased. It has been shown that the alpha-radiation-emitting nuclide Ra-223 is an effective treatment of bone metastases prolonging survival and progression-free interval in castration-resistant prostate cancer patients without visceral metastases [4]. Furthermore, alpha radiation therapy with Ra-223 could prevent the above-mentioned complications of bone metastases like pain progression and spinal compression [4, 5].

Also bone metastases of further tumour entities like breast and lung cancer can be treated

H. Palmedo (✉)
Institute of Radiology and Nuclear Medicine in der Kaiser-Passage Bonn, PET-CT Center, Clinical Cancer Center Johanniter Hospital, Bonn, Germany

H. Ahmadzadehfar et al. (eds.), *Clinical Nuclear Medicine*,
https://doi.org/10.1007/978-3-030-39457-8_31

by radionuclides. Effective pain palliation could be proven for breast cancer patients with osseous metastases by administering beta-radiation-emitting radionuclides [6]. However, evidence for benefits of beta emitters for survival and progression-free interval is only present in phase II but not in phase III trials [7, 8].

Since prostate cancer has come into focus as the most accepted tumour disease for antitumour therapy with radionuclides, it is important that the nuclear medicine community offers a sufficient amount of physicians and facilities necessitated for the treatment of patients. Additionally, high efforts in continuing education in the urologic field should be made by the nuclear medicine physician to appear as a competent member of the prostate cancer tumour board.

Radionuclide therapy is recommended in the actual guidelines for prostate cancer patients [9, 10]. The European as well the German guidelines of highest evidence level (S3 quality) propose alpha radiation therapy with Ra-223 as a first- and second-line treatment of bone metastases in symptomatic, castration-resistant prostate cancer patients without visceral disease [9, 10]. Alternative treatment options recommended by the guidelines and to be discussed with the treating urologist and oncologist are chemotherapy (docetaxel, cabazitaxel) and second-line antihormonal treatment (abiraterone, enzalutamide).

However, due to recent results of an interim analysis of the ERA-223 study, radium-223 chloride is not to be applied before the patient has received two systemic treatments like abiraterone and docetaxel.

31.2 Physical Characteristics

It is important to realize that the physical characteristics of α-emitters are different from those of ß-emitters. Ra-223 decays to stable lead (Pb-207) including four alpha and two beta decays (Table 31.1). The most important alpha decay is that of Ra-223 with a half-life of 11.4 days followed by five short-living radionuclides [11]. The alpha radiation of Ra-223 and its daughter nuclides delivers 95% of the emitted energy in comparison to only 3.6% and 1.1% produced by beta and gamma radiation. The alpha energy ranges between 5.0 and 7.5 MeV; the beta and gamma energy lies between 0.445 and 0.492 MeV and 0.01 and 1.27 MeV, respectively. Alpha radiation has a high linear energy transfer (LET) that is defined as the ionizing capacity per track length unit and ranges between 50 and 100 μm equalizing one to two cell diameters. In comparison to ß-radiation, alpha emitters deliver a markedly higher amount of energy on a much shorter range (Figs. 31.1 and 31.2).

Table 31.1 Characteristics of radium-223 chloride

Half-life	11.4 days
Radiation characteristics	Alpha particles
Specific activity	1.9 MBq/ng
Concentration	1.1 MBq/ml
Application form	Saline solution

A variety of ß-emitters were investigated for therapy of bone metastases. The maximal ß-energy lies between 0.8 and 2.3 MeV, the average ß-energy between 0.27 and 0.8 MeV. The electrons deposit their radiation energy in a field of a few millimetres around the place of decay. The physical half-life of the beta nuclides differs importantly from each other (2–52 days). Therefore, the energy per time unit transferred to the tissue varies from nuclide to nuclide, although the total amount of radiation energy may be the same for two radionuclides. Principally, the radiation dose can be applied over a very short period necessitating a high dose rate (e.g. samarium-153 or rhenium-188) or over a longer time period administering a radionuclide with a low dose rate (e.g. strontium-89) [12, 13]. Since the aspect of killing tumour cells has gained more and more importance, new treatment schemes that use repeated radionuclide applications and that administer radionuclides combined with low-dose chemotherapy are increasingly favourized [12, 13].

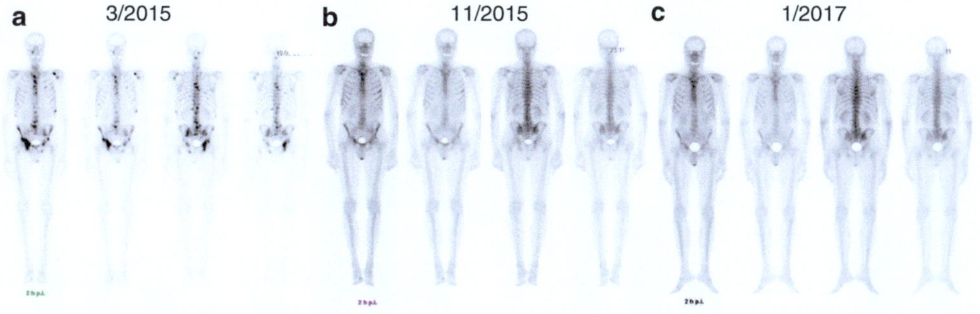

Fig. 31.1 58-year-old patient with castration-resistant prostate cancer that was proven by fine needle biopsy 1 year before the beginning of radionuclide therapy with radium-223 chloride. Multifocal bone metastases were present at the time of initial diagnosis. The patient was treated with a first injection of radium-223 chloride, February 2015. At this time point, the patient received an antihormonal medication with enzalutamide and a treatment with denosumab. Under this medication he developed progressive pain symptoms: he presented significant pain throughout the vertebral column, in the region of the pelvis and the rips and the hips (visual analogue scale 9). Pain medication was ibuprofen 800 4×1 tabl./day. Whole body bone scintigraphy in planar technique shows multifocal metastases of the body stem (**a**). Interestingly, the prostate cancer was PSA negative. Also alkaline phosphatase was within the normal range. The patient received six injections of radium-223 chloride. During the course of radionuclide therapy, pain symptoms were significantly decreased and pain medication could be reduced. It is noteworthy that pain in the right hip was significantly reduced to VAS 1–2 although radiation therapy of this region was done 1 year before. The patient tolerated radionuclide therapy without any side effects. Thrombocytes and leukocytes (neutrophils) did not show significant alterations after therapy. Whole body bone scintigraphy 3 (**b**) and 16 (**c**) months after the last radium-223 injection confirmed a significant improvement of osseous metastases indicating only minor rest activity in the bone metastases

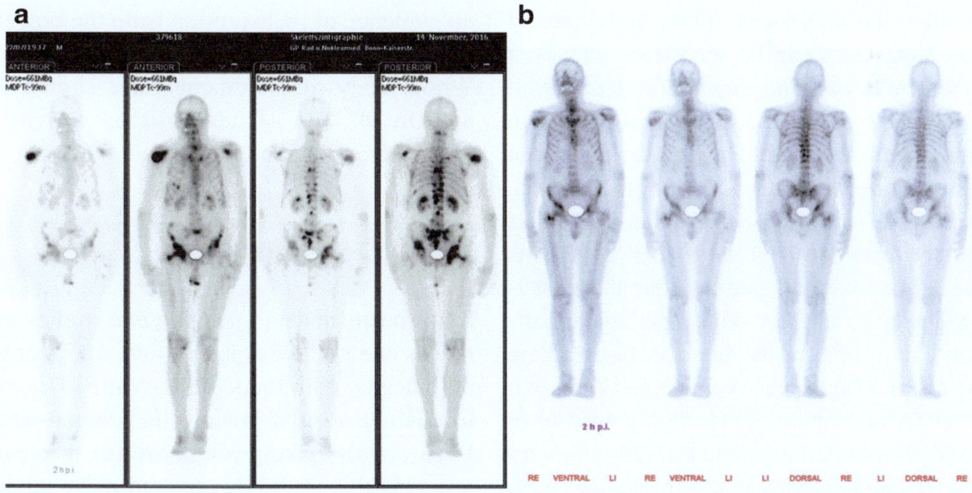

Fig. 31.2 88-year-old patient with multifocal, painful bone metastases (**a**) demonstrating good accumulation in whole body scintigraphy (initial diagnosis pT1c pNx G3 L0 V0 pN0 R1, Gleason score 5 + 4 = 9). Chemotherapy with taxotere was performed for 3 months until February 2016. Secondary antihormonal treatment with abiraterone was started in summer 2015 and was switched to enzalutamide in October 2016. Additionally, the patient received bone therapy with denosumab. Due to clear PSA progression and significant pain symptoms (thorax VAS 4) radionuclide therapy was proposed after the exclusion of visceral metastases. No pain medication was taken. Six injections of radium-223 chloride could be applied. After the second injection of radium-223 chloride pain symptoms disappeared and no pain medication was necessary. The patient remained in a good state during the complete phase of radionuclide treatment. He did not report any side effects; thrombocytes and neutrophils remained stable. However, haemoglobin decreased during the following course of disease. PSA and alkaline phosphatase values showed a significant decrease during therapy (see **c**, **d**). Whole body scintigraphy 2 months after the end of radionuclide therapy showed a significant improvement of osseous disease (**b**)

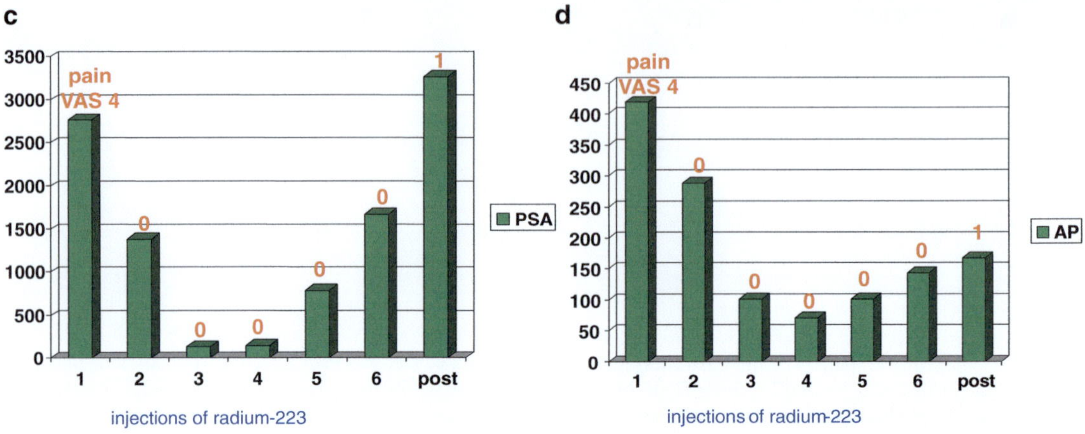

Fig. 31.2 (continued)

31.3 Uptake Mechanism and Biodistribution

Ra-223 is a calcium analogue that is accumulated in high concentration in the area of bone metastases where the osteoblasts induce an increased bone metabolism. Following the principle of theranostics, the high tracer uptake in the area of osseous metastases can be visualized and even quantified by bone scintigraphy correlating well with the uptake of Ra-223 [11]. Already 10 min after the administration of Ra-223, the tracer can be found on bone surface and in the small bowel. The amount of activity bound to the bone after 4 h ranged between 44% and 77%. Ra-223 is complexed to hydroxylapathite after the attachment to the bone surface. With a biological half-time of 1 day, 17% of the bone surface radium will be transferred to bone volume and 83% will be retransferred to blood [14]. Eighty percent of this to-bone-volume integrated Ra-223 will reappear on the bone surface with a biological half-time of 30 days, the remaining 20% is kept as unchangeable in the bones for many years.

After the injection, Ra-223 is rapidly cleared from the vascular compartment. In a phase I study in men with castration-resistant prostate cancer, only 2% of the administered radium activity was left in the vasculature after 4 h [15]. The biodistribution studies showed early passage into the small bowl and subsequent faecal excretion with a median of 52% of applied Ra-223 at 24 h. No relevant hepatobiliary excretion was found. Only about 4% of administered activity will be cleared by urinary excretion [15]. Nilsson et al. supposed main clearing by the hepatobiliary route [16]. However, imaging studies could not confirm this [15]. There was no evidence of reabsorption from the bowel, but further passage via the large bowel was proven. Whole body measurements have shown that a median of 76% of administered activity was cleared from the body.

31.4 Dosimetry

It has been shown in cell survival studies that as few as one to three alpha particle tracks crossing the nucleus may induce cell death [17]). Alpha irradiation results mainly in double-stranded DNA breaks making cellular repair mechanisms less effective [18]. Also tumour cells staying in the inactive G0 phase of the cell cycle may be eliminated by high LET alpha radiation [19].

Lassmann et al. have performed dosimetric calculations for 25 organs or tissues referring to a complete therapy of six Ra-223 injections [14]. The highest organ dose coefficient was found for the bone and red bone marrow followed by liver, colon and intestines. After a completed treatment schedule for a standard 70 kg patient, the absorbed

Table 31.2 Dosimetry of radium-223

Organ	Radiation dose in Gy/MBq
Bone tissue	1.152
Red bone marrow	0.138
Colon	0.007
Small bowel	0.007
Kidneys	0.003
Whole body	0.023

alpha dose for bone and red marrow was 16 Gy and 1.5 Gy, respectively (Table 31.2). However, haematotoxicity was lower than expected what might be due to the short-range radiation and its special microdistribution. The whole body dose for one injection is calculated with 0.023 Gy per MBq resulting in dose equivalent of 80 mSv (for a patient with 70 kg body weight). After six injections of Ra-223, the total radiation dose for the colon, small bowel, kidneys and liver is 0.0078 Gy, 0.0072 Gy, 0.0032 Gy and 0.0029 Gy per MBq, respectively. In bone metastases, one injection of radium-223 could deliver between 5 and 76 Gy [14].

All available radiopharmaceuticals for treatment of bone metastases (Ra-223 chloride, Sr-89 chloride, Re-186/Re-188 HEDP and Sm-153 EDTMP) do not accumulate in the tumour cell itself, but they are deposited in close vicinity in the bone emitting effective radiation to tumour and pain mediator cells. The higher the energy of the radionuclide the longer is the range of the alpha particles and the electrons into tissue. Since bone is characterized by high energy absorption the range of therapeutic electrons emitted by osteotropic radionuclides does not reach more than a few millimetres at a maximum.

The creation of bone tissue takes place around conglomerations of tumour cells in primitive tumour bone or osteoid. If osteolytic metastases are present, a broad resorption line in lacunes is found in a distance of 80–100 μm to the tumour borders. In case of osteoblastic metastases, resorption lacunes are rarely found. Typically, the trabecula is covered by freshly produced bone tissue and the agent is integrated deeply in the bone structure. Therefore, the accumulation of radiopharmaceuticals is much higher in osteoblastic than in osteolytic metastases with ratios of 1:15 and 1:3 (normal bone to osseous metastases), respectively. The uptake of the radionuclide determines the therapeutic dose in the bone metastases and, thus, following the principle of theranostics, the performance of bone scintigraphy previous to treatment is indispensable even if osseous metastases have yet been diagnosed by other imaging modalities like CT or MRI or PSMA-PET [20].

31.5 Pain Documentation

Documentation of pain is important because large inter- and intraindividual variations exist for the parameter 'pain' and, furthermore, patients are not able to remind reliably pain status over a long period, retrospectively. Chronic pain results in important alterations of the patient's behaviour concerning all fields of life. It is recommended to use standardized questionnaires for pain documentation to evaluate the success of the treatment. Pain questionnaires should not be preserved for scientific purposes. Moreover, the clinician should increasingly perform patient interrogations by standardized pain questionnaires to sustain the decisions for further treatment. For the daily routine, such a questionnaire must be short but efficient enough to comprise the fields 'pain', activity of patient' and 'consumption of analgesics'. For prostate cancer patient, standardized pain and quality of life questionnaires are available (e.g. brief pain inventory short form, BPI-SF) [21].

31.6 Clinical Indications

Therapy with Ra-223 is indicated in patients with castration-resistant prostate cancer and symptomatic, metastatic osseous disease without visceral metastases [4]. The presence of lymph node metastases is no contraindication for alpha radiation therapy (Table 31.3). Symptomatic patient means the presence of pain or a reduction of quality of life due to the metastatic disease [22]. If the patient takes pain medication he/she can be considered as symp-

Table 31.3 Checklist for patient selection

– Symptomatic patient (mild to significant symptoms, reduction of quality of life, pain medication)
– Castration-resistant prostate cancer
– No visceral metastases
– Reception of two systemic treatments like chemotherapy or abiraterone

tomatic and therapy with Ra-223 can be applied also if pain is not the predominant symptom at the time of examination.

The existing national and European guidelines recommend alpha radionuclide therapy as a first-line or second-line treatment in patients with mild or moderate or significant clinical symptoms due to bone metastases of prostate cancer in the castration-resistant stage of disease [9, 10].

However, an interim analysis of a phase III study combining radium-223 chloride and abiraterone and prednisolone in chemotherapy-naïve patients has shown a higher risk for fractures and a tendency (not statistically significant) for higher mortality (ERA-223 study). Therefore, the simultaneous treatment of prostate cancer patients with radium-223 and abiraterone/prednisolone is contraindicated. Although there is no further data for the effect of combination of radium-223 and other hormonal treatments like enzalutamide, the use of Xofigo has been restricted to symptomatic patients who show disease progression after having received two systemic treatment modalities (e.g. abiraterone and chemotherapy) or who are not available for the aforementioned second-line treatments. This means that radium-223 chloride can be applied only as second- or third-line treatment in symptomatic prostate cancer patients at a late stage of disease. This decision seems to be inadequate and not data based because efficiency and safety of radium-223 as a monotherapy before and after chemotherapy has been proven in a randomized phase III trial. Furthermore, there are data showing that using chemotherapy or second-line hormonal therapy after or before therapy with Ra-223 is feasible and safe [23, 24]. However, prostate cancer patients can be treated simultaneously by radium-223 and LHRH analogues.

31.7 Effects of Therapy

It has been shown that radionuclide therapy with Ra-223 is an effective antitumour therapy prolonging survival in castration-resistant prostate cancer patients with osseous metastases [4]. In a phase 3, randomized, double-blind, placebo-controlled study, 921 patients were included [4]. The patients received either six injections of Ra-223 or placebo. In the treatment group of 614 patients, 56% of patients received previous chemotherapy with docetaxel. In the placebo group of 307 patients, it was the same situation meaning that 57% of the patients already had chemotherapy before radium-223 injections. Simultaneous use of bisphosphonates was observed in 41% of the treatment group and in 40% of the placebo group, respectively. ECOG performance status of 0 and 1 was observed in 27% and 25%, 60% and 61% in the treatment and placebo group, respectively. Six or more osseous metastases were reported in 84% of patients in the radium-223 treatment group and in 88% of the patients in the placebo group. With regard to the pretreatment and the clinical performance status, it can be stated that both study groups were comparable. Bone scintigraphy was used to show sufficient tracer accumulation in the bone metastases before therapy with Ra-223. Also, the two groups did not show a significant difference with regard to pretreatment PSA, LDH and alkaline phosphatase levels.

In these two comparable patient groups, the patients treated with Ra-223 showed a longer survival of 14.9 months vs. 11.3 months in the placebo group [4]. The median gain of overall survival with 3.6 months was highly statistically significant. The effect of Ra-223 on overall survival was consistent across all subgroups and was not depending on the previous use of docetaxel, the baseline ECOG performance status, the extent of bone disease, the existence of opioid intake or the simultaneous bisphosphonate use.

In the ALSYMPCA study [4], also all main secondary endpoints provided strong support for the benefit of radionuclide treatment over placebo. The results of Ra-223 therapy on symptomatic skeletal events was reported in a special analysis [5]. In this subanalysis, symptomatic skeletal events occurred in 33% of patients in the Ra-223 group and in 38% of patients in the placebo group. Time to first symptomatic skeletal event which was defined as either regular use of analgesic medication for cancer-related bone pain or treatment with external beam radiation therapy for bone pain within the previous 12 weeks was longer with Ra-223 than with placebo (15.6 months vs. 9.8 months). Furthermore, the risk of spinal cord compression was reduced significantly by Ra-223. However, the risk of symptomatic pathological bone fractures or the need of tumour-related orthopaedic surgical intervention was not clearly reduced.

The effect of radionuclide therapy of delaying the development of first symptomatic skeletal events was not depending on the previous use of docetaxel, the baseline ALP value or bisphosphonate use. These results shows clearly that the overall pain situation and quality of life of the patient treated by radionuclide therapy with Ra-223 can be significantly improved and, finally, result also in a gain of quality of life in the prolonged survival time [25].

31.8 Side Effects

Side effects are the result of radiation doses to organs and tissues. Pharmacological effects of Ra-223 are not expected because the amount is very low with 2 ng. When Ra-223 is applied, especially, the intestine and red bone marrow are affected. Most frequent symptoms observed are diarrhoea, nausea, vomiting and thrombocytopenia followed by neutropenia and lymphopenia [4]. Our experience is that diarrhoea and nausea will last for some days and disappear spontaneously. In most cases, these side effects are moderate and will not have a major impact on the patient's quality of life. In the ALSYMPCA study [4], thrombocytopenia was found in only 11.5% of patients which is a rather low rate compared to that observed after chemotherapy. Thrombocytopenia of higher grade [3, 4] was found in 6.3%. If patient did not have previous chemotherapy this rate was even lower with 2.8%. However, after treatment with chemotherapy, the patients showed a significant decrease of thrombocytes (grades 3 and 4) in 8.9% of cases. Patients showing a high extent of metastatic disease ('superscan') also had a somehow higher rate of overall thrombocytopenia with 19.6% including 5.9% grade 3 and 4 toxicities.

Neutropenia of all grades was observed in 5% of patients. Grade 3 and 4 toxicity was found in only 2.2% of patients what compares favourable with chemotherapy. Patients that received docetaxel before Ra-223 therapy versus those that did not showed grade 3 and 4 toxicity in 3.2% vs. 0.8%, respectively. In a phase I study, the nadir of thrombo- and neutropenia was observed 2–3 weeks after a single Ra-223 injection [11].

Due to these potential haematological side effects it is mandatory to check blood counts within 14 days before the start of therapy with radium-223. Counts for neutrophils, thrombocytes and haemoglobin should be higher than 1.5×10^9/l, 100×10^9/l and 10.0 g/dl, respectively. After each injection, further check of blood counts is necessary. During ongoing treatment, counts for neutrophils and thrombocytes should be higher than 1.0×10^9/l and 50×10^9/l, respectively. In patients with extensive metastatic bone disease (e.g. superscan), haematological toxicity is higher. Therefore, it might be necessary to decrease the administered dose of radium-223. Also the administration of chemotherapy given several weeks before the planned radionuclide therapy can result in a limited bone marrow reserve. However, the available data has shown that, in patients with normal blood counts after previous chemotherapy, treatment with radium-223 can be applied without significantly increased risk [24]. Also external beam radiation therapy seems to be no risk factor if it is applied only locally.

In patients with known chronic inflammatory disease of the bowel, decision for treatment should be taken with care because the elimination of radioactivity by the bowel might worsen the inflammation. However, no data is available sustaining this theory.

In the ALSYMPCA study, osteonecrosis of the jaw was observed in 0.67% (4 of 600) of the patients in the radium-233 group compared to 0.33% (1 of 301) patients in the placebo group [4]. It is noteworthy that all patients with osteonecrosis had obtained previous chemotherapy combined with bisphosphonates which are likely to have caused this bone effect.

During a follow-up time of 3 years, no radium-223-induced neoplasia has been reported [26].

31.9 Protocol of Application

How many injections should be given for radionuclide therapy with radium-223 chloride? In the beginning of radionuclide therapy for bone metastases, only single injection treatments were performed [11]. Palmedo et al. showed that the repeated injection of a beta-emitting radiopharmaceutical results in better effect of treatment [7, 27]. It was shown that PSA decline could be achieved in 67% of patients that underwent repeated radionuclide therapy in contrast to only 18% of patients receiving only single injection treatment [7]. In this randomized phase 2 trial, patients receiving rhenium-188 HDP for a second time after 4 weeks showed better overall survival of 16.8 months in comparison to 13.3 months in the control group. Since toxicity in the repeated treatment group was not increased significantly, further research was performed including a treatment protocol with up to 6 injections per patient. In a later study of the same group, Biersack et al. could show that the patient group receiving six injections of rhenium-188 HDP showed significantly better survival than the patient group receiving only one or two injections [27]. There was only moderate toxicity in all three patient groups.

Consecutively, repeated therapy was studied also by using alpha radiation therapy. Nilsson et al. started different application schedules including a patient group receiving up to four injections with a time interval of 4 weeks [12, 13]. They also investigated different activity groups, the one group received 5 kBq/kg radium-223 chloride and the other groups 25, 50 and 100 kBq/kg radium-223 chloride, respectively. They found that toxicity was not significantly increased in

Table 31.4 Patient preparation and treatment

– Contact patient 2 days before therapy
– Calculation of dose
– Indwelling catheter to avoid paravenous infusion
– Prepare application room (radiation protection)
– Prepare radium-223 syringe

the groups that received one injection using an activity up to 100 kBq/kg radium-223 chloride. However, a decline of alkaline phosphatase was observed in the groups with 50 and 100 kBq/kg radium-223 chloride.

Aiming at a low toxicity in the palliative care situation of the patient, a standard dose of 55 KBq radium-223 chloride per kilogram body weight for a single injection is actually recommended [28]. Finally, the standard protocol that was used for the ALSYMPCA study, including six injections of radium-223 chloride with a time interval of 4 weeks between the treatments, is the chosen standard protocol (Table 31.4).

31.10 Patient Preparation

It is essential to select the patients adequately (Table 31.5). Castration resistance has to be proven by determination of testosterone levels.

The patient has to be symptomatic meaning that either pain medication is given or a pain syndrome is present. Also shortcomings due to bone metastases like reduced quality of life or reduced mobility should be defined as a symptomatic situation. It is mandatory to proof accumulating bone metastases by bone scintigraphy. Ideally, bone scintigraphy should be performed in SPECT-CT technique of the body stem because more bone metastases will be detected as shown in recent studies [20]. Following the principle of theranostic, bone scintigraphy gives pretherapeutic estimation of dosimetry and should not be replaced by any other imaging modality like CT, MRI or PSMA-PET/CT. However, CT of the abdomen and ideally of the thorax (alternatively x-ray of the thorax) should be performed and results be available to exclude visceral metastases [28]. The presence of lymph node metastases is no contraindication for radium-223 therapy.

Table 31.5 Checklist for pretreatment documents, diagnostics and laboratory values

– X-ray thorax, CT of thorax/abdomen
– Bone scintigraphy (principle of theranostic)
– Thrombocytes (> 100 × 10^9/l), leukocytes, neutrophils (>1.5 × 10^9/l), haemoglobin creatinine, calcium
– Testosterone
– PSA, alkaline phosphatase, LDH
– Pain documentation (visual analogue scale)
– Pain medication
– Previous medical reports
– Informed consent

Table 31.6 Follow-up of patient

– Pain score, pain medication, further interventions
– Bone scintigraphy after 6–8 weeks
– In case of progression alternative treatments
– PSMA-PET-CT and potentially Lutetium-177 PSMA therapy

However, extraosseous metastases, for example, in the lung or liver should make the treating physician choose another treatment option like chemotherapy or hormonal therapy. Laboratory values including calcium, creatinine, leukocytes, thrombocytes, neutrophils, alkaline phosphatase and PSA must be available before deciding to treat. Progression of disease should be documented by three subsequent PSA measurements or imaging modalities or symptoms of the patient (Table 31.6). Also medical reports must be available and the close contact to the urologist and oncologist is necessary.

References

1. Palmedo H, Guhlke S, Bender H, Sartor J, Schoeneich G, Risse J, Grünwald F, Knapp F.F, Biersack HJ. Dose escalation study with rhenium-188 HEDP in prostate cancer patients with osseous metastases. Eur J Nucl Med 2000;27:123–130.
2. Hillner BE, et al. American society of clinical oncology guideline on the role of bisphosphonates in breast cancer. J Clin Oncol. 2000;18:1378–91.
3. Tu SM, Kim J, Pagliaro LC, Vakar-Lopez F, Wong FC, Wen S, General R, Podoloff DA, Lin SH, Logothetis CJ. Therapy tolerance in selected patients with androgen-independent prostate cancer following strontium-89 combined with chemotherapy. J Clin Oncol. 2005;23(31):7904–10.
4. Parker C, Nilsson S, Heinrich D, et al. Alpha emitter radium-223 and survival in metastatic prostate cancer. N Engl J Med. 2013;369:213–23.
5. Sartor O, Coleman R, Nilsson S, et al. Effect of radium-223 dichloride on symptomatic skeletal events in patients with castration-resistant prostate cancer and bone metastases: results from a phase 3, double-blind, randomised trial. Lancet Oncol. 2014;15:738–46.
6. Palmedo H, Bender H, Dierke-Dzierzon C, Carl UM, Krebs D, Risse J, Biersack HJ. Pain palliation with Rhenium-186 HEDP in breast cancer patients with disseminated bone metastases. Clin Nucl Med. 1999;24:643–8.
7. Palmedo H, Manka-Waluch A, Albers P, Schmidt-Wolf IG, Reinhardt M, Ezziddin S, Joe A, Roedel R, Fimmers R, Knapp FF Jr, Guhlke S, Biersack HJ. Repeated bone-targeted therapy for hormone-refractory prostate carcinoma: tandomized phase II trial with the new, high-energy radiopharmaceutical rhenium-188 hydroxyethylidenediphosphonate. J Clin Oncol. 2003;21(15):2869–75.
8. Tu S, Millikan RE, Mengistu B, et al. Bone targeted therapy for advanced androgen-imdependent carcinoma of the prostate: randomised phase II trial. Lancet. 2001;357:336–41.
9. Interdisziplinäre Leitlinie der Qualität S3 zur Früherkennung, Diagnose und Therapie der verschiedenen Stadien des Prostatakarzinoms 2. Aktualisierung – Oktober 2014 AWMF-Register-Nummer 043/022OL.
10. European guideline, prostate cancer.
11. Nilsson S, Larsen RH, Fosså SD, Balteskard L, Borch KW, Westlin JE, Salberg G, Bruland OS. First clinical experience with alpha-emitting radium-223 in the treatment of skeletal metastases. First clinical experience with alpha-emitting radium-223 in the treatment of skeletal metastases. Clin Cancer Res. 2005;11(12):4451–9.
12. Serafini AN, Houston SJ, Resche I, et al. Palliation of pain associated with metastatic bone cancer using Samarium-153 lexidronam: a double blind placebo-controlled trial. J Clin Oncol. 1998;16:1574–81.
13. Nilsson S, Franzén L, Parker C, Tyrrell C, Blom R, Tennvall J, Lennernäs B, Petersson U, Johannessen DC, Sokal M, Pigott K, Yachnin J, Garkavij M, Strang P, Harmenberg J, Bolstad B, Bruland OS. Bone-targeted radium-223 in symptomatic, hormone-refractory prostate cancer: a randomised, multicentre, placebo-controlled phase II study. Lancet Oncol. 2007;8(7):587–94.
14. Lassmann et al Eur J Nucl Med Mol Imaging 2013;40:207.
15. Carrasquillo Eur J Nucl Med Mol Imaging 2013 EJNM 2013.
16. Clin Canc Res 2005:11;4451.
17. Hobbs RF et al. Phys Med Biol 2012 3207–3222.
18. Ritter MA, et al. Nature. 1977;266:5603.
19. Bruland OS, et al. Clin Cancer Res. 2006;12:6250.

20. Palmedo H, Marx C, Ebert A, Kreft B, Ko Y, Türler A, Vorreuther R, Göhring U, Schild HH, Gerhardt T, Pöge U, Ezziddin S, Biersack HJ, Ahmadzadehfar H. Whole-body SPECT/CT for bone scintigraphy: diagnostic value and effect on patient management in oncological patients. Eur J Nucl Med Mol Imaging. 2014;41(1):59–67.
21. Palmedo H, Eschmann S, Werner A, Selinski I, Möllers MO, Pinkert J, van Crüchten I Neußer T, Pöppel T. First interim analysis of PARABO – a non-interventional study evaluating mCRPC patients with bone metastases treated with radium-223 in a real life german practice setting. Abstract march 2018 European Association of Urology, Kopenhagen.
22. Parker C, Finkelstein SE, Michalski JM, et al. Efficacy and safety of radium-223 dichloride in symptomatic castration-resistant prostate cancer patients with or without baseline opioid use from the phase 3 ALSYMPCA trial. Eur Urol. 2016;70:875–83.
23. Saad F, Carles J, Gillessen S, Heidenreich A, Heinrich D, Gratt J, Lévy J, Miller K, Nilsson S, Petrenciuc O, Tucci M, Wirth M, Federhofer J. O'Sullivan JM; Radium-223 international early access program investigators. Radium-223 and concomitant therapies in patients with metastatic castration-resistant prostate cancer: an international, early access, open-label, single-arm phase 3b trial. Lancet Oncol. 2016;17(9):1306–16.
24. Hoskin P, Sartor O, O'Sullivan JM, et al. Efficacy and safety of radium-223 dichloride in patients with castration-resistant prostate cancer and symptomatic bone metastases, with or without previous docetaxel use: a prespecified subgroup analysis from the randomised, double-blind, phase 3 ALSYMPCA trial. Lancet Oncol. 2014;15:1397–406.
25. Nilsson S, Cislo P, Sartor O, Vogelzang NJ, Coleman RE, O'Sullivan JM, Reuning-Scherer J, Shan M, Zhan L, Parker C. Patient-reported quality-of-life analysis of radium-223 dichloride from the phase III ALSYMPCA study. Ann Oncol. 2016;27(5):868–74.
26. Parker CC, Coleman RE, Sartor O, Vogelzang NJ, Bottomley D, Heinrich D, Helle SI, O'Sullivan JM, Fosså SD, Chodacki A, Wiechno P, Logue J, Seke M, Widmark A, Johannessen DC, Hoskin P, James ND, Solberg A, Syndikus I, Kliment J, Wedel S, Boehmer S, Dall'Oglio M, Franzén L, Bruland ØS, Petrenciuc O, Staudacher K, Li R, Nilsson S. Three-year safety of Radium-223 dichloride in patients with castration-resistant prostate cancer and symptomatic bone metastases from phase 3 randomized Alpharadin in symptomatic prostate cancer trial. Eur Urol. 73(3):427–35.
27. Biersack HJ, Palmedo H, Andris A, Rogenhofer S, Knapp FF, Guhlke S, Ezziddin S, Bucerius J, von Mallek D. Palliation and survival after repeated (188) Re-HEDP therapy of hormone-refractory bone metastases of prostate cancer: a retrospective analysis. J Nucl Med. 2011;52(11):1721.
28. Poeppel TD, Handkiewicz-Junak D, Andreeff M, Becherer A, Bockisch A, Fricke E, Geworski L, Heinzel A, Krause BJ, Krause T, Mitterhauser M, Sonnenschein W, Bodei L, Delgado-Bolton RC, Gabriel M. EANM guideline for radionuclide therapy with radium-223 of metastatic castration-resistant prostate cancer. Eur J Nucl Med Mol Imaging. 2018;45(5):824–45.

32 Peptide Receptor Radionuclide Therapy

Anna Yordanova

32.1 Introduction

Neuroendocrine tumours (NET) are neoplasms, which comprise the features of both endocrine cells and nerve cells. Although they are rare, the incidence is continuously rising. Most of the NETs present with slow proliferation and absent clinical symptoms; for that reason, they are often diagnosed either as incidental finding or at advanced stage with inoperable disease. Most frequent NETs are bronchopulmonary NET and gastroenteropancreatic (GEP) NETs. GEP-NETs originate most frequently from the pancreas, duodenum, midgut (jejunum, ileum and proximal colon), rectum, appendix and colon. Well-differentiated NETs overexpress somatostatin receptors (SSTRs), especially the SSTR-2 subtype [1, 2].

Peptide receptor radionuclide therapy (PRRT) uses, as a therapeutic target, the overexpression of SSTR in NET, and it shows a high affinity for the most frequent receptor subtype, SSTR2. PRRT has been shown to be especially effective in patients with slow-growing, G1–G2 (well-/moderately differentiated) GEP-NETs [3–9]. NETTER-1 is a recent prospective randomized phase III trial which showed a clear benefit from PRRT in comparison to non-radiolabelled somatostatin analogues in patients with advanced midgut NET. The study is pointing this therapy as a promising treatment option in unresectable midgut NET [9]. Another advantage of this therapy is its favourable toxicity profile. Several studies have shown a good tolerability regarding renal function and haematopoiesis of patients [4, 5, 7, 10–15].

32.2 Radiopharmaceuticals

There are several radiopharmaceuticals used for the PRRT in patients with somatostatin receptor-positive advanced non-resectable neuroendocrine tumours. All agents have similar structure and consist of a somatostatin analogue, which binds the target: somatostatin receptors and a linking molecule (chelator), which binds the radioisotope and enables stable connection between the binding molecule and the radionuclide (Fig. 32.1). After the radiolabelled somatostatin analogue binds the G-protein-coupled somatostatin receptor, it mediates the internalization of the radiolabelled somatostatin analogue and the intracellular retention of the radiopeptide. In this way PRRT is able to irradiate the intracellular components of the cancer cells with high doses, resulting in inhibition of the tumour proliferation or tumour shrinkage (Fig. 32.2) [16]. Different conjugates of radioisotopes and somatostatin analogues are used in the practice for targeting somatostatin receptor-positive tumours.

A. Yordanova (✉)
Department of Radiology, St. Marien Hospital, Bonn, Germany

Department of Nuclear Medicine, University Hospital Bonn, Bonn, Germany
e-mail: anna.yordanova@mail.de

H. Ahmadzadehfar et al. (eds.), *Clinical Nuclear Medicine*,
https://doi.org/10.1007/978-3-030-39457-8_32

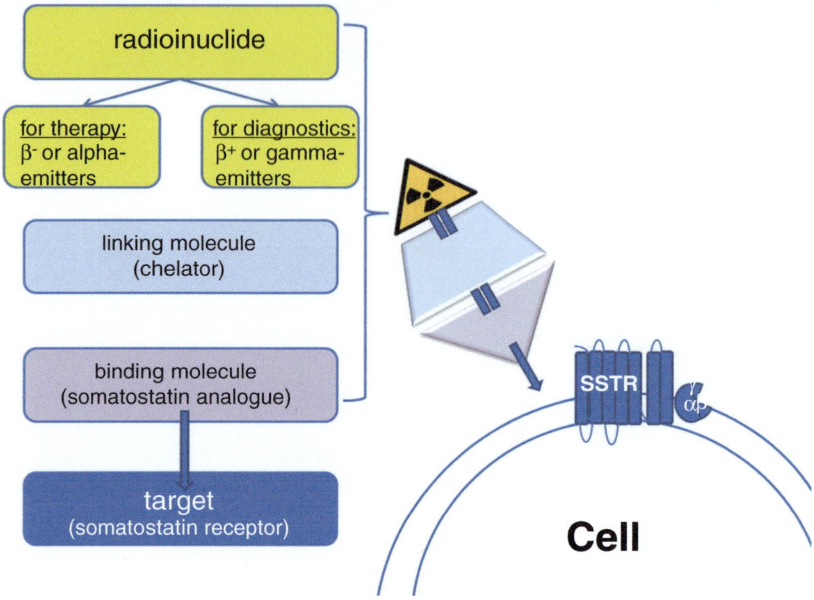

Fig. 32.1 Radiopharmaceutical model. The image shows a simplified model of a radiopharmaceutical, which consists of a binding molecule (somatostatin analogue), which binds the target (somatostatin receptor), and a linking molecule (chelator such as DOTA or DTPA), which binds the radioisotope

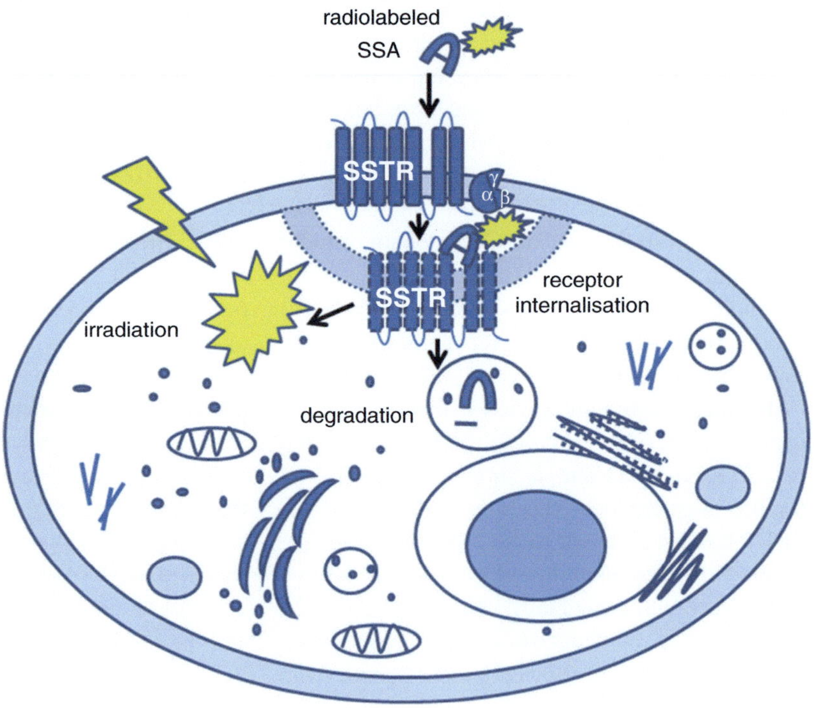

Fig. 32.2 Model of a neuroendocrine cell with a somatostatin receptor, which binds radiolabelled somatostatin analogue. The G-protein-coupled somatostatin receptor (SSTR) mediates the internalization of the radiolabelled somatostatin analogue (SSA) and the intracellular retention of the radiopeptide. In this way PRRT is able to irradiate the intracellular components of the cancer cells with high doses, resulting in inhibition of the tumour proliferation or tumour shrinkage

32.2.1 Somatostatin Receptor Targeting

32.2.1.1 Somatostatin Receptors as Targets

Well-differentiated GEP-NETs overexpress somatostatin receptors [17, 18]. Somatostatin (SST) is a hypothalamic peptide hormone that inhibits the secretion of the pituitary growth hormone. G-protein-coupled SSTRs are widely expressed in various tissues in the body, for example, in islet cells of the pancreas, gastrointestinal tract, endocrine organs and immune and haematopoietic system. Somatostatin inhibits the hormone and growth factor secretion, regulates the immune system and acts anti-proliferative [19–24].

Modulation functions of somatostatin are mediated by G-protein-coupled SSTRs (SST1 to SST5). There are two variants of SST2: unspliced (SST2A) and spliced (SST2B). The most frequent type in well-differentiated GEP-NET is SST2, followed by SST1, SST5 and SST3. The level of expression of SSTRs depends on the grading of the tumour: higher expression in well-differentiated neoplasm than in the poorly differentiated cancer. Technics of the detection of the different SSTR subtypes are the examination of mRNA, autoradiography and immunohistochemistry [18, 23, 25].

SSTRs are mostly localized homogeneously throughout GEP-NETs, making them potential therapeutic targets. However, somatostatin is in vivo rapidly degraded (half-life 1–3 min) and for that reason unsuitable for the therapy. Thus, more stable synthetic analogues, such as Octreotide and Lanreotide, have been developed. They have high affinity for SSTR2 and lower affinities for SSTR3 and SSTR5. The SST analogues are approved for the therapy of functioning neuroendocrine tumours with hormone-related symptoms [26, 27]. Subsequently, radioactive-labelled somatostatin analogues have been developed for the therapy of NETs. 111In-diethylenetriaminepentaacetic acid (DTPA)0-octreotide was the first widely available radiopharmaceutical for the therapy and was then replaced by DOTA-coupled, somatostatin-based radiopeptides [DOTA0,Tyr3]-Octreotide (DOTATOC) and [DOTA0,Tyr3,Thr8]-Octreotide (DOTATATE), which had significant better affinity to SSTR, especially SSTR2 [28]. Another compound with high affinity to SSTR3 and SSTR5 is 1-naphthyl-alanine (1-Nal) (DOTANOC).

Newer development for targeting of SSTR is the application of SSTR antagonists. They have the ability to bind the receptor to multiple sites and seem according to early study results to be more potent than the agonists [29–32].

32.2.1.2 Somatostatin Analogues

There are three available DOTA-conjugated SST analogues which bind specifically SSTRs: DOTATOC (DOTA-D-Phe1-Tyr3-Octreotide), DOTATATE (DOTA-DPhe1,Tyr3-Octreotate) and DOTANOC (DOTA-1-Nal3-Octreotide). However, the affinity of each SSTR subtype is different for the different peptides. For example, DOTATATE and DOTATOC bind preferentially to SSTR-2, but the affinity of DOTATATE to SSTR-2 is nearly tenfold higher [33]. DOTANOC binds with a high affinity to SSTR-5, SSTR-2 and SSTR-3 [34]. Several studies compared the differences in the renal uptake and the renal excretion between radiolabelled DOTATOC and DOTATATE (with Indium-111, Lutetium-177 or Gallium-68). DOTATOC showed the lower renal uptake and therefore is preferred for the diagnostic. DOTATATE had better tumour uptake and therefore is preferred for the therapy [35–37].

32.2.2 Isotopes

There are several isotopes used in PRRT. The pioneer was Indium-111, followed by more potent radionuclides such as Yttrium-90 and Lutetium-177. Newer development is the targeted alpha therapy with Bismuth-213 or Actinium-225. Physical characteristics of the different isotopes are shown in Table 32.1.

32.2.2.1 Indium-111

The pioneer in the therapy with radiolabelled somatostatin analogues in patients with advanced neuroendocrine tumours was Indium-111, linked with the chelator diethylenetriaminepentaacetic acid (DTPA) to D-Phe1-Octreotide ([^{111}In]In-DTPA0-Octreotide). Indium-111 is a gamma emitter, which enables tumour-specific imaging. Furthermore, it emits Auger electrons (tissue penetration range of 0.02–10 μm) and conversion electrons (tissue penetration range of 200–500 μm) with a potentially cytotoxic effect. The tumour response is dependent on internalization of the radiolabelled somatostatin analogues, which allows the Auger electrons to reach the nucleus.

Anthony et al. reported a prolonged survival in patients with GEP neuroendocrine tumours after PRRT with [^{111}In]In-DTPA-Octreotide; however, objective responses were rare (8%) [38]. Eventually, the Indium-111-

Table 32.1 Characteristics of radioisotopes for the PRRT

Radionuclide	Emitted particle	Particle energy (mean MeV)	Maximum tissue penetration range (mm)	Half-life (days)
Indium-111	Auger electron Gamma emission	0.003–0.019 0.1 and 0.2	0.01	2.8
Yttrium-90	Beta emission	0.9	11	2.7
Lutetium-177	Beta emission Gamma emission	0.1 (maximum 0.5) 0.1–0.2	2–3	6.7
Bismuth-213	Beta emission Alpha decay (+ gamma co-emission)	0.4 5.9	0.1	0.03 (46 min)
Actinium-225	Alpha decay	5.1–5.8	0.1	10

labelled somatostatin analogue was replaced by more potent radioisotopes, Yttrium-90 and Lutetium-177 [28].

32.2.2.2 Lutetium-177 and Yttrium-90

Currently, the most frequently applied isotopes for PRRT are Lutetium-177 (maximum beta energy 497 keV (79%), gamma energy 113 KeV (6%) and 208 KeV (11%), half-life: 6.7 days, mean tissue penetration: 0.5–0.6 mm, maximum tissue penetration: 2 mm, betta and gamma emitter) and Yttrium-90 (a pure beta emitter with mean beta particle energy of 935 keV, half-life: 64 h, tissue penetration: mean 2.5 mm, maximum tissue penetration: 11 mm) [39]. Due to the shorter tissue penetration range and lower energy, Lutetium-177 is less toxic than Yttrium-90, which makes it easier to manage and enables the performance of several PRRT cycles without any relevant renal toxicity [2, 40]. Another advantage of Lutetium-177 is the combination of beta and gamma emission. The gamma component enables post-therapeutic imaging, suitable for tumoural uptake assessment and dosimetry purposes [41]. Kratochwil et al. proposed an algorithm for the choice of radionuclide based on the tumour size: larger lesions (>2 cm diameter) should respond better after treatment with Yttrium-90, and smaller lesions (<2 cm diameter) should benefit more from the small-range tissue penetration of Lutetium-177. In heterogeneous and various-sized tumour lesions, a combination of Yttrium-90 and Luterium-177 should be applied [42].

32.2.2.3 Bismuth-213

Bismuth-213 (half-life: 46 min, 98% beta emission, 435 keV, 2% alpha decay, 440 keV gamma emission with an emission probability per decay of 26%) decays to Lead-213 (half-life: 3.7 μs, alpha emitter) and then to Lead-209 (half-life: 3.2 h, beta emitter, 198 keV). Using the gamma co-emission of Bismuth-213, planar imaging (whole body) and SPECT scan can be performed. However, the timeframe is rather short: the scintigraphy should be completed not later than 60 min after [^{213}Bi]Bi-Octreotide administration.

Preclinical data showed a sixfold cell-killing rate in CA20948 in vitro model after exposure of the alpha-particle-labelled somatostatin analogue: [^{213}Bi]Bi-DTPA or [^{213}Bi]Bi-Octreotate compared to [^{177}Lu]Lu-Octreotate [16]. Another survey from the Rotterdam Study Group demonstrated in the mouse model that [^{213}Bi]Bi-Octreotate could significantly decrease tumour burden and improve the overall survival [43].

Kratochwil et al. published in 2014 the first-in-human experience with [^{213}Bi]Bi-Octreotide neuroendocrine tumours refractory to Lutetium-177 or Yttrium-90-labelled PRRT. The study included seven patients. The therapy was administered intravenously except of patients with liver-dominant tumour load: they received intraarterial treatment in the hepatic artery. The majority of patients showed a clinical benefit according to RECIST: 3/7 had stable disease, 2/7 had partial response, 1/7 had complete response, and 2 patients were not accessible for response because of bone marrow carcinosis or disseminated metastases in the liver. The acute haematological toxicity was moderate. One patient developed myelodysplastic syndrome (MDS) 24 months after [^{213}Bi]Bi-Octreotide administration, followed by acute myeloid leukaemia (AML), and eventually the patient died. This patient received previously (5 years before MDS) multiple repeated cycles of [^{90}Y]Y-Octreotide (16 GBq) and [^{177}Lu]Lu-Octreotate (24 GBq) [44].

32.2.2.4 Actinium-225

Actinum-225 is an alpha-emitting isotope with a 10-day half-life and has high cytotoxic activity. Miederer et al. evaluated the biodistribution, toxicity and the efficacy of [^{225}Ac]Ac-Octreotide in pancreatic neuroendocrine tumour-bearing mice. Biodistribution studies showed a good accumulation of [^{225}Ac]Ac-Octreotide in neuroendocrine xenograft tumours. Thirty kBq [^{225}Ac]Ac-Octreotide or higher activities induced tubular necrosis. Activities between 12 and 20 kBq proved to be nontoxic and achieved growth control of neuroendocrine tumours. Furthermore, [^{225}Ac]Ac-Octreotide showed improved efficacy compared to [^{177}Lu]Lu-Octreotate. Therefore, the nuclide Actinium-225 might be an option to improve the response in neuroendocrine tumours [45]. However, even 10 years after the first report from Miederer et al., no clinical data about response and toxicities of PRRT using [^{225}Ac]Ac-Octreotide in patients has been released so far.

32.3 Rationale and Patient Selection

32.3.1 When to Start with PRRT?

According to current guidelines, PRRT can be recommended as second-line therapy in differentiated intestinal NET (SSTR+ status is required) [46, 47]. As a first-line treatment, PRRT can be considered in inoperable midgut NET (G1/G2, SSTR+ status is required) with extended disease and/or extrahepatic disease. In pancreatic NET, PRRT is an option if cytotoxic chemotherapy, everolimus and sunitinib fail or are contraindicated according to current guidelines [46].

The Milan study group published 2004 results of 2 phase I–II studies and retrospective analyses in 141 patients treated with 2–16 cycles [^{90}Y]Y-Octreotide in 4–6 intervals (cumulative dose 7.4–26.4 GBq). The analyses showed that patients with stable disease at baseline had better outcome (objective response in 32%) than patients with progressive disease (objective response in 24%) [48]. Of course, this data needs to be considered cautiously. On the one hand, patients who are stable for a long time with indolent disease progression are hardly comparable to other patients with rapidly progressive disease. On the other hand, waiting until tumour progression might result in more difficult disease control.

Taken together, there is a need of comparative prospective trials to compare the outcome of stable and progressive patients before PRRT. It is important to evaluate not only the response but also the overall survival of patients.

32.3.2 Inclusion and Exclusion Criteria

PRRT is indicated as a palliative treatment in patients with well-differentiated NET with good SSTR expression. Required for the PRRT are good general condition, sufficient bone marrow function and renal function. Table 32.2 summarizes the most important inclusion criteria and contraindications for the PRRT [49].

Laboratory Checklist

- Differential blood count.
- Renal parameters (creatinine, urea, creatinine clearance).
- Liver parameters (bilirubin, albumin, ALP, GGT, ALT, AST, INR).
- Electrolytes (serum potassium and serum calcium).
- LDH.
- Chromogranin A and other secretory products including specific hormones, if elevated at baseline.

Table 32.2 Inclusion and exclusion criteria for PRRT according to the ENETS Consensus Guidelines 2017

Checklist of criteria	Inclusion criteria	Contraindications
Therapeutic options?	Advanced metastatic, unresectable NET, progressive under first-line therapy	Curative operation possible
NET grading	Well-differentiated NET G1/G2 and also G3 NET may be considered	Undifferentiated NEC G3
SSTR imaging	Adequate uptake in SSTR imaging	SSTR-negative lesions/ SSTR-positive lesions in 8-fluorodeoxyglucose (FDG)-PET/CT and combined PRRT with chemotherapy may be considered
Laboratory results	Hb > = 8 g/dl, platelets > = 75 × 10^9/L, WBC > = 2 × 10^9/L creatinine clearance >50 ml/min, bilirubin <3× upper limit of normal, albumin >25 g/dl, prothrombin time increased <1.5 ULN	Hb < 8 g/dl, platelets <75 × 10^9/L, WBC < 2 × 10^9/L creatinine clearance <50 ml/min, bilirubin >3× upper limit or both an albumin <25 g/dl and prothrombin time increased >1.5 ULN
General condition of the patient	Karnofsky Performance Status >50 (ECOG <3) Expected survival >3 months	Severe cardiac/renal/hepatic impairment Karnofsky performance status < = 50 (ECOG > = 3) Expected survival <3 months
General criteria	Signed informed consent	Unable to comprehend and consent for PRRT (e.g. dementia) Pregnancy or ongoing lactation

32.3.3 Dual Molecular Imaging for Better Patient Selection

The indication for PRRT should be discussed for each individual patient in a multidisciplinary tumour board to carefully weigh the advantages and risks of the therapy. Increasing role as a prognostic tool has the so-called theranostics, which means the combination of therapy and diagnostic imaging to "treat what we see" and "to see what we treat" [50]. In this way, potential therapeutic targets could be detected in the imaging, which can help to predict the response of the treatment. Theranostics can be performed by using the same molecule or at least very similar molecules, for example, somatostatin receptor agonists such as DOTATOC and DOTATATE, but differently radiolabelled or molecules labelled with the same isotope, but given in different dosages for diagnostics or therapy [39].

Presupposition for PRRT is the adequate SSTR expression on the molecular imaging such as Octreoscan®/[^{99m}Tc]Tc-EDDA/HYNIC-TOC or Gallium-68-DOTATOC/DOTATATE/DOTANOC. Gallium-68-labelled radiopharmaceuticals have DOTA-conjugated peptides (DOTATOC/DOTATATE/DOTANOC), which bind somatostatin receptors and are used for PET. Compared to SPECT with Octreoscan®/[^{99m}Tc]Tc-EDDA/HYNIC-TOC, the PET imaging with [^{68}Ga]Ga-DOTATOC/DOTATATE/DOTANOC shows better sensitivity and spatial resolution. High uptake in the SSTR imaging correlates with high expression of somatostatin receptors in well-differentiated NET, especially SSTR2 [51, 52]. The tracer uptake in the SSTR imaging can be graded visually using the Krenning score: from 0 (no tracer uptake) to 4 (greater tracer uptake in the tumour than in the spleen) [53]. The Krenning score correlates strongly with the response after PRRT ($p < 0.01$) [54].

Another diagnostic tool used in neuroendocrine tumours is [^{18}F]F-FDG-PET, which shows the metabolic activity of the tumour and is prognostic for the survival. For example, patients with absent/very low uptake in [^{18}F]F-FDG-PET have less aggressive tumours and longer survival than patients with high uptake [55–58]. [^{18}F]F-FDG-PET could be also used for tumour grading similar to the Ki-67 index in the histopathology, which is defined as the proportion of MIB-1-positive cells out of at least 2000 manually counted cells in areas of highest mitotic density. According to the WHO criteria, there are three grades of NET: G1 (Ki-67 < 3%), G2 (Ki-67 3–20%) and G3 (Ki-67 > 20%) [59]. A limiting factor for the determination of the Ki-67 index is the requirement of invasive biopsy. Furthermore, if the NET is diagnosed at late stage with multiple metastases, it is difficult to biopsy all of the tumour sites. Otherwise, randomly selected metastasis might not always be representative for the whole tumour burden. Last, tumour lesions of NET might be very heterogeneous with well- and poor-differentiated tumour cells in the same metastatic site. In this case, a non-invasive metabolic imaging might be useful. Ezziddin and colleagues proposed a metabolic grading score using [^{18}F]F-FDG-PET and the ratio of a reference tumour lesion with the highest tracer uptake and liver uptake: the tumour-to-liver ratio of maximum standardized uptake value (T/L ratio SUVmax). T/L ratio of ≤1.0 corresponded to mG1; mG2 had T/L ratio of 1.0–2.3 and mG3 > 2.3. The metabolic grading seemed in a retrospective analysis to be an independent prognostic factor for the survival of patients (HR, 4.7; $p = 0.015$) [57]. A similar study was conducted in the prospective setting in France from Bahri et al. According to this study, only lesions with SUVmax >4.5 and T/L ratio ≥ 2.5 correlated with poor survival: 4-year survival rate of 0% [55]. [^{18}F]F-FDG-PET can be also useful in low-grade NET or SSTR-positive NET. Binderup et al. showed that G1 tumours with Ki67 < 2% are in 40% of cases FDG-positive, 70% of G1/G2 tumours with Ki-67 between 2% and 15% and 93% of tumours with Ki-67 > 15%. This means that even low-grade NET may be FDG-positive, which indicates poor survival. Therefore, [^{18}F]F-FDG-PET can be a useful tool for the initial staging and follow-up to determine the aggressiveness of the tumour and eventually to initiate a more aggressive treatment.

SSTR imaging and [^{18}F]F-FDG-PET should not be considered as competitive but as complementing diagnostic tools [52, 60]. The combined imaging SSTR-PET and [^{18}F]F-FDG-PET might be the key for personalized medicine improving the tumour grading and helping to choose an individualized treatment. Chan et al. developed a scoring system, dividing subjects according to the tumour uptake in SSTR-PET and [^{18}F]F-FDG-PET: solely SSTR-positive, solely FDG-negative, both SSTR- and FDG-positive and both SSTR- and FDG-negative. This is the so-called NETPET grade, which correlated significantly with the overall survival ($p = 0.0018$ in the univariate analysis) in contrast to the initial WHO grade, which did not seem to be prognostic in this cohort of patients [51] (Table 32.3).

Majority of the studies about PRRT included only G1/G2 tumours, but there is a rising demand for the so-called NET-G3 with a high SSTR expression, especially if they showed no response after chemotherapy or the patients were unsuitable for this treatment. Even though FDG-avidity is associated with a higher tumour grade and poor prognosis, there is data which showed that patients with FDG-avid disease can benefit from a peptide receptor chemo-radionuclide therapy (PRCRT). The results are comparable to the data of other studies with G1/G2 tumours after PRRT [61, 62].

Thus, the role of the differentiation on histopathological examination between well- and poorly differentiated G3 NEN is rising. Furthermore the tracer uptake on SSTR-PET not only correlates with the SSTR expression of the tumour lesions but might be also useful for predicting individual prognosis [63].

Table 32.3 The NETPET score with a relevance of the PRRT indication

Score PET	P0	P1	P2	P3	P4	P5
SSTR	–	+	+	+	+	–
FDG	–	–	+	+	+	+
Correlation SST/FDG uptake	–	–	SST > FDG	SST = FDG	SST < FDG	–
PRRT indicated?	No	Yes	Yes	Yes, but not as monotherapy	No	No

Table 32.4 First-line therapy options in inoperable metastatic neuroendocrine tumours according to the ENET Consensus Guidelines [54]

Drug	Functionality	Grading	Primary site	STTR status	Special considerations
Octreotide	±	G1	Midgut	+	Low tumour burden
Lanreotide	±	G1/G2 (−10%)	Midgut, pancreas	+	Low and high (>25%) liver tumour burden
Interferon alpha	±	G1/G2	Midgut		If SSTR negative
STZ/5-FU	±	G1/G2	Pancreas		Progressive in short-term or high tumour burden or symptomatic
TEM/CAP	±	G2	Pancreas		Progressive in short-term or high tumour burden or symptomatic if STZ is contraindicated or not available
Everolimus	±	G1/G2	Lung		Atypical carcinoid and/or SSTR negative; insulinoma or contraindications for CTX if SSTR negative
Sunitinib	±	G1/G2	Pancreas		Contraindications for CTX
PRRT	±	G1/G2	Midgut	+ (required)	Extended disease; extrahepatic disease, e.g. bone metastases
Cisplatin/ Etoposide	±	G3	Any		All poorly differentiated NEC

Concluding, dual SSTR- and [^{18}F]F-FDG-PET are useful in patients before starting PRRT to evaluate the SSTR status and metabolic activity of the tumour burden and can help to decide whether PRRT should be performed as a monotherapy or combined with more aggressive treatment (Table 32.4). Furthermore, the combined imaging might be predictive for the outcome. The important role has the dual imaging also in the follow-up when the clinical aggressiveness of the tumour does not correspond with the WHO grade. In such cases, the molecular imaging can help to choose the most representative tumour sites for re-biopsy.

32.4 Applications

32.4.1 PPRT as a Palliative Treatment

Since PRRT is mostly performed in trials with progressive metastatic patients, durable complete remission rate was relatively low. This condition leads to an inappropriate concept that considered PRRT merely as a palliative treatment. Current guidelines from the European Neuroendocrine Tumour Society (ENETS), the North American Neuroendocrine Tumour Society (NANETS) and the National Comprehensive Cancer Network (NCCN) discuss the status of PRRT in the palliative treatment of neuroendocrine tumours.

32.4.2 Recommendations in the Guidelines

32.4.2.1 The ENETS Guidelines

The European Neuroendocrine Tumour Society (ENETS) was founded in 2004 "to integrate basic and clinical research with teaching and to establish guidelines for the diagnosis and therapy for gastroenteropancreatic neuroendocrine tumours". In the third version of the guidelines (2016), there is a huge development in treatment and diagnosis of NETs compared with the past version from 2012. More diagnostic accuracy could be achieved by the introduction of the hybrid imaging: computed tomography with positron emission tomography (PET) with Gallium-labelled somatostatin analogues. Furthermore, many novel therapies have been developed, like PRRT or other targeted therapies. In the current guidelines, evidence and indications for the PRRT are discussed [46, 64]. It should be distinguished between intestinal NET and pancreatic NET. PRRT is recommended as a second-line therapy in intestinal NET (Fig. 32.3).

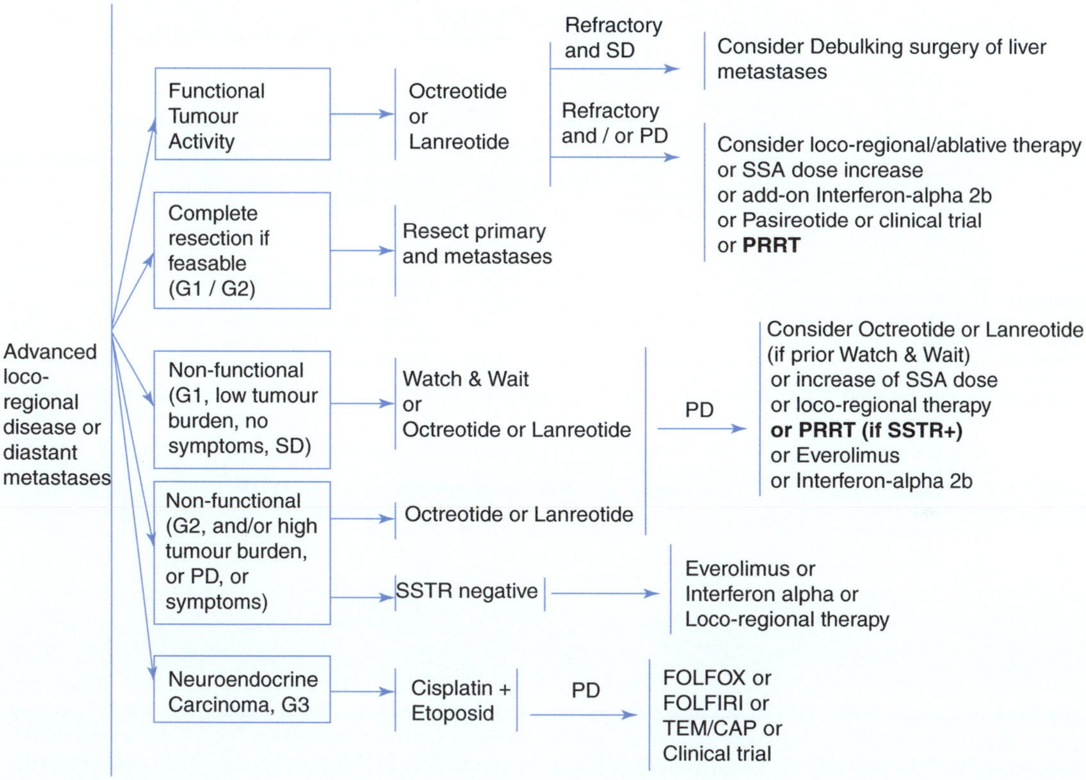

Fig. 32.3 Intestinal (midgut) NEN. This figure shows the therapeutic algorithm for the management of the advanced intestinal (midgut) NEN in the ENETS Consensus Guidelines [46]. *PD* progressive disease, *SD* stable disease, *SSTR* somatostatin receptor, *SSA* somatostatin analogues, *CS* carcinoid syndrome, *PRRT* peptide receptor radionuclide therapy, *LM* liver metastases, *TEM/CAP* temozolomide/capecitabine. *cisplatin may be replaced by carboplatin

In the newest ENETS guidelines, PPRT might be considered as an option in the first line in differentiated SSTR-positive inoperable intestinal midgut NEN with extensive disease (Table 32.3). The PFS of patients with pancreatic NET in a prospective randomized phase III trial was 11.0 months for everolimus (RADIANT-3 study) and 11.4 months for sunitinib. Retrospective studies showed a PFS longer after therapy with 177Lu-DOTATATE: 31–34 months, compared to this data [65, 66]. However, according to the guidelines in pancreatic NET, PRRT could be an option if chemotherapy and targeted therapies such as everolimus/sunitinib fail (Fig. 32.4).

32.4.2.2 The NANETS Guidelines

The North American Neuroendocrine Tumour Society (NANETS) published recently (2017) updated guidelines for the management of midgut neuroendocrine tumours. These guidelines concentrate on the newest findings from prospective phase III trials: the CLARINET trial, which studied Lanreotide in patients with non-functioning enteropancreatic NETs; the RADIANT-2 and RADIANT-4 trials, which tested everolimus in NET of the lungs and of the gastrointestinal tract (functioning and non-functioning); the TELESTAR study, which presents telotristat ethyl in patients with refractory carcinoid syndrome; and the NETTER-1 trial, which evaluated [^{177}Lu]Lu-Octreotate in midgut NETs (the small intestine and proximal colon). In this guideline, PRRT plays a role in the second-line treatment of midgut NET (if somatostatin receptor-positive) and should be favoured over everolimus. The reason is that everolimus in the RADIANT-4

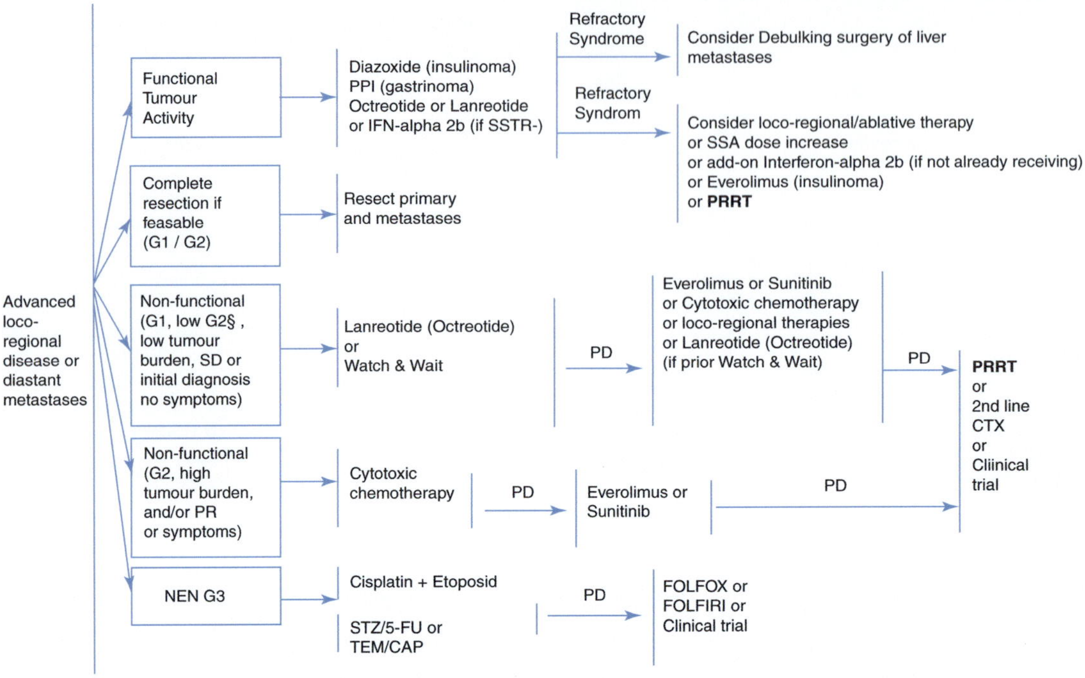

Fig. 32.4 Pancreatic NEN. This figure shows the therapeutic algorithm for the management of the advanced pancreatic NEN in the ENETS Consensus Guidelines [46]. *PD* progressive disease, *SD* stable disease, *SSTR* somatostatin receptor, *SSA* somatostatin analogues, *CS* carcinoid syndrome, *PRRT* peptide receptor radionuclide therapy, *LM* liver metastases, *TEM/CAP* temozolomide/capecitabine, *STZ* streptozotocin, *5-FU* 5-fluorouracil. § Ki-67 20% but well or moderately differentiated morphology

trial was more effective in non-midgut NETs [47]. In 2018 these findings led to the approval of the Food and Drug Administration (FDA) and European Medicines Agency (EMA).

32.4.2.3 The NCCN Guidelines

The guidelines from the National Comprehensive Cancer Network (NCCN) from 2015 discuss the diagnosis and management of NETs, especially which originate from the pancreas, gastrointestinal tract, lung and thymus. In these guidelines, the PRRT does not appear in the therapeutic algorithm for advanced NETs and is described as "investigational". To this point, the only prospective data available was a phase II study in 90 patients with metastatic NET after failure of somatostatin analogues. Although the study showed that PRRT was associated with symptom improvement and tumour control, the majority of patients did not show an objective response in the radiographic imaging. Therefore the expert team from NCCN required more randomized prospective trials to validate the benefit and assess relevant toxicities of radiopeptide therapy in advanced neuroendocrine tumours [67].

32.4.3 Neoadjuvant Treatment with PRRT

In patients with unresectable tumour because of extensive vascular invasion of the tumour, a neoadjuvant treatment with PRRT might be an option. The feasibility of PRRT as a neoadjuvant option was tested in Rotterdam in 29 Dutch patients with borderline or unresectable pancreatic NET without metastases or with oligometastatic disease (≤3 liver metastases). After the PRRT with [^{177}Lu]Lu-Octreotate, about a third of the patients (9 of 29 patients) received a successful surgery of the primary tumour. This led to a significant longer median progression-free survival (PFS) in those patients compared to inoperated patients: 69 months vs. 49 months. In this study, no perioperative mortality was observed, and there were no PRRT-related surgical complications. Five of the patients eventually progressed; in four of the patients, no recurrence of the disease could be observed [68].

32.4.4 Rare Indications

Most clinical data about PRRT include patients with gastroenteropancreatic or pulmonary NET. However, these are also some rare indications, such as phaeochromocytoma, paraganglioma and thyroid cancer, which can also be appropriate for PRRT. Adequate tumour uptake confirmation with SSTR imaging is essential as a prerequisite for considering PRRT in these patients.

32.4.4.1 Phaeochromocytoma and Paraganglioma

Phaeochromocytoma and paraganglioma are neuroendocrine tumours, which can secrete catecholamine, leading to hypertension, palpitations, sweating and other symptoms of increased sympathetic activity. Treatment options for unresectable paraganglioma and phaeochromocytoma are limited. Two centres from Melbourne and Jerusalem tested the efficacy of PPRT in 20 patients with functional metastatic paraganglioma and phaeochromocytoma. The median administered cumulative activity was 22 GBq in a median of four cycles. In more than half of the patients, treated for hypertension, the dose of the anti-hypertension medication could be reduced. Almost 70% of patients had serum chromogranin A reduction. According to RECIST, 36% showed objective response, 29% partial and 7% minor response, and 50% had stable disease. After median follow-up of 28 months, a median progression-free survival of 39 months was reached; only five patients (25%) died, and the median overall survival was not reached. Significant haematotoxicity was rare; lymphopenia grade III occurred in four patients and grade III thrombocytopenia in two patients.

These encouraging results support further prospective evaluation especially because compared to [^{131}I]I-metaiodobenzylguanidine (MIBG) therapy, PRRT is associated with logistic and radiation-safety advantages [69].

A study from London retrospectively compared the outcome of patients with phaeochromocytoma and paraganglioma treated with PRRT ([Lu^{177}]Lu-Octreotate/[Y90]Y-Octreotate) or [^{131}I]I-MIBG. The PRRT group of patients had significantly better PFS and response to treatment compared to the patients treated with [^{131}I]I-MIBG. However, there was significant difference in the overall survival (OS) only in patients with paraganglioma. The incidence of major toxicities was similar between both groups [70].

32.4.4.2 Medullary Thyroid Cancer and Non-iodine Avid Differentiated (Nonmedullary) Thyroid Cancer

There is limited data about PRRT in patients with medullary thyroid cancer or non-radioiodine avid thyroid cancer. However, if there is an adequate SSTR expression on the SSTR imaging, the PRRT might be an effective option.

The majority of medullary thyroid cancers express SSTR, but the density is mostly low to moderate. Therefore, the SSTR-PET/CT imaging with its high sensitivity is more suitable for pretherapeutic evaluation of the SSTR expression [15]. The studies, which evaluated the efficacy of PRRT in medullary thyroid cancer, analysed relatively small number of patients. For example, the Basel study group initiated a pilot study with 12 patients, who received 1–4 injections of 1700–7400 MBq/m2 [^{90}Y]Y-Octreotide at intervals of 6 weeks, followed by a phase II study, which included 31 patients. There are no phase III studies or retrospective studies, which assessed the effect of PRRT in medullary cancer in larger patient groups. In selected patients, the tumour control rate varies according to different studies between 42%([^{90}Y]Y-Octreotide) and 79% ([^{90}Y]Y- or [^{177}Lu]Lu-Octreotate); the median overall survival ranged between 36 months (after [^{90}Y]Y- or [^{177}Lu]Lu-Octreotate if responded with stable disease) and 91 months ([^{90}Y]Y-Octreotide). The incidence of relevant toxicity was low [15, 71, 72].

The fraction of patients with non-iodine avid differentiated thyroid cancer is relatively low but with increased demand of validated effective therapies. Multi-kinase inhibitors such as sorafenib or lenvatinib are indicated in this case, but because of some severe undesirable side effects, sometimes the risk exceeds the treatment benefit [73]. Indeed, the data about patients with differentiated thyroid cancer, treated with PRRT, is limited. However, because of the favourable safety profile of PRRT, an evaluation of the SSTR status using SSTR-PET/CT or SPECT/CT imaging is warrantable. In a prospective study from Reggio Emilia (Italy), 13/41 patients with differentiated thyroid cancer were selected using [^{68}Ga]Ga-DOTATOC-PET/CT suitable for PRRT. Eleven patients received 2–6 administrations of 1.5–3.7 GBq [^{90}Y]Y-Octreotide-injections. 7/11 patients showed a clinical benefit (2 partial response and 5 stabilization) with a progression-free survival of 3.5–11.5 months [74]. In comparison, the response rate in patients treated with sorafenib is 15–23%, 53–56% of patients are stable, and the median progression-free survival is 15–21 months. Relevant toxicity including hand-foot syndrome and dose reduction of the medication was evident in 56–79% of patients [73].

32.5 Patient Preparations and Administration

32.5.1 Discontinuation of Other Somatostatin Analogues

Non-radioactive somatostatin agonists (SSA) are currently applied for treating of hormone-related symptoms. The randomized phase III trials CLARINET (on Lanreotide) and PROMID (on long-acting Octreotide) showed that SSAs were efficient for treating carcinoid syndrome and exerted antitumour effects, with a positive impact on the progression-free survival (PFS) of patients with intestinal and pancreatic NETs [26, 27, 75–77]. These agents have mainly high affinity to SSTR2 and therefore might act competitive to PRRT in binding tumour cells of neuroendocrine tumours. In current practice to avoid interactions with radiolabelled somatostatin analogues, long-acting somatostatin analogues should be discontinued 4–6 weeks before PRRT. If patients have severe carcinoid syndrome, the medication can be switched to short-acting formulations, which can be applied up to 8 hours before PRRT [49]. A recent Dutch study suggests that the discontinuation of somatostatin agonists is not necessary. Two groups of patients were compared. The first group received [^{68}Ga]Ga-DOTATATE PET/CT 1 day before the next injection of Lanreotide and the other group 1 day after the injection. Against the assumption, the images 1 day after the injection showed an increase of tumour uptake and decrease of the liver uptake and other normal tissues. However, the difference is too small to be clinically relevant [78].

32.5.2 Amino Acid Administration for the Renal Protection

Infusions of amino acid solutions with positively charged amino acids such as lysine and arginine are essential for the renal protection after PRRT. They inhibit the renal uptake of radiolabelled peptides and thus reduce the renal radiation-absorbed dose. The recommended duration of infusion can vary between 2 and 10 h depending on the renal function of the patient and the nephrotoxicity of the PRRT ([^{90}Y]Y-Octreotide vs. [^{177}Lu]Lu-Octreotate). There can be also various compositions of the infusion: only lysine and only arginine or combination of lysine and arginine [49].

The Milan study group reported about the therapy with [^{90}Y]Y-Octreotide in association with amino acid infusion in a phase I study. They separated the patients in three groups: the first group of patients received infusion of lysine hydrochloride and arginine hydrochloride over 3–4 h before [^{90}Y]Y-Octreotide administration. The second group received also lysine hydrochloride plus arginine hydrochloride but in smaller amounts over 1–2 h prior therapy, followed by lysine infusion over 2–3 h after therapy. The third group of patients received only lysine hydrochloride over an hour before therapy and over 2 h after therapy. The amino acid infusion is associated with mild gastrointestinal adverse effects, probably induced by metabolic acidosis. In this study, more events of grade I–II nausea and vomiting were observed in the first two protocols (arginine + lysine) than in the third protocol (lysine alone). Arginine seemed to be the main cause of the nausea and vomiting. Finally, there was no relevant difference in the renal protection between the groups [79].

Most departments use for renal protection after Lutetium-177-labelled PRRT the regimen, developed by the Erasmus Medical Center: 25 g lysine and 25 g arginine in 1 litre saline infused over 4 hours, starting 30 min before the administration of the radiopharmaceutical [80]. In NETTER-1 a commercial amino acid solution was used. Premedication with granisetron or ondansetron (5- HT3-antagonists) prevents the most frequent adverse events after amino acid infusion: nausea and vomiting [49]. The duration of the nephroprotective infusion of amino acids after Yttrium-90-labelled PRRT can last between 10 h and 2 days.

32.5.3 Administration of PRRT

It is still controversial which is the optimal therapeutic activity per cycle, optimal interval between cycles or the adequate cumulative administered activity for PRRT (Yttrium-90-labelled or Lutetium-177-labelled). For example, the Basel group have used a weight-adapted administration for [^{90}Y]Y-Octreotide (3.7GBq/m2 body surface area), and the NETTER-1 trial used fixed administered activity of 7.4 GBq [^{177}Lu]Lu-Octreotate per cycle with a total of four cycles in intervals of 2 months [81]. In the current COMPETE study, patients should receive a maximum of four cycles with 7.5 GBq [^{177}Lu]Lu-Edotreotide, 90 days apart (ClinicalTrials.gov Identifier: NCT03049189). Even in the current EANM guidelines, there is no precise information which treatment protocols should be used. This decision should be met for each patient individually. The adjustment of administered activity can be depending on tumour burden, bone marrow reserve, renal function and body weight. Of course, in case of progressive disease during the treatment or CTCAE grade 3 or 4 haematological, renal, or hepatic toxicity, the PRRT should be discontinued [49]. The majority of clinics perform normally four cycles with 7.4 GBq each 2–3 months.

32.5.4 Intravenously Vs Intrarterial Administration

In most centres, PRRT is administered intravenously. The advantage of this approach is the easier and safer placement of a peripheral intravenous catheter than the placement of an arterial catheter. However, especially in liver metastases, the intraarterial PRRT administration might increase the intratumoural uptake.

The Heidelberg study group assessed in 15 patients the effect of the intraarterial administration of [^{90}Y]Y–/ [^{177}Lu]Lu-Octreotate. The choice of radionuclide was based on the tumour size: larger lesions (>2 cm diameter) were treated with Yttrium-90 (maximum tissue range: 11mm), smaller lesions (<2 cm diameter) with Lutetium-177 (maximum tissue range: 3mm) or both Yttrium-90 and Lutetium-177 if the size distribution was heterogeneous.

A complete response could be observed in one (7%) patient, and partial response was achieved in eight (53%) patients. About 40% of patients had stable disease. After a mean follow-up of 20 months, the median progression-free survival was not reached. Limiting factors for the radiopeptide therapy were receptor saturation, which reduces the tumour uptake over time as well as tracer washout and redistribution.

The high response rate of the intraarterial therapy is comparable with responses after chemotherapy and intravenous [^{90}Y]Y–/ [^{177}Lu]Lu-Octreotate. In this study, no acute side effects or impairment of the renal function occurred. One of the treated patients developed relevant pancytopenia with prolonged recovery (> 6 months) [42].

32.6 Efficacy

32.6.1 Efficacy of PPRT in Comparison to Other Systemic Treatments

NETTER-1 study is a milestone study for PRRT, which changed the status of this treatment in the current guidelines for neuroendocrine tumours [46, 47]. This was the first phase III prospective multicentre randomized study to evaluate the effect of PRRT in progressive midgut NET in comparison to the established therapy Octreotide LAR and showed a clear survival benefit from the PRRT [82]. Another current multicentre study is randomizing patients to compare the survival after PRRT and everolimus in GEP-NET patients (COMPETE study, ClinicalTrials.gov Identifier: NCT03049189). More comparative prospective analyses are needed to establish the potential of PRRT. Table 32.5 summarizes data from phase III trials in neuroendocrine tumours. It should be

Table 32.5 Important phase III trials in neuroendocrine tumours

Study	Study arms	Tumour entity/ patients	Median follow-up	Objective response in %	Stable disease in %	Progression-free survival in months	Year—[Reference]
NETTER-1 phase III	[^{177}Lu] Lu-Octreotate 7.4 GBq every 8 weeks + Octreotate LAR 30 mg vs. octreotide LAR 60 mg	Progressive midgut NET (*N* = 230)	14 months	19 vs. 3	66 vs. 62	Not reached vs. 8.4	2017—[82]
PROMID Phase III	Octreotide LAR 30 mg vs. placebo	Midgut NET (*N* = 84)	96	2 vs. 2	67 vs. 37	14.3 vs. 6.0	2009/2017—[27, 83]
CLARINET Phase III	Lanreotide autogel 120 mg vs. placebo	Non-functioning, somatostatin receptor-positive neuroendocrine tumours of grade 1 or 2 (*N* = 204)	24	NA	66 vs. 49	Not reached vs. 18	2014/2016—[26, 76]
RADIANT 2 Phase III	Everolimus + octreotide LAR vs. octreotide LAR + placebo	NET with carcinoid syndrome (*N* = 429)	28	2 vs. 2	84 vs. 81	16.4 vs. 11.3	2011/2017—[84, 85]
RADIANT 3 Phase III	Everolimus vs. placebo	Pancreatic NET (*N* = 420)	17	5 vs. 2	73 vs. 51	11.0 vs. 4.6	2011/2016—[86, 87]
RADIANT 4 Phase III	Everolimus vs. placebo	Non-functional gastrointestinal NET and lung NET (*N* = 302)	21	2 vs. 1	80 vs. 64	11.0 vs. 3.9	2016—[88]
Sunitinib Phase III	Sunitinib malate vs. placebo	Pancreatic NET (*n* = 171)	NA	9 vs. 0	63 vs. 60	11.4 vs. 5.5	2011—[89]
FNCLCC-FFCD 9710 Phase III	Streptozotocin + fluorouracil vs. interferon alpha	Lung NET (*n* = 3), GEP-NET (*n* = 48), CUP-NET (*n* = 11) grade 1 or 2	46	3 vs. 9	56 vs. 63	5.5 vs. 14.1	2009—[90]

taken into account that the inclusion criteria and therefore the patients' collectives are very different in the different studies, which might have affected the outcome of these patients irrespective of the treatment administered. Therefore, the effects of the different therapies are not directly comparable. For example, in both PROMID and CLARINET trials, patients with progressive and not progressive neuroendocrine tumours were included; however the time to progression in the placebo arm of the PROMID study was 6 months and in the CLARINET study 18 months, respectively [26, 27, 76, 83].

32.6.2 Efficacy of PRRT in Different Types of Neuroendocrine Tumours

Most common primary sites of neuroendocrine tumours are the bronchopulmonary (25%), small intestine (18%), large intestine (13%), rectum (12%), pancreas (9%) and stomach (5%). Intestinal NET and rectum NET have better prognosis regarding survival and recurrence of disease compared to bronchopulmonary and pancreas NET [91]. Although the lung/bronchus is the most common site of origin of NET, the PRRT is studied mainly in gastroenteropancreatic NET. The reason might be the relatively low response rate compared to pancreas or intestinal NET [92, 93]. Highest responses showed pancreas NET and the longest survival NET from the small intestine [66, 94]. A large multi-institutional registry study with prospective follow-up compared different PRRT protocols (with Yttrium-90 or Lutetium-177 or combined with both radionuclides) in different neuroendocrine tumour entities: the pancreas, small intestine and cancer of unknown disease. The longest survival had patients with midgut NET (PFS 51 months, OS not reached), followed by pancreas NET (PFS 39 months, OS 53 months), and the shortest survival was observed in CUP-NET (PFS 38 months, OS 47 months) [95].

	Response in % (RECIST 1.1/SWOG criteria)						Survival in months from start of treatment		
Primary site	CR	PR	MR	SD	OR	PD	PFS	OS	References
Bronchopulmonary	–	27	–	41	27	32	27–28	42–59	[92, 93]
Small intestine	–	16/13	–/31	74/48	16/44	10/8	33–51	61-not reached	[94, 95]
Pancreas	–	57/60	12	28/13	57/72	14/15	34–39	53	[66, 95]

32.6.3 Predictive Factors for Efficacy

The assessment of predicative factors for the efficacy of PRRT including response rate und survival data is important for the individual treatment planning and tailored evaluation approach.

Kwekkeboom et al. examined the potential factors that correlated with the outcome after treatment with [^{177}Lu]Lu-Octreotate. Higher SSTR expression seen in the pretherapy [^{111}In]In-DTPA-Octreotide scintigraphy ($p = 0.008$) and limited liver involvement ($p = 0.042$) showed higher remission rates. Associated with progression of disease were low performance status ($p < 0.001$), weight loss ($p < 0.001$) and extensive liver involvement ($p = 0.008$). Significant shorter time to progression showed patients with gastrinoma (20 months vs. 36 months, $p = 0.004$) and bone metastases ($p = 0.037$). Treatment outcome, liver involvement, performance status (cut off 70% Karnofsky status), weight loss, bone metastases and gastrinoma were also factors, which correlated with shorter survival [54, 96]. In another study, an independent marker for the prediction of the survival was also an elevated neuron-specific enolase in plasma at baseline (>15 ng/mL) [6]. There are several studies revealing the high predictive value of the metabolic activity of the tumour detected in FDG-PET/CT [55–58]. With a dual imaging (SSTR and FDG), both response and survival after PRRT could be predicted [51].

32.6.4 Efficacy of PRRT as Single Agent

32.6.4.1 [^{177}Lu]Lu-Octreotate: The First Widely Approved Agent

The agent with the most solid study data is [^{177}Lu]Lu-Octreotate. First reports from the phase I/II study about the toxicity and efficacy of [^{177}Lu]Lu-Octreotate were published in 2011. Included were 51 patients with unresectable SSTR2-positive tumours: mainly NET but also 3 patients with paraganglioma and 1 patient with meningioma. In one of the patients, a leucopenia grade 3 and thrombopenia grade 3 according to CTC were observed.

The study group from Rotterdam tested the response to the PRRT with [^{177}Lu]Lu-Octreotate in 504 GEP-NET patients. In 2% of patients, a complete response could be achieved; 28% of patients had partial response and 16% minor response (tumour reduction >25 < 50%). The largest proportion of patients was stable: 35%. 20% of patients progressed. The achieved median progression-free survival was 40 months. The median overall survival from start of treatment was 46 months and if calculated from the initial diagnosis, 128 months [96].

The NETTER-1 study was the first randomized phase III study to access the effect of ^{177}Lu-Octreotate (Lutathera®) in well-differentiated, metastatic midgut neuroendocrine tumours. Included were 229 patients. One hundred sixteen of the patients were treated with 7.4 GBq Lutathera® every 8 weeks and 30 mg Octreotide long-acting repeatable every 4 weeks. The other group of patients (113 patients) received 60 mg Octreotide LAR alone. The preliminary results were published in 2017. After 20 months of follow-up, 65.2% of patients in the Lutathera® group were progression-free, and 14 patients died; in the control group, only 10.8% of patients were progression-free, and 26 patients died. The differences in progression-free survival and death rate were significant: $p < 0.001$ and $p = 0.004$, respectively. Relevant toxicity (grade 3 or 4) in the Lutathera® arm was 1% neutropenia, 2% thrombocytopenia and 9% lymphopenia. Clinically significant myelosuppression occurred in one of the patients. This patient had a history of monoclonal gammopathy of unknown clinical significance. No significant renal toxicity was observed. Overall, the treatment with Lutathera® resulted in a significantly prolonged progression-free survival with a favourable toxicity profile [82]. On January 26, 2018, the FDA approved Lutetium Lu 177 dotatate (Lutathera®) for the treatment of somatostatin receptor-positive gastroenteropancreatic neuroendocrine tumours (GEP-NETs), including foregut, midgut and hindgut neuroendocrine tumours in adults. Formerly in September 2017, the European Commission (EC) approved the marketing authorization of Lutathera® for the treatment of unresectable or metastatic, progressive, well-differentiated (G1 and G2), somatostatin receptor-positive gastroenteropancreatic neuroendocrine tumours (GEP-NETs) in adults.

32.6.4.2 Efficacy and Safety of [^{177}Lu]Lu-Edotreotide in GEP-NET Patients

A phase II study from Bad Berka evaluated the efficacy of [^{177}Lu]Lu-Edotreotide (also known as [^{177}Lu]Lu-DOTATOC) in patients with neuroendocrine tumours. The PFS and OS were 17 months and 34 months. GEP-NET reached a PFS of 35 months; the objective response in this group was 54%. Patients with other NETs showed much shorter survival (PFS = 12 months) and no objective response. In total, no serious adverse events could be observed [97].

Recently, a phase III study (multicentre, randomized, controlled, open-label) was initiated to assess the effect and safety of [^{177}Lu]Lu-Edotreotide in patients with progressive unresectable GEP-NET. The PRRT consists of four cycles of 7.5 ± 0.7 GBq [^{177}Lu]Lu-Edotreotide, 90 days apart. The control arm consists of patients treated with the targeted molecular agent everolimus (Afinitor®): initial dose of 10 mg/day, which will be administered daily until occurrence of progression. The primary outcome of the study is the progression-free survival under PRRT with [^{177}Lu]Lu-Edotreotide in comparison to everolimus. The secondary outcome is the overall survival. The expected final data collection date for primary outcome measure is end of 2020 (ClinicalTrials.gov Identifier: NCT03049189).

32.6.4.3 Studies with [^{90}Y]Y-Octreotide

Bodei et al. aimed to prospectively determine the maximum tolerated dose of [^{90}Y]Y-Octreotide per cycle in 40 patients with somatostatin receptor-positive neuroendocrine tumours. The PRRT was administered with concomitant amino acid solution for kidney protection. In this phase I study, the determined maximum tolerated dose [^{90}Y]Y-Octreotide was 5.18 GBq; 5 GBq per cycle with concomitant amino acids for kidney protection is the recommended dosage. In the study, no acute kidney toxicity occurred; however because of delayed kidney toxicity, the cumulative dose is limited to 25 Gy [79].

Waldherr et al. reported in a phase II study about the effect of [^{90}Y]Y-Octreotide in 41 patients with neuroendocrine tumours. Tumour response, treatment on the carcinoid syndrome and relief of tumour-associated pain were investigated. The patients received four injections of 6000 MBq/m^2 [^{90}Y]Y-Octreotide each 6 weeks. *Tumour* response was found in 24% of patients: 2% complete remissions, 22% partial remissions and 12% minor response. About 49% of patients had stable disease and 15% progressive disease. At the time of the analyses, the median progression-free survival has not been reached (> 26 months). Symptomatic relief of the malignant carcinoid syndrome was achieved in 83% of patients. All patients in the study with morphine consumption because of tumour-associated pain (5 of 41) experienced significant reduction of symptoms. Significant lymphocytopenia (grade 3) was observed in 5% of patients. Often (27%) but not severe adverse events were post-therapeutic nausea, vomiting and flushing. No severe nephrotoxicity was observed [98].

In Basel 2011 was conducted a phase II single-centre open-label trial in 1109 patients with neuroendocrine tumours. The patients received repeated cycles of [^{90}Y]Y-Octreotide (3.7GBq/m^2 body surface). In total 2472 cycles were administered (median, 2; range, 1 to 10 cycles per patient). Morphological response was seen in 34.1% of patients and biochemical response in 15.5%, and in 29.7% clinical response could be observed. About 5.8% of patients were stable, and 0.6% achieved a complete remission. After a median follow-up of 23 months, 491 patients (44.3%) died. Relevant factors correlated with longer survival were morphologic (44.7 vs. 18.3 months; $p < 0.001$), biochemical (35.3 vs. 25.7 months; $p = 0.023$) and clinical response (36.8 vs. 23.5 months; $p < 0.001$). Also at high initial SSTR expression, the tumour seen as high tracer uptake in tumour lesions was correlated with better overall survival ($p < 0.001$) [81].

A multicentre study included 90 patients from 5 European countries and the United States. The patients were treated with three cycles of 4.4 GBq [^{90}Y]Y-Octreotide. The PFS was in median 16 months, and the OS reached in median 27 months. Patients with diarrhoea improvement had significantly better survival: PFS of 18 months vs. 8 months in patients with no symptomatic response [99].

32.6.4.4 Treatment with [^{90}Y]Y-Octreotate

In Warsaw Cwikla et al. performed a phase II study with [^{90}Y]Y-Octreotate to explore the response in 60 patients with metastatic GEP-NETs. The mean cumulative activity was 11.2 GBq per patient; the mean activity per cycle was 3.7 GBq. According to RECIST-criteria, 13 patients (23%) showed a response, and 77% of patients had a stable disease. Clinical PR was achieved in 43 patients (72%), 9 patients had SD, and 8 patients progressed. The median time to progression was 17 months; the estimated median overall survival was 22 months. Non-responder showed a PFS of 4.5 months and OS of 9.5 months, while in patients who achieved a clinical benefit (objective response and stable disease), time to progression was 19.5 months, and OS was 23.5 months. Significant haematological toxicity (grade 3/4) was observed in 10% of patients (five patients

Table 32.6 Efficacy of different radiopharmaceuticals

	Response in %						Survival in months from start of treatment		Survival in months from diagnosis	Number of patients	
Radiopharmaceutical	CR	PR	MR	SD	OR	PD	PFS	OS	OS		References
[^{177}Lu]Lu-Octreotate	2	27–28	16–26	27–66	18–55	5–20	36–40	46	128	51–504	[82, 95, 96, 107]
[^{90}Y]Y-octreotide	1–22	22–33	12	5–49	39–75	15–61	37	38	94	41–1109	[81, 95, 98]
[^{90}Y]Y-Octreotate	–	23	–	77	23	–	17	22	–	60	[100]
[^{90}Y]Y-Octreotate + [^{177}Lu]Lu-Octreotate	2	22	–	64–65	14–24	6–16	29	–	–	25–59	[104, 105]
[^{90}Y]Y-octreotide + [^{177}Lu]Lu-octreotide	7	16	–	62	23	15	29	–	–	69	[106]

with leucopenia, one patient had thrombocytopenia, six patients developed anaemia) and persisted in 5%. Two patients experienced a delayed grade 3 renal toxicity; therefore careful monitoring of the renal function is recommended [100].

32.6.5 Combination of Lutetium-177 and Yttrium-90-Labelled PRRT

There are several comparative studies, which evaluated the effect and toxicity of combined Lutetium- and Yttrium-labelled radiopharmaceuticals compared to monotherapy. The analyses showed a superior survival of the combined therapy. For example, in a study from Basel, the patients treated with [^{90}Y]Y-Octreotide and [^{177}Lu]Lu-Octreotide reached an overall survival of 5.51 years vs. 3.96 years with [^{90}Y]Y-Octreotide alone ($p = 0.006$). Especially patients with progressive metastasized gastrinoma have a significant survival benefit from a combined treatment [101]. Another study showed a very high response rate after tandem PPRT with Yttrium-90 and Lutetium-177: 42% [102]. The synergistic effect of the combined therapy could be explained in a rat tumour model, which demonstrated that there was no complete absorption of the radiation energy of Yttrium-90 in smaller tumours. On the other hand, Lutetium-177 alone may fail to induce a complete remission in large tumours [103].

Another important issue about the combined treatment is the adverse events. The safety results in patients after monotherapy with Yttrium-90 and combined PRRT seem to be comparable [101, 104]. The study group from Warsaw published results after 6 years follow-up and in patients treated with tandem PRRT: 2% of patients experienced MDS, and another 2% developed serious (grade 3) nephrotoxicity [105]. Severe (grade 3/4) haematotoxicity was observed in 7% of patients [106] (Table 32.6).

32.6.6 Combination Therapies of PRRT with Other Systemic Therapies

PRRT alone results in most of the cases a partial response or stable disease; complete responses are rare. The combination of PRRT with other therapies might enhance the antitumour effect. However, there are just a few studies, which evaluated the feasibility and outcome of combination therapies with PRRT, some of them phase I/II trials with a limited number of patients.

32.6.6.1 PRRT and Somatostatin Analogues

The NETTER-1 trial revealed that the combined PRRT with somatostatin analogues (SSA) resulted in a better survival than the treatment with SSA alone in advanced midgut NET [82].

However, this study does not answer the question whether the combined treatment with PRRT and SSAs can provide a survival benefit compared to monotherapy with PRRT.

A recent study from Bonn reviewed the survival and response rate of patients with GEP-NET treated with SSA as a combination therapy with PRRT and/or as a maintenance therapy after PRRT. In this analysis, a significantly better progression-free survival (48 months vs. 27 months, $p = 0.012$), overall survival (91 months vs. 47 months, $p < 0.001$) and lower death-event rates (26% vs. 63%) could be achieved with the combined treatment compared to PRRT alone. Therefore, SSA as a combined therapy and/or maintenance treatment may play a significant role in tumour control in patients who underwent a PRRT [108].

32.6.6.2 PRRT and Chemotherapy

Minimally cytotoxic doses of chemotherapy may induce a radiosensitizing effect in neuroendocrine tumour cells, increasing the tumour response after PRRT. This effect can be explained with increased DNA damage and inhibition of DNA repair, inhibition of cell proliferation, tumour cell reoxygenation, apoptosis or synchronization of the cell cycle [109]. Common radiosensitizing agents are capecitabine, temozolomide and 5-fluorouracil.

In Rotterdam the combination of [^{177}Lu]Lu-Octreotate and capecitabine was evaluated in seven patients. The treatment included four cycles with 7.4 GBq [^{177}Lu]Lu-Octreotate and capecitabine (1650 mg/m(2) per day) for 2 weeks. The interval between cycles was 6–10 weeks. There were no cases of hand-foot syndrome. Grade 1 stomatitis occurred in one patient. No severe leucopenia or neutropenia occurred. One patient developed grade 3 anaemia; another patient had grade 3 thrombocytopenia. No significant changes in serum creatinine levels were observed. None of the patients had symptoms of cardiac ischaemia [110].

Claringbold et al. investigated in a phase II study the toxicity and outcome of combined capecitabine and [^{177}Lu]Lu-Octreotate in a total of 33 patients with histologically proven NETs. The patients were treated with four cycles of 7.8 GBq [^{177}Lu]Lu-Octreotate each 8 weeks. On the morning of the radionuclide therapy began a chemotherapy of 1650 mg/m(2) capecitabine per day for 14 consecutive days. 76% of patients completed all four cycles. Grade 3 thrombocytopenia occurred 3–4 weeks after the therapy. There were no relevant nephrotoxicity. Only 6% of patients progressed, the majority of patients showed stable disease (70%), and objective response rates (ORR) were 24%. None of the patients achieved a complete remission. As the study results were reported, neither the median progression-free survival nor the median overall survival had been reached. The median follow-up was 16 months (range 5–33 months). Two years after the therapy, 88% of patients were still alive. In summary, capecitabine chemotherapy as radiosensitizer was well tolerated and resulted in tumour control and stabilization of disease in 94% of these patients [111].

Another study published from Claringbold et al. assessed prospectively the effect of the combination of [^{177}Lu]Lu-Octreotate with capecitabine and temozolomide (phase I/II study). All 35 patients received a therapy of 4 cycles with 7.8 GBq [^{177}Lu]Lu-Octreotate each 8 weeks, with 14 days of capecitabine 1500 mg/m(2). Within a phase I trial, escalating doses of temozolomide in groupings of 100, 150 and 200 mg/m(2) were applied, starting in the last 5 days of each capecitabine cycle. In phase II, patients received 200 mg/m(2) temozolomide. The therapy was well tolerated in all dosage groups. No grade 4 toxicities occurred. Transient grade 3 nausea occurred in 3% of patients and neutropenia grade 3 in 6% of patients. With the combination therapy, complete response (CR) in 15% of patients could be achieved. 91% of patients showed a clinical benefit rate (53% objective response and 38% stable disease). Higher response rates were seen in patients with gastropancreatic NETs than in those with bowel primaries [112]. Combined treatment PRRT with capecitabine (14 days of at 1500 mg/m^2) and temozolomide (5 days of at 200 mg/m^2) each 8 weeks was tested in a phase II study in 30 patients with pancreatic NET. None of the patients experienced progressive disease.

A complete remission was achieved in 13% of patients; 70% had partial response. The median PFS was 48 months; the OS was at the time of the analyses (median follow-up 33 months) not reached [113].

A report from Melbourne reviewed 68 patients, who received 4 cycles of [^{177}Lu]Lu-Octreotate, combined with 5-fluorouracil (5-FU) chemotherapy. The treatment protocol included four cycles of PRRT; the first cycle was given alone. 5-FU (200 mg/m^2/24 h) was started approximately 4 days before the administration of the second PRRT and continued for 3 weeks. Clinical benefit in the imaging (objective response or stable disease) showed about 70% of patients; biochemical response was seen in about 60% of patients. No complete response could be achieved [114].

32.6.6.3 Combination with Everolimus

Everolimus is a molecular-targeted therapy, which inhibits the mammalian target of rapamycin (mTOR), with growth-inhibitory activity, and is administered orally. There is evidence from the RADIANT-3 and RADIANT-4 study, which indicate that everolimus is safe and effective in gastroenteropancreatic NETs [86, 88].

A phase I study with 16 patients aimed to determine the optimal safe dose of everolimus in combination with [^{177}Lu]Lu-Octreotate peptide receptor radionuclide therapy. Participants underwent four cycles of 7.8 GBq [^{177}Lu]Lu-Octreotate each 8 weeks. Successive cohorts of three patients were treated with escalating doses of everolimus: 5, 7.5 and 10 mg daily for 24 weeks. The medication with 10 mg everolimus was required in all patients' dose reduction or discontinuation because of neutropenia and thrombocytopenia and reduced creatinine clearance. Thus, the maximum tolerated dose of everolimus in combination with [^{177}Lu]Lu-Octreotate was 7.5 mg daily [115]. In a recent preclinical study was evaluated the response after everolimus alone vs. PRRT alone vs. PRRT combined with PRRT vs. placebo in vivo. The combined therapy induced better responses and longer survival than the placebo group or everolimus alone in mice with SSTR-positive tumours. However, the combined therapy was not significantly superior to PRRT alone [116]. Clinical data comparing the combined treatment PRRT and everolimus with monotherapies is still lacking.

32.6.7 Re-challenge PRRT

Despite the long progression-free survival achieved with PRRT (in median 3 years), most of the patients eventually progress. Re-challenge PRRT might be an option for patients who initially benefited from the therapy a. There are several studies which investigated the use of PRRT as a retreatment: from Rotterdam, Bonn and Meldola. Van Essen et al. from the Rotterdam Study Group concluded that the re-challenge PRRT with [^{177}Lu]Lu-Octreotate is well tolerated with no serious adverse events in selected patients. Repeated cycles with [^{177}Lu]Lu-Octreotate showed antitumour effects with a progression-free survival of 17 months. However the effects were less favourable than for the baseline therapy. The reason may be the worse clinical condition, more extended tumour burden or changed tumour characteristics [117].

Similar results showed retrospective analyses from Bonn. Time to progression from the start of the re-challenge therapy with [^{177}Lu]Lu-Octreotate was 13 months. Interestingly, patients who were durably progression-free after the initial PRRT seemed to have longer PFS after the re-challenge therapy ($p = 0.04$) [14].

In a recently published study from Bonn, patients who received multiple repeated ($\geq$8) cycles of a [^{177}Lu]Lu-Octreotate were analysed. The median administered activity was 63.8 GBq in a median of 9 cycles and ranged up to 96.6 GBq cumulative activity in 13 cycles. Reversible haematotoxicity was recorded in 2 of 15 patients (13%). No CTC-3/4 renal toxicity occurred. The survival of these patients was compared with the survival of patients who received a baseline PRRT (3–4 cycles) in Bonn. In result, there was a survival benefit in patients treated with multiple repeated PRRT (overall survival 85.6 vs. 69.7 months, $p < 0.001$) [2]. Neither in the study from Rotterdam nor in Bonn, a case of MDS after

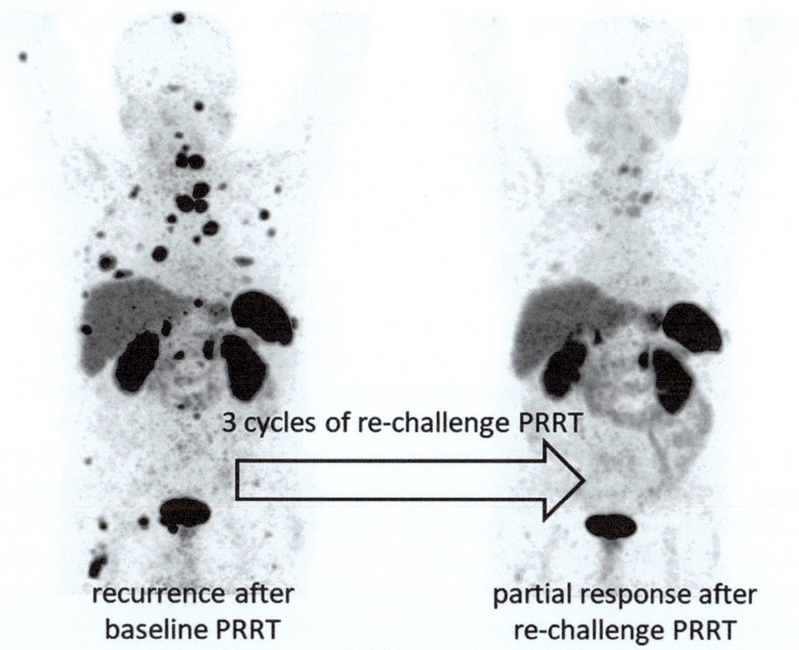

Fig. 32.5 Pre- and post-therapeutic image of patient with metastatic neuroendocrine tumour of unknown primary after re-challenge PRRT. Image A from 09/15 shows a recurrence of disease after 23 months of progression-free survival. After 3 cycles of re-challenge PRRT (cumulative activity, 43.4 GBq), the patient showed in image B from 07/16 a partial response

retreatment with PRRT was reported [2, 14, 117]. Figure 32.5 represents a [^{68}Ga]Ga-DOTATOC image of a male patient with a neuroendocrine tumour of unknown origin. The patient developed a recurrence of the disease nearly 2 years after the baseline PRRT (image A). After a re-challenge therapy of PRRT, the patient had a partial response (image B).

Severi et al. studied the outcome of GEP-NET patients, who relapsed after treatment with [^{90}Y]Y-Octreotide and eventually received a retreatment with [^{177}Lu]Lu-Octreotate. In summary, those patients were suitable candidates for PRRT with [^{177}Lu]Lu-Octreotate as a salvage therapy. The response rates and the progression-free survival were comparable with the outcome after the primary treatment with ^{90}Y-PRRT [118].

32.7 Toxicity

32.7.1 Definition of Toxicity

According to Common Terminology Criteria for Adverse Events v4.0 (CTCAE), an adverse event (AE) is any unfavourable and unintended sign, symptom or disease during or after a medical treatment/procedure. The AE may or may not be related to the medical treatment/procedure. The term AE and its classification are used for medical documentation and study analyses. AEs are graded from 1 to 5 according to the severity of the event [119]:

- Grade 1 Mild; asymptomatic or mild symptoms; clinical or diagnostic observations only; intervention not indicated.
- Grade 2 Moderate; minimal, local or non-invasive intervention indicated; limiting age-appropriate instrumental activities of daily living (e.g., preparing meals, shopping for groceries or clothes, using the telephone, managing money, etc.)
- Grade 3 Severe or medically significant but not immediately life-threatening; hospitalization or prolongation of hospitalization indicated; disabling; limiting self-care and activities of daily living (refer to bathing, dressing and undressing, feeding self, using the toilet, taking medications and not bedridden).
- Grade 4 Life-threatening consequences; urgent intervention indicated.
- Grade 5 Death related to AE.

32.7.2 Acute Toxicity

[^{177}Lu]Lu-Octreotate is a well-tolerated therapy with mostly easily manageable adverse events such as nausea (25%), vomiting (10%) and abdominal pain/discomfort (9%). Radiation-induced swelling of metastases might also lead to local complications compressing other organs or nerves. In such cases, an escalation of analgesia and supportive therapy with corticosteroids might be required. About 1% of patients develop a severe hormonal syndrome, like flushing and diarrhoea, after [^{177}Lu]Lu-Octreotate. This may require a prolonged hospitalization or readmission. Associated with a hormonal crisis is the extensive metastatic disease and liver metastases. Patients should be treated symptomatically with high-dose Octreotide, i.v. fluid replacement and other supportive medications such as corticosteroids, metoclopramide and loperamide [120].

32.7.3 Subacute Toxicity

Severe subacute toxicity after PRRT administration is rarely occurring. To the most common subacute adverse events counts fatigue, mild alopecia, hypo-/azoospermia, mild/moderate renal impairment and hematological abnormalities.

The Rotterdam Study Group investigated 320 patients and the incidence of subacute haematological toxicity after PRRT with [^{177}Lu]Lu-Octreotate. There was an acceptable grade 3/4 haematotoxicity (11%). Relevant risk factors for developing haematotoxicity were impaired renal function, low leucocyte count, extensive tumour mass, high tumour uptake on the Octreoscan® and/or age >70 years. The mean bone marrow radiation dose was 2 Gy in patients who received four cycles of 7.4 GBq PRRT. This means that the limit of 2 Gy bone marrow radiation dose, adopted from Iodine-131, seems not to be valid for PRRT with [^{177}Lu]Lu-Octreotate [121]. Another study from Rotterdam investigated the impact of [^{177}Lu]Lu-Octreotate on the renal function on 323 patients. Only three (1%) patients developed (subacute) renal toxicity grade 2. No subacute grade 3 or 4 nephrotoxicity occurred, and the annual decrease in renal function was <20%. No risk factors for renal toxicity could be observed [122].

32.7.4 Delayed Toxicity

Bodei et al. followed up 807 patients for a median of 30 months, after treatment with [^{177}Lu]Lu-Octreotate or [^{90}Y]Y-Octreotide or combination PRRT. Patients treated with [^{90}Y]Y-Octreotide or combination PRRT were more likely to develop renal toxicity than monotherapy with [^{177}Lu]Lu-Octreotate (33.6%, 25.5% and 13.4% of patients, respectively, $p < 0.0001$). Severe nephrotoxicity (grade 3 + 4) occurred in 1.5%. Although target tissue dosimetry was performed and risk factors were estimated, in <30% of patients, the occurrence of nephrotoxicity could be predicted. Hypertension and anaemia were the most relevant factors. In about a quarter of patients occurred persistent toxicity, mainly in patients with shorter interval between the cycles. Myelodysplastic syndrome occurred in 2.35% of patients and acute leukaemia in 1.1% of patients [4].

In a report from Imhof et al., from 1109 patients, 12.8% developed grade 3 to 4 transient hematologic toxicities after PRRT with [^{90}Y]Y-Octreotide. The median follow-up was 23 months. A single patient developed MDS, there was one case of acute leukaemia, and 103 patients (9.2%) experienced grade 4 to 5 permanent renal toxicity. Suggested risk factors for developing a severe nephrotoxicity were older age (p = 0.02), low baseline glomerular filtration rate ($p < 0.01$) and high kidney uptake score ($p = 0.03$) [81].

A study from Cwikla et al. included 60 patients with a median follow-up of 12 months after PRRT with [^{90}Y]Y-Octreotide. Five patients developed grade 2 or 3 renal toxicity. Haematological toxicity (WHO grade 3 and 4) was noted during therapy in 10% of patients and persisted in 5% [100].

Anterior and posterior lobes of the pituitary gland are proven to express somatostatin receptors, which mean that the adrenal function can be theoretically impaired by PRRT. There is sparse data about the effect of PRRT on the pituitary function. A study from Rotterdam assessed the adrenal function with hormone measurements in serum at baseline and after treatment with [^{177}Lu]Lu-Octreotate. The follicle-stimulating hormone and luteinizing hormone decreased in postmenopausal women after treatment with [^{177}Lu]Lu-Octreotate. In men were detected inhibitory effects on spermatogenesis, but non-SHBG-bound testosterone levels remained unaffected. Two patients from a total of 66 patients developed persistent primary hypothyroidism; 5 patients showed elevated HbA(1c) levels [123].

Radiopharmaceutical	Haematotoxicity grade 3/4 in % Hb	Leu	Thro	HTX	MDS	Acute leukaemia	Renal toxicity grade 3/4 in %	Number of patients	References
[^{177}Lu] Lu-Octreotate	0	2–9	2	2–11	0.9–2	0.5–1	0	203	[4, 13, 82, 107]
[^{90}Y]Y-octreotide	1	5–6	6	13–14	0.2–2	0.1–1	3–9	41–1109	[4, 81, 98]
[^{90}Y]Y-Octreotate	10	8	1	10	–	–	3	60	[100]

32.8 Dosimetry

Dosimetry improves the safety and efficacy of PRRT. The estimation of the accumulated activity in target regions is mostly performed using a region of interest (ROI)-based evaluation of planar whole-body scintigraphy. Dosimetric calculations are analysed according to medical internal radiation dose (MIRD) scheme. The internal radiation dose can be assessed using software such as MIRDOSE or OLINDA/EXM [124, 125]. With the newer software OLINDA/EXM, a 3D mapping using SPECT (with CT) can be performed, which enables even further improvement in dosimetry [126]. Most relevant dose-limiting organs are the kidney and bone marrow.

32.8.1 Tumour Dosimetry

Schuchard et al. demonstrated different absorbed doses in the targeted lesions using Lutetium-177-labelled peptides DOTATATE, DOTANOC and DOTATOC. Lowest absorbed tumour dose and the highest dose in the normal tissues showed [^{177}Lu] Lu-DOTANOC: 2 mGy/MBq in tumour and 0.07 mGy/MBq in the whole body. There were no relevant differences in the tumour kinetics between [^{177}Lu]Lu-Octreotate and [^{177}Lu]Lu-Octreotide: 5.2 vs. 4.9 mGy/MBq. [^{177}Lu]Lu-Octreotide demonstrated the lowest dose in the normal organs and highest tumour-to-kidney ratio [127].

32.8.2 Kidney Dosimetry

According to Gupta et al., up to 40 GBq [^{177}Lu] Lu-Octreotate can be applied safely to patients until reaching the maximum kidney dose of 23 Gy, determined by the National Council on Radiation Protection and Measurements [128] [129]. Pauwels et al. estimated that the maximum tolerable kidney dose for internal radiotherapy with [^{90}Y]Y-Octreotide therapy is 35 ± 7 Gy, which is significantly higher than the dose limit for external beam therapy [130]. Bethesda et al. support the idea that the radiation dose threshold, adopted from the radiotherapy, does not seem valid for PRRT, especially for [^{177}Lu] Lu-Octreotate. A study from Bonn evaluated the safety of PRRT after multiple repeated cycles [^{177}Lu]Lu-Octreotate (range 8–13). In this study, no severe nephrotoxicity (grade 3 or 4 according to the common toxicity criteria) was recorded. The maximum estimated absorbed radiation dose of the kidney was 87 Gy [2].

Guerriero et al. tested if using just 1–2 scans a simplified kidney dosimetry with reliable results could be performed. For the calculation of the renal dose and the time-integrated activity, they used the formula, (MNfix): $y(t) = a_{\text{pt}} \cdot \exp.(-\lambda_{\text{MNfix,TOC}} \cdot t)$; $y(t) = a_{\text{pt}} \cdot \exp.(-\lambda_{\text{MNfix,TATE}} \cdot t)$, which is a monoexponential model with a unique fit for all the data sets for each radiopeptide (DOTA-Octreotide and DOTA-Octreotate labelled with Lutetium-177 or Yttrium-90).

According to the study, dosimetry data should be collected until 100 h for Lutetium-177 therapy and 70 h for Yttrium-90 therapy; otherwise the calculations are significantly influenced by the curve interpolating the data. Risk factors such as hypertension and diabetes result in a substantial increase of 20% of the renal dose. Compared to DOTA-Octreotide, DOTA-Octreotate had a relevant higher renal dose (increase of 25%) [131].

32.8.3 Bone Marrow Dosimetry

To determine the bone marrow dosimetry after treatment with [^{177}Lu]Lu-Octreotate, Forrer et al. compared the accumulated radioactivity of the radiopharmaceutical in the blood with the activity in bone marrow aspirates. They also examined the absorbed cross-dose from organs relevant for the bone marrow function such as the liver, spleen, kidneys and blood, defined as "remainder of the body". The study included in total 15 patients. The measured activities in the bone marrow aspirates correlated strongly with the radioactivity in the blood ($r = 0.914$, $p < 0.001$). Furthermore the "remainder of the body" organs contributed to the bone marrow absorbed dose. The total absorbed dose to the red marrow after application of 3700 MBq [^{177}Lu]Lu-Octreotate was in median 83 mGy and varied between 40 and 466 mGy. In result, the interindividual bone marrow dose differed significantly, which verifies the assumption that individual dosimetry is necessary to reduce the bone marrow toxicity and the risk of developing MDS [132].

Another study from Uppsala aimed to develop an individualized bone marrow dosimetry protocol. After an application of a single cycle of 7.4 GBq [^{177}Lu]Lu-Octreotate, the absorbed dose to the bone marrow ranged from 0.05 to 0.4 Gy. The study group also observed the patients, who first reached the critical accumulated dose of either 2 Gy to the bone marrow or 23 Gy to the kidneys after repeated therapies with 7.4 GBq [^{177}Lu]Lu-Octreotate per cycle. The upper dose limit in these patients was reached after two to ten cycles, in more than 98% because the kidneys accumulated an absorbed dose [133].

32.8.4 Dosimetry of Other Organs

Apart from the kidney, physiological uptake of [^{177}Lu]Lu-Octreotate is also seen in the spleen, liver and pituitary gland. The measured radiation-absorbed doses in the literature are 1.1 to 2.15 mGy/MBq for the spleen (tolerance dose: 30 to 40 Gy) [28, 127, 129, 134], 0.27 to 0.59 mGy/MBq for the liver (tolerance dose to 30–40 Gy [135, 136], 50% probability of 5% injury to the liver in doses greater than 40 Gy) and 0.058 ± 0.011 mGy/MBq for the pituitary gland [129].

32.9 Quality of Life

To choose the appropriate therapy, physicians have always to weigh the risks and benefits. A favourable effect on quality of life is also required for the approval of new drugs [137]. There are several reports about the change in quality of life after PRRT from Vienna, Rotterdam, Meldola and Bonn [138–142]. For the assessment of quality of life, patients had to complete the European Organization for the Research and Treatment of Cancer Quality of Life Questionnaire before and after PRRT. All study groups report an improvement of the quality of life, pain and other tumour-related symptoms. In pancreatic NET, the global health status, emotional functioning and the social functioning significantly improved after the therapy compared to baseline. Also symptoms such as fatigue, nausea, dyspnoea, constipation and appetite loss [139]. The Rotterdam Study Group presented similar results of 265 patients with GEP- or bronchial NET. A good quality of life is very important, especially in patients with metastatic NET in the palliative situation. The health-related quality of life of asymptomatic patients should not also be impaired. The study results confirm that PRRT seems to meet these requirements [138].

32.10 Controls After PRRT Administration and Follow-Up

To evaluate the tumour uptake after PRRT administration, post-therapeutic images are required. The distribution of Yttrium-90-labelled analogues can be detected using bremsstrahlung scintigraphy (planar or SPECT/CT). Lutetium-177-labelled analogues have additional gamma emission, which provides images (planar or quantitative SPECT/CT) with better quality and enables the individual dosimetry.

Laboratory check-ups including blood count should be performed each 2 weeks for at least 6 weeks after each therapy cycle. Closer monitoring is recommended in case of radiosensitizing chemotherapy. If severe haemotoxicity occurs, weekly testing should be performed until recovery. Furthermore, blood product support should be performed, if needed according to national guidelines. Finally, the regular assessment of the quality of life at regular intervals is recommended.

NET patients, treated with PRRT, need lifetime follow-ups. Essential for the follow-up visits are lab tests, including the evaluation of the tumour marker chromogranin A in serum and eventually the urinary excretion of 5-hydroxyindoleacetic acid (5-HIAA) in case of midgut NET [143]. Another vital part of the staging after PRRT is the SSTR imaging, especially with Gallium-68-[DOTATOC/DOTATATE]-PET/CT, because of its high sensitivity (alternatively Octreoscan®/[^{99m}Tc]Tc-EDDA/HYNIC-TOC) [144]. The first imaging after PRRT is recommended 3 months after the last administration. In case of high-grade tumours or suspicion of dedifferentiation, the SSTR imaging should be complemented by [^{18}F]F-FDG-PET/CT [1, 145].

The intervals between the follow-ups are 6–12 monthly for G1- and G2-NET. Patients with G3 tumours should receive follow-ups each 3 months [46, 146, 147].

32.11 New Development: PRRT with Antagonists

A valuable tumour-targeting feature of SSTR agonists is the internalization of the radioligands together with the receptor, which allows a direct irradiation in the tumour cells. However, Ginj et al. was the first study group in 2006 who changed this paradigm showing that SSTR antagonists, even though the majority are not internalized, have superior tumour uptake. The reason may be more binding sites than agonists and the lower dissociation rate of the antagonists [148].

Cescato et al. from Berne compared via autoradiography the in vitro binding of ^{177}Lu-DOTA-SSTR2-antagonist ([^{177}Lu]Lu-DOTA-BASS) with ^{177}Lu-DOTA-SSTR2-agonist ([^{177}Lu]Lu-Octreotate) in five different human cancer entities. The tissue samples included ileum carcinoids ($N = 9$), phaeochromocytoma ($N = 10$), breast carcinoma ($N = 7$), renal cell carcinoma ($N = 10$) and non-Hodgkin lymphoma ($N = 12$). Radiolabelled antagonist showed better binding affinity than the agonist in all the tested tumour types. In detail, the mean ratios of antagonist/agonist were 4.2 in the ileum carcinoid, 12 in phaeochromocytoma, 11 in breast carcinoma, 5.1 in renal cell carcinoma and 4.8 in non-Hodgkin lymphoma. The results show that also in nonneuroendocrine cancers such as breast carcinoma and renal cell carcinoma, a nearly equal number of receptors to phaeochromocytoma with the agonists can be achieved, which makes the agent relevant for the therapy. Also the non-Hodgkin-lymphomas, which are normally radiosensitive but express a small number of SSTR2, have with the antagonists more chances for successful targeted tumour radiotherapy than with the agonists. These data support the testing of SSTR2-antagonists in patients not only with neuroendocrine but also in nonneuroendocrine tumours [149].

Similar results, but investigating the antagonist [^{177}Lu]Lu-DOTA-JR11 in vitro (SSTR2-positive cells) and in vivo (tumour-xenografted mice), published the Rotterdam study group. 88% of the antagonists were membrane bound in contrast to the agonists, which were to 74% internalized. Compared to [^{177}Lu]Lu-Octreotate, [^{177}Lu]Lu-DOTA-JR11 showed 5-times-higher tumour uptake. In vivo studies showed a longer median tumour growth delay time with [^{177}Lu]Lu-DOTA-JR11 than [^{177}Lu]Lu-Octreotate: 26 days vs. 18 days, respectively. Also in the animal model, better survival rates with the antagonist could be reached: 71 days for the [^{177}Lu]

Lu-DOTA-JR11 group and 61 day for [^{177}Lu]Lu-Octreotate-treated group [30].

Recently published by Nicolas et al. from Basel, preclinical study results include biodistribution and dosimetry data from Lutetium-177-, Yttrium-90- and Indium-111-labelled OPS201 (DOTA-JR11) compared to [^{177}Lu]Lu-Octreotate. Best properties revealed the label with Lutetium-177 OPS201, showing higher tumour dose and better tumour-to-kidney dose ratio [150].

Reubi et al. tested the antagonist [^{125}I]I-DOTA-JR11 in nonneuroendocrine tumour tissue samples: breast carcinoma (*N* = 13), renal cell carcinoma (*N* = 12), medullary thyroid cancer (*N* = 5), 15 non-Hodgkin lymphoma (*N* = 15), prostate carcinoma (*N* = 14) and colon carcinoma (*N* = 17). In vitro receptor autoradiography demonstrated in all tumour entities that the antagonist [^{125}I]I-DOTA-JR11 had better binding as the agonist [^{125}I]I-Octreotide. [^{125}I]I-DOTA-JR11 showed high binding affinity in renal cell carcinoma, breast carcinoma, medullary thyroid cancer and non-Hodgkin lymphoma comparable to neuroendocrine tumours with SSTR2 agonists [31].

Wild et al. demonstrated in NET patients that with [^{111}In]In-DOTA-BASS, significantly more tumour lesions of metastatic thyroid carcinoma or neuroendocrine tumours could be detected (25 of 28 lesions) than with [^{111}In]In-DTPA-Octreotide (only 17 of 28 lesions). The new developed antagonist showed higher tumour and lower renal uptake than the routinely used agonist: 3.5% vs. 1.0% of injected activity tumour uptake and 1.5% vs. 2.3% renal uptake at 4 h after injection [151].

Two years later, Wild et al. published clinical data of four patients with advanced neuroendocrine tumours, treated with the antagonist [^{177}Lu]Lu-DOTA-JR11, showing that the therapy was feasible and effective. Two patients achieved partial remission, one patient had stable disease, and the other patient showed mixed response; none of the patients experienced irreversible or severe adverse events. The dosimetry analyses revealed that [^{177}Lu]Lu-DOTA-JR11 had 1.7–10. Sixfold tumour dose compared to [^{177}Lu]Lu-Octreotate. Also tumour-to-kidney dose ratio and tumour-to-bone marrow dose ratio were with the antagonist 1.1–7.2 times higher [32].

In Basel was conducted the first phase I/II open-label study to test the diagnostic value of the antagonist [^{68}Ga]Ga-OPS202 ([^{68}Ga]Ga-NODAGA-JR11) for PET imaging in 12 patients with GEP-NETs. The evaluation included safety assessment, pharmacokinetics, dosimetry studies and efficacy. Patients received two intravenous injections of 150 MBq [^{68}Ga]Ga-OPS202 with an interval of 3–4 weeks in-between. [^{68}Ga]Ga-OPS202 has proven to be safe. The radiopharmaceutical was rapidly cleared from the bloodstream. The highest doses were in the urinary bladder, kidneys and spleen. The calculated effective dose for activity of 150 MBq was 3.6 mSv (2.4E–02 ± 0.2E–02 mSv/MBq). The highest number of malignant lesions could be detected between 1 and 2 h after injection; the best contrast between malignant liver lesions and liver background was 1 h after injection. In conclusion, further imaging studies with [^{68}Ga]Ga-OPS202 in NETs are warranted [152].

In the phase II component of the study, Nicolas et al. compared the diagnostic sensitivity of [^{68}Ga]Ga-OPS202 with the agonist [^{68}Ga]Ga-DOTATOC. Three intravenous injections per patient for the imaging were performed: 15 μg peptide/150 MBq for ^{68}Ga-DOTATOC, 15 μg peptide/150 MBq for [^{68}Ga]Ga-OPS202 and 50 μg peptide/150 MBq for [^{68}Ga]Ga-OPS202. Best sensitivity showed the antagonist [^{68}Ga]Ga-OPS202 with 50 μg peptide (94%), followed by [^{68}Ga]Ga-OPS202 with 15 μg peptide (88%) and the worst sensitivity had 15 μg peptide [^{68}Ga]Ga-DOTATOC (59%). [^{68}Ga]Ga-OPS202 PET/CT and [^{68}Ga]Ga-DOTATOC PET/CT had similar positive predictive values (approximately 98%). Despite the different peptide quantities of [^{68}Ga]Ga-OPS202 (15 μg vs. 50 μg), the difference in terms of image contrast, sensitivity or positive predictive value was not significant.

In November 2015, Bodei et al. initiated a prospective open-label clinical trial in Memorial Sloan Kettering Cancer Center (New York) to evaluate the theranostic pair [^{68}Ga]Ga-DOTA-JR11 and [^{177}Lu]Lu-DOTA-JR11 (ClinicalTrials.gov Identifier: NCT02609737). To this point, 20 patients have been enrolled in the study. Imaging with [^{68}Ga]Ga-DOTA-JR11

(150–200 MBq) should help to select suitable patients with neuroendocrine tumours. If there is an adequate tracer uptake in the imaging, the patients will be treated with two cycles [^{177}Lu]Lu-DOTA-JR11 (1850 MBq) in an interval of approximately 3 months. Dosimetry studies and response assessment will be performed.

32.12 Conclusion and Future Developments

PRRT proved to prolong the survival in patients with neuroendocrine tumours with a favourable side effects profile, which is important for the compliance of the patients and for the quality of life. Although the therapy is known for almost three decades, preliminary survival data from the phase III NETTER-1 trial, which evaluated the effect of PRRT in midgut NET, was quite recently published. These data changed the status of PRRT in many NET guidelines. Currently, the phase III COMPETE trial is randomizing patients, to compare the effect of [^{177}Lu]Lu-Edotreotide with everolimus. However, more randomized prospective trials with head-to-head comparison with other systemic drugs in neuroendocrine tumours are needed.

PRRT is mainly administered in progressive metastatic patients; therefore a lower complete remission rate is not unexpected. However, need for improvement is essential to achieve higher rates of complete response following PRRT. The potential for better tumour targeting might be achieved with combination therapies or with PRRT with SSTR antagonists. Another approach is the targeted alpha therapy. However, more data about long-term side effects such as MDS and the occurrence of acute leukaemia is needed.

References

1. Yordanova A, Ahmadzadehfar H, Gonzalez-Carmona M, et al. A step-by-step clinical approach for the management of neuroendocrine Tumours. Horm Metab Res. 2017;49(2):77–85.
2. Yordanova A, Mayer K, Brossart P, et al. Safety of multiple repeated cycles of (177)Lu-octreotate in patients with recurrent neuroendocrine tumour. Eur J Nucl Med Mol Imaging. 2017;44(7):1207–14.
3. Bodei L, Mueller-Brand J, Baum RP, et al. The joint IAEA, EANM, and SNMMI practical guidance on peptide receptor radionuclide therapy (PRRNT) in neuroendocrine tumours. Eur J Nucl Med Mol Imaging. 2013;40(5):800–16.
4. Bodei L, Kidd M, Paganelli G, et al. Long-term tolerability of PRRT in 807 patients with neuroendocrine tumours: the value and limitations of clinical factors. Eur J Nucl Med Mol Imaging. 2015;42(1):5–19.
5. Delpassand ES, Samarghandi A, Zamanian S, et al. Peptide receptor radionuclide therapy with 177Lu-DOTATATE for patients with somatostatin receptor-expressing neuroendocrine tumors. Pancreas. 2014;43(4):518–25.
6. Ezziddin S, Attassi M, Yong-Hing CJ, et al. Predictors of long-term outcome in patients with well-differentiated gastroenteropancreatic neuroendocrine tumors after peptide receptor radionuclide therapy with 177Lu-octreotate. J Nucl Med. 2014;55(2):183–90.
7. Kwekkeboom DJ, de Herder WW, van Eijck CHJ, et al. Peptide receptor radionuclide therapy in patients with Gastroenteropancreatic neuroendocrine tumors. Semin Nucl Med. 2010;40(2):78–88.
8. Kwekkeboom DJ, de Herder WW, Krenning EP. Somatostatin receptor-targeted radionuclide therapy in patients with Gastroenteropancreatic neuroendocrine tumors. Endocrinol Metab Clin N Am. 2011;40(1):173–85.
9. Strosberg J, Wolin E, Chasen B, et al. NETTER-1 phase III in patients with midgut neuroendocrine tumors treated with 177Lu-Dotatate: efficacy and safety results. J Nucl Med. 2016;57(suppl 2):629.
10. Gupta SK, Singla S, Bal C. Renal and hematological toxicity in patients of neuroendocrine tumors after peptide receptor radionuclide therapy with 177Lu-DOTATATE. Cancer Biother Radiopharm. 2012;27(9):593–9.
11. Kam BLR, Teunissen JJM, Krenning EP, et al. Lutetium-labelled peptides for therapy of neuroendocrine tumours. Eur J Nucl Med Mol Imaging. 2012;39(Suppl 1):S103–12.
12. Sabet A, Ezziddin K, Pape U-F, et al. Long-term hematotoxicity after peptide receptor radionuclide therapy with 177Lu-octreotate. J Nucl Med. 2013;54(11):1857–61.
13. Sabet A, Ezziddin K, Pape U-F, et al. Long-term Hematotoxicity after peptide receptor radionuclide therapy with 177Lu-Octreotate. J Nucl Med. 2013;54(11):1857–61.
14. Sabet A, Haslerud T, Pape U-F, et al. Outcome and toxicity of salvage therapy with 177Lu-octreotate in patients with metastatic gastroenteropancreatic neuroendocrine tumours. Eur J Nucl Med Mol Imaging. 2014;41(2):205–10.
15. Salavati A, Puranik A, Kulkarni HR, et al. Peptide receptor radionuclide therapy (PRRT) of medullary and nonmedullary thyroid Cancer using radio-

labeled somatostatin analogues. Semin Nucl Med. 2016;46(3):215–24.
16. Chan HS, de Blois E, Morgenstern A, et al. In vitro comparison of 213Bi- and 177Lu-radiation for peptide receptor radionuclide therapy. PLoS One. 2017;12(7):e0181473.
17. Kubota A, Yamada Y, Kagimoto S, et al. Identification of somatostatin receptor subtypes and an implication for the efficacy of somatostatin analogue SMS 201-995 in treatment of human endocrine tumors. J Clin Invest. 1994;93(3):1321–5.
18. Papotti M, Bongiovanni M, Volante M, et al. Expression of somatostatin receptor types 1-5 in 81 cases of gastrointestinal and pancreatic endocrine tumors. A correlative immunohistochemical and reverse-transcriptase polymerase chain reaction analysis. Virchows Arch. 2002;440(5):461–75.
19. Basu S, Dasgupta PS. Dopamine, a neurotransmitter, influences the immune system. J Neuroimmunol. 2000;102(2):113–24.
20. Brazeau P, Vale W, Burgus R, et al. Hypothalamic polypeptide that inhibits the secretion of immunoreactive pituitary growth hormone. Science. 1973;179(4068):77–9.
21. Buscail L, Esteve JP, Saint-Laurent N, et al. Inhibition of cell proliferation by the somatostatin analogue RC-160 is mediated by somatostatin receptor subtypes SSTR2 and SSTR5 through different mechanisms. Proc Natl Acad Sci U S A. 1995;92(5):1580–4.
22. Kumar U, Sasi R, Suresh S, et al. Subtype-selective expression of the five somatostatin receptors (hSSTR1-5) in human pancreatic islet cells: a quantitative double-label immunohistochemical analysis. Diabetes. 1999;48(1):77–85.
23. Patel YC. Somatostatin and its receptor family. Front Neuroendocrinol. 1999;20(3):157–98.
24. van Hagen PM, Krenning EP, Kwekkeboom DJ, et al. Somatostatin and the immune and haematopoetic system; a review. Eur J Clin Investig. 1994;24(2):91–9.
25. Oberg KE, Reubi J-C, Kwekkeboom DJ, et al. Role of somatostatins in gastroenteropancreatic neuroendocrine tumor development and therapy. Gastroenterology. 2010;139(3):742–53, 753.e1.
26. Caplin ME, Pavel M, Cwikla JB, et al. Lanreotide in metastatic enteropancreatic neuroendocrine tumors. N Engl J Med. 2014;371(3):224–33.
27. Rinke A, Muller H-H, Schade-Brittinger C, et al. Placebo-controlled, double-blind, prospective, randomized study on the effect of octreotide LAR in the control of tumor growth in patients with metastatic neuroendocrine midgut tumors: a report from the PROMID study group. J Clin Oncol. 2009;27(28):4656–63.
28. Kwekkeboom DJ, Bakker WH, Kooij PP, et al. 177Lu-DOTAOTyr3octreotate: comparison with 111In-DTPAooctreotide in patients. Eur J Nucl Med. 2001;28(9):1319–25.
29. Beykan S, Dam JS, Eberlein U, et al. (177)Lu-OPS201 targeting somatostatin receptors: in vivo biodistribution and dosimetry in a pig model. EJNMMI Res. 2016;6(1):50.
30. Dalm SU, Nonnekens J, Doeswijk GN, et al. Comparison of the therapeutic response to treatment with a 177Lu-labeled somatostatin receptor agonist and antagonist in preclinical models. J Nucl Med. 2016;57(2):260–5.
31. Reubi JC, Waser B, Macke H, et al. Highly increased 125I-JR11 antagonist binding in vitro reveals novel indications for sst2 targeting in human cancers. J Nucl Med. 2017;58(2):300–6.
32. Wild D, Fani M, Fischer R, et al. Comparison of somatostatin receptor agonist and antagonist for peptide receptor radionuclide therapy: a pilot study. J Nucl Med. 2014;55(8):1248–52.
33. Poeppel TD, Binse I, Petersenn S, et al. 68Ga-DOTATOC versus 68Ga-DOTATATE PET/CT in functional imaging of neuroendocrine tumors. J Nucl Med. 2011;52(12):1864–70.
34. Wild D, Schmitt JS, Ginj M, et al. DOTA-NOC, a high-affinity ligand of somatostatin receptor subtypes 2, 3 and 5 for labelling with various radiometals. Eur J Nucl Med Mol Imaging. 2003;30(10):1338–47.
35. Esser JP, Krenning EP, Teunissen JJM, et al. Comparison of (177)Lu-DOTA(0),Tyr(3)octreotate and (177)Lu-DOTA(0),Tyr(3)octreotide. Eur J Nucl Med Mol Imaging. 2006;33(11):1346–51.
36. Forrer F, Uusijärvi H, Waldherr C, et al. A comparison of (111)in-DOTATOC and (111)in-DOTATATE. Eur J Nucl Med Mol Imaging. 2004;31(9):1257–62.
37. Velikyan I, Sundin A, Sörensen J, et al. Quantitative and qualitative intrapatient comparison of 68Ga-DOTATOC and 68Ga-DOTATATE. J Nucl Med. 2014;55(2):204–10.
38. Anthony LB, Woltering EA, Espenan GD, et al. Indium-111-pentetreotide prolongs survival in gastroenteropancreatic malignancies. Semin Nucl Med. 2002;32(2):123–32.
39. Yordanova A, Eppard E, Kurpig S, et al. Theranostics in nuclear medicine practice. Onco Targets Ther. 2017;10:4821–8.
40. Romer A, Seiler D, Marincek N, et al. Somatostatin-based radiopeptide therapy with 177Lu-DOTA-TOC versus 90Y-DOTA-TOC in neuroendocrine tumours. Eur J Nucl Med Mol Imaging. 2014;41(2):214–22.
41. Chinol M, Bodei L, Cremonesi M, et al. Receptor-mediated radiotherapy with 90Y-DOTA-DPhe1-Tyr3-octreotide. Semin Nucl Med. 2002;32(2):141–7.
42. Kratochwil C, López-Benítez R, Mier W, et al. Hepatic arterial infusion enhances DOTATOC radiopeptide therapy in patients with neuroendocrine liver metastases. Endocr Relat Cancer. 2011;18(5):595–602.
43. Chan HS, Konijnenberg MW, Daniels T, et al. Improved safety and efficacy of (213)bi-DOTATATE-targeted alpha therapy of somatostatin receptor-expressing neuroendocrine tumors in mice pre-treated with L-lysine. EJNMMI Res. 2016;6(1):83.
44. Kratochwil C, Giesel FL, Bruchertseifer F, et al. (2)(1)(3)bi-DOTATOC receptor-targeted alpha-radionuclide therapy induces remission in neuroendo-

crine tumours refractory to beta radiation. Eur J Nucl Med Mol Imaging. 2014;41(11):2106–19.
45. Miederer M, Henriksen G, Alke A, et al. Preclinical evaluation of the alpha-particle generator nuclide 225Ac for somatostatin receptor radiotherapy of neuroendocrine tumors. Clin Cancer Res. 2008;14(11):3555–61.
46. Pavel M, O'Toole D, Costa F, et al. ENETS consensus guidelines update for the Management of Distant Metastatic Disease of intestinal, pancreatic, bronchial neuroendocrine neoplasms (NEN) and NEN of unknown primary site. Neuroendocrinology. 2016;103(2):172–85.
47. Strosberg JR, Halfdanarson TR, Bellizzi AM, et al. The north American neuroendocrine tumor society consensus guidelines for surveillance and medical Management of Midgut Neuroendocrine Tumors. Pancreas. 2017;46(6):707–14.
48. Bodei L, Cremonesi M, Grana C, et al. Receptor radionuclide therapy with 90Y-DOTA0-Tyr3-octreotide (90Y-DOTATOC) in neuroendocrine tumours. Eur J Nucl Med Mol Imaging. 2004;31(7):1038–46.
49. Hicks RJ, Kwekkeboom DJ, Krenning E, et al. ENETS consensus guidelines for the standards of Care in Neuroendocrine Neoplasia. Neuroendocrinology. 2017;105(3):295–309.
50. Baum RP, Kulkarni HR. Theranostics. Theranostics. 2012;2(5):437–47.
51. Chan DL, Pavlakis N, Schembri GP, et al. Dual somatostatin receptor/FDG PET/CT imaging in metastatic neuroendocrine Tumours. Theranostics. 2017;7(5):1149–58.
52. Hindié E. The NETPET score. Theranostics. 2017;7(5):1159–63.
53. Krenning EP, Valkema R, Kooij PP, et al. Scintigraphy and radionuclide therapy with indium-111-labelled-diethyl triamine penta-acetic acid-D-Phe1-octreotide. Ital J Gastroenterol Hepatol. 1999;31(Suppl 2):S219–23.
54. Kwekkeboom DJ, Teunissen JJ, Bakker WH, et al. Radiolabeled somatostatin analog 177Lu-DOTA0,Tyr3octreotate in patients with endocrine gastroenteropancreatic tumors. J Clin Oncol. 2005;23(12):2754–62.
55. Bahri H, Laurence L, Edeline J, et al. High prognostic value of 18F-FDG PET for metastatic gastroenteropancreatic neuroendocrine tumors. J Nucl Med. 2014;55(11):1786–90.
56. Binderup T, Knigge U, Loft A, et al. 18F-fluorodeoxyglucose positron emission tomography predicts survival of patients with neuroendocrine tumors. Clin Cancer Res. 2010;16(3):978–85.
57. Ezziddin S, Adler L, Sabet A, et al. Prognostic stratification of metastatic gastroenteropancreatic neuroendocrine neoplasms by 18F-FDG PET. J Nucl Med. 2014;55(8):1260–6.
58. Sansovini M, Severi S, Ianniello A, et al. Long-term follow-up and role of FDG PET in advanced pancreatic neuroendocrine patients treated with 177Lu-D OTATATE. Eur J Nucl Med Mol Imaging. 2017;44(3):490–9.
59. Rindi G, Klöppel G, Couvelard A, et al. TNM staging of midgut and hindgut (neuro) endocrine tumors. Virchows Arch. 2007;451(4):757–62.
60. Garin E, Le Jeune F, Devillers A, et al. Predictive value of 18F-FDG PET and somatostatin receptor scintigraphy in patients with metastatic endocrine tumors. J Nucl Med. 2009;50(6):858–64.
61. Hofman MS, Michael M, Kashyap R, et al. Modifying the poor prognosis associated with 18F-FDG-avid NET with peptide receptor chemo-radionuclide therapy (PRCRT). J Nucl Med. 2015;56(6):968–9.
62. Kashyap R, Hofman MS, Michael M, et al. Favourable outcomes of (177)Lu-octreotate peptide receptor chemoradionuclide therapy in patients with FDG-avid neuroendocrine tumours. Eur J Nucl Med Mol Imaging. 2015;42(2):176–85.
63. Brunner P, Jorg A-C, Glatz K, et al. The prognostic and predictive value of sstr2-immunohistochemistry and sstr2-targeted imaging in neuroendocrine tumors. Eur J Nucl Med Mol Imaging. 2017;44(3):468–75.
64. Zandee WT, de Herder WW. The evolution of neuroendocrine tumor treatment reflected by ENETS guidelines. Neuroendocrinology. 2018;106:357.
65. Brabander T, van der Zwan WA, Teunissen JJM, et al. Long-Term Efficacy, Survival, and Safety of 177Lu-DOTA0,Tyr3octreotate in Patients with Gastroenteropancreatic and Bronchial Neuroendocrine Tumors. Clin Cancer Res. 2017;23(16):4617–24.
66. Ezziddin S, Khalaf F, Vanezi M, et al. Outcome of peptide receptor radionuclide therapy with 177Lu-octreotate in advanced grade 1/2 pancreatic neuroendocrine tumours. Eur J Nucl Med Mol Imaging. 2014;41(5):925–33.
67. Kulke MH, Shah MH, Benson AB, et al. Neuroendocrine tumors, version 1.2015. J Natl Compr Cancer Netw. 2015;13(1):78–108.
68. van Vliet EI, van Eijck CH, de Krijger RR, et al. Neoadjuvant Treatment of Nonfunctioning Pancreatic Neuroendocrine Tumors with 177Lu-DOTA0,Tyr3Octreotate. J Nucl Med. 2015;56(11):1647–53.
69. Kong G, Grozinsky-Glasberg S, Hofman MS, et al. Efficacy of peptide receptor radionuclide therapy for functional metastatic Paraganglioma and Pheochromocytoma. J Clin Endocrinol Metab. 2017;102(9):3278–87.
70. Nastos K, Cheung VTF, Toumpanakis C, et al. Peptide receptor radionuclide treatment and (131)I-MIBG in the management of patients with metastatic/progressive phaeochromocytomas and paragangliomas. J Surg Oncol. 2017;115(4):425–34.
71. Iten F, Muller B, Schindler C, et al. Response to 90Yttrium-DOTA-TOC treatment is associated with long-term survival benefit in metastasized medullary thyroid cancer. Clin Cancer Res. 2007;13(22 Pt 1):6696–702.
72. Waldherr C, Schumacher T, Pless M, et al. Radiopeptide transmitted internal irradiation of non-

iodophil thyroid cancer and conventionally untreatable medullary thyroid cancer using. Nucl Med Commun. 2001;22(6):673–8.
73. Gild ML, Bullock M, Robinson BG, et al. Multikinase inhibitors. Nat Rev Endocrinol. 2011;7(10):617–24.
74. Versari A, Sollini M, Frasoldati A, et al. Differentiated thyroid cancer. Thyroid. 2014;24(4):715–26.
75. Arnold R, Wittenberg M, Rinke A, et al. Placebo controlled, double blind, prospective, randomized study on the effect of octreotide LAR in the control of tumor growth in patients with metastatic neuroendocrine midgut tumors (PROMID): results on long-term survival. JCO. 2013;31(15 suppl):4030.
76. Caplin ME, Pavel M, Cwikla JB, et al. Anti-tumour effects of lanreotide for pancreatic and intestinal neuroendocrine tumours. Endocr Relat Cancer. 2016;23(3):191–9.
77. Rinke A, Wittenberg M, Schade-Brittinger C, et al. Placebo-controlled, double-blind, prospective, randomized study on the effect of octreotide LAR in the control of tumor growth in patients with metastatic neuroendocrine midgut tumors (PROMID): results of long-term survival. Neuroendocrinology. 2017;104(1):26–32.
78. Aalbersberg EA, de wit-van der Veen BJ, Versleijen MWJ, et al. Influence of lanreotide on uptake of 68Ga-DOTATATE in patients with neuroendocrine tumours. Eur J Nucl Med Mol Imaging. 2018;46(3):696–703.
79. Bodei L, Cremonesi M, Zoboli S, et al. Receptor-mediated radionuclide therapy with 90Y-DOTATOC in association with amino acid infusion: a phase I study. Eur J Nucl Med Mol Imaging. 2003;30(2):207–16.
80. Rolleman EJ, Valkema R, de Jong M, et al. Safe and effective inhibition of renal uptake of radiolabelled octreotide by a combination of lysine and arginine. Eur J Nucl Med Mol Imaging. 2003;30(1):9–15.
81. Imhof A, Brunner P, Marincek N, et al. Response, survival, and long-term toxicity after therapy with the radiolabeled somatostatin analogue 90Y-DOTA-TOC in metastasized neuroendocrine cancers. J Clin Oncol. 2011;29(17):2416–23.
82. Strosberg J, El-Haddad G, Wolin E, et al. Phase 3 trial of 177Lu-Dotatate for midgut neuroendocrine tumors. N Engl J Med. 2017;376(2):125–35.
83. Rinke A, Wittenberg M, Schade-Brittinger C, et al. Placebo-controlled, double-blind, prospective, randomized study on the effect of octreotide LAR in the control of tumor growth in patients with metastatic neuroendocrine midgut tumors (PROMID). Neuroendocrinology. 2017;104(1):26–32.
84. Pavel ME, Hainsworth JD, Baudin E, et al. Everolimus plus octreotide long-acting repeatable for the treatment of advanced neuroendocrine tumours associated with carcinoid syndrome (RADIANT-2). Lancet. 2011;378(9808):2005–12.
85. Pavel ME, Baudin E, Oberg KE, et al. Efficacy of everolimus plus octreotide LAR in patients with advanced neuroendocrine tumor and carcinoid syndrome. Ann Oncol. 2017;28(7):1569–75.
86. Yao JC, Shah MH, Ito T, et al. Everolimus for advanced pancreatic neuroendocrine tumors. N Engl J Med. 2011;364(6):514–23.
87. Yao JC, Pavel M, Lombard-Bohas C, et al. Everolimus for the treatment of advanced pancreatic neuroendocrine tumors. J Clin Oncol. 2016;34(32):3906–13.
88. Yao JC, Fazio N, Singh S, et al. Everolimus for the treatment of advanced, non-functional neuroendocrine tumours of the lung or gastrointestinal tract (RADIANT-4). Lancet. 2016;387(10022):968–77.
89. Raymond E, Dahan L, Raoul J-L, et al. Sunitinib malate for the treatment of pancreatic neuroendocrine tumors. N Engl J Med. 2011;364(6):501–13.
90. Dahan L, Bonnetain F, Rougier P, et al. Phase III trial of chemotherapy using 5-fluorouracil and streptozotocin compared with interferon alpha for advanced carcinoid tumors. Endocr Relat Cancer. 2009;16(4):1351–61.
91. Hallet J, Law CHL, Cukier M, et al. Exploring the rising incidence of neuroendocrine tumors. Cancer. 2015;121(4):589–97.
92. Mariniello A, Bodei L, Tinelli C, et al. Long-term results of PRRT in advanced bronchopulmonary carcinoid. Eur J Nucl Med Mol Imaging. 2016;43(3):441–52.
93. Sabet A, Haug AR, Eiden C, et al. Efficacy of peptide receptor radionuclide therapy with 177Lu-octreotate in metastatic pulmonary neuroendocrine tumors. Am J Nucl Med Mol Imaging. 2017;7(2):74–83.
94. Sabet A, Dautzenberg K, Haslerud T, et al. Specific efficacy of peptide receptor radionuclide therapy with (177)Lu-octreotate in advanced neuroendocrine tumours of the small intestine. Eur J Nucl Med Mol Imaging. 2015;42(8):1238–46.
95. Hörsch D, Ezziddin S, Haug A, et al. Effectiveness and side-effects of peptide receptor radionuclide therapy for neuroendocrine neoplasms in Germany. Eur J Cancer. 2016;58:41–51.
96. Kwekkeboom DJ, de Herder WW, Kam BL, et al. Treatment with the radiolabeled somatostatin analog 177 Lu-DOTA 0,Tyr3octreotate. J Clin Oncol. 2008;26(13):2124–30.
97. Baum RP, Kluge AW, Kulkarni H, et al. (177) Lu-DOTA(0)-D-Phe(1)-Tyr(3)-octreotide ((177) Lu-DOTATOC) for peptide receptor radiotherapy in patients with advanced neuroendocrine Tumours. Theranostics. 2016;6(4):501–10.
98. Waldherr C, Pless M, Maecke HR, et al. The clinical value of 90Y-DOTA-D-Phe1-Tyr3-octreotide (90Y-DOTATOC) in the treatment of neuroendocrine tumours. Ann Oncol. 2001;12(7):941–5.
99. Bushnell DL, O'Dorisio TM, O'Dorisio MS, et al. 90Y-edotreotide for metastatic carcinoid refractory to octreotide. J Clin Oncol. 2010;28(10):1652–9.
100. Cwikla JB, Sankowski A, Seklecka N, et al. Efficacy of radionuclide treatment DOTATATE Y-90 in patients with progressive metastatic gastroenteropancreatic neuroendocrine carcinomas (GEP-NETs): a phase II study. Ann Oncol. 2010;21(4):787–94.

101. Villard L, Romer A, Marincek N, et al. Cohort study of somatostatin-based Radiopeptide therapy with [90Y-DOTA]-TOC versus [90Y-DOTA]-TOC plus [177Lu-DOTA]-TOC in neuroendocrine cancers. J Clin Oncol. 2012;30(10):1100–6.
102. Seregni E, Maccauro M, Chiesa C, et al. Treatment with tandem 90YDOTA-TATE and 177LuDOTA-TATE of neuroendocrine tumours refractory to conventional therapy. Eur J Nucl Med Mol Imaging. 2014;41(2):223–30.
103. de Jong M, Breeman WAP, Valkema R, et al. Combination radionuclide therapy using 177Lu- and 90Y-labeled somatostatin analogs. J Nucl Med. 2005;46(Suppl 1):13S–7S.
104. Kunikowska J, Krolicki L, Hubalewska-Dydejczyk A, et al. Clinical results of radionuclide therapy of neuroendocrine tumours with 90Y-DOTATATE and tandem 90Y/177Lu-DOTATATE. Eur J Nucl Med Mol Imaging. 2011;38(10):1788–97.
105. Kunikowska J, Pawlak D, Bak MI, et al. Long-term results and tolerability of tandem peptide receptor radionuclide therapy with (90)Y/(177) Lu-DOTATATE in neuroendocrine tumors with respect to the primary location. Ann Nucl Med. 2017;31(5):347–56.
106. Pfeifer AK, Gregersen T, Gronbaek H, et al. Peptide receptor radionuclide therapy with Y-DOTATOC and (177)Lu-DOTATOC in advanced neuroendocrine tumors. Neuroendocrinology. 2011;93(3):189–96.
107. Bodei L, Cremonesi M, Grana CM, et al. Peptide receptor radionuclide therapy with (1)(7)(7) Lu-DOTATATE. Eur J Nucl Med Mol Imaging. 2011;38(12):2125–35.
108. Yordanova A, Wicharz MM, Mayer K, et al. The role of adding somatostatin analogues to peptide receptor radionuclide therapy as a combination and maintenance therapy. Clin Cancer Res. 2018;24(19):4672–9.
109. Bison SM, Konijnenberg MW, Melis M, et al. Peptide receptor radionuclide therapy using radiolabeled somatostatin analogs. Clin Transl Imaging. 2014;2:55–66.
110. van Essen M, Krenning EP, Kam BL, et al. Report on short-term side effects of treatments with 177Lu-octreotate in combination with capecitabine in seven patients with gastroenteropancreatic neuroendocrine tumours. Eur J Nucl Med Mol Imaging. 2008;35(4):743–8.
111. Claringbold PG, Brayshaw PA, Price RA, et al. Phase II study of radiopeptide 177Lu-octreotate and capecitabine therapy of progressive disseminated neuroendocrine tumours. Eur J Nucl Med Mol Imaging. 2011;38(2):302–11.
112. Claringbold PG, Price RA, Turner JH. Phase I-II study of radiopeptide 177Lu-octreotate in combination with capecitabine and temozolomide in advanced low-grade neuroendocrine tumors. Cancer Biother Radiopharm. 2012;27(9):561–9.
113. Claringbold PG, Turner JH. Pancreatic neuroendocrine tumor control. Neuroendocrinology. 2016;103(5):432–9.
114. Kong G, Thompson M, Collins M, et al. Assessment of predictors of response and long-term survival of patients with neuroendocrine tumour treated with peptide receptor chemoradionuclide therapy (PRCRT). Eur J Nucl Med Mol Imaging. 2014;41(10):1831–44.
115. Claringbold PG, Turner JH. NeuroEndocrine tumor therapy with Lutetium-177-octreotate and Everolimus (NETTLE). Cancer Biother Radiopharm. 2015;30(6):261–9.
116. Zellmer J, Vomacka L, Boening G, et al. Combination of peptide receptor radionuclide therapy with Lu-177 DOTATATE and the m-TOR inhibitor RAD001 (Everolimus) in AR42J tumor bearing mice and response assessment by Ga-68 DOTATATE PET. J Nucl Med. 2018;59(suppl 1):1346b.
117. van Essen M, Krenning EP, Kam BLR, et al. Salvage therapy with (177)Lu-octreotate in patients with bronchial and gastroenteropancreatic neuroendocrine tumors. J Nucl Med. 2010;51(3):383–90.
118. Severi S, Sansovini M, Ianniello A, et al. Feasibility and utility of re-treatment with (177)Lu-DOTATATE in GEP-NENs relapsed after treatment with (90) Y-DOTATOC. Eur J Nucl Med Mol Imaging. 2015;42(13):1955–63.
119. Program N C I C T E. Common terminology criteria for adverse events:(CTCAE). Cancer Therapy Evaluation Program; 2003.
120. de Keizer B, van Aken MO, Feelders RA, et al. Hormonal crises following receptor radionuclide therapy with the radiolabeled somatostatin analogue [(177)Lu-DOTA(0),Tyr(3)]octreotate. Eur J Nucl Med Mol Imaging. 2007;35(4):749–55.
121. Bergsma H, Konijnenberg MW, Kam BLR, et al. Subacute haematotoxicity after PRRT with (177) Lu-DOTA-octreotate: prognostic factors, incidence and course. Eur J Nucl Med Mol Imaging. 2016;43(3):453–63.
122. Bergsma H, Konijnenberg MW, van der Zwan WA, et al. Nephrotoxicity after PRRT with (177) Lu-DOTA-octreotate. Eur J Nucl Med Mol Imaging. 2016;43(10):1802–11.
123. Teunissen JJM, Krenning EP, de Jong FH, et al. Effects of therapy with 177Lu-DOTA 0,Tyr 3octreotate on endocrine function. Eur J Nucl Med Mol Imaging. 2009;36(11):1758–66.
124. Stabin MG. MIRDOSE: personal computer software for internal dose assessment in nuclear medicine. J Nucl Med. 1996;37(3):538–46.
125. Stabin MG, Sparks RB, Crowe E. OLINDA/EXM: the second-generation personal computer software for internal dose assessment in nuclear medicine. J Nucl Med. 2005;46(6):1023–7.
126. Kupitz D, Wetz C, Wissel H, et al. Software-assisted dosimetry in peptide receptor radionuclide therapy with 177Lutetium-DOTATATE for various imaging scenarios. PLoS One. 2017;12(11):e0187570.

127. Schuchardt C, Kulkarni HR, Prasad V, et al. The Bad Berka dose protocol: comparative results of dosimetry in peptide receptor radionuclide therapy using (177)Lu-DOTATATE, (177)Lu-DOTANOC, and (177)Lu-DOTATOC. Recent Results Cancer Res. 2013;194:519–36.
128. Misadministration of radioactive material in medicine. Bethesda, MD: NCRP; 1991.
129. Gupta SK, Singla S, Thakral P, et al. Dosimetric analyses of kidneys, liver, spleen, pituitary gland, and neuroendocrine tumors of patients treated with 177Lu-DOTATATE. Clin Nucl Med. 2013;38(3):188–94.
130. Pauwels S, Barone R, Walrand S, et al. Practical dosimetry of peptide receptor radionuclide therapy with (90)Y-labeled somatostatin analogs. J Nucl Med. 2005;46(Suppl 1):92S–8S.
131. Guerriero F, Ferrari ME, Botta F, et al. Kidney dosimetry in (1)(7)(7)Lu and (9)(0)Y peptide receptor radionuclide therapy. Biomed Res Int. 2013;2013:935351.
132. Forrer F, Krenning EP, Kooij PP, et al. Bone marrow dosimetry in peptide receptor radionuclide therapy with 177Lu-DOTA(0),Tyr(3)octreotate. Eur J Nucl Med Mol Imaging. 2009;36(7):1138–46.
133. Sandstrom M, Garske-Roman U, Granberg D, et al. Individualized dosimetry of kidney and bone marrow in patients undergoing 177Lu-DOTA-octreotate treatment. J Nucl Med. 2013;54(1):33–41.
134. Wehrmann C, Senftleben S, Zachert C, et al. Results of individual patient dosimetry in peptide receptor radionuclide therapy with 177Lu DOTA-TATE and 177Lu DOTA-NOC. Cancer Biother Radiopharm. 2007;22(3):406–16.
135. Emami B, Lyman J, Brown A, et al. Tolerance of normal tissue to therapeutic irradiation. Int J Radiat Oncol Biol Phys. 1991;21(1):109–22.
136. Milano MT, Constine LS, Okunieff P. Normal tissue tolerance dose metrics for radiation therapy of major organs. Semin Radiat Oncol. 2007;17(2):131–40.
137. Johnson JR, Temple R. Food and Drug Administration requirements for approval of new anticancer drugs. Cancer Treat Rep. 1985;69(10):1155–9.
138. Khan S, Krenning EP, van Essen M, et al. Quality of life in 265 patients with gastroenteropancreatic or bronchial neuroendocrine tumors treated with 177Lu-DOTA0,Tyr3octreotate. J Nucl Med. 2011;52(9):1361–8.
139. Marinova M, Mücke M, Mahlberg L, et al. Improving quality of life in patients with pancreatic neuroendocrine tumor following peptide receptor radionuclide therapy assessed by EORTC QLQ-C30. Eur J Nucl Med Mol Imaging. 2018;45(1):38–46.
140. Severi S, Grassi I, Nicolini S, et al. Peptide receptor radionuclide therapy in the management of gastrointestinal neuroendocrine tumors. Onco Targets Ther. 2017;10:551–7.
141. Teunissen JJM, Kwekkeboom DJ, Krenning EP. Quality of life in patients with gastroenteropancreatic tumors treated with 177Lu-DOTA0,Tyr3octreotate. J Clin Oncol. 2004;22(13):2724–9.
142. Traub-Weidinger T, Raderer M, Uffmann M, et al. Improved quality of life in patients treated with peptide radionuclides. World J Nucl Med. 2011;10(2):115–21.
143. O'Toole D, Grossman A, Gross D, et al. ENETS consensus guidelines for the standards of Care in Neuroendocrine Tumors: biochemical markers. Neuroendocrinology. 2009;90(2):194–202.
144. Ruf J, Heuck F, Schiefer J, et al. Impact of multiphase 68Ga-DOTATOC-PET/CT on therapy management in patients with neuroendocrine tumors. Neuroendocrinology. 2010;91(1):101–9.
145. Kayani I, Bomanji JB, Groves A, et al. Functional imaging of neuroendocrine tumors with combined PET/CT using 68Ga-DOTATATE (DOTA-DPhe1,Tyr3-octreotate) and 18F-FDG. Cancer. 2008;112(11):2447–55.
146. Pape U-F, Perren A, Niederle B, et al. ENETS consensus guidelines for the management of patients with neuroendocrine neoplasms from the jejuno-ileum and the appendix including goblet cell carcinomas. Neuroendocrinology. 2011;95(2):135–56.
147. Pavel M, Baudin E, Couvelard A, et al. ENETS consensus guidelines for the management of patients with liver and other distant metastases from neuroendocrine neoplasms of foregut, midgut, hindgut, and unknown primary. Neuroendocrinology. 2012;95(2):157–76.
148. Ginj M, Zhang H, Waser B, et al. Radiolabeled somatostatin receptor antagonists are preferable to agonists for in vivo peptide receptor targeting of tumors. Proc Natl Acad Sci U S A. 2006;103(44):16436–41.
149. Cescato R, Waser B, Fani M, et al. Evaluation of 177Lu-DOTA-sst2 antagonist versus 177Lu-DOTA-sst2 agonist binding in human cancers in vitro. J Nucl Med. 2011;52(12):1886–90.
150. Nicolas GP, Mansi R, McDougall L, et al. Biodistribution, pharmacokinetics, and dosimetry of177Lu-,90Y-, and111In-labeled somatostatin receptor antagonist OPS201 in comparison to the Agonist177Lu-DOTATATE. J Nucl Med. 2017;58(9):1435–41.
151. Wild D, Fani M, Behe M, et al. First clinical evidence that imaging with somatostatin receptor antagonists is feasible. J Nucl Med. 2011;52(9):1412–7.
152. Nicolas GP, Beykan S, Bouterfa H, et al. Safety, biodistribution, and radiation dosimetry of68Ga-OPS202 (68Ga-NODAGA-JR11) in patients with Gastroenteropancreatic neuroendocrine tumors. J Nucl Med. 2018;59(6):909–14.

33 Treatment of Neuroendocrine Tumours (Neuroblastoma Stage III or IV, Metastatic Pheochromocytoma, Etc.) with ^{131}I-mIBG

Matthias Schmidt and Frank Grünwald

33.1 History

While radiopharmaceuticals demonstrating uptake in the adrenal medulla were developed since 1967 [^{14}C-labeled epinephrine and precursors [1], iodinated compound of dopamine [2–4], radioiodinated bretylium analogue [5]], the real clinical success story started with the introduction of iodine-131-meta-iodobenzylguanidine (^{131}I-mIBG), developed by Dr. Donald Wieland, Ann Arbor, Michigan, in 1979. MIBG was primarily intended as a scintigraphic agent to allow imaging of the adrenal medulla [6]. Wieland and colleagues showed that mIBG accumulates in the neurosecretory granules of adrenal chromaffin cells, similarly to norepinephrine.

In 1981, mIBG was used for imaging of pheochromocytoma [7, 8] and in 1983 the first publication appeared dealing with I-131-mIBG treatment in a patient with metastatic pheochromocytoma [9].

MIBG accumulation was observed also in neuroblastoma [10]. The first treatment of a patient suffering from neuroblastoma with I-131-mIBG took place in Europe [11].

In carcinoid tumours, Fischer et al. reported an intense uptake in 1984 [12]. Time has demonstrated that the statement in 1981 of one of the fathers of radionuclide therapy has come true: "The therapeutic approach of internally administered radiopharmaceuticals offers the potential to outmode the present approaches of conventional radiation therapy or chemotherapy" [11].

33.1.1 The Radiopharmaceutical mIBG

Meta-iodobenzylguanidine (mIBG) or" iobenguane" is an aralkylguanidine resulting from the combination of the benzyl group of bretylium and the guanidine group of guanethidine and is radioiodinated in position 3 of the aromatic ring [13]. When labelled with ^{123}I, this radiopharmaceutical is a key tracer in neuroblastoma and pheochromocytoma imaging and when labelled with ^{131}I it can be used for therapy. ^{124}I-labelled mIBG is available in some institutions for PET imaging. No-carrier-added radioiodinated mIBG has been shown to achieve higher levels of specifically incorporated radioactivity than carrier-added mIBG [14]. In an attempt to further improve the specific uptake characteristics, new mIBG derivatives were developed. One compound containing the non-polar methyl group at the 4 position of the aromatic ring, 3-[I-131]iodo-4-methyl-

M. Schmidt (✉)
Department of Nuclear Medicine, University Hospital of Cologne, Cologne, Germany
e-mail: matthias.schmidt@uk-koeln.de

F. Grünwald
Department of Nuclear Medicine, University Hospital of Frankfurt, Frankfurt, Germany

H. Ahmadzadehfar et al. (eds.), *Clinical Nuclear Medicine*,
https://doi.org/10.1007/978-3-030-39457-8_33

benzylguanidine (MeIBG), showed a higher cellular retention in animal and in vitro studies, compared to I-125-MIBG [15], however has not found clinical introduction yet.

33.1.2 MIBG Uptake Mechanisms

Because of structural similarity with noradrenaline (norepinephrine (NE)) [16], mIBG is selectively concentrated by tissues with high adrenergic innervation, essentially neuroectodermal tissue, including tumours of neuroectodermal origin [17]. Meta-iodobenzylguanidine accumulates in the neurosecretory granules of adrenal chromaffin cells, similarly to norepinephrine. The majority of mIBG uptake in neuroblastoma cells occurs by an energy-dependent active transport (type 1 amine transporter uptake mechanism), which is approximately 30 times more efficient than passive transport. A small portion of the tracer passively diffuses into the presynaptic cell. The uptake 1 mechanism is saturable and dependent upon serum sodium and chloride co-transported substrates, temperature, pH, oxygen and vascularity [18]. The vast majority of neuroblastoma cells express the norepinephrine transporter and therefore can take up mIBG [17].

33.1.3 Physiologic Distribution

After intravenous injection, meta-iodobenzylguanidine (mIBG) is mainly cleared from the vascular compartment within about 1 h. MIBG shows physiologic uptake in the parotids and submandibular glands, nasopharynx, myocardium, liver and adrenals and is excreted via the renal collecting system, bladder and sometimes bowel, especially colon [19]. Excretion occurs mainly via the kidneys with visualization of radioactive urine in the bladder. To a little extent bowel uptake is seen, less than 2% had been measured in the faeces. Liver uptake tends to be heterogeneous and may be more prominent in the left lobe [20]. Splenic uptake is either very mild or not present at all [21]. Lacrimal glands can occasionally show low-grade, usually symmetrical mIBG uptake [22]. Uterine uptake during the menstrual cycle is possible [23]. Sites of normal uptake also include brown adipose tissue. Enzymatic deiodination of mIBG produces free radioactive iodide which is taken up in the thyroid. In patients who have undergone resection of a primary tumour involving one adrenal gland, the remaining contralateral adrenal may show prominent mIBG uptake due to hyperplasia which is considered a physiological finding [24]. Uptake in the salivary glands and the heart is due to the sympathetic innervation. Several transporters have been described being responsible for mIBG uptake, such as the norepinephrine transporter (NET), the vesicular monoamine transporter 2 (VMAT2) and the organic cation transporter (OCT), the latter being most likely responsible for physiologic liver uptake of mIBG. For therapeutic purposes, pathophysiologic basis for I-131-mIBG therapy is the expression of the norepinephrine transporter on the tumour cell membrane [17].

33.1.4 Pitfalls

In children under the age of 6 months an intense myocardial mIBG uptake may be visualized leading to a heterogeneous display of the right mediastinal region due to tracer accumulation in the right heart. Furthermore a bilateral symmetrical uptake occurs frequently in the upper thoracic region in brown adipose tissue and may be misinterpreted as representing retro- or supraclavicular lymph nodes. The physiologic high liver uptake can hamper the diagnosis of liver metastases, since they can hardly be distinguished from the background liver activity in some cases [24]. Urinary activity may mask tumours adjacent to the bladder.

33.2 Indications for ^{131}I-mIBG Therapy

33.2.1 Neuroblastoma Stage III or IV

Neuroblastoma is the most common extracranial paediatric solid tumour with about 130 new cases diagnosed each year in Germany and about 650 newly diagnosed patients per year in the United States of America. It commonly presents in children younger than 2 years of age, with 90% being younger than 5 years of age. There is marked variability in clinical behaviour ranging from spontaneous regression or differentiation into benign tumours to rapid and progressive disease with fatal outcome. Approximately 50% of patients will have metastases at the time of presentation. The management is dependent on age, stage of the disease and biological as well as biochemical markers. Current treatment for high-risk neuroblastoma patients consists of induction chemotherapy with combinations of cisplatin, etoposide, doxorubicin, cyclophosphamide, vincristine and topotecan followed by a consolidation therapy with myeloablative cytotoxic agents and autologous stem cell transplantation. Surgery for the primary tumour and/or metastases and external radiation therapy are additional therapeutic modalities. Despite aggressive treatment regimens, high-risk neuroblastoma continues to have a devastating mortality rate of more than 40% and 5-year overall survival of patients with stage IV neuroblastoma is only 30–50% [25]. Since 1984, it is known that neuroblastoma cells accumulate mIBG [10]. ^{131}I-mIBG therapy is an additional treatment option and can be used in case of persistent mIBG-avid lesions at the end of induction chemotherapy, in case of tumour progression or disease relapse or refractory disease or as palliative treatment for pain relief, and in some centres, mainly in the Netherlands, ^{131}I-mIBG was included in upfront protocols [25, 26]. Wilson et al. published a systematic review about ^{131}I-mIBG therapy in neuroblastoma patients and reported about a high heterogeneity of the data without identification of a prospective randomized controlled trial. The objective tumour response rate in 25 studies reported ranged from 0% to 75%, mean 32% [27].

33.2.2 Metastatic Pheochromocytoma/Paraganglioma (Extraadrenal Pheochromocytoma)

In metastatic or inoperable malignant pheochromocytoma there is usually no curative therapy option and ^{131}I-mIBG is a palliative first-line therapy. Szalat et al. reported that ^{131}I-mIBG was the only treatment in their series of patients which led repetitively and for a notable period of time to disease stabilization [28]. The indication for ^{131}I-mIBG therapy is usually non-resectable, progressive pheochromocytoma or paraganglioma (extraadrenal pheochromocytoma) (Fig. 33.1). ^{131}I-mIBG can be used for symptomatic therapy, to reduce hormonal activity and to control hypertension as well as to relieve pain caused by metastases [29, 30]. Apart from paragangliomas being extraadrenal pheochromocytomas, another entity is termed paraganglioma, i.e. head and neck paragangliomas. The latter tumours derive from parasympathetic tissue and are predominantly somatostatin receptor positive and may also be treated with peptide receptor radionuclide therapy in a metastatic situation.

33.2.3 Rare Indications (Metastatic Carcinoid Tumours, mMTC, mMCC)

Metastatic carcinoid tumours are rare indications for ^{131}I-mIBG therapy as these tumours usually display somatostatin receptors and are thus preferentially amenable for peptide receptor radionuclide therapy in case of disease progression despite treatment with somatostatin analogues [31, 32]. Midgut carcinoids, localized in the ileum and cecum, were reported to take up mIBG better than tumours found in the pancreas, stomach and bronchus [33].

Most patients with metastatic medullary thyroid cancer [mMTC] require a multimodal diagnostic and therapeutic approach. Imaging techniques such as MRI, CT, DOPA-PET and FDG-PET play the main role in the diagnosis of mostly recurrent MTC [34]. ^{18}F-FDG-PET has shown a sensitivity of 78% and a specificity of 79% for the detection of metastases or recurrence of MTC and was superior to somatostatin receptor scintigraphy, ^{99m}Tc-DMSA scintigraphy, ^{99m}Tc-MIBI scintigraphy and CT. Only MRI showed comparable results with a sensitivity of 82%, but a specificity of only 67%. MIBG scintigraphy can

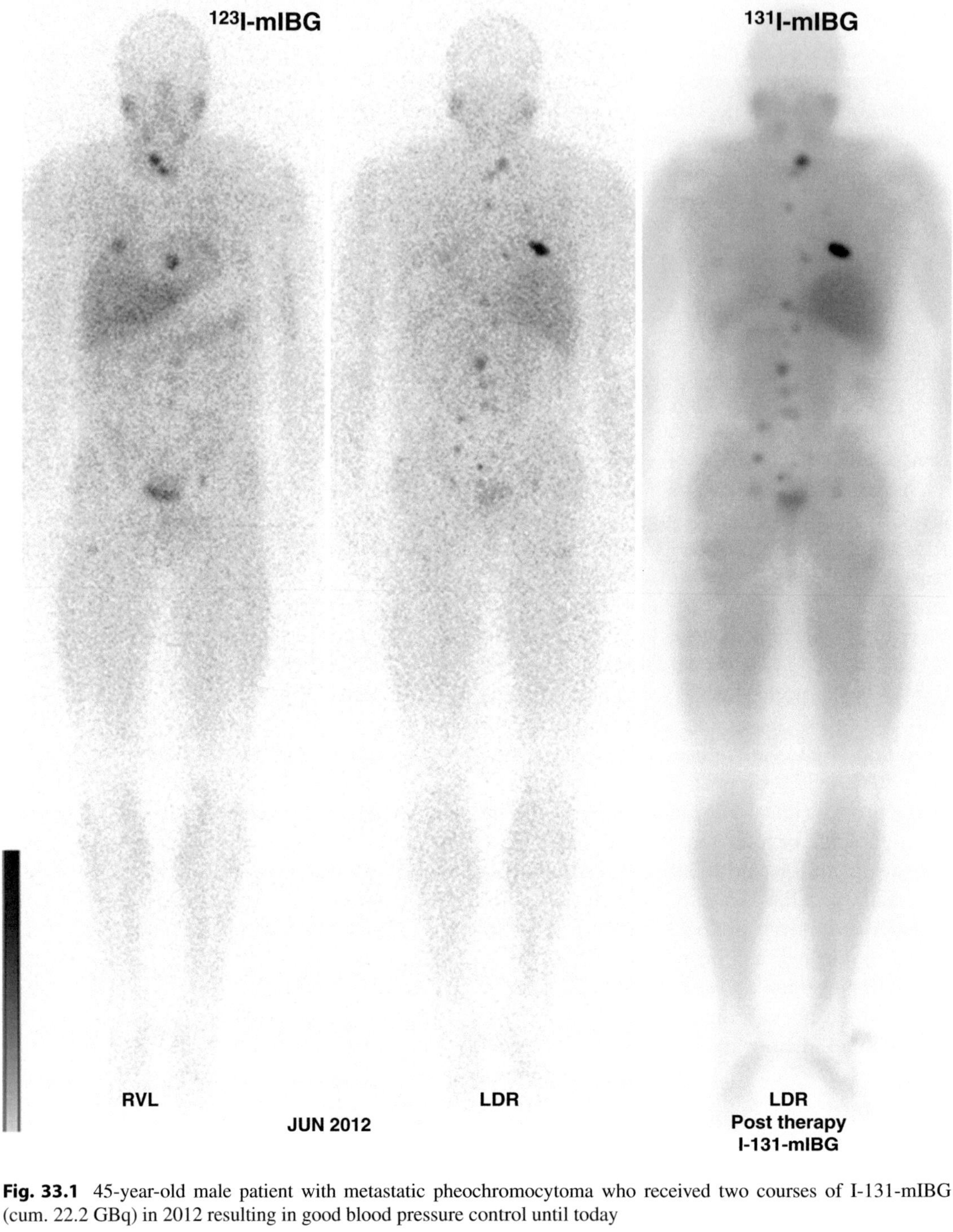

Fig. 33.1 45-year-old male patient with metastatic pheochromocytoma who received two courses of I-131-mIBG (cum. 22.2 GBq) in 2012 resulting in good blood pressure control until today

be useful in restaging recurrent MTC. The sensitivity given in the literature ranges from 11 to 50% [35–37]. MIBG is useful to determine therapeutic options with ^{131}I-mIBG. In case of tumour progression treatment with tyrosine kinase inhibitors is usually indicated. Metastatic medullary thyroid cancer may be treated with ^{131}I-mIBG in selected patients with avid mIBG uptake (Fig. 33.2).

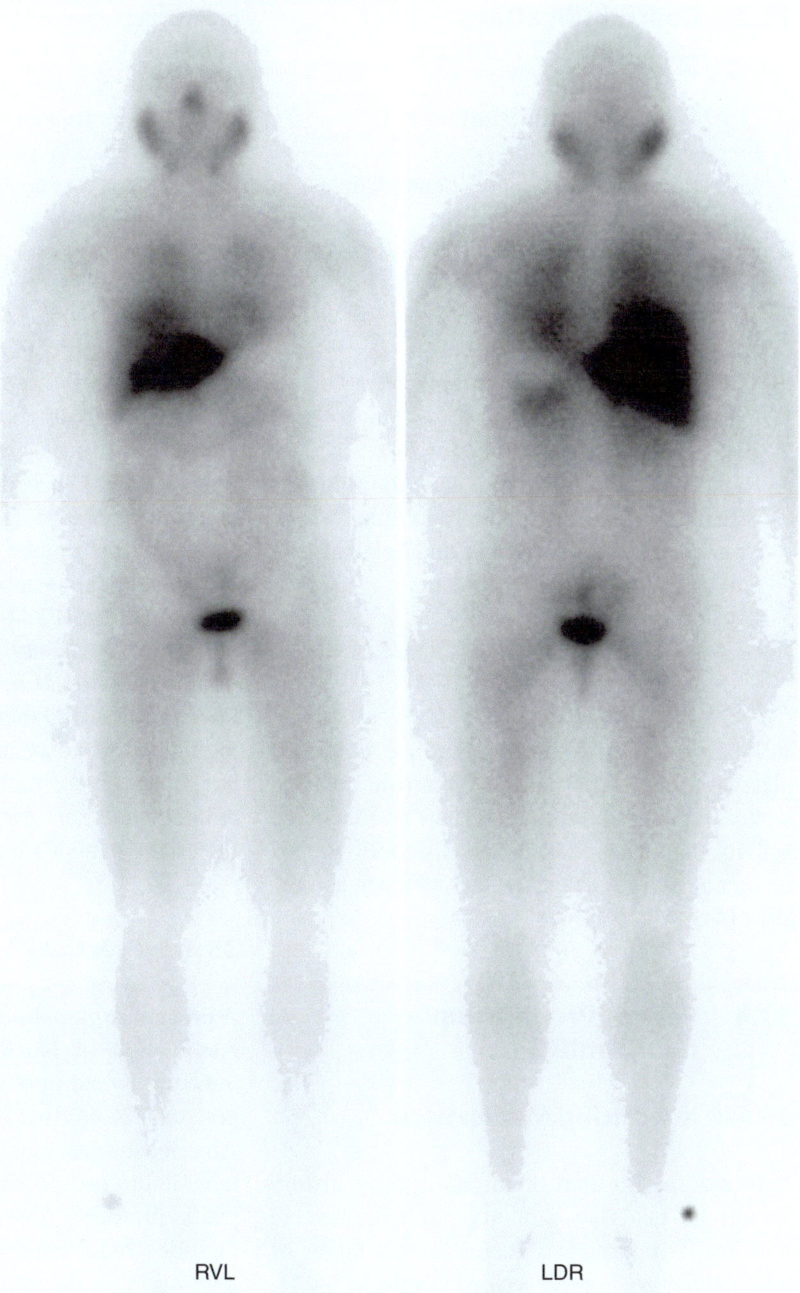

Fig. 33.2 66-year-female patient with liver metastases from medullary thyroid carcinoma. Two courses of I-131-mIBG (cum. 21.1 GBq) in 2014 and 2015 stopped weight loss and improved diarrhoea and blood pressure control. CEA dropped by around 50%

Positive mIBG uptake has also been described in ganglioneuromas, ganglio-neuroblastomas and Merkel cell tumours [38–40]. There are licensed drugs for the treatment of metastatic Merkel cell tumours [mMCC] such as PD-L1- (programmed cell death ligand 1) ligand antibodies or chemotherapy. Merkel cell tumours often display somatostatin receptors. Thus, peptide receptor radionuclide therapy may be a treatment option. ^{131}I-mIBG therapy is a very rare indication nowadays.

33.3 Contraindications for ^{131}I-mIBG Therapy

Absolute contraindications:

1. Pregnancy, breastfeeding.
2. Life expectancy less than 3 months, unless in case of intractable bone pain.
3. Renal insufficiency, requiring dialysis on short term.

Relative contraindications:

1. Unacceptable medical risk for isolation.
2. Unmanageable urinary incontinence.
3. Rapidly deteriorating renal function: glomerular filtration rate less than 30 ml/min.
4. Progressive haematological and/or renal toxicity because of prior treatment.
5. Myelosuppression:
   - Total white cell count less than 3.0×10^9/l.
   - Platelets less than 100×10^9/l.

In case of low white blood cell counts, low platelet counts, massive bone marrow invasion and/or impaired renal function, the administered activity should be reduced, and close follow-up is recommended to detect toxicity as early as possible [41].

33.4 Patient Preparation for ^{131}I-mIBG

33.4.1 Interfering Medications

Before administration of mIBG, a drug history should be taken as numerous drugs interfere with mIBG uptake and various mechanisms of interaction have been described (Table 33.1) [41, 42, 45–49]. Table 33.1 taken from the EANM guideline [17] gives an overview of potential drug interactions [17, 41]. If clinically feasible, interfering drugs should be withdrawn or their dose should be reduced. In most cases four biological half-lives are sufficient; however there are exceptions, such as labetalol [47], which requires a longer withdrawal time. However, the withdrawal of drugs should not harm the patient. The precise percentage of uptake reduction in an individual patient is usually not known or predictable. In some cases withdrawal of drugs before ^{131}I-mIBG is impossible in order not to risk an uncontrolled and potentially seriously harmful high blood pressure. A reduced uptake in salivary glands has been proposed as an indicator of drug interference [50].

33.4.2 Thyroid Protection

Due to the lack of absolute radiochemical purity, thyroid blocking is required before administration of mIBG in order to prevent unnecessary thyroid irradiation and imaging deterioration caused by the uptake of free ^{131}I which emerges from chemical instability and biologic decomposition of mIBG. For diagnostic applications of ^{123}I-mIBG, mostly perchlorate, divided in 3–4 portions per day, is used from day − 1 to day +3. Prior to ^{131}I-mIBG therapy, thyroid blockade with high doses of potassium iodine adjusted to body weight are given. Table 33.2 provides the EANM recommendations for thyroid blockade depending on the patient's body weight [41].

33.4.3 Practical Aspects

A procedure guideline published by the European Association of Nuclear Medicine summarized indications and contraindications and addresses practical issues [41]. In the United States of America the vast majority of ^{131}I-mIBG therapy is done under prospective multi-institutional therapeutic protocols (Personal communication). The facilities requirements will depend on national legislation on the therapeutic use of radioactive-emitting agents. Most of the time, in-patient treatment is required by national legislation; therefore, this should take place in an approved facility with appropriately shielded rooms and ensuite bathroom facilities [41].

A slow intravenous administration over 1–2 h is usually chosen to prevent release of norepinephrine from storage granules due to mIBG, which could result in a hypertensive crisis.

Table 33.1 Drug interactions with mIBG (taken from [17])

Medication category	Subcategory	Most commonly tested medication(s)	Level of evidence	Strength of mIBG-inhibitory effect	Recommendations/Comments
Drugs acting on adrenoreceptors	Beta-blockers	Labetalol	High	Labetalol: Strong	Labetalol should be withheld
		Propranolol		Others: None	Others: Withholding not required
	Beta agonists	Salbutamol	Very low	None	Withdrawal not required
	Alpha antagonists	Phenoxybenzamine	Low	Uncertain	Withdrawal probably not necessary
	Alpha agonists	Clonidine	Very low	Uncertain	Withdrawal probably not necessary
Drugs affecting NE transport, retention or release	Tricyclic antidepressants	Desipramine	Medium	Moderate to strong	Should be withheld (otherwise, an alternative tracer for scanning should be considered)
	SSRIs and SNRIs	Fluvoxamine	Low	Moderate to strong for some agents	Consider withholding agents with documented effect on NET
	Other antidepressants	Trazodone	Very low	None	Insufficient evidence for recommendation
	NE depleters	Reserpine	High	Strong	If still in clinical use, should be withheld
	Sympathomimetics	Phenylpropanolamine	Low	Strong	Should be withheld (otherwise, an alternative tracer for scanning should be considered)
	Monoamines	Cocaine	Moderate	Moderate	In case of suspected use, screen patients prior to mIBG scan
Calcium channel blockers		Nifedipine	Medium	None	Effect (if any) is on release, not on mIBG uptake. Not necessary to withhold
		Cilnidipine			
Miscellaneous	Neuroleptics	Haloperidol	Very low	Uncertain	Uncertain
	Anaesthetics	Ketamine	Very low	Uncertain	Uncertain
		Xylazine			
		Pentobarbital			
	Cardiac glycosides	Digoxin	Very low	Uncertain	Uncertain; withdrawal probably not necessary
	Antiarrhythmics	Amiodarone	Medium	None	Effect (if any) beneficial. Not necessary to withhold

Extensive lists of medications with the theoretical potential to affect mIBG imaging have been previously published ([42],[41], [43], [44]). Several drugs listed in these publications are no longer commercially available. Moreover, the inclusion of drugs in these lists was based on the assumption that all drugs within a category could have the same effect on mIBG uptake as the drugs actually tested (Jacobson et al. 2015). Medications that only indirectly affect circulating levels of norepinephrine, with an unknown specific mechanism of action, should not automatically be considered as likely to affect mIBG imaging results. This table presents the main categories of medications that can potentially affect mIBG uptake, with recommendations and comments regarding withdrawal based on the available evidence

Modified from [45], table from Bar-Sever et al. (EANM guideline [17])

NE norepinephrine, *NET* norepinephrine transporter, *SSRI* selective serotonin reuptake inhibitor, *SNRI* serotonin-norepinephrine reuptake inhibitor. Very low evidence, 1–2 articles; low, 3–4 articles; medium, 5–7 articles; high >7 articles

Table 33.2 Medication regimens for thyroid protection ([41]—www.eanm.org)

Compound	Children (<5 kg)	Children (5–15 kg)	Children (15–50 kg)	Adults (>50 kg)
Capsules				
Potassium iodate	20 mg/day	40 mg/day	80 mg/day	170 mg/day
Potassium iodide (KI)	16 mg/day	32 mg/day	65 mg/day	130 mg/day
Lugol solution 1%	1 drop/kg per day with a maximum of 40 (20 drops twice daily)			
Potassium perchlorate	100 mg/day	200 mg/day	300 mg/day	400 mg/day

During infusion vital signs have to be monitored [41, 51]. In the author's institution a continuous monitoring by pulsoximetry is used for the duration of the infusion and blood pressure is checked every 10–15 min. Vital signs should also be checked twice daily afterwards. More frequent monitoring is recommended in the case of catecholamine-secreting tumours. Short-acting alpha- or beta-blockers must be available for emergency use in the event of catecholamine surge during or immediately after I-131-mIBG administration [41].

33.5 Radionuclide Dosage and Results

33.5.1 Diagnostic Imaging

According to the EANM procedure guidelines 200–400 MBq (5,4–10.8 mCi) ^{123}I-mIBG should be used for adults for diagnostic imaging [52, 53]. The appropriate dosage for children is weight adapted and can be calculated using the schedule of the Paediatric Task Group of the EANM. A minimum dose of 80 MBq ^{123}I-mIBG was recommended for many years, but a more recent publication reduced the recommended dose to 37 MBq ^{123}I-mIBG [54]. This recommendation may be questioned in view of findings from Ladenstein et al.: mIBG image data sets were judged to be of poor quality and/or incomplete in 72/413 (17.4%) patients of the SIOPEN/HRNBL1 trial and in 64/280 (22.9%) patients of the COG A3973 trial [55]. Thus, it is the individual responsibility of the nuclear medicine specialist to inject sufficient ^{123}I-mIBG to come to clinically useful diagnostic images. When injecting ^{123}I-mIBG side effects are rare and mainly due to a release of catecholamines from storage granules and may occur after too rapid injection. Symptoms include tachycardia, hypertension, pallor, vomiting and abdominal pain [43, 56].

33.5.2 Dosage and Results of ^{131}I-mIBG Treatment

For therapeutic use, reported doses vary considerably with respect to treatment intention, the clinical condition of the patient and the availability of stem cell rescue (mostly in neuroblastoma patients). Further aspects have been published by Lewington [57].

33.5.2.1 Neuroblastoma Stage III or IV

^{131}I-mIBG therapy in high-risk neuroblastoma patients started in 1984 and these early studies focused on feasibility and toxicity. Seven studies with a total of 151 patients reported on highly variable ^{131}I-mIBG activities per treatment cycle 2.59–16.65 GBq (70–450 mCi) and on a response rate (complete or mostly partial response) of 17–66%. Subsequent phase I/II studies used ^{131}I-mIBG in progressive, refractory or relapsed high-risk neuroblastoma. In 1998, Matthay et al. reported on the treatment of 30 patients with escalating doses from 96.2 to 673.4 MBq/kg (3.33–30.3 GBq) [2.6 to 18.2 mCi/kg (90–819 mCi)]. None of the patients treated with 444 MBq/kg (12 mCi/kg) or less experienced prolonged neutropenia and therefore did not require autologous stem cell rescue. In contrast, 2 of 5 patients treated with 555 MBq/kg (15 mCi/kg) and 4 of 9 patients treated with 666 MBq/kg (18 mCi/kg) required stem cell rescue. The maximum tolerated dose for patients without stem cell support was 444 MBq/kg (12 mCi/kg) ^{131}I-mIBG. The objective response rate was 37%, with most of the responses observed in patients receiving 444 MBq/kg (12 mCi/kg) or more. Median survival time following ^{131}I-mIBG therapy was 6 months [58]. Other strategies included the combination of ^{131}I-mIBG with other therapies of neuroblastoma and as part of myeloablative therapy/autologous stem cell transplantation (ASCT) [59–61]. In Germany, ^{131}I-mIBG is given at the end of induction chemotherapy in case of persistent mIBG-avid disease before autologous stem cell transplantation with one intravenous infusion of 444 MBq ^{131}I-mIBG/kg body weight (max. Single dose 11.1 GBq I-131-mIBG) [62]. Other indications comprise neuroblastoma relapse or pain palliation [25]. In the Netherlands, ^{131}I-mIBG therapy was also included in first-line treatment protocols [63].

33.5.2.2 Metastatic Pheochromocytoma/Paraganglioma (Extraadrenal Pheochromocytoma)

For treatment with ^{131}I-mIBG adequate tumour uptake must be present. A special subgroup of pheochromocytoma are tumours with SDHB mutations which may be mIBG negative but may display somatostatin receptors allowing peptide receptor radionuclide therapy [64]. A relative contraindication for ^{131}I-mIBG treatment is proteinuria or nephrotic syndrome as these conditions increase the risk for an acute respiratory distress syndrome. A number of treatment cycles and cumulative activities vary considerably for therapy of metastatic pheochromocytoma. Most authors reported on 2–4 treatment cycles using 3.0 to 11.1 [80–300 mCi] ^{131}I-mIBG per cycle and cumulative activities of 11.1 to 31.6 GBq [300–854 mCi] ^{131}I-mIBG. In a report on the treatment of malignant pheochromocytoma, the median single dose was as high as 29.6 GBq (800 mCi) ^{131}I-mIBG [65]. Gedik et al. treated 19 patients with malignant pheochromocytoma or paraganglioma with a median initial dose of 7.4 GBq ^{131}I-mIBG. The median cumulative dose was 22.2 GBq ^{131}I-mIBG. Objective tumour response was achieved in 47% of the patients. Biochemical response rate was 67%, and symptomatic response was seen in 89% of all cases [66].

Postema et al. reported on a symptomatic improvement in the vast majority of patients while biochemical improvement occurs in about 50% and morphological response in about 30% of patients [65]. Thus, imaging results may lag behind clinical improvement; e.g. we have seen a dramatic clinical improvement in a patient with massive pulmonary metastases from pheochromocytoma while I-131-mIBG demonstrated stable disease for many years. In a retrospective series from the Cross Cancer Institute, Edmonton, Alberta (Canada), 5-year overall survival was 63% in 58 patients treated with ^{131}I-mIBG for metastatic pheochromocytoma while it was 47% in 59 patients who did not receive this therapy [65]. At the University Hospital of Cologne mostly two cycles with 444 MBq/kg ^{131}I-mIBG are given with a maximum activity of 11.1. GBq ^{131}I-mIBG per treatment cycle and a maximum whole-body dose of 2 Gy per cycle while treatment cycle intervals are 3–6 months. Thereafter, further treatments may be scheduled in case of tumour progress. In a meta-analysis of 17 publications comprising 243 patients with metastatic pheochromocytoma or paraganglioma treated with 6.9–39.4 GBq ^{131}I-mIBG, mostly partial responses or stable diseases were observed [67].

33.5.2.3 Rare Indications

For the treatment of metastatic carcinoid tumours, median doses of 6.75 GBq (182 mCi) [68] and 14.8 GBq (400 mCi) ^{131}I-mIBG [69] have been described. Ezziddin et al. performed a retrospective analysis of 20 patients with carcinoid tumours treated with 11.1 GBq ^{131}I-mIBG and found a minor response in two patients (10%), stable disease in 16 patients (80%; median time to progression, 34 months) and progressive disease in two patients (10%) [70]. In another publication the same group reported a patient treated with ten therapy cycles and a cumulative activity of 111 GBq ^{131}I-mIBG given over 6 years in metastatic paraganglioma [71].

There are case reports about radionuclide treatment of patients with metastatic medullary thyroid cancer. Gao et al. reported that the therapeutic procedures of targeted internal radiation were performed with 3.33 GBq

^{90}Y-DOTATOC at 6-week intervals or 11.1 GBq ^{131}I-mIBG with a minimum interval of 3 months. After three to five sessions of treatment, three patients with partial remission and six with stable disease were observed. The effective rate was 3/9 (33.3%) and the overall tumour response rate was 9/9 (100%). No relevant toxicity was observed [72]. Castellani et al. from the institute of Milan reported that in patients with medullary thyroid carcinoma a partial response was observed in one patient with mediastinal metastases and two disease stabilisations were seen in another two patients using 3.7–7.4 GBq ^{131}I-mIBG [73]. In an earlier report from Hoefnagel et al. cumulative reported data on the diagnostic use of ^{131}I-mIBG in 178 MTC patients indicated that overall 34.5% of medullary cancers concentrated mIBG. At the Netherlands Cancer Institute ^{131}I-mIBG scintigraphy was positive in 8 of 23 patients with MTC. Four of these patients received therapeutic amounts of ^{131}I-mIBG, resulting in one partial remission and meaningful palliation in three patients with metastatic MTC [29, 30].

For the treatment of metastatic Merkel cell carcinoma drugs have been licenced which are nowadays usually preferred over radionuclide therapy and ^{131}I-mIBG is usually not indicated in these patients. However, there are case reports about the clinical benefit of peptide receptor radionuclide therapy using Lu-177-DotaTATE in combination with capecitabine in metastatic Merkel cell carcinoma [74].

33.6 Complications/Side Effects of ^{131}I-mIBG Therapy

The most important and usually intermediate complication of ^{131}I-mIBG therapy is related to haematotoxicity due to bone marrow irradiation but rarer complications have been reported [25, 41, 75, 76]. Neutropenia and thrombocytopenia are the most likely side effects and can be effectively overcome in combination with autologous stem cell transplantation. Matthay et al. demonstrated in a phase I trial that 30% of patients receiving ≥555 MBq (15 mCi)/kg of ^{131}I-mIBG had prolonged and significant myelosuppression which could be abrogated with infusion of autologous haematopoietic stem cells [58]. Haematological toxicity is more noticeable in patients with bone marrow metastases and patients who received higher whole-body radiation doses [77]. Haematopoietic cell transplantation was required in about one-third of patients treated with 666 MBq (18 mCi)/kg. In contrast, all patients treated with less than 444 MBq (12 mCi)/kg of ^{131}I-mIBG did not need haematopoietic cell transplantation [58, 77].

Early complications can include nausea and vomiting in 10–20% of all patients usually requiring an antiemetic medication. Sialoadenitis is seen with a relatively high frequency, while permanent xerostomia is rare. Modak et al. reported on transient sialoadenitis in nine neuroblastoma patients who had received 444–666 MBq (12–18 mCi)/kg of ^{131}I-mIBG [78].

Blood pressure-related adverse advents are rare: antihypertensive drugs were required in 2.8% of 218 ^{131}I-mIBG administrations [79].

Veno-occlusive liver disease (VOLD) is an important early complication in patients who received ^{131}I-mIBG therapy followed by myeloablative chemotherapy and haematopoietic cell transplantation. The new approaches to neuroblastoma therapy (NANT) consortium reported that 6 of 22 patients had VOLD after the therapies and an apparently high rate of VOLD was seen in the patients with a low glomerular filtration rate [59]. In contrast, no VOLD was seen in patients receiving double infusions of high-dose ^{131}I-mIBG without chemotherapy [60]. A decreased clearance of the chemotherapeutic agents was considered a major cause of VOLD.

Late complications include persistent haematotoxicity and thyroid dysfunction. Hypothyroidism is a frequent long-term side effect despite various protocols for thyroid protection. Van Santen et al. reported about the development of a TSH ≥4.5 mU/L in 16 (64%) out of 25 neuroblastoma patients treated with ^{131}I-mIBG and concluded that occurrence of thyroid dysfunction after treatment with ^{131}I-mIBG for neuroblastoma is high, in spite of potassium iodide prophylaxis requiring close thyroid follow-up [80]. In addition, they reported on an improved thyroid blockade with thyroxine, methimazole and potassium iodide with 19/23 patients (86%) of patients having a normal thyroid function after a mean follow-up of 19 months [81]. Recently, another author from this group reported on long-term efficacy of thyroid prophylaxis. Defining thyroid dysfunction as a plasma TSH > 5.0 mU/l or the use of levothyroxine thyroid disorders were as seen in 12/24 patients available for long-term evaluation with a mean follow-up of 9.0 years after ^{131}I-mIBG treatment demonstrating the significant risk of thyroid damage. Thus, the incidence of thyroid disorders is high and increases with advancing time [82]. As hypothyroidism can be easily treated, this side effect is usually not considered as serious. No deleterious effects of ^{131}I-mIBG therapy on the parathyroid glands were found [82].

Other less likely complications include fatigue secondary to anaemia, sterility and amenorrhoea but these side effects are usually an effect of the combination with other therapies such as chemotherapy. Clement et al. published two patients with ovarian insufficiency after treatment with ^{131}I-mIBG therapy [83]. Hepatic, adrenal or cardiac dysfunction has rarely been reported.

Secondary malignancies have been reported with an incidence of less than 5% [18, 75]. In a report from Italy, two leukaemia, one angiomatoid fibrous histiocytoma, one schwannoma and one rhabdomyosarcoma occurred in 119 patients with neuroblastoma after ^{131}I-mIBG therapy [84]. The University of California group from San Francisco described that leukaemia was observed in 3 of 95 patients with refractory neuroblastoma at 7, 11 and 12 months after ^{131}I-mIBG therapy [85]. It was difficult to clarify the main factors of the secondary malignancies, because all patients received several intensive therapies including chemotherapy and ^{131}I-mIBG therapy. Papillary thyroid carcinomas have been reported in 2 of 9 patients with thyroid nodules [86].

33.7 Image Acquisition

Subsequent to therapy, images can be acquired with a large field gamma camera. For ^{131}I-mIBG, a camera equipped with a high energy, parallel-hole collimator is needed and an energy window of 20% centred at 364 keV should be used.

Most tumours are visible after 24 h; however camera characteristics must be taken into account, e.g. dead time. Due to a decline in liver activity over time, a better contrast may be achieved 48 or even 72 h after injection [51]. Therefore, whole-body images are recommended 24 and 48 h after injection, and an additional scan after 72 h may be helpful in some cases when ^{131}I-mIBG was used. Anterior and posterior views are acquired with a scan speed of 4–8 cm/min for I-131-mIBG [41, 43, 56]. In addition, SPECT images should be performed as it increases the number of detected lesions [87] and the certainty of interpretation [88]. Fukuoka et al. investigated 16 patients with malignant pheochromocytoma/paraganglioma and neuroblastoma, who were referred for ^{131}I-mIBG therapy. Post-therapy high-dose ^{131}I-mIBG scintigraphy was superior over ^{123}I-mIBG scintigraphy in lesion detectability even in comparison with ^{123}I-mIBG SPECT/CT images and high-dose ^{131}I-mIBG planar images in patients with malignant neuroendocrine tumours. SPECT/CT images were helpful for accurate identification of anatomic localization compared with planar images [89].

33.8 Radiation Exposure/Dosimetry

For ^{123}I-mIBG the relative equivalent dose is 14 μSv/MBq (μSv/0.03 mCi), equalling an effective equivalent dose of 5.6 mSv for the use of 400 MBq (10.8 mCi) ^{123}I-mIBG. The relative equivalent dose for ^{131}I-mIBG is 140 μSv/MBq (μSv/0.03 mCi), which leads to an effective equivalent dose of 5.6–11.2 mSv for the use of 40–80 MBq (1.2–2.2 mCi) ^{131}I-mIBG.

According to European standards, dosimetric information must be obtained and is of clinical importance [90–92]. Heterogeneity in ^{131}I-mIBG uptake, tumour characteristics and radiation resistance as well as limitations of the current equipment and methods make correlation of dosimetry with response a continuing challenge [76]. Tumour dosimetry is an extensive topic on which progress has been achieved [90–93].

For therapeutic use, different dosimetric concepts have been reported. One approach was reported by Monsieurs et al. The whole-body absorbed dose can be used as a representation of bone marrow toxicity. To calculate the absorbed dose, ^{131}I-mIBG or ^{123}I-mIBG images can be acquired. Calculation with ^{131}I-labeling has the advantage of allowing measurement of the bi-exponential pattern of whole-body clearance. Monsieurs et al. used a combination of pretherapeutic ^{123}I-mIBG scans and post-therapeutic ^{131}I-mIBG images [94]. Flux et al. described a determination of absorbed dose ratios from 3D dose distributions [95]. The most precise method seems to be the one proposed by Flower et al. An activity of 75 MBq (2 mCi) ^{131}I-mIBG is administered and a series of planar whole-body images acquired starting on day 3 up to 4 weeks. Whole-body retention and organ uptake can be measured using the ROI technique. For decay correction a point source with a defined activity of ^{131}I-mIBG is placed in the field of view for each acquired image [96]. A less time-consuming protocol suggests whole-body images from day 3 through day 7 for post-therapeutic treatment [97]. Another regimen suggested starting image acquisition immediately after injection of 100 MBq (2.7 mCi) ^{131}I-mIBG with a dynamic acquisition of the kidneys in order to calculate renal toxicity. Whole-body planar images in anterior and posterior views were carried out 30 min, 24, 48 and 72 h after injection. From this data the absorbed dose ratios for the whole body, organs and tumour sites could be calculated and the necessary therapeutic activity extrapolated (Kranert et al., unpublished data). Considering these time-consuming protocols it is not astonishing that none of these have gained widespread clinical use. Usually, empirical treatment activities were chosen and post-therapeutic whole-body and SPECT examinations were performed. Without stem cell support, the maximum allowable bone marrow absorbed dose consisted of 2 Gy for adults and 2.5 Gy for children. If stem cell rescue were available, higher bone marrow doses were possible. Thus, some institutions aim to give two cycles of ^{131}I-mIBG respecting 4 Gy whole-body dose. Serial post-therapy measurements during the first treatment cycle were used for calculation of the second therapeutic activity provided that stem cell rescue was available. In addition, the maximal doses for administration can be taken from the tables of the International Commission of Radiological Protection (ICRP). In the author's institution, 16 neuroblastoma patients (and further five patients with other mIBG-positive tumours) were treated with ^{131}I-mIBG between 2004 and 2008 according to a clearly defined protocol. Whole-body absorbed doses were determined by a series of scintillation probe readings. Tumour absorbed doses were calculated on the basis of quantitative imaging for an entity of 25 lesions investigated individually using the ROI technique based on five scans each. With an activity of 444 MBq/kg body weight (and a maximum activity of 11,1 GBq ^{131}I-mIBG per cycle) typical whole-body absorbed doses were found in the region of 2 Gy (range, 1.0–2.9 Gy) whereas tumour absorbed doses in turn covered a span between 10 and 60 Gy [93].

33.9 Potential Future Developments

Combined hyperbaric oxygen (HBO) and ^{131}I-mIBG therapy showed promising results in treatment of neuroblastoma [98]. According to the Frankfurt protocol, patients were administered a weight adapted dose between 2.96 and 7.4 GBq (80 and 200 mCi) ^{131}I-mIBG. On the subsequent 4 days an HBO session was performed. Pressure was increased slowly over 15 min to a total of 2.4 bar. An intermittent oxygen supply of 100% was given for 20-min periods with pauses of 5 min for a total of 95 min. Decompression was then performed slowly over another 15 min [99]. The effect of this combination therapy is based on three mechanisms: (1) mIBG itself has a discrete antiproliferative effect, independent of the iodide isotope, by inhibition of complex I of the respiratory chain. This leads to a discharge of paired electrons, resulting in an increased production of superoxide radicals. Neuroblastoma cells are more vulnerable to these radicals, since they show a decreased activity of enzymes responsible for the metabolism of radicals to water and oxygen. (2) The radiation of ^{131}I shows effects on a cellular basis. (3) Under HBO the oxygen accumulation within the tumour increases, depending on the partial pressure, which further increases the production of radicals.

The combination of ^{131}I-mIBG with radiosensitizing chemotherapy is a therapy option that would deserve further future research [100].

No-carrier-added mIBG: With the standard preparation ^{131}I-mIBG contains significant amounts of nonradiolabelled mIBG with a distribution of 1 radiolabelled in contrast to 2000 nonradiolabelled molecules [18]. Both molecules compete for norepinephrine transporter uptake. One strategy to enhance uptake is therefore to use no-carrier-added mIBG with the aim to improve uptake due to the higher specific activity of this mIBG preparation.

^{125}I-mIBG for microscopic disease: With a beta range of about 0.8 mm I-131 was hypothesized to work suboptimal in patients with submillimeter tumours. Iodine-125 emits very short-range Auger and conversion electrons with a high linear energy transfer and a maximum range of 30 μm. I-125-mIBG was considered as theoretically superior for the treatment of neuroblastoma patients with microscopic disease. Further studies are needed [101].

Alpha-particle therapy: Astatine-211 (^{211}At) generates alpha particles with a high linear energy transfer with a very short range in tissue of only a few cell diameters [102]. Because of their potent cytotoxicity, alpha particles are more suitable than beta particles for targeted radionuclide therapy of microscopic disease which was shown in a study with patients with brain tumours. MIBG analogues labelled with ^{211}At, ^{211}At meta-astatobenzylguanidine (MABG) was shown to have cytotoxic superiority to ^{131}I-mIBG in human neuroblastoma cells which overexpressed NE transporters [102, 103]. Alpha emitters hold great potentials for radionuclide therapy but need also special expertise with respect to handling and waste management. Further studies about ^{211}At-MABG and other alpha emitters in both preclinical and clinical settings would be needed.

Development of antibody therapy may bring further progress. Therapy with unlabelled anti-GD2 antibodies ch 14.18. has already been implemented [104]. Radiolabelled antibodies have also been used for diagnostic purposes [105]. A therapy with radiolabelled antibodies will hopefully be available in the future.

References

1. Morales JO, Beierwaltes WH, Counsell RE, Meier DH. The concentration of radioactivity from labeled epinephrine and its precursors in the dog adrenal medulla. J Nucl Med. 1967;8:800–9.
2. Anderson BG, Beierwaltes WH, Harrison TS, Ansari AN, Buswink AA, Ice RD. Labeled dopamine concentration in pheochromocytomas. J Nucl Med. 1973;14:781–4.
3. Ice RD, Wieland DM, Beirwaltes WH, Lawton RG, Redmond MJ. Concentration of dopamine analogs in the adrenal medulla. J Nucl Med. 1975;16:1147–51.
4. Lieberman LM, Beierwaltes WH, Varma VM, Weinhold P, Ling R. Labeled dopamine concentration in human adrenal medulla and in neuroblastoma. J Nucl Med. 1969;10:93–7.
5. Korn N, Buswink A, Yu T, Carr EA Jr, Carroll M, Counsell RE. A radioiodinated bretylium analog as a potential agent for scanning the adrenal medulla. J Nucl Med. 1977;18:87–9.
6. Wieland DM, Swanson DP, Brown LE, Beierwaltes WH. Imaging the adrenal medulla with an I-131-labeled antiadrenergic agent. J Nucl Med. 1979;20:155–8.
7. Sisson JC, Frager MS, Valk TW, Gross MD, Swanson DP, Wieland DM, Tobes MC, Beierwaltes WH, Thompson NW. Scintigraphic localization of pheochromocytoma. N Engl J Med. 1981;2(305):12–7.
8. Valk TW, Frager MS, Gross MD, Sisson JC, Wieland DM, Swanson DP, Mangner TJ, Beierwaltes WH. Spectrum of pheochromocytoma in multiple endocrine neoplasia. A scintigraphic portrayal using 131I-metaiodobenzylguanidine. Ann Intern Med. 1981;94:762–7.
9. Sisson J, Shapiro B, Beierwaltes WH, Nakajo M, Glowniak J, Mangner T, Carey JE, Swanson DP, Copp J, Satterlee W, et al. Treatment of malignant pheochromocytoma with a new radiopharmaceutical. Trans Assoc Am Phys. 1983;96:209–17.
10. Treuner J, Feine U, Niethammer D, et al. Scintigraphic imaging of neuroblastoma with [131-I] iodobenzylguanidine. Lancet. 1984;1:333–4.
11. Beierwaltes WH. Horizons in radionuclide therapy: 1985 update. J Nucl Med. 1985;26:421–7.
12. Fischer M, Kamanabroo D, Sonderkamp H, Proske T. Scintigraphic imaging of carcinoid tumours with 131I-metaiodobenzylguanidine. Lancet. 1984;2(8395):165.

13. Wieland DM, Wu J, Brown LE, Mangner TJ, Swanson DP, Beierwaltes WH. Radiolabeled adrenergic neuron-blocking agents: adrenomedullary imaging with [131I]iodobenzylguanidine. J Nucl Med. 1980;21:349–53.
14. Franceschini R, Pecorale A, Chinol M, Calcagni ML, Servidei T, Riccardi R, Troncone L. In vitro and in vivo studies with no-carrier added radioiodinated MIBG. Q J Nucl Med. 1995;39:72–7.
15. Vaidyanathan G, Welsh PC, Vitorello KC, Snyder S, Friedman HS, Zalutsky MR. A 4-methyl-substituted meta-iodobenzylguanidine analogue with prolonged retention in human neuroblastoma cells. Eur J Nucl Med Mol Imaging. 2004;31:1362–70.
16. Shapiro B, Gross MD. Radiochemistry, biochemistry, and kinetics of 131I-metaiodobenzylguanidine (MIBG) and 123I-MIBG: clinical implications of the use of 123I-MIBG. Med Pediatr Oncol. 1987;15:170–7.
17. Bar-Sever Z, Biassoni L, Shulkin B, Kong G, Hofman MS, Lopci E, Manea I, Koziorowski J, Castellani R, Boubaker A, Lambert B, Pfluger T, Nadel H, Sharp S, Giammarile F. Guidelines on nuclear medicine imaging in neuroblastoma. Eur J Nucl Med Mol Imaging. 2018;45(11):2009–24.
18. Streby KA, Shah N, Ranalli MA, Kunkler A, Cripe TP. Nothing but NET: a review of norepinephrine transporter expression and efficacy of 131I-mIBG therapy. Pediatr Blood Cancer. 2015;62:5–11.
19. Nakajo M, Shapiro B, Copp J, Kalff V, Gross MD, Sisson JC, Beierwaltes WH. The normal and abnormal distribution of the adrenomedullary imaging agent m-[I-131]iodobenzylguanidine (I-131 MIBG) in man: evaluation by scintigraphy. J Nucl Med. 1983;24:672–82.
20. Jacobsson H, Hellstrom PM, Kogner P, Larsson SA. Different concentrations of I-123 MIBG and in-111 pentetreotide in the two main liver lobes in children: persisting regional functional differences after birth? Clin Nucl Med. 2007;32:24–8.
21. Sharp SE, Trout AT, Weiss BD, Gelfand MJ. MIBG in neuroblastoma diagnostic imaging and therapy. Radiographics: a review publication of the Radiological Society of North America, Inc. 2016;36:258–78.
22. Parisi MT, Sandler ED, Hattner RS. The biodistribution of metaiodobenzylguanidine. Semin Nucl Med. 1992;22:46–8.
23. Bomanji J, Britton KE. Uterine uptake of iodine-123 metaiodobenzylguanidine during the menstrual phase of uterine cycle. Clin Nucl Med. 1987;12:601–803.
24. Bonnin F, Lumbroso J, Tenenbaum F, Hartmann O, Parmentier C. Refining interpretation of MIBG scans in children. J Nucl Med. 1994;35:803–10.
25. Schmidt M, Hero B, Simon T. I-131-mIBG therapy in neuroblastoma: established role and prospective applications. Clin Transl Imaging. 2016;4:87–101.
26. Schmidt M, Baum RP, Simon T, Howman-Giles R. Therapeutic nuclear medicine in pediatric malignancy. Q J Nucl Med Mol Imaging. 2010;54:411–28.
27. Wilson JS, Gains JE, Moroz V, Wheatley K, Gaze MN. A systematic review of 131I-meta iodobenzylguanidine molecular radiotherapy for neuroblastoma. Eur J Cancer. 2014;50:801–15.
28. Szalat A, Fraenkel M, Doviner V, Salmon A, Gross DJ. Malignant pheochromocytoma: predictive factors of malignancy and clinical course in 16 patients at a single tertiary medical center. Endocrine. 2011;39(2):160–6.
29. Hoefnagel CA, Delprat CC, Valdés Olmos RA. Role of [131I]metaiodobenzylguanidine therapy in medullary thyroid carcinoma. J Nucl Biol Med. 1991;35:334–6.
30. Hoefnagel CA, Schornagel J, Valdes Olmos RA. [131I]metaiodobenzylguanidine therapy for malignant phaeochromocytoma: interference of medication. J Nucl Biol Med. 1991;35:308–12.
31. Nocaudie-Calzada M, Huglo D, Carnaille B, Proye C, Marchandise X. Comparison of somatostatin analogue and metaiodobenzylguanidine scintigraphy for the detection of carcinoid tumours. Eur J Nucl Med. 1996;23:1448–54.
32. Oberg K, Eriksson B. Nuclear medicine in the detection, staging and treatment of gastrointestinal carcinoid tumours. Best Pract Res Clin Endocrinol Metab. 2005;19:265–76.
33. Feldman JM, Blinder RA, Lucas KJ, Coleman RE. Iodine- 131 metaiodobenzylguanidine scintigraphy of carcinoid tumors. J Nucl Med. 1986;27:1691–6.
34. Diehl M, Risse JH, Brandt-Mainz K, Dietlein M, Bohuslavizki KH, Matheja P, Lange H, Bredow J, Körber C, Grünwald F. Fluorine-18 fluorodeoxyglucose positron emission tomography in medullary thyroid cancer: results of a multicentre study. Eur J Nucl Med. 2001;28:1671–6.
35. Clarke SE, Lazarus CR, Wraight P, Sampson C, Maisey MN. Pentavalent [99mTc]DMSA, [131I] MIBG, and [99mTc]MDP – an evaluation of three imaging techniques in patients with medullary carcinoma of the thyroid. J Nucl Med. 1988;29:33–8.
36. Troncone L, Rufini V, De Rosa G, Testa A. Diagnostic and therapeutic potential of new radiopharmaceutical agents in medullary thyroid carcinoma. Henry Ford Hosp Med J. 1989;37:178–84.
37. Verga U, Muratori F, Di Sacco G, Banfi F, Libroia A. The role of radiopharmaceuticals MIBG and (V) DMSA in the diagnosis of medullary thyroid carcinoma. Henry Ford Hosp Med J. 1989;37:175–7.
38. Castagnoli A, Biti G, De Cristofaro MT, Ferri P, Magrini SM, Papi MG, Bianchi S. Merkel cell carcinoma and iodine-131 metaiodobenzylguanidine scan. Eur J Nucl Med. 1992;19:913–6.
39. Clerico A, Jenkner A, Castello MA, Ciofetta G, Lucarelli C, Codini M. Functionally active ganglioneuroma with increased plasma and urinary catecholamines and positive iodine 131-metaiodobenzylguanidine scintigraphy. Med Pediatr Oncol. 1991;19:329–33.
40. Watanabe N, Shimizu M, Kageyama M, Kitagawa K, Hayasaka S, Seto H. 123I-MIBG SPECT of Merkel cell carcinoma. Br J Radiol. 1998;71:886–7.

41. Giammarile F, Chiti A, Lassmann M, Brans B, Flux G. EANM procedure guidelines for ^{131}I-metaiodobenzylguanidine (^{131}I-mIBG) therapy. Eur J Nucl Med Mol Imaging. 2008;35:1039–47.
42. Solanki KK, Bomanji J, Moyes J, Mather SJ, Trainer PJ, Britton KE. A pharmacological guide to medicines which interfere with the biodistribution of radiolabelled meta-iodobenzylguanidine (MIBG). Nucl Med Commun. 1992;13:513–21.
43. Bombardieri E, Giammarile F, Aktolun C, Baum RP, Bischof Delaloye A, Maffioli L, et al. 131I/123I-metaiodobenzylguanidine (mIBG) scintigraphy: procedure guidelines for tumour imaging. Eur J Nucl Med Mol Imaging. 2010;37:2436–46.
44. Stefanelli A, Treglia G, Bruno I, Rufini V, Giordano A. Pharmacological interference with 123I-metaiodobenzylguanidine: a limitation to developing cardiac innervation imaging in clinical practice? Eur Rev Med Pharmacol Sci. 2013;17:1326–33.
45. Jacobson AF, Travin MI. Impact of medications on mIBG uptake, with specific attention to the heart: comprehensive review of the literature. J Nucl Cardiol. 2015;22:980–93.
46. Babich JW, Graham W, Fischman AJ. Effect of adrenergic receptor ligands on metaiodobenzylguanidine uptake and storage in neuroblastoma cells. Eur J Nucl Med. 1997;24:538–43.
47. Khafagi FA, Shapiro B, Fig LM, Mallette S, Sisson JC. Labetalol reduces iodine-131 MIBG uptake by pheochromocytoma and normal tissues. J Nucl Med. 1989;30:481–9.
48. Tobes MC, Jaques S Jr, Wieland DM, Sisson JC. Effect of uptake-one inhibitors on the uptake of norepinephrine and metaiodobenzylguanidine. J Nucl Med. 1985;26:897–907.
49. Wafelman AR, Hoefnagel CA, Maes RA, Beijnen JH. Radioiodinated metaiodobenzylguanidine: a review of its biodistribution and pharmacokinetics, drug interactions, cytotoxicity and dosimetry. Eur J Nucl Med. 1994;21:545–59.
50. Zaplatnikov K, Menzel C, Dobert N, Hamscho N, Kranert WT, Gotthard M, Behr TM, Grünwald F. Case report: drug interference with MIBG uptake in a patient with metastatic paraganglioma. Br J Radiol. 2004;77:525–7.
51. McEwan AJ, Shapiro B, Sisson JC, Beierwaltes WH, Ackery DM. Radioiodobenzylguanidine for the scintigraphic location and therapy of adrenergic tumors. Semin Nucl Med. 1985;15:132–53.
52. Olivier P, Colarinha P, Fettich J, et al. (2002) Guidelines for radioiodinated MIBG scintigraphy in children guidelines issued date: December 29, 2002 (www.eanm.org).
53. Taïeb D, Timmers HJ, Hindié E, et al. EANM 2012 guidelines for radionuclide imaging of phaeochromocytoma and paraganglioma. Eur J Nucl Med Mol Imaging. 2012;39:1977–95.
54. Lassmann M, Treves ST. Pediatric Radiopharmaceutical Administration: harmonization of the 2007 EANM Paediatric Dosage Card (Version 1.5.2008) and the 2010 North American consensus guideline. Eur J Nucl Med Mol Imaging. 2014;41(5):1036–41.
55. Ladenstein R, Lambert B, Pötschger U, Castellani MR, Lewington V, Bar-Sever Z, Oudoux A, Śliwińska A, Taborska K, Biassoni L, Yanik GA, Naranjo A, Parisi MT, Shulkin BL, Nadel H, Gelfand MJ, Matthay KK, Park JR, Kreissman SG, Valteau-Couanet D. Boubaker a (2017) validation of the mIBG skeletal SIOPEN scoring method in two independent high-risk neuroblastoma populations: the SIOPEN/HR-NBL1 and COG-A3973 trials. Eur J Nucl Med Mol Imaging. 2017 Sep 23;45:292. https://doi.org/10.1007/s00259-017-3829-7.
56. Bombardieri E, Aktolun C, Baum RP, Bishof-Delaloye A, Bus-combe J, Chatal JF, Maffioli L, Moncayo R, Mortelmans L, Reske SN. 131I/123I-metaiodobenzylguanidine (MIBG) scintigraphy: procedure guidelines for tumour imaging. Eur J Nucl Med Mol Imaging. 2003;30:132–9.
57. Lewington V. I-131 Meta iodobenzylguanidine therapy. In: Baum RP, editor. Therapeutic nuclear medicine. Heidelberg: Springer-Verlag; 2014. p. 571–81.
58. Matthay KK, DeSantes K, Hasegawa B, Huberty J, Hattner RS, Ablin A, et al. Phase I dose escalation of ^{131}I-metaiodobenzylguanidine with autologous bone marrow support in refractory neuroblastoma. J Clin Oncol. 1998;16:229–36.
59. Matthay KK, Tan JC, Villablanca JG, Yanik GA, Veatch J, Franc B, et al. Phase I dose escalation of iodine-131-metaiodobenzylguanidine with myeloablative chemotherapy and autologous stem-cell transplantation in refractory neuroblastoma: a new approaches to neuroblastoma therapy consortium study. J Clin Oncol. 2006;24:500–6.
60. Matthay KK, Yanik G, Messina J, Quach A, Huberty J, Cheng SC, et al. Phase II study on the effect of disease sites, age, and prior therapy on response to iodine-131-metaiodobenzylguanidine therapy in refractory neuroblastoma. J Clin Oncol. 2007;25:1054–60.
61. Yanik GA, Levine JE, Matthay KK, Sisson JC, Shulkin BL, Shapiro B, Hubers D, Spalding S, Braun T, Ferrara JL, Hutchinson RJ. Pilot study of iodine-131-metaiodobenzylguanidine in combination with myeloablative chemotherapy and autologous stem-cell support for the treatment of neuroblastoma. J Clin Oncol. 2002;20:2142–9.
62. Schmidt M, Simon T, Hero B, Eschner W, Dietlein M, Sudbrock F, et al. Is there a benefit of 131 I-MIBG therapy in the treatment of children with stage 4 neuroblastoma? A retrospective evaluation of the German neuroblastoma trial NB97 and implications for the German neuroblastoma trial NB2004. Nuklearmedizin. 2006;45:145–51.
63. Bleeker G, Schoot RA, Caron HN, de Kraker J, Hoefnagel CA, van Eck BL, Tytgat GA. Toxicity of upfront 131Imetaiodobenzylguanidine (131I-MIBG) therapy in newly diagnosed neuroblastoma patients: a retrospective analysis. Eur J Nucl Med Mol Imaging. 2013;40:1711–7.

64. Virgolini I, Ambrosini V, Bomanji JB, et al. Procedure guidelines for PET/CT tumour imaging with 68 Ga-DOTA-conjugated peptides: 68 Ga-DOTA-TOC, 68 Ga-DOTA-NOC, 68 Ga-DOTA-TATE. Eur J Nucl Med Mol Imaging. 2010;37:2004–10.
65. Postema EJ, McEwan AJB. Radioiodinated metaiodobenzylguanidine treatment of neuroendocrine tumors in adults. Cancer Biother Radiopharm. 2009;24:519–24.
66. Gedik GK, Hoefnagel CA, Bais E, Olmos RAV. 131I-MIBG therapy in metastatic phaeochromocytoma and paraganglioma. Eur J Nucl Med Mol Imaging. 2008;35:725–33.
67. Van Hulsteijn LT, Niemeijer ND, Dekkers OM, Corssmit EP. (131)I-MIBG therapy for malignant paraganglioma and phaeochromocytoma: systematic review and meta-analysis. Clin Endocrinol. 2014;80:487–501.
68. Sywak MS, Pasieka JL, McEwan A, Kline G, Rorstad O. 131I-meta-iodobenzylguanidine in the management of met- astatic midgut carcinoid. Tumors World J Surg. 2004;28:1157–62.
69. Safford SD, Coleman RE, Gockerman JP, Moore J, Feldman J, Onaitis MW, Tyler DS, Olson JA Jr. Iodine-131 metaiodobenzylguanidine treatment for metastatic carcinoid. Results in 98 patients. Cancer. 2002;101:1987–93.
70. Ezziddin S, Sabet A, Logvinski T, Alkawaldeh K, Yong-Hing CJ, Ahmadzadehfar H, Grünwald F, Biersack HJ. Long-term outcome and toxicity after dose-intensified treatment with 131I-MIBG for advanced metastatic carcinoid tumors. J Nucl Med. 2013;54:2032–8.
71. Ezziddin S, Sabet A, Ko YD, et al. Repeated radionuclide therapy in metastatic paraganglioma leading to the highest reported cumulative activity of ^{131}I-MIBG. Radiat Oncol. 2012;7:8.
72. Gao ZR, An R, Zhang YX, Biersack HJ. Targeted radionuclide therapy for patients with metastatic medullary thyroid carcinoma. [article in Chinese]. Zhonghua Zhong Liu Za Zhi. 2006;28:621–4.
73. Castellani MR, Chiti A, Seregni E, Bombardieri E. Role of 131I-metaiodobenzylguanidine (MIBG) in the treatment of neuroendocrine tumours. Experience of the National Cancer Institute of Milan. Q J Nucl Med. 2000;44:77–87.
74. Schmidt MC, Uhrhan K, Markiefka B, Hasselbring L, Schlaak M, Cremer B, Kunze S, Baum RP, Dietlein M. ^{68}Ga-DotaTATE PET-CT followed by peptide receptor radiotherapy in combination with capecitabine in two patients with Merkel cell carcinoma. Int J Clin Exp Med. 2012;5(4):363–6.
75. Kayano D, Kinuya S. Iodine-131 metaiodobenzylguanidine therapy for neuroblastoma: reports so far and future perspective. Scientific World J. 2015;189135.
76. Taggart D, Dubois S, Matthay KK. Radiolabeled metaiodobenzylguanidine for imaging and therapy of neuroblastoma. Q J Nucl Med Mol Imaging. 2008;52:403–18.
77. DuBois SG, Messina J, Maris JM, Huberty J, Glidden DV, Veatch J, Charron M, Hawkins R, Matthay KK. Hematologic toxicity of high-dose iodine-131-metaiodobenzylguanidine therapy for advanced neuroblastoma. J Clin Oncol. 2004;22:2452–60.
78. Modak S, Pandit-Taskar N, Kushner BH, Kramer K, Smith-Jones P, Larson S, Cheung NK. Transient sialoadenitis: a complication of 131I-metaiodobenzylguanidine therapy. Pediatr Blood Cancer. 2008;50:1271–3.
79. Wong T, Matthay KK, Boscardin WJ, Hawkins RA, Brakeman PR, Dubois SG. Acute changes in blood pressure in patients with neuroblastoma treated with I-131-metaiodobenzylguanidine (MIBG). Pediatr Blood Cancer. 2013;60:1424–30.
80. van Santen HM, de Kraker J, van Eck BL, de Vijlder JJ, Vulsma T. High incidence of thyroid dysfunction despite prophylaxis with potassium iodide during (131)I-meta-iodobenzylguanidine treatment in children with neuroblastoma. Cancer. 2002;94:2081–9.
81. van Santen HM, de Kraker J, van Eck BL, de Vijlder JJ, Vulsma T. Improved radiation protection of the thyroid gland with thyroxine, methimazole, and potassium iodide during diagnostic and therapeutic use of radiolabeled metaiodobenzylguanidine in children with neuroblastoma. Cancer. 2003;98:389–96.
82. Clement SC, van Rijn RR, van Eck-Smit BL, van Trotsenburg AS, Caron HN, Tytgat GA, van Santen HM. Long-term efficacy of current thyroid prophylaxis and future perspectives on thyroid protection during 131I-metaiodobenzylguanidine treatment in children with neuroblastoma. Eur J Nucl Med Mol Imaging. 2015;42:706–15.
83. Clement SC, Kraal KC, van Eck-Smit BL, van den Bos C, Kremer LC, Tytgat GA, van Santen HM. Primary ovarian insufficiency in children after treatment with 131I-metaiodobenzyl-guanidine for neuroblastoma: report of the first two cases. J Clin Endocrinol Metab. 2014;99:E112–6.
84. Garaventa A, Gambini C, Villavecchia G, Di Cataldo A, Bertolazzi L, Pizzitola MR, et al. Second malignancies in children with neuroblastoma after combined treatment with 131I-metaiodobenzylguanidine. Cancer. 2003;97:1332–8.
85. Weiss B, Vora A, Huberty J, Hawkins RA, Matthay KK. Secondary myelodysplastic syndrome and leukemia following 131I-metaiodobenzylguanidine therapy for relapsed neuroblastoma. J Pediatr Hematol Oncol. 2003;25:543–7.
86. van Santen HM, Tytgat GA, van de Wetering MD, van Eck-Smit BL, Hopman SM, van der Steeg AF, Nieveen van Dijkum EJ, van Trotsenburg AS. Differentiated thyroid carcinoma after 131I-MIBG treatment for neuroblastoma during childhood: description of the first two cases. Thyroid. 2012;22:643–6.
87. Rufini V, Fisher GA, Shulkin BL, Sisson JC, Shapiro B. Io- dine-123-MIBG imaging of neuroblastoma: utility of SPECT and delayed imaging. J Nucl Med. 1996;37:1464–8.

88. Gelfand MJ, Elgazzar AH, Kriss VM, Masters PR, Golsch GJ. Iodine-123-MIBG SPECT versus planar imaging in children with neural crest tumors. J Nucl Med. 1994;35:1753–7.
89. Fukuoka M, Taki J, Mochizuki T, Kinuya S. Comparison of diagnostic value of I-123 MIBG and high-dose I-131 MIBG scintigraphy including incremental value of SPECT/CT over planar image in patients with malignant pheochromocytoma/paraganglioma and neuroblastoma. Clin Nucl Med. 2011;36:1–7.
90. Buckley SE, Chittenden SJ, Saran FH, Meller ST, Flux GD. Whole-body dosimetry for individualized treatment planning of 131I-MIBG radionuclide therapy for neuroblastoma. J Nucl Med. 2009;50:1518–24.
91. Buckley SE, Saran FH, Gaze MN, Chittenden S, Partridge M, Lancaster D, et al. Dosimetry for fractionated (131)I-mIBG therapies in patients with primary resistant high-risk neuroblastoma: preliminary results. Cancer Biother Radiopharm. 2007;22:105–12.
92. Lassmann M, Chiesa C, Flux G, Bardiès M. EANM dosimetry committee guidance document: good practice of clinical dosimetry reporting. Eur J Nucl Med Mol Imaging. 2011;38:192–200.
93. Sudbrock F, Schmidt M, Simon T, Eschner W, Berthold F, Schicha H. Dosimetry for ^{131}I-MIBG therapies in metastatic neuroblastoma, phaeochromocytoma and paraganglioma. Eur J Nucl Med Mol Imaging. 2010;37:1279–90.
94. Monsieurs M, Brans B, Bacher K, Dierckx R, Thierens H. Patient dosimetry for 131I-MIBG therapy for neuroendocrine tumours based on 123I-MIBG scans. Eur J Nucl Med Mol Imaging. 2002;29:1581–7.
95. Flux GD, Guy MJ, Papavasileiou P, South C, Chittenden SJ, Flower MA, Meller ST. Absorbed dose ratios for re- peated therapy of neuroblastoma with I-131 mIBG. Cancer Biother Radiopharm. 2003;18:81–7.
96. Flower MA, Fielding SL. Radiation dosimetry for 131I- mIBG therapy of neuroblastoma. Phys Med Biol. 1996;41:1933–40.
97. Matthay KK, Panina C, Huberty J, Price D, Glidden DV, Tang HR, Hawkins RA, Veatch J, Hasegawa B. Correlation of tumor and whole-body dosimetry with tumor response and toxicity in refractory neuroblastoma treated with (131)I-MIBG. J Nucl Med. 2001;42:1713–21.
98. Voûte PA, van der Kleij AJ, De Kraker J, Hoefnagel CA, Thiel van Buul MMC, Van Gennip H. Clinical experience with radiation enhancement by hyperbaric oxygen in children with recurrent neuroblastoma stage IV. Eur J Cancer. 1995;31:596–600.
99. Diehl M, Fußhoeller G, Menzel C, Kranert WT, Graichen S, Klingebiel T, Grünwald F. Hyperbarer Sauerstoff zur Intensivierung der 131I-MIBG-Therapie beim therapierefraktären Neuroblastom Stadium 4 (case repeort). Nuklearmedizin. 2004;43:N77–80.
100. Gaze MN, Chang YC, Flux GD, Mairs RJ, Saran FH, Meller ST. Feasibility of dosimetry-based high-dose 131I-meta-iodobenzylguanidine with topotecan as a radiosensitizer in children with metastatic neuroblastoma. Cancer Biother Radiopharm. 2005;20: 195–9.
101. Sisson JC, Shapiro B, Hutchinson RJ, Shulkin BL, Zempel S. Survival of patients with neuroblastoma treated with 125-I MIBG. Am J Clin Oncol. 1996;19:144–8.
102. Strickland DK, Vaidyanathan G, Zalutsky MR. Cytotoxicity of α-particle-emitting m-[at-211] astatobenzylguanidine on human neuroblastoma cells. Cancer Res. 1994;54:5414–9.
103. Cunningham SH, Mairs RJ, Wheldon TE, Welsh PC, Vaidyanathan G, Zalutsky MR. Toxicity to neuroblastoma cells and spheroids of benzylguanidine conjugated to radionuclides with short-range emissions. Br J Cancer. 1998;77:2061–8.
104. Klingebiel T, Bader P, Bares R, Beck J, Jürgens H, Lang P, Niethammer D, Rath B, Handgretinger R. Treatment of neuroblastoma stage 4 with ^{131}I-meta-iodo-benzylguani- dine, high-dose chemotherapy and immunotherapy. A pilot study. Eur J Cancer. 1998;34:1398–402.
105. Carrel F, Amstutz H, Novak-Hofer I, Schubiger PA. Evaluation of radioiodinated and radiocopper labeled monovalent fragments of monoclonal antibody chCE7 for targeting of neuroblastoma. Nucl Med Biol. 1997;24:539–46.

Radioimmunotherapy

34

Vikas Prasad, Richard P. Baum, and Juan P. Oliva

34.1 Introduction

Since Paul Ehrlich proposed the hypothesis (*Seitenkettentheorie*) more than a century ago that bacteria can be killed by selective usage of certain compounds having specific affinity to the bacteria and thus acting as a "magic bullet," antibodies have captured the imagination of scientists dealing with diseases. Cancer was and still remains among the most intriguing and challenging of diseases for which the exact cure for its many forms is not available to date. Parallel to the development of certain compounds such as sulfur and nitrogen mustard, with the capacity to modify the DNA and thus retard and kill the growth of cancer cells [1], Pressman and colleagues showed that radiolabeled antibodies had the potential to localize tumors in rabbits [2–4]. This was soon followed by first attempts by Beierwaltes and his colleagues at curing cancer in patients using radiolabeled polyclonal antibodies. An inability to find a way to purify the antitumor globulin from other globulins in order to increase the specificity was the major limitation of the study [3, 5]. The development of monoclonal antibodies (mAbs) using the hybridoma technique was a major breakthrough because mAbs generated by this technique had a very high specificity for antigens [6]. Initial studies for localization of tumor using radioimmunoimaging in humans showed encouraging results in renal cell carcinomas and gliomas [7, 8]. However, the use of mAbs for the treatment of cancer was not very successful in the preliminary studies. Their immunogenicity, due to the murine origin of these mAbs, and their poor ability to generate an effective immune response against the cancer cells marred the promising role of antibody-mediated cancer therapy [9–11]. It was possible to circumvent the problem of antigenicity of murine mAbs by the development of chimeric, humanized, and fully human mAbs [12–15]. These unconjugated mAbs were envisaged to have a high potential for cancer therapy; however, because of certain inherent limitations, even they have failed to live up to their potential. Slow extravasation from the blood, poor tumor vascularization, poor lymphatic drainage, antigen heterogeneity, and interactions between mAbs and their receptors have been thought to be responsible for this lack of prolonged and efficient intratumoral unconjugated mAb uptake [16–20]. The other contributing factor which has led to the limited therapeutic efficacy is the extent to which ADCC (antibody-dependent cell-mediated cytotoxicity), induction of direct signaling events, or complement-dependent cytotoxicity leads to the

V. Prasad (✉)
Department of Nuclear Medicine, University Hospital of Ulm, Ulm, Germany
e-mail: vikas.prasad@uniklinik-ulm.de

R. P. Baum
CURANOSTICUM Wiesbaden-Frankfurt, DKD Helios Klinik, Wiesbaden, Germany

J. P. Oliva
Department of Nuclear Medicine, National Institute of Oncology and Radiobiology, Plaza, Havana, Cuba

H. Ahmadzadehfar et al. (eds.), *Clinical Nuclear Medicine*,
https://doi.org/10.1007/978-3-030-39457-8_34

cancer cell death [21]. These failures of unconjugated mAbs lead to the concept of arming these highly specific molecules with compounds which have additional cell killing properties like drugs, toxins, and radionuclides. Radioimmunotherapy (RIT) has the added advantage over the mAbs labeled with drugs or toxins because (1) radionuclides are not sensitive to multidrug resistance, (2) even those cancer cells which do not express targeted antigen can be sterilized because of the phenomenon of "cross fire" [22], and (3) simultaneous localization of the tumor is possible through radioimmunoscintigraphy [23, 24]. In 1951, Beierwaltes conducted the first clinical trial to investigate the therapeutic potential of ^{131}I-labeled rabbit antibodies in 14 patients having metastatic melanoma and documented the pathologically confirmed complete remission in one patient [25]. Since then numerous studies have been conducted; however, radioimmunotherapy had its major breakthrough with the approval of ibritumomab tiuxetan (Zevalin, murine CD20 mAb conjugated to ^{90}Y) by the FDA in February 2002 [26]. This was immediately followed by the approval of another radioimmunoconjugate, ^{131}I-tositumomab (Bexxar), in the year 2003 [27]. The road to this success was not easy because of several challenges including the possible decay of radionuclide-conjugated mAbs before being delivered to the target site, the possible perturbation of mAb antigen-binding site by the conjugates, and the possible suboptimal pharmacokinetics and biodistribution of the mAb carriers [21]. Even now most of the success that radioimmunotherapy has achieved is mainly in hematological malignancies. Medical scientists are still working on expanding the field of RIT into solid tumors.

In order to understand the rationale used and the complexities associated with the use of these radiopharmaceuticals in radioimmunotherapy for the treatment of some of the indolent carcinomas, it is essential to understand the key steps for the development and manufacture of monoclonal antibodies, the methods and mechanism of action of radionuclides used for conjugation with mAbs, and their pharmacokinetics and normal tissue uptake.

34.2 Radiopharmaceuticals for Radioimmunotherapy

34.2.1 Development and Manufacture of mAbs

The targeting antibodies used for RIT should ideally have the following properties: (1) no or very low immunogenicity for repeated administration, (2) optimal antigen binding, (3) good tumor penetration, (4) good rate of clearance from normal tissues (essential for efficient and specific tumor targeting and thus decreasing the radiation exposure to normal tissues), (5) optimal tumor residence time for delivering therapeutic radiation dose, and (6) optimal tumor accretion. The initial studies of radioimmunoimaging and radioimmunotherapy were performed mostly with animal-derived polyclonal antibodies which lacked specificity [28–33]. The development of the hybridoma technique allowed to produce large amounts of mAbs with predefined specificity but still suffered because of three major factors: (1) immunogenicity of murine origin of the mAbs limiting the administration to one or two cycles, (2) no significant improvement in tumor uptake because of the limited number of tumor-binding sites, and (3) the poor pharmacokinetics for effective usage in RIT [34]. The strategy developed to improve the pharmacokinetics for effective RIT was the development of smaller molecules with faster clearance and better tumor penetration. Radiolabeled antibody fragments and subfragments have been found to have good therapeutic effects in animal models with faster clearance and good tumor penetration. Bivalent F $(ab')_2$ and monovalent F ab′ fragments belong to this class of molecule [35–45]. Various diabodies (M_r 55,000) and minibodies, having molecular weights above the range for rapid renal clearance, have been constructed with the aim of binding to more than two antigen molecules while retaining the property of rapid clearance from the body [45]. However, this improvement in tumor to nontumor uptake was achieved at the cost of lower affinity and decreased tumor residence time leading to lowered absolute tumor uptake as compared to the intact immunoglobulins (IgG).

As of now, the small molecular constructs are being considered for use in pretargeting strategies which deal with separation of tumor targeting from the delivery of therapeutic radionuclides and are discussed in detail later on. These diabodies and minibodies have also found significant usage in the evaluation of biokinetics of certain drugs and tracers using PET and radioimmunoimaging of certain forms of cancer using a gamma camera (SPECT). ^{68}Ga-radiolabeled F ab′ fragments of trastuzumab monitoring Her2 expression [46] and the use of ^{123}I-labeled scFv dimer with specific affinity for the fibronectin extra domain B, which is expressed in tumor neovasculature, are two examples [47]. Whether these fragments and subfragments of antibodies will have any role in RIT is still a matter of debate as is shown by several animal studies [37–40, 43, 44]. Various antibodies and antibody fragments used in immunotherapy/radioimmunotherapy and their salient properties are shown in Table 34.1.

The problem of antigenicity after repeated administration of the initial mAbs was overcome by the development of chimerized, humanized, and fully human antibodies. In gradual steps of development, murine mAbs were first converted into murine/human chimeras which subsequently were turned into murine CDR-grafted human antibodies and ultimately into fully human antibodies. Most of the clinical experience has been exclusively with chimeric and CDR-grafted antibodies. The results have documented less antigenicity as compared to the previous generation mAbs [34, 48]. Future studies are being directed towards resolving the issue of superiority between these three congeners. Chimeric antibodies have been shown to generate immune response [49]. It is also expected that fully human antibodies may generate T cell-dependent or anti-idiotype immune response [34].

One of the most important considerations and constraints in the development and research usage of these mAbs is the implementation of the GMP (Good Manufacturing Practice) law in most parts of the developed world. The legislation requires preclinical testing and management of clinical trials, which will greatly increase the cost of running and reduce the number of such research programs. This law has necessitated the development and awareness of ways and means to use the limited resources for designing manufacture protocols of mAbs. Table 34.2 lists some of the mAbs (conjugated and unconjugated) which are presently approved for use in oncology.

34.2.2 Radioimmunoconjugation for RIT

The following factors have to be taken into consideration for the radionuclides used for conjugation with mAbs for effective RIT: (1) physical and chemical properties, (2) nature of radiation emitted, (3) fate of the radionuclide after the metabolism of antibody in vivo, and (4) the need for a simple, efficient, and reproducible commercial method for radioimmunoconjugation. Some of the clinically relevant properties of radionuclides

Table 34.1 Salient properties of commonly used monoclonal antibodies/antibody fragments (Modified from [34])

Properties	IgG	Fab′	F(ab′)z	scFv	Diabody
Biological					
Capability to induce immune response	Present	Absent	Absent	Absent	Absent
$T_{1/2}$ in blood	2–3days	4 h	1–2 days	1 h	< 4h
Target organ	Liver	Kidney	Liver	Kidney	Kidney
Physical					
Molecular weight	150 K	50 K	100 K	40 K	20 K
Tumor binding					
Optimal accretion time	Days	Hours	Day	Hour	Hours
Duration	++++	+++	++	+	+++
Uptake	++++	+++	++	+	+++

++++ indicates maximum and + indicates minimum, with the rest (++ and +++) being intermediate between these two

Table 34.2 Monoclonal antibodies approved by the FDA for use in oncology (Modified from [50])

Trade name	FDA approval	Source	Format and isotype	Target	Indication
Immunoconjugates					
^{90}Y-Ibritumomab tiuxetan (Zevalin) with rituximab	2002	Murine	^{90}Y-IgGl	CD20	Lymphoma
Tositumomab and ^{131}I-tositumomab	2003	Murine	^{131}I-IgG2a	CD20	Lymphoma
Gemtuzumab (Mylotarg)	2000	Human mAb, drug derived from streptomyces	hIgG4-cali-cheamicin	CD33	Acute myelogenous leukemia
Unconjugated mAbs					
Rituximab (Rituxan)	1997	Murine-human chimeric	hIgG1	CD20	Lymphoma
Trastuzumab (Herceptin)	1998	Humanized	hIgG1	HER2/neu	Breast cancer
Alemtuzumab (Campath-1H)	2001	Humanized	hIgG1	CD52	Chronic lymphocytic leukemia
Cetuximab (Erbitux)	2004	Murine-human chimeric	hIgG1	EGF receptor	Colorectal cancer
Bevacizumab (Avastin)	2004	Murine-human chimeric	hIgG1	VEGF	Colorectal, lung cancer

Table 34.3 Relevant radionuclides presently used in RIT

Radionuclide	t ½ in hours	Emission used in therapy	Emax (keV)	Maximum path length (mm)
^{131}I	193	β	610	2.0
^{90}Y	64	β	2,280	12.0
^{177}Lu	161	β	496	1.5
^{186}Re	91	β	1,080	5.0
^{188}Re	17	β	2,120	11.0
^{67}Cu	62	β	577	1.8
^{225}Ac	240	α	5,935	<0.1
^{211}At	7.2	α	7,450	0.09
^{212}Bi	1	α	8,780	>0.1
^{213}Bi	0.77	α	>6,000	0.08
^{125}I	1442.4	Low energy electrons	350	0.02

used at present in RIT are listed in Table 34.3. In order to deliver the effective killing dose to the cancerous cells, a choice has to be made between alpha particles, beta particles, and Auger electrons. One has to bear in mind that the efficacy of RIT depends not only on the properties of the radionuclides and mAbs but is also very sensitive to the type of tumor, its location, size, physiology, morphology, and radiosensitivity to radionuclides. There has to be an adequate balance between the dose delivered to the normal tissues and the tumor so that there is reduced radiation toxicity with effective radiation killing dose.

The two most commonly used radionuclides in RIT are currently the β-emitters ^{90}Y and ^{177}Lu. Other β-particle-emitting radionuclides that are being used clinically for RIT are ^{131}I,^{67}Cu, ^{186}Re, and ^{188}Re [51–56]. β-particles are available in a wide range of half-lives and emissions and have longer path lengths than α-particles. History suggests that ^{131}I has been used most commonly for radiotherapy because it is readily available, is inexpensive, is capable of being imaged using gamma cameras (thus making it possible to perform dosimetry), has a half-life of only 8 days, and is conjugated with proteins with relative ease. Considering the physical properties of ^{131}I, the Nuclear Regulatory Commission of the United States has approved the RIT of patients using ^{131}I on an outpatient basis [57]. In spite of these advantages, the use of ^{131}I in RIT suffers from certain drawbacks like rapid degradation of radioimmunoconjugates resulting in reduced overall tumor dose and tumor residence time [34]. Compared to ^{131}I, ^{90}Y is a pure β-emitter, and the β-particle emitted has a higher energy and path length (2 mm for ^{131}I vs 12 mm for ^{90}Y), making it suitable for irradiation of tumors having larger dimension. The other favorable property of ^{90}Y is its longer residence time because it is a residualizing label. Radiolabeling of ^{90}Y with mAbs is very effective with high yield and good stability. The most common chelator which is being used for achieving these encouraging results is 1,4,7,10-tetraazacyclododecane-*N,N′N″N‴*-tetraacetic acid (DOTA). Antibody conjugation is achieved by the activation with *N*-hydroxysulfosuccinimide [58].

Lutetium-177 (^{177}Lu) has gained popularity as the therapeutic radionuclide of choice due to its desirable physical properties [59]. Ideally, the emission characteristics of a therapeutic radionuclide should match the lesion size/volume to be treated to ideally focus energy within the tumor rather than in the tissue surrounding the lesion. ^{177}Lu is a medium-energy β-emitter (490 keV) with a maximum energy of 0.5 MeV and a maximal tissue penetration of <2 mm. The shorter β-range of ^{177}Lu provides better irradiation of small tumors, in contrast to the longer β-range of ^{90}Y. ^{177}Lu is a reactor-produced radiometal that emits low-energy γ-rays at 208 and 113 keV with 10 and 6% abundance, respectively. The gamma emission from ^{177}Lu allows for *in vivo* imaging (scintigraphy) and consequently the collection of information pertaining to tumor localization and dosimetry. Furthermore, ^{177}Lu has a relatively long physical half-life of 6.73 days. It is these physical properties that allow for the delivery of high activities of ^{177}Lu PSMA to cancer cells [60, 61].

The use of α-particles for RIT is relatively new but has shown promising results. The development of ^{234}Ra and ^{225}Ac generators, which produce high yields of α-particle-emitting ^{212}Bi and ^{213}Bi, respectively, has opened up the possibility of conjugation with mAbs [62, 63]. The other α-particle-emitting radionuclide, ^{211}At, which is a cyclotron product, has also been used in RIT [64, 65]. These α-particle emitting radionuclides have a high LET (~100 keV μm) and a very short path length (< 0.1 mm). The possibility of delivering high LET radiation from a very short range on DNA, resulting in strand breaks, has been the major cause for this renewed interest. One of the prerequisites for these α-particle-emitting radionuclides being used in RIT is the availability of fast mAb conjugation methods because of the very short life of these particles. Most of the conjugation methods used these days take less than 2 h, which is still not sufficient. These radionuclides find their best usage in the treatment of micrometastases or circulating tumor cells. The radionuclides, ^{125}I emitting low energy electrons, have also been used for RIT.

34.3 Different Strategies for RIT

34.3.1 Factors to Be Considered for Developing an Effective RIT Strategy

As is true for most of the therapy regimes used in cancer, a RIT regime takes into consideration the amount of radioactivity administered and the number of cycles used for achieving an optimal therapeutic effect with minimal toxicity/side effects. Radioimmunotherapy, although it appears simple in principle, becomes complex in achieving the desired effect as it is dependent upon three separate but interdependent variables, i.e., the radionuclide, the antibody, and the characteristics of the tumor and host. In order to achieve a therapeutic effect, minute details concerning these factors have to be taken into consideration, of which of paramount importance is the development of a strategy to deliver an adequate dose of radioactivity for killing the cancer cells without affecting the normal tissues. The potential for high absorbed dose of the bone marrow due to circulating or bone tumor-bound antibody, the fear of developing bone marrow toxicity, prevents the delivery of an adequate amount of radiation dose to the tumor cells. The data from external beam radiotherapy suggests that a minimum cumulative tumor dose of 5,000 cGy should be delivered to provide an adequate therapeutic response. However, even at an accretion as high as 0.01 % of the injected dose/g of tumor, radiolabeled antibodies deliver a cumulative tumor dose of less than 1,500 cGy [34].

The response of the tumor depends upon the type of cells it is composed of, its vascularity, and volume of the tumor. Most of the damaging effects of radiation occur in the presence of an adequate oxygen concentration. This makes the vascularity of the tumor a very important factor in determining the outcome of RIT. Delivery of the radioimmunoconjugates to the tumor also depends on the vascularity. The normal physiologic distribution of the tumor antigens against which the antibodies are prepared also has an important role to play. The toxicity due to RIT may rise if the antibody is not tumor specific. Taking all these factors together, the strategies which have been developed for RIT differ according to whether the tumor is solid and bulky or has a small volume. It has been observed that whereas RIT has gained sufficient therapeutic potential in hematopoietic malignancies, and minimal or micrometastatic disease, it has failed to deliver an adequate radiation dose in solid tumors.

34.3.2 Pretargeting Strategies

The aim of pretargeting strategies (i.e., the use of cold, nonradiolabeled molecules prior to the administration of radioimmunoconjugates) is to increase the amount of radioactivity administered without having serious detrimental side effects on the normal tissues. Almost all the pretargeting strategies use modified mAbs [66]. It is possible to create, chemically or through genetic engineering, from monovalent antibody fragments, other antibody fragments (bispecific monoclonal antibody, bsmAb) which not only bind to the specific antigen but also have the capacity to bind to another hapten chelate. Radiolabeled chelates are prepared that have higher clearance, diffusion rates, and permeation. These radiolabeled chelates are injected after the administration of bsmAbs, which leads to the rapid and highly selective tumor uptake [67–69]. In order to achieve the ideal condition of almost zero background activity and maximal tumor concentration, scientists have added a third step in this concept of pretargeting by the incorporation of another molecule, rightly called the scavenger molecule or chaser, which leads to the removal of tumor-targeted macromolecule from the circulation. Indeed, the use of pretargeting strategies in RIT and radioimmunoimaging has been very successful in delivering a higher amount of radiation to the tumor as compared to those achieved using radiolabeled IgG directly as is documented by several studies [67, 68, 70, 71].

In order to simplify the concept of pretargeting strategies, they can be divided into two broad groups: (1) the two-step method and (2) the three-step method. In the two-step method, bsmAb is constructed, which has one hapten binding site (radiochelate binding site) and one to two target binding sites (tumor antigen detecting site) [72]. The bsmAbs used for RIT are very small-sized molecules equivalent to F $(ab')_2$. The small size of the bsmAbs enables them to penetrate deep into the tumor tissue, making it possible for the radiolabeled components to deliver a uniform radiation dose to the tumor. A sufficient time gap (several days) is given between step 1 (injection of bsmAbs) and step 2 (injection of radiolabeled component) for adequate clearance of the bsmAbs; otherwise, there will be an increase in the nontumor-tumor ratio because of complex formation between the two components in the circulation.

The three-step methods currently being employed in pretargeting strategies for RIT are (1) streptavidin (StAv) or avidin-conjugated mAb and radiolabeled biotin [73–75], (2) avidin-biotin [76–81], and (3) antibody-conjugated DNA and complementary nucleotide sequence [82]. The high affinity of avidin for biotin and availability of four binding sites has been instrumental in bringing forward this concept of using streptavidin or avidin and biotin in pretargeting strategies [83]. In the first method, StAv conjugated to mAb is injected first, followed by administration of a clearing agent for removal of StAv-mAb complex from the circulation, and subsequently, in the third step, radiolabeled biotin (^{90}Y-biotin) is injected. However, rapid trafficking of mAb-StAv conjugate into the liver and kidneys makes its biodistribution unfavorable for RIT, leading to the use of modification of the technique. In the second method, radiolabeled biotin is also used.

However, instead of using Stav-mAb complex, mAb-biotin complex is used first. In the second step, avidin is injected to remove the biotinylated IgG from the circulation, and then StAv is added, which penetrates deep into the tumor and binds to the mAb-biotin complex. The use of avidin prior to the administration of StAv for the clearance of biotinylated IgG from the system is based upon the rationale that avidin is cleared faster from the circulation compared to StAv (because avidin is glycosylated and StAv is nonglycosylated). Most of the biotinylated conjugates are made to withstand the effect of biotinidase, lest there be free radionuclide in the serum due to the breakdown of biotin-radionuclide complex [84–87]. In the third method, target-specific mAb conjugated with oligonucleotides is injected first followed by the administration of complementary oligonucleotide for the clearance of mAb-oligonucleotide complex. In the final step, radiolabeled oligonucleotides are injected. Different clinical conditions in which these strategies have been employed until now will be discussed in the section dealing with clinical studies in this chapter [88–104].

While the uses of bsmAbs and StAv have their own merits and demerits in pretargeting strategies, results have suggested that StAv is immunogenic even after the first exposure [100, 105]. The same is true for the use of murine bsmAbs, prompting scientists to shift to more humanized and fully humanized bsmAbs for pretargeting [98, 106].

34.3.2.1 Proof of Concept of DOTA-PRIT: A Platform Approach in Human Tumors

Chelators can play a significant role in deciding the pharmacokinetics of a radiolabelled moiety. DOTA chelators have revolutionized diagnostics and therapy with radiolabeled peptides. Several studies have renewed the interest in pretargeting radioimmunotherapy using DOTA chelators (DOTA-PRIT). One of the major advantages of such pretargeting is to increase the bioavailability of radiolabeled haptens in and around tumor cells thereby increasing the therapeutic efficacy. In addition, this novel approach reduces nonspecific radiohaptens uptake, e.g., in kidneys and bone marrow and thereby increases the therapeutic index. This kind of approach albeit in nascent stage, developed by pioneering works of Steven Larson and his group from MSKCC, has shown promising results in preclinical studies for several solid tumors like colorectal cancer, neuroblastoma, and breast cancer and also for hematological malignancies, e.g., lymphomas [107–110].

34.3.3 Combination Therapy

The aim of multimodality therapy in the treatment of cancer is to increase the therapeutic efficacy while decreasing the adverse effects. To date there have been few clinical studies which have documented the improved efficacy of RIT if combined with chemotherapy [111–114]. These studies will be discussed briefly in the section concerning clinical studies in this chapter. Another concept which has been in vogue for a few years is the use of radionuclides with different radiation properties for the treatment of both bulky disease and micrometastases [115]. The concept of combining external beam radiation therapy with radionuclide therapy is also being developed, named exclusively by R.P. Baum as COMBIERT (combined internal external radiation therapy). Whether these concepts will remain true to their potential is yet to be seen.

34.3.4 Dosimetry for RIT

The dosimetry approaches for the calculation of tumor, total body, and normal organ radiation-absorbed doses in RIT are similar to those for other radiopharmaceuticals. The readers are suggested to go through the published guidelines by the European Association of Nuclear Medicine and Molecular Imaging.

34.3.5 Nonmyeloablative vs Myeloablative RIT

In general for the delivery of cytocidal radioactivity to the tumor cells, two different approaches of RIT are in vogue: the low-dose or nonmyeloablative approach and the high-dose or myeloablative approach [116, 117]. In the low-dose approach, the dose of radionuclide given does not result in myeloablation. The only significant and dose-limiting toxicity (DLT) of this approach is myelosuppression, which usually occurs 3–6 weeks post-therapy. The nadir of the toxicity is reached at 4–8 weeks, with the full recovery usually happening by 12 weeks. Nonhematological toxicity is minimal with this approach [118–137]. In the high-dose myeloablative RIT approach, the higher amount of radioactivity administered results in a higher probability (sometimes almost certain) of having a bone marrow ablation [138–142]. Therefore, this approach usually requires a hematopoietic, generally autologous, stem cell transplant (HSCT) with peripheral blood stem cells or bone marrow. Apart from this severe toxicity, the myeloablative approach also results in significant nonhematological toxicity to other organs, which usually appears within 1–2 months after therapy, with full recovery usually completed within a few weeks. The DLT for this approach is gastrointestinal and cardiopulmonary toxicity. Hepatic toxicity is also observed.

34.3.6 Dosing Methods for RIT

There are two different methods for prescribing the amount of radioactivity to be administered in the myeloablative or nonmyeloablative approaches of RIT. The first method is dosimetry based, in which the amount of radioactivity to be given is derived from the radiation dose to the critical dose-limiting organ. As already described in the previous section, the maximum tolerated dose (MTD) depends on the critical organs, which are red marrow/total body (as a surrogate to marrow) in the nonmyeloablative regime of RIT [124–126, 131, 143] or the second organ, e.g., the lungs, heart, and gastrointestinal tract, in the myeloablative regime [138, 140–142]. Pre-therapy tracer imaging is used for calculating the radioactivity to be administered taking into account the anticipated radiation dose to the critical organ/MBq of administered activity. This method of calculation of radioactivity to be administered for RIT is patient specific as the mAb pharmacokinetics varies significantly from one individual to another.

The second method is based on the fixed amounts of radioactivity or body weight/body surface corrected radiation dose [119–121, 123, 128–130, 133, 135, 144]. It is the simpler of the two methods and does not require a pre-therapy tracer study but is not patient specific.

34.3.7 Immuno-PET

The concept of immuno-PET is becoming more and more important as through serial quantitative PET/CT, it has become possible to ascertain the labeled mAb concentration in the tumor and thereby facilitate the dosing of the mAb for RIT. It is also possible to perform individualized dosimetry with far more accuracy, which will limit the toxicity and thereby increase the therapeutic index and effectiveness of RIT. Zirconium-89-labeled chimeric monoclonal antibody U36 was one of the first such radiopharmaceuticals [145, 146], and many others meanwhile have been in clinical trials [147]

34.3.8 RIT vs Immunotherapy

There are certain distinct advantages of RIT over immunotherapy, either using unconjugated antibodies or using toxin-conjugated antibodies. In RIT, specifically in the case of B-cell NHL, the cytocidal effect is more pronounced than immunotherapy as both biologic and immunologic mechanisms of the antitumor effects of mAbs, e.g., apoptosis and ADCC, come into play along with the radiation-induced damage to the tumor cells. The "cross fire" or the "bystander" effect of radiation in RIT, which results in damage to the neighboring nontargeted cells and thus obviates the need to target every cell in the tumor, is a definite advantage over immunotherapy, in which the antitumor effect on a tumor cell is apparent only if it is targeted with the mAb [148].

34.4 Clinical Studies

This section will deal with the most common disease conditions in which the utility of RIT has been conducted most often and in which there is a clear-cut advantage of the implementation of RIT for improved prognosis/quality of life of patients. Broadly, the clinical conditions in which RIT has been implemented and studied can be classified into hematological malignancies and solid tumor. This classification is justified because of the different parameters which have to be taken into consideration when using RIT for these conditions.

34.4.1 Hematopoietic Tumors

34.4.1.1 B-Cell Non-Hodgkin's Lymphoma

B-cell non-Hodgkin's lymphoma (NHL) is one of the most common cancers in the United States accounting for 4% of all cancers. According to the American Cancer Society estimate for 2019, nearly 74,200 patients will be diagnosed with NHL. There are numerous histologic variants of NHL, which are best classified using the WHO classification (Blood. 2016;127(20):2375-2390).

Approximately 80 % of lymphomas are of B-cell origin. The Ann-Arbor system previously used for staging of the patients has now been replaced by the Lugano classification which classifies lymphoma disease according to the compartments and extent [149, 150].

B-cell NHL patients not responding to chemotherapy and immunotherapy or who relapse after these therapies are the ideal candidates for the institution of RIT [151].

The potential role of RIT in B-cell NHL was first described by DeNardo et al. in a patient treated with ^{131}I-labeled anti-B-cell lymphoma mAb (called Lym-1). Since then, numerous trials have been conducted, with the majority showing significant improvement in the patient's disease status after treatment with these radioimmunoconjugates. Among various other reasons, the tumor biology of B-cell NHL makes it an ideal candidate for RIT. NHL is radiosensitive and expresses numerous target-specific antigens, making it easier for scientists to create specific mAb against these antigens. The numerous antigens which have been targeted until now for RIT are listed in Table 34.4. However, only ibritumomab tiuxetan (Zevalin, murine mAb against CD20 antigen con-

Table 34.4 Radioimmunoconjugates currently used in oncology

Clinical indications	Radiolabeled antibodies
Hematological malignancies	
NHL	^{90}Y-ibritumomab tiuxetan[a]
	^{131}I-tositumomab[a]
	^{90}Y-epratuzumab anti-CD22 IgG
Leukemia	^{131}I-BCB anti CD45 IgG
	^{90}Y or ^{188}Re-anti-CD66 IgG
	^{213}Bi-HuM195 antiCD33 IgG
NHL, Hodgkin's lLymphoma and T-cell lymphoma	^{90}Y-anti-Tac IgG
Solid malignancies	
Colorectal cancer	^{90}Y-T84.66 anti CEA IgG
	^{131}I- and ^{90}Y-labetuzumab (anti CEA IgG)
	^{131}I-CC49-ΔCH2
	^{125}I/131I-A33 IgG
	^{90}Y-biotin pretargeted with CC49 StAv fusion protiein
Prostate cCancer	^{177}Lu-J591IgG
	^{131}I-murine CC49 mAb
	^{90}Y-CYT-356 capromab peandetdidte
Ovarian cCancer	^{90}Y/177Lu-CC49
	^{90}Y-Hu3S193
	^{131}I-anti-CEA IgG
	^{90}Y-biotin pretargeted by biotinylated mAb cocktail
Glioma	^{90}Y-BC-2 and BC4 anti-tenascin
	^{125}I-425 IgG
	^{131}I labeled anti-tenascin
Pancreatic cCancer	^{90}Y-PAM4 IgG
Lung cCancer	^{131}I-ch TNT
Breast cCancer	^{90}Y-Br-E3
	^{211}At-81C6
	^{131}I-81C6
	^{90}Y-170H.82
	^{131}I-CC49
Renal cCancer	^{131}I-cG250 IgG
Medullary tThyroid cCancer	^{131}I-hapten pretargeted by anti-CEA bsmAb
CNS or leptomeningeal cancer	^{131}I-BH9 IgG
Medulloblastoma	^{131}I-3F8 IgG
Head and nNeck cancer	^{186}Re-bivatuzumab
Hepatocellular cCarcinoma	^{131}I-Hepama IgG
	^{90}Y-hAFP IgG

[a]Approved by FDA for RIT of NHL

jugated to ^{90}Y) and tositumomab (Bexxar, murine mAb against CD20 antigen conjugated to ^{131}I) have been approved by the FDA so far.

34.4.1.2 ^{90}Y-Ibritumomab Tiuxetan (Zevalin)

Zevalin prepared by IDEC pharmaceuticals, San Diego, CA, was the first radioimmunoconjugate to be approved by the FDA for clinical use in February 2002. It consists of ^{90}Y-labeled murine antibody to CD20. Based upon the International Workshop Response Criteria, Zevalin has been found to produce a response rate of 74–83 % in patients with relapsed/refractory low-grade, follicular, or CD20+ transformed NHL [152–154]. It has also been documented based upon the same response criteria that Zevalin has the response rate of 83 % in patients who failed to respond to rituximab.

34.4.1.3 Dosimetry and Dosing

The results of dosimetry and dosing of ^{90}Y-ibritumomab tiuxetan in several studies have come to the following conclusions [155]:

1. ^{90}Y-ibritumomab tiuxetan can be administered safely without significant toxicity if the dose is based upon a patient's body weight and the pretreatment platelet counts. If the pretreatment platelet count is 150 X 10^9/L and more, then a dose of 15 MBq/kg up to a maximum of 1200 MBq can be administered, and if pretreatment platelet count is more than 100×10^9/L but less than 150×10^9/L, then a dose of 11 MBq/kg up to a maximum of 1200 MBq is recommended.
2. Dosimetry was not required if the patients have the desired pretreatment platelet count and < 25 % bone marrow involvement (as determined by bone marrow biopsy).
3. Dosimetry should ideally be performed if the indication for use of ^{90}Y-ibritumomab tiuxetan is different from the one defined in the registration trials in patients with low-grade NHL.
4. Almost the whole of radioactivity administered in the therapeutic dose of ^{90}Y-ibritumomab is retained in the body, with only 7.3 ± 3.25 % being excreted through the kidneys (primary pathway of clearance).
5. As an additional safety measure, ^{111}In-ibritumomab tiuxetan scintigraphy can be performed to confirm the expected biodistribution of ^{90}Y-ibritumomab (in the US the In-111 study must be done).

34.4.1.4 Preparation and Administration

The procedure for radiolabeling of ^{90}Y-ibritumomab tiuxetan begins with 1,480 MBq. The patient dose ranges between 777 and 1,110 MBq, with the maximum administered activity of 1200 MBq. Zevalin is commercially available in solution form, containing 3.2 mg of the immunoconjugate in 2 ml of saline solution. A quantity of 1,480 MBq of ^{90}Y can be incorporated in 1.3 ml of the solution, resulting in a relatively low dose of mAb being administered [155].

The radiochemical purity of the preparation is checked prior to its administration to the patient. If it is 95 %, then the preparation can be used for injection into the patient. For radiation safety measures, the drug is kept in plastic or acrylic shields, and the syringe should also be shielded accordingly. The drug can be prepared at a regional radiopharmacy center and distributed to the user centers.

Prior to therapy with 90Y-ibritumomab tiuxetan, two infusions with rituximab are administered. These rituximab infusions must be performed under the responsibility of an experienced hematologist-oncologist who is familiar with rituximab. Day 1, infusion of 250mg/m^2 rituximab: the volume of normal saline solution, which contains the rituximab stock solution, and the infusion must comply with the recommendations contained in the package insert of the preparation. In Switzerland and the United States, this infusion is followed by IV infusion of ^{111}In-ibritumomab tiuxetan (180 MBq) over 10 minutes. At least one anterior and posterior whole-body scan has to be recorded within 24 hours and 7–9 days after injection. Day 7 or 8 or 9, infusion of 250 mg/m^2 rituximab, followed by administration of 90Yibritumomab tiuxetan as slow IV infusion over 10 minutes: Zevalin® should not be administered as an intravenous bolus [156].

This step is essential to improve tumor targeting by blocking easily accessible CD20 sites in the peripheral blood and preventing indiscriminate uptake of the radioimmunoconjugate in the reticuloendothelial system [157]. ^{90}Y-ibritumomab tiuxetan administration should begin within 4 h of completion of rituximab dose [158]. A slow intravenous push over 10 min rather than a rapid intravenous bolus is the preferred mode of injection. The patients can be injected on an outpatient basis.

34.4.1.5 Adverse Effects and Toxicity

The most common nonhematologic adverse effects of ^{90}Y-ibritumomab tiuxetan therapy are as follows: asthenia, nausea, infection, fever, chills, and abdominal pain [155]. Because of the murine mAb component of Zevalin, anaphylaxis, a potentially serious adverse effect, may develop.

Development of human anti-mouse antibody (HAMA) response to murine antibodies [159] is common, but the intensity of the reaction is not very high in NHL patients who have already received chemotherapy. The most deleterious effect of this reaction to the murine antibody is limitation of the number of therapy cycles which can be instituted in patients already documented to have had HAMA response [34]. Keeping these anaphylactic reactions in mind, it is obligatory to make sure that epinephrine, antihistamines, and corticosteroids are readily available during the administration of Zevalin as well as rituximab.

34.4.1.6 Radiation Safety Measures

As mentioned already, ^{90}Y-ibritumomab tiuxetan can be administered on an outpatient basis. The treatment with Zevalin results in the emission of beta particles and bremsstrahlung radiation. Since there is no emission of penetrating gamma radiation, the risk of radiation exposure to healthcare workers, patients, family members, or other close contacts is minimal. In accordance with US guidelines (*Criteria for the Release of Individuals Administered Radioactive Material*, Nuclear Regulatory Commission, Washington, DC, US, 1997, Title 10 CFR parts 20 and 35:62 FR 4120, and *Release of Patients Administered Radioactive Materials*, Nuclear Regulatory Commission, Washington, DC, US, 1997. Regulatory Guide 8.39), patients can be released immediately after therapy. Minimal risks associated with the use of ^{90}Y-labeled monoclonal antibodies preclude the need for determining activity limits or dose limits for the patients. The recommended instructions to be given to patients who have been treated with ^{90}Y-ibritumomab tiuxetan are as follows [155]:

1. Up to 3 days post-therapy: (a) proper care to be taken during micturition to prevent spilling of urine. Spilled urine should be cleaned up. (b) Good hand washing after using the toilet. (c) Disposal of any body fluid-contaminated material, e.g., in a toilet or in a plastic bag in the household trash.
2. Up to 1 week after therapy: use of condoms for sexual intercourse.

Some patients may be required to be treated as inpatients for medical reasons. These patients should be handled like every other patient, and no precautions other than the universal precautions are needed [155].

34.4.1.7 ^{131}I-Tositumomab (Bexxar)

^{131}I-tositumomab was approved by the FDA for the treatment of relapsed and refractory B-cell NHL patients in June 2003; however, it has gone out of production since 2014.

34.4.1.8 Dosimetry and Dosing

Unlike Zevalin, individualized dosimetry is essential prior to the administration of Bexxar. For dosimetry [160], 450 mg of unlabeled tositumomab is given intravenously over 1 h followed by infusion of 35 mg of (185 MBq) iodine (^{131}I) tositumomab over 20 min. Whole-body images are acquired under the gamma camera at 1 h postinjection and then on the 2nd, 3rd, 4th, 6th, and 7th days. A best fit line derived from a time activity curve of the percentage of residual injected radioactivity is used to calculate the total body residence time. The MTD calculated for ^{131}I-tositumomab is 75 cGy. This value is taken into consideration when calculating the total dose of ^{131}I-tositumomab to be administered to the patient. The rationale for using individualized dosimetry is to increase the *therapeutic index*, which is defined as the ratio of the radiation-absorbed dose delivered to cancerous cells and the dose delivered to normal tissues.

34.4.1.9 Preparation and Administration

Bexxar used to be supplied by a centralized radiopharmacy. For the end users, it used to come in two different forms depending on its use. For the purpose of dosimetry, it is supplied at radioactivity (^{131}I) and protein (tositumomab) concentrations of 22.5 MBq/ml and 0.1 mg/ml, respectively. The therapeutic dosage form consists of 207 MBq/ml and 1.1 mg/ml of radioactivity (^{131}I) and protein (tositumomab), respectively. Free radioiodine and other reactants are removed at the manufacturer's end by chromatographic purification steps. The potential of thyroid damage from Bexxar is high because of ^{131}I [34]. Therefore thyroid blockage is recommended 1 day prior to, to continue up to 14 days after, the administration of ^{131}I-tositumomab. It is essential to monitor the platelet count before prescribing the dose for ^{131}I-tositumomab. Cold, nonradioactive tositumomab (450 mg) is administered intravenously over 1 h followed by a patient-specific whole-body dose of ^{131}I-tositumomab over 20 min. The radioactivity to be administered is calculated with the aim of delivering 75 cGy, provided the patient's platelet count is 150 X 10^9/L. Patients having relative thrombocytopenia (100–149 X 10^9/L) should be given a radioactivity amount equivalent to the delivery of a total body dose of 65 cGy, because of grade IV hematological toxicity, which is observed with high frequency in these patients [160]. If the bone marrow reserve is > 25 %, then the Bexxar regimen should not be administered. It is recommended that the therapeutic dose of ^{131}I-tositumomab should be delivered within 8–14 days of the initiation of dosimetric steps.

34.4.1.10 Adverse Effects and Toxicity

Immediate: As compared to Zevalin, infusional adverse reaction is minimal with Bexxar. Nonhematological toxicity is also minimal [34]. Sometimes a serious hypersensitivity reaction, including anaphylaxis, is observed with ^{131}I-tositumomab. In patients who have not received chemotherapy previously, the incidence of HAMA after Bexxar is as high as approximately 60 % [161]. This is a potential drawback of the regime as the development of HAMA precludes the administration of the second cycle of the regime. It is essential to keep medications to combat these hypersensitivity reactions ready prior to the administration of ^{131}I-tositumomab.

Long-term adverse effects: Because of the usually high release of ^{131}I from Bexxar, the chances of developing hypothyroidism are high even with thyroid blockage [162]. The majority of patients treated with Bexxar develop grade III/IV hematological toxicities across the full range of administered doses [160]. Severe thrombocytopenia and neutropenia are the most common hematological adverse reactions. These hematological adverse effects reach a nadir at 4–6 weeks after therapy and recover to grade II by the 9th week [160]. Some patients treated with Bexxar have also shown myelodysplasia on long-term follow-up. But these patients were heavily pretreated with chemotherapy, which might have been a separate contributory factor [34]. ^{131}I released from Bexxar is cleared from the kidneys, thereby precluding its usage in hydronephrosis or renal dysfunction of another etiology.

34.4.1.11 Radiation Safety Measures

According to the new Nuclear Regulatory Commission regulations for the administration of ^{131}I for therapy, Bexxar can be given to most (but not all) patients on an outpatient basis in the United States [57]. The essential prerequisite for the new regulation is that the total effective dose equivalent to another individual from exposure to a patient treated with ^{131}I containing radiopharmaceutical should be > 500 mrem. *However, in the UK and many other European countries including Germany, the administration is still done on an inpatient basis*. Renal clearance of ^{131}I released from Bexxar makes it mandatory to explain about hygiene and toilet habits to the patients. Healthcare workers should handle the urine or patient's body fluid-contaminated materials in accordance with the set guidelines for handling of ^{131}I.

34.4.1.12 Clinical Experience of Radioimmunotherapy in B-Cell NHL

To date there have been numerous studies and trials done to evaluate the efficacy of RIT in the treatment of B-cell NHL in various clinical settings. It is beyond the scope of this book to elaborate upon all of these studies. The results of some of the studies in various clinical settings of NHL are summarized in Table 34.5.

A brief outline of some of these studies along with their conclusions is mentioned in the following paragraphs.

Table 34.5 RIT in NHL: representative studies

References	No. of patients	Radioimmuno-conjugate	Target	Isotype of mAb	Myeloablative RIT	Dosing schedule	Responses
Behr et al. [163, 164]	3	^{131}I-hLL2	CD22	Humanized IgG2a	1/3	Single	1CR, 1PR, 1PD
	5	^{131}I-C2B8	CD20	Chimeric IgG1	5/5	RID/RIT	3CR, 1PR, 1NA
	7	^{131}I-C2B8	CD20	Chimeric IgG1	7/7	RID/RIT	6CR, 1PR
Czuczman et al. [165]	18	^{131}I-OKB7	CD21	Murine IgG2b	Not given	Quadruple	1PR, 12SD, 5NA
DeNardo et al. [121, 166][a]	18	^{131}I-Lym-l	HLA-DRIO	Murine IgG2a	Not given	Multiple	2CR, 8PR, 3SD, 1PD
	21	^{131}I-Lym-l	HLA-DRIO	Murine IgG2a	Not given	RID/RIT at 1–4 weeks	7CR, 4PR, 9SD, 1PD
Davis et al. [167]	42	^{131}I-anti-Bl	CD20	Murine IgG2a	Not given	RID/RIT	14CR, 9PR
Goldenberg et al. [168]	7	^{131}I-LL2	CD22	Murine IgG2a	Not given	Double	2PR, 3SD
Juweid et al. [123, 124]	7	^{131}I-LL2	CD22	MurineIgG2a	Not given	Multiple	1CR, 1PR, 5 unk
	13	^{131}I-LL2 F(ab)$_2$	CD22	Murine F(ab)$_2$	Not given	Multiple	1CR, 1PR, 11unk
	1	^{131}I-cLL2	CD22	Chimeric IgG2a	Not given	Multiple	1 unk
	3	^{131}I-LL2	CD22	Murine IgG2a	3/3	Multiple	2PR, 1 NE
	13	^{131}I-hLL2	CD22	HumanizedIgG2a	Not given	RID/RIT	1CR, 1PR, 5SD, 6PD
	7	^{90}Y-hLL2	CD22	Humanized IgG2a	Not given	RID/RIT	2PR, 5PD
Kaminski et al. (2005)[b]	76	^{131}I-anti-B1	CD20	Murine IgG2a	Not given	RID/RIT	57CR, 15PR
Linden et al. [169]	8	^{131}I-LL2	CD22	Murine IgG22a	Not given	RID/RIT at 1–3 weeks	3PR, 1SD, 4PD
O'Donnell et al. [170]	12	^{67}Cu-Lym-l	HLA-DRIO	Murine IgG2a	Not given	Multiple	1CR,6PR
Press et al. [141]	6	^{131}I-MB-l	CD37	Murine IgG1	3/6	RID/RIT	6CR
	1	^{131}I-1FS	CD20	Murine IgG2a	l/l	RID/RIT	1PR
	12	^{131}I-anti-B1	CD20	Murine IgG2a	11/12	RID/RIT	10CR, 1PD, 1SD
Postema et al. (2003)[c]	15	^{186}Re-hLL2	CD22	Humanized IgG2a	Not given	RID/RIT	1CR, 4PR, 4SD, 6PD
Scheidhauer et al. [171]	26	^{131}I-C2B8	CD22	Chimeric IgGI	Not given	RID/RIT	9CR, SPR
	25	^{131}J-C2B8	CD22	Chimeric IgGI	25/25	RID/RIT	12CR, 7PR
Witzig et al. [136, 137]	143	^{90}Y-ibritumomab tiuxetan	CD20	Murine IgG2a	Not given	RID/RIT	80% ORR, 30%CR
	54	^{90}Y-ibritumomab tiuxetan	CD20	Murine IgG2a	Not given	Multiple, RID/RIT	74%ORR, 15%CR, 59%PR
Wiseman and Witzig [172]	211	^{90}Y-ibritumomab tiuxetan	CD20	Murine IgG2a		Multiple	TTP 29.3 months. Median TTP was 53.9 months in patients with ongoing response

CR complete remission, *PR* partial remission, *SD* stable disease, *PD* progressive disease, *unk* unknown, *TTP* time to progression, *ORR* overall response rate, *RIT* radioimmunotherapy, *NA* not available, *RID* radioimmunodosimetry

[a]DeNardo GL, DeNardo SJ, Goldstein DS, Kroger LA, Lamborn KR, Levy NB, McGahan JP, Salako Q, Shen S, Lewis JP Maximum-tolerated dose, toxicity, and efficacy of (131)I-Lym-1 antibody for fractionated radioimmunotherapy of non-Hodgkin's lymphoma J Clin Oncol. 1998 Oct; 16(10):3246–56

[b]Kaminski MS, Tuck M, Estes J, et al. I-131 tositumomab therapy as initial treatment for follicular lymphoma. N Engl J Med. 2005; 352:496–498

[c]Postema EJ, Raemaekers JM, Oyen WJ, Boerman OC, Mandigers CM, Goldenberg DM, van Dongen GA, Corstens FH Final results of a phase I radioimmunotherapy trial using (186)Re-epratuzumab for the treatment of patients with non-Hodgkin's lymphoma Clin Cancer Res. 2003 Sep 1; 9(10 Pt 2)3995S–4002S

34.4.1.13 RIT in Relapsed/Refractory B-Cell NHL or Transformed Lymphoma

In a prospective randomized trial of Zevalin in 143 patients with refractory/relapsed low-grade follicular lymphoma or transformed NHL, Zevalin was found to have an overall objective response rate (ORR) and a completion rate (CR) of 80 % and 30 %, respectively, as compared to 56 % and 16 % in the group that received unlabeled rituximab [173]. This study also showed that Zevalin when given at a nonmyeloablative dose of 15 MBq/kg delivered acceptable radiation-absorbed doses to normal organs without performing pre-therapy dosimetry with ^{111}In-labeled Zevalin. In a similar study, in patients with relapsed or refractory NHL, Bexxar was found to have an overall ORR and CR of 55 % and 33 %, respectively, as against 19 % (ORR) and 8 % (CR) in patients treated with unconjugated tositumomab [174]. The median duration of response was not reached in the patient group treated with Bexxar as compared to 28.1 months for those treated with tositumomab. In a phase II study in patients with indolent (the majority follicular) or transformed indolent lymphoma at the time of 1st or 2nd recurrence, 76 % of the patients were found to respond to Bexxar, with 49 % achieving a CR [175]. The response rate was highest in patients with follicular lymphoma (OR 79 %). In the results of a phase I/II study in patients with relapsed or refractory B-cell NHL treated with Zevalin published by Witzig et al. [135] and Wiseman et al. [133], it was observed that Zevalin was able to achieve an ORR of 67 %, with low-grade lymphoma showing the maximum ORR of 82 % as compared to 43 % for intermediate grade lymphoma. Time to disease progression and the duration of response as estimated by Kaplan-Meier estimates were found to be 12.7 months and 11.6 months, respectively. In patients with transformed indolent lymphoma, Bexxar has been reported to have an ORR and a CR of 39 % and 25 %, respectively [176]. The majority of the patients enrolled in this study had a poor prognosis. The median duration of response of patients achieving CR was 36 months.

34.4.1.14 RIT Following Failure of Rituximab

The initial results of a phase II multicenter study in patients who failed to respond to rituximab and were later treated with Bexxar showed that 68 % of patients with follicular lymphoma responded, with 30 % achieving CR [177]. In this subgroup of NHL patients, in a separate study, Zevalin was found to have an ORR of 74 %, with 15 % achieving CR in accordance with the Cheson criteria [173, 178], or an ORR of 59 % and a CR of 4 % by the IDEC criteria. Duration of response was also significantly longer (7.7 months vs 4 months) in patients receiving Zevalin after rituximab failure. The Kaplan-Meier estimated time to progression of disease was found to be 6.8 months for all patients and 8.7 patients for responders.

34.4.1.15 First-Line Therapy

In order to evaluate the efficacy of RIT in patients of B-cell NHL who were not treated previously with chemotherapy or immunotherapy, Wahl et al. conducted a phase II study in patients in stage III or stage IV of low-grade or transformed NHL [161]. These patients were treated with dosimetry-based radioactivity doses of Bexxar reaching 75 cGy to the total body. It was found that 97 % of the patients showed a PR or CR, 63 % achieved CR, and the median duration of response was not reached until 38 months of follow-up, with median duration of follow-up being 16.2 %. However, the potential drawback of the use of Bexxar as the first-line therapy is the high incidence of HAMA response observed due to the murine origin of tositumomab. The use of humanized chimeric or hyperchimeric mAb regimens containing very small amounts of murine mAb is being contemplated.

Summary of Results of Phase II and Phase III Studies with Nonmyeloablative Doses of ^{131}I-Tositumomab and ^{90}Y-Ibritumomab Tiuxetan.

The reported studies have clearly demonstrated that both of these radionuclide-conjugated mAbs are quite effective in the treatment of relapsed/refractory low-grade and transformed NHL with an ORR and CR of 60–80 % and

20–30 %, respectively [148]. The median duration of response observed with both these radioimmunoconjugates is 1 year. In aggressive NHL, phase I/II studies in a limited number of patients have shown that RIT causes ORR and CR in 30–40 % and 10–30 % of patients, respectively [126, 127, 135].

34.4.1.16 Results of Phase II Myeloablative Dose of RIT

Most of the limited number of studies evaluating the myeloablative dose regime of RIT have been performed with Bexxar [139, 142]. The limited experience has suggested that this treatment approach results in higher CR and longer duration of response compared with nonmyeloablative RIT in patients with relapsed/refractory low-grade B-cell NHL. However, there are numerous merits and demerits of these studies, and conclusions about the efficacy of a myeloablative dose regime of RIT can only be ascertained with future studies.

34.4.1.17 RIT Combined with Chemotherapy

In an effort to improve the outcome of patients, studies have been conducted to evaluate the efficacy of combining chemotherapy with RIT. Two approaches have been used: (1) a nonmyeloablative approach (low-dose RIT combined with standard or low-dose chemotherapy) and (2) a myeloablative approach (high-dose RIT combined with either standard or high-dose chemotherapy, HDC). The second approach usually requires HSCT to control myelotoxicity. Leonard et al. [179] demonstrated in their study that sequential standard-dose chemotherapy (fludarabine), when combined with low-dose ^{131}I-tositumomab in patients with previously untreated low-grade, transformed, or follicular NHL, results in increased efficacy with acceptable toxicity level as compared to fludarabine alone. None of the patients in this study showed a HAMA response, probably due to the prior administration of fludarabine, which suppresses the immune response. Future studies are being designed to evaluate the efficacy of concurrent administration of RIT and chemotherapy to exploit the potential radiosensitizing effect of chemotherapy.

The myeloablative approach was evaluated by Press et al. [180]. It was observed that sequential high-dose RIT (up to 2,500 cGy of 2.5 mg/kg ^{131}I-tositumomab) and HDC (60 mg/kg etoposide and 100 mg/kg cyclophosphamide) when administered in relapsed/refractory cases of B-cell NHL results in progression-free survival and overall survival in 73 % and 85 % of patients followed up to 2 years. The mortality rate in this group was 8 %, which was due to opportunistic infections and nonhematological toxicities; the data is similar to that observed with combination of HDC and total body irradiation (TBI). By this approach, it was possible to deliver a median tumor dose of 38 Gy with RIT as compared to only 12 Gy with TBI (this data was arrived at on the assumption that the median tumor-to-lung radiation-absorbed dose ratio was 1.5) [148]. Puronen CE et al. have shown that ^{90}Y-ibritumomab tiuxetan-based allografting is an option in patients with indolent histologies [181]. In follow-up of nearly 9 years, the graft versus lymphoma effect that resulted in the 5-year overall and progression-free survival for patients with indolent B-NHL was 40% and 27.5%, respectively. Authors concluded that improved strategies are needed for aggressive B-NHL.

34.4.1.18 Summary of RIT in B-Cell NHL

The following conclusions can be drawn from various trials on the use of RIT in NHL [34]:

1. RIT can achieve a significant and durable response in patients who relapse after chemotherapy/have bulky disease.
2. Even a low radiation dose can achieve an objective tumor response.
3. As compared to the nonmyeloablative dose, a myeloablative dose combined with autologous bone marrow or peripheral stem cell transplantation can result in overall response rates with significant longer duration of response.
4. Patients having low-tumor burden with low bone marrow involvement and without splenomegaly are better responders.

5. The combined approach of using RIT and chemotherapy may be more effective than any single modality.
6. RIT appears superior to unconjugated mAb in the therapy of patients with relapsed B-cell NHL.
7. Hypothyroidism, myelodysplasia, and possible secondary neoplasms are the expected long-term adverse effects of RIT.
8. Unconjugated antibodies may improve the biodistribution of radioimmunoconjugates.
9. The tumor dosimetry of mAbs conjugated with ^{90}Y appears superior to ^{131}I conjugated mAbs.

34.4.1.19 RIT in Other Hematological Malignancies

Efficacy of RIT in other hematological malignancies like cutaneous T-cell lymphoma, chronic lymphocytic leukemia (CLL), acute leukemia, and multiple myeloma have been documented in a few studies [34]. The most promising results have been documented in acute leukemia, in which RIT was shown to improve the outcome of bone marrow grafting by decreasing the relapse rate [182, 183]. In the study, ^{131}I-labeled anti-CD45 murine antibody (BC8) for RIT was combined with cyclophosphamide and 12 Gy total body irradiation as a bone marrow conditioning regimen. The disease-free survival significantly improved in AML/myelodysplastic syndrome or acute lymphoblastic leukemia [183]. Mention should be made of the use of ^{213}Bi, an alpha emitter with an LET of 8 MeV and a half-life of 45.6 min which was conjugated with humanized anti-CD33 antibody and used for treatment of leukemia [63]. The results, although in a very small group of patients, showed that alpha particle radioimmunoconjugates can deliver a several fold higher amount of radiation dose to the liver, spleen, and marrow as compared to beta particle radioimmunoconjugates.

34.4.2 RIT in Solid Tumors

The popularity achieved by RIT in the successful treatment of B-cell NHL encouraged clinical scientists to venture into and expand the field of RIT in solid tumors. However, the inherent radioresistant property of these tumors as well as the immunogenicity of murine proteins and relatively slow clearance of humanized intact immunoglobulins has meant that scientists have not had a major success as was achieved with NHL [34, 184]. At the same time, a better understanding of the methodology essential for delivering significant amounts of radioactivity to tumor has opened up new avenues for expanding the role of RIT in solid tumors [185]. The main tumor antigens against which the target antibodies (either chimeric or humanized form) have been used are CEA, TAG-72, MUC1, tenascin, and prostate-specific membrane antigen (PSMA). Along with the other factors which govern the outcome of treatment with radioimmunoconjugates, the main concern in RIT of solid tumor is to develop a radioimmunoconjugate which matches the heterogeneity of antigen expression of these tumors and also has a high penetration (Jhan war and Divgi 2005). The following sections will briefly cover some of the solid tumors for which RIT has achieved some sort of success in phase I/II dose escalation studies in which suboptimal doses were used. One of the major limitations in coming to a definite conclusion from these studies is that the majority of the studies were conducted on patients having advanced stage disease in which the prognosis was poor in any case [34].

34.4.2.1 Colon Cancer

In the past, colon cancer has been most commonly used as a model for use of RIT in solid tumors (Table 34.6). Carcinoembryonic antigen (CEA), which is expressed in a number of cancers, has been used for the localization of tumors using immunoscintigraphy [197]. RIT with ^{131}I-labeled murine and humanized anti-CEA antibodies in colorectal and other cancers has been performed (Fig. 34.1). A phase II study using humanized ^{131}I-labeled anti-CEA mAb (hMN-14) in patients with small volume metastasis refractory to treatment and patients who have had curative surgical resection of metachronous liver metastases has shown an overall response rate of 58 % with a mean duration response of 9 months in both

Table 34.6 RIT in colorectal cancer: representative phase I/II studies

Reference studies	No. of patients	Radioimmunoconjugate	Target	Isotype of mAb	Responses	Comments
Behr et al. [186–188]	12	^{131}I-MN-14	CEA	Humanized IgG1	2PR, 4 mixed/minimum response/SD, CEA reduction in 9	
	30	^{131}I-MN-14	CEA	Humanized IgG1	3PR, 8 mixed response	Adjuvant RIT in 9 patients after surgical removal of metastases
	57	^{131}I-NP4 (IMMU-4)	CEA	Murine F(ab′)z	1PR, 4 mixed/minor response and 7 stabilization disease after previously progressive disease	
Divgi et al. [189][a]	24	^{131}I-CC-49	TAG72	Murine IgG1	No response	
Juweid et al. [42]	13	^{131}I-NP4 (IMMU-4)	CEA	Murine F(ab′)z	7SD	
Meredith et al. [190–192]	12	^{131}I-B72.3	TAG72	Chimeric IgG4	3SD, 1 minimum response 4SD	
	14	^{131}I-COL-1 +	CEA/	Murine IgG1		Dual antibody combined with IFNa-2b
		^{131}I-CC49	TAG72			
	28	^{125}I-17 – 1A	Ep-CAM	Chimeric IgG2a	10SD	
Mittal et al. [193]	9	^{131}I-IMMU-4	CEA	Murine IgG1	1PR	Hyperthermia used
Welt et al. [194, 195]	21	^{125}I-A33	A33	Murine IgG2a	1 mixed response, 12SD	
	23	^{131}I-A33	A33	Murine IgG2a	3 mixed response	
Wong et al. [114]	21	^{90}Y-T84.66	CEA	Chimeric IgG 1	11 SD, 1 mixed response	
Ychou et al. [196]	10	^{131}I-F6	CEA	Murine F(ab′)z	1PR, 2SD, 6PD	

[a]Divgi CR, Scott AM, Dantis L, Capitelli P, Siler K, Hilton S, Finn RD, Kemeny N, Kelsen D, Kostakoglu L, et al. Phase I radioimmunotherapy trial with iodine-131-CC49 in metastatic colon carcinoma. J Nucl Med. 1995 Apr; 36(4):586-92

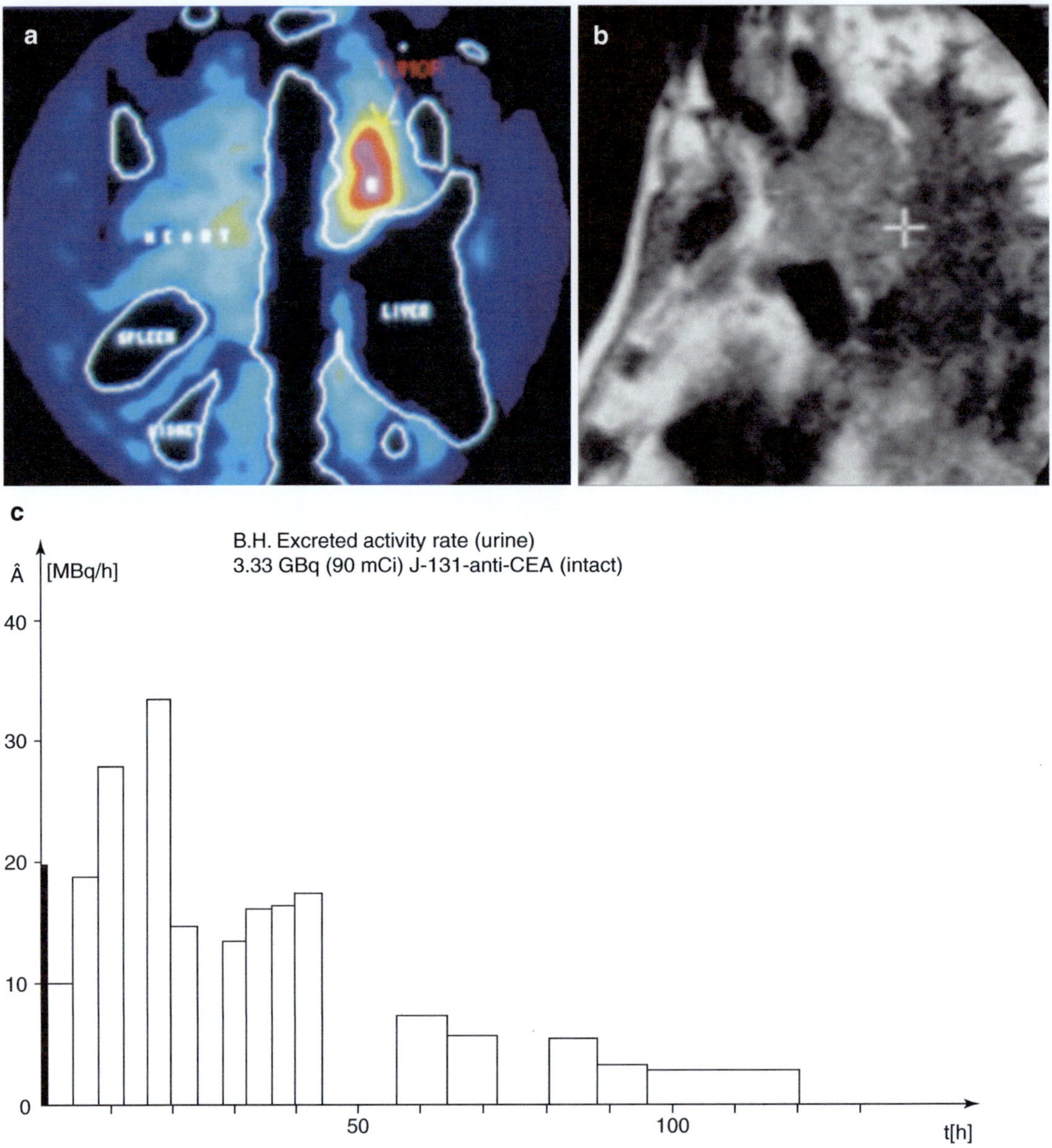

Fig. 34.1 Radioimmunotherapy using an intact anti-CEA antibody, labeled with I-131 (3.33 GBq, 90 mCi) in a patient with recurrent, irresectable squamous cell carcinoma of the lung. Serum CEA was strongly elevated (679 ng/ml). Posterior image of the thorax (**a**) using a double tracer isocontour technique (DTICT) after subtraction of a Tc-99mcolloid scan from the I-131 scan for outlining the anatomical structures (early image fusion technique); **b** MRI scan of the thorax outlining the infiltrating tumor; **c** excreted activity in urine (in MBq/h) over 4 days after therapy

groups [188]. The study, although meant to evaluate the efficacy of RIT in solid tumor, again proves that the present methodology of RIT is suitable for small volume disease rather than bulky disease. Another phase 1 study [114] conducted in patients with metastatic CEA-producing malignancies for evaluating the efficacy of ^{90}Y-anti-CEA chimeric T84.66 antibodies demonstrated that there was no response in these patients and that the toxicity of the radioimmunoconjugate was radionuclide-dependent. This observation has given an edge to the unconjugated antibodies as a separate treatment modality rather than the conjugated ones. However, contrary to this study, several earlier studies using ^{131}I-labeled CEA have documented a modest response [42, 186, 198].

Other radioimmunoconjugates like ^{131}I-anti-CEA/19-9 (Fig. 34.2), ^{131}I-anti-CA125 (Fig. 34.3), ^{131}I-CC49, ^{90}Y-CC49, and ^{131}I-A33 have been targeted without any objective response (Table 34.6). Intra-arterial administration of radiolabeled antibodies (Fig. 34.4) was tried but did not result in much greater success. Pretargeting strategies using streptavidin conjugates of the NR-LU-10 pancarcinoma antibody and ^{90}Y-biotin have shown only a modest response of 8 % along with

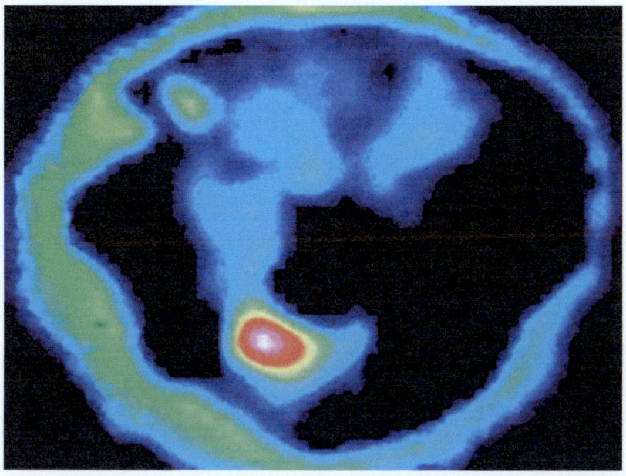

Fig. 34.2 First radioimmunotherapy using a cocktail of I-131-labeled anti-CEA/CA19-9 F(ab′)$_2$ antibodies (2.33 GBq, 63 mCi) in a 13-year-old girl with recurrent sigmoid carcinoma and peritoneal carcinosis (University Medical Center, Frankfurt/Main, Germany, July 1985). Transversal SPECT slice (DTICT) showing high uptake in an abdominal lesion. Tumor dosimetry/half-life: whole body 0.46 Gy/2.2 days; liver 2.9 Gy/ 2.2 days; tumor abdomen 14 Gy/2.3 days

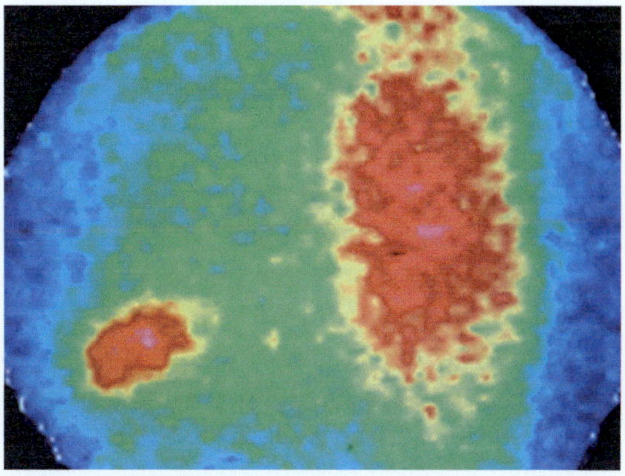

Fig. 34.3 Radioimmunotherapy using I-131-OC 125 F(ab′)$_2$ antibodies for treatment of a diffuse, infiltrating mucinous adenocarcinoma with lymphangiosis carcinomatosa of both lungs expressing the CA125 antigen (as shown by immunohistochemistry, serum CA125 800 U/ml) in a 39-year-old male. Planar posterior image of thorax/abdomen revealing significant uptake in the right hemithorax as well as uptake in the spleen (antibody complexation due to HAMA formation after the diagnostic study)

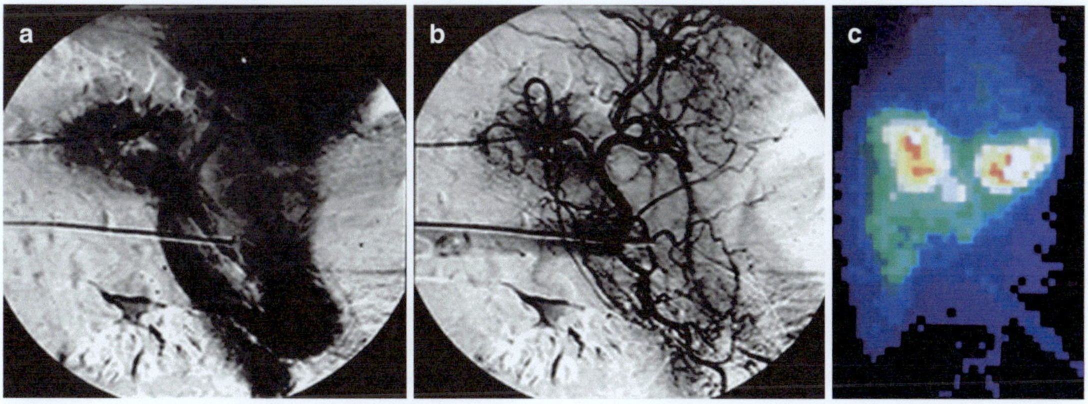

Fig. 34.4 Intra-arterial radioimmunotherapy (intact anti-CEA antibody injected together with DSM particles to slow down the blood flow) via the hepatic artery in a patient with colorectal liver metastases. Arterial (**a**) and late (**b**) phase of digital subtraction angiography (DSA) shows hyperperfused lesions in the right hepatic lobe; dynamic immunoscintigraphy (**c**) reveals high uptake in the CEA-positive metastases 2 min after starting the intra-arterial infusion

diarrhea as the grade IV nonhematological toxicity, the results being much inferior as to what was suggested by preclinical studies [96].

34.4.2.2 Prostate Cancer

The success of diagnostic markers in prostate cancer prompted scientists to target them for RIT. However, most of the radioimmunoconjugates used in the past, like ^{131}I-murine CC49 mAb and ^{90}Y-CYT-356 capromab pendetide antibody, have not shown significant response rates [152, 190, 199, 200]. PSMA, which is not a secreted antigen, has also been targeted for RIT of prostate cancer. ^{90}Y-labeled PSMA mAb 7E11/CY356 has demonstrated no therapeutic efficacy. The possible explanation for this failure is the targeting of the internal epitope of PSMA by this agent [201].

Tagawa et al. have used ^{177}Lu labeled-mAb J591, which targets the external domain of PSMA. Radioimmunotherapy was well tolerated with reversible myelosuppression [202]. The maximum tolerated dose of 70 mCi/m^2 resulted in longer overall survival of 21.8 months in patient showing more than 30% PSA decrease; however, grade 4 hematologic toxicity and platelet transfusions were also high.

To overcome the issue of early relapse after initial response and to find the optimal dose of RIT with J591, Tagawa et al. performed a phase I dose escalation trial in 49 patients using ^{177}Lu J591 (ClinicalTrials.gov Identifier NCT00538668). The authors found a significant dose-response relationship with more PSA declines and longer survival (87.5% PSA decline, 58.8% >30% decline, 29.4% >50% decline); lower intensity of PSMA expression was associated with poorer responses. Median OS was 43.9 months in patients who received the recommended phase II dose versus 15.3 months in patients who received lower doses [203]. In another study, the researchers also found that the combination of ^{177}Lu-J591 RIT with docetaxel (75 mg/m^2) is also feasible and relatively well tolerated with significant antitumor activity [204]. Overall, these trials demonstrated that RIT with ^{177}Lu J591 in mCRPC can successfully target metastatic disease in ~90% of patients, albeit with dose-limiting toxicities, particularly reversible myelosuppression [205].

34.4.2.3 Ovarian Cancer

The success story of RIT in ovarian cancer has been a bit different from that in other solid tumors. It has been documented that ^{90}Y-labeled MUC1 antibody when given intraperitoneally in patients with ovarian cancer stage IC–IV without any evidence of disease after debulking and platinum-based chemotherapy results in significant prolongation of duration of disease-free survival (80 % 5 year survival rate as compared to 55 % for nonrandomized chemotherapy controls without RIT) [206]. The same group has also demonstrated that this therapy is more effective when used in patients with tumor nodules less than 2 cm, and no response is observed when the tumors are larger [207]. The success of ^{186}Re-NR-LU-10 and ^{177}Lu-CC49 given intraperitoneally in patients having tumor nodules > 5 mm or micrometastatic disease supports the previous notion that RIT is mainly useful in nonbulky tumors [54, 55]. However, preliminary studies by Baum et al. (unpublished) using ^{188}Re-B43.13 antibody in patients with small volume recurrences of ovarian cancer (Fig. 34.5) did not show a significant improvement as compared to conventional chemotherapy. Although the development of HAMA is a potential limitation for RIT in ovarian carcinomas [208], in some of the studies [209–211], it has been documented that development of immune response to murine monoclonal antibody-B43.13 correlates well with the survival of patients with recurrent ovarian cancer; patients developing immune response had significantly prolonged survival compared to the ones not showing any immune response.

34.4.2.4 Brain and Other CNS Tumors

Brain and other CNS tumors have been treated successfully using locoregional RIT. ^{90}Y- and ^{131}I-labeled anti-tenascin antibodies have been used for this purpose [212]. These radioimmunoconjugates have been shown to significantly prolong the median survival for patients with glioblastoma when injected directly into the tumor bed after surgery. Among the two radionuclides, ^{90}Y has been shown to have better results in bulky disease with fewer radioprotection problems [34].

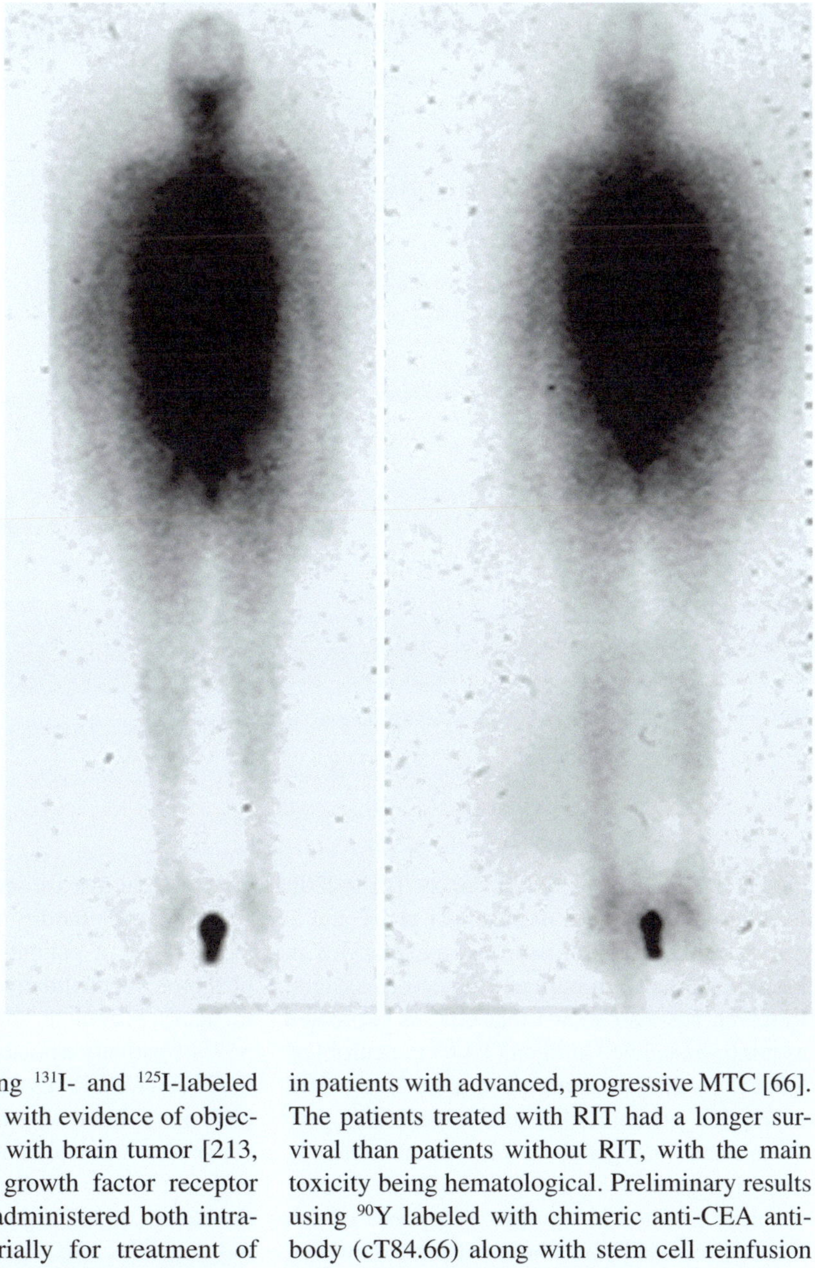

Fig. 34.5 First radioimmunotherapy (September 1997) using a Re-188 labeled anti-CA125 antibody for treatment of a patient with recurrent ovarian cancer [whole-body scan 24 h after therapy with 3.7 GBq (100 mCi) B43.13 antibody]

Intra-arterial RIT using ^{131}I- and ^{125}I-labeled antibodies has been used with evidence of objective response in patients with brain tumor [213, 214]. ^{125}I-antiepidermal growth factor receptor antibody 425 has been administered both intravenously and intra-arterially for treatment of patients with glioblastoma multiforme with similar results [213, 215]. Some other tumors which have been treated using locoregional injections are medulloblastoma and neuroblastoma [216].

Other solid tumors for which RIT is being employed are neuroblastoma (Fig. 34.6), renal cell carcinoma, breast cancer, urinary bladder carcinoma, and medullary thyroid cancer. A recent study has shown the efficacy of pretargeted RIT with bsmAb and ^{131}I-labeled bivalent hapten in patients with advanced, progressive MTC [66]. The patients treated with RIT had a longer survival than patients without RIT, with the main toxicity being hematological. Preliminary results using ^{90}Y labeled with chimeric anti-CEA antibody (cT84.66) along with stem cell reinfusion have shown promising evidence of antitumor activity in patients with breast cancer [217].

34.5 Novel Radioimmunotherapy Targeting Gangliosides

Disialoganglioside (GD2) is expressed in the fetus and hence is an oncofetal antigen. In addition GD is also found on several stem cells like neural,

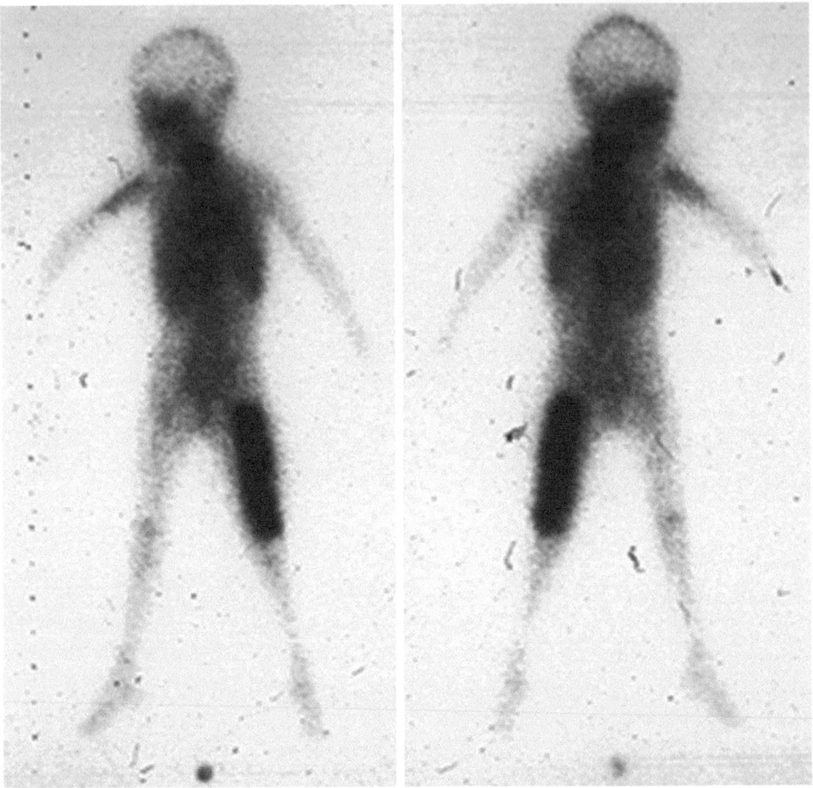

Fig. 34.6 First radioimmunotherapy (March 1994) of a 4-year-old child with metastatic neuroblastoma using 12 mg of the I-131-labeled (2.26 GBq, 61 mCi) chimeric anti-NCAM antibody ch14.18 antibody showing strong uptake in bone metastases in the left femur (whole-body anterior/posterior scan 8 days after therapy)

mesenchymal, and of breast cancer [218–220]. Its expression expands in postnatal phase and is detected on peripheral neurons, melanocytes in the skin, and also in our central nervous system. Research has also shown that GD2 is expressed as tumor-associated antigen (TAA) in neuroblastoma [221–223]. In contrast to other TAA, GD2 expression on neuroblastoma is generally very intense and homogeneous. Radioimmunotherapy with high-dose (6–8 mCi/kg) ^{131}I-3F8 given intravenously resulted in significant response of soft tissue lesions and bone marrow disease; however, the myeloablative dose (20 mCi/kg) did not lead to any significant improvement in overall survival [224, 225]. ^{131}I-3F8 combined with bevacizumab in phase 1 clinical trial (NCT00450827) did not lead to any significant response benefit in comparison to ^{131} I-3F8 alone. Despite its rather non-enthusiastic results through intravenous route of application, when applied intraventricularly (compartmental radioimmunotherapy, cRIT) in patients with brain metastases or leptomeningeal disease seems to be promising with acceptable tolerability in terms of toxicity [226, 227]. Even in patients with relapsed medulloblastoma, consolidative cRIT has been shown to achieve durable survival benefit in roughly 53% of patients who achieve complete remission (NCT00445965). Even more remarkable is that cRIT in children with relapsed medulloblastoma can lead to survival of at least 6 months in 89% of patients. Future research is going on to ascertain the benefit of RIT with 3F8 by using more potent radionuclides like alpha emitters and using better dosimetry protocols and better pretargeting methods [228].

34.6 Novel Dosimetry Method

A novel method for calculation of the appropriate dosage for radioimmunotherapy is using physiologically based pharmacokinetic modeling (PBPK). Kletting P et al. used two new

PBPK models considering fully, half, and non-immunoreactive antibodies and constraints for estimating the red marrow (RM) antigen number [229]. The authors fitted both models to gamma camera and serum measurements of 27 patients. For model averaging, Akaike weights were used. Total body, liver, spleen, RM, and serum time-integrated activity coefficients were calculated. Model-based predictions of the serum biokinetics during therapy were compared to actual measurements. They showed variability in the RM time activity coefficients suggesting need for patient-specific dosimetry. This new approach based on PBPK has the potential to perform individualized dosimetry, e.g., for radioimmunotherapy (RIT) with ^{90}Y-labeled anti-CD66 antibody which is used to selectively irradiate the red marrow (RM) prior to blood stem cell transplantation of acute leukemia patients.

34.7 Conclusions

In the recent past, immense interest has been generated in RIT because of the wide success of immunotherapy and targeted radionuclide therapy. However, success of RIT is primarily dependent on the delivery of adequate amount of radiolabeled monoclonal antibodies in a tumor lesion, especially if lesions are bulky. There are several techniques to deliver this dose to the target lesions with an optimal therapeutic index, e.g., using pretargeting (DOTA-PRIT), increasing the immunoreactivity of the antigen, using an appropriate radionuclide with adequate half-life and path length, selecting the route of administration, optimizing dosimetry, using novel chelators, etc. In future, it would be interesting to assess the clinical benefit of combinations of RIT with other therapies, e.g., in fractionated dose with chemotherapy and/or immunotherapy to maximize the cytotoxic effect of body's immune cells.

References

1. Sausville EA, Longo DL. Principles of cancer treatment: surgery, chemotherapy, and biologic therapy. In: Kasper DL, Braunwald E, Fauci AS, Hauser SL, Longo DL, Jameson JL, editors. Harrison's principles of internal medicine. 16th ed. New York: McGraw Hill; 2005. p. 464–82.
2. Pressman D, Keighley G. The zone of activities of antibodies as determined by the use of radioactive tracers; the zone of activity of nephrotoxic anti kidney serum. J Immunol. 1948;59:141–6.
3. Pressman D, Korngold L. The in vivo localisation of anti-Wagner-osteogenic-sarcoma antibodies. Cancer. 1953;6:619–23.
4. Pressman D, Day ED, Blau M. The use of paired labeling in the determination of tumor-localizing antibodies. Cancer Res. 1957;17:845–50.
5. Bale WF, Spar IL. Studies directed towards use of antibodies as carriers of radioactivity for therapy. Adv Biol Med Phys. 1957;5:285–356.
6. Kohler G, Milstein C. Continuous cultures of fused cells secreting antibody of predefined specificity. Nature. 1975;256:495–7.
7. Belitsky P, Ghose T, Aquino J, Norvell ST, Blair AH. Radionuclide imaging of primary renal-cell carcinoma by I-131-labeled antitumor antibody. J Nucl Med. 1978;19:427–30.
8. Day ED, Lassiter S, Woodhall B, Mahaley JL, Mahaley MS Jr. The localization of radioantibodies in human brain tumors. I. Preliminary exploration. Cancer Res. 1965;25:773–8.
9. Badger CC, Anasetti C, Davis J, Bernstein ID. Treatment of malignancy with unmodified antibody. Pathol Immunopathol Res. 1987;6:419–34.
10. Khazaeli MB, Conry RM, LoBuglio AF. Human immune response to monoclonal antibodies. J Immunother. 1994;15:42–52.
11. Lee J, Fenton BM, Koch CJ, Frelinger JG, Lord EM. Interleukin 2 expression by tumor cells alters both the immune response and the tumor microenvironment. Cancer Res. 1998;58:1478–85.
12. Feldhaus MJ, Siegel RW. Yeast display of antibody fragments: a discovery and characterization platform. J Immunol Methods. 2004;290:69–80.
13. Hoogenboom HR, Chames P. Natural and designer binding sites made by phage display technology. Immunol Today. 2000;21:371–8.
14. Irving RA, Coia G, Roberts A, Nuttall SD, Hudson PJ. Ribosome display and affinity maturation: from antibodies to single V-domains and steps towards cancer therapeutics. J Immunol Methods. 2001;248:31–45.
15. Lipovsek D, Pluckthun A. In-vitro protein evolution by ribosome display and mRNA display. J Immunol Methods. 2004;290:51–67.
16. Green LL, Hardy MC, Maynard-Currie CE, Tsuda H, Louie DM, Mendez MJ, Abderrahim H, Noguchi M, Smith DH, Zeng Y, et al. Antigen-specific human monoclonal antibodies from mice engineered with human Ig heavy and light chain YACs. Nat Genet. 1994;7:13–21.
17. Jain RK. Tumor physiology and antibody delivery. Front Radiat Ther Oncol. 1990;24:32–46. discussion 64–8
18. Lonberg N, Taylor LD, Harding FA, Trounstine M, Higgins KM, Schramm SR, Kuo CC, Mashayekh

R, Wymore K, McCabe JG, et al. Antigen-specific human antibodies from mice comprising four distinct genetic modifications. Nature. 1994;368:856–9.
19. Ruiz-Cabello F, Cabrera T, Lopez-Nevot MA, Garrido F. Impaired surface antigen presentation in tumors: implications for T cell-based immunotherapy. Semin Cancer Biol. 2002;12:15–24.
20. Saga T, Neumann RD, Heya T, Sato J, Kinuya S, Le N, Paik CH, Weinstein JN. Targeting cancer micrometastases with monoclonal antibodies: a binding-site barrier. Proc Natl Acad Sci U S A. 1995;92:8999–9003.
21. Wu AM, Senter PD. Arming antibodies: prospects and challenges for immunoconjugates. Nat Biotechnol. 2005;23:1137–46.
22. Dixon KL. The radiation biology of radioimmunotherapy. Nucl Med Commun. 2003;24:951–7.
23. Baum RP, Lorenz M, Senekowitsch R, Albrecht M, Hor G. Clinical results of immunoscintigraphy and radioimmunotherapy. Nuklearmedizin. 1987;26:68–78.
24. Perkins AC, Baum RP. Immunoscintigraphy and immunotherapy 1988. Report of the 3rd IRIST Meeting, Frankfurt/Main, March 1988. Int J Biol Markers. 1988;3:265–72.
25. Beierwaltes WH. Radioiodine-labelled compounds previously or currently used for tumour localisation. In: Proceedings of an Advisory Group Meeting on Tumour Localisation with Radioactive Agents. Austria: Panel Proceedings Series. International Atomic Energy Agency Vienna; 1974. p. 47–56.
26. Borghaei H, Schilder RJ. Safety and efficacy of radioimmunotherapy with yttrium 90 ibritumomab tiuxetan (Zevalin). Semin Nucl Med. 2004;34:4–9.
27. Wahl RL. Tositumomab and (131) therapy in non-Hodgkins lymphoma. J Nucl Med. 2005;46(Suppl):128s–40s.
28. Goldenberg DM, DeLand F, Kim E, Bennett S, Primus FJ, van Nagell JR, Jr EN, DeSimone P, Rayburn P. Use of radiolabeled antibodies to carcinoembryonic antigen for the detection and localization of diverse cancers by external photoscanning. N Engl J Med. 1978;298:1384–6.
29. Order SE, Stillwagon GB, Klein JL, Leichner PK, Siegelman SS, Fishman EK, Ettinger DS, Haulk T, Kopher K, Finney K, et al. Iodine 131 antiferritin, a new treatment modality in hepatoma: a Radiation Therapy Oncology Group study. J Clin Oncol. 1985;3:1573–82.
30. Order SE, Sleeper AM, Stillwagon GB, Klein JL, Leichner PK. Current status of radioimmunoglobulins in the treatment of human malignancy. Oncology (Williston Park). 1989;3:115–20; discussion 122, 129–30.
31. Order S, Pajak T, Leibel S, Asbell S, Leichner P, Ettinger D, Stillwagon G, Herpst J, Haulk T, Kopher K, et al. A randomized prospective trial comparing full dose chemotherapy to 131I antiferritin: an RTOG study. Int J Radiat Oncol Biol Phys. 1991;20:953–63.
32. Primus FJ, Goldenberg DM. Immunological considerations in the use of goat antibodies to carcinoembryonic antigen for the radioimmunodetection of cancer. Cancer Res. 1980;40:2979–83.
33. Vriesendorp HM, Quadri SM, Wyllie CT, Lai J, Borchardt PE, Harris L, Wucher R, Askew E, Schweichler L. Fractionated radiolabeled antiferritin therapy for patients with recurrent Hodgkin's disease. Clin Cancer Res. 1999;5:3324s–9s.
34. Goldenberg DM. Targeted therapy of cancer with radiolabeled antibodies. J Nucl Med. 2002;43:693–713.
35. Baum RP. At the crossroads: from cancer imaging and therapy using radiolabeled monoclonal antibodies to metabolic tumour imaging with positron emission tomography (PET). Ind J Nucl Med. 1999:51–66.
36. Behr TM, Goldenberg DM. Improved prospects for cancer therapy with radiolabeled antibody fragments and peptides? J Nucl Med. 1996;37:834–6.
37. Behr TM, Blumenthal RD, Memtsoudis S, Sharkey RM, Gratz S, Becker W, Goldenberg DM. Cure of metastatic human colonic cancer in mice with radiolabeled monoclonal antibody fragments. Clin Cancer Res. 2000;6:4900–7.
38. Buchegger F, Pfister C, Fournier K, Prevel F, Schreyer M, Carrel S, Mach JP. Ablation of human colon carcinoma in nude mice by 131I-labeled monoclonal anti-carcinoembryonic antigen antibody F(ab′)2 fragments. J Clin Invest. 1989;83:1449–56.
39. Buchegger F, Pelegrin A, Delaloye B, Bischof-Delaloye A, Mach JP. Iodine-131-labeled MAb F(ab′)2 fragments are more efficient and less toxic than intact anti-CEA antibodies in radioimmunotherapy of large human colon carcinoma grafted in nude mice. J Nucl Med. 1990;31:1035–44.
40. Buchegger F, Mach JP, Folli S, Delaloye B, Bischof-Delaloye A, Pelegrin A. Higher efficiency of 131I-labeled anti-carcinoembryonic antigen-monoclonal antibody F(ab′)2 as compared to intact antibodies in radioimmunotherapy of established human colon carcinoma grafted in nude mice. Recent Res Cancer Res. 1996;141:19–35.
41. Buchegger F, Allal AS, Roth A, Papazyan JP, Dupertuis Y, Mirimanoff RO, Gillet M, Pelegrin A, Mach JP, Slosman DO. Combined radioimmunotherapy and radiotherapy of liver metastases from colorectal cancer: a feasibility study. Anticancer Res. 2000;20:1889–96.
42. Juweid ME, Sharkey RM, Behr T, Swayne LC, Dunn R, Siegel J, Goldenberg DM. Radioimmunotherapy of patients with small-volume tumors using iodine-131-labeled anti-CEA monoclonal antibody NP-4 F(ab′)2. J Nucl Med. 1996;37:1504–10.
43. Larson SM, Carrasquillo JA, Krohn KA, Brown JP, McGuffin RW, Ferens JM, Graham MM, Hill LD, Beaumier PL, Hellstrom KE, et al. Localization of 131I-labeled p97-specific Fab fragments in human melanoma as a basis for radiotherapy. J Clin Invest. 1983;72:2101–14.
44. Larson SM, Carrasquillo JA, McGuffin RW, Krohn KA, Ferens JM, Hill LD, Beaumier PL, Reynolds JC, Hellstrom KE, Hellstrom I. Use of I-131 labeled,

murine Fab against a high molecular weight antigen of human melanoma: preliminary experience. Radiology. 1985;155:487–92.
45. Milenic DE. Radioimmunotherapy: designer molecules to potentiate effective therapy. Semin Radiat Oncol. 2000;10:139–55.
46. Smith-Jones PM, Solit DB, Akhurst T, Afroze F, Rosen N, Larson SM. Imaging the pharmacodynamics of HER2 degradation in response to Hsp90 inhibitors. Nat Biotechnol. 2004;22:701–6.
47. Santimaria M, Moscatelli G, Viale GL, Giovannoni L, Neri G, Viti F, Leprini A, Borsi L, Castellani P, Zardi L, Neri D, Riva P. Immunoscintigraphic detection of the ED-B domain of fibronectin, a marker of angiogenesis, in patients with cancer. Clin Cancer Res. 2003;9:571–9.
48. McQuarrie SA, Baum RP, Golberg L, Niesen A, Golberg K, Noujaim AA, McEwan AJ. A pharmacokinetic comparison of murine and chimeric forms of the 99mTc-labelled 174H.64 monoclonal antibody. J Nucl Biol Med. 1994;38:140–4.
49. Meredith RF, Khazaeli MB, Plott WE, et al. Effect of human immune response on repeat course of 131I-chimeric b72.3 antibody therapy. Antibody Immunoconj Radiopharm. 1993;6:39–46.
50. Adams GP, Weiner LM. Monoclonal antibody therapy of cancer. Nature Biotechnol. 2005;23:1147–57.
51. Alvarez RD, Partridge EE, Khazaeli MB, Plott G, Austin M, Kilgore L, Russell CD, Liu T, Grizzle WE, Schlom J, LoBuglio AF, Meredith RF. Intraperitoneal radioimmunotherapy of ovarian cancer with 177Lu-CC49: a phase I/II study. Gynecol Oncol. 1997;65:94–101.
52. DeNardo GL, Kukis DL, Shen S, DeNardo DA, Meares CF, DeNardo SJ. 67Cu-versus 131I-labeled Lym-1 antibody: comparative pharmacokinetics and dosimetry in patients with non-Hodgkin's lymphoma. Clin Cancer Res. 1999;5:533–41.
53. Hughes OD, Bishop MC, Perkins AC, Wastie ML, Denton G, Price MR, Frier M, Denley H, Rutherford R, Schubiger PA. Targeting superficial bladder cancer by the intravesical administration of copper-67-labeled anti-MUC1 mucin monoclonal antibody C595. J Clin Oncol. 2000;18:363–70.
54. Jacobs AJ, Fer M, Su FM, Breitz H, Thompson J, Goodgold H, Cain J, Heaps J, Weiden P. A phase I trial of a rhenium 186-labeled monoclonal antibody administered intraperitoneally in ovarian carcinoma: toxicity and clinical response. Obstet Gynecol. 1993;82:586–93.
55. Meredith RF, Partridge EE, Alvarez RD, Khazaeli MB, Plott G, Russell CD, Wheeler RH, Liu T, Grizzle WE, Schlom J, LoBuglio AF. Intraperitoneal radioimmunotherapy of ovarian cancer with lutetium-177-CC49. J Nucl Med. 1996;37:1491–6.
56. Seitz U, Neumaier B, Glatting G, Kotzerke J, Bunjes D, Reske SN. Preparation and evaluation of the rhenium-188-labelled anti-NCA antigen monoclonal antibody BW 250/183 for radioimmunotherapy of leukaemia. Eur J Nucl Med. 1999;26:1265–73.
57. Siegel JA. Revised Nuclear Regulatory Commission regulations for release of patients administered radioactive materials: outpatient iodine-131 anti-B1 therapy. J Nucl Med. 1998;39:28S–33S.
58. Govindan SV, Shih LB, Goldenberg DM, Sharkey RM, Karacay H, Donnelly JE, Losman MJ, Hansen HJ, Griffiths GL. 90Yttrium-labeled complementarity-determining-region-grafted monoclonal antibodies for radioimmunotherapy: radiolabeling and animal biodistribution studies. Bioconjug Chem. 1998;9:773–82.
59. Baum RP (Handbook Editor). Therapeutic nuclear medicine. Berlin: Springer; 2014. eBook ISBN: 978-3-540-36719-2; https://doi.org/10.1007/978-3-540-36719-2; Hardcover ISBN: 978-3-540-36718-5 (951 pages).
60. Baum RP, Kulkarni HR, Schuchardt C, Singh A, Wirtz M, Wiessalla S, Schottelius M, Mueller D, Klette I, Wester HJ. Lu-177 labeled prostate-specific membrane antigen radioligand therapy of metastatic castration-resistant prostate cancer: safety and efficacy. J Nucl Med. 2016;57:1006–13.
61. Emmett L, Willowson K, Violet J, Shin J, Blanks A, Lee J. Lutetium 177 PSMA radionuclide therapy for men with prostate cancer: a review of the current literature and discussion of practical aspects of therapy. J Med Radiat Sci. 2017;64:52–60.
62. McDevitt MR, Sgouros G, Finn RD, Humm JL, Jurcic JG, Larson SM, Scheinberg DA. Radioimmunotherapy with alpha-emitting nuclides. Eur J Nucl Med. 1998;25:1341–51.
63. Sgouros G, Ballangrud AM, Jurcic JG, McDevitt MR, Humm JL, Erdi YE, Mehta BM, Finn RD, Larson SM, Scheinberg DA. Pharmacokinetics and dosimetry of an alpha-particle emitter labeled antibody: 213Bi-HuM195 (anti-CD33) in patients with leukemia. J Nucl Med. 1999;40:1935–46.
64. Aurlien E, Larsen RH, Kvalheim G, Bruland OS. Demonstration of highly specific toxicity of the alpha-emitting radioimmunoconjugate^{211}At-rituximab against non-Hodgkin's lymphoma cells. Br J Cancer. 2000;83:1375–9.
65. Zalutsky MR, Vaidyanathan G. Astatine-211-labeled radiotherapeutics: an emerging approach to targeted alpha-particle radiotherapy. Curr Pharm Des. 2000;6:1433–55.
66. Goldenberg DM, Sharkey RM, Paganelli G, Barbet J, Chatal JF. Antibody pretargeting advances cancer radioimmunodetection and radioimmunotherapy. J Clin Oncol. 2006;24:823–34.
67. Boerman OC, van Schaijk FG, Oyen WJ, Corstens FH. Pretargeted radioimmunotherapy of cancer: progress step by step. J Nucl Med. 2003;44:400–11.
68. Chang CH, Sharkey RM, Rossi EA, Karacay H, McBride W, Hansen HJ, Chatal JF, Barbet J, Goldenberg DM. Molecular advances in pretargeting radioimmunotherapy with bispecific antibodies. Mol Cancer Ther. 2002;1:553–63.
69. Goodwin DA, Meares CF. Advances in pretargeting biotechnology. Biotechnol Adv. 2001;19:435–50.

70. Axworthy DB, Reno JM, Hylarides MD, Mallett RW, Theodore LJ, Gustavson LM, Su F, Hobson LJ, Beaumier PL, Fritzberg AR. Cure of human carcinoma xenografts by a single dose of pretargeted yttrium-90 with negligible toxicity. Proc Natl Acad Sci U S A. 2000;97:1802–7.
71. Sharkey RM, Karacay H, Richel H, McBride WJ, Rossi EA, Chang K, Yeldell D, Griffiths GL, Hansen HJ, Goldenberg DM. Optimizing bispecific antibody pretargeting for use in radioimmunotherapy. Clin Cancer Res. 2003;9:3897S–913S.
72. Le Doussal JM, Martin M, Gautherot E, Delaage M, Barbet J. In vitro and in vivo targeting of radiolabeled monovalent and divalent haptens with dual specificity monoclonal antibody conjugates: enhanced divalent hapten affinity for cell-bound antibody conjugate. J Nucl Med. 1989;30:1358–66.
73. Axworthy DB, Fritzberg AR, Hylarides MD, et al. Preclinical evaluation of anti-tumor monoclonal antibody/streptavidin conjugate for pretargeted 90Y radioimmunotherapy in a mouse xenograft model. J Immunother. 1994;16:158.
74. Moro M, Pelagi M, Fulci G, Paganelli G, Dellabona P, Casorati G, Siccardi AG, Corti A. Tumor cell targeting with antibody-avidin complexes and biotinylated tumor necrosis factor alpha. Cancer Res. 1997;57:1922–8.
75. Waldmann TA. Immunotherapy: past, present and future. Nat Med. 2003;9:269–77.
76. Casadevall A. Antibody-based therapies as anti-infective agents. Expert Opin Investig Drugs. 1998;7:307–21.
77. Chinol M, De Cobelli O, Trifiro G, Scardino E, Bartolomei M, Verweij F, Papi S, Matei DV, Paganelli G. Localization of avidin in superficial bladder cancer: a potentially new approach for radionuclide therapy. Eur Urol. 2003;44:556–9.
78. Paganelli G, Pervez S, Siccardi AG, Rowlinson G, Deleide G, Chiolerio F, Malcovati M, Scassellati GA, Epenetos AA. Intraperitoneal radio-localization of tumors pre-targeted by biotinylated monoclonal antibodies. Int J Cancer. 1990;45:1184–9.
79. Paganelli G, Magnani P, Zito F, Villa E, Sudati F, Lopalco L, Rossetti C, Malcovati M, Chiolerio F, Seccamani E, et al. Three-step monoclonal antibody tumor targeting in carcinoembryonic antigen-positive patients. Cancer Res. 1991;51:5960–6.
80. Saga T, Weinstein JN, Jeong JM, Heya T, Lee JT, Le N, Paik CH, Sung C, Neumann RD. Two-step targeting of experimental lung metastases with biotinylated antibody and radiolabeled streptavidin. Cancer Res. 1994;54:2160–5.
81. Yao Z, Zhang M, Kobayashi H, Sakahara H, Nakada H, Yamashina I, Konishi J. Improved targeting of radiolabeled streptavidin in tumors pretargeted with biotinylated monoclonal antibodies through an avidin chase. J Nucl Med. 1995;36:837–41.
82. He J, Liu G, Gupta S, Zhang Y, Rusckowski M, Hnatowich DJ. Amplification targeting: a modified pretargeting approach with potential for signal amplification – proof of a concept. J Nucl Med. 2004;45:1087–95.
83. Hnatowich DJ, Virzi F, Rusckowski M. Investigations of avidin and biotin for imaging applications. J Nucl Med. 1987;28:1294–302.
84. Chauhan J, Dakshinamurti K. Purification and characterization of human serum biotinidase. J Biol Chem. 1986;261:4268–75.
85. Goodwin DA, Meares CF, Osen M. Biological properties of biotin-chelate conjugates for pretargeted diagnosis and therapy with the avidin/biotin system. J Nucl Med. 1998;39:1813–8.
86. Karacay H, Sharkey RM, Govindan SV, McBride WJ, Goldenberg DM, Hansen HJ, Griffiths GL. Development of a streptavidin-anti-carcinoembryonic antigen antibody, radiolabeled biotin pretargeting method for radioimmunotherapy of colorectal cancer. Reagent development. Bioconjug Chem. 1997;8:585–94.
87. Sabatino G, Chinol M, Paganelli G, Papi S, Chelli M, Leone G, Papini AM, De Luca A, Ginanneschi M. A new biotin derivative-DOTA conjugate as a candidate for pretargeted diagnosis and therapy of tumors. J Med Chem. 2003;46:3170–3.
88. Barbet J, Peltier P, Bardet S, Vuillez JP, Bachelot I, Denet S, Olivier P, Leccia F, Corcuff B, Huglo D, Proye C, Rouvier E, Meyer P, Chatal JF. Radioimmunodetection of medullary thyroid carcinoma using indium-111 bivalent hapten and anti-CEA x anti-DTPA-indium bispecific antibody. J Nucl Med. 1998;39:1172–8.
89. Bardies M, Bardet S, Faivre-Chauvet A, Peltier P, Douillard JY, Mahe M, Fiche M, Lisbona A, Giacalone F, Meyer P, Gautherot E, Rouvier E, Barbet J, Chatal JF. Bispecific antibody and iodine-131-labeled bivalent hapten dosimetry in patients with medullary thyroid or small-cell lung cancer. J Nucl Med. 1996;37:1853–9.
90. Breitz HB, Fisher DR, Wessels BW. Marrow toxicity and radiation absorbed dose estimates from rhenium-186-labeled monoclonal antibody. J Nucl Med. 1998;39:1746–51.
91. Breitz HB, Fisher DR, Goris ML, Knox S, Ratliff B, Murtha AD, Weiden PL. Radiation absorbed dose estimation for 90Y-DOTA-biotin with pretargeted NR-LU-10/streptavidin. Cancer Biother Radiopharm. 1999;14:381–95.
92. Chetanneau A, Barbet J, Peltier P, Le Doussal JM, Gruaz-Guyon A, Bernard AM, Resche I, Rouvier E, Bourguet P, Delaage M, et al. Pretargeted imaging of colorectal cancer recurrences using an 111In-labelled bivalent hapten and a bispecific antibody conjugate. Nucl Med Commun. 1994;15: 972–80.
93. Cremonesi M, Ferrari M, Chinol M, Stabin MG, Grana C, Prisco G, Robertson C, Tosi G, Paganelli G. Three-step radioimmunotherapy with yttrium-90 biotin: dosimetry and pharmacokinetics in cancer patients. Eur J Nucl Med. 1999;26: 110–20.
94. Gruaz-Guyon A, Janevik-Ivanovska E, Raguin O, De Labriolle-Vaylet C, Barbet J. Radiolabeled bivalent haptens for tumor immunodetection and radioimmunotherapy. Q J Nucl Med. 2001;45:201–6.

95. Kalofonos HP, Rusckowski M, Siebecker DA, Sivolapenko GB, Snook D, Lavender JP, Epenetos AA, Hnatowich DJ. Imaging of tumor in patients with indium-111-labeled biotin and streptavidin-conjugated antibodies: preliminary communication. J Nucl Med. 1990;31:1791–6.
96. Knox SJ, Goris ML, Tempero M, Weiden PL, Gentner L, Breitz H, Adams GP, Axworthy D, Gaffigan S, Bryan K, Fisher DR, Colcher D, Horak ID, Weiner LM. Phase II trial of yttrium-90-DOTA-biotin pretargeted by NR-LU-10 antibody/streptavidin in patients with metastatic colon cancer. Clin Cancer Res. 2000;6:406–14.
97. Kraeber-Bodere F, Bardet S, Hoefnagel CA, Vieira MR, Vuillez JP, Murat A, Ferreira TC, Bardies M, Ferrer L, Resche I, Gautherot E, Rouvier E, Barbet J, Chatal JF. Radioimmunotherapy in medullary thyroid cancer using bispecific antibody and iodine 131-labeled bivalent hapten: preliminary results of a phase I/II clinical trial. Clin Cancer Res. 1999;5:3190s–8s.
98. Le Doussal JM, Chetanneau A, Gruaz-Guyon A, Martin M, Gautherot E, Lehur PA, Chatal JF, Delaage M, Barbet J. Bispecific monoclonal antibody-mediated targeting of an indium-111-labeled DTPA dimer to primary colorectal tumors: pharmacokinetics, biodistribution, scintigraphy and immune response. J Nucl Med. 1993;34:1662–71.
99. Magnani P, Paganelli G, Modorati G, Zito F, Songini C, Sudati F, Koch P, Maecke HR, Brancato R, Siccardi AG, Fazio F. Quantitative comparison of direct antibody labeling and tumor pretargeting in uveal melanoma. J Nucl Med. 1996;37:967–71.
100. Paganelli G, Grana C, Chinol M, Cremonesi M, De Cicco C, De Braud F, Robertson C, Zurrida S, Casadio C, Zoboli S, Siccardi AG, Veronesi U. Antibody-guided three-step therapy for high grade glioma with yttrium-90 biotin. Eur J Nucl Med. 1999;26:348–57.
101. Shen S, Forero A, LoBuglio AF, Breitz H, Khazaeli MB, Fisher DR, Wang W, Meredith RF. Patient-specific dosimetry of pretargeted radioimmunotherapy using CC49 fusion protein in patients with gastrointestinal malignancies. J Nucl Med. 2005;46:642–51.
102. Stickney DR, Anderson LD, Slater JB, Ahlem CN, Kirk GA, Schweighardt SA, Frincke JM. Bifunctional antibody: a binary radiopharmaceutical delivery system for imaging colorectal carcinoma. Cancer Res. 1991;51:6650–5.
103. Vuillez JP, Moro D, Brichon PY, Rouvier E, Brambilla E, Barbet J, Peltier P, Meyer P, Sarrazin R, Brambilla C. Two-step immunoscintigraphy for non-small-cell lung cancer staging using a bispecific anti-CEA/anti-indium-DTPA antibody and an indium-111-labeled DTPA dimer. J Nucl Med. 1997;38:507–11.
104. Vuillez JP, Kraeber-Bodere F, Moro D, Bardies M, Douillard JY, Gautherot E, Rouvier E, Barbet J, Garban F, Moreau P, Chatal JF. Radioimmunotherapy of small cell lung carcinoma with the two-step method using a bispecific anti-carcinoembryonic antigen/anti-diethylenetriaminepentaacetic acid (DTPA) antibody and iodine-131 Di-DTPA hapten: results of a phase I/II trial. Clin Cancer Res. 1999;5:3259s–67s.
105. Breitz HB, Weiden PL, Beaumier PL, Axworthy DB, Seiler C, Su FM, Graves S, Bryan K, Reno JM. Clinical optimization of pretargeted radioimmunotherapy with antibody-streptavidin conjugate and 90Y-DOTA-biotin. J Nucl Med. 2000;41:131–40.
106. Kraeber-Bodere F, Faivre-Chauvet A, Ferrer L, Vuillez JP, Brard PY, Rousseau C, Resche I, Devillers A, Laffont S, Bardies M, Chang K, Sharkey RM, Goldenberg DM, Chatal JF, Barbet J. Pharmacokinetics and dosimetry studies for optimization of anti-carcinoembryonic antigen x anti-hapten bispecific antibody-mediated pretargeting of iodine-131-labeled hapten in a phase I radioimmunotherapy trial. Clin Cancer Res. 2003;9:3973S–81S.
107. Cheal SM, Fung EK, Patel M, Xu H, Guo HF, Zanzonico PB, Wittrup KD MS, Cheung NV, Larson SM. Curative Multicycle Radioimmunotherapy Monitored by Quantitative SPECT/CT-Based Theranostics, Using Bispecific Antibody Pretargeting Strategy in Colorectal Cancer. J Nucl Med. 2017;58(11):1735–42. https://doi.org/10.2967/jnumed.117.193250.
108. Cheal SM, Xu H, Guo HF, Zanzonico PB, Larson SM, Cheung NK. Preclinical evaluation of multi-step targeting of disialoganglioside GD2 using an IgG-scFv bispecific antibody with high affinity for GD2 and DOTA metal complex. Mol Cancer Ther. 2014;13(7):1803–12. https://doi.org/10.1158/1535-7163.MCT-13-0933.
109. Cheal SM, Xu H, Guo HF, Patel M, Punzalan B, Fung EK, Lee SG, Bell M, Singh M, Jungbluth AA, Zanzonico PB, Piersigilli A, Larson SM, Cheung NV. Theranostic pretargeted radioimmunotherapy of internalizing solid tumor antigens in human tumor xenografts in mice: Curative treatment of HER2-positive breast carcinoma. Theranostics. 2018;8(18):5106–25. https://doi.org/10.7150/thno.26585.
110. Green DJ, Frayo SL, Lin Y, Hamlin DK, Fisher DR, Frost SH, Kenoyer AL, Hylarides MD, Gopal AK, Gooley TA, Orozco JJ, Till BG, O'Steen S, Orcutt KD, Wilbur DS, Wittrup KD, Press OW. Comparative analysis of bispecific antibody and streptavidin-targeted radioimmunotherapy for b-cell cancers. Cancer Res. 2016;76(22):6669–79. https://doi.org/10.1158/0008-5472.CAN-16-0571.
111. Press OW, Unger JM, Braziel RM, Maloney DG, Miller TP, LeBlanc M, Gaynor ER, Rivkin SE, Fisher RI. A phase 2 trial of CHOP chemotherapy followed by tositumomab/iodine I 131 tositumomab for previously untreated follicular non-Hodgkin lymphoma: Southwest Oncology Group Protocol S9911. Blood. 2003;102:1606–12.
112. Vose JM, Bierman PJ, Enke C, Hankins J, Bociek G, Lynch JC, Armitage JO. Phase I trial of iodine-131 tositumomab with high-dose chemotherapy and autologous stem-cell transplantation for

relapsed non-Hodgkin's lymphoma. J Clin Oncol. 2005;23:461–7.
113. Winter JN. Combining yttrium 90-labeled ibritumomab tiuxetan with high-dose chemotherapy and stem cell support in patients with relapsed non-Hodgkin's lymphoma. Clin Lymphoma. 2004;5(Suppl 1):S22–6.
114. Wong JY, Shibata S, Williams LE, Kwok CS, Liu A, Chu DZ, Yamauchi DM, Wilczynski S, Ikle DN, Wu AM, Yazaki PJ, Shively JE, Doroshow JH, Raubitschek AA. A Phase I trial of 90Y-anti-carcinoembryonic antigen chimeric T84.66 radioimmunotherapy with 5-fluorouracil in patients with metastatic colorectal cancer. Clin Cancer Res. 2003;9:5842–52.
115. O'Donoghue JA, Bardies M, Wheldon TE. Relationships between tumor size and curability for uniformly targeted therapy with beta-emitting radionuclides. J Nucl Med. 1995;36:1902–9.
116. DeNardo GL, Juweid ME, White CA, Wiseman GA, DeNardo SJ. Role of radiation dosimetry in radioimmunotherapy planning and treatment dosing. Crit Rev Oncol Hematol. 2001;39:203–18.
117. Juweid M, Sharkey RM, Goldenberg DM. Radioimmunotherapy of non-Hodgkins lymphoma with non-myeloablative doses of radiolabeled monoclonal antibodies. Philadelphia: Harwood Academic; 1999.
118. Cheson BD. Some like it hot! J Clin Oncol. 2001;19:3908–11.
119. DeNardo SJ, DeNardo GL, O'Grady LF, Macey DJ, Mills SL, Epstein AL, Peng JS, McGahan JP. Treatment of a patient with B cell lymphoma by I-131 LYM-1 monoclonal antibodies. Int J Biol Markers. 1987;2:49–53.
120. DeNardo GL, Lewis JP, DeNardo SJ, O'Grady LF. Effect of Lym-1 radioimmunoconjugate on refractory chronic lymphocytic leukemia. Cancer. 1994;73:1425–32.
121. DeNardo GL, DeNardo SJ, Goldstein DS, Kroger LA, Lamborn KR, Levy NB, McGahan JP, Salako Q, Shen S, Lewis JP. Maximum-tolerated dose, toxicity, and efficacy of (131)I-Lym-1 antibody for fractionated radioimmunotherapy of non-Hodgkin's lymphoma. J Clin Oncol. 1998;16:3246–56.
122. Gelman R, Gelber R, Henderson IC, Coleman CN, Harris JR. Improved methodology for analyzing local and distant recurrence. J Clin Oncol. 1990;8:548–55.
123. Juweid M, Sharkey RM, Markowitz A, Behr T, Swayne LC, Dunn R, Hansen HJ, Shevitz J, Leung SO, Rubin AD, et al. Treatment of non-Hodgkin's lymphoma with radiolabeled murine, chimeric, or humanized LL2, an anti-CD22 monoclonal antibody. Cancer Res. 1995;55:5899s–907s.
124. Juweid ME, Stadtmauer E, Hajjar G, Sharkey RM, Suleiman S, Luger S, Swayne LC, Alavi A, Goldenberg DM. Pharmacokinetics, dosimetry, and initial therapeutic results with 131I- and (111) In-/90Y-labeled humanized LL2 anti-CD22 monoclonal antibody in patients with relapsed, refractory non-Hodgkin's lymphoma. Clin Cancer Res. 1999;5:3292s–303s.
125. Kaminski MS, Fig LM, Zasadny KR, Koral KF, Del Rosario RB, Francis IR, Hanson CA, Normolle DP, Mudgett E, Liu CP, et al. Imaging, dosimetry, and radioimmunotherapy with iodine 131-labeled anti-CD37 antibody in B-cell lymphoma. J Clin Oncol. 1992;10:1696–711.
126. Kaminski MS, Zasadny KR, Francis IR, Fenner MC, Ross CW, Milik AW, Estes J, Tuck M, Regan D, Fisher S, Glenn SD, Wahl RL. Iodine-131-anti-B1 radioimmunotherapy for B-cell lymphoma. J Clin Oncol. 1996;14:1974–81.
127. Kaminski MS, Estes J, Zasadny KR, Francis IR, Ross CW, Tuck M, Regan D, Fisher S, Gutierrez J, Kroll S, Stagg R, Tidmarsh G, Wahl RL. Radioimmunotherapy with iodine (131)I tositumomab for relapsed or refractory B-cell non-Hodgkin lymphoma: updated results and long-term follow-up of the University of Michigan experience. Blood. 2000;96:1259–66.
128. O'Donnell RT, Shen S, Denardo SJ, Wun T, Kukis DL, Goldstein DS, Denardo GL. A phase I study of 90Y-2IT-BAD-Lym-1 in patients with non-Hodgkin's lymphoma. Anticancer Res. 2000;20:3647–55.
129. Scheinberg DA, Straus DJ, Yeh SD, Divgi C, Garin-Chesa P, Graham M, Pentlow K, Coit D, Oettgen HF, Old LJ. A phase I toxicity, pharmacology, and dosimetry trial of monoclonal antibody OKB7 in patients with non-Hodgkin's lymphoma: effects of tumor burden and antigen expression. J Clin Oncol. 1990;8:792–803.
130. Vose JM, Colcher D, Gobar L, Bierman PJ, Augustine S, Tempero M, Leichner P, Lynch JC, Goldenberg D, Armitage JO. Phase I/II trial of multiple dose 131Iodine-MAb LL2 (CD22) in patients with recurrent non-Hodgkin's lymphoma. Leuk Lymphoma. 2000;38:91–101.
131. Vose JM, Wahl RL, Saleh M, Rohatiner AZ, Knox SJ, Radford JA, Zelenetz AD, Tidmarsh GF, Stagg RJ, Kaminski MS. Multicenter phase II study of iodine-131 tositumomab for chemotherapy-relapsed/refractory low-grade and transformed low-grade B-cell non-Hodgkin's lymphomas. J Clin Oncol. 2000;18:1316–23.
132. Weiden PL, Breitz HB, Press O, Appelbaum JW, Bryan JK, Gaffigan S, Stone D, Axworthy D, Fisher D, Reno J. Pretargeted radioimmunotherapy (PRIT) for treatment of non-Hodgkin's lymphoma (NHL): initial phase I/II study results. Cancer Biother Radiopharm. 2000;15:15–29.
133. Wiseman GA, White CA, Witzig TE, Gordon LI, Emmanouilides C, Raubitschek A, Janakiraman N, Gutheil J, Schilder RJ, Spies S, Silverman DH, Grillo-Lopez AJ. Radioimmunotherapy of relapsed non-Hodgkin's lymphoma with zevalin, a 90Y-labeled anti-CD20 monoclonal antibody. Clin Cancer Res. 1999;5:3281s–6s.

134. Wiseman GA, Gordon LI, Multani PS, Witzig TE, Spies S, Bartlett NL, Schilder RJ, Murray JL, Saleh M, Allen RS, Grillo-Lopez AJ, White CA. Ibritumomab tiuxetan radioimmunotherapy for patients with relapsed or refractory non-Hodgkin lymphoma and mild thrombocytopenia: a phase II multicenter trial. Blood. 2002;99:4336–42.
135. Witzig TE, White CA, Wiseman GA, Gordon LI, Emmanouilides C, Raubitschek A, Janakiraman N, Gutheil J, Schilder RJ, Spies S, Silverman DH, Parker E, Grillo-Lopez AJ. Phase I/II trial of IDEC-Y2B8 radioimmunotherapy for treatment of relapsed or refractory CD20(+) B-cell non-Hodgkin's lymphoma. J Clin Oncol. 1999;17:3793–803.
136. Witzig TE, Flinn IW, Gordon LI, Emmanouilides C, Czuczman MS, Saleh MN, Cripe L, Wiseman G, Olejnik T, Multani PS, White CA. Treatment with ibritumomab tiuxetan radioimmunotherapy in patients with rituximab-refractory follicular non-Hodgkin's lymphoma. J Clin Oncol. 2002;20:3262–9.
137. Witzig TE, Gordon LI, Cabanillas F, Czuczman MS, Emmanouilides C, Joyce R, Pohlman BL, Bartlett NL, Wiseman GA, Padre N, Grillo-Lopez AJ, Multani P, White CA. Randomized controlled trial of yttrium-90-labeled ibritumomab tiuxetan radioimmunotherapy versus rituximab immunotherapy for patients with relapsed or refractory low-grade, follicular, or transformed B-cell non-Hodgkin's lymphoma. J Clin Oncol. 2002;20:2453–63.
138. Juweid ME, Hajjar G, Stein R, Sharkey RM, Herskovic T, Swayne LC, Suleiman S, Pereira M, Rubin AD, Goldenberg DM. Initial experience with high-dose radioimmunotherapy of metastatic medullary thyroid cancer using 131I-MN-14 F(ab)2 anti-carcinoembryonic antigen MAb and AHSCR. J Nucl Med. 2000;41:93–103.
139. Liu SY, Eary JF, Petersdorf SH, Martin PJ, Maloney DG, Appelbaum FR, Matthews DC, Bush SA, Durack LD, Fisher DR, Gooley TA, Bernstein ID, Press OW. Follow-up of relapsed B-cell lymphoma patients treated with iodine-131-labeled anti-CD20 antibody and autologous stem-cell rescue. J Clin Oncol. 1998;16:3270–8.
140. Press OW, Eary JF, Badger CC, Martin PJ, Appelbaum FR, Levy R, Miller R, Brown S, Nelp WB, Krohn KA, et al. Treatment of refractory non-Hodgkin's lymphoma with radiolabeled MB-1 (anti-CD37) antibody. J Clin Oncol. 1989;7:1027–38.
141. Press OW, Eary JF, Appelbaum FR, Martin PJ, Badger CC, Nelp WB, Glenn S, Butchko G, Fisher D, Porter B, et al. Radiolabeled-antibody therapy of B-cell lymphoma with autologous bone marrow support. N Engl J Med. 1993;329:1219–24.
142. Press OW, Eary JF, Appelbaum FR, Martin PJ, Nelp WB, Glenn S, Fisher DR, Porter B, Matthews DC, Gooley T, et al. Phase II trial of 131I-B1 (anti-CD20) antibody therapy with autologous stem cell transplantation for relapsed B cell lymphomas. Lancet. 1995;346:336–40.
143. Kaminski MS, Zasadny KR, Francis IR, Milik AW, Ross CW, Moon SD, Crawford SM, Burgess JM, Petry NA, Butchko GM, et al. Radioimmunotherapy of B-cell lymphoma with [131I]anti-B1 (anti-CD20) antibody. N Engl J Med. 1993;329:459–65.
144. Parker BA, Vassos AB, Halpern SE, Miller RA, Hupf H, Amox DG, Simoni JL, Starr RJ, Green MR, Royston I. Radioimmunotherapy of human B-cell lymphoma with 90Y-conjugated anti idiotype monoclonal antibody. Cancer Res. 1990;50:1022s–8s.
145. Borjesson PK, Jauw YW, Boellaard R, de Bree R, Comans EF, Roos JC, Castelijns JA, Vosjan MJ, Kummer JA, Leemans CR, Lammertsma AA, van Dongen GA. Performance of immuno-positron emission tomography with zirconium-89-labeled chimeric monoclonal antibody U36 in the detection of lymph node metastases in head and neck cancer patients. Clin Cancer Res. 2006;12:2133–40.
146. Zalutsky MR. Potential of immuno-positron emission tomography for tumor imaging and immunotherapy planning. Clin Cancer Res. 2006;12:1958–60.
147. Heskamp S, Raave Ŕ, Boerman O, Rijpkema M, Goncalves V, Denat F. ^{89}Zr-Immuno-Positron Emission Tomography in Oncology: State-of-the-Art ^{89}Zr Radiochemistry. Bioconjug Chem. 2017;28:2211–23.
148. Juweid ME. Radioimmunotherapy of B-cell non-Hodgkin's lymphoma: from clinical trials to clinical practice. J Nucl Med. 2002;43:1507–29.
149. Armitage JO, Mauch PM, Harris NL, Bierman P. Non-Hodgkin's lymphoma. Philadelphia: Lippincott, Williams & Wilkins; 2001.
150. Cheson BD, Fisher RI, Barrington SF, Cavalli F, Schwartz LH, Zucca E, Lister TA. Recommendations for initial evaluation, staging, and response assessment of Hodgkin and non-Hodgkin lymphoma: the Lugano classification. J Clin Oncol. 2014;32(27):3059–68.
151. NCCN Guideline Version 1. 2019 B-Cell lymphomas.
152. Knox SJ, Goris ML, Trisler K, Negrin R, Davis T, Liles TM, Grillo-Lopez A, Chinn P, Varns C, Ning SC, Fowler S, Deb N, Becker M, Marquez C, Levy R. Yttrium-90-labeled anti-CD20 monoclonal antibody therapy of recurrent B-cell lymphoma. Clin Cancer Res. 1996;2:457–70.
153. Witzig TE, Gordon LI, Wiseman GA, et al. Reduced dose Zevalin is safe and effective in patients with relapsed or refractory, low grade, follicular or CD20+ transformed B cell non-Hodgkin's lymphoma (L/F/T NHL) and mild thrombocytopenia. Blood. 2000;96:728a.
154. Witzig TE, White CA, Flinn IW, et al. Zevalin radioimmunotherapy of rituximab refractory follicular non-Hodgkin's lymphoma. Blood. 2000;96:507a.
155. Wagner HN Jr, Wiseman GA, Marcus CS, Nabi HA, Nagle CE, Fink-Bennett DM, Lamonica DM, Conti PS. Administration guidelines for radioimmunotherapy of non-Hodgkin's lymphoma with (90) Y-labeled anti-CD20 monoclonal antibody. J Nucl Med. 2002;43:267–72.

156. Tennvall J, Fischer M, Bischof Delaloye A, Bombardieri E, Bodei L, Giammarile F, Lassmann M, Oyen W, Brans B. EANM procedure guideline for radio-immunotherapy for B-cell lymphoma with 90Y-radiolabelled ibritumomab tiuxetan (Zevalin). Eur J Nucl Med Mol Imag. 2007;34(4):616–22.
157. Zelenetz AD. Radioimmunotherapy for lymphoma. Curr Opin Oncol. 1999;11:375–80.
158. Wiseman G, Gordon L, Leigh BR, et al. Safety and efficacy of the Zevalin radioimmunotherapy regimen are not diminished by extending the time interval between rituximab infusion and zevalin injection. Blood. 2000;96:251b.
159. Konig T, Baum RP, Radtke M, Franke D. HAMA-ELISA medac: a new assay for the quantitation of human anti-mouse antibodies. Clin Lab. 2002;48:207–10.
160. Davies AJ. Tositumomab and iodine [131I] tositumomab in the management of follicular lymphoma. An oncologist's view. Q J Nucl Med Mol Imaging. 2004;48:305–16.
161. Wahl RL, Zasadny KR, Estes J, et al. Single center experience with iodine 131I tositumomab radioimmunotherapy for previously untreated follicular lymphoma (FL). J Nucl Med. 2000;41(Suppl):79.
162. Gregory SA, Leonard JP, Knox SJ, Zelenetz AD, Armitage JO, Kaminski MS. The iodine I131 tositumomab therapeutic regimen: summary of safety in 995 patients with relapsed/refractory low grade (LG) and transformed LG non-Hodgkin's lymphoma (NHL). American Society of Clinical Oncology, Annual Meeting Proceedings (post-meeting edition). J Clin Oncol. 2004;22(14S):6732.
163. Behr TM, Wormann B, Gramatzki M, Riggert J, Gratz S, Behe M, Griesinger F, Sharkey RM, Kolb HJ, Hiddemann W, Goldenberg DM, Becker W. Low- versus high-dose radioimmunotherapy with humanized anti-CD22 or chimeric anti-CD20 antibodies in a broad spectrum of B cell-associated malignancies. Clin Cancer Res. 1999;5:3304s–14s.
164. Behr TM, Griesinger F, Riggert J, Gratz S, Behe M, Kaufmann CC, Wormann B, Brittinger G, Becker W. High-dose myeloablative radioimmunotherapy of mantle cell non-Hodgkin lymphoma with the iodine-131-labeled chimeric anti-CD20 antibody C2B8 and autologous stem cell support. Results of a pilot study. Cancer. 2002;94:1363–72.
165. Czuczman MS, Straus DJ, Divgi CR, Graham M, Garin-Chesa P, Finn R, Myers J, Old LJ, Larson SM, Scheinberg DA. Phase I dose-escalation trial of iodine 131-labeled monoclonal antibody OKB7 in patients with non-Hodgkin's lymphoma. J Clin Oncol. 1993;11:2021–9.
166. DeNardo GL, DeNardo SJ, O'Grady LF, Levy NB, Adams GP, Mills SL. Fractionated radioimmunotherapy of B-cell malignancies with 131I-Lym-1. Cancer Res. 1990;50:1014s–6s.
167. Davis TA, Kaminski MS, Leonard JP, Gregory SA, Wahl RL, Hsu FJ, Wilkinson M, Frankel SR, Serafini A, Zelenetz AD, Kroll S, Coleman M, Levy R, Knox SJ. Results of a randomized study of Bexxar (tositumomab or iodine I-131 tositumomab) versus unlabeled tositumomab in patients with relapsed or refractory low-grade or transformed non-Hodgkin's lymphoma (NHL). In: Proc Am Soc Hematology; 2001. p. 3503.
168. Goldenberg DM, Horowitz JA, Sharkey RM, Hall TC, Murthy S, Goldenberg H, Lee RE, Stein R, Siegel JA, Izon DO, et al. Targeting, dosimetry, and radioimmunotherapy of B-cell lymphomas with iodine-131-labeled LL2 monoclonal antibody. J Clin Oncol. 1991;9:548–64.
169. Linden O, Tennvall J, Cavallin-Stahl E, Darte L, Garkavij M, Lindner KJ, Ljungberg M, Ohlsson T, Sjogreen K, Wingardh K, Strand SE. Radioimmunotherapy using 131I-labeled anti-CD22 monoclonal antibody (LL2) in patients with previously treated B-cell lymphomas. Clin Cancer Res. 1999;5:3287s–91s.
170. O'Donnell RT, DeNardo GL, Kukis DL, Lamborn KR, Shen S, Yuan A, Goldstein DS, Mirick GR, DeNardo SJ. 67Copper-2-iminothiolane-6-[p-(bromoacetamido)benzyl-TETA-Lym-1] for radioimmunotherapy of non-Hodgkin's lymphoma. Clin Cancer Res. 1999;5:3330s–6s.
171. Scheidhauer K, Schwarz K, von Schilling C, Schmidt B, Wolf I, Peschel C, Schwaiger M. Pradiktion von Remission und ereignisfereim Uberleben nach Radioimmunotherapie (RIT) von Non-Hodgkin's-Lymphomen. In: 41 Jahrestagung DGN; 2003. p V152 (abstract).
172. Wiseman GA, Witzig TE. Yttrium-90 (90Y) ibritumomab tiuxetan (Zevalin) induces long-term durable responses in patients with relapsed or refractory B-cell non-Hodgkin's lymphoma. Cancer Biother Radiopharm. 2005;20:185–8.
173. Witzig TE, White CA, Gordon LI, et al. Final results of a randomized controlled study of the Zevalin radioimmunotherapy regimen versus a standard course of rituximab immunotherapy for B-cell NHL. Blood. 2000;96(abstract):3591.
174. Davis T, Kaminski MS, Leonard JP, Hsu FJ, Wilkinson M, Wahl RL. Long-term results of a randomised trial comparing tositumomab and iodine I131-tositumomab (BEXXAR) with tositumomab alone in patients with relapsed or refractory low-grade (lg) or transformed low grade (t-lg) non-Hodgkin's lymphoma (NHL). Blood. 2003;102:405a.
175. Davies AJ, Rohatiner AZ, Howell S, Britton KE, Owens SE, Micallef IN, Deakin DP, Carrington BM, Lawrance JA, Vinnicombe S, Mather SJ, Clayton J, Foley R, Jan H, Kroll S, Harris M, Amess J, Norton AJ, Lister TA, Radford JA. Tositumomab and iodine I 131 tositumomab for recurrent indolent and transformed B-cell non-Hodgkin's lymphoma. J Clin Oncol. 2004;22:1469–79.
176. Zelenetz AD, Saleh M, Vose J, Younes A, Kaminski MS. Patients with transformed low grade follicular lymphoma attain durable responses following outpatient radioimmunotherapy with tositumomab and iodine (131I) tositumomab (Bexxar). Blood. 2002;100:357a.

177. Horning SJ, Younes A, Lucas J, Podoloff D, Jain V. Rituximab treatment failures: tositumomab and iodine (131I) tositumomab (Bexxar) can produce meaningful durable responses. Blood. 2002;100:357a.
178. Cheson BD, Horning SJ, Coiffier B, Shipp MA, Fisher RI, Connors JM, Lister TA, Vose J, Grillo-Lopez A, Hagenbeek A, Cabanillas F, Klippensten D, Hiddemann W, Castellino R, Harris NL, Armitage JO, Carter W, Hoppe R, Canellos GP. Report of an international workshop to standardize response criteria for non-Hodgkin's lymphomas. NCI Sponsored International Working Group. J Clin Oncol. 1999;17:1244.
179. Leonard JP, Coleman CN, Kostakoglu K, et al. Fludarabine monophosphate followed by iodine 131I tositumomab for untreated low grade and follicular non-Hodgkin's lymphoma (NHL). Blood. 1999;94(Suppl):90a.
180. Press OW, Eary JF, Gooley T, Gopal AK, Liu S, Rajendran JG, Maloney DG, Petersdorf S, Bush SA, Durack LD, Martin PJ, Fisher DR, Wood B, Borrow JW, Porter B, Smith JP, Matthews DC, Appelbaum FR, Bernstein ID. A phase I/II trial of iodine-131-tositumomab (anti-CD20), etoposide, cyclophosphamide, and autologous stem cell transplantation for relapsed B-cell lymphomas. Blood. 2000;96:2934–42.
181. Puronen CE, Cassaday RD, Stevenson PA, et al. Long-Term Follow-Up of 90Y-Ibritumomab Tiuxetan, Fludarabine, and Total Body Irradiation-Based Nonmyeloablative Allogeneic Transplant Conditioning for Persistent High-Risk B Cell Lymphoma. Biol Blood Marrow Transplant. 2018;24:2211–5.
182. Corcoran MC, Press OW, Matthews DC, Appelbaum FR, Bernstein ID. The role of radioimmunotherapy in bone marrow transplantation. Curr Opin Hematol. 1996;3:438–45.
183. Matthews DC, Appelbaum FR, Eary JF, Fisher DR, Durack LD, Hui TE, Martin PJ, Mitchell D, Press OW, Storb R, Bernstein ID. Phase I study of (131)I-anti-CD45 antibody plus cyclophosphamide and total body irradiation for advanced acute leukemia and myelodysplastic syndrome. Blood. 1999;94:1237–47.
184. Jhanwar YS, Divgi C. Current status of therapy of solid tumors. J Nucl Med. 2005;46(Suppl 1):141S–50S.
185. Divgi C. Editorial: what ails solid tumor radioimmunotherapy? Cancer Biother Radiopharm. 2006;21:81–4.
186. Behr TM, Sharkey RM, Juweid ME, Dunn RM, Vagg RC, Ying Z, Zhang CH, Swayne LC, Vardi Y, Siegel JA, Goldenberg DM. Phase I/II clinical radioimmunotherapy with an iodine-131-labeled anti-carcinoembryonic antigen murine monoclonal antibody IgG. J Nucl Med. 1997;38:858–70.
187. Behr TM, Salib AL, Liersch T, Behe M, Angerstein C, Blumenthal RD, Fayyazi A, Sharkey RM, Ringe B, Becker H, Wormann B, Hiddemann W, Goldenberg DM, Becker W. Radioimmunotherapy of small volume disease of colorectal cancer metastatic to the liver: preclinical evaluation in comparison to standard chemotherapy and initial results of a phase I clinical study. Clin Cancer Res. 1999;5:3232s–42s.
188. Behr TM, Liersch T, Greiner-Bechert L, Griesinger F, Behe M, Markus PM, Gratz S, Angerstein C, Brittinger G, Becker H, Goldenberg DM, Becker W. Radioimmunotherapy of small-volume disease of metastatic colorectal cancer. Cancer. 2002;94:1373–81.
189. Divgi CR, Scott AM, Dantis L, Capitelli P, Siler K, Hilton S, Finn RD, Kemeny N, Kelsen D, Kostakoglu L, et al. Phase I radioimmunotherapy trial with iodine-131-CC49 in metastatic colon carcinoma. J Nucl Med. 1995;36:586–92.
190. Meredith RF, Khazaeli MB, Macey DJ, Grizzle WE, Mayo M, Schlom J, Russell CD, LoBuglio AF. Phase II study of interferon-enhanced 131I-labeled high affinity CC49 monoclonal antibody therapy in patients with metastatic prostate cancer. Clin Cancer Res. 1999;5:3254s–8s.
191. Meredith RF, Khazaeli MB, Plott WE, Spencer SA, Wheeler RH, Brady LW, Woo DV, LoBuglio AF. Initial clinical evaluation of iodine-125-labeled chimeric 17–1A for metastatic colon cancer. J Nucl Med. 1995;36:2229–33.
192. Nanus DM, Milowsky MI, Kostakoglu L, Smith-Jones PM, Vallabahajosula S, Goldsmith SJ, Bander NH. Clinical use of monoclonal antibody HuJ591 therapy: targeting prostate specific membrane antigen. J Urol. 2003;170:S84–8. discussion S88–9
193. Mittal BB, Zimmer MA, Sathiaseelan V, Benson AB 3rd, Mittal RR, Dutta S, Rosen ST, Spies SM, Mettler JM, Groch MW. Phase I/II trial of combined 131I anti-CEA monoclonal antibody and hyperthermia in patients with advanced colorectal adenocarcinoma. Cancer. 1996;78:1861–70.
194. Welt S, Divgi CR, Kemeny N, Finn RD, Scott AM, Graham M, Germain JS, Richards EC, Larson SM, Oettgen HF, et al. Phase I/II study of iodine 131-labeled monoclonal antibody A33 in patients with advanced colon cancer. J Clin Oncol. 1994;12:1561–71.
195. Welt S, Scott AM, Divgi CR, Kemeny NE, Finn RD, Daghighian F, Germain JS, Richards EC, Larson SM, Old LJ. Phase I/II study of iodine 125-labeled monoclonal antibody A33 in patients with advanced colon cancer. J Clin Oncol. 1996;14:1787–97.
196. Ychou M, Pelegrin A, Faurous P, Robert B, Saccavini JC, Guerreau D, Rossi JF, Fabbro M, Buchegger F, Mach JP, Artus JC. Phase-I/II radio-immunotherapy study with iodine-131-labeled anti-CEA monoclonal antibody F6 F(ab′)2 in patients with non-resectable liver metastases from colorectal cancer. Int J Cancer. 1998;75:615–9.
197. Baum RP, Hertel A, Lorenz M, Schwarz A, Encke A, Hör G. ^{99m}Tc-labelled anti-CEA monoclonal antibody for tumour immunoscintigraphy: first clinical results. Nucl Med Commun. 1989;10:345–52.

198. Behr TM, Sharkey RM, Juweid ME, Dunn RM, Ying Z, Zhang CH, Siegel JA, Goldenberg DM. Variables influencing tumor dosimetry in radioimmunotherapy of CEA-expressing cancers with anti-CEA and antimucin monoclonal antibodies. J Nucl Med. 1997;38:409–18.
199. Dillman RO. Why event-free survival is better than tumor response or other measures of survival as an endpoint in cancer trials. Cancer Biother Radiopharm. 1996;11:99–104.
200. Meredith RF, Bueschen AJ, Khazaeli MB, Plott WE, Grizzle WE, Wheeler RH, Schlom J, Russell CD, Liu T, LoBuglio AF. Treatment of metastatic prostate carcinoma with radiolabeled antibody CC49. J Nucl Med. 1994;35:1017–22.
201. McDevitt MR, Ma D, Lai LT, Simon J, Borchardt P, Frank RK, Wu K, Pellegrini V, Curcio MJ, Miederer M, Bander NH, Scheinberg DA. Tumor therapy with targeted atomic nanogenerators. Science. 2001;294:1537–40.
202. Tagawa ST, Milowsky M, Morris M, Vallabhajosula S, Christos P, Akhtar NH, Osborne J, Goldsmith SJ, Larson S, Taskar NP, Scher HI, Bander NH, Nanus DM. Phase II study of Lutetium-177-labeled anti-prostate-specific membrane antigen monoclonal antibody J591 for metastatic castration-resistant prostate cancer. Clin Cancer Res. 2013;19(18):5182–91. https://doi.org/10.1158/1078-0432.CCR-13-0231. Epub 2013 May 28
203. Tagawa ST, Batra J, Vallabhajosula S, et al. Final results of 2-dose fractionation of 177Lu-J591 for progressive metastatic castration resistant prostate cancer (mCRPC). J Clin Oncol. 2016;34:5022.
204. Tagawa ST, Whang YE, Kaur G, et al. Phase I trial of docetaxel/prednisone plus fractionated dose radiolabeled anti-prostate-specific membrane antigen (PSMA) monoclonal antibody 177lu-J591 in patients with metastatic, castration-resistant prostate cancer (mCRPC). J Clin Oncol. 2014;32:5064.
205. Miyahira AK, Pienta KJ, Morris MJ, Bander NH, Baum RP, Fendler WP, Goeckeler W, Gorin MA, Hennekes H, Pomper MG, Sartor O, Tagawa ST, Williams S, Soule HR. Meeting report from the Prostate Cancer Foundation PSMA-directed radionuclide scientific working group. Prostate. 2018;78(11):775–89. https://doi.org/10.1002/pros.23642.
206. Nicholson S, Gooden CS, Hird V, Maraveyas A, Mason P, Lambert HE, Meares CF, Epenetos AA. Radioimmunotherapy after chemotherapy compared to chemotherapy alone in the treatment of advanced ovarian cancer: a matched analysis. Oncol Rep. 1998;5:223–6.
207. Epenetos AA, Munro AJ, Stewart S, Rampling R, Lambert HE, McKenzie CG, Soutter P, Rahemtulla A, Hooker G, Sivolapenko GB, et al. Antibody-guided irradiation of advanced ovarian cancer with intraperitoneally administered radiolabeled monoclonal antibodies. J Clin Oncol. 1987;5:1890–9.
208. Oltrogge JB, Baum RP, Lema KN, Donnerstag B, Hor G. How to overcome the disturbing effects of human anti-mouse antibodies (HAMA) on in vitro assays. Int J Biol Markers. 1997;12:15–7.
209. Mobus VJ, Baum RP, Bolle M, Kreienberg R, Noujaim AA, Schultes BC, Nicodemus CF. Immune responses to murine monoclonal antibody-B43.13 correlate with prolonged survival of women with recurrent ovarian cancer. Am J Obstet Gynecol. 2003;189:28–36.
210. Noujaim AA, Schultes BC, Baum RP, Madiyalakan R. Induction of CA125-specific B and T cell responses in patients injected with MAb-B43.13 – evidence for antibody-mediated antigen-processing and presentation of CA125 in vivo. Cancer Biother Radiopharm. 2001;16:187–203.
211. Schultes BC, Baum RP, Niesen A, Noujaim AA, Madiyalakan R. Anti-idiotype induction therapy: anti-CA125 antibodies (Ab3) mediated tumor killing in patients treated with Ovarex mAb B43.13 (Ab1). Cancer Immunol Immunother. 1998;46:201–12.
212. Riva P, Franceschi G, Riva N, Casi M, Santimaria M, Adamo M. Role of nuclear medicine in the treatment of malignant gliomas: the locoregional radioimmunotherapy approach. Eur J Nucl Med. 2000;27:601–9.
213. Brady LW, Markoe AM, Woo DV, Rackover MA, Koprowski H, Steplewski Z, Peyster RG. Iodine125 labeled anti-epidermal growth factor receptor-425 in the treatment of malignant astrocytomas. A pilot study. J Neurosurg Sci. 1990;34:243–9.
214. Kalofonos HP, Pawlikowska TR, Hemingway A, Courtenay-Luck N, Dhokia B, Snook D, Sivolapenko GB, Hooker GR, McKenzie CG, Lavender PJ, et al. Antibody guided diagnosis and therapy of brain gliomas using radiolabeled monoclonal antibodies against epidermal growth factor receptor and placental alkaline phosphatase. J Nucl Med. 1989;30:1636–45.
215. Zalutsky MR, Moseley RP, Benjamin JC, Colapinto EV, Fuller GN, Coakham HP, Bigner DD. Monoclonal antibody and F(ab′)2 fragment delivery to tumor in patients with glioma: comparison of intracarotid and intravenous administration. Cancer Res. 1990;50:4105–10.
216. Kemshead JT, Papanastassiou V, Coakham HB, Pizer BL. Monoclonal antibodies in the treatment of central nervous system malignancies. Eur J Cancer. 1992;28:511–3.
217. Wong JY, Somlo G, Odom-Maryon T, Williams LE, Liu A, Yamauchi D, Wu AM, Yazaki P, Wilczynski S, Shively JE, Forman S, Doroshow JH, Raubitschek AA. Initial clinical experience evaluating Yttrium-90-chimeric T84.66 anticarcinoembryonic antigen antibody and autologous hematopoietic stem cell support in patients with carcinoembryonic antigen-producing metastatic breast cancer. Clin Cancer Res. 1999;5:3224s–31s.
218. Battula VL, Shi Y, Evans KW, et al. Ganglioside GD2 identifies breast cancer stem cells and promotes tumorigenesis. J Clin Invest. 2012;122:2066–78.

219. Martinez C, Hofmann TJ, Marino R, et al. Human bone marrow mesenchymal stromal cells express the neural ganglioside GD2: anovel surface marker for the identification of MSCs. Blood. 2007;109:4245–8.
220. Yanagisawa M, Yoshimura S, Yu RK. Expression of GD2 and GD3 gangliosides in human embryonic neural stem cells. ASN Neuro. 2011;3.
221. Cheresh DA, Pierschbacher MD, Herzig MA, et al. Disialogangliosides D2 and GD3 are involved in the attachment of human melanoma and neuroblastoma cells to extracellular matrix proteins. J Cell Biol. 1986;102:688–96.
222. Lammie G, Cheung N, Gerald W, et al. Ganglioside gd(2) expression in the human nervous-system and in neuroblastomas—an immunohistochemical study. Int J Oncol. 1993;3:909–15.
223. Shochat SJ, Abt AB. Schengrund CL.VCN-releasable sialic acid and gangliosides in human neuroblastomas. J Pediatr Surg. 1977;12:413–8.
224. Croog VJ, Kramer K, Cheung NK, et al. Whole neuraxis irradiation to address central nervous system relapse in high-risk neuroblastoma. Int J Radiat Oncol Biol Phys. 2010;78(3):849–54.
225. Larson SM, Divgi C, Sgouros G, et al. Monoclonal antibodies: basic principles— radioisotope conjugates. In: De Vita VT, Hellman S, Rosenberg SA, editors. Biologic therapy of cancer—principles and practice. Philadelphia: Lippincott; 2000. p. 396–412.
226. Kramer K, Humm JL, Souweidane MM, et al. Phase I study of targeted radioimmunotherapy for leptomeningeal cancers using intra-Ommaya 131-I-3F8. J Clin Oncol. 2007;25:5465–70.
227. Kramer K, Kushner BH, Modak S, et al. Compartmental intrathecal radioimmunotherapy: results for treatment for metastatic CNS neuroblastoma. J Neurooncol. 2010;97:409–18.
228. Miederer M, McDevitt MR, Borchardt P, et al. Treatment of neuroblastoma meningeal carcinomatosis with intrathecal application of alpha-emitting atomic nanogenerators targeting disialo-ganglioside GD2. Clin Cancer Res. 2004;10:6985–92.
229. Kletting P, Maaß C, Reske S, Beer AJ, Glatting G. Physiologically based pharmacokinetic modeling is essential in 90Y-labeled anti-CD66 radioimmunotherapy. PLoS One. 2015;10(5):e0127934.

35 Radioactive Microspheres

Gerd Wunderlich

35.1 Introduction and Overview

Radioactive microspheres are mostly aqueous dispersions of nanometre or micrometre size particles that carry preferable β-emitting radionuclides. The main advantage of radiolabelled microspheres over external radiation is that they can be placed in a defined body area in which they can remain for a period of time regarding their radioactivity half time. An attractive possibility for the delivery of therapeutic microspheres is the application of them via an artery that supplies the tumour. Hepatic tumours usually have a high arteriolar density and particle deposition is proportional to blood flow. A higher proportion of hepatic arterial vessels surround a metastatic lesion than the normal liver tissue. Advantageously, the ratio of tumour vessels to normal-tissue vessels is estimated to be about 3:1. Moreover, if radioactive microspheres are released into the hepatic artery, a therapeutic dose will preferentially be absorbed by the tumour as opposed to the normal liver [1]. The transportation away from the vascular bed is hindered for particles with a mean diameter of more than 10 μm. The endoradiotherapy of tumours by selective catheterisation has been proven to be an effective therapy for the local cure of cancer. This is one possibility for achieving a high radionuclide concentration in the tumour after intra-arterial injection, overcoming the disadvantages of systemic application, which is limited by accumulation in target tissue and the radiosensitivity of non-target tissues.

Ideal properties of radiolabelled microparticles for sufficient intra-arterial therapy are [2–4]:

- The preparation should be easily labelled and resistant to elution of the radioactive label, macrophage removal or radiolysis.
- Uniform particle size and density comparable to that of blood are necessary to prevent settling and ensure uniform uptake.
- For effective radiotherapy, the radionuclide label must be a high-energy β-emitter with low γ-emission and an intermediate half-life of a few days. In contrast to nanoparticles, the physicochemical carrier surface properties of microspheres with a diameter > 10 μm are not as important.
- The microparticles can be based on polymers, polymeric resins, albumin or inorganic materials.

Earlier endoradiotherapy studies applied ^{32}P colloid nanoparticles (Phosphocol) [5–7] and ^{198}Au [8]. An overview of the preclinical investigations of intra-arterial brachytherapy in the liver was presented by Kennedy and co-workers [1].

G. Wunderlich (✉)
Department of Nuclear Medicine, University Hospital Carl Gustav Carus, Technical University Dresden, Dresden, Germany
e-mail: Gerd.Wunderlich@uniklinikum-dresden.de

H. Ahmadzadehfar et al. (eds.), *Clinical Nuclear Medicine*,
https://doi.org/10.1007/978-3-030-39457-8_35

In 1960, most of the experience with intra-arterial radiolabelled microspheres was from Italy, published by Badellino and colleagues, using ^{32}P resin microspheres. The resin was a strong acid cation exchanger and was labelled with ^{32}P and sometimes with ^{51}Cr. The microspheres had a diameter of 45–55 µm. ^{32}P was bound to the resin as a colloidal complex with chromium. By using γ-emitting ^{51}Cr as a tracer, the distribution of the particles could be followed with the aid of a scintillation counter [5, 9].

Also in the 1960s, ^{131}I-labelled macroaggregated HSA (human serum albumin) was introduced for intra-arterial tracer studies. Since then, ^{99m}Tc macroaggregated albumin (MAA) has been used almost exclusively for particle distribution studies.

The first reports about the use of ^{90}Y microparticles in liver malignancies dated from 1962 and 1963 [10, 11].

An alternative intra-arterial therapy option today is treatment with ^{131}I-Lipiodol (Lipiocis®, IBA, Brussels, Belgium), i.e. ^{131}I-labelled iodine-rich fatty acid esters in a poppy seed oil originally used as a contrast medium for the detection of hepatocellular carcinoma (HCC). Ahmadzadehfar et al. presented the basis for the clinical use of ^{131}I-Lipidol as an effective treatment both in the treatment of HCC with portal thrombosis and as an adjuvant therapy after the resection of HCC [12]. ^{131}I-Lipidol may represent a possible therapy option in patients with severe liver dysfunction in whom radioembolisation with ^{90}Y-microspheres may be contraindicated [13].

Radionuclides used in the last decades for intra-arterial therapy with microspheres are preferential ^{90}Y and in some cases ^{166}Ho [14–19] and ^{186}Re and ^{188}Re [20, 21]. The mean energy of the β^--particles of these radionuclides is listed in Table 35.1.

35.2 ^{90}Y Microspheres: Commercial Preparations for Intra-arterial Therapy

Initial studies with ^{90}Y resins in the 1980s met with several problems, including difficulties in accurately measuring the absorbed dose, monitoring regional perfusion and excessive leakage of radionuclide from particles and myelosuppression due to ^{90}Y deposition in bone [22]. More recent preparations of ^{90}Y-labelled microspheres have significantly reduced leakage in glass- and resin-based microspheres [23]. Combinations of different imaging techniques enable the more accurate monitoring of absorbed doses and safer delivery to the tumour without excessive shunting to the gastrointestinal tract or lung. For relevant information see the EANM guidelines for the treatment of liver cancer with intra-arterial radioactive compounds [24].

Generally, shunting must be determined by a test infusion of ^{99m}Tc-MAA or ^{99m}Tc microspheres, assuming that these particles distribute in a similar way to therapeutic ^{90}Y microspheres. In principle, ^{86}Y microspheres can be used as surrogates of ^{90}Y SIR-spheres in PET (positron emission tomography) studies [25], but the main problem is the rare availability of ^{86}Y.

^{90}Y is a pure β^--emitter that decays to stable ^{90}Zr with an average β-energy of 0.934 MeV and a half-life of 64.2 hours. It is produced by neutron bombardment of ^{89}Y in a commercial reactor or by a $^{90}Sr/^{90}Y$ generator. The mean tissue penetration is approximately 2.5 mm and the maximum range in tissue is 1.1 cm. Imaging of ^{90}Y is possible by using the bremsstrahlung with minor quality images [26, 27] and also the emitted positrons, which can further be used for PET/CT imaging [28].

Two commercially available ^{90}Y-labelled microspheres are currently on the market:

- Glass microspheres (TheraSphere®, BTG international Medicine).
- Resin microspheres (SIR-Spheres®, SIRTEX Medical Limited).

TheraSphere®

- ^{90}Y is permanently embedded in the glass.
- Each glass sphere has a diameter of 20–30 µm.
- ^{89}Y Yttrium oxide is stably incorporated. For labelling, the microspheres are irradiated with neutrons in a nuclear reactor [29].
- TheraSphere® has a high specific gravity and density (3.3 g/cm³).

Table 35.1 Characteristics of selected radiolabeled microparticles for endoradiotherapy

Radionuclide	Matrix material	$T_{1/2}$ nuclide	Emission	Mean β^- energy (keV)
^{32}P	Resin	14.3 day	β^-	695
^{68}Ga	HSA	68 min	$\beta^+ + \gamma$	–
^{90}Y	Resin	2.7 day	β^- +	934
	Glass		$\beta^-\beta^+$ internal pair production	
^{99m}Tc	HSA	6 h	γ	–
^{166}Ho	PLLA	26.8 h	$\beta^- + \gamma$	665
^{188}Re	HSA	17 h	$\beta^- + \gamma$	763

– Typical dose range from 3 to 5 million microspheres.
– The standard dose of TheraSphere® in water for injection is 5 GBq per patient; doses of 3 GBq to 20 GBq are available.

SIR-Spheres®

– ^{90}Y is permanently embedded in an acrylic polymer resin [30].
– Each resin sphere has a diameter of 20–60 μm.
– The microspheres are labelled with ^{90}Y via cation exchange with sufficiently strong binding. ^{90}Y is a decay product of ^{90}Sr obtained from a generator.
– SIR-Spheres® have a low specific gravity and density (1.4 g/cm^3).
– Typical dose range from 40 to 80 million microspheres.
– The standard dose of SIR-Spheres® is 3 GBq per patient in 5 ml water for injection.

Regarding the amount of radioactivity, the difference between the two ^{90}Y microsphere types is estimated to be 2500 Bq per particle (glass) vs. 50 Bq per particle (resin).

35.3 ^{188}Re Microspheres

^{188}Re seems to be a promising short-lived β^--emitter ($T_{1/2}$ = 17 h, average β-energy is 0.763 MeV, maximum range in tissue 3 mm) for the in-house production of radiopharmaceuticals for therapeutic purposes. The convenient availability of carrier-free (n.c.a.) ^{188}Re from the $^{188}W/^{188}Re$ generator allows a prompt response to clinical demands. The γ-emission (155 keV) enables imaging and dosimetric studies with conventional SPECT imaging equipment.

Different particles could be labelled with ^{188}Re and applied for endotherapeutic purposes in a promising manner [4]. HSA microspheres are the most appropriate carriers. Hafeli and Wunderlich proposed ^{186}Re and ^{188}Re microspheres [20, 21, 31]. Radioactive HSA microspheres have been widely used in clinical nuclear medicine since 1969, especially for lung scanning [32]. One advantage of HSA microspheres compared to other particle-radiopharmaceuticals (e.g. MAA) is the uniformity of their size with a mean particle diameter of 25 μm. Another advantage is the biocompatibility and degradability in vivo of the albumin preparation. In contrast to other preparations proposed for endoradiotherapy or synovectomy (glass, styrene divinylbenzene copolymer resin, rhenium sulphur colloid) [33, 34], the occlusion of blood vessels is only temporary.

Wunderlich et al. have succeeded in labelling HSA microspheres ROTOP B20® (ROTOP, Radeberg, Germany) with ^{188}Re in an advantageous manner. Yields depend on the reaction conditions considerably. They presented data on an efficient kit technique for labelling ^{188}Re HSA microspheres for radiotherapeutic purposes [3].

35.3.1 Example: In-House Kit Preparation of ^{188}Re Microspheres (Fig. 35.1)

Highly pure carrier-free [^{188}Re] $NaReO_4$ was obtained in 25 ml of normal saline from an alumina-based $^{188}W/^{188}Re$ generator [35] (Oak Ridge National Laboratory, TN, USA and ITG,

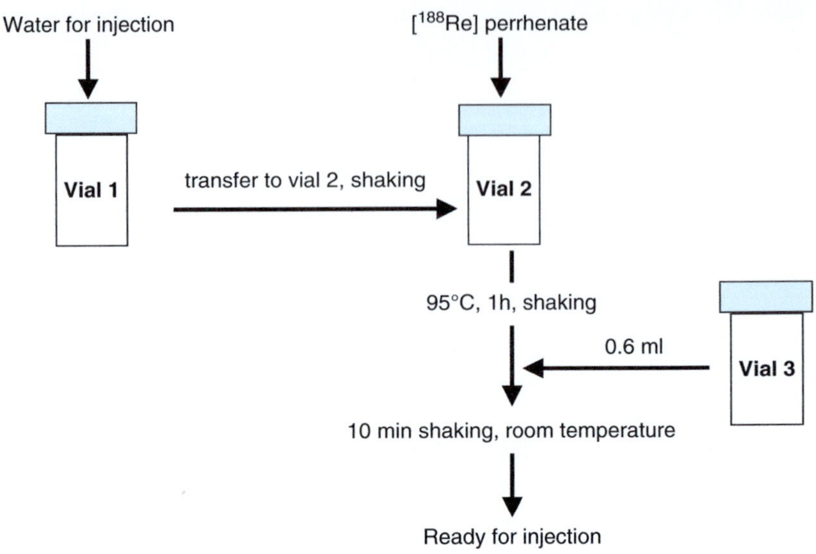

Fig. 35.1 Kit scheme of ^{188}Re labelled HSA microspheres [3], vial 1: gentisic acid, $SnCl_2 \cdot 2H_2O$, vial 2: 10^6 HSA microspheres, vial 3: potassium sodium tartrate solution (see text)

Garching (München), Germany) and concentrated with a system of tandem cation/anion exchange columns to 2 ml solution [36]. To minimise the radiation risk for laboratory staff, it would be desirable to have a shielded and software-controlled arrangement for generator elution and eluate concentration [37].

The labelling process was carried out in the presence of stannous chloride at pH 2. The particle labelling process is time-consuming and depends upon the $SnCl_2 \bullet 2H_2O$ concentration [20]. The particle labelling (coating) may be achieved by a combination of the reduction reaction of Re(VII) with Sn(II) and a particle surface-related co-precipitation effect of tin hydroxide colloid with high adsorption capacity and reduced, hydrolysed rhenium (Fig. 35.2). Above the optimum concentration of 20 μmol $SnCl_2 \bullet 2H_2O$ per mL, the solution becomes increasingly cloudy and the product is visibly mixed with tin hydroxide colloid. The particle-bound radioactivity did not reach more than 85–90% in a 90-min reaction time under optimised reaction conditions. To avoid the washing steps with their higher radiation risk for the laboratory staff, we added 150 μmol tartrate solution after 1 h of the reaction had passed. Subsequently, the pH increased from pH 2 to pH 4–5, resulting in a near-quantita-

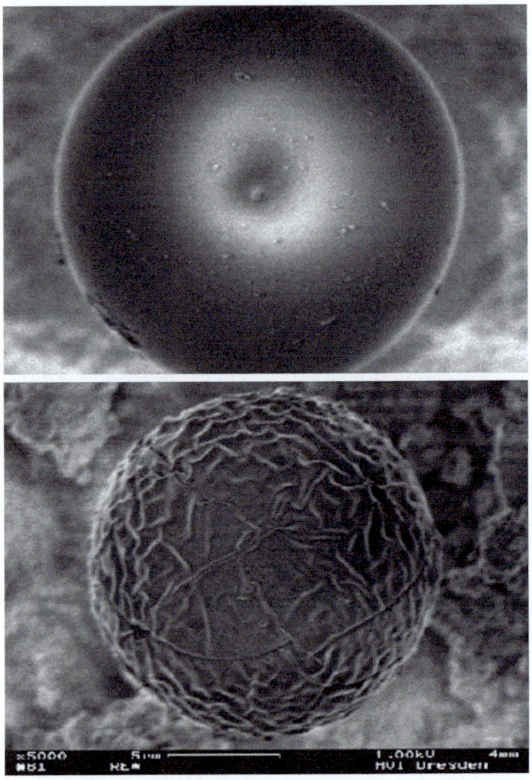

Fig. 35.2 Scanning electron micrographs of HSA microspheres B20 before (above) and after (bottom) labelling with rhenium-188. The tin hydroxide precipitate is responsible for the shrunken surface [20]

tive yield of the used ^{188}Re. Before labelling, the microspheres are distributed between 12 μm and 32 μm particle size (modal value 17 μm). After labelling, the microspheres remained in a narrow particle size distribution. Here, 90% of the surface area to be labelled included those particles with a diameter between 14 and 40 μm (modal value 22 μm) (Fig. 35.3). The particle labelling was found to be stable in vitro in human plasma, blood and saline for 30 h as >88% of the ^{188}Re was bound to the microspheres.

Maximum labelling-specific activity was found to be 2 GBq/mg HSA microspheres (10–16 kBq/particle). Thus, for therapeutic purposes, the radiation dose per particle is adjustable over a wide range. The kit permits a simple and reliable quantitative method of labelling for MS with high radionuclide activities on the particle surface. It requires the minimal handling of ^{188}Re, which markedly lowers the radiation burden for laboratory staff.

The biodistribution results revealed excellent in vivo stability with low uptake in the non-target tissues (Table 35.2). After i.v. injection in Wistar rats, the microspheres were effectively trapped in the pre-capillary arterioles of the lungs. Fine material would be collected in the RES of liver and spleen. There is only a very slow decrease of radioactivity in the lungs. At 96 h p.i., about >90% of the total ^{188}Re available at that time in the body was found in the region of the lungs. The effective half-life of ^{188}Re of the particle

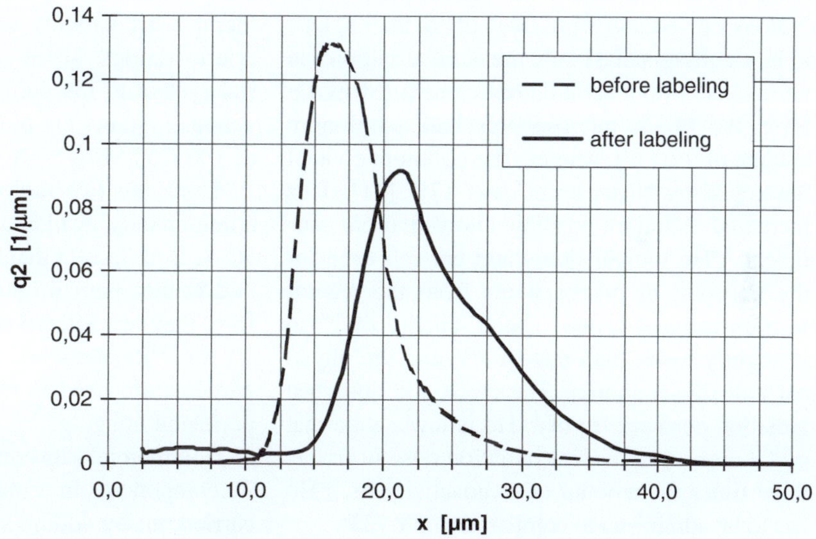

Fig. 35.3 Particle diameter-related surface distribution of the HSA microspheres before and after labelling with ^{188}Re [3]

Table 35.2 Biodistribution of ^{188}Re HSA microspheres B20 (% of injected dose/whole organ) in selected organs and whole body (gamma camera) after i.v. injection in Wistar rats, mean of 3 animals for each time; in addition, the biodistribution of Tc-99 m-labelled microspheres 48 h p.i. (approved radiopharmaceutical) and ^{188}Re perrhenate (all data corrected to the time of injection), $T_{b1/2}$ biological half-life, standard error of the mean < 20% [20]

Time p.i. (h)	Lungs	Liver	Spleen	Kidneys	Stomach	Femur	Bowel	Blood	Thyroid	Body	$T_{b\,1/2}$
0.33	99	0.42	0.02	0.28	0.05	<0.01	0.08	0.06	<0.01	100	–
4	97	1.95	0.23	0.41	0.32	<0.01	0.20	0.04	<0.01	98	–
24	94	1.15	0.10	0.85	0.11	<0.01	0.21	0.02	<0.01	97	–
48	94	0.82	0.07	1.36	0.12	0.01	0.17	0.03	<0.01	89	>250
96	93	0.90	0.10	1.23	0.05	0.01	0.12	0.01	<0.01	96	–
$^{188}Re-ReO_4'$, 48 h	<0.01	0.03	<0.01	0.01	0.30	<0.01	0.06	0.02	<0.01	17	23
^{99}Tc-B20, 48 h	69	0.90	0.06	2.92	0.12	0.01	0.81	0.07	0.01	69	75

preparations is 15.9 h, based on a biological half-life of >250 h. The first studies in man were reported by Liepe et al. [38]. To obtain an equivalent radiation dose, four- to five-fold higher activities of ^{188}Re need to be administered compared to ^{90}Y.

35.4 ^{166}Ho Microparticles

Mumper et al. have described biodegradable microspheres made of poly(L)lactic acid (PLLA) [39–41]. These polymer MS are prepared by dissolving the lipophilic complex holmium acetylacetonate and PLLA in chloroform, followed by the emulsification and subsequent evaporation of chloroform. The microspheres are made radioactive by neutron activation of ^{165}Ho to yield ^{166}Ho. ^{166}Ho is a β^--emitter with a half-life of 26.9 h. Due to its γ-emission of 81 keV, the biodistribution can be imaged with a scintillation camera (SPECT). First, the PLLA microspheres had a holmium content of 9% [39], whereas the holmium content developed by Nijsen et al. was 17% [41]. This increased holmium loading allowed more sufficient ^{166}Ho tumour doses and enough time for the transport of microspheres from the reactor to the treatment centre. The β^--energy of ^{166}Ho is slightly lower than that of ^{90}Y and the physical half-life is shorter. Therefore, the absorbed radiation dose per Bq of ^{166}Ho is lower than that of ^{90}Y. For an equivalent radiation dose in tissue, three times the amount of radioactivity of ^{166}Ho has to be administered compared to ^{90}Y [23].

The polylactic microspheres are slowly biodegradable to holmium lactate, but not until the incorporated ^{166}Ho has completely decayed [42].

In addition to the nuclear characteristics, holmium is highly paramagnetic and can be visualised by magnetic resonance imaging [43]. This multimodal approach has previously been demonstrated in preclinical animal studies [44]. The first MRI data of patients treated with ^{166}Ho PLLA MS show the feasibility of MRI-based dosimetry for radioembolisation therapy [45]. Intrahepatic microsphere biodistribution can be visualised with great detail; quantitative calculations of the absorbed radiation dose can be obtained within minutes during the radioembolisation procedure.

One commercially available ^{166}Ho microspheres preparation is currently on the market: PLLA microspheres (QuiremSpheres®, Quirem Medical).

35.5 Microparticles for Pre-therapeutic Use

35.5.1 ^{99m}Tc Microparticles

^{99m}Tc microparticles with a similar diameter as the particles for endoradiotherapy are used as a surrogate to estimate the distribution of microspheres in the hepatic circulation. Prior to the administration of particles for an intra-arterial therapy, all patients were tested for an occult arterio-venous shunt from the hepatic arterial system to the pulmonary or gastrointestinal venous systems via planar and SPECT imaging of 100–150 MBq ^{99m}Tc particles [46].

There are two radiopharmaceuticals that are commercially available: ^{99m}Tc-MAA and ^{99m}Tc-HSA. Both have a diameter of more than 10 µm and cannot pass through the capillaries; therefore, they are filtered out of circulation like the ^{90}Y or ^{188}Re particles. Routinely, ^{99m}Tc-labelled particles are used in nuclear medicine for lung perfusion imaging.

Commercial kits contain the lyophilised, sterile components in a multidose vial. Labelling is carried out by adding sterile ^{99m}Tc pertechnetate from a ^{99}Mo/^{99m}Tc generator with high radiochemical yield. The lyophilised material will be dissolved by agitating the reaction vial. After 5–20 min, the suspension is ready for injection.

35.5.1.1 Macroaggregates

Macroaggregates are obtained by the aggregation of HSA at acidic pH under controlled conditions. Macroaggregates are irregularly formed and have a relatively wide particle size distribution after filtration of between 10 µm and 50 µm in commercial kits. For instance, 2 mg of MAA correspond to 1.5–2 million particles [47].

35.5.1.2 Microspheres

Microspheres are obtained by heat denaturation of HSA in vegetable oil under controlled conditions. The size distribution of HSA microspheres depends on the degree of dispersion in oil. An advantage of albumin microspheres over other particle-radiopharmaceuticals (e.g. HSA macroaggregates) is the uniformity of their size after sieving with a mean particle diameter of 25 μm [48]. In commercial kits, 2.5 mg microspheres correspond to 300,000–500,000 microspheres per vial.

35.5.2 ^{68}Ga Particles

An alternative to ^{99m}Tc microparticles are ^{68}Ga-labelled microparticles.

With these particles, imaging of liver and liver tumour perfusion is possible with PET. Prior selective intra-arterial therapy commercial HSA microspheres can be labelled and used to estimate the distribution of microspheres in the hepatic circulation. For example, ^{68}Ga can be eluted from a commercially available ^{68}Ge/^{68}Ga generator. Labelling is simply achieved by mixing 1 mL 0.5 M ammonium acetate buffer pH 5 and ^{68}Ga generator eluate (100-300 MBq in 98/2 acetone/1 M hydrochloric acid eluate) with microspheres in the commercial vial. After 15 min of heating (90 °C) in a shaker, labelling is completed [49, 50].

35.6 Particles Loading with Alpha Emitters

Alpha emitters can deliver an extremely high linear energy transfer (LET) to tissues. For example, the α-emitter ^{211}At ($T_{1/2}$ 7.2 h, E_{α} = 6.8 MeV) proposed for therapeutic use has a mean LET of about 100 keV/μm, compared with 0.2 keV/μm of the typical β-emitter ^{90}Y. The accompanying gamma emission makes SPECT distribution studies possible. Goddu et al. calculated the cellular absorbed dose per unit radioactivity for a variety of β- and α-emitting radionuclides, and found that α-emitters produce about 100 times more absorption [51]. However, the short range of α-emission has the disadvantage that only two or three cell diameters can be penetrated by one α-particle.

Bloomer et al. showed that ^{211}At tellurium particles (3–5 μm) are effective on an ascites mouse model [52]. Larsen et al. labelled amine-functionalised polymer particles with ^{211}At [53]. The labelled particles were tested in an intraperitoneal tumour model in mouse and led to increased survival. One general problem is the leakage of the radioactive label from the particle surface and the radiotoxicity of "free" ^{211}At. To overcome this lack, Wunderlich and co-workers coated the surface of HSA B20 microspheres with silver and generated a stable radioactive label of the particles with ^{211}At that could be verified by injection in mice and after application in the tongue of pigs [54]. First clinical experiences were obtained in 1990 with the endoarterial therapy of a lingual carcinoma with ^{211}At-labelled HSA microspheres [12, 55, 56]; these data showed that α-emitters are potentially effective as therapeutic agents, but their major handicaps are the short penetration in tissue, rare availability, and the often low stability of the label in vivo.

References

1. Kennedy AS, Nutting C, Coldwell D, Gaiser J, Drachenberg C. Pathologic response and microdosimetry of (90)Y microspheres in man: review of four explanted whole livers. Int J Radiat Oncol Biol Phys. 2004;60:1552–63.
2. Harbert J. Nuclear medicine diagnosis and therapy. In: Harbert J, editor. Therapy with intra-arterial radioactive particles. New York: Thieme Medical Publishers, Inc.; 1996. p. 1141–55.
3. Wunderlich G, Drews A, Kotzerke J. A kit for labeling of [188Re] human serum albumin microspheres for therapeutic use in nuclear medicine. Appl Radiat Isot. 2005;62:915–8.
4. Wunderlich G, Pinkert J, Stintz M, Kotzerke J. Labeling and biodistribution of different particle materials for radioembolization therapy with 188Re. Appl Radiat Isot. 2005;62:745–50.
5. Dogliotti AM, Caldarola L, Badellino F, Cavalli A, Calderini P. Endo-arterial regional injection of radioisotopes in the treatment of malignant tumours. Int J Appl Radiat Isot. 1966;17:51–9.

6. Caldarola L, Badellino F, Cavalli A, et al. Intra-hepatic localisation of P-32-Labelled particles administered by Endoportal and intra-splenic injection. Panminerva Med. 1965;34:176–84.
7. Caldarola L, Badellino F, Del Fante FM, Roccia L, Del Boca R. The use of P32 in the surgical treatment of malignant oro-maxillofacial tumors. Minerva Stomatol. 1966;15:471–3.
8. Muller JH, Rossier PH. A new method for the treatment of cancer of the lungs by means of artificial radioactivity. Acta Radiol. 1951;35:449–68.
9. Caldarola L, Sosi S, Badellino F, Calderini P, Cavalli A. Preliminary experimental observations on endoarterial introduction of radiating resin microspheres. Int J Appl Radiat Isot. 1968;19:135–9.
10. Grady ED, Sale WT, Rollins LC. Localization of radioactivity by intravascular injection of large radioactive particles. Ann Surg. 1963;157:97–114.
11. Kim YS, Lafave JW, Maclean LD. The use of radiating microspheres in the treatment of experimental and human malignancy. Surgery. 1962;52:220–31.
12. Ahmadzadehfar H, Sabet A, Wilhelm K, Biersack HJ, Risse J. Iodine-131-lipiodol therapy in hepatic tumours. Methods. 2011;55:246–52.
13. Ahmadzadehfar H, Habibi E, Ezziddin S, et al. Survival after 131I-labeled lipiodol therapy for hepatocellular carcinoma. A single-center study based on a long-term follow-up. Nuklearmedizin Nucl Med. 2014;53:46–53.
14. Salem R, Thurston KG. Radioembolization with 90Yttrium microspheres: a state-of-the-art brachytherapy treatment for primary and secondary liver malignancies. Part 1: technical and methodologic considerations. J Vasc Intervent Radiol. 2006;17:1251–78.
15. Vente MA, Hobbelink MG, van Het Schip AD, Zonnenberg BA, Nijsen JF. Radionuclide liver cancer therapies: from concept to current clinical status. Anti Cancer Agents Med Chem. 2007;7:441–59.
16. Vente MA, Wondergem M, van der Tweel I, et al. Yttrium-90 microsphere radioembolization for the treatment of liver malignancies: a structured meta-analysis. Eur Radiol. 2009;19:951–9.
17. Welsh JS, Kennedy AS, Thomadsen B. Selective internal radiation therapy (SIRT) for liver metastases secondary to colorectal adenocarcinoma. Int J Radiat Oncol Biol Phys. 2006;66:S62–73.
18. Gulec SA, Fong Y. Yttrium 90 microsphere selective internal radiation treatment of hepatic colorectal metastases. Arch Surg. 2007;142:675–82.
19. Kennedy AS, Coldwell D, Nutting C, et al. Resin 90Y-microsphere brachytherapy for unresectable colorectal liver metastases: modern USA experience. Int J Radiat Oncol Biol Phys. 2006;65:412–25.
20. Wunderlich G, Pinkert J, Andreeff M, et al. Preparation and biodistribution of rhenium-188 labeled albumin microspheres B 20: a promising new agent for radiotherapy. Appl Radiat Isot. 2000;52:63–8.
21. Hafeli UO, Casillas S, Dietz DW, et al. Hepatic tumor radioembolization in a rat model using radioactive rhenium (186Re/188Re) glass microspheres. Int J Radiat Oncol Biol Phys. 1999;44:189–99.
22. Mantravadi RV, Spigos DG, Tan WS, Felix EL. Intraarterial yttrium 90 in the treatment of hepatic malignancy. Radiology. 1982;142:783–6.
23. Bult W, Vente MA, Zonnenberg BA, Van Het Schip AD, Nijsen JF. Microsphere radioembolization of liver malignancies: current developments. Q J Nucl Med Mol Imaging. 2009;53:325–35.
24. Giammarile F, Bodei L, Chiesa C, et al. EANM procedure guideline for the treatment of liver cancer and liver metastases with intra-arterial radioactive compounds. Eur J Nucl Med Mol Imaging. 2011;38:1393–406.
25. Avila-Rodriguez MA, Selwyn RG, Hampel JA, et al. Positron-emitting resin microspheres as surrogates of 90Y SIR-spheres: a radiolabeling and stability study. Nucl Med Biol. 2007;34:585–90.
26. Ahmadzadehfar H, Muckle M, Sabet A, et al. The significance of bremsstrahlung SPECT/CT after yttrium-90 radioembolization treatment in the prediction of extrahepatic side effects. Eur J Nucl Med Mol Imaging. 2012;39(2):309–15.
27. Wang XD, Yang RJ, Cao XC, Tan J, Li B. Dose delivery estimated by bremsstrahlung imaging and partition model correlated with response following intra-arterial radioembolization with 32P-glass microspheres for the treatment of hepatocellular carcinoma. J Gastrointest Surg. 2010;14:858–66.
28. Gates VL, Esmail AA, Marshall K, Spies S, Salem R. Internal pair production of 90Y permits hepatic localization of microspheres using routine PET: proof of concept. J Nucl Med. 2011;52:72–6.
29. Andrews JC, Walker SC, Ackermann RJ, et al. Hepatic radioembolization with yttrium-90 containing glass microspheres: preliminary results and clinical follow-up. J Nucl Med. 1994;35:1637–44.
30. Gray B. Patent application WO 02/34300 A1. Polymer based radionuclide containing particulate material. 2002.
31. Hafeli UO, Roberts WK, Pauer GJ, Kraeft SK, Macklis RM. Stability of biodegradable radioactive rhenium (re-186 and re-188) microspheres after neutron-activation. Appl Radiat Isot. 2001;54:869–79.
32. Rhodes BA, Zolle I, Buchanan JW, Wagner HN Jr. Radioactive albumin microspheres for studies of the pulmonary circulation. Radiology. 1969;92:1453–60.
33. Wang SJ, Lin WY, Chen MN, et al. Rhenium-188 microspheres: a new radiation synovectomy agent. Nucl Med Commun. 1998;19:427–33.
34. Wang SJ, Lin WY, Hsieh BT, et al. Rhenium-188 Sulphur colloid as a radiation synovectomy agent. Eur J Nucl Med. 1995;22:505–7.
35. Knapp FF Jr, Beets AL, Guhlke S, et al. Availability of rhenium-188 from the alumina-based tungsten-188/rhenium-188 generator for preparation of rhenium-188-labeled radiopharmaceuticals for cancer treatment. Anticancer Res. 1997;17:1783–95.
36. Guhlke S, Beets AL, Oetjen K, et al. Simple new method for effective concentration of 188Re solutions

from alumina-based 188W-188Re generator. J Nucl Med. 2000;41:1271–8.
37. Wunderlich G, Hartmann H, Andreeff M, Kotzerke J. A semi-automated system for concentration of rhenium-188 for radiopharmaceutical applications. Appl Radiat Isot. 2008;66:1876–80.
38. Liepe K, Brogsitter C, Leonhard J, et al. Feasibility of high activity rhenium-188-microsphere in hepatic radioembolization. Jpn J Clin Oncol. 2007;37:942–50.
39. Mumper RJ, Ryo UY, Jay M. Neutron-activated holmium-166-poly (L-lactic acid) microspheres: a potential agent for the internal radiation therapy of hepatic tumors. J Nucl Med. 1991;32:2139–43.
40. Nijsen JF, van Steenbergen MJ, Kooijman H, et al. Characterization of poly(L-lactic acid) microspheres loaded with holmium acetylacetonate. Biomaterials. 2001;22:3073–81.
41. Nijsen JF, Zonnenberg BA, Woittiez JR, et al. Holmium-166 poly lactic acid microspheres applicable for intra-arterial radionuclide therapy of hepatic malignancies: effects of preparation and neutron activation techniques. Eur J Nucl Med. 1999;26:699–704.
42. Zielhuis SW, Nijsen JF, de Roos R, et al. Production of GMP-grade radioactive holmium loaded poly(L-lactic acid) microspheres for clinical application. Int J Pharm. 2006;311:69–74.
43. Seevinck PR, Seppenwoolde JH, de Wit TC, et al. Factors affecting the sensitivity and detection limits of MRI, CT, and SPECT for multimodal diagnostic and therapeutic agents. Anti Cancer Agents Med Chem. 2007;7:317–34.
44. Nijsen JF, Seppenwoolde JH, Havenith T, et al. Liver tumors: MR imaging of radioactive holmium microspheres--phantom and rabbit study. Radiology. 2004;231:491–9.
45. van de Maat GH, Seevinck PR, Elschot M, et al. MRI-based biodistribution assessment of holmium-166 poly(L-lactic acid) microspheres after radioembolisation. Eur Radiol. 2013;23:827–35.
46. Ahmadzadehfar H, Biersack HJ, Ezziddin S. Radioembolization of liver tumors with yttrium-90 microspheres. Semin Nucl Med. 2010;40:105–21.
47. Zolle I, Janoki G. Tc-99m Albumin Macroaggregates. In: Zolle I, editor. Tc-99m pharmaceuticals Berlin. Heidelberg, New York: Springer; 2007. p. 187–93.
48. Zolle I. Tc-99m albumin microspheres. In: Zolle I, editor. Tc-99m radiopharmaceuticals. Berlin: Springer; 2007. p. 194–202.
49. Kotzerke J, Andreeff M, Wunderlich G, Wiggermann P, Zophel K. Ventilation-perfusion-lungscintigraphy using PET and 68Ga-labeled radiopharmaceuticals. Nuklearmedizin Nuclear medicine. 2010;49: 203–8.
50. Wunderlich G, Schiller E, Bergmann R, Pietzsch HJ. Comparison of the stability of Y-90-, Lu-177- and Ga-68- labeled human serum albumin microspheres (DOTA-HSAM). Nucl Med Biol. 2010;37: 861–7.
51. Goddu SM, Howell RW, Rao DV. Cellular dosimetry: absorbed fractions for monoenergetic electron and alpha particle sources and S-values for radionuclides uniformly distributed in different cell compartments. J Nucl Med. 1994;35:303–16.
52. Bloomer WD, McLaughlin WH, Lambrecht RM, et al. 211At radiocolloid therapy: further observations and comparison with radiocolloids of 32P, 165Dy, and 90Y. Int J Radiat Oncol Biol Phys. 1984;10: 341–8.
53. Larsen RH, Hoff P, Vergote IB, et al. Alpha-particle radiotherapy with 211At-labeled monodisperse polymer particles, 211At-labeled IgG proteins, and free 211At in a murine intraperitoneal tumor model. Gynecol Oncol. 1995;57:9–15.
54. Wunderlich G, Henke E, Iwe B, et al. Animal studies on the in vivo stability of 211At-labelled albumin particles. Nucl Med Commun. 1986;7:211–4.
55. Wunderlich G, Franke WG, Doberenz I, Fischer S. Two ways to establish potential at-211 radiopharmaceuticals. Anticancer Res. 1997;17:1809–13.
56. Doberenz I, Doberenz W, Wunderlich G, Franke WG, Heidelbach JG, Fischer S. Endoarterial therapy of lingual carcinoma using at-211 labeled HSA microspheres - preliminary clinical experience. NUCCompact. 1990;21:124–7.

Radioembolization

36

Caren van Roekel, Arthur J. A. T. Braat, Maarten L. J. Smits, Rutger C. G. Bruijnen, Bart de Keizer, and Marnix G. E. H. Lam

Abbreviations

^{166}Ho	Holmium-166
^{18}FDG	Fluorodeoxyglucose
^{68}Ga	Gallium-68
^{89}Y	Yttrium-89
^{90}Sr	Strontium-90
^{90}Y	Yttrium-90
^{90}Zr	Zirconium-90
^{99m}Tc-MAA	^{99m}technetium macro-accregated albumin
ADC	Apparent diffusion coefficient
AE	Adverse event
BCLC	Barcelona Clinic Liver Cancer
BED_{ave}	Biologically effective dose averaged over voxel values
Bq	Becquerel
BSA	Body surface area
CA	Cystic artery
CBCT	C-arm cone beam CT
CEA	Carcinoembryonic antigen
CHA	Common hepatic artery
CMR	Complete metabolic response
CT	Computed tomography
D	Mean absorbed dose
DCE	Dynamic contrast-enhanced
DEB-TACE	Chemoembolization with drug-eluting beads
dPET	Digital photon counting PET
DSA	Digital subtraction angiography
DWI	Diffusion-weighted imaging
EBRT	External beam radiation therapy
ECOG performance status	Eastern Cooperative Oncology Group performance status
EUBED	Equivalent uniform biologically effective dose
EUD	Equivalent uniform dose
FLR	Future liver remnant
FWHM	Full width at half maximum
G5W	Glucose 5% water
GBq	Giga Becquerel
GDA	Gastroduodenal artery
Gy	Gray
HCC	Hepatocellular carcinoma
HFA	Hepatic falciform artery
IA	Injected activity
keV	Kiloelectron volt
LHA	Left hepatic artery
LSF	Lung shunt fraction
MBq	Megabecquerel
mCRC	Metastatic colorectal carcinoma
MeV	Megaelectron volt

C. van Roekel · A. J. A. T. Braat · M. L. J. Smits
R. C. G. Bruijnen · B. de Keizer · M. G. E. H. Lam (✉)
Department of Radiology and Nuclear Medicine, University Medical Center Utrecht, Utrecht, The Netherlands
e-mail: j.vanroekel@umcutrecht.nl; a.j.a.t.braat@umcutrecht.nl; m.l.j.smits-3@umcutrecht.nl; r.bruijnen@umcutrecht.nl; b.dekeizer@umcutrecht.nl; m.lam@umcutrecht.nl

H. Ahmadzadehfar et al. (eds.), *Clinical Nuclear Medicine*,
https://doi.org/10.1007/978-3-030-39457-8_36

MIRD	Medical Internal Radiation Dose
mRECIST	Modified RECIST
MRI	Magnetic resonance imaging
MWA	Microwave ablation
NEN	Neuroendocrine neoplasm
OS	Overall survival
PERCIST	Positron emission tomography response criteria in solid tumors
PET	Positron emission tomography
PHA	Proper hepatic artery
PSI	Pound-force per square inch
PVE	Portal vein embolization
PVT	Portal vein thrombosis
RECIST	Response Evaluation Criteria In Solid Tumors
REILD	Radioembolization-induced liver disease
RGA	Right gastric artery
RHA	Right hepatic artery
SIRT	Selective internal radiation therapy
SPECT	Single-photon emission computed tomography
SUL	SUV corrected for lean body mass
SUV	Standardized uptake value
T/N ratio	Tumor-to-non-tumor ratio
TACE	Transarterial chemoembolization
TAE	Transarterial embolization
WHO	World Health Organization

36.1 Basic Principles and Indications

36.1.1 Radioembolization

Also known as selective internal radiation therapy (SIRT), radioembolization is a therapy during which radioactive microspheres are injected into the hepatic artery. A microcatheter is placed in the hepatic arterial vasculature, and millions of microspheres are administered. Hepatic malignancies are fed mainly by arterial blood, and because of preferential arterial flow, the microspheres lodge in small tumor arterioles. There, they emit high-energy β-radiation to induce cell death. In this way, the hepatic tumors are selectively irradiated, and the healthy liver tissue is relatively spared, which is a great advantage over conventional external beam radiation therapy (EBRT) [1]. Radioembolization is a fast developing field of expertise, and therefore, in this chapter, we will confine ourselves to the basics. The essential steps for radioembolization include (1) visceral angiography to map tumor-feeding vessels, embolize collateral vessels, and assess portal vein patency, (2) assessment of pulmonary and gastrointestinal shunts by intra-arterial administration of a scout dose, and (3) determination of the optimal therapeutic activity, e.g., dosimetry [2].

36.1.2 Types of Microspheres

Ideal properties of radiolabeled microparticles for sufficient intra-arterial therapy are the following [3–5]:

- The microspheres should be easily labeled and resistant to elution of the radioactive label, macrophage removal, or radiolysis.
- Uniform microsphere size (i.e., greater than microcapillary diameter of around 8 micron and small enough to lodge as distal as possible) and density comparable to that of blood are necessary to prevent settling and ensure uniform distribution.
- For efficacy, the radionuclide label must be a high-energy β-emitter with sufficient range and an intermediate half-life of a few days.
- The microspheres should be visible by PET (positron emission), SPECT (γ-emission), CT (sufficient density), or MRI (paramagnetic properties), to assess distribution.
- The microspheres can be based on polymers, polymeric resins, albumin, or inorganic materials.

Currently, three different types of radioactive microspheres are commercially available. The type of microspheres can be divided based on the embedded radioactive isotope (yttrium-90 (^{90}Y) or holmium-166 (^{166}Ho)) or microsphere material (resin, glass, or poly-L-lactic acid).

36.1.2.1 ^{90}Y Microspheres

^{90}Y is a pure (99.99%) β^--emitter that decays to stable zirconium-90 (^{90}Zr) with an average β-energy of 0.9 MeV and a half-life of 64.2 h [6, 7]. ^{90}Y can either be produced by neutron bombardment of stable yttrium-89 (^{89}Y) in a commercial reactor or by chemical separation from the parent isotope strontium-90 (^{90}Sr), a fission product of uranium [7]. The mean tissue penetration is approximately 2.5 mm, and the maximum range in tissue is 1.1 cm [8, 9]. Imaging of ^{90}Y is possible by using either the bremsstrahlung for single-photon emission computed tomography/computed tomography (SPECT/CT) [10, 11] or the emitted positrons (32 positrons per one million decays) for positron emission tomography/computed tomography (PET/CT) imaging [6].

Two commercially available ^{90}Y-labeled microspheres are currently on the market:

- Glass microspheres (TheraSphere®, BTG international Medicine).
- Resin microspheres (SIR-Spheres®, SIRTEX Medical Limited).

TheraSphere®

^{90}Y is permanently embedded in the glass. Each glass sphere has a diameter of 20–30 μm. ^{89}Y yttriumoxide is stable incorporated. For labeling, the microspheres are irradiated with neutrons in a nuclear reactor [12]. TheraSphere® has a high specific gravity and density (3.3 g/cm^3). A typical injected activity ranges from 3 to 5 million microspheres with a high specific activity of 2500 Bq/sphere. An extended shelf-life activity ranges from 5 to 10 million microspheres with a high specific activity of approximately 1250 Bq/sphere. The standard activity of TheraSphere® in water for injection is 5 GBq per patient; activities of 3 GBq up to 20 GBq are available.

SIR-Spheres®

^{90}Y is permanently embedded in an acrylic polymer resin [13]. Each resin microsphere has a diameter of 20–60 μm. The microspheres are labeled with ^{90}Y via cation-exchange with sufficiently strong binding. ^{90}Y is a decay product of ^{90}Sr obtained from a generator. SIR-Spheres® have a low specific gravity and density (1.4 g/cm^3) and a specific activity of 50 Bq/sphere. A typical injected activity ranges from 40 to 80 million microspheres. The standard activity of SIR-Spheres® is 3 GBq per patient in 5 ml water for injection.

36.1.2.2 ^{166}Ho Microspheres (QuiremSpheres®)

^{166}Ho is a high-energy beta-emitting isotope for therapeutic use and emits primary gamma photons. The maximum energy of the beta particles is 1.85 MeV (50.0%) and 1.77 MeV (48.7%) with a half-life of 26.8 h. The maximum range of emissions of the beta particles in tissue is 9 mm (mean 3.2 mm). They were developed by the University Medical Center Utrecht (the Netherlands) and are commercialized under the name QuiremSpheres® (Quirem Medical, Deventer, The Netherlands).

Just like ^{90}Y microspheres, ^{166}Ho emits an electron to reach a stable state (beta radiation). Furthermore, it emits gamma photons (81 keV, 6%), which are useful for SPECT/CT imaging [14]. ^{166}Ho is part of the metallic chemical elements known as lanthanides, which have paramagnetic properties, so magnetic resonance imaging (MRI) can also be used to image the distribution in the liver and quantify the dose in the tumors [15, 16]. ^{166}Ho microspheres decay is faster due to a shorter half-life (26.8 vs 64.2 h) but deposits less energy than ^{90}Y microspheres per decay (16 vs 49 J/GBq). This results in a higher administered activity to reach the same dose deposition. As a result, a higher dose rate is achieved.

Microspheres loaded with Ho are irradiated per patient dose in one of the predetermined neutron reactors with a suitable irradiation profile: the reactor must have a high neutron flux without being accompanied by extensive gamma heating, as this detriments the structural integrity of ^{166}Ho microspheres [17]. In the current commercially available product, the specific activity is 450 Bq/sphere with a density of 1.4 g/mL.

36.1.3 Patient Selection

Currently, radioembolization is mainly indicated in a palliative setting for unresectable, chemorefractory primary and secondary hepatic malignancies [1]. Several studies investigate(d) the role of radioembolization combined with systemic therapy in the first- and second-line treatment of colorectal cancer liver metastases [18, 19].

Work-up for radioembolization includes clinical status, hematologic and biochemical status, anatomic assessment with CT/MR imaging, and, when appropriate, molecular imaging with SPECT/CT or PET/CT. Indications and contraindications for radioembolization are listed in Table 36.1, according to Braat et al. [1]. Since a higher age has no influence on prognosis, age is not a contraindication [20]. In patients with hepatocellular carcinoma (HCC), radioembolization is reserved for patients with intermediate and early advanced disease stages (with Barcelona Clinic Liver Cancer [BCLC] stage B–C, liver-dominant disease, Eastern Cooperative Oncology Group [ECOG] status 1–2, and a portal vein thrombosis [PVT]). Patients with a Child-Pugh score > B7 and a main portal vein tumor thrombus tend to have a limited potential survival benefit after radioembolization; thus patient selection should be done carefully [1]. It should be noted that, as clinical experience accumulates over the years, indications and contraindications may change over time.

36.2 Work-Up

36.2.1 Clinical Investigations

During clinical investigation, a detailed medical history of the patient should be obtained. Previous treatments, current use of medication, chronic diseases, allergies, and recent periods of acute illness should be recorded. Also, the performance status (as defined by the World Health Organization(WHO)/ECOG [21]) should be defined: 0, asymptomatic; 1, symptomatic but completely ambulatory; 2, symptomatic and < 50% of time in bed; 3, symptomatic and > 50% of time in bed but not bedbound; 4, bedbound; and 5, dead. A performance status >2 is considered an exclusion criterion for radioembolization.

Table 36.1 Common indications and relative and absolute contraindications for radioembolization

Indication	Relative contraindication	Absolute contraindication
Disease not amenable to surgical resection, liver transplantation, or curative ablative strategies	Portal vein thrombosis of main branch (no contraindication in HCC)	Extensive and untreated portal hypertension
Disease not amenable to or refractory to chemotherapeutic alternatives, or patient not willing to receive these alternatives	Abnormalities of bile ducts or stents; exceptions: Papillotomy and cholecystectomy	Life expectancy <3 months
Compensated or early decompensated liver cirrhosis (child-Pugh ≤B7)	Serum bilirubin >34.2 μmol/L (2 mg/dL)	Active hepatitis
Performance state (ECOG) ≤2	Leukocytes $<2 \times 10^9$/L or platelet count $<50 \times 10^9$/L	
Liver-only or liver-dominant disease	Glomerular filtration rate <35 mL/min	Uncorrectable gastrointestinal microsphere deposition; expected lung dose >30 Gy (or 50 Gy cumulative)
Preoperative indications, such as downstaging before surgery or the inducement of contralateral hypertrophy before surgery	INR (internationalized normalized ratio) >1.5	Active use of antiangiogenic agents (bevacizumab, aflibercept)
	Celiac axis and superior mesenteric artery occluded	Occluded intrahepatic arterial network
	Interval since last dose of systemic therapy <4 weeks	

36.2.2 Laboratory Investigations

The laboratory investigations are needed to assess hepatobiliary function (aspartate aminotransferase, alanine aminotransferase, alkaline phosphatase, gamma-glutamyl transferase, total bilirubin, lactate dehydrogenase, and albumin), renal function (creatinine, estimated glomerular filtration ratio), hematological function (white cell count, hemoglobin, and hematocrit), and coagulation status (internationalized normalized ratio, thrombin time, prothrombin time, activated partial thromboplastin time, and platelet count).

36.2.3 Imaging

Before treatment, it is essential to perform cross-sectional imaging of the patient, to identify all sites of (metastatic) disease, and to assess the vascular anatomy. For this purpose, various imaging modalities can be used.

36.2.3.1 Liver CT/MRI and ^{18}FDG-PET

In general, three-phase CT images are made: late arterial phase for the detection of hypervascular tumors, a portal venous phase for the detection of hypovascular tumors, and a late venous phase for the detection of washout [22]. An early arterial phase may be preferable for vascular evaluation in the work-up for radioembolization. Compared to the late arterial phase, the contrast-to-noise ratio of the hepatic artery relative to the portal vein is higher in this early arterial phase [23]. MRI is superior to CT in terms of soft tissue contrast, but inferior regarding the detection of small arteries, due to the higher resolution of CT. Dynamic contrast-enhanced sequences can be used to assess tumor hypervascularity and washout in a large number of phases. Diffusion-weighted and T2-weighted imaging provide options for high-sensitivity tumor detection.

The added value of ^{18}FDG-PET-imaging in the work-up for radioembolization is widely accepted. The most important benefit in the work-up is the visualization of extrahepatic disease. The study of Rosenbaum et al. found a change of management in 17% of patients with metastatic colorectal carcinoma, based on imaging with ^{18}FDG-PET [24]. Metastases from uveal melanoma, breast cancer, and colorectal carcinoma are generally FDG-avid. HCC, however, accumulates FDG to varying degrees, limiting the sensitivity of PET for primary tumors [25]. Despite this lower sensitivity, the studies of Nagaoka et al. and Cho et al. show that ^{18}FDG-PET does have a role in initial staging of hepatocellular carcinoma [26, 27]. Well-differentiated HCC lesions show very little uptake on ^{18}FDG-PET imaging, whereas poorly differentiated HCCs show much more uptake. Park et al. reported that patients with ^{18}FDG-positive tumors have lower survival compared to patients with ^{18}FDG-negative tumors [28]. Thus, ^{18}FDG-PET may be useful for characterization of cancer biology [29].

Over 90% of gastroenteropancreatic neuroendocrine tumors have high concentrations of somatostatin receptors. A 68-gallium-labeled somatostatin receptor analog (i.e., DOTATATE/DOTATOC/DOTANOC) PET/CT is the most sensitive imaging modality to detect neuroendocrine tumors and metastases [30, 31].

36.2.3.2 Vascular Anatomy

The functional anatomy of the liver is based on the branching pattern of the portal vein. According to the Couinaud model of segmental anatomy, eight liver segments can be distinguished with a distinct vascularization and biliary drainage (Fig. 36.1).

The standard arterial anatomy of the adult liver is described as a common hepatic artery (CHA) originating from a celiac trifurcation that gives off the gastroduodenal artery branch (GDA) and then continues as the proper hepatic artery (PHA). The PHA then splits into the left hepatic artery (LHA), vascularizing segments 2–4, and the right hepatic artery (RHA), vascularizing segments 5–8. However, in as much as 21–45% of patients, there are anatomic variants of the hepatic arterial configuration [32–35]. The vascularization of the caudate lobe (segment 1 according to Couinaud) is particularly varied, with a range of 1–5 arteries supplying

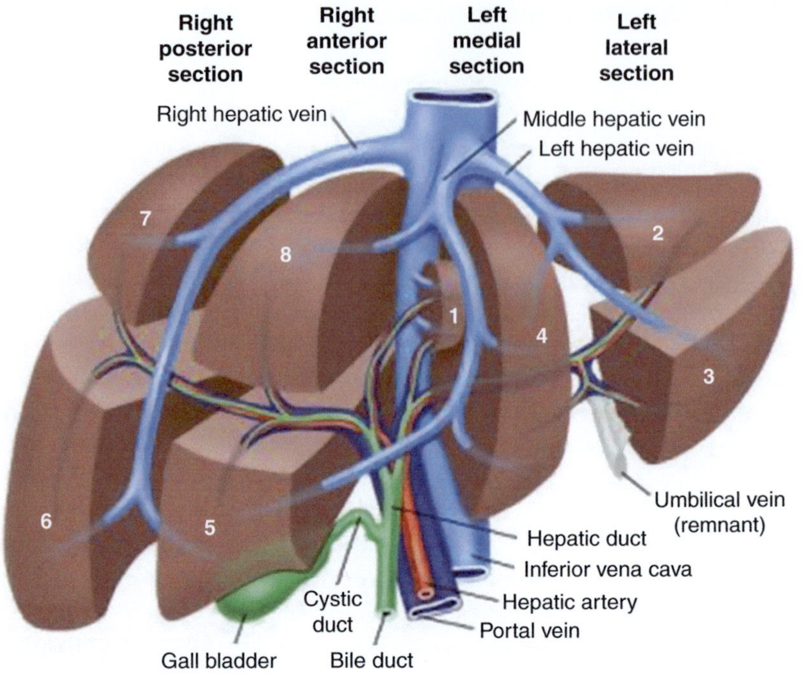

Fig. 36.1 Segmental hepatic anatomy according to Couinaud

this lobe. Most often, this segment is supplied by two branches, originating from the RHA and LHA. Although resection of caudate lobe tumors is associated with high complication and mortality rates and techniques such as radiofrequency ablation (RFA) are hindered by the nearby large vessels, radioembolization is a good alternative for treatment of caudate lobe tumors [36]. Van den Hoven et al. described as many as 16 different hepatic arterial segmental vascularization patterns, differing by the presence of accessory or replaced hepatic arteries, their respective vascular territory, and the origin of the artery vascularizing liver segment 4 [37]. An accessory hepatic artery is an aberrant hepatic artery that vascularizes the left (segment 2) or right hemiliver partially (any segments), existing in addition to a normally derived LHA and RHA. A replaced hepatic artery is an (aberrant) hepatic artery with a different origin (not the PHA) that vascularizes the left (segments 2–3 or segments 2–4) or right hemiliver (segments 5–8). Timely assessment of the anatomy enables the establishment of a personalized treatment strategy ahead of time, including coil embolization of aberrant arteries, planning the number of injection positions and pretreatment activity calculation [37, 38]. It is important to localize the segment 4 artery: it can be decided to use the segment 4 artery as a separate site of administration, include it in a more proximal injection position, or coil embolize it to induce intrahepatic redistribution of blood flow [39, 40]. Knowledge of the location of the segment 4 artery can also be used in pretreatment activity calculation and avoidance of over- or underdosing of segment 4 [23].

36.3 Preparatory Angiography and Intraprocedural Imaging

Before treatment, a preparatory angiography is performed for several reasons: (1) to map the arterial anatomy, (2) to assess the necessity of coil embolization of arterial branches, (3) to determine optimal catheter positioning, and (4) to administer a simulation scout tracer. Traditionally, a transcutaneous transfemoral approach using the Seldinger technique was mostly used to gain intra-arterial access. Recently, there has been a rapid increase in the use of the radial artery as

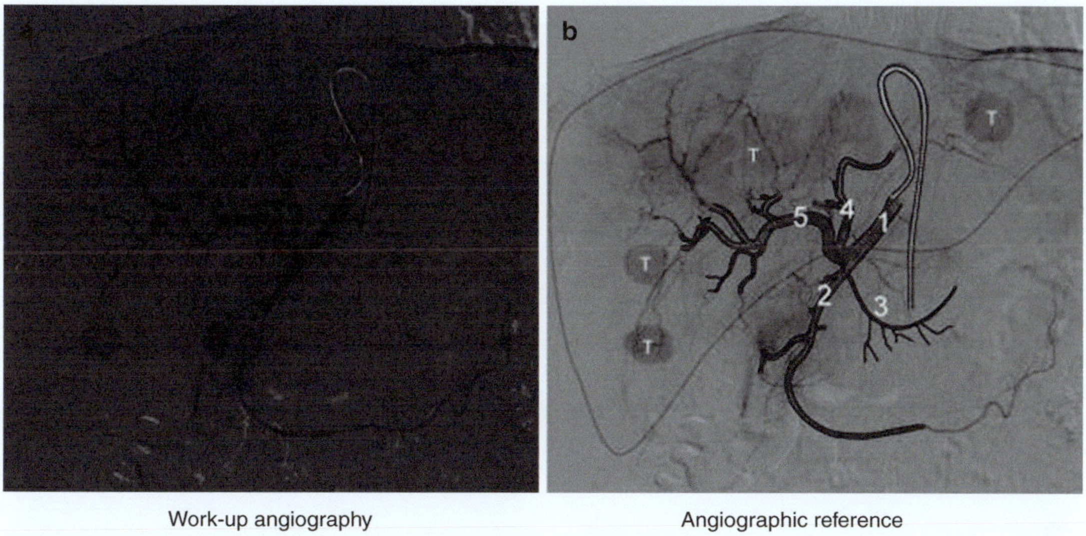

Fig. 36.2 (**a** and **b**) (**a**) shows a digital subtraction angiography with contrast injection in the common hepatic artery. (**b**) shows the angiographic reference: (1) common hepatic artery, (2) gastroduodenal artery, (3) right gastric artery, (4) left hepatic artery, (5) right hepatic artery. (Image reproduced from angiofellow.com, with permission from M. Smits)

access site. Bishay et al. found that the transradial approach is a safe and feasible access option for radioembolization and that it is associated with a low complication rate [41]. After securing the access site, a pre-shaped catheter is used to enter the source of the hepatic arterial vasculature (usually the celiac axis). A standard end-hole microcatheter is advanced over an atraumatic microguidewire for further selectively catheterization (Fig. 36.2).

36.3.1 Intraprocedural Imaging

During angiography, digital subtraction angiography (DSA) is performed (Fig. 36.3). DSA provides two-dimensional images of the vasculature at a high spatial resolution. Moreover, it is possible to acquire cinematic DSA images during high-rate contrast administration with a power injector. The study of Theysohn et al. shows that with DSA as much as 6.5% of extrahepatic shunt vessels is missed, leading to possible extrahepatic deposition of the microspheres. Therefore, other imaging modalities are needed in the work-up for radioembolization [42].

Cone beam computed tomography (CBCT) is a relatively new imaging modality that has been integrated into the angiography suite and that provides 3D images. CBCT is based on the rotational movement of a C-arm equipped with a flat panel detector around the patient [43]. It can be used to acquire, reconstruct, and display 3D images of selective contrast-enhanced vessels and the surrounding soft tissue. During radioembolization, CBCT is used to map the hepatic arterial anatomy, to identify extrahepatic branches, and to rule out extrahepatic shunting or non-perfusion of a target volume [44]. There are various CBCT protocols. The CBCT acquisitions in the liver are mostly obtained following intravascular contrast administration through a catheter that is placed in the vessel of interest. Several types of 3D images can be obtained: unenhanced, angiographic, and images of the liver parenchyma during arterial, portal venous, and delayed phases [43]. Van den Hoven et al. developed an acquisition protocol for CBCT imaging that provides a combination of these images. In their study, a continuous infusion of contrast agent, a variable scan delay based on the time to parenchymal enhancement on DSA, and a 10-s

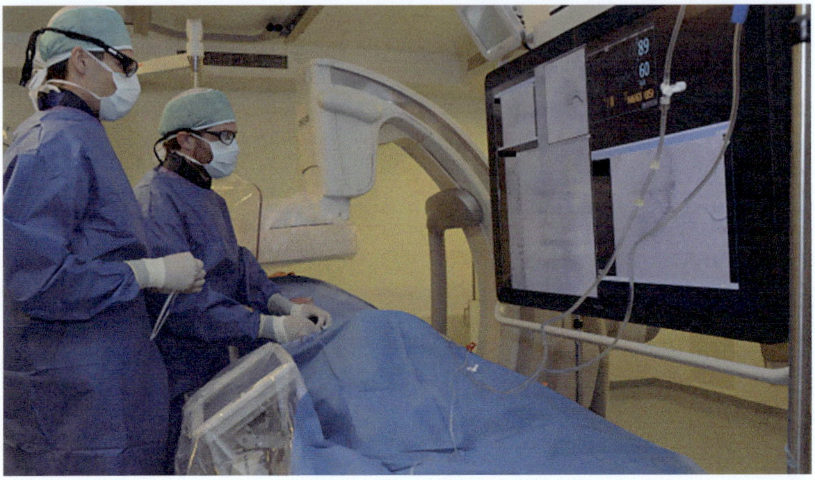

Fig. 36.3 Work-up procedure in the angiography suite. (Image reproduced from angiofellow.com, with permission from M. Smits)

high-dose scan setting resulted in images that contain both contrast enhancement of the arterial tree and liver parenchyma. They also show gastrointestinal shunting and provide sufficient contrast between perfused and non-perfused liver territories [44]. The study of Grözinger et al. showed that the CBCT approach is superior to the angiographic determination of vascular supply of specific segments, mainly segments 1 and 4 [45]. The main limitation of CBCT is the limited field of view compared to conventional CT. Other limitations are the greater risk of motion artifacts and the increased procedural time [43].

36.3.2 Coil Embolization of Culprit Vessels

Since extrahepatic deposition of radioactive microspheres may cause serious complications, it should be assessed whether arterial branches pose a risk. The three most common culprit vessels that cause extrahepatic deposition are the gastroduodenal artery, the cystic artery, and the right gastric artery. Previously, it was advised to preventively coil embolize these arteries. However, there are quite some disadvantages to coil embolization: there is an increased radiation dose and an increase of procedure time and complexity, potential vessel damage, and complications of coil deployment. Moreover, in the time between the preparatory angiography and treatment, new collateral vessels may develop. Nowadays, most centers try to avoid coil embolization unless extrahepatic deposition of activity is found on pretreatment simulation scout dose SPECT/CT. Sometimes, a more distal injection position or the use of an antireflux catheter can provide a safe treatment procedure without the need for coil embolization [1].

36.4 Scout Dose Imaging and Pretreatment Dosimetry

36.4.1 ^{99m}Tc-MAA

Worldwide, pretreatment simulation of radioembolization with ^{90}Y is currently based on ^{99m}Tc-MAA planar imaging and SPECT/CT for assessment of extrahepatic depositions and lung shunting. MAA are biodegradable particles. Their size is not well-calibrated, estimated at between 10 and 150 μm, with 90% of the particles falling between 10 and 40 μm, and 1–2% below 15 μm [46]. Typically, between 150 and 250 MBq of ^{99m}Tc-MAA are injected into the hepatic artery for therapy simulation, with around 1.5×10^6 MAA particles [47]. As a comparison, normally around $3–5 \times 10^6$ spheres for 3 GBq of glass microspheres are injected and around $40–80 \times 10^6$ spheres for 1.5 GBq of resin microspheres.

The size, density, and number of injected particles differ between ^{99m}Tc-MAA particles and glass/resin microspheres (Fig. 36.4). Thus far, ^{99m}Tc-MAA particles are the only particles used for the pretreatment simulation of radioembolization with ^{90}Y, but there are controversies regarding the predictive value. Wondergem et al. studied the relation between pretreatment ^{99m}Tc-MAA distribution and posttreatment ^{90}Y distribution. They found a difference of >10% in 68% of the hepatic segments analyzed [48]. Haste et al. have evaluated the value of ^{99m}Tc-MAA in predicting subsequent ^{90}Y glass microspheres distribution in patients with hepatocellular carcinoma. ^{99m}Tc-MAA was a poor surrogate to quantitatively predict the tumor absorbed dose of ^{90}Y, but there was a correlation between ^{99m}Tc-MAA and ^{90}Y in the distribution in normal liver tissue [49]. Ilhan et al. analyzed the predictive value of ^{99m}Tc-MAA SPECT for radioembolization with ^{90}Y resin microspheres, by comparing uptake on pretherapeutic ^{99m}Tc-MAA SPECT with uptake on posttherapeutic ^{90}Y bremsstrahlung SPECT. They analyzed 502 patients who underwent radioembolization for primary and secondary liver tumors. They found a significant but quite low correlation between the ^{99m}Tc-MAA and ^{90}Y-microsphere tumor-to-background ratio [50]. Another study, however, evaluated the agreement between ^{99m}Tc-MAA SPECT/CT-based predictive dosimetry and posttreatment ^{90}Y PET/CT-based dosimetry in patients with hepatocellular carcinoma, treated with both glass and resin spheres. They found that predictive dosimetry based on ^{99m}Tc-MAA SPECT/CT provides good estimates of absorbed doses as calculated on posttreatment ^{90}Y PET/CT, for tumor and non-tumor tissues [51]. However, the majority of the treatments analyzed (25/27) was selective, which may have led to more positive results and a better correlation between ^{99m}Tc-MAA and ^{90}Y. Not only the size, density, and number of the injected particles play a role in the different distributions of ^{99m}Tc-MAA and ^{90}Y-microspheres. Other confounding factors are tumor type, tumor vascularization, tumor size, prior therapy, ^{99m}Tc-MAA injection parameters, and angiographic considerations such as catheter position and vasoactive arterial status. There are large differences in ^{99m}Tc-MAA uptake between hepatocellular carcinomas that are generally large and hypervascular and liver metastases such as colorectal cancer liver metastases, which are often smaller and hypovascular. Prior therapy can also have an influence, because it can induce arterial disorders and weaknesses. There is no established protocol for the injection of ^{99m}Tc-MAA, but guidelines indicate that the injection time should be 20–30 s.

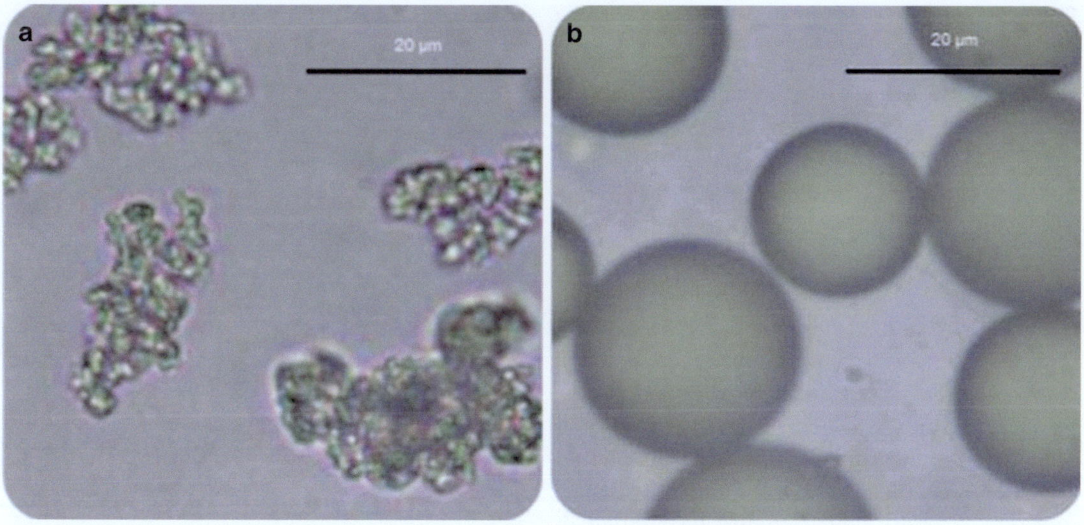

Fig. 36.4 (**a**) Microscopic image of ^{99m}Tc-MAA particles. (**b**) Microscopic image of ^{90}Y-microspheres

This is quite comparable to a bolus injection, which is significantly different from the pulsing method used during the actual administration of resin- and ^{166}Ho-microspheres.

The most important factor is the injection position of the catheter during ^{99m}Tc-MAA infusion and ^{90}Y-microsphere infusion. This catheter position should be exactly the same, with the same distance to bifurcations and the same orientation in the vascular lumen [48]. Another important factor is the vasoactive status of the hepatic arteries at the time of injection, since vasospasm may occur during radioembolization procedures and may impact the distribution of microspheres [46].

Because of the discrepancies between ^{99m}Tc-MAA and ^{90}Y-microsphere distribution, several alternatives to ^{99m}Tc-MAA are currently under investigation [52].

36.4.2 ^{166}Ho Scout Dose

When planning radioembolization with ^{166}Ho, a small batch of ^{166}Ho-microspheres with limited radioactivity (200–250 MBq) can be used as a scout dose, instead of ^{99m}Tc-MAA. This ^{166}Ho scout dose is sufficient to be visualized and quantified on SPECT imaging, but limited enough not to cause tissue damage in case of shunting to the gastrointestinal organs or the lungs. To prevent embolization of the arteries before treatment, only 60 mg is administered, whereas a treatment dose consists of 540–600 mg of microspheres. Because the same particles are used, lung shunting can be estimated more accurately [53]. The safety of the ^{166}Ho scout dose has been established recently by Braat et al. [54].

36.4.3 Lung Shunt Calculation

Lung shunting is caused by arteriovenous anastomoses or shunts in the liver parenchyma or in a tumor. Excessive activity deposition in the lungs can result in radiation pneumonitis after radioembolization. Based on experience with external beam radiation therapy (EBRT), the highest tolerable lung shunt was defined as 30 Gy after a single treatment and a cumulative dose of 50 Gy after repeated treatments [1].

The lung shunt fraction (LSF) is defined as [2, 46]:

$$\text{LSF} = \frac{\sqrt{\text{lungs}_{\text{anterior}} * \text{lungs}_{\text{posterior}}}}{\sqrt{\text{lungs}_{\text{anterior}} * \text{lungs}_{\text{posterior}}}) + \sqrt{\text{liver}_{\text{anterior}} * \text{liver}_{\text{posterior}}}}$$

Planar imaging can be used to calculate the lung shunt after administration of ^{99m}Tc-MAA (Fig. 36.5). However, Elschot et al. and Yu et al. have demonstrated that the lung absorbed doses are significantly overestimated by pretreatment ^{99m}Tc-MAA imaging [53, 55].

There are several factors that may have an influence on LSF calculation. LSF estimation without attenuation correction gives a large overestimation with respect to attenuation-corrected evaluations. There is reduced photon attenuation in the lungs compared to the photon attenuation in the abdomen. Another factor is scatter correction, which should be applied in order to avoid overestimations of the

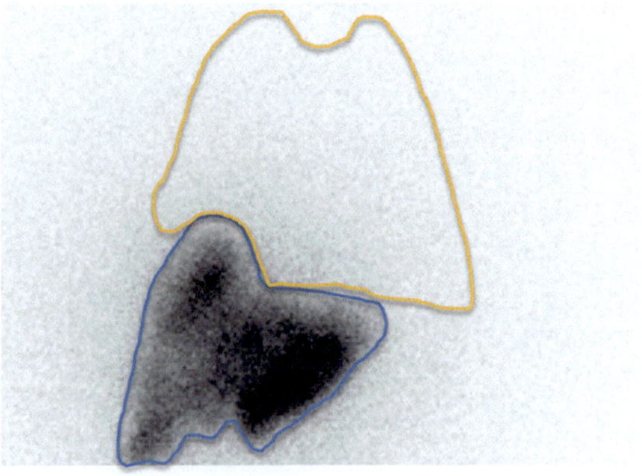

Fig. 36.5 Figure shows a planar scan with lung and liver ROIs to calculate lung shunt. In this example, there was visually no lung shunt and calculation showed 9%

LSF. Moreover, ^{99m}Tc-MAA degrades after several hours, which increases the LSF. Therefore, it is important to perform the image acquisition as soon as possible after administration of ^{99m}Tc-MAA [2, 46]. The studies of Yu et al. and Kao et al. proved that SPECT/CT leads to more accurate calculation of lung shunt absorbed dose than planar imaging [55, 56].

However, lung shunting differs significantly between different tumor types. Gaba et al. published a study of 141 patients with primary and secondary hepatic malignancies who underwent radioembolization. The LSF was calculated for every patient and LSF > 20% occurred much more often in HCC patients than in patients with other tumor types (14% versus 3%). In HCC patients, a high LSF was associated with infiltrative morphologic structure, tumor burden >50%, portal vein invasion, and arterioportal shunting. In other tumor types, such as colorectal carcinoma metastases, neuroendocrine tumors, and cholangiocarcinomas, a larger tumor size and greater tumor burden were associated with lung shunting [57]. In patients with these factors, care should be taken to avoid deposition of radioactive microspheres in the lungs.

36.4.4 Extrahepatic Activity and Non-tumor Dose in the Liver

Pretreatment simulation with ^{99m}Tc-MAA is useful not only to establish the LSF but also to give an impression of the total absorbed radiation dose in the healthy liver parenchyma: the non-tumor dose. It is widely known that with an increasing non-tumor dose, the risk of complications such as radioembolization-induced liver disease (REILD) is higher, but the maximum tolerable non-tumor dose is not well established. It is dependent on the type of tumor, the condition of the liver, prior treatments (e.g., bevacizumab), and the distribution of radiation within the non-tumor volume. With radioembolization, the absorbed dose in the liver is never uniform, which makes higher average absorbed doses tolerable. A non-tumor dose limit of <70 Gy in normal liver tissue and a non-tumor dose limit of <50 Gy in cirrhotic livers is proposed, but this is highly dependent on microspheres used and the number of microspheres administered [1, 46]. Thresholds for an acceptable average normal liver absorbed dose have yet to be established.

36.4.5 Pretreatment Dosimetry

Different methods for pretreatment activity calculations for the different types of microspheres have been proposed. The first method that was used was the so-called "empirical" method, based on the tumor burden. The used activity ranged between 2 and 3 GBq. This method was abandoned because it was associated with unacceptable clinical toxicity [58].

For resin microspheres, the body surface area (BSA) method is mostly used. This method adjusts the prescribed activity for the patient's BSA and the fractional tumor burden. The formula for BSA in square meter is:

$$\text{BSA} = 0.2024 * \text{height}(\text{m})^{0.725} * \text{weight}(\text{kg})^{0.425}$$

The formula for the injected activity (IA) is:

$$\text{IA}_{(\text{GBq})} = (\text{BSA} - 0{,}2) + \frac{\text{tumor volume}}{(\text{tumor volume} + \text{liver volume})}[1,2]$$

The prescribed activity is reduced in case of lung shunting, depending on the percentage of lung shunting: 20% activity reduction with 10–15% LSF, 40% activity reduction with 15–20% LSF, and no treatment with >20% LSF [52]. The BSA method assumes a correlation between BSA and liver weight. However, this is not necessarily true and may result in an undertreatment of small patients with large livers and an overtreatment of large patients with small livers. Another limitation of this method is that it does not take into account the degree of tumor uptake [1, 2].

For glass microspheres, Salem et al. developed the Medical Internal Radiation Dose (MIRD) method [59–61]. With this method, the prescribed activity is determined by calculating the activity required to achieve a desired absorbed dose (between 80 and 150 Gy). The MIRD method assumes a homogenous intrahepatic microsphere distribution throughout the treated portion of the liver and an assumed yield of 50 Gy per GBq ^{90}Y per kilogram of liver tissue. This method also does not take into account the degree of tumor uptake, nor does it account for fractional or total tumor burden. The formula for the IA is:

$$\mathrm{IA}_{(\mathrm{GBq})} = \frac{\left(\text{Desired average absorbed dose}(\mathrm{Gy}) * M_{\mathrm{Target}}(\mathrm{kg})\right)}{50(\mathrm{J}/\mathrm{GBq})}$$

where M_{Target} is the mass of the target volume. The MIRD method is especially useful for radiation segmentectomy, where a large absorbed dose (e.g., 200 Gy) is administered to a limited target volume in order to ablate both the tumorous and non-tumorous liver tissue within that target volume while sparing the untreated part of the liver [52].

For ^{166}Ho, a method comparable to the MIRD method for ^{90}Y is currently used. Based on findings of the HEPAR I trial, a phase I dose escalation study, a maximum tolerable absorbed dose for the whole liver is set at 60 Gy [62]. The absorbed dose in Gy delivered by 1 GBq in 1 kg tissue is 15.87 Gy for ^{166}Ho, under the assumption of homogenous distribution in the target volume and absorption of all energy within that volume. The formula for the IA is:

$$\mathrm{IA}_{(\mathrm{MBq})} = \text{liver weight}(\mathrm{kg}) * 3780(\mathrm{MBq}/\mathrm{kg})$$

Another method, which can be used for pretreatment dosimetry for both resin and glass spheres, is the partition model. In general, the tumor and healthy liver tissue are delineated on anatomical imaging modalities. The anticipated activity in these delineated compartments is calculated on ^{99m}Tc-MAA SPECT/CT. The tumor to non-tumor (T/N) ratio on MAA is calculated as:

$$\frac{T}{N} = \frac{\mathrm{Activity}_{\mathrm{tumor}}(\mathrm{GBq}) / \mathrm{Mass}_{\mathrm{tumor}}(\mathrm{kg})}{\mathrm{Activity}_{\mathrm{liver}}(\mathrm{Gbq}) / \mathrm{Mass}_{\mathrm{liver}}(\mathrm{kg})}$$

The formula for the IA is:

$$A(\mathrm{GBq}) = \frac{\mathrm{Dose}(\mathrm{Gy}) * \left(\left[\frac{T}{N} * \mathrm{Mass}_{\mathrm{tumor}}(\mathrm{kg})\right] + \mathrm{Mass}_{\mathrm{tumor}}(\mathrm{kg})\right)}{49{,}670 * (1 - \text{lung shunt fraction})}$$

The partition method does correct for the difference in tumor and non-tumor dose. Limitations of this model are that it is more time-consuming and that it is problematic in patients with ill-defined tumors [1, 52]. Furthermore, neither the acceptable absorbed dose in the healthy liver nor the effective absorbed tumor dose is defined yet.

Recently, Chiesa et al. developed a method for activity calculation that does take nonuniformity of the absorbed dose into account. In a cohort of 52 patients with HCC, treated with glass microspheres, they studied lesion and parenchymal absorbed dose at voxel level on ^{99m}Tc-MAA SPECT images. The biodistribution of the ^{99m}Tc-MAA and ^{90}Y-microspheres was assumed to be identical. The degree of agreement between clinical observations of response and several dosimetric variables was compared. A dosimetric variable that accounts for both non-uniformity of absorbed dose deposition and the dose-rate effect was the best variable to predict response of a lesion. The 50% tumor control probability was different for small (<10 cc) and large (>10 cc) lesions, with much higher absorbed doses needed for larger lesions, which weakens the predictive power of planning on lesions. There was a high tolerance of the healthy liver tissue to glass microspheres. The best prediction method was found to be the parenchymal mean dose, with a limit of 75 Gy at a 15% toxicity risk [63]. Drawbacks of a voxel-based dosimetry approach can be divided in physical factors, such as attenuation, scatter, noise, and partial-volume effects, and in clinical factors, such as respiration. Corrections for these factors should be implemented in the reconstruction protocol [64].

36.5 Treatment

36.5.1 Treatment Angiography

Usually, within 2 weeks after the scout procedure, the treatment procedure takes place. Similar to the angiography procedure for the scout dose administration, intra-arterial access is obtained via the femoral artery. Before infusion of the microspheres, the vascular tree should be investigated carefully. The exact same injection position as during the scout procedure should be chosen to avoid a different intrahepatic distribution. Wondergem et al. found a relative difference of >30% in absorbed activity per milliliter in as many as 24 of 68 analyzed segments, due to a difference in injection position of >5 mm [48]. It is important to make sure that no new hepaticoenteric collaterals have been recruited in the time interval between the scout and therapy procedures. In a study of 122 patients with primary and metastatic hepatic tumors, Abdelmaksoud et al. investigated the development of new hepatoenteric collaterals. These patients underwent a preparatory angiography before treatment with radioembolization, during which hepaticoenteric collaterals were embolized. At the time of radioembolization, new collaterals had developed in 42 patients (34.4%), requiring adjunctive embolization. The mean time interval between the preparatory and treatment angiography in this subgroup was 14.7 days (range 1–72) [40]. In 2007, one of the official recommendations of the radioembolization brachytherapy oncology consortium was that "all extrahepatic vessels originating from the hepatic arteries that supply the gastrointestinal tract should, under most circumstances, be embolized to exclude extrahepatic deposition of the ^{90}Y microspheres" [65]. However, the rapid development of new hepatico-enteric collaterals opposes this so-called skeletonization and brings it benefit into question. In a review, Borggreve et al. looked into the evidence supporting prophylactic embolization. They found that refraining from embolization of the GDA, right gastric artery (RGA), and the cystic artery (CA) is justified when the catheter tip can be placed distal to the origin of these arteries [66]. It is recommended to use a more distal injection position, already during the scout procedure.

36.5.2 Medication

During treatment, it is common practice to monitor vital signs (blood pressure, pulse, and saturation). Recently, a large study was published on adjuvant medications that improve survival after locoregional therapy, such as radioembolization. The medications were taken at the time of embolization. Beta-blockers and aspirin were associated with improved survival in HCC patients. These medications were not associated with improved survival when taken by patients with neuroendocrine tumors or colorectal cancer liver metastases [67]. The authors provided the following hypotheses for the mechanisms behind this survival benefit: (1) aspirin inhibits hypoxia-induced angiogenesis, which might prevent radioembolization-induced ischemia from promoting angiogenesis and growth of the residual viable tumor. It also inhibits glycolysis, which may make tumor cells less likely to survive radioembolization-induced ischemia. Furthermore, aspirin is a COX inhibitor, and COX-2 inhibition promotes an antitumor immune response. (2) Beta-blockers decrease blood flow in the portal vein, which is associated with improved response after radioembolization of colorectal cancer liver metastases. Moreover, beta-blockers can reduce stress hormone-mediated invasion of tumor cells [67].

Besides beta-blockers and aspirin, proton-pump inhibitors are often given during the first week before and continued up to a month after treatment, as prophylaxis for gastrointestinal ulcer formation. Heparin, according to local guidelines in interventional radiology, is given for thrombosis prophylaxis during treatment. If a vasospasm occurs during the procedure, it is indicated to give a vasodilator intra-arterially.

Neuroendocrine tumors can rapidly release a large amount of vasoactive substances after radioembolization. This may lead to a carcinoid crisis with flushing, hypertension, and tachycardia, followed by hypotension and possibly death [68]. To prevent a carcinoid crisis, somatostatin analog prophylaxis intravenously may be indicated.

When patients are in pain, intravenous analgesia should be considered during the procedure, according to local interventional radiology guidelines.

36.5.3 Dose Administration

All three types of microspheres are provided in a vial. The administration systems are quite different from each other, but they all have two lines: one that connects the vial with the microcatheter and one through which the nuclear physician can inject a diluting solution in the vial (i.e., saline, sterile water, or 5% glucose) [9, 69, 70].

There are significant differences in administration techniques between ^{90}Y resin microspheres, ^{90}Y glass microspheres, and ^{166}Ho microspheres.

^{90}Y resin microspheres should be administered very carefully with a flow rate of no more than 5 mL per min, to allow for optimal distribution in the tumor microvasculature. The administration usually takes up to 20 min. While administrating, the interventional radiologist should check for slow flow or stasis, by administrating small aliquots of contrast fluid and microspheres alternately. When stasis occurs, the procedure should be terminated to prevent reflux [9]. It was hypothesized that sterile water, which was injected with the microspheres, caused a temporary change in the osmolality of the blood, leading to vascular endothelial injury and vasospasm, causing stasis. Two studies were published regarding the replacement of sterile water with glucose 5% water (G5W). Ahmadzadehfar et al. report about 78 patients treated with resin microspheres. Fifty procedures were performed with sterile water, and 54 procedures were performed with G5W. A significantly higher proportion of the calculated activity was administered with G5W (96.1% versus 77.4%), and there was a significantly lower incidence of stasis (28% versus 11%) and significantly less abdominal pain during the procedure (1.8% versus 44%) [70]. The findings of Paprottka et al. confirm the positive effects of using G5W as a diluting solution, as they also showed a significantly reduced need for periprocedural analgesia [71]. ^{90}Y glass microspheres are less prone to stasis because the number of microspheres is much lower. Administration of ^{90}Y glass microspheres is much faster, because they are injected in one bolus [69]. To prevent high injection pressures, a small pressure relief valve is included in the administration set, limiting the injection pressure to 30 pound-force per square inch (PSI) [69].

^{166}Ho microspheres are administered in the same way as ^{90}Y resin microspheres, carefully with a low flow rate in a pulsatile manner, to avoid stasis and reflux [72]. However, simultaneous injection with a diluted contrast agent is possible.

36.5.4 Possible Side Effects and Adverse Events

In the literature, controversy exists on the term "toxicity" after radioembolization. It is graded in multiple ways on diverse time points after treatment. To compare data on toxicity, it is essential this is graded according to the same definition. Most often, side effects after treatment are scored according to the Common Terminology Criteria for Adverse Events (CTCAE) version 4.0. Adverse events (AEs) are defined as "any unfavorable and unintended sign, symptom, or disease temporally associated with the use of a medical treatment or procedure that may or may not be considered related to the medical treatment or procedure." Five grades are used to classify the adverse events, referring to the severity of the AEs, with grade 1 being mild and grade 5 indicating death related to the AE [73].

Hepatotoxicity is the most important adverse event after radioembolization, but a clear definition is often lacking. Braat et al. proposed the following grading for hepatotoxicity after radioembolization [74]:

- Grade 0: no liver toxicity (i.e., no CTCAE toxicity grade changes over baseline).
- Grade 1: minor liver toxicity, limited to increased aspartate aminotransferase, alanine aminotransferase, alkaline phosphatase, and/or gamma-glutamyl transpeptidase levels (all not exceedingly newly developed grade 1 CTCAE toxicity).
- Grade 2: moderate liver toxicity, with a self-limiting course. No medical intervention necessary.
- Grade 3: REILD, manageable with noninvasive treatments such as diuretics, ursodeoxycholic acid, and steroids.
- Grade 4: REILD necessitating invasive medical treatment such as paracentesis, transfusions, hemodialysis, or a transjugular intrahepatic portosystemic shunt.
- Grade 5: fatal REILD.

The most frequent side effect of radioembolization is the post-embolization syndrome, which consists of fatigue, nausea, vomiting, anorexia, fever, and abdominal pain. These effects are usually mild and self-limiting within 2 weeks. The post-embolization syndrome occurs in up to 55% of patients [75]. Another common side effect is a transient elevation of liver enzymes [75]. In a retrospective analysis of 58 patients with diverse hepatic malignancies, Roberson et al. found that a decreased pretreatment albumin and an elevated pretreatment INR were associated with the development of severe liver toxicity after radioembolization [76]. Gabrielson et al. evaluated toxicity after radioembolization in patients with hepatocellular carcinoma. They found that a pretreatment elevation of bilirubin and an elevation of the transaminases were associated with a higher risk of a decline in liver function after treatment [77].

Laboratory abnormalities usually go without associated clinical side effects [78]. However, when laboratory toxicities are associated with ascites, this may be a sign of a much more serious complication: radioembolization-induced liver disease (REILD) (Fig. 36.6).

REILD is usually defined as "a symptomatic post-radioembolization deterioration in the ability of the liver to maintain its (normal or preprocedural) synthetic, excretory and detoxifying functions. It is characterized by jaundice and the development of or increase in ascites, hyperbilirubinemia and hypoalbuminemia developing at least two weeks – four months after radioembolization, in the absence of tumor progression or biliary obstruction" [74]. Histopathologically, REILD is characterized by veno-occlusive disease with congestion of the central veins and sinusoids [78]. The incidence of REILD is reported to be 0–5.4%. The natural course of REILD is highly variable: it can either result in fulminant hepatic failure and death, or it can be transient and self-limiting. Reported risk factors for REILD include previous liver-directed therapies, such as chemotherapy, external beam radiation therapy (EBRT), radioembolization, and other intra-arterial therapies. Furthermore, a high absorbed dose and single-session whole liver treatment also increase the risk of hepatotoxicity [74]. Other risk factors are exposure to chemotherapy within 2 months after radioembolization, a liver volume < 1.5 L, and increased baseline bilirubin and aspartate aminotransferase [79]. Treatment options consist mainly of supportive measures, such as the reduction of ascites or pleural effusion and the avoidance of hepatotoxic drugs [74]. To reduce the excessive extravascular volume, diuretics (spironolactone 100 mg and/or furosemide 40 mg daily) can be tried. When liver function starts to decline, 10 mg/day defibrotide intravenously or oral steroids can be considered. If medical treatment is ineffective, a transjugular intrahepatic portosystemic stent-shunt (TIPS) could be placed. Based on an expert panel and literature review, prevention of REILD can be pursued by excluding patients with poor liver functional reserve (such as total bilirubin >2 mg/dL or ascites) from radioembolization.

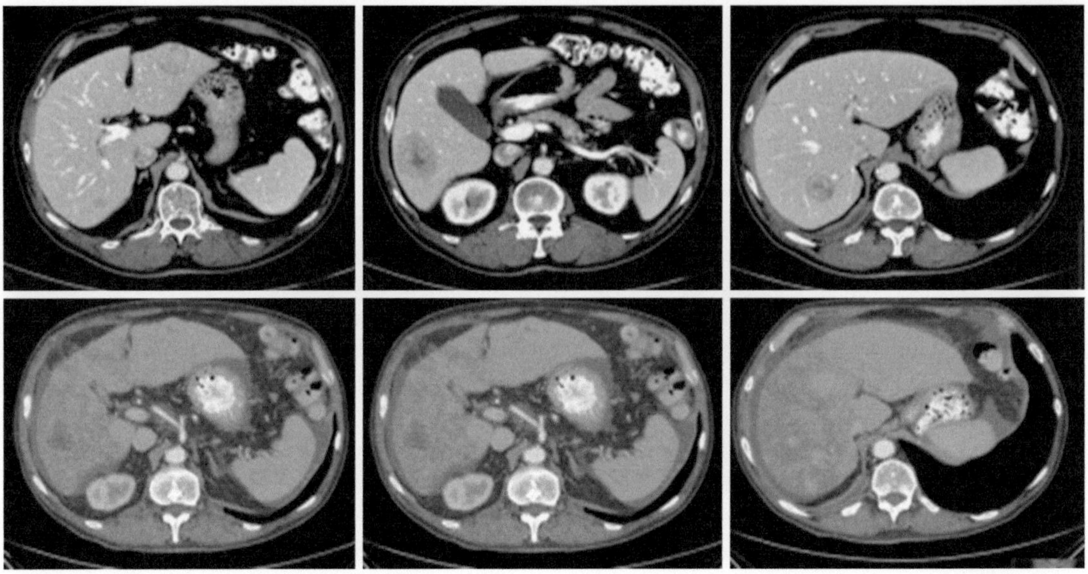

Fig. 36.6 The upper row shows contrast-enhanced CT images of a 60-year-old woman with hepatic metastases of a neuroendocrine carcinoma, before treatment with radioembolization. The lower row shows contrast-enhanced CT images after treatment with ^{166}Ho-radioembolization, with the development of REILD (impaired hepatic function and ascites)

Furthermore, it is recommended to adapt the calculated activity in patients with steatosis, steatohepatitis, hepatitis, cirrhosis, a liver volume <1.5 L, and multiple lines of prior chemotherapy. Also, sequential lobar treatment may improve liver tolerance to radioembolization [79]. Since a high absorbed dose is an important cause of hepatotoxicity, a personalized dosimetric approach, as proposed by Chiesa et al., should be implemented in clinical practice, especially in patients with known risk factors. The most vital aspect in the prevention of REILD should be the healthy-liver tissue absorbed dose. Therefore, the parenchymal mean dose should be taken into account in treatment planning [63].

Another relatively uncommon complication of radioembolization is gastrointestinal ulceration, caused by nontarget delivery of microspheres [75]. Gastrointestinal ulceration usually presents 2–6 weeks after treatment with symptoms of acute epigastric pain, nausea, vomiting, dyspepsia, and anorexia. The incidence is about 2–3%. Symptoms can last up to 10 months despite adequate treatment with proton pump inhibitors. Normally, full recovery occurs. Prevention of ulceration by using proton pump inhibitors around treatment is often advocated but lacks scientific evidence [79]. Lam et al. performed a root cause analysis to identify risk factors for the development of gastrointestinal ulceration. In their cohort of 278 treatments in 247 patients, the following risk factors were identified: stasis, proximal administration site, young age, and distal origin of the GDA. To prevent gastrointestinal ulceration, it is advised to administer microspheres exclusively distally [80]. Although much attention is paid to its prevention by calculating lung shunt, radiation pneumonitis is rarely seen. It is characterized by exertional dyspnea, dry cough, restrictive ventilator dysfunction, and bilateral lung infiltrates. The lung shunt is estimated based on the fraction of ^{99m}Tc-MAA that is deposited in the lung vasculature after the pretreatment work-up. However, Elschot et al. showed that ^{99m}Tc-MAA usually overestimates the lung shunt, with an absolute error range of 9.4–12.1 Gy [53]. The manufacturer of resin microspheres

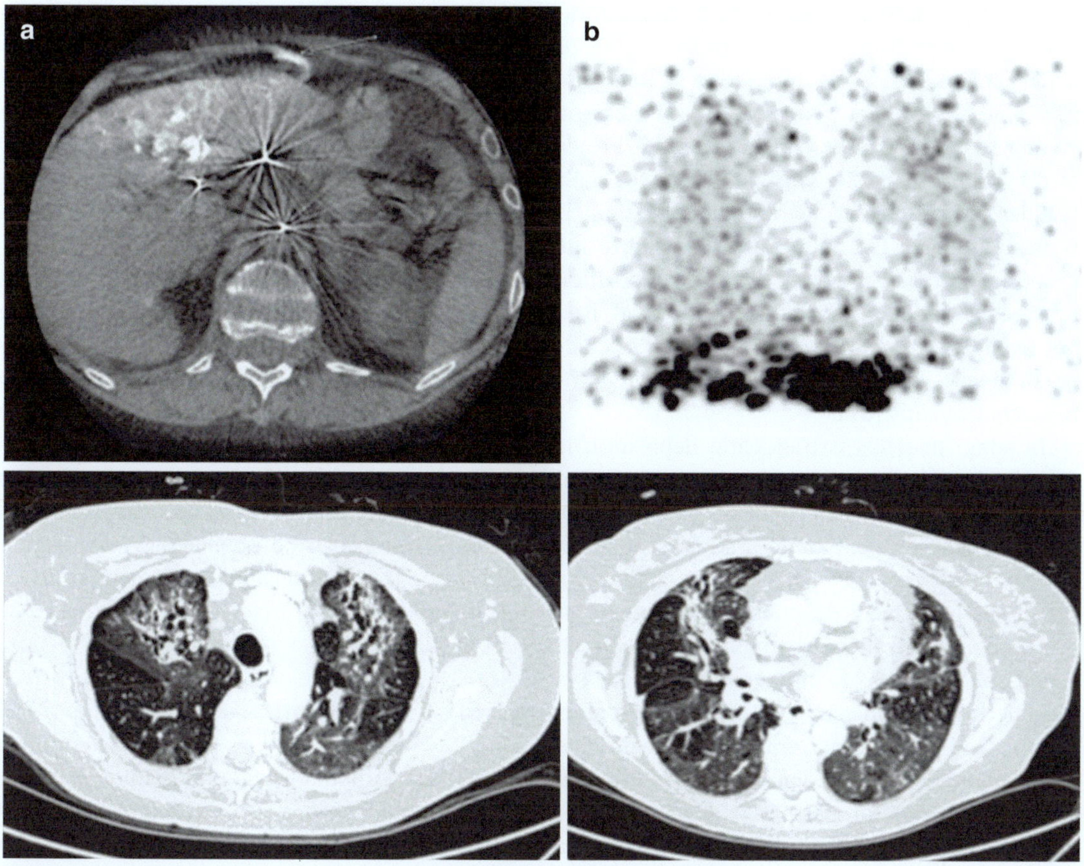

Fig. 36.7 (**a–d**) (**a**): cone beam CT of a 65-year-old woman with HCC, with arteriovenous shunt (arrow). (**b**) shows the lung shunt on ^{90}Y-PET. (**c–d**) show high-resolution CT images of the lungs with ground-glass nodularities and fibrosis

recommends dose reductions of 20%, 40%, and 100% if the LSF exceeds 10, 15, or 20% [79]. A maximum tolerated dose of 30 Gy in one treatment or 50 Gy in sequential treatments to the lungs is widely used, but due to the very low incidence of radiation pneumonitis, it is difficult to establish an endorsed threshold. Sangro et al. propose to refrain from treatment with radioembolization if the LSF is ≥15%, rather than adjusting the amount of injected activity. However, since lung shunt doses are often overestimated, this would result in withholding patients from what can be their last treatment option. Radiation pneumonitis is characterized by bilateral symmetric ill-defined patchy opacities and ground-glass nodularities on CT (Fig. 36.7a–d). Treatment consists of steroids and supportive measures [79].

Other complications that may arise are portal hypertension and biliary tree damage. Portal hypertension can develop months to years after radioembolization. Symptoms consist of an increased spleen volume and possibly gastroesophageal varices. Bile duct necrosis and strictures are often asymptomatic and seen in about 2–4% of patients [79].

Furthermore, radiation cholecystitis is occasionally reported. The incidence ranges from 0 to 7%. It is characterized by upper right quadrant abdominal pain, nausea, vomiting, malaise, and occasional fever [81]. The diagnosis is confirmed by the presence of a thickened, hyperenhanced gallbladder wall with pericholecystic fluid, intramural gas, or hydrops, seen on ultrasound, CT, or MRI. The mainstay of treatment is analgetic treatment. However, in severe cases, a cholecystectomy can be considered [79]. Prince et al. propose the following strategies for gallbladder protection during radioembolization: if possible, placing the microcatheter distal to the cystic artery or adjustment of the catheter position to alter the direction of blood flow. It is advised not to apply temporarily or permanently occluding of the cystic artery, since this can lead to ischemic cholecystitis [81].

In some patients, extrahepatic deposition is seen in the falciform ligament, due to a patent hepatic falciform artery (HFA). Theoretically, this could cause radiation dermatitis or abdominal pain. However, this is rarely seen, and only a few cases have been described. In a review of 410 radioembolization treatments, Braat et al. found only 16 cases of extrahepatic deposition in the falciform ligament. None of these patients experienced symptoms compatible with the extrahepatic deposition. These results show that there is no need for prophylactic measures or even exclusion from therapy of patients with a patent HFA [82].

36.5.5 Long-Term Hepatic Changes

Su et al. investigated the long-term hepatotoxicity after radioembolization in patients with NENs. The median follow-up time was 3.5 years. Twenty-six of 54 evaluated patients developed cirrhosis-like morphology after a median time of 1.8 years, but only 5 of them exhibited clinical symptoms that were attributable to radioembolization. Splenic volume increased by 64.7% in patients treated with whole-liver radioembolization and by 21.9% in patients treated with unilobar radioembolization. Findings of portal hypertension, such as ascites and varices, also developed more frequently in patients who received a whole-liver treatment [83]. This study shows that the long-term hepatotoxicity is mild. Long-term hepatotoxicity will become more and more important, since in the future, (combination) treatment with radioembolization may be applied in first- or second-line settings.

36.6 Posttreatment Imaging and Dosimetry

Posttreatment Imaging

Currently, posttreatment imaging serves two purposes: the evaluation of technical success and the prediction of treatment efficacy. Technical success is evaluated by checking for extrahepatic deposition of microspheres and assessing the intrahepatic distribution.

The heterogeneity of microsphere distribution within a lesion and the absorbed radiation dose within a lesion can be obtained. By evaluating dose-response relationships, treatment efficacy can be predicted [84].

36.6.1 ^{90}Y Imaging

^{90}Y decays without emission of gamma photons. Bremsstrahlung x-rays are emitted along a continuous decreasing energy spectrum ranging up to 2.3 MeV. Positron emission, which produces two annihilation gamma rays, happens only in 32 out of one million decays.

Thus, the quantitative imaging is limited to bremsstrahlung SPECT/CT and PET/CT.

36.6.1.1 ^{90}Y SPECT/CT

The emitted bremsstrahlung x-rays have energies that can range up to 2.3 MeV. The maximal energy usable by a gamma camera with a mechanical collimator is approximately 0.5 MeV. As a result, all acquisitions are corrupted by high-energy x-rays scattering down into the acquisition window.

There are five different image-degrading effects: scattering inside the patient body, penetration through collimator septa, scattering from a collimator septa, the lead fluorescence K_α and K_β emissions, and the backscattering from the photomultiplier tube, electronic boards, and lead housing of the camera [85]. The shape and magnitude of these effects depend on photon energy, tissue composition, collimator, and detector characteristics, the distance between the source and the collimator, and the energy window settings [86]. Elschot et al. developed a new method for ^{90}Y SPECT reconstruction. This Monte Carlo-based reconstruction algorithm compensates for scatter and attenuation effects and improves the quantitative accuracy of bremsstrahlung SPECT images [86]. Because of the wide range of photon energy, the energy window for bremsstrahlung SPECT/CT should be wide. However, because of the high focal uptake in the liver after radioembolization, a single-window approach is sufficient [87]. Reported ranges in the literature are 105–195 keV and 50–250 keV [86–88]. A high-energy collimator is proven to be better than a medium-energy collimator by Elschot et al. [14]. The specifications of the SPECT/CT are defined by Elschot et al.: a radius of rotation of camera of 260 mm, 120 projections/360°, 40-min acquisition time, 256 × 256 matrix size, and 1.6 × 1.6 mm^2 pixel size [88, 89].

A largely neglected issue in clinical SPECT is respiratory motion. Bastiaannet et al. showed that respiratory motion has a very large effect on dosimetry on the spatial scale of individual tumors, with an average decrease in activity recovery and tumor-to-non-tumor ratio from 90% to 66%. Thus, respiratory motion leads to an underestimation of tumor dose. This can partially be solved by using retrospective gating schemes [90].

36.6.1.2 ^{90}Y PET/CT

Although annihilation photon pairs are produced about 700 times less often than bremsstrahlung photons, ^{90}Y PET/CT was found to be superior over bremsstrahlung SPECT/CT for the assessment of the microsphere distribution after radioembolization [88, 91]. One of the first post-infusion clinical ^{90}Y PET/CT scans was performed in 2009. Since then, many studies have described results from both patient and phantom imaging. There are two major issues in ^{90}Y PET/CT imaging: the low true-coincidence rate and the high single rate due to bremsstrahlung x-rays. The first issue may result in noisy images, long scan times, and background noise from scintillator decay. The single-count rate from bremsstrahlung is much higher than the positron emission rate and may cause saturation of the detector, leading to a limited quantitative accuracy [84]. However, this latter issue is not found in recent investigations [92]. Regarding the first problem, the full width at half maximum (FWHM) of ^{90}Y PET/CT is around 5 mm, and scan times of about 20 min are enough for dosimetry. The background noise is worse in organs where the ^{90}Y activity concentration is lower [84].

Due to the higher intrinsic resolution of ^{90}Y PET/CT compared to ^{90}Y SPECT/CT, intrahepatic distribution is more accurately visualized by ^{90}Y PET/CT imaging.

In the next-generation PET/CT systems, the photomultiplier tubes are replaced with solid-state digital photon counting detectors. Wright et al. showed that detection of internal pair production is feasible with this digital photon counting (dPET) technology. dPET images provided increased contrast and allow for more precise localization of microsphere distribution [93]. There is no guideline as to when patients should undergo ^{90}Y PET/CT imaging. Due to the limited sensitivity, it is advised to perform these scans the day of treatment or 1 day later.

36.6.1.3 ^{90}Y PET/MRI

The next development in ^{90}Y imaging is PET/MRI. PET/MRI provides a better soft tissue contrast than PET/CT. The first clinical study of ^{90}Y radioembolization with posttreatment PET/MRI imaging was conducted by Fowler et al. Twenty-four patients with tumors of diverse origin were treated with radioembolization with either glass or resin microspheres. Images were qualitatively assessed for microsphere distribution, and the absorbed doses per lesion were calculated, as well as dose volume histograms, to measure the dose distribution within a tumor. The duration of PET/MR imaging ranged from 42 to 60 min. They found that the average dose per lesion, as well as the minimum dose to 70% of the lesion, were significant predictors of response [94].

Simultaneous PET/MRI offers the opportunity to directly image liver motion due to respiration during the PET acquisition and correct for it during the PET reconstruction. Eldib et al. have performed phantom experiments with PET/MRI. They found that motion resulted in a large loss of contrast recovery, but this was successfully corrected by MR-based data correction [95].

36.6.2 ^{166}Ho Imaging

Because ^{166}Ho emits gamma photons, is paramagnetic, and has a high attenuation coefficient, it can be detected during and after administration. While radioactive, the gamma photons emitted by ^{166}Ho can be measured using single-photon emission computed tomography (SPECT) (Fig. 36.8a–c). Independent of radioactivity, holmium is a lanthanide and with its paramagnetic properties allows visualization and quantification using MR imaging, while the high atom weight attenuates x-rays [15, 16].

36.6.2.1 ^{166}Ho SPECT/CT

Upon decay, ^{166}Ho emits several gamma photons, most of which are 81 keV (abundance 6.7%), 1379 keV (0.9%), or 1581 keV (0.2%). To quantify ^{166}Ho accurately, the SPECT detector has to be set to register photons with an energy window of 7.5% around the photon peak of 81 keV [14]. However, the bremsstrahlung photons and other photons with high energies scatter and become part of the photo peak window, limiting accurate quantification. Also, the higher keV gamma photons from ^{166}Ho decay interact with the patient and the detector. Both these effects are partially corrected for by a downscatter window of 118 ± 6% keV, as well as the use of a medium-energy collimator. Furthermore, attenuation of the patient's body causes a decrease in the photons. A Monte Carlo simulation compensates for attenuation, scatter, and collimator-detector response and was developed to improve quantification [86].

Acquisition of a ^{166}Ho SPECT/CT takes about 30 min. When all ^{166}Ho has decayed to erbium, there are no more gamma photons to image, so there is a time constraint on the imaging procedure. Conversely, just after administration of ^{166}Ho, the gamma photons are so abundant, that they invoke detector dead time; the recorded photon produces a pulse of a certain duration during which no second pulse can be detected. Detector dead time is seen when the activity in the scanner is greater than 1420 MBq [14]. In practice, patients undergo a SPECT when the activity of their ^{166}Ho microspheres is between 250 and 500 MBq and between 3 and 6 days after treatment, depending on the infused activity.

36.6.2.2 ^{166}Ho MRI

Quantification of ^{166}Ho using MR techniques is possible because of the local field inhomogeneities it induces. It allows for imaging of higher resolution, is independent of radioactivity, and can be combined with anatomical scans of different kinds to show tumor boundaries and deposition of microspheres, but its application is limited

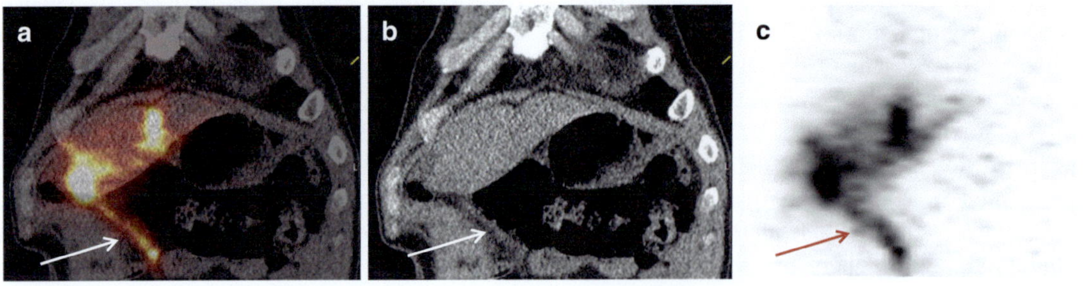

Fig. 36.8 (**a**–**c**) show extrahepatic deposition in the falciform ligament (arrows) in a 53-year-old patient with hepatic metastases of a neuroendocrine neoplasm who was treated with ^{166}Ho-radioembolization. (**a**–**c**) show the ^{166}Ho SPECT/CT, the low-dose CT, and a planar image of the ^{166}Ho SPECT/CT

to tissue without air (i.e., not in the lungs and gastrointestinal organs) and metal (staples from prior hepatectomies).

In MR imaging, the nuclear magnetic moment of the nuclei of hydrogen atoms is aligned along a constantly applied magnetic field, after which a radiofrequency pulse disturbs its alignment. The resulting realignment of the nuclei after this pulse induces an electrical current in the receiver coil, which can be reconstructed to form an image. The realignment can be separated in a longitudinal (expressed in T_1) and a transversal vector (T_2). The T_2 vector from tissue decays quickly (several milliseconds) which is accelerated by the presence of Ho, while its effect on the T_1 is little to none. The decrease in T_2* invokes a lower signal on gradient echo MR images; the microspheres show up as dark areas on these images. A linear relation was shown between the disturbance in the T_2 signal decay and the concentration of Ho present [16]. This relationship, called the relaxivity (R_2*), depends on the strength of the main magnetic field of the scanner and the Ho content.

A calibration phantom with known Ho microspheres concentrations enables the translation of the differences in R_2* into units of microsphere concentrations, which convert into local activity using the activity per sphere.

As MR imaging of Ho is independent of radioactivity, it is possible during or immediately after infusion, but also after several months. The first enables real-time estimation of damage to tumors or healthy liver, which could, in the future, lead to MR-guided radioembolization with simultaneous quantification for treatment optimization. The latter is useful for research into the dynamics and stability of implanted microspheres. The first human MR quantification was performed as part of the phase 1 HEPAR I trial [15]. Of the injected mean total of 523 mg (range, 438–640 mg), MR quantification detected a mean of 431 mg (range, 236–666 mg) of microspheres in the liver or 89 ± 19%. As surgical clips distorted the quantification, the detection improved to 96 ± 13% when these patients (5/14) were excluded. For this quantification, a map of T_2* values of the liver was made before and after radioembolization. After subtraction (with inherent registration errors), the amount of microspheres was computed.

36.7 Follow-Up Imaging and Response Identification

36.7.1 Imaging with CT and MRI

After radioembolization, follow-up imaging is usually performed at 3-month intervals [2]. It is important to consider the changes in tumor appearance that may be a consequence of radioembolization treatment itself. For example, the tumor may increase shortly after therapy, due to acute necrosis, edema, and hemorrhage. Also, inflammation and fibrosis adjacent to the tumor may be falsely interpreted. These changes may lead to a rim enhancement around the tumor, which resembles vital tumor. Furthermore, the presence of tumor necrosis has to be taken into account when measuring tumor size.

Because of these typical radioembolization-induced changes, CT and MRI protocols should at least include contrast-enhanced imaging, using an arterial and portal-venous contrast delay. Unenhanced images can be helpful to distinguish between hemorrhage and vital tumor tissue.

With MRI, different sequences add to the diagnosis of a lesion. T1 sequences allow for the detection of fat and other substances with a high T1 signal, such as hemorrhage. T2 sequences are used to distinguish between solid and cystic lesions. Diffusion-weighted imaging (DWI) evaluates the free motility of water molecules. The mobility is restricted by cell membranes, and tissues with different cellularities have differences in water molecule movement. Malignancies are generally highly cellular, and water molecule motility is restricted, so malignancies appear hyperintense on DWI. DWI can be quantified by apparent diffusion coefficient (ADC). Changes of DWI under therapy are applied for response evaluation and can be used as a surrogate for the degree of tumor necrosis: necrotic tissue reveals an increased ADC because the free water mobility is increased. However, drawbacks of DWI sequences are a lack of reproducibility and no uniform DWI protocol [96].

DWI can also be used as a prognostic factor: Schmeel et al. investigated the prognostic value of the pretreatment mean ADC in predicting treatment response, progression-free survival, and overall survival in 46 patients who underwent radioembolization for unresectable colorectal cancer liver metastases. The mean posttreatment ADC values were increased by 23% on average. Patients with progressive disease had significantly lower tumor ADC values than patients with tumor response ($p = 0.04$). A cutoff value for distinguishing long- and short-term survivors was estimated to be a tumor ADC value of 935. The difference in survival between patients below and above this threshold was significant (3 months versus 5 months) [97]. These findings seem to be of great potential, but they have to be confirmed in larger prospective series. Due to the absence of uniform DWI protocols, these results cannot be translated to DWI assessments in other centers.

Recently, the use of perfusion imaging has emerged. This is based on the assumption that tumors with a higher arterial flow would receive a greater number of microspheres and respond better to treatment. CT perfusion parameters are well correlated with histopathologically determined tumor vascularity. Morsbach et al. analyzed 40 patients who underwent radioembolization for hepatic metastases of various tumors. They found a significant difference between responders and non-responders in arterial perfusion, with the latter being much higher in responders [98].

Using dynamic contrast-enhanced (DCE) sequences, tumor perfusion can also be quantified on MRI images [96]. In a multivariate analysis of prognostic factors in 45 patients with neuroendocrine neoplasms, Sommer et al. found that the vascularization of hepatic metastases is of great prognostic significance, with hypervascularized metastases showing a significantly longer progression-free survival [99].

36.7.2 Functional Imaging with ^{18}FDG-PET CT and Somatostatin Receptor Analogue

Functional imaging modalities may overcome the drawbacks of morphologic-based treatment assessment. The backbone of oncologic imaging is ^{18}FDG-PET. Most malignancies have a high FDG uptake, and this can be assessed both qualitatively and quantitatively during follow-up.

However, not all tumors show a high FDG uptake. Neuroendocrine neoplasms G1/2 (Ki67 < 20%) are not well visualized by ^{18}FDG-PET imaging. These tumors express somatostatin receptors, and this led to the development of molecular imaging with radiolabeled somatostatin analogues. Gallium-68 is a positron-emitting isotope, and a ^{68}Ga-somatostatin analogue (^{68}Ga-DOTATATE/-TOC/-NOC) PET scan proved to be superior to ^{18}FDG-PET imaging in the detection and follow-up of neuroendocrine neoplasms [100, 101].

36.7.3 Response Evaluation

There is a variety of established response criteria. Most are based on the change in size of lesions, but since the rise of functional imaging, also quantitative response criteria are determined. The most widely used criteria, the RECIST, mRECIST, and PERCIST, will be briefly discussed.

36.7.3.1 RECIST 1.1

The Response Evaluation Criteria In Solid Tumors (RECIST) were developed in 2000 and were revised in 2009. The rationale behind these criteria is that objective response (shrinkage of the tumor) and time to progression are important endpoints in clinical trials. These endpoints are used to measure treatment effect, and tumor shrinkage is believed to positively influence overall survival.

At baseline, two target lesions per organ, with a maximum of five lesions in total, have to be chosen. The longest diameter of the lesions must be measured, and the lesions should be at least 10 mm in size if the CT scan has a slice thickness ≤ 5 mm. Usually, the biggest and most well-defined lesions are chosen as target lesions.

The sum of diameters should be recorded, and this parameter is used as a reference. At follow-up evaluation, the same target lesions must be evaluated. Complete response is defined as a disappearance of all target lesions. Partial response is classified as a ≥ 30% decrease in the sum of diameters of target lesions. Progressive disease is characterized by a ≥ 20% increase in the sum of diameters of target lesions. The sum must also demonstrate an absolute increase of ≥5 mm, and the appearance of a new lesion denotes progression as well. Stable disease, at last, is depicted by an increase in diameter of target lesions of <20% or a decrease of <30% [102].

Limitations of the RECIST criteria are that the thresholds for response and progression are arbitrarily chosen (sometimes a small change in size can already have quite some influence on overall survival) and that there is a large interobserver variability [103]. Furthermore, necrosis (i.e., an effect that regularly occurs after locoregional treatments) is included in the target lesion, leading to an overestimation of remaining tumor load [104].

36.7.3.2 mRECIST

The modified RECIST (mRECIST) criteria were developed for the evaluation of hepatocellular carcinoma (HCC). They take into account the tumor necrosis induced by treatment. Viable tumor shows an uptake of contrast agent in the arterial phase on contrast-enhanced CT or MRI.

Just as the RECIST criteria, target lesions are defined at baseline. An HCC lesion should be ≥10 mm, measurable, and well-defined and should have intratumoral arterial enhancement on contrast-enhanced CT or MRI. Response categories are defined like the RECIST response categories with the alteration that only the viable, enhancing part of the lesions should be measured. Not all HCC lesions show arterial enhancement or are well-defined. For those lesions, conventional RECIST criteria must be used [103, 105]. mRECIST could also be used for other hypervascular tumors, like neuroendocrine neoplasms, however need to be validated in future studies.

36.7.3.3 PERCIST 1.0

Metabolic tumor response can be assessed using the positron emission tomography (PET) response criteria in solid tumor (PERCIST 1.0) criteria. At baseline, measurement of the "hottest" single tumor and background area is required. The background data are needed to establish the right threshold for the standardized uptake value (SUV) of a lesion at baseline. The SUV is corrected for lean body mass and abbreviated as "SUL." A single target lesion is chosen at each time point during follow-up, because the most metabolically active tumor focus corresponds to the most aggressive portion of the tumor. The tumor portion with the highest average SUL value, along with the activity in the surrounding 1 cm^3, is recorded as SULpeak. PERCIST 1.1. categories for response are a bit more elaborate than the RECIST response categories. Complete response is the complete resolution of FDG uptake of the target lesion, with the uptake of all other lesions returning to background values as well. Partial metabolic response is a decrease of ≥30% and of ≥0.8 SUL units between the most intense lesion at follow-up and the most intense lesion at baseline. This is not necessarily the same lesion. Furthermore, there should be no new lesions compared to baseline and no increase of ≥30% in size of a nontarget lesion. Stable metabolic disease is defined as an increase or decrease in SULpeak of <30%. Progressive disease, finally, is characterized by an increase ≥30% and of ≥0.8 SUL units in a target lesion or by the development of a new lesion [106].

36.7.3.4 Comparison of RECIST and PERCIST Criteria

In a recent review, Min et al. analyzed six studies that compared RECIST and PERCIST response criteria. Overall, there was moderate agreement of tumor response between the two criteria (linear weighted kappa 0.59, 95% CI 0.52–0.66), and in almost 38% there was discordance in

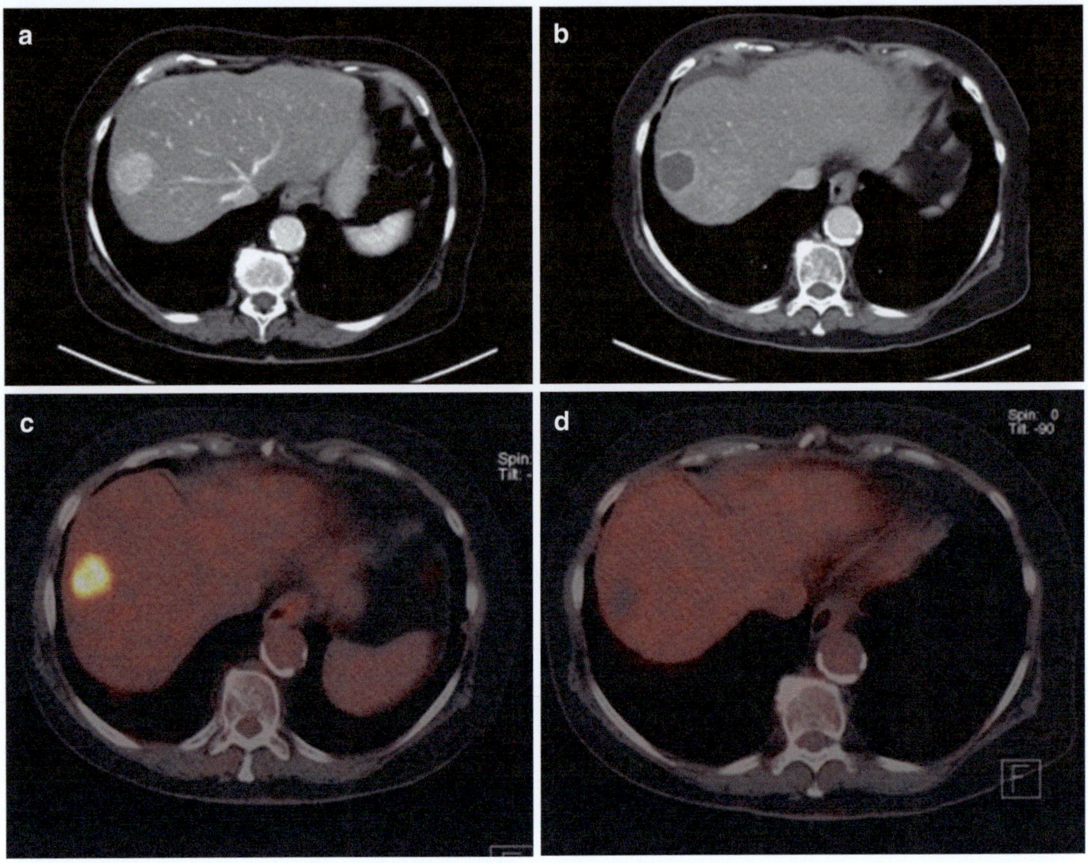

Fig. 36.9 (**a–d**) Figure (**a**) shows a contrast-enhanced CT image of a metastasis of an intrahepatic cholangiocarcinoma in an 80-year-old woman. Figure (**b**) shows a contrast-enhanced CT image of the same metastasis 3 months later, after treatment with radioembolization (120 Gy TheraSpheres). Figure (**c**) shows a baseline PET/CT image of the same metastases. Figure (**d**) shows a PET/CT image of the same metastasis 3 months after treatment

response category. Overall response rates were 35.1% by the RECIST and 54.1% by the PERCIST criteria. Thus, the PERCIST criteria significantly increased the overall tumor response rate. An example of a difference in response according to the RECIST and PERCIST criteria after radioembolization is depicted in Fig. 36.9. This figure shows images of an 80-year-old woman with metastases of an intrahepatic cholangiocarcinoma who was treated with radioembolization. According to the RECIST 1.1 criteria, the response to treatment would be characterized as SD (stable disease). According to the mRECIST and PERCIST criteria, however, the response to treatment would be characterized as CR (complete response) and CMR (complete metabolic response). Since functional imaging can detect metabolic changes when there are no morphological changes yet, response evaluation using the PERCIST criteria may be a better mainstay for clinicians [107]. However, PERCIST comes with several logistical challenges before allowing physicians to compare baseline and follow-up imaging [108].

36.8 Response

Hepatocellular carcinoma (HCC) is the fifth most common type of cancer and the third cancer-related cause of death worldwide. The incidence is highest in Asia and rising in the USA. Risk factors of HCC are hepatitis C virus infection, hepatitis B virus infection, and alcohol abuse.

These risk factors can cause chronic liver disease, possibly leading to the development of fibrosis and/or cirrhosis and HCC. [109].

Patients with HCC are classified according to the BCLC staging system. This system is divided in five categories: 0-D, based on performance status, liver function, and tumor dimensions. Patients are treated according to the proposed treatment strategy for each BCLC stage [110]. Although radioembolization is not incorporated in the treatment algorithm yet, several trials on radioembolization in HCC patients have been conducted. For selected patients, radioembolization could be positioned between TACE and sorafenib (Fig. 36.10).

For patients with BCLC stage 0-A, ablation, resection, and liver transplantation are the treatment options of choice. There is a possible role for radioembolization in these stages in the form of radiation segmentectomy. Padia et al. described superselective radioembolization for patients with unresectable HCC, with a median dose to the treated segments of 254 Gy. Response rates were excellent, with 95% CR and 5% PR. There was no significant hepatoxicity [111]. Recently, a retrospective analysis of Biederman et al. was published. In a cohort of 121 patients with solitary HCC up to 3 cm, 41 patients were treated with radiation segmentectomy, and 80 patients were treated with a combination of TACE and microwave ablation (MWA). Target lesion complete response was 87.5% in both groups. Median time to progression was 11.6 months in the TACE MWA group and 11.1 months in the radiation segmentectomy group (p = 0.83). Overall progression and overall survival rates were similar in both groups. These findings show that radiation segmentectomy is just as effective as the combination of TACE and MWA in BCLC stage A patients [112].

Radioembolization can be used for downstaging or as a bridge to transplantation. Many patients do not meet the Milan criteria for transplantation (≤5 cm for single lesion or no more than three lesions with the largest measuring ≤3 cm) [113]. Radioembolization can be used to induce a shrinkage of the lesions to render patients eligible for transplantation. Since waiting times for the transplantation list are long, many patients develop progressive disease and are no longer candidates for transplantation. To overcome this, radioembolization can be used to delay progression.

Tohme et al. describe 20 patients with HCC who were treated with radioembolization as a bridge to transplantation. Radioembolization

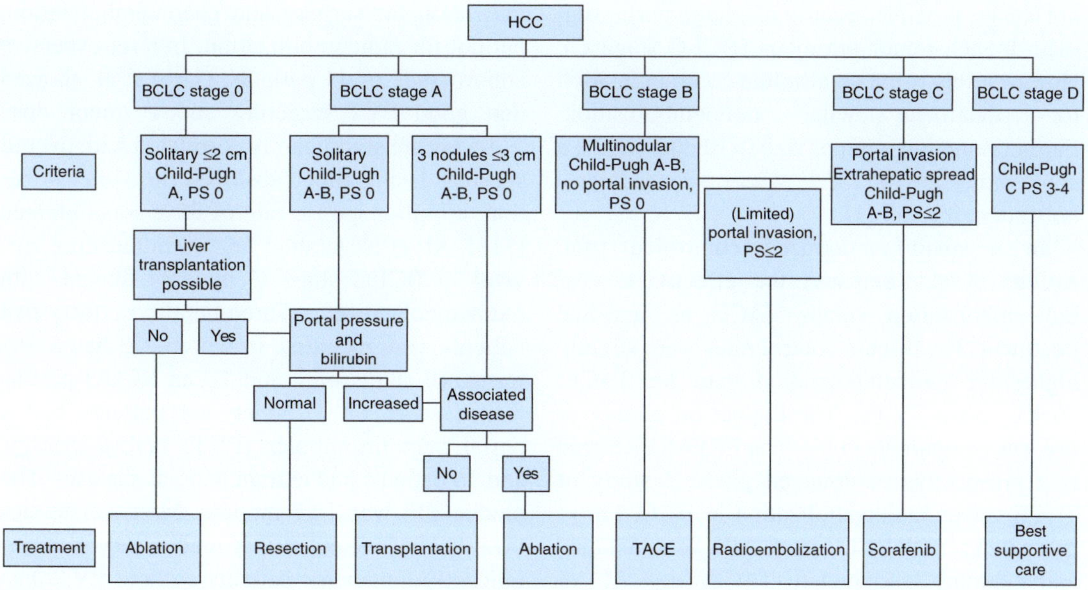

Fig. 36.10 Barcelona Clinic Liver Cancer (BCLC) staging system with proposal for radioembolization in the treatment algorithm. *PS* performance score

induced a complete or partial response in 9 of 16 evaluable patients. Histopathologic analysis of the explanted livers showed complete tumor necrosis in 5 cases, 50–99% necrosis in 6 cases, and <50% necrosis in 9 cases. Median survival was 75.1 months, and there were four patients with disease recurrence, of whom one had cancer in the new liver [113]. Mohamed et al. reported their center's experience in using several therapeutic modalities before liver transplantation. In comparison with stereotactic radiotherapy, TACE, and RFA, treatment with radioembolization yielded the highest radiologic complete response rate (33% versus 25% for TACE, 8.6% for stereotactic radiotherapy, and 22% for RFA) and also the highest proportion of pathologic necrosis (75% versus 41% for TACE, 28.5% for stereotactic radiotherapy, and 60% for RFA). There were seven patients with disease recurrence after transplantation, but none of them were treated with radioembolization [114].

These findings show that radioembolization can enable patients to remain on the waiting list for transplantation by stabilizing or even downstaging their disease.

To date, several trials with radioembolization were performed with BCLC stage B and C patients. Transarterial chemoembolization (TACE), the gold standard for BCLC stage B, is not always possible because of a large portal vein main branch tumor thrombus (BCLC stage C). However, this is not an absolute contraindication for treatment with radioembolization. Furthermore, large tumor size (>10 cm) can be a contraindication for TACE, whereas for radioembolization, it is not [1].

In a small randomized controlled trial, Kolligs et al. compared the effectiveness of radioembolization versus TACE as first-line treatment. The disease control rates were slightly higher for radioembolization than for TACE: 76.9% versus 73.3%. The impact on quality of life was comparable [115]. The PREMIERE trial is a prospective randomized phase 2 study of TACE versus radioembolization in HCC. Forty-five patients with BCLC stage A/B were included and randomly assigned to TACE (n = 21) or radioembolization (n = 24). Clinical toxicities and objective response rates were similar in both patient groups. Median time to progression was 6.4 months in the TACE group and not reached in the radioembolization group (p = 0.002). However, this significantly longer time to progression did not translate into a significant difference in overall survival [116].

Katsanos et al. compared the effectiveness of different transarterial embolization therapies, alone or in combination with local ablative or adjuvant systemic treatments, in patients with HCC. They compared studies investigating bland transarterial embolization (TAE), TACE, chemoembolization with drug-eluting beads (DEB-TACE), TACE+radiotherapy, TACE+ablation, TACE+adjuvant, DEB-TACE+adjuvant, and radioembolization with control series. TACE combined with external radiation therapy or percutaneous tumor ablation was the most effective treatment strategies, in terms of overall survival. Radioembolization was the safest treatment modality with less adverse events and side effects than the other locoregional therapies. Median survival of patients treated with radioembolization was 24.3 months, compared to 13.9 months in the control series with best supportive treatment [117].

In BCLC stage C patients, a portal vein thrombosis (PVT) is present, which is a contraindication for surgery and chemoembolization, but not for radioembolization. In a retrospective cohort study of 41 patients, Garin et al. showed that good PVT targeting and a tumor dose ≥205 Gy are significantly correlated with overall survival. Using aimed absorbed dose intensification, a high response rate of 85% was obtained [118]. Ali et al. studied factors influencing survival in BCLC stage C patients treated with radioembolization. Three-hundred forty-five patients were included, of whom 223 had a performance status of 1 and 10 an ECOG performance score of 2. Ninety-six patients had a portal vein thrombosis (PVT) before therapy, and 16 patients had extrahepatic metastases. The median OS was 10.7 months. Multivariate survival analysis showed that median OS was significantly longer for patients without PVT than for patients with PVT: 15.6 versus 7.3 months,

$p < 0.0001$. Extrahepatic disease at baseline also significantly influenced median OS: 7.4 versus 12.6 months for patients with and without extrahepatic metastases [119]. The presence of PVT as a prognostic factor is confirmed by Floridi et al. who studied radioembolization in patients with mainly BCLC stage B. These patients had a longer median OS of 22.7 months after radioembolization [120].

Recently, two trials have compared radioembolization with sorafenib: the Study to Compare Selective Internal Radiation Therapy (SIRT) Versus Sorafenib in Locally Advanced Hepatocellular Carcinoma (SIRveNIB) and the SorAfenib Versus Radioembolization in Advanced Hepatocellular carcinoma (SARAH) trial (clinicaltrials.gov identifiers NCT01135056 and NCT01482442). The results of the SIRveNIB trial are not published yet, but they have been presented at an international congress. Both trials were developed to identify whether radioembolization improves OS compared to the standard treatment with sorafenib. The results from the SARAH trial showed no significant difference in OS (median OS 8.0 months for radioembolization and 9.9 months for sorafenib in the intention-to-treat groups, and median OS 9.9 months for radioembolization and 9.9 months for sorafenib in the per protocol analysis). Median progression-free survival was a bit longer for the radioembolization group (4.1 versus 3.7 months), but this was not significantly different. However, progression in the liver as first site was significantly lower in the radioembolization group (HR 0.72, 95% CI 0.56–0.93, $p = 0.01$), and tumor response rate was significantly better (19% of evaluable patients in the radioembolization group achieved a complete or partial response versus 12% of evaluable patients in the sorafenib group ($p = 0.04$)). Most important, the number of adverse events was lower with radioembolization, and the quality of life over time was significantly better (Fig. 36.11) [121].

In the SIRveNIB trial, there was no significant difference in OS either. Median OS was 8.8 months for radioembolization and 10 months for sorafenib. Tumor-response rate was much better for the radioembolization group: 16.5% versus 1.7% ($p < 0.001$). Like the SARAH trial, patients who received radioembolization had significantly fewer (serious) adverse events when compared with those treated with sorafenib [122].

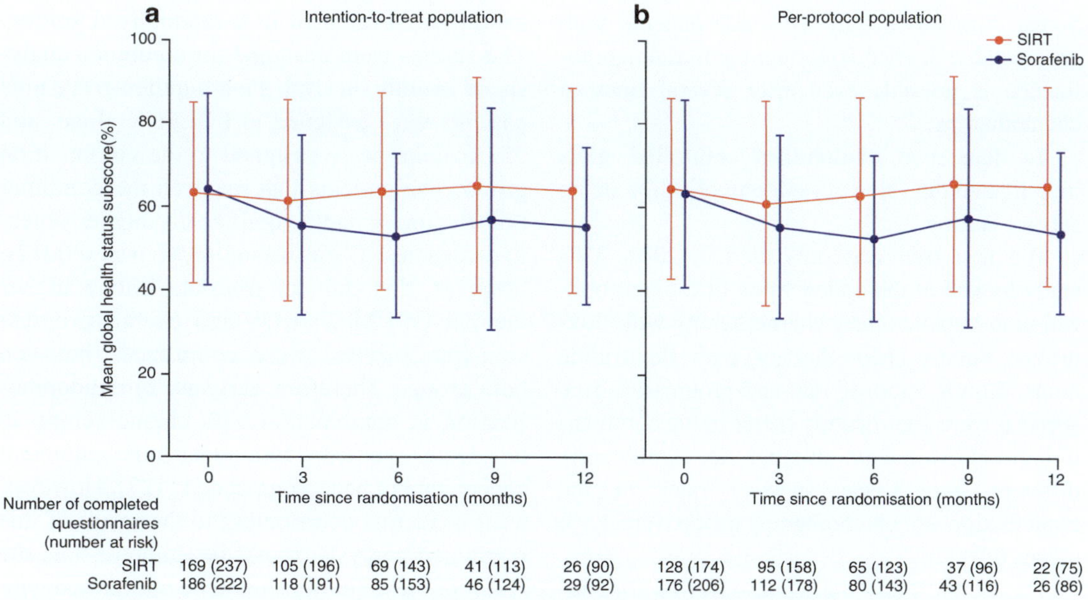

Fig. 36.11 Quality of life (as depicted by the mean global health status subscore from the EORTC QLQ-C30 questionnaire) over time of patients treated in the SARAH trial: in the intention-to-treat population (**a**) and in the per-protocol population (**b**). (Reprinted with permission from Elsevier)

Unfortunately, these trials are not without limitations. In both studies, a larger proportion of patients in radioembolization group did not receive the allocated intervention compared to the patients randomized to sorafenib (SARAH trial, 22.0% versus 4.6%; SIRveNIB trial, 28.6% versus 9.0%) [121, 122]. Furthermore, in both studies, the BSA method was used for activity calculation. This method often leads to over- or underdosing and does not differentiate between tumorous and non-tumorous tissue, which may have led to suboptimal treatment outcomes. Also, time to progression in the liver was significantly longer in the radioembolization groups, but progression at any site was comparable or shorter in the radioembolization group. This is not unexpected when comparing a regional versus a systemic therapy, and one may advocate the addition of a systemic therapy to radioembolization.

36.8.1 Metastatic Colorectal Carcinoma

The majority of patients with hepatic metastases of colorectal carcinoma are not suitable for surgical therapy. Resection of hepatic metastases is the only possible curative treatment option. The 5-year survival is only 10% for patients with unresectable disease. Treatment with radioembolization is possible even after several lines of chemotherapy.

To date, two randomized controlled trials investigated the value of radioembolization in the salvage setting.

The first trial was published in 2001. This study looked at the added value of radioembolization to hepatic artery chemotherapy with floxuridine versus chemotherapy with floxuridine alone. Tumor response rate and progression-free survival were significantly better in the combination group. Moreover, although not significantly different, the 5-year survival rates in the combination and chemotherapy group were 3.5% versus 0% [58].

The second study was a phase III trial comparing intravenous fluorouracil infusion alone or with radioembolization in patients with liver-limited metastatic colorectal carcinoma (mCRC). Forty-four patients were treated, and median time to liver progression was 2.1 months in the chemotherapy arm versus 5.5 months in the combination arm. Median OS rates in the treatment arms were 7.3 and 10.0 months, respectively, but this was not significantly different [123].

The MORE study was a large retrospective study of mCRC patients treated with radioembolization. The main findings of this study were that radioembolization offered favorable survival benefits for patients with unresectable mCRC, even after several lines of chemotherapy [124].

Prognostic factors for poorer survival after radioembolization in this salvage setting were ECOG performance status ≥1, baseline extrahepatic metastases, elevated levels of carcinoembryonic antigen (CEA), high tumor-to-non-tumor ratio, increased lines of chemotherapy, ascites, impaired liver function, lymphovascular invasion of the primary tumor, and KRAS mutation [67, 125, 126].

In the first-line setting, three trials investigating the role of radioembolization were performed. In the SIRFLOX, FOXFIRE, and FOXFIRE-Global studies, the efficacy of combining first-line chemotherapy (FOLFOX with or without targeted therapy) with radioembolization was evaluated in a randomized setting. The studies were designed for combined analysis of overall survival. Five-hundred forty-nine patients were assigned to FOLFOX alone, and 554 patients were assigned to the combination group. The patients that received the combination treatment had a significantly higher objective response (72% versus 63%, $p = 0.0012$); however, this did not translate into a higher median OS. Median OS and overall progression-free survival were comparable between both groups. Therefore, early use of radioembolization in combination with chemotherapy in unselected patients with metastatic colorectal cancer cannot be recommended [127]. However, a lot of factors contributing to the result of this combined analysis cannot be ignored; thus the result of these studies should be interpreted with caution. The most important factor is the dosimetry. In their study, Wasan et al. used the BSA method for activity calculation. However, this method often leads to over- or underdosing. Furthermore, the BSA method does not differentiate between tumorous and non-tumorous tissue, leading to undetermined absorbed doses in these tissues. In the SIRFLOX, FOXFIRE, and FOXFIRE-Global studies, the tumor-absorbed dose was not optimized, leading to an uncertainty about the true effect of radioembolization in the first-line setting [128].

36.8.2 Neuroendocrine Neoplasms

Neuroendocrine neoplasms (NENs) metastasize to the liver in 50–95% of patients [83]. Neuroendocrine neoplasm metastases generally have a high arterial uptake and are therefore excellent candidates for radioembolization [99]. To date, several studies about radioembolization for NEN metastases are published. A meta-analysis of 12 studies showed that median OS ranged from 14 to 70 months, with a median of 28.5 months. The pooled disease control rate was 86%. The wide range in OS may be due to the inclusion of pancreatic NENs in the analysis, because pancreatic NENs generally have a lower survival than NENs from other primary sites [129]. Jia et al. analyzed the outcome of radioembolization in 36 patients with hepatic metastases of NENs. At 3-month follow-up, overall disease control rate (CR, PR, or SD) was 88.9%. There were 16 patients with carcinoid syndrome (flushing, diarrhea), and 15 of them experienced symptomatic improvement after treatment. Side effects were mild, with the exception of two patients who developed duodenal ulcers. Median OS was 41 months [130].

In a retrospective study, Chansanti et al. analyzed the tumor-dose relationship in NENs. They included 15 patients with a total of 55 tumors. Primary tumors were located in the pancreas ($n = 8$), the gastrointestinal tract ($n = 6$), and the lung ($n = 1$). The majority of tumors were hypervascular (80%). Tumor-absorbed dose was estimated using the partition model, as predicted by uptake of ^{99m}Tc-MAA. Mean tumor-absorbed dose was 231.4 Gy, and a cutoff value of ≥191 Gy predicted tumor response with 93% specificity. These results show that tumor-absorbed dose estimation based on ^{99m}Tc-MAA uptake is predictive of tumor response and that the partition model can be used for optimal treatment planning [131]. Prognostic factors that may influence OS after radioembolization are ECOG score ≥ 1, higher tumor grade and tumor burden >50% [132].

36.8.3 Other Tumor Types

Radioembolization is also increasingly used for hepatic metastases of other primary tumors, such as intrahepatic cholangiocarcinoma, breast carcinoma, pancreatic adenocarcinoma, renal cell carcinoma, and uveal melanoma. In all these tumor types, radioembolization shows promising results with limited toxicity [133–137].

36.9 Future Directions

36.9.1 Retreatment

Radioembolization is usually performed as a monotherapy (i.e., one shot), after failure of other therapeutic options. However, sometimes there is an indication for repeated radioembolization. Patients may have an impaired liver function after a previous radioembolization treatment, which raises questions regarding safety. Two studies investigated the safety of repeated radioembolization. Lam et al. describe eight patients that underwent repeated treatment, defined as multiple treatments to the same target volume. The second procedure was done with a reduced radioactivity dose. The interval between treatments was 203–968 days. After the second treatment, three patients had stable disease, four patients partial response, and one patient complete response. After the second radioembolization procedure, two patients developed REILD and deceased shortly after treatment. The authors concluded that a higher administered activity per target volume increased the risk of REILD [138].

Zarva et al. analyzed repeated radioembolization in 21 patients with HCC or hepatic metastases from different primary tumors. Sixteen patients received 3 lobar treatments, 4 patients received 4 lobar treatments and 1 patient received 5 lobar treatments. The interval between sessions was 4–6 weeks. The most frequent adverse events were ascites, elevation of bilirubin or liver enzymes, and decrease of serum albumin levels. There were no grade IV or V toxicities. Median time to progression after the first treatment session was 3 months and median OS was 18 months [139].

Despite the possible increased risk of REILD, repeated radioembolization may be a good option for patients with progressive disease after radioembolization. Careful patient selection should be applied, and doses should be calculated with taking into account the administered activity per target volume.

36.9.2 Advances in Dosimetry

The need for optimized dosimetry is more and more emphasized. A huge step forward from the BSA and the MIRD method was made with the invention of the partition method for activity calculation. This method takes into account the mass of the tumors and the liver. However, it does not correct for the difference in tumor and non-tumor expected absorbed dose. Another limitation is that it is difficult to delineate ill-defined tumors. As stated above, a voxel-based method for activity calculation is proposed by Chiesa et al. [63]. This method uses the ^{99m}Tc-MAA quantification as a surrogate of microsphere distribution and takes nonuniformity of the absorbed dose into account. However, limitations of this voxel-based approach are physical factors such as attenuation, scatter, noise, and partial-volume effects, which should be corrected for [64]. Garin et al. have developed a personalized dosimetry approach, with an aimed absorbed tumor dose of ≥205 Gy. They evaluated the ^{99m}Tc-MAA volume of distribution in the injected liver and tumor and the total injected activity. The injected activities in the tumors and liver were calculated with the MIRD formula, with the endpoints of attaining a tumor-absorbed dose of ≥205 Gy, a healthy liver absorbed dose of <120 Gy, and a lung absorbed dose of <30 Gy. Treatment intensification was performed when the estimated tumor dose would not reach 205 Gy as calculated with the MIRD method [118]. In a study of 85 patients with HCC, this method was used for activity calculation. Response rate was 80.3% on lesion-based analysis and 77.5% on patient-based analysis. There was a clear dose-response relationship, with a response rate of 89.7% for tumors with an absorbed dose of ≥205 Gy versus a response rate of 9.1% in tumors with an absorbed dose <205 Gy. Tumor-absorbed dose was also significantly associated with overall survival ($p = 0.005$ on multivariate analysis) [140].

A personalized dosimetric approach is advocated for the treatment of not only HCC patients but also for patients with hepatic metastases. Optimal tumor-absorbed doses and maximum tolerable dose to the healthy liver have to be defined for multiple tumor types.

36.9.3 Radioembolization as a Bridge to Surgery

Surgical resection of hepatic tumors offers the best chance of survival. Still, in many patients, the future liver remnant (FLR) is deemed too small to preserve enough liver function, and often patients die because of liver failure. To overcome this hepatic failure, different strategies were developed to increase the FLR, such as portal vein embolization (PVE). The FLR increases with 44–69% already 6–8 weeks after PVE. However, there are reports of patients developing tumors in the embolized and non-embolized lobes, which make them ineligible for surgery.

Radioembolization also induces hypertrophy of the untreated liver lobe, but this develops at a slower pace. This slower pace allows for the discovery of possible new lesions in the treated lobe and new lesions in the FLR (i.e., biological test of time). Furthermore, contrary to PVE, there is a tumoricidal effect in the treated lobe [141]. Goebel et al. found a mean increase of 36% in

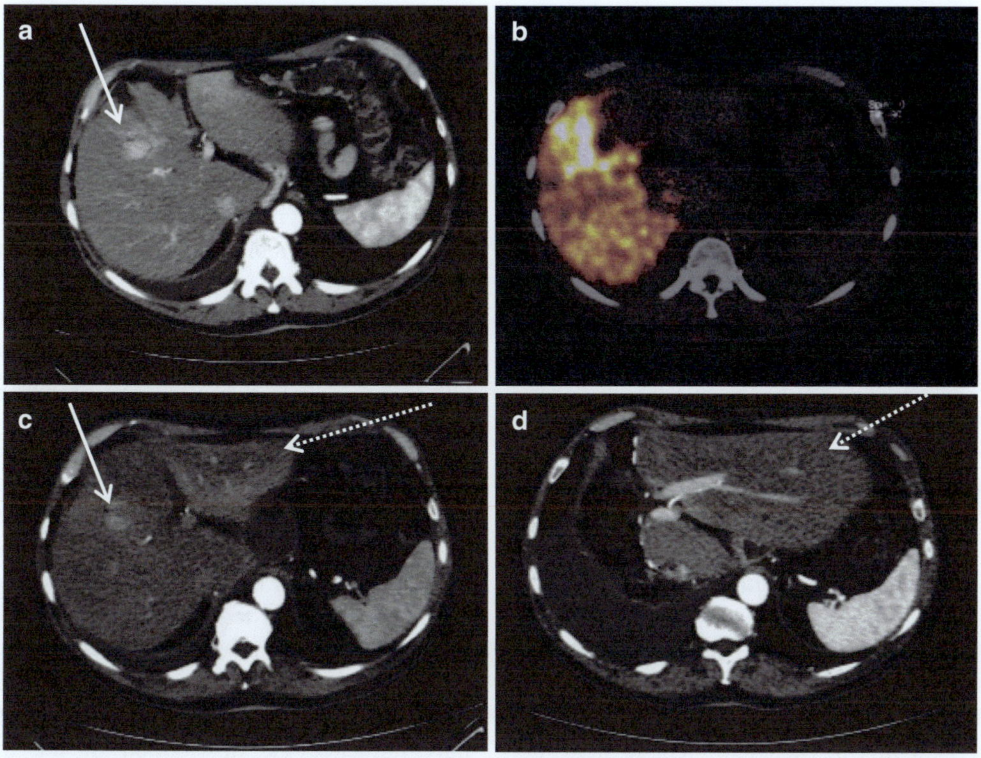

Fig. 36.12 (**a–d**) (**a**) shows a contrast-enhanced CT image of a 60-year-old man with an HCC (white arrow). (**b**) shows the ^{90}Y-PET CT after treatment with radioembolization of the right hemiliver (120 Gy, TheraSpheres). (**c**) shows a CT image of a hypertrophied left hemiliver (dotted white arrow), 3 months after radioembolization. (**d**) shows a contrast-enhanced CT image of the left hemiliver (dotted white arrow) 4 months after right hemihepatectomy

FLR volume in a series of 27 patients with HCC. A lower tumor burden, lower Child-Pugh score, and lower age were associated with a larger increase in FLR volume [142]. An example of a patient who underwent radioembolization to induce hypertrophy of the FLR is shown in Fig. 36.12a–d.

36.9.4 Single-Day Sessions

Currently, the standard radioembolization treatment algorithm is a work-up with ^{99m}Tc-MAA, followed by administration of the ^{90}Y-microspheres about 2 weeks later. This can be quite burdensome for patients, as they have to visit the hospital multiple times. Furthermore, it is expensive, since in most hospitals, radioembolization is not performed as an outpatient procedure so patients will have to stay the night after treatment.

Gates et al. described the outpatient single-session radioembolization with ^{90}Y-glass microspheres of 14 patients. Before the patients arrived, the hepatic volume and number of primary vessels supplying the treatment volume were acquired using CT images. Activity vials were ordered assuming a 10% LSF for HCC and 5% LSF for metastatic disease. At the day of treatment, patients underwent the work-up angiographic procedure with administration of ^{99m}Tc-MAA. Within 2 hours, planar scintigraphy was performed, and LSF was calculated. Activity was calculated according to the MIRD method, and this was done between the scan and the transfer back to the angiography suite, where patients received treatment. Cone beam CT was used for the evaluation of possible enterohepatic vessels.

The mean total procedure time was 2.7 hours. This study shows that single-day treatment is feasible [143]. In a letter to the editor, Van den Hoven et al. even advocate to eliminate the LSF calculation in patients with colorectal carcinoma metastases, since these patients seldom have a high LSF [144]. However, if one leaves out this work-up procedure, personalized dosimetry based on the distribution of ^{99m}Tc-MAA becomes impossible.

Radioembolization with ^{166}Ho is always performed on a single day in the current clinical trials. Between the work-up procedure and the treatment procedure, the angiography suite is used for other treatments, to increase cost-effectiveness.

36.9.5 Technical Advances

Another option to shorten treatment time is to use simultaneous x-ray and nuclear imaging. This would allow the intervention radiologist to directly identify possible extrahepatic deposition of the microspheres and render the possibility of, e.g., adjusting the injection position. A prototype was built with a mobile C-arm and a gamma camera with a four-pinhole collimator (Fig. 36.13). The x-ray detector, the x-ray tube, and the gamma camera were all placed in one line to enable imaging of the same field of view. Measurements with this prototype demonstrated the feasibility of simultaneous x-ray and nuclear imaging [145, 146].

Recently, much effort is being put into the development of different catheter types, such as anti-reflux catheters. Advantages of anti-reflux catheters, such as the Surefire catheters with an expandable tip or the Occlusafe catheters with an expandable balloon tip, are the anti-reflux capacities and the fixed catheter tip in the middle of the lumen [147, 148]. The anti-reflux mechanism may obliterate the need for coil embolization of proximal branches, leading to a reduced procedure time, radiation dose, and even costs [149, 150]. Furthermore, by affecting the fluid-particle hemodynamics, the fixed catheter tip position may influence the distribution of the microspheres [151, 152].

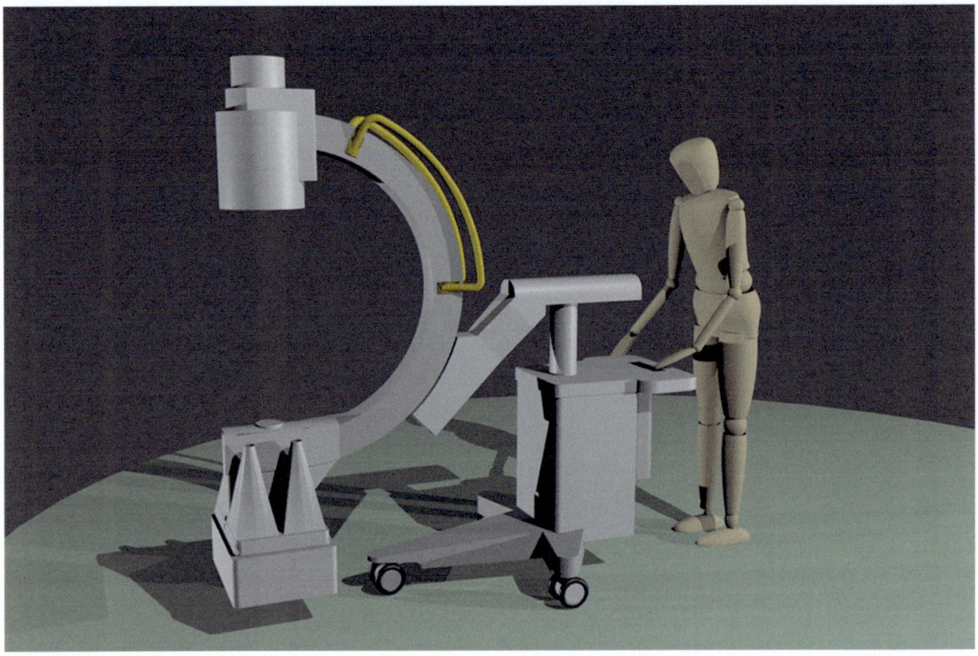

Fig. 36.13 This image shows a prototype of the hybrid fluoroscopic and nuclear imaging device. (With courtesy to Van der Velden et al.)

36.10 Conclusion

Radioembolization is a minimal invasive therapy during which radioactive microspheres are injected into the hepatic artery. A microcatheter is placed in the hepatic arterial vasculature, and millions of microspheres are administered that selectively irradiate the tumors and relatively spare the healthy liver tissue. The essential steps for radioembolization are a visceral angiography to map the vascular anatomy, followed by a SPECT/CT after administration of a scout dose to assess lung shunt, exclude extrahepatic depositions, and assess intrahepatic particle distribution, after which the optimal therapeutic activity is calculated and administered during a second visceral angiography.

Radioembolization is a safe and effective treatment and currently mainly indicated in a palliative setting for unresectable, chemorefractory primary and secondary hepatic malignancies.

Side effects of radioembolization are usually mild and self-limiting.

Within nuclear medicine and interventional oncology, radioembolization is a fast developing field of expertise.

References

1. Braat AJ, Smits ML, Braat MN, van den Hoven AF, Prince JF, de Jong HW, et al. (9)(0)Y hepatic Radioembolization: an update on current practice and recent developments. J Nucl Med. 2015;56(7):1079–87. Epub 2015/05/09.
2. Giammarile F, Bodei L, Chiesa C, Flux G, Forrer F, Kraeber-Bodere F, et al. EANM procedure guideline for the treatment of liver cancer and liver metastases with intra-arterial radioactive compounds. Eur J Nucl Med Mol Imaging. 2011;38(7):1393–406. Epub 2011/04/16.
3. Harbert J. In: Harbert J, editor. Nuclear medicine diagnosis and therapy. New York: Thieme Medical; 1996. p. 1141–55.
4. Wunderlich G, Drews A, Kotzerke J. A kit for labeling of [188Re] human serum albumin microspheres for therapeutic use in nuclear medicine. Appl Radiat Isot. 2005;62(6):915–8. Epub 2005/04/01.
5. Wunderlich G, Pinkert J, Stintz M, Kotzerke J. Labeling and biodistribution of different particle materials for radioembolization therapy with 188Re. Appl Radiat Isot. 2005;62(5):745–50. Epub 2005/03/15.
6. Gates VL, Esmail AA, Marshall K, Spies S, Salem R. Internal pair production of 90Y permits hepatic localization of microspheres using routine PET: proof of concept. J Nucl Med. 2011;52(1):72–6. Epub 2010/12/15.
7. Walker LA. Radioactive yttrium 90: a review of its properties, biological behavior, and clinical uses. Acta Radiol Ther Phys Biol. 1964;2(4):302–14.
8. Lewandowski RJ, Salem R. Yttrium-90 radioembolization of hepatocellular carcinoma and metastatic disease to the liver. Semin Interv Radiol. 2006;23(1):64–72.
9. Sirtex. SIR-Spheres Y-90 resin microspheres. Sirtex Medical Limited; 2017. https://www.sirtex.com/media/155126/ssl-us-13.pdf.
10. Ahmadzadehfar H, Muckle M, Sabet A, Wilhelm K, Kuhl C, Biermann K, et al. The significance of bremsstrahlung SPECT/CT after yttrium-90 radioembolization treatment in the prediction of extrahepatic side effects. Eur J Nucl Med Mol Imaging. 2011;39:309–15. Epub 2011/10/07.
11. Wang XD, Yang RJ, Cao XC, Tan J, Li B. Dose delivery estimated by bremsstrahlung imaging and partition model correlated with response following intra-arterial radioembolization with 32P-glass microspheres for the treatment of hepatocellular carcinoma. J Gastrointest Surg. 2010;14(5):858–66. Epub 2010/03/13.
12. Andrews JC, Walker SC, Ackermann RJ, Cotton LA, Ensminger WD, Shapiro B. Hepatic radioembolization with yttrium-90 containing glass microspheres: preliminary results and clinical follow-up. J Nucl Med. 1994;35(10):1637–44. Epub 1994/10/01.
13. Gray B. Patent application WO 02/34300 A1. Polymer based radionuclide containing particulate material. 2002.
14. Elschot M, Nijsen JF, Dam AJ, de Jong HW. Quantitative evaluation of scintillation camera imaging characteristics of isotopes used in liver radioembolization. PLoS One. 2011;6.
15. van de Maat GH, Seevinck PR, Elschot M, Smits ML, de Leeuw H, van Het Schip AD, et al. MRI-based biodistribution assessment of holmium-166 poly(L-lactic acid) microspheres after radioembolisation. Eur Radiol. 2013;23(3):827–35. Epub 2012/09/28.
16. Nijsen JF, Seppenwoolde JH, Havenith T, Bos C, Bakker CJ, van het Schip AD. Liver tumors: MR imaging of radioactive holmium microspheres--phantom and rabbit study. Radiology. 2004;231(2):491–9. Epub 2004/03/20.
17. Vente MA, Nijsen JF, de Roos R, van Steenbergen MJ, Kaaijk CN, Koster-Ammerlaan MJ, et al. Neutron activation of holmium poly(L-lactic acid) microspheres for hepatic arterial radio-embolization: a validation study. Biomed Microdevices. 2009;11(4):763–72. Epub 2009/02/26.
18. Virdee PS, Moschandreas J, Gebski V, Love SB, Francis EA, Wasan HS, et al. Protocol for com-

bined analysis of FOXFIRE, SIRFLOX, and FOXFIRE-global randomized phase III trials of chemotherapy +/− selective internal radiation therapy as first-line treatment for patients with metastatic colorectal cancer. JMIR Res Protocol. 2017;6(3):e43. Epub 2017/03/30.
19. van Hazel GA, Heinemann V, Sharma NK, Findlay MP, Ricke J, Peeters M, et al. SIRFLOX: randomized phase III trial comparing first-line mFOLFOX6 (plus or minus bevacizumab) versus mFOLFOX6 (plus or minus bevacizumab) plus selective internal radiation therapy in patients with metastatic colorectal Cancer. J Clin Oncol. 2016;34(15):1723–31. Epub 2016/02/24.
20. Golfieri R, Bilbao JI, Carpanese L, Cianni R, Gasparini D, Ezziddin S, et al. Comparison of the survival and tolerability of radioembolization in elderly vs. younger patients with unresectable hepatocellular carcinoma. J Hepatol. 2013;59: 753–61.
21. Oken MM, Creech RH, Tormey DC, Horton J, Davis TE, McFadden ET, et al. Toxicity and response criteria of the Eastern Cooperative Oncology Group. Am J Clin Oncol. 1982;5(6):649–55.
22. Radiology ACo. CT/MRI LI-RADS v2017. 2017.
23. van den Hoven AF, Braat MN, Prince JF, van Doormaal PJ, van Leeuwen MS, Lam MG, et al. Liver CT for vascular mapping during radioembolisation workup: comparison of an early and late arterial phase protocol. Eur Radiol. 2017;27(1):61–9. Epub 2016/04/25.
24. Rosenbaum CE, van den Bosch MA, Veldhuis WB, Huijbregts JE, Koopman M, Lam MG. Added value of FDG-PET imaging in the diagnostic workup for yttrium-90 radioembolisation in patients with colorectal cancer liver metastases. Eur Radiol. 2013;23(4):931–7. Epub 2012/11/01.
25. Yoon KT, Kim JK, Kim DY, Ahn SH, Lee JD, Yun M, et al. Role of 18F-fluorodeoxyglucose positron emission tomography in detecting extrahepatic metastasis in pretreatment staging of hepatocellular carcinoma. Oncology. 2007;72(Suppl 1):104–10. Epub 2007/12/22.
26. Cho Y, Lee DH, Lee YB, Lee M, Yoo JJ, Choi WM, et al. Does 18F-FDG positron emission tomography-computed tomography have a role in initial staging of hepatocellular carcinoma? PLoS One. 2014;9(8):e105679. Epub 2014/08/26.
27. Nagaoka S, Itano S, Ishibashi M, Torimura T, Baba K, Akiyoshi J, et al. Value of fusing PET plus CT images in hepatocellular carcinoma and combined hepatocellular and cholangiocarcinoma patients with extrahepatic metastases: preliminary findings. Liver Int. 2006;26(7):781–8. Epub 2006/08/17.
28. Park JW, Kim JH, Kim SK, Kang KW, Park KW, Choi JI, et al. A prospective evaluation of 18F-FDG and 11C-acetate PET/CT for detection of primary and metastatic hepatocellular carcinoma. J Nucl Med. 2008;49(12):1912–21. Epub 2008/11/11.
29. Lam MG, Kwee TC, Basu S, Alavi A. Underestimated role of 18F-FDG PET for HCC evaluation and promise of 18F-FDG PET/MR imaging in this setting. J Nucl Med. 2013;54(8):1510–1. Epub 2013/06/20.
30. Sadowski SM, Millo C, Cottle-Delisle C, Merkel R, Yang LA, Herscovitch P, et al. Results of (68)gallium-DOTATATE PET/CT scanning in patients with multiple endocrine neoplasia type 1. J Am Coll Surg. 2015;221(2):509–17. Epub 2015/07/25.
31. van Binnebeek S, Vanbilloen B, Baete K, Terwinghe C, Koole M, Mottaghy FM, et al. Comparison of diagnostic accuracy of (111)in-pentetreotide SPECT and (68)Ga-DOTATOC PET/CT: a lesion-by-lesion analysis in patients with metastatic neuroendocrine tumours. Eur Radiol. 2016;26(3):900–9. Epub 2015/07/15.
32. Michels NA. Newer anatomy of the liver and its variant blood supply and collateral circulation. Am J Surg. 1966;112(3):337–47.
33. Koops A, Wojciechowski B, Broering DC, Adam G, Krupski-Berdien G. Anatomic variations of the hepatic arteries in 604 selective celiac and superior mesenteric angiographies. Surg Radiol Anat. 2004;26(3):239–44. Epub 2004/02/18.
34. Hiatt JR, Gabbay J, Busuttil RW. Surgical anatomy of the hepatic arteries in 1000 cases. Ann Surg. 1994;220(1):50–2.
35. Gruttadauria S, Foglienie S, Doria C, Luca A, Lauro A, Marino IR. The hepatic artery in liver transplantation and surgery: vascular anomalies in 701 cases. Clin Transpl. 2001;15:359–63.
36. Braat MN, van den Hoven AF, van Doormaal PJ, Bruijnen RC, Lam MG, van den Bosch MA. The caudate lobe: the blind spot in Radioembolization or an overlooked opportunity? Cardiovasc Intervent Radiol. 2016;39(6):847–54. Epub 2016/03/24.
37. van den Hoven AF, van Leeuwen MS, Lam MG, van den Bosch MA. Hepatic arterial configuration in relation to the segmental anatomy of the liver; observations on MDCT and DSA relevant to radioembolization treatment. Cardiovasc Intervent Radiol. 2015;38(1):100–11. Epub 2014/03/08.
38. van den Hoven AF, Smits ML, de Keizer B, van Leeuwen MS, van den Bosch MA, Lam MG. Identifying aberrant hepatic arteries prior to intra-arterial radioembolization. Cardiovasc Intervent Radiol. 2014;37(6):1482–93. Epub 2014/01/29.
39. Spreafico C, Morosi C, Maccauro M, Romito R, Lanocita R, Civelli EM, et al. Intrahepatic flow redistribution in patients treated with radioembolization. Cardiovasc Intervent Radiol. 2015;38(2):322–8. Epub 2014/06/15.
40. Abdelmaksoud MH, Hwang GL, Louie JD, Kothary N, Hofmann LV, Kuo WT, et al. Development of new hepaticoenteric collateral pathways after hepatic arterial skeletonization in preparation for yttrium-90 radioembolization. J Vasc Interv Radiol. 2010;21(9):1385–95. Epub 2010/08/07.
41. Bishay VL, Biederman DM, Ward TJ, van der Bom IMJ, Patel RS, Kim E, et al. Transradial approach for hepatic Radioembolization: initial results and technique. Am J Roentgenol. 2016;207(5):1112–21.

42. Theysohn JM, Ruhlmann M, Muller S, Dechene A, Best J, Haubold J, et al. Radioembolization with Y-90 glass microspheres: do we really need SPECT-CT to identify extrahepatic shunts? PLoS One. 2015;10(9):e0137587. Epub 2015/09/04.
43. Bapst B, Lagadec M, Breguet R, Vilgrain V, Ronot M. Cone Beam Computed Tomography (CBCT) in the field of interventional oncology of the liver. Cardiovasc Intervent Radiol. 2016;39(1):8–20. Epub 2015/07/17.
44. van den Hoven AF, Prince JF, de Keizer B, Vonken EJ, Bruijnen RC, Verkooijen HM, et al. Use of C-arm cone beam CT during hepatic Radioembolization: protocol optimization for extrahepatic shunting and parenchymal enhancement. Cardiovasc Intervent Radiol. 2016;39(1):64–73. Epub 2015/06/13.
45. Grozinger G, Kupferschlager J, Dittmann H, Maurer M, Grosse U, la Fougere C, et al. Assessment of the parenchymal blood volume by C-arm computed tomography for radioembolization dosimetry. Eur J Radiol. 2016;85(9):1525–31. Epub 2016/08/10.
46. Garin E, Rolland Y, Laffont S, Edeline J. Clinical impact of (99m)Tc-MAA SPECT/CT-based dosimetry in the radioembolization of liver malignancies with (90)Y-loaded microspheres. Eur J Nucl Med Mol Imaging. 2016;43(3):559–75. Epub 2015/09/05.
47. van de Wiele C, Maes A, Brugman E, D'Asseler Y, De Spiegeleer B, Mees G, et al. SIRT of liver metastases: physiological and pathophysiological considerations. Eur J Nucl Med Mol Imaging. 2012;39(10):1646–55. Epub 2012/07/18.
48. Wondergem M, Smits ML, Elschot M, de Jong HW, Verkooijen HM, van den Bosch MA, et al. 99mTc-macroaggregated albumin poorly predicts the intrahepatic distribution of 90Y resin microspheres in hepatic radioembolization. J Nucl Med. 2013;54(8):1294–301. Epub 2013/06/12.
49. Haste P, Tann M, Persohn S, LaRoche T, Aaron V, Mauxion T, et al. Correlation of technetium-99m macroaggregated albumin and Yttrium-90 glass microsphere biodistribution in hepatocellular carcinoma: a retrospective review of pretreatment single photon emission CT and posttreatment positron emission tomography/CT. J Vasc Interv Radiol. 2017;28(5):722–30.e1. Epub 2017/02/28.
50. Ilhan H, Goritschan A, Paprottka P, Jakobs TF, Fendler WP, Todica A, et al. Predictive value of 99mTc-MAA SPECT for 90Y-labeled resin microsphere distribution in Radioembolization of primary and secondary hepatic tumors. J Nucl Med. 2015;56(11):1654–60. Epub 2015/09/01.
51. Gnesin S, Canetti L, Adib S, Cherbuin N, Silva Monteiro M, Bize P, et al. Partition model-based 99mTc-MAA SPECT/CT predictive dosimetry compared with 90Y TOF PET/CT posttreatment dosimetry in Radioembolization of hepatocellular carcinoma: a quantitative agreement comparison. J Nucl Med. 2016;57(11):1672–8. Epub 2016/11/03.
52. Smits ML, Elschot M, Sze DY, Kao YH, Nijsen JF, Iagaru AH, et al. Radioembolization dosimetry: the road ahead. Cardiovasc Intervent Radiol. 2015;38(2):261–9. Epub 2014/12/30.
53. Elschot M, Nijsen JF, Lam MG, Smits ML, Prince JF, Viergever MA, et al. ((9)(9)m)Tc-MAA overestimates the absorbed dose to the lungs in radioembolization: a quantitative evaluation in patients treated with (1)(6)(6)Ho-microspheres. Eur J Nucl Med Mol Imaging. 2014;41(10):1965–75. Epub 2014/05/14.
54. Braat A, Prince JF, van Rooij R, Bruijnen RCG, van den Bosch M, Lam M. Safety analysis of holmium-166 microsphere scout dose imaging during radioembolisation work-up: a cohort study. Eur Radiol. 2017. Epub 2017/08/09.
55. Yu N, Srinivas SM, Difilippo FP, Shrikanthan S, Levitin A, McLennan G, et al. Lung dose calculation with SPECT/CT for (9)(0)Yittrium radioembolization of liver cancer. Int J Radiat Oncol Biol Phys. 2013;85(3):834–9. Epub 2012/08/09.
56. Kao YH, Magsombol BM, Toh Y, Tay KH, Chow PKH, Goh ASW, et al. Personalized predictive lung dosimetry by technetium-99m macroaggregated albumin SPECT/CT for yttrium-90 radioembolization. EJNMMI Res. 2014;4(33).
57. Gaba RC, Zivin SP, Dikopf MS, Parvinian A, Casadaban LC, Lu Y, et al. Characteristics of primary and secondary hepatic malignancies associated with hepatopulmonary shunting. Radiology. 2014;271(2):602–12.
58. Gray B, van Hazel G, Hope M, Burton M, Moroz P, Anderson J, et al. Randomised trial of SIR-spheres plus chemotherapy vs. chemotherapy alone for treating patients with liver metastases from primary large bowel cancer. Ann Oncol. 2001;12(12):1711–20.
59. Salem R, Thurston KG. Radioembolization with 90Yttrium microspheres: a state-of-the-art brachytherapy treatment for primary and secondary liver malignancies. Part 1: technical and methodologic considerations. J Vasc Interv Radiol. 2006;17(8):1251–78. Epub 2006/08/23.
60. Salem R, Thurston KG. Radioembolization with 90yttrium microspheres: a state-of-the-art brachytherapy treatment for primary and secondary liver malignancies. Part 2: special topics. J Vasc Interv Radiol. 2006;17(9):1425–39. Epub 2006/09/23.
61. Salem R, Thurston KG. Radioembolization with yttrium-90 microspheres: a state-of-the-art brachytherapy treatment for primary and secondary liver malignancies: part 3: comprehensive literature review and future direction. J Vasc Interv Radiol. 2006;17(10):1571–93. Epub 2006/10/24.
62. Smits MLJ, Nijsen JFW, van den Bosch MAAJ, Lam MGEH, Vente MAD, Mali WPTM, et al. Holmium-166 radioembolisation in patients with unresectable, chemorefractory liver metastases (HEPAR trial): a phase 1, dose-escalation study. Lancet Oncol. 2012;13(10):1025–34.
63. Chiesa C, Mira M, Maccauro M, Spreafico C, Romito R, Morosi C, et al. Radioembolization of hepatocarcinoma with (90)Y glass microspheres: development of an individualized treatment planning strategy based

on dosimetry and radiobiology. Eur J Nucl Med Mol Imaging. 2015;42(11):1718–38. Epub 2015/06/27.
64. Pacilio M, Ferrari M, Chiesa C, Lorenzon L, Mira M, Botta F, et al. Impact of SPECT corrections on 3D-dosimetry for liver transarterial radioembolization using the patient relative calibration methodology. Med Phys. 2016;43(7).
65. Kennedy A, Nag S, Salem R, Murthy R, McEwan AJ, Nutting C, et al. Recommendations for radioembolization of hepatic malignancies using yttrium-90 microsphere brachytherapy: a consensus panel report from the radioembolization brachytherapy oncology consortium. Int J Radiat Oncol Biol Phys. 2007;68(1):13–23. Epub 2007/04/24.
66. Borggreve AS, Landman AJ, Vissers CM, de Jong CD, Lam MG, Monninkhof EM, et al. Radioembolization: is prophylactic embolization of Hepaticoenteric arteries necessary? A systematic review. Cardiovasc Intervent Radiol. 2016;39(5):696–704. Epub 2016/03/05.
67. Boas FE, Ziv E, Yarmohammadi H, Brown KT, Erinjeri JP, Sofocleous CT, et al. Adjuvant medications that improve survival after Locoregional therapy. J Vasc Interv Radiol. 2017;28(7):971–7.e4. Epub 2017/05/22.
68. Yarmohammadi H, Erinjeri JP, Brown KT. Embolization of metastatic neuroendocrine tumor resulting in clinical manifestations of syndrome of inappropriate secretion of antidiuretic hormone. J Vasc Interv Radiol. 2015;26(4):533–7. Epub 2015/03/26.
69. BTG. TheraSphere Yttrium-90 Glass Microspheres Instructions for Use. 2017. https://www.btg-im.com/BTG/media/TheraSphere-Documents/PDF/10093509-Rev8_English-searchable.pdf.
70. Ahmadzadehfar H, Meyer C, Pieper CC, Bundschuh R, Muckle M, Gartner F, et al. Evaluation of the delivered activity of yttrium-90 resin microspheres using sterile water and 5% glucose during administration. EJNMMI Res. 2015;5(1):54. Epub 2015/10/16.
71. Paprottka KJ, Lehner S, Fendler WP, Ilhan H, Rominger A, Sommer W, et al. Reduced Periprocedural analgesia after replacement of water for injection with glucose 5% solution as the infusion medium for 90Y-resin microspheres. J Nucl Med. 2016;57(11):1679–84. Epub 2016/11/03.
72. Customer Kit and Delivery Set. QuiremSpheres; 2017. http://www.quiremspheres.com/customer-kit.html.
73. Services UDoHaH. Common Terminology Criteria for Adverse Events (CTCAE) Version 4.0. National Cancer Institute. 2010.
74. Braat MN, van Erpecum KJ, Zonnenberg BA, van den Bosch MA, Lam MG. Radioembolization-induced liver disease: a systematic review. Eur J Gastroenterol Hepatol. 2017;29(2):144–52. Epub 2016/12/08.
75. Mahnken AH. Current status of transarterial radioembolization. World J Radiol. 2016;8(5):449–59. Epub 2016/06/02.
76. Roberson Ii JD, McDonald AM, Baden CJ, Lin CP, Jacob R, Burnett Iii OL. Factors associated with increased incidence of severe toxicities following yttrium-90 resin microspheres in the treatment of hepatic malignancies. World J Gastroenterol. 2016;22(10):3006–14. Epub 2016/03/15.
77. Gabrielson A, Miller A, Banovac F, Kim A, He AR, Unger K. Outcomes and predictors of toxicity after selective internal radiation therapy using Yttrium-90 resin microspheres for Unresectable hepatocellular carcinoma. Front Oncol. 2015;5:292. Epub 2016/01/19.
78. Smits ML, van den Hoven AF, Rosenbaum CE, Zonnenberg BA, Lam MG, Nijsen JF, et al. Clinical and laboratory toxicity after intra-arterial radioembolization with (90)y-microspheres for unresectable liver metastases. PLoS One. 2013;8(7):e69448. Epub 2013/07/31.
79. Sangro B, Martínez-Urbistondo D, Bester L, Bilbao JI, Coldwell DM, Flamen P, et al. Prevention and treatment of complications of selective internal radiation therapy: expert guidance and systematic review. Hepatology. 2017;66(3).
80. Lam MG, Banerjee S, Louie JD, Abdelmaksoud MH, Iagaru AH, Ennen RE, et al. Root cause analysis of gastroduodenal ulceration after yttrium-90 radioembolization. Cardiovasc Intervent Radiol. 2013;36(6):1536–47. Epub 2013/02/26.
81. Prince JF, van den Hoven AF, van den Bosch MA, Elschot M, de Jong HW, Lam MG. Radiation-induced cholecystitis after hepatic radioembolization: do we need to take precautionary measures? J Vasc Interv Radiol. 2014;25(11):1717–23. Epub 2014/12/03.
82. Braat A, Lam M. No need for prophylactic abdominal ice packing during radioembolization. Cardiovasc Intervent Radiol. 2017.
83. Su YK, Mackey RV, Riaz A, Gates VL, Benson AB, 3rd, Miller FH, et al. Long-term hepatotoxicity of yttrium-90 radioembolization as treatment of metastatic neuroendocrine tumor to the liver. J Vascu Interv Radiol. 2017. Epub 2017/07/05.
84. Pasciak AS, Bourgeois AC, McKinney JM, Chang TT, Osborne DR, Acuff SN, et al. Radioembolization and the dynamic role of (90)Y PET/CT. Front Oncol. 2014;4:38. Epub 2014/03/01.
85. Yue J, Mauxion T, Reyes D, Lodge M, Hobbs R, Rong X, et al. Comparison of quantitative Y-90 SPECT and non-time-of-flight PET imaging in post-therapy radioembolization of liver cancer. Med Phys. 2016;43(10):5779.
86. Elschot M, Lam MG, van den Bosch MA, Viergever MA, de Jong HW. Quantitative Monte Carlo-based 90Y SPECT reconstruction. J Nucl Med. 2013;54(9):1557–63. Epub 2013/08/03.
87. Dewaraja YK, Chun SY, Srinivasa RN, Kaza RK, Cuneo KC, Majdalany BS, et al. Improved quantitative 90Y bremsstrahlung SPECT/CT reconstruction with Monte Carlo scatter modeling. Med Phys. 2017;44(12):6364–76.

88. Elschot M, Vermolen BJ, Lam MG, de Keizer B, van den Bosch MA, de Jong HW. Quantitative comparison of PET and bremsstrahlung SPECT for imaging the in vivo yttrium-90 microsphere distribution after liver radioembolization. PLoS One. 2013;8(2):e55742. Epub 2013/02/14.
89. Takahashi A, Himuro K, Yamashita Y, Komiya I, Baba S, Sasaki M. Monte Carlo simulation of PET and SPECT imaging of 90Y. Med Phys. 2015;42(4):1926–35. Epub 2015/04/04.
90. Bastiaannet R, Viergever MA, de Jong H. Impact of respiratory motion and acquisition settings on SPECT liver dosimetry for radioembolization. Med Phys. 2017. Epub 2017/07/25;44:5270.
91. Zade AA, Rangarajan V, Purandare NC, Shah SA, Agrawal AR, Kulkarni SS, et al. 90Y microsphere therapy: does 90Y PET/CT imaging obviate the need for 90Y bremsstrahlung SPECT/CT imaging? Nucl Med Commun. 2013;34(11):1090–6. Epub 2013/08/15.
92. Willowson KP, Tapner M, Bailey DL. A multicentre comparison of quantitative (90)Y PET/CT for dosimetric purposes after radioembolization with resin microspheres: the QUEST phantom study. Eur J Nucl Med Mol Imaging. 2015;42(8):1202–22. Epub 2015/05/15.
93. Wright CL, Binzel K, Zhang J, Wuthrick EJ, Knopp MV. Clinical feasibility of 90Y digital PET/CT for imaging microsphere biodistribution following radioembolization. Eur J Nucl Med Mol Imaging. 2017;44(7):1194–7. Epub 2017/04/14.
94. Fowler KJ, Maughan NM, Laforest R, Saad NE, Sharma A, Olsen J, et al. PET/MRI of hepatic 90Y microsphere deposition determines individual tumor response. Cardiovasc Intervent Radiol. 2016;39(6):855–64. Epub 2016/01/02.
95. Eldib M, Oesingmann N, Faul DD, Kostakoglu L, Knesaurek K, Fayad ZA. Optimization of yttrium-90 PET for simultaneous PET/MR imaging: a phantom study. Med Phys. 2016;43(8):4768. Epub 2016/08/05.
96. Donato H, Franca M, Candelaria I, Caseiro-Alves F. Liver MRI: from basic protocol to advanced techniques. Eur J Radiol. 2017;93:30–9. Epub 2017/07/03.
97. Schmeel FC, Simon B, Luetkens JA, Traber F, Meyer C, Schmeel LC, et al. Prognostic value of pretreatment diffusion-weighted magnetic resonance imaging for outcome prediction of colorectal cancer liver metastases undergoing 90Y-microsphere radioembolization. J Cancer Res Clin Oncol. 2017;143(8):1531–41. Epub 2017/03/21.
98. Morsbach F, Sah BR, Spring L, Puippe G, Gordic S, Seifert B, et al. Perfusion CT best predicts outcome after radioembolization of liver metastases: a comparison of radionuclide and CT imaging techniques. Eur Radiol. 2014;24(7):1455–65. Epub 2014/05/13.
99. Sommer WH, Ceelen F, Garcia-Albeniz X, Paprottka PM, Auernhammer CJ, Armbruster M, et al. Defining predictors for long progression-free survival after radioembolisation of hepatic metastases of neuroendocrine origin. Eur Radiol. 2013;23(11):3094–103. Epub 2013/06/29.
100. Mojtahedi A, Thamake S, Tworowska I, Ranganathan D, Delpassand ES. The value of 68Ga DOTATATE PET/CT in diagnosis and management of neuroendocrine tumors compared to current FDA approved imaging modalities: a review of literature. Am J Nucl Med Mol Imaging. 2014;4(5):426–34.
101. Kayani I, Bomanji JB, Groves A, Conway G, Gacinovic S, Win T, et al. Functional imaging of neuroendocrine tumors with combined PET/CT using 68Ga-DOTATATE (DOTA-DPhe1,Tyr3-octreotate) and 18F-FDG. Cancer. 2008;112(11):2447–55. Epub 2008/04/03.
102. Eisenhauer EA, Therasse P, Bogaerts J, Schwartz LH, Sargent D, Ford R, et al. New response evaluation criteria in solid tumours: revised RECIST guideline (version 1.1). Eur J Cancer. 2009;45(2):228–47. Epub 2008/12/23.
103. Fournier L, Ammari S, Thiam R, Cuenod CA. Imaging criteria for assessing tumour response: RECIST, mRECIST, Cheson. Diagn Interv Imaging. 2014;95(7–8):689–703. Epub 2014/06/22.
104. Tirkes T, Hollar MA, Tann M, Kohli MD, Akisik F, Sandrasegaran K. Response criteria in oncologic imaging: review of traditional and new criteria. Radiographics. 2013;33:1323–41.
105. Lencioni R, Llovet JM. Modified RECIST (mRECIST) assessment for hepatocellular carcinoma. Semin Liver Dis. 2010;30(1):52–60. Epub 2010/02/23.
106. Hyun O, Lodge M, Wahl R. Practical PERCIST: a simplified guide to PET response criteria in solid tumors 1.0. Radiology. 2016;280(2):576–84.
107. Min SJ, Jang HJ, Kim JH. Comparison of the RECIST and PERCIST criteria in solid tumours: a pooled analysis and review. Oncotarget. 2016;7(19).
108. Hyun O, Lodge M, Wahl R. Practical PERCIST: a simplified guid to PET response criteria in solid tumors 1.0. Radiology. 2016;280(2):576–84.
109. Magistri P, Tarantino G, Ballarin R, Berretta M, Pecchi A, Ramacciato G, et al. The evolving role of local treatments for HCC in the third millennium. Anticancer Res. 2017;37(2):389–401. Epub 2017/02/10.
110. Bruix J, Reig M, Sherman M. Evidence-based diagnosis, staging, and treatment of patients with hepatocellular carcinoma. Gastroenterology. 2016;150(4):835–53. Epub 2016/01/23.
111. Padia SA, Kwan SW, Roudsari B, Monsky WL, Coveler A, Harris WP. Superselective yttrium-90 radioembolization for hepatocellular carcinoma yields high response rates with minimal toxicity. J Vasc Interv Radiol. 2014;25(7):1067–73. Epub 2014/05/20.
112. Biederman DM, Titano JJ, Bishay VL, Durrani RJ, Dayan E, Tabori N, et al. Radiation Segmentectomy

versus TACE combined with microwave ablation for Unresectable solitary hepatocellular carcinoma up to 3 cm: a propensity score matching study. Radiology. 2017;283(3):895–905.
113. Tohme S, Sukato D, Chen HW, Amesur N, Zajko AB, Humar A, et al. Yttrium-90 radioembolization as a bridge to liver transplantation: a single-institution experience. J Vasc Interv Radiol. 2013;24(11):1632–8. Epub 2013/10/29.
114. Mohamed M, Katz AW, Tejani MA, Sharma AK, Kashyap R, Noel MS, et al. Comparison of outcomes between SBRT, yttrium-90 radioembolization, transarterial chemoembolization, and radiofrequency ablation as bridge to transplant for hepatocellular carcinoma. Adv Radiat Oncol. 2016;1(1):35–42. Epub 2015/12/29.
115. Kolligs FT, Bilbao JI, Jakobs T, Inarrairaegui M, Nagel JM, Rodriguez M, et al. Pilot randomized trial of selective internal radiation therapy vs. chemoembolization in unresectable hepatocellular carcinoma. Liver Int. 2015;35(6):1715–21. Epub 2014/12/03.
116. Gordon A, Lewandowski R, Hickey R, Kallini J, Gabr A, Sato K, et al. Prospective randomized phase 2 study of chemoembolization versus radioembolization in hepatocellular carcinoma: results from the PREMIERE trial. J Vasc Interv Radiol. 2016;27(3):S61–S2.
117. Katsanos K, Kitrou P, Spiliopoulos S, Maroulis I, Petsas T, Karnabatidis D. Comparative effectiveness of different transarterial embolization therapies alone or in combination with local ablative or adjuvant systemic treatments for unresectable hepatocellular carcinoma: a network meta-analysis of randomized controlled trials. PLoS One. 2017;12(9):e0184597. Epub 2017/09/22.
118. Garin E, Rolland Y, Edeline J, Icard N, Lenoir L, Laffont S, et al. Personalized dosimetry with intensification using 90Y-loaded glass microsphere radioembolization induces prolonged overall survival in hepatocellular carcinoma patients with portal vein thrombosis. J Nucl Med. 2015;56(3):339–46. Epub 2015/02/14.
119. Ali R, Gabr A, Abouchaleh N, Al Asadi A, Mora RA, Kulik L, et al. Survival analysis of advanced HCC treated with Radioembolization: comparing impact of clinical performance status versus vascular invasion/metastases. Cardiovasc Intervent Radiol. 2017. Epub 2017/09/08.
120. Floridi C, Pesapane F, Angileri SA, de Palma D, Fontana F, Caspani F, et al. Yttrium-90 radioembolization treatment for unresectable hepatocellular carcinoma: a single-Centre prognostic factors analysis. Med Oncol. 2017;34(10):174. Epub 2017/09/07.
121. Vilgrain V, Pereira H, Assenat E, Guiu B, Ilonca AD, Pageaux G-P, et al. Efficacy and safety of selective internal radiotherapy with yttrium-90 resin microspheres compared with sorafenib in locally advanced and inoperable hepatocellular carcinoma (SARAH): an open-label randomised controlled phase 3 trial. Lancet Oncol. 2017;18:1624.
122. Chow PK, Gandhi M. SIRveNIB clinical study ASCO oral abstract presentation. 2017.
123. Hendlisz A, van den Eynde M, Peeters M, Maleux G, Lambert B, Vannoote J, et al. Phase III trial comparing protracted intravenous fluorouracil infusion alone or with yttrium-90 resin microspheres radioembolization for liver-limited metastatic colorectal cancer refractory to standard chemotherapy. J Clin Oncol. 2010;28(23):3687–94. Epub 2010/06/23.
124. Kennedy A, Cohn M, Coldwell DM, Drooz A, Ehrenwald E, Kaiser A, et al. Updated survival outcomes and analysis of long-term survivors from the MORE study on safety and efficacy of radioembolization in patients with unresectable colorectal cancer liver metastases. J Gastrointest Oncol. 2017;8(4):614–24. Epub 2017/09/12.
125. Kennedy AS, Nutting C, Coldwell D, Gaiser J, Drachenberg C. Pathologic response and microdosimetry of (90)Y microspheres in man: review of four explanted whole livers. Int J Radiat Oncol Biol Phys. 2004;60(5):1552–63. Epub 2004/12/14.
126. Sofocleous CT, Violari EG, Sotirchos VS, Shady W, Gonen M, Pandit-Taskar N, et al. Radioembolization as a salvage therapy for heavily pretreated patients with colorectal Cancer liver metastases: factors that affect outcomes. Clin Colorectal Cancer. 2015;14(4):296–305. Epub 2015/08/19.
127. Wasan HS, Gibbs P, Sharma NK, Taieb J, Heinemann V, Ricke J, et al. First-line selective internal radiotherapy plus chemotherapy versus chemotherapy alone in patients with liver metastases from colorectal cancer (FOXFIRE, SIRFLOX and FOXFIRE-Global): a combined analysis of three multicentre, randomised, phase 3 trials. Lancet Oncol. 2017;18:1159.
128. Braat AJAT, Kappadath SC, Bruijnen RCG, van den Hoven AF, Mahvash A, de Jong HWAM, et al. Adequate SIRT activity dose is as important as adequate chemotherapy dose. Lancet Oncol. 2017;18(11):e636.
129. Devcic Z, Rosenberg J, Braat AJ, Techasith T, Banerjee A, Sze DY, et al. The efficacy of hepatic 90Y resin radioembolization for metastatic neuroendocrine tumors: a meta-analysis. J Nucl Med. 2014;55(9):1404–10. Epub 2014/07/12.
130. Jia Z, Paz-Fumagalli R, Frey G, Sella DM, McKinney JM, Wang W. Single-institution experience of radioembolization with yttrium-90 microspheres for unresectable metastatic neuroendocrine liver tumors. J Gastroenterol Hepatol. 2017;32(9):1617–23. Epub 2017/01/31.
131. Chansanti O, Jahangiri Y, Matsui Y, Adachi A, Geeratikun Y, Kaufman JA, et al. Tumor dose response in Yttrium-90 resin microsphere embolization for neuroendocrine liver metastases: a tumor-specific analysis with dose estimation using SPECT-CT. J Vasc Interv Radiol. 2017;28:1528. Epub 2017/09/11.
132. Chen JX, Rose S, White SB, El-Haddad G, Fidelman N, Yarmohammadi H, et al. Embolotherapy for neuroendocrine tumor liver metastases: prognos-

tic factors for hepatic progression-free survival and overall survival. Cardiovasc Intervent Radiol. 2017;40(1):69–80. Epub 2016/10/16.
133. Jia Z, Jiang G, Zhu C, Wang K, Li S, Qin X. A systematic review of yttrium-90 radioembolization for unresectable liver metastases of melanoma. Eur J Radiol. 2017;92:111–5. Epub 2017/06/19.
134. Michl M, Haug AR, Jakobs TF, Paprottka P, Hoffmann RT, Bartenstein P, et al. Radioembolization with Yttrium-90 microspheres (SIRT) in pancreatic cancer patients with liver metastases: efficacy, safety and prognostic factors. Oncology. 2014;86(1):24–32. Epub 2014/01/10.
135. Kim AY, Unger K, Wang H, Pishvaian MJ. Incorporating Yttrium-90 trans-arterial radioembolization (TARE) in the treatment of metastatic pancreatic adenocarcioma: a single center experience. BMC Cancer. 2016;16:492. Epub 2016/07/20.
136. Kis B, Shah J, Choi J, El-Haddad G, Sweeney J, Biebel B, et al. Transarterial Yttrium-90 Radioembolization treatment of patients with liver-dominant metastatic renal cell carcinoma. J Vasc Interv Radiol. 2017;28(2):254–9. Epub 2016/12/14.
137. Kuei A, Saab S, Cho SK, Kee ST, Lee EW. Effects of Yttrium-90 selective internal radiation therapy on non-conventional liver tumors. World J Gastroenterol. 2015;21(27):8271–83. Epub 2015/07/29.
138. Lam MG, Louie JD, Iagaru AH, Goris ML, Sze DY. Safety of repeated yttrium-90 radioembolization. Cardiovasc Intervent Radiol. 2013;36(5):1320–8. Epub 2013/01/29.
139. Zarva A, Mohnike K, Damm R, Ruf J, Seidensticker R, Ulrich G, et al. Safety of repeated radioembolizations in patients with advanced primary and secondary liver tumors and progressive disease after first selective internal radiotherapy. J Nucl Med. 2014;55(3):360–6. Epub 2014/02/12.
140. Garin E, Rolland Y, Pracht M, Le Sourd S, Laffont S, Mesbah H, et al. High impact of macroaggregated albumin-based tumour dose on response and overall survival in hepatocellular carcinoma patients treated with (90) Y-loaded glass microsphere radioembolization. Liver Int. 2017;37(1):101–10. Epub 2016/08/16.
141. Braat MN, Samim M, van den Bosch MA, Lam MG. The role of 90Y-radioembolization in downstaging primary and secondary hepatic malignancies: a systematic review. Clin Trans Imaging. 2016;4:283–95. Epub 2016/08/12.
142. Goebel J, Sulke M, Lazik-Palm A, Goebel T, Dechene A, Bellendorf A, et al. Factors associated with contralateral liver hypertrophy after unilateral radioembolization for hepatocellular carcinoma. PLoS One. 2017;12(7):e0181488. Epub 2017/07/15.
143. Gates VL, Marshall KG, Salzig K, Williams M, Lewandowski RJ, Salem R. Outpatient single-session yttrium-90 glass microsphere radioembolization. J Vasc Interv Radiol. 2014;25(2):266–70. Epub 2013/12/18.
144. van den Hoven AF, Prince JF, Van den Bosch MA, Lam MGEH. Hepatic radioembolization as a true single-session treatment. J Vasc Interv Radiol. 2014;25(7):1143–4.
145. van der Velden S, Beijst C, Viergever MA, de Jong HW. Simultaneous fluoroscopic and nuclear imaging: impact of collimator choice on nuclear image quality. Med Phys. 2017;44(1):249–61. Epub 2017/01/04.
146. Beijst C, Elschot M, Viergever MA, de Jong HWAM. Toward simultaneous real-time fluoroscopic and nuclear imaging in the intervention room. Radiology. 2015;278(1):232–8.
147. Occlusafe-Occlusive Micro Balloon Catheter. Terumo Interventional Systems; 2017. http://www.terumo-europe.com/en-emea/interventional-oncology/access-diagnostic-products/balloon-occlusive-catheter/occlusafe%C2%AE-occlusive-micro-balloon-catheter.
148. The Surefire Infusion System. Surefire Medical; 2017. https://surefiremedical.com/products/.
149. Fischman AM, Ward TJ, Patel RS, Arepally A, Kim E, Nowakowski FS, et al. Prospective, randomized study of coil embolization versus surefire infusion system during yttrium-90 radioembolization with resin microspheres. J Vasc Interv Radiol. 2014;25(11):1709–16. Epub 2014/09/23.
150. Morshedi MM, Bauman M, Rose SC, Kikolski SG. Yttrium-90 resin microsphere radioembolization using an antireflux catheter: an alternative to traditional coil embolization for nontarget protection. Cardiovasc Intervent Radiol. 2015;38(2):381–8. Epub 2014/07/06.
151. van den Hoven AF, Lam MG, Jernigan S, van den Bosch MA, Buckner GD. Innovation in catheter design for intra-arterial liver cancer treatments results in favorable particle-fluid dynamics. J Exp Clin Cancer Res. 2015;34:74. Epub 2015/08/02.
152. Aramburu J, Anton R, Rivas A, Ramos JC, Sangro B, Bilbao JI. Computational particle-haemodynamics analysis of liver radioembolization pretreatment as an actual treatment surrogate. Int J Numer Methods Biomed Eng. 2017;33(2). Epub 2016/04/03.

Assessment of Tumor Response with MRI and CT After Radioembolization

37

Thomas C. Lauenstein, Juliane Schelhorn, and Sonja Kinner

37.1 Introduction

The assessment of therapeutic success is crucial for any form of therapy in patients with malignant disease. The general key issue is to distinguish between responders and non-responders. The rationale to identify the latter group as early as possible is twofold: (a) these patients can be prevented from receiving unsuccessful therapeutic pathways potentially coupled with harmful side-effects and (b) another alternative therapy line can be initiated. Thus, an optimal patient management can be guaranteed.

As selective internal radiotherapy (SIRT) is a relatively new therapeutic option in patients with advanced hepatic tumor disease, there is still no general consensus about the best way to assess tumor response. Cross-sectional imaging including computed tomography (CT) and magnetic resonance imaging (MRI) plays an important role for the initial diagnosis and staging of liver tumors. Hence, it is obvious that these modalities also can be utilized for therapeutic assessment—beyond parameters such as clinical status of the patient, tumor and laboratory markers, and other imaging tool as positron emission tomography (PET).

In the context of SIRT, it is important to adapt the CT or MRI protocols to the primary tumor in question. Many of the tumor entities that are treated with SIRT are hypervascular including hepatocellular carcinoma (HCC) or metastases of neuroendocrine tumors. Hence, it is mandatory to integrate contrast-enhanced imaging with an arterial contrast delay to the examination protocol. This allows for a most accurate delineation of the tumor and the evaluation of changing enhancement patterns, which may be basic markers for therapy success. In this chapter, we discuss current strategies for therapy monitoring based on morphologic/anatomic as well as functional/biologic cross-sectional imaging. Furthermore, literature is reviewed with regards to the most common tumor entities treated with SIRT.

37.2 Assessment of Tumor Morphology

Follow-up imaging using CT or MRI is typically performed at 1 and 3 months after SIRT and subsequently every 3 months or as clinically indicated. The comparison of size and/or tumor morphology with the status prior to SIRT can be used as an indicator for therapy response. Interestingly, first size changes can often only be visualized 3 months post SIRT (Fig. 37.1). Hence, a constant tumor size at 1 month post SIRT does not necessarily mean a

T. C. Lauenstein (✉)
Department of Radiology, Evangelisches Krankenhaus Düsseldorf, Düsseldorf, Germany
e-mail: thomas.lauenstein@uni-due.de

J. Schelhorn · S. Kinner
Department of Diagnostic and Interventional Radiology and Neuroradiology, University Hospital Essenn, Essen, Germany

H. Ahmadzadehfar et al. (eds.), *Clinical Nuclear Medicine*,
https://doi.org/10.1007/978-3-030-39457-8_37

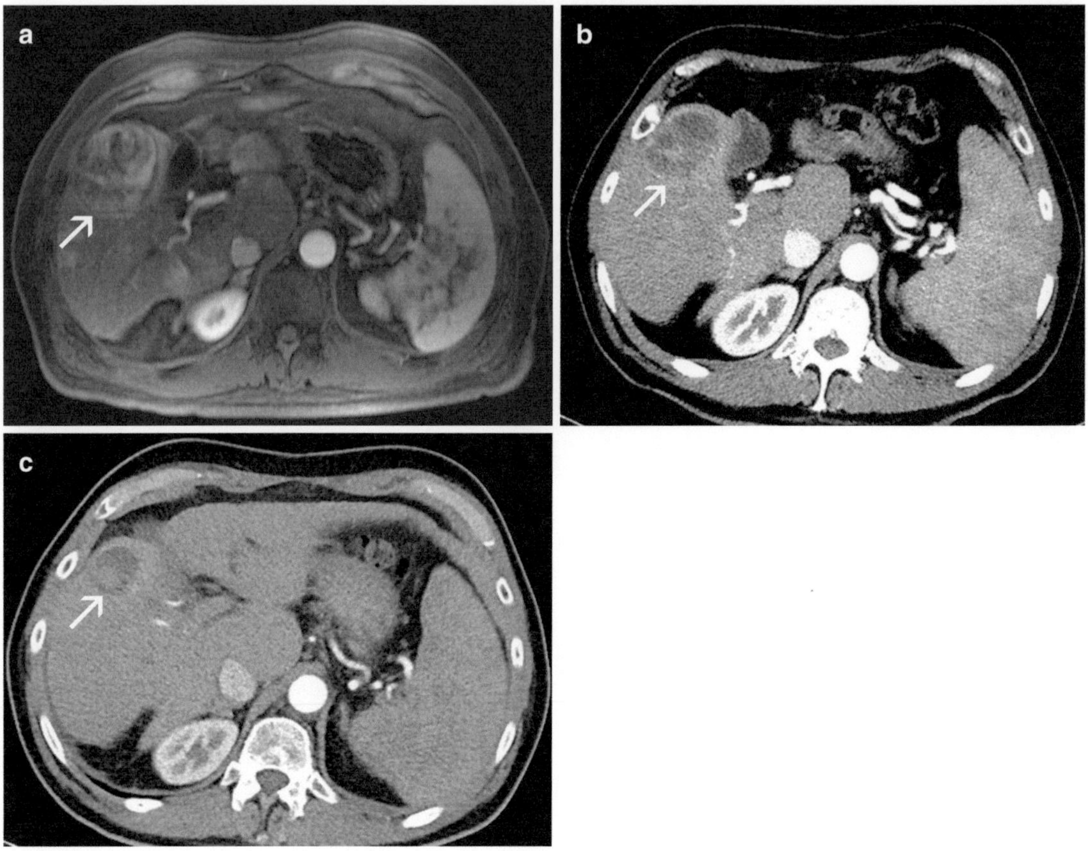

Fig. 37.1 Patient with HCC manifestation in the right liver lobe, which is displayed on the arterial phase contrast-enhanced MRI pre therapy (**a**; arrow). At 1 month post SIRT hardly any size changes are seen on the respective arterial phase CT scan (**b**; arrow). Only 3 months post therapy a tumor response is seen based on size parameters (**c**; CT scan; arrow)

failing response to therapy. In some cases, the tumor may even increase in size during the first 4 weeks after SIRT due to acute necrosis, edema, and hemorrhage. These changes are different from the therapy response assessment following traditional systemic therapy. CT and MRI protocols should therefore always include unenhanced imaging in addition to contrast-enhanced imaging using an arterial and portal-venous contrast delay. Unenhanced CT or MRI may help to distinguish between hemorrhage and vital tumor tissue.

Furthermore, malignancies treated with SIRT may exhibit some morphologic imaging characteristics that can be easily mistaken as tumor progress or recurrence. Particularly post-treatment changes including edema, inflammation, and fibrosis adjacent to the primary tumor may be falsely interpreted. These changes may lead to a rim enhancement around the tumor (Fig. 37.2), which is difficult to be distinguished from vital tumor. As a rule of thumb, edema/inflammation/fibrosis lead to a homogenous enhancement around the lesion whereas vital tumor shows a more nodular and focal appearance.

37.2.1 RECIST/WHO

RECIST and WHO criteria were initially utilized for the evaluation of therapy response to cytotoxic treatments in solid tumors. WHO criteria introduced in 1979 involve two-dimensional measurements of tumor size [1]. To that, the longest tumor diameter is multiplied with the longest

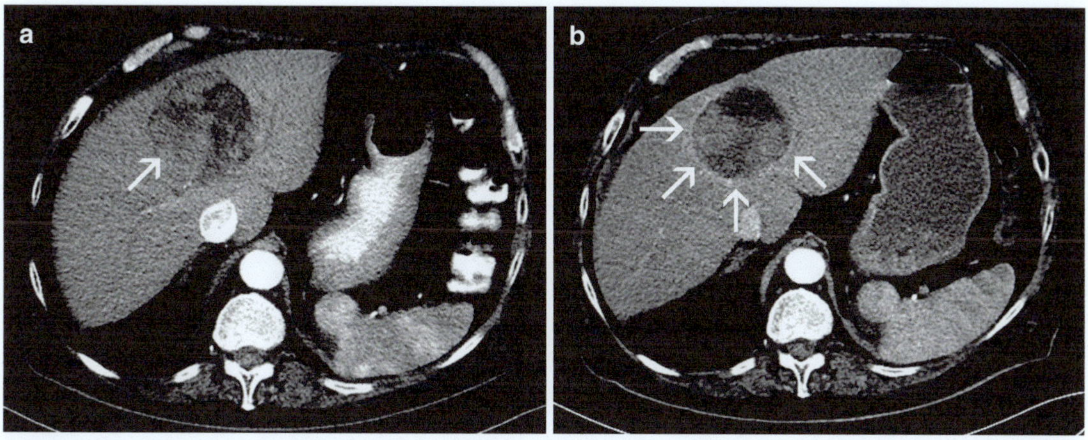

Fig. 37.2 HCC at the border of left and right liver lobe before (**a**; arrow) and 3 months after SIRT (**b**). Post therapy there is a homogenous rim enhancement at the tumor margin in keeping with granulomatous inflammation/fibrosis (**b**; arrows)

Table 37.1 Criteria for the assessment of tumor response

	Complete response (CR)	Partialresponse (PR)	Stable disease(SD)	Progressivedisease (PD)
WHO	Tumor disappearance	≥50% decrease in size	No CR/PR/PD	≥25% increase in size
RECIST	Tumor disappearance	≥30% decrease in size	No CR/PR/PD	≥20% increase in size
EASL	Disappearance of arterial enhancement	≥ 50% decrease in the sum of the arterially enhancing areas	No CR/PR/PD	≥ 25% increase in the size of the arterially enhancing areas
Choi	Tumor disappearance	≥ 10% decrease in size or 15% decrease in density on contrast-enhanced CT	No CR/PR/PD	≥ 10% increase in size and no PR criteria by tumor density

perpendicular diameter. Using WHO criteria, therapeutic success can be categorized as complete response (CR), partial response (PR), stable disease (SD), and progressive disease (PD) (Table 37.1). However, WHO criteria are coupled with some practical limitations. There is neither consensus about the type of imaging modality nor the number of lesions that should be assessed nor the minimum lesion size. Thus, WHO criteria can result in inconsistencies and different response findings [2].

In 2000, RECIST tumor evaluation was introduced to overcome the limitations of the WHO system and to unify the report system of tumor response [3]. Rather than using two-dimensional measurements, RECIST only focuses on the longest uni-dimensional tumor diameter. Furthermore, RECIST criteria define the type of imaging modality and terms such as "target lesion," "non-target-lesion," and "measurable lesion." RECIST is widely used as it is simple, convenient, and reproducible. Further developments of RECIST include RECIST 1.1 [4]. RECIST 1.1 takes criteria into account such as the number of lesions to be assessed and also evaluation of lymph node metastases.

37.2.2 EASL Criteria

An important feature of SIRT is the induction of tumor necrosis, which can be depicted as a lack of contrast enhancement in CT or MRI. Necrosis usually can be seen shortly after SIRT and before changes in tumor size. WHO and RECIST criteria, however, do not take induction of necrosis

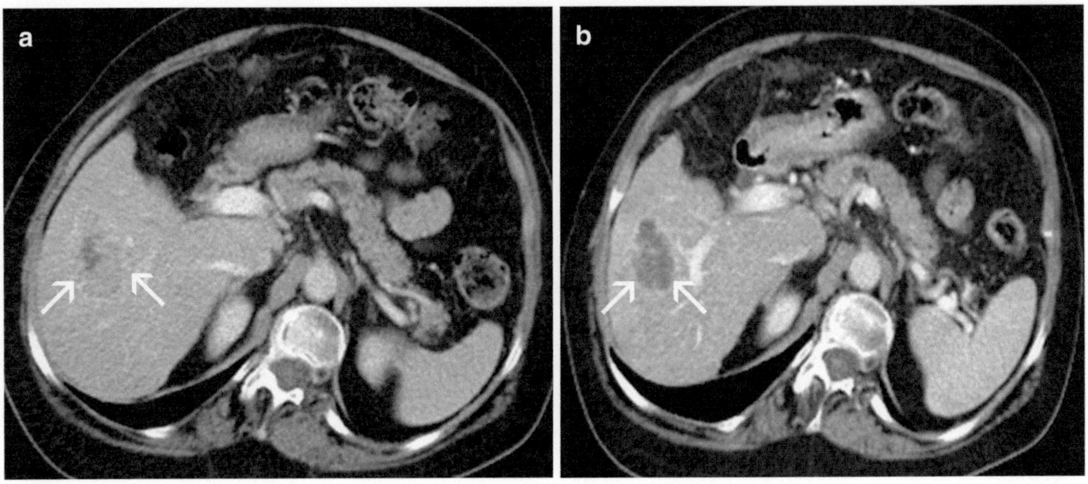

Fig. 37.3 HCC in the right liver lobe. The tumor margins are hard to delineate on the pre therapy CT scan (**a**; arrows). Three months after SIRT, the tumor shows necrotic transformation on the CT scan as a marker for tumor response (**b**; arrows). However, one might misinterpret the better delineation as a tumor growth and as a sign of therapy failure

into account. Thus, the EASL amendments were proposed in order to evaluate viable vs. non-viable tumor (Table 37.1) [5]. The EASL criteria are mainly utilized in patients with HCC (Fig. 37.3). A further development of RECIST applies similar features as EASL: (modified) mRECIST takes arterial enhancement patterns as tumor viability into account. Hence, complete response in mRECIST would represent a total loss of arterial enhancement of all HCC target lesions.

The measurement of tumor necrosis is not trivial. Necrosis can be very irregular in distribution throughout the tumor and may represent not clearly defined, but patchy areas. Hence, the quantification of necrosis is time-consuming and lacks consistency. Monsky et al. [6] introduced a semiautomated software for the determination of tumor necrosis. They evaluated the software in 23 patients with either HCC or hepatic metastases. The volumetric analysis of liver, tumor, and necrosis volume could be performed with a high intra- and interobserver reproducibility. The mean evaluation time amounted to 6 min. The authors found a correlation between necrotic tumor volume and patient survival when a > 10% increase of necrosis was shown on contrast-enhanced CT scans at 1 month after SIRT.

37.2.3 Choi Criteria

The Choi criteria were initiated to assess therapeutic response in patients with gastrointestinal stromal tumors (GIST) to tyrosine kinase inhibitors [7]. To that, changes in tumor density were evaluated by measuring Hounsfield units on CT images. Responders showed a decrease in tumor density interpreted as a feature of necrotic transformation. Similar criteria also have been utilized to predict tumor response after SIRT in patients with hepatic metastases of colorectal cancer (Table 37.1) [8]. Hereby, changes in attenuation based on CT corresponded well with metabolic tumor activity in PET. There are drawbacks of this approach as changes in tumor density may be heterogeneous throughout a lesion and may not be applicable for all tumor entities. Therefore, Choi criteria are not widely used for therapy response evaluation after SIRT.

37.3 Assessment of Tumor Biology

Morphologic changes in tumor size are widely accepted as an imaging marker for the evaluation of therapeutic response in systemic chemotherapy. However, there are differences when local/regional therapies for liver malignancies are employed. Hence, the mere morphologic assessment of tumor after SIRT may lead to false-positive or -negative findings. Therefore, new parameters allowing for an insight into tumor biology rather than tumor morphology are currently investigated regarding their usefulness for therapy assessment.

37.3.1 DWI

Diffusion-weighted imaging (DWI) is a tool to evaluate the free motility of water molecules (Brownian movement). Free water molecules show a random motion. However, cell membranes restrict this motion. Thus, DWI may be used as a marker for tumor cellularity and cell membrane integrity. DWI can be quantified by apparent diffusion coefficient (ADC). The initial ADC pre SIRT is used for the prediction of possible therapy response. Furthermore, changes of DWI under therapy are applied for therapy response evaluation (Fig. 37.4). In this context, ADC measurements can be used as a surrogate for the degree of tumor necrosis: while vital tumor often is associated with restricted diffusion and low ADC, necrotic tissue reveals increased ADC as free water mobility is increased. A successful therapy also results in increased free water mobility as cell density and cell membrane integrity decreases. DWI has been used particularly to monitor SIRT in patients with HCC [9]. Significant changes of DWI in responders precede morphologic changes and can be observed as early as 1 month after SIRT.

Although being a promising tool, DWI is coupled with some limitations. There is a lack of reproducibility of DWI analysis. It is not fully understood if DWI assessment and ADC values can be compared when the MR examinations are performed at different field strengths (e.g., at 1.5 T or 3.0 T) or even at different MR systems with the same field strength. In addition, there are different techniques on how to perform DWI and there is no consensus about a uniform DWI protocol. It will be challenging to overcome these limitations and to standardize the way DWI is performed at different centers worldwide.

37.3.2 Perfusion Imaging

Contrast-enhanced CT or MRI acquired with a high temporal resolution may allow for an insight into tumor perfusion. This may be used as a biomarker for therapy monitoring and even as a predictor for therapy response. In this context, arterial flow can represent a marker for the accumulation of microspheres in a hypervascular tumor. Morsbach et al. examined 38 patients with liver metastases [10]. Responders and non-responders were retrospectively analyzed with regards to perfusion characteristics of the tumor before SIRT. A significant difference in perfusion characteristics was found for the two patient groups. The authors concluded that perfusion analysis enables prediction of therapy response of SIRT with regards to morphologic tumor changes and overall survival.

One of the main drawbacks of perfusion analysis is related to its complexity. Dedicated software tools are needed to perform perfusion analyses. Furthermore, it is not fully clear whether arterial data are sufficient or whether portal-venous and venous enhanced CT or MRI images are needed for the assessment of therapy response as well. Hence, perfusion should be considered a preliminary tool with some potential that needs further evaluation.

37.3.3 Use of Liver-Specific MR Contrast Agents

There are two commercially available MR contrast agents with specific characteristics for liver imaging: Gd-EOB-DTPA (gadoexetic acid, Primovist® or Eovist®; Bayer Healthcare) and Gd-BOPTA (gadobenate dimeglumine, Multihance®; Bracco). These contrast agents show a delayed uptake by hepatocytes and therefore may help to differentiate between liver tissue and non-hepatic tissue (i.e., liver metastases or HCC).

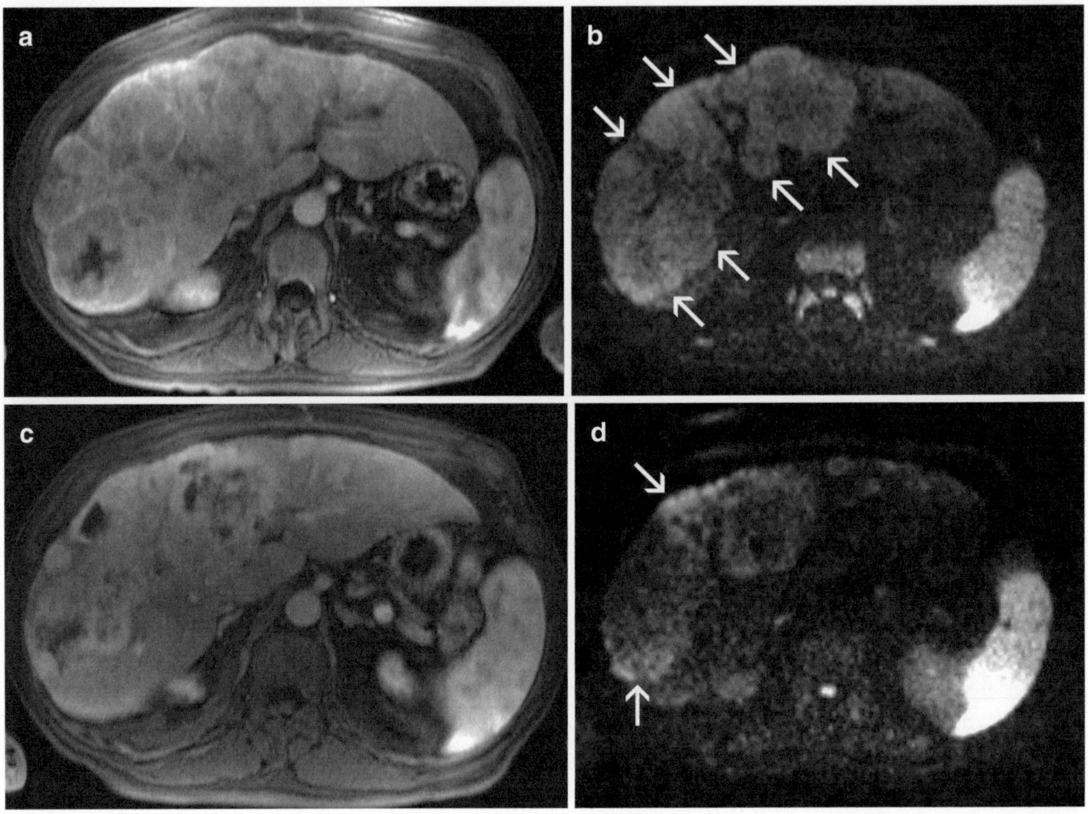

Fig. 37.4 DWI may help to identify responders earlier than morphologic tumor evaluation. Contrast-enhanced MRI shows diffuse tumor disease before (**a**) and 1 month after SIRT (c) with hardly any size changes. DWI, however, exhibits a strong restriction of diffusion in the tumor before SIRT (**b**; arrows; high signal). One month post SIRT, there is a decline of diffusion restriction in the tumor (**d**; arrows)

Thus, they are useful to distinguish between benign perilesional enhancement adjacent to the treated tumor (as described before as inflammation and fibrosis) and vital recurrent or residual tumor lesions. Overall, it may help to avoid false-positive and false-negative findings after SIRT. However, there is still no evidence that the use of this kind of contrast agent may be a marker for therapy response itself.

37.4 Outcome for Different Tumor Entities

37.4.1 HCC

There are several trials evaluating therapy success of SIRT in patients with HCC. Hilgard et al. examined 108 patients undergoing SIRT with glass microspheres [11]. The response to treatment was assessed using CT data pre and post therapy and applying the EASL criteria. Time to progression and overall survival was documented. Complete response was determined in 3%, partial response in 37%, stable disease in 53%, and disease progression in 6% of all cases. Time to progression amounted to 10 months, while median survival was 16.4 months.

Memon et al. addressed another aspect of therapy response evaluation [12]. In their study, they analyzed the association between tumor response and survival times. Furthermore, they addressed the question whether patients responding to tumor therapy live longer than non-responders. One hundred and fifty-nine patients with HCC were evaluated after SIRT and/or transarterial chemoembolization (TACE). Both MRI and CT were used as image modalities and EASL and WHO criteria were applied. Survival times of responders were compared to those of patients with stable disease and progressive disease. Interestingly, survival in responders was only statistically significant longer when EASL criteria were applied. However, WHO criteria failed to prove any statistically significant difference. Hence, EASL criteria more consistently predict the survival time than WHO criteria.

Rhee et al. compared diffusion-weighted imaging with anatomic imaging features [9]. They addressed the question whether response based on DWI actually precedes response based on anatomic changes after therapy. Twenty patients with HCC underwent SIRT. Both morphologic data based on MRI as well as DWI were analyzed before and at 1 and 3 months after SIRT. HCC tumor response could be revealed already 1 month post SIRT using DWI. However, there were no anatomic size changes before 3 months post therapy. These results were confirmed by Kinner et al. [13]. In their trial, 42 patients with histopathologically proven HCC underwent MRI including DWI before and 30 days after SIRT. Changes of tumor size as well as changes in DWI were analyzed. Response to SIRT could be documented by DWI at 1 month post SIRT, while morphologic changes failed to discriminate between responders and non-responders at this time. Hence, DWI may assist in the early determination of response or non-response of SIRT for HCC.

37.4.2 Metastases of Neuroendocrine Tumors (NET)

Neperud et al. analyzed different radiologic features including RECIST, WHO, EASL, and Choi criteria [14]. A total number of 65 liver metastases were assessed in 17 patients who had undergone SIRT with resin microspheres. Interestingly, there was no statistically significant difference for response comparing lesions >2 cm and < 2 cm in diameter. While most evaluation criteria failed to prove a good differentiation between responders and non-responders, only the CHOI criteria were statistically significantly different for both groups.

Saxena et al. evaluated the prognostic variables that may influence radiologic response and survival [15]. Forty-eight patients with NET metastases undergoing SIRT were evaluated. Patients were analyzed radiologically using CT and RECIST criteria and serologically at 1 month and 3 months post SIRT. Complete response was determined in 15%, partial response in 40%, stable disease in 23%, and disease progression in 23% of all cases. The following prognostic factors were associated with an improved survival: low hepatic tumor burden, well-differentiated tumor, female gender, and no extrahepatic disease.

37.4.3 Metastases of Colorectal Carcinoma (CRC)

Most recent studies regarding SIRT in patients with CRC metastases focused on strategies beyond WHO and RECIST to assess therapy response. Tochetto et al. examined 20 patients with colorectal liver metastases [8]. CT scans and DFG PET data (serving as the standard of reference) were acquired before as well as 1 and 3 months after therapy. Attenuation changes based on CT according to the Choi criteria were used to assess therapy response. While morphologic changes including WHO and RECIST only helped to identify 13.3% of responders at 1 month after SIRT, Choi criteria were correct in 53.3%. Choi criteria at 3 months post SIRT even helped to discriminate responders from non-responders in all patients. The authors found that a 15% decrease in attenuation was associated with response with a sensitivity of 93.3% and a specificity of 100%.

Also DWI has been evaluated in patients with colorectal liver metastases undergoing SIRT. Dudeck et al. assessed 41 metastases in 21 patients [16]. DWI was performed before, 48 h after and 6 weeks after SIRT. Metastases were categorized as responding ($n = 33$) or non-responding lesions ($n = 8$) with tumor volume serving as the standard or reference. Interestingly, ADC decreased already 2 days after SIRT in responding lesions, while ADC increased in non-responding lesions. The authors concluded that DWI may be a very early predictor for therapy response.

37.5 Conclusions

CT is a very robust and widely available imaging tool that can be used for tumor staging and follow-up based on size criteria in patients with hepatic malignancies. The analysis of mere anatomic size features for the assessment of therapy response after SIRT may yet lead to false-positive, false–negative, or delayed results. Hence, characteristics such as quantification of tumor necrosis, enhancement pattern, and changes in diffusion restriction are alternatives for therapy monitoring. Thus, MRI is evolving as an attractive surrogate to CT for tumor response evaluation. However, all tools that have been proposed for tumor response assessment after SIRT are coupled with two limitations: (a) Current data are based on only small patient cohorts and further prospective studies are needed. (b) There is no clear evidence if tumor response based on imaging is associated with clinical benefit such as prolonged survival rates of the patients or longer time-to-progression of disease.

Overall, the application of a multiparametric analysis will be a promising approach to monitor therapeutic success in patients after SIRT. As different imaging tools (morphologic and functional) may be helpful depending on the tumor type but also within one group of primary malignancies, a combination of these parameters will be applied in the future for therapy monitoring. The evaluation of a sole imaging technique should rather be avoided.

References

1. Miller AB, Hoogstraten B, Staquet M, Winkler A. Reporting results of cancer treatment. Cancer. 1981;47(1):207–14.
2. Suzuki C, Jacobsson H, Hatschek T, Torkzad MR, Boden K, Eriksson-Alm Y, Berg E, Fujii H, Kubo A, Blomqvist L. Radiologic measurements of tumor response to treatment: practical approaches and limitations. Radiographics. 2008;28(2):329–44.
3. Therasse P, Arbuck SG, Eisenhauer EA, Wanders J, Kaplan RS, Rubinstein L, Verweij J, Van Glabbeke M, van Oosterom AT, Christian MC, et al. New guidelines to evaluate the response to treatment in solid tumors. European Organization for Research and Treatment of Cancer, National Cancer Institute of the United States, National Cancer Institute of Canada. J Natl Cancer Inst. 2000;92(3):205–16.
4. Shanbhogue AK, Karnad AB, Prasad SR. Tumor response evaluation in oncology: current update. J Comput Assist Tomogr. 2010;34(4):479–84.
5. Duke E, Deng J, Ibrahim SM, Lewandowski RJ, Ryu RK, Sato KT, Miller FH, Kulik L, Mulcahy MF, Larson AC, et al. Agreement between competing imaging measures of response of hepatocellular carcinoma to yttrium-90 radioembolization. J Vasc Interv Radiol. 2010;21(4):515–21.
6. Monsky WL, Garza AS, Kim I, Loh S, Lin TC, Li CS, Fisher J, Sandhu P, Sidhar V, Chaudhari AJ, et al. Treatment planning and volumetric response assessment for Yttrium-90 radioembolization: semiautomated determination of liver volume and volume of tumor necrosis in patients with hepatic malignancy. Cardiovasc Intervent Radiol. 2011;34(2):306–18.
7. Choi H, Charnsangavej C, Faria SC, Macapinlac HA, Burgess MA, Patel SR, Chen LL, Podoloff DA, Benjamin RS. Correlation of computed tomography and positron emission tomography in patients with metastatic gastrointestinal stromal tumor treated at a single institution with imatinib mesylate: proposal of new computed tomography response criteria. J Clin Oncol. 2007;25(13):1753–9.
8. Tochetto SM, Tore HG, Chalian H, Yaghmai V. Colorectal liver metastasis after 90Y radioembolization therapy: pilot study of change in MDCT attenuation as a surrogate marker for future FDG PET response. AJR Am J Roentgenol. 2012;198(5):1093–9.
9. Rhee TK, Naik NK, Deng J, Atassi B, Mulcahy MF, Kulik LM, Ryu RK, Miller FH, Larson AC, Salem R, et al. Tumor response after yttrium-90 radioembolization for hepatocellular carcinoma: comparison of diffusion-weighted functional MR imaging with anatomic MR imaging. J Vasc Interv Radiol. 2008;19(8):1180–6.
10. Morsbach F, Pfammatter T, Reiner CS, Fischer MA, Sah BR, Winklhofer S, Klotz E, Frauenfelder T, Knuth A, Seifert B, et al. Computed tomographic perfusion imaging for the prediction of response and survival to Transarterial Radioembolization of liver metastases. Investig Radiol. 2013;48:787.
11. Hilgard P, Hamami M, Fouly AE, Scherag A, Muller S, Ertle J, Heusner T, Cicinnati VR, Paul A, Bockisch A, et al. Radioembolization with yttrium-90 glass microspheres in hepatocellular carcinoma: European expe-

rience on safety and long-term survival. Hepatology. 2010;52(5):1741–9.
12. Memon K, Kulik L, Lewandowski RJ, Wang E, Riaz A, Ryu RK, Sato KT, Marshall K, Gupta R, Nikolaidis P, et al. Radiographic response to locoregional therapy in hepatocellular carcinoma predicts patient survival times. Gastroenterology. 2011;141(2):526–35, 535. e521–522.
13. Kinner S, Theysohn JM, Erle J, Gerken G, Lauenstein TC: DWI in patients with hepatocellular carcinoma after selective internal radiation therapy (SIRT): can it predict early therapy response? In: RSNA. Chicago; 2013.
14. Neperud J, Mahvash A, Garg N, Murthy R, Szklaruk J. Can imaging patterns of neuroendocrine hepatic metastases predict response yttruim-90 radioembolotherapy? World J Radiol. 2013;5(6):241–7.
15. Saxena A, Chua TC, Bester L, Kokandi A, Morris DL. Factors predicting response and survival after yttrium-90 radioembolization of unresectable neuroendocrine tumor liver metastases: a critical appraisal of 48 cases. Ann Surg. 2010;251(5):910–6.
16. Dudeck O, Zeile M, Wybranski C, Schulmeister A, Fischbach F, Pech M, Wieners G, Ruhl R, Grosser O, Amthauer H, et al. Early prediction of anticancer effects with diffusion-weighted MR imaging in patients with colorectal liver metastases following selective internal radiotherapy. Eur Radiol. 2010;20(11):2699–706.

38 Radioisotope Therapy of Malignant Pleural and Peritoneal Effusions

Jan Bucerius and Hans-Jürgen Biersack

Treatment of malignant pleural or peritoneal effusions belongs to one of the "oldest" therapies with radioactive isotopes and was firstly described by J. H. Müller more than 50 years ago [1].

For the first therapeutical experiments, radioactive zinc (^{63}Zn) was used as zinc sulfide, which was dissolved in pectin solution. With the beginning in 1949, Müller applied gold colloid (^{198}Au) in patients suffering from malignant pleural- and peritoneal effusions [2]. The main benefit as compared to zinc was a simplified production of a greater amount of the radioisotope which made its wider distribution possible. Beginning in the middle of the fifties, therapy with ^{32}P as colloidal chromic phosphate or ^{90}Yttrium as fluoride, chloride, or silicate became more and more popular for the treatment of malignant pleural and peritoneal effusions [3–5]. Few years later, the application of ^{177}Lutetium-chloride for these diseases was described [6, 7].

J. Bucerius (✉)
Department of Nuclear Medicine, University Medicine Göttingen, Georg-August-University Göttingen, Göttingen, Germany
e-mail: jan.bucerius@med.uni-goettingen.de

H.-J. Biersack
Department of Nuclear Medicine, Beta Klinik Bonn, Bonn, Germany

38.1 Indications and Contraindications for Intracavitary Therapies with Radioisotopes

Intracavitary treatment with radioisotopes, as a palliative procedure can be basically applied for all malignant pleural- and peritoneal effusions. However, the effusion has to be doubtlessly related to the carcinomatosis of the visceral cavity.

For effusions related to cardiovascular, metabolic, or rheumatic diseases, treatment with radioisotopes is not indicated. Furthermore, closed effusions are a contraindication for the treatment with radioisotopes due to the missing distribution of the radioisotope and, therefore, the high risk of radiation-induced necroses.

38.2 Application of Intracavitary Therapies with Radioisotopes

Before the application of the therapy isotope, an effusion chamber has to be excluded. For this purpose, a chest-X-ray during standing and laying has to be performed. Furthermore, the free distribution of a diagnostic isotope in the pleura or the peritoneum needs to be documented. The latter can be performed after intrapleural or -peritoneal installation of approximately 185 MBq ^{99m}Tc-sulfur or tin colloid using a

H. Ahmadzadehfar et al. (eds.), *Clinical Nuclear Medicine*,
https://doi.org/10.1007/978-3-030-39457-8_38

gamma-camera for imaging [8]. In cases of free distribution of the effusion both in the horizontal and vertical direction, a chamber formation of the effusion can sufficiently be excluded. Afterwards, the intrapleural or -peritoneal installation of the therapy radioisotope can be safely applied.

For puncture of the pleura, a commercially available puncture set can be used. Firstly, the pleural effusion should be released as much as possible, whereas a residual volume of the effusion of approximately 250–500 ml should remain in situ. This volume should be documented with a chest X-ray or an ultrasound examination of the pleura. The residual volume of the effusion is mandatory for a homogenous distribution of the therapy radioisotope in the pleura or the peritoneum. Subsequently, the treatment radioisotope can be injected. After the injection and sterile covering of the site of puncture, the patient should change his body position each 15 min during the first 6–8 h in order to achieve a homogenous distribution of the radioisotope over the whole serosa. This should be carried out under the supervision of an experienced physician. After 24 h approximately 90% of the applied activity is fixed in the pleura or peritoneum [9].

38.3 Side Effects of Radioisotope Therapy

Basically, a radiation of the bone marrow, with a reduction of the leukocytes and/or the thrombocytes, cannot be excluded. However, these side effects are rather rare [10]. Additionally, adhesions or necroses are uncommon.

38.4 Radiation Protection

No special radiation protection procedures are required for pure β-radiation as yttrium (^{90}Y) or phosphor (^{32}P) do not reach the environment. According to the German law for radiation protection, patients have to stay for at least 48 h on the ward after each therapy with radioisotopes. As radio-colloids are reabsorbed only to a very small extent, no special protection procedures are necessary with regard to possible radioactivity in the urine or feces.

38.5 Results of Intracavitary Therapies with Radioisotopes

Comparability of the results of the different protocols for the treatment of malignant pleural or peritoneal effusions is limited as patient characteristics, study designs, and endpoints of the studies are mostly very different. However, there are several previously published studies, indicating a temporary cessation of the effusion reflow in 50–70% of treated patients [3, 10–12]. Best results could be achieved in patients suffering from ovarian or breast cancer.

Lang and Riccabona reported an extension of the time interval between two indicated punctures from 10 to 68 days after intracavitary treatment [10]. An improvement of the general condition of the patients could be observed in up to 55% of patients. Austgen and associates reported the application of ^{90}Yttrium silicate for intracavitary treatment [13]. They found a cessation of effusion reflow in 9 of 20 treated patients for an average of 3.5 months.

Kramer and associates reported a single case of developing a malignant pleural mesothelioma as a late complication of radiotherapy for Hodgkin's disease. After primary treatment and to relieve symptoms of dyspnea secondary to pleural effusion, a thoracic drain was installed, followed by intracavitary application of ^{90}Yttrium [14]. The patients remained in good clinical conditions for at least 6 years after diagnosis. The authors conclude that considering the few therapeutic options the use of ^{90}Yttrium-silicate intrapleural installation could be propagated as a safe and effective antitumor treatment for a selected group of patients with malignant pleural mesothelioma.

During the last decades, the number of intracavitary treatments with radioisotopes is strongly declining, mainly in cases of pleural carcinomatosis with effusion. This is mainly due to the promising results of thoracoscopically intrapleural application of magnesium-silicate (talcum) in patients suffering from persistent malignant pleura effusions. This palliative therapy can be applied in general anesthesia and is associated with a success rate of approximately 90% [15]. However, together with further therapy alternatives (e.g., intrapleural application of 5-Fluorouracil, Bleomycin, Novantrone, etc.), treatment with radioactive isotopes may play a certain role in refractory effusions after the described application of talcum, especially in patients with severely impaired general conditions or contraindications for general anesthesia due to concomitant diseases.

In contrast to malignant pleural effusions, there is a different situation in patients suffering from malignant effusions due to peritoneal carcinomatosis. Usually, no surgical options (with the exception of "tumor debulking") are existing in those patients, mainly in higher grades of tumor growth. This is mainly relevant for the palliative treatment of peritoneal carcinomatosis of ovarian cancer. Primarily for this type of cancer, a growing interest of treatment with radioisotopes could be observed during the last years. In a prospective study, Young and associates reported an identical 5-year survival rate of patients with ovarian cancer (tumor stage FIGO II, i.e., tumor restricted to the pelvis) and treatment with intraperitoneal application of ^{32}P as compared to the standard chemotherapy with Melphalan [16].

However, the effect of radiation application is not solely restricted to tumor cells, limiting necessarily the antineoplastic effect of the treatment with radioisotopes. As such, much effort is made to evaluate concepts for a more effective distribution of the ionizing radiation. During the last years, research focused primarily on the application of radioactive labeled antibodies. In 1986, Pectasides and associates reported an antibody-guided irradiation of malignant pleural and pericardial effusions [17]. The tumor-associated antibodies were radiolabelled with ^{131}Iodine and subsequently applied intrapleurally and -pericardially in patients suffering from malignant effusions. Ten out of 13 effusions (3 pericardial and 7 pleural) responded completely with no fluid reflow between 3 and 18 months. Furthermore, they found no clinical or hematological toxicity. In a report of three cases, ^{131}Iodine radiolabeled tumor-associated monoclonal antibodies were given to a patient with malignant pleural effusion, intrapericardially to a patient with pericardial effusion and a tumor mass invading the pericardium, and intraperitoneally to a patient with stage III ovarian cancer resistant to chemotherapy [18]. Cytological examination after antibody-guided therapy showed no neoplastic cells in the residual fluid from patient 1 or peritoneal washings from patient 3. In patient 2, computerized tomography of the pericardium showed that the tumor mass had diminished and the pericardial effusion had resolved. Once again, no clinical or other toxicity was observed.

In a previously published study, Epenetos and associates reported on a long-term evaluation of patients with ovarian cancer and intraperitoneal application of ^{90}Y-labeled monoclonal antibodies [19]. The preliminary results of this study suggest that a substantial proportion of patients who achieve complete remission with conventional therapy can achieve a long-term benefit when treated with intraperitoneal radioimmunotherapy with ^{90}Y-labeled antibodies.

References

1. Müller JH. Über die Verwendung von künstlich radioaktiven Isotopen zur Erzielung von lokalisierten Strahlenwirkungen. Experientia. 1945;1:199.
2. Müller JH. Weitere Entwicklung der Therapie von Peritonealkarzinosen bei Ovarialkarzinom mit künstlicher Radioaktivität (Au-198). Gynaecologica. 1950;129:298.
3. Jaffe HL. Treatment of malignant serous effusions with radioactive colloidal chromic phosphate. Am J Roentgenol. 1955;74:657.
4. Kent EM, Moses C. Radioactive isotopes in the palliative management of carcinomatosis of the pleura. J Thorac Surg. 1951;22:503.
5. Root SW, Tyror MP, Andrews GA, Kniseley RM. Distribution of colloidal radioactive chromic phosphate after intracavitary administration. Radiology. 1954;63:251.
6. Kyker GC, Cress EA, Gleason GL. Fed Proc. 1954;13:245. (cited by Lang and Riccabona).

7. Yamashita HS, Igari S, Lino Y. Fundamental studies and clinical experience on the lutetium (Lu-177) therapy. Int J Appl Radiat. 1960;8:113.
8. Tally TE, Goldberg ME, Loken MK. The use of 99mTc Sulphur colloid to assess the distribution of 32Pchromic phosphate. J Nucl Med. 1974;15:190.
9. zum Winkel K, Chone B, Hermann HJ, Schenk P. Möglichkeiten und Grenzen der Therapie mit offenen radioaktiven Substanzen. Dtsch Ärztebl. 1979;76:619.
10. Lang T, Riccabona G. Langzeitergebnisse der intrakavitären Isotopentherapie maligner Ergüsse. Nuklearmedizin. 1974;12:245.
11. Chang CA, Janzen AH, Shorneck AB, Rosenbaum PJ. Treatment of malignant effusions by intracavitary injection of radioactive colloidal gold. Am J Roentgenol. 1957;77:486.
12. Kligerman MM, Habif DV. The use of radioactive gold in the treatment of effusion due to carcinomatosis of the pleura and the peritoneum. Am J Roentgenol. 1995;75:651.
13. Austgen M, Schlimmer P, Wilhelm H, Trendelenburg F. Palliative therapy of tumor-induced pleural effusions with 90Yttrium-silicate. Eur J Respir Dis. 1984;65:64.
14. Kramer G, Gans S, Rijnders A, Leer J. Long term survival of a patient with malignant pleural mesothelioma as a late complication of radiotherapy for Hodgkin's disease treated with 90yttrium-silicate. Lung Cancer. 2000;27:205.
15. Daniel TM, Tribble CG, Rodgers BM. Thoracoscopy and talc poudrage for pneumothoraces and effusions. Ann Thorac Surg. 1990;50:186.
16. Young RC, Walton LA, Ellenberg SS, et al. Adjuvant therapy in stage I and stage II epithelial ovarian cancer. N Engl J Med. 1990;322:1021.
17. Pectasides D, Stewart S, Courtenay-Luck N, et al. Antibody-guided irradiation of malignant pleural and pericardial effusions. Br J Cancer. 1986;53:727.
18. Hammersmith Oncology Group and the Imperial Cancer Research Fund. Antibody-guided irradiation of malignant lesions: three cases illustrating a new method if treatment. A report from the Hammersmith Oncology Group and the Imperial Cancer Research Fund. Lancet. 1984;30:1441.
19. Epenetos AA, Hird V, Lambert H, Mason P, Coulter C. Long-term survival of patients with advanced ovarian cancer treated with intraperitoneal radioimmunotherapy. Int J Gynecol Cancer. 2000;10(S1):44.

Radiosynoviorthesis (Radiation Synovectomy)

39

Gynter Mödder

39.1 Introduction

Radiosynoviorthesis (RSO) is a proven important instrument for local treatment of chronic inflammatory joint diseases in the context of medical and orthopaedic efforts. The term radiosynoviorthesis was created by Delbarre et al. [1], meaning the restoration (*orthesis*) of the *synov*ium by means of *radio*nuclides. By local administration of radioactive agents, an attempt is made to influence the synovial process favourably as an alternative to surgical synovectomy. In the Anglo-American literature the term "radiosynovectomy" or "radiation synovectomy" came into use.

The first descriptions of the method go back to Ishido [2] and Fellinger and Schmid [3].

In Germany, RSO nowadays is performed in about 63,000 joints per year, as much as radioiodine therapy in thyroid diseases.

39.2 Indications

Basically, RSO is indicated for the local treatment of almost all kinds of chronic synovitis [4–6]. The *main indications* for radiosynoviorthesis are (modified according to German and European guidelines) [7, 8]:

- Rheumatoid arthritis.
- Seronegative spondyloarthropathy (i.e., reactive arthritis, psoriatic arthritis).
- Haemarthrosis in haemophiliacs.
- Recurrent joint effusions (i.e., after arthroscopy).
- Pigmented villonodular synovitis (PVNS).
- Osteoarthritis (activated arthrosis).
- After joint prosthesis: persistent effusions, polyethylene disease.
- Undifferentiated arthritis (where the arthritis is characterized by synovitis, synovial thickening or effusion).

Absolute contraindications:
- Pregnancy.
- Breast feeding.
- Local skin infection.
- Acute rupture of popliteal cyst (Baker's cyst).

Relative contraindications:
- RSO should only be used in children and young patients (<20 years) if the benefit of treatment is likely to outweigh the potential hazards. Taking this into account, it is routinely applied in children with haemophilic arthropathy.
- Extensive joint instability with bone destruction.

G. Mödder (✉)
NURAMED, Praxis für Nuklearmedizin und Radiologie, Deutsches Zentrum für Radiosynoviorthese, Köln, Germany

H. Ahmadzadehfar et al. (eds.), *Clinical Nuclear Medicine*,
https://doi.org/10.1007/978-3-030-39457-8_39

The approvals may be different in different countries. Therefore, the respective national regulations should be taken into account.

39.3 Radiopharmaceuticals

The most common and approved radiopharmaceuticals used for RSO are:

- [^{90}Y]yttrium citrate or silicate ([^{90}Y]colloid), only used for RSO of knee joints
- [^{186}Re]rhenium sulphide ([^{186}Re]colloid), used for RSO of middle sized joints
- [^{169}Er]erbium citrate ([^{169}Er]colloid), used for RSO of small joints.

The physical characteristics of these radioisotopes are shown in Fig. 39.1. Proven dosages are listed in Table 39.1. These radiopharmaceuticals are beta-emitters in colloidal suspensions.

Other radiopharmaceuticals rarely used for RSO are dysprosium-165 ferric hydroxide, holmium-166 hydroxyapatite and samarium-153 hydroxyapatite.

39.4 Mechanism of Action

"Synovitis is the villain of the drama" (Mannerfeldt), in rheumatic diseases causing brutal destruction of cartilage, bone, tendons and ligaments correlated with pain, swelling and loss of function. After intra-articular administration, the radioactive particles in colloidal form are taken up by phagocytosis in synovial macrophages. A particle size of about 5 ± 10 nm is essential to avoid leakage and provide homogenous distribution on the surface of the synovium. β-radiation leads to coagulation necrosis, sclerosis and fibrosis of the synovial tissue including vessels and pain receptors, resulting in reducing effusion, swelling and pain of the joint. Due to the fact that cartilage has no ability to phagocytose, this tissue is not a target for the radiation effects [2].

The remark "synovitis is the villain of the drama" is not only valid for rheumatic diseases but also for osteoarthritis (activated arthrosis). Arthrosis with typical joint space narrowing as a result of cartilage defects is not associated with pain because cartilage has no nerves and vessels. Only after detritus leads to synovitis does simple

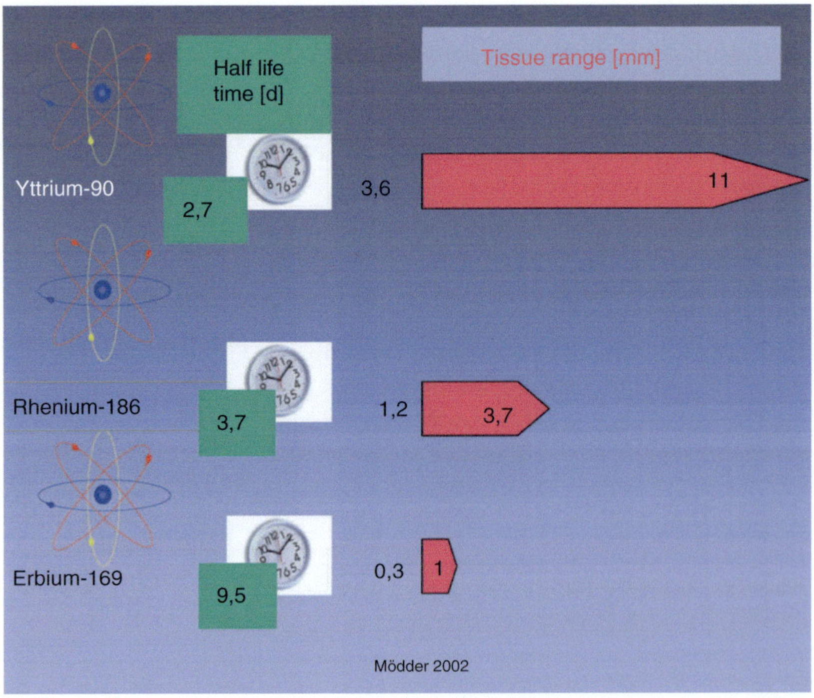

Fig. 39.1 Radioisotopes for radiosynoviorthesis

Table 39.1 Proven dosages for the most frequently treated joints

Joint	Radioisotope	Dose (MBq)
Knee joint	Yttrium-90	185–222
Glenohumeral joint	Rhenium-186	74
Acromioclavicular joint	Erbium-169	30–40
Elbow joint	Rhenium-186	74
Wrist joint	Rhenium-186	55–74
Hip joint	Rhenium-186	111–185
Ankle joint	Rhenium-186	74
Talonavicular/subtalar joint	Rhenium-186	55
Metacarpophalangeal joint (MCP)	Erbium-169	20–40
Proximal interphalangeal joint (PIP)	Erbium-169	10–20
Distal interphalangeal joint (DIP)	Erbium-169	10–15
Metatarsophalangeal joint (MTP)	Erbium-169	30–40
Thumb base	Erbium-169	30

arthrosis escalate to inflammation (activated arthrosis = osteoarthritis) with pain, swelling and effusions [4, 9]. By depleting synovial macrophages that drive synovial inflammation through their respective cytokines, RSO is likely to be effective in both RA and OA. The rather good effects of RSO in early osteoarthritis (i.e., knee joint) will be lacking in late-stage OA, if mechanical problems such as severe instability and axe deviation predominate.

In early-stage OA RSO functions as an excellent tool due to the fact that the origin of pain in most cases then is synovitis and not cartilage, because cartilage has no vessels and nerves and thus never is able to inflict pain [4, 10–12].

Simultaneous intra-articular injection of corticosteroids (i.e., triamcinolone hexacetonide or triamcinolone acetonide) is recommended because this might reduce local inflammation due to radionuclide instillation and prolong residence time of the radiopharmaceutical agent in the joint [11]. An additional reason is the reduction of the often superposed layer of oedema on the synovium so that the thin film of radioisotopes gets closer to the destructing pannus – resulting in improvement of the effect of RSO.

39.5 Local Complications After RSO

Transient increased swelling or pain: mostly rapid relief by local application of ice. Due to incompetent injection technique or too early (<48 h) movement of the treated joint: superficial skin or needle track ulceration may happen, even more rarely local radionecrosis in surroundings of the injection site.

Thromboembolic complications due to posttreatment joint immobilization (48 h) may be prevented by routine anticoagulation pharmacotherapy.

RSO is a safe method. In the everyday routine of RSO in a specialized centre all these complications are regarded as extreme exceptions: 3–5/100.000 treated joints [4, 11, 13, 14].

39.6 Methodology

39.6.1 Patient Selection

Rheumatic patients need systemic treatment with antirheumatoid drugs because rheumatism is a systemic disease. If after at least 6 months a few joints do not show adequate improvement even after corticosteroid injections into the affected joints, these joints are selected for RSO, thus avoiding escalation of systemic therapy with its possible side effects. In monoarthritis or oligoarthritis RSO could be the therapy of first choice, after the failure of locally administered corticosteroids [4, 15].

Orthopaedic patients should be selected after the failure of local corticoid injection and/or ineffective conservative treatment. But also after plenty of surgical interventions, RSO might improve the complaints of the patient, i.e., after total knee replacement [16] or effusions after arthroscopy. Some authors recommend RSO after arthroscopy as a routine method to improve results [17, 18]. The time interval between arthroscopy or joint surgery (i.e., villonodular synovitis) and RSO should be planned as (4-) 6 weeks.

39.6.2 Diagnostic Studies Prior to RSO

- Medical history, clinical inspection, examination of joint function (complaints, effusion, pain, restricted joint motion?)
- *X-ray images* provide basic information about the joint.
- *Ultrasound study* evaluates joint space, synovial structure and thickness and extent of effusion, and assesses tenosynovialitis or rotator cuff tear (shoulder).
  Ultrasound is obligatory prior to performing RSO to rule out a **Baker's cyst** (Fig. 39.2). Immediately before starting RSO procedure make sure that no current rupture has happened. In this case: absolute contraindication for RSO! In all other cases with a big Baker's cyst the effusion should be aspired (in prone position of the patient), and after that typical method of knee-RSO should follow [10, 11, 19].
- *Multiphase scintigraphy* with ^{99m}Tc-MDP (or similar radiopharmaceuticals) is the best diagnostic tool for detecting and demonstrating inflammation of the synovium, thus – including findings of the clinical examination – selecting joints for RSO. In the first step (10 min after injection) *soft tissue scintigraphy* detects the degree of active inflammation of the synovium. In the second step (3 h p.i.) *bone scintigraphy* assesses the bone involvement in the painful process. The study reveals nearly indispensable information in activated arthrosis (osteoarthritis) and gives the best overview over multiple joint involvement especially in (also seronegative) polyarthritis [4, 20] (Figs. 39.3 and 39.4).
- Magnetic resonance imaging might be suitable for additional information in a few patients (i.e., bone oedema, femur head necrosis).

39.6.3 Performance of RSO

39.6.3.1 Joint Puncture

A suitable room and strict asepsis are necessary. A good puncture technique is essential (for details see Ref. [4]). The best puncture technique for the knee joint is shown in Fig. 39.5.

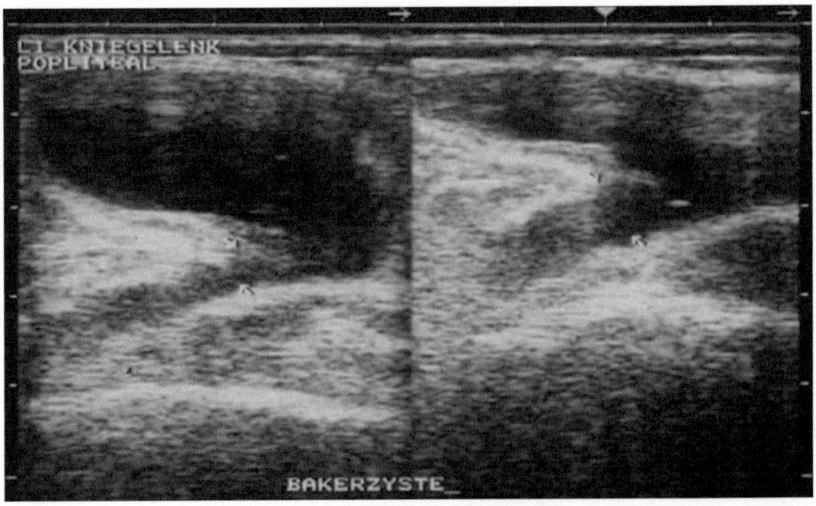

Fig. 39.2 Ultrasound of a Baker's cyst (transverse). Check for valve mechanism. *Left* The connecting duct between the knee joint (*below*) and Baker's cyst is seen. *Right* By soundhead pressure the cyst is decreased in size and the duct dilates. There is no valve mechanism

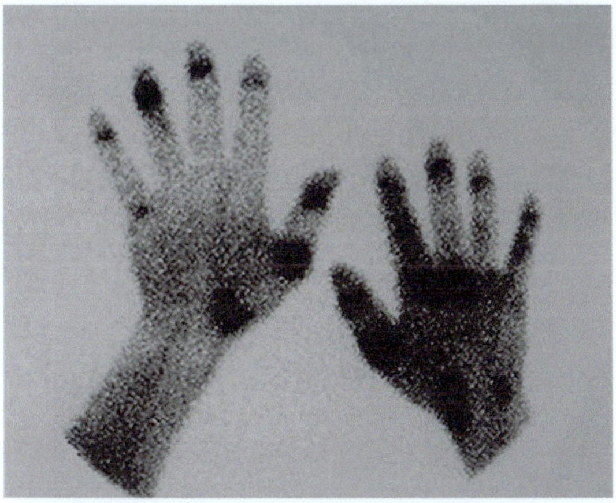

Fig. 39.3 The hands as the "visiting card" of the rheumatic patient. Soft tissue scintigram with ^{99m}Tc-MDP shows a typical pattern in psoriatic arthritis

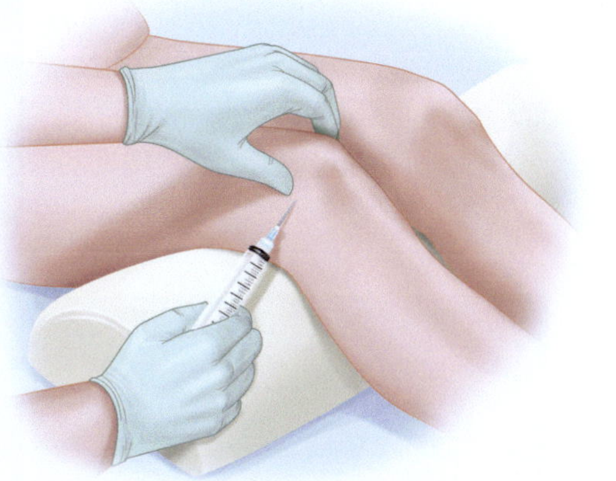

Fig. 39.5 Injection technique for the knee joint. Beware of injecting beside the ligamentum patellae with the patient in the sitting position, because then there is the danger of injecting yttrium-90 into the crucial ligaments or into Hoffa's fat body

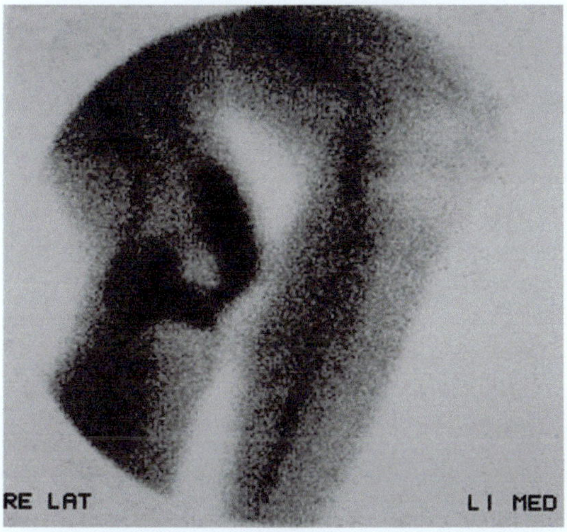

Fig. 39.4 Non-specific but highly sensitive synovitis—typical increased accumulation above the right knee joint in a patient with knee osteoarthritis. In rheumatoid arthritis the scintigram would look identical

39.6.3.2 Fluoroscopy

Apart from the knee, all joints have to be punctured for RSO by fluoroscopy and often by arthrography. Dye distribution predicts the distribution of radionuclide which is injected immediately afterwards. Using this procedure perfect needle position in the cavity of the joint is ensured (Fig. 39.6a, b).

Examples of the importance of fluoroscopic control for an absolutely exact injection technique are given in Figs. 39.7 and 39.8.

Figure 39.9 illustrates (a) a soft tissue scintigram, (b) an arthrogram and (c) a distribution scintigram as a proof for a perfect performance.

39.6.3.3 Radiation Safety Considerations

For the patient: Very late radiation-induced stochastic hazards have not been observed [21, 22]. The effective dose to the whole body is estimated to be 30 times lower than in iodine-131 therapy of benign thyroid diseases [23, 24]. The risk of radiation-induced genetic alterations is negligible [13].

For the personnel: To avoid high radiation exposure for the fingers during preparation and administration of yttrium-90 radiation, protection has to be provided by the use of acrylic syringe protectors, nitrile or vinyl gloves, finger dosimeters, etc. [25, 26] (Fig. 39.10).

39.6.4 After RSO/Follow-Up

- *A distribution scintigram* confirms the appropriate intra-articular distribution of the radiopharmaceutical. Scintigraphy is enabled

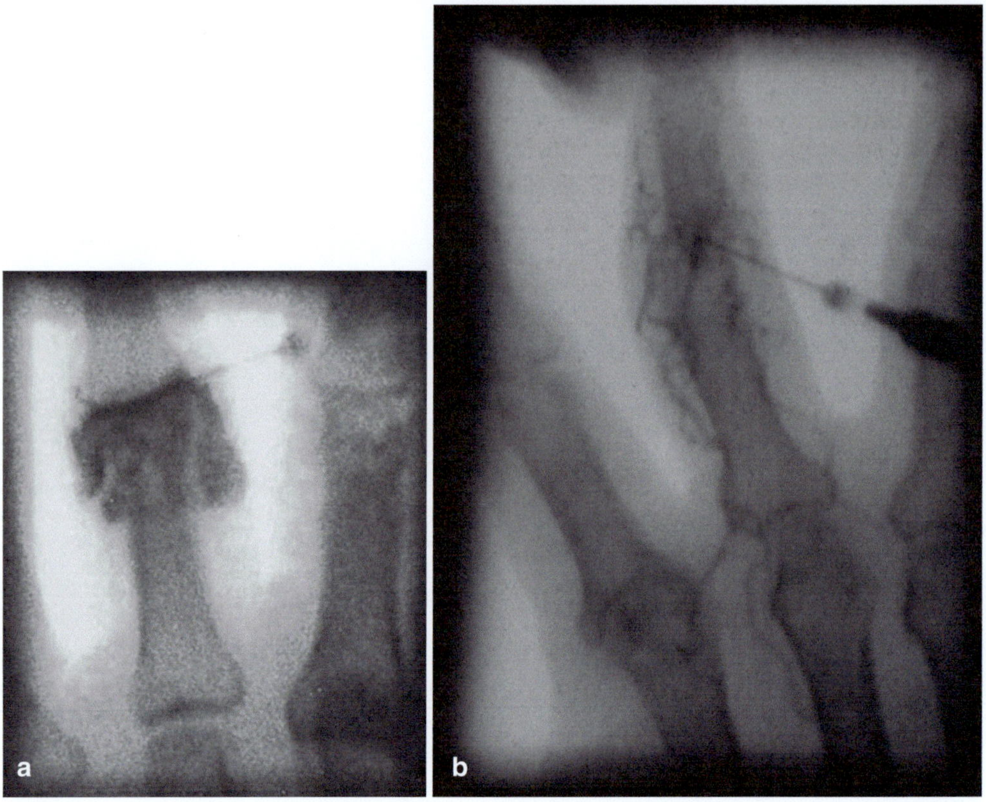

Fig. 39.6 (**a**) Arthrogram after perfect injection into a proximal interphalangeal joint (PIP) joint. (**b**) Arthrogram of a PIP joint. Intra-articular position of the needle, but *not in the cavity*. The contrast medium is injected into a villus with transportation by vessels. If this occurred with injection of erbium-169, it would be followed by side effects

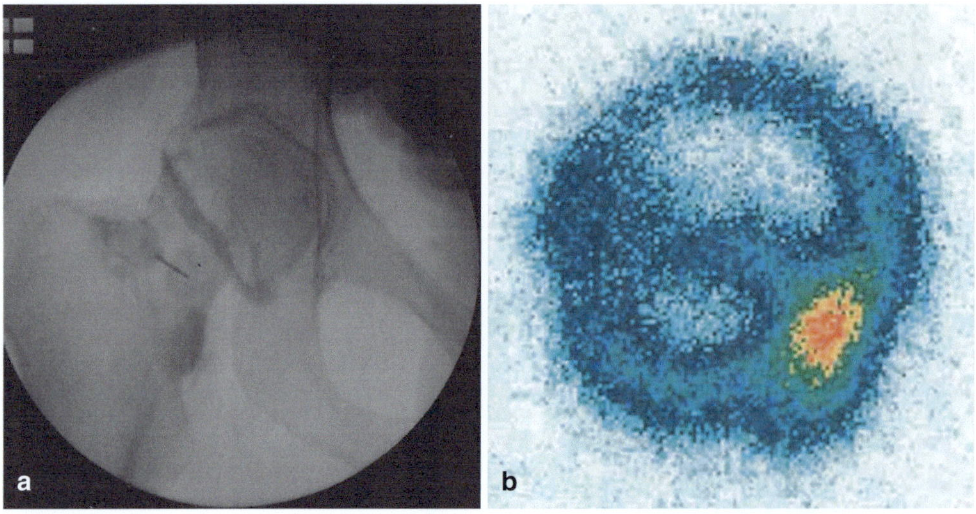

Fig. 39.7 (**a**) Arthrogram of a hip joint. The image shows the perfect and safe needle position. Beware of injecting into the joint space as usually recommended! You would risk destroying the ligamentum capitis femoris and thus cause femur head necrosis. (**b**) Distribution scintigram after injection of rhenium-186 colloid into the hip joint

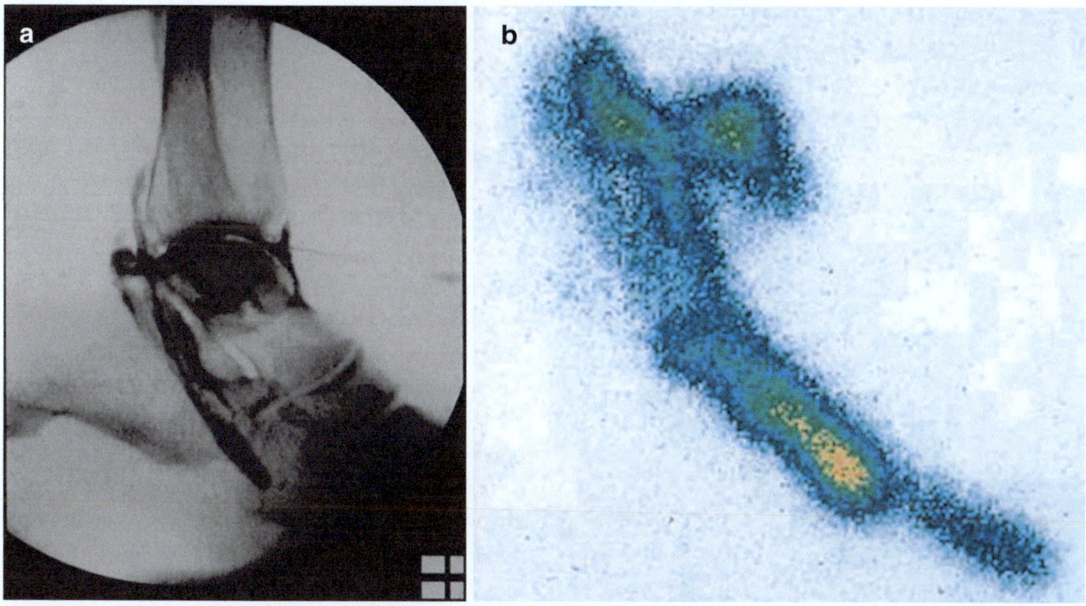

Fig. 39.8 (**a**) Arthrogram during RSO of ankle joint. Also a peroneal tenosynovialitis is involved in the psoriatic process. (**b**) The distribution scintigram demonstrates the distribution of rhenium-186 within the ankle joint and within the peroneal sheet, indicating a good RSO effect for both structures

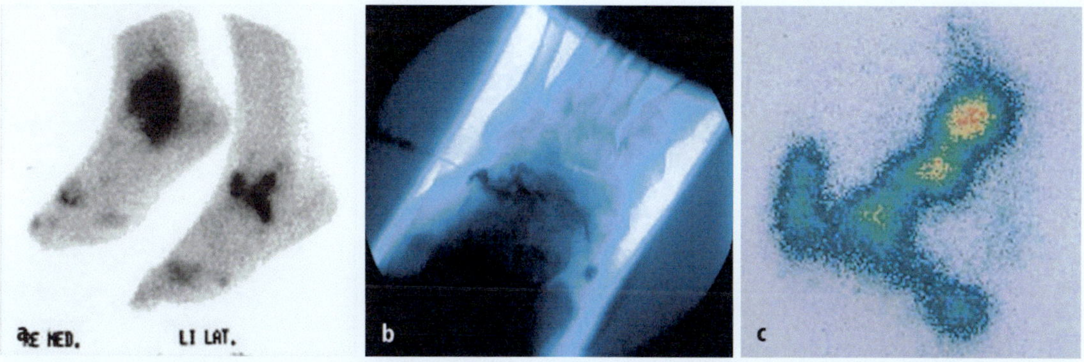

Fig. 39.9 Patient with rheumatoid arthritis was submitted for RSO of the left ankle. (**a**) Soft tissue scintigram detected no inflammatory involvement in the ankle but in the talonavicular, subtalar and calcaneocuboid joint. (**b**) Arthrogram after injection in the calcaneocuboid joint. (**c**) Distribution scintigram demonstrating perfect distribution in all joints marked in the diagnostic scintigram (**a**)

after use of yttrium-90 by its *bremsstrahlung*, after use of Rhenium-186 by its gamma portion (140 keV). After the use of erbium-169 no scintigram is available.

- The joint has to be immobilized to avoid necrosis of injection channel or skin caused by reflux and to avoid transport of radioactive particles through the lymphatic vessels (leakage). A splint is required for 48 h. After removal of the splint the joint should be treated with care for 1 week, but then the patient should go into training of the joint and muscles.
- In our experience, the first *follow-up* is recommended about 6 months after RSO, or of course earlier when problems (reactive inflammation, suspected infection, swelling of Baker's cyst) occur. Clinical evaluation, possibly ultrasound scans of the joints and also checking that sufficient active joint training has been done, belong to the basic control steps.

Sometimes an effusion fluid or a Baker's cyst has to be punctured before the development of the definitive effect of RSO. Clinical examination and ultrasound scans, sometimes control of scintigraphy, should take place 12 months after treatment.

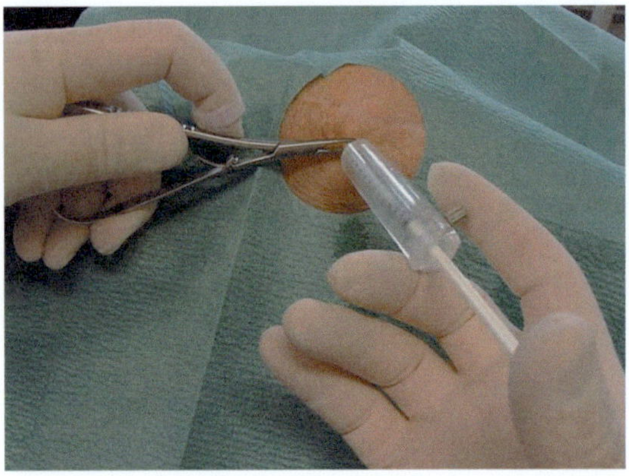

Fig. 39.10 Radiation protection for the RSO performing doctor: sterile gloves, forceps and finger ring dosimeter (see text)

39.7 Repetition of Radiosynoviorthesis

Radiosynoviorthesis should be performed at an early stage of the disease, when cartilage damage is minimal. Reasons for non-satisfactory results of RSO might be, e.g., rapidly recurrent effusions, strongly developed thickness of synovial villus, enlargement of the joint cavity by additional cavities (Baker's cyst, bursa subdeltoidea), unfavourable Larsen stage, etc. Then a repetition of RSO (Re-RSO) may be indicated, normally not earlier than 6 months after the previous procedure [4]. Re-RSO of the wrist will not only treat the proximal wrist joint but will additionally reach the intercarpal compartments. And after total knee replacement, the deeper layers of polyethylene disease can be attacked by Re-RSO. A new fraction is more effective than a primarily enhanced dose (Fig. 39.11a, b).

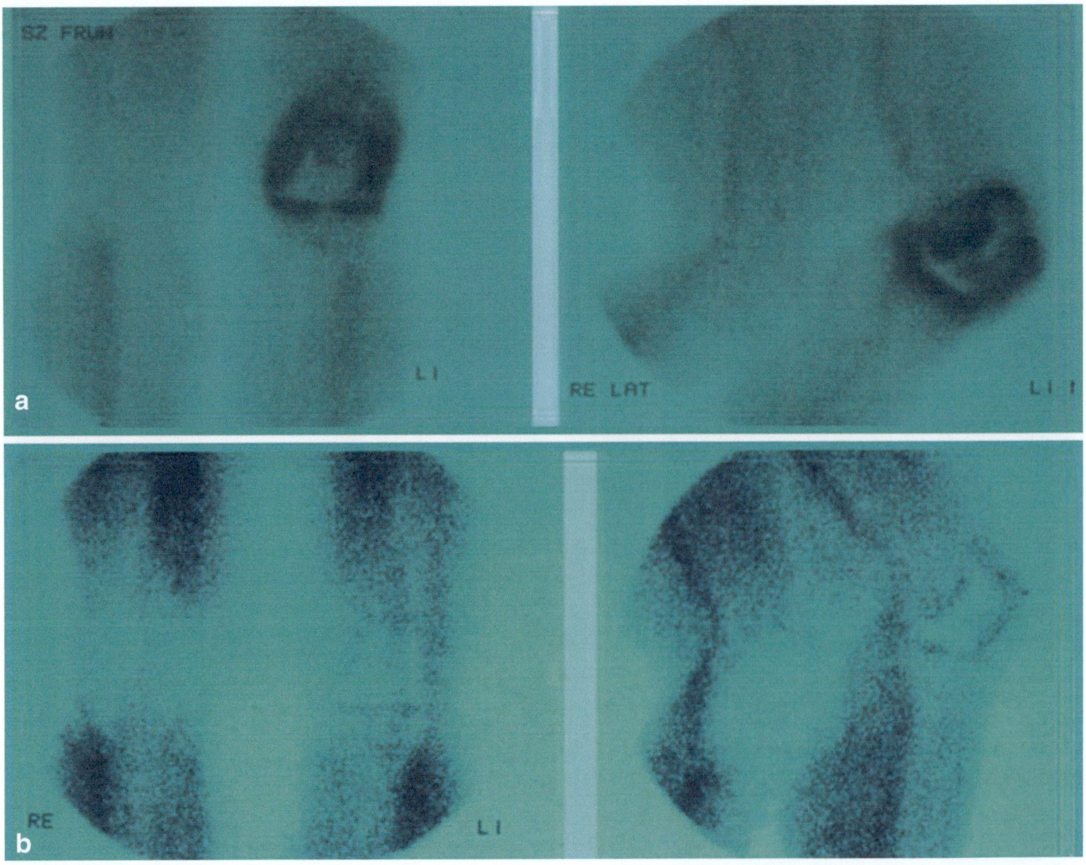

Fig. 39.11 Patient with total knee replacement of the right knee. (**a**) Prior to RSO: left knee joint with polyethylene disease, pain and recurrent effusions. (**b**) After RSO: improvement with regard to symptoms and scintigraphic findings [16]

39.8 Results

In principle, any chronic inflammatory joint with proven synovitis can be treated with RSO. RSO-response rates reported in an abundant literature range from about 60% to >90% for all joints, depending on the advanced stage of the joint disease, often with greater success for rheumatoid diseases than for osteoarthritis. Most of the studies relating to RSO in the last 40 years do not fulfil the criteria of modern evidence-based medicine, but recently a number of well-designed trials have been carried out in order to evaluate the efficacy of RSO. In a multicentre prospective study, an improvement of 78% without a significant difference in rheumatoid arthritis or osteoarthritis was found [7, 27]. In a prospective study on rheumatoid arthritis, Göbel et al. [28] found a significant improvement in terms of pain and swelling after 3 years and a reduced progression of radiological destruction compared to triamcinolone. More recently two prospective multicentre studies carried out under strict evidence-based medicine criteria demonstrated a significant improvement (pain, swelling, joint mobility) for erbium-169 versus placebo [29] and after 2 years for rhenium-186 versus high dose corticosteroid [30].

In a recent study, Jahangier et al. [31] drew unfavourable conclusions about the performance of RSO with yttrium-90. But it could be demonstrated that their conclusions were wrong because the results in fact provided evidence for the efficacy of RSO with yttrium-90 [24, 32, 33].

Kresnik et al. [34] investigated the clinical outcome of radiosynoviorthesis in a meta-analysis including 2190 treated joints. They found an overall response rate of 72.5 ± 17%. In rheumatoid arthritis, RSO was successful in 66.7 ± 15.4%. There was a difference according to the Steinbrocker stages (Steinbrocker I: 72.8 ± 12.3%; Steinbrocker II: 64 ± 17.3%; Steinbrocker III and IV: 52.4 ± 23.6%). The response rate in osteoarthritis was 56 ± 11%, with better results in the case of minimal radiological changes. Improvement in haemophilia and Willebrand's disease was 91 ± 4.3%, and in pigmented villonodular synovitis it was 77.3 ± 25.3%.

The conclusion of this study was that radiosynoviorthesis provides better results in rheumatoid arthritis than in osteoarthritis. Minimal or moderate changes according to Steinbrocker stages I and II respond better to radionuclide therapy than do stages III and IV. Deformed or unstable joints might fail treatment and therefore surgical interventions should be considered. Close cooperation with orthopaedists and rheumatologists is necessary in the consideration of RSO for each patient to ensure optimal medical care.

Zuderman et al. [20] demonstrated success rates from 70% for knees with OA to 90% for finger joints with RA. Independent of the type of joint, the response rate to RSO was significantly higher in patients with RA than in patients with – not communicated stages of – OA (89% vs. 79%).

Haemophilic arthropathy: RSO with the overall improvement of 80–92% must be the procedure of choice for haemophiliacs with repeated bleeding and in those where surgery cannot be done. The greatest advantage is the prevention of joint deformities especially when intervention is done early and the cartilage damage is yet minimal [35].

References

1. Delbarre F, Cayla J, Menkes C, Aignan J, Roucayrol J, Ingrand J. La synoviorthèse par les radioisotopes. Presse Med. 1968;76:1045–50.
2. Ishido C. Über die Wirkung des Radiothoriums auf die Gelenke. Strahlentherapie. 1923;15:537–44.
3. Fellinger K, Schmid J. Die lokale Behandlung der rheumatischen Erkrankungen. Wiener Z Inn Med. 1952;33:351–63.
4. Mödder G. Radiosynoviorthesis. Involvement of nuclear medicine in rheumatology and orthopaedics. Warlich: Meckenheim; 2001.
5. Mödder G. Radiosynoviorthese, Radium-224-Therapie und Röntgenstrahlentherapie. In: Zeidler H, Zacher J, Hiepe F, editors. Interdisziplinäre klinische Rheumatologie. Berlin: Springer; 2001. p. 361–77.
6. Kampen WU, Brenner W, Kroeger S, Sawula JA, Bohuslavizki KH, Henze E. Long-term results of radiation synovectomy: a clinical follow-up study. Nucl Med Commun. 2001;22:239–46.
7. Farahati J, Reiners C, Fischer M, Mödder G, Franke C, Mahlstedt J, et al. Guidelines for radiosynorviorthesis. Nuklearmedizin. 1999;38:254–5.
8. Clunie G, Fischer M, EANM. EANM procedure guidelines for radiosynovectomy. Eur J Nucl Med Mol Imaging. 2003;30:BP12–6.

9. Otte P. Der Arthrose-Prozeß. Gelenkerhaltung—Gefährdung—Destruktion, Teil 1: Osteochondrale Strukturen. Nürnberg: Novartis Pharma Verlag; 2000.
10. Mödder G. Radiosynoviorthesis (radiation Synovectomy) of knee joint. In: Fogelman I, Gnanasegaran G, Van der Wall H, editors. Radionuclide and hybrid bone imaging. New York: Springer; 2012. p. 935–51.
11. Mödder G. Radionuclide therapy of inflammatory joint diseases (radiation Synovectomy, Radiosynoviorthesis). In: Baum R, editor. Therapeutic nuclear medicine. New York: Springer; 2014. p. 459–93.
12. Mödder G, Mödder-Reese R. Radiosynoviorthesis. In: Aktolun C, Goldsmith S, editors. Nuclear medicine therapy—principles and clinical applications. Springer; 2013. p. 315–35.
13. Fischer M, Czech N, Kampen W. Nuklearmedizinische Schmerztherapie bei Knochen- und Gelenkerkrankungen. In: Baron R, Koppert W, Strumpf M, Willweber-Strumpf A, editors. Praktische Schmerzmedizin. Springer; 2019. p. 1–19.
14. Kampen W. Local complications after Radiosynovectomy and possible treatment strategies: a literature survey. In: Kampen W, Fischer M, editors. Local treatment of inflammatory joint diseases – benefits and risks. Switzerland: Springer; 2015. p. 115–25.
15. Fischer M, Mödder G. Radionuclide therapy of inflammatory joint diseases. Nucl Med Commun. 2002;23:829–31.
16. Mödder G, Mödder-Reese R. Radiosynoviorthese nach Knieendoprothesen: Effektive Therapie bei "polyethylene disease". Der Nuklearmediziner. 2001;24:97–103.
17. Kerschbaumer F, Herresthal J. Arthroskopische Synovektomie und Radiosynoviorthese. Z Rheumatol. 1996;55:388–93.
18. Thabe H. Operative Behandlungskonzepte, Kapitel 5.3. In: Thabe H, editor. Praktische Rheumatherapie. Weinheim: Chapman & Hall; 1997.
19. Klett R. Baker's cysts: a relevant contraindication? In: Kampen W, Fischer M, editors. Local treatment of inflammatory joint diseases – benefits and risks. Switzerland: Springer; 2015. p. 135–42.
20. Zuderman L, Liepe K, Zophel K, Andreeff M, Kotzerke J, Luboldt W. Radiosynoviorthesis (RSO): influencing factors and therapy monitoring. Ann Nucl Med. 2008;22:735–41. https://doi.org/10.1007/s12149-008-0167-7.
21. Turkmen C. Risk of cancer induction. In: Kampen W, Fischer M, editors. Local treatment of inflammatory joint diseases—benefits and risks. Switzerland: Springer; 2015. p. 127–34.
22. Vuorela J, Sokka T, Pukkala E, Hannonen P. Does yttrium radiosynovectomy increase the risk of cancer in patients with rheumatoid arthritis? Ann Rheum Dis. 2003;62:251–3.
23. Manil L, Voisin P, Aubert B, Guerreau D, Verrier P, Lebegue L, et al. Physical and biological dosimetry in patients undergoing radiosynoviorthesis with erbium-169 and rhenium-186. Nucl Med Commun. 2001;22:405–16.
24. Mödder G. Radiosynoviorthese. In: Kuwert T, Grünwald F, Haberkorn U, Krause T, editors. Nuklearmedizin. Stuttgart: Thieme; 2008. p. 401–9.
25. Barth I, Rimpler A. Radiation exposure of medical staff and radiation protection measures. In: Kampen W, Fischer M, editors. Local treatment of inflammatory joint diseases—benefits and risks. Switzerland: Springer 2015. p. 103–114.
26. Brenner W. Grundlagen und Technik der Radiosynoviorthese. Der Nuklearmediziner. 2006;29:5–14.
27. Farahati J, Kenn W, Körber C, Schulz G, Reidemeister C, Mödder G, et al. Zeit bis zur Remission nach Radiosynovektomie (RSV). Nuklearmedizin; 1999. p. A98.
28. Göbel D, Gratz S, von Rothkirch T, Becker W. Chronische Polyarthritis und Radiosynoviorthese: Eine prospektive, kontrollierte Studie der Injektionstherapie mit Erbium-169 und Rhenium-186. Z Rheumatol. 1997;56:207–13.
29. Kahan A, Mödder G, Menkes CJ, Verrier P, Devaux JY, Bonmartin A, et al. 169Erbium-citrate synoviorthesis after failure of local corticosteroid injections to treat rheumatoid arthritis-affected finger joints. Clin Exp Rheumatol. 2004;22:722–6.
30. Tebib JG, Manil LM, Mödder G, Verrier P, De Rycke Y, Bonmartin A, et al. Better results with rhenium-186 radiosynoviorthesis than with cortivazol in rheumatoid arthritis (RA): a two-year follow-up randomized controlled multicentre study. Clin Exp Rheumatol. 2004;22:609–16.
31. Jahangier ZN, Jacobs JW, Lafeber FP, Moolenburgh JD, Swen WA, Bruyn GA, et al. Is radiation synovectomy for arthritis of the knee more effective than intraarticular treatment with glucocorticoids? Results of an eighteen-month, randomized, double-blind, placebo-controlled, crossover trial. Arthritis Rheum. 2005;52:3391–402. https://doi.org/10.1002/art.21376.
32. Kampen WU, Czech N. Methodologic issues in the assessment of the efficacy of radiation synovectomy for arthritis of the knee: comment on the article by Janangier et al. Arthritis Rheum. 2007;56:385. https://doi.org/10.1002/art.22287.
33. Mödder G, Langer HE. Evidence of the efficacy of radiation synovectomy with yttrium-90: comment on the article by Jahangier et al. Arthritis Rheum. 2007;56:386. https://doi.org/10.1002/art.22288.
34. Kresnik E, Mikosch P, Gallowitsch HJ, Jesenko R, Just H, Kogler D, et al. Clinical outcome of radiosynoviorthesis: a meta-analysis including 2190 treated joints. Nucl Med Commun. 2002;23:683–8.
35. Andres-Barrenechia E, Chua M, Navarra S. Radionuclide therapy for bleeding joints in hemophilia. In: Baum R, editor. Therapeutic nuclear medicine. Berlin: Springer; 2014. p. 495–502.

Radioligand Therapy in Prostate Cancer Using PSMA Ligands

40

Robert Seifert and Kambiz Rahbar

40.1 Introduction

Prostate cancer is the most common cancer in men in the United States [1]. Therefore, new therapy strategies, especially after failing standard therapies, are urgently needed.

In localized prostate cancer, the 5-year survival rate is nearly 100%, but in the case of metastasized disease the survival rate decreases to 29% [1]. The androgen deprivation therapy (ADT) is, besides radical prostatectomy (RPE) and external beam radiation, one of the most important therapy strategies of metastasized and progressive prostate cancer. Nearly all patients treated with ADT show a good initial response [2]. But in the course of the disease, an androgen independence can occur, which is mainly called castration resistance. During the last decade, several therapeutics have been developed and approved for metastasized castration-resistant prostate cancer (mCRPC), such as first- and second-line chemotherapeutics (Docetaxel and Cabazitaxel) and new age antihormonal therapies (abiraterone and enzalutamide). Finally, an alpha-emitting compound, Radium-223, has been approved for the treatment of symptomatic bone metastatic CRPC in men without soft tissue metastases [3].

R. Seifert · K. Rahbar (✉)
Department of Nuclear Medicine, University Hospital Muenster, Muenster, Germany
e-mail: Kambiz.Rahbar@ukmuenster.de

In the recent years, prostate-specific membrane antigen (PSMA)-targeted radioligands have been developed and used as compassionate therapy if the above-mentioned therapies have failed in patients with no other therapy option. PSMA seems to be the most promising molecular target in the radioligand therapy of mCRPC.

The Yttrium-90-labelled CYT-356 monoclonal antibody (mAb) that binds to the intracellular domain of PSMA was one of the first unsuccessful attempts. Phase 1 and 2 clinical trials using PSMA mAb J591 [4–6], labelled with Lutetium-177 or Yttrium-90, showed high ratios of hematologic toxicities, reporting of grade 4 thrombocytopenia and neutropenia in 46.8% and 25.5% of the patients treated but reported of promising response rates. The high toxicity might be due to the large size of mAb and its long half-life in blood without binding.

Mild toxicities were reported by Zechman et al. in the first experience with Iodine-131-labelled PSMA ligand, showing promising response rate with a PSA decline ≥ 50% in 60% of the treated patients [7]. Despite all these ligands, the Lutetium-177-labelled PSMA-617, a small molecule developed by German Cancer Research Centre in Heidelberg, seems to be the most promising ligand to receive an approval in the treatment of patients with progressive mCRPC. The first patient was reported end of 2014 [8] and the first patient series was published in 2015 [9]. This chapter will give an overview of the current development of PSMA-targeted

H. Ahmadzadehfar et al. (eds.), *Clinical Nuclear Medicine*,
https://doi.org/10.1007/978-3-030-39457-8_40

radioligand therapy using ^{177}Lutetium-PSMA-617 (Lu-PSMA).

40.2 Indications and Procedure

The current indication for Lu-PSMA radioligand therapy is mCRPC being progressive after first- and/or second-line chemotherapy and at least one line of abiraterone and/or enzalutamide as standard therapy course according to guidelines. Additionally, the following conditions of patients must be given:

1. Showing high PSMA expression in PSMA-targeted imaging (PET or SPECT).
2. Leucocytes >2000/μl, platelets >75.000/μl and haemoglobin >8 g/dl.
3. Creatinine <2 mg/dl and no obstructive renal disease.
4. Liver transaminase <5× of the upper limit.
5. > 6 weeks delay after other myelosuppressive therapy
6. ECOG ≤2.

Lu-PSMA radioligand therapy, later referred to as PSMA-therapy, is administered 4–6 cycles in an interval of 6–8 weeks. In the case of disease progression (biochemical or imaging), therapy ought to be stopped. Progression should be assessed after several cycles, as a percentage of patients not responding to the first will respond to the second or third administration [10]. We propose the following therapy protocol:

- Cooling of salivary glands 30 min prior up to 4 h after the administration of Lu-PSMA. This aims at a reduction of salivary glands' radiation injuries.
- Utilization of a urinary catheter in incontinent patients for 48 h after therapy administration to minimise the risk of contamination.
- Use of a dosage of 6–7.5 GBq ^{177}Lu-PSMA-617.
- Inject Lu-PSMA slowly as bolus using a venous catheter followed by 1000 ml of NaCl or equivalent physiologic solution.
- Administration of Lu-PSMA therapy is repeated every 6–8 weeks. If therapy response is maintained, a set of Lu-therapy cycles usually consists of six administrations.

A revaluation of patient health condition should be performed after the administration of every Lu-PSMA cycle:

- Blood test should be carried out every two weeks (blood cell counts, creatinine and liver panel).
- Continuation of therapy is dependent on PSMA imaging, PSA levels and clinical situation.

40.3 Response

In analogy to the recommendations of the Prostate Cancer Clinical Trials Working Group, response to PSMA radioligand therapy is defined as relieve of disease manifestations or prevention of disease manifestations anticipated to occur [11]. Recent retrospective studies on PSMA radioligand therapy primarily focus on the elimination of present disease features, as patients enrolled have been refractory to above-mentioned standard therapy regimes, suffering from end-stage prostate cancer. Thereby a ≥ 50% decline of PSA levels compared to baseline is most commonly regarded as treatment response. However, due to their arbitrary nature, fixed limits of PSA decline should not be used to define therapy response [10, 11].

A German multicentre study enrolling 145 patients suffering from mCRPC could provide proof that $^{\text{Lu-PSMA}}$-617 radioligand therapy is safe and of high efficacy (mean dose: 5.9 GBq; median amount of cycles: 1). The biochemical response rate was 45%, whereas toxicity effects were modest [11, 12]. Several negative predictors could be revealed, among them were the presence of visceral metastases and high levels of alkaline phosphatase (≥ 220 U/l). In order to provide a more detailed patient stratification, prostate cancer's bone and lymphatic metastases ^{68}Ga-PSMA-11 uptake assessed by PET were evaluated as predictors [13]. Interestingly, the evaluation of prior anti-cancer treatments did not

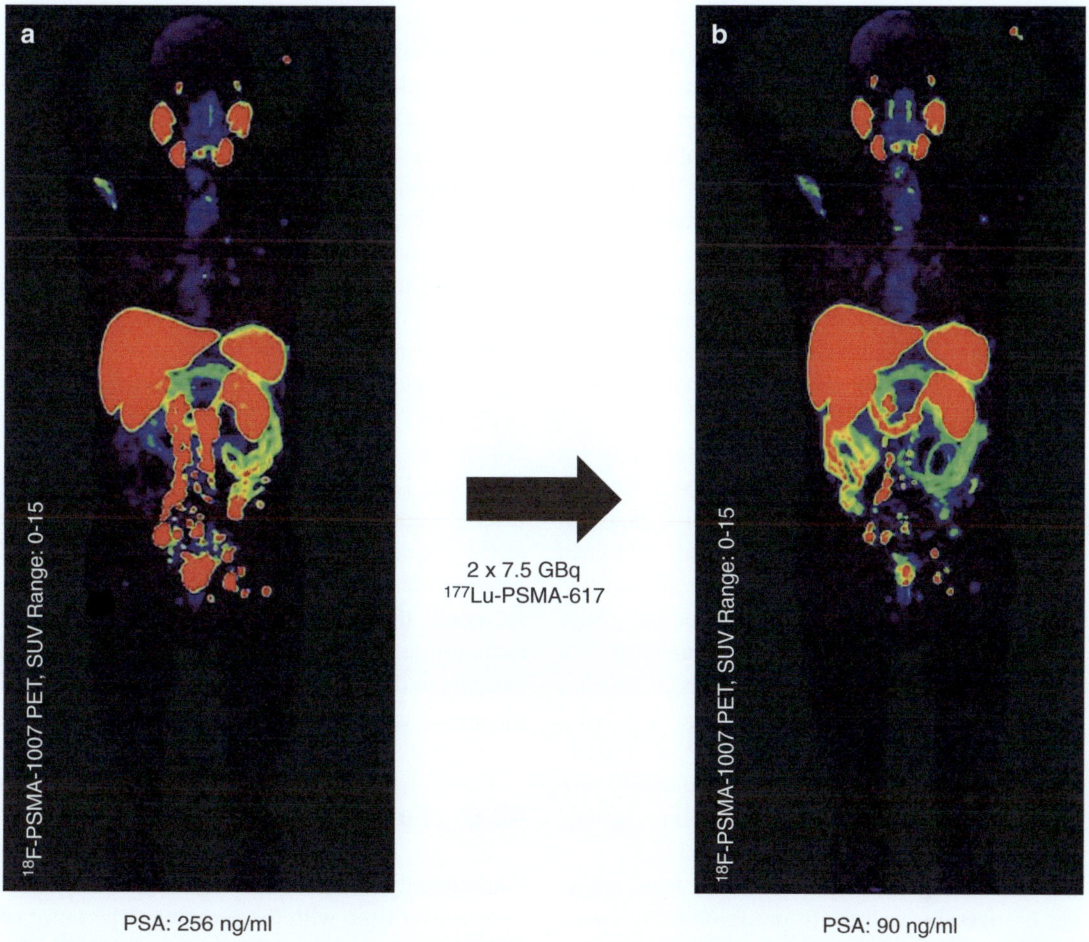

Fig. 40.1 We present a patient (age 64) with metastatic castration-resistant prostate cancer (mCRPC) being refractory to androgen depression therapy, abiateron and first-line chemotherapy (docetaxel). Panel A depicts the maximum intensity projection of a ^{18}F-PSMA-1007 PET, demonstrating the extensive spread of retroperitoneal lymphatic metastases. After the first two cycles of 7.5 GBq ^{177}Lu-PSMA-617, PSA declined from 256 to 90 ng/ml. Accordingly, Panel B reveals the reduction in tumour size as correlative to therapy response

significantly predict any therapy effects. This underlines PSMA therapy's fundamentally different mechanism of action compared commonly used anti-cancer treatments like chemotherapeutics or androgen withdrawal. Figure 40.1 shows an example of reduced lymph node metastatic burden in PSMA-targeted PET.

It is important to note that delayed responses to PSMA therapy have been reported [10, 14]. Up to 50% of patients without any PSA decline after the first cycle responded to the second or third administration of PSMA therapy. This is in line with recommendations of the Prostate Cancer Clinical Trials Working Group, according to which therapy response should be assessed 12 weeks after the start of treatment.

40.4 Survival

Current standard therapy regimes serve as reference in the evaluation of overall survival accounted to PSMA therapy. To date, after the failure of chemotherapy and enzalutamide or abiraterone, the standard treatment of mCRPC is predominantly based on best supportive care strategies. No randomized prospective study analysed the benefit of PSMA therapy compared to this standard treatment. However, to assess the survival benefit of PSMA therapy, historic control groups providing best supportive care can be utilized. Following such approaches, extended survival rates could be verified [15]: The survival of a comparable historic group (best supportive care) was 4.9 months, whereas the PSMA-therapy group accounted for an overall survival of 7.4 months (28 treated patients; mean dose: 5.89 GBq; median amount of cycles: 2; $P = 0.031$). Notably, in the mentioned study, 78% of patients were pretreated with chemotherapy, 75% with abiraterone and 86% with enzalutamide.

PSA response to Lu-PSMA is a predictor for the survival benefit, enabling patient stratification under treatment. The first prospective phase II study presented by Hofman et al. obtained a ≥ 30% PSA decline in 70% of the 30 enrolled patients [16]. Patients with a PSA decline ≥50% exhibited a progression-free survival of 9.9 months, compared to 4.1 months in patients with <50% PSA decline (mean dose: 7.5 GBq; median amount of cycles: 3; $P = 0.014$). Moreover, overall survival was significantly prolonged in the >50% PSA decline group: 17.0 months vs. 9.9 months ($P = 0.038$).

Considering larger patient collectives, analysis of overall survival is predominantly based retro-perspective data. In a retrospectively analysed cohort of 104 patients suffering from mCRPC, patients with a PSA decline of ≥20.9% had an overall survival of 14.5 months, compared to 11.5 months (mean dose: 6.1 GBq; median amount of cycles:3; $P < 0.001$) in case of otherwise PSA response [17].

40.5 Toxicity

PSMA therapy is wildly well tolerated, exhibiting a modest extend of adverse effects. This is mainly because of the beneficial pharmacokinetic of the small PSMA molecule, particularly compared to labelled antibodies. Adverse effects are generally reported using the Common Terminology Criteria for Adverse Events (CTCAE) v4 (impairment grade 1–4). Dosimetry studies revealed that salivary glands and kidneys are exposed to the highest levels of radiation besides the tumour manifestations. However, the impairment of organ function did not reach a critical extend [18]. Absorbed doses of salivary glands and kidneys vary in publications, typically in the range of 0.6 Gy/GBq and 1.4 Gy/GBq, respectively. Even repeated administrations of PSMA therapy did not cause grade 3/4 renal toxicity, eye dryness or Xerostomia [19, 20].

Bone marrow's absorbed dose accounts approximately 12 mGy/GBq. Despite the relatively low absorbed radiation energy, adverse effects concerning the haematopoietic system are common. Due to the impaired haematopoietic reserve capacity caused by bone metastases, a grade 3/4 anaemia has been reported in 19% of patients treated with 3 cycles in median [19]. However, thrombopoiesis is known to be most radiation sensitive, but is impaired in only 3% of patients, indicating that anaemia is caused by the metastatic cancer extend.

40.6 Future Perspectives

Undoubtedly, the presented therapy regimes will evolve over time with the growing experience of PSMA-therapy. The utilization of PSMA for diagnostics and RLT is presenting promising results; however, in order to straighten its practical significance, some issues need to be resolved. These include the choice of either alpha or beta radiation and discovering the most suited patient collective. To this end, Endocyte, Inc. announced the VISION trial as principle Phase III study evaluating the efficacy and safety of ^{177}Lu-PSMA-617 early 2018. This trial continues the exciting journey of nuclear medicine treatment for patients suffering from prostate cancer. Yet whether PSMA therapy should be used in earlier prostate cancer stages or in combination with antiandrogen treatments should be studied in future trials. This is of particular importance, as antiandrogen therapy can promote PSMA expression, potentially offering synergistic treatment effects. For this purpose, large multicentre studies are needed, evaluating the potential of

PSMA therapy with regard to long-term toxicity effects and other available treatment regimes.

Not only is the development of PSMA-617 a paramount example of theranostics approaches, revealing the unparalleled acceleration enabled by direct visualization and quantification of treatment-action. Far more importantly, for the first time, nuclear medicine specialists are directly contributing to the fight against a leading cause of death. Carried by the promising preliminary results, we are optimistic that PSMA therapy is a potential tool controlling cancer for the good of patients. In this way, PSMA therapy will decisively shape the next decade of nuclear medicine clinical progress.

References

1. Siegel RL, Miller KD, Jemal A. Cancer statistics, 2017. CA Cancer J Clin. 2017;67:7–30.
2. Mongiat-Artus P, Teillac P. Role of Luteinising Hormone Releasing Hormone (LHRH) agonists and hormonal treatment in the management of prostate cancer. Prostate Cancer Testosterone Suppr Levels Eligard®. 2005;4:4–13.
3. Parker C, Nilsson S, Heinrich D, et al. Alpha emitter Radium-223 and survival in metastatic prostate Cancer. N Engl J Med. 2013;369:213–23.
4. Bander NH, Milowsky MI, Nanus DM, Kostakoglu L, Vallabhajosula S, Goldsmith SJ. Phase I trial of 177lutetium-labeled J591, a monoclonal antibody to prostate-specific membrane antigen, in patients with androgen-independent prostate cancer. J Clin Oncol. 2005;23:4591–601.
5. Tagawa ST, Milowsky MI, Morris M, et al. Phase II study of Lutetium-177-labeled anti-prostate-specific membrane antigen monoclonal antibody J591 for metastatic castration-resistant prostate cancer. Clin Cancer Res. 2013;19:5182–91.
6. Vallabhajosula S. Radioimmunotherapy of prostate cancer using 90Y- and 177Lu-labeled J591 monoclonal antibodies: effect of multiple treatments on myelotoxicity. Clin Cancer Res. 2005;11:7195s–200s.
7. Zechmann CM, Afshar-Oromieh A, Armor T, et al. Radiation dosimetry and first therapy results with a (124)I/ (131)I-labeled small molecule (MIP-1095) targeting PSMA for prostate cancer therapy. Eur J Nucl Med Mol Imaging. 2014;41:1280–92.
8. Kratochwil C, Giesel FL, Eder M, et al. [177Lu] Lutetium-labelled PSMA ligand-induced remission in a patient with metastatic prostate cancer. Eur J Nucl Med Mol Imaging. 2015;42:987–8.
9. Ahmadzadehfar H, Rahbar K, Kürpig S, et al. Early side effects and first results of radioligand therapy with (177)Lu-DKFZ-617 PSMA of castrate-resistant metastatic prostate cancer: a two-Centre study. EJNMMI Res. 2015;5:114.
10. Rahbar K, Bögeman M, Yordanova A, et al. Delayed response after repeated^{177}Lu-PSMA-617 radioligand therapy in patients with metastatic castration resistant prostate cancer. Eur J Nucl Med Mol Imaging. 2017:243–6.
11. Scher HI, Halabi S, Tannock I, et al. Design and end points of clinical trials for patients with progressive prostate cancer and castrate levels of testosterone: recommendations of the prostate Cancer clinical trials working group. J Clin Oncol. 2008;26:1148–59.
12. Rahbar K, Ahmadzadehfar H, Kratochwil C, et al. German multicenter study investigating 177Lu-PSMA-617 Radioligand therapy in advanced prostate Cancer patients. J Nucl Med. 2017;58:85–90.
13. Ferdinandus J, Eppard E, Gaertner FC, et al. Predictors of response to Radioligand therapy of metastatic castrate-resistant prostate Cancer with 177Lu-PSMA-617. J Nucl Med. 2017;58:312–9.
14. Ahmadzadehfar H, Wegen S, Yordanova A, et al. Overall survival and response pattern of castration-resistant metastatic prostate cancer to multiple cycles of radioligand therapy using [(177)Lu]Lu-PSMA-617. Eur J Nucl Med Mol Imaging. 2017;44:1448–54.
15. Rahbar K, Bode A, Weckesser M, et al. Radioligand therapy with 177Lu-PSMA-617 as a novel therapeutic option in patients with metastatic castration resistant prostate Cancer. Clin Nucl Med. 2016;41:522–8.
16. Hofman MS, Violet J, Hicks RJ, et al. [177Lu]-PSMA-617 radionuclide treatment in patients with metastatic castration-resistant prostate cancer (LuPSMA trial): a single-Centre, single-arm, phase 2 study. Lancet Oncol. 2018;19:825–33.
17. Rahbar K, Boegemann M, Yordanova A, et al. PSMA targeted radioligand therapy in metastatic castration resistant prostate cancer after chemotherapy, abiraterone and/or enzalutamide. A retrospective analysis of overall survival. Eur J Nucl Med Mol Imaging. 2018;45:12–9.
18. Delker A, Fendler WP, Kratochwil C, et al. Dosimetry for 177Lu-DKFZ-PSMA-617: a new radiopharmaceutical for the treatment of metastatic prostate cancer. Eur J Nucl Med Mol Imaging. 2016;43:42–51.
19. Bräuer A, Grubert LS, Roll W, et al. 177Lu-PSMA-617 radioligand therapy and outcome in patients with metastasized castration-resistant prostate cancer. Eur J Nucl Med Mol Imaging. 2017;44:1663–70.
20. Yordanova A, Becker A, Eppard E, et al. The impact of repeated cycles of radioligand therapy using [(177) Lu]Lu-PSMA-617 on renal function in patients with hormone refractory metastatic prostate cancer. Eur J Nucl Med Mol Imaging. 2017;44:1473–9.

MIX
Papier aus verantwortungsvollen Quellen
Paper from responsible sources
FSC® C105338

If you have any concerns about our products,
you can contact us on
ProductSafety@springernature.com

In case Publisher is established outside the EU,
the EU authorized representative is:
Springer Nature Customer Service Center GmbH
Europaplatz 3, 69115 Heidelberg, Germany

Printed by Libri Plureos GmbH
in Hamburg, Germany